CONTEMPORARY
Nutrition

Ninth Edition

Gordon M. Wardlaw PH.D.
Formerly of Department of Human Nutrition,
College of Education and Human Ecology
The Ohio State University

Anne M. Smith PH.D., R.D., L.D.
Department of Human Nutrition,
College of Education and Human Ecology
The Ohio State University

With contributions by
Angela L. Collene M.S., R.D., L.D.
Dietetics Program
Department of Family and Consumer Sciences
Ashland University

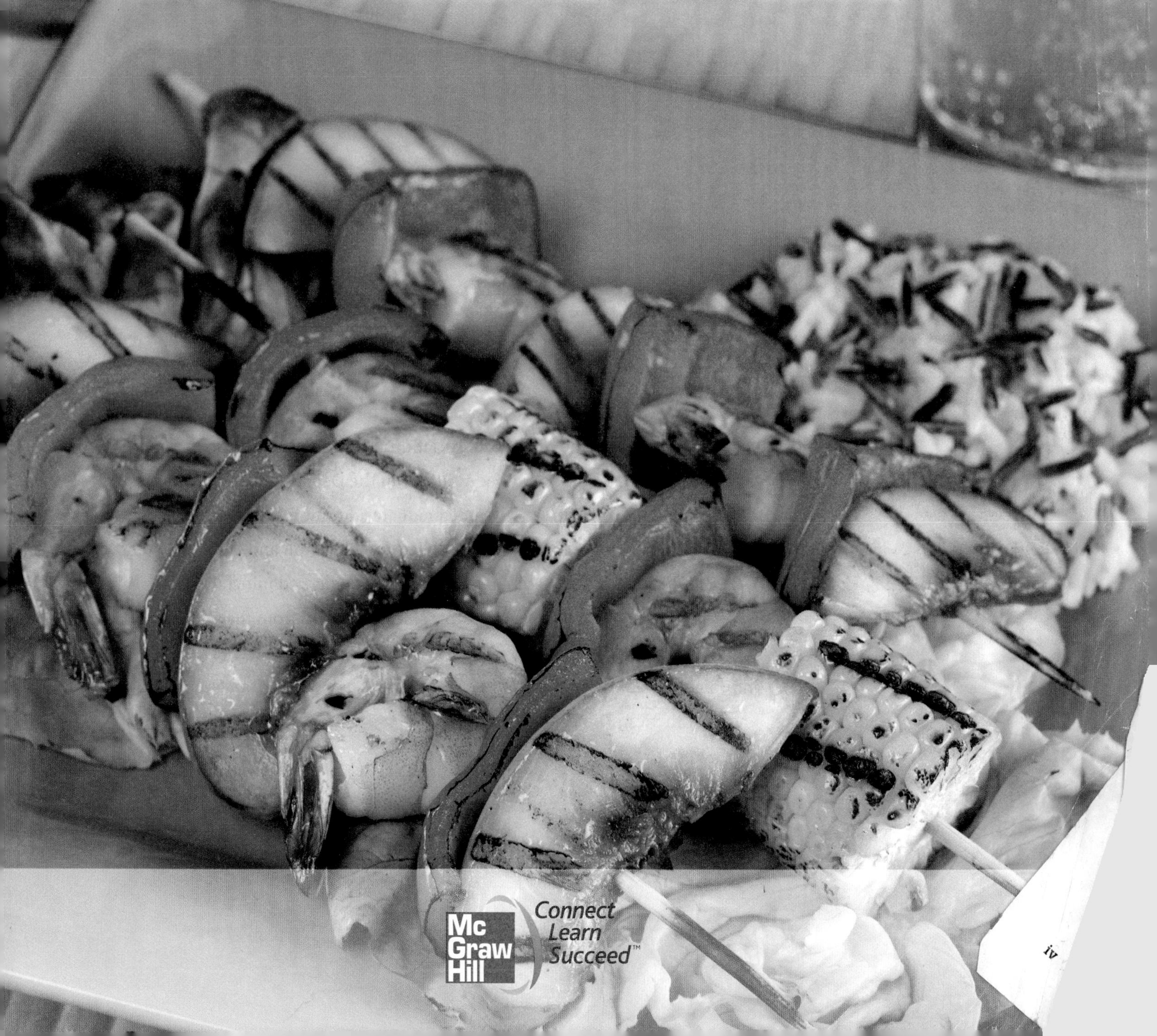

McGraw Hill
Connect
Learn
Succeed™

iv

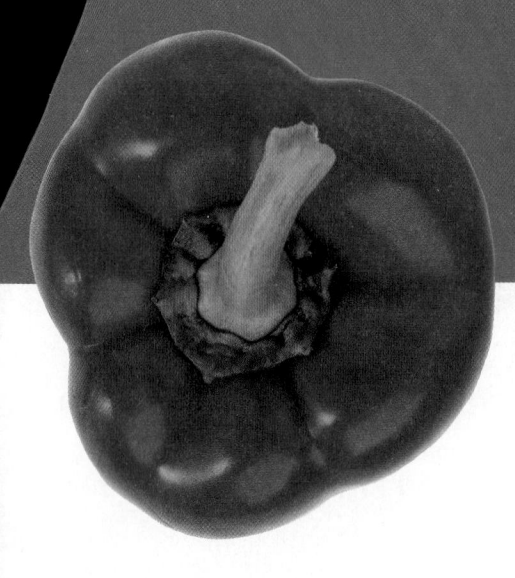

About the Authors

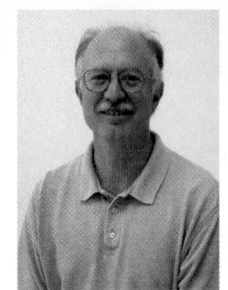

GORDON M. WARDLAW, Ph.D., has taught introductory nutrition courses to students in the Department of Human Nutrition at The Ohio State University and at other colleges and universities. Dr. Wardlaw is the author of many articles that have appeared in prominent nutrition, biology, physiology, and biochemistry journals and was the 1985 recipient of the American Dietetic Association's Mary P. Huddleson Award. Dr. Wardlaw is a member of the American Society for Nutritional Sciences and is certified as a Specialist in Human Nutrition by the American Board of Nutrition. Dr. Wardlaw is currently retired from academia.

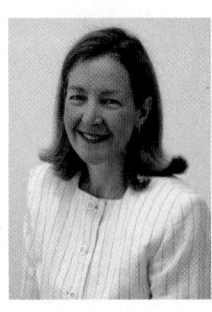

ANNE M. SMITH, Ph.D., R.D., L.D., currently teaches nutrition majors and nonmajors at The Ohio State University and was the recipient of the 1995 Outstanding Teacher Award from the College of Human Ecology. Dr. Smith is the Director of the Didactic Program in Dietetics in the Department of Human Nutrition, College of Education and Human Ecology, of The Ohio State University and received the 2008 Outstanding Dietetic Educator Award from the Ohio Dietetic Association and the 1998 Emerging Dietetic Leader Award from the American Dietetic Association. She also was the recipient of the 2006 Outstanding Faculty Member Award from the Department of Human Nutrition for her commitment to undergraduate education in nutrition and the 2011 Distinquished Service Award from the College of Education and Human Ecology. Dr. Smith has conducted research in the area of vitamin and mineral metabolism and was awarded the 1996 Departmental Research Award from the Ohio Agricultural Research and Development Center. Dr. Smith's research articles have appeared in prominent nutrition journals. She is a member of the American Nutrition Society and the American Dietetic Association.

BLACKBOARD®

The next big thing in digital education!

Ingredients

1 Single sign-on with Blackboard Learn

1 Deeply integrated McGraw-Hill content and tools

1 Automatic Roster/Gradebook synchronization

1 Company—first to use Learning Technology Interoperability (LTI) Standards

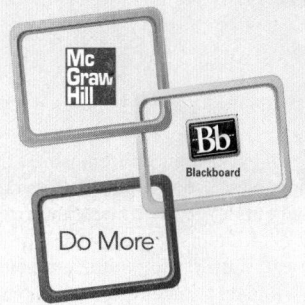

Directions

1. Go to **www.domorenow.com**.

2. Customize and integrate McGraw-Hill content and ground-breaking learning tools into your Bb courses.

3. Increase student retention and satisfaction.

4. Less building and managing. More teaching!

5. More integration on the way—ask us about the LMS used on your campus.

McGRAW-HILL CREATE™

Customize your perfect course solution!

Ingredients

1 New, self-service website that allows you to quickly and easily create custom course materials with McGraw-Hill's comprehensive, cross-disciplinary content and other third party resources

1 Place to create, edit, view, and purchase customized products

1 eBook or print text—you choose the best format for your students

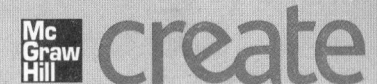

Directions

1. Go to **www.mcgrawhillcreate.com**.

2. Select, then arrange the content in a way that makes sense for your course.

3. Combine material from different sources and even upload your own content.

4. Edit and update your course materials as often as you'd like.

5. Receive your pdf review copy in minutes!

6. Create what you've only imagined!

McGRAW-HILL TEGRITY®

Students can focus on your lectures with digital lecture capture!

Ingredients

1 Ability to record from anywhere, anytime, with or without an Internet connection

1 Key word search allows students to search for exactly what they need to review

1 Highly personalized learning environment makes study time incredibly efficient

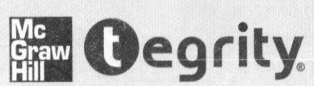

Directions

1. You need nothing more than a computer and microphone to quickly and easily record lectures.

2. Tegrity captures synchronized audio, video, and computer screen activity with the click of a button.

3. View recordings on a PC, Mac, or mobile device 24/7. Tegrity's intuitive interface with a detailed timeline and associated thumbnails makes it easy to find exactly what you're looking for.

4. Help students retain more and achieve higher levels of performance!

*Tip: Learn more at **www.tegrity.com***

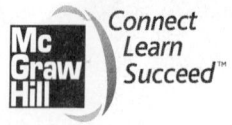

The McGraw·Hill Companies

Connect
Learn
Succeed™

CONTEMPORARY NUTRITION, NINTH EDITION

Published by McGraw-Hill, a business unit of The McGraw-Hill Companies, Inc., 1221 Avenue of the Americas, New York, NY 10020. Copyright © 2013 by The McGraw-Hill Companies, Inc. All rights reserved. Printed in the United States of America. Previous editions © 2011, 2009, and 2006. No part of this publication may be reproduced or distributed in any form or by any means, or stored in a database or retrieval system, without the prior written consent of The McGraw-Hill Companies, Inc., including, but not limited to, in any network or other electronic storage or transmission, or broadcast for distance learning.

Some ancillaries, including electronic and print components, may not be available to customers outside the United States.

This book is printed on acid-free paper.

4 5 6 7 8 9 0 RMN/RMN 1 0 9 8 7 6 5 4

ISBN 978-0-07-340254-3
MHID 0-07-340254-0

Vice President, Editor-in-Chief: *Marty Lange*
Vice President, EDP: *Kimberly Meriwether David*
Senior Director of Development: *Kristine Tibbetts*
Publisher: *Michael S. Hackett*
Sponsoring Editor: *Lynn M. Breithaupt*
Director of Digital Content Development: *Barbekka Hurtt, Ph.D.*
Senior Developmental Editor: *Lynne M. Meyers*
Marketing Manager: *Amy L. Reed*
Lead Project Manager: *Sheila M. Frank*
Senior Buyer: *Kara Kudronowicz*
Senior Media Project Manager: *Tammy Juran*
Manager, Creative Services: *Michelle D. Whitaker*
Cover/Interior Designer: *Ellen Pettengell*
Cover Image: © *The McGraw-Hill Companies, Inc., Kevin May Photography*
Senior Photo Research Coordinator: *John C. Leland*
Photo Research: *Mary Reeg*
Compositor: *Laserwords Private Limited*
Typeface: *10/12 Giovanni Book*
Printer: *RR Donnelley*

All credits appearing on page or at the end of the book are considered to be an extension of the copyright page.

Library of Congress Cataloging-in-Publication Data
Wardlaw, Gordon M.
    Contemporary nutrition / Gordon M. Wardlaw, Anne M. Smith, Angela Collene.—9th ed.
        p. cm.
    Includes index.
    ISBN 978-0-07-340254-3 — ISBN 0-07-340254-0 (hard copy : alk. paper) 1. Nutrition—Textbooks.
I. Smith, Anne M., 1955– II. Collene, Angela. III. Title.
    QP141.W378 2013
    612.3—dc23
                                                                    2011036913

Brief Contents

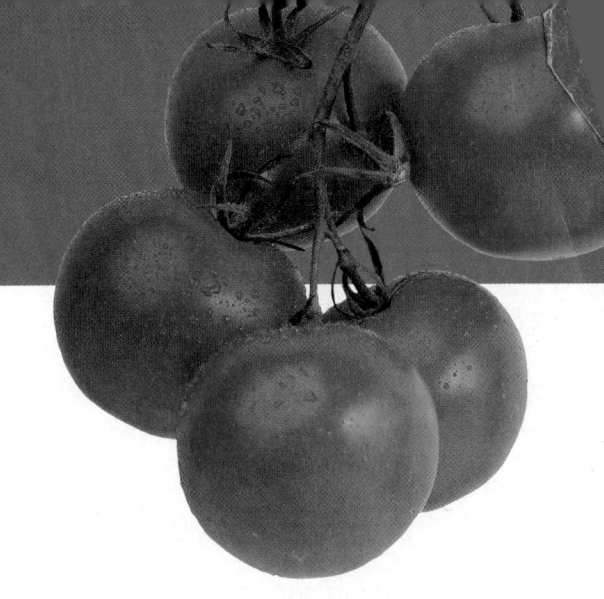

Preface

Dear Students,

Welcome to the fascinating world of nutrition! We are all nutrition experts, in a sense, because we all eat—several times a day. At the same time, though, nutrition can seem a bit confusing. One reason for all the confusion is that it seems like "good nutrition" is a moving target: different authorities have different ideas of how we should eat and nutrition recommendations are subject to change! Are eggs good for us or not? Should we model our diets after a pyramid or a plate? Second, there are so many choices. Did you know that the average supermarket carries about 40,000 food and beverage products? Food manufacturers and grocery chains have one purpose—to make as large a profit as possible. Typically, the most aggressively marketed items are not the healthiest. This has made shopping very complicated. In addition, as a nation, we eat out a lot. When we eat foods that someone else has prepared for us, we surrender control over how much salt and fat is in our food and how much food goes on our plates. There is a lot yet to learn, and you are undoubtedly interested in what you personally should be eating and how the food you eat affects you.

Contemporary Nutrition is designed to accurately convey changing and seemingly conflicting messages to all kinds of students. Our students commonly have misconceptions about nutrition, and many have a limited background in biology or chemistry. Contemporary Nutrition teaches complex scientific concepts at a level that will enable you to meaningfully apply the material to your own life.

We have written Contemporary Nutrition to help you make informed choices about the food you eat. We will take you through explanations of the nutrients in food and their relationship to health, but will also make you aware of the multitude of other factors that drive food choices. To guide you, we refer to many reputable research studies, books, policies, and web sites throughout the book. With this information at your fingertips, you will be well equipped to make your own informed choices about what and how much to eat. There is much to learn, so let's get started!

-Anne Smith

Connecting Students to Course Concepts

Introducing McGraw-Hill ConnectPlus™ Nutrition

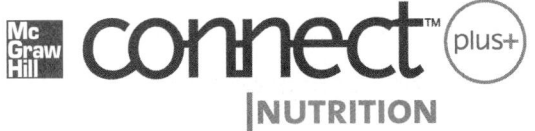

McGraw-Hill Connect® is a web-based assignment and assessment platform that gives students the means to better connect with coursework, instructors, and important concepts that they will need to know for success now and in the future. Connect Nutrition includes high quality interactive questions and tutorials, LearnSmart, digital lecture capture, eBook, and more!

Save time with auto-graded assessments and tutorials.

You can easily create customized assessments that will be automatically graded. All Connect content is created by nutrition instructors so it is pedagogical, instructional, and at the appropriate level. Interactive questions using high-quality art from the textbook, animations and videos from a variety of sources, take you way beyond multiple choice.

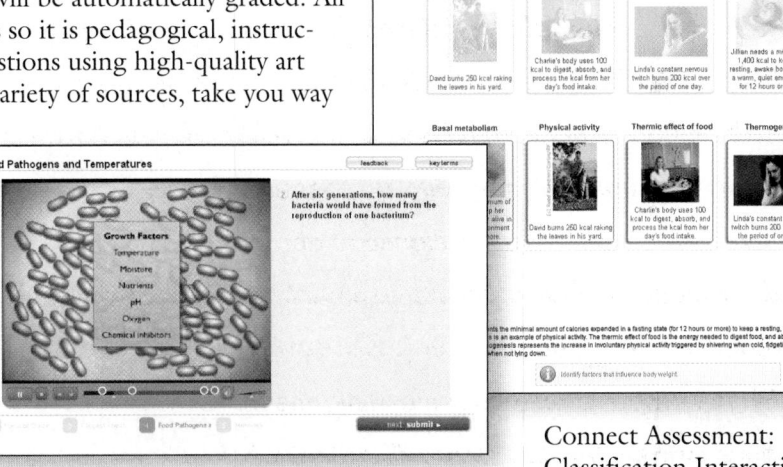

Connect Assessment: Classification Interactive

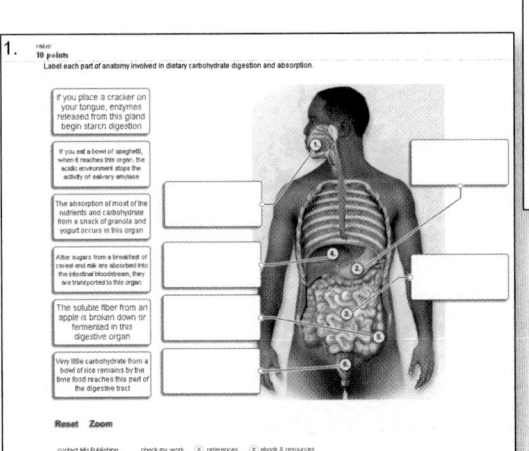

Connect Assessment: Labeling Interactive

Connect Assessment: Animation Tutorial

"… I and my adjuncts have reduced the time we spend on grading by 90 percent and student test scores have risen, on average, 10 points since we began using Connect!"

—William Hoover, Bunker Hill Community College

Gather assessment information

All Connect questions are tagged to learning outcome, specific topics, level of difficulty, and allow you to tag your own learning outcomes—so you can easily track assessment data!

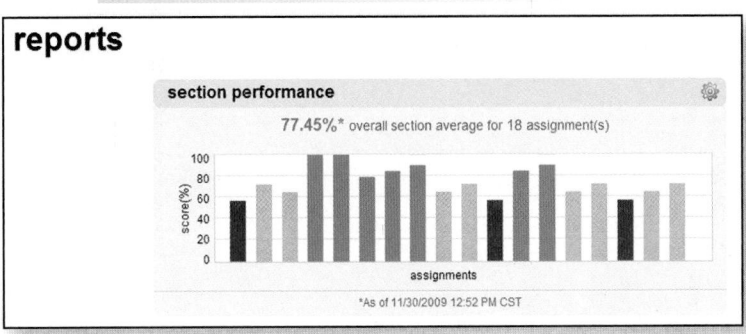

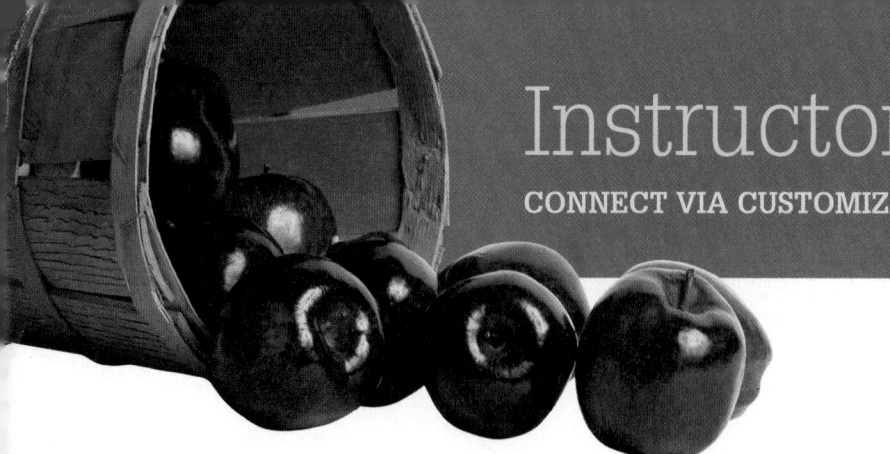

Instructors

CONNECT VIA CUSTOMIZATION

Presentation Tools allow you to customize your lectures.

Enhanced Lecture Presentations contain lecture outlines, art, photos, tables, and animations embedded where appropriate. Fully customizable, complete and ready to use, these presentations will streamline your work and let you spend less time preparing for lecture!

Editable Art   Fully editable (labels and leaders) line art from the text.

Animations   Over 50 animations bringing key concepts to life, available for instructors *and* students.

Animation PPTs   Animations are truly embedded in PowerPoint® for ultimate ease of use! Just copy and paste into your custom slideshow and you're done!

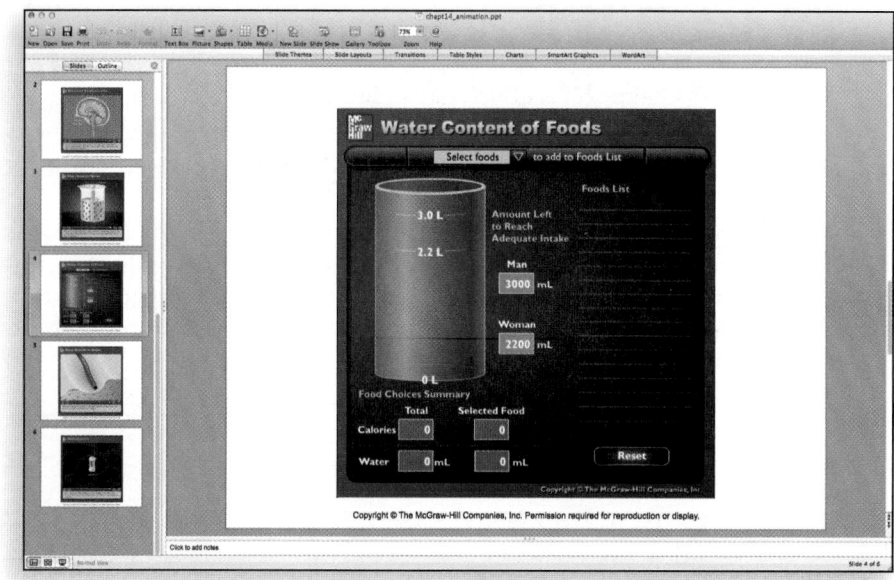

Take your course online—*easily and quickly* with one-click Digital Lecture Capture.

McGraw-Hill Tegrity® records and distributes your lectures with just a click of a button. Students can view them anytime/anywhere via computer, iPod, or mobile device. Tegrity® indexes and records your slideshow presentations, and anything shown on your computer, so **students can use keywords to find exactly what they want to study.**

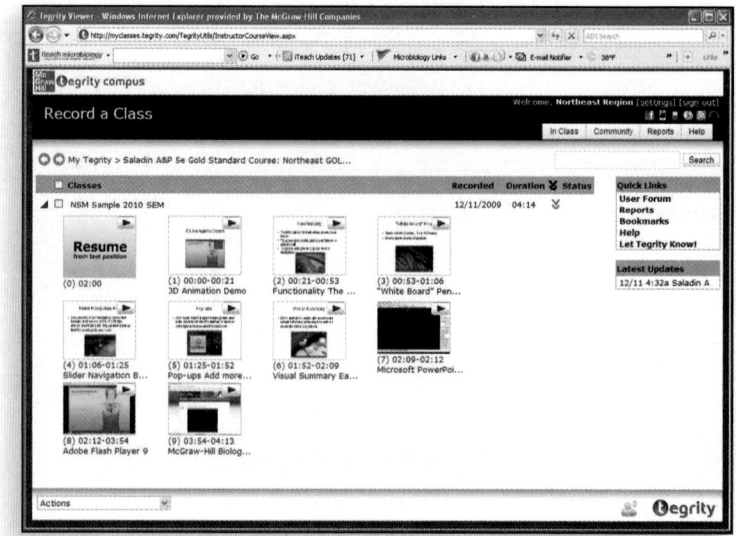

Students

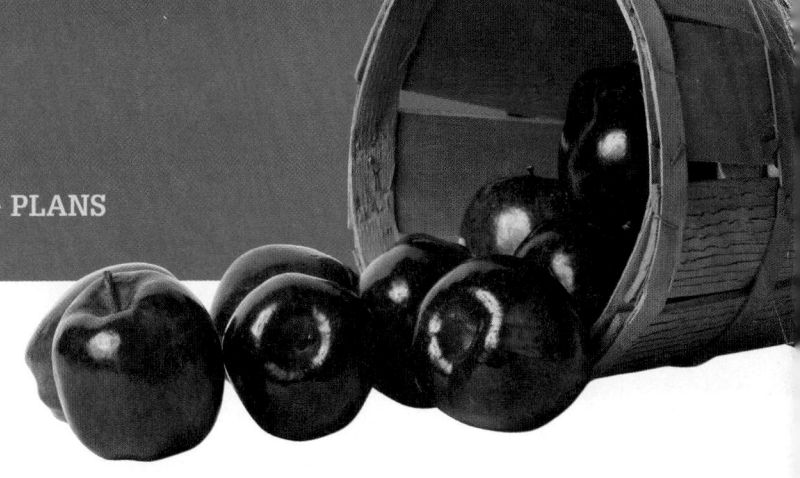

Access content anywhere, any time, with a customizable, interactive eBook.

McGraw-Hill ConnectPlus eBook takes digital texts beyond a simple PDF. With the same content as the printed book, but optimized for the screen, ConnectPlus has embedded animations and videos, which bring concepts to life and provide "just in time" learning for students. Fully integrated self-study questions allow students to interact with the questions in the text and determine if they're gaining mastery of the content.

> **"Use of technology, especially LEARNSMART, assisted greatly in keeping on track and keeping up with the material."**
>
> —*student, Triton College*

McGraw-Hill LearnSmart™
A Diagnostic, Adaptive Learning System

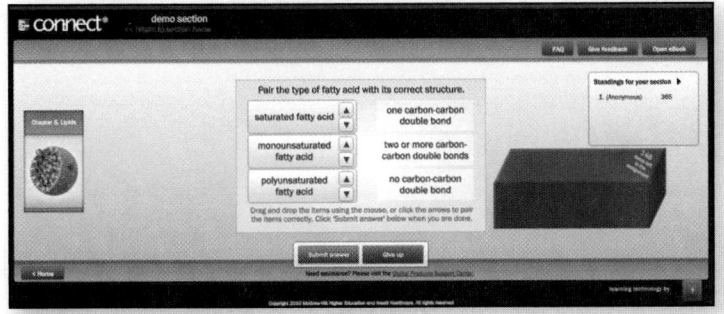

McGraw-Hill *LearnSmart* is an adaptive learning system designed to help students learn faster, study more efficiently, and retain more knowledge for greater success.

LearnSmart effectively assesses students' skill levels to determine which topics students have mastered and which require further practice. A personalized learning path based upon student strengths and weaknesses gives students exactly the help they need, when they need it.

Self-study resources are also available at www.mhhe.com/wardlawcont9.

> **"I love LearnSmart. Without it, I would not be doing as well."**
>
> —*student, Triton College*

ix

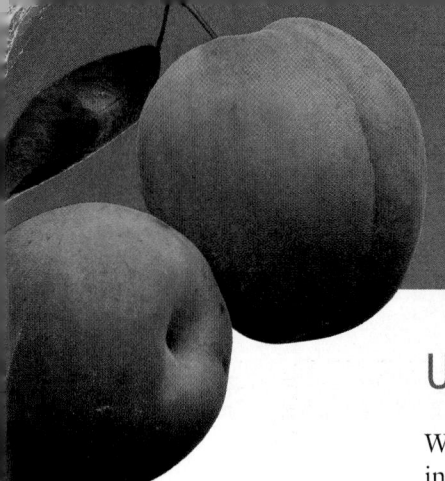

Connecting Today's Students to Today's Nutrition

Understanding Our Audience

We have written *Contemporary Nutrition* assuming that our students have a limited background in college-level biology, chemistry, or physiology. We have been careful to include the essential science foundation needed to adequately comprehend certain topics in nutrition, such as protein synthesis in Chapter 6. The science in this text has been presented in a simple, straightforward manner so that undergraduate students can master the material and apply it to their own lives. The Concept Maps that provide a visual depiction of macronutrient functions and characteristics are an additional aid to help students grasp nutrition science.

Featuring the Latest Guidelines and Research

The vast amount of published research is constantly reshaping our knowledge of nutritional science. The ninth edition has been carefully updated to reflect current scientific understanding, as well as the latest health and nutrition guidelines. Students will learn about the Dietary Guidelines for Americans, 2010, MyPlate, and Healthy People 2020.

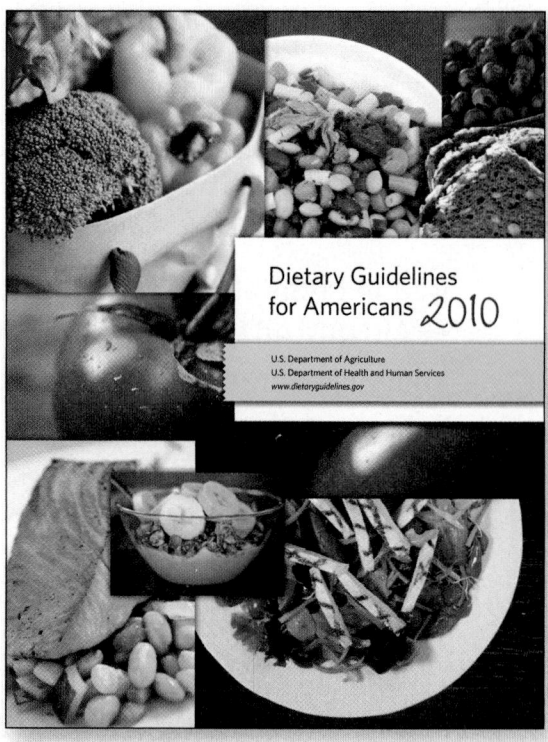

Dietary Guidelines for Americans 2010

U.S. Department of Agriculture
U.S. Department of Health and Human Services
www.dietaryguidelines.gov

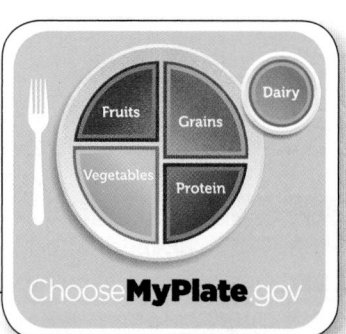

Choose **MyPlate**.gov

Healthy People 2020

Connecting with a Personal Focus

Applying Nutrition on a Personal Level

Throughout the ninth edition we reinforce the fact that each person responds differently to nutrients. To further convey the importance of applying nutrition to their personal lives, we include many examples of people and situations that resonate with college students. We also stress the importance of learning to intelligently sort through the seemingly endless range of nutrition messages to recognize reliable information and to sensibly apply it to their own lives. Our goal is to provide students the tools they need to eat healthy and make informed nutrition decisions after they leave this course.

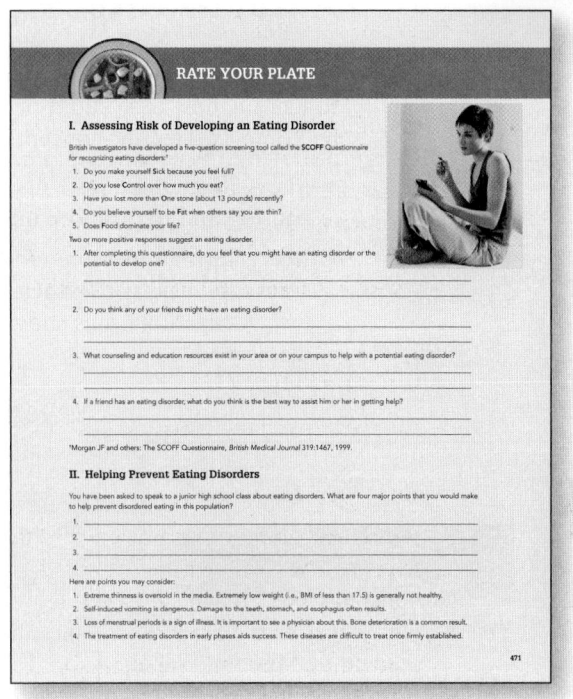

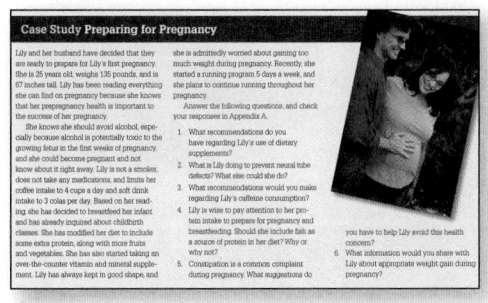

Challenging Students to Think Critically

The pages of *Contemporary Nutrition* contain numerous opportunities for students to learn more about themselves and their diet and to use their new knowledge of nutrition to improve their health. In the ninth edition, pedagogical elements, such as Making Decisions, Critical Thinking, Case Studies, and Nutrition and Your Health, are further enhanced by the addition of What Would You Choose? and Newsworthy Nutrition. Many of the thought-provoking topics highlighted in these features are expanded upon in the online resources found in Connect Nutrition.

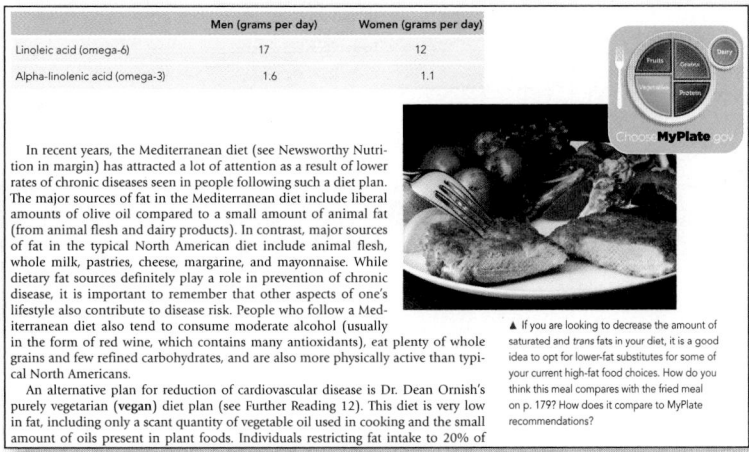

	Men (grams per day)	Women (grams per day)
Linoleic acid (omega-6)	17	12
Alpha-linolenic acid (omega-3)	1.6	1.1

In recent years, the Mediterranean diet (see Newsworthy Nutrition in margin) has attracted a lot of attention as a result of lower rates of chronic diseases seen in people following such a diet plan. The major sources of fat in the Mediterranean diet include liberal amounts of olive oil compared to a small amount of animal fat (from animal flesh and dairy products). In contrast, major sources of fat in the typical North American diet include animal flesh, whole milk, pastries, cheese, margarine, and mayonnaise. While dietary fat sources definitely play a role in prevention of chronic disease, it is important to remember that other aspects of one's lifestyle also contribute to disease risk. People who follow a Mediterranean diet also tend to consume moderate alcohol (usually in the form of red wine, which contains many antioxidants), eat plenty of whole grains and few refined carbohydrates, and are also more physically active than typical North Americans.

An alternative plan for reduction of cardiovascular disease is Dr. Dean Ornish's purely vegetarian (vegan) diet plan (see Further Reading 12). This diet is very low in fat, including only a scant quantity of vegetable oil used in cooking and the small amount of oils present in plant foods. Individuals restricting fat intake to 20% of

▲ If you are looking to decrease the amount of saturated and trans fats in your diet, it is a good idea to opt for lower-fat substitutes for some of your current high-fat food choices. How do you think this meal compares with the fried meal on p. 179? How does it compare to MyPlate recommendations?

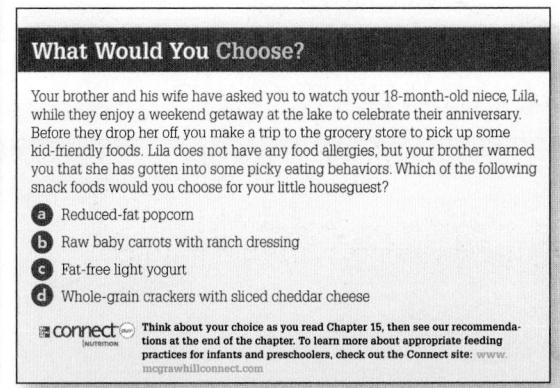

What Would You Choose?

Your brother and his wife have asked you to watch your 18-month-old niece, Lila, while they enjoy a weekend getaway at the lake to celebrate their anniversary. Before they drop her off, you make a trip to the grocery store to pick up some kid-friendly foods. Lila does not have any food allergies, but your brother warned you that she has gotten into some picky eating behaviors. Which of the following snack foods would you choose for your little houseguest?

ⓐ Reduced-fat popcorn

ⓑ Raw baby carrots with ranch dressing

ⓒ Fat-free light yogurt

ⓓ Whole-grain crackers with sliced cheddar cheese

connect NUTRITION Think about your choice as you read Chapter 15, then see our recommendations at the end of the chapter. To learn more about appropriate feeding practices for infants and preschoolers, check out the Connect site: www. mcgrawhillconnect.com

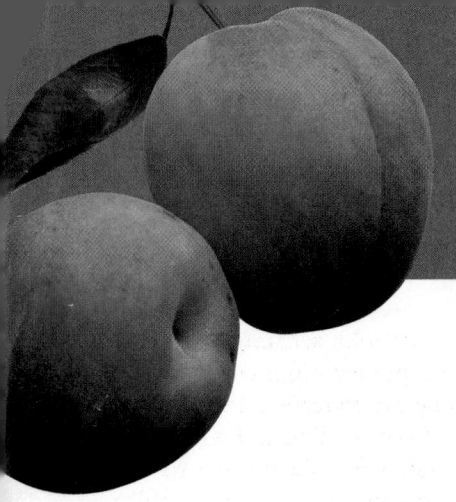

Making Visual Connections

Attractive, Accurate Artwork

More than 1000 drawings, photographs, and tables in the text were critically analyzed to identify how each could be enhanced and refined to help students more easily master complex scientific concepts.

- Many illustrations were updated or replaced to inspire student inquiry and comprehension and to promote interest and retention of information.
- Many illustrations were redesigned to use brighter colors and a more attractive, contemporary style. Others were fine-tuned to make them clearer and easier to follow. Navigational aids show where a function occurs and put it in perspective of the whole body.

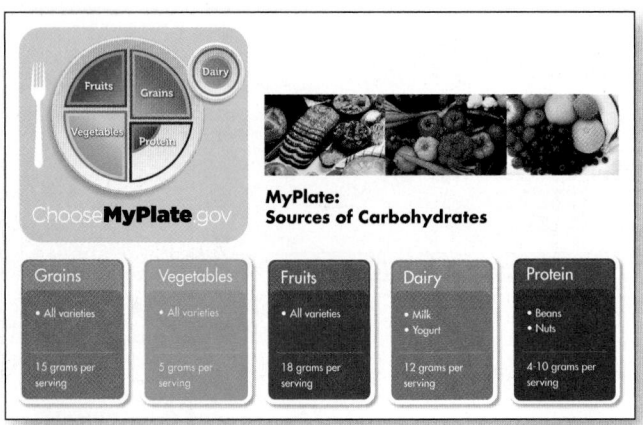

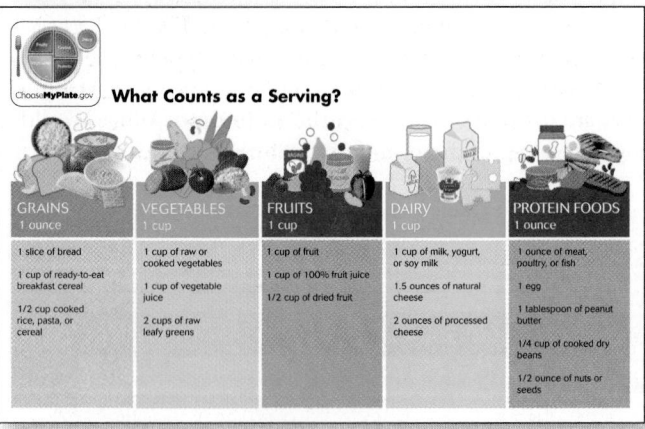

TABLE 2-5 Recommended Diet Changes Based on the Dietary Guidelines

If You Usually Eat This,	Try This Instead	Benefit
White bread	Whole-wheat bread	• Higher nutrient density, due to less processing • More fiber
Sugary breakfast cereal	Low-sugar, high-fiber cereal with fresh fruit	• Higher nutrient density • More fiber • More phytochemicals
Cheeseburger with French fries	Hamburger and baked beans	• Less saturated fat and trans fat • Less cholesterol • More fiber • More phytochemicals
Potato salad	Three-bean salad	• More fiber • More phytochemicals
Doughnuts	Bran muffin/bagel with light cream cheese	• More fiber • Less fat
Regular soft drinks	Diet soft drinks	• Fewer calories
Boiled vegetables	Steamed vegetables	• Higher nutrient density, due to reduced loss of water-soluble vitamins
Canned vegetables	Fresh or frozen vegetables	• Higher nutrient density, due to reduced loss of heat-sensitive vitamins • Lower in sodium
Fried meats	Broiled meats	• Less saturated fat
Fatty meats, such as ribs or bacon	Lean meats, such as ground round, chicken, or fish	• Less saturated fat
Whole milk	Low-fat or fat-free milk	• Less saturated fat • Fewer calories • More calcium
Ice cream	Sherbet or frozen yogurt	• Less saturated fat • Fewer calories
Mayonnaise or sour cream salad dressing	Oil-and-vinegar dressings or light creamy dressings	• Less saturated fat • Less cholesterol • Fewer calories
Cookies	Popcorn (air popped with minimal margarine or butter)	• Fewer calories and trans fat
Heavily salted foods	Foods flavored primarily with herbs, spices, lemon juice	• Lower in sodium
Chips	Pretzels	• Less fat

▲ Choose low-sugar, high-fiber cereal with fresh fruit instead of sugary breakfast cereal.

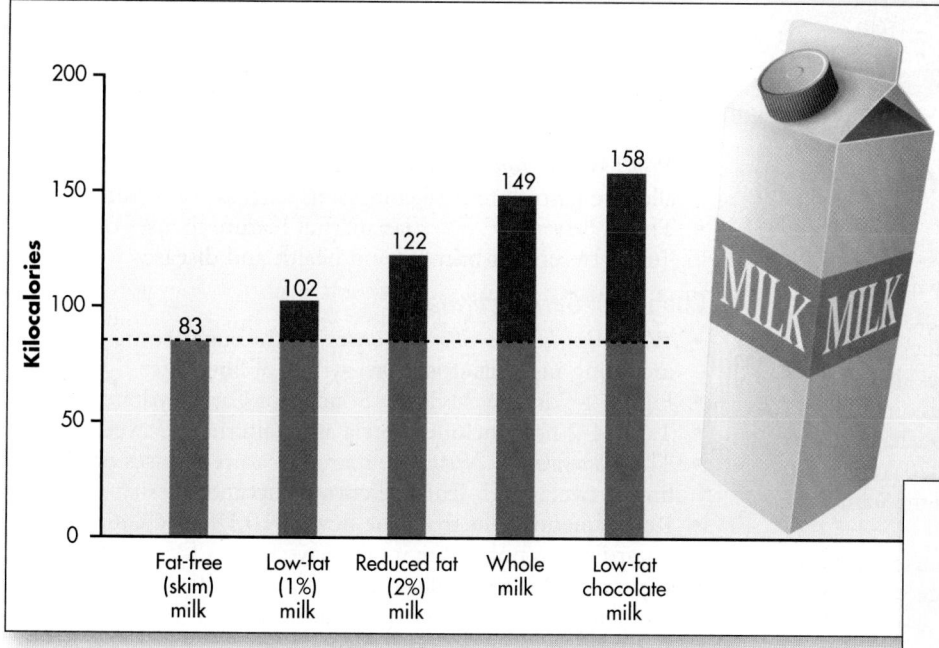

- Coordinated color schemes and drawing styles keep presentations consistent and strengthen the educational value of the artwork. Color-coding and directional arrows in figures make it easier to follow events and reinforce interrelationships.
- In many figures, process descriptions appear in the body of the figures. This pairing of the action and an explanation walks students step-by-step through the process and increases the teaching effectiveness of these figures.

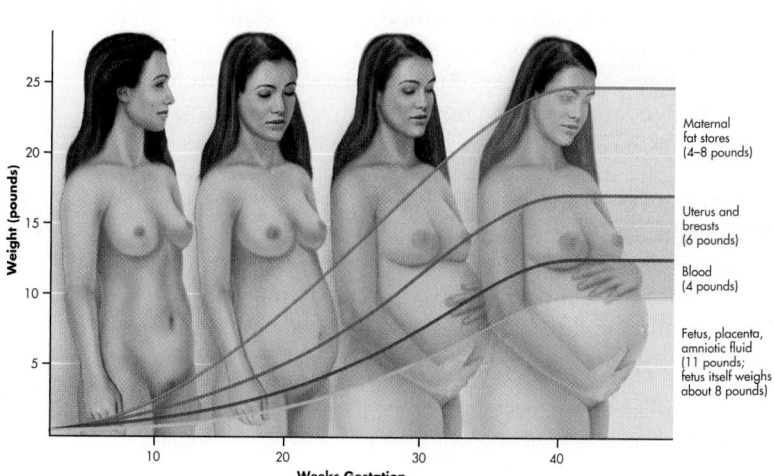

Finally, a careful comparison of artwork with its corresponding text was done to ensure that they are completely coordinated and consistent. The final result is a striking visual program that holds readers' attention and supports the goals of clarity, ease of comprehension, and critical thinking. The attractive layout and design of this edition are clean, bright, and inviting. This creative presentation of the material is geared toward engaging today's visually oriented students.

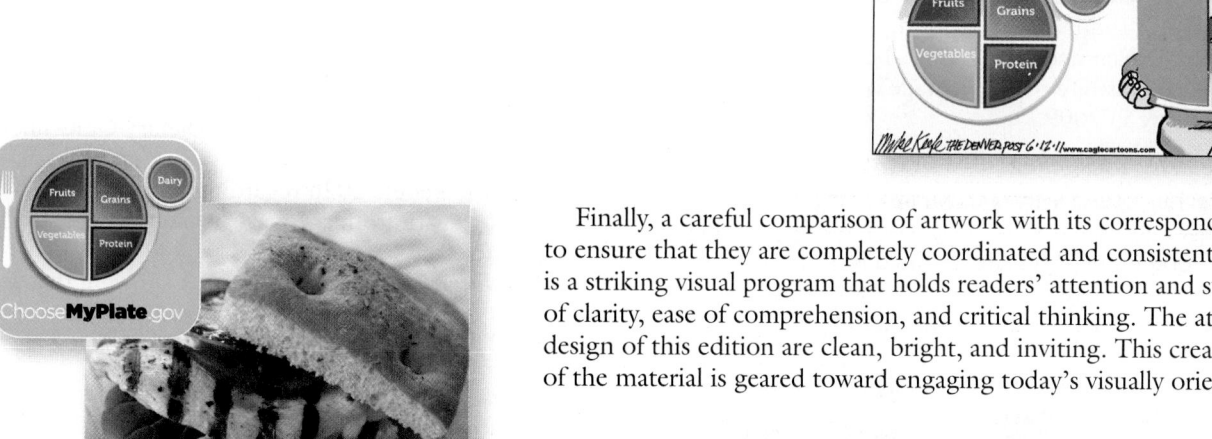

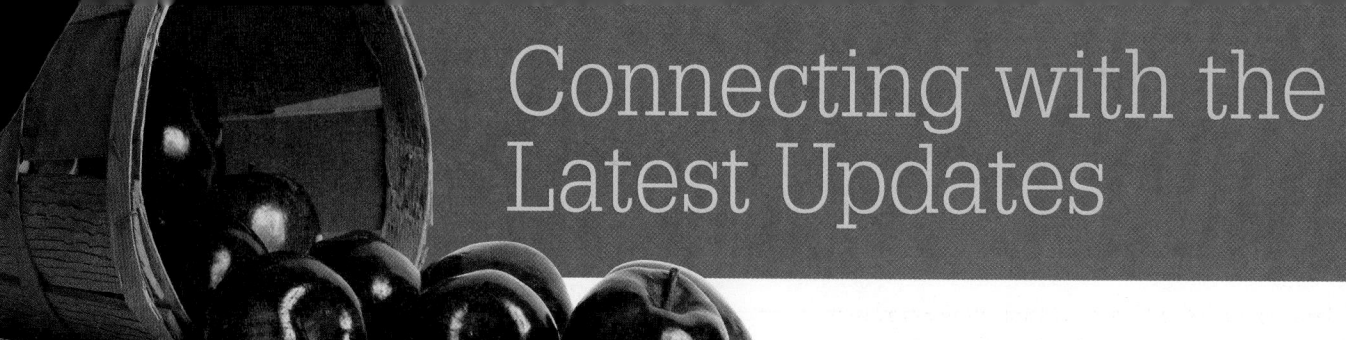

Connecting with the Latest Updates

Chapter-by-Chapter Revisions

Chapter 1: *Choosing What You Eat and Why*

- Chapter 1 has been reorganized beginning with a discussion of factors that influence our food choices and ending with a conversation about eating well in college.
- Chemical details of nutrients (e.g., dissacharides) have been moved to chapters on specific nutrients. Details on the hormonal control of appetite have been moved to Chapter 7.
- The newly released *Healthy People 2020* (HP2020) report is discussed, including its key "Nutrition and Weight Status" objectives.
- The new *What Would You Choose* feature focuses on time-saving breakfast options, especially for college students.
- Two *Newsworthy Nutrition* margin features are included in Chapter 1. One describes the link between TV food ads and childhood obesity and the other the link between a healthy diet and risk of sudden cardiac death.
- Causes of Death have been updated in Table 1-2.
- Added Figure 1-4 to illustrate the percentage of adults who are obese by state in 2009.

Chapter 2: *Guidelines for Designing a Healthy Diet*

- The *What Would You Choose* feature illustrates nutrient density and energy density.
- The new USDA food guide, MyPlate, released in June 2011, has been included with references to www.Choose MyPlate.gov and the Daily Food Plans that accompany MyPlate.
- The new Dietary Guidelines for Americans, 2010, released in January 2011, are fully discussed.
- Discussion of the scientific method, nutrient standards, and recommendations for healthy eating have been reorganized.
- New Figure 2-8 compares American intakes to current recommendations and Figure 2-11 shows what counts as a serving with MyPlate.
- New Figure 2-26 illustrates the concept of empty calories from solid fats and/or added sugars. *Newsworthy Nutrition* highlights the increasing costs of healthy eating.
- The new Rate Your Plate, "Are you putting health advice into practice?" reflects the 2010 Dietary Guidelines for Americans and 2008 Physical Activity Guidelines.

Chapter 3: *The Human Body: A Nutrition Perspective*

- Figure 3-7 is a new illustration of the pancreas and the function of endocrine cells secreting hormones into the bloodstream.

- *What Would You Choose* focuses on the best menu options to alleviate gastrointestinal complaints such as constipation.
- The *Newsworthy Nutrition* margin feature focuses on the link between gut bacteria and health and disease.

Chapter 4: *Carbohydrates*

- *What Would You Choose* focuses on the sugar content, including high-fructose corn syrup, of beverages.
- Figure 4-7 is now MyPlate: Sources of Carbohydrates.
- Table 4-2 now includes Stevia as an alternative sweetener.
- The *Newsworthy Nutrition* margin feature focuses on the link between high-fructose corn syrup and obesity.
- Recommendations from the new 2010 Dietary Guidelines regarding carbohydrate intake have been added.
- Figure 4-12 is a new illustration from the 2010 Dietary Guidelines of the sources of added sugars in U.S. diets.

Chapter 5: *Lipids*

- The new *What Would You Choose* feature focuses on the fat content of ground beef.
- Figure 5-5 has been revised to MyPlate: Sources of Fats.
- Peanut Butter: Is it "good fat?," has been included.
- Recommendations from the new 2010 Dietary Guidelines regarding fat intake have been added.
- Goals of Healthy People 2020 regarding reducing saturated fat intake, death from coronary heart disease, and total blood cholesterol are included.
- *Newsworthy Nutrition* focuses on research showing that a low-fat diet is not necessary for weight loss.

Chapter 6: *Proteins*

- The new *What Would You Choose* feature focuses on protein and amino acid intake and weight training.
- Figure 6-4 is now MyPlate: Sources of Protein.
- Recommendations from the new 2010 Dietary Guidelines regarding protein intake have been added.
- *Newsworthy Nutrition* focuses on the link between colon cancer and recent fat, protein, and red meat consumption.

Chapter 7: *Energy Balance and Weight Control*

- The new *What Would You Choose* feature focuses on the calorie content of frozen desserts.
- Figure 7-1 has been updated with obesity trends for 2009.
- New Weight Status Objectives from Healthy People 2020 are included.
- Recommendations from the new 2010 Dietary Guidelines regarding "Balancing Calories to Manage Weight," have been added.

- Two *Newsworthy Nutrition* features are included. One focuses on research indicating that small changes result in large weight changes and the other on a popular weight loss drug that has been withdrawn from the market.

Chapter 8: *Vitamins*

- The new *What Would You Choose* feature focuses on rich sources of folic acid, especially for pregnant women.
- Food group sources of the vitamins are now illustrated using the MyPlate graphic.
- The new Recommended Dietary Allowances for vitamin D, released in 2010, are discussed.
- Recommendations from the new 2010 Dietary Guidelines regarding vitamin intake have been added.
- Figure 8-27, Supplement Sales, has been updated to include sales for 2009 and 2010, and the Top Five Dietary Supplements have been updated for 2010.
- *Newsworthy Nutrition* focuses on research showing that folic acid added to cereal reduces neural-tube defects.

Chapter 9: *Water and Minerals*

- The new *What Would You Choose* feature focuses on the best choice of bottled water, especially when working out.
- Food group sources of the vitamins are now illustrated using the MyPlate graphic.
- *Newsworthy Nutrition* focuses on research indicating that lower sodium and higher potassium intakes reduce risk of cardiovascular disease.

Chapter 10: *Nutrition: Fitness and Sports*

- The *What Would You Choose* feature compares and contrasts some popular sports nutrition products.
- Discussion of the 2008 Physical Activity Guidelines for Americans has been expanded.
- Table 10-5 has been updated with protein needs of athletes.
- New products have been added to Table 10-6, Popular Energy Drinks and Table 10-8, Popular Energy Bars and Gels. Table 10-6 now includes caffeine, energy, and sugar content of energy drinks.
- The *Newsworthy Nutrition* feature distinguishes between sports drinks and energy drinks for athletic performance.

Chapter 11: *Eating Disorders*

- The *What Would You Choose* feature addresses how to approach a friend with a suspected eating disorder.
- The upcoming revisions to the *Diagnostic and Statistical Manual of Mental Disorders* related to eating disorders have been discussed, including the probable reclassification of Binge-Eating Disorder as an eating disorder.
- Discussion of genetics and eating disorders has been enhanced.
- Information on Muscle Dysmorphia has been included.
- The *Newsworthy Nutrition* feature points out common threads between binge eating and binge drinking.

Chapter 12: *Undernutrition Throughout the World*

- The new *What Would You Choose* feature focuses on choices to help put an end to world hunger.
- The content has been updated with current statistics on food insecurity, homelessness, hunger, and malnutrition.
- Table 12-2 has been updated to include new federally subsidized programs that supply food for people in the U.S.

- A New section, "Access to Healthy Food," includes discussion of food deserts in low income neighborhoods.
- The global impact of HIV/AIDS has been updated and illustrated in Figure 12-4.
- The *Newsworthy Nutrition* margin feature focuses on whether HIV-positive women should choose to breastfeed.
- Prevalence of genetically modified crops is updated.

Chapter 13: *Safety of Our Food Supply*

- *What Would You Choose* focuses on choosing fruits and vegetables with the best nutritional value, fewest preservatives and pesticides, and lowest risk for foodborne illness.
- The content has been updated with information about the most recent outbreaks of foodborne illnesses.
- Discussion of the new FDA Food Safety Modernization Act, signed into law in 2011 is included.
- The Food Safety Danger Zone has been updated.
- *Newsworthy Nutrition* focuses on the *E. coli* outbreak that was linked to German organic sprouts.

Chapter 14: *Pregnancy and Breastfeeding*

- The *What Would You Choose* feature addresses food choices to meet the needs of a pregnant vegetarian.
- Physical Activity Guidelines for pregnancy are included.
- New figures have been added to illustrate how nutrient requirements for pregnancy and breastfeeding differ from those of the RDAs/AIs of adult women.
- The *Newsworthy Nutrition* feature explores a proposed increase in vitamin D recommendations during pregnancy.
- Recommendations from the new 2010 Dietary Guidelines pertinent to pregnancy and breastfeeding have been added.
- Advice on maternal dietary restrictions to prevent food allergies has been updated to reflect the updated position of the American Academy of Pediatrics.
- Discussion of Fetal Alcohol Syndrome has been updated with the updated Fetal Alcohol Spectrum Disorders.

Chapter 15: *Nutrition from Infancy through Adolescence*

- The *What Would You Choose* feature looks into healthy and age-appropriate food choices for children.
- Throughout the chapter, including the *Newsworthy Nutrition* feature, the importance of family meals is emphasized.
- The latest American Academy of Pediatrics (AAP) recommendations on infant feeding have been included.
- Revised recommendations from the AAP and National Institute of Allergy and Infectious Disease for preventing food allergies and atopic disease have been included.
- New Figure 15-3 shows examples of meals that comply with MyPlate for children, ages 2, 4, 8, and 16.

Chapter 16: *Nutrition During Adulthood*

- The *What Would You Choose* feature explores nutritional approaches for reducing cancer risk.
- Recommendations from the new 2010 Dietary Guidelines and the 2008 Physical Activity Guidelines pertaining to older adults have been included.
- Figures have been added comparing nutrient requirements for older adults with those of the young adults.
- The *Newsworthy Nutrition* feature focuses on research regarding caloric restriction and longevity.

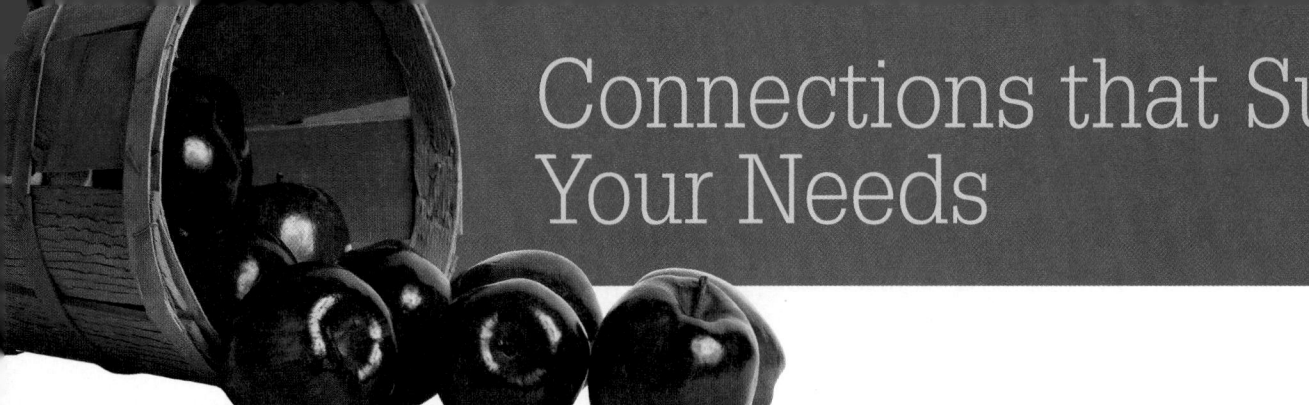

Connections that Suit Your Needs

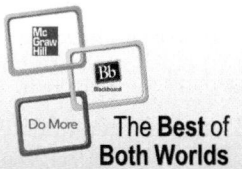

The **Best** of
Both Worlds

McGraw-Hill Higher Education and Blackboard® have teamed up!

What does this mean for you?

- **Life simplified.** Now, all McGraw-Hill content (text, tools, & homework) can be accessed directly from within your Blackboard course. All with one sign-on.

- **Deep integration.** McGraw-Hill's content and content engines are seamlessly woven within your Blackboard course.

- **No more manual synching!** Connect® assignments within Blackboard automatically (and instantly) feed grades directly to your Blackboard grade center. No more keeping track of two gradebooks!

- **A solution for everyone.** Even if your institution is not currently using Blackboard, we have a solution for you. Ask your McGraw-Hill representative for details.

Customize your course materials to your learning outcomes!

Create what you've only imagined.

Introducing McGraw-Hill Create™—a new, self-service website that allows you to create custom course materials—print and eBooks—by drawing upon McGraw-Hill's comprehensive, cross-disciplinary content. Add your own content quickly and easily. Tap into other rights-secured third-party sources as well. Then, arrange the content in a way that makes the most sense for your course. Even personalize your book with your course name and information! Choose the best format for your course: color print, black-and-white print, or eBook. The eBook is now even viewable on an iPad! And, when you are done, you will receive a free PDF review copy in just minutes!

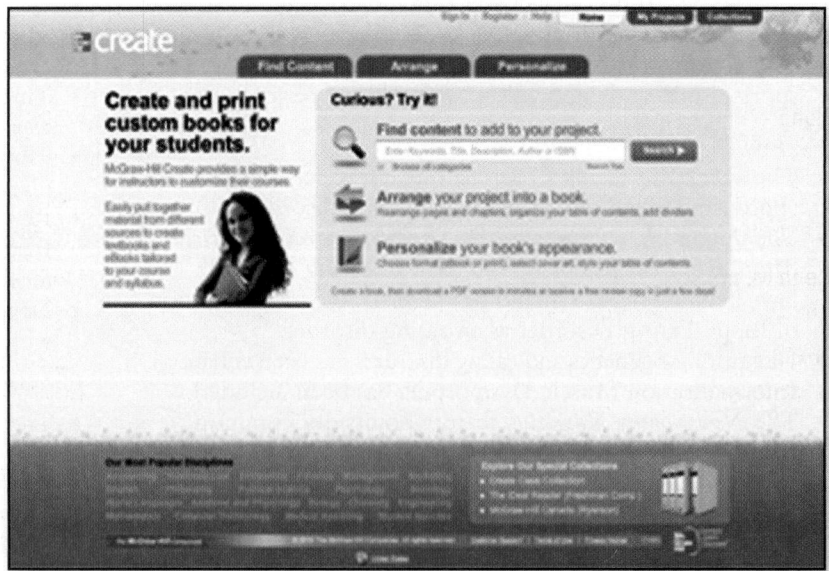

Finally, a way to quickly and easily create the course materials you've always wanted.

Imagine that.

Visit McGraw-Hill Create—www.mcgrawhillcreate.com—**today and begin building your perfect book.**

Acknowledgments

Special Acknowledgements

Writing a textbook requires much energy and constant support. We are indebted to several individuals for their creative abilities and generous interest in the production of this book. First, our deepest gratitude to our long-time editor Lynne Meyers, whose commitment, patience and encouragement has been extraordinary. She and her staff at McGraw-Hill have guided and assisted us through every phase of this and several previous revisions of Contemporary Nutrition. This edition is also much improved by the written contributions of Angela Collene, M.S., R.D. We thank her for always being ready at a moment's notice, especially with the recent updates to the Dietary Guidelines, MyPlate, and Healthy People 2020. Finally, we are grateful to Sheila Frank and her staff for the meticulous coordination of the many production efforts needed to produce the very appealing yet accurate ninth edition.

Thank you to reviewers

Our goal is to provide students and educators with the most accurate, up-to-date, and useful textbook possible. As with earlier editions, the quality of the ninth edition of *Contemporary Nutrition* is largely dependent on the thorough, professional assistance of nutrition educators from academic institutions across the nation. We are indebted to these colleagues who reviewed the eighth edition, evaluated new material for the ninth edition, participated in instructional symposia, and responded to surveys. The advice and suggestions from these colleagues have been used in every chapter and have resulted in a textbook that is current and inviting.

Gregory Avellana
Ohio University

Alena Clark
University of Northern Colorado

Robert DiSilvestro
The Ohio State University

Mary Jeanne Doyle
The University of Montana Missoula College of Technology

Keith M. Erikson
The University of North Carolina, Greensboro

Leslie Sisson Goudarzi
Kilgore College

Megan Govindan
West Virginia University

Charlene Harkins
University of Minnesota, Duluth

Maureen Baun Jamgochian
College of the Canyons

Gail L. Kaye
The Ohio State University

Molly Michelman
University of Nevada

Maria Montemagni
College of the Sequoias

Cheryl Neudauer
Minneapolis Community and Technical College

Janet Tou
West Virginia University

Ann M. Volk
Antelope Valley College

Mary Watson
University of Nebraska, Omaha

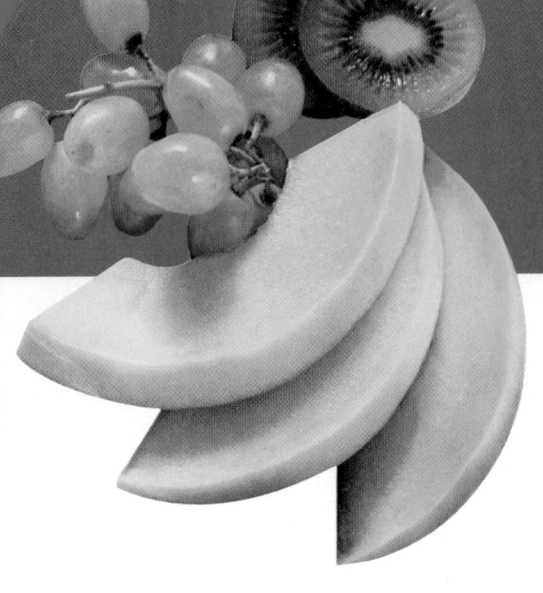

Contents

Preface vi

Part One Nutrition: A Key to Health 2

Chapter 1 Choosing What You Eat and Why 2

Chapter 2 Guidelines for Designing a Healthy Diet 34

Chapter 3 The Human Body: A Nutrition
Perspective 80

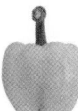

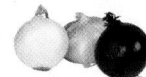

Part Three Vitamins, Minerals, and Water 288

Chapter 8 Vitamins 288

Part Four Nutrition: Beyond the Nutrients 406

Chapter 10 Nutrition: Fitness and Sports 406

Part Five Nutrition: A Focus on Life Stages 540

Chapter 1 Choosing What You Eat and Why

Student Learning Outcomes

Chapter 1 is designed to allow you to:

1.1 Describe how our food habits are affected by the flavor, texture, and appearance of food; routines and habits; early experiences and customs; advertising; nutrition and health concerns; restaurants; social changes; and economic, as well as physiological processes affected by meal size and composition.

1.2 Identify diet and lifestyle factors that contribute to the 15 leading causes of death in North America.

1.3 Define the terms *nutrition, carbohydrate, protein, lipid (fat), alcohol, vitamin, mineral, water, kilocalorie (kcal)*, and *fiber*.

1.4 Determine the total calories (kcal) of a food or diet using the weight and calorie content of the energy-yielding nutrients and use the basic units of the metric system to calculate percentages, such as percent of calories from fat in a diet.

1.5 List the major characteristics of the North American diet, the food habits that often need improvement, and the key "Nutrition and Weight Status" objectives of the *Healthy People 2020* report.

1.6 Describe a basic plan for health promotion and disease prevention and what to expect from good nutrition and a healthy lifestyle.

1.7 Identify food and nutrition issues relevant to college students.

What Would You Choose?

You were awake last night until 2:30 A.M. finishing a group project. Unfortunately, your Psychology 101 class meets at 9:00 this morning. When your alarm goes off at 7:30 A.M., you decide to sleep those extra 20 minutes it would take to sit down and enjoy breakfast at the dining hall. What's your best time-saving breakfast option?

a Skip breakfast, but plan to consume a few extra calories at lunch and dinner.

b Eat a low-fat granola bar and iced coffee from the vending machines in your dorm.

c Fix yourself a quick bowl of Wheaties with a banana and low-fat milk along with a yogurt, all from your dorm room "pantry."

d Pick up a ham, egg, and cheese bagel.

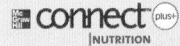 **Think about your choice as you read Chapter 1, then see our recommendations at the end of the chapter. To learn more about breakfast choices, check out the Connect site:** www.mcgrawhillconnect.com

Part One
Nutrition: A Key to Health

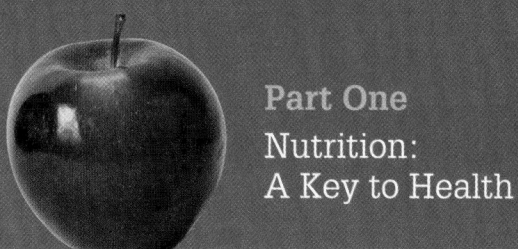

Research has clearly shown that a lifestyle that includes a diet rich in fruits, vegetables, and whole grains, coupled with regular exercise, can enhance our quality of life in the short term and keep us healthy for many years to come. Unfortunately, this healthy lifestyle is not always easy to follow. When it comes to "nutrition," it is clear that some of our diets are out of balance with our metabolism, physiology, and physical activity level.

We begin Chapter 1 with some questions. What influences your daily food choices? How important are factors such as taste, appearance, convenience, cost or value? Is nutrition one of the factors you consider? Are your food choices influencing your quality of life and long-term health? By making optimal dietary choices, we can bring the goal of a long, healthy life within reach. This is the primary theme of Chapter 1 and throughout this book.

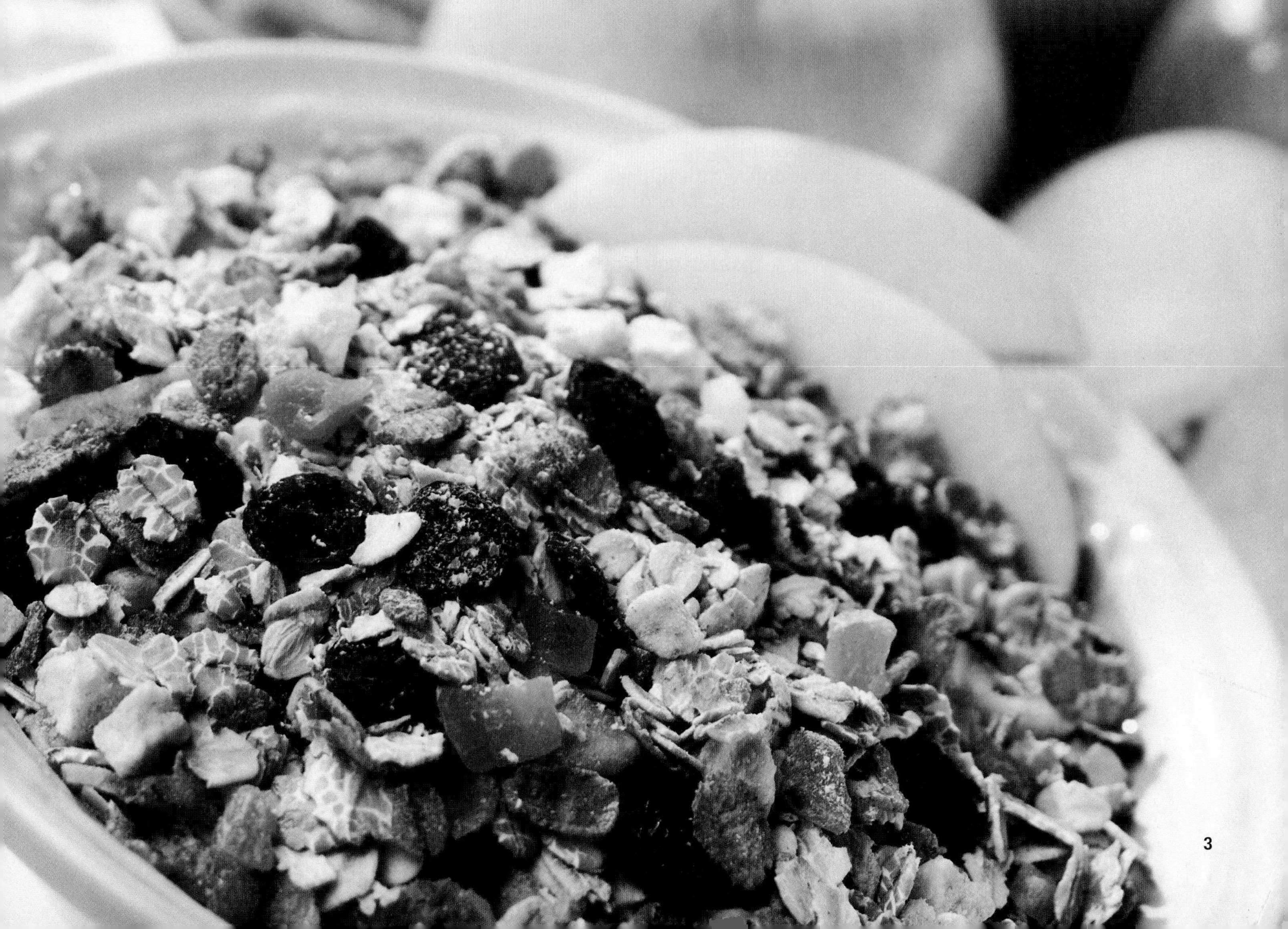

The ultimate goal of this book is to help you find the best path to good nutrition. The information presented is based on emerging science that is translated into everyday actions that improve health. After completion of your nutrition course you should understand the knowledge behind the food choices you make and recommend to others. We call this achievement of making food choices that are right for you "nutrition literacy."

 Refresh Your Memory

As you begin your study of choosing what you eat and why in Chapter 1, you may want to review:

- The metric system in Appendix I.

1.1 Why Do You Choose the Food You Eat?

In your lifetime, you will eat about 70,000 meals and 60 tons of food. Many factors influence our food choices including celebrations (see the comic below). Chapter 1 begins with a discussion of these factors and ends with a conversation specifically about eating well as a college student. In between, we examine the powerful effect of dietary habits in determining overall health and take a close look at the general classes of nutrients—as well as the calories—supplied by the food we eat, the major characteristics of the North American diet, the food habits that often need improvement, and the key "Nutrition and Weight Status" objectives in the *Healthy People 2020* report.

Understanding what drives us to eat and what affects food choice will help you understand the complexity of factors that influence eating, especially the effects of our routines and food advertising (Fig. 1-1). You can then appreciate why foods may have different meanings to different people and thus why food habits and preferences of others may differ from yours.

What Influences Your Food Choices?

Food means so much more to us than nourishment—it reflects much of what we think about ourselves. In the course of our lives, we spend the equivalent of 3 to 4 years eating. Yes, the Bureau of Labor Statistics estimated that in 2010 Americans spent the equivalent of 17 days eating and drinking. If we live to be 80 years old, that will add up to 3.7 years of eating and drinking. Overall, our daily food choices stem

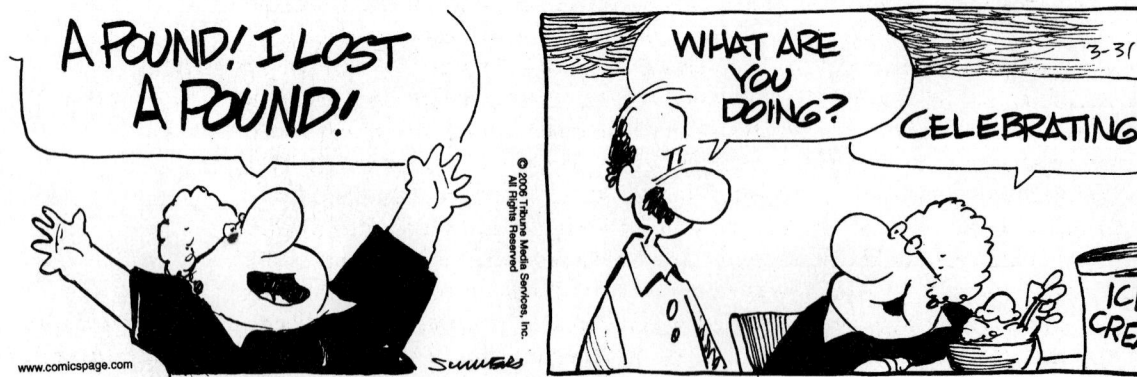

Copyright, 2002, Tribune Media Services. Reprinted with permission.

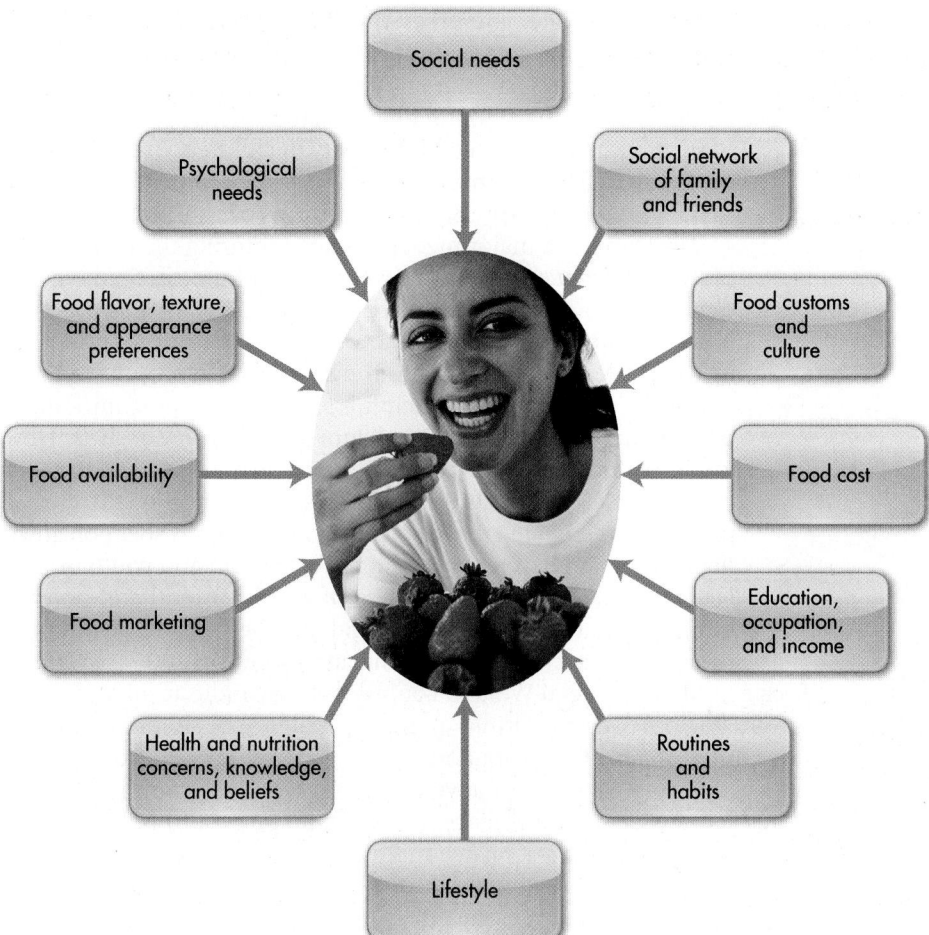

FIGURE 1-1 ▶ Food choices are affected by many factors. Which have the greatest impact on your food choices?

from a complicated mix of biological and social influences (see Fig. 1-1). Let's examine some of the key reasons we choose what we eat.

Flavor, texture, and *appearance* are the most important factors determining our food choices. Creating more flavorful foods that are both healthy and profitable is a major focus of the food industry. These foods are often referred to as "healthy" choices or "better for you" products. The challenge to the food industry is to match the "taste" of the foods we prefer with the nutrition and health characteristics of these products.

Early influences that expose us to various people, places, and events have a continuing impact on our food choices. Many ethnic diet patterns begin as we are introduced to foods during childhood. Developing healthy patterns during childhood, therefore, will go a long way to ensuring healthy preferences and choices when we are teenagers and adults. Food advertising and marketing have been shown to have a definite effect on weight gain in children and adolescents. Read more about the effect of television advertising and the development of obesity in childhood in the Newsworthy Nutrition margin note.

Routines and habits are tied to some food choices. Food habits, food availability, and convenience strongly influence choices. Most of us eat from a core group of foods with about 100 basic items accounting for 75% of an individual's total food intake. Recent surveys indicate that the most commonly purchased foods in America are milk (about 30 gallons yearly), ready-to-eat cereal, bottled water (about 25 gallons per year), soft drinks (nearly 50 gallons per year), and bread. It is no surprise that milk and cereal are both on the top-five list because they are eaten together as the daily breakfast for many Americans. Bottled water has become the drink of choice for business meetings and other large-group gatherings, including outdoor activities. Despite the

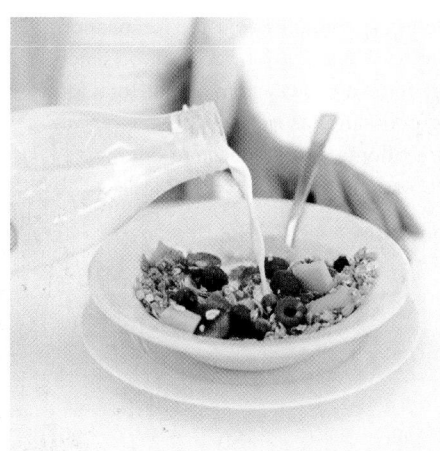

▲ Cereal and milk are two of the most commonly purchased foods in America largely because they are eaten together for breakfast every day by many.

NEWSWORTHY NUTRITION | **Link found between TV food ads and childhood obesity**

The higher prevalence of childhood obesity in the United States compared to other countries could be explained by greater exposure to TV food advertising. Scientists estimated the exposure of children ages 6 to 11 years in six countries to TV food advertising and its connection with obesity. The contribution of TV food ads to the occurrence of childhood obesity was greatest for the United States at 16% to 40%; lower in Australia and Italy at 10% to 28%; and lowest in Great Britain, Sweden, and the Netherlands at 4% to 18%. Children in the United States were exposed to 11.5 min/day of TV food ads compared to only 1.8 min/day in the Netherlands. Conclusions are that the contribution of TV food ads to the prevalence of childhood obesity is significant in some countries and greatest in the United States.

Source: Goris JM and others: Television food advertising and the prevalence of childhood overweight and obesity: A multicountry comparison. *Public Health Nutrition* 13: 1003, July 2010 (see Further Reading 7).

connect Check out the Connect site www.mcgrawhillconnect.com to further explore TV food ads and childhood obesity.

popularity of water and milk, Americans still drink nearly twice as many carbonated soft drinks per year as either water or milk. The large amount of sugar in many soft drinks is of particular concern because studies have found an association between consumption of sugar-sweetened drinks and obesity in children. Bread is also on the list because it is typically consumed at every meal in America, making it one of the most common forms of grain eaten.

Advertising is a major media tool for capturing the food interest of the consumer. Consumers have more food choices than ever and these choices are well advertised in newspapers, magazines, billboards, radio, television, and now the Internet. The food industry in the United States spends well over $33 billion on advertising. Some of this advertising is helpful, as it promotes the importance of food components such as calcium and fiber in our diets. However, the food industry also advertises highly sweetened cereals, cookies, cakes, and soft drinks because they bring in the greatest profits. It is estimated that as much as $10 billion is spent on advertising food and beverages to America's children and youth. A 2008 Federal Trade Commission survey of 44 major food and beverage marketers in the United States found that they spent $1.6 billion to promote products to children and adolescents in 2006 (see Further Reading 6). Recent studies in several Western countries clearly indicate an association between TV advertising of foods and drinks and the prevalence of childhood obesity, especially in the United States. (Read about one of these studies in Newsworthy Nutrition.) Concern for the negative effect of advertising and marketing on the diets and health of children led the Center for Science in the Public Interest to publish *Guidelines for Responsible Food Marketing to Children* in 2005 (see Further Reading 2). These guidelines provide criteria for marketing food to children in a manner that does not undermine children's diets or harm their health.

Restaurant dining plays a significant role in our food choices, although the recession caused a 11.5 percent decline in food eaten away from home between 2006 and 2009 (Fig 1-2). Restaurant food is often calorie-dense, in large portions, and of poorer nutritional quality compared to foods made at home. Fast-food and pizza restaurant menus typically emphasize meat, cheese, fried foods, and carbonated beverages. I response to recent consumer demands, restaurants have placed healthier items on

FIGURE 1-2 ▶ This chart shows the total food expenditures adjusted for inflation from 1990 to 2009 including food eaten at home and away from home. Total food expenditures as well as food eaten away from home dipped declined during the recession from 2006 to 2009.

Source: http://www.ers.usda.gov/AmberWaves/September11/Features/FoodSpending.htm

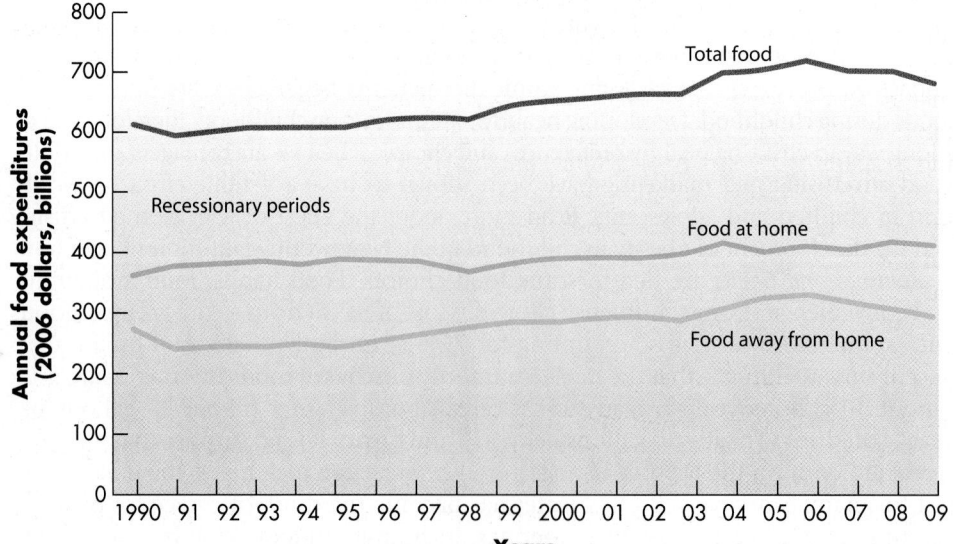

Total food expenditures adjusted for inflation dipped during the 2007–09 recession

their menus and many are listing nutritional content on their menus. Mandatory posting of the calorie content of restaurant items is expected to go into effect soon as a result of the health care reform bill that President Obama signed into law in March 2010. The law requires that chain restaurants with 20 or more locations post the calorie content of their offerings on menus or menu boards with other nutritional information available upon request.

Social changes are leading to a general time shortage for many of us. This creates the need for *convenience*. Supermarkets now supply prepared meals, microwavable entrees, and various quick-prep frozen products.

Economics play a minor role in our food choices. Increases in personal income have exceeded increases in dollars spent for food. This has resulted in the average North American spending only about 12% of after-tax income on food (greater for low-income people). However, as income increases, so do meals eaten away from home and preferences for foods such as cookies, chocolate, cheese, and meat. Also keep in mind that as calorie intake increases so does the food bill.

Last but not least, *nutrition*—or what we think of as "healthy foods"—also directs our food purchases. North Americans who tend to make health-related food choices are often well-educated, middle-class professionals. These same people are generally health-oriented, have active lifestyles, and focus on weight control. In the 2008 Health and Diet Survey (a snapshot of the nation's dietary habits), the Food and Drug Administration (FDA) found that more than half (54%) of consumers in the United States read the food label when buying a product for the first time. This number was an increase since 2002. Among those who are reading the Nutrition Facts, 67% use the label "often" to check how high or low a food is in calories and in substances such as salt, vitamins, and fat; 55% "often" use the label to get a general idea of the food's nutritional content; and 46% "often" use the calorie information on the label. Their key findings also indicate that consumers are increasingly aware of the link between diet and heart disease. Of those surveyed, 91% knew of this link, 81% knew that certain foods or drinks may help prevent heart disease or heart attacks, and 62% mentioned fats as a factor related to heart disease (see Further Reading 4).

Why Are You So Hungry?

Two drives, **hunger** and **appetite,** influence our desire to eat. These drives differ dramatically. Hunger is primarily our physical biological drive to eat and is controlled by internal body mechanisms. For example, as foods are digested and absorbed by the stomach and small intestine, these organs send signals to the liver and brain to reduce further food intake.

Appetite, our primarily psychological drive to eat, is affected by many of the external food choice mechanisms we discussed in the last section, such as environmental and psychological factors and social customs (see Fig. 1-1). Appetite can be triggered simply by seeing a tempting dessert or smelling popcorn popping at the movie theater. Fulfilling either or both drives by eating sufficient food normally brings a state of **satiety,** a feeling of satisfaction that temporarily halts our desire to continue eating.

A region of the brain helps regulate satiety. Imagine a game of tug-of-war in the brain. The *feeding center* and the *satiety center* work in opposite ways to promote adequate availability of nutrients at all times. When stimulated, cells in the feeding center signal us to eat. As we eat, cells in the satiety center are stimulated and we stop eating. For example, when we haven't eaten for a while, stimulation of the feeding center signals

hunger The primarily physiological (internal) drive to find and eat food, mostly regulated by internal cues to eating.

appetite The primarily psychological (external) influences that encourage us to find and eat food, often in the absence of obvious hunger.

satiety State in which there is no longer a desire to eat; a feeling of satisfaction.

MAKING DECISIONS

Putting Our Food Choices into Perspective

The next time you pick up a candy bar or reach for a second helping, remember the internal and external influences on eating behavior. You should now understand that daily food intake is a complicated mix of biological and social influences. Body cells, nutrients in the blood, hormones, brain chemicals, and our social and family customs all influence food choices. When food is abundant, appetite—not hunger—most likely triggers eating. Satiety associated with consuming a meal may reside primarily in our psychological frame of mind. Also, because satiety regulation is not perfect, body weight can fluctuate. We become accustomed to a certain amount of food at a meal. Providing less than that amount leaves us wanting more. One way to use this observation for weight-loss purposes is to train your eye to expect less food by slowly decreasing serving sizes to more appropriate amounts. Your appetite then readjusts as you expect less food. Keep track of what triggers your eating for a few days. Is it primarily hunger or appetite? The Rate Your Plate activity in this chapter also asks you to keep track of what influences your food intake on a daily basis.

CRITICAL THINKING

Sarah is majoring in nutrition and is well aware of the importance of a healthy diet. She has recently been analyzing her diet and is confused. She notices that she eats a great deal of high-fat foods, such as peanut butter, cheese, chips, ice cream, and chocolate, and few fruits, vegetables, and whole grains. She also has become hooked on her daily cappuccino with lots of whipped cream. What three factors may be influencing Sarah's food choices? What advice would you give her on how to have her diet match her needs?

nutrients Chemical substances in food that contribute to health, many of which are essential parts of a diet. Nutrients nourish us by providing calories to fulfill energy needs, materials for building body parts, and factors to regulate necessary chemical processes in the body.

essential nutrient In nutritional terms, a substance that, when left out of a diet, leads to signs of poor health. The body either cannot produce this nutrient or cannot produce enough of it to meet its needs. Then, if added back to a diet before permanent damage occurs, the affected aspects of health are restored.

us to eat. When the nutrient content in the blood rises after a meal, the satiety center is stimulated and we no longer have a strong desire to seek food. Admittedly, this concept of a tug-of-war between the feeding and satiety centers is an oversimplification of a complex process. The various feeding and satiety messages from body cells to the brain do not single-handedly determine what we eat. We often eat because food confronts us (see Further Reading 17). Almost everyone has encountered a mouthwatering dessert and devoured it, even on a full stomach. It smells, tastes, and looks good. We might eat because it is the right time of day, we are celebrating (see the cartoon in this section), or we are seeking emotional comfort to overcome the blues. After a meal, memories of pleasant tastes and feelings reinforce appetite. If stress or depression sends you to the refrigerator, you are mostly seeking comfort, not food calories. Appetite may not be a physical process, but it does influence food intake. We will discuss more about this mechanism, including the effect of meal size and composition on satiety, in Chapter 7 on energy balance and weight control.

CONCEPT CHECK

Hunger is the primarily physical or internal desire to find and eat food. Fulfilling it creates satiety—no further desire to eat exists. Satiety is influenced by hunger-related (internal) signals from the brain and other organs, as well as the content of the foods in the meal. Food intake is also affected by appetite-related (external) forces like social customs, time of day, and being with others. Factors such as flavor, appearance, and texture; early influences, routines, and habits; advertising and restaurant menus; economics and convenience; seeking emotional comfort; social changes; and hopefully, nutrition and health concerns, also greatly influence our food choices. North Americans probably respond more to external, appetite-related forces than to hunger-related ones in choosing when and what to eat.

1.2 How Is Nutrition Connected to Good Health?

Fortunately the foods we eat can support good health in many ways depending on their components. You just learned, however, that lifestyle habits and other factors may have a bigger impact on our food choices than the food components themselves. Unfortunately many North Americans suffer from diseases that could have been prevented if they had known more about the foods and, more importantly, had applied this knowledge to planning meals and designing their diet. We will now look at the effect these choices are having on our health both today and in the future.

What Is Nutrition?

Nutrition is the science that links foods to health and disease. It includes the processes by which the human organism ingests, digests, absorbs, transports, and excretes food substances.

Nutrients Come from Food

What is the difference between food and **nutrients**? Food provides the energy (in the form of calories) as well as the materials needed to build and maintain all body cells. Nutrients are the substances obtained from food that are vital for growth and maintenance of a healthy body throughout life. For a substance to be considered an **essential nutrient**, three characteristics are needed:

- First, at least one specific biological function of the nutrient in the body must be identified.

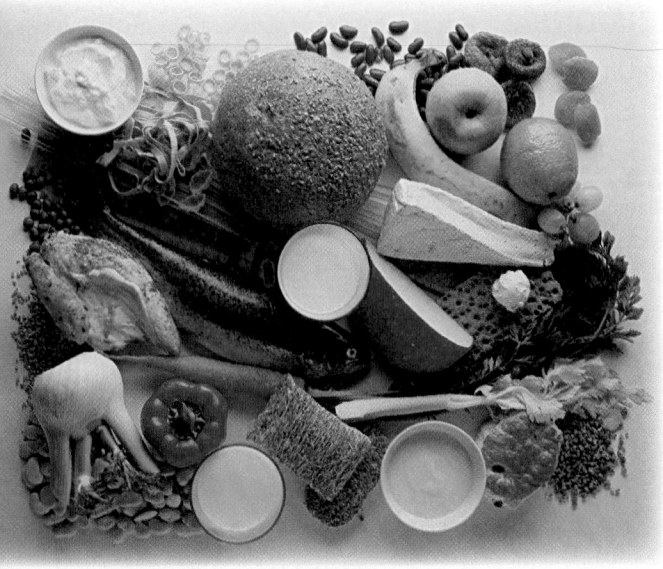

▲ Many foods are rich sources of nutrients.

- Second, omission of the nutrient from the diet must lead to a decline in certain biological functions, such as production of blood cells.
- Third, replacing the omitted nutrient in the diet before permanent damage occurs will restore those normal biological functions.

Why Study Nutrition?

Nutrition is a lifestyle factor that is a key to developing and maintaining an optimal state of health for you. A poor diet and a sedentary lifestyle are known to be **risk factors** for life-threatening **chronic** diseases such as **cardiovascular (heart) disease, hypertension, diabetes,** and some forms of **cancer** (Table 1-1). Together, these and related disorders account for two-thirds of all deaths in North America (Table 1-2)

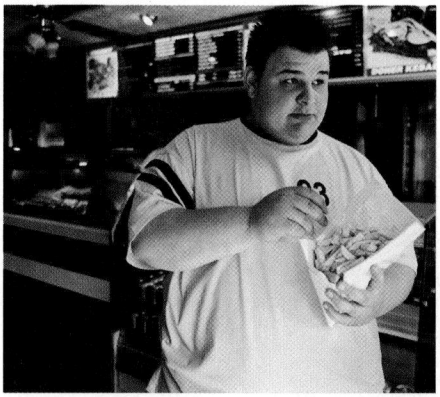

▲ Major health problems are largely caused by a poor diet, excessive calorie intake, and not enough physical activity.

TABLE 1-1 Glossary Terms to Aid Your Introduction to Nutrition*

Cancer	A condition characterized by uncontrolled growth of abnormal cells.
Cardiovascular (heart) disease	A general term that refers to any disease of the heart and circulatory system. This disease is generally characterized by the deposition of fatty material in the blood vessels (hardening of the arteries), which in turn can lead to organ damage and death. Also termed coronary heart disease (CHD), as the vessels of the heart are the primary sites of the disease.
Cholesterol	A waxy lipid found in all body cells; it has a structure containing multiple chemical rings. Cholesterol is found only in foods of animal origin.
Chronic	Long-standing, developing over time. When referring to disease, this term indicates that the disease process, once developed, is slow and lasting. A good example is cardiovascular disease.
Diabetes	A group of diseases characterized by high blood **glucose.** Type 1 diabetes involves insufficient or no release of the hormone insulin by the pancreas and therefore requires daily insulin therapy. Type 2 diabetes results from either insufficient release of insulin or general inability of insulin to act on certain body cells, such as muscle cells. Persons with type 2 diabetes may or may not require insulin therapy.
Hypertension	A condition in which blood pressure remains persistently elevated. Obesity, inactivity, alcohol intake, excess salt intake, and genetics may each contribute to the problem.
Kilocalorie (kcal)	Unit that describes the energy content of food. Specifically, a kilocalorie (kcal) is the heat energy needed to raise the temperature of 1000 grams (1 liter) of water 1° Celsius. Kcal refers to a 1000 calorie unit of measurement, but is commonly referred to as calories. It is a familiar term for the energy content of a food, so we will use it in this book.
Obesity	A condition characterized by excess body fat.
Osteoporosis	Decreased bone mass related to the effects of aging (including estrogen loss during menopause in women), genetic background, and poor diet.
Risk factor	A term used frequently when discussing the factors contributing to the development of a disease. A risk factor is an aspect of our lives—such as heredity, lifestyle choices (e.g., smoking), or nutritional habits.

glucose A six-carbon sugar that exists in a ring form; found as such in blood, and in table sugar bound to fructose; also known as *dextrose,* it is one of the simple sugars.

*Many bold terms are also defined in the page margins within each chapter and in the glossary at the end of this book.

TABLE 1-2 Fifteen Leading Causes of Death in the United States

Rank	Cause of Death	Percent of Total Deaths
	All causes	100
1	Heart disease*†#	24.6
2	Cancer*‡	23.3
3	Chronic lower respiratory diseases‡	5.6
4	Stroke (cerebrovascular diseases)*†‡#	5.3
5	Accidents (unintentional injuries)	4.8
6	Alzheimer's disease*	3.2
7	Diabetes mellitus*	2.8
8	Influenza and pneumonia	2.2
9	Kidney disease*‡	2.0
10	Intentional self harm (suicide)	1.5
11	Blood-borne infections (septicemia)	1.4
12	Chronic liver disease and cirrhosis†	1.2
13	Essential hypertension*	1.1
14	Parkinson's disease	0.8
15	Assault (homicide)	0.7

From Centers for Disease Control and Prevention, *National Vital Statistics Report,* Preliminary Data for 2009, March 16, 2011. Canadian statistics are quite similar.

*Causes of death in which diet plays a part.

†Causes of death in which excessive alcohol consumption plays a part.

‡Causes of death in which tobacco use plays a part.

#Diseases of the heart and cerebrovascular disease are included in the more global term "cardiovascular disease."

stroke A decrease or loss in blood flow to the brain that results from a blood clot or other change in arteries in the brain. This in turn causes the death of brain tissue. Also called a *cerebrovascular accident.*

NEWSWORTHY NUTRITION

Healthy diet lowers women's risk of sudden cardiac death

Sudden cardiac death (death occurring within 1 hour after symptom onset) is the cause of more than half of all heart-related deaths and usually occurs as the first sign of heart disease, especially in women. Lifestyle information from the Nurses' Health Study (81,722 women) was used to determine if adherence to a healthy lifestyle lowers the risk of sudden cardiac death among women. Low-risk lifestyle was considered as not smoking, not overweight, exercising 30 minutes/day or longer, and following the Mediterranean Diet. Risk of sudden cardiac death dropped by 92% with a combination of the four healthy lifestyles; and women who ate a diet most similar to the Mediterranean Diet with a high proportion of vegetables, fruits, nuts, omega-3 fats, and fish, along with moderate amounts of alcohol and small amounts of red meat, had a 40% less risk than women whose diets least resembled this diet. The conclusion is that a healthy diet along with other healthy lifestyle factors can protect women from sudden cardiac death.

Source: Chiuve SE, and others: Adherence to a low-risk, healthy lifestyle and risk of sudden cardiac death among women. *Journal of the American Medical Association,* 306:62, 2011 (see Further Reading 3).

Check out the Connect site www.mcgrawhillconnect.com **to further explore women's risk of sudden cardiac death.**

(see Further Reading 9). Not meeting nutrient needs in younger years makes us more likely to suffer health consequences, such as bone fractures from the disease **osteoporosis,** in later years. At the same time, taking too much of a nutrient—such as a vitamin A supplement—can be harmful. Another dietary problem, drinking too much alcohol, is associated with many health problems.

U.S. government scientists have calculated that a poor diet combined with a lack of sufficient physical activity contributes to hundreds of thousands of fatal cases of cardiovascular disease, cancer, and diabetes each year among adults in the United States. Thus, the combination of poor diet and too little physical activity may be the second leading cause of death in the United States. In addition, **obesity** is considered the second leading cause of preventable death in North America (smoking is the first). When they occur together, obesity and smoking cause even more health problems. Obesity and chronic diseases are often preventable. An important key to good health and more health care dollars in your pocket, is to realize that the cost of prevention, usually when we are children and young adults, is a small fraction of the cost of treating these diseases when we are older.

3

The good news is that the increased interest in health, fitness, and nutrition shown by Americans has been associated with long-term decreasing trends for heart disease, cancer, and stroke (the three leading causes of death) that continued in 2009. Mortality from heart disease, the leading cause of death, has been declining steadily since 1980. As you gain understanding about your nutritional habits and increase your knowledge about optimal nutrition, you will have the opportunity to dramatically reduce your risk for many common health problems. Read more about research on the link between eating a healthy diet and protection against death from heart disease in Newsworthy Nutrition. For additional help, the U.S. federal government provides two websites that contain links to many sources of health and nutrition information (www.healthfinder.gov and www.nutrition.gov). Other useful sites are www.webmd.com and www.eatright.org.

1.3 What Are the Classes and Sources of Nutrients?

To begin the study of nutrition, let's start with an overview of the six classes of nutrients. You are probably already familiar with the terms **carbohydrates, lipids** (fats and oils), **proteins, vitamins,** and **minerals.** These, plus **water,** make up the six classes of nutrients found in food.

Nutrients can then be assigned to three functional categories: (1) those that primarily provide us with calories to meet energy needs (expressed in **kilocalories [kcal]**); (2) those important for growth, development, and maintenance; and (3) those that act to keep body functions running smoothly. Some function overlap exists among these categories. The energy-yielding nutrients, carbohydrate, fat, and protein, make up a major portion of most foods (Table 1-3).

Let's now look more closely at these six classes of nutrients.

Carbohydrates

Chemically, carbohydrates can exist in foods as simple sugars and complex carbohydrates. **Simple sugars,** frequently referred to as *sugars,* are relatively small molecules. These sugars are found naturally in fruits, vegetables, and dairy products. Table sugar, sucrose, is an example of a simple sugar that is added to many foods we eat. Glucose, also known as blood sugar or dextrose, is an example of a simple sugar in your blood. **Complex carbohydrates** are formed when many simple sugars are joined together. For example, plants store carbohydrates in the form of **starch,** a complex carbohydrate made up of hundreds of sugar units. Breads, cereals, grains, and starchy vegetables are the main sources of complex carbohydrates.

TABLE 1-3 Major Functions of the Various Classes of Nutrients

Nutrient Classes That Provide Energy	Nutrient Classes That Promote Growth, Development, and Maintenance	Nutrient Classes That Regulate Body Processes
Most carbohydrates	Proteins	Proteins
Proteins	Lipids	Some lipids
Most lipids	Some vitamins	Some vitamins
	Some minerals	Some minerals
	Water	Water

Carbohydrates, proteins, lipids, and water are needed in relatively large amounts, so they are called **macronutrients.** Vitamins and minerals are needed in such small amounts in the diet that they are called **micronutrients.**

carbohydrate A compound containing carbon, hydrogen, and oxygen atoms. Most are known as *sugars, starches,* and *fibers.*

lipid A compound containing much carbon and hydrogen, little oxygen, and sometimes other atoms. Lipids do not dissolve in water, and include fats, oils, and cholesterol.

protein Food and body compounds made of amino acids; proteins contain carbon, hydrogen, oxygen, nitrogen, and sometimes other atoms, in a specific configuration. Proteins contain the form of nitrogen most easily used by the human body.

vitamin Compound needed in very small amounts in the diet to help regulate and support chemical reactions in the body.

mineral Element used to promote chemical reactions and to form body structures.

water The universal solvent; chemically, H_2O. The body is composed of about 60% water. Water (fluid) needs are about 9 (women) or 13 (men) cups per day; needs are greater if one exercises heavily.

kilocalorie (kcal) Heat energy needed to raise the temperature of 1000 grams (1 L) of water 1 degree Celsius; also written as *Calories.*

simple sugar Monosaccharide or disaccharide in the diet.

complex carbohydrate Carbohydrate composed of many monosaccharide molecules. Examples include glycogen, starch, and fiber.

macronutrient A nutrient needed in gram quantities in a diet.

micronutrient A nutrient needed in milligram or microgram quantities in a diet.

cell The structural basis of plant and animal organization. Cells contain genetic material and systems for synthesizing energy-yielding compounds. Cells have the ability to take up compounds from and excrete compounds into their surroundings.

bond A linkage between two atoms formed by the sharing of electrons, or attractions.

fiber Substances in plant foods not digested by the processes that take place in the human stomach or small intestine. These add bulk to feces. Fiber naturally found in foods is also called dietary fiber.

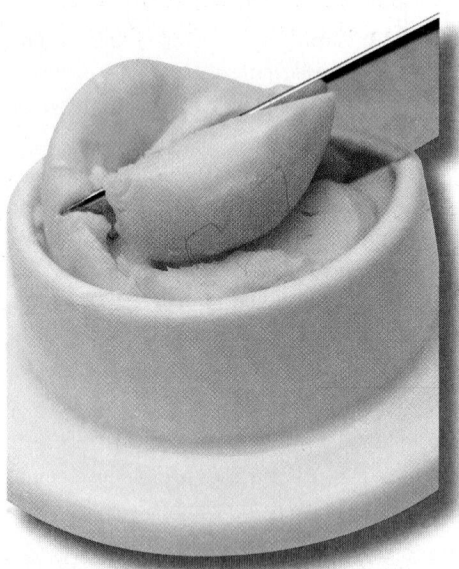

▲ Butter is an animal fat made from milk fat and is solid at room temperature.

enzyme A compound that speeds the rate of a chemical reaction but is not altered by the reaction. Almost all enzymes are proteins (some are made of genetic material).

amino acid The building block for proteins containing a central carbon atom with nitrogen and other atoms attached.

During digestion, complex carbohydrates are broken down into single sugar molecules (such as glucose), and absorbed via **cells** lining the small intestine into the bloodstream (see Chapter 3 for more on digestion and absorption). However, the **bonds** between the sugar molecules in certain complex carbohydrates, called **fiber,** cannot be broken down by human digestive processes. Fiber passes through the small intestine undigested to provide bulk for the stool (feces) formed in the large intestine (colon).

Aside from enjoying their taste, we need sugars and other carbohydrates in our diets primarily to help satisfy the calorie needs of our body cells. Carbohydrates provide a major source of calories for the body, on average 4 kcal per gram. Glucose, a simple sugar that the body can derive from most carbohydrates, is a major source of calories for most cells. When not enough carbohydrate is consumed to supply sufficient glucose, the body is forced to make glucose from proteins—not a healthy change. Chapter 4 focuses on carbohydrates.

Lipids

Lipids (mostly fats and oils) in the foods we eat also provide energy. Lipids yield more calories per gram than do carbohydrates—on the average, 9 kcal per gram—because of differences in their chemical composition. They are also the main form for energy storage in the body.

Lipids dissolve in certain chemical solvents (e.g., ether and benzene) but not in water. In this book, the more familiar terms *fats* and *oils* will generally be used, rather than lipids or triglycerides. Generally, fats are lipids that are solid at room temperature and oils are lipids that are liquid at room temperature. We obtain fats and oils from animal and plant sources. Animal fats, such as butter or lard, are solid at room temperature. Plant oils, such as corn or olive oil, tend to be liquid at room temperature. Solid fat should be limited in our diet because it can raise blood **cholesterol.** High blood cholesterol leads to clogged arteries and can eventually lead to cardiovascular disease (see Chapter 5).

Certain fats are essential nutrients that must come from our diet. These key fats that the body cannot produce, called essential fatty acids, perform several important functions in the body: they help regulate blood pressure and play a role in the synthesis and repair of vital cell parts. However, we need only about 4 tablespoons of a common plant oil (such as the canola or soybean oil) each day to supply these essential fatty acids. A serving of fatty fish, such as salmon or tuna, at least twice a week is another healthy source of essential fatty acids. The unique fatty acids in these fish complement the healthy aspects of common vegetable oils. This will be explained in greater detail in Chapter 5, which focuses on lipids.

Proteins

Proteins are the main structural material in the body. For example, proteins constitute a major part of bone and muscle; they are also important components in blood, body cells, **enzymes,** and immune factors. Proteins can also provide calories for the body—on average, 4 kcal per gram. Typically, however, the body uses little protein for the purpose of meeting daily calorie needs. Proteins are formed when **amino acids** are bonded together. Some of these are essential nutrients.

Protein in our diet also comes from animal and plant sources. The animal products meat, poultry, fish, dairy products, and eggs are significant sources of protein in most diets. Beans, grains, and some vegetables are good plant protein sources. Plant protein is important to include in vegetarian diets.

Most North Americans eat up to two times as much protein as the body needs to maintain health. This amount of extra protein in the diet reflects the standard of living and the dietary habits of most North Americans and is generally not harmful for healthy persons with no evidence of heart or kidney disease, diabetes, or family history of colon cancer or kidney stones. The excess is used for calorie needs and carbohydrate production but ultimately can contribute to storage of fat. Chapter 6 focuses on proteins.

Vitamins

The main function of vitamins is to enable many <u>chemical reactions</u> to occur in the body. Some of these reactions help release the energy trapped in carbohydrates, lipids, and proteins. Remember, however, that vitamins themselves contain no usable calories for the body.

The 13 vitamins are divided into two groups: four are **fat-soluble** because they dissolve in fat (vitamins A, D, E, and K); nine are **water-soluble** because they dissolve in water (the B vitamins and vitamin C). The two groups of vitamins have different sources, functions, and characteristics. Water-soluble vitamins are found mainly in fruits and vegetables, whereas dairy products, nuts, seeds, oils, and breakfast cereals are good sources of fat-soluble vitamins. Cooking destroys water-soluble vitamins much more readily than it does fat-soluble vitamins. Water-soluble vitamins are also excreted from the body much more readily than are fat-soluble vitamins. Thus, the fat-soluble vitamins, especially vitamin A, are much more likely to accumulate in excessive amounts in the body, which then can lead to toxicity. Vitamins are the focus of Chapter 8.

Minerals

Minerals are structurally simple, **inorganic** substances, which do not contain carbon atoms. Minerals such as sodium and potassium typically function independently in the body, whereas minerals such as calcium and phosphorus function as parts of simple mineral combinations, such as bone mineral. Because of their simple structure, minerals are not destroyed during cooking, but they can still be lost if they dissolve in the water used for cooking and that water is then discarded. Minerals are critical players in nervous system functioning, water balance, structural (e.g., skeletal) systems, and many other cellular processes, but produce no calories as such for the body.

The 16 or more essential minerals required in the diet for good health are divided into two groups: **major minerals** and **trace minerals** because dietary needs vary enormously. If daily needs are less than 100 milligrams, the mineral is classified as a trace mineral; otherwise, it is a major mineral. Minerals that function based on their electrical charge when dissolved in water are also called **electrolytes;** these include sodium, potassium, and chloride. Many major minerals are found naturally in dairy products and fruits, whereas many trace minerals are found in meats, poultry, fish, and nuts. Minerals are the focus of Chapter 9.

Water

Water makes up the sixth class of nutrients. Although sometimes overlooked as a nutrient, water (chemically, H_2O) has numerous vital functions in the body. It acts as a **solvent** and lubricant, as a vehicle for transporting nutrients and waste, and as a medium for temperature regulation and chemical processes. For these reasons, and because the human body is approximately 60% water, the average man should consume about 3 liters—equivalent to 3000 grams or about 13 cups—of water and/or other fluids containing water every day. Women need closer to 2200 grams or about 9 cups per day.

Water is not only available from the obvious sources, but it is also the major component in some foods, such as many fruits and vegetables (e.g., lettuce, grapes, and melons). The body even makes some water as a by-product of **metabolism.** Water is examined in detail in Chapter 2.

Other Important Components in Food

Another group of compounds in foods from plant sources, especially within the fruit and vegetable groups, is what scientists call **phytochemicals.** Although these plant components are not considered essential nutrients in the diet, many of these substances provide significant health benefits. Considerable research attention is focused on various phytochemicals in reducing the risk for certain diseases. For example, evidence from animal and laboratory studies indicate that compounds in blueberries and

chemical reaction An interaction between two chemicals that changes both chemicals.

inorganic Any substance lacking carbon atoms bonded to hydrogen atoms in the chemical structure.

electrolytes Substances that separate into ions in water and, in turn, are able to conduct an electrical current. These include sodium, chloride, and potassium.

solvent A liquid substance in which other substances dissolve.

metabolism Chemical processes in the body by which energy is provided in useful forms and vital activities are sustained.

phytochemical A chemical found in plants. Some phytochemicals may contribute to a reduced risk of cancer or cardiovascular disease in people who consume them regularly.

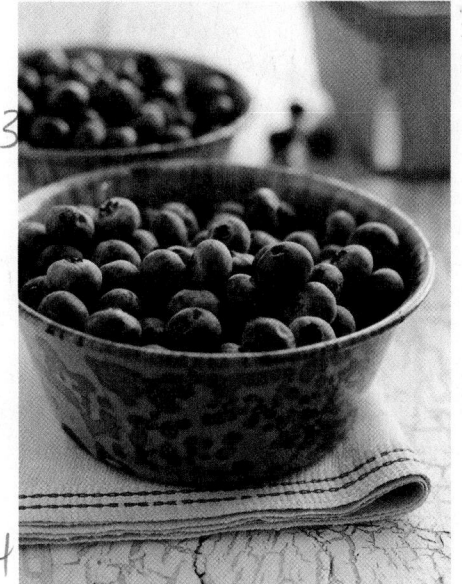

▲ Blueberries are among the fruits, vegetables, beans, and whole-grain breads and cereals that are typically rich in phytochemicals.

TABLE 1-4 Food Sources of Some Phytochemical Compounds under Study

Phytochemical	Food Sources
Allyl sulfides/organosulfurs	Garlic, onions, leeks
Saponins	Garlic, onions, licorice, legumes
Carotenoids (e.g., lycopene)	Orange, red, yellow fruits and vegetables (egg yolks are a source as well)
Monoterpenes	Oranges, lemons, grapefruit
Capsaicin	Chili peppers
Lignans	Flaxseed, berries, whole grains
Indoles	Cruciferous vegetables (broccoli, cabbage, kale)
Isothiocyanates	Cruciferous vegetables, especially broccoli
Phytosterols	Soybeans, other legumes, cucumbers, other fruits and vegetables
Flavonoids	Citrus fruit, onions, apples, grapes, red wine, tea, chocolate, tomatoes
Isoflavones	Soybeans, other legumes
Catechins	Tea
Polyphenols	Blueberries, strawberries, raspberries, grapes, apples, bananas, nuts
Anthocyanosides	Red, blue, and purple plants (blueberries, eggplant)
Fructooligosaccharides	Onions, bananas, oranges (small amounts)
Resveratrol	Grapes, peanuts, red wine

Some related compounds under study are found in animal products, such as sphingolipids (meat and dairy products) and conjugated linoleic acid (meat and cheese). These are not phytochemicals per se because they are not from plant sources, but they have been shown to have health benefits.

strawberries prevent the growth of certain cancer cells. Although certain phytochemicals are available as dietary supplements, research suggests that their health benefits are best obtained through the consumption of whole foods. Foods with high phytochemical content are sometimes called "superfoods" because of the health benefits they are thought to confer. There is no legal definition of the term superfood, however, and there is concern that it is being over-used in marketing certain foods. Table 1-4 lists some noteworthy phytochemicals with their common food sources. Tips for boosting the phytochemical content of your diet will be discussed in Chapter 2.

Sources of Nutrients

Now that we know the six classes of nutrients, it is important to understand that the quantities of the various nutrients that people consume in different foods vary widely. On a daily basis we consume about 500 grams, or about 1 pound, of protein, fat, and carbohydrate. In contrast, the typical daily mineral intake totals about 20 grams (about 4 teaspoons), and the daily vitamin intake totals less than 300 milligrams (1/15 of a teaspoon). Although we require a gram or so of some minerals, such as calcium and phosphorus, we need only a few milligrams or less of other minerals each day. For example, we need about 10 milligrams of zinc per day, which is just a few specks of the mineral.

 The nutrient content of the foods we eat also differs from the nutrient composition of the human body. This is because growth, development, and later maintenance of the human body are directed by the genetic material (DNA) inside body cells. This genetic blueprint determines how each cell uses the essential nutrients to perform body functions. These nutrients can come from a variety of sources. Cells are not concerned about whether available amino acids come from animal or plant sources. The carbohydrate glucose can come from sugars or starches. The food that you eat provides cells with basic materials to function according to the directions supplied by the genetic material (**genes**) housed in body cells. Genetics and nutrition will be discussed in Chapter 3.

1.4 What Are Your Sources of Energy?

Calories

Humans obtain the energy we need for involuntary body functions and voluntary physical activity from various calorie sources: carbohydrates (4 kcal per gram), fats (9 kcal per gram), and proteins (4 kcal per gram). Foods generally provide more than one calorie source. Plant oils, such as soybean or canola oil are one exception; these are 100% fat at 9 kcal per gram.

Alcohol is also a source of calories for some of us, supplying about 7 kcal per gram. It is not considered an essential nutrient, however, because it has no required function. Still, alcoholic beverages, such as beer—also rich in carbohydrate—are a contributor of calories to the diet of many adults.

The body releases the energy from the chemical bonds in carbohydrate, protein, and fat (and alcohol) into other forms of energy in order to:

- Build new **compounds.**
- Perform muscular movements.
- Promote nerve transmissions.
- Maintain electrolyte balance within cells.

Chapters 7 and 12 describe how that energy is released from the chemical bonds in energy-yielding nutrients and then used by body cells to support the processes just described.

The energy in food is often expressed in terms of calories on food labels. As defined earlier, a calorie is the amount of heat energy it takes to raise the temperature of 1 gram of water 1 degree Celsius (1°C, centigrade scale). (Chapter 7 has a diagram of the bomb calorimeter that can be used to measure calories in foods.) A calorie is a tiny measure of heat, so food energy is more conveniently expressed in terms of the kilocalorie (kcal), which equals 1000 calories. (If the "c" in calories is capitalized, this also signifies kilocalories.) A kcal is the amount of heat energy it takes to raise the temperature of 1000 grams (1 liter) of water 1°C. The abbreviation *kcal* is used throughout this book. On food labels, the word *calorie* (without a capital "C") is also used loosely to mean *kilocalorie*. Any values given on food labels in calories are actually in kilocalories (Fig. 1-3). A suggested intake of 2000 calories per day on a food label is technically 2000 kcal.

genes A specific segment on a chromosome. Genes provide the blueprints for the production of all body proteins.

alcohol Ethyl alcohol or ethanol (CH_3CH_2OH) is the compound in alcoholic beverages.

compound A group of different types of atoms bonded together in definite proportion.

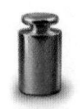

Carbohydrate
4 kcal per gram

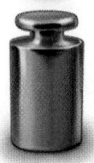

Fat
9 kcal per gram

Protein
4 kcal per gram

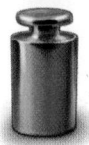

Alcohol
7 kcal per gram

▲ Calorie content of energy nutrients and alcohol.

Nutrition Facts			
Serving Size 1 slice (36g)		Servings Per Container 19	
Amount Per Serving			
Calories 80		Calories from Fat 10	
	% Daily Value*		**% Daily Value***
Total Fat 1g	**2%**	**Total Carbohydrate** 15g	**5%**
Saturated Fat 0g	**0%**	Dietary Fiber 2g	**8%**
Trans Fat less than 1g	**		
Cholesterol 0mg	**0%**	Sugars less than 1g	
Sodium 200mg	**8%**	**Protein** 3g	
Vitamin A 0%	Vitamin C 0%	Calcium 0%	Iron 4%
HONEY WHEAT BREAD			

*Percent Daily Values (DV) are based on a 2,000 calorie diet. Your daily values may be higher or lower depending on your calorie needs:

		Calories:	2,000	2,500
Total Fat	Less than		65g	80g
Sat Fat	Less than		20g	25g
Cholesterol	Less than		300mg	300mg
Sodium	Less than		2,400mg	2,400mg
Total Carbohydrate			300g	375g
Dietary Fiber			25g	30g

** Intake of *trans* fat should be as low as possible.

INGREDIENTS: WHOLE WHEAT, WATER, ENRICHED WHEAT FLOUR [FLOUR, MALTED BARLEY, NIACIN, REDUCED IRON, THIAMINE MONONITRATE (VITAMIN B1) AND RIBOFLAVIN (VITAMIN B2)], CORN SYRUP, PARTIALLY HYDROGENATED COTTONSEED OIL, SALT, YEAST.

FIGURE 1-3 ▶ Use the nutrient values on the Nutrition Facts label to calculate calorie content of a food. Based on carbohydrate, fat, and protein content, a serving of this food (Honey Wheat Bread) contains 81 kcal ([15 × 4] + [1 × 9] + [3 × 4] = 81). The label lists 80, suggesting that the calorie value was rounded down.

Calculating Calories

Use the 4-9-4 estimates for the calorie content of carbohydrate, fat, and protein introduced over the last few pages to determine calorie content of a food. Consider these foods:

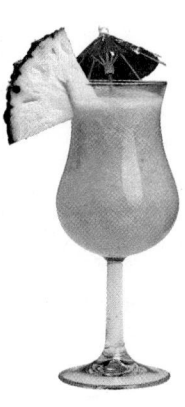 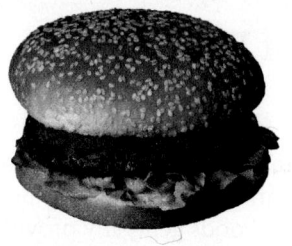

1 Large Hamburger

Carbohydrate	39 grams × 4 = 156 kcal
Fat	32 grams × 9 = 288 kcal
Protein	30 grams × 4 = 120 kcal
Alcohol	0 grams × 7 = 0 kcal
Total	**564 kcal**

8-ounce Piña Colada

Carbohydrate	57 grams × 4 = 228 kcal
Fat	5 grams × 9 = 45 kcal
Protein	1 gram × 4 = 4 kcal
Alcohol	23 grams × 7 = 161 kcal
Total	**438 kcal**

You can also use the 4-9-4 estimates to determine what portion of total calorie intake is contributed by the various calorie-yielding nutrients. Assume that one day you consume 290 grams of carbohydrates, 60 grams of fat, and 70 grams of protein. This consumption yields a total of 1980 kcal ([290 × 4] + [60 × 9] + [70 × 4]5 = 1980). The percentage of your total calorie intake derived from each nutrient can then be determined:

$$\text{\% of kcal as carbohydrate} = (290 × 4) ÷ 1980 = 0.59 \ (×100 = 59\%)$$
$$\text{\% of kcal as fat} = (\ 60 × 9) ÷ 1980 = 0.27 \ (×100 = 27\%)$$
$$\text{\% of kcal as protein} = (\ 70 × 4) ÷ 1980 = 0.14 \ (×100 = 14\%)$$

Check your calculations by adding the percentages together. Do they total 100?

MAKING DECISIONS

Percentages and the Metric System

You will use a few mathematical concepts in studying nutrition. Besides performing addition, subtraction, multiplication, and division, you need to know how to calculate percentages and convert English units of measurement to metric units.

Percentages

The term percent (%) refers to a part of the total when the total represents 100 parts. For example, if you earn 80% on your first nutrition examination, you will have answered the equivalent of 80 out of 100 questions correctly. This equivalent could be 8 correct answers out of 10; 80% also describes 16 of 20 (16/20 = 0.80 or 80%). The decimal form of percents is based on 100% being equal to 1.00. It is difficult to succeed in a nutrition course unless you know what a percentage means and how to calculate one. Percentages are used frequently when referring to menus and nutrient composition. The best way to master this concept is to calculate some percentages. Some examples follow:

Question	Answer
What is 6% of 45?	6% = 0.06 or 0.06 × 45 = 2.7
What percent of 99 is 3?	3/99 = 0.03 or 3% (0.03 × 100)

Joe ate 15% of the adult Recommended Dietary Allowance (RDA = 8 milligrams) for iron at lunch. How many milligrams did he eat?

$$0.15 × 8 \text{ milligrams} = 1.2 \text{ milligrams}$$

The Metric System

The basic units of the metric system are the meter, which indicates length; the gram, which indicates weight; and the liter, which indicates volume. Appendix I in this textbook lists conversions from the metric system to the English system (pounds, feet, cups) and vice versa. Here is a brief summary:

A gram (g) is about 1/30 of an ounce (28 grams to the ounce).
5 grams of sugar or salt is about 1 teaspoon.
A pound (lb) weighs 454 grams.
A kilogram (kg) is 1000 grams, equivalent to 2.2 pounds.
To convert your weight to kilograms, divide it by 2.2.
A 154-pound man weighs 70 kilograms (154/2.2 = 70).
A gram can be divided into 1000 milligrams (mg) or 1,000,000 micrograms (μg or mcg).
    10 milligrams of zinc (approximate adult needs) would be a few grains of zinc.
Liters are divided into 1000 units called milliliters (ml).
One teaspoon equals about 5 milliliters (ml), 1 cup is about 240 milliliters, and 1 quart
    (4 cups) equals almost 1 liter (L) (0.946 liter to be exact).

If you plan to work in any scientific field, you will need to learn the metric system. *For now, remember that a kilogram equals 2.2 pounds, an ounce weighs 28 grams, 2.54 centimeters equals 1 inch, and a liter is almost the same as a quart.* In addition, know the fractions that the following prefixes represent: micro (1/1,000,000), milli (1/1000), centi (1/100), and kilo (1000).

CONCEPT CHECK

Nutrition is the study of food and nutrients—their digestion, absorption, and metabolism, and their effect on health and disease. Food contains the vital nutrients essential for good health: carbohydrates, lipids (fats and oils), proteins, vitamins, minerals, and water. Nutrients have three general functions in the body: (1) to provide materials for building and maintaining the body; (2) to act as regulators for key metabolic reactions; and (3) to participate in metabolic reactions that provide the energy necessary to sustain life. A common unit of measurement for this energy is the kilocalorie (kcal). On average, carbohydrates and protein provide 4 kcal per gram of energy to the body, while lipids provide 9 kcal per gram. Although not considered a nutrient, alcohol provides about 7 kcal per gram. The other classes of nutrients (vitamins, minerals, and water) do not supply calories but are essential for proper body functioning.

1.5 What Is the Current State of the North American Diet and Health?

Does Obesity Threaten Our Future?

In 2001, the U.S. Surgeon General issued a Call to Action about the obesity epidemic in America. Over the past 10 years, however, the problem has worsened. Whereas in 2001 61% of U.S. adults were overweight or obese, in 2010 the rates were even higher with 68%, or 190 million people, overweight or obese. A recent report from the Trust for America's Health and the Robert Wood Johnson Foundation indicated that between 2009 and 2010 the percentage of obese adults increased in 16 states and did not decline in any states. Their report, "F as in Fat: How Obesity Threatens America's Future 2011" (July 2011), also revealed that 12 states now have obesity rates above 30%, compared to 2006, when only one state was above 30%. This recent report (Fig. 1-4) is based on self-reported state-by-state obesity data from the Centers for Disease Control and Prevention (CDC) (see Further Reading 16). Because we tend to underreport our

FIGURE 1-4 ▶ Percentage of adults who are obese,* by state, 2009.

*Body mass index (BMI) ≥ 30, or about 30 pounds overweight for a 5′ 4″ person, based on self-reported weight and height.

Source: CDC, Behavioral Risk Factor Surveillance System.

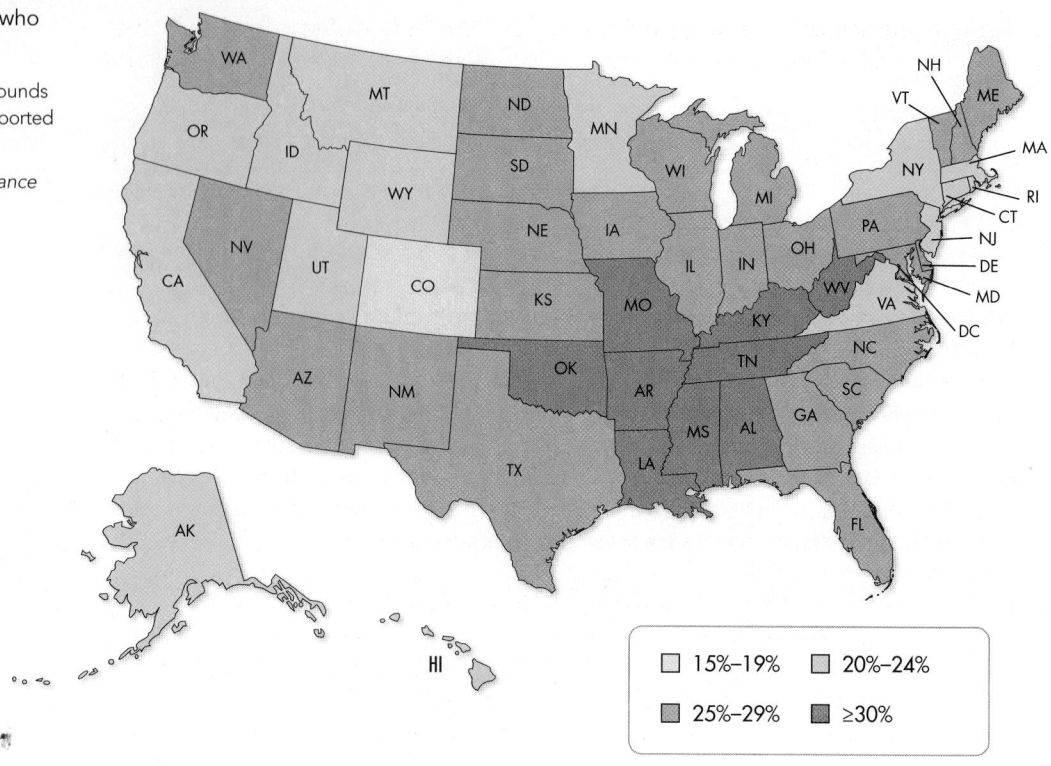

Legend	
☐ 15%–19%	☐ 20%–24%
☐ 25%–29%	■ ≥30%

weight, the percentage of Americans who are obese is probably greater than reported. Even more alarming are the statistics for children. In 2001 nearly 12% of children and adolescents were overweight, whereas in 2010 nearly one-third of children and teens fell into these categories.

It is well documented that this extra weight of more than 4.5 billion extra pounds has and will continue to have dangerous consequences. In an earlier section of this chapter, we already pointed out that obesity plays a role in chronic illness, including heart disease, stroke, high blood pressure, high cholesterol, diabetes, arthritis, and certain cancers. It is estimated that obesity kills more than 110,000 Americans a year. Because of its role in so many chronic disorders, obesity is also an expensive condition. More than $150 billion is spent annually on health care related to obesity, and obesity costs U.S. employers $73 billion in lost productivity every year. It has become obvious that the answers to the obesity crisis are not simple. From a nutrition perspective, however, the problem can be clearly stated. Most of us continue to eat too much, especially foods with a high number of calories and a low number of nutrients, and we do not engage in enough physical activity.

Assessing the Current North American Diet

With the aim of finding out what North Americans eat, federal agencies conduct surveys to collect data about food and nutrient consumption, as well as connections between diet and health. In the United States, the U.S. Department of Health and Human Services monitors food consumption with the National Health and Nutrition Examination Survey (NHANES). In Canada, this information is gathered by Health Canada in conjunction with Agriculture and Agrifood Canada. Survey data indicate that North American adults consume about 15% of their calorie intake as proteins, 52% as carbohydrates, and 33% as fats. These percentages, which do not consider alcohol, fall within the ranges recommended by the Food and Nutrition Board (FNB) of the National Academy of Sciences. The FNB advocates that 10%

to 35% of calories come from protein, 45% to 65% from carbohydrate, and 20% to 35% from fat. These standards apply to people in both the United States and Canada.

Food-consumption data also indicate that animal sources supply about two-thirds of protein intake for most North Americans, whereas plant sources supply only about one-third. In many other parts of the world, it is just the opposite: plant proteins—from rice, beans, corn, and other grains and vegetables—dominate protein intake. About half the carbohydrate in North American diets comes from simple sugars; the other half comes from starches (such as in pastas, breads, and potatoes). About 60% of dietary fat comes from animal sources and 40% from plant sources.

Results from national nutrition surveys and other studies show that North Americans consume more calories than ever before and from a wide variety of foods. Individuals, however, often do not choose the foods that will meet all their nutrient needs. Food availability data from 1909 to 2007 confirm that the major contributors to increased energy intake over the last century are oils, shortening, meat, cheese, and frozen desserts. Since 1970 there has been an increase in added sweeteners, and carbonated beverage availability has increased at the expense of milk.

In the next section, we discuss recommendations to consume a variety of nutrient-dense foods within and across the food groups, especially whole grains, fruits, vegetables, low-fat or fat-free milk or milk products, and lean meats and other protein sources. These foods will provide nutrients that are often overlooked, including various B vitamins, vitamin C (especially for smokers), vitamin D, vitamin E, calcium, potassium, magnesium, iron, fiber, and many phytonutrients. Daily intake of a balanced multivitamin and mineral supplement is another strategy to help meet nutrient needs but does not make up for a poor diet, particularly for calcium, potassium, and fiber intake. Also keep in mind that taking numerous dietary supplements can lead to health problems (see Chapter 8).

Routinely, experts also recommend that we pay more attention to balancing calorie intake with needs. An excess intake of calories is usually tied to overindulgence in sugar, fat, and alcoholic beverages. African-Americans and Hispanics have a greater chance of developing hypertension than do other ethnic groups in North America and therefore may need to decrease the amount of **salt** (sodium chloride) and alcohol in their diets. These substances are two of the many factors linked to hypertension. Moderation of salt and alcohol intake—along with certain fats, cholesterol, and total calorie intake—is a recommended practice for all adults.

Many North Americans would benefit from a healthier balance of food in their diets. Moderation is the key for some foods, such as sugared soft drinks and fried foods. For other foods, such as fruits and vegetables, increased quantity and variety are warranted. Few adults currently meet the new recommendation to "fill half your plate with fruits and vegetables" promoted in the new USDA MyPlate guidelines for total servings of vegetables and fruits.

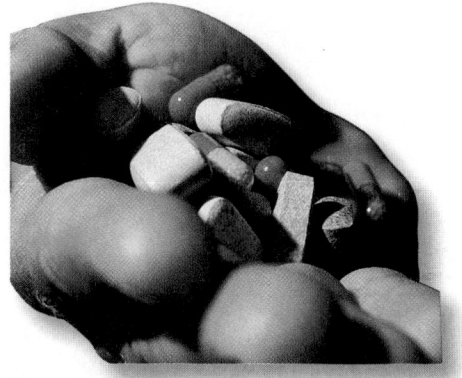

▲ Taking numerous nutrient supplements can lead to health problems. Chapter 8 will explore the appropriate and safe use of nutrient supplements in detail.

salt Compound of sodium and chloride in a 40:60 ratio.

Health Objectives for the United States for the Year 2020

Health promotion and disease prevention have been public health strategies in North America for the past three decades. One part of this strategy is *Healthy People 2020*, a report issued in December 2010 by the U.S. Department of Health and Human Services' (DHHS) Public Health Service. Every 10 years, DHHS issues a collection of health objectives for the nation. These objectives are developed by experts in federal agencies and target major public health concerns, setting goals for the coming decade. *Healthy People 2020* sets forth more than 600 health objectives across 42 topic areas and outlines national standards to eliminate health disparities, improve access to health education and quality health care, and strengthen public health services. The vision for 2020 is a society in which all people live long, healthy lives. Important new features of *Healthy People 2020* include a focus on health equity and social determinants of health, and a move to an interactive, personalized website at www.HealthyPeople.gov.

The overarching goals of *Healthy People 2020* aim to:

- Attain high-quality, longer lives free of preventable disease, disability, injury, and premature death.
- Achieve health equity, eliminate disparities, and improve health of all groups.
- Create social and physical environments that promote good health for all.
- Promote quality of life, healthy development, and healthy behaviors across all life stages.

Healthy People 2020, like earlier versions, includes a topic area specific to nutrition. This topic is called Nutrition and Weight Status, and its objectives target individual behaviors, as well as the policies and environments that support these behaviors. Nutrition and weight status is important because a healthful diet helps us reduce our risks for numerous health conditions that burden the public health system, including heart disease, high blood pressure, diabetes, osteoporosis, and some cancers. Good nutrition for children is also emphasized in this report because of its importance for growth and development. The goal of this topic is to promote health and reduce chronic disease risk through the consumption of healthful diets and achievement and maintenance of healthy body weights. This goal also includes increasing household food security and eliminating hunger.

The Nutrition and Weight Status objectives are based on strong science that supports the health benefits of eating a healthful diet and maintaining a healthy body weight. A healthful diet is described as one that includes:

- Consuming a variety of nutrient-dense foods within and across the food groups, especially whole grains, fruits, vegetables, low-fat or fat-free milk or milk products, and lean meats and other protein sources
- Limiting intake of solid fats, cholesterol, added sugars, sodium (salt), and alcohol
- Limiting intake of calories to meet needs for calories

The objectives also emphasize that individual behaviors, as well as the policies and environments that support these behaviors in settings such as schools, worksites, health care organizations, and communities, should be addressed in any efforts to change diet and weight.

Table 1-5 is a list of the six categories of objectives for the Nutrition and Weight Status topic, along with the the 22 specific objectives. Table 1-6 provides a more detailed sample of nine of the specific Nutrition and Weight Status objectives along with the current status of these objectives and their targets for 2020.

Other new topic areas highlight changes in the health needs of specific segments of the population: Early and Middle Childhood, Adolescence, and Older Adults. Because young people develop habits, including eating and physical activity behaviors, which are likely to persist throughout life, new objectives promote strengthened health education in schools and communities and fostering an environment in which young people can develop healthy habits. Older adults are the fastest-growing segment of the American population and are at high risk for experiencing the chronic health problems that so severely impact our health care system. The objectives for Older Adults include improving access to health care, helping older adults to manage their own health conditions, and ensuring proper training and support of professionals and nonprofessionals who care for this population.

A scientifically exciting new topic area is **Genomics.** Nine of the ten leading causes of death have a strong genetic component. Genetic testing is becoming a

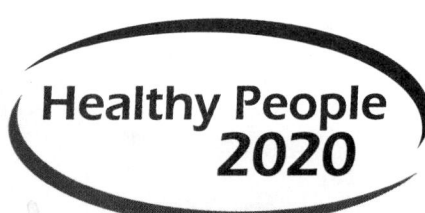

▲ Many nutrition-related objectives are part of the *Healthy People 2020* report. The report outlines health promotion and disease prevention objectives for the United States for the year 2020.

TABLE 1-5 *Healthy People 2020*: Nutrition and Weight Status Objectives

Category 1: Healthier Food Access

1. Increase the number of states with nutrition standards for child care.

2. Increase the proportion of schools that offer nutritious foods and beverages outside of school meals.

3. Increase the number of states that have incentive policies for food retail to provide foods that are encouraged by the 2010 Dietary Guidelines for Americans.

4. Increase the proportion of Americans who have retail access to foods recommended by the 2010 Dietary Guidelines for Americans.

Category 2: Health Care and Worksite Settings

5. Increase the proportion of primary care physicians who measure patients' body mass index (BMI).

6. Increase the proportion of physician office visits that include nutrition or weight counseling or education.

7. Increase the proportion of worksites that offer nutrition and weight-management classes and counseling.

Category 3: Weight Status

8. Increase the proportion of adults who are at a healthy weight.

9. Reduce the proportion of adults who are obese.

10. Reduce the proportion of children and adolescents who are considered obese.

11. Prevent inappropriate weight gain in youth and adults.

Category 4: Food Insecurity

12. Eliminate very low food security among children.

13. Reduce household food insecurity and in so doing reduce hunger.

Category 5: Food and Nutrient Consumption

14. Increase the contribution of fruits to the diets of the population ages 2 years and older.

15. Increase the variety and contribution of vegetables to the diets of the population ages 2 years and older.

16. Increase the contribution of whole grains to the diets of the population ages 2 years and older.

17. Reduce consumption of calories from solid fats and added sugars in the population ages 2 years and older.

18. Reduce consumption of saturated fat in the population ages 2 years and older.

19. Reduce consumption of sodium in the population ages 2 years and older.

Category 6: Iron Deficiency

20. Increase consumption of calcium in the population ages 2 years and older.

21. Reduce iron deficiency among young children and females of childbearing age.

22. Reduce iron deficiency among pregnant females.

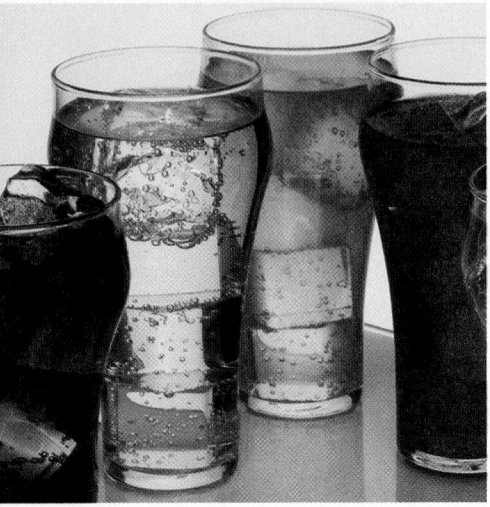

▲ Moderation in the intake of some foods, such as sugared soft drinks and fried foods, can lead to a healthier balance of food in the North American diet.

TABLE 1-6 A Sample of Nutrition and Weight Status Objectives from *Healthy People 2020* along with Details about the Current Status and Targets for 2020

	Target	Current Estimate
Increase the proportion of adults at a healthy weight.	33.9%	30.8%
Reduce the proportion of overweight or obese children and adolescents.	14.6%	16.2%
Increase the contribution of the following to the diets of the population ages 2 years and older (per 1000 calories).		
• Fruits	0.9 cup	0.5 cup
• Total vegetables	1.1 cups	0.8 cup
• Whole grains	0.6 ounce	0.3 ounce
Reduce consumption of calories from solid fats (of total calorie intake).	16.7%	18.9%
Reduce consumption of calories from added sugars (of total calorie intake).	10.8%	15.7%
Increase consumption of calcium in the population ages 2 years and older.	1300 mg	1118 mg
Reduce iron deficiency among females of childbearing age.	9.4%	10.4%

Note: In later chapters, we will explore additional nutrition-related objectives, such as those addressing osteoporosis, various forms of cancer, diabetes prevention and treatment, food allergies, cardiovascular disease, low birth weight, nutrition during pregnancy, breastfeeding, eating disorders, physical activity, and alcohol use.

valuable tool for improving diagnosis and treatment of chronic diseases, especially for cancers of the breast and colon. In combination with family history, genetic testing can help health care professionals guide patients in treatment options, including lifestyle changes. The relationship between genetics and nutrition will be discussed in Chapter 3.

1.6 What Can You Expect from Good Nutrition and a Healthy Lifestyle?

The obesity epidemic in the United States illustrates that something is not right with many of our diets and/or lifestyles. The strong association between obesity and poor health is clear. The reverse is also well documented—when an obese or overweight person loses just 5% to 10% of body weight, that person's risks of many chronic diseases are greatly reduced.

Because weight gain is one of the greatest lifelong nutrition challenges we face, we encourage you to seek a lifestyle that will make gaining weight more difficult and maintaining a healthy weight easier. Believe it or not, preventing obesity in the first place is the easiest approach. Unfortunately, many aspects of our society make it hard for us not to gain weight. The earlier (preferably in childhood) we develop lifestyle habits of good nutrition, regular physical activity, and the avoidance of addictions to salt, fat, sweets, high-calorie foods, and sedentary lifestyles, the better (see

Further Readings 14 and 15). As you enter the workforce, seek out employers who offer wellness programs that encourage weight management and weight loss among their employees. Aim to live in a city or town that has opportunities for physical activity such as bike paths, walking trails, and parks, as well as access to fresh fruits and vegetables through farmers' markets and community gardens. Seek out organizations that offer running or walking clubs. Make a habit of shopping at grocery stores that offer a good selection of fruits, vegetables, and other healthy foods. When dining out, choose restaurants that have tasty but healthy options on their menu. While we still are choosing foods with too many calories, many other dietary habits have improved during the past decade. Today we can choose from a tremendous variety of food products, the result of continual innovation by food manufacturers. We are eating more breakfast cereals, pizza, pasta entrees, stir-fried meats and vegetables served on rice, salads, tacos, burritos, and fajitas than ever before. Sales of whole milk are down, and sales of fat-free and 1% low-fat milk have increased. Consumption of frozen vegetables rather than canned vegetables is also on the rise. Despite the alarming problem of overweight and obesity, our cultural diversity, varied cuisines, and general lack of nutrient deficiencies should be points of pride for North Americans.

Today, North Americans live longer than ever and enjoy better general health. Many also have more money and more diverse food and lifestyle choices to consider. The nutritional consequences of these trends are varied. Deaths from cardiovascular disease, for example, have dropped dramatically since the late 1960s, partly because of better medical care and diets. Affluence, however, has also led to sedentary lifestyles and high intakes of animal fat, cholesterol, salt, and alcohol. This lifestyle pattern has led to problems such as cardiovascular disease, hypertension, diabetes, and, of course, obesity. Greater efforts are needed by the general public to lower intake of animal fat and cholesterol and to improve variety in our diets, especially from fruits, vegetables, and whole grains. With better technology and greater choices, we can have a much better diet today than ever before—if we know what choices to make.

Nutrition experts generally agree that there are no "good" or "bad" foods, but some foods provide relatively few nutrients in comparison to calorie content. In Chapter 2, you will learn that an individual's total diet is the proper focus in a nutritional evaluation. Health experts have prepared many reports and outlined numerous objectives to get us closer to being a *Healthy People* as soon as 2020. In Chapter 2, we will discuss the new "Dietary Guidelines" that were published in 2010, and the new interactive program called "ChooseMyPlate.gov" that was unveiled in 2011. As you reexamine your nutritional habits, remember your health is largely your responsibility. Your body has a natural ability to heal itself. Offer it what it needs, and it will serve you well. Confusing and conflicting health messages hinder diet change. Nutrition science does not have all the answers, but as you will see, enough is known to help you set a path to good health and put diet-related recommendations you hear in the future into perspective. Table 1-7 summarizes several diet, physical activity, and general lifestyle recommendations to promote your health and prevent chronic diseases in the future. In total, these contribute to maximal health and prevention of the diseases listed. The final section in Chapter 1, Nutrition and Your Health: Eating Well in College, elaborates on several nutrition issues very relevant to most college students, including the "freshman 15," vegetarianism, fuel for athletes, eating disorders, and alcohol and binge drinking. This section gives you a "sneak peek" at issues that will be covered more fully later in the book.

▼ A healthy diet benefits people of all ages.

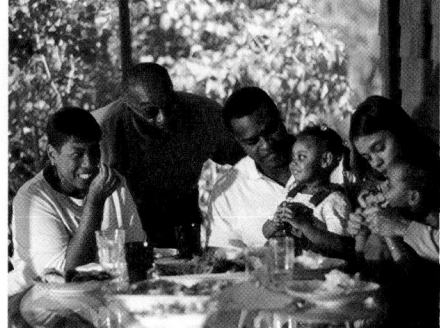

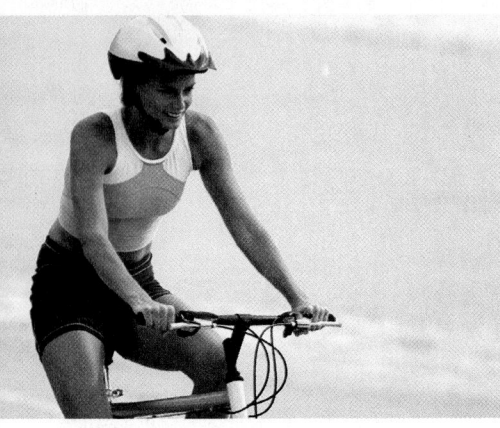

▲ Regular physical activity complements a healthy diet. Whether it is all at once or in segments throughout the day, incorporate 30 to 60 minutes or more of such activity into your daily routine.

TABLE 1-7 Recommendations for Health Promotion and Disease Prevention

Diet

Consuming enough essential nutrients, including fiber, while moderating energy, solid fat, cholesterol, added sugar, and alcohol intake can result in:

- Increased bone mass during childhood and adolescence
- Prevention of some adult bone loss and osteoporosis, especially in older adults
- Fewer dental caries
- Prevention of digestive problems, such as constipation
- Decreased susceptibility to some cancers
- Decreased degradation of the retina (intake of green and orange vegetables, in particular)
- Lower risk of obesity and related diseases, such as type 2 diabetes and cardiovascular disease
- Reduced risk for deficiency diseases, such as cretinism (lack of iodide), scurvy (lack of vitamin C), and anemia (lack of iron, folate, or other nutrients)

Physical Activity

Adequate, regular physical activity (at least 30 minutes on most or all days) helps reduce the risk of:

- Obesity
- Type 2 diabetes
- Cardiovascular disease
- Some adult bone loss and loss of muscle tone
- Premature aging
- Certain cancers

Lifestyle

Minimizing alcohol intake (no more than two drinks per day for men and one drink for both women and all adults age 65 years and older) helps prevent:

- Liver disease
- Accidents

Not smoking cigarettes or cigars helps prevent:

- Lung cancer, other lung disease, kidney disease, cardiovascular disease, and degenerative eye diseases

In addition, minimum use of medication, no illicit drug use, adequate sleep (7 to 8 hours), adequate water and related fluid intake (9 to 13 cups per day), and a reduction in stress (practice better time management, relax, listen to music, have a massage, and stay physically active) provide a more complete approach to good nutrition and health. Add to this maintaining close relationships with others and a positive outlook on life. Finally, consultation with health care professionals on a regular basis is important. This is because early diagnosis is especially useful for controlling the damaging effects of many diseases. Prevention of disease is an important investment of one's time, including during the college years.

CONCEPT CHECK

Surveys in the United States and Canada show that we generally have a variety of foods available to us. However, some of us could improve our diets by focusing on food sources rich in various vitamins, minerals, and fiber. In addition, many of us should reduce our consumption of calories, added sugar, protein, solid fat, cholesterol, salt, and alcoholic beverages. These recommendations are consistent with an overall goal to attain and maintain good health.

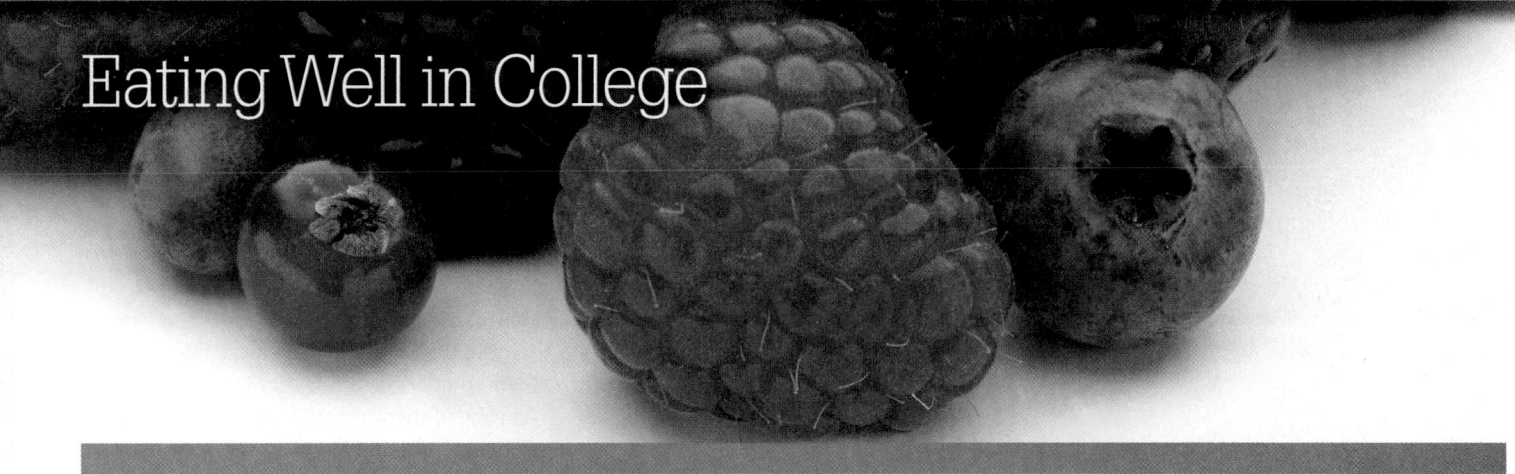

Eating Well in College

The college years are a time for freedom and a chance to make personal lifestyle decisions. Studies show that the diets of college students are not optimal. Typically, students fall short of diet recommendations for whole grains, vegetables, fruits, milk, and meat, opting instead to max out on fats, sweets, and alcohol. This information is disturbing because young adulthood is the time when many health behaviors are formed that will persist throughout life.

What is it about the college lifestyle that makes it so difficult to build healthy habits? In this section we will discuss several topics and provide possible solutions.

Food Choices

College students face changes in academic requirements, interpersonal relationships, and living environment. These stressful situations contribute to poor health behaviors. For example, when writing papers and cramming for exams, balanced meals are all-too-easily replaced by high-fat and

▼ Late-night pizza can add extra calories to the college student's daily intake.

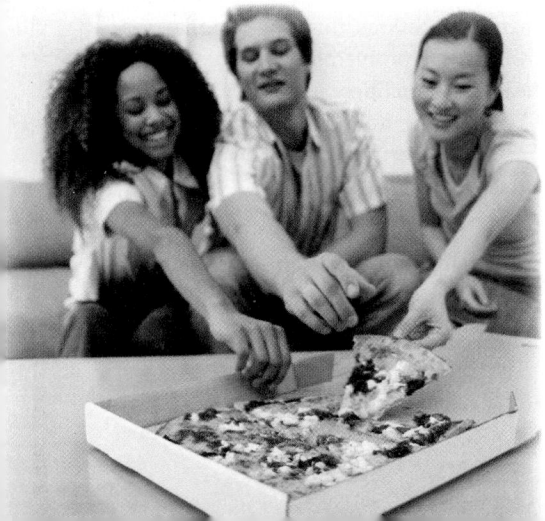

high-calorie fast-foods; convenience items; and sugary, caffeinated beverages. Physical activity is sacrificed in favor of study time.

Also consider that on campus, you are faced with a wide variety of dining choices. Dining halls, fast-food establishments, bars, and vending machines combine to offer food 24 hours per day. While it is certainly possible to make wise food choices at each of these outlets, the temptations of convenience, taste, and value (i.e., inexpensive, oversized portions) may persuade the college student to select unhealthy options.

Meals and snacks are also times to socialize. You may feel pressured to eat a big lunch at noon without regard to hunger if your peers are meeting in the dining hall to catch up. While chatting, it is easy to lose track of portions and to overeat. In addition, food may be a source of familiarity and comfort in a new and stressful place.

Weight Control and the "Freshman Fifteen"

Studies show that most college students gain weight during their first year (see Further Reading 5). The "freshman fifteen" is a term used to describe the weight gained by students during their first year of college. Although most freshman do not gain the fifteen pounds, a recent study of U.S. and Canadian college students found that students pack on 6 to 9 pounds their first year away from home. Although calorie intake does not increase significantly, dramatic increases in beer drinking and significant decreases in physical activity are key reasons for the weight gain (see Further Reading 8).

There are several reasons to maintain a healthy weight. Over the long term, risk of chronic diseases goes up as weight increases. In the short term, losing excess weight can improve how you feel and perform. Detecting "flab" around your midsection or feeling that your clothes are getting tighter are two good indicators that you are carrying excess weight. If weight loss is necessary, with some knowledge and perseverance, you can safely lose excess pounds.

Behavioral research clearly demonstrates that setting several small, achievable goals will spur motivation. As you will learn in Chapter 7, body weight is a balancing act between calories in and calories burned. Try keeping track of your calorie consumption for several days and comparing that to your energy needs, based on your age, gender, and activity level. You can use one of the equations presented in Chapter 7 or take advantage of the interactive tools on www.Choose MyPlate.gov to estimate your energy needs.

A healthy rate of weight loss is one to two pounds per week. Greater rates of weight loss will not likely be sustained over time. Remember that the numbers on the scale are not as important as your body composition—the amount of fat in relation to lean mass. One pound of weight loss requires a deficit of 3500 kilocalories. Thus, to lose one pound per week, you will need to cut back on food intake and/or increase your exercise routine to shift the energy balance equation by 500 kilocalories per day.

Although many students skip breakfast, breakfast is the *most* important meal of the day. Starting the day off with a fortified,

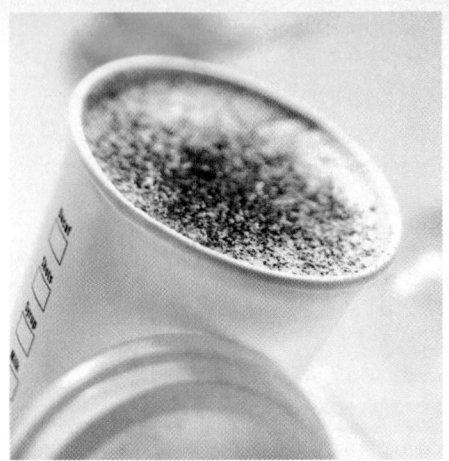

▲ Research (see Further Reading 13) has shown that gourmet coffee beverages, such as lattes and cappuccinos, can increase calorie consumption by about 200 kcal per day.

whole-grain breakfast cereal, skim milk, and a serving of fruit puts you on the right path for meeting recommendations for fiber, calcium, and fruit intake. Even though it may seem that coffee gets your brain going in the morning, your brain is fueled best by carbohydrates, not caffeine. Studies also show that eating breakfast prevents overeating later in the day. Read more about breakfast choices in the *What Would You Choose* recommendations at the end of this chapter.

One of the biggest contributors to weight gain for college students is consuming several hundred calories per day

▶ **Five Simple Tips to Avert Weight Gain**

- *Eat breakfast.* Rev up your metabolism with a protein source such as an egg or low-fat yogurt, at least one serving of whole grains such as a breakfast cereal, and a fruit such as a banana.

- *Plan ahead.* Eat a balanced meal or snack every 3 to 4 hours.

- *Limit liquid calories.* Drink water instead of high-calorie soft drinks, fruit juice, alcohol, or coffee; if you drink alcohol, limit it to 1 or 2 drinks per day.

- *Stock the fridge.* Keep a stash of low-calorie, nutritious snacks, such as pretzels, light microwave popcorn, fruit (fresh, canned, or dried).

- *Exercise regularly.* Find a friend to work out with you. Experts recommend 30 minutes of moderate exercise at least 5 days a week.

in sugary or alcoholic beverages. One 12-ounce can of regular cola contains about 140 kcal. A 12-ounce can of regular beer has 150 kcal. Consuming gourmet coffee beverages, such as lattes and cappuccinos can increase average calorie consumption by about 200 kilocalories per day (see Further Reading 13). Even fruit juices have at least 100 kcal per 8-ounce glass. Furthermore, a 24-ounce mug of a soft drink makes you feel no fuller than an equal volume of water, yet the soft drink adds 300 kcal more. A convenient stash of water is the best way to quench your thirst.

Exercise is very important to any weight loss and weight maintenance plan but sticking with it is hard to do. When you find yourself short on time, exercise is often the first thing we sacrifice. To ensure your success at boosting daily activity, choose activities you enjoy such as working out with friends at the campus recreation center, participating in intramural sports, or taking an activity class like dancing. Don't forget the brisk walking to and from classes. For more information on planning an exercise program, see Chapter 10.

Alcohol and Binge Drinking

Excessive alcohol consumption is a big problem on college campuses. Legal or not, many college students consider drinking alcohol to be a "rite of passage" into adulthood. On campuses, binge drinking—consuming five or more drinks in a row for men, or four drinks or more for women—has become an epidemic. A new level of "extreme drinking" goes far beyond binge drinking. For example, recent studies indicate that college students celebrate twenty-first birthdays with an average of 12 drinks for men and nine for women (see Further Reading 12).

The statistics on the impact of binge drinking on college campuses are sobering. An estimated two of every five students on college campuses participates in binge drinking. Each year, 1400 college students between the ages of 18 and 24 die from alcohol-related unintentional injuries, including motor vehicle crashes. In addition to deaths and injuries, other problems stemming from binge drinking include unsafe sex and its consequences, long-term health problems, suicides, academic problems, legal troubles, and

alcohol abuse or dependence. Thirty-one percent of college students meet the criteria for a diagnosis of alcohol abuse.

In addition alcohol consumption definitely contributes to weight gain—by virtue of its own calories and the increased food consumption at events where drinking occurs. If you choose to drink alcohol, do so in moderation—no more than two drinks per day for men and one drink per day for women. Be aware of the warning signs and dangers of alcohol poisoning shown in the margin. Excessive alcohol intake, has many long-term health and nutrition implications that are covered in Chapter 16.

Eating Disorders

As many as 30% of college students are at risk of developing an eating disorder. As you will learn in Chapter 13, disordered eating is a mild and short-term change in eating patterns that typically occurs in response to life stress, a desire to change appearance, or a bad habit. Sometimes, disordered eating habits may lead to an eating disorder, such as anorexia nervosa, bulimia nervosa, or binge-eating disorder. Chapter 13 includes advice on what to do if you suspect that your roommate or friend is suffering from an eating disorder.

Starving the body also starves the brain, limiting performance in academics and beyond, and the negative consequences of disordered eating may last a lifetime. Ultimately, eating disorders do not arise from problems with food but rather from problems with self-esteem, control, and abusive relationships. Frequently, what begins as a diet spirals into a much larger problem. Eating disorders are not just diets gone bad—they require professional intervention. Left unchecked, eating disorders lead to serious adverse effects, such as loss of menstrual periods, thinning of bones, gastrointestinal problems, kidney problems, heart abnormalities, and eventually death.

Choosing a Vegetarian Lifestyle

Many college students experiment with or adopt a vegetarian eating pattern. Plant-based diets can meet nutrition needs and decrease risk of many chronic diseases, but they require appropriate planning at all life stages.

Protein is not typically deficient, even with a vegan diet, which contains no animal products. However, vegetarians, and especially vegans, may be at risk for deficiencies of several vitamins and minerals. Consuming a ready-to-eat breakfast cereal is an easy and inexpensive way to obtain these nutrients. See Chapter 6 for more information on vegetarian food planning.

Restaurants and campus dining services have responded to the growing interest in vegetarian meals by offering a variety of vegetarian options. For optimal health benefits, choose foods that are baked, steamed, or stir-fried rather than deep-fried; select whole grains rather than refined carbohydrates; and consume food fortified with vitamins and minerals. Even if you do not follow a plant-based diet all the time, choosing several plant-based meals each week can help with weight control and boost intake of fiber and healthy phytochemicals. You will learn in Chapter 2 that the new ChooseMyPlate program recommends that the largest portion of your plate be filled with plant foods, including whole grains, fruits and vegetables.

Fuel for Competition: Student Athletes

Students who compete in sports such as intramural and intercollegiate athletics need to consume more calories and nutrients. Despite an emphasis on a lean physique athletes at all levels must take care not to severely restrict calories, as this could impact performance and health. Muscles require adequate carbohydrates for fuel and protein for growth and repair. Fat, as well, is an important source of stored energy for use during exercise. Low levels of body fat in women may lead to amenorrhea (cease menstruating), a condition costly to long-term bone health.

In addition to fueling the body with calories, fluids are essential for health and performance. While water is adequate for events lasting less than 60 minutes, sports drinks are ideal for longer events because they supply carbohydrates to fuel fatigued muscles as well as electrolytes to replenish those lost in perspiration. Intentional fluid losses to "make weight" for a competition are detrimental to health and performance.

Athletes also should take care not to be wooed by the supplement industry.

Increasing food intake to meet the energy demands of athletic training is usually sufficient to also meet vitamin and mineral needs. As an exception, athletes may be at risk for iron-deficiency anemia. Consuming a balanced multivitamin and mineral supplement is adequate for most people. Individual vitamin, mineral, amino acid, or herbal supplements are not advised, in spite of the hype of supplement makers.

Tips for Eating Well on a College Student's Budget

Because higher education can be hard on the wallet it is good to know that it is possible to eat well on campus on a budget. If you live on campus, participate in a pre-paid campus meal plan (see Further Reading 1). These are generally designed to offer great food value with a variety of healthy foods. If you live off campus or have your own kitchen, plan ahead. Packing a lunch from home will save a lot of cash compared to grabbing lunch on the run and puts you more in control of healthy choices. For example, preparing a sandwich at home costs less than half as much as purchasing one at a fast-food restaurant or deli.

Never go grocery shopping on an empty stomach—everything will look good and you'll buy more. Also, go to the store with a list in hand and stick to it, because impulse buys tend to drain your wallet. Buy store-brand foods rather than name-brand items. Make use of canned and frozen fruits and vegetables—they are just as nutritious as fresh fruits and vegetables, particularly if you choose low-sodium and low-sugar varieties. Rather than buying cartons of fruit juice, select cans of fruit juice concentrate and mix with water at home. Likewise, preparing other drinks, such as iced tea, from store-brand powder (look for sugar-free) will save over gallon jugs or vending machine containers of drinks. Canned (fruits, tuna) and dry (oatmeal) foods can be nutritious and last a long time, so you can avoid throwing out spoiled items. Finally, eggs and peanut butter are inexpensive and simple sources of protein.

In conclusion, *The College Student's Guide to Eating Well on Campus* (see Further Reading 10) and *The Dorm Room Diet* (see Further Reading 11) are excellent books with more details on ways college students can plan a healthy diet and stay fit.

▶ **The warning signs and symptoms of alcohol poisoning**

- Semiconsciousness or unconsciousness
- Slow respiration of eight or fewer breaths per minute or lapses between breaths of more than 8 seconds
- Cold, clammy, pale, or bluish skin
- Strong odor of alcohol, which usually accompanies these symptoms

Some calorie traps for college students:

Number of Calories	
Six-pack of regular beer	900
Two handfuls of almonds	500
Two handfuls of granola	330
Personal-size pizza	500 to 600
1 cup of ice cream	300
Two handfuls of frosted cereal	250

Source: Ann Litt, *The College Student's Guide to Eating Well on Campus*

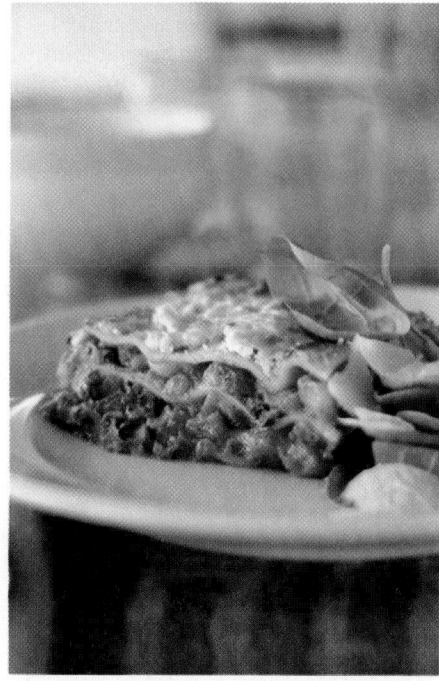

▲ Many students adopt a vegetarian diet during college. Guidelines for planning a nutritious vegetarian diet, with items such as this veggie lasagna, and spinach salad are presented in Chapter 6.

Case Study Typical College Student

Andy is like many other college students. He grew up on a quick bowl of cereal and milk for breakfast and a hamburger, French fries, and cola for lunch, either in the school cafeteria or at a local fast-food restaurant. At dinner, he generally avoided eating any of his salad or vegetables, and by 9 o'clock he was deep into bags of chips and cookies. Andy has taken most of these habits to college. He prefers coffee for breakfast and possibly a chocolate bar. Lunch is still mainly a hamburger, French fries, and cola, but pizza and tacos now alternate more frequently than when he was in high school. One thing Andy really likes about the restaurants surrounding campus is that, for less than a dollar more, he can make his hamburger a double or get extra cheese and pepperoni on his pizza. This helps him stretch his food dollar; searching out large-portion value meals for lunch and dinner now has become part of a typical day.

Provide some dietary advice for Andy. Start with his positive habits and then provide some constructive criticism, based on what you now know.

Answer the following questions, and check your responses in Appendix A.

1. **Start with Andy's positive habits:** What healthy choices are being made when Andy eats at local restaurants?

2. **Now provide some constructive criticisms:**

   a. What are some of the negative aspects of items available at fast-food restaurants?
   b. Why is ordering the "value meals" a dangerous habit?

   c. What healthier substitutions could he make at each meal?
   d. List some healthier choices he could make at fast-food restaurants on campus.

Summary (Numbers refer to numbered sections in the chapter.)

1. The flavor, texture, and appearance of foods primarily influence our food choices. Several other factors also help determine food habits and choices: food availability and convenience; early childhood experiences and ethnic customs; nutrition and health concerns; advertising; restaurants; social changes; and economics. A variety of external (appetite-related) forces affect satiety (feeling of satisfaction that halts our desire to continue eating). Hunger cues combine with appetite cues, such as easy availability of food, to promote food intake.

2. Nutrition is a lifestyle factor that is a key to developing and maintaining an optimal state of health. A poor diet and a sedentary lifestyle are known to be risk factors for life-threatening chronic diseases such as heart disease, hypertension, diabetes, and cancer. Not meeting nutrient needs in younger years makes us more likely to suffer health consequences in later years. Too much of a nutrient also can be harmful. Drinking too much alcohol is another dietary problem associated with many health problems.

3. Nutrition is the study of the food substances vital for health and the study of how the body uses these substances to promote and support growth, maintenance, and reproduction of cells. Nutrients in foods fall into six classes: (1) carbohydrates, (2) lipids (mostly fats and oils), (3) proteins, (4) vitamins, (5) minerals, and (6) water. The first three, along with alcohol, provide calories for the body to use.

4. The body transforms the energy contained in carbohydrate, protein, and fat into other forms of energy that in turn allow the body to function. Fat provides, on average, 9 kcal per gram, whereas both protein and carbohydrate provide, on average, 4 kcal per gram. Vitamins, minerals, and water do not supply calories to the body but are essential for proper body function.

5. The overweight and obesity problem has worsened with 68% of people in the United States (190 million people) reported to be overweight or obese in 2010. This increase is a result of eating too much, especially foods with a high number of

calories and a low number of nutrients, and not engaging in enough physical activity. Results from large nutrition surveys in the United States and Canada suggest that some of us need to concentrate on consuming foods that supply more of certain vitamins, minerals, and fiber. *Healthy People 2020* is a national initiative that includes Nutrition and Weight Status objectives related to eating a healthful diet and maintaining a healthy body weight. A healthful diet includes consuming a variety of nutrient-dense foods within and across the food groups, especially whole grains, fruits, vegetables, low-fat or fat-free milk or milk products, and lean meats and other protein sources; limiting intake of solid fats, cholesterol, added sugars, sodium (salt), and alcohol; and limiting intake of calories to meet energy needs.

6. A basic plan for health promotion and disease prevention includes eating a varied diet, performing regular physical activity, not smoking, not abusing nutrient supplements (if used), consuming adequate water and other fluids, getting enough sleep, limiting alcohol intake (if consumed), and limiting or appropriately coping with stress. The primary focus of nutrition planning should be on food, not on dietary supplements. The focus on foods to supply nutrient needs avoids the possibility of severe nutrient imbalances.

7. Studies show that the diets and other health habits of college students are not optimal. Students fall short of recommendations for servings of grains, vegetables, fruits, milk, and meat, opting instead for fats, sweets, and alcohol. This information is disturbing from a public health

standpoint, because young adulthood is the time when many health behaviors are formed and will likely persist throughout life. Issues of particular importance on college campuses are weight control, making healthy meal choices, alcohol and binge drinking, and eating disorders.

Check Your Knowledge (Answers to the following multiple choice questions are below.)

1. Our primary psychological drive to eat that is affected by many external food-choice mechanisms is called
   a. hunger.   c. satiety.
   b. appetite.   d. feeding.

2. Energy-yielding nutrients include
   a. vitamins, minerals, and water.
   b. carbohydrates, proteins, and fats.
   c. trace minerals and fat-soluble vitamins.
   d. iron, vitamin C, and potassium.

3. The *essential* nutrients
   a. must be consumed at every meal.
   b. are required for infants but not adults.
   c. can be made in the body when they are needed.
   d. cannot be made by the body and therefore must be consumed to maintain health.

4. Sugars, starches, and dietary fibers are examples of
   a. proteins.   c. carbohydrates.
   b. vitamins.   d. minerals.

5. Which nutrient classes are most important in the regulation of body processes?
   a. vitamins
   b. carbohydrates
   c. minerals
   d. lipids
   e. Both a and c.

6. A kcal is a
   a. measure of heat energy.
   b. measure of fat in food.
   c. heating device.
   d. term used to describe the amount of sugar and fat in foods.

7. A food that contains 10 grams of fat would yield _____ kcal.
   a. 40   c. 90
   b. 70   d. 120

8. If you consume 300 grams of carbohydrate in a day that you consume 2400 kcal, the carbohydrates will provide _____% of your total energy intake.
   a. 12.5   c. 50
   b. 30   d. 60

9. Which of the following is true about the North American diet?
   a. Most of our protein comes from plant sources.
   b. About half of the carbohydrates come from simple sugars.
   c. Most of our fats come from plant sources.
   d. Most of our carbohydrates come from starches.

10. The _____ is a term used to describe the amount of weight college students gain during the first year of college.
    a. varsity 8
    b. stadium 7
    c. dormitory 12
    d. freshman 15

Answer Key: 1. b (LO 1.1), 2. b (LO 1.3), 3. d (LO 1.3), 4. c (LO 1.3), 5. e (LO 1.3), 6. a (LO 1.4), 7. c (LO 1.4), 8. c (LO 1.4), 9. b (LO 1.5), 10. d (LO 1.7)

Study Questions (Numbers refer to Learning Outcomes)

1. Describe the process that controls hunger and satiety in the body. List other factors that influence our food choices. (**LO 1.1**)

2. Describe how your food preferences have been shaped by the following factors:
   a. Exposure to foods at an early age
   b. Advertising (what is the newest food you have tried?)
   c. Eating out
   d. Peer pressure
   e. Economic factors (**LO 1.1**)

3. What products in your supermarket reflect the consumer demand for healthier foods? For convenience? (**LO 1.1**)

4. Name one chronic disease associated with poor nutrition habits. Now list a few corresponding risk factors. (**LO 1.2**)

5. Describe two sources of fat and explain why the differences are important in terms of overall health. (**LO 1.3**)

6. Identify three ways that water is used in the body. (**LO 1.3**)

7. Explain the concept of calories as it relates to foods. What are the values used to calculate kcals from grams of carbohydrate, fat, protein, and alcohol? (**LO 1.4**)

8. Wendy's Big Bacon Classic contains 44 grams carbohydrate, 36 grams fat, and 37 grams protein. Calculate the percentage of calories derived from fat. (**LO 1.4**)

9. According to national nutrition surveys, which nutrients tend to be underconsumed by many North Americans? Why do you think this is the case? (**LO 1.5**)

10. List four *Healthy People 2020* objectives for the United States. How would you rate yourself in each area? Why? (**LO 1.5 & 1.6**)

11. List five strategies to avoid weight gain during college. (**LO 1.7**)

What Would You Choose Recommendations

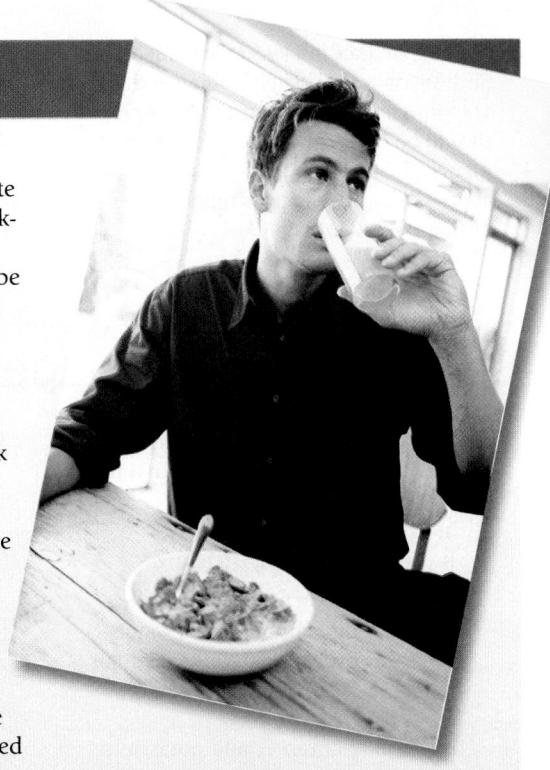

Even bleary-eyed procrastinators can fuel their bodies for a new day of higher education! *Skipping breakfast is not a smart plan.* After a period of fasting (i.e., overnight), the body and the brain need fuel to operate at peak efficiency. In addition, many research studies demonstrate that eating a sensible breakfast is a good way to control weight. Compared to those who eat breakfast, people who skip breakfast tend to crave higher-calorie foods, snack more throughout the day, and eat more at subsequent meals. Consider eating breakfast each day as part of your plan to fend off the freshman fifteen.

Grab-and-go food options, such as those available in vending machines or from fast-food establishments, are often high in calories but low in nutrients. For example, a low-fat granola bar has only 100 kcal and 3 grams of fat but offers little else in terms of nutrition. Also, a granola bar is not likely to stave off hunger for very long.

On the other hand, a fast-food breakfast sandwich will probably promote satiety but its calorie, fat, and sodium contents are too high. This type of sandwich provides 550 kcal, 23 grams of fat (38% of a day's total kcal in the sandwich and 35% of the whole day's limit for fat), and 1490 mg sodium (just under the 1500 mg Adequate Intake for this nutrient). A fast-food breakfast sandwich can fit into an otherwise healthy diet on occasion but should not be part of your normal routine.

Keeping nutritious but convenient breakfast options accessible is a good strategy for any time-pressed college student. Whole-grain, fortified, ready-to-eat breakfast cereal with fat-free milk is a great choice: it is quick, provides a wide variety of vitamins and minerals, and boosts fiber intake. Adding a source of protein will help to support body processes and make you feel full for a longer time. Hard-boiled eggs or a handful of dry-roasted nuts provide protein in ready-to-eat form. A cup of low-fat yogurt offers protein with the added benefit of calcium. Fresh and dried fruit are portable and nutritious options for breakfast. Many fruit choices are loaded with potassium and vitamin C, plus they provide fiber. A 1.5-ounce box of raisins, which can be stored for months without a refrigerator, provides about 130 kcal, no fat or cholesterol, very little sodium, 2 grams of fiber, and 320 mg potassium.

▲ With a little bit of planning, breakfast can be both quick and healthy.

So, the bowl of Wheaties with a banana and low-fat milk along with a yogurt, all from your dorm room "pantry," would be the healthiest choice for most.

Further Readings

1. Brown LB and others: College students can benefit by participating in a prepaid meal plan. *Journal of the American Dietetic Association* 105:445, 2005.

   Participation in a prepaid campus meal plan resulted in modest nutritional benefits to students through an increase in servings of foods from fruit, vegetable, and meat groups.

2. Center for Science in the Public Interest: *Guidelines for Responsible Food Marketing to Children.* Washington, DC, 2005. *www.cspinet.org/marketingguidelines.pdf.*

   These guidelines are written for all companies or organizations who manufacture, sell, market, advertise, or promote food to children. Criteria are provided for marketing food to children in a manner that does not undermine children's diets or harm their health. The guidelines address not only how food is marketed but also which foods are marketed to children.

3. Chiuve SE and others: Adherence to a low-risk, healthy lifestyle and risk of sudden cardiac death among women. *Journal of the American Medical Association* 306: 62, 2011.

   Sudden cardiac death causes more than half of all heart-related deaths and usually occurs as the first sign of heart disease, especially in women. Adherence to a healthy lifestyle and the risk of sudden cardiac death was studied in women from the Nurses' Health Study. Risk of sudden cardiac death dropped by 92% with a combination of the four healthy lifestyles (not smoking, not overweight, exercising 30 minutes/day or longer, and following the Mediterranean Diet). Women who ate a high proportion of vegetables, fruits, nuts, omega-3 fats, and fish, along with moderate amounts of alcohol and small amounts of red meat, had a 40% less risk than women whose diets least resembled this diet. Therefore, a healthy diet along with other healthy lifestyle factors appears to protect women from sudden cardiac death.

4. Choinière CJ, Lando A: *2008 Health and Diet Survey,* Food and Drug Administration, March 2010. *www.fda.gov/Food/Science-Research/ResearchAreas/ConsumerResearch/ucm193895.htm.*

   This report is a snapshot of the nations dietary habits based on the FDA 2008 telephone survey of more than 2500 adults in every state and the District of Columbia. One of the key findings was that more than half of consumers in the United States often read the food label when buying a product for the first time, and they are increasingly aware of the link between diet and heart disease..

5. Edmonds MJ and others: Body weight and percent body fat increase during the transition from high school to university in females. *Journal of the American Dietetic Association* 108:1033, 2008.

   The notion that weight gain occurs during the first year of university was studied in Canadian females making the transition from high school to university. There was a significant increase in body weight of 2.4 kg (5.28 pounds) during the first 6 to 7 months of university. Percent body fat also increased from 23.8% to 25.6%. Although dietary energy (calorie) intake did not increase, a decrease in moderate physical activity was an important predictor of weight. Body weight, therefore, may be modified by lifestyle factors during this formative period.

6. Federal Trade Commission: Marketing food to children and adolescents: A review of industry expenditures, activities, and self-regulation, a report to Congress. July 2008. http://www.ftc.gov/opa/2008/07/foodmkting.shtm.

   This study by the Federal Trade Commission found that 44 major food and beverage marketers spent $1.6 billion to promote their products to children under 12 and adolescents ages 12 to 17 in the United States in 2006. The report states that food advertising to youth is dominated by advertising campaigns that combine traditional media, such as television, with previously unmeasured forms of marketing, such as packaging, in-store advertising, sweepstakes, and Internet. This advertising often involves cross-promotion with a new movie or popular television program. The report calls for all food companies "to adopt and adhere to meaningful, nutrition-based standards for marketing their products to children under 12."

7. Goris JM and others: Television food advertising and the prevalence of childhood overweight and obesity: A multicountry comparison. *Public Health Nutrition* 13:1003, 2010.

   The higher prevalence of childhood obesity in the United States compared to other countries could be explained by greater exposure to TV food advertising. In a study of children ages 6 to 11 years in six countries, the contribution of TV food ads to the occurrence of childhood obesity was greatest for the United States at 16% to 40% and lowest in Great Britain, Sweden, and the Netherlands at 4% to 18%. Children in the United States were exposed to 11.5 minutes/day of TV food ads compared to only 1.8 minutes/day in the Netherlands. The authors conclude that the contribution of TV food ads to the prevalence of childhood obesity is significant in some countries and greatest in the United States.

8. Hoffman DY and others: Changes in body weight and fat mass of men and women in the first year of college: A study of the "freshman 15." *Journal of American College of Health* 55:41, 2006.

   It is commonly thought that there is a high risk of gaining 15 pounds of weight during freshman year of college. In this study, changes in body weight and percentage of body fat were measured in first-year college students. Body weight increased by an average of almost 3 pounds (1.3 kilograms) and body fat increased an average of 0.7%. This study, therefore, found that weight and fat gain may occur during the first year of college.

9. Kochanek KD and others: *National Vital Statistics Reports*, Deaths: Preliminary Data for 2009: 59, 2011.

   Preliminary U.S. data on deaths, death rates, life expectancy, leading causes of death, and infant mortality for 2009 are presented. Death rates decreased significantly from 2008 to 2009 for 10 of the 15 leading causes of death: heart diseases, cancer, chronic lower respiratory diseases, cerebrovascular diseases, accidents (unintentional injuries), Alzheimer's disease, diabetes mellitus, influenza and pneumonia, septicemia, and assault (homicide).

10. Litt, AS: *The College Student's Guide to Eating Well on Campus.* Tulip Hill Press, Glen Echo, MD, 2005.

    This book provides important information on how to survive and eat well during your college years and covers how to avoid and spot eating disorders.

11. Oz D: *The Dorm Room Diet: The 10-Step Program for Creating a Healthy Lifestyle Plan That Really Works.* Newmarket Press, 2010.

    This book is written to help students stay fit while at college. The 10-step program shows students how to stop eating out of emotional need; navigate the most common danger zones at school for unhealthy eating; get the exercise you need, even in your small dorm room; choose vitamins and supplements wisely; and relax and rejuvenate amid the stress of college life.

12. Rutledge PC and others: 21st birthday drinking: Extremely extreme. *Journal of Consulting and Clinical Psychology* 76:511, 2008.

    A new level of extreme drinking goes beyond the four or five drinks in one sitting defined as "bingeing." At the University of Missouri, a study of 2518 students found 34% of men and 24% of women who imbibed on their 21st birthdays drank 21 alcoholic drinks or more. The authors conclude that interventions shown to be effective with general risky drinking may prove effective in reducing 21st birthday excess.

13. Shields DH and others: Gourmet coffee beverage consumption among college women. *Journal of the American Dietetic Association* 104:650, 2004.

    A significant percentage of college women were shown to consume gourmet coffee beverages, which contributed additional calories and fat to their daily dietary intake.

14. Woolf K and others: Physical activity is associated with risk factors for chronic disease across adult women's life cycle. *Journal of the American Dietetic Association* 108:948, 2008.

    The results of this study confirm that younger age and greater physical activity across the adult women's life cycle are associated with more favorable serum lipid levels; less inflammation; lower concentrations of insulin, glucose, and leptin in serum; and more favorable body composition. These factors are associated with reduced risk for several chronic diseases including cardiovascular disease, type 2 diabetes, and obesity.

15. U.S. Department of Health and Human Services. 2008 Physical Activity Guidelines for Americans. www.health.gov/paguidelines.

    Inactivity remains relatively high among American children, adolescents, and adults. These science-based guidelines are designed to help Americans aged six and older use appropriate physical activity to improve their health. The guidelines include information about the health benefits of physical activity; how to do physical activity in a manner that meets the guidelines; how to reduce the risks of activity-related injury; and how to assist others in participating regularly in physical activity.

16. Vital Signs: State-Specific Obesity Prevalence Among Adults—United States, 2009. *Morbidity and Mortality Weekly Report* 59(30), 2010.

    Each year state health departments collect obesity data through a series of telephone interviews with U.S. adults. Obesity is defined as body mass index (BMI) of 30 or higher. Prevalence of obesity has increased significantly since 1985. In 2009, nine of these states (Alabama, Arkansas, Kentucky, Louisiana, Mississippi, Missouri, Oklahoma, Tennessee, and West Virginia) had a prevalence of obesity equal to or greater than 30%; 33 states had a prevalence equal to or greater than 25%; only Colorado and the District of Columbia had a prevalence of obesity less than 20%.

17. Yanover T, Sacco WP: Eating beyond satiety and body mass index. *Eating and Weight Disorders* 13:119, 2008.

    Eating beyond satiety (EBS), snacking, night eating, and hunger were examined in undergraduate females. EBS was the strongest predictor of body mass and therefore may be a variable to target in interventions to prevent and treat overweight and obesity.

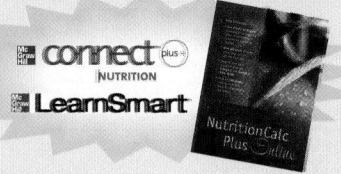

To get the most out of your study of nutrition, go to McGraw-Hill's online resources: Connect www.mcgrawhillconnect.com **, where you will find NutritionCalc Plus, LearnSmart, and many other dynamic tools.**

I. Examine Your Eating Habits More Closely

Choose one day of the week that is typical of your eating pattern. Using the first table found in Appendix E, list all foods and drinks you consumed for 24 hours. In addition, write down the approximate amounts of food you ate in units, such as cups, ounces, teaspoons, and tablespoons. After you record the amount of each food and drink consumed, indicate in the table why you chose to consume the item. Place the corresponding abbreviation in the space provided to indicate why you picked that food or drink.

FLVR	Flavor/texture	ADV	Advertisement	PEER	Peers
CONV	Convenience	WTCL	Weight control	NUTR	Nutritive value
EMO	Emotions	HUNG	Hunger	$	Cost
AVA	Availability	FAM	Family/cultural	HLTH	Health

There can be more than one reason for choosing a particular food or drink.

Application

Ask yourself what your most frequent reason is for eating or drinking. To what degree is health or nutritive value a reason for your food choices? Should you make these higher priorities?

II. Observe the Supermarket Explosion

Today's supermarkets carry up to 60,000 items, compared to 20,000 items 10 years ago. Think about your last grocery shopping trip and the items you purchased to eat. Following is a list of 20 newer food products added to supermarket shelves. Check the items that you have tried. Then use the key from Part I of the Rate Your Plate exercise to identify why you might have chosen these products.

_____ Prepackaged salad greens (variety packs other than iceberg lettuce) _____

_____ Gourmet or sprayable salad oils (e.g., walnut, almond, olive, or sesame oil) _____

_____ Gourmet vinegars (e.g., balsamic or rice) _____

_____ Prepackaged lunch products (e.g., nacho, pizza, taco, and tortilla Lunchables) _____

_____ Precooked frozen turkey patties, precooked bacon _____

_____ Bean soup mixes (e.g., lentil, black bean, combination bean soups) _____

_____ Microwavable sandwiches (e.g., Hotpockets, frozen sandwiches) _____

_____ Microwavable meals in a bowl (e.g., mac and cheese, soup) _____

_____ Refrigerated, precooked pasta (e.g., tortellini, fettucini) and accompanying sauces (e.g., pesto, tomato basil) _____
_____

_____ Imported grain products (e.g., risotto, farfalline, gnocchi, fusilli) _____

_____ Whole-grain pasta or rice _____

_____ Frozen dinners (list your favorite of any of the wide variety) _____

_____ Imported sauces for food preparation (e.g., hoisin or brown bean sauce; mandarin marinade, sesame, curry, or fire oils) _____

_____ Bottled waters (flavored or unflavored) _____

_____ Trendy juices (e.g., draft apple cider, acai, pomegranate) _____

_____ Roasted and/or flavored coffees (e.g., beans, ground, instant, or k-cups) _____

_____ Gourmet jelly beans and candies (e.g., gummi coca-colas or imported chocolates) _____

_____ Instant hot cereal in a bowl (add water and go!) _____

_____ "Fast-shake" pancake mix (add water, shake, and ready to cook) _____

_____ Breakfast bars or cookies (e.g., granola or fruit-flavored bars) _____

_____ Meal replacement/fitness products (e.g., "energy" bars, high-protein bars, sports drinks) _____

_____ Low-carbohydrate meat and pasta dishes _____

_____ Low-calorie muffin tops, bagel thins _____

_____ Packaged yogurt smoothies _____

_____ Milk substitutes (e.g., rice milk, soy milk) _____

Finally, identify three new food products not on this list that you have seen in the past year. Discuss the appeal of these products to the North American consumer.

Chapter 2 Guidelines for Designing a Healthy Diet

Student Learning Outcomes

Chapter 2 is designed to allow you to:

2.1 Develop a healthy eating plan.

2.2 Outline the measurements used (ABCDEs) in nutrition assessment: **A**nthropometric, **B**iochemical, **C**linical, **D**ietary, and **E**nvironmental status.

2.3 Understand the basis of the scientific method as it is used in developing hypotheses and theories in the field of nutrition, including the determination of nutrient needs.

2.4 Describe what the Recommended Dietary Allowances (RDAs) and other dietary standards represent.

2.5 List the purpose and key recommendations of the Dietary Guidelines and the 2008 Physical Activity Guidelines for Americans.

2.6 Exemplify a meal that conforms to MyPlate recommendations.

2.7 Describe the components of the Nutrition Facts panel and the various health claims and label descriptors that are allowed.

2.8 Identify reliable sources of nutrition information.

What Would You Choose?

Living and learning in close quarters make it easy to share germs when flu season rolls around. You have heard that vitamin C supports the immune system, helping your body to fight infections. Many varieties of fruit juice and other beverages contain 100% of the Daily Value of vitamin C. In terms of nutrient density, is it better to get your vitamin C from a glass of orange juice or by eating a whole orange? How do oranges compare to orange juice in terms of energy density?

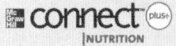 **Think about your choice as you read chapter 2, then see our recommendations at the end of the chapter. To learn more about nutrient density and energy density, check out the Connect site:** www.mcgrawhillconnect.com

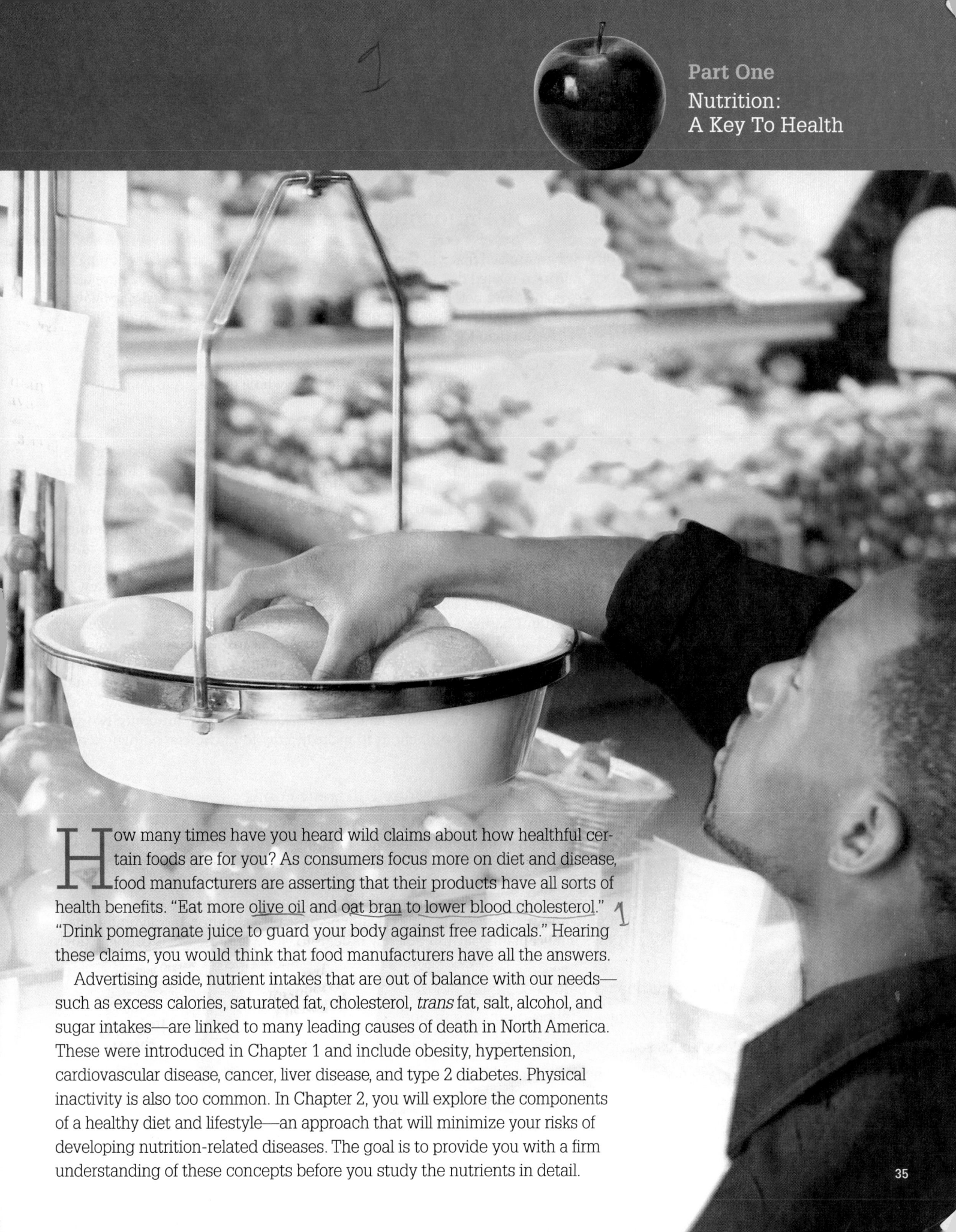

How many times have you heard wild claims about how healthful certain foods are for you? As consumers focus more on diet and disease, food manufacturers are asserting that their products have all sorts of health benefits. "Eat more <u>olive oil</u> and <u>oat bran</u> to lower blood cholesterol." "Drink pomegranate juice to guard your body against free radicals." Hearing these claims, you would think that food manufacturers have all the answers.

Advertising aside, nutrient intakes that are out of balance with our needs— such as excess calories, saturated fat, cholesterol, *trans* fat, salt, alcohol, and sugar intakes—are linked to many leading causes of death in North America. These were introduced in Chapter 1 and include obesity, hypertension, cardiovascular disease, cancer, liver disease, and type 2 diabetes. Physical inactivity is also too common. In Chapter 2, you will explore the components of a healthy diet and lifestyle—an approach that will minimize your risks of developing nutrition-related diseases. The goal is to provide you with a firm understanding of these concepts before you study the nutrients in detail.

Refresh Your Memory

As you begin your study of diet planning in Chapter 2, you may want to review:

▪ The terms in the margin in Chapter 1 and Table 1-1.

2.1 A Food Philosophy That Works

You may be surprised that what you should eat to minimize the risk of developing the nutrition-related diseases seen in North America is exactly what you have heard many times before: *Consume a variety of foods balanced by a moderate intake of each food.* Health professionals have recommended the same basic diet and health plan for the past 50 years:

- Control *how much* you eat.
- Pay attention to *what* you eat—choose whole grains, fruits, and vegetables.
- Stay physically active.

It is disappointing, however, that according to a recent survey conducted by the American Dietetic Association, two of five people in the United States believe that following a healthful diet means completely giving up foods they enjoy. To the contrary, a healthful diet does not have to mean deprivation and misery; it simply requires some basic nutrition know-how and planning. Besides, eliminating favorite foods typically does not work for "dieters" in the long run. The best plan consists of learning the basics of a healthful diet: variety, balance, and moderation. Monitoring total calorie intake is also important for many of us, especially if unwanted weight gain is taking place.

As noted in Chapter 1, many nutrition experts agree that there are no exclusively "good" or "bad" foods. Even so, many North Americans have diets that miss the mark when it comes to the foundations of healthy eating. Diets overloaded with fatty meats, fried foods, sugared soft drinks, and refined starches can result in substantial risk for nutrition-related chronic diseases.

Let's now define *variety, balance,* and *moderation.* We will also introduce two very important concepts that will help us to make healthy food choices: nutrient density and energy density.

Variety Means Eating Many Different Foods

Variety in your diet means choosing a number of different foods within any given food group rather than eating the "same old thing" day after day. Variety makes meals more interesting and helps ensure that a diet contains sufficient nutrients. A variety of foods is best because no one food meets all your nutrient needs. For example, meat provides protein and iron but little calcium and no vitamin C. Eggs are a source of protein, but they provide little calcium because the calcium is mostly in the shell. Cow's milk contains calcium but very little iron. None of these foods contains fiber.

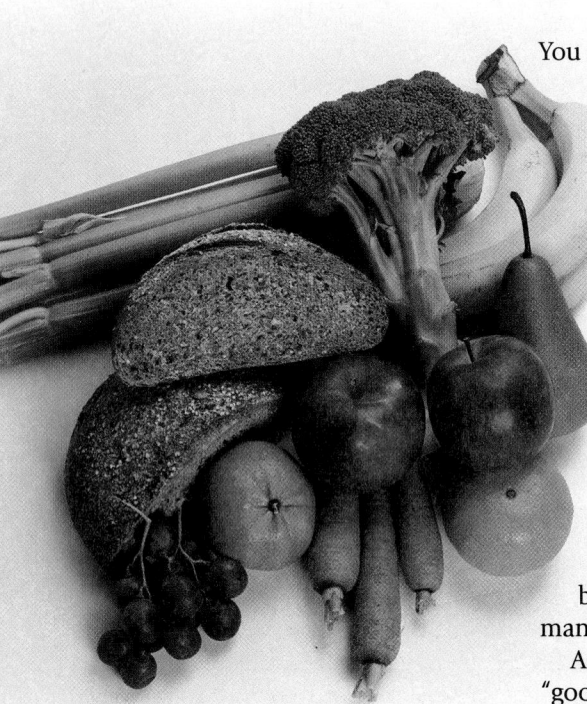

▲ A plate mostly full of fruits, vegetables, and whole-grain breads and cereals will help ward off disease and control body weight.

What do nutrition experts recommend for a healthy diet? Why are whole grains, fruits, and vegetables so important? How many servings do we need from each food group? How big is a serving? Are North Americans generally following the advice of the Dietary Guidelines? Chapter 2 provides some answers.

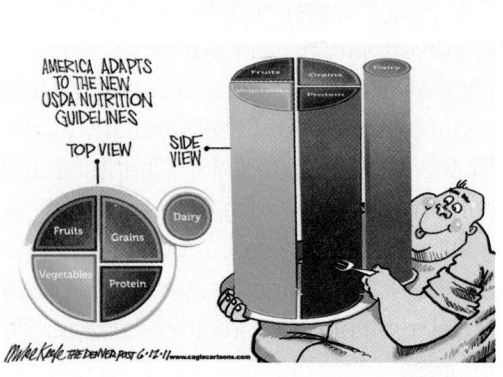

Carrots—a source of fiber and a pigment that forms vitamin A—may be your favorite vegetable. However, if you choose carrots every day as your only vegetable source, you may miss out on the vitamin folate. Other vegetables, such as broccoli and asparagus, are rich sources of this nutrient. Hopefully, you're beginning to get a sense of how different foods and food groups vary in the nutrients they contain. You'll learn much more about this in Chapters 8 and 9. For now, just recognize that you need a variety of foods in your diet because the required nutrients are scattered among many foods.

An added bonus of variety in the diet, especially within the fruit and vegetable groups, is the inclusion of a rich supply of **phytochemicals.** Recall from Chapter 1 that phytochemicals were discussed along with the nutrient classes. Many of these substances provide significant health benefits. Considerable research attention is focused on various phytochemicals in reducing the risk for certain diseases (e.g., cancer). You can't just buy a bottle of phytochemicals—they are generally available only within whole foods. Current multivitamin and mineral supplements contain few or none of these beneficial plant chemicals.

Numerous population studies show reduced cancer risk among people who regularly consume fruits and vegetables (see Further Reading 9). Researchers suspect that some phytochemicals present in the fruits and vegetables block the cancer process. Links between cancer and nutrition are described more thoroughly in the Nutrition and Your Health section in Chapter 16. Some phytochemicals also have been linked to a reduced risk of cardiovascular disease. Could it be that, because humans evolved eating a wide variety of plant-based foods, the body developed with a need for these phytochemicals, along with the various nutrients present, to maintain optimal health?

Foods rich in phytochemicals are now part of a family of foods referred to as **functional foods.** A functional food provides health benefits beyond those supplied by the traditional nutrients it contains. For example, a tomato contains the phytochemical lycopene, so it can be called a functional food. You may hear this term more from the food industry in the future.

It will likely take many years for scientists to unravel all of the important effects of the myriad of phytochemicals in foods, and it is unlikely that all will ever be available or effective in supplement form. For this reason, leading nutrition and medical experts suggest that a diet rich in fruits, vegetables, and whole-grain breads and cereals is the most reliable way to obtain the potential benefits of phytochemicals.

A note of caution: Some research suggests that increasing dietary variety can lead to overeating. Thus, as one incorporates a wide variety of foods in a diet, attention to total calorie intake is also important to consider. Table 2-1 provides a number of suggestions for including more phytochemicals in your diet, as do the websites www.fruitsandveggiesmorematters.org and www.fruitsandveggiesmatter.gov.

functional foods Foods that provide health benefits beyond those supplied by the traditional nutrients they contain. For example, a tomato contains the phytochemical lycopene, so it can be called a functional food.

Balance Means Consuming Food from Each Group

One way to balance your diet as you consume a variety of foods is to select foods from each of these five major food groups every day:

- Grains
- Vegetables
- Fruits
- Dairy
- Protein

MyPlate, a food guide plan discussed later in this chapter, offers a visual reminder and advice to help you make smart choices from each of these food groups. A dinner consisting of a bean burrito, lettuce and tomato salad with oil-and-vinegar dressing, a glass of milk, and an apple covers all groups.

Balance also refers to matching your energy intake (how many total calories you consume) with energy expenditure (calories burned by metabolism and physical activity) over time. As you will see in Chapter 7, a prolonged imbalance between energy intake and energy expenditure leads to fluctuations in body weight.

CRITICAL THINKING

Andy would benefit from more variety in his diet. What are some practical tips he can use to increase his fruit and vegetable intake?

TABLE 2-1 Tips for Boosting the Phytochemical Content of a Diet

- Include vegetables in main and side dishes. Add these to rice, omelets, potato salad, and pastas. Try broccoli or cauliflower florets, mushrooms, peas, carrots, corn, or peppers.
- Look for quick-to-fix grain side dishes in the supermarket. Pilafs, couscous, rice mixes, and tabbouleh are just a few that you'll find.
- Choose fruit-filled cookies, such as fig bars, instead of sugar-rich cookies. Use fresh or canned fruit as a topping for pudding, hot or cold cereal, pancakes, and frozen desserts.
- Put raisins, grapes, apple chunks, pineapples, grated carrots, zucchini, or cucumber into coleslaw, chicken salad, or tuna salad.
- Be creative at the salad bar: Try fresh spinach, leaf lettuce, red cabbage, zucchini, yellow squash, cauliflower, peas, mushrooms, or red or yellow peppers.
- Pack fresh or dried fruit for snacks away from home instead of grabbing a candy bar or going hungry.
- Add slices of cucumber, zucchini, spinach, or carrot slivers to the lettuce and tomato on your sandwiches.
- Each week try one or two vegetarian meals, such as beans and rice or pasta; vegetable stir fry; or spaghetti and tomato sauce.
- If your daily protein intake exceeds the recommended amounts, reduce the meat, fish, or poultry in casseroles, stews, and soups by one-third to one-half and add more vegetables and legumes.
- Keep a container of fresh vegetables in the refrigerator for snacks.
- Choose fruit or vegetable juices (preferably 100% juice varieties) instead of soft drinks.
- Substitute tea for coffee or soft drinks on a regular basis.
- Have a bowl of fresh fruit on hand.
- Switch from crisp head lettuce to leaf lettuce, such as romaine.
- Use salsa as a dip for chips in place of creamy dips.
- Choose whole-grain breakfast cereals, breads, and crackers.
- Add flavor to your plate with ginger, rosemary, basil, thyme, garlic, onions, parsley, and chives in place of salt.
- Incorporate soy products, such as tofu, soy milk, soy protein isolate, and roasted soybeans into your meals (see Chapter 6).

Moderation Refers Mostly to Portion Size

nutrient density The ratio derived by dividing a food's nutrient content by its calorie content. When the food's contribution to our nutrient need for that nutrient exceeds its contribution to our calorie need, the food is considered to have a favorable nutrient density.

Eating in moderation requires paying attention to portion sizes and planning your day's diet so that you do not overconsume any nutrients. This is especially important for fat, salt, and sugar because Americans typically consume too much of these food components—and too many calories overall. For example, if you plan to eat a bacon cheeseburger (relatively high in fat, salt, and calories) at lunch, you should eat foods such as fruits and salad greens (less concentrated sources of these nutrients) at other meals that same day. If you prefer whole milk to low-fat or fat-free milk, reduce the fat elsewhere in your meals. Try low-fat salad dressings, or use jam rather than butter or margarine on toast. Overall, it is more feasible to consume moderate portions of foods that supply lots of fat, salt, and sugar than to try to eliminate these foods altogether.

Let's be clear that moderation is important for all food components, not just fat, salt, and sugar. For example, many North Americans do not consume enough

4

vitamin E, which is found in plant oils, nuts, and some fruits and vegetables. However, taking large doses of vitamin E (e.g., from supplements) can lead to excessive bleeding because of its effects on blood clotting. You *can* get too much of a good thing!

Nutrient Density Focuses on Nutrient Content

The **nutrient density** of a food is a characteristic used to determine its nutritional quality. Nutrient density of a food is determined by comparing its protein, vitamin, or mineral content with the amount of calories it provides. A food is deemed nutrient dense if it provides a large amount of a nutrient for a relatively small amount of calories when compared with other food sources. The higher a food's nutrient density, the better it is as a nutrient source. Comparing the nutrient density of different foods is an easy way to estimate their relative nutritional quality.

Generally, nutrient density is determined with respect to individual nutrients (see Further Reading 4). For example, many fruits and vegetables have a high content of vitamin C compared with their modest calorie content; that is, they are nutrient-dense foods for vitamin C. Figure 2-1 shows that fat-free milk is much more nutrient dense than sugared soft drinks for many nutrients, especially protein, vitamin A, riboflavin, and calcium.

As noted previously, menu planning should focus mainly on the total diet—not on the selection of one critical food as the key to an adequate diet. Nutrient-dense foods—such as fat-free and low-fat milk, lean meats, legumes (beans), oranges, carrots, broccoli, whole-wheat bread, and whole-grain breakfast cereals—do help balance less nutrient-dense foods—such as cookies and potato chips, which many people like to eat. The latter are often called empty-calorie foods because they tend to be high in sugar and/or fat but provide few other nutrients.

Eating nutrient-dense foods is especially important for people who consume diets relatively low in calories. This includes some older people and those following weight-loss diets. This is because nutrient needs remain high even though calorie needs may be diminished.

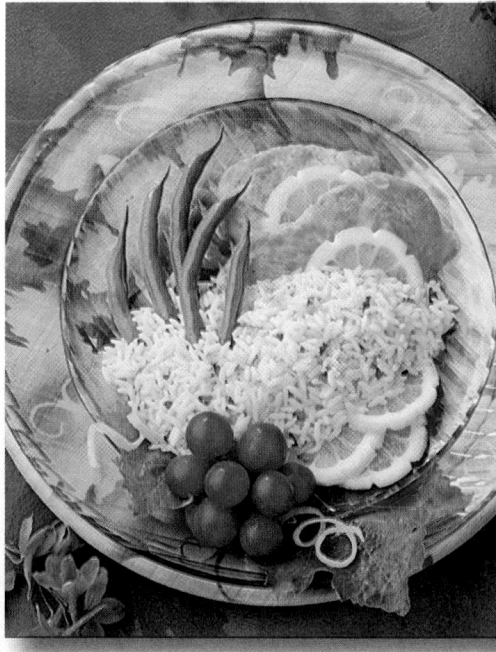

▲ Focus on nutrient-rich foods as you strive to meet your nutrient needs. The more colorful the food on your plate, the greater the content of nutrients and phytochemicals.

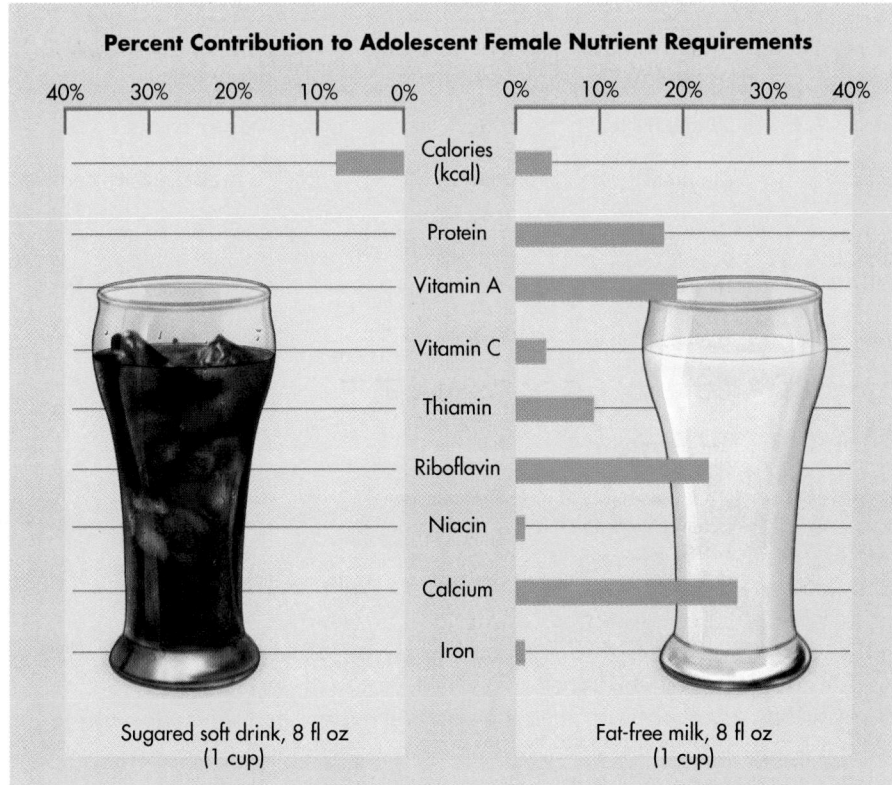

Sugared soft drink, 8 fl oz (1 cup)

Fat-free milk, 8 fl oz (1 cup)

FIGURE 2-1 ▶ Comparison of the nutrient contributions of a sugared soft drink with that of fat-free (i.e., nonfat or skim) milk. Choosing a glass of fat-free milk makes a significantly greater contribution to nutrient intake than does a sugared soft drink. An easy way to determine nutrient density from this chart is to compare the lengths of the bars indicating vitamin or mineral contribution with the bar that represents calorie contribution. For the soft drink, no nutrient surpasses calorie content. Fat-free milk, in contrast, has longer nutrient bars for protein, vitamin A, the vitamins thiamin and riboflavin, and the mineral calcium than it does for calories. Including many nutrient-dense foods in your diet is a good way to meet nutrient needs without exceeding calorie needs.

energy density A comparison of the calorie (kcal) content of a food with the weight of the food. An energy-dense food is high in calories but weighs very little (e.g., potato chips), whereas a food low in energy density has few calories but weighs a lot, such as an orange.

Energy (kcal) Density Affects Calorie Intake

Energy density is a measurement that best describes the calorie content of a food. Energy density of a food is determined by comparing the calorie (kcal) content with the weight of food. A food that is rich in calories but weighs relatively little is considered energy dense. Examples include nuts; cookies; fried foods in general; and even fat-free snacks, such as fat-free pretzels. Foods with low energy density include fruits, vegetables, and any food that incorporates lots of water during cooking, such as oatmeal (Table 2-2).

Researchers have shown that eating a meal with many foods of low energy density promotes satiety without contributing many calories (see Further Reading 6). This is probably because we typically consume a constant weight of food at a meal rather than a constant number of calories. How this constant weight of food is regulated is not known, but careful laboratory studies show that people consume fewer calories in a meal if most of the food choices are low in energy density, compared with foods high in energy density. Eating a diet low in energy density can aid in losing (or maintaining) weight.

Overall, foods with lots of water and fiber (i.e., low-energy-density foods) contribute few calories even though they help one feel full. Alternatively, foods with high energy density must be eaten in greater amounts to promote fullness. This is one more reason to eat a diet rich in fruits, vegetables, and whole-grain breads and cereals, a pattern that is typical of many ethnic diets throughout rural areas of the world.

Still, favorite foods, even if they are high in energy density, can have a place in your dietary pattern, but you will have to plan for them. For example, chocolate is a very energy-dense food, but a small portion at the end of a meal can supply a satisfying finale. In addition, foods with high energy density can help people with poor appetites, such as some older people, to maintain or gain weight.

The following sections of Chapter 2 describe various states of nutritional health and provide tools and nutrient guidelines for planning healthy diets to support overall health.

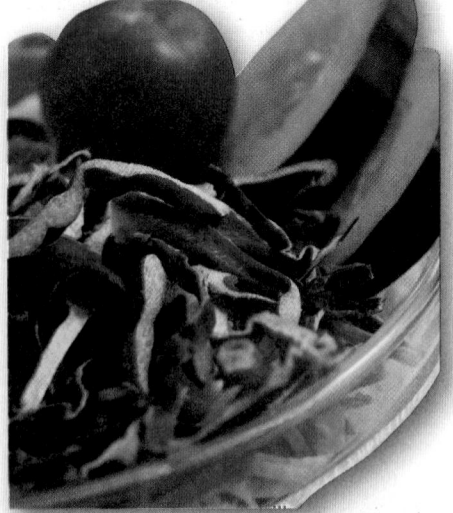

▲ Salads are low in energy density if we limit additional calories from salad dressing, bacon bits, cheese crumbles or cubes, and croutons.

TABLE 2-2 Energy Density of Common Foods (Listed in Relative Order)

Very Low Energy Density (less than 0.6 kcal per gram)	Low Energy Density (0.6 to 1.5 kcal per gram)	Medium Energy Density (1.5 to 4 kcal per gram)	High Energy Density (greater than 4 kcal per gram)
Lettuce	Whole milk	Eggs	Graham crackers
Tomatoes	Oatmeal	Ham	Fat-free sandwich cookies
Strawberries	Cottage cheese	Pumpkin pie	Chocolate
Broccoli	Beans	Whole-wheat bread	Chocolate chip cookies
Salsa	Bananas	Bagels	Tortilla chips
Grapefruit	Broiled fish	White bread	Bacon
Fat-free milk	Fat-free yogurt	Raisins	Potato chips
Carrots	Ready-to-eat breakfast cereals with 1% low-fat milk	Cream cheese	Peanuts
Vegetable soup		Cake with frosting	Peanut butter
		Pretzels	Mayonnaise
	Plain baked potato	Rice cakes	Butter or margarine
	Cooked rice		Vegetable oils
	Spaghetti noodles		

Data adapted from Rolls B, *The Volumetrics Eating Plan.* New York: HarperCollins, 2005.

TABLE 2-3 Conducting an Evaluation of Nutritional Health

Parameters	Example
Background	Medical history (e.g., current diseases, past surgeries, current weight, weight history, and current medications)
	Social history (marital status, living conditions)
	Family health history
	Education level
	Economic status
Nutritional	Anthropometric assessment: height, weight, skinfold thickness, arm muscle circumference, and other parameters
	Biochemical (laboratory) assessment of blood and urine: enzyme activities, concentrations of nutrients or their by-products
	Clinical assessment (physical examination): general appearance of skin, eyes, and tongue; rapid hair loss; sense of touch; ability to walk
	Dietary assessment: usual intake or record of previous days' meals

A **clinical assessment** would follow, during which a health professional would search for any physical evidence (e.g., high blood pressure) of diet-related diseases or deficiencies. Then, a close look at the person's diet (**dietary assessment**), including a record of at least the previous few days' food intake, would help to determine any possible problem areas.

Finally, adding the **environmental assessment** (from the background analysis) provides further details about the living conditions, education level, and ability to purchase and prepare foods needed to maintain health. Now the true nutritional state of a person emerges. Taken together, these five assessments form the ABCDEs of nutritional assessment: anthropometric, biochemical, clinical, dietary, and environmental (Fig. 2-3).

MAKING DECISIONS

Nutritional Assessment

A practical example using the ABCDEs for evaluating nutritional status can be illustrated in a person who chronically abuses alcohol. Upon evaluation, the physician notes:

(A) Low weight for height, recent 10-pound weight loss, muscle wasting in the upper body
(B) Low amounts of the vitamins thiamin and folate in the blood
(C) Psychological confusion, facial sores, and uncoordinated movement
(D) Dietary intake of little more than wine and hamburgers for the last week
(E) Currently residing in a homeless shelter; $35.00 in wallet; unemployed

Evaluation: This person needs medical attention, including nutrient repletion.

Recognizing the Limitations of Nutritional Assessment

A long time may elapse between the initial development of poor nutritional health and the first clinical evidence of a problem. A diet high in saturated (typically solid) fat often increases blood cholesterol but without producing any clinical evidence for years. However, when the blood vessels become sufficiently blocked by cholesterol and other materials, chest pain during physical activity or a **heart attack** may occur. An active area of nutrition research is the development of better methods for early detection of nutrition-related problems such as heart attack risk.

clinical assessment Examination of general appearance of skin, eyes, and tongue; evidence of rapid hair loss; sense of touch; and ability to cough and walk.

dietary assessment Estimation of typical food choices relying mostly on the recounting of one's usual intake or a record of one's previous days' intake.

environmental assessment Includes details about living conditions, education level, and the ability of the person to purchase, transport, and cook food. The person's weekly budget for food purchases is also a key factor to consider.

heart attack Rapid fall in heart function caused by reduced blood flow through the heart's blood vessels. Often part of the heart dies in the process. Technically called a myocardial infarction.

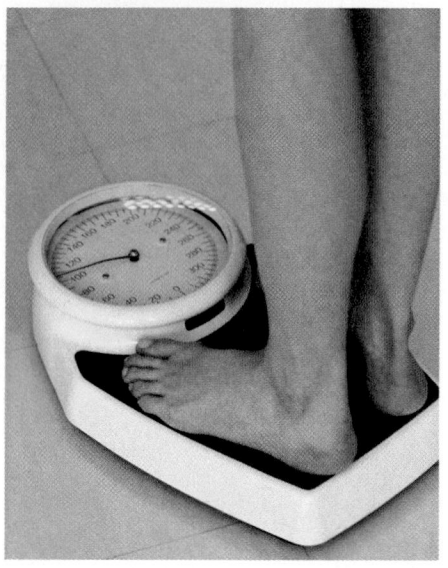

Anthropometric

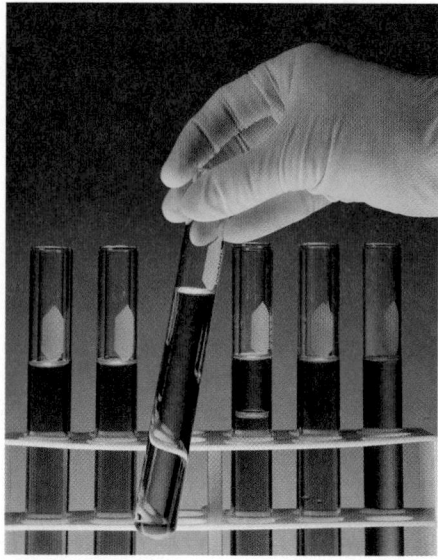

Biochemical

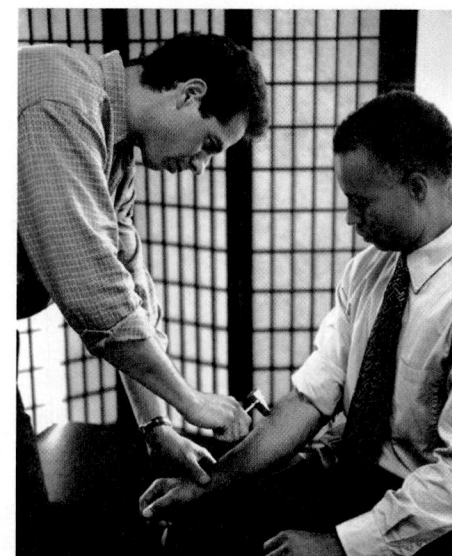

Clinical

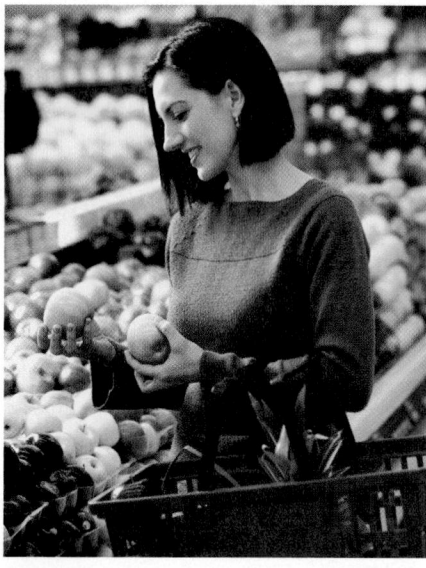

Dietary

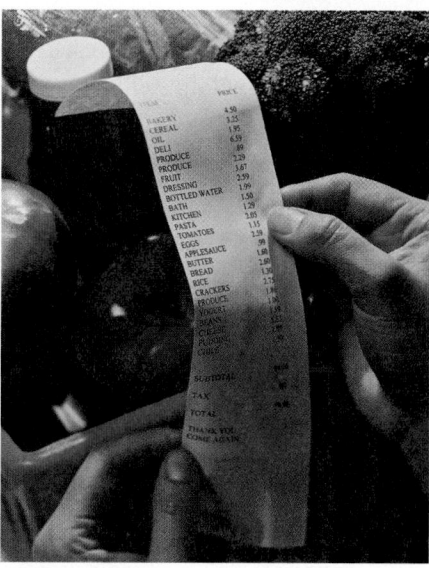

Environmental

FIGURE 2-3 ▶ A complete nutritional assessment includes anthropometric, biochemical, clinical, and dietary information. Environmental status adds further information, rounding out the ABCDEs of nutritional assessment.

Another example of a serious health condition with delayed symptoms is low bone density resulting from a calcium deficiency—a particularly relevant issue for adolescent and young adult females. Many young women do not consume the needed amount of calcium but suffer no obvious effects in their younger years. However, the bone structures of these women with low calcium intakes do not reach full potential during the years of growth, making osteoporosis more likely later in life.

Furthermore, clinical symptoms of some nutritional deficiencies (e.g., diarrhea, inability to walk normally, and facial sores) are not very specific. These may have causes other than poor nutrition. The long time it takes for symptoms to develop and their potential to be vague often make it difficult to establish a link between an individual's current diet and nutritional state.

Concern About the State of Your Nutritional Health Is Important

Table 1-7 in Chapter 1 portrayed the close relationship between nutrition and health. The good news is that people who focus on maintaining nutritional health are apt to enjoy a long, vigorous life. For example, a recent study found that women with a healthy lifestyle had a decreased risk for heart attacks (80% reduction) compared to women without such healthy practices. The healthy habits included:

- Consumed a healthy diet
  - Varied
  - Rich in fiber
  - Included some fish
  - Low in animal fat and *trans* fat
- Maintained a healthy weight
- Occasionally consumed alcohol in small amounts
- Exercised for at least 30 minutes daily
- Avoided use of tobacco

Should all adults follow this example (with optional use of alcohol)?

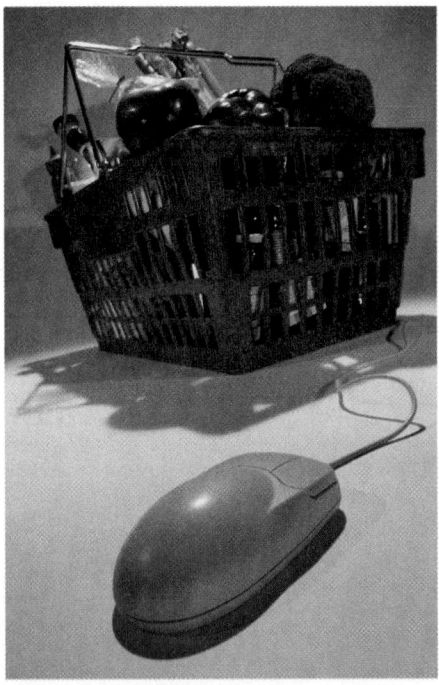

▲ Is there an app for that? Yes, there is! Health-conscious consumers can tap into a growing number of smartphone applications to help them stay on track with a healthy lifestyle. From calorie counters to pedometers to gentle reminders to get up and stretch, smartphone users have access to a virtual arsenal against diet-related disease. Log onto the Connect site to find links to apps from reputable sources.

CONCEPT CHECK

A desirable nutritional state results when the body has enough nutrients to function fully and contains stores to use in times of increased needs. When nutrient intake fails to meet body needs, undernutrition develops. Symptoms of such an inadequate nutrient intake can take months or years to develop. Overloading the body with nutrients, leading to overnutrition, is another potential problem to avoid. Nutritional state can be assessed by using anthropometric, biochemical, clinical, dietary, and economic assessments (ABCDEs).

2.4 Using the Scientific Method to Determine Nutrient Needs

How do we know what we know about nutrient needs? In a word, research. Like other sciences, the research that sets the foundation for nutrition knowledge has developed through the use of the *scientific method,* a testing procedure designed to detect and eliminate error.

MAKING DECISIONS

Research on Stomach Ulcers

Overall, the scientific method requires a skeptical attitude. A recent example of this need for skepticism involves stomach **ulcers.** Not so many years ago, everyone "knew" that stomach ulcers were caused by a stressful lifestyle and a poor diet. Then, in 1983, an Australian physician, Dr. Barry Marshall, reported in a respected medical journal that ulcers are usually caused by a common **microorganism** called *Helicobacter pylori.* Furthermore, he stated that a cure is possible using antibiotics. At first, other physicians were skeptical about this finding and continued to prescribe medications such as antacids that reduce stomach acid. But, as more studies were published demonstrating that patients using antibiotics were cured of ulcers, the medical profession eventually accepted the findings. Today, ulcers are managed for the most part by medications that destroy the microorganism. (We will discuss the treatment of stomach ulcers in more detail in Chapter 3.) Sound scientific discoveries will always be subject to challenge and change.

ulcer Erosion of the tissue lining, usually in the stomach (gastric ulcer) or the upper small intestine (duodenal ulcer). As a group these are generally referred to as peptic ulcers.

microorganism Bacterium virus, or other organism invisible to the naked eye, some of which cause diseases. Also called *microbe.*

hypotheses Tentative explanations by a scientist to explain a phenomenon.

scurvy The deficiency disease that results after a few weeks to months of consuming a diet that lacks vitamin C; pinpoint sites of bleeding on the skin are an early sign.

epidemiology The study of how disease rates vary among different population groups.

The first step of the scientific method is the observation of a natural phenomenon. Scientists then suggest possible explanations, called **hypotheses,** about its cause. At times, historical events can provide clues to important relationships in nutrition science, such as the link between vitamin C and **scurvy** (see Chapter 8). In a related approach, scientists may study diet and disease patterns among various populations, a research method called **epidemiology.**

Historical and epidemiological findings can *suggest* hypotheses about the role of diet in various health problems. *Proving* the role of particular dietary components, however, requires controlled experiments. The data gathered from experiments may either support or refute each hypothesis. If the results of many experiments support a hypothesis, scientists accept the hypothesis as a **theory** (such as the theory of gravity). Often, the results from one experiment suggest a new set of questions (Fig. 2-4).

The most rigorous type of controlled experiment follows a randomized, double-blind, placebo-controlled study design. In this type of study, a group of participants—the experimental group—follows a specific protocol (e.g., consuming a certain food or nutrient), and participants in a corresponding **control group** follow their normal habits or consume a **placebo**. People are randomly assigned to each group, such as by the flip of a coin. Scientists then observe the experimental group over time to see if there is any effect not found in the control group.

theory An explanation for a phenomenon that has numerous lines of evidence to support it.

control group Participants in an experiment who are not given the treatment being tested.

placebo Generally a fake medicine or treatment used to disguise the treatments given to the participants in an experiment.

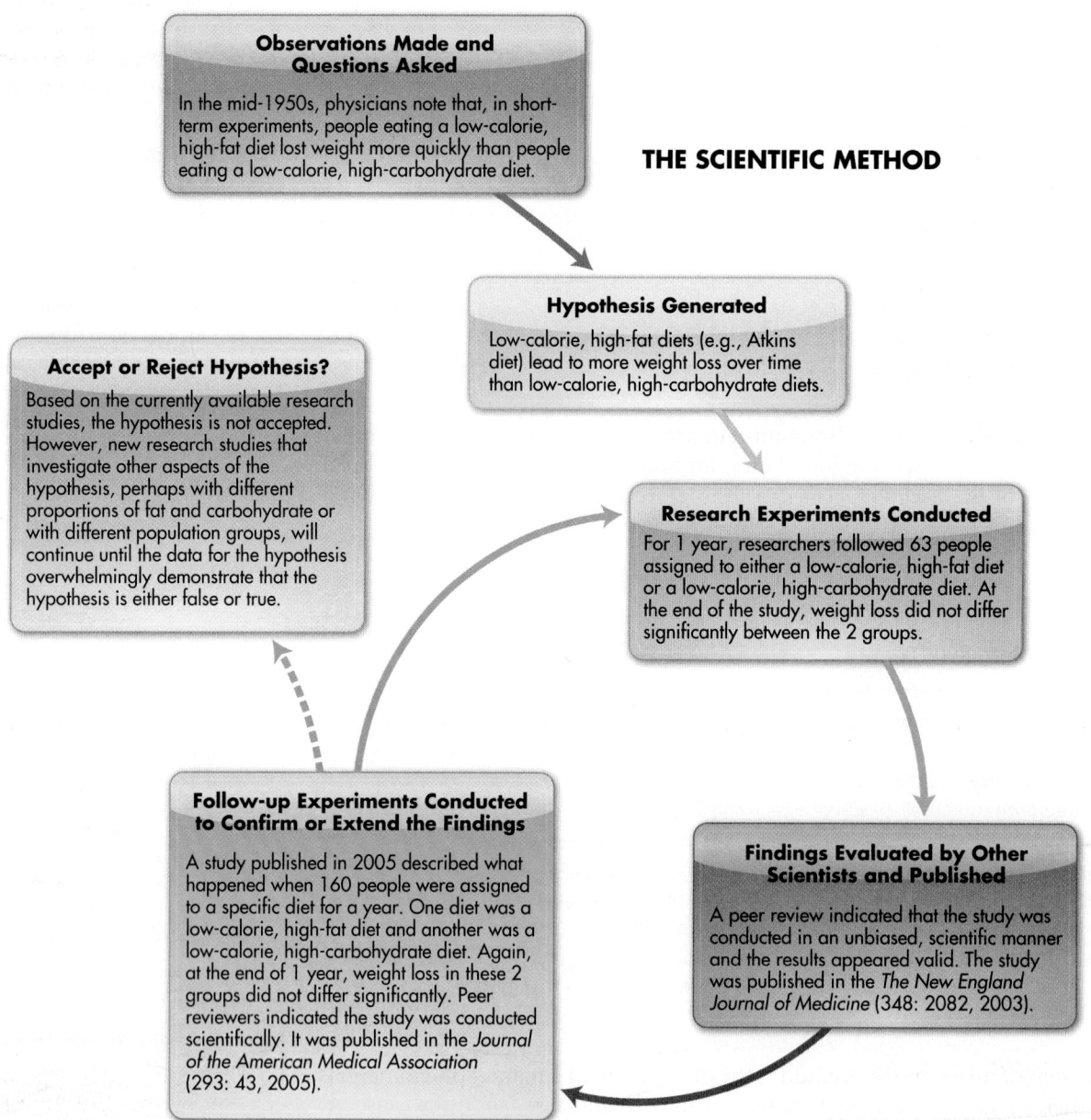

THE SCIENTIFIC METHOD

Observations Made and Questions Asked

In the mid-1950s, physicians note that, in short-term experiments, people eating a low-calorie, high-fat diet lost weight more quickly than people eating a low-calorie, high-carbohydrate diet.

Hypothesis Generated

Low-calorie, high-fat diets (e.g., Atkins diet) lead to more weight loss over time than low-calorie, high-carbohydrate diets.

Accept or Reject Hypothesis?

Based on the currently available research studies, the hypothesis is not accepted. However, new research studies that investigate other aspects of the hypothesis, perhaps with different proportions of fat and carbohydrate or with different population groups, will continue until the data for the hypothesis overwhelmingly demonstrate that the hypothesis is either false or true.

Research Experiments Conducted

For 1 year, researchers followed 63 people assigned to either a low-calorie, high-fat diet or a low-calorie, high-carbohydrate diet. At the end of the study, weight loss did not differ significantly between the 2 groups.

Follow-up Experiments Conducted to Confirm or Extend the Findings

A study published in 2005 described what happened when 160 people were assigned to a specific diet for a year. One diet was a low-calorie, high-fat diet and another was a low-calorie, high-carbohydrate diet. Again, at the end of 1 year, weight loss in these 2 groups did not differ significantly. Peer reviewers indicated the study was conducted scientifically. It was published in the *Journal of the American Medical Association* (293: 43, 2005).

Findings Evaluated by Other Scientists and Published

A peer review indicated that the study was conducted in an unbiased, scientific manner and the results appeared valid. The study was published in the *The New England Journal of Medicine* (348: 2082, 2003).

FIGURE 2-4 ▶ This example shows how the scientific method was used to test a hypothesis about the effects of low-calorie, high-fat diets on weight loss. Scientists consistently follow these steps when testing all types of hypotheses. Scientists do not accept a nutrition or another scientific hypothesis until it has been thoroughly tested using the scientific method.

Human experiments provide the most convincing evidence about relationships between nutrients and health, but they are often not practical or ethical. Thus, much of what we know about human nutritional needs and functions has been gleaned from animal experiments. The use of animal experiments to study the role of nutrition in certain human diseases depends on the availability of an **animal model**—a disease in laboratory animals that closely mimics a particular human disease. Often, however, if no animal model is available and human experiments are ruled out, scientific knowledge cannot advance beyond what can be learned from epidemiological studies.

Once an experiment is complete, scientists summarize the findings and seek to publish the results in scientific journals. Generally, before articles are published in scientific journals, they are critically reviewed by other scientists familiar with the subject, which helps to ensure that only high-quality, objective research findings are published.

Keep in mind, one experiment is never enough to prove a particular hypothesis or provide a basis for nutritional recommendations. Rather, through follow-up studies, the results obtained in one laboratory must be confirmed by experiments conducted in other laboratories and, possibly, under varying circumstances. Only then can we really trust and use the results. The more lines of evidence available to support an idea, the more likely it is to be true (Fig. 2-5).

Epidemiological studies may suggest hypotheses, but controlled experiments are needed to rigorously test hypotheses before nutrition recommendations can be made. For example, epidemiologists found that smokers who regularly consumed fruits and vegetables had a lower risk for lung cancer than smokers who ate few fruits and vegetables. Some scientists proposed that beta-carotene, a pigment present in many fruits and vegetables, may be responsible for reducing the damage that tobacco smoke creates in the lungs. However, in **double-blind studies** involving heavy smokers, the risk of lung cancer was found to be *higher* for those who took beta-carotene supplements than for those who did not (this is not true for the small amount of beta-carotene found naturally in foods). Soon after these results were reported, the U.S. federal agency supporting two other large ongoing studies that employed beta-carotene supplements called a halt to the research, stating that these supplements are ineffective in preventing both lung cancer and cardiovascular disease.

animal model Use of animals to study disease to understand more about human disease.

case-control study A study in which individuals who have a disease or condition, such as lung cancer, are compared with individuals who do not have the condition.

double-blind study An experimental design in which neither the participants nor the researchers are aware of each participant's assignment (test or placebo) or the outcome of the study until it is completed. An independent third party holds the code and the data until the study has been completed.

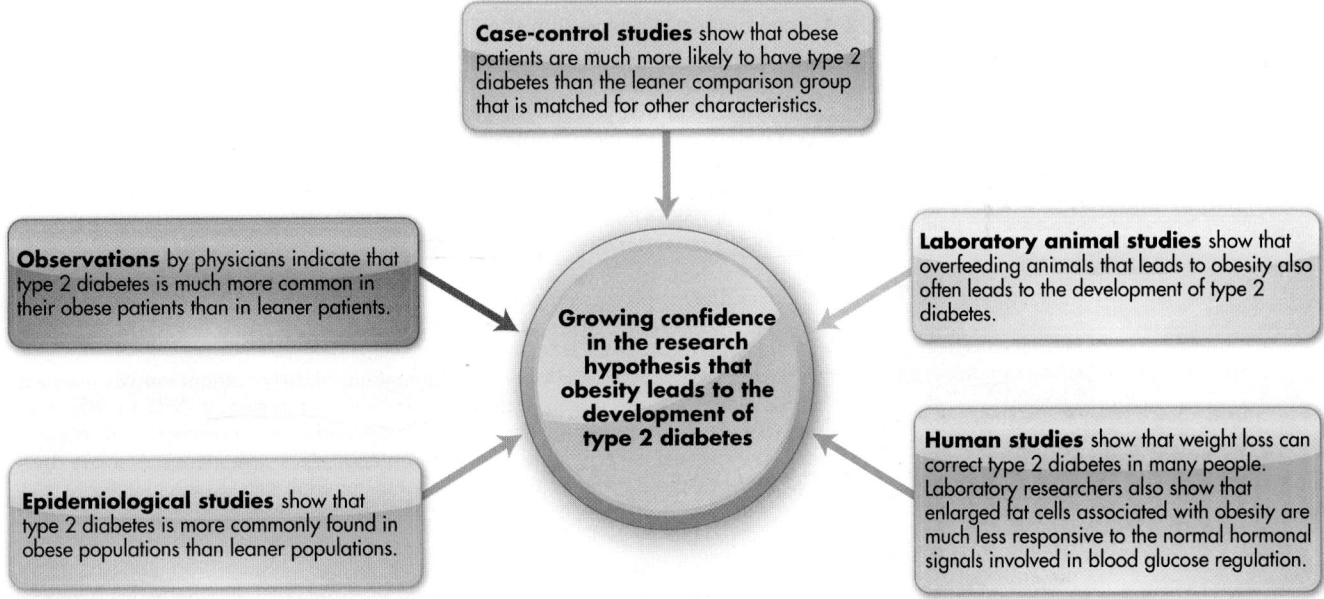

FIGURE 2-5 ▶ Data from a variety of sources can come together to support a research hypothesis. This diagram shows how various types of research data support the hypothesis that obesity leads to the development of type 2 diabetes (see Chapter 4).

2.5 Specific Nutrient Standards and Recommendations

The overarching goal of any healthy diet plan is to meet nutrient needs. To begin, we must determine what amount of each essential nutrient is necessary to maintain health. Most of the terms that describe nutrient needs fall under one umbrella term— **Dietary Reference Intakes (DRIs).** The development of DRIs is an ongoing, collaborative effort between the Food and Nutrition Board of the Institute of Medicine in the United States and Health Canada (see Further Reading 2). Included under the DRI umbrella are **Recommended Dietary Allowances (RDAs), Adequate Intakes (AIs), Estimated Energy Requirements (EERs),** and **Tolerable Upper Intake Levels (Upper Levels or ULs).**

As you begin your study of nutrition, all these acronyms can seem like an alphabet soup of abbreviations! However, you can more easily sift through these nutrient standards if you have some basic knowledge about their development and use (summarized in Table 2-4).

Recommended Dietary Allowance

A Recommended Dietary Allowance (RDA) is the amount of a nutrient that will meet the needs of nearly all individuals (about 97%) in a particular age and gender group. A person can compare his or her individual intake of specific nutrients to the RDA. Although an intake slightly above or below the RDA for a particular nutrient is no reason for concern, a significant deviation below (about 70%) or above (about three times or more for some nutrients) the RDA for an extended time can eventually result in a deficiency or toxicity of that nutrient, respectively.

Adequate Intake

An RDA can be set for a nutrient only if there is sufficient information on the human needs for that particular nutrient. Today, there is not enough information on some nutrients, such as chromium, to set such a precise standard as an RDA. For this and other nutrients, the DRIs include a category called an Adequate Intake (AI). This standard is based on the dietary intakes of people that appear to be maintaining nutritional health. That amount of intake is assumed to be adequate, as no evidence of a nutritional deficiency is apparent.

Although nutrition recommendations are often made for the entire healthy population, each of us have individual needs based on our particular health status and genetic background. It would be more appropriate, but also more expensive, if recommendations were made on an individual basis once a person's health status is known.

Dietary Reference Intakes (DRIs) Term used to encompass nutrient recommendations made by the Food and Nutrition Board of the National Academy of Sciences. These include RDAs, EARs, AIs, EERs, and ULs.

Recommended Dietary Allowance (RDA) Nutrient intake amount sufficient to meet the needs of 97% to 98% of the individuals in a specific life stage.

Adequate Intake (AI) Nutrient intake amount set for any nutrient for which insufficient research is available to establish an RDA. AIs are based on estimates of intakes that appear to maintain a defined nutritional state in a specific life stage.

Estimated Energy Requirement (EER) Estimate of the energy (kcal) intake needed to match the energy use of an average person in a specific life stage.

Tolerable Upper Intake Level (UL) Maximum chronic daily intake level of a nutrient that is unlikely to cause adverse health effects in almost all people in a specific life stage.

TABLE 2-4 Recommendations within the Dietary Reference Intakes

RDA	Recommended Dietary Allowance. Use to evaluate your current intake for a specific nutrient. The further you stray above or below this value, the greater your chances of developing nutritional problems.
AI	Adequate Intake. Use to evaluate your current intake of nutrients, but realize that an AI designation implies that further research is required before scientists can establish a more definitive recommendation.
EER	Estimated Energy Requirement. Use to estimate calorie needs of the average person within a specific height, weight, gender, age, and physical activity pattern.
UL	Upper Level. Use to evaluate the highest amount of daily nutrient intake unlikely to cause adverse health effects in the long run in almost all people (97% to 98%) in a population. This number applies to chronic use and is set to protect even very susceptible people in the healthy general population. As intake increases above the Upper Level, the potential for adverse effects generally increases.
DV	Daily Value. Use as a rough guide for comparing the nutrient content of a food to approximate human needs. Typically, the Daily Value used on food labels refers to ages 4 years through adulthood. It is based on a 2000 kcal diet. Some Daily Values also increase slightly with higher calorie intakes (see Fig. 2-16 in the section on food labeling).

Estimated Energy Requirement

For calorie needs, we use the Estimated Energy Requirement (EER) instead of an RDA or AI. As described, the RDAs are set somewhat higher than the average needs for nutrients. This is fine for nutrients other than calories because a slight excess of vitamins and minerals is not harmful. However, a long-term excess of even a small amount of calories will lead to weight gain. Therefore, the calculation of EER needs to be more specific, taking into account age, gender, height, weight, and physical activity (e.g., sedentary or moderately active). In some cases, the additional calorie needs for growth and lactation are also included (see Chapters 7, 14, and 15 for the specific formulas used). Note that the EER is based on the "average" person. Thus, it can only serve as a starting point for estimating calorie needs.

Tolerable Upper Intake Level

A Tolerable Upper Intake Level (Upper Level or UL) has been set for some vitamins and minerals (see the inside cover). The UL is the highest amount of a nutrient unlikely to cause adverse health effects in the long run. As intake exceeds the UL, the risk of ill effects increases. These amounts generally should not be exceeded day after day, as toxicity could develop. For people eating a varied diet and/or using a balanced multivitamin and mineral supplement, exceeding the UL is unusual. Problems are more likely to arise with diets that promote excessive intakes of a limited variety of foods, with the use of many fortified foods, or with excessive doses of individual vitamins or minerals.

Daily Value

A nutrition standard more relevant to everyday life is the Daily Value (DV). This is a generic standard used on food labels. It is applicable to both genders from 4 years of age through adulthood, and is based on consuming a 2000 kcal diet. DVs are mostly set at or close to the highest RDA value or related nutrient standard seen in the various age and gender categories for a specific nutrient (see Appendix B). DVs have been set for vitamins, minerals, protein, and other dietary components. For fat and cholesterol, the DVs represent a maximum level, not a goal one should strive to reach. DVs allow consumers to compare their intake from a specific food to desirable (or maximum) intakes.

How Should These Nutrient Standards Be Used?

To sum up the acronyms described so far, the type of standard set for nutrients depends on the quality of available evidence. A nutrient recommendation backed by lots of experimental research will have an RDA. For a nutrient that still requires more research, only an AI is presented. We use the EER as a starting point for determining calorie needs. Some nutrients also have a UL if information on toxicity or adverse health effects is available. Periodically, new DRIs become available as expert committees review and interpret the available research.

RDAs and related standards are intended mainly for diet planning. Specifically, a diet plan should aim to meet the RDA or AI as appropriate and not to exceed the UL over the long term (Fig. 2-6). Specific RDA, AI, EER, and UL standards are printed on the inside cover of this book. To learn more about these nutrient standards, visit the link for Food and Nutrition on the Institute of Medicine's website (www.iom.edu).

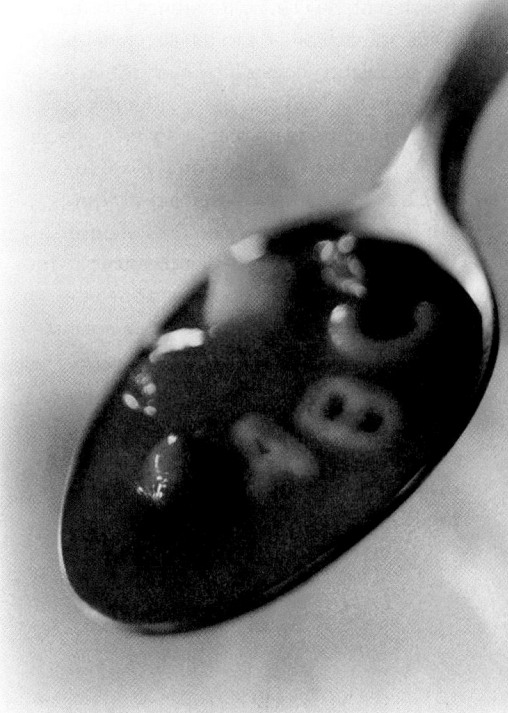

▲ With a little bit of study, you can master the alphabet soup of nutrition recommendations.

MAKING DECISIONS

Using Nutrient Recommendations

As nutrient intake increases, the Recommended Dietary Allowance (RDA) for the nutrient, if set, is eventually met and a deficient state is no longer present. An individual's needs most likely will be met since RDAs are set high to include almost all people. Related to the RDA concept of meeting an individual's needs are the standards of Adequate Intake (AI) and the Estimated Energy Requirement (EER). These can be used to estimate an individual's needs for some nutrients and calories, respectively. Still, keep in mind that these standards do not share the same degree of accuracy as the RDA. For example, EER may have to be adjusted upward if the individual is very physically active. Finally, as nutrient intake increases above the Upper Level (UL), poor nutritional health is again likely. However, this poor health is due now to the toxic effects of a nutrient, rather than those of a deficiency.

CONCEPT CHECK

Standards for nutrient intake are included in the broad category of Dietary Reference Intakes (DRIs). The Recommended Dietary Allowances (RDAs) are the amounts of each nutrient that will meet the needs of healthy individuals within specific gender and age categories. If not enough information is available to set an RDA, an Adequate Intake (AI) value is used. Tolerable Upper Intake Levels (ULs) are the highest amounts of a nutrient unlikely to cause adverse health effects. ULs have been set for some vitamins and minerals.

FIGURE 2-6 ▶ This figure shows the relationship of the Dietary Reference Intakes (DRIs) to each other and the percentage of the population covered by each. At intakes between the RDA and the UL, the risk of either an inadequate diet or adverse effects from the nutrient in question is close to 0. The UL is then the highest level of nutrient intake likely to pose no risks of adverse health effects to almost all individuals in the general population. At intakes above the UL, the margin of safety to protect against adverse effects is reduced. The AI is set for some nutrients instead of an RDA. The Food and Nutrition Board states that there is no established benefit for healthy individuals if they consume nutrient intakes above the RDA or AI.

Recommended Dietary Allowance (RDA): The dietary intake level that is sufficient to meet the nutrient requirement of nearly all (97% to 98%) healthy individuals in a particular life stage and gender group. When set for a nutrient, aim for this intake.

Adequate Intake (AI): A recommended intake value based on observed or experimentally determined approximations or estimates of nutrient intake by a group (or groups) of healthy people that is assumed to be adequate—used when an RDA cannot be determined. When set for a nutrient, aim for this intake.

Tolerable Upper Intake Level (Upper Level or UL): The highest level of nutrient intake that is likely to pose no risk of adverse health effects for almost all individuals in the general population. As intake increases above the Upper Level, the risk of adverse effects increases.

2.6 Recommendations for Healthy Living

Since the early twentieth century, researchers have worked to translate the science of nutrition into practical terms so that people with no special training could estimate whether their nutritional needs were being met. Early food guidance systems aimed to reduce risk for nutrient deficiencies, but severe deficiency diseases are no longer common. Marginal deficiencies of calcium, iron, folate and other B vitamins, vitamin C, vitamin D, vitamin E, potassium, magnesium, and fiber are still a problem; but for many North Americans, major health problems stem from overconsumption of one or more of the following: calories, saturated fat, cholesterol, *trans* fat, alcohol, and sodium (see Further Reading 18).

The following sections of Chapter 2 will describe guidelines and tools for planning healthy lifestyles. You will notice how those core concepts of variety, balance, and moderation keep showing up throughout our discussions of the Dietary Guidelines, MyPlate, and the Physical Activity Guidelines.

Dietary Guidelines—The Basis for Menu Planning

The 2010 **Dietary Guidelines for Americans** provide nutrition and physical activity advice based on the latest and strongest scientific information to improve the health of all Americans age 2 and older (see Further Readings 12 and 14). The USDA and U.S. Department of Health and Human Services (DHHS) have published Dietary Guidelines since 1980 to aid diet planning. In light of the current epidemic of overweight and obesity—pressing health issues that now affect two-thirds of adults and one-third of children and adolescents—the message of calorie balance is woven throughout this seventh edition of the Dietary Guidelines.

The most important changes from the 2005 edition of the Dietary Guidelines include powerful emphases on reduction of total calories, sugar-sweetened beverages, saturated fat, and sodium. In addition, the report calls for a much-needed increase in physical activity among all population groups. Previous editions of the Dietary Guidelines have targeted healthy Americans, but these latest recommendations also include those at risk of developing chronic diseases. The health of children is highlighted. The new recommendations are also more culturally sensitive to reflect the

Dietary Guidelines for Americans General goals for nutrient intakes and diet composition set by the USDA and the U.S. Department of Health and Human Services.

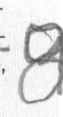

Losing weight is a challenge that takes time and continual awareness of calorie balance. We live in an *obesogenic* environment. With around-the-clock access to an increasing variety of super-sized, energy-dense foods, the typical American consumes about 600 more kilocalories per day than in 1970. Furthermore, out of convenience or necessity, our work, school, and home lives are dominated by sedentary activities.

growing diversity and varied health concerns of the American population. Finally, the new Dietary Guidelines recognize the prevalence of food insecurity (see Chapter 12), aiming to help populations with limited access to food optimize the nutritional content of meals within their resource constraints.

The Dietary Guidelines give direction for the development of educational materials, aid policy makers, and serve as the basis for consumer nutrition messages (see Further Reading 7). Overall, Americans should use this information along with related tools, such as MyPlate and the Physical Activity Guidelines for Americans, to form lifestyle patterns that optimize health.

The report identifies 29 key recommendations (outlined in Figure 2-7) to support three major goals:

- Balance calories with physical activity to manage weight.
- Consume more of certain foods and nutrients, such as fruits, vegetables, whole grains, fat-free and low-fat dairy products, and seafood.
- Consume fewer foods with sodium (salt), saturated fats, *trans* fats, cholesterol, added sugars, and refined grains.

Appendix C contains nutrient guidelines for Canadians.

CRITICAL THINKING

Shannon has grown up eating the typical American diet. Having recently read and heard many media reports about the relationship between nutrition and health, she is beginning to look critically at her diet and is considering making changes. However, she doesn't know where to begin. What advice would you give her?

FIGURE 2-7 ▶ Key Recommendations from the 2010 Dietary Guidelines for Americans

BALANCING CALORIES TO MANAGE WEIGHT

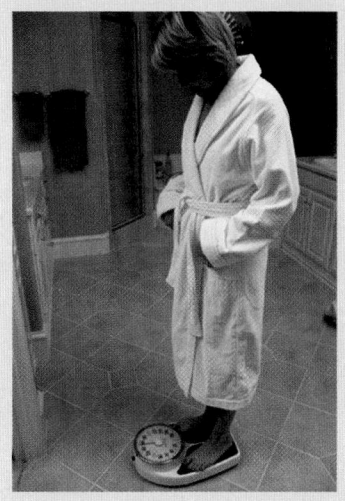

- Prevent and/or reduce overweight and obesity through improved eating and physical activity behaviors.
- Control total calorie intake to manage body weight. For people who are overweight or obese, this will mean consuming fewer calories from foods and beverages.
- Increase physical activity and reduce time spent in sedentary behaviors.
- Maintain appropriate calorie balance during each stage of life—childhood, adolescence, adulthood, pregnancy and breastfeeding, and older age.

Key Recommendations for Specific Population Groups

- Women of childbearing age: Achieve and maintain a healthy weight before becoming pregnant.
- *Pregnant women*: Gain weight within the 2009 Institute of Medicine gestational weight-gain guidelines.
- Adults ages 65 years and older: If overweight, avoid additional weight gain. For those with cardiovascular disease risk factors, lose weight to improve quality of life and reduce risk of chronic diseases and associated disabilities.

FOODS AND FOOD COMPONENTS TO REDUCE

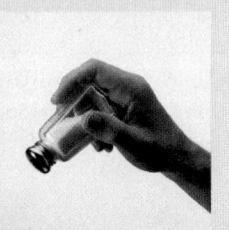

- Reduce daily sodium intake to less than 2300 mg and further reduce intake to 1500 mg among persons who are 51 and older and those of any age who are African-American or have hypertension, diabetes, or chronic kidney disease. The 1500-mg recommendation applies to about half of the U.S. population, including children, and the majority of adults.
- Consume less than 10% of calories from saturated fatty acids by replacing them with monounsaturated and polyunsaturated fatty acids.
- Consume less than 300 mg per day of dietary cholesterol.
- Keep *trans* fatty acid consumption as low as possible by limiting foods that contain synthetic sources of *trans* fats, such as partially hydrogenated oils, and by limiting other solid fats.
- Reduce the intake of calories from solid fats and added sugars.
- Limit the consumption of foods that contain refined grains, especially refined grain foods that contain solid fats, added sugars, and sodium.
- If alcohol is consumed, it should be consumed in moderation—up to one drink per day for women and two drinks per day for men—and only by adults of legal drinking age.

continued on next page

10, 11, 12, 13, 14

FIGURE 2-7 ▶ continued

FOODS AND NUTRIENTS TO INCREASE

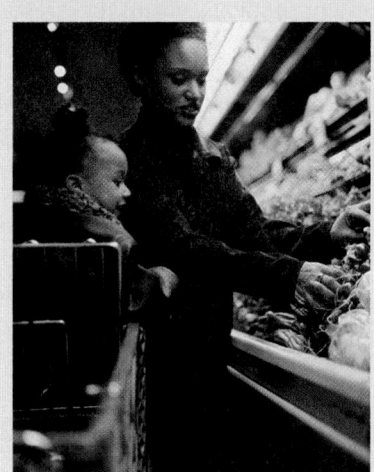

- Increase vegetable and fruit intake.

- Eat a variety of vegetables, especially dark-green and red and orange vegetables and beans and peas.

- Consume at least half of all grains as whole gains. Increase whole-grain intake by replacing refined grains with whole grains.

- Increase intake of fat-free or low-fat milk and milk products, such as milk, yogurt, cheese, or fortified soy beverages.

- Choose a variety of protein foods, which include seafood, lean meat and poultry, eggs, beans and peas, soy products, and unsalted nuts and seeds.

- Increase the amount and variety of seafood consumed by choosing seafood in place of some meat and poultry.

- Replace protein foods that are higher in solid fats with choices that are lower in solid fat and calories and/or sources of oils.

- Use oils to replace solid fats where possible.

10

- Choose foods that provide more potassium, dietary fiber, calcium, and vitamin D, which are nutrients of concern in American diets. These foods include vegetables, fruits, whole grains, and milk and milk products.

For women capable of becoming pregnant:

11

- Choose foods that supply heme iron (e.g., lean red meat), which is more readily absorbed by the body, additional iron sources, and enhancers of iron absorption, such as vitamin C-rich foods.

12

- Consume 400 micrograms per day of synthetic folic acid (from fortified foods and/or supplements) in addition to food forms of folate from a varied diet.

For women who are pregnant or breastfeeding:

13

- Consume 8 to 12 ounces of seafood per week from a variety of seafood types.

- Due to their high methyl mercury content, limit white (albacore) tuna to 6 ounces per week and do not eat the following four types of fish: tilefish, shark, swordfish, and king mackerel.

14

- If pregnant, take an iron supplement, as recommended by an obstetrician or other health care provider.

For individuals ages 50 years and older:

- Consume foods fortified with vitamin B-12, such as fortified cereals, or dietary supplements.

	Calorie Range (kcal)	
Children	Sedentary ⟶	Active
2–3 years	1000 ⟶	1400
Females		
4–8 years	1200 ⟶	1800
9–13	1400 ⟶	2200
14–18	1800 ⟶	2400
19–30	1800 ⟶	2400
31–50	1800 ⟶	2200
51+	1600 ⟶	2200
Males		
4–8 years	1200 ⟶	2000
9–13	1600 ⟶	2600
14–18	2000 ⟶	3200
19–30	2400 ⟶	3000
31–50	2200 ⟶	3000
51+	2000 ⟶	2800

FIGURE 2-8 ▶ Estimates of calorie needs (kcals).

The full report contains background on the development of the Dietary Guidelines, many informative tables and charts to support the recommendations, and a comprehensive list of consumer behaviors and key strategies for achieving each recommendation. This information is available at www.health.gov/dietaryguidelines.

Balancing Calories to Manage Weight. As you will see in Chapter 7, the balance between calories consumed (from foods and beverages) and calories expended (through physical activity and metabolic processes) determines body weight. Consuming too many calories without increasing physical activity will inevitably lead to weight gain, which exacts an enormous toll on individuals and communities. Many chronic diseases, especially cardiovascular disease, type 2 diabetes, and osteoporosis, could be alleviated by meeting nutrient needs within calorie limits.

The Dietary Guidelines encourage all Americans to achieve and maintain a healthy body weight. Knowing how many calories you need each day is a good place to start (Fig. 2-8). You can calculate your EER on your own (see Chapter 7) or use an online calculator such as the one at www.ChooseMyPlate.gov. Once calorie needs are known, the next step is to become familiar with the calorie content of foods and beverages. Chapters 4, 5, and 6 will cover sources of calories in the diet. Finally, monitoring weight over time will allow you to see how your food and physical activity choices are balancing out.

Foods and Food Components to Reduce. Typical American diets contain too much sodium (salt), **solid fats** (e.g., butter), **added sugars,** and refined grains. Diets predominated by these food components especially increase risk for obesity, type 2 diabetes, hypertension, cardiovascular disease, and cancer.

Moderate alcohol consumption is associated with reduced risk of cardiovascular disease, deaths, and cognitive decline. However, those who do not drink should not begin drinking to attain these health benefits, because there are risks associated with even moderate alcohol consumption, including increased risk of breast cancer, violence, drowning, and injuries from falls and motor vehicle crashes. Heavy drinking is inherently risky and should be avoided altogether. More information about alcohol is presented in Chapter 16.

Foods and Nutrients to Increase. The Dietary Guidelines urge Americans to replace the problem foods we have discussed with nutrient-dense foods. Emphasize vegetables, fruits, whole grains, fat-free or low-fat milk and milk products, seafood, lean meats and poultry, eggs, beans and peas, and nuts and seeds. Instead of solid fats, choose foods made with vegetable oils.

These recommendations reflect the nutrient inadequacies of greatest public health concern: potassium, dietary fiber, calcium, and vitamin D. Individuals should strive to meet these goals without exceeding their calorie needs. Focusing on vegetables, fruits, whole grains, lean sources of protein, and low-fat or fat-free dairy products will not only contribute to nutrient adequacy but will also lower intake of problem nutrients, improve gastrointestinal function, aid in weight management, and decrease risk for a variety of chronic diseases.

A basic premise of the Dietary Guidelines is that nutrient needs should be met primarily through consuming foods. Foods provide an array of nutrients and other compounds that may benefit health. In certain cases, fortified foods and dietary supplements may be useful sources of one or more nutrients that otherwise might be consumed in less than recommended amounts. These are especially important for people whose typical food choices lead to a diet that cannot meet one or more nutrient recommendations, such as for vitamin D, vitamin E, or calcium. However, dietary supplements cannot and should not replace a healthy diet.

Building Healthy Eating Patterns. The Dietary Guidelines steer clear of a rigid prescription and, instead, promote an array of healthful options that can accommodate cultural, ethnic, traditional, and personal preferences, as well as food cost and availability factors. Well-studied examples of **eating patterns** consistent with the Dietary Guidelines include Dietary Approaches to Stop Hypertension (DASH), the USDA Food Patterns that accompanied MyPyramid (now MyPlate), vegetarian eating patterns, and Mediterranean-style eating patterns (see Further Reading 5). Common among these patterns are an abundance of vegetables and fruits, emphasis on whole grains, moderate amounts and varied sources of protein-rich foods, limited added sugars and solid fats, a high proportion of unsaturated fats compared to saturated fats, high potassium, and lower sodium.

The Dietary Guidelines and You. When applying the Dietary Guidelines, you need to consider your own state of health. Make specific changes and see whether they are effective for you. Note that results do not occur overnight and may not meet your expectations. Even when carefully following a diet low in saturated fat, some people continue to have high blood cholesterol. Other people can eat greater amounts of saturated fats and keep their blood cholesterol under control. Differences in genetic background are a key reason for these different responses, as you will learn in Chapter 3. Each of us must take into consideration our individual nutritional needs and

solid fats Fats that are solid at room temperature, such as butter and margarine. Foods containing solid fats tend to be high in saturated fatty acids or *trans* fatty acids.

added sugars Sugars or syrups that are added to foods during processing or preparation.

eating pattern A combination of foods and beverages that constitute an individual's complete dietary intake over time.

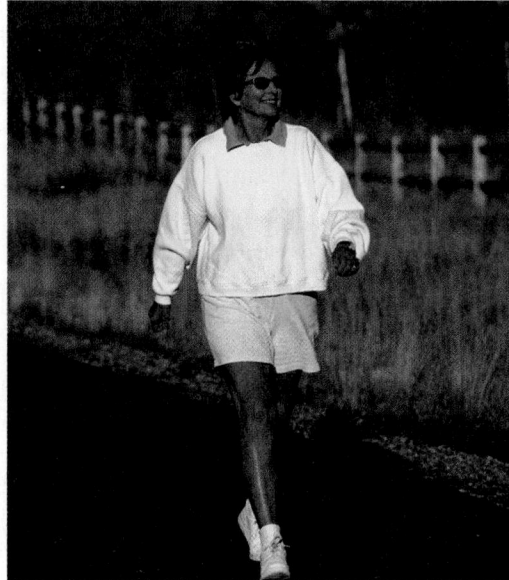

▲ Active means a lifestyle that includes physical activity equivalent to walking more than 3 miles per day at 3 to 4 miles per hour, in addition to the light physical activity associated with typical day-to-day life.

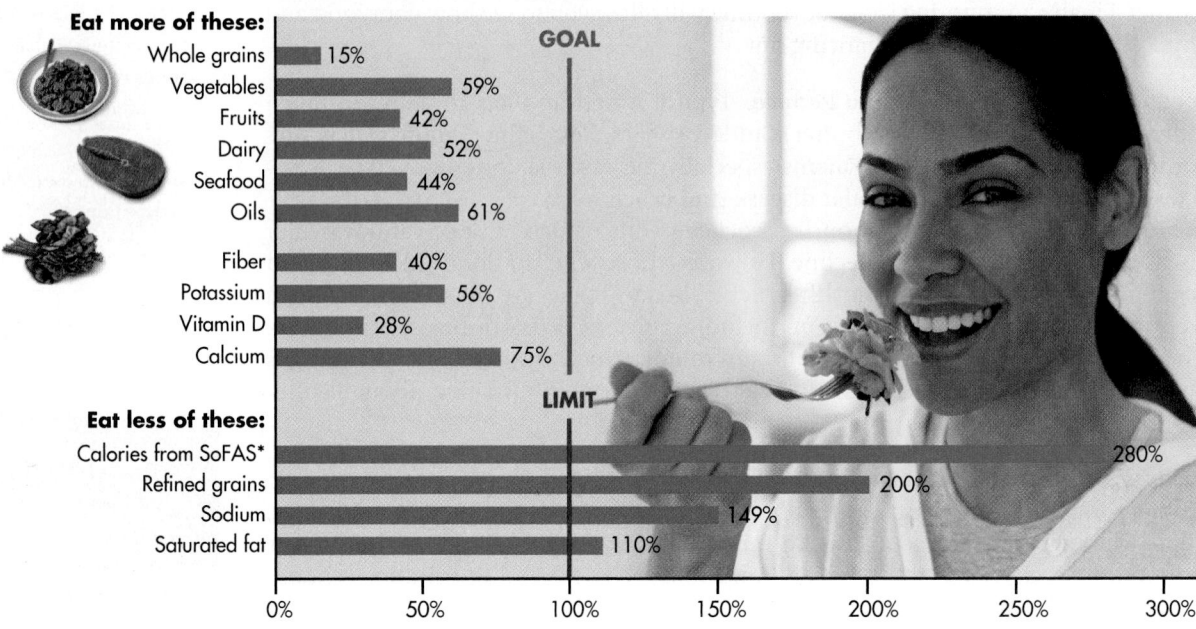

Usual Intake as a Percent of Goal or Limit

Eat more of these:

Whole grains	15%
Vegetables	59%
Fruits	42%
Dairy	52%
Seafood	44%
Oils	61%
Fiber	40%
Potassium	56%
Vitamin D	28%
Calcium	75%

Eat less of these:

Calories from SoFAS*	280%
Refined grains	200%
Sodium	149%
Saturated fat	110%

Percent of goal or limit

FIGURE 2-9 ▶

Comparing American Dietary habits to the Dietary Guidelines.

Source: Based on data from: U.S. Department of Agriculture, Agricultural Research Service and U.S. Department of Health and Human Services, Centers for Disease Control and Prevention. What We Eat in America, NHANES 2001–2004 or 2005–2006.

*SoFAS = solid fats and added sugars.
Note: Bars show average intakes for all individuals (ages 1 or 2 years or older, depending on the data source) as a percent of the recommended intake level or limit. Recommended intakes for food groups and limits for refined grains and solid fats and added sugars are based on amounts in the USDA 2000-calorie food pattern. Recommended intakes for fiber, potassium, vitamin D, and calcium are based on the highest AI or RDA for age 14 to 70 years. Limits for sodium are based on the UL and for saturated fat on 10% of calories. The protein foods group is not shown here because, on average, intake is close to recommended levels.

our risks of developing certain diseases (see Further Reading 3). Plan your diet with your specific needs in mind, taking into account your current health status and family history.

Whereas the Dietary Guidelines are not able to tailor a unique nutrition program for every North American citizen, they do provide adults with simple nutritional advice, which can be implemented by anyone willing to take a step toward good health. Table 2-5 provides examples of recommended diet changes based on the Dietary Guidelines. Although the cost of healthy eating is on the rise, you can make good choices and stay within your budget—canned or frozen fruits and vegetables and non-fat dry milk are a few of the available lower-cost foods.

Diet recommendations for adults have been issued by other scientific groups, such as the American Heart Association, U.S. Surgeon General, National Academy of Sciences, American Cancer Society, Canadian Ministries of Health (see Appendix C), and World Health Organization. All are consistent with the spirit of the Dietary Guidelines. These groups encourage people to modify their eating behaviors in ways that are both healthful and pleasurable.

MyPlate—A Menu-Planning Tool

The titles, food groupings, and shapes of food guides have evolved since the first edition published by the U.S. Department of Agriculture (USDA) nearly a century ago. The most recent food-guidance systems have incorporated physical activity and provided a means for individualization of dietary advice via interactive technology available on the Internet.

To keep pace with updated nutrition advice presented by the 2010 Dietary Guidelines for Americans and *Healthy People 2020* (see Chapter 1), MyPlate was released in 2011 as the leading depiction of healthy eating for Americans (Fig. 2-10). MyPlate,

FIGURE 2-10 ▶ MyPlate is a visual representation of the advice contained in the 2010 Dietary Guidelines for Americans.

TABLE 2-5 Recommended Diet Changes Based on the Dietary Guidelines

If You Usually Eat This,	Try This Instead	Benefit
White bread	Whole-wheat bread	• Higher nutrient density, due to less processing • More fiber
Sugary breakfast cereal	Low-sugar, high-fiber cereal with fresh fruit	• Higher nutrient density • More fiber • More phytochemicals
Cheeseburger with French fries	Hamburger and baked beans	• Less saturated fat and *trans* fat • Less cholesterol • More fiber • More phytochemicals
Potato salad	Three-bean salad	• More fiber • More phytochemicals
Doughnuts	Bran muffin/bagel with light cream cheese	• More fiber • Less fat
Regular soft drinks	Diet soft drinks	• Fewer calories
Boiled vegetables	Steamed vegetables	• Higher nutrient density, due to reduced loss of water-soluble vitamins
Canned vegetables	Fresh or frozen vegetables	• Higher nutrient density, due to reduced loss of heat-sensitive vitamins • Lower in sodium
Fried meats	Broiled meats	• Less saturated fat
Fatty meats, such as ribs or bacon	Lean meats, such as ground round, chicken, or fish	• Less saturated fat
Whole milk	Low-fat or fat-free milk	• Less saturated fat • Fewer calories • More calcium
Ice cream	Sherbet or frozen yogurt	• Less saturated fat • Fewer calories
Mayonnaise or sour cream salad dressing	Oil-and-vinegar dressings or light creamy dressings	• Less saturated fat • Less cholesterol • Fewer calories
Cookies	Popcorn (air popped with minimal margarine or butter)	• Fewer calories and *trans* fat
Heavily salted foods	Foods flavored primarily with herbs, spices, lemon juice	• Lower in sodium
Chips	Pretzels	• Less fat

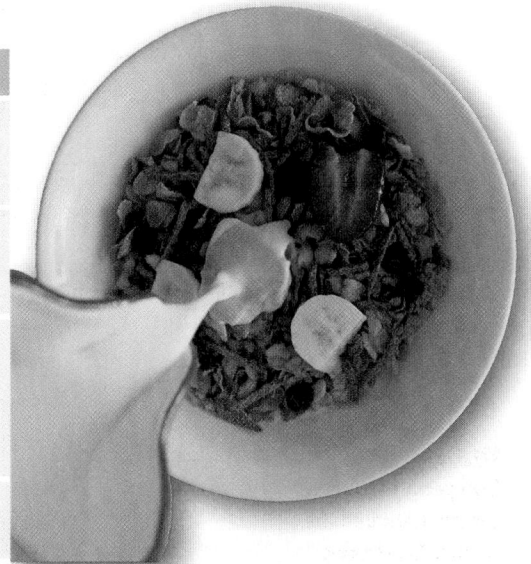

▲ Choose low-sugar, high-fiber cereal with fresh fruit instead of sugary breakfast cereal.

which replaces the familiar MyPyramid, shapes the key recommendations from the Dietary Guidelines into an easily recognizable and universally applicable visual: a place setting.

empty calories Calories from solid fats and/or added sugars. Foods with empty calories supply energy but few or no other nutrients.

17

NEWSWORTHY
NUTRITION

Diet quality impacts waistlines and wallets

Diets with low energy density are associated with higher intakes of nutrients but also with higher food costs. Researchers used food-frequency questionnaires to assess dietary intake and food costs among 164 men and women in Seattle, Washington. Dietary data were compared with components of socioeconomic status. Household income and especially education were strong predictors of dietary energy density. The association between food spending and energy density was particularly strong for women. Nutrition advice to consume foods with lower energy density may be difficult to follow for people with limited financial resources. The increasing cost of consuming foods with low energy density and high nutrient density may play a role in the correlations between socioeconomic status (e.g., income and education) and rates of obesity and diet-related chronic diseases.

Source: Monsivais P, Drewnowski A. Lower-energy-density diets are associated with higher monetary costs per kilocalorie and are consumed by women of higher socioeconomic status. *Journal of the American Dietetic Association* 109:804, 2009.

connect NUTRITION
Check out the Connect site
www.mcgrawhillconnect.com
to further explore energy density and food costs.

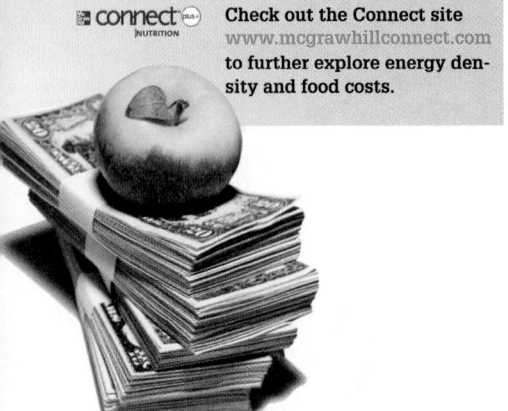

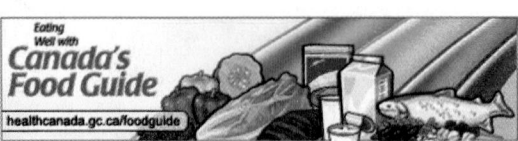

▲ In 1942, Canada released its first set of Official Food Rules. Since then, food guidance has evolved based on nutrition research and the changing needs of the population. Now, Health Canada publishes *Canada's Food Guide to Healthy Eating*, available in Appendix C.

Dishing Up MyPlate. Although it is not intended to stand alone as a source of dietary advice, MyPlate serves as a reminder of how to build a healthy plate at mealtimes (see Further Reading 13). It emphasizes important areas of the American diet that are in need of improvement. Recall from the discussion of the Dietary Guidelines that Americans need to increase the relative proportions of fruits, vegetables, whole grains, and fat-free or low-fat dairy products while simultaneously decreasing consumption of refined grains and high-fat meats.

The new MyPlate icon emphasizes five food groups:

- **Fruits** and **vegetables** cover half of the plate. These foods are dense sources of nutrients and health-promoting phytochemicals despite their low calorie contents.
- **Grains** occupy slightly more than one-fourth of the plate. The message to make half your grains whole is stressed throughout accompanying consumer-education materials.
- The remaining space on the plate is reserved for sources of **protein**. Specifically, the Dietary Guidelines recommend lean meats and poultry, plant sources of protein, and inclusion of fish twice a week.
- A cup of **dairy** appears next to the plate. Depending on personalized calorie recommendations, users should have 2 to 3 cups per day of low-fat or fat-free dairy products or other rich sources of calcium.

Unlike MyPyramid, MyPlate does not display a separate group for fats and oils, as they are mostly incorporated into other foods. Consumer messages tied to the MyPlate campaign reinforce recommendations to limit solid fats and focus instead *17* on plant oils, which are sources of essential fatty acids and vitamin E.

Actionable Health Messages. Consumer research points to the need for simple, actionable health messages to capture the attention of the public and achieve successful behavior change. Accordingly, ChooseMyPlate.gov provides a series of succinct imperatives to help Americans make healthier food choices. Consumer messages include:

Balancing Calories

- Enjoy your food, but eat less.
- Avoid oversized portions.

Foods to Increase

- Make half your plate fruits and vegetables.
- Make at least half your grains whole.
- Switch to skim or 1% milk.

Foods to Reduce

- Compare sodium in foods like soup, bread, and frozen meals—and choose the foods with lower numbers.
- Drink water instead of sugary drinks.

Daily Food Plan. The Daily Food Plan is an interactive tool that estimates your calorie needs and suggests a food pattern based on your age, gender, height, and weight (Table 2-6). The Daily Food Plan provides useful information for each food group, including recommended daily amounts in common household measures, suggested oil intake, limits for **empty calories** and sodium, as well as advice for physical activity.

The recommended numbers of servings are given in cups for vegetables, fruits, and dairy foods. Grains and protein foods are listed in ounces. See Figure 2-11 for a description of what counts as a MyPlate serving. Pay close attention to the stated serving size for each choice when following your Daily Food Plan to help control calorie intake. Figure 2-12 provides a convenient guide to estimating common serving size measurements.

Modified daily food plans are also available for preschoolers, pregnant or breast-feeding mothers, and those interested in losing weight. Be sure to visit www.Choose MyPlate.gov to generate your own Daily Food Plan.

TABLE 2-6 MyPlate Food-Intake Patterns Based on Calorie Needs

Daily Amount of Food from Each Group

Calorie Level	1000	1200	1400	1600	1800	2000	2200	2400	2600	2800	3000	3200
Fruits	1 cup	1 cup	1.5 cups	1.5 cups	1.5 cups	2 cups	2 cups	2 cups	2 cups	2.5 cups	2.5 cups	2.5 cups
Vegetables[1,2]	1 cup	1.5 cups	1.5 cups	2 cups	2.5 cups	2.5 cups	3 cups	3 cups	3.5 cups	3.5 cups	4 cups	4 cups
Grains[3]	3 oz-eq	4 oz-eq	5 oz-eq	5 oz-eq	6 oz-eq	6 oz-eq	7 oz-eq	8 oz-eq	9 oz-eq	10 oz-eq	10 oz-eq	10 oz-eq
Protein Foods	2 oz-eq	3 oz-eq	4 oz-eq	5 oz-eq	5 oz-eq	5.5 oz-eq	6 oz-eq	6.5 oz-eq	6.5 oz-eq	7 oz-eq	7 oz-eq	7 oz-eq
Dairy[4]	2 cups	2 cups	2 cups	3 cups	3 cups	3 cups	3 cups	3 cups	3 cups	3 cups	3 cups	3 cups
Oils[5]	3 tsp	4 tsp	4 tsp	5 tsp	5 tsp	6 tsp	6 tsp	7 tsp	8 tsp	8 tsp	10 tsp	11 tsp
Empty Calorie Limit[6]	140	120	120	120	160	260	270	330	360	400	460	600

oz-eq stands for ounce equivalent; tsp stands for teaspoon.

[1]Vegetables are divided into five subgroups (dark green, orange, legumes, starchy, and other). Over a week's time, a variety of vegetables should be eaten, especially green and orange vegetables.

[2]Dry beans and peas can be counted *either* as vegetables (dry beans and peas subgroup), *or* in the protein foods group. Generally, individuals who regularly eat meat, poultry, and fish would count dry beans and peas in the vegetable group. Individuals who seldom eat meat, poultry, or fish (vegetarians) would consume more dry beans and peas and count some of them in the protein foods group until enough servings from that group are chosen for the day.

[3]At least half of the grain servings should be whole-grain varieties.

[4]Most of the dairy servings should be fat-free or low-fat.

[5]Limit solid fats such as butter, stick margarine, shortening, and meat fat, as well as foods that contain these.

[6]Empty calories refers to added sugars and/or solid fats.

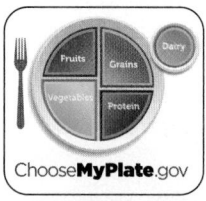

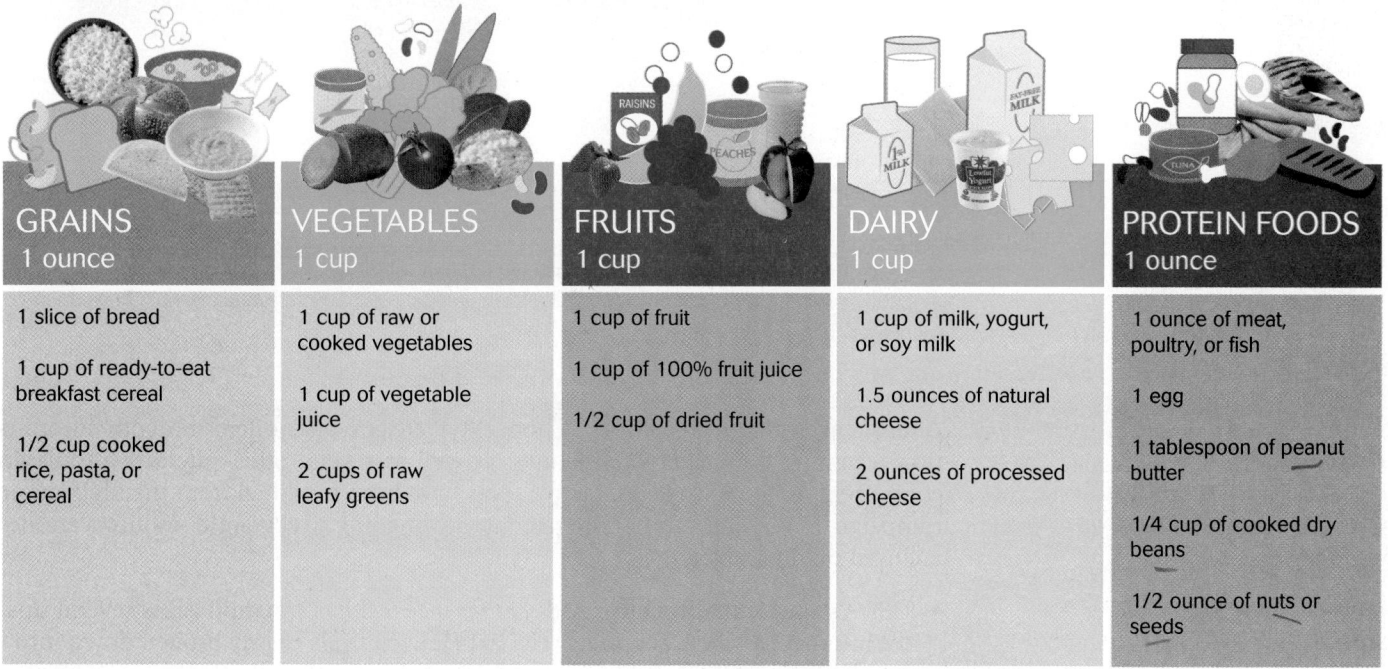

What Counts as a Serving?

GRAINS 1 ounce	VEGETABLES 1 cup	FRUITS 1 cup	DAIRY 1 cup	PROTEIN FOODS 1 ounce
1 slice of bread	1 cup of raw or cooked vegetables	1 cup of fruit	1 cup of milk, yogurt, or soy milk	1 ounce of meat, poultry, or fish
1 cup of ready-to-eat breakfast cereal	1 cup of vegetable juice	1 cup of 100% fruit juice	1.5 ounces of natural cheese	1 egg
1/2 cup cooked rice, pasta, or cereal	2 cups of raw leafy greens	1/2 cup of dried fruit	2 ounces of processed cheese	1 tablespoon of peanut butter
				1/4 cup of cooked dry beans
				1/2 ounce of nuts or seeds

FIGURE 2-11 ▶ MyPlate: What counts as a serving?

Portion sizes

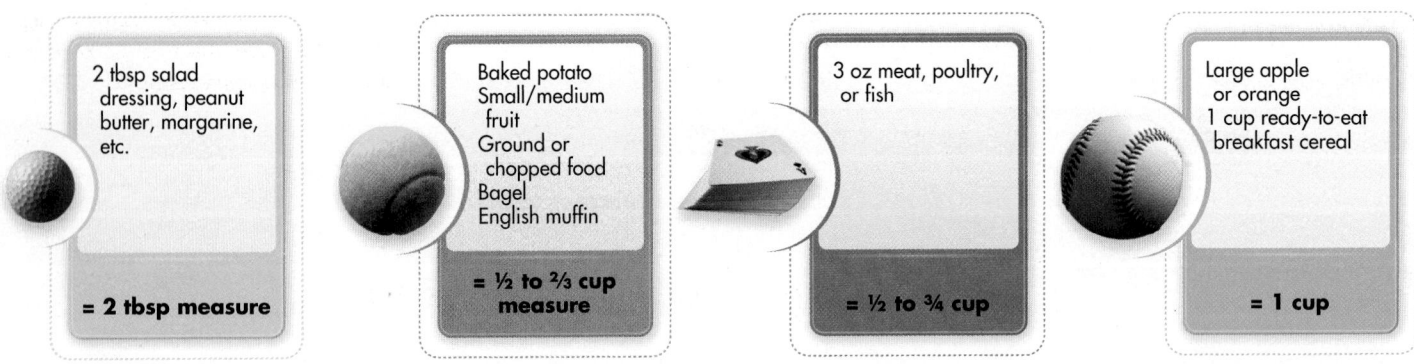

2 tbsp salad dressing, peanut butter, margarine, etc.	Baked potato Small/medium fruit Ground or chopped food Bagel English muffin	3 oz meat, poultry, or fish	Large apple or orange 1 cup ready-to-eat breakfast cereal
= 2 tbsp measure	**= ½ to ⅔ cup measure**	**= ½ to ¾ cup**	**= 1 cup**

FIGURE 2-12 ▶ A golf ball, tennis ball, deck of cards, and baseball are standard-size objects that make convenient guides for judging serving sizes. Your hand provides an additional handy guide (for the greatest accuracy, compare your fist with a baseball, and adjust the following guides accordingly).

Fist = 1 cup
Thumb = 1 oz of cheese
Thumb tip to first joint = 1 tsp

Palm of hand = 3 oz
Handful = 1 or 2 oz of a snack food

MAKING DECISIONS

Measuring Your Portion Size

How familiar are you with serving size measurements? Common household units are listed in Appendix I with their metric equivalents. Ounces and fluid ounces differ. Ounces are a measure of weight, while fluid ounces are a measure of volume. Fluid ounces are based on the corresponding volume of water as the standard; 1 ounce of water by weight equals 1 fluid ounce. Any fluid more or less dense than water will yield a different number of fluid ounces per ounce of material.

The International Food Information Council, available online at www.ific.org, is another great resource for current nutrition information.

MAKING DECISIONS

Empty Calories

MyPlate sets limits for empty calories, which come from solid fats and/or added sugars (Fig. 2-13). Solid fats and added sugars add calories to the diet but contribute few nutrients. Solid fats are solid at room temperature and include butter, beef fat, and shortening. Some solid fats, such as the marbling in a cut of ribeye steak, are naturally present in foods. Others, such as the shortening used to make a flaky croissant, are added during food processing or preparation. Added sugars include sugars and syrups that are added to foods during processing or preparation. Examples of foods that are major contributors of empty calories in the American diet are cakes, cookies, pastries, soft drinks, energy drinks, cheese, pizza, ice cream, and processed meats. The Daily Food Plans available on www.ChooseMyPlate.gov allow for 120 to 600 empty calories per day, depending on total energy needs:

Calorie Intake (kcal)	Empty Calories (kcal)	Calorie Intake (kcal)	Empty Calories (kcal)
1000*	140	2200	270
1200*	120	2400	330
1400*	120	2600	360
1600	120	2800	400
1800	160	3000	460
2000	260	3200	600

*Calorie intakes below 1600 kcal per day are generally intended for children 2 to 8 years of age. Unless under the guidance of a physician or registered dietitian, adults should consume at least 1600 kcal per day.

Additional MyPlate Resources. ChooseMyPlate.gov also offers in-depth information regarding the Dietary Guidelines, as well as several other interactive tools for consumers. Many of these interactive tools have been modified from the MyPyramid campaign, but updates and improvements are ongoing. MyPyramid resources are also archived on the website.

• USDA's consumer brochure, *Let's Eat for the Health of It*, emphasizes several tips for improving Americans' diets (Fig. 2-14). Each tip is clearly broken down into specific actions the consumer can take. For example, one key recommendation

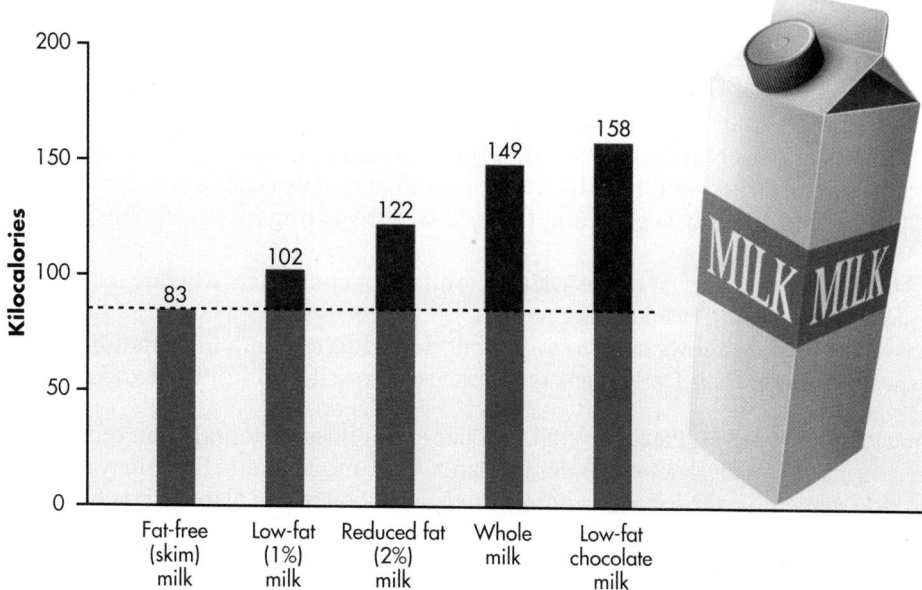

FIGURE 2-13 ▶ Empty calories come from solid fats and/or added sugars. This bar graph compares the amounts of empty calories in various types of milk.

Grains	Vegetables	Fruits	Dairy	Protein
Make half your grains whole grains	**Vary your veggies**	**Focus on fruits**	**Get your calcium-rich foods**	**Go lean with protein**

Grains

Use whole grains in mixed dishes, such as barley in vegetable soup or stews and bulgur wheat in casseroles or stir-fries.

Add whole-grain flour or oatmeal when making cookies or other baked treats.

Use the Nutrition Facts label and choose whole-grain products with a higher % Daily Value (%DV) for fiber. Many, but not all, whole-grain products are good or excellent sources of fiber.

Vegetables

Buy fresh vegetables in season. They cost less and are likely to be at their peak flavor.

Include chopped vegetables in pasta sauce or lasagna.

Allow children to pick a new vegetable to try while shopping.

Fruits

Make most of your choices whole or cut-up fruit rather than fruit juice, for the benefits dietary fiber provides.

Select fruits with more potassium often, such as bananas, prunes and prune juice, dried peaches and apricots, and orange juice.

Add fruits like pineapple or peaches to kabobs as part of a barbeque meal.

Dairy

Include milk or calcium-fortified soymilk as a beverage at meals. Choose fat-free or low-fat milk.

If you avoid milk because of lactose intolerance, the most reliable way to get the health benefits of dairy products is to choose lactose-free alternatives within the Dairy Group, such as cheese, yogurt, lactose-free milk, or calcium-fortified soy milk or to consume the enzyme lactase before consuming milk.

Protein

The leanest beef cuts include round steaks and roasts (eye of round, top round, bottom round, round tip), top loin, sirloin, and chuck shoulder and arm roasts.

Trim away all of the visible fat from meats and poultry before cooking.

Choose beans, peas, or soy products as a main dish or part of a meal often.

Physical Activity

Find your balance between food and physical activity
- Do stretches, exercises, or pedal a stationary bike while watching television.
- Replace a coffee break with a brisk 10-minute walk. Ask a friend to go with you.
- Get the whole family involved—enjoy an afternoon bike ride with your kids.

Food Safety

Keep food safe to eat
- Wash your hands with warm water and soap for at least 20 seconds before and after handling food and after using the bathroom or changing diapers.
- Separate raw meat, poultry, seafood, and eggs from other foods in your grocery shopping cart, grocery bags, and in your refrigerator.
- Use a food thermometer, which measures the internal temperature of cooked meat, poultry, and egg dishes, to make sure that the food is cooked to a safe internal temperature.

FIGURE 2-14 ▶ These consumer tips have been developed by the USDA to help you build healthy meals with MyPlate. Many more tips are available at www.ChooseMyPlate.gov.

is "Cut back on foods high in solid fats, added sugars, and salt." One way a consumer can put this message into practice is to choose foods and drinks with little or no added sugars. Specific techniques associated with this recommendation include "Drink water instead of sugary drinks," "Select fruit for dessert," and "Choose 100% fruit juice instead of fruit-flavored drinks."

- USDA's Ten Tips Nutrition Education series provides access to one-page handouts for consumers and health educators. The materials cover a variety of topics, such as "Kid-friendly veggies and fruits," "Healthy eating for vegetarians," and "Got your dairy today?"
- Sample menus and recipes are available online for consumers who are ready to make a change and need a place to start.
- MyFood-a-Pedia allows users to locate calorie and food group information for specific food entries. Daily trackers enable users to self-monitor food and activity.

Menu Planning with MyPlate. Overall, MyPlate exemplifies the foundations of a healthy diet you have already learned: variety, balance, and moderation. To achieve optimal nutrition, remember the following points when using MyPlate to plan your daily menus:

- The guide does not apply to infants or children under 2 years of age. Daily Food Plans for children from ages 2 to 8 are based on average height and weight for age and gender.
- Variety is key to successful implementation of MyPlate. There is no single, perfect food that is absolutely essential to good nutrition. Each food is rich in some nutrients but deficient in at least one essential nutrient. Likewise, no food group is more important than another; each food group makes an important, distinctive contribution to nutritional intake (Table 2-7). Choose foods from each food group and also choose different foods within each food group. For a sample meal plan, see Table 2-8.
- The foods within a group may vary widely with respect to nutrients and calories. For example, the calorie content of 3 ounces of baked potato is 98 kcal, whereas that of 3 ounces of potato chips is 470 kcal. With respect to vitamin C, an orange has 70 mg and an apple has 10 mg.

Solid fats contribute almost 20% of total calories in typical American diets, but they have little to offer in terms of essential nutrients and dietary fiber. Instead of solid fats, choose foods containing plant oils.

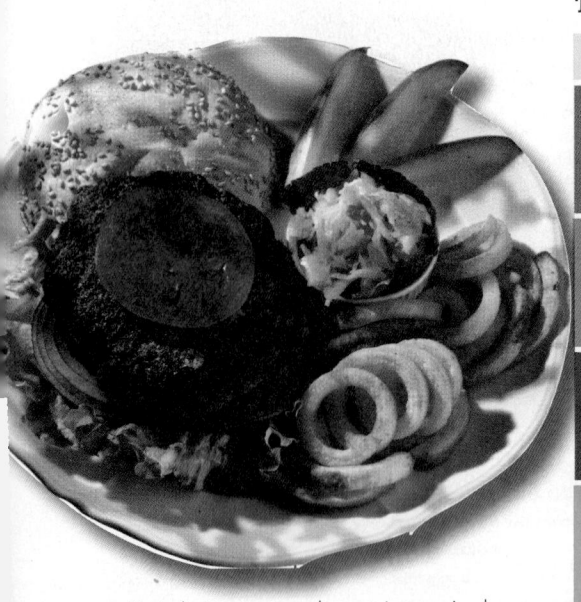

▲ Typical restaurant meals contain oversized portions that do not align with MyPlate.

TABLE 2-7 Nutrient Contributions of MyPlate Food Groups

Food Category	Major Nutrient Contributions
Grains	Carbohydrate Vitamins such as thiamin Minerals such as iron Fiber*
Vegetables	Carbohydrate Vitamins such as plant pigments that form vitamin A Minerals such as magnesium Fiber
Fruits	Carbohydrate Vitamins such as folate and vitamin C Minerals such as potassium Fiber
Dairy	Carbohydrate Protein Vitamins such as vitamin D Minerals such as calcium and phosphorus
Protein Foods	Protein Vitamins such as vitamin B-6 Minerals such as iron and zinc

*Whole-grain varieties

TABLE 2-8 Putting MyPlate into Practice.

Meal	Food Group
Breakfast	
1 small orange	Fruits
¾ cup Healthy Choice Low-fat Granola	Grains
with ½ cup fat-free milk	Dairy
½ toasted, small raisin bagel	Grains
with 1 tsp soft margarine	Oils
Optional: coffee or tea	
Lunch	
Turkey sandwich	
2 slices whole-wheat bread	Grains
2 oz turkey	Protein Foods
2 tsp mustard	
1 small apple	Fruits
2 oatmeal-raisin cookies (small)	Empty Calories
Optional: diet soft drink	
3 P.M. Study Break	
6 whole-wheat crackers	Grains
1 tbsp peanut butter	Protein Foods
½ cup fat-free milk	Dairy
Dinner	
Tossed salad	
1 cup romaine lettuce	Vegetables
½ cup sliced tomatoes	Vegetables
1½ tbsp Italian dressing	Oils
½ carrot, grated	Vegetables
3 oz broiled salmon	Protein Foods
½ cup rice	Grains
½ cup green beans	Vegetables
with 1 tsp soft margarine	Oils
Optional: coffee or tea	
Late-Night Snack	
1 cup "light" fruit yogurt	Dairy
Nutrient Breakdown	
1800 kcal	
Carbohydrate	56% of kcal
Protein	18% of kcal
Fat	26% of kcal

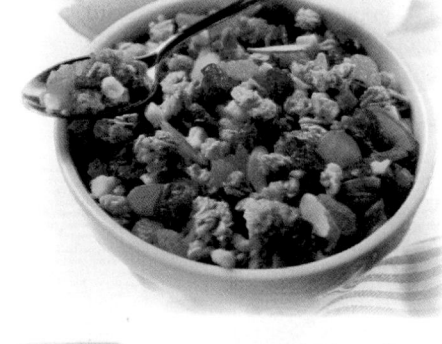
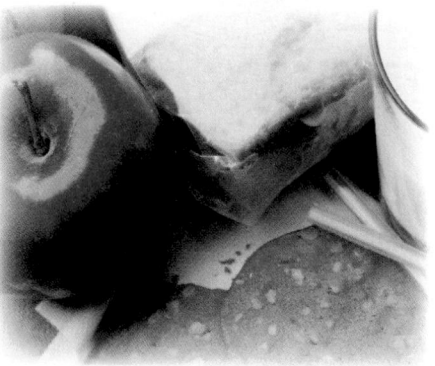
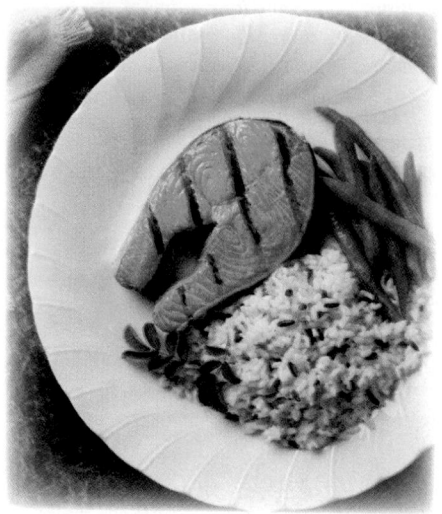

This menu meets nutrient needs for all vitamins and minerals for an average adult who needs 1800 kcal. For adolescents, teenagers, and older adults, add one additional serving of milk or other calcium-rich sources.

- •Choose primarily low-fat and fat-free items from the dairy group. By reducing calorie intake in this way, you can select more items from other food groups. If milk causes intestinal gas and bloating, emphasize yogurt and cheese (see Chapter 4 for details on the problem of lactose maldigestion and lactose intolerance).

Check out CONNECT for links to alternative menu planning tools, such as the Healthy Eating Plate from Harvard School of Public Health. ■■connect NUTRITION

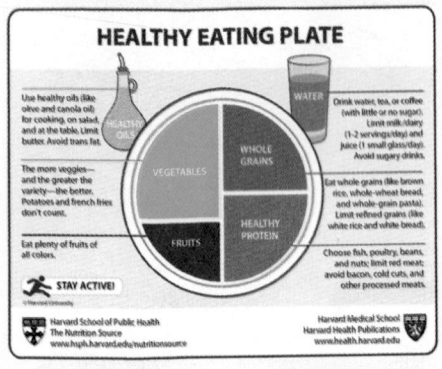

HEALTHY EATING PLATE

Use healthy oils (like olive and canola oil) for cooking, on salad, and at the table. Limit butter. Avoid trans fat.

HEALTHY OILS

WATER

Drink water, tea, or coffee (with little or no sugar). Limit milk/dairy (1-2 servings/day) and juice (1 small glass/day). Avoid sugary drinks.

The more veggies— and the greater the variety—the better. Potatoes and french fries don't count.

VEGETABLES

WHOLE GRAINS

Eat whole grains (like brown rice, whole-wheat bread, and whole-grain pasta). Limit refined grains (like white rice and white bread).

Eat plenty of fruits of all colors.

FRUITS

HEALTHY PROTEIN

Choose fish, poultry, beans, and nuts; limit red meat; avoid bacon, cold cuts, and other processed meats.

🏃 STAY ACTIVE!

Harvard School of Public Health
The Nutrition Source
www.hsph.harvard.edu/nutritionsource

Harvard Medical School
Harvard Health Publications
www.health.harvard.edu

The **Exchange System** is an alternative menu-planning tool. This tool organizes foods based on calorie, protein, carbohydrate, and fat content. The result is a manageable framework for designing diets, especially for treatment of diabetes. For more information on the Exchange System, see Appendix D.

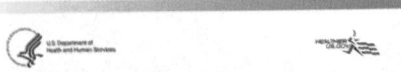

U.S. Department of
Health and Human Services

HEALTHIER·US·GOV

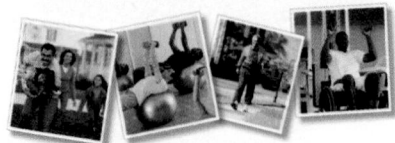

2008 Physical Activity Guidelines for Americans

Be Active, Healthy, and Happy!

www.health.gov/paguidelines

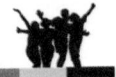

▲ http://www.health.gov/PAGuidelines/.

- Include plant foods that are good sources of proteins, such as beans and nuts, at least several times a week because many are rich in vitamins (such as vitamin E), minerals (such as magnesium), and fiber.
- For vegetables and fruits, try to include a dark-green or orange vegetable for vitamin A and a vitamin-C rich fruit, such as an orange, every day. Do not focus primarily on potatoes (e.g., French fries) for your vegetable choices. Surveys show that fewer than 5% of adults eat a full serving of a dark-green vegetable on any given day. Increased consumption of these foods is important because they contribute vitamins, minerals, fiber, and phytochemicals.
- Choose whole-grain varieties of breads, cereals, rice, and pasta because they contribute vitamin E and fiber. A daily serving of a whole-grain, ready-to-eat breakfast cereal is an excellent choice because the vitamins (such as vitamin B-6) and minerals (such as zinc) typically added to it, along with fiber, help fill in common nutritional gaps.
- Include some plant oils on a daily basis, such as those in salad dressing, and eat fish at least twice a week. This supplies you with health-promoting essential fatty acids.

Reviews of MyPlate. Although MyPlate will promote important changes in American diets, it does have some limitations. Some critics say that the new icon is too simple. For example, it does not immediately provide information about overall calories, serving sizes, or number of servings to choose from each food group (recall the comic at the beginning of this chapter). However, many of these details will vary by person. Users will need to access the accompanying materials available on www.ChooseMyPlate.gov to obtain a personally tailored Daily Food Plan.

Food *quality* is just as important as food *quantity* when it comes to good nutrition. Consider the difference in calorie contents of the following two meals, both of which fit the proportions suggested by MyPlate:

Fried chicken fillet sandwich with mayonnaise on a white sandwich roll, 1 each
French fries, 1 medium order
Apple-filled pastry, 1 each
Whole milk, 1 cup
1293 kcal

Skinless grilled chicken breast, 3 ounces
Brown rice, prepared with reduced-fat tub margarine, 1 cup
Steamed green beans, 1 cup
Cubed watermelon, 1 cup
Skim milk, 1 cup
513 kcal

The MyPlate icon does not address the types of foods to choose within each food group. Making appropriate food choices for weight management and prevention of diet-related chronic diseases requires consumers to have some nutrition knowledge. Fortunately, public health messages and online content related to MyPlate are available to educate Americans.

MyPlate shows how to build a healthy plate at mealtimes, but it does not adequately address the total diet, which, in reality, includes many snacks between meals. Consumer messages about healthy snacking will be a part of the consumer communications initiative over the next few years.

As with any public health campaign, it is possible that the people who need it most will overlook the MyPlate message. Educated consumers with access to interactive MyPlate tools likely already comply with many of the Dietary Guidelines. Populations with poor diets may be unlikely or unable to click through to find a personalized Daily Food Plan. The USDA's best response is to rely on the coordinated partnership of the National Communicator's Network to spread those actionable MyPlate messages, such as "Switch to fat-free or low-fat (1%) milk."

Overall, the new MyPlate icon is an attractive and relevant tool that immediately shows us how to build a healthy plate at meals. The strength of MyPlate lies in its simplicity. It conveys the major messages that are needed when shopping, cooking, and eating and can be enhanced with the details provided on www.ChooseMyPlate.gov and in forthcoming materials.

MAKING DECISIONS

The Mediterranean Diet Pyramid

Recently updated in 2009, the Mediterranean Diet Pyramid (Fig. 2-15) is a useful alternative to MyPlate. It is based on the dietary patterns of the southern Mediterranean region, which has enjoyed the lowest recorded rates of chronic diseases and the highest adult life expectancy. An abundance of research supports the health benefits of following the Mediterranean Diet (see Further Reading 9). Characteristics include:

- Foods from plant sources form the foundation of every meal.
- A variety of minimally processed and, wherever possible, seasonally fresh and locally grown foods are emphasized.
- Olive oil is the principal fat.
- Total fat ranges from less than 25% to over 35% of energy, with saturated fat no more than 7% to 8% of calories.
- Fish and seafood are consumed at least twice weekly.
- Lean or low-fat sources of protein, such as cheese, yogurt, poultry, and eggs, should be consumed in moderation.
- Red meats and sweet desserts are consumed less often.
- Regular physical activity is performed at a level that promotes a healthy weight, fitness, and well-being.
- Moderate wine drinking has health benefits.
- Water is the beverage of choice.

Oldways—a respected, international, nonprofit culinary think tank—also publishes the Latin-American Diet Pyramid and was the force behind development of the Whole Grain stamp seen on food packages.

Source: Oldways Food Issues Think Tank, 266 Beacon St., Boston, MA 02116, www.oldwayspt.org.

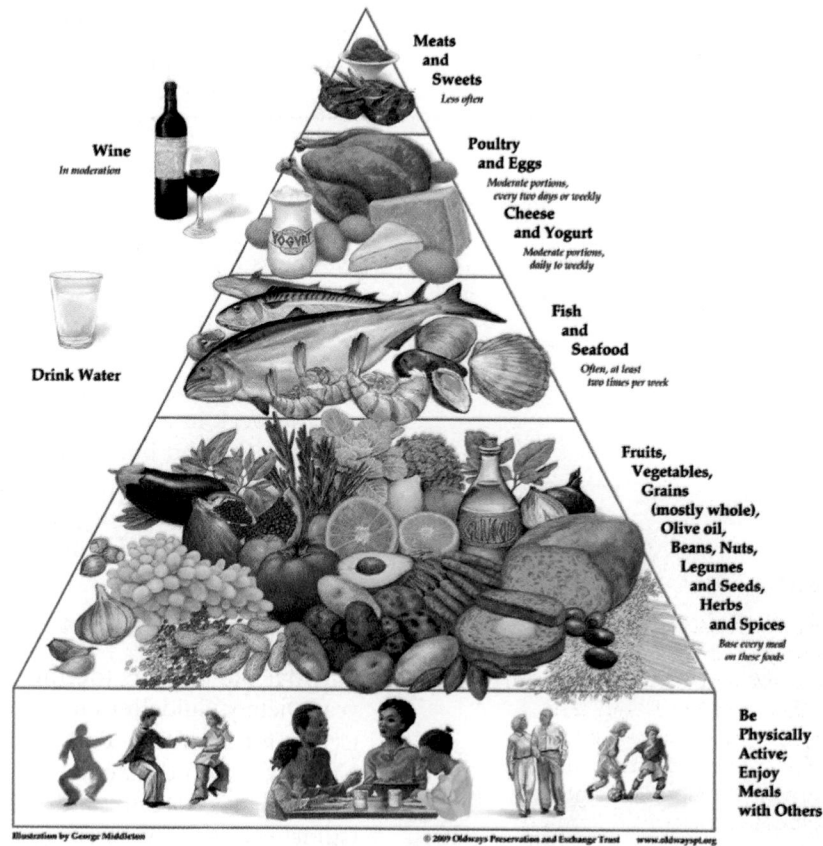

FIGURE 2-15 ▶ The Mediterranean Diet Pyramid is based on dietary patterns from the Mediterranean region, which has low rates of chronic diseases and high life expectancy.

How Does Your Plate Rate?   Regularly comparing your daily food intake with your personalized Daily Food Plan recommendations is a relatively simple way to evaluate the quality of your overall diet. Identify the nutrients that are low in your diet based on the nutrients found in each food group (review Table 2-7). For example, if you do not consume enough servings from the milk group, your calcium intake is most likely too low. Look for foods that you enjoy that supply calcium, such as calcium-fortified orange juice.

For a more detailed analysis of your current diet, use the Food Tracker tool on www.ChooseMyPlate.gov. Your NutritionCalc software also helps you compare your food choices to MyPlate. With a detailed dietary analysis, you can compare your intakes of individual nutrients to the DRI standards and clearly see the areas that need improvement. Even small diet and exercise changes can have positive results.

Physical Activity Guidelines for Americans

In line with its goal for all Americans to live healthier, more prosperous, and more productive lives, the U.S. Department of Health and Human Services issued its first Physical Activity Guidelines for Americans in 2008 as a complement to the Dietary Guidelines (see Further Reading 11). The overarching idea is that regular physical activity—for people of all ages, races, ethnicities, and physical abilities—produces long-term health benefits. The guidelines are truly meant to inform the work of health professionals and policy makers, but consumer materials are available. *Be Active Your Way: A Guide for Adults*, available at www.health.gov, translates the guidelines into consumer-friendly, practical advice.

The key guidelines, listed in Table 2-9, provide measurable physical activity standards for Americans age 6 and older. Specific recommendations (not listed in Table 2-9) also apply to special population groups, including pregnant women, adults with disabilities, and people with chronic medical conditions. For adults, the guidelines emphasize that health benefits occur with at least 150 minutes per week of moderate-intensity physical activity. Adults may accumulate activity throughout the week in a variety of ways—extended sessions (e.g., 50 minutes on 3 days a week) or in short bursts throughout the week that amount to at least 150 minutes. Children and adolescents should strive to include 60 minutes of physical activity per day. For optimum benefits, include both aerobic and muscle-strengthening activities. Overall, physical activity should be enjoyable and safe for each individual.

A Coordinated Effort

The MyPlate icon fits together with a variety of educational tools as part of a multi-year Dietary Guidelines for Americans consumer communications initiative. USDA's Center for Nutrition Policy and Promotion heads up a National Communicator's Network to coordinate the efforts of public and private organizations, including the Department of Health and Human Services (sponsors of the 2008 Physical Activity Guidelines) as well as city governments, educational institutions, health networks, fitness centers, grocery chains, and a growing list of other organizations throughout the nation.

The Partnership program promotes a series of nutrition messages, starting with "Make half your plate fruits and vegetables." The campaign also incorporates the physical activity theme, "Be Active Your Way." The Dietary Guidelines Communications Message Calendar is available at http://www.choosemyplate.gov/downloads/MyPlate/DGCommunicationsMessageCalendar.pdf. Through a multifaceted media approach, this coordinated effort will help to expand the reach of the Dietary Guidelines, MyPlate, and Physical Activity Guidelines to individuals who, despite needing health improvements, may not be likely to access these tools.

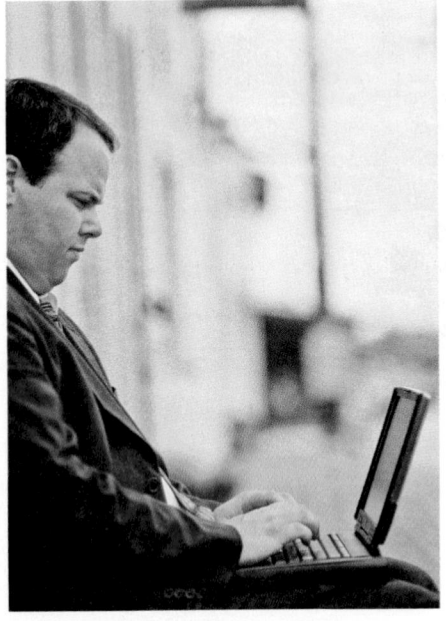

▲ Americans of all ages should limit screen time—hours spent watching TV, at the computer, or playing video games.

CONCEPT CHECK

The 2010 Dietary Guidelines for Americans aim to improve the health of all Americans, ages 2 and older. Three major goals include: (1) balancing calories with physical activity to manage weight; (2) increasing intake of fruits, vegetables, whole grains, fat-free and low-fat dairy products, and seafood; and (3) reducing intake of foods with sodium, saturated fats, *trans* fats, cholesterol, added sugars, and refined grains. MyPlate and associated tools found at www.ChooseMyPlate.gov embody the Dietary Guidelines with a plate icon that serves as a reminder for healthy eating. Grains, fruits, vegetables, protein, and dairy are the five major food groups represented on MyPlate. The 2008 Physical Activity Guidelines for Americans advise a minimum of 150 minutes per week of moderate-intensity physical activity for adults or at least 60 minutes daily for children and adolescents.

TABLE 2-9 Selected Recommendations of the 2008 Physical Activity Guidelines for Americans*

Key Guidelines for Children and Adolescents

- Children and adolescents should do 60 minutes or more of physical activity daily.

  - Aerobic: Most of the 60 or more minutes a day should be either moderate- or vigorous-intensity aerobic physical activity and should include vigorous-intensity activity at least 3 days a week.

  - Muscle-strengthening: As part of their 60 or more minutes of daily physical activity, children and adolescents should include muscle-strengthening physical activity on at least 3 days of the week.

  - Bone-strengthening: As part of their 60 or more minutes of daily physical activity, children and adolescents should include bone-strengthening physical activity on at least 3 days of the week.

- It is important to encourage young people to participate in physical activities that are appropriate for their age, that are enjoyable, and that offer variety.

Key Guidelines for Adults

- All adults should avoid inactivity. Some physical activity is better than none, and adults who participate in any amount of physical activity gain some health benefits.

- For substantial health benefits, adults should do at least 150 minutes a week of moderate-intensity, or 75 minutes a week of vigorous-intensity aerobic physical activity, or an equivalent combination of moderate- and vigorous-intensity aerobic activity. Aerobic activity should be performed in episodes of at least 10 minutes, and preferably, it should be spread throughout the week.

- For additional and more extensive health benefits, adults should increase their aerobic physical activity to 300 minutes a week of moderate-intensity, or 150 minutes a week of vigorous-intensity aerobic physical activity, or an equivalent combination of moderate- and vigorous-intensity activity. Additional health benefits are gained by engaging in physical activity beyond this amount.

- Adults should also do muscle-strengthening activities that are moderate or high intensity and involve all major muscle groups on 2 or more days a week, as these activities provide additional health benefits.

Key Guidelines for Older Adults

- When older adults cannot do 150 minutes of moderate-intensity aerobic activity a week because of chronic conditions, they should be as physically active as their abilities and conditions allow.

- Older adults should do exercises that maintain or improve balance if they are at risk of falling.

- Older adults should determine their level of effort for physical activity relative to their level of fitness.

- Older adults with chronic conditions should understand whether and how their conditions affect their ability to do regular physical activity safely.

Key Guidelines for Safe Physical Activity

To do physical activity safely and reduce the risk of injuries and other adverse events, people should:

- Understand the risks and yet be confident that physical activity is safe for almost everyone.

- Choose to do types of physical activity that are appropriate for their current fitness level and health goals, because some activities are safer than others.

- Increase physical activity gradually over time whenever more activity is necessary to meet guidelines or health goals. Inactive people should "start low and go slow" by gradually increasing how often and how long activities are done.

- Protect themselves by using appropriate gear and sports equipment; looking for safe environments; following rules and policies; and making sensible choices about when, where, and how to be active.

- Be under the care of a health care provider if they have chronic conditions or symptoms. People with chronic conditions and symptoms should consult their health care provider about the types and amounts of activity appropriate for them.

*The 2008 Physical Activity Guidelines for Americans also include recommendations for pregnant women, adults with disabilities, and people with chronic medical conditions. These are available at www.health.gov.

2.7 Food Labels and Diet Planning

Today, nearly all foods sold in stores must be in a package that has a label containing the following information: the product name, name and address of the manufacturer, amount of product in the package, and ingredients listed in descending order by weight. This food and beverage labeling is monitored in North America by government agencies such as the Food and Drug Administration (FDA) in the United States (see Further Reading 10). The listing of certain food constituents also is required—specifically, on a Nutrition Facts panel (Fig. 2-16). Use the information in the Nutrition Facts panel to learn more about what you eat. The following components must be listed: total calories (kcal), calories from fat, total fat, saturated fat, *trans* fat, cholesterol, sodium, total carbohydrate, fiber, sugars, protein, vitamin A, vitamin C, calcium, and iron. In addition to these required components, manufacturers can choose to list polyunsaturated and monounsaturated fat, potassium, and others. Listing these components becomes *required* if the food is fortified with that nutrient or if a claim is made about the health benefits of the specific nutrient (see the upcoming section in Chapter 2 entitled "Health Claims on Food Labels").

Remember that the Daily Value is a generic standard used on the food label. The percentage of the Daily Value (% Daily Value or % DV) is usually given for each nutrient per serving. These percentages are based on a 2000 kcal diet. In other words, they are not as applicable to people who require considerably more or less than 2000 kcal per day with respect to fat and carbohydrate intake. DVs are mostly set at or close to the highest RDA value or related nutrient standard seen in the various age and gender categories for a specific nutrient.

Serving sizes on the Nutrition Facts panel must be consistent among similar foods. This means that all brands of ice cream, for example, must use the same serving size on their label. (These serving sizes may differ from those of MyPlate because those on food labels are based on typical serving sizes.) In addition, food claims made on packages must follow legal definitions (Table 2-10). For example, if a product claims to be "low sodium," it must have 140 milligrams of sodium or less per serving.

Many manufacturers list the Daily Values set for dietary components such as fat, cholesterol, and carbohydrate on the Nutrition Facts panel. This can be useful as a reference point. As noted, they are based on 2000 kcal; if the label is large enough, amounts based on 2500 kcal are listed as well for total fat, saturated fat, carbohydrate, and other components. As mentioned, DVs allow consumers to compare their intake from a specific food to desirable (or maximum) intakes.

Exceptions to Food Labeling

Foods such as fresh fruits and vegetables and fish currently are not required to have Nutrition Facts labels. However, many grocers have voluntarily chosen to provide their customers with information about these products. The next time you are at the grocery store, ask where you might find information on the fresh products that do not have a Nutrition Facts panel. You will likely find a poster or pamphlet near the product; often, these pamphlets contain recipes that use your favorite fruit, vegetable, or fish fillet. They may even assist you in your endeavor to improve your diet.

Protein deficiency is not a public health concern in the United States, so declaration of the % Daily Value for protein is not mandatory on foods for people over 4 years of age. If the % Daily Value for protein is given on a label, FDA requires that the product be analyzed for protein quality. This procedure is expensive and time-consuming, so many companies opt not to list a % Daily Value for protein. However, labels on food for infants and children under 4 years of age must

The Nutrition Facts label uses the term "calorie" to express energy content in some cases, but kilocalorie (kcal) values are actually listed.

Nutrient and herbal supplement labels have a different layout with a "Supplement Facts" heading. The Nutrition and Your Health section at the end of this chapter and Chapter 8 show examples of these labels.

▼ Use the Nutrition Facts label to learn more about the nutrient content of the foods you eat. Nutrient content is expressed as a percent of Daily Value. Canadian food laws and related food labels have a slightly different format (review Appendix C).

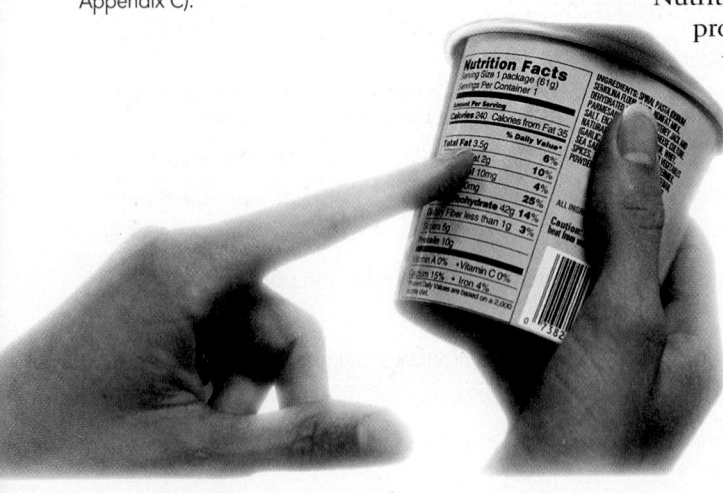

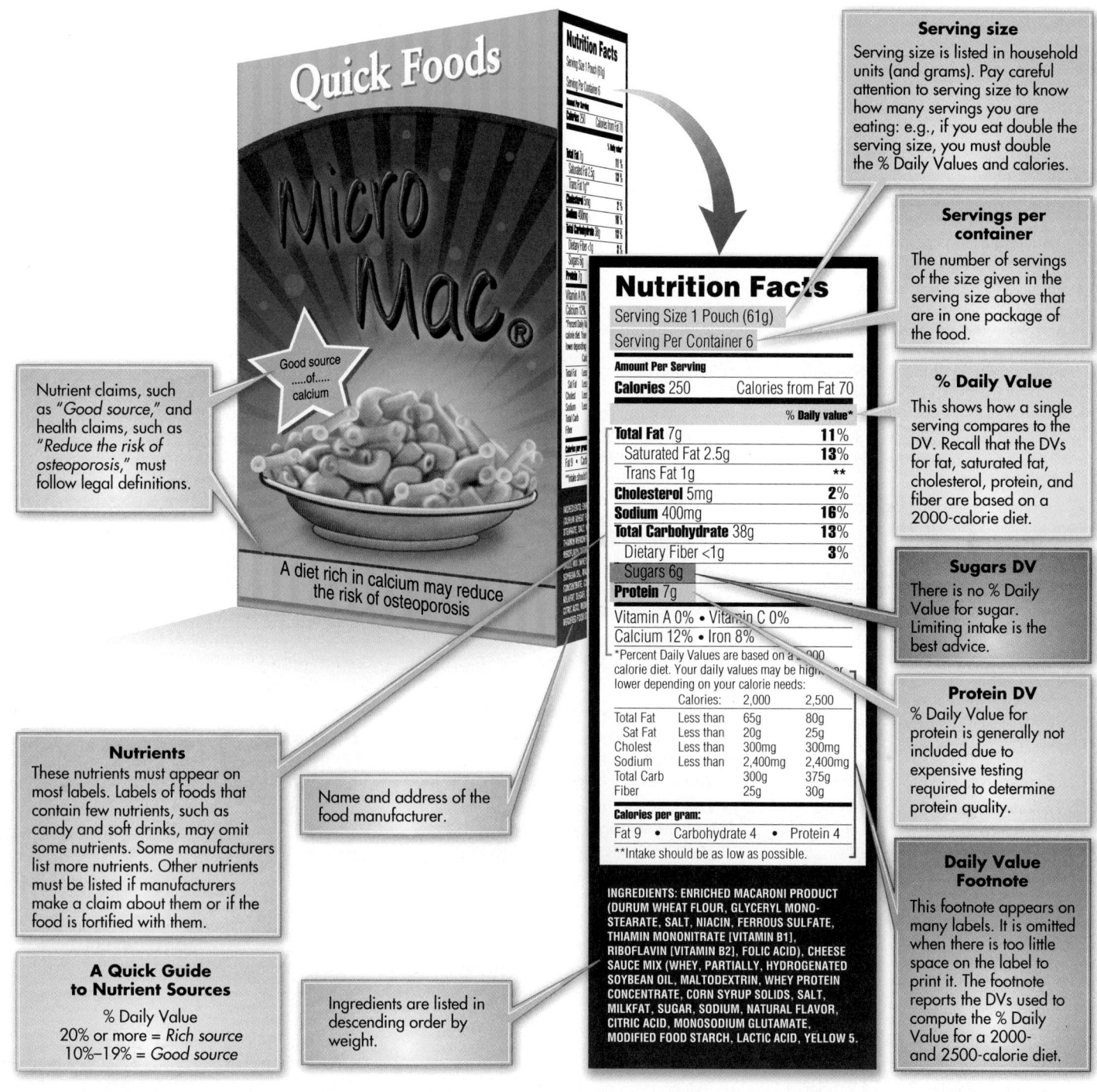

Serving size

Serving size is listed in household units (and grams). Pay careful attention to serving size to know how many servings you are eating: e.g., if you eat double the serving size, you must double the % Daily Values and calories.

Servings per container

The number of servings of the size given in the serving size above that are in one package of the food.

% Daily Value

This shows how a single serving compares to the DV. Recall that the DVs for fat, saturated fat, cholesterol, protein, and fiber are based on a 2000-calorie diet.

Sugars DV

There is no % Daily Value for sugar. Limiting intake is the best advice.

Protein DV

% Daily Value for protein is generally not included due to expensive testing required to determine protein quality.

Daily Value Footnote

This footnote appears on many labels. It is omitted when there is too little space on the label to print it. The footnote reports the DVs used to compute the % Daily Value for a 2000- and 2500-calorie diet.

Nutrient claims, such as "*Good source,*" and health claims, such as "*Reduce the risk of osteoporosis,*" must follow legal definitions.

Nutrients

These nutrients must appear on most labels. Labels of foods that contain few nutrients, such as candy and soft drinks, may omit some nutrients. Some manufacturers list more nutrients. Other nutrients must be listed if manufacturers make a claim about them or if the food is fortified with them.

A Quick Guide to Nutrient Sources

% Daily Value
20% or more = *Rich source*
10%–19% = *Good source*

Name and address of the food manufacturer.

Ingredients are listed in descending order by weight.

Nutrition Facts

Serving Size 1 Pouch (61g)

Serving Per Container 6

Amount Per Serving

Calories 250	Calories from Fat 70

	% Daily value*
Total Fat 7g	**11**%
Saturated Fat 2.5g	**13**%
Trans Fat 1g	**
Cholesterol 5mg	**2**%
Sodium 400mg	**16**%
Total Carbohydrate 38g	**13**%
Dietary Fiber <1g	**3**%
Sugars 6g	
Protein 7g	

Vitamin A 0% • Vitamin C 0%

Calcium 12% • Iron 8%

*Percent Daily Values are based on a 2,000 calorie diet. Your daily values may be higher or lower depending on your calorie needs:

		Calories:	2,000	2,500
Total Fat	Less than		65g	80g
Sat Fat	Less than		20g	25g
Cholest	Less than		300mg	300mg
Sodium	Less than		2,400mg	2,400mg
Total Carb			300g	375g
Fiber			25g	30g

Calories per gram:

Fat 9 • Carbohydrate 4 • Protein 4

**Intake should be as low as possible.

INGREDIENTS: ENRICHED MACARONI PRODUCT (DURUM WHEAT FLOUR, GLYCERYL MONO-STEARATE, SALT, NIACIN, FERROUS SULFATE, THIAMIN MONONITRATE [VITAMIN B1], RIBOFLAVIN [VITAMIN B2], FOLIC ACID), CHEESE SAUCE MIX (WHEY, PARTIALLY, HYDROGENATED SOYBEAN OIL, MALTODEXTRIN, WHEY PROTEIN CONCENTRATE, CORN SYRUP SOLIDS, SALT, MILKFAT, SUGAR, SODIUM, NATURAL FLAVOR, CITRIC ACID, MONOSODIUM GLUTAMATE, MODIFIED FOOD STARCH, LACTIC ACID, YELLOW 5.

FIGURE 2-16 ▶ Food packages must list product name, name and address of the manufacturer, amount of product in the package, and ingredients. The Nutrition Facts panel is required on virtually all packaged food products. The % Daily Value listed on the label is the percent of the amount of a nutrient needed daily that is provided by a single serving of the product. Canadian food labels use a slightly different group of health claims and label descriptors (see Appendix C).

include the % Daily Value for protein, as must the labels on any food carrying a claim about protein content (see Chapter 15).

Health Claims on Food Labels

As a marketing tool directed toward the health-conscious consumer, food manufacturers like to claim that their products have all sorts of health benefits. The FDA has

TABLE 2-10 Definitions for Nutrient Claims Allowed on Food Labels

Sugar

- **Sugar free:** less than 0.5 grams (g) per serving.
- **No added sugar; without added sugar; no sugar added:**
  - No sugars were added during processing or packing, including ingredients that contain sugars (for example, fruit juices, applesauce, or jam).
  - Processing does not increase the sugar content above the amount naturally present in the ingredients. (A functionally insignificant increase in sugars is acceptable for processes used for purposes other than increasing sugar content.)
  - The food that it resembles and for which it substitutes normally contains added sugars.
  - If the food doesn't meet the requirements for a low- or reduced-calorie food, the product bears a statement that the food is not low calorie or calorie reduced and directs consumers' attention to the Nutrition Facts panel for further information on sugars and calorie content.
- **Reduced sugar:** at least 25% less sugar per serving than reference food

Calories

- **Calorie free:** fewer than 5 kcal per serving
- **Low calorie:** 40 kcal or less per serving and, if the serving is 30 g or less or 2 tablespoons or less, per 50 g of the food
- **Reduced or fewer calories:** at least 25% fewer kcal per serving than reference food

Fiber

- **High fiber:** 5 g or more per serving. (Foods making high-fiber claims must meet the definition for low fat, or the level of total fat must appear next to the high-fiber claim.)
- **Good source of fiber:** 2.5 to 4.9 g per serving
- **More or added fiber:** at least 2.5 g more per serving than reference food

Fat

- **Fat free:** less than 0.5 g of fat per serving
- **Saturated fat free:** less than 0.5 g per serving, and the level of *trans* fatty acids does not exceed 0.5 g per serving

- **Low fat:** 3 g or less per serving and, if the serving is 30 g or less or 2 tablespoons or less, per 50 g of the food. 2% milk can no longer be labeled low fat, as it exceeds 3 g per serving. *Reduced fat* will be the term used instead.
- **Low saturated fat:** 1 g or less per serving and not more than 15% of kcal from saturated fatty acids
- **Reduced or less fat:** at least 25% less per serving than reference food
- **Reduced or less saturated fat:** at least 25% less per serving than reference food

Cholesterol

- **Cholesterol free:** less than 2 milligrams (mg) of cholesterol and 2 g or less of saturated fat per serving
- **Low cholesterol:** 20 mg or less of cholesterol and 2 g or less of saturated fat per serving or, if the serving is 30 g or less or 2 tablespoons or less, per 50 g of the food
- **Reduced or less cholesterol:** at least 25% less cholesterol than reference food and 2 g or less of saturated fat per serving

Sodium

- **Sodium free:** less than 5 mg per serving
- **Very low sodium:** 35 mg or less per serving and, if the serving is 30 g or less or 2 tablespoons or less, per 50 g of the food
- **Low sodium:** 140 mg or less per serving or, if the serving is 30 g or less or 2 tablespoons or less, per 50 g of the food
- **Light in sodium:** at least 50% less per serving than reference food
- **Reduced or less sodium:** at least 25% less per serving than reference food

Other Terms

- **Fortified or enriched:** Vitamins and/or minerals have been added to the product in amounts in excess of at least 10% of that normally present in the usual product. Enriched generally refers to replacing nutrients lost in processing, whereas fortified refers to adding nutrients not originally present in the specific food.
- **Healthy:** An individual food that is low fat and low saturated fat and has no more than 360 to 480 mg of sodium or 60 mg of cholesterol per serving can be labeled "healthy" if it provides at least 10% of the Daily Value for vitamin A, vitamin C, protein, calcium, iron, or fiber.

- **Light or lite:** The descriptor *light* or *lite* can mean two things: first, that a nutritionally altered product contains one-third fewer kcal or half the fat of reference food (if the food derives 50% or more of its kcal from fat, the reduction must be 50% of the fat) and, second, that the sodium content of a low-calorie, low-fat food has been reduced by 50%. In addition, "light in sodium" may be used for foods in which the sodium content has been reduced by at least 50%. The term *light* may still be used to describe such properties as texture and color, as long as the label explains the intent—for example, "light brown sugar" and "light and fluffy."

Diet: A food may be labeled with terms such as *diet, dietetic, artificially sweetened,* or *sweetened with nonnutritive sweetener* only if the claim is not false or misleading. The food can also be labeled *low calorie* or *reduced calorie.*

Good source: *Good source* means that a serving of the food contains 10% to 19% of the Daily Value for a particular nutrient. If 5% or less, it is a *low source.*

High: *High* means that a serving of the food contains 20% or more of the Daily Value for a particular nutrient.

Organic: Federal standards for organic foods allow claims when much of the ingredients do not use chemical fertilizers or pesticides, genetic engineering, sewage sludge, antibiotics, or irradiation in their production. At least 95% of ingredients (by weight) must meet these guidelines to be labeled "organic" on the front of the package. If the front label instead says "made with organic ingredients," only 70% of the ingredients must be organic. For animal products, the animals must graze outdoors, be fed organic feed, and cannot be exposed to large amounts of antibiotics or growth hormones.

Natural: The food must be free of food colors, synthetic flavors, or any other synthetic substance.

The following terms apply only to meat and poultry products regulated by USDA.

Extra lean: less than 5 g of fat, 2 g of saturated fat, and 95 mg of cholesterol per serving (or 100 g of an individual food)

Lean: less than 10 g of fat, 4.5 g of saturated fat, and 95 mg of cholesterol per serving (or 100 g of an individual food)

Many definitions are from FDA's *Dictionary of Terms,* as established in conjunction with the 1990 Nutrition Labeling and Education Act (NLEA).
g = grams; mg = milligrams

legal oversight over most food products and permits some health claims with certain restrictions.

Overall, claims on foods fall into one of four categories:

- Health claims—closely regulated by FDA
- Preliminary health claims—regulated by FDA but evidence may be scant for the claim
- Nutrient claims—closely regulated by FDA (review Table 2-10)
- Structure/function claims—as discussed in the Nutrition and Your Health section at the end of this chapter, these are not FDA-approved or necessarily valid

Table 2-10 lists the definitions for nutrient claims on food labels. Currently, FDA limits the use of health messages to specific instances in which there is significant scientific agreement that a relationship exists between a nutrient, food, or food constituent and the disease. The claims allowed at this time may show a link between the following:

- A diet with enough calcium and vitamin D and a reduced risk of osteoporosis
- A diet low in total fat and a reduced risk of some cancers
- A diet low in saturated fat and cholesterol and a reduced risk of cardiovascular disease (typically referred to as heart disease on the label)
- A diet rich in fiber—containing grain products, fruits, and vegetables—and a reduced risk of some cancers
- A diet low in sodium and high in potassium and a reduced risk of hypertension and stroke
- A diet rich in fruits and vegetables and a reduced risk of some cancers
- A diet adequate in the synthetic form of the vitamin folate (called folic acid) and a reduced risk of neural tube defects (a type of birth defect) (see Chapter 8)
- Use of sugarless gum and a reduced risk of tooth decay, especially when compared with foods high in sugars and starches
- A diet rich in fruits, vegetables, and grain products that contain fiber and a reduced risk of cardiovascular disease. Oats (oatmeal, oat bran, and oat flour) and psyllium are two fiber-rich ingredients that can be singled out in reducing the risk of cardiovascular disease, as long as the statement also says the diet should also be low in saturated fat and cholesterol.
- A diet rich in whole-grain foods and other plant foods, as well as low in total fat, saturated fat, and cholesterol, and a reduced risk of cardiovascular disease and certain cancers
- A diet low in saturated fat and cholesterol that also includes 25 grams of soy protein and a reduced risk of cardiovascular disease. The statement "one serving of the (name of food) provides _____ grams of soy protein" must also appear as part of the health claim.
- Fatty acids from oils present in fish and a reduced risk of cardiovascular disease
- Margarines containing plant stanols and sterols and a reduced risk of cardiovascular disease (see Chapter 5 for more details on plant stanols and sterols)

A "may" or "might" qualifier must be used in the statement.

In addition, before a health claim can be made for a food product, it must meet two general requirements. First, the food must be a "good source" (before any fortification) of fiber, protein, vitamin A, vitamin C, calcium, or iron. The legal definition of "good source" appears in Table 2-10. Second, a single serving of the food product cannot contain more than 13 grams of fat, 4 grams of saturated fat, 60 milligrams of cholesterol, or 480 milligrams of sodium. If a food exceeds any one of these requirements, no health claim can be made for it, despite its other nutritional qualities. For example, even though whole milk is high in calcium, its label can't make the health

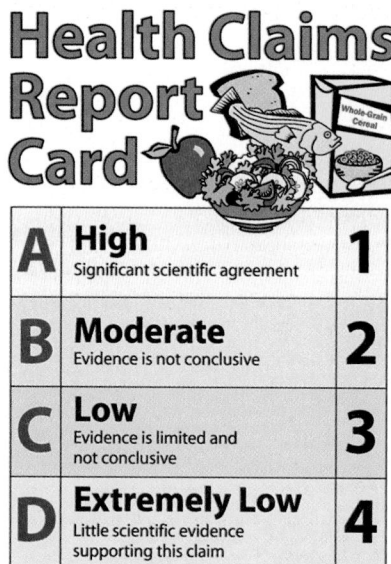

A	**High** Significant scientific agreement	**1**
B	**Moderate** Evidence is not conclusive	**2**
C	**Low** Evidence is limited and not conclusive	**3**
D	**Extremely Low** Little scientific evidence supporting this claim	**4**

▲ In 2003, FDA unveiled a new process, including the Health Claims Report card, to provide more science-based, FDA-regulated health information on food product labels. This process is used to rank the claim based on the amount of scientific evidence and agreement. Only the first three classes are allowed.

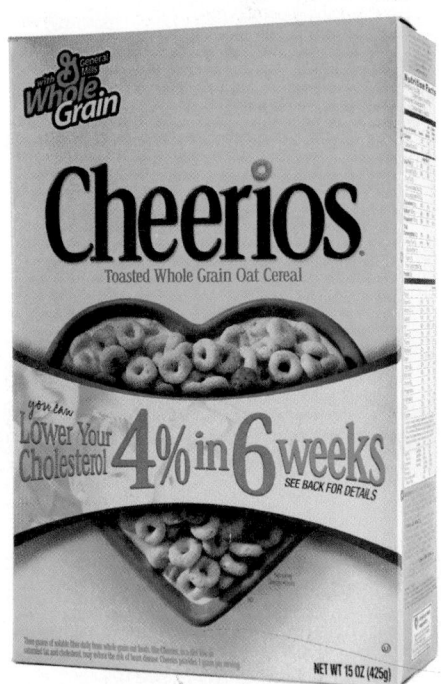

▲ Specific health claims can be made on food labels for whole-grain cereals.

claim about calcium and osteoporosis because whole milk contains 5 grams of saturated fat per serving. In another example, a health claim regarding fat and cancer can be made only if the product contains 3 grams or less of fat per serving, the standard for low-fat foods.

MAKING DECISIONS

Health Claims

FDA allows the three preliminary classes of health claims shown in the preceding section as long as the label qualifies the food with a disclaimer such as "this evidence is not conclusive." These preliminary health claims haven't shown up on many foods at this time (nuts, such as walnuts, and fish have been some of the first examples). These claims also cannot be used on foods considered unhealthy (review Table 2-10 for the definition of healthy with regard to a food).

CONCEPT CHECK

The Nutrition Facts panel on a food label provides key information for helping track one's food intake. Nutrient quantities are compared with the Daily Values and expressed on a percentage basis (% Daily Value). This information can be used to either increase or reduce intake of specific nutrients. Health and nutrient claims on food labels are closely regulated by FDA. Fruits, vegetables, whole-grain breads and cereals, soy, and good sources of calcium are prominent among the foods that can make specific health claims.

2.8 Epilogue

The tools discussed in Chapter 2 greatly aid in menu planning. Menu planning can start with MyPlate. The totality of choices made within the groups can then be evaluated using the Dietary Guidelines. Individual foods that make up a diet can be examined more closely using the Daily Values listed on the Nutrition Facts panel of the product. For the most part, these Daily Values are in line with the Recommended Dietary Allowances and related nutrient standards. The Nutrition Facts panel is especially useful in identifying nutrient-dense foods—foods high in a specific nutrient, such as the vitamin folate, but low in the relative amount of calories provided—and the energy-dense foods—foods that fill you up without providing a lot of calories. Generally speaking, the more you learn about and use these tools, the more they will benefit your diet.

Evaluating Nutrition Claims and Dietary Supplements

The following suggestions should help you make healthful and logical nutrition decisions:

1. Apply the basic principles of nutrition as outlined in this chapter (along with the 2010 Dietary Guidelines for Americans and related resources in Chapter 2) to any nutrition claim including those on websites. Do you note any inconsistencies? Do reliable references support the claims? Beware of the following:
   - Testimonials about personal experience
   - Disreputable publication sources
   - Promises of dramatic results (rarely true)
   - Lack of evidence from other scientific studies

2. Examine the background and scientific credentials of the individual, organizations, or publication making the nutritional claim. Usually, a reputable author is one whose educational background or present affiliation is with a nationally recognized university or medical center that offers programs or courses in the field of nutrition, medicine, or a closely allied specialty.

3. Be wary if the answer is "Yes" to any of the following questions about a health-related nutrition claim:
   - Are only advantages discussed and possible disadvantages ignored?
   - Are claims made about "curing" disease? Do they sound too good to be true?
   - Is extreme bias against the medical community or traditional medical treatments evident? Physicians as a group strive to cure diseases in their patients, using what proven techniques are available. They do not ignore reliable cures.
   - Is the claim touted as a new or secret scientific breakthrough?

4. Note the size and duration of any study cited in support of a nutrition claim. The larger it is and the longer it went on, the more dependable its findings. Also consider the type of study: epidemiology versus case-control versus double-blind. Check out the group studied; a study of men or women in Sweden may be less relevant than one of men or women of Southern European, African, or Hispanic descent, for example. Keep in mind that "contributes to," "is linked to," or "is associated with" does not mean "causes."

5. Beware of press conferences and other hype regarding the latest findings. Much of this will not survive more detailed scientific evaluation.

6. When you meet with a nutrition professional, you should expect that he or she will do the following:
   - Ask questions about your medical history, lifestyle, and current eating habits.
   - Formulate a diet plan tailored to your needs, as opposed to simply tearing a form from a tablet that could apply to almost anyone.
   - Schedule follow-up visits to track your progress, answer any questions, and help keep you motivated.
   - Involve family members in the diet plan, when appropriate.
   - Consult directly with your physician and readily refer you back to your physician for those health problems a nutrition professional is not trained to treat.

7. Avoid practitioners who prescribe **megadoses** of vitamin and mineral supplements for everyone.

8. Examine product labels carefully. Be skeptical of any promotional information about a product that is not clearly stated on the label. A product is not likely to do something not specifically claimed on its label or package insert (legally part of the label).

Dietary Supplements

A cautious approach to nutrition-related advice and products is even more important today because of broad changes in U.S. federal law passed in 1994.

The Dietary Supplement Health and Education Act (DSHEA) of 1994 classified vitamins, minerals, amino acids, and herbal remedies as "foods," which restrains the U.S. Food and Drug Administration (FDA) from regulating them as tightly as drugs and food additives. According to this act, rather than the manufacturer having to prove a dietary supplement is safe, FDA must prove it is unsafe before preventing its sale. In contrast, the safety of food additives and drugs must be demonstrated to FDA's satisfaction before they are marketed.

megadose Large intake of a nutrient beyond estimates of needs or what would be found in a balanced diet; 2 to 10 times human needs is a starting point.

▶ Recently, major nutrition organizations put together 10 red flags that they consider signals for poor nutrition advice:

1. Recommendations that promise a quick fix
2. Dire warnings of dangers from a single product or regimen
3. Claims that sound too good to be true
4. Simplistic conclusions drawn from a complex study
5. Recommendations based on a single study
6. Dramatic statements refuted by reputable scientific organizations
7. Lists of "good" and "bad" foods
8. Recommendations made to help sell a product
9. Recommendations based on studies published without peer review
10. Recommendations from studies that ignore differences among individuals or groups

▶ The FDA can act if evidence accumulates showing that a product is harmful. This has been true for some herbal remedies marketed as dietary supplements, such as ephedra.

Currently, a dietary supplement (or herbal product) can be marketed in the United States without FDA approval if (1) there is a history of its use or other evidence that it is expected to be reasonably safe when used under the conditions recommended or suggested in its labeling, and (2) the product is labeled as a dietary supplement. The Supplement Facts panel resembles the Nutrition Facts panel on foods and is required on all dietary supplements. It is permissible for the labels on such products to claim a benefit related to a classic nutrient-deficiency disease, describe how a nutrient affects human body structure or function (called structure/function claims), and claim that general well-being results from consumption of the ingredient(s). Examples could be "maintains bone health" or "improves blood circulation." However, the label of products bearing such claims also must prominently display in boldface type the following disclaimer: "This statement has not been evaluated by the Food and Drug Administration. This product is not intended to diagnose, treat, cure, or prevent disease" (Fig. 2-17). Despite this warning, when consumers find these products on the shelves of supermarkets,

health-food stores, and pharmacies, they may mistakenly assume FDA has carefully evaluated the products.

Many of us are willing to try untested nutrition products and believe in their miraculous actions. Popular products claim to increase muscle growth, enhance sexuality, boost energy, reduce body fat, increase strength, supply missing nutrients, increase longevity, and even improve brain function. Clearly, many nutritional products commonly found in stores are not strictly regulated in terms of effectiveness and safety (see Further Reading 8). The amount and potency of dietary supplements have also been in question. In June 2007, FDA issued long-awaited standards that require supplement manufacturers to test the purity, strength, and composition of all their products. The usefulness of supplements is discussed further in the Nutrition and Your Health section in Chapter 8, "Dietary Supplements—Who Needs Them?"

If you embark on a self-cure by means of such products, you will probably waste money and possibly risk ill health. A better approach is to consult a physician or **registered dietitian** first (see Further Reading 1). You can find a registered dietitian in North America by consulting the Yellow Pages in the telephone directory, contacting the local dietetic association, calling the dietary department of a local hospital, or visiting www.eatright.org/ or www.dietitians.ca. Make sure the person has the credentials "R.D." after his/her name ("R.D.N." is also used in Canada). This indicates the person has completed rigorous classroom and clinical training in nutrition and participates in continuing education. Appendix H also lists many reputable sources of nutrition advice for your use. Finally, the following websites can help you evaluate ongoing nutrition and health claims:

Supplement Facts

Serving Size 1 Softgel

Each Softgel Contains	% DV
Ginseng Extract *(Panax ginseng)* (root) 100 mg (Standardized to 4% Ginsenosides)	*

*Daily Value (DV) not established.

INGREDIENTS: Gelatin, Soybean Oil, Panax Ginseng Extract, Vegetable Oil, Lecithin, Palm Oil, Glycerin, Sorbitol, Yellow Beeswax, Hydrogenated Coconut Oil, Titanium Dioxide, Yellow 5, Blue 1, Red 40, Green 3, Chlorophyll.

DIST. BY NUTRA ASSOC., INC.
4411 WHITE POINT RD., SPRING CITY, IL 12345

Suggested use: Adults- 1 to 2 capsules daily taken with a full glass of water, or as a tea, add one to two capsules to a cup of hot water.

When you need to perform your best, take ginseng.

This statement has not been evaluated by the Food and Drug Administration. This product is not intended to diagnose, treat, cure, or prevent disease.

- Suggested serving size
- Product and amount
- Name and address of manufacturer
- Suggested use
- Structure/function claim
- Standard FDA disclaimer

FIGURE 2-17 ▶ Supplement Facts label on an herbal product. Note the structure/function claim and the FDA disclaimer. Any nutrients or other food constituents would also be listed if contained in the product.

registered dietitian (R.D.) A person who has completed a baccalaureate degree program approved by the American Dietetic Association, performed at least 1200 hours of supervised professional practice, passed a registration examination, and complies with continuing education requirements.

www.acsh.org/
American Council on Science and Health

www.quackwatch.org/
Quackwatch: Your Guide to Quackery,
Health Fraud, and Intelligent Decisions

www.ncahf.org/
National Council Against Health Fraud

http://dietary-supplements.info.nih.gov/
National Institutes of Health, Office
of Dietary Supplements

www.fda.gov/
U.S. Food and Drug Administration

Overall, nutrition is a rapidly advancing
field and there are always new findings.

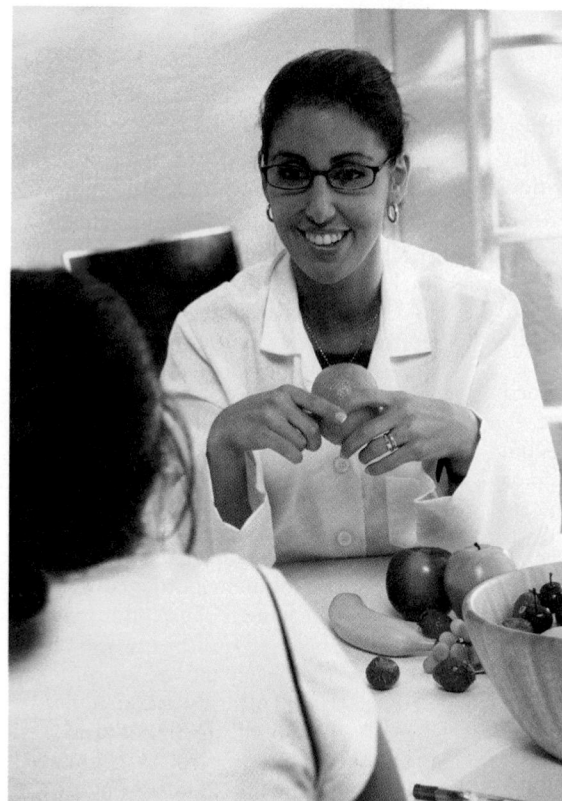

◀ Registered dietitians are a reliable source of nutrition advice.

Case Study Dietary Supplements

While Whitney was driving to campus last week, she heard an advertisement for a supplement containing a plant substance recently imported from China. It supposedly gives people more energy and helps one cope with the stress of daily life. This advertisement caught Whitney's attention because she has been feeling run-down lately. She is taking a full-course load and has been working 30 hours a week at a local restaurant to try to make ends meet. Whitney doesn't have a lot of extra money. Still, she likes to try new things and this recent breakthrough from China sounded almost too good to be true. After searching for more information about this supplement on the Internet, she discovered that the recommended dose would cost $60 per month. Because Whitney is looking for some help with her low energy level, she decides to order a 1-month supply.

Answer the following questions, and check your response in Appendix A.

1. Is the advertised supplement regulated by the FDA or other government agency?

2. What type of label claim is the phrase "increases energy," and does it require government approval?

3. Can Whitney feel confident that the supplement is safe and effective?

4. Is the amount of active ingredients in supplements tightly controlled?

5. Does it make sense for Whitney to spend the extra $60 per month for this supplement?

6. What advice would you give Whitney about the fact that she has been feeling run-down lately?

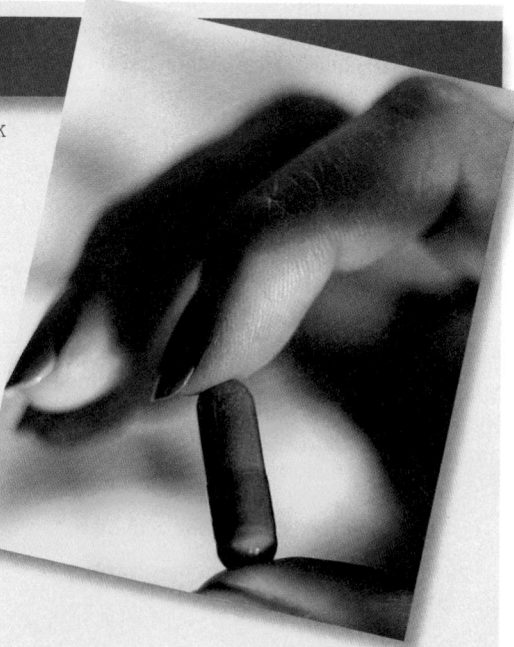

▲ Do you agree with Whitney's decision to try this supplement?

Summary (Numbers refer to numbered sections in the chapter.)

2.1 A healthy eating plan is based on consuming a *variety* of foods *balanced* by a moderate intake of each food and will minimize the risk of developing nutrition-related diseases.

Nutrient density reflects the nutrient content of a food in relation to its calorie content. Nutrient-dense foods are relatively rich in nutrients, in comparison with calorie content.

Energy density of a food is determined by comparing calorie content with the weight of food. A food rich in calories but weighing relatively very little, such as nuts, cookies, fried foods in general, and most snack foods (including fat-free brands), is considered energy dense. Foods with low energy density include fruits, vegetables, and any food that incorporates lots of water during cooking, such as oatmeal.

2.2 A person's nutritional state can be categorized as *desirable nutrition,* in which the body has adequate stores for times of increased needs; *undernutrition,* which may be present with or without clinical symptoms; and *overnutrition,* which can lead to vitamin and mineral toxicities and various chronic diseases.

2.3 Evaluation of nutritional state involves analyzing background factors, as well as anthropometric, biochemical, clinical, dietary, and environmental assessments. It is not always possible to detect nutritional inadequacies via nutrition assessment because symptoms of deficiencies are often nonspecific and may not appear for many years.

2.4 The scientific method is the procedure for testing the validity of possible explanations of a phenomenon, called hypotheses. Experiments are conducted to either support or refute a specific hypothesis. Once we have enough experimental information to support a specific hypothesis, it then can be called a theory. All of us need to be skeptical of new ideas in the nutrition field, waiting until many lines of experimental evidence support a concept before adopting any suggested dietary practice.

2.5 Recommended Dietary Allowances (RDAs) are set for many nutrients. These amounts yield enough of each nutrient to meet the needs of healthy individuals within specific gender and age categories. Adequate Intake (AI) is the standard used when not enough information is available to set a more specific RDA. Estimated Energy Requirements (EERs) set calorie needs for both genders at various ages and physical activity patterns. Tolerable Upper Intake Levels (Upper Levels or ULs) for nutrient intake have been set for some vitamins and minerals.

All of the many dietary standards fall under the term *Dietary Reference Intakes (DRIs).* Daily Values are used as a basis for expressing the nutrient content of foods on the Nutrition Facts panel and are based for the most part on the RDAs.

2.6 Dietary Guidelines for Americans have been issued to help improve the health of all Americans ages 2 and older. The guidelines emphasize balancing calories to manange weight; performing regular physical activity; moderating consumption of fat, *trans* fat, cholesterol, sugar, salt, and alcohol; eating plenty of whole-grain products, fruits, and vegetables; and safely preparing and storing foods, especially perishable foods.

MyPlate and accompanying online tools are designed to translate nutrient recommendations into a food plan that exhibits variety, balance, and moderation. The best results are obtained by using low-fat or fat-free dairy products; incorporating some vegetable proteins in the diet in addition to animal-protein foods; including citrus fruits and dark-green vegetables; and emphasizing whole-grain breads and cereals.

2.7 Food labels, especially the Nutrition Facts panels, are a useful tool to track your nutrient intake and learn more about the nutritional characteristics of the foods you eat. Any health claims listed must follow criteria set by FDA.

N&YH Apply the basic principles of nutrition to evaluate any nutrition claim. Dietary supplements can be marketed in the United States without FDA approval. Certain health claims can be made on supplement labels, although few have been thoroughly evaluated by reputable scientists.

Check Your Knowledge (Answers to the following questions are below.)

1. Anthropometric measurements include
   a. height, weight, skinfolds, and body circumferences.
   b. blood concentrations of nutrients.
   c. a diet history of the previous days' intake.
   d. blood levels of enzyme activities.

2. Foods with *high* nutrient density offer the _____ nutrients for the _____ calories.
   a. least, lowest
   b. least, most
   c. most, lowest
   d. most, most

3. A meal of a bean burrito, tossed salad, and glass of milk represents foods from all MyPlate food groups except
   a. dairy.   c. vegetables.
   b. protein.   d. fruits.

4. The Dietary Guidelines for Americans were recently revised in
   a. 2000   c. 2008
   b. 2005   d. 2010

5. The term Daily Value is used on
   a. restaurant menus.
   b. food labels.
   c. medical charts.
   d. None of the above.

6. The Tolerable Upper Intake Level, or UL, is used to
   a. estimate calorie needs of the average person.
   b. evaluate the highest amount of daily nutrient intake unlikely to cause adverse health effects.
   c. evaluate your current intake for a specific nutrient.
   d. compare the nutrient content of a food to approximate human needs.

7. The current food label must list
   a. a picture of the product.
   b. a uniform and realistic serving size.

c. the RDA for each age group.
d. ingredients alphabetically.

8. Dietary supplements are tightly regulated by the
   a. FDA.
   b. USDA.
   c. FTC.
   d. None of the above.

9. The scientific method begins with
   a. a hypothesis.
   b. research experiments.
   c. publication of research findings.
   d. observations made and questions asked.

10. The most common type of undernutrition in industrialized nations, such as the United States, is

a. anorexia.
b. protein deficiency.
c. obesity.
d. iron deficiency.

Answer Key: 1. a (LO 2.2), 2. c (LO 2.1), 3. d (LO 2.6), 4. d (LO 2.5), 5. b (LO 2.4), 6. b (LO 2.4), 7. b (LO 2.7), 8. d (LO 2.8), 9. d (LO 2.3), 10. d (LO 2.2).

Study Questions (Numbers refer to Learning Outcomes)

1. Among your classmates, you observe that students who consume coffee get better grades. Provide an example of how you could use the scientific method to examine the effects of coffee consumption on academic performance **(LO 2.3)**.

2. How would you explain the concepts of nutrient density and energy density to a fourth-grade class **(LO 2.1)**?

3. Trace the progression, in terms of physical results, of a person who went from an overnourished to an undernourished state **(LO 2.2)**.

4. How could the nutritional state of the person at each state in question 3 be evaluated **(LO 2.2)**?

5. Describe the philosophy underlying the creation of MyPlate. What dietary changes would you need to make to comply with the healthy eating guidelines exemplified by MyPlate on a regular basis **(LO 2.6)**?

6. Describe the intent of the Dietary Guidelines for Americans. Point out one criticism for their general application to all North American adults **(LO 2.5)**.

7. Based on the discussion of the Dietary Guidelines for Americans, suggest two key dietary changes the typical North American adult should consider making **(LO 2.5)**.

8. How do RDAs and AIs differ from Daily Values in intention and application **(LO 2.4)**?

9. Dietitians encourage all people to read labels on food packages to learn more about what they eat. What four nutrients could easily be tracked in your diet if you read the Nutrition Facts panels regularly on food products **(LO 2.7)**?

10. What would you list as the top five sources of reliable nutrition information? What makes these sources reliable **(LO 2.8)**?

What Would You Choose Recommendations

An 8-ounce glass of orange juice provides 114 kcal, 24 grams of sugar, 0 grams of fiber, and 72 mg of vitamin C. The weight of this serving of orange juice is about 250 grams, or almost 9 ounces (there are about 28 grams in 1 ounce). To estimate energy density, compare the calorie content of this food to its weight: 114 kcal/250 grams = 0.456 kcal/gram. To find nutrient density for vitamin C, calculate a ratio of vitamin C content to the calorie content of the food: 72 milligrams of vitamin C/114 kcal = 0.63 mg vitamin C/kcal.

A whole, fresh, medium orange has about 60 kcal, 12 grams of sugar, 3 grams of fiber, and 70 mg of vitamin C. The weight of an orange is about 130 grams. Comparing calorie content to weight of the food results in 60 kcal/130 grams = 0.462 kcal/gram for energy density. Nutrient density for vitamin C is calculated as 70 milligrams of vitamin C/60 kcal = 1.17 mg vitamin C/kcal.

Oranges and orange juice have about the same energy density, but the nutrient density for vitamin C is almost twice as high as that for orange juice. Oranges and 100% orange juice are both good choices in terms of energy density, and both are rich sources of vitamin C. The RDA for vitamin C is 75 mg/day for women and 90 mg/day for men. A person who is trying to restrict calorie intake while still consuming adequate nutrients should choose the whole, fresh orange instead of the orange juice as a source of vitamin C because it has higher nutrient density—it provides excellent nutrition in fewer calories than the serving of orange juice. Whole fruits also provide more fiber and phytochemicals than juice. Be assured that 100% fruit juice is still a healthy choice. When choosing your servings of fruit, choose whole fruits more often than fruit juice to get the best nutrition in the fewest calories.

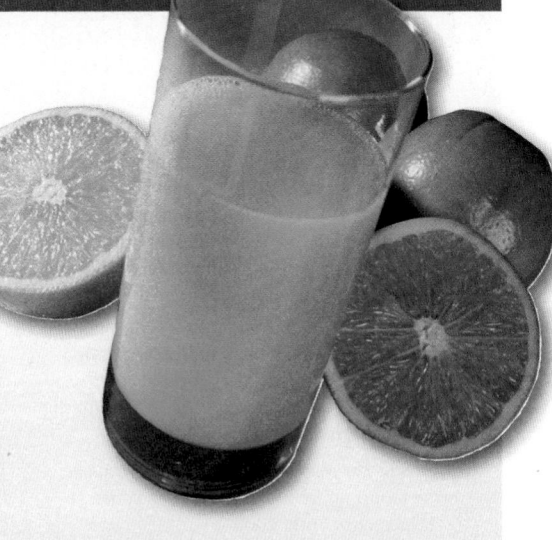

▲ The nutrient density of whole oranges surpasses that of orange juice.

Further Readings

1. ADA Reports: Position of the American Dietetic Association: Food and nutrition misinformation. *Journal of the American Dietetic Association* 106:601, 2006.

   Much food and nutrition misinformation pervades North American society. Individuals should carefully consider the training of those who give advice and be assured that registered dietitians are credible and reliable resources.

2. Barr SI: Introduction to dietary reference intakes. *Applied Physiology, Nutrition, and Metabolism* 31:61, 2006.

   The development of the Dietary Reference Intakes (DRIs) was a joint initiative by the United States and Canada to update and replace the former Recommended Nutrient Intakes for Canadians and the Recommended Dietary Allowances for Americans. The new DRIs are described.

3. Kennedy ET: Evidence for nutritional benefits in prolonging wellness. *American Journal of Clinical Nutrition* 83:410S, 2006.

   The interaction between genes; the environment; and lifestyle factors, especially diet and physical activity, are involved in healthy aging. The need to consider all the lifestyle and environmental factors contributing to suboptimal eating and lifestyle patterns is discussed.

4. Mobley AR and others: Putting the nutrient-rich foods index into practice. *Journal of the American College of Nutrition* 28:427S, 2009.

   In response to a need for a standardized definition of nutrient density as well as a growing interest among consumers and food manufacturers in front-of-pack labeling to convey nutrient information in a glance, the Nutrient Rich Foods Coalition formulated a Nutrient-Rich Foods educational tool and a symbol, called My5, which conveys nutrient content of a food within the context of a healthy diet.

5. Reedy J, Krebs-Smith SM: A comparison of food-based recommendations and nutrient values of three food guides: USDA's MyPyramid, NHLBI's dietary approaches to stop hypertension eating plan, and Harvard's healthy eating pyramid. *Journal of the American Dietetic Association* 108: 522, 2008.

   The three food guides share consistent messages to eat more fruits, vegetables, legumes, and whole grains; eat less added sugar and saturated fat; and emphasize plant oils.

6. Rolls B: *The volumetric eating plan: Techniques and recipes for feeling full on fewer calories.* Harper, New York, 2005.

   Energy density of food choices strongly affects total calories consumed at a meal and throughout the day. The volumetric eating plan includes techniques and recipes that decrease energy density of the diet—incorporating more fiber and water—which helps people lower their calories without feeling deprived.

7. Rowe S and others: Translating the Dietary Guidelines for Americans 2010 to bring about real behavior change. *Journal of the American Dietetic Association* 111:28, 2011.

   Nutition experts devised a set of recommendations to assist health professionals, government authorities, and food manufacturers in implementing the Dietary Guidelines for Americans, 2010. The coordination of efforts of educators, health care providers, policy makers, and industry leaders is needed to reach the public. Nutrition messages should be simple and targeted. Along with efforts to encourage people to want to change their habits, food manufacturers should make gradual changes in food composition to better align products with the goals of the Dietary Guidelines. Education efforts should begin at an early age and should be sensitive to differences in culure and ethnic background.

8. Sheth A and others: Potential liver damage associated with over-the-counter vitamin supplements. *Journal of the American Dietetic Association* 108:1536, 2008.

   This case report provides an example of the potential for liver damage associated with long-term intakes of megadose dietary supplements. In this case, a patient developed liver cirrhosis after long-term (2 years) daily ingestion of over-the-counter dietary supplements containing 13,000 micrograms of vitamin A. Such adverse effects indicate the need for medical supervision of use of these products.

9. Sofi F and others: Adherence to Mediterranean Diet and health status: Meta-analysis. *British Medical Journal* 337:a1344, 2008.

   A systematic review found that greater adherence to a Mediterranean Diet is associated with a significant reduction in overall mortality (9%), mortality from cardiovascular diseases (9%), incidence of mortality from cancer (6%), and incidence of Parkinson's disease and Alzheimer's disease (13%). These results indicate that a Mediterranean-like dietary pattern should be encouraged for primary prevention of major chronic diseases.

10. Taylor CL, Wilkening VL: How the nutrition food label was developed, Part 1: The nutrition facts panel. Part 2: The purpose and promise of nutrition claims. *The Journal of the American Dietetic Association* 108: 437, 618, 2008.

    These articles offer insight into the development of the nutrition label and discuss its role in improving the diet and health of Americans. The issues discussed highlight the fact that the nutrition label is a "work in progress."

11. U.S. Department of Health and Human Services. *2008 Physical Activity Guidelines for Americans.* 2008. www.health.gov/PAGuidelines/.

    Inactivity remains high among American children, adolescents, and adults, putting Americans at unnecessary risk of disease. The Guidelines provide science-based guidance to help Americans aged six and older improve their health through appropriate physical activity.

12. U.S. Department of Health and Human Services. *Dietary Guidelines for Americans, 2010.* 2011. www.health.gov/dietaryguidelines/2010.

    The most recent Dietary Guidelines have three overarching goals. 1.) balance calories with physical activity to manage weight; 2.) consume more fruits, vegetables, whole grains, fat-free and low-fat dairy products, and seafoods; and 3.) consume fewer foods with sodium, saturated fats, trans fats, cholesterol, added sugars, and refined grains.

13. United States Department of Agriculture. *USDA's MyPlate.* 2011. www.choosemyplate.gov.

    MyPlate replaces MyPyramid as the icon depicting healthy eating for Americans. In addition to the graphic representations of MyPlate, www.ChooseMyPlate.gov. provides Daily Food Plans specific to individual energy needs, several interactive tools for consumers, and resources for health educators. Building a healthy meal with balanced proportions of fruits, vegetables, grains, protein, and dairy will help Americans reach the goals set forth by the Dietary Guidelines.

14. Watts ML and others: The art of translating nutritional science into dietary guidance: History and evolution of the Dietary Guidelines for Americans. *Nutrition Reviews* 69:404, 2011.

    The U.S. government has issued dietary guidance for more than 100 years. Over time, the guidelines have become more firmly rooted in scientific evidence and more specific to the target audience. There is widespread recognition that successful implementation of dietary guidance requires the coordination of stakeholders at all levels—policy makers, health care providers, educators, industry, and consumers.

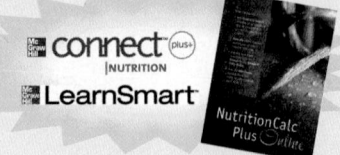

To get the most out of your study of nutrition, go to McGraw-Hill's online resources: Connect www.mcgrawhillconnect.com, **where you will find NutritionCalc Plus, LearnSmart, and many other dynamic tools.**

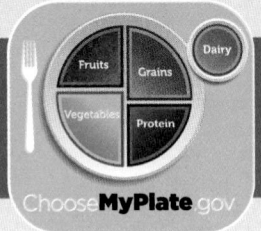
I. Does your Diet Compare to MyPlate?

Using your food-intake record from Chapter 1, place each food item in the appropriate group of the accompanying MyPlate chart. That is, for each food item, indicate how many servings it contributes to each group based on the amount you ate (see Food Composition Table Supplement for serving sizes). Many of your food choices may contribute to more than one group. For example, spaghetti with meat sauce contributes to three categories; grains, vegetables, and protein. After entering all the values, add the number of servings consumed in each group. Finally, compare your total in each food group with the recommended number of servings shown in Table 2-6 or obtained from the www.ChooseMyPlate.gov website. Enter a minus sign (−) if your total falls below the recommendation or a plus sign (+) if it equals or exceeds the recommendation.

   Indicate the number of servings from MyPlate that each food yields:

Food or Beverage	Amount Eaten	Grains	Vegetables	Fruits	Dairy	Protein	Oils
Group totals							
Recommended servings							
Shortages/overages in numbers of servings							

II. Are You Putting Health Advice into Practice?

The broad range of diet and physical activity advice provided by the 2010 Dietary Guidelines for Americans, 2008 Physical Activity Guidelines for Americans, and MyPlate can seem overwhelming. Fill out the following inventory to see how well you comply with the basic intent of these consumer health guidelines and identify areas in which you need improvement.

Build a Healthy Plate

Y N Do fruits and vegetables cover at least half of your plate at meal times?

Y N Do you use fruits, vegetables, or unsalted nuts as snacks?

Y N Do you use either skim or 1% milk?

Y N Do you consume at least three servings of whole grains per day?

Y N Do you include seafood as your source of protein at least twice per week?

Y N Do you include beans as your source of protein at least once per week?

Y N Do you consume alcohol in moderation (≤1 drink/day for women; ≤2 drinks/day for men)?

Y N Do you use a meat thermometer to determine if your foods are thoroughly cooked?

Y N Do you clean hands, food contact surfaces, and fruits and vegetables before preparation?

Cut Back on Foods High in Solid Fats, Added Sugars, and Salt

Y N Do you choose water or other calorie-free beverages to drink most of the time?

Y N When you drink juice, do you choose 100% fruit juice?

Y N Do you use the Nutrition Facts panel to select foods low in sodium?

Y N Do you use spices and herbs instead of salt to season your food?

Y N Do you use vegetable oils rather than butter, lard, or shortening when preparing foods?

Y N Do you select foods that are reduced-fat, low-fat, or fat-free?

Eat the Right Amount of Calories for You

Y N Is your weight within a healthy range?

Y N Do you know how many calories you need per day?

Y N Do you limit your portions to one serving (i.e., as listed on food labels) of most foods?

Y N Do you stop eating when you are satisfied rather than uncomfortably full?

Y N Do you prepare most of your own foods?

Y N When eating out, do you seek out nutrition information on menu items?

Y N Do you take home leftovers or share meals with a friend when dining out?

Be Physically Active Your Way

| Y | N | Do you exercise at least 150 minutes per week? |

| Y | N | Do you include aerobic and muscle-strengthening activities into your exercise routine? |

| Y | N | Do you protect yourself from injury when participating in physical activity? |

| Y | N | Does your exercise routine match your current level of fitness, ability, and health? |

III. Applying the Nutrition Facts Label to Your Daily Food Choices

Imagine that you are at the supermarket looking for a quick meal before a busy evening. In the frozen food section, you find two brands of frozen cheese manicotti (see labels a and b). Which of the two brands would you choose? What information on the Nutrition Facts label in the figure contributed to this decision?

_____

_____

_____

_____

(a)

Nutrition Facts
Serving Size 1 Package (260g)
Servings Per Container 1

Amount Per Serving

Calories 390   Calories from Fat 160

	% Daily Value*
Total Fat 18g	**27**%
Saturated Fat 9g	**45**%
Trans Fat 2g	**
Cholesterol 45mg	**14**%
Sodium 880mg	**36**%
Total Carbohydrate 38g	**13**%
Dietary Fiber 4g	**15**%
Sugars 12g	
Protein 17g	

Vitamin A 10% • Vitamin C 4%

Calcium 40% • Iron 8%

*Percent Daily Values are based on a 2,000 calorie diet. Your daily values may be higher or lower depending on your calorie needs:

	Calories:	2,000	2,500
Total Fat	Less than	65g	80g
Sat Fat	Less than	20g	25g
Cholesterol	Less than	300mg	300mg
Sodium	Less than	2,400mg	2,400mg
Total Carbohydrate		300g	375g
Dietary Fiber		25g	30g

Calories per gram:
Fat 9 • Carbohydrate 4 • Protein 4

**Intake of *trans* fat should be as low as possible.

(b)

Nutrition Facts
Serving Size 1 Package (260g)
Servings Per Container 1

Amount Per Serving

Calories 230   Calories from Fat 35

	% Daily Value*
Total Fat 4g	**6**%
Saturated Fat 2g	**10**%
Trans Fat 1g	**
Cholesterol 15mg	**4**%
Sodium 590mg	**24**%
Total Carbohydrate 28g	**9**%
Dietary Fiber 3g	**12**%
Sugars 10g	
Protein 19g	

Vitamin A 10% • Vitamin C 10%

Calcium 35% • Iron 4%

*Percent Daily Values are based on a 2,000 calorie diet. Your daily values may be higher or lower depending on your calorie needs:

	Calories:	2,000	2,500
Total Fat	Less than	65g	80g
Sat Fat	Less than	20g	25g
Cholesterol	Less than	300mg	300mg
Sodium	Less than	2,400mg	2,400mg
Potassium		3,500mg	3,500mg
Total Carbohydrate		300g	375g
Dietary Fiber		25g	30g

Calories per gram:
Fat 9 • Carbohydrate 4 • Protein 4

**Intake of *trans* fat should be as low as possible.

Chapter 3 The Human Body: A Nutrition Perspective

Student Learning Outcomes

Chapter 3 is designed to allow you to:

3.1 Understand some basic roles of nutrients in human physiology.

3.2 Identify the functions of the common cellular components.

3.3 Define tissue, organ, and organ system.

3.4 Identify the role of the cardiovascular and lymphatic systems in nutrition.

3.5 List basic characteristics of the nervous system and its role in nutrition.

3.6 List basic characteristics of the endocrine system, especially the pancreas, and its role in nutrition.

3.7 List basic characteristics of the immune system and its role in nutrition.

3.8 Outline the overall processes of digestion and absorption in the mouth, stomach, small intestine, and large intestine, as well as the roles played by the liver, gallbladder, and pancreas.

3.9 List basic characteristics of the urinary system and its role in nutrition.

3.10 Understand the importance of the body storage areas for nutrients.

3.11 Understand the emerging field of nutrigenomics.

3.12 Identify the major nutrition-related gastrointestinal health problems and approaches to treatment.

What Would You Choose?

For spring break, you are volunteering to help build a house with Habitat for Humanity. You are carpooling with some friends and staying in a retreat house. Unfortunately, the travel, budget, living accommodations, and your building schedule won't allow for home-cooked meals this week. Being out of your normal routine and relying on fast-food sandwiches and pizza have left you feeling constipated. This reminds you that you will need to make smarter choices at fast-food establishments. To decrease your constipation which menu combination would you choose from a pizza buffet?

ⓐ 2 slices of pepperoni pizza, 2 cups of tossed salad

ⓑ 2 slices of veggie pizza, 1 cup of bean and pasta soup

ⓒ 2 slices of ham and pineapple pizza, 1 cup of pasta with Alfredo sauce

ⓓ 2 slices of cheese pizza, 1 garlic breadstick with marinara sauce

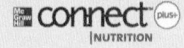 **NUTRITION**

Think about your choices as you read Chapter 3, then see our recommendations at the end of the chapter. To learn more about the connection between our diets and our bodies, check out the Connect site: www.mcgrawhillconnect.com

Part One
Nutrition: A Key to Health

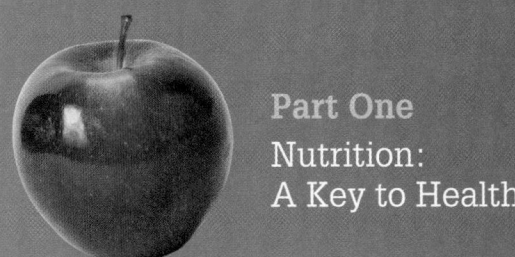

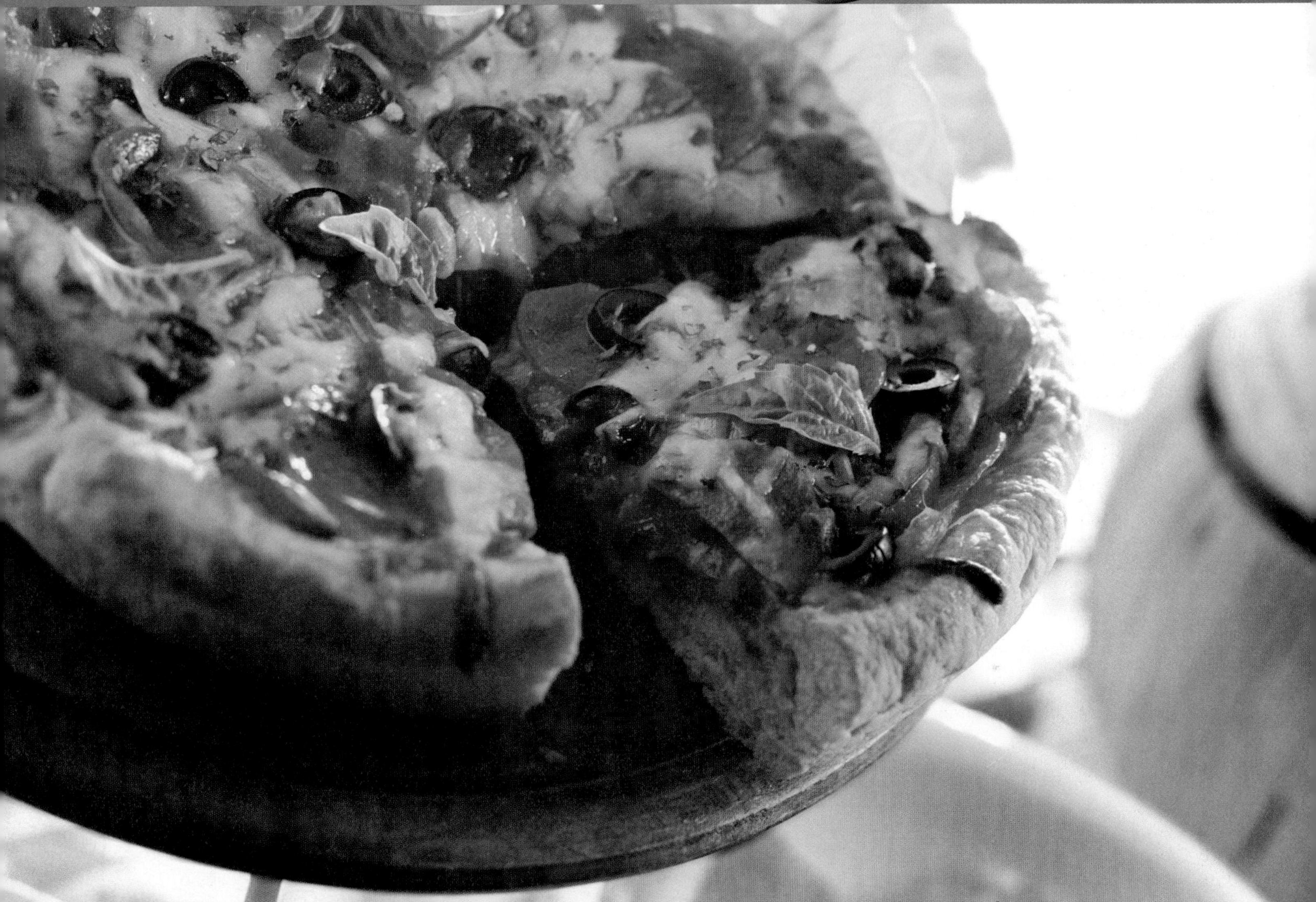

Merely eating food won't nourish you. You must first digest the food by breaking it down into usable forms of the essential nutrients that can be absorbed into the bloodstream. Once nutrients are taken up by the bloodstream, they can be distributed to and used by body cells.

We rarely think about, let alone control, digesting and absorbing foods. Except for a few voluntary responses—such as deciding what and when to eat, how well to chew food, and when to eliminate the remains—most digestion and absorption processes control themselves. As suggested in the comic in this chapter, we don't consciously decide when the pancreas will secrete digestive substances into the small intestine or how quickly foodstuffs will be propelled down the intestinal tract. Various hormones and the nervous system mostly control these functions. Your only awareness of these involuntary responses may be a hunger pang right before lunch or a "full" feeling after eating that last slice of pizza.

Let's examine digestion and absorption as well as other aspects of human physiology that support nutritional health. In the process you will become acquainted with the basic anatomy (structure) and physiology (function) of the circulatory system, nervous system, endocrine system, immune system, digestive system, urinary system, and storage capabilities of the human body.

Refresh Your Memory

As you begin your study of human physiology in Chapter 3, you may want to review:

- Cell structure and function from previous coursework in university-level biology courses
- Each of the body's organ systems from any previous biology training

3.1 Nutrition's Role in Human Physiology

Overall, the human body is a coordinated unit of many highly structured organ systems (Fig. 3-1). Together, these system are composed of trillions of cells. Each cell is a self-contained, living entity. Cells of the same type normally join together, using intercellular substances to form **tissues,** such as muscle tissue. One, two, or more tissues then combine in a particular way to form more complex structures, called **organs.** All organs contribute to nutritional health, and a person's overall nutritional state determines how well each organ functions. At a still higher level of coordination, several organs can cooperate for a common purpose to form an **organ system,** such as the digestive system.

Chemical processes (reactions) occur constantly in every living cell: The production of new substances is balanced by the breaking down of older ones. An example is the constant formation and degradation of bone. For this turnover of substances to occur, cells require a continuous supply of energy in the form of dietary carbohydrate, protein, and/or fat. Cells also need water; building supplies, especially protein and minerals; and chemical regulators, such as the vitamins. Almost all cells also need a steady supply of oxygen. These substances enable the tissues, made from individual cells, to function properly.

Getting an adequate supply of all nutrients to the body's cells begins with a healthy diet. To assure optimal use of nutrients, the body's cells, tissues, organs, and organ systems also must work efficiently.

tissues Collections of cells adapted to perform a specific function.

organ A group of tissues designed to perform a specific function—for example, the heart, which contains muscle tissue, nerve tissue, and so on.

organ system A collection of organs that work together to perform an overall function.

FRANK & ERNEST® by Bob Thaves

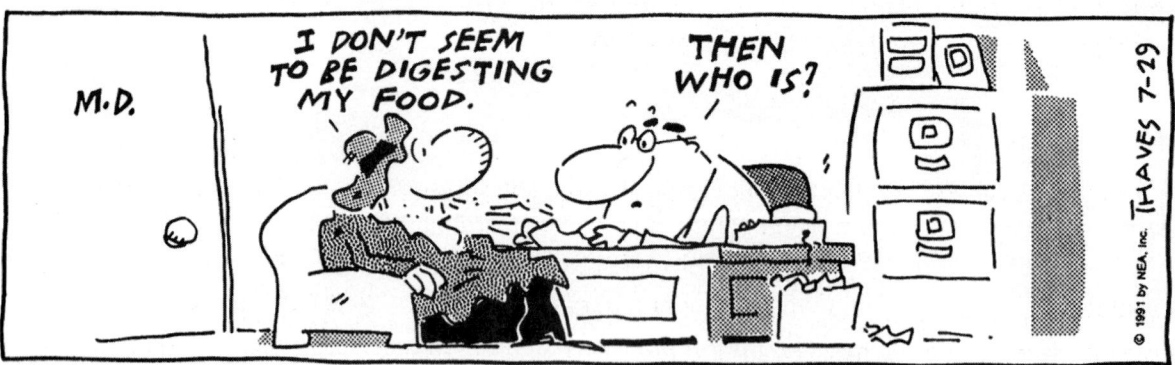

Some popular (fad) diets suggest not combining meat and potatoes to improve digestion and that fruit should only be eaten before noon. These diets might also claim that foods get stuck in the body and in turn putrefy and create toxins. Are there any scientific reasons to suggest that the timing of our food intake should optimize digestion? Do certain food practices improve digestion and subsequent absorption? This chapter provides some answers.

FRANK AND ERNEST reprinted by permission of Newspaper Enterprise Association, Inc.

1 **Chemical level.** Atoms combine to form molecules.

2 **Cell level.** Molecules form organelles, such as the nucleus and mitochondria, which make up cells.

3 **Tissue level.** Similar cells and surrounding materials make up tissues.

4 **Organ level.** Different tissues combine to form organs, such as the stomach.

5 **Organ system level.** Organs such as the stomach and intestines make up an organ system.

6 **Organism level.** Organ systems make up an organism.

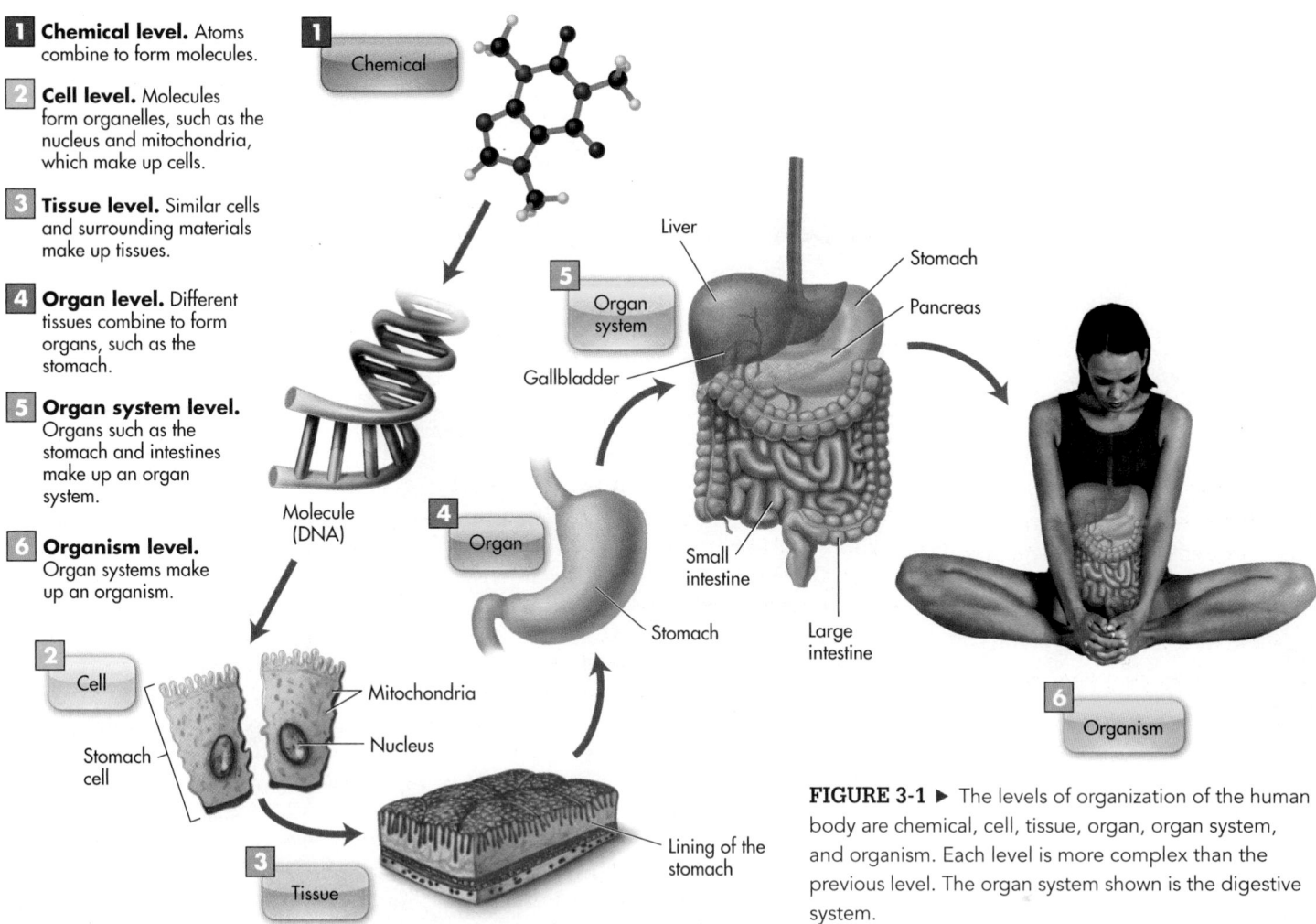

FIGURE 3-1 ▶ The levels of organization of the human body are chemical, cell, tissue, organ, organ system, and organism. Each level is more complex than the previous level. The organ system shown is the digestive system.

Chapter 3 covers the anatomy and physiology of the cell and major organ systems, especially as they relate to human nutrition. The information you are about to study is limited to the components of the various organ systems specifically influenced by the more than 45 essential nutrients discussed in this text.

3.2 The Cell: Structure, Function, and Metabolism

The cell is the basic structural and functional component of life. Living organisms are made of many different kinds of cells specialized to perform particular functions, and all cells are derived from preexisting cells. In the human body, all cells have certain common features. These cells have compartments and specialized structures that perform particular functions; these components are called **organelles** (Fig. 3-2). There are at least 15 different organelles. Eight of the most important organelles will be discussed. The numbers following the names of the cell structures correspond to the structures illustrated in Figure 3-2. Metabolism, the chemical processes that take place in body cells, will also be discussed.

organelles Compartments, particles, or filaments that perform specialized functions within a cell.

Cell (Plasma) Membrane 1

There is an outside and inside to every cell, separated by the cell (plasma) membrane. This membrane holds the cellular contents together and regulates the direction and flow of substances into and out of the cell. Cell-to-cell communication also occurs by way of this membrane.

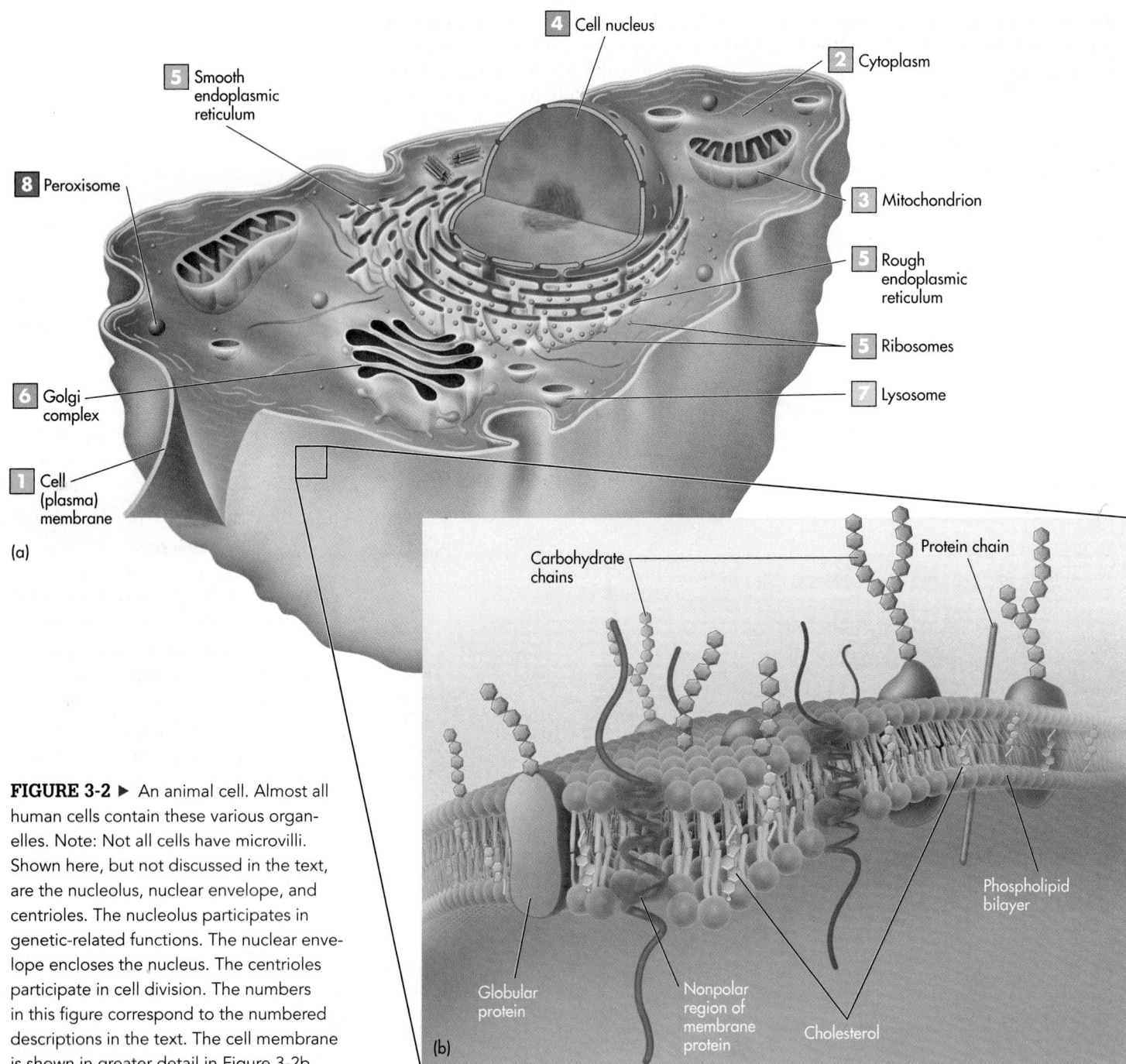

4 Cell nucleus

2 Cytoplasm

5 Smooth endoplasmic reticulum

8 Peroxisome

3 Mitochondrion

5 Rough endoplasmic reticulum

5 Ribosomes

6 Golgi complex

7 Lysosome

1 Cell (plasma) membrane

(a)

Carbohydrate chains

Protein chain

Phospholipid bilayer

Globular protein

Nonpolar region of membrane protein

Cholesterol

(b)

FIGURE 3-2 ▶ An animal cell. Almost all human cells contain these various organelles. Note: Not all cells have microvilli. Shown here, but not discussed in the text, are the nucleolus, nuclear envelope, and centrioles. The nucleolus participates in genetic-related functions. The nuclear envelope encloses the nucleus. The centrioles participate in cell division. The numbers in this figure correspond to the numbered descriptions in the text. The cell membrane is shown in greater detail in Figure 3-2b.

phospholipid Any of a class of fat-related substances that contain phosphorus, fatty acids, and a nitrogen-containing component. Phospholipids are an essential part of every cell.

enzyme A compound that speeds the rate of a chemical process but is not altered by that process. Almost all enzymes are proteins.

The cell membrane, illustrated in Figure 3-2(b), is a lipid bilayer (or double membrane) of **phospholipids** with their water-soluble heads facing both the interior of the cell and the exterior of the cell. Their water-insoluble tails are tucked into the center portion of the cell membrane.

Cholesterol is another component of the cell membrane. It is fat soluble, so it is embedded within the bilayer. This cholesterol provides rigidity and thus stability to the membrane.

There are also various proteins embedded in the cell membrane. Proteins provide structural support, act as transport vehicles, and function as **enzymes** that affect chemical processes within the membrane (see the later section on digestion for more about enzymes). Some proteins form open channels that allow water-soluble substances to pass into and out of the cell. Proteins on the outside surface of the membrane act as receptors, snagging essential substances that the cell needs and drawing them into the cell. Other proteins act as gates that open and close to control the flow of various particles into and out of the cell.

In addition to the lipid and protein, the membrane also contains carbohydrates that mark the exterior of the cell. These carbohydrates are combined either with protein or fat, and they help send messages to the cell's organelles and act as identification markers for the cell. In addition, they detect invaders and initiate defensive actions. In sum, these carbohydrates provide tags that are important to cellular identity and interaction.

Cytoplasm 2

The **cytoplasm** is the combination of fluid material and organelles within the cell, not including the nucleus. A small amount of energy for use by the cell can be produced by chemical processes that occur in the cytoplasm. This contributes to the survival of all cells and is the sole source of energy production in red blood cells. This energy production is called **anaerobic** metabolism because it doesn't require oxygen.

Organelles. Included within the cytoplasm are organelles. As described in the next two pages, they carry out vital roles in cell functions.

Mitochondria 3

Mitochondria are sometimes called the "power plants," or the powerhouse of the cell. These organelles are capable of converting the food energy in energy-yielding nutrients (carbohydrate, protein, and fat) to a form of energy that cells can use. This is an **aerobic** process that uses the oxygen we inhale, as well as water, enzymes, and other compounds (see Chapter 10 for details). With the exception of red blood cells, all cells contain mitochondria; only the size, shape, and quantity vary.

Cell Nucleus 4

With the exception of the red blood cell, all cells have one or more nuclei. The **cell nucleus** is bounded by its own double membrane. The nucleus contains the genetic material responsible for controlling actions that occur in the cell. The genetic material consists of **genes** on **chromosomes** made up of **deoxyribonucleic acid (DNA).** DNA is the "code book" that contains directions for making substances, specifically proteins, the cell needs. This code book remains in the nucleus of the cell, but sends its information to other cell organelles by way of a similar "messenger" molecule called **ribonucleic acid (RNA).** The information on the DNA is copied onto the RNA through the process of **transcription** and then moves out to the cytoplasm through pores in the nuclear membrane. The RNA carries the transcribed DNA code to protein-synthesizing sites called **ribosomes.** There, the RNA code is used in the process of **translation** to make a specific protein (see Chapter 6 for details on protein synthesis). This process is also known as **gene expression.**

All of the DNA in a cell is copied during cell replication. DNA is a double-stranded molecule, and when the cell begins to divide, each strand is separated and an identical copy of each is made. Thus, each new DNA contains one new strand of DNA and one strand from the original DNA. In this way, the genetic code is preserved from one cell generation to the next. (The mitochondria contain their own DNA, so they reproduce themselves within a cell independent of action in the cell's nucleus.)

cytoplasm The fluid and organelles (except the nucleus) in a cell.

anaerobic Not requiring oxygen.

mitochondria The main sites of energy production in a cell. They contain the pathway for oxidizing fat for fuel, among other metabolic pathways.

aerobic Requiring oxygen.

cell nucleus An organelle bound by its own double membrane and containing chromosomes, the genetic information for cell protein synthesis and cell replication.

gene A specific segment on a chromosome. Genes provide the blueprint for the production of cell proteins.

chromosome A single, large DNA molecule and its associated proteins; contains many genes to store and transmit genetic information.

deoxyribonucleic acid (DNA) The site of hereditary information in cells; DNA directs the synthesis of cell proteins.

ribonucleic acid (RNA) The single-stranded nucleic acid involved in the transcription of genetic information and translation of that information into protein structure.

transcription Information on DNA needed to make a protein is copied onto RNA.

ribosomes Cytoplasmic particles that mediate the linking together of amino acids to form proteins; may exist freely in the cytoplasm or attached to endoplasmic reticulum.

translation The information contained in RNA is used to determine the amino acids in a protein.

gene expression Use of DNA information on a gene to produce a protein. Thought to be a major determination of cell development.

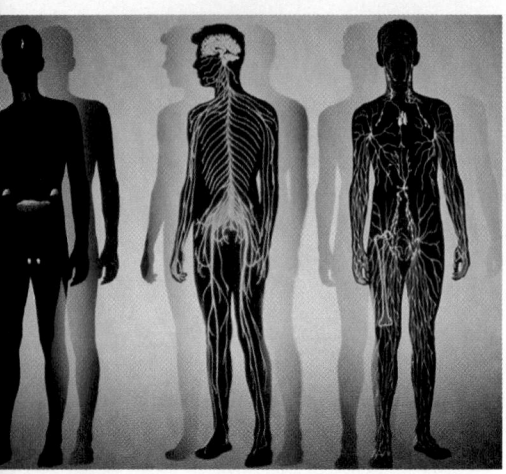

▲ The body is made up of numerous organ systems including the endocrine, nervous, and circulatory systems shown here.

endoplasmic reticulum (ER) An organelle in the cytoplasm composed of a network of canals running through the cytoplasm. Part of the endoplasmic reticulum contains ribosomes.

Golgi complex The cell organelle near the nucleus that processes newly synthesized protein for secretion or distribution to other organelles.

secretory vesicles Membrane-bound vesicles produced by the Golgi apparatus; contain protein and other compounds to be secreted by the cell.

lysosome A cellular organelle that contains digestive enzymes for use inside the cell for turnover of cell parts.

peroxisome A cell organelle that destroys toxic products within the cell.

adenosine triphosphate (ATP) The main energy currency for cells. ATP energy is used to promote ion pumping, enzyme activity, and muscular contraction.

Endoplasmic Reticulum (ER) 5

The outer membrane of the cell nucleus is continuous with a network of tubes called the **endoplasmic reticulum (ER)**. Part of the endoplasmic reticulum (termed the rough [as opposed to smooth] endoplasmic reticulum) contains the ribosomes, where the RNA code is translated into proteins during protein synthesis. Many of these proteins play a central role in human nutrition. Parts of the endoplasmic reticulum also are involved in lipid synthesis, detoxification of toxic substances, and calcium storage and release in the cell.

Golgi Complex 6

The **Golgi complex** is a packaging site for proteins used in the cytoplasm or exported from the cell. It consists of sacs within the cytoplasm in which proteins are "packaged" as **secretory vesicles** for secretion by the cell.

Lysosomes 7

Lysosomes are the cell's digestive system. They are sacs that contain enzymes for the digestion of foreign material. Sometimes known as "suicide bags," they are responsible for digesting worn-out or damaged cell components. Certain cells associated with immune functions contain many lysosomes (see the later section on the immune system).

Peroxisomes 8

Peroxisomes contain enzymes that detoxify harmful chemicals. Peroxisomes get their name from the fact that hydrogen peroxide (H_2O_2) is formed as a result of such enzyme action. Peroxisomes also contain a protective enzyme called *catalase*, which prevents excessive accumulation of hydrogen peroxide in the cell, which would be very damaging. Peroxisomes also play a minor role in metabolizing one possible source of energy for cells—alcohol.

Cell Metabolism

Metabolism refers to the entire network of chemical processes involved in maintaining life. It encompasses all the sequences of chemical reactions that occur in the body's cells. These biochemical reactions take place in the cell cytoplasm and organelles that we have just discussed. They enable us to release and use energy from foods, synthesize one substance from another, and prepare waste products for excretion.

The reactions of metabolism that take place within your body can be categorized into one of two types. One type of reaction, anabolic, puts different molecules together and, therefore, requires energy. The other type of reaction, catabolic, takes molecules apart and, therefore, releases energy. The metabolism of the nutrients, carbohydrates, proteins, and fats are interrelated and yield energy. The other nutrients, vitamins and minerals, contribute to the enzyme activity that supports metabolic reactions in the cell.

The metabolism of energy production begins in the cytoplasm with the initial anaerobic breakdown of glucose. The remaining aerobic steps of energy production take place in the mitochondria. Ultimately, the cells of the body use these interconnected processes to convert the energy found in food to energy stored in the high-energy compound, **adenosine triphosphate (ATP)**. You will learn more about the metabolism of energy sources in Chapter 10, "Nutrition: Fitness and Sports."

CONCEPT CHECK

In Chapter 1, you learned that fat (lipids), protein, and carbohydrate function as fuels. Now you recognize that these nutrients also serve as structural materials in the cell membrane. This is typical of many nutrients; they can carry out multiple functions. The cell receives nutrients and other substances through the cell membrane by using various transport systems.

The basic structural unit in the body is the cell. Within the cell are a variety of organelles with unique functions to perform. Although there is no typical cell, virtually all cells have the same organelles, each performing the same essential task.

3.3 Body Systems

As noted earlier, when groups of similar cells work together to accomplish a specialized task, the arrangement is referred to as a tissue. Humans are composed of four primary types of tissue: **epithelial, connective, muscle,** and **nervous.** Epithelial tissue is composed of cells that cover surfaces both inside and outside the body. For example, the lining of the respiratory tract is made up of epithelial cells. These cells of epithelial tissue secrete important substances, absorb nutrients, and excrete waste. Connective tissue supports and protects the body, stores fat, and produces blood cells. Muscle tissue is designed for movement. Nervous tissue found in the brain and spinal cord is designed for communication. These four types of tissues then go on to form various organs, and ultimately, organ systems (Table 3-1).

We will focus primarily on the digestive system in Chapter 3. The nutrients we consume in food are unavailable until such time as they have been processed by the digestive system. This employs chemical and mechanical means to alter food so that the nutrients can be released and absorbed into the body for distribution to body tissues.

Sometimes organs within a system can serve another system. For example, the basic function of the digestive system is to convert the food we eat into absorbable nutrients. At the same time, the digestive system serves the immune system by preventing dangerous pathogens from invading the body and causing illness. As you study nutrition, you will note the multiple roles played by many organs (Fig. 3-3).

The overriding theme of human nutrition is to understand the actions of nutrients as they affect different cells, tissues, organs, and organ systems. Each type of organ system is impacted by nutrient intake and simultaneously determines how each nutrient is used.

Our task now is to explore the key systems in the body as they specifically relate to the study of human nutrition: circulatory (cardiovascular and lymphatic), nervous, endocrine, immune, digestive, and urinary systems. This part of Chapter 3 will set the stage for a more detailed look at these and other organ systems in later chapters covering various aspects of human nutrition.

Also in this chapter, we will introduce the emerging area of genetics and nutrition. Throughout this book, discussions will point out how you can personalize nutrition advice based on your genetic background. In this way, you can identify and avoid the "controllable" risk factors that would contribute to development of genetically linked diseases present in your family.

3.4 Cardiovascular System and Lymphatic System

The body has two separate organ systems that circulate fluids in the body: the **cardiovascular system** and the **lymphatic system.** The cardiovascular system consists of the heart and blood vessels. The lymphatic system consists of lymphatic vessels and

epithelial tissue The surface cells that line the outside of the body and all external passages within it.

connective tissue Protein tissue that holds different structures in the body together. Some body structures are made up of connective tissue—notably, tendons and cartilage. Connective tissue also forms part of bone and the nonmuscular structures of arteries and veins.

muscle tissue A type of tissue adapted to contract to cause movement.

nervous tissue Tissue composed of highly branched, elongated cells, which transport nerve impulses from one part of the body to another.

cardiovascular system The body system consisting of the heart, blood vessels, and blood. This system transports nutrients, waste products, gases, and hormones throughout the body and plays an important role in immune responses and regulation of body temperature.

lymphatic system A system of vessels and lymph that accepts fluid surrounding cells and large particles, such as products of fat absorption. Lymph eventually passes into the bloodstream from the lymphatic system.

TABLE 3-1 Organ Systems of the Body

System	Major Components	Functions Related to Nutrition
Cardiovascular	Heart, blood vessels, and blood	Transports nutrients, waste products, gases, and hormones throughout the body and plays a role in the immune response and the regulation of body temperature
Lymphatic	Lymph vessels, lymph nodes, and other lymph organs	Removes foreign substances from the blood and lymph, combats disease, maintains tissue fluid balance, and aids in fat absorption
Nervous	Brain, spinal cord, nerves, and sensory receptors	A major regulatory system: detects sensation, controls movements, and controls physiological and intellectual functions
Endocrine	Endocrine glands, such as the pituitary, thyroid, and adrenal glands	A major regulatory system: participates in the regulation of metabolism, reproduction, and many other functions through the action of hormones
Immune	White blood cells, lymph vessels and nodes, spleen, thymus gland, and other lymph tissues	Provides defense against foreign invaders; formation of white blood cells
Digestive	Mouth, esophagus, stomach, intestines, and accessory structures (liver, gallbladder, and pancreas)	Performs the mechanical and chemical processes of digestion, absorption of nutrients, and elimination of wastes
Urinary	Kidneys, urinary bladder, and the ducts that carry urine	Removes waste products from the circulatory system and regulates the acidity, chemical composition, and water content of the blood
Integumentary	Skin, hair, nails, and sweat glands	Protects the body, regulates temperature, prevents water loss, and produces a substance that converts to vitamin D upon sun exposure
Skeletal	Bones, associated cartilage, and joints	Supports the body, and allows for body movement, produces blood cells, and stores minerals
Muscular	Smooth, cardiac, and skeletal muscle	Produces body movement, maintains posture, and produces body heat
Respiratory	Lungs and respiratory passages	Exchanges gases (oxygen and carbon dioxide) between the blood and the atmosphere and regulates blood acid-base (pH) balance
Reproductive	Gonads, accessory structures, and genitals of males and females	Performs the processes of reproduction and influences sexual functions and behaviors

lymph A clear fluid that flows through lymph vessels; carries most forms of fat after their absorption by the small intestine.

plasma The fluid, extracellular portion of the circulating blood. This includes the blood serum plus all blood-clotting factors. In contrast, serum is the fluid that remains after clotting factors have been removed from plasma.

a number of lymph tissues. Blood flows through the cardiovascular system, while **lymph** flows through the lymphatic system.

Cardiovascular System

The heart is a muscular pump that normally contracts and relaxes 50 to 90 times per minute when the body is at rest. This continual pumping, measured by taking your pulse, keeps blood moving through the blood vessels. The blood that flows through the cardiovascular system is composed of **plasma**, red blood cells, white blood cells, platelets, and many other substances. It travels two basic routes. In the first route, blood circulates from the right side of the heart, through the lungs, and then back to the heart. In the lungs, blood picks up oxygen and releases carbon dioxide. After this exchange of gases has taken place, blood is said to be *oxygenated* and returns to the left side of your heart. In the second route, the oxygenated blood circulates from the left side of the heart to all other body cells, eventually returning back to the right side of the heart (Fig. 3-4). After blood has circulated throughout the body, it is *deoxygenated*. (As you review the cardiovascular system, recall from your previous studies of biology that *left* and *right* designations of the heart refer to the left and right sides of your body, not of the page in your textbook.)

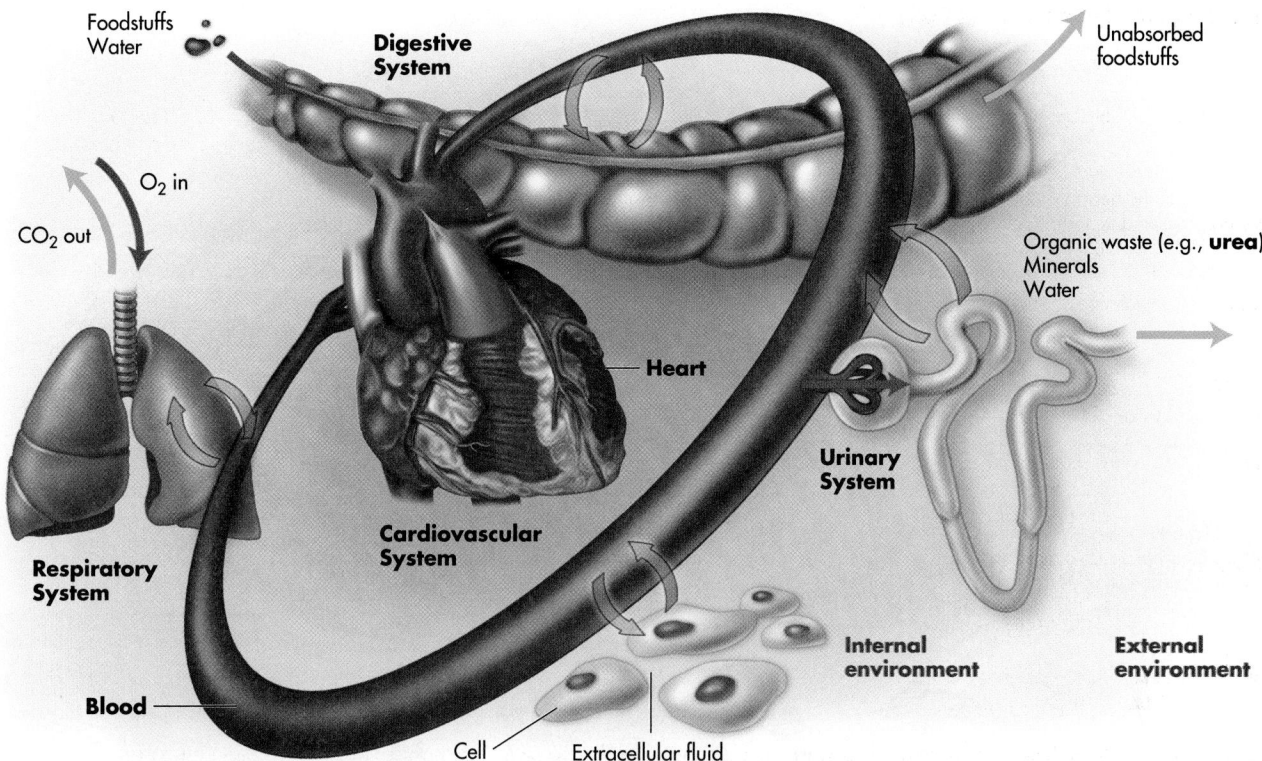

FIGURE 3-3 ▶ Exchanges of nutrients occur between our external environment and the internal environment of the circulatory system via the digestive, respiratory, and urinary systems. Overall, the human body is a combination of 12 systems working together to support cell needs.

In the cardiovascular system, blood leaves the heart via **arteries,** which branch into **capillaries,** a network of tiny blood vessels. Exchange of nutrients, oxygen, and waste products between the blood and cells occurs through the minute, web-like pores of the capillaries (Fig. 3-5). Capillaries service every region of the body via individual capillary beds only one cell layer thick. The blood then returns to the heart via the **veins.**

The cardiovascular system distributes nutrients absorbed from food and oxygen from the air to all body cells (review Fig. 3-3). Other functions include delivery of hormones to their target cells, maintenance of a constant body temperature, and distribution of white blood cells throughout the body to protect against pathogens as part of the immune system (see the later section, "Immune System").

Portal Circulation in the Gastrointestinal Tract. Water and nutrients are transferred to the circulatory system through capillary beds. Once absorbed through the stomach or intestinal wall, nutrients reach one of two destinations. Some nutrients are taken up by cells in the intestines and portions of the stomach to nourish those organs. Most of the nutrients from recently eaten foods, however, are transferred into **portal circulation.** To enter portal circulation, the nutrients pass from the intestinal capillaries into veins that eventually merge into a very large vein called a **portal vein.** Unlike most veins in the body—which carry blood back to the heart—this portal vein leads directly to the liver. This enables the liver to process absorbed nutrients before they enter the general circulation of the bloodstream. Overall, portal circulation represents a special form of circulation in the cardiovascular system.

Lymphatic System

The **lymphatic system** is also a circulatory system. It consists of a network of lymphatic vessels and the fluid (lymph) that moves through them. Lymph is similar to

artery A blood vessel that carries blood away from the heart.

capillary A microscopic blood vessel that connects the smallest arteries and veins; site of nutrient, oxygen, and waste exchange between body cells and the blood.

vein A blood vessel that carries blood to the heart.

portal circulation The portion of the circulatory system that uses a large vein (portal vein) to carry nutrient-rich blood from capillaries in the intestines and portions of the stomach to the liver.

urea Nitrogenous waste product of protein metabolism; major source of nitrogen in the urine.

portal vein Large vein leaving the intestine and stomach and connecting to the liver.

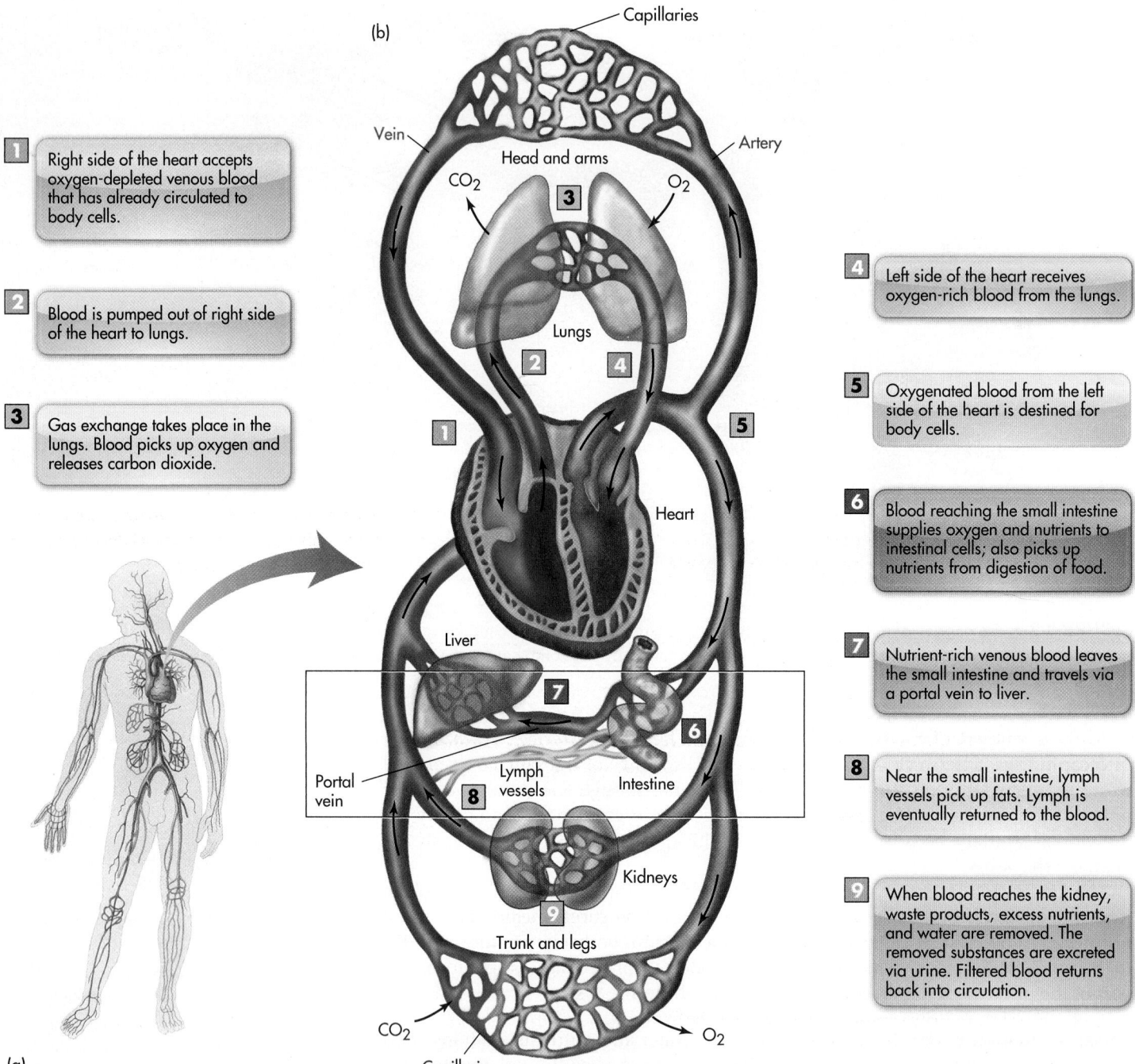

(b)

Capillaries

1 Right side of the heart accepts oxygen-depleted venous blood that has already circulated to body cells.

2 Blood is pumped out of right side of the heart to lungs.

3 Gas exchange takes place in the lungs. Blood picks up oxygen and releases carbon dioxide.

Vein

Head and arms

Artery

CO_2 **3** O_2

Lungs

2 **4**

1

Heart

5

4 Left side of the heart receives oxygen-rich blood from the lungs.

5 Oxygenated blood from the left side of the heart is destined for body cells.

6 Blood reaching the small intestine supplies oxygen and nutrients to intestinal cells; also picks up nutrients from digestion of food.

7 Nutrient-rich venous blood leaves the small intestine and travels via a portal vein to liver.

8 Near the small intestine, lymph vessels pick up fats. Lymph is eventually returned to the blood.

9 When blood reaches the kidney, waste products, excess nutrients, and water are removed. The removed substances are excreted via urine. Filtered blood returns back into circulation.

Liver

7

6

Portal vein

Lymph vessels

8

Intestine

Kidneys

9

Trunk and legs

CO_2 O_2

Capillaries

(a)

FIGURE 3-4 ▶ Blood circulation through the body. Figure (a) shows the heart and some examples of the major arteries and veins of the cardiovascular system. Figure (b) shows the paths that blood takes from the heart to the lungs (**1**–**3**), back to the heart (**4**), and through the rest of the body (**5**–**9**). The red color indicates blood richer in oxygen; blue is for blood carrying more carbon dioxide. Keep in mind that arteries and veins go to all parts of the body.

blood, consisting largely of blood plasma that has found its way out of capillaries and into the spaces between cells. It contains a full array of the various white blood cells that play an important role in the immune system. However, neither red blood cells nor platelets are present. Lymph is collected in tiny lymph vessels all over the body and moves through even larger vessels until it eventually enters the cardiovascular system through major veins near the heart. This flow is driven by muscle contractions arising from normal body movements.

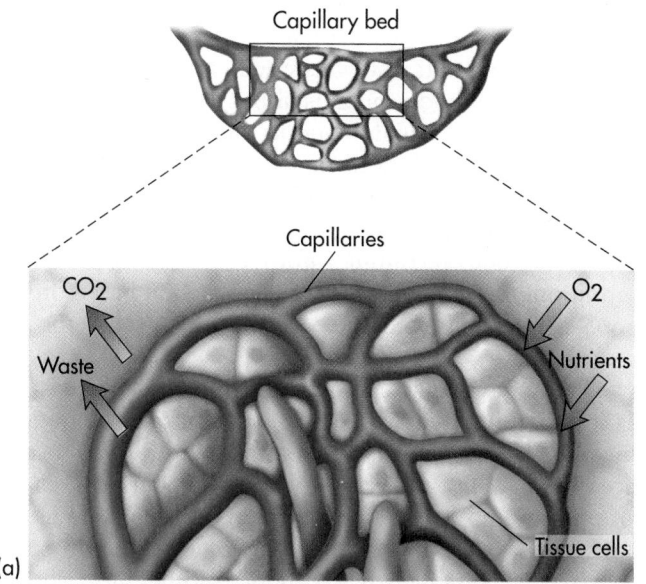

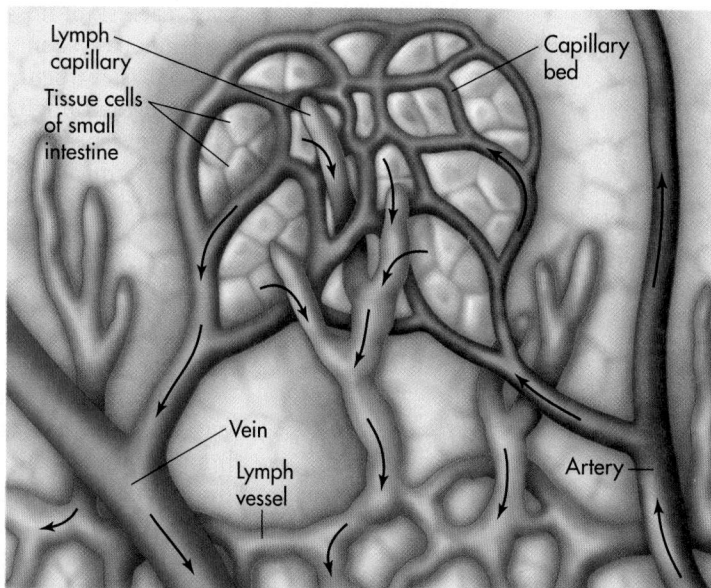

FIGURE 3-5 ▶ Capillary and lymph vessels. (a) Exchange of oxygen (O_2) and nutrients for carbon dioxide (CO_2) and waste products occurs between the capillaries and the surrounding tissue cells. (b) Lymph vessels are also present in capillary beds, such as in the small intestine. Lymph vessels in the small intestine are also called lacteals. The lymph vessels have closed ends and are important for fat absorption.

Lymphatic Circulation in the Gastrointestinal Tract. Besides contributing to the defense of the body against invading pathogens, lymphatic vessels that serve the small intestine play an important role in nutrition. These vessels pick up and transport the majority of products of fat digestion and fat absorption. These fat-related products are too large to enter the bloodstream directly and therefore are generally emptied into the bloodstream only after passing through the lymphatic system. The lymph vessels also take up excess fluid that collects between cells and returns it to the bloodstream.

_____ **CONCEPT CHECK** _____

Blood is transported from the right side of the heart to the capillaries in the lungs. Carbon dioxide is removed and oxygen is taken up by red blood cells. The oxygenated blood returns to the left side of the heart. Here it is pumped into general circulation. In the capillaries, oxygen is released from the red blood cells and delivered through pores in the capillaries to the surrounding cells. Nutrients also are distributed from the bloodstream to body cells via the capillaries. Carbon dioxide released from cells travels through the capillary pores to the blood.

The lymph system serves several purposes: the transport of absorbed dietary fats, the uptake and return to the bloodstream of excess fluid that collects between cells, and the defense of the body against invading pathogens.

3.5 Nervous System

The **nervous system** is a regulatory system that centrally controls most body functions. The nervous system can detect changes occurring in various organs and the external environment and initiate corrective action when needed to maintain a constant internal body environment. The nervous system also regulates activities that change almost instantly, such as muscle contractions and perception of danger. The body has many receptors that receive information about what is happening within the body and in the outside environment. For the most part these receptors are found in our

nervous system The body system consisting of the brain, spinal cord, nerves, and sensory receptors. This system detects sensations, directs movements, and controls physiological and intellectual functions.

neuron The structural and functional unit of the nervous system. Consists of a cell body, dendrites, and an axon.

synapse The space between one neuron and another neuron (or cell).

neurotransmitter A compound made by a nerve cell that allows for communication between it and other cells.

eyes, ears, skin, nose, and stomach. We act on information from these receptors via the nervous system.

The basic structural and functional unit of the nervous system is the **neuron.** These are elongated, highly branched cells. The body contains about 100 billion neurons. Neurons respond to electrical and chemical signals, conduct electrical impulses, and release chemical regulators. Overall, neurons allow us to perceive what is occurring in our environment, engage in learning, store vital information in memory, and control the body's voluntary (and involuntary) actions.

The brain stores information, reacts to incoming information, solves problems, and generates thoughts. In addition, the brain plans a course of action based on the other sensory inputs. Responses to the stimuli are carried out mostly through the rest of the nervous system.

Simply put, the nervous system receives information through stimulation of various receptors, processes this information, and sends out signals through its various branches for an action that needs to be taken. Actual transmission of the signal occurs through a change in the concentration of two nutrients, sodium and potassium, in the neuron. There is an influx of sodium into the neuron and a loss of potassium as the message is sent. Concentrations of these minerals are then restored to normal amounts in the neuron after the signal passes, making it ready to conduct another message.

When the signal must bridge a gap **(synapse)** between the branches of different neurons, the message is generally converted to a chemical signal called a **neurotransmitter.** The neurotransmitter is then released into the gap, and its target may be another neuron or another type of cell, such as a muscle cell (Fig. 3-6). If the signal is sent to another neuron, this allows it to continue on to its final destination. The neurotransmitters

FIGURE 3-6 ▶ Transmission of a message from one neuron to another neuron or to another type of cell that relies on neurotransmitters. Vesicles containing neurotransmitters, formed within the neuron, fuse with the membrane of the neuron and the neurotransmitter is released into the synapse. The neurotransmitter then binds to the receptors on the nearby neuron (or cell). In this way, the message is transmitted from one neuron to another or to the cell that ultimately performs the action directed by the message.

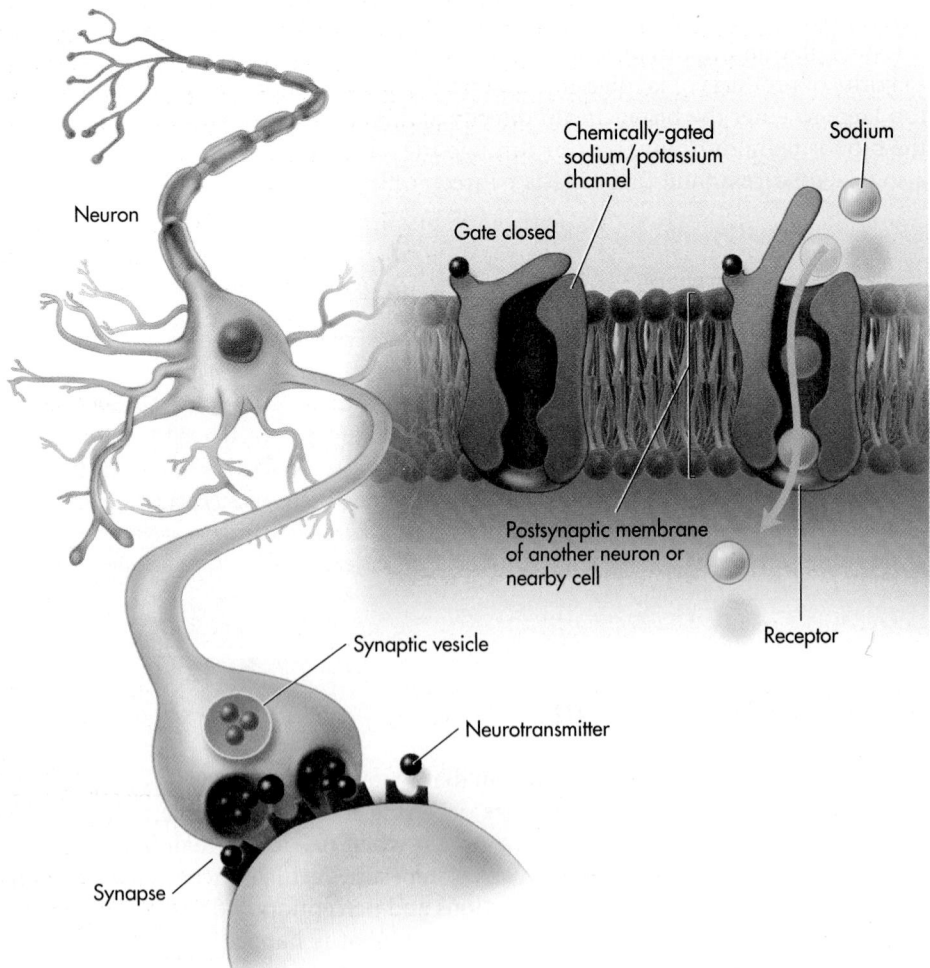

used in this process are often made from common nutrients found in foods, such as amino acids. The amino acid tryptophan is converted to the neurotransmitter serotonin, and the amino acid tyrosine is converted to the neurotransmitters **norepinephrine** and **epinephrine** (also called adrenaline).

Other nutrients also play a role in the nervous system. Calcium is needed for the release of neurotransmitters from neurons. Vitamin B-12 plays a role in the formation of the **myelin sheath,** which provides insulation around specific parts of most neurons. Finally, a regular supply of carbohydrate in the form of glucose is important for supplying fuel for the brain. The brain can use other calorie sources, but generally relies on glucose.

3.6 Endocrine System

The **endocrine system** plays a major role in the regulation of metabolism, reproduction, water balance, and many other functions by producing hormones in the **endocrine glands** of the body and subsequently releasing them into the blood (Table 3-2). The term *hormone* comes from the Greek word for "to stir or excite." A true hormone is a regulatory compound that has a specific site of synthesis from which it then enters the bloodstream to reach target cells. Hormones are the messengers of the body. They can be permissive (turn on), antagonistic (turn off), or synergistic (work in cooperation with another hormone) in performing a task. Some compounds must undergo chemical changes before they can function as hormones. For example, vitamin D, synthesized in the skin or obtained from food, is converted into an active hormone by chemical changes made in the liver and kidneys.

The hormone **insulin,** synthesized in and released from the pancreas, helps control the amount of glucose in the blood (Fig. 3-7). Insulin is mostly produced when glucose in the blood rises to a certain level, usually after a meal. At this point, insulin is released and it travels to the muscle, adipose, and liver cells of the body. Among its many functions, insulin allows for the movement of glucose from the blood into muscle and adipose cells. In the liver cells, insulin causes an increase in stored glycogen by stimulating the synthesis of glycogen from glucose. Once a sufficient amount of glucose has been cleared from the blood, the production of insulin lessens. The hormones epinephrine, norepinephrine, glucagon, and growth hormone have just the opposite effect on blood glucose. They all cause an increase in blood glucose through a variety of actions (Table 3-2). **Thyroid hormones,** synthesized in and released from the thyroid gland

norepinephrine A neurotransmitter from nerve endings and a hormone from the adrenal gland. It is released in times of stress and is involved in hunger regulation, blood glucose regulation, and other body processes.

epinephrine A hormone also known as *adrenaline;* it is released by the adrenal glands (located on each kidney) at times of stress. It acts to increase glycogen breakdown in the liver, among other functions.

myelin sheath A lipid and protein combination (lipoprotein) that covers nerve fibers.

endocrine system The body system consisting of the various glands and the hormones these glands secrete. This system has major regulatory functions in the body, such as reproduction and cell metabolism.

endocrine gland A hormone-producing gland.

thyroid hormones Hormones produced by the thyroid gland that among their functions increase the rate of overall metabolism in the body.

TABLE 3-2 Some Hormones of the Endocrine System with Nutritional Significance

Hormone	Gland/Organ	Target	Effect	Role in Nutrition
Insulin	Pancreas	Adipose (fat) and muscle cells	Decreased blood glucose	Uptake and storage of glucose, fat, and amino acids by cells
Glucagon	Pancreas	Liver	Increased blood glucose	Release of glucose from liver stores, release of fat from adipose tissue
Epinephrine, Norepinephrine	Adrenal glands	Heart, blood vessels, brain, lungs	Increased body metabolism and blood glucose	Release of glucose and fat into the blood
Growth hormone	Pituitary gland	Most cells	Promotion of amino acid uptake by cells, increased blood glucose	Promotion of protein synthesis and growth, increased fat use for energy
Thyroid hormones	Thyroid gland	Most organs	Increased oxygen consumption, overall growth, brain development of the nervous system	Protein synthesis, increased body metabolism

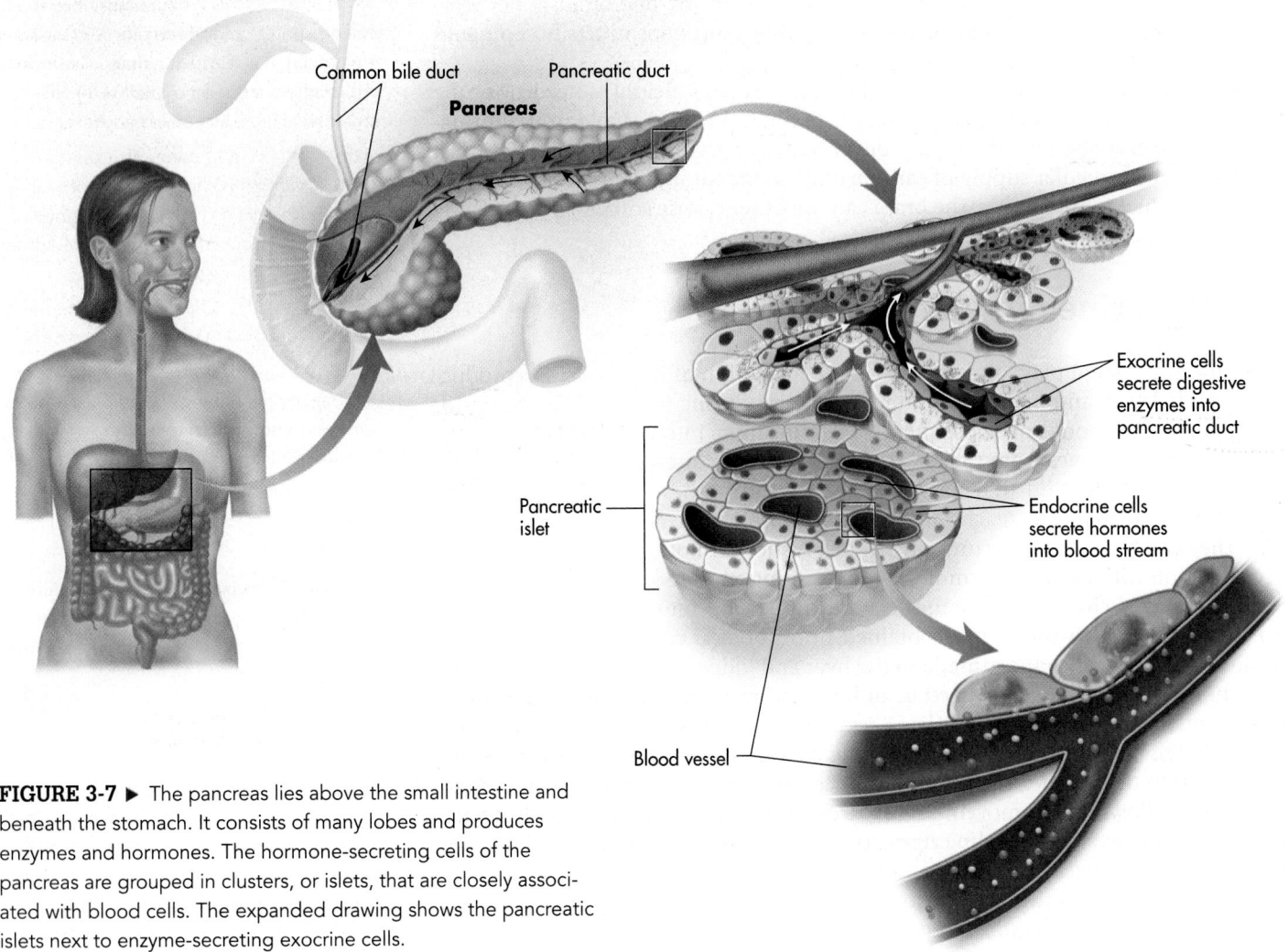

FIGURE 3-7 ▶ The pancreas lies above the small intestine and beneath the stomach. It consists of many lobes and produces enzymes and hormones. The hormone-secreting cells of the pancreas are grouped in clusters, or islets, that are closely associated with blood cells. The expanded drawing shows the pancreatic islets next to enzyme-secreting exocrine cells.

help to control the body's rate of metabolism. Other hormones are especially important in regulating digestive processes (see the later section, "Digestive System").

Hormones are not taken up by all cells in the body, but only those with the correct **receptor** protein. These binding sites are highly specific for a certain hormone. They are generally found on the cell membrane. The hormone attaches to its receptor on the cell membrane. This binding activates additional compounds called second messengers within the cell to carry out the assigned task. This is true of insulin. A few hormones can penetrate the cell membrane and eventually bind to receptors on the DNA in the nucleus (e.g., thyroid hormone and estrogen).

receptor A site in a cell at which compounds (such as hormones) bind. Cells that contain receptors for a specific compound are partially controlled by that compound.

CONCEPT CHECK

The functional unit of the nervous system is the neuron. Communication between neurons themselves, and other types of cells, is via neurotransmitters released into the synapse between the cells.

In the endocrine system, hormones are produced by glands in response to a change in the internal or external environment of the body. The gland secretes the hormone into the blood, and the blood delivers it to target cells. The hormone either attaches to receptors in the cell membrane and, through the action of second messengers, causes changes within the cell, or enters the cell and binds to the DNA in the cell to cause changes within the cell.

3.7 Immune System

Many types of body cells and body components work in cooperation as part of the **immune system** to maintain a defense against infection (Fig. 3-8). The components that work as part of the immune system include the skin, intestinal cells, and white blood cells. Several nutrients, including protein; minerals iron, copper, and zinc; and vitamins A, B-6, B-12, C, and folate have important roles in the immune system. These nutrients are key factors in the synthesis, growth, development, and activity of immune cells and additional factors that kill pathogens. It is easy to demonstrate the importance of nutritional health for immune function. Early humans were plagued by famine and thus, malnutrition; this contributed to infections, often leading to death. Today, largely because of better nutrition, most of the world avoids that cycle.

We are born with most aspects of immune function; these are termed **non-specific** (or innate) because the targets are a variety of microorganisms. In contrast, white blood cells produce **immunoglobulins,** also called **antibodies,** that target specific organisms or foreign proteins called **antigens.** These immunoglobulins constitute **specific** (or adaptive) immune function. Once exposed, a memory is created such that a second exposure to the substance will produce a more vigorous and rapid attack.

Skin

The skin is a large component of the immune system, forming an almost continuous barrier surrounding the body. Invading microorganisms have difficulty penetrating the skin. However, if the skin is split by lesions, bacteria can easily penetrate this barrier. Skin health is poor during deficiencies of such nutrients as essential fatty acids, vitamin A, niacin, and zinc. Vitamin A deficiency also decreases gland secretions in the skin that contain the enzyme **lysozyme,** capable of killing bacteria. Bacterial eye infections are common in developing countries, often as a result of a vitamin A deficiency.

Intestinal Cells

The cells of the intestines form an important barrier to invading microorganisms. The cells are packed closely together, producing a physical barrier to microorganisms. In addition, specialized cells that produce immune factors—such as immunoglobulins—are scattered throughout the intestinal tract. These immune factors bind to the invading microorganisms, preventing them from entering the bloodstream. These factors are part of the mucosal membrane aspect of immunity.

Nutrient deficiencies can cause the intestinal cells to break down weakening the mucosal membrane so that microorganisms more easily enter the body and cause infections. Thus, two common results of undernutrition related to an impaired immune system are diarrhea and bacterial infections of the bloodstream. To protect the health of the intestinal tract, an adequate nutrient intake is necessary—especially of protein, vitamin A, vitamin B-6, vitamin B-12, vitamin C, folate, and zinc.

MAKING DECISIONS

Immune Status

Although many studies show that a healthy nutritional state is associated with good immune status, other studies show that an overabundance of certain nutrients can harm the immune system. For example, taking too much zinc may decrease immune function (see Chapter 9).

FIGURE 3-8 ▶ Just as the roof and other external structures of a house protect the inside environment from outside elements, host protective factors (shown on the bricks) of the immune system "shelter" humans from threats such as diseases and toxins (shown in the rain).

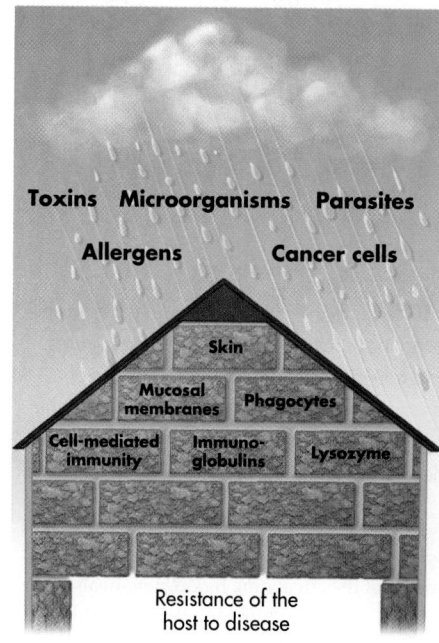

immune system The body system consisting of white blood cells, lymph glands and vessels, and various other body tissues. The immune system provides defense against foreign invaders, primarily due to the action of various types of white blood cells.

non-specific immunity Defenses that stop the invasion of pathogens; requires no previous encounter with a pathogen.

immunoglobulins Proteins found in the blood that bind to specific antigens; also called antibodies. The five major classes of immunoglobulins play different roles in antibody-mediated immunity.

antigen Any substance that induces a state of sensitivity and/or resistance to microorganisms or toxic substances after a lag period; foreign substance that stimulates a specific aspect of the immune system.

antibody Blood protein (immunoglobulin) that binds foreign proteins found in the body. This helps to prevent and control infections.

specific immunity Function of lymphocytes directed at specific antigens.

lysozyme An enzyme produced by a variety of cells; it can destroy bacteria by rupturing their cell membranes.

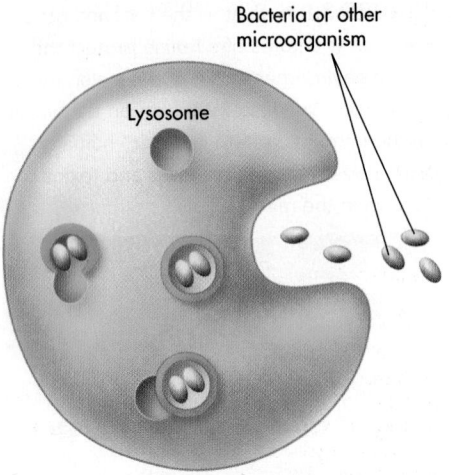

Bacteria or other microorganism

Lysosome

Phagocyte

FIGURE 3-9 ▶ One class of white blood cell, phagocytes, can ingest bacteria, fungi, viruses, and other foreign particles in the process of phagocytosis. An indentation is formed and the particle is engulfed by the cell. The foreign material is eventually digested by lysosomes in the cell.

white blood cells One of the formed elements of the circulating blood system; also called *leukocytes*. White blood cells are able to squeeze through intracellular spaces and migrate. They phagocytize bacteria, fungi, and viruses, as well as detoxify proteins that may result from allergic reactions, cellular injury, and other immune system cells.

phagocytes Cells that engulf substances; include neutrophils and macrophages.

phagocytosis Process in which a cell forms an indentation, and particles or fluids enter the indentation and are engulfed by the cell.

cell-mediated immunity A process in which certain white blood cells come in contact with the invading cells to destroy them.

digestive system System consisting of the gastrointestinal tract and accessory structures (liver, gallbladder, and pancreas). This system performs the mechanical and chemical processes of digestion, absorption of nutrients, and elimination of wastes.

digestion Process by which large ingested molecules are mechanically and chemically broken down to produce basic nutrients that can be absorbed across the wall of the GI tract.

absorption The process by which substances are taken up from the GI tract and enter the bloodstream or the lymph.

White Blood Cells

Once a microorganism enters the bloodstream, **white blood cells** move in to attack it. Several types of white blood cells participate in this response and function in unique ways. For example, a class called **phagocytes** circulates throughout the circulatory system and ingests and sometimes digests microorganisms and foreign particles (via lysosomes present in the cells) in a process called **phagocytosis** (Fig. 3-9). Other white blood cells participate in **cell-mediated immunity**, achieved when certain immune cells recognize foreign cells or proteins and directly attack and destroy them. Immunoglobulins, also known as antibodies and made by these cells, elicit an antibody-antigen response that binds microorganisms and proteins that are foreign to the body and destroys them, and then creates a template (memory) that allows future recognition of the microorganism or foreign protein. Recognition allows more rapid attacks in the future.

Some white blood cells live only a few days. Their constant resynthesis requires steady nutrient intake. The immune system needs the following nutrients: (1) iron to produce an important killing factor; (2) copper for synthesis of a specific type of white blood cell; and (3) protein, vitamin B-6, vitamin B-12, vitamin C, and folate for general cell synthesis and, later, cell activity. Zinc and vitamin A are also needed for the overall growth and development of immune cells.

CONCEPT CHECK

Many types of body cells and body components work in cooperation as part of the immune system to maintain a defense against infection. The skin forms an almost continuous barrier surrounding the body. Cell secretions contain the enzyme lysozyme. Specialized cells in the intestines and certain white blood cells secrete antibodies (immunoglobulins). Phagocytes roam throughout the circulatory system and ingest and sometimes digest microorganisms and foreign particles. Other white blood cells participate in cell-mediated immunity. This occurs when certain immune cells recognize foreign cells and directly attack them. Many nutrients, including protein, iron, copper, zinc, vitamin B-6, B-12, C, and folate, are needed for the overall growth and development of immune cells.

3.8 Digestive System

The foods and beverages we consume, for the most part, must undergo extensive alteration by the **digestive system** to provide us with usable nutrients. The processes of **digestion** and **absorption** take place in a long tube that is open at both ends and extends from the mouth to the anus. This tube is called the **gastrointestinal (GI) tract** (Fig. 3-10). Nutrients from the food we eat must pass through the walls of the GI tract—from the inside to the outside—to be absorbed into the bloodstream. The organs that make up the GI tract, as well as some additional accessory organs located nearby, are collectively known as the digestive system.

In the digestive system, food is broken down mechanically and chemically. Mechanical digestion takes place as soon as you begin chewing your food and continues as muscular contractions simultaneously mix and move food through the length of the GI tract (as part of a process known as **motility**). Chemical digestion refers to the chemical breakdown of foods by substances secreted into the GI tract. Finally, the digestive system eliminates wastes. In addition to nutrients that arise from digestion of food, the bacteria that live in the large intestine produce vitamin K and the vitamin biotin, some of which we can absorb and use.

Most of the processes of digestion and absorption are under autonomic control; that is, they are involuntary. Almost all of the functions involved in digestion and absorption are controlled by signals from the nervous system, hormones from the

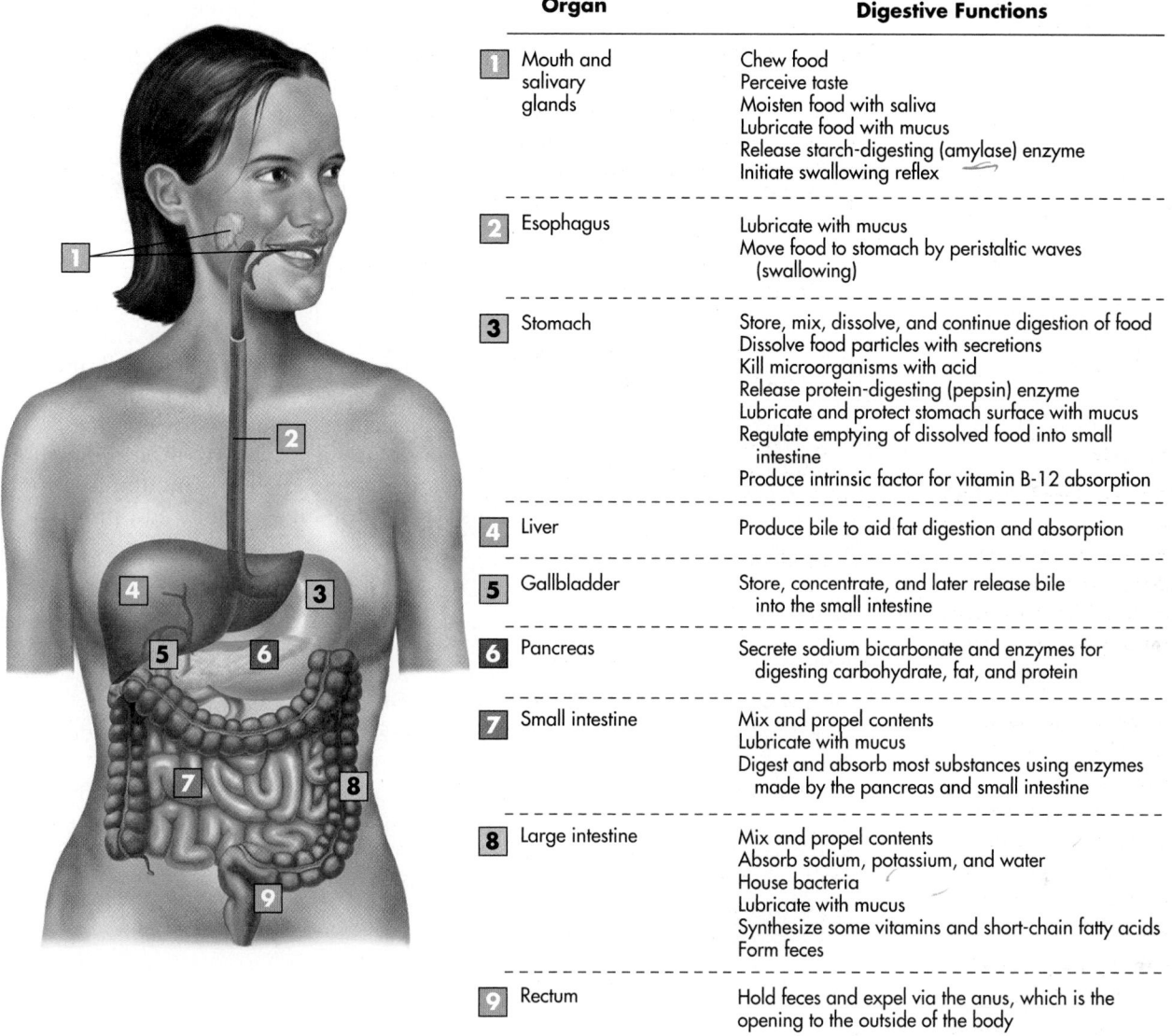

Organ	Digestive Functions
1 Mouth and salivary glands	Chew food Perceive taste Moisten food with saliva Lubricate food with mucus Release starch-digesting (amylase) enzyme Initiate swallowing reflex
2 Esophagus	Lubricate with mucus Move food to stomach by peristaltic waves (swallowing)
3 Stomach	Store, mix, dissolve, and continue digestion of food Dissolve food particles with secretions Kill microorganisms with acid Release protein-digesting (pepsin) enzyme Lubricate and protect stomach surface with mucus Regulate emptying of dissolved food into small intestine Produce intrinsic factor for vitamin B-12 absorption
4 Liver	Produce bile to aid fat digestion and absorption
5 Gallbladder	Store, concentrate, and later release bile into the small intestine
6 Pancreas	Secrete sodium bicarbonate and enzymes for digesting carbohydrate, fat, and protein
7 Small intestine	Mix and propel contents Lubricate with mucus Digest and absorb most substances using enzymes made by the pancreas and small intestine
8 Large intestine	Mix and propel contents Absorb sodium, potassium, and water House bacteria Lubricate with mucus Synthesize some vitamins and short-chain fatty acids Form feces
9 Rectum	Hold feces and expel via the anus, which is the opening to the outside of the body

FIGURE 3-10 ▶ Physiology of the GI tract. Many organs cooperate in a regulated fashion to allow the digestion and absorption of nutrients in foods.

endocrine system, and hormone-like compounds. Many common ailments arise from problems with the digestive system. Several of these digestive problems are discussed in the "Nutrition and Your Health" section at the end of this chapter.

The digestive system is composed of six separate organs; each organ performs one, or more, specific job(s). Let's look briefly at the role of each organ. These organs are listed in Figure 3-10 and in the flowchart on the next page. More detailed descriptions of digestive processes will be explained in later chapters as each nutrient is introduced.

Mouth

The mouth performs many functions in the digestion of food. Besides chewing food to reduce it to smaller particles, the mouth also senses the taste of the foods we consume. The tongue, through the use of its taste buds, identifies foods on the basis of their specific flavor(s). Sweet, sour, salty, bitter, and **umami** comprise the primary taste sensations we experience. Surprisingly, the nose and our sense of smell greatly contribute to our ability to sense the taste of food. When we chew a food, chemicals are released that stimulate the nasal passages. Thus, it makes perfect sense that when

gastrointestinal (GI) tract The main sites in the body used for digestion and absorption of nutrients. It consists of the mouth, esophagus, stomach, small intestine, large intestine, rectum, and anus. Also called the *digestive tract*.

motility Generally, the ability to move spontaneously. It also refers to movement of food through the GI tract.

umami A brothy, meaty, savory flavor in some foods. Monosodium glutamate enhances this flavor when added to foods.

GI Tract Components and Flow

Mouth

↓

Esophagus (10 inches long)

↓

Stomach—4-cup (1-liter) capacity. Food remains about 2 to 3 hours, or longer for large meals.

↓

Small intestine—duodenum (10 in long), jejunum (4 ft long), ileum (5 ft long)—about 10 ft (3.1 meters) in total length. Food remains about 3 to 10 hours.

↓

Large intestine (colon)—cecum, ascending colon, transverse colon, descending colon, sigmoid colon—3½ ft (1.1 meters) in total length. Food can remain up to 72 hours.

↓

Rectum

↓

Anus

saliva Watery fluid, produced by the salivary glands in the mouth, that contains lubricants, enzymes, and other substances.

salivary amylase A starch-digesting enzyme produced by salivary glands.

we have a cold and our noses are stuffed up and congested, even our most favorite foods will not taste as good as they normally do.

The taste of food, or the anticipation of it, signals the rest of the GI tract to prepare for the digestion of food. Once in the mouth, mechanical and chemical digestion begins. Salivary glands produce **saliva,** which functions as a solvent so that food particles can be further separated and tasted. In addition, saliva contains a starch-digesting enzyme, **salivary amylase** (see Chapter 4 for more on starch-digesting enzymes).

Enzymes are a key part of digestion. Each enzyme is specific to one type of chemical process. For example, enzymes that recognize and digest table sugar (sucrose) ignore milk sugar (lactose). Besides working on only specific types of chemicals, enzymes are sensitive to acidic and alkaline conditions, temperature, and the types of vitamins and minerals they require. Digestive enzymes that work in the acidic environment of the stomach do not work well in the alkaline environment of the small intestine. Overall, enzymes work to hasten certain events that take place in the body (Fig. 3-11).

The pancreas and the small intestine produce most of the digestive enzymes; however, the mouth and the stomach also contribute their own enzymes to digestion. **Mucus,** another component of saliva, makes it easy to swallow a mouthful of food. The food then travels to the esophagus. The important secretions and products of digestion are listed in Table 3-3.

MAKING DECISIONS

Enzymes and Digestion

The authors of some popular (fad) diet books contend that eating certain combinations of foods, such as meats and fruits together, hinders the digestive process. However, does this make sense in light of our newly gained knowledge about GI tract physiology? The body is able to increase the production of certain digestive enzymes in response to the type of diet consumed. The GI tract can respond to the nutritional makeup and amount of food consumed because of this fine-tuning. Once consumed, foods are attacked by multiple enzymes to release nutrients and other compounds for absorption.

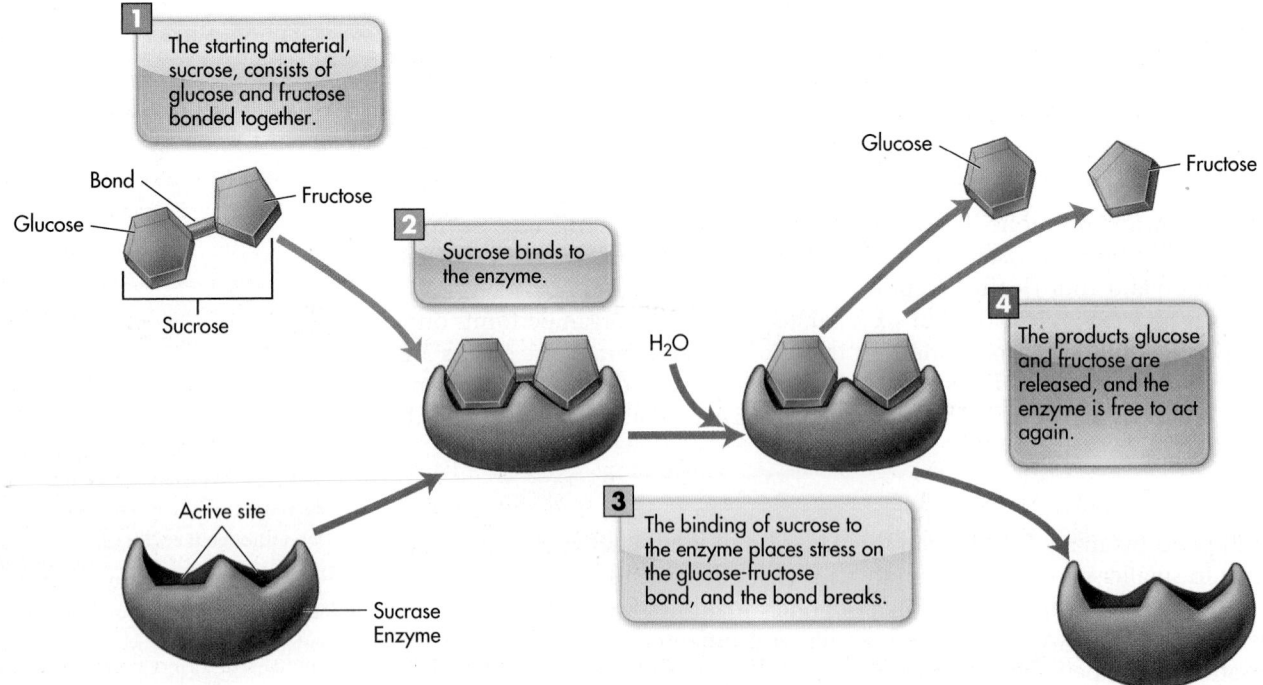

1 The starting material, sucrose, consists of glucose and fructose bonded together.

Bond

Fructose

Glucose

Sucrose

2 Sucrose binds to the enzyme.

H_2O

Glucose

Fructose

4 The products glucose and fructose are released, and the enzyme is free to act again.

Active site

Sucrase Enzyme

3 The binding of sucrose to the enzyme places stress on the glucose-fructose bond, and the bond breaks.

FIGURE 3-11 ▶ A model of enzyme action. The enzyme sucrase splits the sugar sucrose into two simpler sugars; glucose and fructose. [Note that sometimes energy input is needed to make reactions occur.]

TABLE 3-3 Important Secretions and Products of the Digestive Tract

Secretion	Site of Production	Purpose
Saliva	Mouth	Partial starch digestion using **salivary amylase,** lubrication of food for swallowing
Mucus	Mouth, stomach, small intestine, large intestine	Protects GI tract cells, lubricates food as it travels through the GI tract
Enzymes	Mouth, stomach, small intestine, pancreas	Promote digestion of carbohydrates, fats, and proteins into forms small enough for absorption (Examples: **amylases, lipases, proteases)**
Acid	Stomach	Promotes digestion of protein among other functions
Bile	Liver (stored in gallbladder)	Aids fat digestion in the small intestine by suspending fat in water using **bile acids, cholesterol,** and **lecithin**
Bicarbonate	Pancreas, small intestine	Neutralizes stomach acid when it reaches the small intestine
Hormones	Stomach, small intestine, pancreas	Stimulate production and/or release of acid, enzymes, bile, and bicarbonate; help regulate peristalsis and overall GI tract flow (Examples: gastrin, secretin, insulin, cholecystokinin, glucagon)

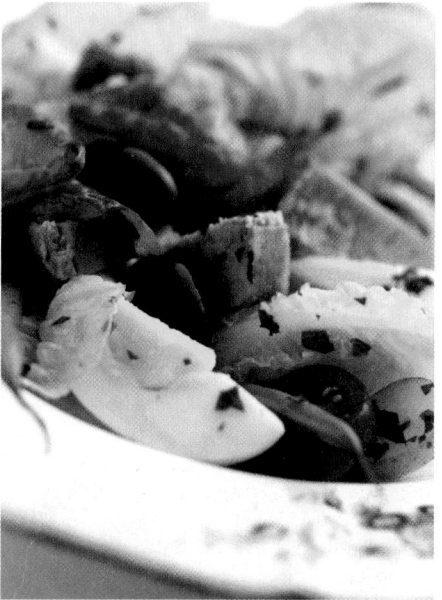

▲ The body digests the foods as they are presented—the order in which foods are eaten plays no role in digestion.

Esophagus

The **esophagus** is a long tube that connects the **pharynx** with the stomach. Near the pharynx is a flap of tissue (called the **epiglottis**) that prevents the **bolus** of swallowed food from entering the trachea (wind pipe) (Fig. 3-12). During swallowing, food lands on the epiglottis, folding it down to cover the opening of the trachea. Breathing also stops automatically. These responses ensure that swallowed food will only travel down the esophagus. If food instead travels down the trachea, choking may occur (the victim will not be able to speak or breathe). A group of techniques to treat such a person are called the Heimlich maneuver (see www.heimlichinstitute.org for details).

At the top of the esophagus, nerve fibers release signals to tell the GI tract that food has been consumed. This results in an increase in gastrointestinal muscle action, called **peristalsis.** These continual waves of muscle contractions, followed by muscle relaxation, force the food down the digestive tract from the esophagus onward (Fig. 3-13).

At the end of the esophagus is the **lower esophageal sphincter,** a muscle that constricts (closes) after food enters the stomach. The main function of sphincters is to prevent the backflow of GI tract contents. Sphincters respond to various stimuli, such as signals from the nervous system, hormones, acidic versus alkaline conditions, and pressure that builds up around the sphincter. The primary function of the lower esophageal sphincter is to prevent the acidic contents of the stomach from flowing back up into the esophagus—which can cause some of the health problems we will discuss in the "Nutrition and Your Health" section at the end of Chapter 3.

Stomach

The stomach is a large sac that can hold up to 4 cups (or 1 quart) of food for several hours until all of the food is able to enter the small intestine. Stomach size varies individually and can be reduced surgically as a radical treatment for obesity (more on this in Chapter 7). While in the stomach, the food is mixed with gastric juice,

mucus A thick fluid secreted by many cells throughout the body. It contains a compound that has both carbohydrate and protein parts. It acts as a lubricant and means of protection for cells.

amylase Starch-digesting enzyme produced by the salivary glands and pancreas.

lipase Fat-digesting enzyme produced by the salivary glands, stomach, and pancreas.

protease Protein-digesting enzyme produced by the stomach, small intestine, and pancreas.

esophagus A tube in the GI tract that connects the pharynx with the stomach.

pharynx The organ of the digestive tract and respiratory tract located at the back of the oral and nasal cavities, commonly known as the throat.

epiglottis The flap that folds down over the trachea during swallowing.

bolus A moistened mass of food swallowed from the oral cavity into the pharynx.

peristalsis A coordinated muscular contraction used to propel food down the gastrointestinal tract.

lower esophageal sphincter A circular muscle that constricts the opening of the esophagus to the stomach. Also called the *gastroesophageal sphincter.*

FIGURE 3-12 ▶ The process of swallowing. (a) During swallowing, food does not normally enter the trachea because the epiglottis closes over the larynx. (b) The closed epiglottis allows food to proceed down the esophagus. When a person chokes, food becomes lodged in the trachea, blocking air flow to the lungs. (c) The food should move down the esophagus.

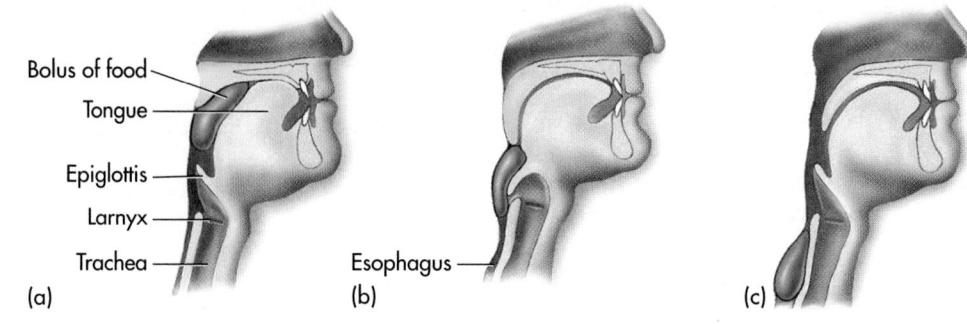

Bolus of food
Tongue
Epiglottis
Larnyx
Trachea
(a)
Esophagus
(b)
(c)

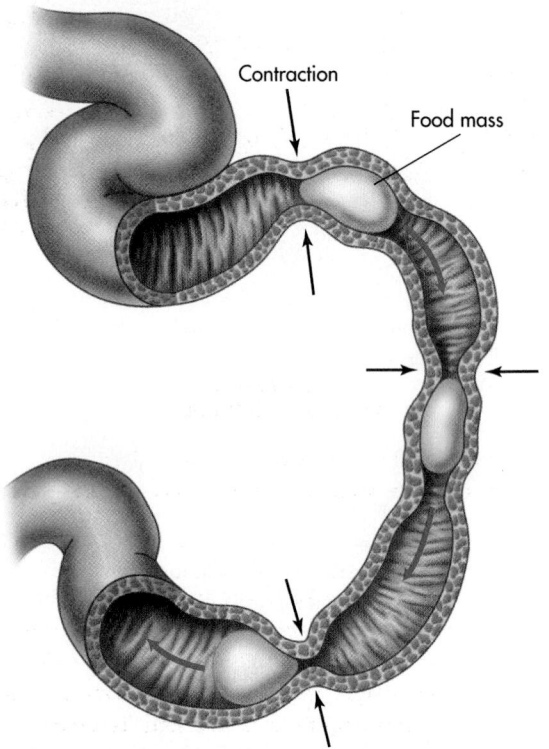

Contraction
Food mass

FIGURE 3-13 ▶ Peristalsis. Peristalsis is a progressive type of movement, propelling material from point to point along the GI tract. To begin this, a ring of contraction occurs where the GI wall is stretched, passing the food mass forward. The moving food mass triggers a ring of contraction in the next region, which pushes the food mass even farther along. The result is a ring of contraction that moves like a wave along the GI tract, pushing the food mass down the tract.

chyme A mixture of stomach secretions and partially digested food.

pyloric sphincter Ring of smooth muscle between stomach and small intestine.

intrinsic factor A proteinlike compound produced by the stomach that enhances vitamin B-12 absorption.

villi (singular, **villus**) The fingerlike protrusions into the small intestine that participate in digestion and absorption of food.

which contains water, a very strong acid, and enzymes. (Gastric is a term pertaining to the stomach.) The acid in the gastric juice maintains the acidity of the stomach contents and, thereby destroys the biological activity of proteins, converts inactive digestive enzymes to their active form, partially digests food protein, and makes dietary minerals soluble so that they can be absorbed. The mixing that takes place in the stomach produces a watery food mixture, called **chyme,** which slowly leaves the stomach a teaspoon (5 milliliters) at a time and enters the small intestine. Following a meal, the stomach contents are emptied into the small intestine over the course of 1 to 4 hours. The **pyloric sphincter,** located at the base of the stomach, controls the rate at which the chyme is released into the small intestine (Fig. 3-14). There is very little absorption of nutrients from the stomach, except for some alcohol.

You might wonder how the stomach prevents itself from being digested by the acid and enzymes it produces. First, the stomach has a thick layer of mucus that lines and protects it. The production of acid and enzymes also requires the release of a specific hormone (gastrin). This release happens primarily when we are eating or thinking about eating. Last, as the concentration of acid in the stomach increases, hormonal control causes acid production to taper off.

One other important function of the stomach is the production of a substance called **intrinsic factor.** This vital proteinlike compound is essential for the absorption of vitamin B-12.

Small Intestine

The small intestine is about 10 feet (3 meters) long, beginning at the stomach and ending at the large intestine (colon) (Fig. 3-15). The small intestine is considered "small" because of its narrow (1 inch [2.5 centimeters]) diameter. Most of the digestion and absorption of food occurs in the small intestine. The chyme secreted from the stomach is moved through the small intestine by peristaltic contractions so that it can be well mixed with the digestive juices of the small intestine (review Fig. 3-13). These juices contain many enzymes that function in the breakdown of carbohydrates, protein, and fat, as well as in the preparation of vitamins and minerals for absorption.

The physical structure of the small intestine is very important to the body's ability to digest and absorb the nutrients it needs. The lining of the small intestine is called the mucosa and is folded many times; within these folds are fingerlike projections called **villi.** These "fingers" are constantly moving, which helps them trap food to enhance absorption. Each individual villus (singular) is made up of many **absorptive cells,** and each of these cells has a highly folded cap. The combined folds, villi, and caps in the small intestine increase its surface area 600 times beyond that of a simple tube (Fig. 3-16).

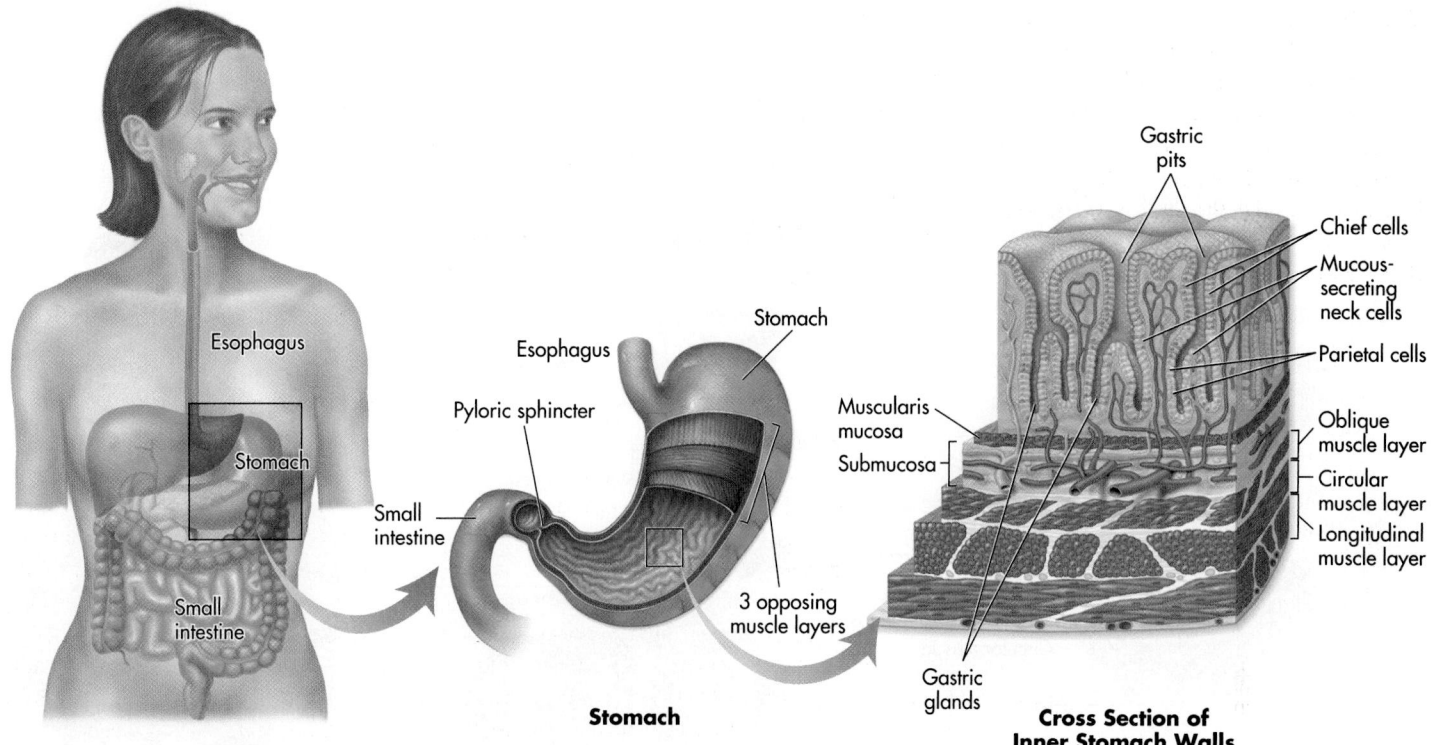

Stomach

Cross Section of Inner Stomach Walls

FIGURE 3-14 ▶ Physiology of the stomach. The interior surface mucous cells produce mucus for protection from stomach acid and enzymes. Parietal cells produce the hydrochloric acid (HCL), and chief cells produce the enzymes. Mucous neck cells, scattered among the cells in the gastric pits, also produce mucus. The exterior surface is made up of three types of muscle layers.

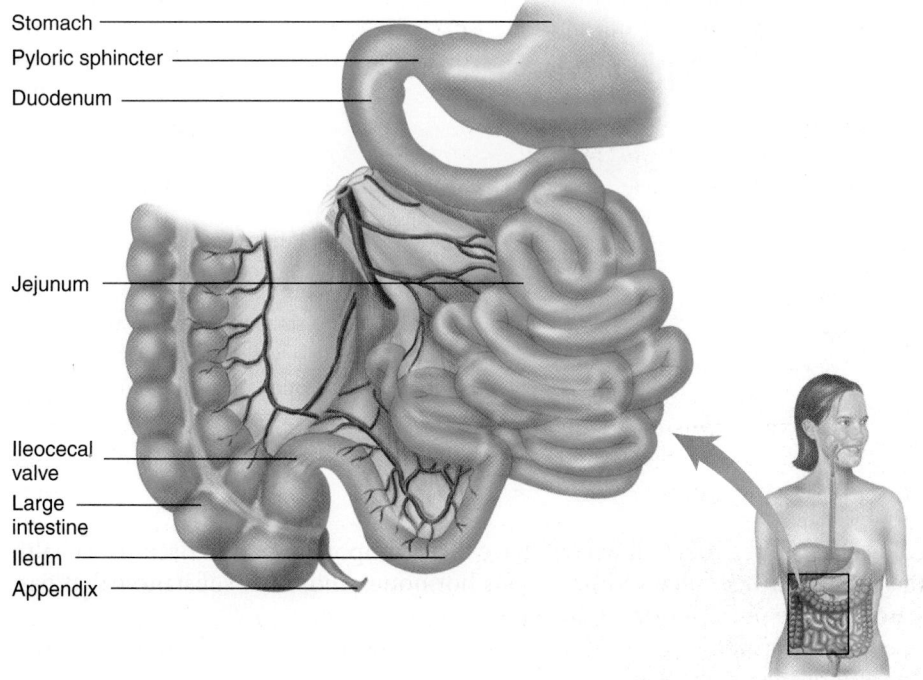

FIGURE 3-15 ▶ The small intestine and beginning of the large intestine. The three parts of the small intestine are the duodenum, jejunum, and ileum. Notice the smaller diameter of the small intestine, compared with the large intestine.

The absorptive cells have a short life. New intestinal absorptive cells are constantly produced in the crypts of the small intestine (Fig. 3-16) and appear daily along the surface of each villus "finger." This is probably because absorptive cells are subjected to a harsh environment, so renewal of the intestinal cell lining is necessary. This rapid cell turnover leads to high nutrient needs for the small intestine. Fortunately, many of

absorptive cells Intestinal cells that line the villi; and participate in nutrient absorption.

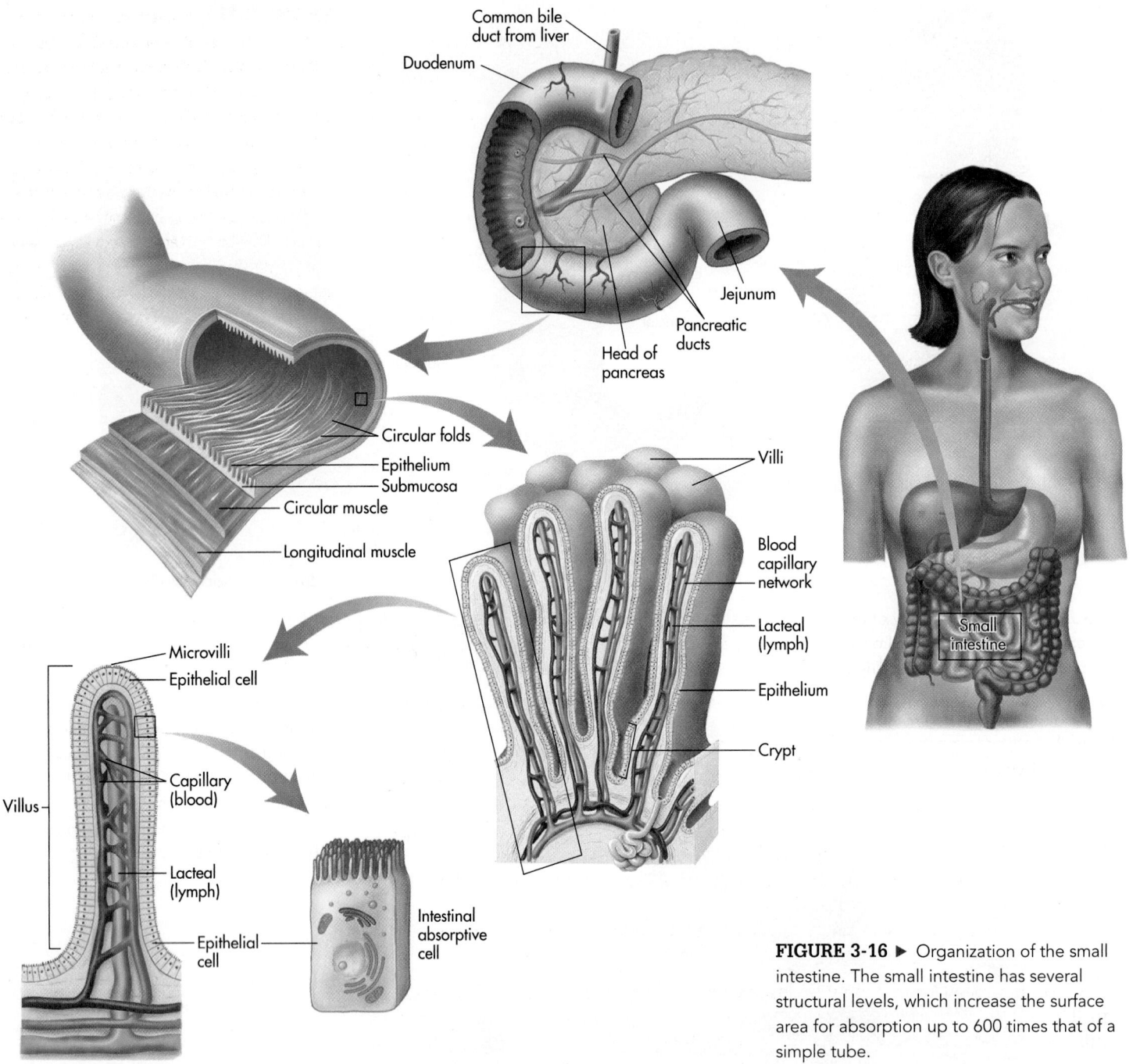

FIGURE 3-16 ▶ Organization of the small intestine. The small intestine has several structural levels, which increase the surface area for absorption up to 600 times that of a simple tube.

the old cells can be broken down and have their component parts reused. The health of the cells is further enhanced by various hormones and other substances that participate in or are produced as part of the digestive process.

The small intestine absorbs nutrients through the intestinal wall through various means and processes, as illustrated in Figure 3-17:

- **Passive diffusion:** When the nutrient concentration is higher in the cavity (lumen) of the small intestine than in the absorptive cells, the difference in nutrient concentration drives the nutrient into the absorptive cells by diffusion. Fats, water, and some minerals are absorbed by passive diffusion.

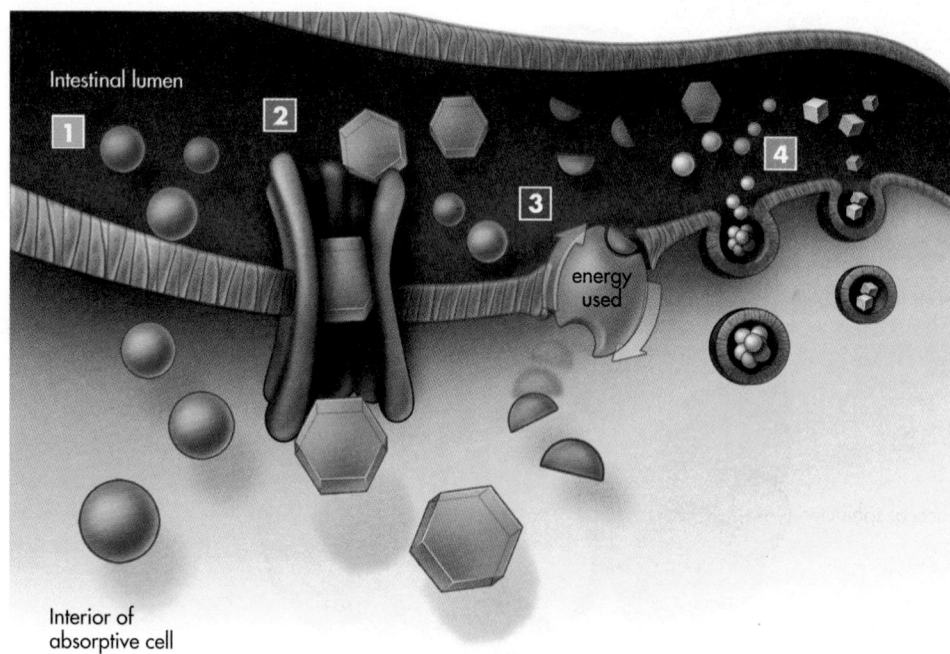

Intestinal lumen

Interior of
absorptive cell

FIGURE 3-17 ▶ Nutrient absorption relies on four major absorptive processes. **1** Passive diffusion (in blue) is diffusion of nutrients across the absorptive cell membranes. **2** Facilitated diffusion (in green) uses a carrier protein to move nutrients down a concentration gradient. **3** Active absorption (in purple) involves a carrier protein as well as energy to move nutrients (against a concentration gradient) into absorptive cells. **4** Phagocytosis and pinocytosis (in green and brown) are forms of active transport in which the absorptive cell membrane forms an indentation that engulfs a nutrient to bring it into the cell.

- **Facilitated diffusion:** Some compounds require a carrier protein to drive them into absorptive cells. This type of absorption is called faciliated diffusion. Fructose is one example of a compound that makes use of such a carrier to allow for facilitated diffusion.
- **Active absorption:** In addition to the need for a carrier protein, some nutrients also require energy input to move from the lumen of the small intestine into the absorptive cells. This mechanism makes it possible for cells to take up nutrients even when they are consumed in low concentrations. Some sugars, such as glucose, are actively absorbed, as are amino acids.
- **Phagocytosis** and **pinocytosis:** In a further means of active absorption, absorptive cells literally engulf compounds (phagocytosis) or liquids (pinocytosis). As described earlier, a cell membrane can form an indentation of itself so that when particles or fluids move into the indentation, the cell membrane surrounds and engulfs them. This process is used when an infant absorbs immune substances from human milk (see Chapter 14).

Once absorbed, water-soluble compounds such as glucose and amino acids go to the capillaries and then on to the portal vein. Recall that the liver is the end of this process. Most fats eventually go into the lymph vessels. In doing so, they can eventually enter the bloodstream (see the earlier section on the circulatory system for details; and review Figs. 3-4 and 3-5).

Undigested food cannot be absorbed into cells of the small intestine. Any undigested food that reaches the end of the small intestine must pass through the **ileocecal sphincter** on the way to the large intestine (Fig. 3-18). This sphincter prevents the contents of the large intestine from reentering the small intestine.

ileocecal sphincter The ring of smooth muscle between the end of the small intestine and the large intestine.

Large Intestine

When the contents of the small intestine enter the large intestine, the material left bears little resemblance to the food originally eaten. Under normal circumstances, only a minor amount (5%) of carbohydrate, protein, and fat escape absorption to reach the large intestine (Table 3-4).

FIGURE 3-18 ▶ The parts of the colon: cecum ascending colon, transverse colon, descending colon, and sigmoid colon.

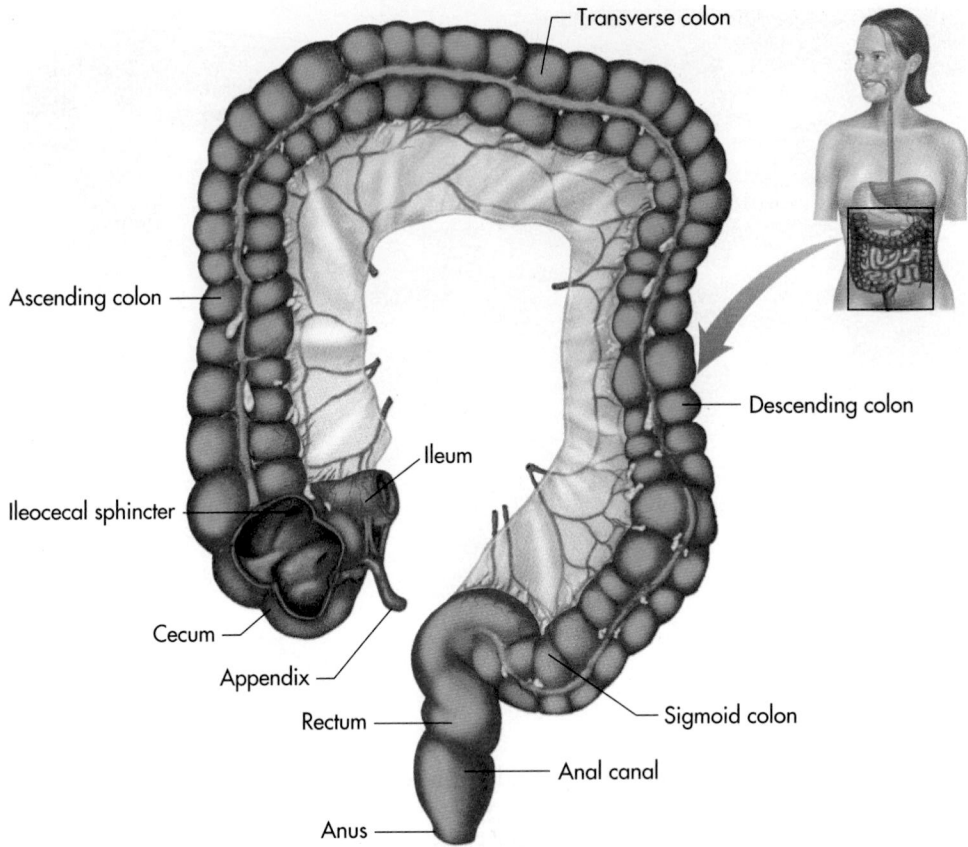

Transverse colon

Ascending colon

Descending colon

Ileum

Ileocecal sphincter

Cecum

Appendix

Rectum

Sigmoid colon

Anal canal

Anus

Physiologically, the large intestine differs from the small intestine in that there are no villi or digestive enzymes. The absence of villi means that little absorption takes place in the large intestine in comparison to the small intestine. Nutrients absorbed from the large intestine include water, some vitamins, some fatty acids, and the minerals sodium and potassium. Unlike the small intestine, the large intestine has a number of mucus-producing cells. The mucus secreted by these cells functions to hold the feces together and to protect the large intestine from the bacterial activity within it. The large intestine is home to a large population of bacteria (over 500 different species). Whereas the stomach and small intestine have some bacterial activity, the large intestine is the organ most heavily colonized with bacteria. Starting at infancy, the diet plays a major part in determining the type of bacteria in our digestive tracts. The number and type of bacteria in the human colon recently has become of great interest. Research has shown that intestinal bacteria play a significant role in the maintenance of health, especially health of the colon. It is speculated that higher levels of beneficial organisms can reduce the activity of disease-causing bacteria. This is another illustration of the intestinal tract working as an important immune organ. The strains *bifidobacteria* and *lactobacilli* are typically associated with health, whereas *clostridia* are considered problematic. These bacteria are able to break down some of the remaining food products that enter the large intestine, such as the milk sugar lactose (in lactose intolerant people), and some components of fiber. The products of bacterial metabolism in the large intestine, which include various acids, can then be absorbed.

Foods containing certain live microorganisms such as lactobacilli have been linked to some health benefits, such as improving intestinal tract health. These microorganisms are called **probiotics** because once consumed, they take up residence in the large

probiotic Product that contains specific types of bacteria. Use is intended to colonize the large intestine with the specific bacteria in the product. An example is yogurt.

TABLE 3-4 Major Sites of Absorption Along the GI Tract

Organ	Primary Nutrients Absorbed
Stomach	Alcohol (20% of total)
	Water (minor amount)
Small intestine	Calcium, magnesium, iron, and other minerals
	Glucose
	Amino acids
	Fats
	Vitamins
	Water (70% to 90% of total)
	Alcohol (80% of total)
	Bile acids
Large intestine	Sodium
	Potassium
	Some fatty acids
	Gases
	Water (10% to 30% of total)

NEWSWORTHY NUTRITION

Link between gut bacteria and health and disease

The benefits of probiotics and prebiotics have been confirmed in over 700 research studies. Probiotics, especially, are now recommended for the prevention and treatment of gastrointestinal tract disorders including inflammation, infections, and allergy. Evidence is available to support the growing interest in these microorganisms and to aid the development of intervention strategies and practical guidelines for their use.

Source: Wallace TC and others al. Human gut microbiota and its relationship to health and disease. *Nutrition Reviews* 69(7):392 2011 (see Further Reading 16).

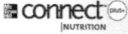 **Check out the Connect site** www.mcgrawhillconnect.com **to further explore probiotics.**

intestine and confer a health benefit. You can find these probiotic microorganisms in certain forms of fluid milk, fermented milk, yogurt, and in pill form (see Further Reading 13). A related term is **prebiotic**. These are substances that increase growth of probiotic microorganisms. One example is fructooligosaccharides (see Table 1-5 in Chapter 1 for dietary sources). The beneficial organisms of the large intestine and their use as probiotics are highlighted in "Newsworthy Nutrition" and will be discussed further in Chapter 4 when we explore their use as probiotics.

Some water remains in the material that enters the large intestine because the small intestine absorbs only 70% to 90% of the fluid it receives, which includes large amounts of GI-tract secretions produced during digestion. The remnants of a meal also contain some minerals and some fiber. Because water is removed from the large intestine, its contents become semisolid by the time they have passed through the first two-thirds of it. What remains in the **feces**, besides water and undigested fiber, is tough connective tissues (from animal foods); bacteria from the large intestine; and some body wastes, such as parts of dead intestinal cells.

Rectum

The feces or stool remains in the last portion of the large intestine, the **rectum**, until muscular movements push it into the **anus** to be eliminated. The presence of feces in the rectum stimulates elimination. The anus contains two **anal sphincters** (internal and external), one of which is under voluntary control (external sphincter). Relaxation of this sphincter allows for elimination.

prebiotic Substance that stimulates bacterial growth in the large intestines.

rectum Terminal portion of the large intestine.

anus Last portion of the GI tract; serves as an outlet for that organ.

anal sphincters A group of two sphincters (inner and outer) that help control expulsion of feces from the body.

gallbladder An organ attached to the underside of the liver; site of bile storage, concentration, and eventual secretion.

bile A liver secretion stored in the gallbladder and released through the common bile duct into the first segment of the small intestine. It is essential for the digestion and absorption of fat.

See Nutrition and Your Health: Common Problems with Digestion at the end of Chapter 3.

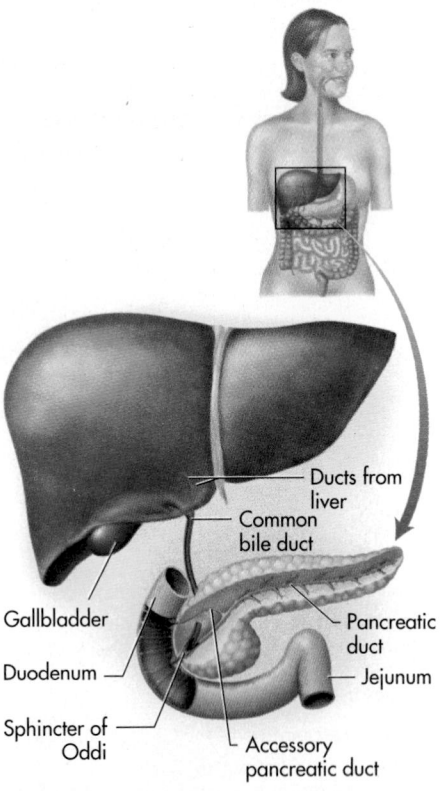

Gallbladder

Duodenum

Sphincter of Oddi

Ducts from liver

Common bile duct

Pancreatic duct

Jejunum

Accessory pancreatic duct

FIGURE 3-19 ▶ The liver, gallbladder, and pancreas are accessory organs that work with the GI tract. The liver produces bile, stored in the gallbladder and released into the duodenum portion of the small intestine, via the common bile duct, to help digest fat. The pancreas secretes pancreatic juice containing water, bicarbonate, and digestive enzymes into the duodenum via the common bile duct. The common bile duct from the liver and gallbladder and the pancreatic duct join together at the sphincter of Oddi to deliver bile, pancreatic enzymes, and bicarbonate to the duodenum.

Accessory Organs

The liver, **gallbladder,** and pancreas work with the GI tract and are considered accessory organs to the process of digestion (review Fig. 3-10). These accessory organs are not part of the GI tract through which food passes, but they play necessary roles in the process of digestion. These organs secrete digestive fluids into the GI tract and enable the process of converting food into absorbable nutrients.

The liver produces a substance called **bile.** The bile is stored and concentrated in the gallbladder until the gallbladder receives a hormonal signal to release the bile. This signal is induced by the presence of fat in the small intestine. Bile is released and delivered to the small intestine via a tube called the bile duct (Fig. 3-19).

In action, bile is like soap. Components of the bile enable large portions of fat to break into smaller bits so that they can be suspended in water (Chapter 5 will cover this process in detail). Interestingly, some of the bile constituents can be "recycled" in a process known as **enterohepatic circulation.** These components of bile are reabsorbed from the small intestine, returned to the liver via the portal vein, and reused.

In addition to bile, the liver releases a number of other unwanted substances that travel with the bile to the gallbladder and end up in the small intestine and eventually in the large intestine for excretion. The liver functions in this manner to remove unwanted substances from the blood. (Other byproducts are excreted via the urine; see the next section, "Urinary System.")

The pancreas manufactures hormones and pancreatic juice. The hormones include glucagon and insulin, which as noted earlier function in glucose regulation (review Fig. 3-7). Pancreatic juice contains water, bicarbonate, and a variety of digestive enzymes capable of breaking apart carbohydrates, proteins, and fats into small fragments. Bicarbonate is a base that neutralizes the acidity of chyme as it moves from the stomach into the small intestine. In contrast to the stomach, the small intestine, does not have a protective layer of mucus, because mucus would impede nutrient absorption. Instead, the neutralizing capacity of bicarbonate from the pancreas protects the walls of the small intestine from erosion by acid, which would otherwise lead to formation of an ulcer (see the "Nutrition and Your Health" section at the end of Chapter 3).

CONCEPT CHECK

Digestion is a mechanical and chemical process mediated by enzymes and coordinated by hormones and nerves. Whereas swallowing and ultimate elimination of feces from the anus are voluntary, the majority of the digestive processes are involuntary. The stomach initiates the process of digestion by mixing food with gastric juice and converting this partially digested food into chyme. The products of digestion are molecules of the original food or beverage small enough to be absorbed into the villi of the small intestine and transferred to the blood or lymph. For the most part, nutrients are absorbed in the small intestine; only a few are absorbed in the large intestine. Any dietary component that escapes digestion by human or bacterial enzymes exits the body as feces.

3.9 Urinary System

The **urinary system** is composed of two kidneys, one on each side of the spinal column. Each kidney is connected to the bladder by a **ureter.** The bladder is emptied by way of the **urethra** (Fig. 3-20). The main function of the kidneys is to remove waste from the body. The kidneys are constantly filtering blood to control its composition. This results in the formation of urine, mostly water, along with dissolved waste products of metabolism such as urea, and excess and unneeded water-soluble vitamins and various minerals.

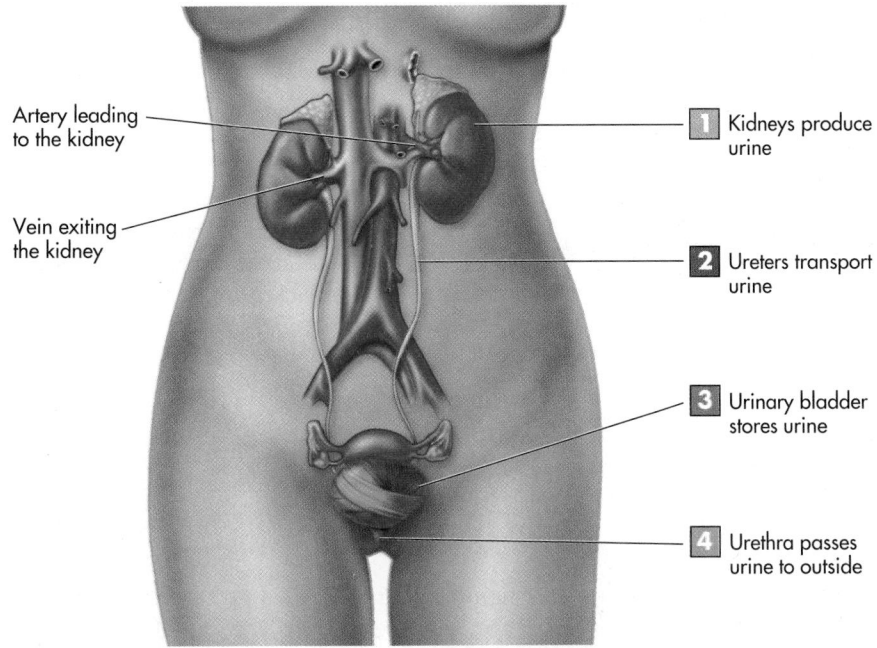

Artery leading to the kidney

Vein exiting the kidney

1 Kidneys produce urine

2 Ureters transport urine

3 Urinary bladder stores urine

4 Urethra passes urine to outside

FIGURE 3-20 ▶ Organs of the urinary system. The kidneys, 1 bean-shaped organs located on either side of the spinal column, filter waste from the blood and form urine, which is transported to the bladder by the ureters 2 and stored in the bladder 3 as urine. The urethra 4 transports the urine to outside the body. The urinary system of the female is shown. The male's urinary system is the same, except that the urethra extends through the penis.

enterohepatic circulation A continual recycling of compounds such as bile acid between the small intestine and the liver.

urinary system The body system consisting of the kidneys, urinary bladder, and the ducts that carry urine. This system removes waste products from the circulatory system and regulates blood acid-base balance, overall chemical balance, and water balance in the body.

ureter Tube that transports urine from the kidney to the urinary bladder.

urethra Tube that transports urine from the urinary bladder to the outside of the body.

pH A measure of relative acidity or alkalinity of a solution. The pH scale is 0 to 14. A pH of 7 is neutral; A pH below 7 is acidic; a pH above 7 is alkaline.

erythropoietin A hormone secreted mostly by the kidneys that enhances red blood cell synthesis and stimulates red blood cell release from bone marrow.

Together with the lungs, the kidneys also maintain the acid-base balance **(pH)** of the blood. The kidneys also convert a form of vitamin D into its active hormone form and produce a hormone that stimulates red blood cell synthesis (**erythropoietin;** see Chapter 12 for information on misuse of this hormone by some athletes). During times of fasting, the kidneys even produce glucose from certain amino acids. Thus, the kidneys perform many important functions related to nutrition and are a vital component of the body.

The proper function of the kidneys is closely tied to the strength of the cardio-vascular system, particularly its ability to maintain adequate blood pressure, and the consumption of sufficient fluid. Uncontrolled diabetes, hypertension, and drug abuse are harmful to the kidneys.

3.10 Nutrient Storage Capabilities

The human body must maintain reserves of nutrients, otherwise we would need to eat continuously. Storage capacity varies for each different nutrient. Most fat is stored in adipose tissue, made up of cells designed specifically for this. Short-term storage of carbohydrate occurs in muscle and liver in the form of glycogen. The blood maintains a small reserve of glucose and amino acids. Many vitamins and minerals are stored in the liver, while other nutrient stores are found in other sites in the body.

When people do not meet certain nutrient needs, these nutrients are obtained by breaking down a tissue that contains high concentrations of the nutrient. For example, calcium is taken from bone and protein is taken from muscle. In cases of long-term deficiency, these nutrient losses weaken and harm these tissues.

Many people believe that if too much of a nutrient is obtained—for example, from a vitamin or mineral supplement—only what is needed is stored and the rest is excreted by the body. Though true for some nutrients, such as vitamin C, the large dosages of other nutrients frequently found in supplements, such as vitamin A and iron, can cause harmful side effects because they are not readily excreted. This is one reason why obtaining your nutrients primarily (or exclusively) from a balanced diet is the safest means to acquire the building blocks you need to maintain the good health of all organ systems.

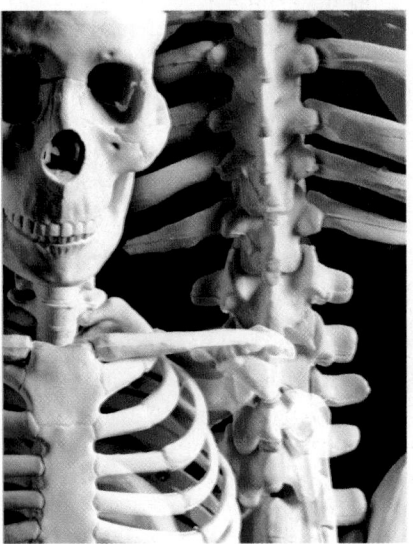

▲ The skeletal system provides a reserve of calcium for day-to-day needs when dietary intake is inadequate. Long-term use of this reserve, however, reduces bone strength.

CONCEPT CHECK

The urinary system removes the wastes produced by the body and many nutrients ingested in excess of storage capacity and need. The kidneys maintain the chemical composition and acidity of the blood. In addition, the kidneys help convert vitamin D to its active form and produce a hormone needed for red blood cell synthesis.

In well-nourished individuals, nutrients are constantly present in the blood for immediate use and are stored in the body tissues for later use when sufficient amounts are not consumed from food. However, when the body suffers a nutrient deficiency after an inadequate diet is consumed over a long period, vital tissues will be broken down for their nutrients, which can lead to ill health. Additionally, too much of any nutrient can be detrimental. It's best to focus primarily (or exclusively) on obtaining all essential nutrients from a balanced diet rather than mostly from dietary supplements.

3.11 Nutrition and Genetics

Once nutrients and other dietary components are taken up by cells, they may interact with our genes and have an effect on gene expression. The growth, development, and maintenance of cells, and ultimately of the entire organism, are directed by genes present in the cells. Each gene essentially represents a recipe, noting the ingredients (amino acids) and how those ingredients should be put together (to make proteins). The products (proteins) of all the recipes in the cookbook (the human genome) would then make up the human organism. The genome and the **epigenome**, the way the genome is marked and packaged inside a cell's nucleus, control the expression of individual traits, such as height, eye color, and susceptibility to many diseases. **Epigenetics** refers to inherited changes in gene expression caused by mechanisms other than changes in the underlying DNA sequence. While our genome contains the code for the proteins that can be made by our bodies, our epigenome is an extra layer of instructions that influences gene activity. In many cases it is the epigenome that can be repaired by treatments, or affected by diet, rather than the genetics.

The causes of chronic diseases are complex and include a significant genetic component. Fortunately, the science of genetics is moving swiftly such that medical breakthroughs are beginning to touch our lives. Genetic discoveries are leading to new drugs that disrupt disease processes at the molecular level and to tests that predict our risk for disease. In 2008, scientists discovered more than 100 genetic variations associated with many medical conditions associated with aging, including type 2 diabetes, Alzheimer's disease, osteoporosis, high blood pressure, and heart disease.

The Emerging Field of Nutrigenomics

In the near future, genetic information will enhance the ability of health professionals to help individuals manage diseases and optimize health. Nutritional genomics or **nutrigenomics** is the study of how food impacts health through its interaction with our genes and its subsequent effect on gene expression. Nutrigenomics also includes the study of how genes determine our nutritional requirements. Research in this area highlights the fallacy of a "one-size-fits-all" approach to nutrition interventions for disease prevention and management. It is becoming clear that the general nutrient requirements do not apply to certain genetic subgroups. Research is very active in identifying these subgroups and classifying the human genetic variation that may affect nutrient utilization and physiological function and therefore their unique nutrient requirements (see Further Readings 5, 14, and 15).

In addition to the direct effect of genes on disease risk, in many cases, genes influence the effect of diet and nutrition on disease development and progression. In some cases, a food component can cause a gene to be turned on or off, thus manipulating the production of proteins that can affect—positively or negatively—development

---

epigenome The way that the genome is marked and packaged inside the cell nucleus.

epigenetics Inherited changes in gene expression caused by mechanisms other than changes in the DNA sequence.

A genetic variation can directly affect the proteins encoded by our genes and result in different:

- nutrient requirements among individuals.
- susceptibilities to diseases.
- effects of environmental factors (such as our diet) on our genes and their proteins.

nutrigenomics Study of how food impacts health through its interaction with our genes and its subsequent effect on gene expression.

or progression of diseases. With a better understanding of the interactions between genes and our diet, it will not be long before dietary recommendations may be personalized to help those with various genetically-linked diseases (see Further Reading 7).

Nutritional Diseases with a Genetic Link

Studies of families, including those with twins and adopted children, provide strong support for the effects of genetics in various disorders. In fact, family history is considered to be an important risk factor in the development of many nutrition-related diseases.

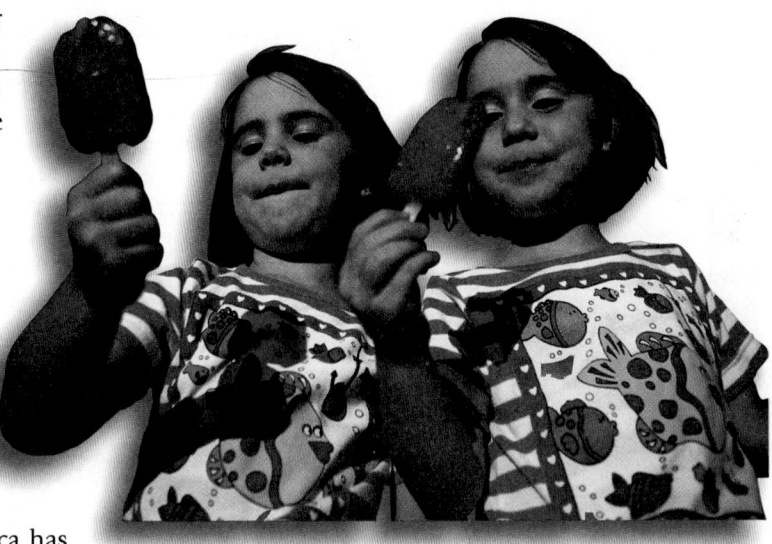

▲ Studies of twins have provided strong evidence for the interaction between genes and diet and their combined effects on disease risk.

Cardiovascular Disease. There is strong evidence that cardiovascular disease is the result of gene-environment interactions. About 1 of every 500 people in North America has a defective gene that greatly delays cholesterol removal from the bloodstream. As discussed in Chapter 1, elevated blood cholesterol is one major risk factor for development of cardiovascular disease. The gene-diet interactions being discovered for cardiovascular disease, particularly the cases of high blood lipid levels, will likely be the first to lead to nutrition plans personalized to decrease cardiovascular disease risk. Another genetic variation can cause abnormally high levels of an amino acid called homocysteine, which increases cardiovascular disease risk. Diet changes can help these people, but medications and even surgery are needed to address these problems.

Obesity. Most obese North Americans have at least one obese parent. This strongly suggests a genetic link. Findings from many human studies suggest that a variety of genes (likely 60 or more) are involved in the regulation of body weight. Little is known, however, about the specific nature of these genes in humans or how the actual changes in body metabolism (such as lower calorie-burning in general or fat use in particular) are produced.

Still, although some individuals may be genetically predisposed to store body fat, whether they do so depends on how many calories they consume relative to their needs. A common concept in nutrition is that *nurture*—how people live and the environmental factors that influence them—allows *nature*—each person's genetic potential—to be expressed. Although not every person with a genetic tendency toward obesity becomes obese, those genetically predisposed to weight gain have a higher lifetime risk than individuals without a genetic predisposition to obesity.

Diabetes. Both of the two common types of diabetes—type 1 and type 2—have genetic links. Evidence for these genetic links comes from studies of families, including twins, and from the high incidence of diabetes among certain population groups (e.g., South Asians or Pima Indians). Diabetes, in fact, is a complex disease with more than 200 genes identified as possible causes. Only sensitive and expensive testing can determine who is at risk. Type 2 diabetes is the most common form of diabetes (90% of all cases), and also has a strong link to obesity. Typically a genetic tendency for type 2 diabetes is expressed once a person becomes obese but often not before, again illustrating that nurture affects nature.

Cancer. A few types of cancer (e.g., some forms of colon [large intestine] and breast cancer) have a strong genetic link, and genetics may play a role in others, such as **prostate cancer.** Because obesity increases the risk of several forms of cancer, a long-standing excess calorie intake is also a risk factor. Although genes are an important determinant in the development of cancer, environmental and lifestyle factors, such as excessive sun exposure and a poor diet, also contribute significantly to the risk profile.

CRITICAL THINKING

Wesley notices that at family gatherings his parents, uncles, aunts, and older siblings typically drink excessive amounts of alcohol. His father has been arrested for driving while intoxicated, as has one of his aunts. Two of his uncles died before the age of 60 from alcohol abuse. As Wesley approaches the age of legal drinking, he wonders if he is destined to fall into the pattern of alcohol abuse. What advice would you give to Wesley concerning his future use of alcohol?

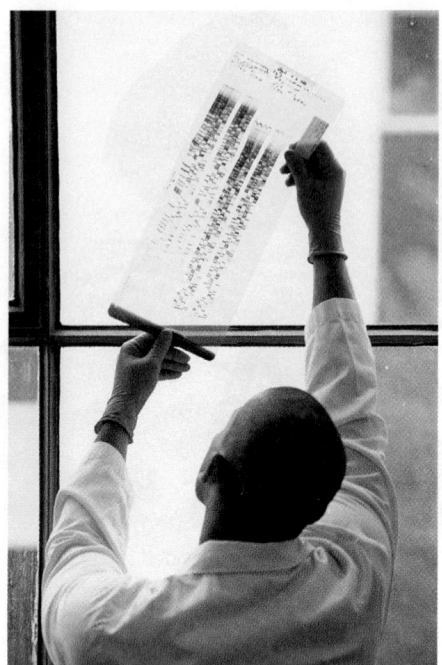

▲ Genetic testing for disease susceptibility will be more common in the future as the genes that increase the risk of developing various diseases are isolated and decoded.

The following weblinks will help you gather more information about genetic conditions and testing:

http://nutrigenomics.ucdavis.edu/
Center for Excellence for Nutritional Genomics. Website dedicated to promoting the new science of nutritional genomics

www.geneticalliance.org
Alliance of Genetic Support Groups

www.kumc.edu/gec/support
Information on genetic and rare conditions

www.cancer.gov/cancertopics/
prevention-genetics-causes
Genetics information from the National Cancer Institute

http://www.genome.gov/
National Human Genome Research Institute (at the National Institutes of Health) website. Describes the latest research finding, discusses some ethical issues, and provides a talking glossary.

http://history.nih.gov/exhibits/genetics/
Revolution in Progress: Human Genetics and Medical Research

MAKING DECISIONS

Research is opening the way for "personalized nutrition" that uses the results of genetic testing to determine which diet will work most effectively with the person's genetic makeup. There are genetic tests available for at least 1500 diseases and conditions, but mechanisms are not in place to ensure that the tests are based on adequate evidence or that marketing claims are truthful. Many companies are already tailoring genetic testing services and products for certain genetic profiles even though there are insufficient data on which to base genotype-specific recommendations. Most of these offers are online. As we discussed in Chapter 2, caution is always needed when evaluating nutrition information and claims. Genetic testing is no exception. Some DNA-testing companies are responsible organizations, and some are not. Some are offering DNA tests to determine the best weight-loss diets or the best supplements. These marketing schemes belittle the science of genetics to consumers. Use the principles outlined in Chapter 2 to evaluate any genetic testing services or products.

Your Genetic Profile

From this discussion, you can see that your genes can greatly influence your risk of developing certain diseases. By recognizing your potential for developing a particular disease, you can avoid behavior that further raises your risk. How can you figure out your genetic profile? Genetic testing can be valuable if it confirms that you carry a gene for a disease that you can do something about in terms of protecting against it. Testing is also of interest when you do not know your family medical history or there are gaps in your family tree. About 1000 genetic tests have become available in recent years. It typically costs about $1000 to have your DNA read to reveal the diseases to which you are most susceptible. Many tests are covered by health insurance plans. The Genetic Information Nondiscrimination Act (GINA) became a law in May 2008, and prohibits health insurers from raising premiums or denying coverage based on genetic information and applies to people who have genes that carry the risk of disease. DNA testing includes providing a saliva sample from which your DNA will be separated. Certain areas of the genome are then read and measured in the process known as genotyping. After this 1-to 2-month process, you receive your DNA profile, which will supplement what you already know about your family history. You can also compare your DNA profile to future findings from DNA research.

Many of the genes involved in common diseases, such as diabetes, are still unknown. Although there are genetic tests available for some diseases, your family history of certain diseases is still a much better indicator of your genetic profile and risk of disease. Put together a family tree of illnesses and deaths by compiling a few key facts on your primary relatives: siblings, parents, aunts and uncles, and grandparents, as suggested in the "Rate Your Plate" section. In general, the greater number of your relatives who had a genetically transmitted disease and the closer they are related to you, the greater your risk. If there is a significant family history of a certain disease, lifestyle changes may be appropriate. For example, women with a family history of breast cancer should avoid becoming obese, should minimize alcohol use, and should obtain mammograms regularly.

Figure 3-22 shows an example of a family tree (also called a *genogram*). High-risk conditions include two or more first-degree relatives in a family with a specific disease (first-degree relatives include one's parents, siblings, and offspring). Another sign of risk of inherited disease is development of the disease in a first-degree relative before the age of 50 to 60 years. In the family depicted in Figure 3-21, prostate cancer killed the man's father. Knowing this, the man should be tested regularly for prostate cancer. His sisters should have frequent mammograms and other preventive practices because their mother died of breast cancer. Because heart attack and stroke are also common in the family, all the children should adopt a lifestyle that minimizes the risk of developing these conditions, such as avoiding excessive animal fat and salt intake. Colon cancer is also evident, so careful screening throughout life is important.

Information about our genetic makeup will increasingly influence our dietary and lifestyle choices. Throughout this book we will discuss "controllable" risk factors that could contribute to development of genetically linked diseases present in your family. This information will help you personalize nutrition advice based on your genetic background and identify and avoid the risk factors that could lead to the diseases present in your family.

This review of human anatomy, physiology, and genetics from a nutrition perspective sets the stage for developing a more detailed understanding of the nutrients. Chapters 4, 5, and 6 will build on this information.

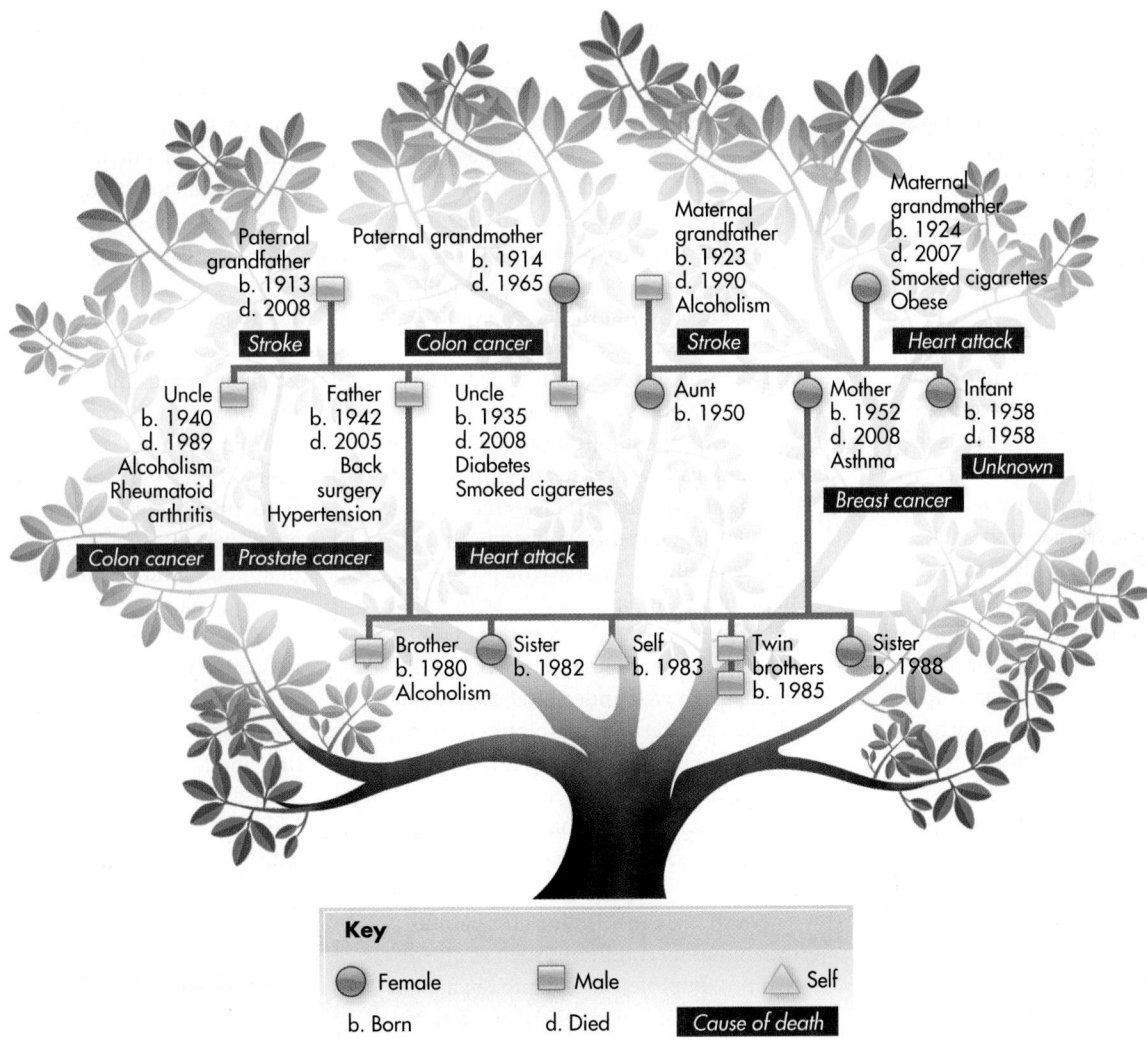

FIGURE 3-21 ▶ Example of a family tree for Justin, designated as "Self" at the trunk of the tree. The gender of each family member is identified by color (blue squares for males, orange circles for females). Dates of birth (b) and death (d) are listed below each family member. If deceased, the cause of death is highlighted using white text against a red background. Other medical conditions the family members experienced are noted beneath each name. Create your own family tree of frequent diseases using the diagram in "Rate Your Plate" and this figure as a guide. Then show your family tree to your physician to get a more complete picture of what the information means for your health.

Common Problems with Digestion

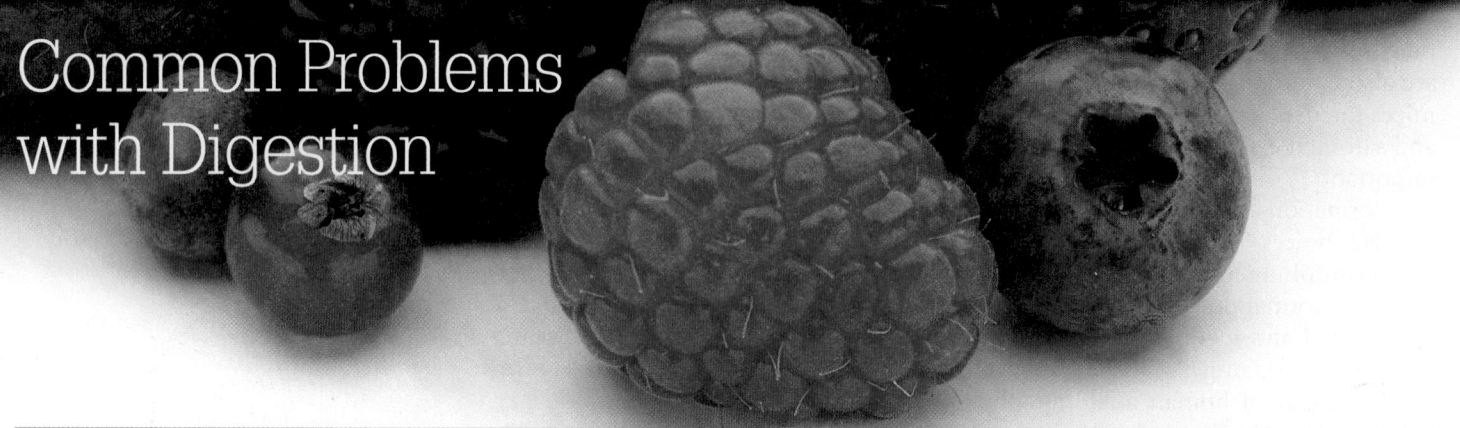

The fine-tuned organ system we call the digestive system can develop problems. Knowing about these common problems can help you avoid or lessen them. Two common GI tract-related problems are diverticulosis and lactose maldigestion and intolerance. These disorders will be discussed in Chapter 4 after you learn more about carbohydrates.

Ulcers

A peptic **ulcer** can occur when the lining of the esophagus, stomach, or small intestine is eroded by the acid secreted by the stomach cells (Fig. 3-22). As the stomach lining deteriorates in ulcer development, it loses its protective mucus layer, and the acid further erodes the stomach tissue. Acid can also erode the lining of the esophagus and the first part of the small intestine, the duodenum. In young people, most ulcers occur in the small intestine, wheras in older people they occur primarily in the stomach.

Millions of North Americans develop ulcers during their lifetimes. As a result, billions of healthcare dollars are spent annually on the treatment of peptic ulcers and their complications. Fortunately, our understanding of ulcer formation has increased, resulting in a variety of improved treatment options. The typical symptom of an ulcer is pain about 2 hours after eating. Stomach acid acting on a meal irritates the ulcer after most of the meal has moved from the site of the ulcer.

Not long ago, the major cause of ulcer disease was thought to be excess acid. Therefore, neutralizing and curtailing the secretion of stomach acid were the logical treatment choices. Although acid is still a significant player in ulcer formation, the principal causes of ulcer disease are currently thought to be infection of the stomach by the acid-resistant bacteria, *Helicobacter pylori (H. pylori);* heavy use of nonsteroidal anti-inflammatory drugs **(NSAIDS),** such as aspirin; and disorders that cause excessive acid production in the stomach. Stress is regarded as a predisposing factor for ulcers, especially if the person is infected with *H. pylori* or has certain anxiety disorders. Cigarette smoking is also known to cause ulcers, increase ulcer complications such as bleeding, and lead to ulcer treatment failure.

The *H. pylori* bacteria is found in more than 80% of patients with stomach and duodenal ulcers. The bacteria is common but results in ulcer disease in only 10% to 15% of those infected. Although the mechanism of how *H. pylori* causes ulcers is not well understood, treatment of the infection with antibiotics heals the ulcers and prevents their recurrence. Two Australian physicians were awarded the Nobel Prize in 2005 "for their discovery of the bacterium *Helicobacter pylori* and its role in gastritis and peptic ulcer disease."

NSAIDs are medications for painful inflammatory conditions such as arthritis. Aspirin, ibuprofen, and naproxen are the most commonly used NSAIDs. NSAIDs reduce the mucus secreted by the stomach. Newer medications, called "Cox-2 inhibitors" (e.g., celecoxib [Celebrex]), have been used as a replacement for NSAIDs because they are less likely to cause stomach ulcers. They do offer some advantages over NSAIDs, but they may not be totally safe for some people, especially those with a history of cardiovascular disease or strokes.

The primary risk associated with an ulcer is the possibility that it will erode entirely through the stomach or intestinal wall. The GI contents could then spill into the body cavities, causing a massive infection. In addition, an ulcer may erode a blood vessel, leading to substantial blood loss. For these reasons, it is important not to ignore the early warning signs of ulcer development, including a persistent gnawing or burning near the stomach that may occur immediately following a meal or awaken you at night. In addition to the pain that may improve with food, other signs and symptoms of ulcers are weight loss, nausea, vomiting, loss of appetite, and abdominal bloating.

In the past, milk and cream therapy was used to help cure ulcers. Clinicians now know that milk and cream are two of the worst foods for an ulcer. The calcium in these foods stimulates stomach acid secretion and actually inhibits ulcer healing.

Today, a combination of approaches is used for ulcer therapy. People infected with *H. pylori* are given antibiotics as well as stomach acid-blocking medica-

ulcer Erosion of the tissue lining, usually in the stomach or the upper small intestine. As a group these are generally referred to as *peptic ulcers.*

NSAIDs Nonsteroidal anti-inflammatory drugs; includes aspirin, ibuprofen (Advil®), and naproxen (Aleve®).

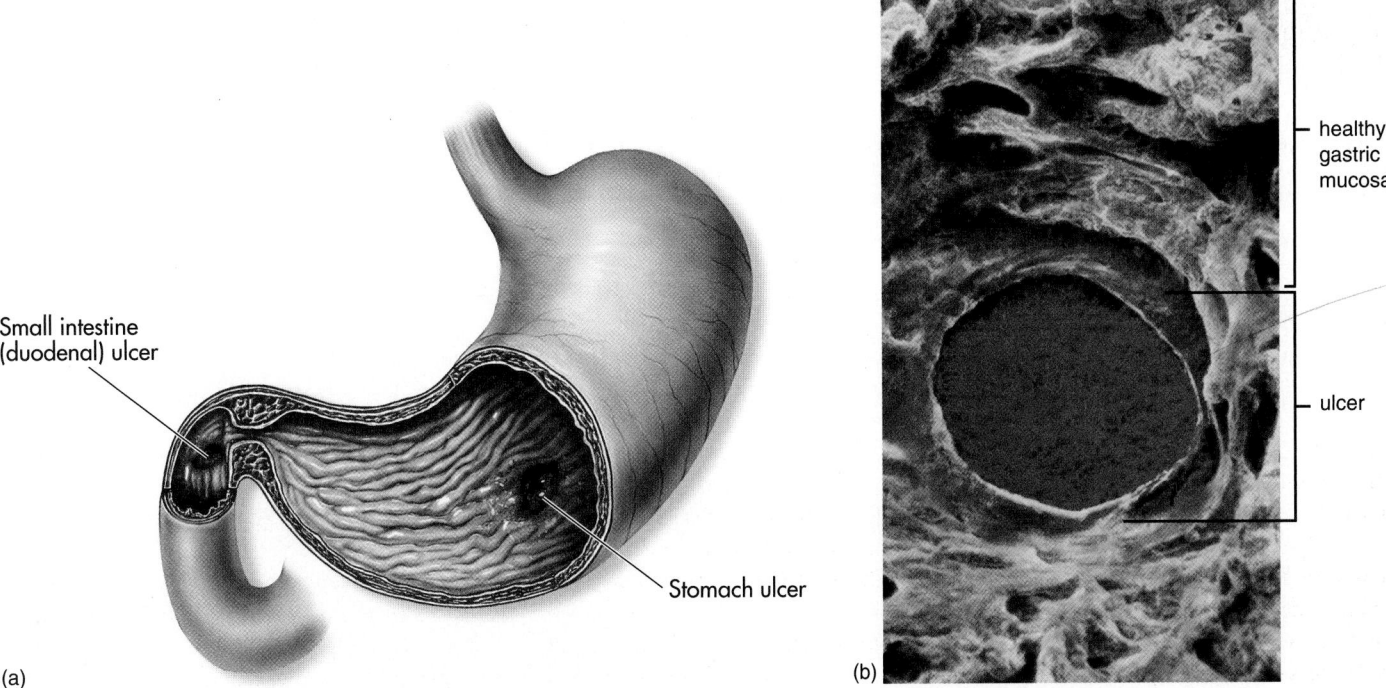

Small intestine (duodenal) ulcer

Stomach ulcer

(a)

healthy gastric mucosa

ulcer

(b)

FIGURE 3-22 ▶ (a) A peptic ulcer in the stomach or small intestine. *H. pylori* bacteria and NSAIDs (e.g., aspirin) cause ulcers by impairing mucosal defense, especially in the stomach. In the same way, smoking, genetics, and stress can impair mucosal defense, as well as cause an increase in the release of pepsin and stomach acid. All of these factors can contribute to ulcers. (b) Close-up of a stomach ulcer. This needs to be treated or eventual perforation of the stomach is possible.

▶ When suffering from persistent heartburn or GERD, see a doctor if you have:

- Difficulty swallowing or pain when swallowing
- Heartburn that has persisted for more than 10 years
- Initial onset of heartburn after age 50
- Heartburn that resists treatment with medications
- Sudden, unexplained weight loss
- Chest pain
- Blood loss or anemia
- Blood in stool or vomit

tions called **proton** (proton is another name for the hydrogen ion that creates acidity) **pump inhibitors** (e.g., omeprazole [Prilosec], esomeprazole [Nexium], and lansoprazole [Prevacid]). In many cases, there is a 90% cure rate for *H. pylori* infections in the first week of this treatment. Recurrence is unlikely if the infection is cured, but an incomplete cure almost certainly leads to repeated ulcer formation (see Further Reading 2).

Antacid medications may also be part of ulcer care, as is a class of medicines called **H2 blockers.** These include cimetidine (Tagamet), ranitidine (Zantac), nizatidine (Axid), and famotidine (Pepcid), all of which prevent **histamine**-related acid secretion in the stomach. Medications that coat the ulcer, such as sucralfate (Carafate), are also commonly used.

People with ulcers should refrain from smoking and minimize the use of NSAIDs. These practices reduce the mucus secreted by the stomach. Overall, a combination of lifestyle therapy and medical treatment has so revolutionized ulcer

therapy that dietary changes are of minor importance today. Current diet-therapy approaches recommend avoiding foods that increase ulcer symptoms (Table 3-5).

proton pump inhibitor A medication that inhibits the ability of gastric cells to secrete hydrogen ions. Low doses of this class of medications are also available without prescription (e.g., omeprazole [Prilosec]).

H₂ blocker Medication, such as cimetidine (Tagamet®), that blocks the increase of stomach acid production caused by histamine.

histamine A breakdown product of the amino acid histidine that stimulates acid secretion by the stomach and has other effects on the body, such as contraction of smooth muscles, increased nasal secretions, relaxation of blood vessels, and changes in relaxation of airways.

TABLE 3-5 Recommendations to Prevent Ulcers and Heartburn from Occurring or Recurring

Ulcers
1. Stop smoking if you are now a smoker.
2. Avoid large doses of aspirin, ibuprofen, and other NSAID compounds unless a physician advises otherwise. For people who must use these medications, FDA has approved an NSAID combined with a medication to reduce gastric damage. The medication reduces gastric acid production and enhances mucus secretion.
3. Limit consumption of coffee, tea, and alcohol (especially wine), if this helps.
4. Limit consumption of pepper, chili powder, and other strong spices, if this helps.
5. Eat nutritious meals on a regular schedule; include enough fiber (see Chapter 4 for sources of fiber).
6. Chew foods well.
7. Lose weight if you are currently overweight.

Heartburn
1. Follow ulcer prevention recommendations.
2. Wait about 2 hours after a meal before lying down.
3. Don't overeat. Eat smaller meals that are low in fat.
4. Elevate the head of the bed at least 6 inches.

Heartburn

About half of North American adults experience occasional heartburn, also known as acid reflux (Fig. 3-23). This gnawing pain in the upper chest is caused by the movement of acid from the stomach into the esophagus. The recurrent and therefore more serious form of the problem is called **gastroesophageal reflux disease (GERD)**. Unlike the stomach, the esophagus has very little mucus lining to protect it, so acid quickly erodes the lining of the esophagus, causing pain. Symptoms may also include nausea, gagging, cough, or hoarseness. GERD is characterized by the occurrence of such symptoms of acid reflux two or more times per week. People who have GERD experience occasional relaxation of the gastroesophageal sphincter. Typically it should be relaxed only during swallowing, but in individuals with GERD it is relaxed at other times as well.

The majority of heartburn sufferers say it significantly affects their quality of life, particularly their enjoyment of many favorite foods. On a more serious note, however, if left untreated, heartburn can, over time, damage the lining of the esophagus, leading to chronic esophageal inflammation and an increased risk of esophageal cancer (see Further Reading 8). Heartburn sufferers should follow the general recommendations given in Table 3-5. For occasional heartburn, quick relief can be found with over-the-counter (OTC) antacids. Taking antacids will reduce the acid in the stomach but will not stop the acid reflux. For more persistent (few days a week or everyday) heartburn or GERD, the H2 blockers or PPIs, discussed in the previous section on ulcers, may be needed. PPIs provide long-lasting relief by reducing stomach acid production and should be taken before the first meal of the day because they take longer to work. If the proper medications are not effective at controlling GERD, surgery may be

gastroesophageal reflux disease (GERD) Disease that results from stomach acid backing up into the esophagus. The acid irritates the lining of the esophagus, causing pain.

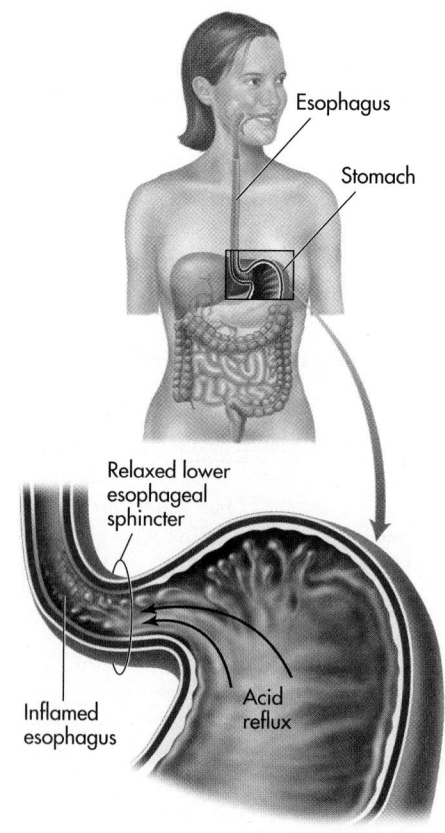

FIGURE 3-23 ▶ Heartburn results from stomach acid refluxing into the esophagus.

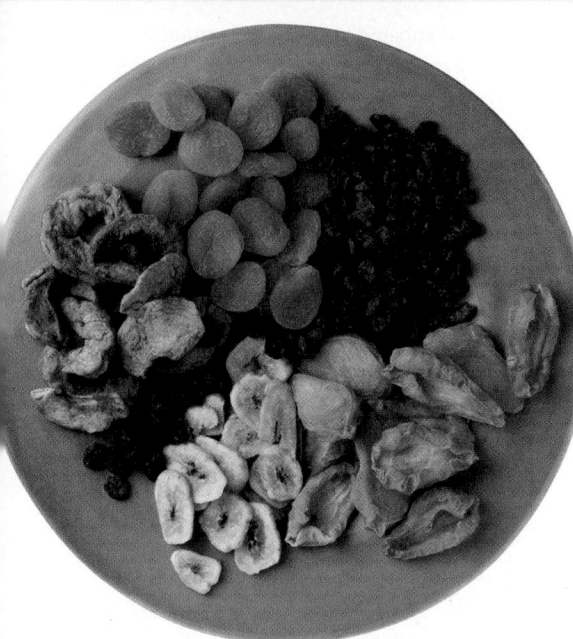

▲ Dried fruits are a natural source of fiber and can help prevent constipation when consumed with an adequate amount of fluid.

MAKING DECISIONS

Use of Laxatives

Perhaps you have heard that taking laxatives after overeating prevents deposition of body fat from excess calorie intake. This erroneous and dangerous premise has gained popularity among followers of numerous fad diets. You may temporarily feel less full after using a laxative because laxatives hasten emptying of the large intestine and increase fluid loss. Most laxatives, however, do not speed the passage of food through the small intestine, where digestion and most nutrient absorption take place. As a result, do you think you can count on laxatives to prevent fat gain from excess calorie intake?

needed to strengthen the weakened esophageal sphincter (see Further Reading 3). A popular theory is that relaxation of the lower esophageal sphincter allows acid and stomach contents to flow back into the esophagus. This situation will be more of a problem when lying down.

Both pregnancy and obesity can lead to heartburn (see Further Reading 6). These conditions result in increased production of estrogen and progesterone, which relax the lower esophageal sphincter, making heartburn more likely. In obesity, adipose tissue turns certain circulating hormones into estrogen; thus, the more adipose tissue one has, the more estrogen produced.

Constipation and Laxatives

Constipation, difficult or infrequent evacuation of the bowels, is commonly reported by adults. Slow movement of fecal material through the large intestine causes constipation. As more fluid is absorbed during the extended time the feces stay in the large intestine, they become dry and hard.

Constipation can result when people regularly ignore their normal bowel reflexes for long periods. People may ignore normal urges when it is inconvenient to interrupt occupational or social activities. Muscle spasms of an irritated large intestine can also slow the movement of feces and contribute to constipation. Calcium, iron supplements, and medications such as antacids can also cause constipation.

Eating foods with plenty of fiber, such as whole-grain breads, cereals, and beans, along with drinking adequate fluid to avoid dehydration, is the best method for treating mild cases of constipation. Fiber stimulates peristalsis by drawing water into the large intestine and helping form a bulky, soft fecal output. Dried fruits are a good source of fiber and therefore can also help stimulate the bowel. Additional fluid should be consumed to facilitate fiber's action in the large intestine. In addition, people with constipation may need to develop more regular bowel habits; allowing the same time each day for a bowel move-

ment can help train the large intestine to respond routinely. Finally, relaxation facilitates regular bowel movements, as does regular physical activity.

Laxatives, as well as various other medications, can also lessen constipation. Some laxatives work by irritating the intestinal nerve junctions to stimulate the peristaltic muscles, while others that contain fiber draw water into the intestine to enlarge fecal output. The larger output stretches the peristaltic muscles, making them rebound and then constrict. Regular use of laxatives, however, should be supervised by a physician. Overall the bulk-forming fiber laxatives are the safest to use.

Hemorrhoids

Hemorrhoids, also called *piles,* are swollen veins of the rectum and anus. The blood vessels in this area are subject to intense pressure, especially during bowel movements. Added stress to the vessels from pregnancy, obesity, prolonged sitting, violent coughing or sneezing, or straining during bowel movements, particularly with constipation, can lead to a hemorrhoid. Hemorrhoids can develop unnoticed until a strained bowel movement precipitates symptoms, which may include pain, itching, and bleeding.

Itching, caused by moisture in the anal canal, swelling, or other irritation, is perhaps the most common symptom. Pain, if present, is usually aching and steady. Bleeding may result from a hemorrhoid and appear in the toilet as a bright red streak in the feces. The sensation of a mass in the anal canal after a bowel movement is symptomatic of an internal hemorrhoid that protrudes through the anus.

Anyone can develop a hemorrhoid, and about half of adults over age 50 do. Diet, lifestyle, and possibly heredity play

constipation A condition characterized by infrequent bowel movements.

laxative A medication or other substance that stimulates evacuation of the intestinal tract.

a role. For example, a low-fiber diet can lead to hemorrhoids as a result of straining during bowel movements. If you think you have a hemorrhoid, you should consult your physician. Rectal bleeding, although usually caused by hemorrhoids, may also indicate other problems, such as cancer.

A physician may suggest a variety of self-care measures for hemorrhoids. Pain can be lessened by applying warm, soft compresses or sitting in a tub of warm water for 15 to 20 minutes. Dietary recommendations are the same as those for treating constipation, emphasizing the need to consume adequate fiber and fluid. Over-the-counter remedies, such as Preparation H, can also offer relief of symptoms.

Irritable Bowel Syndrome

Many adults (25 million or more in the United States alone) have irritable bowel syndrome, noted as a combination of cramps, gassiness, bloating, and irregular bowel function (diarrhea, constipation, or alternating episodes of both). It is more common in younger women than in younger men. In older adults the ratio is closer to 50:50. The disease leads to about 3.5 million visits to physicians in the United States each year.

Symptoms associated with irritable bowel syndrome include visible abdominal distention, pain relief after a bowel movement, increased stool frequency, loose stools with pain onset, mucus in stool, and a feeling of incomplete elimination even after a bowel movement.

The cause is thought to be altered intestinal peristalsis coupled with a decreased pain threshold for abdominal distension—in other words, a minor amount of abdominal bloating causes pain that the average person would not sense. It is also noteworthy that up to 50% of sufferers report a history of verbal or sexual abuse.

Therapy is individualized and can include a trial of high-fiber foods (soluble fiber is more effective than insoluble fiber) or elimination diets that focus on avoiding dairy products and gas-forming foods, such as legumes, certain vegetables (cabbage, beans, and broccoli), and some fruits (grapes, raisins, cherries, and cantaloupe). Herbal formulations, certain probiotics, and cognitive behavioral therapy have been shown to decrease symptoms of irritable bowel syndrome and improve overall quality of life (see Further Reading 1). The patient should moderate or eliminate caffeine-containing foods/beverages altogether. Low-fat and more frequent, small meals may help because large meals can trigger contractions of the large intestine. Other strategies include a reduction in stress, psychological counseling, and certain antidepressant and other medications. Hypnosis has been shown to relieve symptoms in severe cases.

Referral to a registered dietitian can be beneficial, as many patients experience improvement with the elimination of specific problem foods. A good patient/physician relationship is also necessary for the treatment of irritable bowel syndrome; however, before any single treatment is applauded, note that response to placebos alone has been as high as 70% in this population. Although irritable bowel syndrome can be uncomfortable and upsetting, it is harmless as it carries no risk for cancer or other serious digestive problems. The website www.ibsgroup.org provides further information.

Diarrhea

Diarrhea, a GI tract disease that generally lasts only a few days, is defined as increased fluidity, frequency, or amount of bowel movements compared to a person's usual pattern. Most cases of diarrhea result from infections in the intestines, with bacteria and viruses the usual offending agents. They produce substances that cause the intestinal cells to secrete fluid rather than absorb fluid. Another form of diarrhea can be caused by consumption of substances not readily absorbed, such as the sugar alcohol sorbitol found in sugarless gum (see Chapter 4) or large amounts of a high-fiber source such as bran. When consumed in large amounts, the unabsorbed substance draws much water into the intestines, in turn leading to diarrhea. Treatment of diarrhea generally requires drinking lots of fluid during the affected stage; reduced intake of the poorly absorbed substance also is important if that is a cause. Prompt treatment—within 24 to 48 hours—is especially important for infants and older people, as they are more susceptible to the effects of dehydration associated with diarrhea (see Chapters 15 and 16). Diarrhea that lasts more than 7 days in adults should be investigated by a physician as it can be a symptom of more serious intestinal disease, especially if there is also blood in the stool.

Gallstones

Gallstones are a major cause of illness and surgery, affecting 10% to 20% of U.S. adults. Gallstones are pieces of solid material that develop in the gallbladder when substances in the bile—primarily cholesterol (80% of gallstones)—form crystal-like particles. They may be as small as a grain of sand or as large as a golf ball. These stones are caused by a combination of factors, with excess weight being the primary modifiable factor, especially in women 20 to 60 years old. Other factors include genetic background (e.g., Native Americans), advanced age (> 60 years for both women and men), reduced activity of the gallbladder (contracts less than normal), altered bile composition (e.g., too much cholesterol or not enough bile salts), diabetes, and diet (e.g., low-fiber diets). In addition, gallstones may develop during rapid weight loss or prolonged fasting (as the liver metabolizes more fat, it secretes more cholesterol into the bile).

Attacks due to gallstones include intermittent pain in the upper right abdomen, gas and bloating, nausea or vomiting, or other health problems. Surgical removal of the gallbladder is the most common method for treating gallstones (500,000 surgeries per year in the United States).

Prevention of gallstones revolves around avoiding becoming overweight, especially for women. Avoiding rapid weight loss (> 3 pounds per week), limiting animal protein and focusing more on plant protein intake (especially some nut intake), and following a high-fiber diet can help as well. Regular physical activity is also recommended, as is moderate to no caffeine and alcohol intake.

Less Common Digestive Disorders

In **cystic fibrosis**—an inherited disease of infants, children, and sometimes adults—the pancreas often develops thick mucus that blocks its ducts, and active cells then die. As a result, the pancreas is not able to effectively deliver its digestive enzymes into the small intestine. Digestion of carbohydrate, protein, and—most notably—fat then is impaired. Often the missing enzymes must be ingested in capsule form with meals to aid in digestion. Another intestinal problem gaining attention is **celiac disease.** People with this disease experience an allergic reaction to the protein gluten in certain cereals, such as wheat and rye. This reaction damages the absorptive cells, resulting in a much-reduced surface area due to flattening of the villi. Elimination of wheat, rye, and certain other grains from the diet typically cures the problem.

Summary

Overall, typical medical disorders of the GI tract arise from differences in anatomical features and lifestyle habits among individuals. Because of the importance of various nutrition and lifestyle habits, such as adequate fiber and fluid intake, as well as not smoking or abusing NSAID medications, nutrition and lifestyle therapy is often effective in helping treat GI tract disorders.

cystic fibrosis Inherited disease that can cause overproduction of mucus. Mucus can block the pancreatic duct, decreasing enzyme output.

celiac disease Immunological or allergic reaction to the protein gluten in certain grains, such as wheat and rye. The effect is to destroy the intestinal enterocytes, resulting in a much reduced surface area due to flattening of the villi. Elimination of wheat, rye, and certain other grains from the diet restores the intestinal surface.

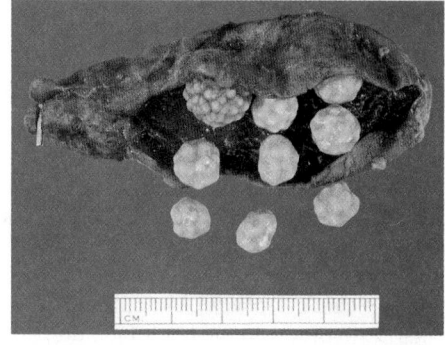

▲ Gallbladder and gallstones seen after surgical removal from the body. Size and composition of the stones vary from one case to another.

Case Study Gastroesophageal Reflux Disease

Caitlin is a 20-year-old college sophomore. Over the last few months, she has been experiencing regular bouts of heartburn. This usually happens after a large lunch or dinner. Occasionally she has even bent down after dinner to pick up something and had some stomach contents travel back up her esophagus and into her mouth. This especially frightened Caitlin, so she visited the University Health Center.

The nurse practitioner at the Center told Caitlin it was good that she came in for a checkup because she suspects Caitlin has a disease called gastroesophageal reflux disease (GERD). She tells Caitlin that this can lead to serious problems, such as a rare form of cancer if not controlled. She provides Caitlin with a pamphlet describing GERD and schedules an appointment with a physician for further evaluation.

Answer the following questions, and check your response in Appendix A.

1. What dietary and lifestyle habits likely contribute to Caitlin's symptoms of GERD?
2. What is the dietary and lifestyle management advice that will help Caitlin cope with this health problem?
3. What types of medications have been especially useful for treating this problem?
4. Overall, how will Caitlin cope with this health problem, and will it ever go away?
5. Why is management of GERD so important?

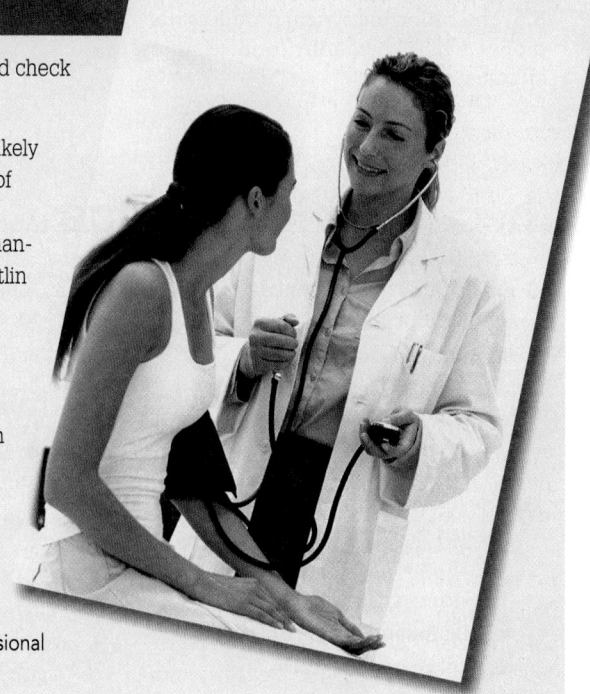

▶ Caitlin was wise to see a health professional about her persistent heartburn.

Summary (Numbers refer to numbered sections in the chapter.)

3.1 Cells join together to make up tissues, tissues unite to form organs, and organs work together as an organ system.

3.2 The basic structural unit of the human body is the cell. A most all cells contain the same organelles (nucleus, mitochondria, endoplasmic reticulum, lysosomes, peroxisomes, and cytoplasm), but cell structure varies according to the type of job they must perform.

3.3 Epithelial, connective, muscle, and nervous, are the four primary types of tissues in the human body. Each type of organ system is affected by nutrient intake.

3.4 Blood is pumped from the heart to the lungs, picking up oxygen. Blood delivers essential nutrients, oxygen, and water to all body cells. Nutrients and wastes are exchanged between blood and cells across the cell membrane. This exchange occurs in the capillaries. Water-soluble compounds absorbed by the small intestine cells enter the portal vein and travel to the liver. Fat-soluble compounds enter the lymphatic system, which eventually connects to the bloodstream.

3.5 The nervous system's neurons are the body's communication network. They control and manage all other organ systems of the body. Neurotransmitters are used to carry the message from one neuron to another (or to another cell).

3.6 The endocrine system produces hormones, which chemically regulate almost all other cells.

3.7 The immune system protects the body from invading pathogens. We activate immunity, such as production of antibodies (immunoglobulins), when we come in contact with a pathogen.

3.8 The gastrointestinal (GI) tract consists of the mouth, esophagus, stomach, small intestine, large intestine (colon), rectum, and anus.

Spaced along the GI tract are ring-like valves (sphincters) that regulate the flow of foodstuffs. Muscular contractions, called *peristalsis*, move the foodstuffs down the GI tract. A variety of nerves, hormones, and other substances control the activity of sphincters and peristaltic muscles.

Digestive enzymes are secreted by the mouth, stomach, wall of the small intestine, and pancreas. The presence of food in the small intestine stimulates the release of pancreatic enzymes.

The major absorptive sites consist of fingerlike projections called *villi*, located in the small intestine. Absorptive cells cover the villi. This intestinal lining is continually renewed. Absorptive cells can perform various forms of passive diffusion and active absorption.

Little digestion and absorption occur in the stomach or large intestine, but some protein is digested in the stomach. Some constituents of fiber and undigested starch are broken down by bacteria in the large intestine and some of the products are absorbed; any undigested fiber that remains is eliminated in the feces.

Final water and mineral absorption takes place in the large intestine. Products from bacterial breakdown of some fibers and other substances are also absorbed here. The presence of feces in the rectum provides the impetus for elimination.

The liver, gallbladder, and pancreas participate in digestion and absorption. Products from these organs, such as enzymes and bile, enter the small intestine help in digesting protein, fat, and carbohydrate.

3.9 The urinary system, including the kidneys, is responsible for filtering the blood, removing body wastes, and maintaining the chemical composition of the blood.

3.10 Limited stores of nutrients are present in the blood for immediate use and stored to a greater or lesser extent in body tissues for later use when sufficient food is unavailable. When the body suffers a nutrient deficiency caused by a poor diet, it breaks down vital tissues for their nutrients, which can lead to ill health. Additionally, too much of any nutrient can be detrimental.

3.11 Genetic background influences the risk for many health-related diseases. Examining one's family tree provides clues for an individual to such risks. Preventative measures are then import ant to implement, especially with respect to diet.

N&YH Common GI-tract diseases, such as heartburn, constipation, and irritable bowel syndrome, can be treated with diet changes. These can include increasing fiber intake and avoiding large meals high in fat. Medications are also very helpful in many cases.

Check Your Knowledge (Answers to the following questions are below.)

1. The stomach is protected from digesting itself by producing
   a. bicarbonate.
   b. a thick layer of mucus.
   c. hydroxyl ions to neutralize acid.
   d. antipepsin that destroys enzymes.

2. The lower esophageal sphincter is located between the
   a. stomach and esophagus.
   b. stomach and duodenum.
   c. ileum and the cecum.
   d. colon and the anus.

3. A muscular contraction that propels food down the GI tract is called
   a. a sphincter.
   b. enterohepatic circulation.
   c. gravitational pull.
   d. peristalsis.

4. Bicarbonate ions (HCO_3-) from the pancreas
   a. neutralize acid in the stomach.
   b. are synthesized in the pyloric sphincter.
   c. neutralize bile in the duodenum.
   d. neutralize the acid in the duodenum.

5. Most digestive processes occur in the
   a. mouth.
   b. stomach.
   c. small intestine.
   d. large intestine.
   e. colon.

6. Bile is formed in the _____ and stored in the _____.
   a. stomach, pancreas
   b. duodenum, kidney
   c. liver, gallbladder
   d. gallbladder, liver

7. Much of the digestion that occurs in the large intestine is caused by
   a. lipase.
   b. pepsin.
   c. saliva.
   d. bacteria.

8. Nexium ("the purple pill") acts as a(n)
   a. H₂ blocker.
   b. laxative.
   c. analgesic.
   d. proton pump inhibitor.

9. The study of how food impacts health through interaction with genes is
   a. nutrigenomics.
   b. epidemiology.
   c. immunology.
   d. genetics.

10. Energy production that takes place in the cytoplasm is anaerobic metabolism because it does not require
    a. water.
    b. oxygen.
    c. anabolic steroids.
    d. anaerobic bacteria.

Answer Keys: 1. b (LO 3.11), 2. a (LO 3.8), 3. d (LO 3.8), 4. d (LO 3.8), 5. c (LO 3.8), 6. c (LO 3.8), 7. d (LO 3.8), 8. d (LO 3.12), 9. a, 10. b (LO 3.2)

Study Questions (Numbers refer to Learning Outcomes)

1. Identify at least one function of the 12 organ systems related to nutrition (LO 3.3)

2. Draw and label parts of the cell, and explain the function of each organelle as it relates to human nutrition. (LO 3.2)

3. Trace the flow of blood from the right side of the heart and back to the same site. How is blood routed through the small intestine? Which class of nutrients enters the body via the blood? Via the lymph? (LO 3.4)

4. Explain why the small intestine is better suited than the other GI tract organs to carry out the absorptive process. (LO 3.8)

5. Identify the four basic tastes. Give an example of one food that exemplifies each of these basic taste sensations. (LO 3.8)

6. What is one role of acid in the process of digestion? Where is it secreted? (LO 3.8)

7. Contrast the processes of active absorption and passive diffusion of nutrients. (LO 3.8)

8. Identify two accessory organs that empty their contents into the small intestine. How do the digestive substances secreted by these organs contribute to the digestion of food? (LO 3.8)

9. In which organ systems would the following substances be found?
   chyme (LO 3.8), plasma (LO 3.4), lymph (LO 3.4), urine (LO 3.9)

10. Describe the nutrition-related diseases for which genetics or family history is considered to be an important risk factor. (LO 3.11)

What Would You Choose Recommendations

Constipation results from slow movement of fecal material through the large intestine. Increasing fiber and water in your diet can often relieve constipation without the aid of an over-the-counter laxative. To boost your fiber intake, choose whole grains, fruits, vegetables, and legumes (beans). This can be a tough task when most of the menu options you will find in fast-food restaurants and convenience stores are low in fiber.

As you select your pizza, look for slices with extra vegetables or fruit. This will increase the fiber content by about 1 gram per slice. Pizza with whole-grain crust, would add another 1 gram of fiber per slice. These are small improvements, so you will probably still need to look for additional fiber sources.

What about your side dish? Unless they are made with whole grains, the pasta and breadsticks will not add much fiber to your meal. A breadstick and a cup of pasta with Alfredo sauce provide about 1 and 2 grams of fiber, respectively. These carbohydrate-rich add-ons are supplying extra calories and would be better off skipped. The salad provides about 1 to 3 grams of fiber, depending on its size and ingredients. The core ingredients of tossed salad—lettuce, cucumbers, tomato—are mostly water and not particularly high in fiber. Toppings such as cheese, egg, or diced meat will not help relieve constipation. Instead, dried fruit (e.g., dried cranberries or raisins) and nuts supply some additional fiber.

An even better choice, however, is the soup! A cup of bean and pasta soup is just what the doctor ordered to help relieve constipation. It provides about 6 grams of fiber and some extra water, as well.

Lastly, be sure to drink plenty of water. Dehydration is an often overlooked cause of constipation. Water helps lubricate the digestive tract and adds bulk to the feces when absorbed by fiber in the large intestine.

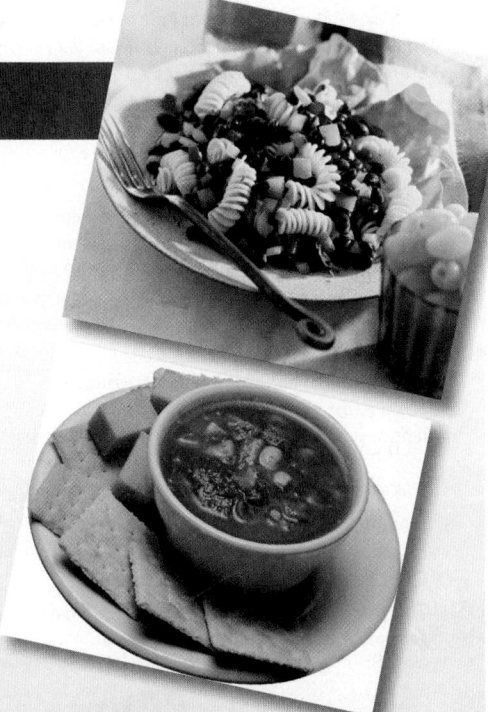

▶ Whole-grain pasta and beans used in salads and soups are good sources of fiber that can prevent intestinal issues such as constipation.

Further Readings

1. Camilleri M: Probiotics and irritable bowel syndrome: Rationale, putative mechanisms, and evidence of clinical efficacy. *Journal of Clinical Gastroenterology* 40:264, 2006.

   The evidence that Bifidobacteria or Lactobacilli species alone or in the specific probiotic combination of VSL#3 are beneficial for treatment of symptoms in IBS is discussed.

2. Consumers Union : Drugs to treat heartburn and stomach acid reflux: The proton pump inhibitors—comparing effectiveness, safety, and price ConsumerReportHealth.org/Best Buy Drugs, 16 pp. May 2010. www.consumer reports.org/health/resources/pdf/best-buy-drugs/PPlsUpdate-FINAL.pdf

   PPls are the most widely prescribed medicines in the United States to treat heartburn and GERD in individuals who have symptoms that persist, are chronic or severe, or are unrelieved by antacids or H2 blockers. The seven available PPl medicines were found to be roughly equal in effectiveness and safety but differed in cost. The report recommended three of the less expensive drugs that are available without a prescription.

3. Galmiche J-P, Deshpande AR: Laparoscopic antireflux surgery versus esomeprazole treatment for chronic GERD: The LOTUS Randomized Clinical Trial. *Journal of the American Medical Association* 305(19): 1969, 2011.

   Study Taking daily medication (Nexium) or undergoing a minimally invasive surgery to treat acid reflux disease control the worst symptoms of the disease in many people. More than 500 persons were studied and after 5 years, 92% of people in the medication group and 85% in the surgery group reported having no GERD symptoms, or symptoms that were easy to live with.

4. Gosden RG, Feinberg AP: Genetics and epigenetics, Nature's pen-and-pencil set. *New England Journal of Medicine* 356:731; 2007.

   Epigenetics refers to inherited changes in gene expression caused by mechanisms other than changes in the underlying DNA sequence. Epigenetic information is like a code written in pencil in the margins around the DNA, which is written in indelible ink. In many cases it is the epigenome that can be repaired by treatments, or affected by diet.

5. Institute of Medicine: *Nutrigenomics and beyond: Informing the future.* Washington, DC: The National Academy Press, 2007.

   This report summarizes the state of nutritional genomics research and policy. It includes guidance for further development and translation of this knowledge into nutrition practice and policy.

6. Jacobson BC and others: Body mass index and symptoms of gastroesophageal reflux in women. *New England Journal of Medicine* 354:2340, 2006.

   BMI was associated with symptoms of GERD in 10,545 participants in the Nurses' Health Study. Even moderate weight gain caused or exacerbated symptoms of reflux.

7. Katsanis SH and others: A case study of personalized medicine. *Science* 320:53, 2008.

   Personalized medicine promises to revolutionize health care by tailoring treatments based on individual genetic information. The need for regulating personalized genomic medicine in a manner beneficial to public health is discussed. Currently, in most states companies are not required to demonstrate clinical validity before offering new genetic tests.

8. Layke JC, Lopez PP: Esophageal cancer. A review and update. *American Family Physician* 73:2187, 2006.

   Esophageal cancer is aggressive and is commonly diagnosed at an advanced stage with a poor prognosis. Associations among the development of esophageal cancer, Helicobacter pylori infection and GERD are discussed. Despite increased use of proton pump inhibitors and eradication of H. pylori, the number of new cases of esophageal cancer continues to grow.

9. Lynch A, Webb C: What are the most effective nonpharmacologic therapies for irritable bowel syndrome? *Journal of Family Practice* 57:57, 2008.

   Herbal formulations, certain probiotics, elimination diets based on immunoglobulin G antibodies, cognitive behavioral therapy, and self-help books are discussed because they have been shown to decrease global symptoms of irritable bowel syndrome (IBS) and improve overall quality of life. Soluble fiber is more effective than insoluble fiber at improving IBS symptoms.

10. Muller-Lisser and others: Myths and misconceptions about constipation. *American Journal of Gastroenterology* 100:232, 2005.

    Increasing fiber intake and avoiding dehydration help in mild cases of constipation. More difficult cases require physician evaluation and likely the use of laxatives and other medications.

11. Niewinski MM: Advances in celiac disease and gluten-free diet. *Journal of the American Dietetic Association* 108:661, 2008.

    Recognition of celiac disease as a disorder, is increasing. This review focuses on the gluten-free diet and the importance for all patients with celiac disease to receive expert dietary counseling. Recent advances in the gluten-free diet are discussed.

12. Omoruyi O, Holten KB: How should we manage GERD? *Journal of Family Practice* 55:410, 2006.

    Guidelines for the use of proton pump inhibitors, H2 blockers, and surgery for the treatment of GERD are presented.

13. Santosa S and others: Probiotics and their potential health claims. *Nutrition Reviews* 64:265, 2006.

    This paper provides strong evidence of the ability of different probiotic strains to prevent and treat diarrhea, and some forms of irritable bowel syndrome.

14. Stover PJ: Influence of human genetic variation on nutritional requirements. *American Journal of Clinical Nutrition* 83:436S, 2006.

    The complexity of the interaction between genes and diet is discussed as well as the reevaluation of criteria used to determine RDAs relative to the contribution of genetic variation to optimal nutrition for individuals.

15. Stover PJ, Caudill MA: Genetic and epigenetic contributions to human nutrition and health: Managing genome-diet interactions. *Journal of the American Dietetic Association* 108:1480, 2008.

    This article discusses ways that nutritional genomics will facilitate the establishment of genome-informed nutrient and food-based dietary guidelines for disease prevention and healthful aging, individualized medical nutrition therapy for disease management, and targeted public health nutrition interventions that maximize benefits and minimize adverse outcomes within genetically diverse human populations.

16. Wallace TC and others: Human gut microbiota and its relationship to health and disease. *Nutrition Review* 69 (7): 392, 2011.

    Evidence is available from over 700 research studies to support the growing interest in the benefits of probiotics and prebiotics and to aid the development of intervention strategies and practical guidelines for their use in the prevention and treatment of gastrointestinal tract disorders.

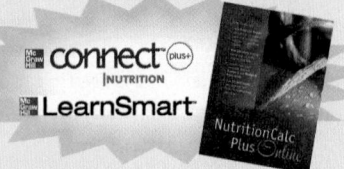

To get the most out of your study of nutrition, go to McGraw-Hill's online resources: Connect www.mcgrawhillconnect.com, **where you will find NutritionCalc Plus, LearnSmart, and many other dynamic tools.**

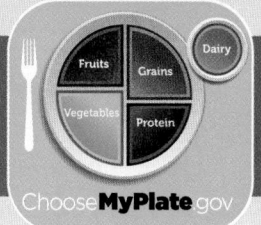

I. Are You Taking Care of Your Digestive Tract?

People need to think about the health of their digestive tracts. There are symptoms we need to notice, as well as habits we need to practice to protect it. The following assessment is designed to help you examine your habits and symptoms associated with the health of your digestive tract. Put a *Y* in the blank to the left of the question to indicate yes and an *N* to indicate no.

_____ 1. Are you currently experiencing greater than normal stress and tension?

_____ 2. Do you have a family history of digestive tract problems (e.g., ulcers, hemorrhoids, recurrent heartburn, constipation)?

_____ 3. Do you experience pain in your stomach region about 2 hours after you eat?

_____ 4. Do you smoke cigarettes?

_____ 5. Do you take aspirin frequently?

_____ 6. Do you have heartburn at least once per week?

_____ 7. Do you commonly lie down after eating a large meal?

_____ 8. Do you drink alcoholic beverages more than two or three times per day?

_____ 9. Do you experience abdominal pain, bloating, or gas 1½ to 2 hours after consuming milk products?

_____ 10. Do you often have to strain while having a bowel movement?

_____ 11. Do you consume less than 9 (women) or 13 (men) cups of a combination of water and other fluids per day?

_____ 12. Do you perform physical activity for less than 60 minutes on most or all days of the week (e.g., jog, swim, walk briskly, row, stair climb)?

_____ 13. Do you eat a diet relatively low in fiber (recall that significant fiber is found in whole fruits, vegetables, legumes, nuts and seeds, whole-grain breads, and whole-grain cereals)?

_____ 14. Do you frequently have diarrhea?

_____ 15. Do you frequently use laxatives or antacids?

Add up the number of yes answers and record the total. If your score is from 8 to 15, your habits and symptoms put you at risk for experiencing future digestive tract problems. Take particular note of the habits to which you answered yes. Consider trying to cooperate more with your digestive tract.

II. Create Your Family Tree for Health-Related Concerns

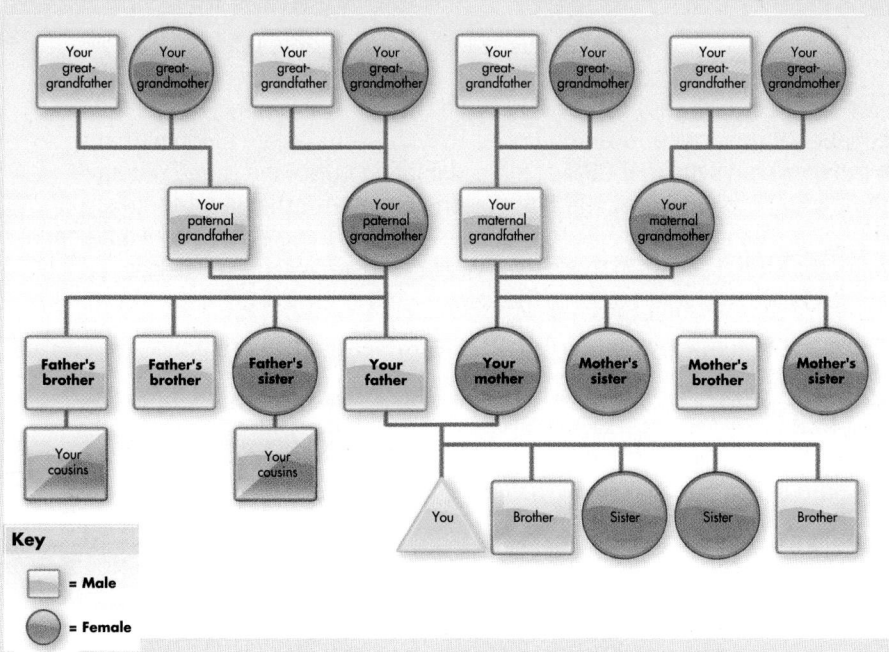

Adapt this diagram to your family tree. Under each heading, list year born, year died (if applicable), major diseases that developed during the person's lifetime, and cause of death (if applicable). Figure 3-21 provides one such example.

You are likely to be at risk for any diseases listed. Creating a plan for preventing such diseases when possible, especially those that developed in your family members before age 50 to 60 years, is advised. Speak with your physician about any concerns arising from this exercise.

Chapter 4 Carbohydrates

Student Learning Outcomes

Chapter 4 is designed to allow you to:

4.1 Identify the basic structures and food sources of the major carbohydrates—monosaccharides, disaccharides, polysaccharides (e.g., starches), and fiber.

4.2 Describe food sources of carbohydrate and list some alternative sweeteners.

4.3 Explain how carbohydrates are digested and absorbed, including the consequences of lactose maldigestion (and lactose intolerance).

4.4 List the functions of carbohydrate in the body and the problems that result from not eating enough carbohydrate.

4.5 Describe the regulation of blood glucose and discuss how other nutrients can be converted to blood glucose.

4.6 Outline the beneficial effects of fiber on the body.

4.7 State the RDA for carbohydrate and various guidelines for carbohydrate intake.

4.8 Identify the consequences of diabetes, and explain appropriate dietary measures that will reduce the adverse effects of this health problem.

What Would You Choose?

In between classes, you stop at a nearby convenience store to pick up a cold drink that will quench your thirst and fill your growling stomach. Immediately, you reach for your favorite cola but the Jones Soda Co.® display with its personalized labels catches your eye. You notice that these sodas are made with no high-fructose corn syrup (HFCS) but instead contain pure cane sugar. You have heard news reports that liken HFCS to poison, but on the other hand, there are commercials saying HFCS is just the same as sugar. Is there a nutritional difference between the added sugars in these two types of sodas? What is the better beverage choice that could provide the calories and energy of an afternoon snack?

a 20-ounce bottle of regular cola (e.g., Coca-Cola®) containing high-fructose corn syrup

b 20-ounce bottle of diet cola (e.g., Coke Zero®) containing aspartame

c 12-ounce bottle of Jones Soda Co.® Pure Cane Root Beer Soda

d ½ pint (8 fluid ounces) of low-fat (1%) chocolate milk

e 16-ounce bottle of water

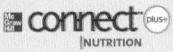 **Think about your choice as you read Chapter 4, then see our recommendations at the end of the chapter. To learn more about various sweeteners, including how HFCS is made and arguments for and against use of HFCS, check out the Connect site:** www.mcgrawhillconnect.com

Part Two

Energy Nutrients and Energy Balance

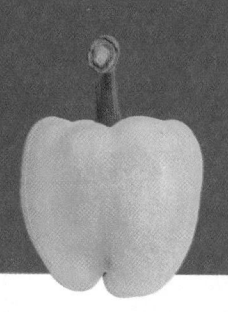

What did you eat to obtain the energy you are using right now? Chapters 4, 5, and 6 will examine this question by focusing on the main nutrients the human body uses for fuel. These nutrients are carbohydrates (on average, 4 kcal per gram) and fats and oils (on average, 9 kcal per gram). Although protein (on average, 4 kcal per gram) *can* be used for energy needs, the body typically reserves this nutrient for other processes.

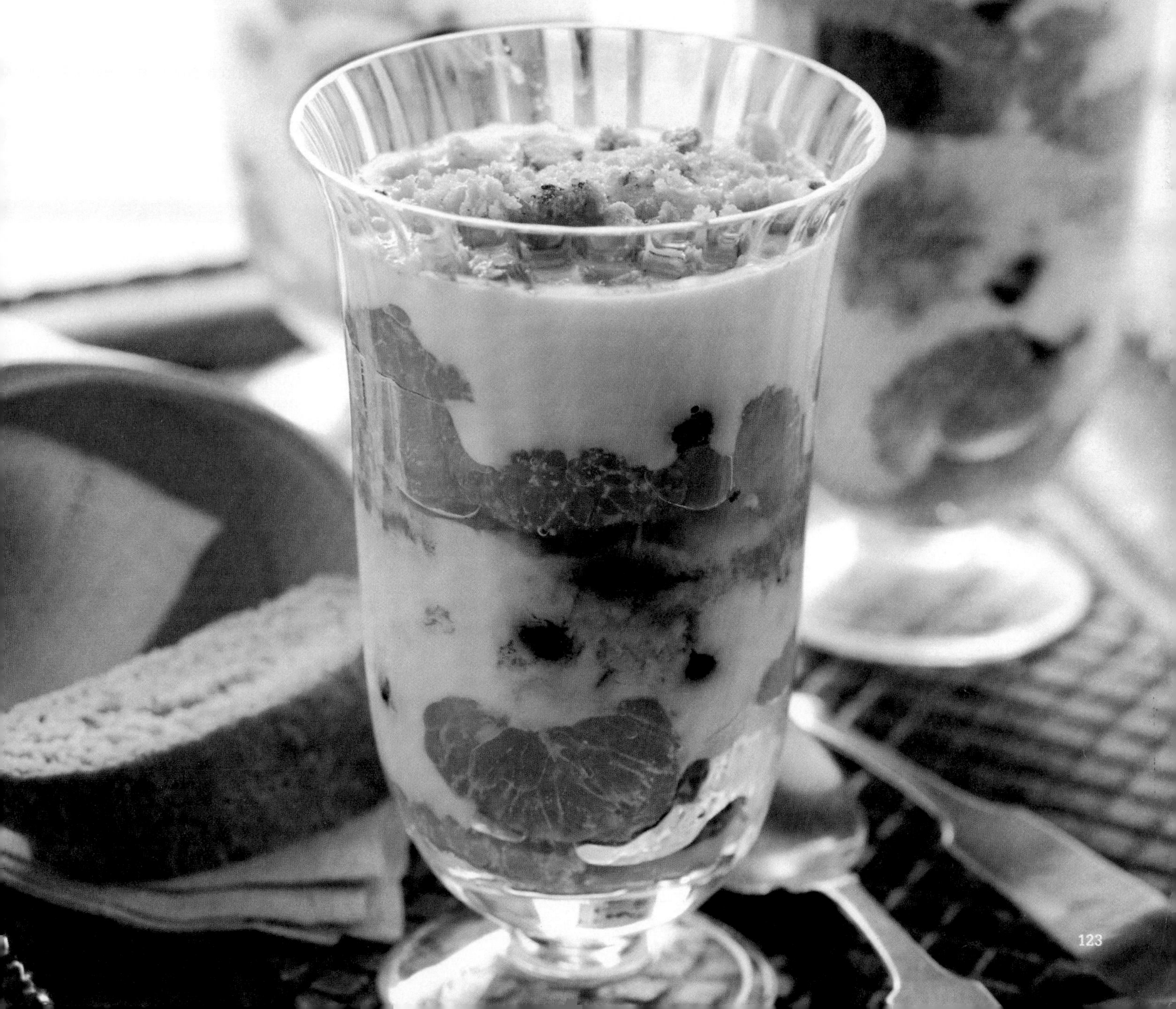

It is likely that you have recently consumed fruits, vegetables, dairy products, cereal, breads, and pasta. These foods supply carbohydrates. Although some carbohydrate sources are more beneficial than others (for example, whole-grain bread compared to white bread, as suggested in the Ziggy comic in this chapter), carbohydrates should be a major part of our diets. Many people think carbohydrate-rich foods cause weight gain but they do not any more so than fat or protein. In fact, pound for pound, carbohydrates are much less fattening than fats and oils. Furthermore, high-carbohydrate foods, especially fiber-rich foods such as fruits, vegetables, whole-grain breads and cereals, and legumes, provide many important health benefits in addition to the calories they contain. Almost all carbohydrate-rich foods, except pure sugars, provide several essential nutrients and should generally constitute 45% to 65% of our daily calorie intake. Let's take a closer look at carbohydrates.

Refresh Your Memory

As you begin your study of carbohydrates in Chapter 4, you may want to review:

- The concept of energy density and the health claims for various carbohydrates in Chapter 2
- The processes of digestion and absorption in Chapter 3
- The hormones that regulate blood glucose in Chapter 3

4.1 Carbohydrates—An Introduction

Carbohydrates are a main fuel source for some cells, especially those in the brain, nervous system, and red blood cells. Muscles also rely on a dependable supply of carbohydrates to fuel intense physical activity. Carbohydrates provide on average 4 kcal per gram and are a readily available fuel for all cells, both in the form of blood glucose and **glycogen** stored in the liver and muscles. The glycogen stored in the liver can be used to maintain blood glucose concentrations in times when you have not eaten for several hours or the diet does not supply enough carbohydrates. Regular intake of carbohydrates is important, because liver glycogen stores are depleted in about 18 hours if no carbohydrate is consumed. After that point, the body is forced to produce carbohydrates, largely from breakdown of proteins in the body. This eventually leads

glycogen A carbohydrate made of multiple units of glucose with a highly branched structure. It is the storage form of glucose in humans and is synthesized (and stored) in the liver and muscles.

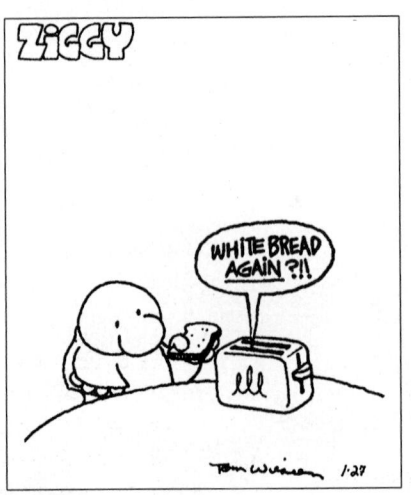

A class of carbohydrate that needs more attention in our diet is fiber. Why is this so? As Ziggy is reminded, white bread is a poor source of fiber. Which health problems typically result from a limited intake of fiber? Which foods are good sources of fiber? How much fiber is enough? Too much? Chapter 4 provides some answers.

ZIGGY © ZIGGY AND FRIENDS, INC. Reprinted with permission of UNIVERSAL PRESS SYNDICATE. All rights reserved.

to health problems including the loss of muscle tissue. To obtain adequate energy, the Food and Nutrition Board recommends that 45% to 65% of the calories we consume each day be from carbohydrates. (See the Acceptable Macronutrient Distribution Range table in the DRI charts in the back pages of this book.)

Despite their important role as a calorie source, some forms of carbohydrate promote health more than others. As you will see in this chapter, whole-grain breads and cereals have greater health benefits than refined and processed forms of carbohydrate. Choosing the healthiest carbohydrate sources most often, while moderating intake of less healthful sources, contributes to a healthy diet. It is difficult to eat so little carbohydrate that body fuel needs are not met, but it is easy to overconsume the simple carbohydrates that can contribute to health problems. Let's explore this concept further as we look at carbohydrates in detail.

Green plants create the carbohydrates in our foods. Leaves capture the sun's solar energy in their cells and transform it to chemical energy. This energy is then stored in the chemical bonds of the carbohydrate glucose as it is produced from carbon dioxide from the air and water from the soil. This complex process is called **photosynthesis** (Fig. 4-1).

$$\text{6 carbon dioxide + 6 water (solar energy)} \rightarrow \text{glucose + 6 oxygen}$$
$$(CO_2) \qquad\qquad (H_2O) \qquad\qquad (C_6H_{12}O_6) \qquad (O_2)$$

Translated into English, this reads: 6 molecules of carbon dioxide combine with 6 molecules of water to form one molecule of **glucose**. Converting solar energy into chemical bonds in the sugar is a key part of the process. Six molecules of oxygen are then released into the air.

4.2 Simple Carbohydrates

As the name suggests, most carbohydrate molecules are composed of carbon, hydrogen, and oxygen atoms. Simple forms of carbohydrates are called **sugars**. Larger, more complex forms are primarily called either **starches** or **fibers**, depending on their digestibility by human GI tract enzymes. Starches are the digestible form. The Concept Map on page 127 summarizes the forms and characteristics of carbohydrates.

Monosaccharides and disaccharides are often referred to as *simple sugars* because they contain only one or two sugar units. Food labels lump all of these sugars under one category, listing them as "sugars."

▲ Fruits such as oranges and pears are an excellent source of carbohydrate, including sugar, starch, and fiber.

photosynthesis Process by which plants use energy from the sun to synthesize energy-yielding compounds, such as glucose.

glucose A six-carbon monosaccharide that usually exists in a ring form; found as such in blood, and in table sugar bonded to fructose; also known as *dextrose*.

sugar A simple carbohydrate with the chemical composition $(CH_2O)_n$. The basic unit of all sugars is glucose, a six-carbon ring structure. The primary sugar in the diet is sucrose, which is made up of glucose and fructose.

starch A carbohydrate made of multiple units of glucose attached together in a form the body can digest; also known as *complex carbohydrate*.

fiber Substances in plant foods not digested by the processes that take place in the stomach or small intestine. These add bulk to feces. Fibers naturally found in foods are also called dietary fiber.

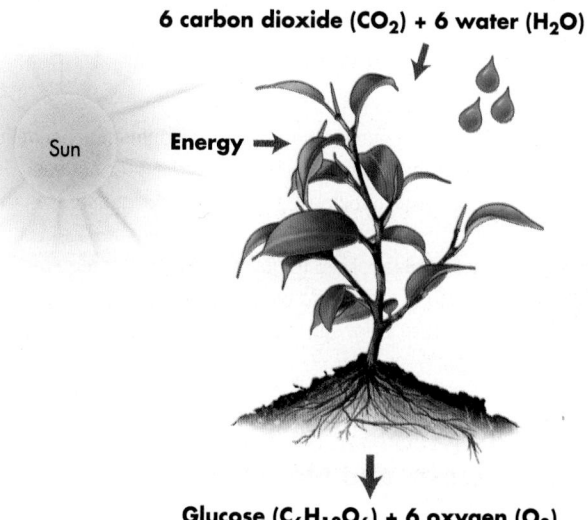

6 carbon dioxide (CO$_2$) + 6 water (H$_2$O)

Sun

Energy →

Glucose (C$_6$H$_{12}$O$_6$) + 6 oxygen (O$_2$)

FIGURE 4-1 ▶ A summary of photosynthesis. Plants use carbon dioxide, water, and energy to produce glucose. Glucose is then stored in the leaf but can also undergo further metabolism to form starch and fiber in the plant. With the addition of nitrogen from soil or air, glucose also can be transformed into protein.

FIGURE 4-2 ▶ Chemical forms of the important monosaccharides.

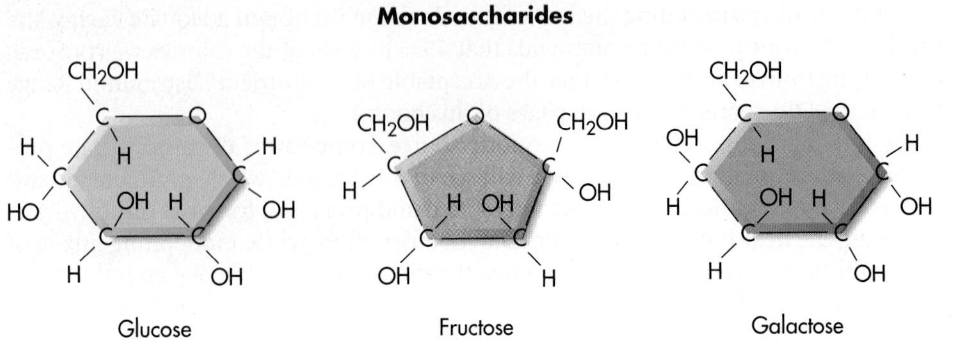

Monosaccharides

Glucose   Fructose   Galactose

monosaccharide Simple sugar, such as glucose, that is not broken down further during digestion.

simple sugar Monosaccharide or disaccharide in the diet.

sucrose Fructose bonded to glucose; table sugar.

fructose A six-carbon monosaccharide that usually exists in a ring form; found in fruits and honey; also known as *fruit sugar*.

high-fructose corn syrup Corn syrup that has been manufactured to contain 42 and 90% fructose.

galactose A six-carbon monosaccharide that usually exists in a ring form; closely related to glucose.

lactose Glucose bonded to galactose; also known as *milk sugar*.

disaccharide Class of sugars formed by the chemical bonding of two monosaccharides.

maltose Glucose bonded to glucose.

Monosaccharides—Glucose, Fructose, and Galactose

Monosaccharides are the **simple sugar** units (*mono* means one) that serve as the basic unit of all carbohydrate structures. The most common monosaccharides in foods are glucose, fructose, and galactose (Fig. 4-2).

Glucose is the major monosaccharide found in the body. Glucose is also known as *dextrose*, and glucose in the bloodstream may be called blood sugar. Glucose is an important source of energy for human cells, although foods contain very little carbohydrate as this single sugar. Most glucose comes from the digestion of starches and **sucrose** (common table sugar) from our food. The latter is made up of the monosaccharides glucose and fructose. For the most part, sugars and other carbohydrates in foods are eventually converted to glucose in the liver. This glucose then goes on to serve as a source of fuel for cells.

Fructose, also called *fruit sugar*, is another common monosaccharide. After it is consumed, fructose is absorbed by the small intestine and then transported to the liver, where it is quickly metabolized. Much is converted to glucose, but the rest goes on to form other compounds, such as fat, if fructose is consumed in very high amounts. Most of the free fructose in our diets comes from the use of **high-fructose corn syrup** in soft drinks, candies, jams, jellies, and many other fruit products and desserts (see the later discussion on nutritive sweeteners and in What Would You Choose?). Fructose also is found naturally in fruits and forms half of each sucrose molecule.

The sugar **galactose** has nearly the same structure as glucose. Large quantities of pure galactose do not exist in nature. Instead, galactose is usually found bonded to glucose in **lactose**, a sugar found in milk and other milk products. After lactose is digested and absorbed, galactose arrives in the liver. There it is either transformed into glucose or further metabolized into glycogen.

MAKING **DECISIONS**

Nutrient Metabolism

Now is a good time to begin emphasizing a key concept in nutrition: the difference between *intake* of a substance and the body's *use* of that substance. The body often does not use all nutrients in their original states. Some of these substances are broken down and later reassembled into the same or a different substance when and where they are needed. For example, much of the galactose in the diet is metabolized to glucose. When later required for the production of milk in the mammary gland of a lactating female, galactose is resynthesized from glucose to help form the milk sugar lactose. Knowing this, do you think it is necessary for a lactating women to drink milk to make milk?

Disaccharides—Sucrose, Lactose, and Maltose

Disaccharides are formed when two monosaccharides combine (*di* means two). The disaccharides in food are sucrose, lactose, and **maltose**. All contain glucose.

Disaccharides

Sucrose: glucose + fructose
Lactose: glucose + galactose
Maltose: glucose + glucose

Sucrose

FIGURE 4-3 ▶ Chemical form of the disaccharide sucrose.

Sucrose forms when the two sugars glucose and fructose bond together (Fig. 4-3). Sucrose is found naturally in sugarcane, sugar beets, honey, and maple sugar. These products are processed to varying degrees to make brown, white, and powdered sugars. Animals do not produce sucrose or much of any carbohydrate except glycogen.

Lactose forms when glucose bonds with galactose during the synthesis of milk. Again, our major food source for lactose is milk products. A later section on lactose maldigestion and lactose intolerance discusses the problems that result when a person can't readily digest lactose.

◀ This Concept Map summarizes the various forms and characteristics of the simple and complex carbohydrates.

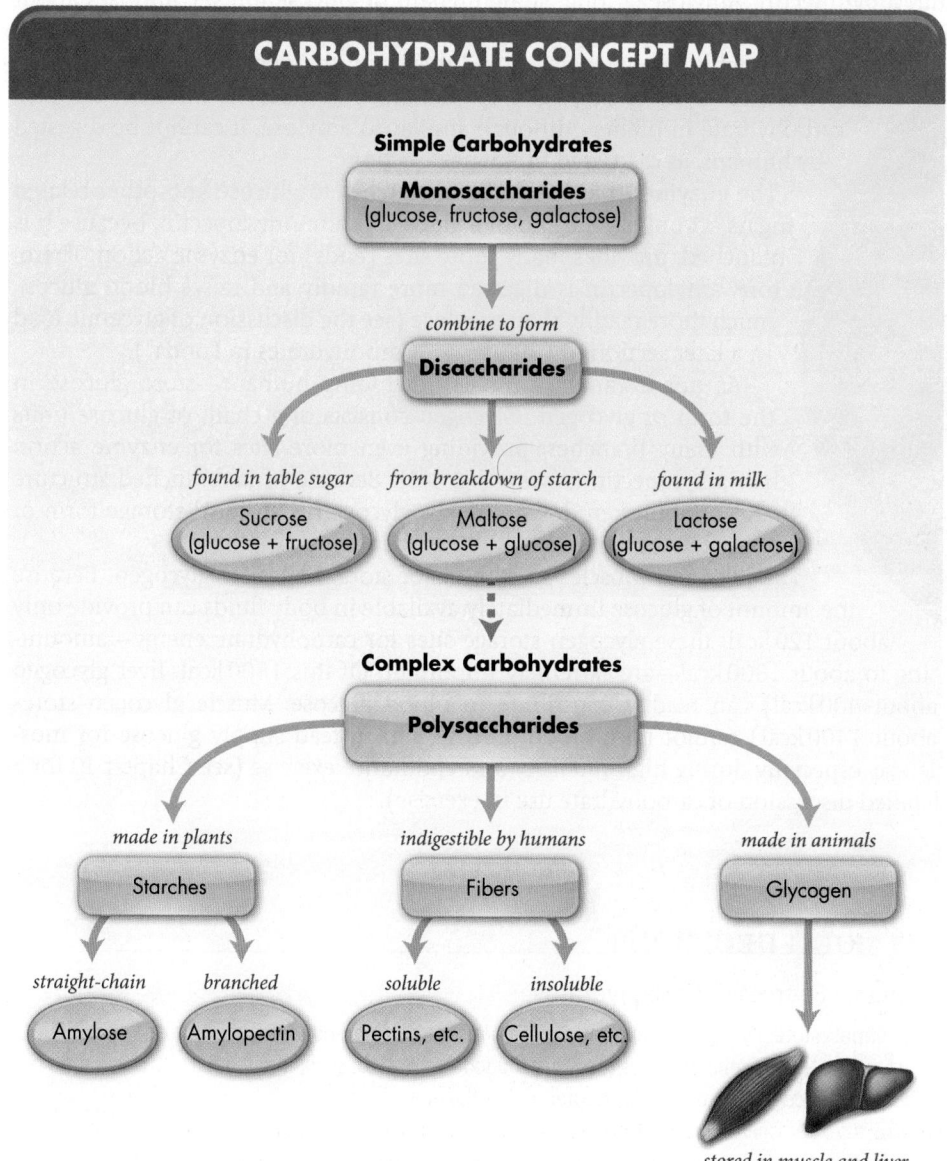

CARBOHYDRATE CONCEPT MAP

Simple Carbohydrates

Monosaccharides
(glucose, fructose, galactose)

combine to form

Disaccharides

found in table sugar — Sucrose (glucose + fructose)
from breakdown of starch — Maltose (glucose + glucose)
found in milk — Lactose (glucose + galactose)

Complex Carbohydrates

Polysaccharides

made in plants — Starches
indigestible by humans — Fibers
made in animals — Glycogen

straight-chain — Amylose
branched — Amylopectin
soluble — Pectins, etc.
insoluble — Cellulose, etc.

stored in muscle and liver

Maltose results when starch is broken down to just two glucose molecules bonded together. Maltose plays an important role in the beer and liquor industry. In the production of alcoholic beverages, starches in various cereal grains are first converted to simpler carbohydrates by enzymes present in the grains. The products of this step—maltose, glucose, and other sugars—are then mixed with yeast cells in the absence of oxygen. The yeast cells convert most of the sugars to alcohol (ethanol) and carbon dioxide, a process called **fermentation**. Little maltose remains in the final product. Few other food products or beverages contain maltose. In fact, most maltose that we ultimately digest in the small intestine is produced during our own digestion of starch.

4.3 Complex Carbohydrates

In many foods, single-sugar units are bonded together to form a chain, known as a polysaccharide (*poly* means many). **Polysaccharides**, also called *complex carbohydrates* or *starch*, may contain 1000 or more glucose units and are found chiefly in grains, vegetables, and fruits. When food labels list "Other Carbohydrates," this primarily refers to starch content.

Plants store carbohydrate in two forms of starch digestible by humans: **amylose** and **amylopectin**. Amylose, a long, straight chain of glucose units, comprises about 20% of the digestible starch found in vegetables, beans, breads, pasta, and rice. Amylopectin is a highly branched chain and makes up the remaining 80% of digestible starches in the diet (Fig. 4-4). Cellulose (a fiber) is another complex carbohydrate in plants. Although similar to amylose, it cannot be digested by humans, as discussed in the next section.

The enzymes that break down starches to glucose and other related sugars act only at the end of a glucose chain. Amylopectin, because it is branched, provides many more sites (ends) for enzyme action. Therefore, amylopectin is digested more rapidly and raises blood glucose much more readily than amylose (see the discussion of glycemic load in a later section of Chapter 4, "Carbohydrates in Foods").

As noted earlier, animals—including humans—store glucose in the form of glycogen. Glycogen consists of a chain of glucose units with many branches, providing even more sites for enzyme action than amylopectin (review Fig. 4-4). Because of its branched structure that can be broken down quickly, glycogen is an ideal storage form of carbohydrate in the body.

The liver and muscles are the major storage sites for glycogen. Because the amount of glucose immediately available in body fluids can provide only about 120 kcal, these glycogen storage sites for carbohydrate energy—amounting to about 1800 kcal—are extremely important. Of this 1800 kcal, liver glycogen (about 400 kcal) can readily contribute to blood glucose. Muscle glycogen stores (about 1400 kcal) cannot raise blood glucose, but instead supply glucose for muscle use, especially during high-intensity and endurance exercise (see Chapter 10 for a detailed discussion of carbohydrate use in exercise).

fermentation The conversion of carbohydrates to alcohols, acids, and carbon dioxide without the use of oxygen.

polysaccharides Carbohydrates containing many glucose units, from 10 to 1000 or more.

amylose A digestible straight-chain type of starch composed of glucose units.

amylopectin A digestible branched-chain type of starch composed of glucose units.

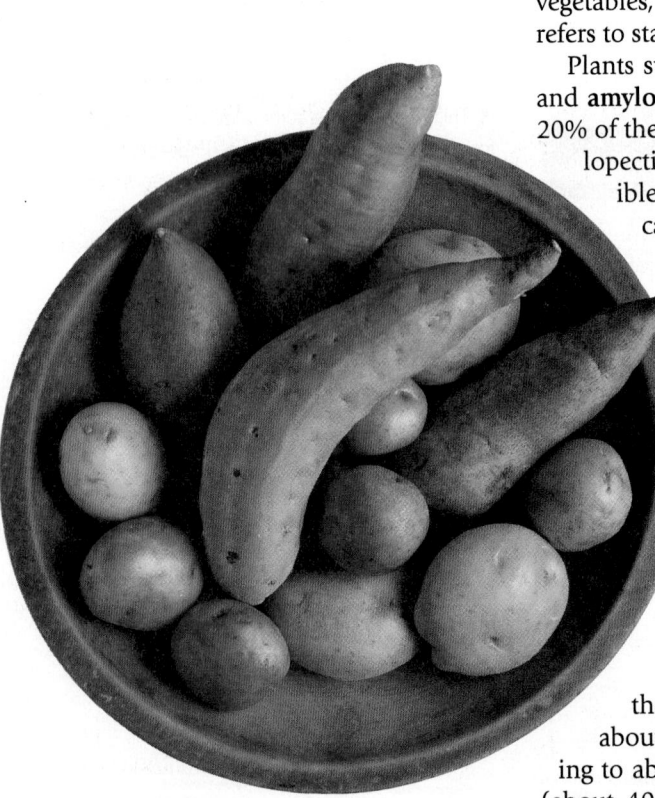

▲ Root vegetables such as potato, yams, and tapioca are high in amylopectin starch.

MAKING **DECISIONS**

Animal Sources of Carbohydrates

If animals store glycogen in their muscles, are meats, fish, and poultry a good source of carbohydrates? No—animal products are not good food sources of this (or any other) carbohydrate because glycogen stores quickly degrade after the animal dies.

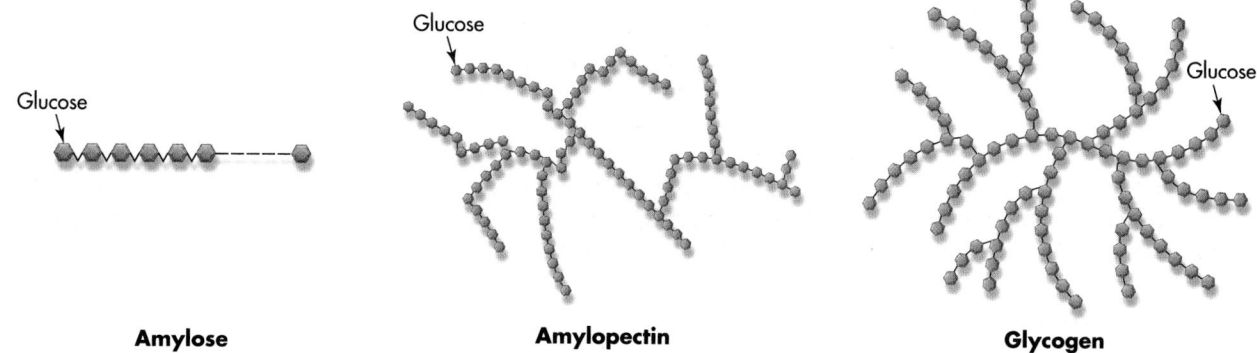

FIGURE 4-4 ▶ Some common starches, amylose and amylopectin, and glycogen. We consume essentially no glycogen. All glycogen found in the body is made by our cells, primarily in the liver and muscles.

4.4 Fiber

Fiber as a class is mostly made up of polysaccharides, but they differ from starches insofar as the chemical links that join the individual sugar units cannot be digested by human enzymes in the GI tract. This prevents the small intestine from absorbing the sugars that make up the various fibers. Fiber is not a single substance but a group of substances with similar characteristics (Table 4-1). The group is comprised of the carbohydrates **cellulose**, **hemicelluloses**, **pectins**, **gums**, and **mucilages**, as well as the noncarbohydrate, **lignin**. In total, these constitute all the nonstarch polysaccharides in foods. Nutrition Facts labels generally do not list these individual forms of fiber, but instead lump them together under the term **dietary fiber**.

Cellulose, hemicelluloses, and lignin form the structural parts of plants. Bran fiber is rich in hemicelluloses and lignin. (The woody fibers in broccoli are partly lignin.) Bran layers form the outer covering of all grains, so **whole grains** (i.e., unrefined) are good sources of bran fiber (Fig. 4-5). Because the majority of these fibers neither readily dissolve in water nor are easily metabolized by intestinal bacteria, they are called **nonfermentable** or insoluble fibers.

Pectins, gums, and mucilages are contained around and inside plant cells. These fibers either dissolve or swell when put into water and are therefore called **viscous** or soluble fibers. They also are readily fermented by bacteria in the large intestine. These fibers are found in salad dressings, some frozen desserts, jams, and jellies as gum arabic, guar gum, locust bean gum, and various pectin forms. Some forms of hemicelluloses also fall into the soluble category.

Most foods contain mixtures of soluble and insoluble fibers. Food labels do not generally distinguish between the two types, but, manufacturers have the option to do so. Often, if food is listed as a good source of one type of fiber, it usually contains some

cellulose An undigestible nonfermentable straight-chain polysaccharide made of glucose molecules.

hemicellulose A nonfermentable fiber containing xylose, galactose, glucose, and other monosaccharides bonded together.

pectin A viscous fiber containing chains of galacturonic acid and other monosaccharides; characteristically found between plant cell walls.

mucilages A viscous fiber consisting of chains of galactose, mannose, and other monosaccharides; characteristically found in seaweed.

lignins A nonfermentable fiber made up of a multiringed alcohol (noncarbohydrate) structure.

dietary fiber Fiber found in food.

whole grains Grains containing the entire seed of the plant, including the bran, germ, and endosperm (starchy interior). Examples are whole wheat and brown rice.

nonfermentable fiber A fiber that is not easily metabolized by intestinal bacteria.

TABLE 4-1 Classification of Fibers

Type	Component(s)	Physiological Effects	Major Food Sources
Nonfermentable or Insoluble			
Noncarbohydrate form	Lignin	Increases fecal bulk	Whole grains, wheat bran
Carbohydrate form	Cellulose, hemicelluloses	Increases fecal bulk Decreases intestinal transit time	All plants, wheat products Wheat, rye, rice, vegetables
Viscous or Soluble			
Carbohydrate form	Pectins, gums, mucilages, some hemicelluloses	Delays stomach emptying; slows glucose absorption; can lower blood cholesterol	Citrus fruits, apples, bananas, oat products, carrots, barley, beans, thickeners added to foods

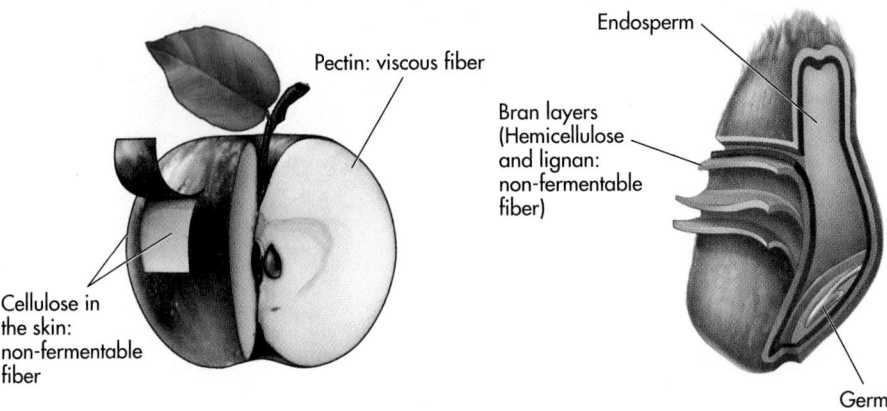

FIGURE 4-5 ▶ Viscous and nonfermentable fiber. (a) The skin of an apple consists of the nonfermentable fiber cellulose, which provides structure for the fruit. The viscous fiber pectin "glues" the fruit cells together. (b) The outside layer of a wheat kernel is made of layers of bran—primarily hemicellulose, a nonfermentable fiber—making this whole grain a good source of fiber. Overall, fruits, vegetables, whole-grain breads and cereals, and beans are rich in fiber.

viscous fiber A fiber that is readily fermented by bacteria in the large intestine.

functional fiber Fiber added to foods that has been shown to provide health benefits.

total fiber Combination of dietary fiber and functional fiber in a food. Also just called *fiber*.

of the other type of fiber as well. The definition of fiber has recently been expanded to include both the dietary fiber found naturally in foods and additional fiber that is added to foods. This second category is called **functional fiber;** a fiber of this type must show beneficial effects in humans to be included in the category. **Total fiber** (or just the term *fiber*) is then the combination of dietary fiber and functional fiber in the food product. Currently the Nutrition Facts label only includes the category dietary fiber; the label has yet to be updated to reflect the latest definition of fiber.

A newly studied category of functional fiber are the prebiotics. Prebiotics include a group of short-chain carbohydrates or oligosaccharides, resistant to digestion, but fermented by bacteria in the colon. They are thought to stimulate the growth or activity of beneficial bacteria in the large intestine and therefore promote the host's health.

CONCEPT CHECK

Important monosaccharides in nutrition are glucose, fructose, and galactose. Glucose is a primary energy source for body cells. Disaccharides form when two monosaccharides bond together. Important disaccharides in nutrition are sucrose (glucose + fructose), maltose (glucose + glucose), and lactose (glucose + galactose). Once digested into monosaccharides and absorbed, most carbohydrates are transformed into glucose by the liver.

Amylose, amylopectin, and glycogen are all polysaccharides, which function as storage forms of glucose. Amylose and amylopectin are the major digestible plant polysaccharides and contain multiple glucose units bonded together. Glycogen is a storage form of glucose in our liver and muscle cells.

Fiber is essentially the portion of plant food that remains undigested as it enters the large intestine. There are two general classes of fiber: nonfermentable and viscous. Nonfermentable (insoluble) fibers are mostly made up of cellulose, hemicelluloses, and lignins. Viscous (soluble) fibers are made up mostly of pectins, gums, and mucilages. Both nonfermentable and viscous fibers are resistant to human digestive enzymes, but bacteria in the large intestine can break down viscous fibers.

4.5 Carbohydrates in Foods

The food components that yield the highest percentage of calories from carbohydrates are table sugar, honey, jam, jelly, fruit, and plain baked potatoes (Fig. 4-6). Corn flakes, rice, bread, and noodles all contain at least 75% of calories as carbohydrates. Foods with moderate amounts of carbohydrate calories are peas, broccoli, oatmeal, dry beans and other legumes, cream pies, French fries, and fat-free milk. In these foods, the carbohydrate content is diluted either by protein, as in the case of fat-free milk, or by fat, as in the case of a cream pie. Foods with essentially no carbohydrates include beef, eggs, chicken, fish, vegetable oils, butter, and margarine.

Food Sources of Carbohydrate

FIGURE 4-6 ▶ Food sources of carbohydrates compared to the RDA of 130 grams for carbohydrate.

Food Item	Carbohydrate (grams)	% RDA
RDA	130	100%
Baked potato, 1 each	51	39%
Cola drink, 12 fluid oz	39	30%
Plain M&M's, ½ oz	30	23%
Banana, 1 each	28	22%
Cooked rice, ½ cup	22	17%
Cooked corn, ½ cup	21	16%
Light yogurt, 1 cup	19	15%
Kidney beans, ½ cup	19	15%
Spaghetti noodles, ½ cup	19	15%
Orange, 1 each	16	12%
Seven grain bread, 1 slice	12	9%
Fat-free milk, 1 cup	12	9%
Pineapple chunks, ½ cup	10	8%
Cooked carrots, ½ cup	8	6%
Peanuts, 1 ounce	6	5%

Key:
- ■ Grains
- ■ Vegetables
- ■ Fruits
- ■ Dairy
- ■ Protein
- ■ Empty calories
- ■ Oils

ChooseMyPlate.gov

The percentage of calories from carbohydrate is more important than the total amount of carbohydrate in a food when planning a healthy high-carbohydrate diet. Figure 4-7 shows that the grain, vegetable, fruit, and dairy groups contain the most nutrient-dense sources of carbohydrate. In planning a healthy high-carbohydrate diet, you need to emphasize whole grains, fruits, and vegetables, rather than potato chips and French fries, because these foods contain too much fat. Currently, the top five carbohydrate sources for U.S. adults are white bread, soft drinks, cookies and cakes (including doughnuts), sugars/syrups/jams, and potatoes. Clearly, many North Americans (teenagers included) should take a closer look at their main carbohydrate sources and strive to improve them from a nutritional standpoint by including more whole-grain versions of breads, pasta, rice, and cereals, as well as fruits and vegetables.

Starch

Starches contribute much of the carbohydrate in our diets. Recall that plants store glucose as polysaccharides in the form of starches. Thus, plant-based foods, such as beans, potatos, and the grains (wheat, rye, corn, oats, barley, and rice) used to make breads, cereals, and pasta, are the best sources of starch. A diet rich in these starches provides ample carbohydrate, as well as many micronutrients.

Fiber

Fiber can be found in many of the same foods as starch, so a diet rich in grains, beans, and potatoes also can provide significant amounts of dietary fiber (especially insoluble cellulose, hemicellulose, and lignins). Because much of the fiber in whole grains

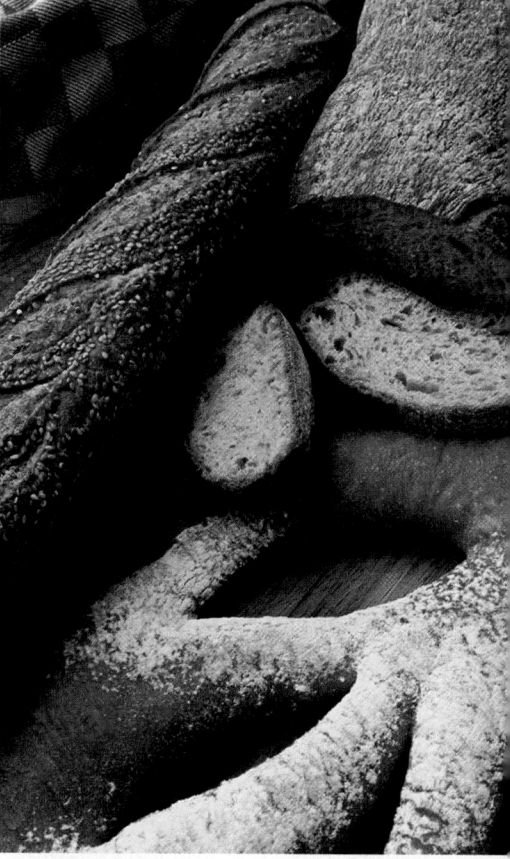

▲ Breads are a rich source of carbohydrate, especially starch and fiber.

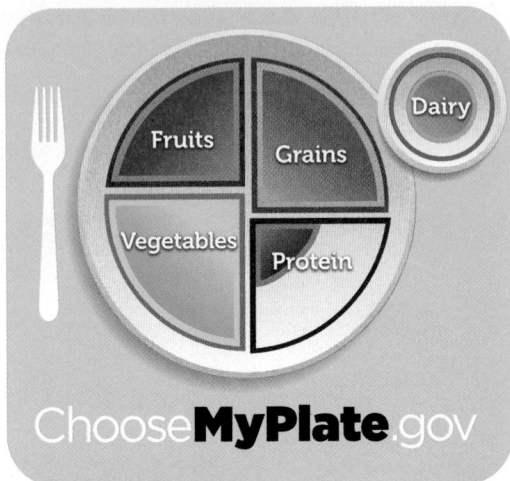

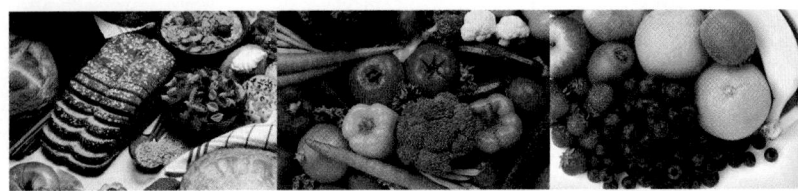

MyPlate:
Sources of Carbohydrates

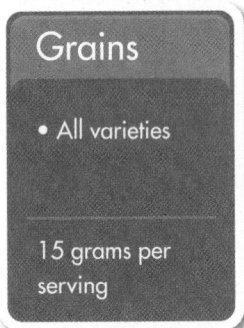

Grains

• All varieties

15 grams per serving

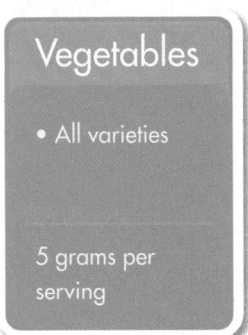

Vegetables

• All varieties

5 grams per serving

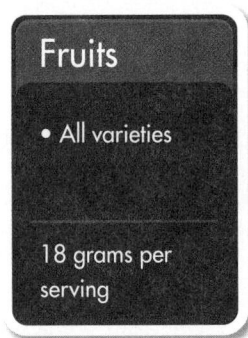

Fruits

• All varieties

18 grams per serving

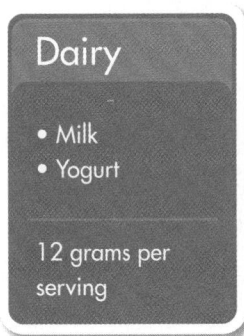

Dairy

• Milk
• Yogurt

12 grams per serving

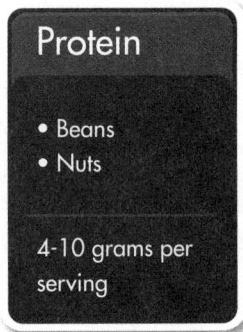

Protein

• Beans
• Nuts

4-10 grams per serving

FIGURE 4-7 ▶ Sources of carbohydrates from MyPlate. The fill of the background color (none, 1/3, 2/3, or completely covered) within each group in the plate indicates the average nutrient density for carbohydrate in that group. Overall, the grain group, vegetable group, fruit group, and dairy group contain many foods that are nutrient-dense sources of carbohydrate. With regard to physical activity, carbohydrates are a key fuel in most endeavors.

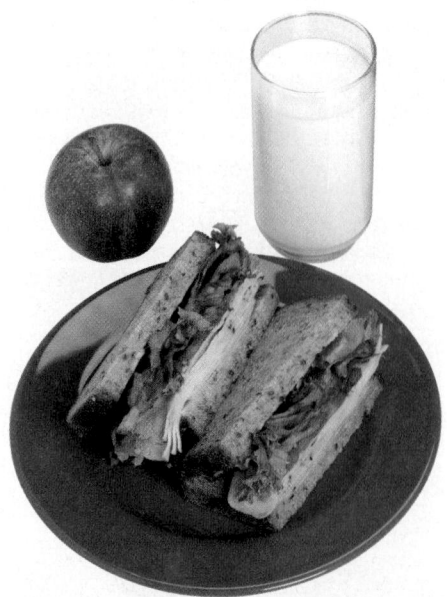

▲ This turkey, cheese, lettuce, and tomato sandwich on whole-grain bread with an apple and glass of low-fat milk fits on **MyPlate** in the right proportions and offers excellent carbohydrate sources of fruits, vegetables, whole grains, and low-fat dairy.

is found in the outer layers, which are removed in processing, highly processed grains are low in fiber. Soluble fibers (pectin, gums, mucilages) are found in the skins and flesh of many fruits and berries; as thickeners and stabilizers in jams, yogurts, sauces, and fillings; and in products that contain psyllium and seaweed.

For individuals who have difficulties consuming adequate dietary fiber, fiber is available as a supplement or as an additive to certain foods (functional fiber). In this way, individuals with relatively low dietary fiber intakes can still obtain the health benefits of fiber.

Nutritive Sweeteners

The various substances that impart sweetness to foods fall into two broad classes: nutritive sweeteners, which can provide calories for the body; and alternative sweeteners, which for the most part provide no calories. As shown in Table 4-2, the alternative sweeteners are much sweeter on a per-gram basis than the nutritive sweeteners. The taste and sweetness of sucrose make it the benchmark against which all other sweeteners are measured. Sucrose is obtained from sugar cane and sugar beet plants. Both sugars and sugar alcohols provide calories along with sweetness. Sugars are found in many different food products, whereas sugar alcohols have rather limited uses.

Sugars. All of the monosaccharides (glucose, fructose, and galactose) and disaccharides (sucrose, lactose, and maltose) discussed earlier are designated *nutritive sweeteners* (Table 4-3). Many forms of sugar are used in food products and result in an intake of about 82 grams or 16 teaspoons of sugar per day.

TABLE 4-2 The Sweetness of Sugars (Nutritive) and Alternative Sweeteners

Type of Sweetener	Relative Sweetness* (Sucrose = 1)	Typical Sources
Sugars		
Lactose	0.2	Dairy products
Maltose	0.4	Sprouted seeds
Glucose	0.7	Corn syrup
Sucrose	1.0	Table sugar, most sweets
Invert sugar[†]	1.3	Some candies, honey
Fructose	1.2–1.8	Fruit, honey, some soft drinks
Sugar Alcohols		
Sorbitol	0.6	Dietetic candies, sugarless gum
Mannitol	0.7	Dietetic candies
Xylitol	0.9	Sugarless gum
Maltitol	0.9	Baked goods, chocolate, candies
Alternative Sweeteners		
Tagatose (Naturlose™)	0.9	Ready-to-eat breakfast cereals, diet soft drinks, meal replacement bars, frozen desserts, candy, frosting
Cyclamate[‡]	30	Tabletop sweetener, medicines
Stevia (Truvia®)	100–300	Tabletop sweetener, food ingredient
Aspartame (Equal®)	180	Diet soft drinks, diet fruit drinks, sugarless gum, tabletop sweetener
Acesulfame-K (Sunette®)	200	Sugarless gum, diet drink mixes, tabletop sweetener, puddings, gelatin desserts
Saccharin (Sweet'N Low®)	300	Diet soft drinks, tabletop sweetener
Sucralose (Splenda®)	600	Diet soft drinks, tabletop sweetener, sugarless gums, jams, frozen desserts
Neotame	7000 to 13,000	Tabletop sweetener, baked goods, frozen desserts, jams

*On a per gram basis.

[†]Sucrose broken down into glucose and fructose.

[‡]Not available in the United States, but available in Canada.

From the *American Dietetic Association*, 2004, and other sources (see Further Reading 1).

High-fructose corn syrup (HFCS) is made by an enzymatic process that converts some of the glucose in cornstarch into fructose, which tastes sweeter than glucose. It is called "high-fructose" corn syrup because it contains 55% fructose, compared to sucrose, which contains only 50% fructose. In the United States, corn is abundant and inexpensive compared to sugar cane or sugar beets, much of which is imported. Food manufacturers prefer HFCS because it is easy to transport, has better shelf-stability, and improves food properties. Because of its low cost and broad range of food-processing applications, HFCS is now used in all kinds of foods, from soft drinks to barbecue sauce. An average American consumes about 60 pounds of HFCS each year. The dramatic rise in obesity has paralleled the increase in HFCS consumption over the past 40 years, and some researchers speculate that properties of the HFCS are to blame. Read more about this in the Newsworthy Nutrition column in the margin and in our recommendations for What Would You Choose?

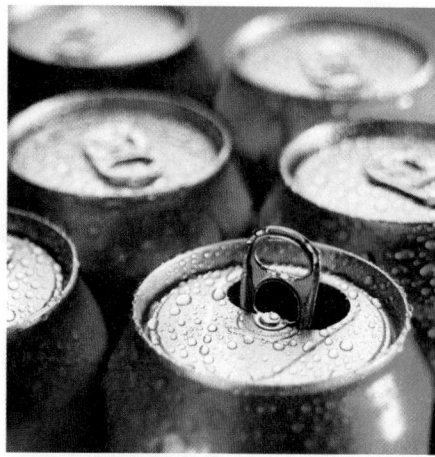

▲ Soft drinks are typical sources of either sugars or alternative sweeteners, depending on the type of soft drink chosen.

NEWSWORTHY NUTRITION

Link between high-fructose corn syrup and obesity

The intake of high-fructose corn syrup (HFCS) from 1967 to 2000 was studied and compared to the development of obesity. HFCS consumption increased >1000% between 1970 and 1990. It was estimated that Americans consume 132 to 316 kcal daily from HFCS. The increase in HFCS use has paralleled the increase in obesity. Differences in the digestion, absorption, and metabolism of fructose compared to glucose have been suggested as explanations for the relationship between HFCS and obesity. Studies of HFCS in humans, however, have been unable to separate the effects of the widely consumed sweetener from the impact of physical inactivity, large portion sizes, smoking cessation, increased consumption of foods prepared outside the home, and other environmental factors.

Source: Bray GA and others. Consumption of high-fructose corn syrup in beverages may play a role in the epidemic of obesity. *American Journal of Clinical Nutrition*, 79(4):537, 2004 (see Further Reading 4).

connect NUTRITION **Check out the Connect site** www.mcgrawhillconnect.com **to further explore HFCS and obesity.**

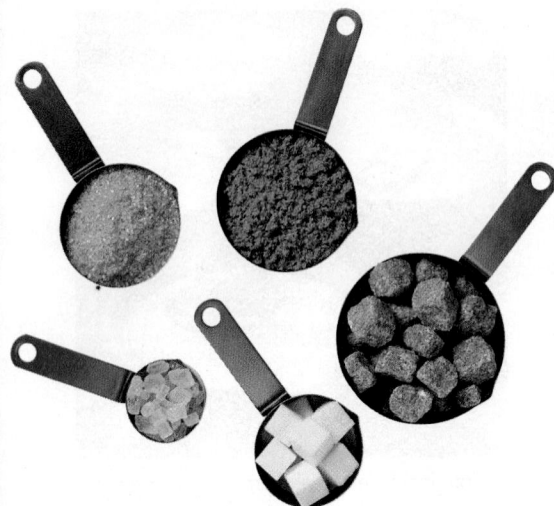

▲ There are many forms of sugar on the market. Used in many foods, together they contribute to our daily intake of approximately 82 grams (16 teaspoons) of sugars in our diets.

TABLE 4-3 Names of Sugars Used in Foods

Sugar	Invert sugar	Honey	Maple syrup
Sucrose	Glucose	Corn syrup or sweeteners	Dextrose
Brown sugar	Sorbitol	High-fructose corn syrup	Fructose
Confectioner's sugar (powdered sugar)	Levulose		Maltodextrins
	Polydextrose	Molasses	Caramel
Turbinado sugar	Lactose	Date sugar	Fruit sugar

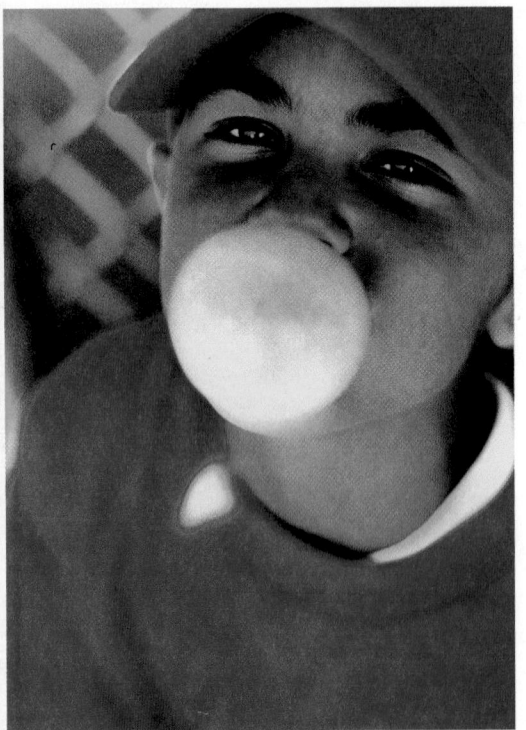

▲ Sugarless gum is typically sweetened with sugar alcohols.

sorbitol Alcohol derivative of glucose that yields about 3 kcal/g but is slowly absorbed from the small intestine; used in some sugarless gums and dietetic foods.

xylitol Alcohol derivative of the 5-carbon monosaccharide xylose.

In addition to sucrose and high-fructose corn syrup, brown sugar, turbinado sugar (sold as raw sugar), honey, maple syrup, and other sugars are also added to foods. Brown sugar is essentially sucrose containing some molasses that is not totally removed from the sucrose during processing or is added to the sucrose crystals. Turbinado sugar is a partially refined version of raw sucrose. Maple syrup is made by boiling down and concentrating the sap that runs during the late winter in sugar maple trees. Because pure maple syrup is expensive, most pancake syrup is primarily corn syrup and high-fructose corn syrup with maple flavor added.

Honey is a product of plant nectar that has been altered by bee enzymes. The enzymes break down much of the nectar's sucrose into fructose and glucose. Honey offers essentially the same nutritional value as other simple sugars—a source of energy and little else. However, honey is not safe to feed to infants because it can contain spores of the bacterium *Clostridium botulinum* that causes fatal food-borne illness. Unlike the acidic environment of an adult's stomach, which inhibits the growth of the bacteria, an infant's stomach does not produce much acid, making infants susceptible to the threat that this bacterium poses.

Sugar Alcohols. Food manufacturers and consumers have numerous options for obtaining sweetness while consuming less sugar and calories. Overall, sugar alcohols and alternative sweeteners enable people with diabetes to enjoy the flavor of sweetness while controlling sugars in their diets; they also provide noncaloric or very-low-calorie sugar substitutes for persons trying to lose (or control) body weight.

Sugar alcohols such as **sorbitol** and **xylitol** are used as nutritive sweeteners. Sugar alcohols contribute fewer calories (about 2.6 kcal per gram) than sugars. They also are absorbed and metabolized to glucose more slowly than are simple sugars. Because of this, they remain in the intestinal tract for a longer time and in large quantities can cause diarrhea. In fact, any products that may be consumed in amounts that may result in a daily ingestion of 50 grams of sugar alcohols, must bear this labeling statement: "Excess consumption may have a laxative effect."

Sugar alcohols are used in sugarless gum, breath mints, and candy. Unlike sucrose, sugar alcohols are not readily metabolized by bacteria to acids in the mouth and thus do not promote tooth decay (see the later section on problems linked to carbohydrate intake).

Sugar alcohols must be listed on labels. If only one sugar alcohol is used in a product, its name must be listed. However, if two or more are used in one product, they are grouped together under the heading "sugar alcohols." The caloric value of each sugar alcohol used in a food product is calculated so that when one reads the total amount of calories a product provides, it includes the sugar alcohols in the overall amount.

Alternative Sweeteners

Alternative sweeteners in increasing order of sweetness include **tagatose**, **cyclamate**, **stevia**, **aspartame**, **acesulfame-K**, **saccharin**, **sucralose**, and **neotame**. Unlike sugar alcohols, alternative sweeteners yield little or no calories when consumed in amounts typically used in food products. All except cyclamate are currently available in the United States. Cyclamate was banned for use in the United States in 1970, although it has never been conclusively proven to cause health problems when used appropriately. Cyclamate is used in Canada as a sweetener in medicines and as a tabletop sweetener.

The safety of sweeteners is determined by the FDA and is indicated by an **Acceptable Daily Intake (ADI)** guideline. The ADI is the amount of alternative sweetener considered safe for daily use over one's lifetime. ADIs are based on studies in laboratory animals and are set at a level 100 times less than the level at which no harmful effects were noted in animal studies. Alternative sweeteners can be used safely by adults and children. Although general use is considered safe during pregnancy, pregnant women may want to discuss this issue with their health-care providers.

Saccharin. The oldest alternative sweetener, saccharin, was first produced in 1879 and is currently approved for use in more than 90 countries. It represents about half of the alternative sweetener market in North America (typically packaged in pink packets, including Sweet 'N Low®). Based on laboratory animal studies, saccharin was once thought to increase the risk of bladder cancer but it is no longer listed as a potential cause of cancer.

Aspartame. Aspartame is in widespread use throughout the world (typically packaged in blue packets, including Equal®). It has been approved for use by more than 90 countries, and its use has been endorsed by the World Health Organization, the American Medical Association, the American Diabetes Association, and other groups.

The components of aspartame are the amino acids phenylalanine and aspartic acid, along with methanol. Recall that amino acids are the building blocks of proteins, so aspartame is more of a protein than a carbohydrate. Aspartame yields about 4 kcal per gram, but it is about 200 times sweeter than sucrose. Thus, only a small amount of aspartame is needed to obtain the desired sweetness, and the amount of calories added is insignificant unless the product is consumed in unusually high amounts. Aspartame is used in beverages, gelatin desserts, chewing gum, toppings and fillings in precooked bakery goods, and cookies. Aspartame does not cause tooth decay. Like other proteins, however, aspartame is damaged when heated for a long time and thus would lose its sweetness if used in products requiring cooking.

Some complaints have been filed with FDA by people claiming to have had adverse reactions to aspartame: headaches, dizziness, seizures, nausea, and other side effects. It is important for people who are sensitive to aspartame to avoid it, but the percentage of sensitive people is likely to be extremely small.

The acceptable daily intake of aspartame set by FDA is 50 milligrams per kilogram of body weight. This is equivalent to the aspartame in about 14 cans of diet soft drink for an adult or about 80 packets of Equal®. Aspartame appears to be safe for pregnant women and children, but some scientists suggest cautious use by these groups, especially young children, who need ample calories to grow.

Sucralose. Sucralose (Splenda®) is 600 times sweeter than sucrose. It is made by adding three chlorines to sucrose. Sucralose is approved for use as an additive to foods such as soft drinks, gum, baked goods, syrups, gelatins, frozen dairy desserts such as ice cream, jams, processed fruits and fruit juices, and for tabletop use. Sucralose doesn't break down under high heat conditions and can be used in cooking and baking. It is also excreted as such in the feces. The small amount absorbed is excreted in the urine.

Sugar alcohols as a class are also called polyols.

stevia Alternative sweetener derived from South American shrub; 100 to 300 times sweeter than sucrose.

aspartame Alternative sweetener made of 2 amino acids and methanol; about 200 times sweeter than sucrose.

sucralose Alternative sweetener that has chlorines in place of 3 hydroxyl (—OH) groups on sucrose; 600 times sweeter than sucrose.

acesulfame K Alternative sweetener that yields no energy to the body; 200 times sweeter than sucrose.

saccharin Alternative sweetener that yields no energy to the body; 300 times sweeter than sucrose.

neotame General-purpose, nonnutritive sweetener that is approximately 7000 to 13,000 times sweeter than table sugar. It has a chemical structure similar to aspartame's.

Persons with an uncommon disease called **phenylketonuria (PKU),** which interferes with the metabolism of phenylalanine, should avoid aspartame because of its high phenylalanine content. A warning label is required on products containing aspartame, alerting people with PKU that a product with aspartame contains phenylalanine.

INGREDIENTS: SORBITOL, GUM BASE, MANNITOL, GLYCEROL, HYDROGENATED GLUCOSE SYRUP, XYLITOL, ARTIFICIAL AND NATURAL FLAVORS, ASPARTAME, RED 40, YELLOW 6 AND BHT (TO MAINTAIN FRESHNESS). PHENYLKETONURICS: CONTAINS PHENYLALANINE.

Sugarless Gum

▲ Sugar alcohols and the alternative sweetener aspartame are used to sweeten this product. Note the warning for people with phenylketonuria PKU that this product is made with aspartame and, thus, contains phenylalanine.

Acceptable Daily Intake (ADI) Estimate of the amount of a sweetener that an individual can safely consume daily over a lifetime. ADIs are given as mg per kg of body weight per day.

phenylketonuria (PKU) Disease caused by a defect in the liver's ability to metabolize the amino acid phenylalanine into the amino acid tyrosine; untreated, toxic byproducts of phenylalanine build up in the body and lead to mental retardation.

Neotame. Neotame was recently approved by FDA for use as a general-purpose sweetener in a wide variety of food products, other than meat and poultry. Neotame is a nonnutritive, high-intensity sweetener that, depending on its food application, is approximately 7000 to 13,000 times sweeter than table sugar. It has a chemical structure similar to aspartame. Neotame is heat stable and can be used as a tabletop sweetener as well as in cooking applications. Examples of uses for which it has been approved include baked goods, nonalcoholic beverages (including soft drinks), chewing gum, confections and frostings, frozen desserts, gelatins and puddings, jams and jellies, processed fruits and fruit juices, toppings, and syrups. Neotame is safe for use by the general population, including children, pregnant and lactating women, and people with diabetes. In addition, no special labeling for people with phenylketonuria is needed because neotame is not broken down in the body to its amino acid components.

Acesulfame-K. The alternative sweetener acesulfame-K (the *K* stands for potassium; Sunette®) was approved by the FDA in July 1988. It is approved for use in more than 40 countries and has been in use in Europe since 1983. Acesulfame-K is 200 times sweeter than sucrose. It contributes no calories to the diet because it is not digested by the body, and it does not cause dental caries.

Unlike aspartame, acesulfame-K can be used in baking because it does not lose its sweetness when heated. In the United States, it is currently approved for use in chewing gum, powdered drink mixes, gelatins, puddings, baked goods, tabletop sweeteners, candy, throat lozenges, yogurt, and nondairy creamers; additional uses may soon be approved. One recent trend is to combine it with aspartame in soft drinks.

Tagatose. Tagatose, sold as Naturlose,® is a slightly altered form of the simple sugar fructose. It is approved for use in ready-to-eat breakfast cereals, diet soft drinks, meal replacement bars, frozen desserts, candy, frosting, and chewing gum. Tagatose is poorly absorbed, so it yields only 1.5 kcal per gram to the body. Use also does not raise the risk for dental caries, nor does it increase blood glucose. Eventual fermentation in the large intestine may even lead to a beneficial effect on that organ (i.e., a prebiotic effect, covered in Chapter 3).

Stevia. Stevia, sold as the dietary supplement Sweet Leaf®, is an alternative sweetener derived from a South American shrub. Stevia extracts are 100 to 300 times sweeter than sucrose but provide no energy. It has been used in teas and as a sweetener in Japan since the 1970s, and the FDA recently (December 2008) stated that stevia is considered generally recognized as safe (GRAS) for use in foods. Stevia can be purchased as a dietary supplement in natural and health food stores and as an alternative sweetener in grocery stores.

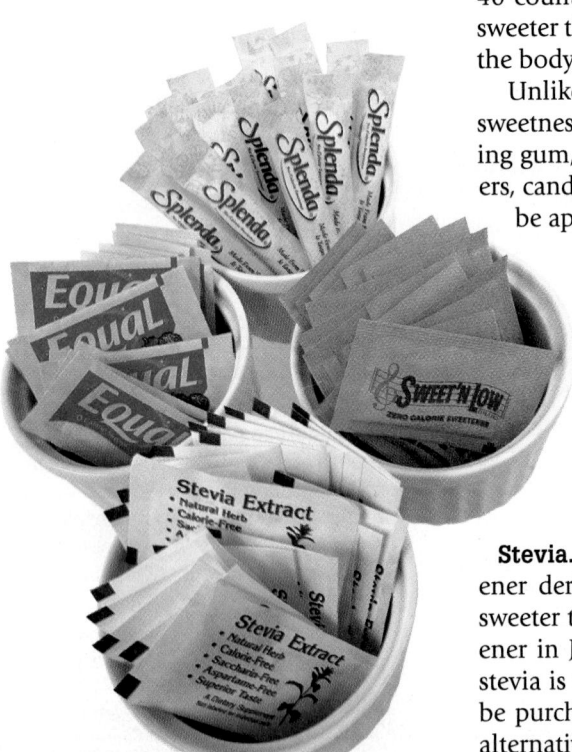

▲ A variety of alternative sweeteners are available.

CONCEPT CHECK

Table sugar, honey, jam, fruit, and plain baked potatoes contain the highest percentage of calories from carbohydrates. Foods such as cream pies, potato chips, whole milk, and oatmeal contain moderate amounts of carbohydrate. Common nutritive sweeteners added to foods include sucrose, maple sugar, honey, brown sugar, and high-fructose corn syrup. For people who want to limit calories from sugar intake, other sweeteners are available and include the sugar alcohols, saccharin, aspartame, sucralose, neotame, acesulfame-K, tagatose, and stevia. Of these, aspartame is the most common alternative sweetener in use.

4.6 Making Carbohydrates Available for Body Use

As discussed in Chapter 3, simply eating a food does not supply nutrients to body cells. Digestion and absorption must occur first.

Digestion

Food preparation can be viewed as the start of carbohydrate digestion because cooking softens tough connective structures in the fibrous parts of plants, such as broccoli stalks. When starches are heated, the starch granules swell as they soak up water, making them much easier to digest. All of these effects of cooking generally make carbohydrate-containing foods easier to chew, swallow, and break down during digestion.

The enzymatic digestion of starch begins in the mouth, when the saliva, which contains an enzyme called salivary **amylase**, mixes with the starchy products during the chewing of the food. This amylase breaks down starch into many smaller units, primarily disaccharides, such as maltose (Fig. 4-8). You can taste this conversion while chewing a saltine cracker. Prolonged chewing of the cracker causes it to taste sweeter as some starch breaks down into the sweeter disaccharides, such as maltose. Still, food is in the mouth for such a short amount of time that this phase of digestion is negligible. In addition, once the food moves down the esophagus and reaches the stomach, the acidic environment inactivates salivary amylase.

amylase Starch-digesting enzyme from the salivary glands or pancreas.

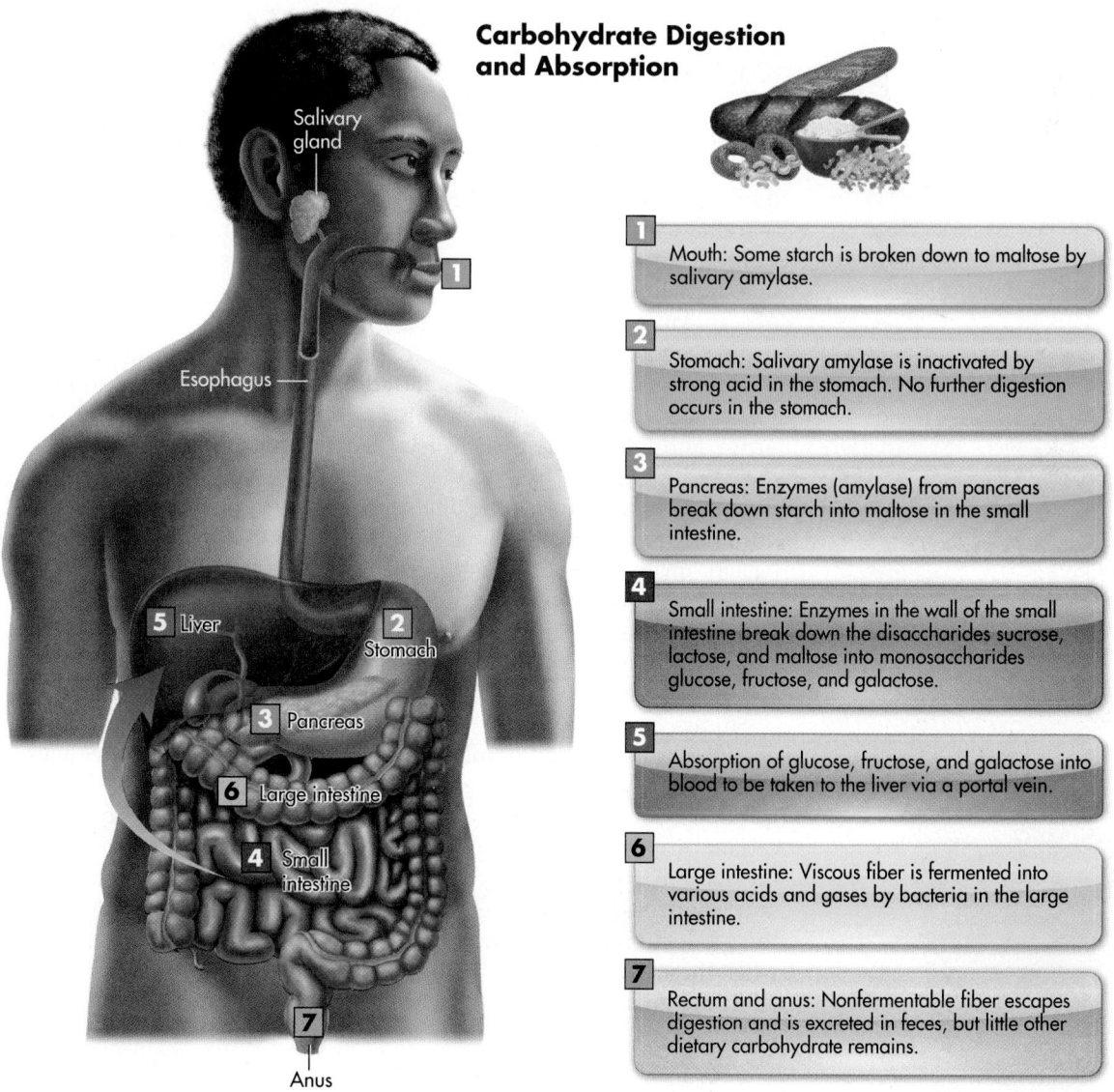

Carbohydrate Digestion and Absorption

1 Mouth: Some starch is broken down to maltose by salivary amylase.

2 Stomach: Salivary amylase is inactivated by strong acid in the stomach. No further digestion occurs in the stomach.

3 Pancreas: Enzymes (amylase) from pancreas break down starch into maltose in the small intestine.

4 Small intestine: Enzymes in the wall of the small intestine break down the disaccharides sucrose, lactose, and maltose into monosaccharides glucose, fructose, and galactose.

5 Absorption of glucose, fructose, and galactose into blood to be taken to the liver via a portal vein.

6 Large intestine: Viscous fiber is fermented into various acids and gases by bacteria in the large intestine.

7 Rectum and anus: Nonfermentable fiber escapes digestion and is excreted in feces, but little other dietary carbohydrate remains.

FIGURE 4-8 ▶ Carbohydrate digestion and absorption. Enzymes made by the mouth, pancreas, and small intestine participate in the process of digestion. Most carbohydrate digestion and absorption take place in the small intestine. Chapter 3 covered the physiology of digestion and absorption in detail.

When the carbohydrates reach the small intestine, the more alkaline environment of the intestine is better suited for further carbohydrate digestion. The pancreas releases enzymes, such as pancreatic amylase, to aid the last stage of starch digestion. After amylase action, the original carbohydrates in a food are now present in the small intestine as the monosaccharides glucose and fructose, originally present as such in food, and disaccharides (maltose from starch breakdown, lactose mainly from dairy products, and sucrose from food and that added at the table).

The disaccharides are digested to their monosaccharide units once they reach the wall of the small intestine, where the specialized enzymes on the absorptive cells digest each disaccharide into monosaccharides. The enzyme **maltase** acts on maltose to produce two glucose molecules. **Sucrase** acts on sucrose to produce glucose and fructose. **Lactase** acts on lactose to produce glucose and galactose.

Lactose Maldigestion and Lactose Intolerance. **Lactose maldigestion** is a normal pattern of physiology that often begins to develop after early childhood, at about ages 3 to 5 years. It can lead to symptoms of abdominal pain, gas, and diarrhea after consuming lactose, generally when eaten in large amounts. This *primary* form of lactose maldigestion is estimated to be present in about 75% of the world's population, although not all of these individuals experience symptoms. (When significant symptoms develop after lactose intake, it is then called **lactose intolerance**.) Another form of the problem, *secondary* lactose maldigestion, is a temporary condition in which lactase production is decreased in response to another condition, such as intestinal diarrhea. The symptoms of lactose intolerance include gas, abdominal bloating, cramps, and diarrhea. The bloating and gas are caused by bacterial fermentation of lactose in the large intestine. The diarrhea is caused by undigested lactose in the large intestine as it draws water from the circulatory system into the large intestine.

In North America, approximately 25% of adults show signs of decreased lactose digestion in the small intestine. Many lactose maldigesters are Asian Americans, African Americans, and Latino/Hispanic Americans, and the occurrence increases as people age. It is hypothesized that approximately 3000 to 5000 years ago, a genetic mutation occurred in regions that relied on milk and dairy foods as a main food source, allowing those individuals (mostly in northern Europe, pastoral tribes in Africa, and the Middle East) to retain the ability to maintain high lactase output for their entire lifetime.

Still, many of these individuals can consume moderate amounts of lactose with minimal or no gastrointestinal discomfort because of eventual lactose breakdown by bacteria in the large intestine (see Further Reading 12). Thus, it is unnecessary for these people to greatly restrict their intake of lactose-containing foods, such as milk and milk products. These calcium-rich food products are important for maintaining bone health. Obtaining enough calcium and vitamin D from the diet is much easier if milk and milk products are included in a diet.

Studies have shown that nearly all individuals with decreased lactase production can tolerate ½ to 1 cup of milk with meals, and that most individuals adapt to intestinal gas production resulting from the fermentation of lactose by bacteria in the large intestine. Combining lactose-containing foods with other foods also helps because certain properties of foods can have positive effects on rates of digestion. For example, fat in a meal slows digestion, leaving more time for lactase action. Hard cheese and yogurt also are more easily tolerated than milk. Much of the lactose is lost in the production of cheese, and the active bacteria cultures in yogurt digest the lactose when these bacteria are broken apart in the small intestine and release their lactase. In addition, an array of products, such as low-lactose milk (Lactaid®, Dairy Ease®) and lactase pills, is available to assist lactose maldigesters when needed.

Absorption

Monosaccharides found naturally in foods and those formed as by-products of starch and disaccharide digestion in the mouth and small intestine generally follow an

maltase An enzyme made by absorptive cells of the small intestine; this enzyme digests maltose to two glucoses.

sucrase An enzyme made by absorptive cells of the small intestine; this enzyme digests sucrose to glucose and fructose.

lactase An enzyme made by absorptive cells of the small intestine; this enzyme digests lactose to glucose and galactose.

lactose maldigestion (primary and secondary) Primary lactose maldigestion occurs when production of the enzyme lactase declines for no apparent reason. Secondary lactose maldigestion occurs when a specific cause, such as long-standing diarrhea, results in a decline in lactase production. When significant symptoms develop after lactose intake, it is then called lactose intolerance.

lactose intolerance A condition in which symptoms such as abdominal gas and bloating appear as a result of severe lactose maldigestion.

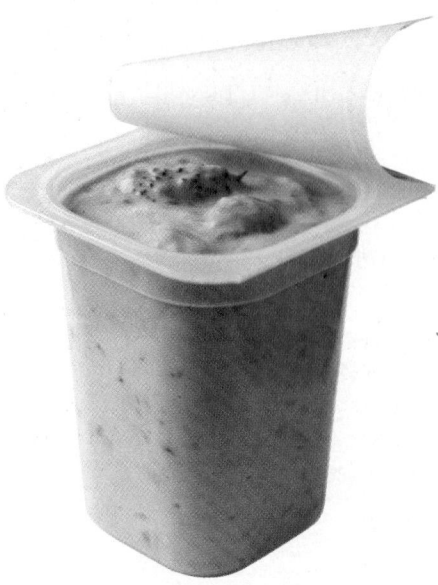
▲ Use of yogurt helps lactose maldigesters meet calcium needs.

active absorption process. Recall from Chapter 3 that this is a process that requires a specific carrier and energy input for the substance to be taken up by the absorptive cells in the small intestine. Glucose and its close relative, galactose, undergo active absorption. They are pumped into the absorptive cells along with sodium.

Fructose is taken up by the absorptive cells via facilitated diffusion. In this case, a carrier is used, but no energy input is needed. This absorptive process is thus slower than that seen with glucose or galactose. So, large doses of fructose are not readily absorbed and can contribute to diarrhea as the monosaccharide remains in the small intestine and attracts water.

Once glucose, galactose, and fructose enter the absorptive cells, some fructose is metabolized into glucose. The single sugars in the absorptive cells are then transferred to the portal vein that goes directly to the liver. The liver then metabolizes those sugars by transforming the monosaccharides galactose and fructose into glucose and:

- Releasing it directly into the bloodstream for transport to organs such as the brain, muscles, kidneys, and adipose tissues
- Producing glycogen for storage of carbohydrate
- Producing fat (minor amount, if any)

Of these three options, producing fat is the least likely, except when carbohydrates are consumed in high amounts and overall calorie needs are exceeded.

Unless an individual has a disease that causes malabsorption, or an intolerance to a carbohydrate such as lactose (or fructose), only a minor amount of some sugars (about 10%) escapes digestion. Any undigested carbohydrate travels to the large intestine and is fermented there by bacteria. The acids and gases produced by bacterial metabolism of the undigested carbohydrate are absorbed into the bloodstream. Scientists suspect that some of these products of bacterial metabolism promote the health of the large intestine by providing it with a source of calories.

MAKING DECISIONS

Fermentable Fiber

Bacteria in the large intestine ferment soluble fibers into such products as acids and gases. The acids, once absorbed, also provide calories for the body. In this way, soluble fibers provide about 1.5 to 2.5 kcal per gram. Although the intestinal gas (flatulence) produced by this bacterial fermentation is not harmful, it can be painful and sometimes embarrassing. Over time, however, the body tends to adapt to a high-fiber intake, eventually producing less gas.

Name some potentially gas-forming foods. Are these foods good sources of soluble fiber?

CONCEPT CHECK

Carbohydrate digestion is the process of breaking down larger carbohydrates into smaller units, and eventually to monosaccharide forms. The enzymatic digestion of starches in the body begins in the mouth with salivary amylase. Enzymes made by the pancreas and small intestine complete the digestion of carbohydrates to single sugars in the small intestine. Lactose maldigestion is a condition that results when cells of the intestine do not make sufficient lactase, the enzyme necessary to digest lactose, resulting in symptoms such as abdominal gas, pain, and diarrhea. Most people with lactose maldigestion can tolerate cheeses and yogurt, as well as moderate amounts of milk. When significant symptoms develop after lactose intake, it is called lactose intolerance. Following primarily an active absorption process, glucose and galactose (resulting from the digestive process or present in the meal) are taken up by absorptive cells in the intestine. Fructose undergoes facilitated absorption. All of the monosaccharides then enter the portal vein that goes directly to the liver. The liver finally exercises its metabolic options, producing glucose, glycogen, and even fat if carbohydrates are consumed in great excess and overall calorie needs are exceeded.

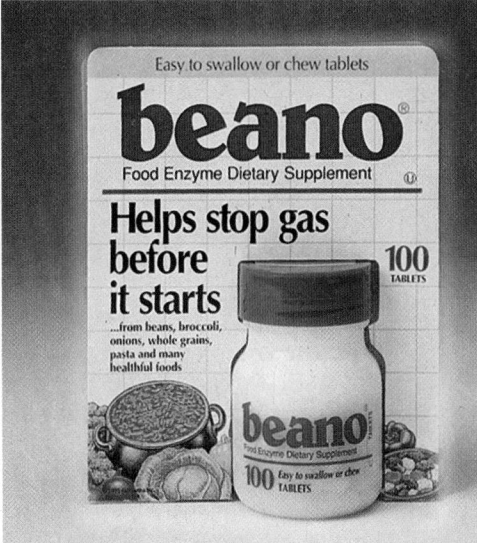

▲ Beano® is a dietary supplement that contains natural digestive enzymes. Such products can be used to reduce intestinal gas produced by bacterial metabolism of undigested sugars in beans and some vegetables in the large intestine.

4.7 Putting Simple Carbohydrates to Work in the Body

As just discussed, all of the digestible carbohydrate that we eat is eventually converted to glucose. Glucose then is the form of carbohydrate that goes on to function in body metabolism. The other sugars can generally be converted to glucose and the starches are broken down to yield glucose, so the functions described here apply to most carbohydrates. The functions of glucose in the body start with supplying calories to fuel the body.

Yielding Energy

The main function of glucose is to supply calories for use by the body. Certain tissues in the body, such as red blood cells, can use only glucose and other simple carbohydrate forms for fuel. Most parts of the brain and central nervous system also derive energy only from glucose, unless the diet contains almost none. In that case, much of the brain can use partial breakdown products of fat—called **ketone bodies**—for energy needs. Other body cells, including muscle cells, can use simple carbohydrates as fuel but many of these cells can also use fat or protein for energy needs.

Sparing Protein from Use as an Energy Source and Preventing Ketosis

A diet that supplies enough digestible carbohydrates to prevent breakdown of proteins for energy needs is considered *protein sparing*. Under normal circumstances, digestible carbohydrates in the diet mostly end up as blood glucose, and protein is reserved for functions such as building and maintaining muscles and vital organs. However, if you don't eat enough carbohydrates, your body is forced to make glucose from body proteins, draining the pool of amino acids available in cells for other critical functions. During long-term starvation, the continuous withdrawal of proteins from the muscles, heart, liver, kidneys, and other vital organs can result in weakness, poor function, and even failure of body systems.

In addition to the loss of protein, when you don't eat enough carbohydrates, the metabolism of fats is inefficient. In the absence of adequate carbohydrate, fats don't break down completely in metabolism and instead form ketone bodies. This condition, known as **ketosis**, should be avoided because it disturbs the body's normal acid-base balance and leads to other health problems. This is a good reason to question the long-term safety of the low-carbohydrate diets that have been popular.

ketone bodies Partial breakdown products of fat that contain three or four carbons.

ketosis The condition of having a high concentration of ketone bodies and related breakdown products in the bloodstream and tissues.

MAKING **DECISIONS**

Carbohydrates and Protein Sparing

The wasting of protein that occurs during long-term fasting can be life threatening. This has prompted companies that make formulas for rapid weight loss to include sufficient carbohydrate in the products to decrease protein breakdown and thereby protect vital tissues and organs, including the heart. Most of these very low-calorie products are powders that can be mixed with different types of fluids and are consumed five or six times per day. When considering any weight-loss products, be sure that your total diet provides at least the RDA for carbohydrate.

Regulating Glucose

Under normal circumstances, a person's blood glucose concentration is regulated within a narrow range. Recall from Chapter 3 that when carbohydrates are digested

▲ When following a weight-loss diet, be sure that your diet provides at least the RDA for carbohydrate.

and taken up by the absorptive cells of the small intestine, the resulting monosaccharides are transported directly to the liver. One of the liver's roles, then, is to guard against excess glucose entering the bloodstream after a meal. The liver works in concert with the pancreas to regulate blood glucose.

When the concentration of glucose in the blood is high, such as during and immediately after a meal, the pancreas releases the hormone **insulin** into the bloodstream. Insulin delivers two different messages to various body cells to cause the level of glucose in the blood to fall. First, insulin directs the liver to store the glucose as glycogen. Second, insulin directs muscle, adipose, and other cells to remove glucose from the bloodstream by taking it into those cells. By triggering both glycogen synthesis in the liver and glucose movement out of the bloodstream into certain cells, insulin keeps the concentration of glucose from rising too high in the blood (Fig. 4-9).

On the other hand, when a person has not eaten for a few hours and blood glucose begins to fall, the pancreas releases the hormone **glucagon**. This hormone has the opposite effect of insulin. It prompts the breakdown of liver glycogen into glucose, which is then released into the bloodstream. In this way, glucagon keeps blood glucose from falling too low.

A different mechanism increases blood glucose during times of stress. **Epinephrine** (adrenaline) is the hormone responsible for the "flight or fight" reaction. Epinephrine and a related compound are released in large amounts from the adrenal glands (located on each kidney) and various nerve endings in response to a perceived threat, such as a car approaching head-on. These hormones cause glycogen in the liver to be quickly broken down into glucose. The resulting rapid flood of glucose from the liver into the bloodstream helps promote quick mental and physical reactions.

In essence, the actions of insulin on blood glucose are balanced by the actions of glucagon, epinephrine, and other hormones. If hormonal balance is not maintained, such as during over- or underproduction of insulin or glucagon, major changes in blood glucose concentrations occur. The disease, type 1 diabetes, is an example of the underproduction of insulin. To maintain blood glucose within an acceptable range, the body relies on a complex regulatory system. This provides a safeguard against extremely high blood glucose (**hyperglycemia**) or low blood glucose (**hypoglycemia**). The failure of blood glucose regulation will be discussed in the Nutrition and Your Health section at the end of this chapter.

insulin A hormone produced by the pancreas. Among other processes, insulin increases the synthesis of glycogen in the liver and the movement of glucose from the bloodstream into body cells.

glucagon A hormone made by the pancreas that stimulates the breakdown of glycogen in the liver into glucose; this ends up increasing blood glucose. Glucagon also performs other functions.

epinephrine A hormone also known as *adrenaline*; it is released by the adrenal glands (located on each kidney) and various nerve endings in the body. It acts to increase glycogen breakdown in the liver, among other functions.

hyperglycemia High blood glucose, above 125 milligrams per 100 milliliters of blood.

hypoglycemia Low blood glucose, below 40 to 50 milligrams per 100 milliliters of blood.

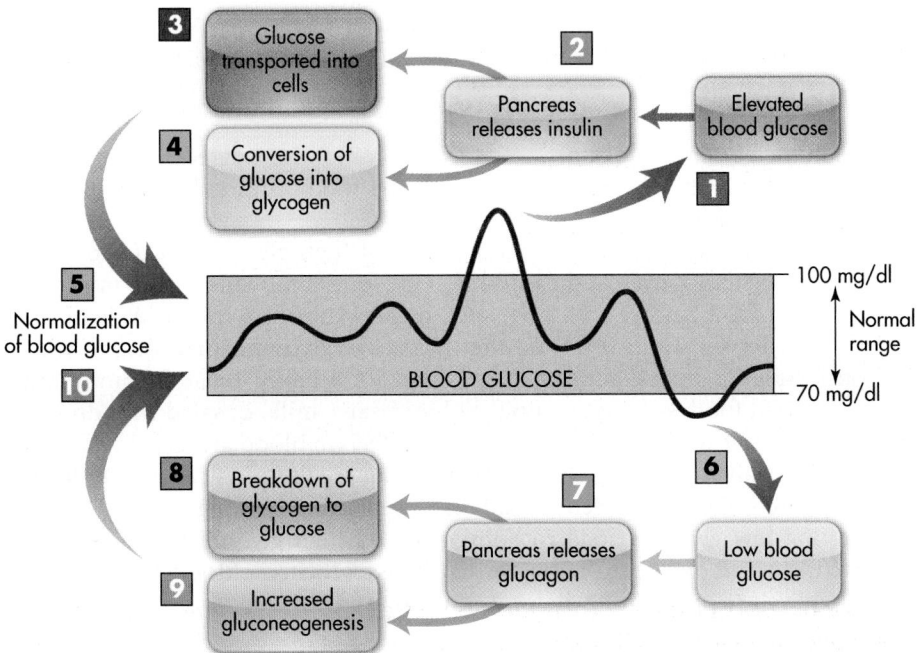

FIGURE 4-9 ▶ Regulation of blood glucose. Insulin and glucagon are key factors in controlling blood glucose. When blood glucose rises above the normal range of 70 to 90 milligrams per deciliter (mg/dl) **1**, insulin is released **2** to lower it **3** and **4** blood glucose then falls back into the normal range **5**. When blood glucose falls below the normal range **6**, glucagon is released **7**, which has the opposite effect of insulin **8**, and **9** this then restores blood glucose to the normal range **10**. Other hormones, such as epinephrine, norepinephrine, cortisol, and growth hormone, also contribute to blood glucose regulation.

See Nutrition and Your Health: Diabetes—
When Blood Glucose Regulation Fails at the
end of Chapter 4.

A term you might see on food labels
is *net carbs*. Although this term is not
FDA-approved, sometimes it is used to
describe the carbohydrates that increase
blood glucose. Fiber and sugar alcohol
content are subtracted from the total
carbohydrate content to yield net carbs
because they have a negligible effect on
blood glucose.

glycemic index (GI) The blood glucose
response of a given food, compared to a
standard (typically, glucose or white bread).
Glycemic index is influenced by starch structure; fiber content; food processing; physical
structure; and macronutrients in the meal,
such as fat.

glycemic load (GL) The amount of carbohydrate in a serving of food multiplied by
the glycemic index of that carbohydrate. The
result is then divided by 100.

The Glycemic Index and Glycemic Load of Carbohydrate Sources

Our bodies react uniquely to different sources of carbohydrates, such that a serving of a high-fiber food, such as baked beans, results in lower blood glucose levels compared to the same size serving of mashed potatoes. Why are we concerned with the effects of various foods on blood glucose? Foods that result in a high blood glucose elicit a large release of insulin from the pancreas. Chronically high insulin output leads to many deleterious effects on the body: high blood triglycerides, increased fat deposition in the adipose tissue, increased tendency for blood to clot, increased fat synthesis in the liver, and a more rapid return of hunger after a meal (insulin rapidly lowers the macronutrients in the blood as it stimulates their storage, signaling hunger). Over time, this increase in insulin output may cause the muscles to become resistant to the action of insulin, and eventually lead to type 2 diabetes in some people. Two food measurements have been developed that are useful in predicting the blood sugar response to various foods and for planning a diet to avoid hyperglycemia (high blood glucose).

The first of these tools is **glycemic index (GI)**. Glycemic index is a ratio of the blood glucose response to a given food compared to a standard (typically, glucose or white bread) (Table 4-4). Glycemic index is influenced by starch structure, fiber content, food processing, physical structure, and other macronutrients in the meal, such as fat. Foods with particularly high glycemic index values are potatoes, especially baking potatoes (due to higher amylopectin content compared to red potatoes), mashed potatoes (due to greater surface area exposed), short-grain white rice, honey, and jelly beans. A major shortcoming of glycemic index is that the measurement is based on a serving of food that would provide 50 grams of carbohydrate. As you can imagine, this amount of food may not reflect the amount typically consumed.

Another way of describing how different foods affect blood glucose (and insulin) levels is **glycemic load (GL)**. The glycemic load is more useful because it takes into account the glycemic index and the amount of carbohydrate consumed. Glycemic load, therefore, better reflects a food's effect on one's blood glucose than either number alone. To calculate the glycemic load of a food, the amount (in grams) of carbohydrate in a serving of the food is multiplied by the glycemic index of that food, and then divided by 100 (because glycemic index is a percentage). For example, vanilla wafers have a glycemic index of 77, and a small serving contains 15 grams of carbohydrate:

$$(\text{Glycemic Index} \times \text{Grams of Carbohydrate}) \div 100 = \text{Glycemic Load}$$
$$(77 \times 15) \div 100 = 12$$

Even though the glycemic index of vanilla wafers (77) is considered high, the glycemic load calculation shows that the impact of this food on blood glucose levels is fairly low (review Table 4-4).

There are many ways to address this problem of high glycemic load foods. The most important is to not overeat these foods at any one meal. This greatly minimizes their effects on blood glucose and the related increased insulin release. At least once per meal, consider substituting a food that has a low glycemic load for one with a higher value, such as long-grain rice or spaghetti for a baked potato. Combining a low glycemic load food, such as an apple, kidney beans, milk, or salad with dressing, with a high glycemic load food also reduces the effect on blood glucose. In addition, maintaining a healthy body weight and performing regular physical activity further reduces the effects of a high glycemic load diet (see Further Reading 9).

Substituting low glycemic load carbohydrates for high glycemic load foods can help in the treatment of diabetes; Chapter 10 discusses the use of foods with different glycemic load values in planning diets for athletes.

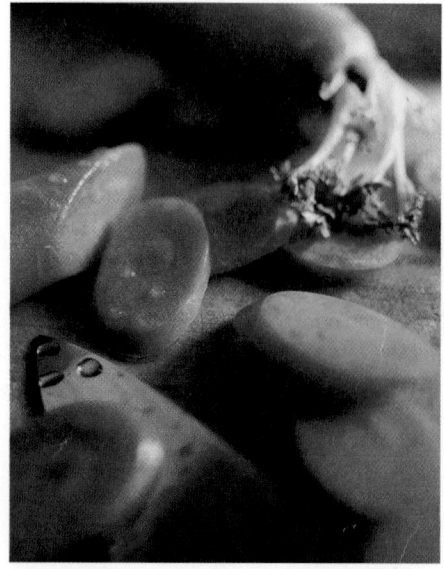

▲ Carrots, criticized in the popular press for having a high glycemic index (which isn't even true),
actually contribute a low glycemic load to a diet.

TABLE 4-4 Glycemic Index (GI) and Glycemic Load (GL) of Common Foods

Reference food glucose = 100
Low GI foods—below 55   Low GL foods—below 15
Intermediate GI foods—between 55 and 70   Intermediate GL foods—between 15 and 20
High GI foods—more than 70   High GL foods—more than 20

	Serving Size (grams)	Glycemic Index (GI)	Carbohydrate (grams)	Glycemic Load (GL)
Pastas/Grains				
White, long grain	1 cup	56	45	25
White, short grain	1 cup	72	53	38
Spaghetti	1 cup	41	40	16
Vegetables				
Carrots, boiled	1 cup	49	16	8
Sweet corn	1 cup	55	39	21
Potato, baked	1 cup	85	57	48
Dairy Foods				
Milk, skim	1 cup	32	12	4
Yogurt, low-fat	1 cup	33	17	6
Ice cream	1 cup	61	31	19
Legumes				
Baked beans	1 cup	48	54	26
Kidney beans	1 cup	27	38	10
Navy beans	1 cup	38	54	21
Sugars				
Honey	1 tsp	73	6	4
Sucrose	1 tsp	65	5	3
Fructose	1 tsp	23	5	1
Breads and Muffins				
Bagel	1 small	72	30	22
Whole-wheat bread	1 slice	69	13	9
White bread	1 slice	70	10	7
Fruits				
Apple	1 medium	38	22	8
Banana	1 medium	55	29	16
Orange	1 medium	44	15	7
Beverages				
Orange juice	1 cup	46	26	13
Gatorade	1 cup	78	15	12
Coca-Cola	1 cup	63	26	16
Snack Foods				
Potato chips	1 oz	54	15	8
Vanilla wafers	5 cookies	77	15	12
Jelly beans	1 oz	80	26	21

Source: Foster-Powell K. and others: International table of glycemic index and glycemic load. *American Journal of Clinical Nutrition* 76:5, 2002.

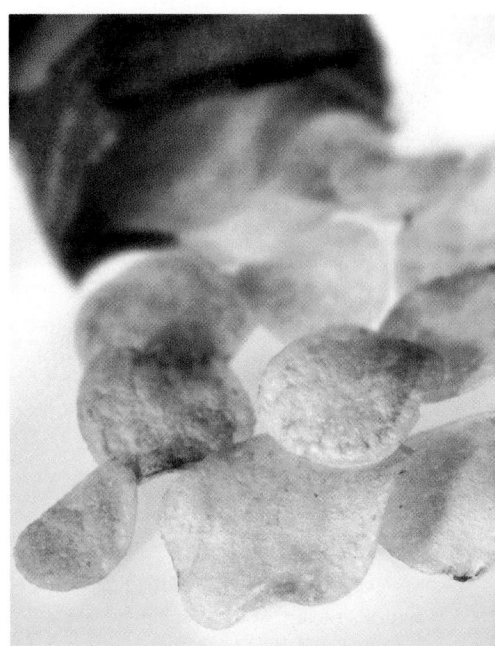

▲ A food such as potato chips, with a low glycemic index, can still have a high glycemic load if eaten in large portions.

You might wonder why the glycemic index and glycemic load of white bread and whole wheat are similar. This is because whole-wheat flour is typically so finely ground that it is quickly digested. Thus the effect of fiber in slowing digestion and related absorption of glucose is no longer present. Some experts suggest we focus more on minimally processed (e.g., coarsely ground, steel cut, or rolled) grains, such as with whole-wheat flour and oatmeal, to get the full benefits of these fiber sources in reducing blood glucose levels.

Recall from Chapter 2 that FDA has approved the following claim: "Diets rich in whole-grain foods and other plant foods and low in total fat, saturated fat, and cholesterol may decrease the risk for cardiovascular (heart) disease and certain cancers."

diverticula Pouches that protrude through the exterior wall of the large intestine.

hemorrhoid A pronounced swelling of a large vein, particularly veins found in the anal region.

diverticulosis The condition of having many diverticula in the large intestine.

diverticulitis An inflammation of the diverticula caused by acids produced by bacterial metabolism inside the diverticula.

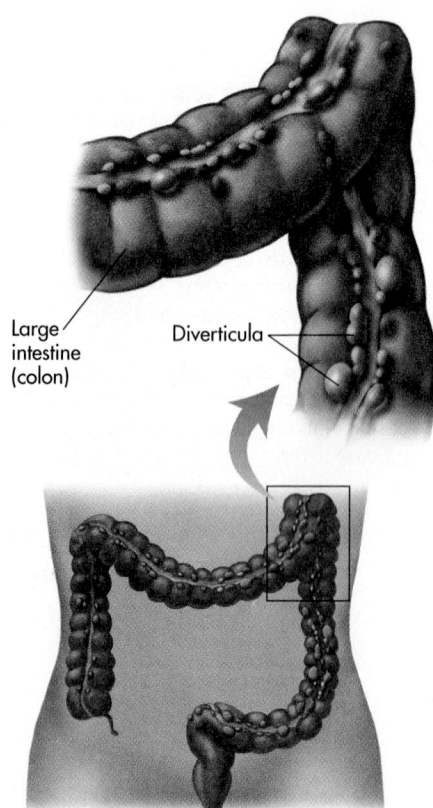

FIGURE 4-10 ▶ Diverticula in the large intestine. A low-fiber diet increases the risk of developing diverticula. About one-third of people over age 45 have diverticulosis, while two-thirds of people over 85 do.

CONCEPT CHECK

Carbohydrates provide glucose for the energy needs of red blood cells and parts of the brain and nervous system. Eating too little carbohydrates forces the body to make glucose using primarily amino acids from proteins found in muscles and other vital organs. A low glucose supply in cells also inhibits efficient metabolism of fats. Ketosis can then result.

Blood glucose concentration is maintained within a narrow range. When blood glucose rises after a meal, the hormone insulin is released in great amounts from the pancreas. Insulin acts to lower blood glucose by increasing glucose storage in the liver and glucose up-take by other body cells. If blood glucose falls during fasting, glucagon and other hormones increase the liver's release of glucose into the bloodstream to restore normal blood glucose concentrations. In a similar way, the hormone epinephrine can make more glucose available in response to stress. This balance in hormone activity helps maintain blood glucose within a healthy range.

4.8 Putting Fiber to Work

Promoting Bowel Health

Fiber supplies mass to the feces, making elimination much easier. This is especially true for insoluble fibers. When enough fiber is consumed, the stool is large and soft because many types of plant fibers attract water. The larger size stimulates the intestinal muscles to contract, which aids elimination. Consequently, less pressure is necessary to expel the stool.

When too little fiber is eaten, the opposite can occur: very little water is present in the feces, making it small and hard. Constipation may result, which forces one to exert excessive pressure in the large intestine during defecation. This high pressure can force parts of the large intestine (colon) wall out from between the surrounding bands of muscle, forming many small pouches called **diverticula** (Fig. 4-10). **Hemorrhoids** may also result from excessive straining during defecation (review Chapter 3).

Diverticula are asymptomatic in about 80% of affected people; that is, they are not noticeable. The asymptomatic form of this disease is called **diverticulosis**. If the diverticula become filled with food particles, such as hulls and seeds, they may eventually become inflamed and painful, a condition known as **diverticulitis**. Surprisingly, intake of fiber then should be reduced to limit further bacterial activity. Once the inflammation subsides, a high-fiber diet is resumed to ease stool elimination and reduce the risk of a future attack.

Over the past 30 years, many population studies have shown a link between increased fiber intake and a decrease in colon cancer development (see Further Reading 10). Most of the research on diet and colon cancer is focusing on the potential preventive effects of fruits, vegetables, whole-grain breads and cereals, and beans (rather than just fiber). Smoking, obesity in men, excessive alcohol use, starch- and sugar-rich foods, and processed meat intake are under study as potential causes of colon cancer. Overall, the health benefits to the colon that stem from a high-fiber diet are partially due to the nutrients that are commonly present in most high-fiber foods, such as vitamins, minerals, phytochemicals, and in some cases essential fatty acids. Thus it is more advisable to increase fiber intake using fiber-rich foods, rather than mostly relying on fiber supplements.

Reducing Obesity Risk

Aside from its role in maintaining bowel regularity, the consumption of fiber has many additional health benefits. A diet high in fiber likely controls weight and reduces the risk of developing obesity (see Further Reading 13). The bulky nature of high-fiber foods requires more time to chew and fills us up without yielding many calories. Increasing intake of foods rich in fiber is one strategy for feeling satisfied or full after a meal (review the discussion of energy density in Chapter 2). This is still another reason to question the low-carbohydrate diets—where is the whole-grain fiber going to come from?

Enhancing Blood Glucose Control

Consuming large amounts of viscous fibers, such as oat fiber, slows glucose absorption from the small intestine, and so contributes to better blood glucose regulation. This effect can be helpful in the treatment of diabetes. In fact, adults whose main carbohydrate source is low-fiber foods are much more likely to develop diabetes than those who have high-fiber diets.

Reducing Cholesterol Absorption

Recall that good sources of viscous fiber are apples, bananas, oranges, carrots, barley, oats, and kidney beans. A high intake of viscous fiber also inhibits absorption of cholesterol and cholesterol-rich bile acids from the small intestine, thereby reducing blood cholesterol and possibly reducing the risk of cardiovascular disease and gallstones. The beneficial bacteria in the large intestine degrade soluble fiber and produce certain fatty acids that probably also reduce cholesterol synthesis in the liver. In addition, the slower glucose absorption that occurs with diets high in viscous fiber is linked to a decrease in insulin release. One of the effects of insulin is to stimulate cholesterol synthesis in the liver, so this reduction in insulin may contribute to the ability of viscous fiber to lower blood cholesterol. Overall, a fiber-rich diet containing fruits, vegetables, beans, and whole-grain breads and cereals (including whole-grain breakfast cereals) is advocated as part of a strategy to reduce cardiovascular disease (coronary heart disease and stroke) risk. And again, this is something that a low-carbohydrate diet can't promise.

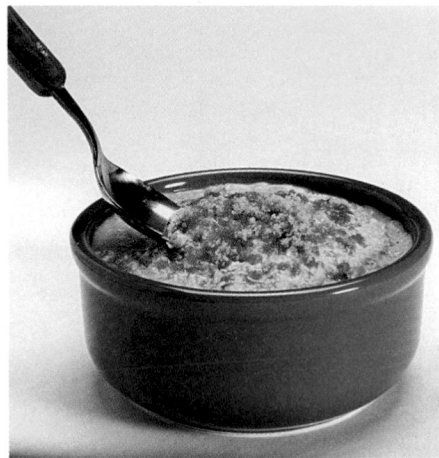

▲ Oatmeal is a rich source of viscous fiber. FDA allows a health claim for the benefits of oatmeal to lower blood cholesterol that arise from the effects of this viscous fiber.

CONCEPT CHECK

Fiber forms a vital part of the diet by adding mass to the stool, which eases elimination. Fiber-rich foods also help in weight control and reduce the risk of developing obesity and cardiovascular disease, and possibly colon cancer. Soluble fiber can also be useful for controlling blood glucose in patients with diabetes and in lowering blood cholesterol. Whole-grain breads and cereals, vegetables, beans, and fruits are excellent sources of fiber.

4.9 Carbohydrate Needs

Currently, recommendations for carbohydrate intake vary widely in the scientific literature and popular press. The RDA for carbohydrates is 130 grams per day for adults (see Further Reading 6). This is based on the amount needed to supply adequate glucose for the brain and nervous system, without having to rely on ketone bodies from incomplete fat breakdown as a calorie source. Somewhat exceeding this amount is fine; the Food and Nutrition Board recommends that carbohydrate intake should range from 45% to 65% of total calorie intake. The Nutrition Facts panel on food labels uses 60% of calorie intake as the standard for recommended carbohydrate intake. This would be 300 grams of carbohydrate when consuming a 2000-calorie diet.

North American adults consume about 180 to 330 grams of carbohydrates per day, which supply about 50% of calorie intake. Worldwide, however, carbohydrates account for about 70% of all calories consumed, and in some countries, up to 80% of the calories consumed. One recommendation on which almost all experts agree is that one's carbohydrate intake should be based primarily on fruits, vegetables, whole-grain breads and cereals, and beans, rather than on refined grains, potatoes, and sugar.

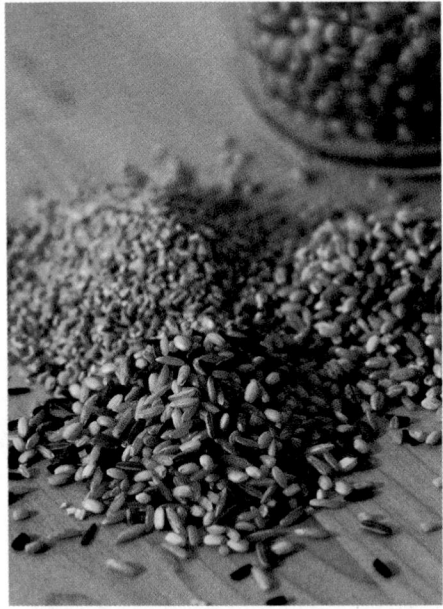

▲ The 2010 Dietary Guidelines define whole grain as the entire grain seed or kernel made of three components: bran, germ, and endosperm.

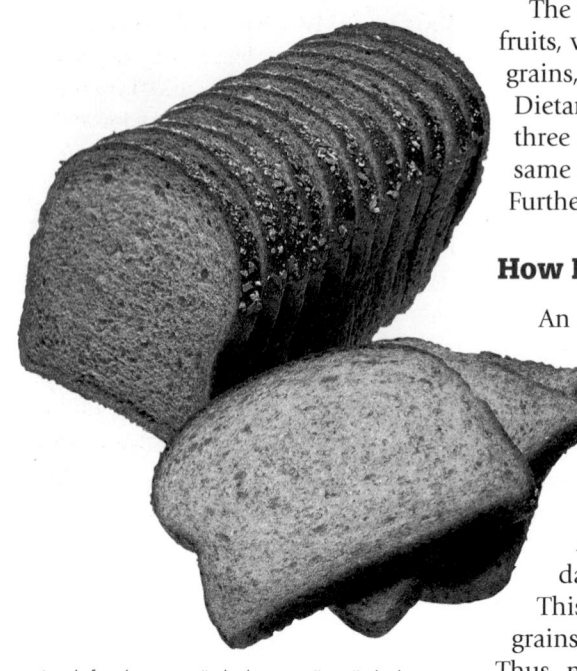

▲ Look for the term "whole-grain" or "whole-wheat" flour on the label for breads that are an excellent source of fiber.

The 2010 Dietary Guidelines for Americans recommend that we choose fiber-rich fruits, vegetables, and whole grains often. More specifically, three or more ounces of grains, roughly one-half of one's grains, should be whole. Remember that the 2010 Dietary Guidelines define whole grain as the entire grain seed or kernel made of three components: the bran, germ, and endosperm, which must be in nearly the same relative proportions as the original grain if cracked, crushed, or flaked (see Further Reading 14).

How Much Fiber Do We Need?

An Adequate Intake for fiber has been set based on the ability of fiber to reduce risk of cardiovascular disease (and likely many cases of diabetes). The Adequate Intake for fiber for adults is 25 grams per day for women and 38 grams per day for men. The goal is to provide at least 14 grams per 1000 kcal in a diet. After age 50, the Adequate Intake falls to 21 grams per day and 30 grams per day, respectively. The Daily Value used for fiber on food and supplement labels is 25 grams for a 2000 kcal diet. In North America, fiber intake averages 13 grams per day for women and 17 grams per day for men and the average whole-grain intake is less than one serving per day. This low intake is attributed to the lack of knowledge on the benefits of whole grains, and the inability to recognize whole-grain products at the time of purchase. Thus, most of us should increase our fiber intake. At least three servings of whole grains per day is recommended. Eating a high-fiber cereal (at least 3 grams of fiber per serving) for breakfast is one easy way to increase fiber intake (Fig. 4-11).

The "Rate Your Plate" exercise shows a diet containing 25 or 38 grams of fiber within moderate calorie intakes. Diets to meet the fiber recommendations are possible and enjoyable if you incorporate plenty of whole-wheat bread, fruits, vegetables, and beans. Use the "Rate Your Plate" exercise to estimate the fiber content of your diet. What is *your* fiber score?

The 2010 Dietary Guidelines for Americans provide the following recommendations regarding carbohydrate intake as part of a healthy eating pattern while staying within their calorie needs:

- Limit the consumption of foods that contain refined grains, especially refined grain foods that contain solid fats, added sugars, and sodium.

- Increase vegetable and fruit intake.

- Eat a variety of vegetables, especially dark-green and red and orange vegetables and beans and peas.

- Consume at least half of all grains as whole grains. Increase whole-grain intake by replacing refined grains with whole grains.

- Choose foods that provide more potassium, dietary fiber, calcium, and vitamin D, which are nutrients of concern in American diets. These foods include vegetables, fruits, whole grains, and milk and milk products.

MAKING DECISIONS

Whole Grains

When buying bread, if you see the name "wheat bread" on the label, do you think you are buying a whole-wheat product? Most people do. The flour is from the wheat plant, so manufacturers correctly list enriched white (refined) flour as wheat flour on food labels. However, if the label does not list "whole-wheat flour" first, then the product is not primarily a whole-wheat bread and thus does not contain as much fiber as it could. Careful reading of labels is important in the search for more fiber. Look especially for the term whole grains on the food label to ensure that you are getting a good source of natural fiber.

In the final analysis, keep in mind that any nutrient can lead to health problems when consumed in excess. High carbohydrate, high fiber, and low fat do not mean zero calories. Carbohydrates help moderate calorie intake in comparison with fats, but high-carbohydrate foods also contribute to total calorie intake.

4.10 Health Concerns Related to Carbohydrate Intake

Aside from the health risks related to ketosis, both excessive fiber and sugar intakes can pose health problems. Too much lactose in the diet is also a problem for some people.

Problems with High-Fiber Diets

Very high intakes of fiber—for example, 60 grams per day—can pose some health risks and therefore should be followed only under the guidance of a physician. Increased

Nutrition Facts

Serving Size — 1 cup (55g/2.0 oz.)
Servings Per Container — 10

Amount Per Serving	Cereal	Cereal with ½ Cup Vitamins A & D Skim Milk
Calories	170	210
Calories from Fat	10	10
	% Daily Value**	
Total Fat 1.0g*	2%	2%
Sat. Fat 0g	0%	0%
Trans Fat 0g		*
Cholesterol 0mg	0%	0%
Sodium 300mg	13%	15%
Potassium 340mg	10%	16%
Total Carbohydrate 43g	14%	16%
Dietary Fiber 7g	**28%**	**28%**
Sugars 16g		
Other Carbohydrate 20g		
Protein 4g		
Vitamin A	15%	20%
Vitamin C	20%	22%
Calcium	2%	15%
Iron	65%	65%
Vitamin D	10%	25%
Thiamin	25%	30%
Riboflavin	25%	35%
Niacin	25%	25%
Vitamin B$_6$	25%	25%
Folic acid	30%	30%
Vitamin B$_{12}$	25%	35%
Phosphorus	20%	30%
Magnesium	20%	25%
Zinc	25%	25%
Copper	10%	10%

*Amount in cereal. One half cup skim milk contributes an additional 40 calories, 65mg sodium, 6g total carbohydrate (6g sugars), and 4g protein.
**Percent Daily Values are based on a 2,000 calorie diet. Your daily values may be higher or lower depending on your calorie needs:

	Calories:	2,000	2,500
Total Fat	Less than	65g	80g
Sat Fat	Less than	20g	25g
Cholesterol	Less than	300mg	300mg
Sodium	Less than	2,400mg	2,400mg
Potassium		3,500mg	3,500mg
Total Carbohydrate		300g	375g
Dietary Fiber		25g	30g

Calories per gram:
Fat 9 • Carbohydrate 4 • Protein 4
*Intake of *trans* fat should be as low as possible.

Ingredients: Wheat bran with other parts of wheat, raisins, sugar, corn syrup, salt, malt flavoring, glycerin, iron, niacinamide, zinc oxide, pyridoxine hydrochloride (vitamin B$_6$), riboflavin (vitamin B$_2$), vitamin A palmitate, thiamin hydrochloride (vitamin B$_1$), folic acid, vitamin B$_{12}$, and vitamin D.

Nutrition Facts

Serving Size: ¾ Cup (30g)
Servings Per Package: About 17

Amount Per Serving	Cereal	Cereal With ½ Cup Skim Milk
Calories	170	210
Calories from Fat	0	5
	%Daily Value**	
Total Fat 0g*	0%	1%
Saturated Fat 0g	0%	1%
Trans Fat 0g		*
Cholesterol 0mg	0%	1%
Sodium 60mg	2%	4%
Potassium 80mg	2%	8%
Total Carbohydrate 35g	9%	11%
Dietary Fiber 1g	4%	4%
Sugars 20g		
Other Carbohydrate 13g		
Protein 3g		
Vitamin A	25%	30%
Vitamin C	0%	2%
Calcium	0%	15%
Iron	10%	10%
Vitamin D	10%	20%
Thiamin	25%	25%
Riboflavin	25%	35%
Niacin	25%	25%
Vitamin B$_6$	25%	25%
Folic acid	25%	25%
Vitamin B$_{12}$	25%	30%
Phosphorus	4%	15%
Magnesium	4%	8%
Zinc	10%	10%
Copper	2%	2%

*Amount in Cereal. One-half cup skim milk contributes an additional 65mg sodium, 6g total carbohydrate (6g sugars), and 4g protein.
**Percent Daily Values are based on a 2,000 calorie diet. Your daily values may be higher or lower depending on your calorie needs:

	Calories:	2,000	2,500
Total Fat	Less than	65g	80g
Sat. Fat	Less than	20g	25g
Cholesterol	Less than	300mg	300mg
Sodium	Less than	2,400mg	2,400mg
Potassium		3,500mg	3,500mg
Total Carbohydrate		300g	375g
Dietary Fiber		25g	30g

Calories per gram:
Fat 9 • Carbohydrate 4 • Protein 4
*Intake of *trans* fat should be as low as possible.

Ingredients: Wheat, Sugar, Corn Syrup, Honey, Caramel Color, Partially Hydrogenated Soybean Oil, Salt, Ferric Phosphate, Niacinamide (Niacin), Zinc Oxide, Vitamin A (Palmitate), Pyridoxine Hydrochloride (Vitamin B6), Riboflavin, Thiamin Mononitrate, Folic Acid (Folate),Vitamin B12 and Vitamin D.

FIGURE 4-11 ▶ Reading the Nutrition Facts on food labels helps us choose more nutritious foods. Based on the information from these nutrition labels, which cereal is the better choice for breakfast? Consider the amount of fiber in each cereal. Did the ingredient lists give you any clues? (Note: Ingredients are always listed in descending order by weight on a label.) When choosing a breakfast cereal, it is generally wise to focus on those that are rich sources of fiber. Sugar content can also be used for evaluation. However, sometimes this number does not reflect added sugar but simply the addition of fruits, such as raisins, complicating the evaluation.

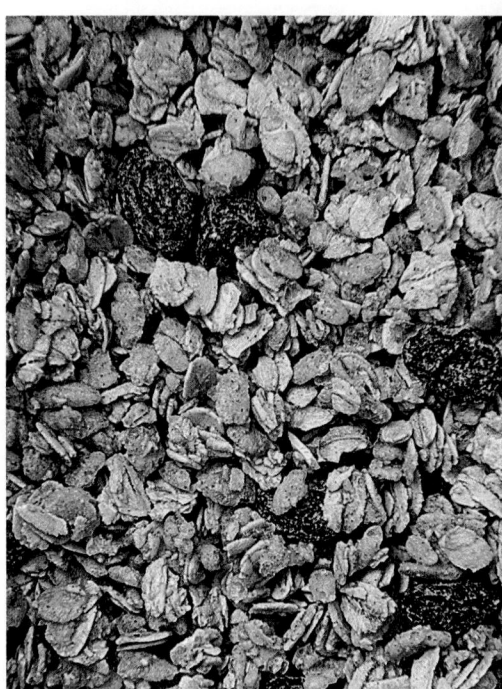

▲ Whole-grain foods, such as granola, are excellent sources of fiber.

fluid intake is extremely important with a high-fiber diet. Inadequate fluid intake can leave the stool very hard and painful to eliminate. In more severe cases, the combination of excess fiber and insufficient fluid may contribute to blockages in the intestine, which may require surgery.

Aside from problems with the passage of materials through the GI tract, a high-fiber diet may also decrease the availability of nutrients. Certain components of fiber may bind to essential minerals, keeping them from being absorbed. For example, when fiber is consumed in large amounts, zinc and iron absorption may be hindered. In children, a very high fiber intake may reduce overall calorie intake, because fiber can quickly fill a child's small stomach before food intake meets energy needs.

Problems with High-Sugar Diets

The main problems with consuming an excess amount of sugar are that it provides empty calories and increases the risk for dental decay.

An excess intake of sugared soft drinks has recently been linked to a risk for both weight gain and type 2 diabetes in adults.

Diet Quality Declines When Sugar Intake Is Excessive. Overcrowding the diet with sweet treats can leave little room for important, nutrient-dense foods, such as fruits and vegetables. Children and teenagers are at the highest risk for overconsuming empty calories in place of nutrients essential for growth. Many children and teenagers are drinking an excess of sugared soft drinks and other sugar-containing beverages and much less milk than ever before. This exchange of soft drinks for milk can compromise bone health because milk contains calcium and vitamin D, both essential for bone health.

Supersizing sugar-rich beverages is also a growing problem; for example, in the 1950s a typical serving size of a soft drink was a 6½-ounce bottle, and now a 20-ounce plastic bottle is a typical serving. This one change in serving size contributes 170 extra kcal of sugars to the diet. Most convenience stores now offer cups that will hold 64 ounces of soft drinks. Filling up on sugared soft drinks in place of foods is not a healthy practice, but enjoying an occasional soft drink or limiting intake to one 12-ounce serving a day is generally fine. Switching to diet soft drinks would spare the simple sugar calories but still lacks nutritional value except for the fluid.

The sugar found in cakes, cookies, and ice cream also supplies many extra calories that promote weight gain, unless an individual is physically active. Today's low-fat and fat-free snack products usually contain lots of added sugar to produce a product with an acceptable taste. The result is to produce a high-calorie food equal to or greater in calorie content than the high-fat food product it was designed to replace.

With regard to sugar intake, an upper limit of 25% of total calorie intake from "added sugars" has been set by the Food and Nutrition Board (sugars added to foods during processing and preparation). Diets that go beyond this upper limit are likely to be deficient in vitamins and minerals. The World Health Organization suggests that added sugars provide no more than 10% of total daily calorie intake.

A moderate intake of about 10% of calorie intake corresponds to a maximum of approximately 50 grams (or 12 tsp) of sugars per day, based on a 2000 kcal diet. Most of the sugars we eat come from foods and beverages to which sugar has been added during processing and/or manufacture. On average, North Americans eat about 82 grams of added sugars daily, amounting to about 16% of calorie intake. Major sources of added sugars include soft drinks; cakes; cookies; fruit drinks; and dairy desserts, such as ice cream (Fig. 4-12). Following the recommendation of having no more than 10% of added calories from sugars is easier if sweet desserts such as cakes, cookies, and ice cream (full and reduced fat) are consumed sparingly (Table 4-5).

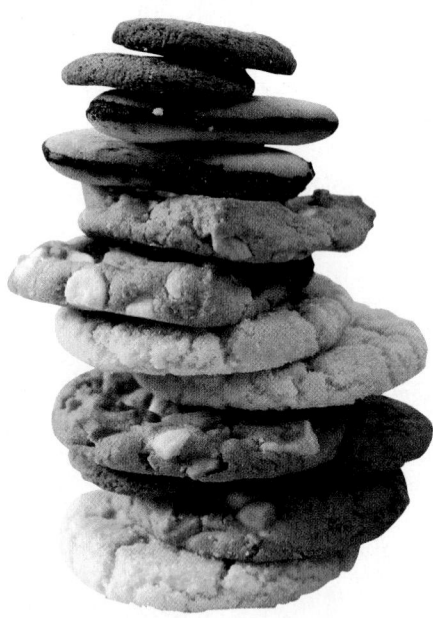

▲ Cookies and cakes are one of the top five carbohydrate sources for U.S. adults.

MAKING **DECISIONS**

Sugar and Hyperactivity

There is a widespread notion that high sugar intake by children causes hyperactivity, typically part of the syndrome called *attention deficit hyperactivity disorder (ADHD)*. However, most researchers find that sucrose may have the opposite effect. A high-carbohydrate meal, if also low in protein and fat, has a calming effect and induces sleep; this effect may be linked to changes in the synthesis of certain neurotransmitters in the brain, such as serotonin. If there is a problem, it is probably the excitement or tension in situations in which sugar-rich foods are served, such as at birthday parties and on Halloween.

TABLE 4-5 Suggestions for Reducing Simple-Sugar Intake

Many foods we enjoy are sweet. These should be eaten in moderation.

At the Supermarket

- Read ingredient labels. Identify all the added sugars in a product. Select items lower in total sugar when possible.
- Buy fresh fruits or fruits packed in water, juice, or light syrup rather than those packed in heavy syrup.
- Buy fewer foods that are high in sugar, such as prepared baked goods, candies, sugared cereals, sweet desserts, soft drinks, and fruit-flavored punches. Substitute vanilla wafers, graham crackers, bagels, English muffins, diet soft drinks, and other low-sugar alternatives.
- Buy reduced-fat microwave popcorn to replace candy for snacks.

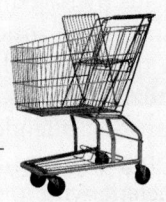

In the Kitchen

- Reduce the sugar in foods prepared at home. Try new low-sugar recipes or adjust your own. Start by reducing the sugar gradually until you've decreased it by one-third or more.
- Experiment with spices, such as cinnamon, cardamom, coriander, nutmeg, ginger, and mace, to enhance the flavor of foods.
- Use home-prepared items with less sugar instead of commercially prepared ones that are higher in sugar.

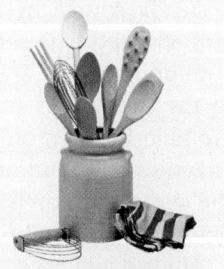

At the Table

- Reduce your use of white and brown sugars, honey, molasses, syrups, jams, and jellies.
- Choose fewer foods high in sugar, such as prepared baked goods, candies, and sweet desserts.
- Reach for fresh fruit instead of cookies or candy for dessert and between-meal snacks.
- Add less sugar to foods—coffee, tea, cereal, and fruit. Cut back gradually to a quarter or half the amount. Consider using sugar alternatives to substitute for some sugar.
- Reduce the number of sugared soft drinks, punches, and fruit juices you drink. Substitute water, diet soft drinks, and whole fruits.

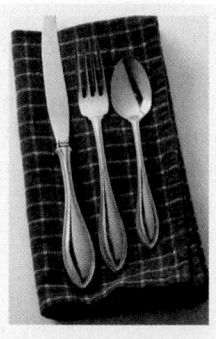

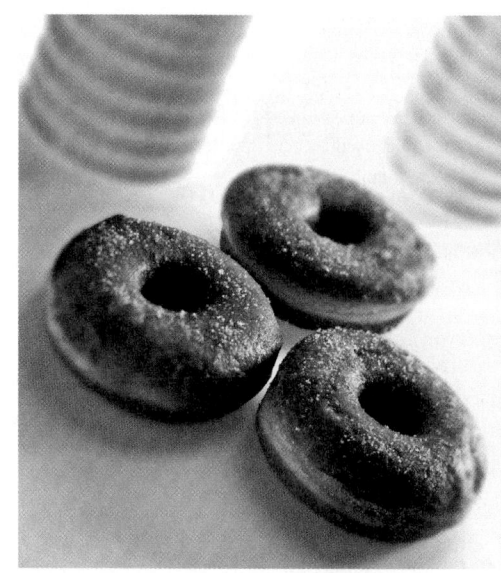

▲ Many foods we enjoy are sweet. These should be eaten in moderation.

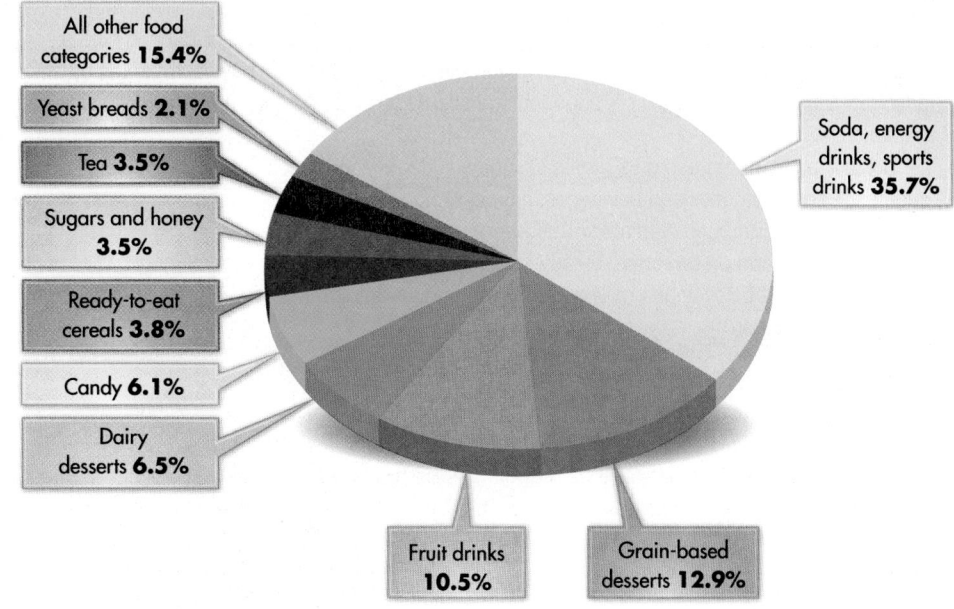

All other food categories **15.4%** • Yeast breads **2.1%** • Tea **3.5%** • Sugars and honey **3.5%** • Ready-to-eat cereals **3.8%** • Candy **6.1%** • Dairy desserts **6.5%** • Fruit drinks **10.5%** • Grain-based desserts **12.9%** • Soda, energy drinks, sports drinks **35.7%**

FIGURE 4-12 ▶ Sources of added sugars in the diets of the U.S. population ages 2 years and olders.

Sources: Dietary Guidelines for Americans Chapter Three.

National Cancer Institute. Sources of added sugars in the diets of the U.S. population ages 2 years and older, NHANES 2005–2006. Risk Factor Monitoring and Methods. Cancer Control and Population Sciences. http://riskfactor.cancer.gov/diet/foodsources/added_sugars/table5a.html. Accessed August 11, 2010.

dental caries Erosions in the surface of a tooth caused by acids made by bacteria as they metabolize sugars.

Dental Caries

Sugars in the diet (and starches readily fermented in the mouth, such as crackers and white bread) also increase the risk of developing **dental caries**. Recall that caries, also known as cavities, are formed when sugars and other carbohydrates are metabolized into acids by bacteria that live in the mouth. These acids dissolve the tooth enamel and underlying structure. Bacteria also use the sugars to make plaque, a sticky substance that both adheres acid-producing bacteria to teeth and diminishes the acid-neutralizing effect of saliva.

The worst offenders in terms of promoting dental caries are sticky and gummy foods high in sugars, such as caramel, because they stick to the teeth and supply the bacteria with a long-lived carbohydrate source. Frequent consumption of liquid sugar sources (e.g., fruit juices) can also cause dental caries. Snacking regularly on sugary foods is also likely to cause caries because it gives the bacteria on the teeth a steady source of carbohydrate from which to continually make acid. Sugared gum chewed between meals is a prime example of a poor dental habit. Still, sugar-containing foods are not the only foods that promote acid production by bacteria in the mouth. As mentioned, if starch-containing foods (e.g., crackers and bread) are held in the mouth for a long time, the starch will be broken down to sugars by enzymes in the mouth; bacteria can then produce acid from these sugars. Overall, the sugar and starch content of a food and its ability to remain in the mouth largely determine its potential to cause caries.

Fluoridated water and toothpaste have contributed to fewer dental caries in North American children over the past 20 years due to fluoride's tooth-strengthening effect (see Chapter 10). Research has also indicated that certain foods—such as cheese, peanuts, and sugar-free chewing gum—can help reduce the amount of acid on teeth. In addition, rinsing the mouth after meals and snacks reduces the acidity in the mouth. Certainly, good nutrition, habits that do not present an overwhelming challenge to oral health (e.g., chewing sugar-free gum), and routine visits to the dentist all contribute to improved dental health.

CRITICAL THINKING

John and Mike are identical twins who like the same games, sports, and foods. However, John likes to chew sugar-free gum and Mike doesn't. At their last dental visit, John had no cavities but Mike had two. Mike wants to know why John, who chews gum after eating, doesn't have cavities and he does. How would you explain this to him?

CONCEPT CHECK

The RDA for carbohydrate is 130 grams per day. The typical North American diet provides 180 to 330 grams per day. A reasonable goal is to have about half of our calorie intake coming from starch and our total carbohydrate intake making up about 60% of our calorie intake, with a range of 45% to 65%. This should allow for the recommended intake of 25 to 38 grams of fiber per day for women and men, respectively. High-fiber diets must be accompanied by adequate fluid intakes to avoid constipation and should be followed only under a physician's guidance.

North Americans eat about 82 grams of sugars added to foods each day. Most of these sugars are added to foods and beverages in processing. To reduce consumption of sugars, one must reduce consumption of items with added sugars, such as some baked goods, sweetened beverages, and presweetened ready-to-eat breakfast cereals. This is one practice that can help reduce the development of dental caries and likely improve diet quality and various aspects of health.

Diabetes—When Blood Glucose Regulation Fails

Improper regulation of blood glucose results in either hyperglycemia (high blood glucose) or hypoglycemia (low blood glucose) as noted in this chapter. High blood glucose is most commonly associated with diabetes (technically, *diabetes mellitus*), a disease that affects 6.5% of the North American population (see Further Reading 5). Of these, it is estimated one-third to one-half of these people do not know that they have the disease. Diabetes leads to about 200,000 deaths each year in North America. Diabetes is currently increasing in epidemic proportions in North America. New recommendations promote testing fasting blood glucose in adults over age 45 every 3 years to help diagnose the problem. Diabetes is diagnosed when one's fasting blood glucose is 126 milligrams per 100 milliliters of blood or greater. In contrast, low blood glucose is a much rarer condition.

Diabetes

There are two major forms of diabetes: **type 1** (formerly called insulin-dependent or juvenile-onset diabetes), and **type 2 diabetes** (formerly called non–insulin-dependent or adult-onset diabetes) (Table 4-6). The change in names to type 1 and type 2 diabetes stems from the fact that many type 2 diabetics eventually must also rely on insulin injections as a part of their treatment. In addition, many children today have type 2 diabetes. A third form, called gestational diabetes, occurs in some pregnant women (see Chapter 16). It is usually treated with an insulin regimen and diet and resolves after delivery of the baby. However, women who have gestational diabetes during pregnancy are at high risk for developing type 2 diabetes later in life.

Traditional symptoms of diabetes are excessive urination, excessive thirst, and excessive hunger. No one symptom is diagnostic of diabetes, and other

TABLE 4-6 Comparison of Type 1 and Type 2 Diabetes

	Type 1 Diabetes	Type 2 Diabetes
Occurrence	5%–10% of cases of diabetes	90% of cases of diabetes
Cause	Autoimmune attack on the pancreas	Insulin resistance
Risk Factors	Moderate genetic predisposition	Strong genetic predisposition Obesity and physical inactivity Ethnicity Metabolic Syndrome Pre-diabetes
Characteristics	Distinct symptoms (frequent thirst, hunger, and urination) Ketosis Weight loss	Mild symptoms, especially in early phases of the disease (fatigue and nighttime urination) Ketosis does not generally occur.
Treatment	Insulin Diet Exercise	Diet Exercise Oral medications to lower blood glucose Insulin (in advanced cases)
Complications	Cardiovascular disease Kidney disease Nerve disease Blindness Infections	Cardiovascular disease Kidney disease Nerve damage Blindness Infections
Monitoring	Blood glucose Urine ketones HbA1c*	Blood glucose HbA1c

*Hemoglobin Alc.

type 1 diabetes A form of diabetes prone to ketosis and that requires insulin therapy.

type 2 diabetes A form of diabetes characterized by insulin resistance and often associated with obesity. Insulin therapy can be used but is often not required.

symptoms—such as unexplained weight loss, exhaustion, blurred vision, tingling in hands and feet, frequent infections, poor wound healing, and impotence—often accompany traditional symptoms.

Type 1 Diabetes

Type 1 diabetes often begins in late childhood, around the age of 8 to 12 years, but can occur at any age. The disease runs in certain families, indicating a clear genetic link. Children usually are admitted to the hospital with abnormally high blood glucose after eating, as well as evidence of ketosis.

The onset of type 1 diabetes is generally associated with decreased release of insulin from the pancreas. As insulin in the blood declines, blood glucose increases, especially after eating. Figure 4-13 shows a typical glucose tolerance curve observed in a patient with this form of diabetes after consuming about 75 grams of glucose. When blood glucose levels are high, the kidneys let excess glucose spill into the urine, resulting in frequent urination of urine high in sugar.

A common clinical method to determine a person's success in controlling blood glucose is to measure glycated (also termed glycosylated) hemoglobin (hemoglobin A1c). Over time, blood glucose attaches to (glycates) hemoglobin in red blood cells and more so when blood glucose remains elevated. A hemoglobin A1c value of over 7% indicates poor blood glucose control. Maintaining near-normal hemoglobin A1c levels (6% or less) greatly reduces the risk of death and developing other diseases in people with diabetes. Elevated blood glucose also leads to glycation of other proteins and fats in the body, forming what are called advanced glycation endproducts (AGEs). These have been shown to be toxic to cells, especially those of the immune system and kidneys.

Most cases of type 1 diabetes begin with an immune system disorder, which causes destruction of the insulin-producing cells in the pancreas. Most likely, a virus or protein foreign to the body sets off the destruction. In response to their damage, the affected pancreatic cells release other proteins, which stimulate a more furious

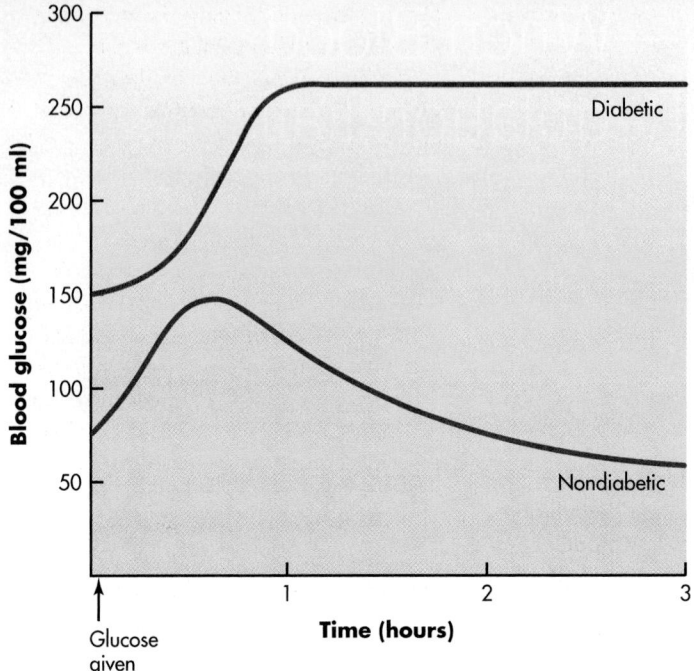

FIGURE 4-13 ▶ Glucose tolerance test. A comparison of blood glucose concentrations in untreated diabetic and healthy nondiabetic persons after consuming a 75 g test load of glucose.

attack. Eventually, the pancreas loses its ability to synthesize insulin, and the clinical stage of the disease begins. Consequently, early treatment to stop the immune-linked destruction in children may be important. Research into this area is ongoing.

Type 1 diabetes is treated primarily by insulin therapy, either with injections two to six times per day or with an insulin pump. The pump dispenses insulin at a steady rate into the body, with greater amounts delivered after each meal. Inhaled forms of insulin also are available. Dietary therapy includes three regular meals and one or more snacks (including one at bedtime) and having a regulated ratio of carbohydrate:protein:fat to maximize insulin action and minimize swings in blood glucose (see Further Reading 2 and 3 for more information on nutrition treatment of diabetes). If one does not eat often enough, the injected insulin can cause a severe drop in blood glucose or hypoglycemia, because it acts on whatever glucose is available. The diet should be moderate in simple carbohydrates, include ample fiber and polyunsaturated fat, but be low in both animal and *trans* fats, supply an amount of calories in balance with needs, and include fish twice a week.

▶ **Symptoms of Diabetes**

The symptoms of diabetes may occur suddenly, and include one or more of the following:

- Extreme thirst
- Frequent urination
- Drowsiness, lethargy
- Sudden vision changes
- Increased appetite
- Sudden weight loss
- Sugar in urine
- Fruity, sweet, or winelike odor on breath
- Heavy, labored breathing
- Stupor, unconsciousness

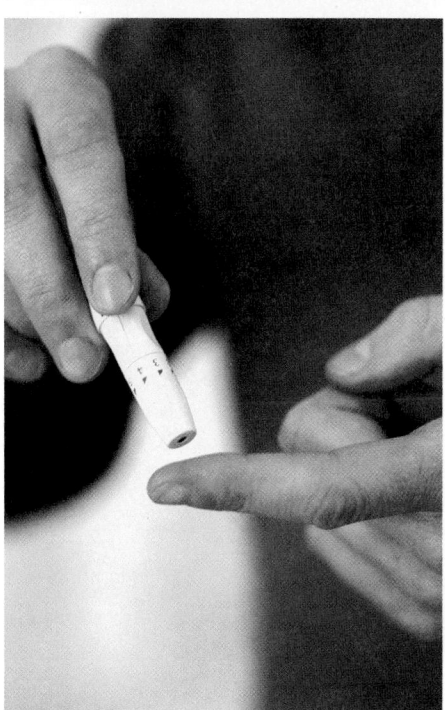

▲ Regularly checking blood glucose is part of diabetes therapy.

MAKING DECISIONS

Are You Prediabetic?

Often people with type 2 diabetes did not develop the disease suddenly. It may develop for years before symptoms are noticed. Prediabetes is a condition in which the concentration of blood glucose has drifts up higher than normal. By the time symptoms are noticeable, organs and tissues may be damaged. Simple tests of your fasting blood glucose level can determine if you are prediabetic. Early detection of diabetes risk can help prevent diabetes if you make lifestyle changes. If you have a family history of diabetes or if your habits (being physically inactive and overweight, and having a poor diet) put you at risk, it is fortunate to discover if your blood glucose is still in the prediabetic stage. Prediabetes, also called impaired fasting glucose, is diagnosed if the fasting blood glucose is 100–125 mg/dL.

Meeting magnesium needs is also helpful, as well as a moderate intake of coffee.

If a high carbohydrate intake raises triglycerides and cholesterol in the blood beyond desired ranges, carbohydrate intake can be reduced and replaced with unsaturated fat. Surprisingly, this change tends to reduce blood triglycerides and cholesterol. Chapter 5 discusses how to implement such a diet (as well as when certain related medications may be beneficial). Some consumption of sugars with meals is fine, as long as blood glucose regulation is preserved and the sugars replace other carbohydrates in the meal, so that undesirable weight gain does not take place.

The latest evidence suggests that diabetes essentially guarantees development of cardiovascular disease. Because people with diabetes (type 1, as well as type 2) are at a high risk for cardiovascular disease and related heart attacks, they should take an aspirin each day (generally 80 to 160 milligrams per day) if their physicians find no reason not to do so. Blood cholesterol lowering medications also may be prescribed. As discussed in Chapter 5, these practices reduce the risk of heart attack.

The hormone imbalances that occur in people with untreated type 1 diabetes—chiefly, not enough insulin—lead to mobilization of body fat, taken up by liver cells. Ketosis is the result because the fat is partially broken down to ketone bodies. Ketone bodies can rise excessively in the blood, eventually forcing ketone bodies into the urine. These pull sodium and potassium ions and water with them into the urine. This series of events also causes frequent urination and can contribute to a chain reaction that eventually leads to dehydration; ion imbalance; coma; and even death, especially in patients with poorly controlled type 1 diabetes. Treatment includes provision of insulin, fluids, and minerals such as sodium and potassium.

In addition to cardiovascular disease, other degenerative complications that result from poor blood glucose regulation, specifically long-term hyperglycemia, include blindness, kidney disease, and deterioration of nerves. The high blood sugar concentration physically deteriorates small blood vessels (capillaries) and nerves. When improper nerve stimulation occurs in the intestinal tract, intermittent diarrhea and constipation result. Because of nerve deterioration in the extremities, many people with diabetes lose the sensation of pain associated with injuries or infections. They do not have as much pain, so they often delay treatment of hand or foot problems. This delay, combined with a rich environment for bacterial growth (bacteria thrive on glucose) sets the stage for damage and death of tissues in the extremities, sometimes leading to the need for amputation of feet and legs. Current research has shown that the development of blood vessel and nerve complications of diabetes can be slowed with aggressive treatment directed at keeping blood glucose within the normal range. The therapy poses some risks of its own, such as hypoglycemia, so it must be implemented under the close supervision of a physician.

A person with diabetes generally must work closely with a physician and registered dietitian to make the correct alterations in diet and medications and to perform physical activity safely. Physical activity enhances glucose uptake by muscles independent of insulin action, which in turn can lower blood glucose. This outcome is beneficial, but people with type 1 diabetes need to be aware of their blood glucose response to physical activity and compensate appropriately.

Type 2 Diabetes

Type 2 diabetes usually begins after age 40. This is the most common type of diabetes, accounting for about 90% of the cases diagnosed in North America. Minority populations such as Latino/Hispanic Americans, African Americans, Asian Americans, Native Americans, and those from Pacific Islands are at particular risk. As noted in the introduction, the overall number of people affected also is on the rise, primarily because of widespread inactivity and obesity in our population. There has been a substantial increase in type 2 diabetes in children, due mostly to an increase in overweight in this population (coupled with limited physical activity). Type 2 diabetes is also genetically linked, so family history is an important risk factor. However, the initial problem is not with the insulin-secreting cells of the pancreas. Instead, type 2 diabetes arises when the insulin receptors on the cell surfaces of certain body tissues, especially muscle tissue, become insulin resistant. In this case, blood glucose is not readily transferred into cells, so the person develops high blood glucose as a result of the glucose remaining in the bloodstream. The pancreas attempts to increase insulin output to compensate, but there is a limit to its ability to do this. Thus, rather than insufficient insulin production, there is an abundance of insulin, particularly during the onset of the disease. As the disease develops, pancreatic function can fail, leading to reduced insulin output. Because of the genetic link for type 2 diabetes, those who have a family history should schedule regular blood glucose tests and be careful to avoid risk factors such as obesity, inactivity, a diet rich in animal and *trans* fats, and simple carbohydrates.

Many cases of type 2 diabetes (about 80%) are associated with obesity (especially with fat located in the abdominal region), but high blood glucose is not directly caused by the obesity. In fact, some lean people also develop this type of diabetes. Obesity associated with oversized adipose cells increases the risk for insulin resistance by the body as more fat is added to these cells during weight gain.

Type 2 diabetes linked to obesity often disappears if the obesity is corrected. Achieving a healthy weight therefore should be a primary goal of treatment, but even limited weight loss can lead to better blood glucose regulation. Although many cases of type 2 diabetes can be relieved by reducing excess adipose tissue stores, many people are not able to lose weight. They remain affected with diabetes and may experience the degenerative complications seen in the type 1 form of the disease. Ketosis, however, is not usually seen in type 2 diabetes. Certain oral medications can also help control blood glucose. Adequate chromium intake is also important for blood glucose regulation (see Chapter 11). Patients with type 2 diabetes may experience decreased effectiveness of their treatments over time resulting in spikes in blood glucose after meals and weight gain. New classes of drugs that mimic gut hormones are helping diabetic patients overcome the chronic

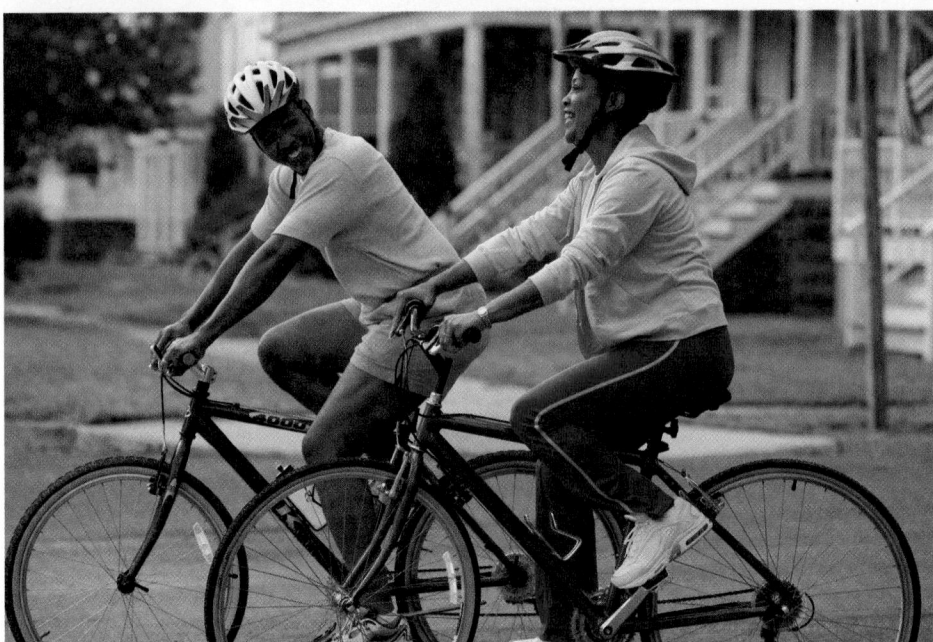

▲ Regular exercise is a key part of a plan to prevent (and control) type 2 diabetes (see Further Reading 8).

problems that conventional treatments alone have been unable to control.

Sometimes it may be necessary to provide insulin injections in type 2 diabetes because nothing else is able to control the disease. (This eventually becomes true in about half of all cases of type 2 diabetes.) Regular physical activity also helps the muscles take up more glucose. And regular meal patterns, with an emphasis on control of calorie intake and consumption of mostly fiber-rich carbohydrates, as well as regular fish intake, is important therapy. Nuts help fulfill the goal of increased fiber consumption. (An almost daily intake of nuts was even shown to reduce the risk of developing type 2 diabetes in one study.) Some sugar consumption is fine with meals, but again these must be substituted for other carbohydrates, not simply added to the meal plan. Distributing carbohydrates throughout the day is also important, as this helps minimize the high and low swings in blood glucose concentrations. Moderate alcohol use is acceptable (1 serving per day) and has been shown to substantially reduce heart attack risk in people with type 2 diabetes. Still, the person must be warned that alcohol can lead to hypoglycemia and that regular testing for this possibility is necessary. And, as mentioned

before, meeting magnesium needs and moderate coffee intake are also helpful.

People with type 2 diabetes who have high blood triglycerides should moderate their carbohydrate intake and increase their intake of unsaturated fat and fiber, as noted earlier for people with type 1 diabetes.

Hypoglycemia

As noted earlier, people with diabetes who are taking insulin sometimes have hypoglycemia if they do not eat frequently enough. Hypoglycemia can also develop in nondiabetic individuals. The two common forms of nondiabetic hypoglycemia are termed *reactive* and *fasting*.

Reactive hypoglycemia occurs 2 to 4 hours after eating a meal, especially a meal high in simple sugars. It results

▶ For more information on diabetes, consult the following websites: **www.diabetes.org** and **www.ndep.nih.gov**.

reactive hypoglycemia Low blood glucose that follows a meal high in simple sugars, with corresponding symptoms of irritability, headache, nervousness, sweating, and confusion; also called *postprandial hypoglycemia*.

in irritability, nervousness, headache, sweating, and confusion. The cause of reactive hypoglycemia is unclear, but it may be overproduction of insulin by the pancreas in response to rising blood glucose. In **fasting hypoglycemia**, blood glucose falls to low concentrations after fasting for about 8 hours to 1 day. It usually is caused by pancreatic cancer, which may lead to excessive insulin secretion. This form of hypoglycemia is rare.

The diagnosis of hypoglycemia requires the simultaneous presence of low blood glucose and the typical hypoglycemic symptoms. Blood glucose of 40 to

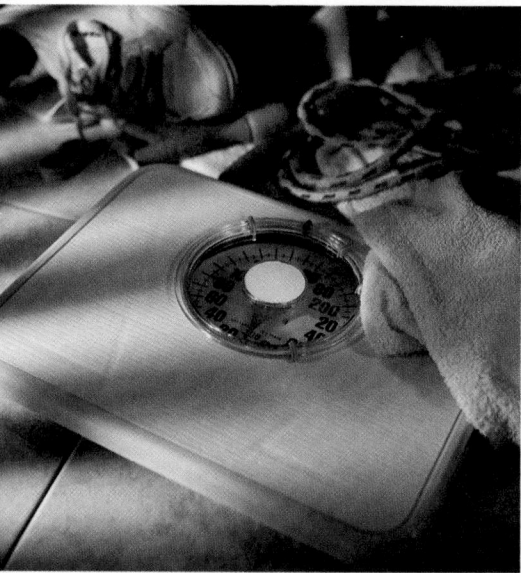

▲ Decreasing body weight and increasing physical activity are interventions to help prevent metabolic syndrome.

fasting hypoglycemia Low blood glucose that follows about a day of fasting.

metabolic syndrome A condition in which a person has poor blood glucose regulation, hypertension, increased blood triglycerides, and other health problems. This condition is usually accompanied by obesity, lack of physical activity, and a diet high in refined carbohydrates. Also called Syndrome X.

50 milligrams per 100 milliliters is suggestive, but just having low blood glucose after eating is not enough evidence to make the diagnosis of hypoglycemia. Although many people think they have hypoglycemia, few actually do.

It is normal for healthy people to have some hypoglycemic symptoms, such as irritability, headache, and shakiness, if they have not eaten for a prolonged period. If you sometimes have symptoms of hypoglycemia, you need to eat regular meals, make sure you have some protein and fat in each meal, and eat complex carbohydrates with ample soluble fiber. Avoid meals or snacks that contain little more than simple carbohydrates. This standard nutrition therapy is one we all could follow. If symptoms continue, try small protein-containing snacks or fruits and juice between meals. Fat, protein, and viscous fiber in the diet tend to moderate swings in blood glucose. Last, moderate caffeine and alcohol intake.

Metabolic Syndrome

Metabolic syndrome, also known as Syndrome X, is characterized by the occurrence of several risk factors for diabetes and cardiovascular disease. The precise definition and criteria for diagnosis have recently been debated by health scholars (see Further Readings 7 and 11). A person with metabolic syndrome has several or all of the following conditions: abdominal obesity (accumulation of fat around and within the midsection), high blood triglycerides, low HDL or "good" cholesterol, hypertension, high fasting blood glucose, increased blood clotting, and increased inflammation (Fig. 4-14). Each aspect of metabolic syndrome is a unique health problem with its own treatment. In metabolic syndrome, however, these risk factors are clustered together, making a person twice as likely to develop cardiovascular disease and five times more likely to develop diabetes.

It is generally accepted that one key element unifies all the aspects of metabolic syndrome: *insulin resistance*. As you learned in this chapter, insulin is a hormone that directs tissues to pull glucose out of the blood and into cells for storage or fuel. With insulin resistance, the pancreas

produces plenty of insulin, but the cells of the body do not respond to it effectively. Instead, excess glucose stays in the bloodstream. For a while the pancreas may be able to compensate for the resistance of cells to insulin by overproducing insulin. Over time, however, the pancreas is unable to keep up the accelerated insulin production and blood glucose levels remain elevated. With metabolic syndrome, blood glucose is not high enough to be classified as diabetes ($\geq$ 126 milligrams per deciliter), but without intervention, it is likely to get worse and eventually lead to diabetes.

Genetics and aging contribute to the development of insulin resistance and the other elements of metabolic syndrome, but environmental factors such as diet and activity play an important role. Obesity, particularly abdominal obesity, is highly related to insulin resistance. More than half of adults in the United States are overweight, 30% are obese, and these numbers continue to climb year after year. Increases in body weight among children and adolescents are of great concern because it places them at high risk for these health problems. This increase in body weight has precipitated a dramatic surge in cardiovascular disease and diabetes risk—an estimated 50 million Americans now have metabolic syndrome.

There is controversy among health professionals over whether to treat each risk factor uniquely or to attempt to integrate therapies to treat all the risk factors simultaneously. For example, the chief culprits contributing to the high blood triglycerides of metabolic syndrome are excessively large meals full of foods rich in simple sugars and refined starches and low in fiber, coupled with little physical activity. Nutrition and lifestyle changes are key strategies in addressing all of the unhealthy conditions of metabolic syndrome as a whole. Suggested interventions include:

- Decrease body weight. Even small improvements (e.g., 5% weight loss) for overweight and obese individuals can lessen disease risk. The most successful weight-loss and weight-maintenance programs include moderate dietary restriction combined with physical activity.

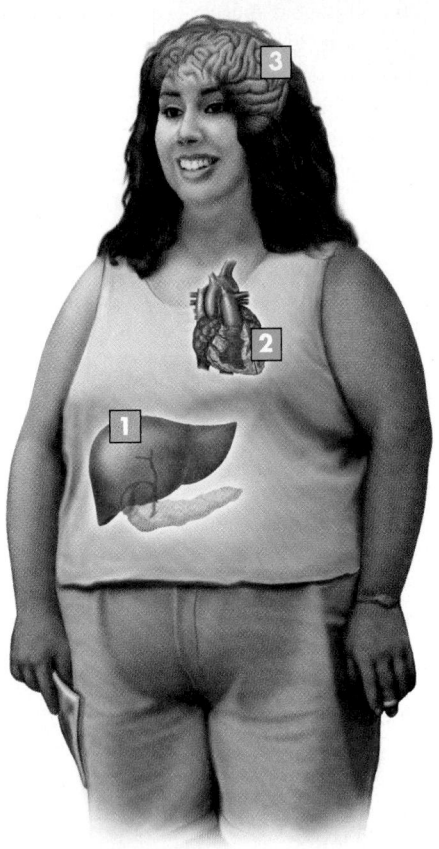

Metabolic Syndrome Risk Indicators

- **High blood pressure**
  130/85 mmHg or higher

- **Low HDL cholesterol**
  - Men with HDL level less than 40 mg/dl
  - Women with HDL level less than 50 mg/dl

- **Elevated glucose**
  Fasting level of 100 mg/dl or higher

- **Elevated triglycerides (blood fat)**
  150 mg/dl or higher

- **Abdominal obesity**
  - Men with waist circumference greater than 40 inches
  - Women with waist circumference greater than 35 inches

Medical Conditions Related to Metabolic Syndrome

1 Type 2 diabetes
Over time, insulin resistance can increase blood glucose levels, which can lead to type 2 diabetes.

2 Coronary artery disease
Elevated blood pressure and cholesterol levels can cause plaque to build up inside coronary arteries, which may eventually lead to a heart attack.

3 Stroke
Plaque buildup in arteries can lead to blood clots that prevent blood flow to the brain, causing damage to brain tissue.

FIGURE 4-14 ▶ For a patient to be diagnosed with metabolic syndrome, he or she must have three of the five risk factors listed above.

- Increase physical activity. To alleviate risks for chronic diseases, the 2010 Dietary Guidelines for Americans include a recommendation to do the equivalent of 150 minutes of moderate-intensity physical activity each week.
- Choose healthy fats. Limiting intakes of total fat, saturated fat, and *trans* fat are generally recommended for improving blood lipids. Including omega-3 fats, such as those found in fish and nuts, is another way to combat chronic disease.
- For those with particularly high risk for cardiovascular disease, medications may be warranted.

Case Study Problems with Milk Intake

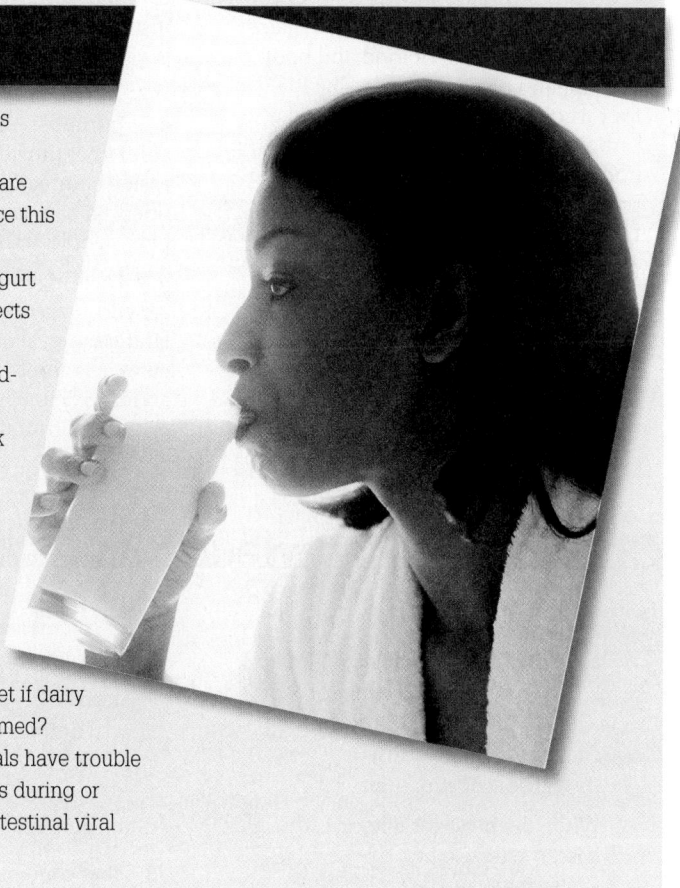

Myeshia is a 19-year-old African-American female who recently read about the health benefits of calcium and decided to increase her intake of dairy products. To start, she drank a cup of 1% milk at lunch. Not long afterward, she experienced bloating, cramping, and increased gas production. She suspected that the culprit of this pain was the milk she consumed, especially because her parents and her sister complain of the same problem. She wanted to determine if other milk products were, in fact, the cause of her discomfort so the next day she substituted a cup of yogurt for the glass of milk at lunch. Subsequently, she did not have any pain.

Answer the following questions, and check your response in Appendix A.

1. Why did Myeshia believe that she was sensitive to milk?
2. What component of milk is likely causing the problems that Myeshia experiences after drinking milk?
3. Why does this component cause intestinal discomfort in some individuals?
4. What is the name of this condition?
5. What groups of people are most likely to experience this condition?
6. Why did consuming yogurt not cause the same effects for Myeshia?
7. Are there any other products on the market that can replace regular milk or otherwise alleviate symptoms for individuals with this problem?
8. Can people with this condition ever drink regular milk?
9. What nutrients may be inadequate in the diet if dairy products are not consumed?
10. Why do some individuals have trouble tolerating milk products during or immediately after an intestinal viral infection?

Summary (Numbers refer to numbered sections in the chapter.)

4.1. Carbohydrates are created in plants through photosynthesis. They are our main fuel source for body cells. Some carbohydrates promote health more than others.

4.2 The common monosaccharides in food are glucose, fructose, and galactose. Once these are absorbed from the small intestine and delivered to the liver, much of the fructose and galactose is converted to glucose.

The major disaccharides are sucrose (glucose + fructose), maltose (glucose + glucose), and lactose (glucose + galactose). When digested, these yield their component monosaccharides.

4.3 One major group of polysaccharides consists of storage forms of glucose: starches in plants and glycogen in humans. These can be broken down by human digestive enzymes, releasing the glucose units. The main plant starches—straight-chain amylose and branched-chain amylopectin—are digested by enzymes in the mouth and small intestine. In humans, glycogen is synthesized in the liver and muscle tissue from glucose. Under the influence of hormones, liver glycogen is readily broken down to glucose, which can enter the bloodstream.

4.4 Fiber is composed primarily of the polysaccharides cellulose, hemicellulose, pectin, gum, and mucilage, as well as the noncarbohydrate lignins. These substances are not broken down by human digestive enzymes. However, soluble (also called viscous) fiber is fermented by bacteria in the large intestine.

4.5 Table sugar, honey, jelly, fruit, and plain baked potatoes are some of the most concentrated sources of carbohydrates. Other high-carbohydrate foods, such as pie and fat-free milk, are diluted by either fat or protein. Nutritive sweeners in food include sucrose, high-fructose corn syrup, brown sugar, and maple syrup. Several alternative sweeteners are approved for use by FDA: saccharin, aspartame, sucralose, neotame, acesulfame-K, and tagatose.

4.6 Some starch digestion occurs in the mouth. Carbohydrate digestion is completed in the small intestine. Some plant fibers are digested by the bacteria present in the large intestine; undigested plant fibers become part of the feces. Monosaccharides in the intestinal contents mostly follow an active absorption process. They are then transported via the portal vein that leads directly to the liver.

The ability to digest large amounts of lactose often diminishes with age. People in some ethnic groups are especially affected. This condition often develops early in childhood and is referred to as *lactose maldigestion*. Undigested lactose travels to the large intestine, resulting in such symptoms as abdominal gas, pain, and diarrhea. Most people with lactose maldigestion can tolerate cheese, yogurt, and moderate amounts of milk.

4.7 Carbohydrates provide calories (on average, 4 kcal per gram), protect against wasteful breakdown of food and body protein, and prevent ketosis. The RDA for carbohydrate is 130 grams per day. If carbohydrate intake is inadequate for the body's needs, protein is metabolized to provide glucose for energy needs. However, the price is loss of body protein, ketosis, and eventually a general body weakening. For this reason, low-carbohydrate diets are not recommended for extended periods.

Blood glucose concentration is regulated within a narrow range of 70 to 99 mg/dl. Insulin and glucagon are hormones that control blood glucose concentration. When we eat a meal, insulin promotes glucose uptake by cells. When fasting, glucagon promotes glucose release from glycogen stores in the liver.

4.8 Insoluble (also called nonfermentable) fiber provides mass to the feces, thus easing elimination. In high doses, soluble fiber can help control blood glucose in diabetic people and lower blood cholesterol.

4.9 Diets high in complex carbohydrates are encouraged as a replacement for high-fat diets. A goal of about half of calories as complex carbohydrates is a good one, with about 45% to 65% of total calories coming from carbohydrates in general. Foods to consume are whole-grain cereal products, pasta, legumes, fruits, and vegetables. Many of these foods are rich in fiber.

4.10 Moderating sugar intake, especially between meals, reduces the risk of dental caries. Alternative sweeteners, such as aspartame, aid in reducing intake of sugars.

N&YH Diabetes is characterized by a persistent high blood glucose concentration. A healthy diet and regular physical activity are helpful in treating both type 1 and type 2 diabetes. Insulin is the main medication employed—it is required in type 1 diabetes and may be used in type 2 diabetes.

Check Your Knowledge (Answers to the following questions are below.)

1. Dietary fiber
   a. raises blood cholesterol levels.
   b. speeds up transit time for food through the digestive tract.
   c. causes diverticulosis.
   d. causes constipation.

2. When the pancreas detects excess glucose, it releases the
   a. enzyme amylase.
   b. monosaccharide glucose.
   c. hormone insulin.
   d. hormone glucagon.

3. Cellulose is a(n)
   a. indigestible fiber.
   b. simple carbohydrate.
   c. energy-yielding nutrient.
   d. animal polysaccharide.

4. Digested white sugar is broken into _____ and _____.
   a. glucose, lactose
   b. glucose, fructose

   c. sucrose, maltose
   d. fructose, sucrose

5. Starch is a
   a. complex carbohydrate.
   b. fiber.
   c. simple carbohydrate.
   d. gluten.

6. Fiber content of the diet can be increased by adding
   a. fresh fruits.
   b. fish and poultry.
   c. eggs.
   d. whole grains and cereals.
   e. Both a and d.

7. Which form of diabetes is most common?
   a. type 1
   b. type 2
   c. type 3
   d. gestational

8. The recommended daily intake for fiber is approximately _____ grams.
   a. 5   c. 100
   b. 30   d. 450

9. Glucose, galactose, and fructose are
   a. disaccharides.
   b. sugar alcohols.
   c. monosaccharides.
   d. polysaccharides.

10. One of the components of metabolic syndrome is
    a. obesity.
    b. diabetes.
    c. low blood sugar.
    d. low blood pressure.

Answer Key: 1. b (LO 4.6), 2. c (LO 4.5), 3. a (LO 4.1), 4. b (LO 4.1), 5. a (LO 4.1), 6. e (LO 4.2), 7. b (LO 4.8), 8. b (LO 4.7), 9. c (LO 4.1), 10. b (LO 4.8)

Study Questions (Numbers refer to Learning Outcomes)

1. Why do we need carbohydrates in the diet? **(LO 4.3)**

2. What are the three major monosaccharides and the three major disaccharides? Describe how each plays a part in the human diet. **(LO 4.3)**

3. Why are some foods that are high in carbohydrates, such as cookies and fat-free milk, not considered to be concentrated sources of carbohydrates? **(LO 4.3)**

4. Describe the digestion of the various types of carbohydrates in the body. **(LO 4.3)**

5. Describe the reason why some people are unable to tolerate high intakes of milk. **(LO 4.3)**

6. List three alternatives to simple sugars for adding sweetness to the diet. **(LO 4.3)**

7. Outline the basic steps in blood glucose regulation, including the roles of insulin and glucagon. **(LO 4.3)**

8. What are the important roles that fiber plays in the diet? **(LO 4.3)**

9. Summarize current carbohydrate intake recommendations. **(LO 4.3)**

10. What, if any, are the proven ill effects of sugar in the diet? **(LO 4.3)**

What Would You Choose Recommendations

It is smart to reach for a carbohydrate-containing beverage when needing quick energy. Some of us also rely on caffeine in drinks to give us a boost. Many beverages on the market contain high concentrations of carbohydrate as "added sugar." This added sugar has recently been the subject of many debates because the consumption of added sugars, especially high-fructose corn syrup (HFCS), has been on the rise since 1970 and excessive sugar intake has been linked to several adverse health conditions. The major sources of added sugars are sodas, energy drinks, and sports drinks (review Fig. 4-12). Sugar intake has been of concern based on total consumption and source of the sugar.

Does the source of the added sugar matter? As we discussed in Chapter 4, the glucose and fructose in HFCS exist in free form, compared to their bound form in cane sugar, sucrose. Sucrose is quickly and completely digested to glucose and fructose in the small intestine so that nearly equal amounts of glucose and fructose are being absorbed from beverages containing HFCS and pure cane sugar. Once absorbed, fructose is more easily converted to and stored as fat than glucose. Researchers speculate that the extra 5% of fructose in HFCS may be responsible for increased body fatness. Also, fructose does not stimulate the release of chemical signals that help to regulate appetite, in the same way glucose does. Changes in appetite can dramatically affect how much of a particular sweetener is consumed. It is still unclear whether altering the type of sweetener in soft drinks will impact our nation's obesity epidemic.

The larger issue here is the abundance of empty calories supplied by soft drinks—regardless of whether these calories come from HFCS or pure cane sugar (sucrose). HFCS represents nearly 100% of sweeteners in all soft drinks, and since soft drink consumption has skyrocketed, so has HFCS consumption. Studies show that liquid calories do not promote satiety in the same way that food calories do. In other words, consuming 250 kcal of cola does not mean that you will feel full enough to eat one less slice of pizza to compensate for those extra kcal. Excess calories from any source will lead to weight gain over time.

Clearly, portion size is an issue. A 20-ounce bottle of regular cola contains about 68 grams (about 15 teaspoons) of sweeteners. This means that a soft drink sweetened with HFCS has 37 grams of fructose compared to 34 grams in a 20-ounce soft drink made with pure cane sugar. Both types of soft drink provide about 250 kcal. Is 3 grams of fructose a big deal? In terms of a soft drink, a 12-ounce soda, such as the Jones Root Beer Soda, will have proportionally less sugar (48 grams) due to its smaller volume. If you consume one soft drink per day or less, the type of sweetener is not likely to make a big difference. If you consume several soft drinks per day, you would be better off choosing a beverage that does not contain calories, such as diet cola or water.

Beverages, such as Coke Zero®, with artificial sweeteners such as aspartame, typically are calorie-free and therefore provide you with no energy when you need a boost. You may feel a temporary lift from the caffeine in some of these products. Water is the perfect drink to restore fluid losses and prevent dehydration but also contains no calories for energy.

Your best choice when needing a quick energy boost in this case is the low-fat chocolate milk. The chocolate milk not only

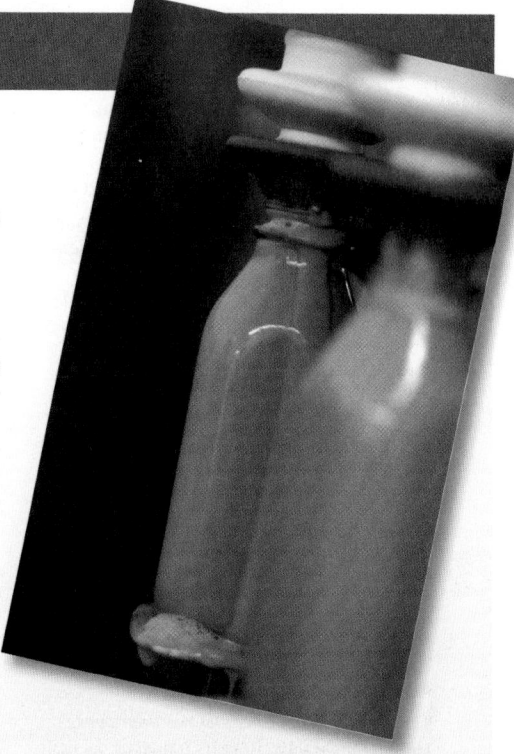

▲ Chocolate milk is a very nutritious beverage that provides protein, vitamins, and minerals, along with calories.

provides less sugar than the sodas on our list but is also the best source of total nutrition. Most convenience stores sell chocolate milk in pint bottles or ½-pint (8-ounce) cartons (similar to those served in school cafeterias). The 8-ounce carton of chocolate milk provides a good amount of calories (150 kcal) as well as 8 grams of protein, 2.5 grams of fat, and 25 grams of sugar. It also provides calcium (290 mg), vitamin A (490 IU), and vitamin D (2.8 micrograms), as well as other vitamins and minerals. A pint bottle (16 ounces) would provide twice the amount of calories and other nutrients. In addition, the chocolate provides a source of caffeine that you may be looking for.

Further Readings

1. ADA Reports: Position of the American Dietetic Association: Use of nutritive and nonnutritive sweeteners. *Journal of the American Dietetic Association* 104:225, 2004.

   When currently recommended diet practices are met, such as the Dietary Guidelines for Americans, use of some nutritive and nonnutritive sweeteners is acceptable. The text of the article explores in detail both classes of sweeteners, in turn supporting this overall conclusion.

2. American Diabetes Association: Nutrition recommendations and interventions for diabetes: A position statement of the American Diabetes Association. *Diabetes Care* 31 (suppl 1):S61, 2008.

   This article provides a comprehensive look at the treatment of diabetes. Goals for therapy and medical tools to help reach those goals are highlighted.

3. American Diabetes Association and American Dietetic Association: *Choose your foods: Exchange lists for diabetes.* 2008.

   This update of a booklet that has been in existence for more than 50 years is used as the basis for nutrition education for diabetes meal planning. Foods are grouped into general categories (or lists) that, per serving size, are similar in macronutrients and calories. Changes have been made so they are easier to use and foods within the lists have been updated.

4. Bray GA and others: Consumption of high-fructose corn syrup in beverages may play a role in the epidemic of obesity. *American Journal of Clinical Nutrition*, 79(4):537, 2004.

   The intake of high-fructose corn syrup (HFCS) was studied and compared to the development of obesity. The increase in HFCS use has paralleled the increase in obesity. Although differences in the digestion, absorption, and metabolism of fructose compared to glucose have been suggested as explanations for the relationship between HFCS and obesity, studies have been unable to separate the effects of the widely consumed sweetener from the impact of other environmental factors.

5. Cowie CC and others: Prevalence of diabetes and impaired fasting glucose in adults in the U.S. population. *Diabetes Care* 29:1263, 2006.

   The results of this study of the National Health And Nutrition Examination Survey (NHANES) suggest that 73 million Americans have diabetes or are at risk based on higher-than-normal blood glucose levels. The prevalence of diagnosed diabetes increased significantly over the last decade, and minority groups remain disproportionately affected. The overall prevalence of total diabetes in 1999–2002 was 9.3% (19.3 million), consisting of 6.5% diagnosed and 2.8% undiagnosed.

   The prevalence of diagnosed diabetes rose from 5.1% in 1988–1994 to 6.5% in 1999–2002. The prevalence of total diabetes was much greater (21.6%) in older individuals aged ≥ 65 years. Diagnosed diabetes was twice as prevalent in non-Hispanic blacks and Mexican-Americans compared with non-Hispanic whites.

6. Food and Nutrition Board: *Dietary reference intakes for energy, carbohydrate, fiber, fat, fatty acids, cholesterol, protein, and amino acids.* Washington, DC: National Academy Press, 2005.

   This report provides the latest guidance for macronutrient intakes. With regard to carbohydrate, the RDA has been set at 130 grams per day. Carbohydrate intake should range from 45% to 65% of calorie intake. Sugars added to foods should constitute no more than 25% of calorie intake.

7. Grundy SM: Does a diagnosis of metabolic syndrome have a value in clinical practice? *American Journal of Clinical Nutrition* 83:1248, 2006.

   The metabolic syndrome concept has led to the development of clinical guidelines by the World Health Organization and the National Cholesterol Education Program. These guidelines have been well accepted by medical professionals. This article reviews the new diagnosis of metabolic syndrome and discusses why organizations including the American Diabetes Association and many diabetes specialists have not embraced the clustering of its risk factors.

8. Hayes C, Kriska A: Role of physical activity in diabetes management and prevention. *Journal of the American Dietetic Association* 108:S19, 2008.

   Evidence supporting the important role of physical activity in the prevention and treatment of diabetes has accumulated. Despite the benefits of physical activity, many people are physically inactive. As the prevalence of overweight and obesity, prediabetes, and type 2 diabetes rises, physical inactivity has become an urgent public health concern. This article reviews research about physical activity/exercise in diabetes and summarizes the current exercise recommendations. This information can be used by health professionals to make safe and effective recommendations for integrating physical activity/exercise into plans for individuals with or at risk of developing diabetes.

9. McMillan-Price J and others: Comparison of 4 diets of varying glycemic load on weight loss and cardiovascular risk reduction in overweight and obese young adults. *Archives of Internal Medicine* 166:1466, 2006.

   In this study of 128 overweight or obese young adults, both high-protein and low-glycemic index diets increased body fat loss. Cardiovascular disease risk was decreased best with a high-carbohydrate, low-glycemic index diet.

10. Park Y and others: Dietary fiber intake and risk of colorectal cancer. *Journal of the American Medical Association* 294:2849, 2005.

    In this large analysis of pooled data from 13 prospective studies, dietary fiber was inversely associated with risk of colorectal cancer when data were adjusted for age. However, when other dietary risk factors (red meat, total milk, and alcohol intake) were accounted for, high-dietary fiber intake was not associated with a decreased risk of colorectal cancer. The authors conclude that a diet high in dietary fiber from whole plant foods can still be advised because this has been related to lower risks of other chronic conditions, including heart disease and diabetes.

11. Pastors JG: Metabolic syndrome—is obesity the culprit? *Today's Dietitian* 8(3):12, 2006.

    Metabolic syndrome, especially its link to obesity, has become better understood in recent years. This article reviews the role of obesity, the dilemmas of diagnosis, new diet and activity guidelines, and the need for a combination of therapeutic approaches for metabolic syndrome.

12. Savaiano DA and others: Lactose intolerance symptoms assessed by meta-analysis: A grain of truth that leads to exaggeration. *Journal of Nutrition* 136:1107, 2006.

    An analysis of the results of 21 studies of lactose intolerance revealed that lactose is not a major cause of symptoms for lactose maldigesters after a moderate intake of dairy foods equaling about 1 cup.

13. Slavin J and others: How fiber affects weight regulation. *Food Technology*, p. 34, February 2008.

    High-fiber diets are linked to lower body weight. This article discusses the effect of different fibers on satiety and food intake. Dietary fiber has intrinsic, hormonal, and intestinal effects that decrease food intake by promoting satiety. Examples of these effects include decreased gastric emptying and/or slowed energy and nutrient absorption.

14. Swann L: Educate your brain about whole grain. *Today's Dietitian* 8(6):36, 2006.

    The 2005 Dietary Guidelines recommend 3 or more ounces of whole-grain products per day. This equals about one-half of one's intake from the grain group. Recent surveys, however, have found that only 5% of American adults eat one-half of their grains as whole grains. This article discusses the need to better educate consumers about whole grain including better definitions and ways of measuring these foods.

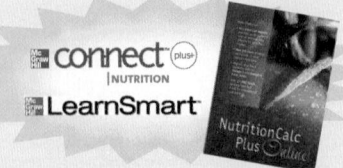

To get the most out of your study of nutrition, go to McGraw-Hill's online resources: Connect www.mcgrawhillconnect.com, **where you will find NutritionCalc Plus, LearnSmart, and many other dynamic tools.**

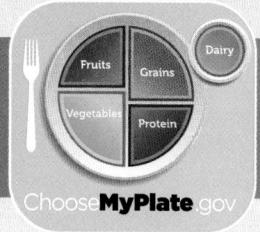

RATE YOUR PLATE

I. Estimate Your Fiber Intake

Review the sample menus shown in Table 4-7. The first menu contains 1600 kcal and 25 grams of fiber (AI for women); the second menu contains 2100 kcal and 38 grams of fiber (AI for men).

TABLE 4-7 Sample Menus Containing 1600 kcal with 25 g of Fiber and 2000 kcal with 38 g of Fiber*

Menu	25 g Fiber			38 g Fiber		
	Serving Size	Carbohydrate Content (g)	Fiber Content (g)	Serving Size	Carbohydrate Content (g)	Fiber Content (g)
Breakfast						
Muesli cereal	1 cup	60	6	1 cup	60	6
Raspberries	½ cup	11	2	½ cup	11	2
Whole-wheat toast	1 slice	13	2	2 slices	26	4
Margarine	1 tsp	0	0	1 tsp	0	0
Orange juice	1 cup	28	0	1 cup	28	0
1% milk	1 cup	24	0	1 cup	24	0
Coffee	1 cup	0	0	1 cup	0	0
Lunch						
Bean and vegetable burrito	2 small	50	4.5	3 small	75	7
Guacamole	¼ cup	5	4	¼ cup	5	4
Monterey Jack cheese	1 oz	0	0	1 oz	0	0
Pear (with skin)	1	25	4	1	25	4
Carrot sticks	—	—	—	¾ cup	6	3
Sparkling water	2 cups	0	0	2 cups	0	0
Dinner						
Grilled chicken (no skin)	3 oz	0	0	3 oz	0	0
Salad	½ cup red cabbage ½ cup romaine ¼ cup peach slices	7	3	½ cup red cabbage ½ cup romaine 1 cup peach slices	19	6
Toasted almonds	—	—	—	½ oz	3	2
Fat-free salad dressing	2 tbsp	0	0	2 tbsp	0	0
1% milk	1 cup	24	0	1 cup	24	0
Total		247	25		306	38

*The overall diet is based on MyPlate Breakdown of approximate energy content: carbohydrate 58%; protein 12%; fat 30%.

To roughly estimate your daily fiber consumption, determine the number of servings that you ate yesterday from each food category listed here. If you are not meeting your needs, how could you do so? Multiply the serving amount by the value listed and then add up the total amount of fiber.

Food	Servings	Grams
Vegetables (serving size: 1 cup raw leafy greens or 1/2 cup other vegetables)	_____ × 2	_____
Fruits (serving size: 1 whole fruit; 1/2 grapefruit; 1/2 cup berries or cubed fruit; 1/4 cup dried fruit)	_____ × 2.5	_____
Beans, lentils, split peas (serving size: 1/2 cup cooked)	_____ × 7	_____
Nuts, seeds (serving size: 1/4 cup; 2 tbsp peanut butter)	_____ × 2.5	_____
Whole grains (serving size: 1 slice whole-wheat bread; 1/2 cup whole-wheat pasta, brown rice, or other whole grain; 1/2 each bran or whole-grain muffin)	_____ × 2.5	_____
Refined grains (serving size: 1 slice bread, 1/2 cup pasta, rice, or other processed grains; and 1/2 each refined bagels or muffins)	_____ × 1	_____
Breakfast cereals (serving size: check package for serving size and amount of fiber per serving)	_____ × grams of fiber per serving	_____
Total Grams of Fiber =		_____

Adapted from Fiber: Strands of protection. *Consumer Reports on Health*, p. 1, August 1999.

How does your total fiber intake for yesterday compare with the general recommendation of 25 to 38 g of fiber per day for women and men, respectively? If you are not meeting your needs, how could you do so?

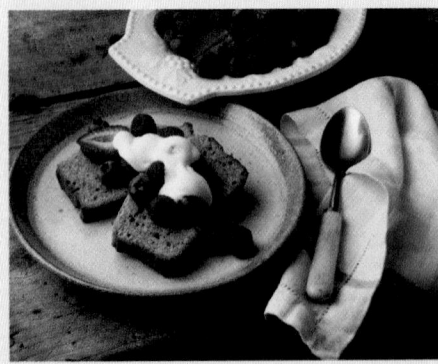

▲ This dessert is an excellent source of fiber from 2 slices of whole-wheat banana bread (7 grams) with ½ cup of berries (1.8 grams) and 2 ounces of yogurt for a total of 8.8 grams of fiber.

II. Can You Choose the Sandwich with the Most Fiber?

Assume the sandwiches on this blackboard are available at your local deli and sandwich shop. All of the sandwiches provide about 350 kcal. The fiber content ranges from about 1 gram to about 7.5 grams. Rank the sandwiches from highest amount of fiber to lowest amount; then check your answers at the bottom of the page.

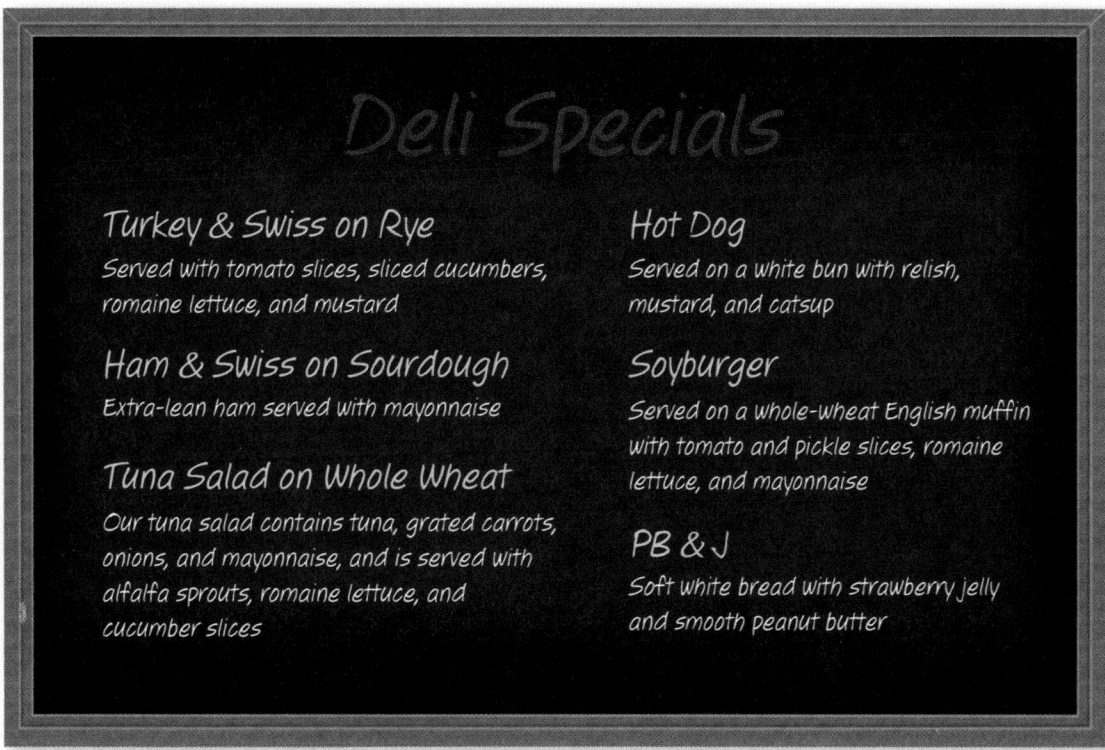

Deli Specials

Turkey & Swiss on Rye
Served with tomato slices, sliced cucumbers, romaine lettuce, and mustard

Ham & Swiss on Sourdough
Extra-lean ham served with mayonnaise

Tuna Salad on Whole Wheat
Our tuna salad contains tuna, grated carrots, onions, and mayonnaise, and is served with alfalfa sprouts, romaine lettuce, and cucumber slices

Hot Dog
Served on a white bun with relish, mustard, and catsup

Soyburger
Served on a whole-wheat English muffin with tomato and pickle slices, romaine lettuce, and mayonnaise

PB & J
Soft white bread with strawberry jelly and smooth peanut butter

Answer Key:
1. Soyburger: 7.5 grams
2. Tuna Salad on Whole Wheat: 7 grams
3. Turkey & Swiss on Rye: 4 grams
4. PB & J: 3 grams
5. Ham & Swiss on Sourdough: 1.5 grams
6. Hot Dog: 1 gram

Chapter 5 Lipids

Student Learning Outcomes

Chapter 5 is designed to allow you to:

5.1 Understand the common properties of lipids.

5.2 List four classes of lipids (fats) and the role of each in nutritional health. Distinguish between fatty acids and triglycerides.

5.3 Differentiate among saturated, monounsaturated, and polyunsaturated fatty acids in terms of structure and food sources.

5.4 Explain how lipids are digested and absorbed.

5.5 Name the classes of lipoproteins and classify them according to their functions.

5.6 Discuss the implications of various fats, including omega-3 fatty acids, with respect to cardiovascular disease.

5.7 List the function of lipids, including the two essential fatty acids.

5.8 Explain the roles of phospholipids in the body.

5.9 Discuss the functions of cholesterol in the body.

5.10 Explain the recommendations for fat intake.

5.11 Characterize the symptoms of cardiovascular disease and highlight some known risk factors.

What Would You Choose?

Several of your friends are getting together for a cookout and you have volunteered to be the grill master. Hamburgers will be the main "protein" portion of your meal. (Remember the size of that group on MyPlate?) You have heard that eating red meat is bad for your heart. Is all red meat bad for your heart? In the meat section of the grocery store, you see several varieties of ground beef. Which of the following types of ground beef would you choose for heart health?

a Ground round

b Ground chuck

c Ground sirloin

d Ground beef

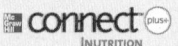 **Think about your choice as you read Chapter 5, then see our recommendations at the end of the chapter. To learn more about ground beef choices, check out the Connect site: www.mcgrawhillconnect.com**

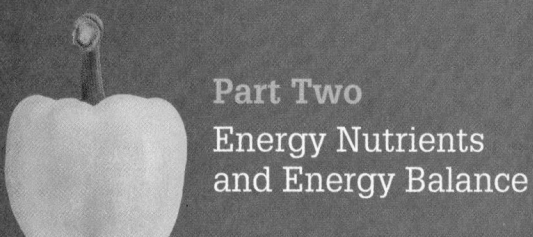

Lipids contain more than twice the calories per gram (on average, 9 kcal) as proteins and carbohydrates (on average, 4 kcal each). Consumption of common solid fats also contributes to the risk of cardiovascular disease. As the comic in this chapter suggests, for these reasons, some concern about certain lipids is warranted, but lipids also play vital roles both in the body and in foods. Their presence in the diet is essential to good health, and in general, lipids such as those found in plant oils and fish, such as the salmon pictured here, should comprise 20% to 35% of an adult's total calorie intake.

Let's look at lipids in detail—their forms, functions, metabolism, and food sources. Chapter 5 will also look at the link between various lipids and the major "killer" disease in North America: cardiovascular disease, which involves the heart, including the coronary arteries (coronary heart disease), as well as other arteries in the body.

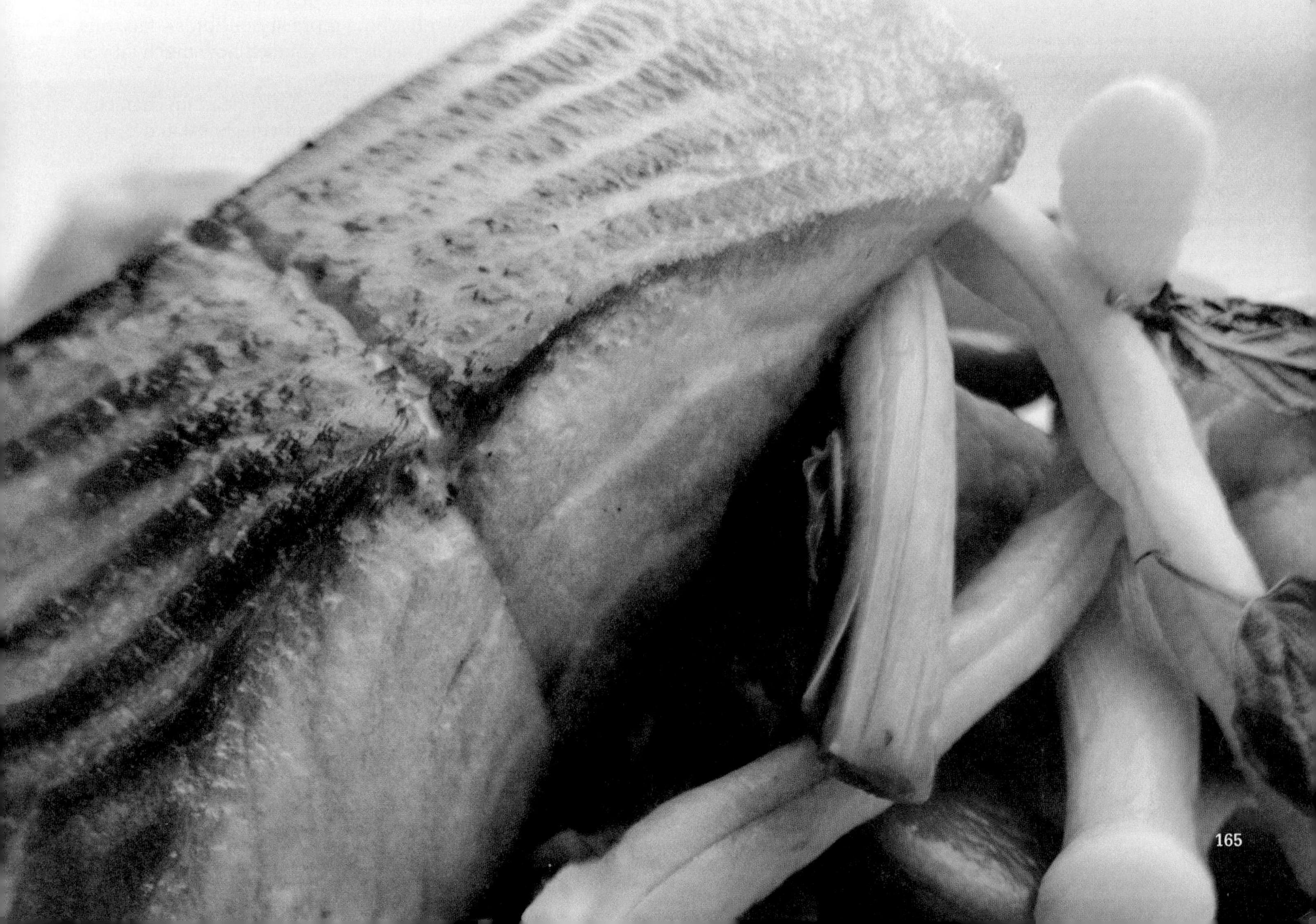

Refresh Your Memory

As you begin your study of lipids in Chapter 5, you may want to review:

- Legal definitions for various label descriptors, such as low fat and fat free in Chapter 2
- The concept of energy density in Chapter 2
- The processes of digestion and absorption in Chapter 3
- The metabolic syndrome in Chapter 4

5.1 Lipids: Common Properties

Humans need very little fat in their diet to maintain health. In fact, the body's need for the essential fatty acids can be met by daily consumption of about 2 to 4 tablespoons of plant oil incorporated into foods and consumption of fatty fish such as salmon or tuna at least twice weekly. If fish is not consumed, the essential fatty acids in canola oil, soybean oil, and walnuts contribute much of the same health benefits as those found in fish. Thus, one could follow a purely vegetarian diet containing about 10% of calories from fat and still maintain health. However, as long as animal fat, cholesterol, and other solid fat are minimized, fat intake can safely be higher than that 10% allotment. The Food and Nutrition Board suggests that fat intake can be as high as 35% of calories consumed for an adult (the Acceptable Macronutrient Distribution Range for fat is 20%–35% of calories consumed for adults). Some experts suggest that an intake as high as 40% of calories is appropriate. After learning more about lipids—fats, oils, and related compounds—in Chapter 5, you can decide for yourself how much fat you want to consume, as well as how to track your daily intake.

Lipids are a diverse group of chemical compounds. They share one main characteristic: They do not readily dissolve in water. Think of an oil and vinegar salad dressing. The oil is not soluble in the water-based vinegar; on standing, the two separate into distinct layers, with oil on top and vinegar on the bottom.

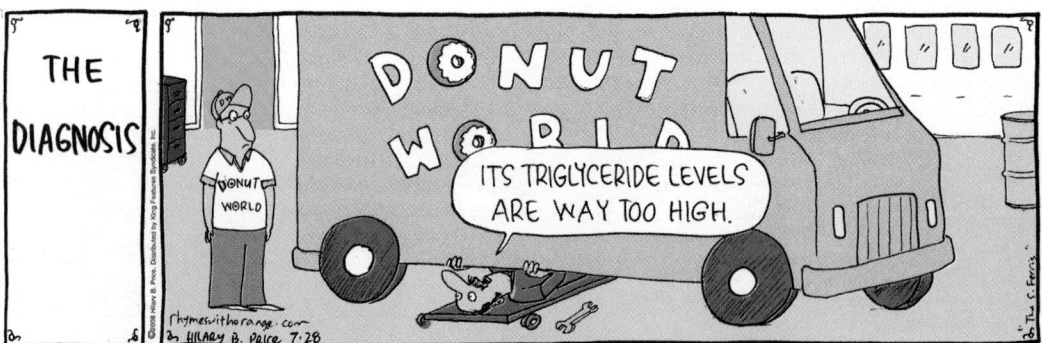

High fat, low fat, no fat—which is best? And why is there such a debate? Would it be easier just to avoid fat altogether? Doesn't a high-fat diet lead to obesity? To cardiovascular disease? Overall, which are the "best" fats, and why are French fries, "donuts," stick margarine, and crackers getting such a bad rap? Chapter 5 provides some answers.

© 2001 Batiuk, Inc. Distributed by North American Syndicates, Inc. All rights reserved.

5.2 Lipids: Main Types

The chemical structure of lipids is diverse. Lipids (mostly fats and oils) are composed primarily of the elements carbon and hydrogen; they contain fewer oxygen **atoms** than do carbohydrates. Lipids yield more calories per gram than do carbohydrates—on the average, 9 kcal per gram—because of this difference in composition. **Triglycerides** are the most common type of lipid found in the body and in foods. Each triglyceride molecule consists of three fatty acids bonded to **glycerol. Phospholipids** and **sterols,** including **cholesterol,** are also classified as lipids, although their structures can be quite different from the structure of triglycerides. All of these lipid compounds are described in Chapter 5.

Food experts, such as chefs, call lipids that are solid at room temperature *fats,* and lipids that are liquid *oils.* Most people use the word *fat* to refer to all lipids because they don't realize there is a difference. However, *lipid* is a generic term that includes triglycerides and many other substances. To simplify our discussion, Chapter 5 primarily uses the term *fat.* When necessary for clarity, the name of a specific lipid, such as cholesterol, will be used. This word use is consistent with the way many people use these terms.

Fatty Acids: The Simplest Form of Lipids

In the body and in foods, fatty acids are found in the main form of lipids, triglycerides. A fatty acid is basically a long chain of carbons bonded together and flanked by hydrogens. At one end of the molecule (the alpha end), is an **acid group.** At the other end (the omega end) is a **methyl group** (Fig. 5-1).

Fats in foods are not composed of a single type of fatty acid. Rather, each dietary fat, or triglyceride, is a complex mixture of many different fatty acids, the combination of which provides each food its unique taste and smell.

Fatty acids can be saturated or unsaturated. Chemically speaking, a carbon atom can form four bonds. Within the carbon chain of a fatty acid, the carbons bond to other carbons and to hydrogens. The carbons that make up the chain of a **saturated fatty acid** are all connected to each other by single bonds. This allows for the maximum number of hydrogens to be bound. Just as a sponge can be saturated (full) with water, a saturated fatty acid such as stearic acid is saturated with hydrogen (Fig. 5-1a).

Most fats high in saturated fatty acids, such as animal fats, remain solid at room temperature. A good example is the solid fat surrounding a piece of uncooked steak. Chicken fat, semisolid at room temperature, contains less saturated fat than beef fat. However, in some foods, saturated fats are suspended in liquid, such as the butterfat in whole milk, so the solid nature of these fats at room temperature is less apparent.

If the carbon chain of a fatty acid contains a double bond, those carbons in the chain have fewer bonds to share with hydrogen, and the chain is said to be *unsaturated.* A fatty acid with only one double bond is **monounsaturated** (Fig. 5-1b). Canola and olive oils contain a high percentage of monounsaturated fatty acids. Likewise, if two or more of the bonds between the carbons are double bonds, the fatty acid is even less saturated with hydrogens, and so it is **polyunsaturated** (Fig. 5-1c, d). Corn, soybean, sunflower, and safflower oils are rich in polyunsaturated fatty acids.

Unsaturated fatty acids can exist in two different structural forms, the *cis* and *trans* forms. In their natural form, monounsaturated and polyunsaturated fatty acids usually are in the *cis* form (Fig. 5-2). By definition, the resulting *cis* fatty acid has the hydrogens on the same side of the carbon-carbon double bond. During certain types of food processing (discussed later in this chapter), some hydrogens are

triglyceride The major form of lipid in the body and in food. It is composed of three fatty acids bonded to glycerol, an alcohol.

glycerol A three-carbon alcohol used to form triglycerides.

phospholipid Any of a class of fat-related substances that contain phosphorus, fatty acids, and a nitrogen-containing base. The phospholipids are an essential part of every cell.

sterol A compound containing a multi-ring (steroid) structure and a hydroxyl group (–OH). Cholesterol is a typical example.

cholesterol A waxy lipid found in all body cells. It has a structure containing multiple chemical rings that is found only in foods that contain animal products.

saturated fatty acid A fatty acid containing no carbon-carbon double bonds.

monounsaturated fatty acid A fatty acid containing one carbon-carbon double bond.

polyunsaturated fatty acid A fatty acid containing two or more carbon-carbon double bonds.

cis **fatty acid** A form of an unsaturated fatty acid that has the hydrogens lying on the same side of the carbon-carbon double bond.

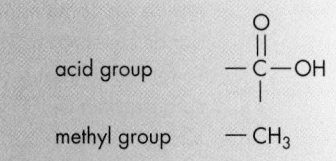

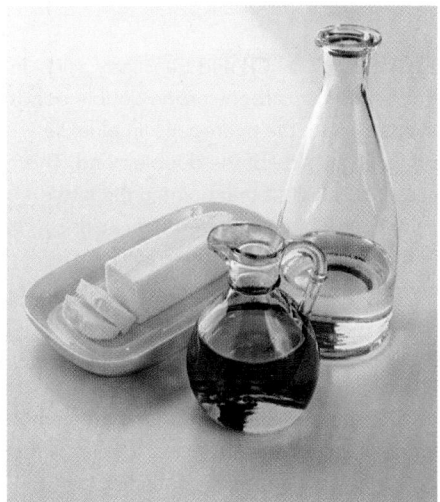

▲ Saturated fats, such as butter, are solid at room temperature, whereas unsaturated fats, such as olive and corn oil, are liquid at room temperature.

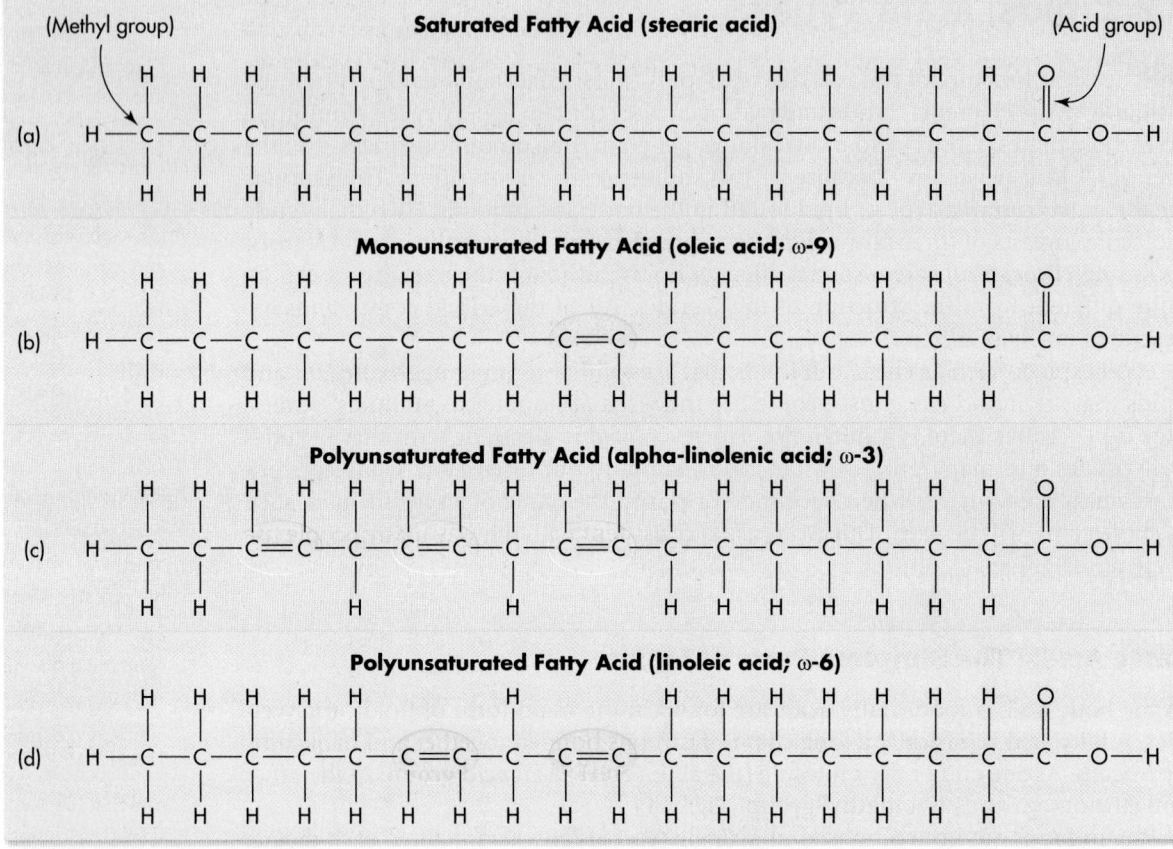

FIGURE 5-1 ▶ Chemical forms of saturated, monounsaturated, and polyunsaturated fatty acids. Each of the depicted fatty acids contains 18 carbons, but they differ from each other in the number and location of double bonds. The double bonds are shaded. The linear shape of saturated fatty acids, as shown in (a), allows them to pack tightly together and so form a solid at room temperature. In contrast, unsaturated fatty acids have "kinks" where double bonds interrupt the carbon chain (see Figure 5-2). Thus, unsaturated fatty acids pack together only loosely, and are usually liquid at room temperature.

FIGURE 5-2 ▶ *Cis* and *trans* fatty acids. In the *cis* form at carbon-carbon double bonds in a fatty acid, the hydrogens (in blue) lie on the same side of the double bond. This causes a "kink" at that point in the fatty acid, typical of unsaturated fatty acids in foods. In contrast, in the *trans* form at carbon-carbon double bonds in a fatty acid, the hydrogens lie across from each other at the double bond. This causes the fatty acid to exist in a linear form, like a saturated fatty acid. *Cis* fatty acids are much more common in foods than *trans* fatty acids. The latter are primarily found in foods containing partially-hydrogenated fats, notably stick margarine, shortening, and deep-fat fried foods.

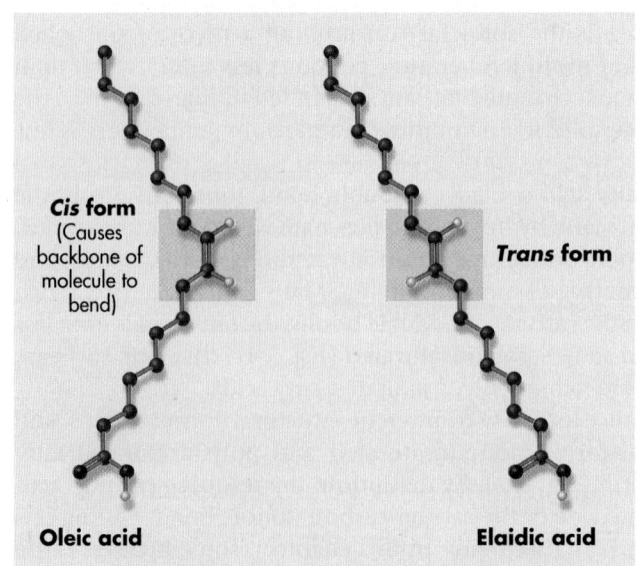

transferred to opposite sides of the carbon-carbon double bond, creating the *trans* form, or a ***trans* fatty acid.** As seen in Figure 5-2, the *cis* bond causes the fatty acid backbone to bend, whereas the *trans* bond allows the backbone to remain straighter. This makes it similar to the shape of a saturated fatty acid. The Food and Nutrition Board suggests limiting intake of *trans* fatty acids in processed foods (also referred to as *trans* fats) as much as possible. Later you will see why.

You may be surprised to learn that some *trans* fatty acids, known as conjugated linoleic acid (CLA), occur naturally. CLA is a family of derivatives of the fatty acid linoleic acid. The bacteria that live in the rumens of some animals (cows, sheep, and goats, for example) produce *trans* fatty acids that eventually appear in foods such as beef, milk, and butter. These naturally occurring *trans* fats are currently under study for possible health benefits, including prevention of cancer, decreasing body fat, and improvement in insulin levels in diabetics. About 20% of *trans* fatty acids in our diets come from this source. Dietary supplements of CLA are available but are highly variable in their quality.

Overall, a fat or an oil is classified as saturated, monounsaturated, or polyunsaturated based on the type of fatty acids present in the greatest concentration (Fig. 5-3). Fats in foods that contain primarily saturated fatty acids are solid at room temperature, especially if the fatty acids have long carbon chains (i.e., a **long-chain fatty acid**), as opposed to shorter versions. In contrast, fats containing primarily polyunsaturated or monounsaturated fatty acids (long chain or shorter) are usually liquid at room temperature. Almost all fatty acids in the body and in foods are long-chain varieties.

An important characteristic of unsaturated fatty acids is the location of the double bonds. If the first double bond starts three carbons from the methyl (omega) end of the fatty acid, it is an **omega-3 (ω-3) fatty acid** (review Fig. 5-1c). If the first double bond is located six carbons from the omega end, it is an **omega-6 (ω-6) fatty acid** (review Fig. 5-1d). Following this scheme, an omega-9 fatty acid has its first double bond starting at the ninth carbon from the methyl end (review Fig. 5-1b). In foods, **alpha-linolenic acid** is the major omega-3 fatty acid; **linoleic acid** is the major omega-6 fatty acid. These are also the **essential fatty acids** we need to consume (more on this in the later section about putting lipids to work in the body). **Oleic acid** is the major omega-9 fatty acid.

Triglycerides

Fats and oils in foods are mostly in the form of triglycerides. The same is true for fats found in body structures. Although some fatty acids are transported in the bloodstream attached to proteins, most fatty acids are formed into triglycerides by cells in the body.

As noted before, triglycerides contain a simple three-carbon alcohol, glycerol, which serves as a backbone for the three attached fatty acids (Fig. 5-4a). Removing one fatty acid from a triglyceride forms a **diglyceride.** Removing two fatty acids from a triglyceride forms a **monoglyceride.** Later you will see that before most dietary fats are absorbed in the small intestine, the two outer fatty acids are typically removed from the triglyceride. This produces a mixture of fatty acids and monoglycerides, absorbed into the intestinal cells. After absorption, the fatty acids and monoglycerides are mostly re-formed into triglycerides.

Phospholipids

Phospholipids are another class of lipid. Like triglycerides, they are built on a backbone of glycerol. However, at least one fatty acid is replaced with a compound containing phosphorus (and often other elements, such as nitrogen) (Fig. 5-4b).

***trans* fatty acid** A form of an unsaturated fatty acid, usually a monounsaturated one when found in food, in which the hydrogens on both carbons forming the double bond lie on opposite sides of that bond.

long-chain fatty acid A fatty acid that contains 12 or more carbons.

omega-3 (ω-3) fatty acid An unsaturated fatty acid with the first double bond on the third carbon from the methyl end (—CH₃).

omega-6 (ω-6) fatty acid An unsaturated fatty acid with the first double bond on the sixth carbon from the methyl end (—CH₃).

alpha-linolenic acid An essential omega-3 fatty acid with 18 carbons and three double bonds.

linoleic acid An essential omega-6 fatty acid with 18 carbons and two double bonds.

essential fatty acids Fatty acids that must be supplied by the diet to maintain health. Currently, only linoleic acid and alpha-linolenic acid are classified as essential.

oleic acid An omega-9 fatty acid with 18 carbons and one double bond.

diglyceride A breakdown product of a triglyceride consisting of two fatty acids bonded to a glycerol backbone.

monoglyceride A breakdown product of a triglyceride consisting of one fatty acid attached to a glycerol backbone.

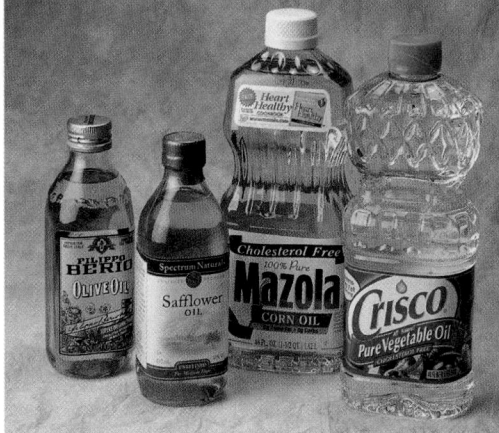

▲ Plant oils vary in their content of specific fatty acids. Oils similar in appearance may vary significantly in fatty acid composition. Olive and canola oils are rich in monounsaturated fat; olive oil has been awarded much attention in recent years. Canola oil, however, is a much less expensive choice of monounsaturated fat. Safflower oil is rich in polyunsaturated fat.

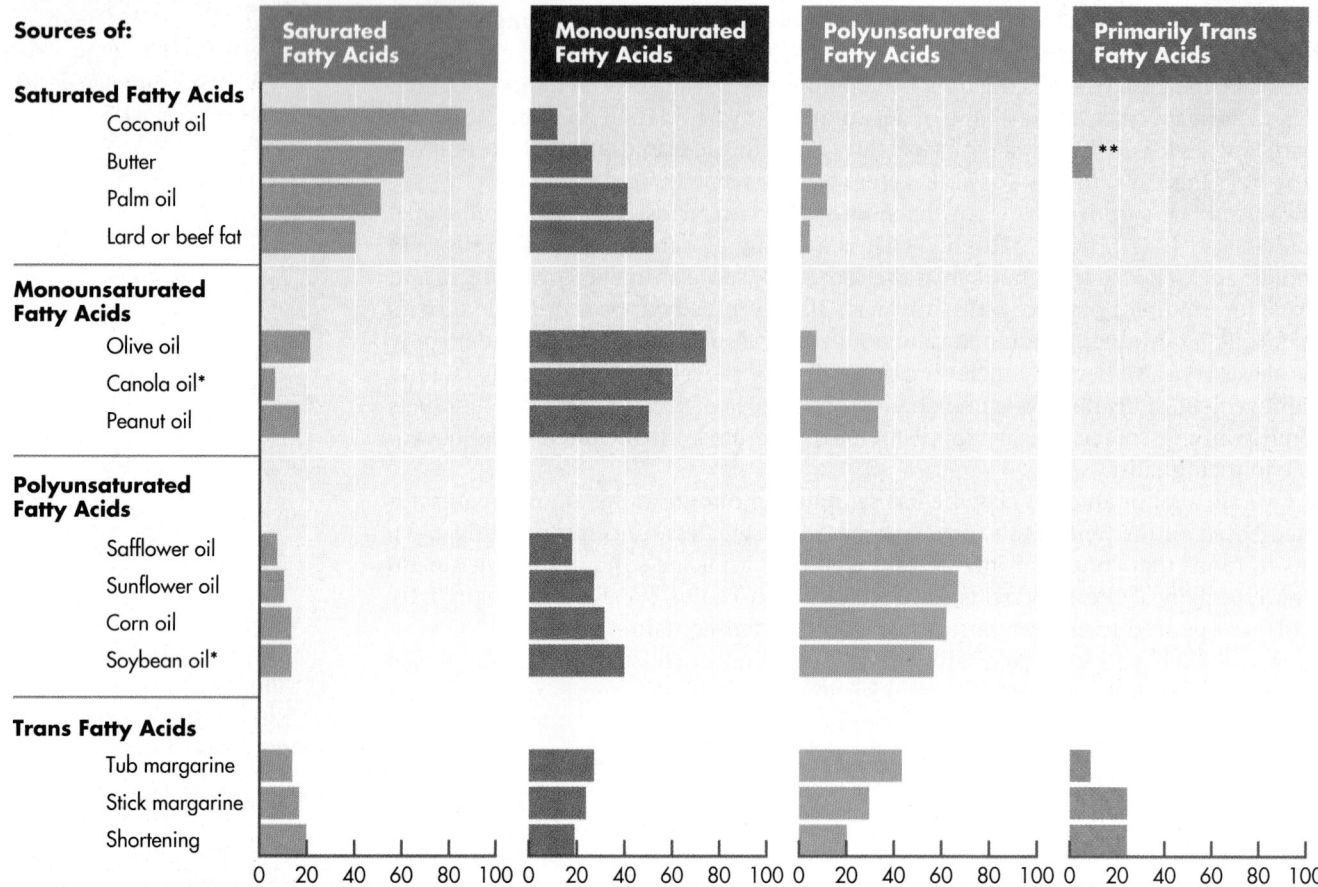

*Rich source of the omega-3 fatty acid alpha-linolenic acid (7% and 12% of total fatty acid content for soybean oil and canola oil, respectively).

**The natural *trans* fatty acids in butter are not harmful and may even have health-promoting properties, such as preventing certain forms of cancer.

FIGURE 5-3 ▶ Saturated, monounsaturated, polyunsaturated, and *trans* fatty acid composition of common fats and oils (expressed as % of all fatty acids in the product).

lecithin A group of compounds that are major components of cell membranes.

Many types of phospholipids exist in the body, especially in the brain. They form important parts of cell membranes. **Lecithin** is a common example of a phospholipid. Various forms are found in body cells and they participate in fat digestion, absorption, and transport. The body is able to produce all the phospholipids it needs. Even though lecithin is sold as a dietary supplement and is present as an additive in many foods, phospholipids such as this one are not essential components of the diet.

Sterols

Sterols are a class of lipids with a characteristic multi-ringed structure that makes them different from the other lipids already discussed (Fig. 5-4c). The most common example of a sterol is cholesterol. This waxy substance doesn't look like a triglyceride—it doesn't have a glycerol backbone or any fatty acids. Still, because it doesn't readily dissolve in water, it is a lipid. Among other functions, cholesterol is used to form certain hormones and bile acids and is incorporated into cell structures. The body can make all the cholesterol it needs.

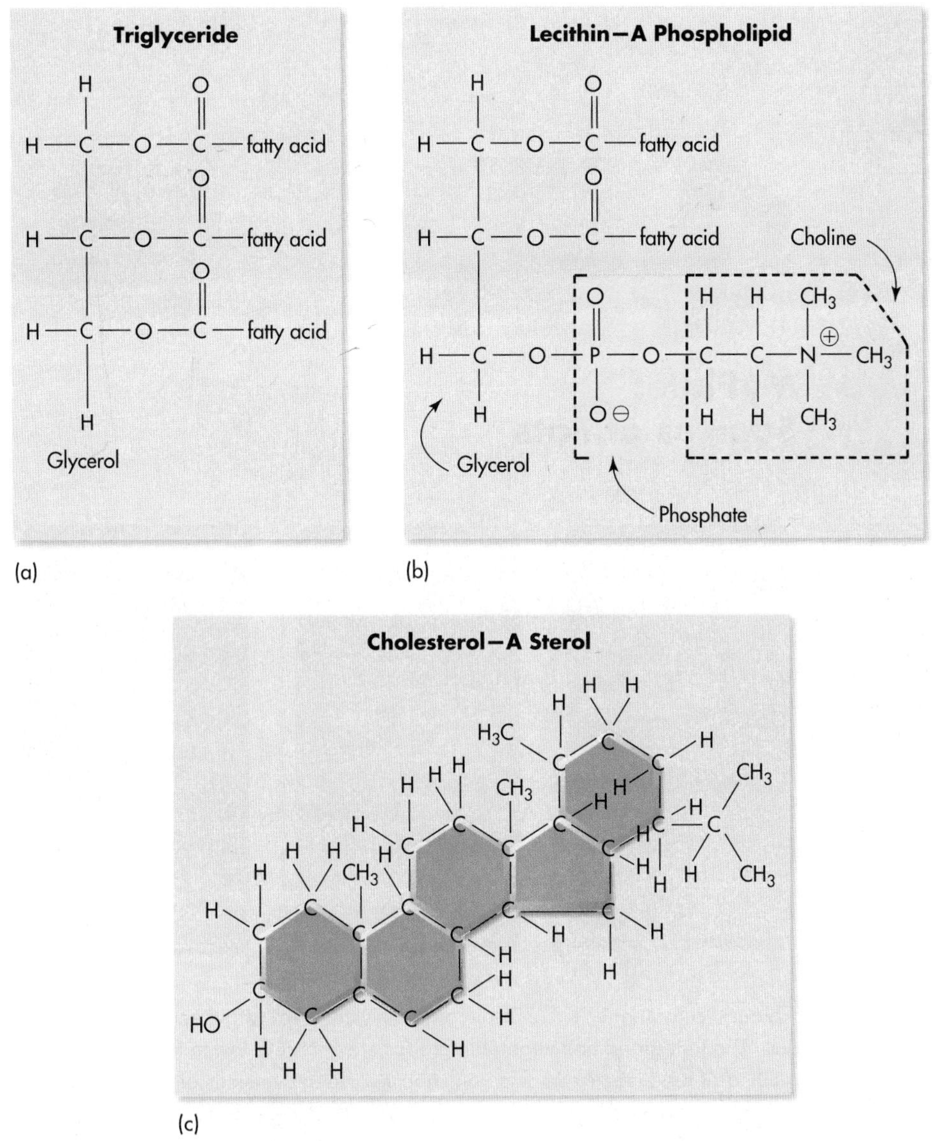

FIGURE 5-4 ▶ Chemical forms of common lipids: (a) triglyceride, (b) phospholipid (in this case, lecithin), and (c) sterol (in this case, cholesterol).

Triglyceride

(a)

Lecithin—A Phospholipid

(b)

Cholesterol—A Sterol

(c)

CONCEPT CHECK

Lipids are a group of compounds that do not dissolve readily in water. Included in this group are fatty acids, triglycerides, phospholipids, and sterols. Fatty acids can be distinguished from one another by the length of the carbon skeleton and the number and position of double bonds along that skeleton. Saturated fatty acids contain no double bonds within their carbon skeleton; that is, they are fully saturated with hydrogens. Monounsaturated fatty acids contain one carbon-carbon double bond, and polyunsaturated fatty acids contain two or more of these bonds. Certain omega-3 and omega-6 fatty acids are essential in the human diet.

Triglycerides are the major form of fat in the body and in foods. These consist of three fatty acids bonded to a glycerol backbone. Phospholipids are similar to triglycerides in structure, but at least one fatty acid is replaced by another compound containing phosphorus. Phospholipids play an important structural role in cell membranes. Sterols, another class of lipids, do not resemble either triglycerides or phospholipids, but instead have a multi-ringed structure. Cholesterol, one example of a sterol, forms parts of cells, some hormones, and bile acids. Whereas certain essential fatty acids (as components of triglycerides) are needed in the diet, the body produces all the triglycerides, phospholipids, and cholesterol it needs. Next we will discuss the sources of fat in foods (Fig. 5-5).

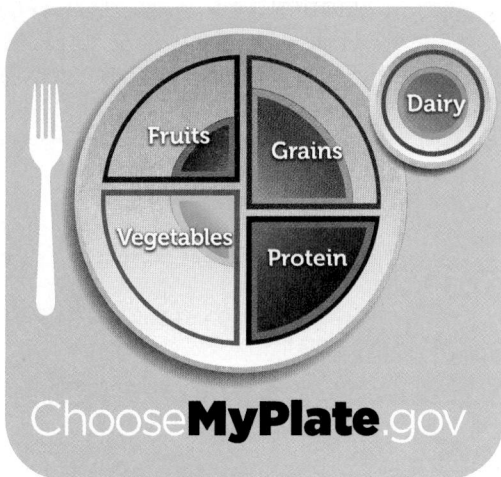

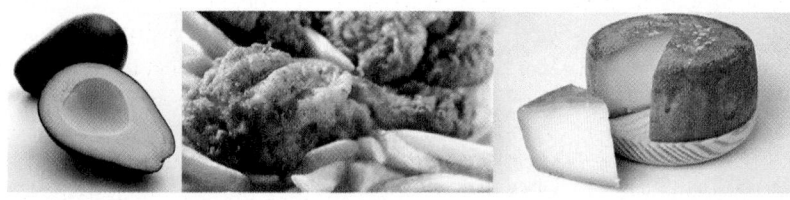

MyPlate: Sources of Fats

Grains	Vegetables	Fruits	Dairy	Protein
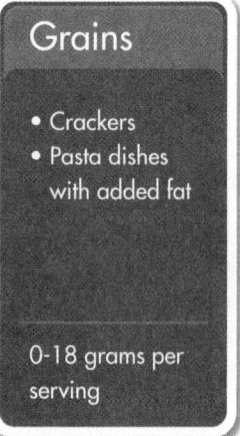	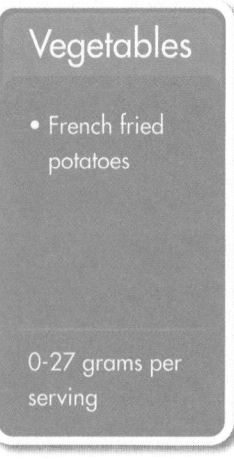	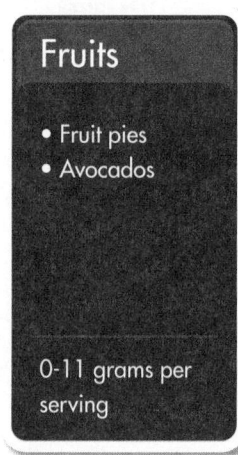	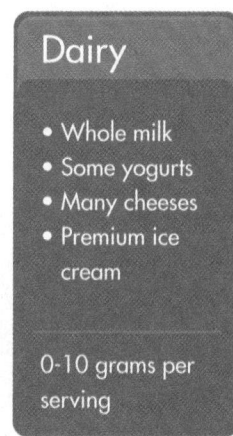	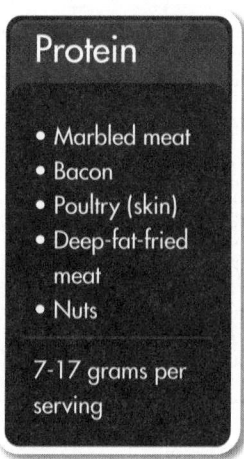
• Crackers • Pasta dishes with added fat	• French fried potatoes	• Fruit pies • Avocados	• Whole milk • Some yogurts • Many cheeses • Premium ice cream	• Marbled meat • Bacon • Poultry (skin) • Deep-fat-fried meat • Nuts
0-18 grams per serving	0-27 grams per serving	0-11 grams per serving	0-10 grams per serving	7-17 grams per serving

FIGURE 5-5 ▶ Sources of fats from MyPlate. The fill of the background color (none, 1/3, 2/3, or completely covered) within each group in the plate indicates the average nutrient density for fat in that group. The fruit group and vegetable groups are generally low in fat. In the other groups, both high-fat and low-fat choices are available. Careful reading of food labels can help you choose lower-fat versions of some foods. In general, any type of frying adds significant amounts of fat to a product, as with French fries and fried chicken. With regard to physical activity, fats are a key fuel in prolonged events, such as long-distance cycling, long-distance running, and prolonged slow to brisk walking.

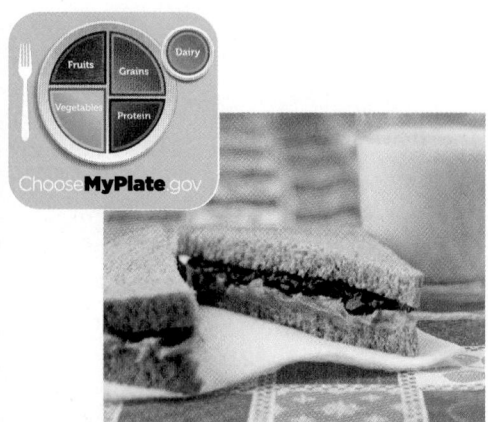

▲ This peanut butter (**protein**) and jelly (**fruit**) sandwich on whole-grain bread (**grain**) with low-fat milk (**dairy**) follows **MyPlate** guidelines well and provides a healthy source of plant fat from the peanut butter. Which section are we missing?

5.3 Fats and Oils in Foods

Lipids in the form of triglycerides are abundant in the North American diet. The foods highest in fat (and therefore energy dense) include salad oils and spreads such as butter, margarine, and mayonnaise. All of these foods contain close to 100% of calories as fat. In reduced-fat margarines, water replaces some of the fat. Whereas regular margarines are 80% fat by weight (11 grams per tablespoon), some reduced-fat margarines are as low as 30% fat by weight (4 grams per tablespoon). When used in recipes, the extra water added to these margarines can cause texture and volume changes in the finished product. Cookbooks can suggest alterations in recipes to compensate for the increased water content of these products.

Still considering the overall fat content, whole foods highest in fat include nuts, bologna, avocados, and bacon, which have about 80% of calories as fat. Next, peanut butter and cheddar cheese have about 75%. Marbled steak and hamburgers (ground chuck) have about 60%, and chocolate bars, ice cream, doughnuts, and whole milk have about 50% of calories as fat. Eggs, pumpkin pie, and cupcakes have 35%, as do lean cuts of meat, such as top round (and ground round) and sirloin. Bread contains about 15%. Finally, foods such as cornflakes, sugar, and fat-free milk have essentially no fat. Figure 5-6 shows examples of food sources of fat. Label reading is necessary to determine the true fat content of food.

The type of fat in food is important to consider along with the total amount of fat. Animal fats are the chief contributors of saturated fatty acids to the North American diet. About 40% to 60% of total fat in dairy and meat products is in the form of saturated fatty acids. In contrast, plant oils contain mostly unsaturated fatty acids, ranging from 73% to 94% of total fat. A moderate to high proportion of total fat (49% to 77%) is supplied by monounsaturated fatty acids in canola oil, olive oil, and peanut oil. Some animal fats are also good sources of monounsaturated fatty acids (30% to 47%) (review Fig. 5-3). Corn, cottonseed, sunflower, soybean, and safflower oils contain mostly polyunsaturated fatty acids (54% to 77%). These plant oils supply the majority of the linoleic and alpha-linolenic acid in the North American food supply.

Wheat germ, peanuts, egg yolk, soy beans, and organ meats are rich sources of phospholipids. Phospholipids such as lecithin, a component of egg yolks, are often added to salad dressing. Lecithin is used as an **emulsifier** in these and other products because of its ability to keep mixtures of lipids and water from separating (see Fig. 5-7). Emulsifiers are added to salad dressings to keep the vegetable oil suspended in water. Eggs added to cake batters likewise emulsify the fat with the milk.

Cholesterol is found only in animal foods. An egg yolk contains about 210 milligrams of cholesterol. Eggs are our main dietary source of cholesterol, along with

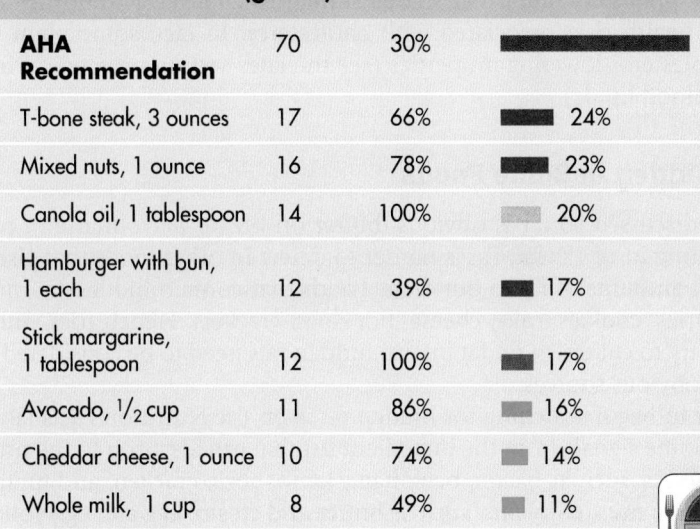

▲ Peanuts are a source of lecithins, as are wheat germ and egg yolks.

emulsifier A compound that can suspend fat in water by isolating individual fat droplets, using a shell of water molecules or other substances to prevent the fat from coalescing.

FIGURE 5-6 ▶ Food sources of fat compared to the American Heart Association (AHA) recommendation of 70 grams per day, or 30% of calories from fat for a 2100 kcal diet.

Food Sources of Fat

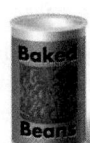

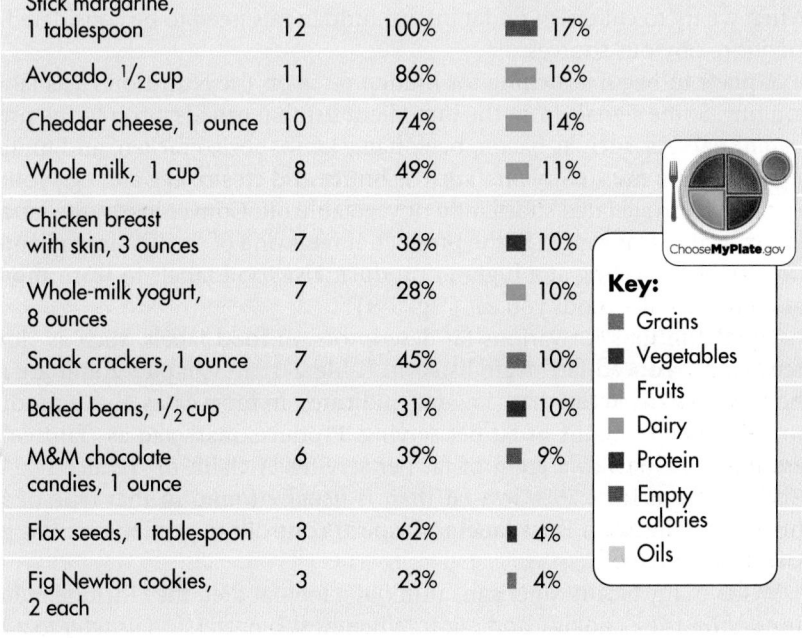

Food Item	Fat (grams)	Calories from Fat %	% AHA Recommendation
AHA Recommendation	70	30%	100%
T-bone steak, 3 ounces	17	66%	24%
Mixed nuts, 1 ounce	16	78%	23%
Canola oil, 1 tablespoon	14	100%	20%
Hamburger with bun, 1 each	12	39%	17%
Stick margarine, 1 tablespoon	12	100%	17%
Avocado, 1/2 cup	11	86%	16%
Cheddar cheese, 1 ounce	10	74%	14%
Whole milk, 1 cup	8	49%	11%
Chicken breast with skin, 3 ounces	7	36%	10%
Whole-milk yogurt, 8 ounces	7	28%	10%
Snack crackers, 1 ounce	7	45%	10%
Baked beans, 1/2 cup	7	31%	10%
M&M chocolate candies, 1 ounce	6	39%	9%
Flax seeds, 1 tablespoon	3	62%	4%
Fig Newton cookies, 2 each	3	23%	4%

Key:
- ■ Grains
- ■ Vegetables
- ■ Fruits
- ■ Dairy
- ■ Protein
- ■ Empty calories
- ■ Oils

FIGURE 5-7 ▶ Emulsifiers in action. Emulsifiers prevent many brands of salad dressings and other condiments from separating into layers of water and fat. Emulsifiers attract fatty acids inside and have a water-attracting group on the outside. Add them to salad dressing, shake well, and they hold the oil in the dressing away from the water. Emulsification is important in both food production and fat digestion/absorption.

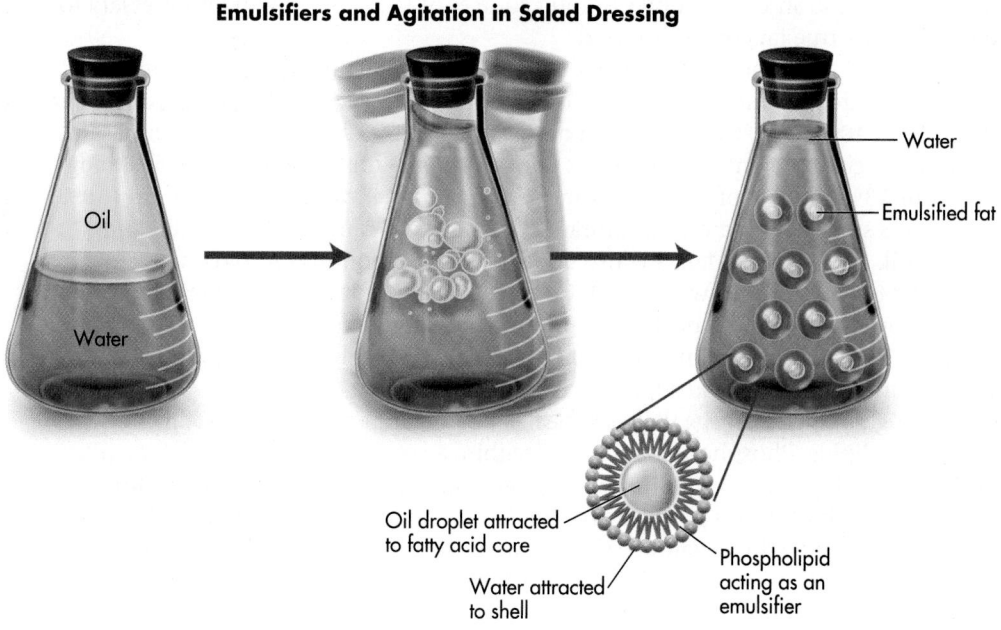

Emulsifiers and Agitation in Salad Dressing

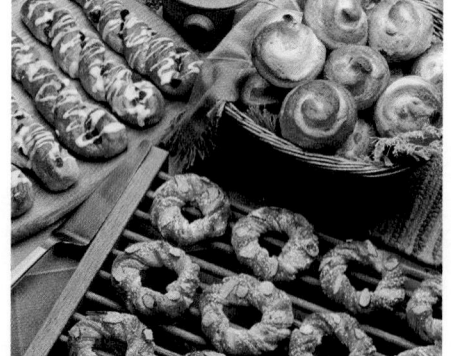

▲ The North American diet contains many high-fat foods—including typical pastry choices. Portion control with these foods is thus important, especially if one is trying to control calorie intake.

meats and whole milk. Manufacturers who advertise their brand of peanut butter, vegetable shortening, margarines, and vegetable oils as "cholesterol-free" are taking advantage of uninformed consumers—all of these products are naturally cholesterol-free. Some plants contain other sterols similar to cholesterol, but they do not pose the heart health risks associated with cholesterol. In fact, some plant sterols have blood cholesterol-lowering properties (see the later section on medical interventions to lower blood lipids).

Fat Is Hidden in Some Foods

Some fat discussed so far is obvious: butter on bread, mayonnaise in potato salad, and marbling in raw meat. Fat is harder to detect in other foods that also contribute significant amounts of fat to our diets. Foods that contain hidden fat include whole milk, pastries, cookies, cake, cheese, hot dogs, crackers, French fries, and ice cream. When we try to cut down on fat intake, hidden fats need to be considered, along with the more obvious sources.

A place to begin searching for hidden fat is on the Nutrition Facts labels of foods you buy. Some signals from the ingredient list that can alert you to the presence of fat are animal fats, such as bacon, beef, ham, lamb, pork, chicken, and turkey fats; lard; vegetable oils; nuts; dairy fats, such as butter and cream; egg and egg-yolk solids; and partially-hydrogenated shortening or vegetable oil. Conveniently, the label lists ingredients by order of weight in the product. If fat is one of the first ingredients listed, you are probably looking at a high-fat product. Use food labels to learn more about the fat content of the foods you eat (Fig. 5-8).

The definitions for various fat descriptors on food labels, such as "low-fat," "fat-free," and "reduced-fat," were listed in Table 2-11 in Chapter 2 and are reprinted in the margin here. Recall that "low-fat" indicates, in most cases, that a product contains no more than 3 grams of fat per serving. Products marketed as "fat-free" must have less than one-half of a gram of fat per serving. A claim of "reduced-fat" means the product has at least 25% less fat than is usually found in that type of food. When there is no Nutrition Facts label to inspect, controlling portion size is a good way to control fat intake.

When many North Americans think of a low-fat diet, they include reduced-fat versions of pastries, cookies, and cakes. When health professionals refer to a low-fat diet,

life, manufacturers often add partially-hydrogenated plant oils to products. Foods most likely to become rancid are deep-fried foods and foods with a large amount of exposed surface. The fat in fish is also susceptible to rancidity because it is highly polyunsaturated.

Antioxidants such as vitamin E help protect foods against rancidity by guarding against fat breakdown. The vitamin E naturally occurring in plant oils reduces the breakdown of double bonds in fatty acids. When food manufacturers want to prevent rancidity in polyunsaturated fats, they often add the synthetic antioxidants **BHA** and **BHT** or vitamin C to products that contain fat such as salad dressings and cake mixes. Manufacturers also tightly seal products and use other methods to reduce oxygen levels inside packages.

Hydrogenation of Fatty Acids in Food Production Increases *Trans* Fatty Acid Content

As mentioned previously, most fats with long-chain saturated fatty acids are solid at room temperature, and those with unsaturated fatty acids are liquid at room temperature. In some kinds of food production, solid fats work better than liquid oils. In pie crust, for example, solid fats yield a flaky product, whereas crusts made with liquid oils tend to be greasy and more crumbly. If oils with unsaturated fatty acids are used to replace solid fats, they often must be made more saturated (with hydrogen), as this solidifies the vegetable oils into shortenings and margarines. Hydrogen is added by bubbling hydrogen gas under pressure into liquid vegetable oils in a process called **hydrogenation** (Fig. 5-9). The fatty acids aren't fully hydrogenated to the saturated fatty acid form, as this would make the product too hard and brittle. Partial hydrogenation—leaving some monounsaturated fatty acids—creates a semi-solid product.

The process of hydrogenation produces *trans* fatty acids as was described earlier in this chapter. Most natural monounsaturated and polyunsaturated fatty acids exist in the *cis* form, causing a bend in the carbon chain, whereas the straighter carbon forms of *trans* fat more closely resemble saturated fatty acids. This may be the mechanism

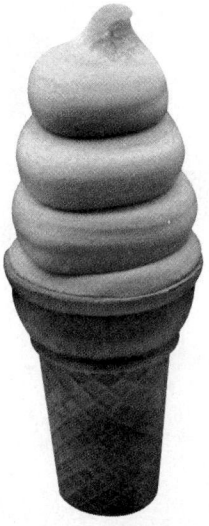

▲ Fat replacements such as gum fiber are typically seen in soft serve ice cream.

Canada has not approved the use of olestra in food products; the United States is the sole country that permits the use of this fat substitute in foods.

BHA, BHT Butylated hydroxyanisole and butylated hydroxytoluene—two common synthetic antioxidants added to foods.

hydrogenation The addition of hydrogen to a carbon-carbon double bond, producing a single carbon-carbon bond with two hydrogens attached to each carbon. Hydrogenation of unsaturated fatty acids in a vegetable oil increases its hardness, so this process is used to convert liquid oils into more solid fats, used in making margarine and shortening. *Trans* fatty acids are a by-product of hydrogenation of vegetable oils.

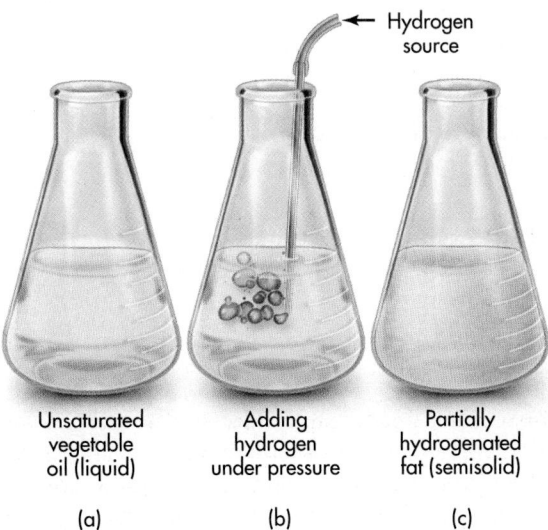

Hydrogen source

Unsaturated vegetable oil (liquid)
(a)

Adding hydrogen under pressure
(b)

Partially hydrogenated fat (semisolid)
(c)

FIGURE 5-9 ▶ How liquid oils become solid fats. (a) Unsaturated fatty acids are present in liquid form. (b) Hydrogens are added (hydrogenation), changing some carbon-carbon double bonds to single bonds and producing some *trans* fatty acids. (c) The partially hydrogenated product is likely to be used in margarine, shortening, or for deep-fat frying.

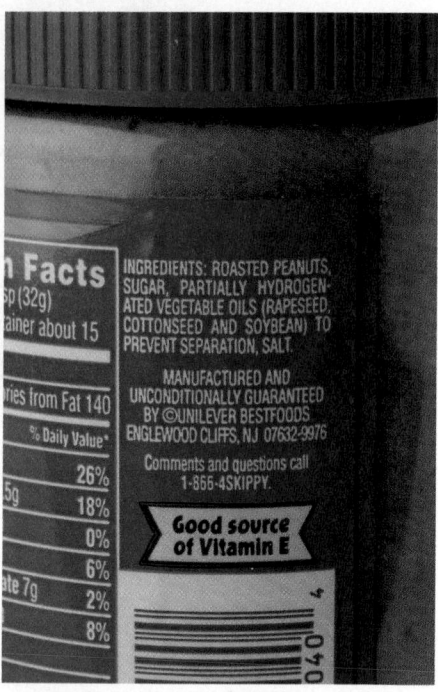

Peanut Butter: Is It "Good" Fat ?

At the grocery store, there are several brands of peanut butter on the shelf. The label on one brand of peanut butter indicates that the product is "cholesterol free," whereas none of the other brands make the same claim. A jar of "natural" peanut butter claims to have no hydrogenated fats. Which jar of peanut butter is best for heart health?

Cholesterol is a type of lipid that is only found in animal products. Therefore, all peanut butter is cholesterol free! Hydrogenated oils are used to increase shelf life of many products, including peanut butter. The process of hydrogenation can produce *trans* fats, which have many of the same detrimental health effects as saturated fat. *Trans* fats increase levels of "bad" blood cholesterol (LDL) and decrease "good" blood cholesterol (HDL). If hydrogenated oils appear in the list of ingredients as in the label shown here, there is a good chance the product contains *trans* fats. As you learned in Chapter 2, a product may claim to be free of *trans* fats as long as the product contains no more than 0.5 g of *trans* fats per serving. Therefore, the only guarantee to avoiding *trans* fat in peanut butter is to buy the "natural" peanut butter made from only peanuts.

whereby *trans* fat increases the risk for heart disease. Studies also indicate that *trans* fats increase overall inflammation in the body, which is not healthful. Thus, people should limit intake of partially-hydrogenated fat and thus *trans* fat. This may not be such a concern for the average person, as long as *trans* fat intake is not excessive and the diet is adequate in polyunsaturated fat. However, because *trans* fatty acids serve no particular role in maintaining body health, the latest Dietary Guidelines for Americans, the American Heart Association, and the Food and Nutrition Board each recommend minimal *trans* fat intake.

Not so long ago, public pressure persuaded manufacturers to eliminate the tropical oils rich in saturated fat (palm, palm olein, and coconut) from food processing. Partially-hydrogenated soybean oil—rich in *trans* fat—became the major replacement. Currently, *trans* fat intake in North America is estimated to contribute about 3% to 4% of total calories, amounting to 10 grams per day, on average. Table 5-1 lists typical sources.

FDA is now requiring the *trans* fat content of foods on food labels (review Fig. 5-8). The food labels in Canada also must list *trans* fat content. FDA hopes to make consumers more aware of the amounts of *trans* fat in foods as well as the negative health consequences associated with their excessive consumption. North American companies are already responding to this issue by creating products free of *trans* fat. For example, Promise, Smart Beat, and some Fleischmann's margarines are lower in or free of *trans* fat (less than 0.5 grams per serving) compared to typical margarines.

This addition of the *trans* fat listing on labels helps consumers at the supermarket, but when dining out, consumers are "left in the dark" as to which foods contain *trans* fat. Knowing which foods are low in *trans* fat when ordering at a restaurant is difficult because information about preparation methods and precise fat

TABLE 5-1 Main Sources of Fatty acids and Their State at Room Temperature

Type and Health Effects	Main Sources	State at Room Temperature
Saturated Fatty Acids Increase blood levels of cholesterol		
Long Chain	Lard; fat in beef, pork, and lamb	Solid
Medium and Short Chain	Milk fat (butter), coconut oil, palm oil, palm kernel oil	Soft or liquid
Monounsaturated Fatty Acids Decrease blood levels of cholesterol	Olive oil, canola oil, peanut oil	Liquid
Polyunsaturated Fatty Acids Decrease blood levels of cholesterol	Sunflower oil, corn oil, safflower oil, fish oil	Liquid
Essential Fatty Acids Omega 3: alpha–linolenic acid Reduces inflammation responses, blood clotting, and plasma triglycerides	Cold-water fish (salmon, tuna, sardines, mackerel), walnuts, flaxseed, hemp oil, canola oil, soybean oil	Liquid
Omega 6: Linoleic Acid Regulates blood pressure and increases blood clotting	Beef, poultry, safflower oil, sunflower oil, corn oil	Solid to liquid
***Trans* Fatty Acids** Increase blood cholesterol more than saturated fat	Margarine (squeeze, tub, stick), shortening	Soft to very solid

composition is rarely available. Many cities, including New York, Philadelphia, and Boston, have banned *trans* fat use in restaurants (see Further Reading 2). To minimize *trans* fat intake, a general guideline is to limit consumption of fried (especially deep-fat fried) food items, any pastries or flaky bread products (such as pie crusts, crackers, croissants, and biscuits), and cookies.

Until all foods are labeled with *trans* fat content, consumers can also make educated guesses on the *trans* fat content of foods by examining the list of ingredients on the food label. If partially-hydrogenated vegetable oil is one of the first three ingredients on the label, you can assume there is a significant amount of *trans* fat in the product.

Limiting *trans* fat at home is a much easier task. Most importantly, use little or no stick margarine or shortening. Instead, substitute vegetable oils and softer tub margarines (whose labels list vegetable oil or water as the first ingredient). Avoid deep-fat frying any food in shortening. Substitute baking, panfrying, broiling, steaming, grilling, or deep-fat frying in unhydrogenated vegetable oils. Replace nondairy creamers with reduced-fat or fat-free milk, since most nondairy creamers are rich in partially-hydrogenated vegetable oils. Finally, read the ingredients on food labels, using the previous tips to estimate *trans* fat content.

▲ Fried foods are a rich source of fat and *trans* fats. Reducing the intake of these foods can help lower blood lipid levels.

CONCEPT CHECK

Hydrogenation of unsaturated fatty acids is the process of adding hydrogen to carbon-carbon double bonds to produce single bonds. This results in the creation of some *trans* fatty acids. Hydrogenation changes vegetable oil to solid fat. It is wise to monitor *trans* fat intake, as this form of fat increases the risk for heart disease.

The carbon-carbon double bonds in polyunsaturated fatty acids are easily broken, yielding products responsible for rancidity. The presence of antioxidants, such as vitamin E in oils, naturally protects unsaturated fatty acids against oxidative destruction. Manufacturers can use hydrogenated fats and add natural or synthetic antioxidants to reduce the likelihood of rancidity.

5.4 Making Lipids Available for Body Use

It's no secret that fats and oils make foods more appealing. Their presence in foods adds flavor, lubrication, and texture. What happens to lipids once they are eaten? Let's take a closer look at the digestion, absorption, and physiological roles of lipids in the body.

Digestion

In the first phase of fat digestion, the stomach (and salivary glands to some extent) secretes **lipase.** This enzyme acts primarily on triglycerides that have fatty acids with short chain lengths, such as those found in butterfat. The action of salivary and stomach lipase, however, is usually dwarfed by that of the lipase enzyme released from the pancreas and active in the small intestine. Triglycerides and other lipids found in common vegetable oils and meats have longer chain lengths and are generally not digested until they reach the small intestine (Fig. 5-10).

In the small intestine, triglycerides are broken down by lipase into smaller products, namely monoglycerides (glycerol backbones with a single fatty acid attached) and fatty acids. Under the right circumstances, digestion is rapid and thorough. The "right" circumstances include the presence of bile from the gallbladder. Bile acids present in the bile act as emulsifiers on the digestive products of lipase action, suspending the monoglycerides and fatty acids in the watery digestive juices. This emulsification improves digestion and absorption because as large fat globules are broken down into smaller ones, the total surface area for lipase action increases (Fig. 5-11).

lipase Fat-digesting enzyme produced by the salivary glands, stomach, and pancreas.

FIGURE 5-10 ▶ A summary of fat digestion and absorption. Chapter 3 covered
general aspects of this process.

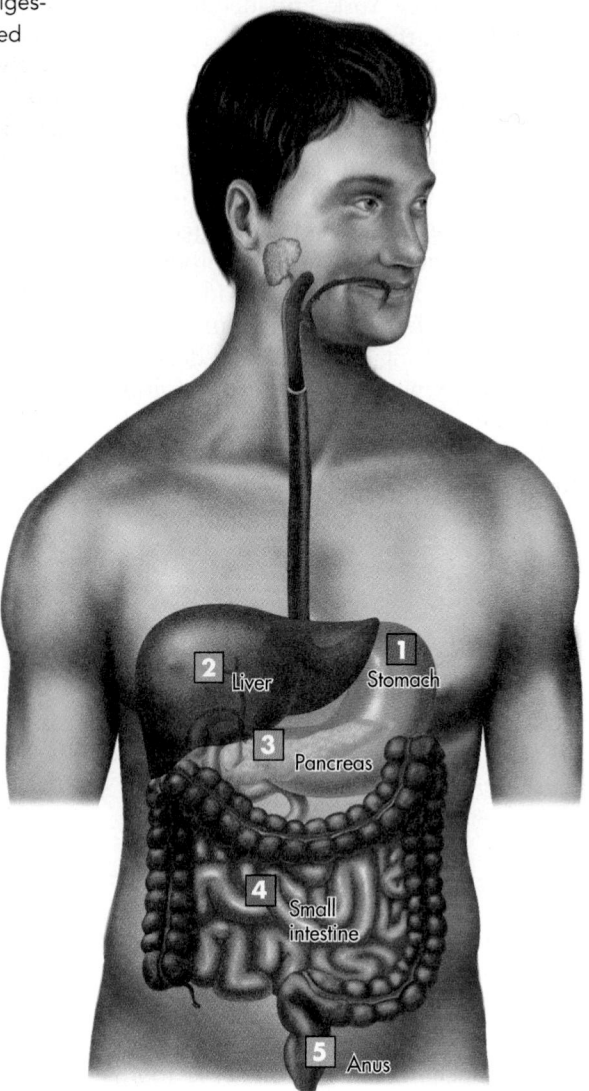

Fat Digestion and Absorption

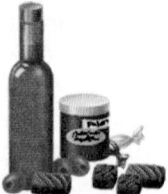

1 Stomach: Only minor digestion of fat
takes place in the stomach through the
action of lipase enzymes.

2 Liver: The liver produces bile, stored in
the gallbladder and released through
the bile duct into the small intestine.
Bile aids in fat digestion and
absorption by emulsifying lipids in the
digestive juices.

3 Pancreas: The pancreas secretes a
mixture of enzymes, including lipase,
into the small intestine.

4 Small intestine: The small intestine
is the primary site for digestion and
absorption of lipids. Once absorbed,
long-chain fatty acids are packaged
for transport through the lymph and
bloodstream. (Shorter-chain fatty acids
are absorbed directly into portal
circulation.)

5 Large intestine: Less than 5% of
ingested fat is normally excreted in the
feces.

If the gallbladder is surgically removed
(e.g., in cases of gallstone formation),
bile will enter the small intestine directly
from the liver.

With regard to phospholipid digestion, certain enzymes from the pancreas and
cells in the wall of the small intestine digest phospholipids. The eventual products
are glycerol, fatty acids, and remaining parts. With regard to cholesterol digestion,
any cholesterol with a fatty acid attached is broken down to free cholesterol and fatty
acids by certain enzymes released from the pancreas.

MAKING **DECISIONS**

Bile Acids

During meals, bile acids circulate in a path that begins in the liver, goes on to the gallbladder,
and then moves to the small intestine. After participating in fat digestion, most bile acids are
absorbed and end up back at the liver. Approximately 98% of the bile acids are recycled. Only
1% to 2% ends up in the large intestine to be eliminated in the feces. Using medicines that
block some of this reabsorption of bile acids is one way to treat high blood cholesterol. The
liver takes cholesterol from the bloodstream to form replacement bile acids. Viscous fiber in
the diet can also bind to bile acids to produce the same effect (see a later section on medical
interventions related to cardiovascular disease for details).

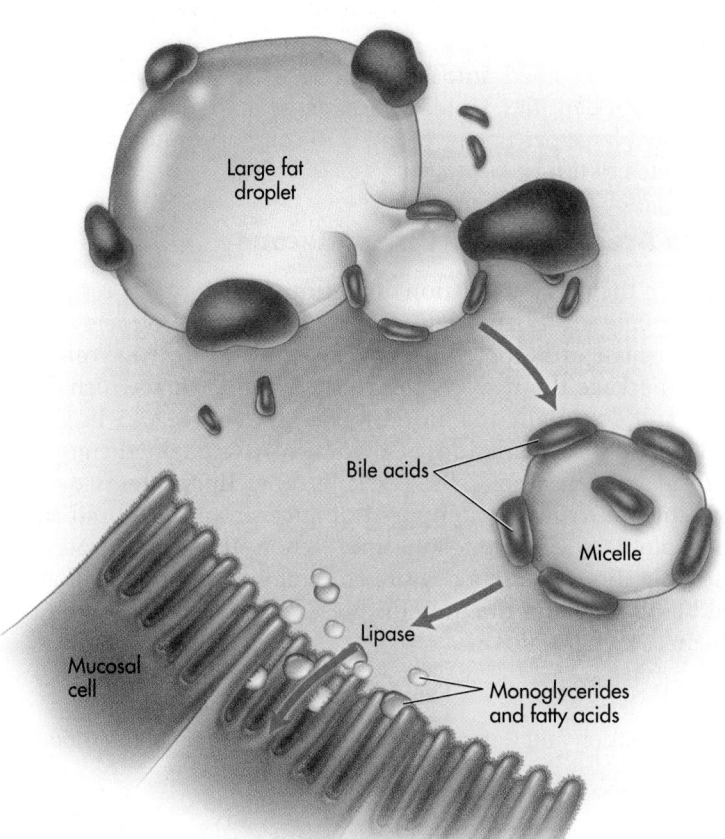

FIGURE 5-11 ▶ Bile acids mix with fats to form small droplets called micelles that facilitate the absorption of monoglycerides and fatty acids into the mucosal cells of the small intestine.

Absorption

The products of fat digestion in the small intestine are fatty acids and monoglycerides. These products diffuse into the absorptive cells of the small intestine. About 95% of dietary fat is absorbed in this way. The chain length of fatty acids affects the ultimate fate of fatty acids and monoglycerides after absorption. If the chain length of a fatty acid is less than 12 carbon atoms, it is water soluble and will therefore probably travel as such through the portal vein that connects directly to the liver. If the fatty acid is a more typical long-chain variety, it must be reformed into a triglyceride in the intestinal absorptive cell and eventually enter circulation via the lymphatic system (review Chapter 3 for an overview of this process).

CONCEPT CHECK

In the small intestine, a lipase enzyme released from the pancreas digests dietary triglycerides into monoglycerides (glycerol backbones with single fatty acids attached) and fatty acids. These breakdown products then diffuse into the absorptive cells of the small intestine. Long-chain fatty acids are transported through the lymphatic system, whereas fatty acids with shorter carbon chains are absorbed directly into the portal vein that connects directly to the liver. Other lipids are prepared for absorption by different enzymes.

5.5 Carrying Lipids in the Bloodstream

As noted earlier, fat and water don't mix easily. This incompatibility presents a challenge for the transport of fats through the watery media of the blood and lymph.

lipoprotein A compound found in the bloodstream containing a core of lipids with a shell composed of protein, phospholipid, and cholesterol.

chylomicron Lipoprotein made of dietary fats surrounded by a shell of cholesterol, phospholipids, and protein. Chylomicrons are formed in the absorptive cells of the small intestine after fat absorption and travel through the lymphatic system to the bloodstream.

Lipoproteins serve as vehicles for transport of lipids from the small intestine and liver to the body tissues (Table 5-2).

Lipoproteins are classified into four groups—chylomicrons, VLDL, LDL, and HDL—based on their densities. Lipids are less dense than proteins. Therefore, lipoproteins that contain a large percentage of lipids in comparison to protein are less dense than those depleted of lipids.

Dietary Fats Are Carried by Chylomicrons

As you learned in the previous section, digestion of dietary fats results in a mixture of glycerol, monoglycerides, and fatty acids. Once these products are absorbed by the cells of the small intestine, they are reassembled into triglycerides. Then, the intestinal cells package the triglycerides into **chylomicrons,** which enter the lymphatic system and eventually the bloodstream (review Fig. 3-5 in Chapter 3 for a depiction of lymphatic circulation). Chylomicrons contain dietary fat and originate only from the intestinal cells. Like the other lipoproteins described in the next section, chylomicrons are composed of large droplets of lipid surrounded by a thin, water-soluble shell of phospholipids, cholesterol, and protein (Fig. 5-12). The water-soluble shell around a chylomicron allows the lipid to float freely in the water-based blood. Some of the proteins present may also help other cells identify the lipoprotein as a chylomicron.

TABLE 5-2 Composition and Roles of the Major Lipoproteins in the Blood

Lipoprotein	Primary Component	Key Role
Chylomicron	Triglyceride	Carries dietary fat from the small intestine to cells
VLDL	Triglyceride	Carries lipids made and taken up by the liver to cells
LDL	Cholesterol	Carries cholesterol made by the liver and from other sources to cells
HDL	Protein	Contributes to cholesterol removal from cells and, in turn, excretion of it from the body

FIGURE 5-12 ▶ The structure of a lipoprotein, in this case an LDL. This structure allows fats to circulate in the water-based bloodstream. Various lipoproteins are found in the bloodstream. The primary component of LDL is cholesterol.

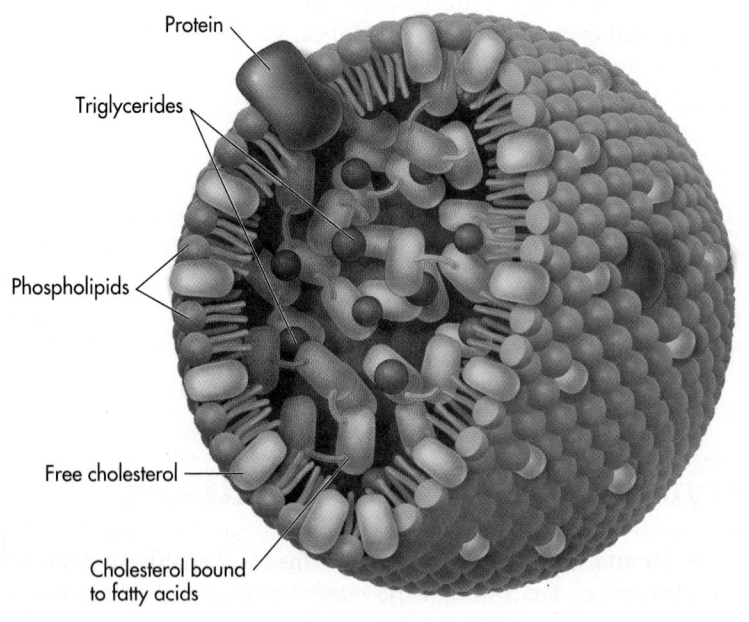

Protein

Triglycerides

Phospholipids

Free cholesterol

Cholesterol bound to fatty acids

Once a chylomicron enters the bloodstream, the triglycerides in its core are broken down into fatty acids and glycerol by an enzyme called **lipoprotein lipase,** attached to the inside walls of the blood vessels (Fig. 5-13). As soon as the fatty acids are released to the bloodstream, they are absorbed by cells in the vicinity, while much of the glycerol circulates back to the liver. Muscle cells can immediately use the absorbed fatty acids for fuel. Adipose cells, on the other hand, tend to re-form the fatty acids into triglycerides for storage. After triglycerides have been removed, a chylomicron remnant remains. Chylomicron remnants are removed from circulation by the liver and their components are recycled to make other lipoproteins and bile acids.

lipoprotein lipase An enzyme attached to the cells that form the inner lining of blood vessels; it breaks down triglycerides into free fatty acids and glycerol.

Other Lipoproteins Transport Lipids from the Liver to the Body Cells

The liver takes up various lipids from the blood. The liver also is the manufacturing site for lipids and cholesterol. The raw materials for lipid and cholesterol synthesis include free fatty acids taken up from the bloodstream, as well as carbon and hydrogen derived from carbohydrates, protein, and alcohol. The liver then must package these synthesized lipids as lipoproteins for transport in the blood to body tissues.

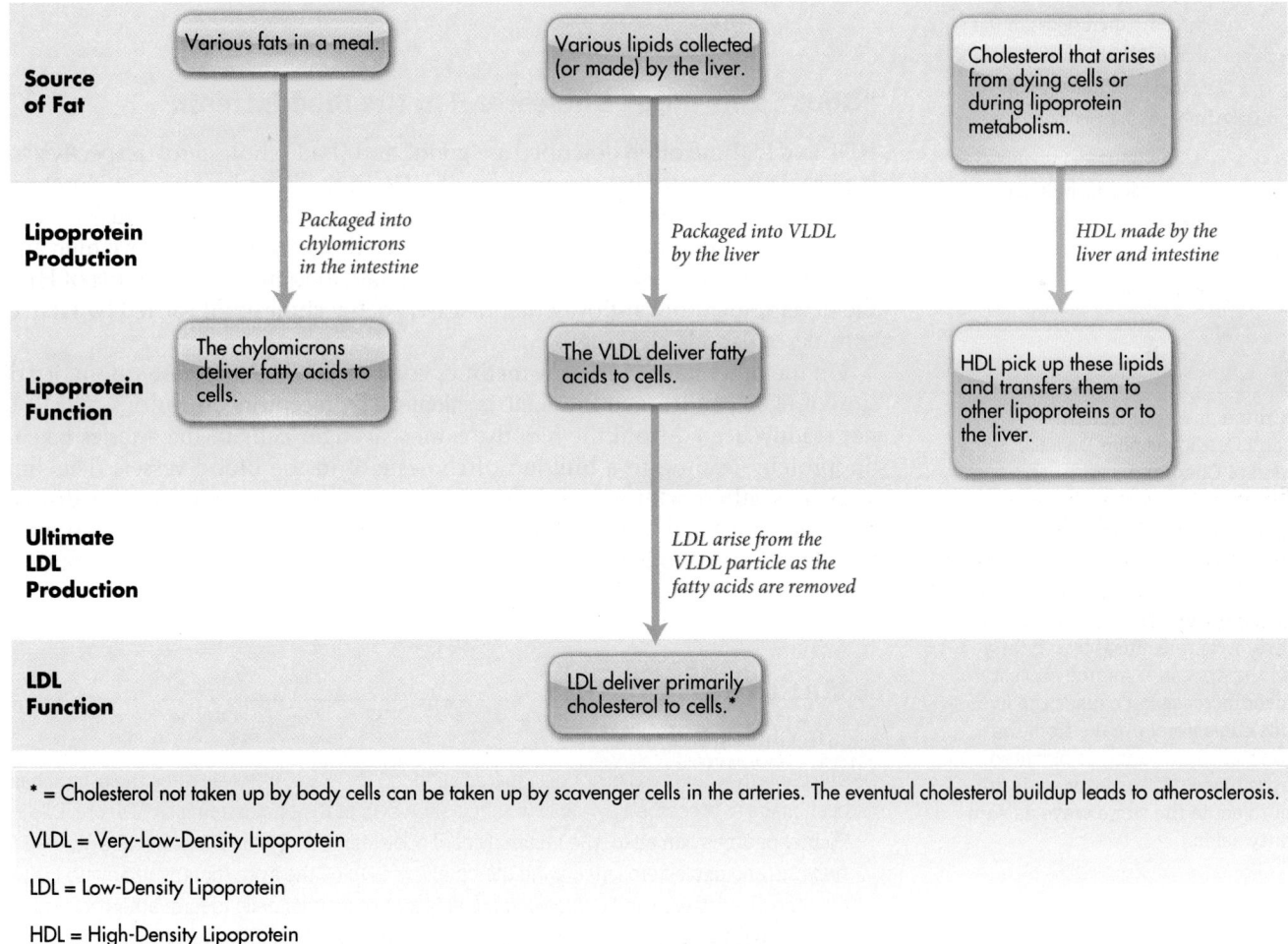

Source of Fat
- Various fats in a meal.
- Various lipids collected (or made) by the liver.
- Cholesterol that arises from dying cells or during lipoprotein metabolism.

Lipoprotein Production
- *Packaged into chylomicrons in the intestine*
- *Packaged into VLDL by the liver*
- *HDL made by the liver and intestine*

Lipoprotein Function
- The chylomicrons deliver fatty acids to cells.
- The VLDL deliver fatty acids to cells.
- HDL pick up these lipids and transfers them to other lipoproteins or to the liver.

Ultimate LDL Production
- *LDL arise from the VLDL particle as the fatty acids are removed*

LDL Function
- LDL deliver primarily cholesterol to cells.*

* = Cholesterol not taken up by body cells can be taken up by scavenger cells in the arteries. The eventual cholesterol buildup leads to atherosclerosis.

VLDL = Very-Low-Density Lipoprotein

LDL = Low-Density Lipoprotein

HDL = High-Density Lipoprotein

FIGURE 5-13 ▶ Lipoprotein production and function. Chylomicrons carry absorbed fat to body cells. VLDL carries fat taken up from the bloodstream by the liver, as well as any fat made by the liver, to body cells. LDL arises from VLDL and carries mostly cholesterol to cells. HDL arises mostly from the liver and intestine. HDL carries cholesterol from cells to other lipoproteins and to the liver for excretion.

very-low-density lipoprotein (VLDL) The lipoprotein created in the liver that carries cholesterol and lipids that have been taken up or newly synthesized by the liver.

low-density lipoprotein (LDL) The lipoprotein in the blood containing primarily cholesterol; elevated LDL is strongly linked to cardiovascular disease risk.

high-density lipoprotein (HDL) The lipoprotein in the blood that picks up cholesterol from dying cells and other sources and transfers it to the other lipoproteins in the bloodstream, as well as directly to the liver; low HDL increases the risk for cardiovascular disease.

menopause The cessation of the menstrual cycle in women, usually beginning at about 50 years of age.

scavenger cells Specific form of white blood cells that can bury themselves in the artery wall and accumulate LDL. As these cells take up LDL, they contribute to the development of atherosclerosis.

atherosclerosis A buildup of fatty material (plaque) in the arteries, including those surrounding the heart.

See Nutrition and Your Health: Lipids and Cardiovascular Disease at the end of Chapter 5.

It appears that saturated fatty acids promote an increase in the amount of free cholesterol (not attached to fatty acids) in the liver, whereas unsaturated fatty acids do the opposite. As free cholesterol in the liver increases, it causes the liver to reduce cholesterol uptake from the bloodstream, contributing to elevated LDL in the blood. (*Trans* fatty acids are thought to act in the same ways as saturated fatty acids.)

First in our discussion of lipoproteins made by the liver are **very-low-density lipoproteins (VLDL).** These particles are composed of cholesterol and triglycerides surrounded by a water-soluble shell. VLDLs are rich in triglycerides and thus are very low in density. Once in the bloodstream, lipoprotein lipase on the inner surface of the blood vessels breaks down the triglyceride in the VLDL into fatty acids and glycerol. Fatty acids and glycerol are released into the bloodstream and taken up by the body cells.

As its triglycerides are released, the VLDL becomes proportionately denser. Much of what eventually remains of the VLDL fraction is then called **low-density lipoprotein (LDL);** this is composed primarily of the remaining cholesterol. The primary function of LDL is to transport cholesterol to tissues. LDL particles are taken up from the bloodstream by specific receptors on cells, especially liver cells, and are then broken down. The cholesterol and protein components of LDL provide some of the building blocks necessary for cell growth and development, such as synthesis of cell membranes and hormones.

The final group of lipoproteins, **high-density lipoproteins (HDL),** is a critical and beneficial participant in this process of lipid transport. Its high proportion of protein makes it the densest lipoprotein. The liver and intestine produce most of the HDL in the blood. It roams the bloodstream, picking up cholesterol from dying cells and other sources. HDL donates the cholesterol primarily to other lipoproteins for transport back to the liver to be excreted. Some HDL travels directly back to the liver.

"Good" and "Bad" Cholesterol in the Bloodstream

HDL and LDL are often described as "good" and "bad" cholesterol, respectively. Many studies demonstrate that the amount of HDL in the bloodstream can closely predict the risk for cardiovascular disease. Risk increases with low HDL because little cholesterol is transported back to the liver and excreted. Women tend to have high amounts of HDL, especially before **menopause,** compared to men. High amounts of HDL slow the development of cardiovascular disease, so any cholesterol carried by HDL can be considered "good" cholesterol.

On the other hand, LDL is sometimes considered "bad" cholesterol. In our discussion of LDL, you learned that LDL is taken up by receptors on various cells. If LDL is not readily cleared from the bloodstream, **scavenger cells** in the arteries take up the lipoprotein, leading to a buildup of cholesterol in the blood vessels. This buildup, known as **atherosclerosis,** greatly increases the risk for cardiovascular disease (see the following Nutrition and Your Health section). LDL is only a problem when it is too high in the bloodstream because low amounts are needed as part of routine body functions.

MAKING DECISIONS

LDL Cholesterol

The cholesterol in foods is not designated as "good" or "bad." It is only after cholesterol has been made or processed by the liver that it shows up in the bloodstream as LDL or HDL. Dietary patterns can affect the metabolism of cholesterol, however. Diets low in saturated fat, *trans* fat, and cholesterol encourage the uptake of LDL by the liver, thereby removing LDL from the bloodstream and decreasing the ability of scavenger cells to form atherosclerotic plaques in the blood vessels. Likewise, diets high in saturated fat, *trans* fat, and cholesterol reduce the uptake of LDL by the liver, increasing cholesterol in the blood and the risk for cardiovascular disease. What foods in your diet are high in saturated fat, *trans* fat, or cholesterol?

CONCEPT CHECK

Lipids generally move through the bloodstream as part of lipoproteins. Dietary fats absorbed from the small intestine are packaged and transported as chylomicrons, whereas lipids synthesized in the liver are packaged as very-low-density lipoproteins (VLDL). Lipoprotein lipase removes triglycerides from the interiors of both chylomicrons and VLDL, breaking the triglycerides down into glycerol and fatty acids, which are taken up by tissues for energy needs or storage. What remains after the action of lipoprotein lipase are chylomicron remnants (from chylomicrons), the components of which are recycled by the liver, or low-density lipoproteins (LDL, from VLDL), rich in cholesterol. LDL is picked up by receptors on body cells, especially liver cells. Scavenger cells in the arteries may do the same, speeding the development of atherosclerosis. High-density lipoprotein (HDL), also produced in part by the liver, picks up cholesterol from cells and transports it primarily to other lipoproteins for eventual transport back to the liver. Risk factors for cardiovascular disease include an elevated level of LDL and/or low amounts of HDL in the blood.

5.6 Essential Functions of Fatty Acids

The various classes of lipids have diverse functions in the body. All are necessary for health, but, as mentioned earlier, many can be made by the body and therefore are not needed in our diet. Of all the classes of lipids, only certain polyunsaturated fatty acids are essential parts of a diet.

The Essential Fatty Acids

We must obtain linoleic acid (an omega-6 fatty acid) and alpha-linolenic acid (an omega-3 fatty acid) from foods to maintain health, so they are called *essential* fatty acids (Fig. 5-14). These omega-6 and omega-3 fatty acids form parts of vital body structures, perform important roles in immune system function and vision, help form cell membranes, and produce hormonelike compounds. Omega-6 and omega-3 fatty acids must be obtained through the diet because human cells lack the enzymes needed to produce these fatty acids. Other fatty acids, such as omega-9 fatty acids, can be synthesized in the body, and therefore are not essential components of the diet.

Omega-3 Fatty Acids in Fish (grams per 3 ounce serving)	
Atlantic salmon	1.8
Anchovy	1.7
Sardines	1.4
Rainbow trout	1.0
Coho salmon	0.9
Bluefish	0.8
Striped bass	0.8
Tuna, white, canned	0.7
Halibut	0.4
Catfish, channel	0.2

Recommended omega-3 fatty acid (alpha-linolenic acid) intake per day:	
Men	1.6 grams
Women	1.1 grams

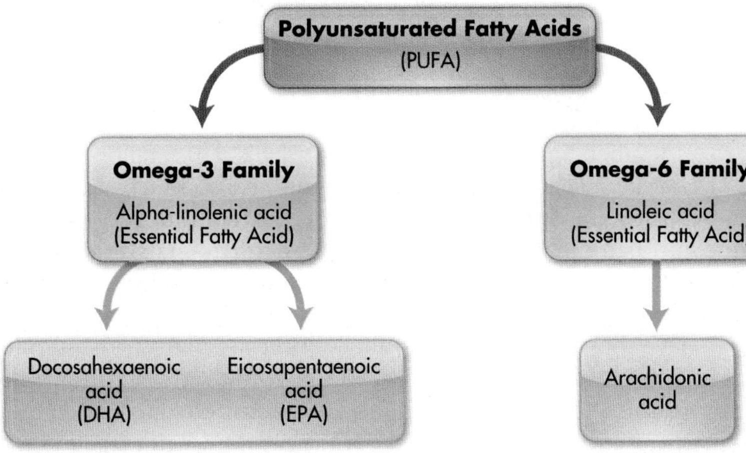

FIGURE 5-14 ▶ The essential fatty acid (EFA) family. Linoleic acid and alpha-linolenic acid are available from dietary sources, and must be consumed as body synthesis does not take place. These are the essential fatty acids. The other fatty acids in this figure can be synthesized from the essential fatty acids.

eicosapentaenoic acid (EPA) An omega-3 fatty acid with 20 carbons and five carbon-carbon double bonds. It is present in large amounts in fatty fish and is slowly synthesized in the body from alpha-linolenic acid.

docosahexaenoic acid (DHA) An omega-3 fatty acid with 22 carbons and six carbon-carbon double bonds. It is present in large amounts in fatty fish and is slowly synthesized in the body from alpha-linolenic acid. DHA is especially present in the retina and brain.

arachidonic acid An omega-6 fatty acid made from linoleic acid with 20 carbon atoms and four carbon-carbon double bonds.

hemorrhagic stroke Damage to part of the brain resulting from rupture of a blood vessel and subsequent bleeding within or over the internal surface of the brain.

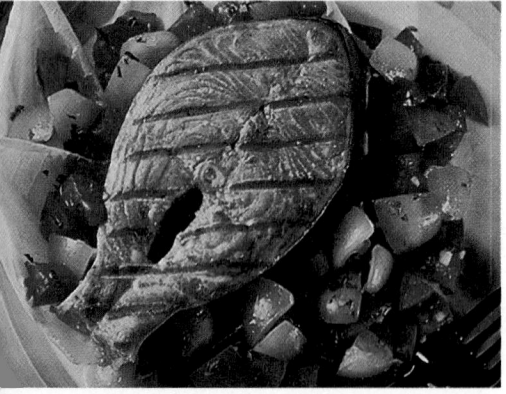

▲ The American Heart Association recommends eating fatty fish such as salmon at least twice a week. As a source of omega-3 fatty acids, fish is a heart-healthy alternative to other animal sources of protein, which can be high in saturated fat and cholesterol.

See Nutrition and Your Health: Lipids and Cardiovascular Disease at the end of Chapter 5.

Still, we need to consume only about 5% of our total calories per day from essential fatty acids. That corresponds to about 2 to 4 tablespoons of plant oil each day. We can easily get that much—from mayonnaise, salad dressings, and other foods—without much effort. Regular consumption of vegetables and whole-grain breads and cereals also helps to supply enough essential fatty acids.

Research also suggests that we include a regular intake of the omega-3 fatty acids, **eicosapentaenoic acid (EPA)** and **docosahexaenoic acid (DHA),** which can be made from alpha-linolenic acid. EPA and DHA are naturally high in fatty fish such as salmon, tuna, sardines, anchovies, striped bass, catfish, herring, mackerel, trout, or halibut. Consumption of one or more of these fish at least twice a week is recommended to obtain EPA and DHA. Additional sources of omega-3 fatty acids include canola and soybean oils, walnuts, flax seeds, mussels, crab, and shrimp (see Further Readings 4, 5, and 15).

MAKING DECISIONS

Mercury in Fish

Consumption of fatty fish at least twice a week is recommended as a good source of the omega-3 fatty acids. Some fish can be a source of mercury, toxic in high amounts, especially swordfish, shark, king mackerel, and tile fish (see Chapter 13). Albacore tuna also is a potential source, while other forms of tuna are much lower in mercury. Those fish low in mercury are salmon, sardines, bluefish, and herring. Shrimp is also low in mercury. For others, varying your choices rather than always eating the same species of fish and limiting overall intake to 12 ounces per week (on average 2 to 3 meals of fish or shellfish per week) is recommended to reduce mercury exposure, especially for pregnant women and children. Existing research indicates that the benefits of fish intake, especially in reducing the risk of cardiovascular disease, outweigh the possible risks of mercury contamination.

The recommendation to consume omega-3 fatty acids stems from the observation that compounds made from omega-3 fatty acids tend to decrease blood clotting and inflammatory processes in the body. The omega-6 fatty acids, notably **arachidonic acid** made from linoleic acid, generally increase clotting and inflammation, and saturated fatty acids also increase blood clotting.

Some studies show that people who eat fish at least twice a week (total weekly intake: 8 ounces [240 grams]) run lower risks for heart attack than do people who rarely eat fish. In these cases, the omega-3 fatty acids in fish oil are probably acting to reduce blood clotting. As will be covered in detail in the "Nutrition and Your Health" section, blood clots are part of the heart attack process. In addition, these omega-3 fatty acids have a favorable effect on heart rhythm. Consequently, the risk of heart attack decreases with the consumption of omega-3 fatty acids from fish, especially for people already at high risk.

We need to remember, however, that blood clotting is a normal body process. Certain groups of people, such as Eskimos in Greenland, eat so much seafood that their normal blood-clotting ability can be impaired. An excess of omega-3 fatty acid intake can allow uncontrolled bleeding and may cause **hemorrhagic stroke.** However, no increase in risk of stroke has been observed in studies using moderate amounts of omega-3 fatty acids.

Studies also have shown that large amounts of omega-3 fatty acids from fish (2 to 4 grams per day) can lower blood triglycerides in people with high triglyceride concentrations. In addition, these omega-3 fatty acids are suspected to be helpful in managing the pain of inflammation associated with rheumatoid arthritis by suppressing immune system responses. This may also help with certain behavioral disorders and cases of mild depression.

In some instances, fish oil capsules can be safely substituted for fish consumption if a person does not like fish. Generally, about 1 gram of omega-3 fatty acids (about three capsules) from fish oil per day is recommended, especially for people with evidence of cardiovascular disease. (Freezing fish oil capsules before consumption or using enteric coated capsules will reduce the fishy aftertaste.) The American Heart Association also recently suggested that fish oil supplements (providing 2 to 4 grams of omega-3 fatty acids per day) could be employed to treat elevated blood triglycerides, as previously noted. However, fish oil capsules should be limited for individuals who have bleeding disorders, take anticoagulant medications, or anticipate surgery, because they may increase risk of uncontrollable bleeding and hemorrhagic stroke. Thus for fish oil capsules, as well as other dietary supplements, it is important to follow a physician's recommendations. Remember that fish oil supplements are not regulated by the FDA. The quality of these supplements, therefore, is not standardized, and contaminants naturally present in the fish oil may not have been removed.

In summary, the regular consumption of fatty fish is advised. Consuming whole fish is thought to have greater benefits and be safer than using fish oil supplements. Fish is not only a rich source of omega-3 fatty acids, but is also a valuable source of protein and trace elements that may also provide protective effects for the cardiovascular system. Broiled or baked fish is recommended rather than fried fish because frying may decrease the ratio of omega-3 to omega-6 fatty acids and may produce *trans* fatty acids and oxidized lipid products that may increase cardiovascular disease risk.

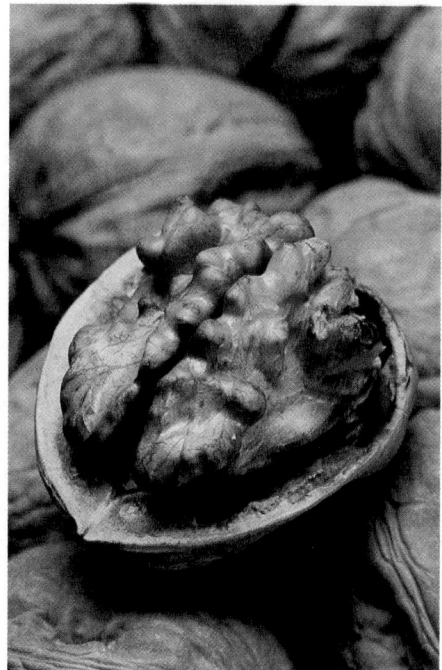

▲ Walnuts are one of the richest plant sources of the omega-3 fatty acid, alpha-linolenic acid, and are also a good source of plant sterols (see Further Reading 8).

MAKING DECISIONS

Flax Seeds or Walnuts?

Flax seeds and walnuts are getting attention today because they are rich vegetable sources of the omega-3 alpha-linolenic acid. About 2 tablespoons of flax seed per day is typically recommended if used as an omega-3 fatty acid source. Flax seeds can be purchased in many natural food stores rather inexpensively. These need to be chewed thoroughly or they will pass through the GI tract undigested. Many people find it easier to grind them in a coffee grinder before eating them. Flax seed oil is also available, but it turns **rancid** very quickly, especially if not refrigerated. Compared to other nuts and seeds, walnuts are one of the richest sources of alpha-linolenic acid (2.6 grams per 1-ounce serving or 14 walnut halves). The DRI for alpha-linolenic acid is 1.6 grams/day for men and 1.1 grams/day for women. In addition, walnuts are a rich source of plant sterols known to inhibit intestinal absorption of cholesterol.

CRITICAL THINKING

Advertisements often claim that fats are bad. Your classmate Mike asks, "If fats are so bad for us, why do we need to have any in our diets?" How would you answer him?

rancid Containing products of decomposed fatty acids that have an unpleasant flavor and odor.

total parenteral nutrition The intravenous feeding of all necessary nutrients, including the most basic forms of protein, carbohydrates, lipids, vitamins, minerals, and electrolytes.

Effects of a Deficiency of Essential Fatty Acids

If humans fail to consume enough essential fatty acids, their skin becomes flaky and itchy, and diarrhea and other symptoms such as infections often are seen. Growth and wound healing may be restricted. These signs of deficiency have been seen in people fed intravenously by **total parenteral nutrition** containing little or no fat for 2 to 3 weeks, as well as in infants receiving formulas low in fat. However, because our bodies need the equivalent of only about 2 to 4 tablespoons of plant oils a day, even a low fat diet will provide enough essential fatty acids if it follows a balanced plan such as MyPyramid and includes a serving of fatty fish at least twice a week.

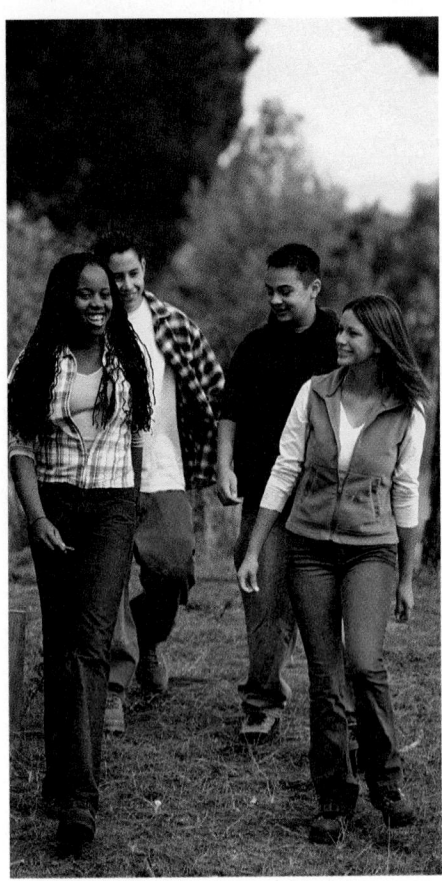

▲ When at rest or during light activity, the body uses mostly fatty acids for fuel.

CONCEPT CHECK

Because humans can't make either omega-3 or omega-6 fatty acids, which perform vital functions in the body, they must be obtained from the diet and therefore are called essential fatty acids. Plant oils are generally rich in omega-6 fatty acids. Eating fatty fish at least twice a week is a good way to meet omega-3 fatty acid needs. Fish oil supplementation (about 1 gram per day of the related omega-3 fatty acids) is generally acceptable under a physician's guidance if a person does not like fish; however, people with certain medical conditions (e.g., taking anti-coagulant medications) should be cautious with use of fish oil supplements due to increased risk of hemorrhagic stroke. Essential fatty acid deficiency can occur after 2 to 3 weeks if fat is omitted from total parenteral nutrition solutions, which in turn can lead to skin disorders, diarrhea, and other health problems.

5.7 Broader Roles for Fatty Acids and Triglycerides in the Body

Many key functions of fat in the body require the use of fatty acids in the form of triglycerides. Triglycerides are used for energy storage, insulation, and transportation of fat-soluble vitamins.

Providing Energy

Triglycerides contained in the diet and stored in adipose tissue provide the fatty acids that are the main fuel for muscles while at rest and during light activity. Muscles use carbohydrate for fuel in addition to fatty acids supplied by triglycerides only in endurance exercise, such as long-distance running and cycling, or in short bursts of intense activity, such as a 200-meter run. Other body tissues also use fatty acids for energy needs. Overall, about half of the energy used by the entire body at rest and during light activity comes from fatty acids. When considering the whole-body, the use of fatty acids by skeletal and heart muscle is balanced by the use of glucose by the nervous system and red blood cells. Recall from Chapter 4 that cells need a supply of carbohydrate to efficiently process fatty acids for fuel. The details about how we burn fat as a fuel will be discussed in Chapter 7.

Storing Energy for Later Use

We store energy mainly in the form of triglycerides. The body's ability to store fat is essentially limitless. Its fat storage sites, adipose cells, can increase about 50 times in weight. If the amount of fat to be stored exceeds the ability of the existing cells to expand, the body can form new adipose cells.

An important advantage of using triglycerides to store energy in the body is that they are energy dense. Recall that these yield, on average, 9 kcal per gram, whereas proteins and carbohydrates yield only about 4 kcal per gram. In addition, triglycerides are chemically stable, so they are not likely to react with other cell constituents, making them a safe form for storing energy. Finally, when we store triglycerides in adipose cells, we store little else, especially water. Adipose cells contain about 80% lipid and only 20% water and protein. In contrast, imagine if we were to store energy as muscle tissue, which is about 73% water. Body weight linked to energy storage would increase dramatically. The same would be true if we stored energy primarily as glycogen, as about 3 grams of water are stored for every gram of glycogen.

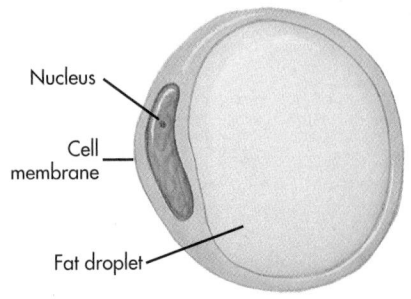

Nucleus

Cell membrane

Fat droplet

Adipose cell

Insulating and Protecting the Body

The insulating layer of fat just beneath the skin is made mostly of triglycerides. Fat tissue also surrounds and protects some organs—kidneys, for example—from injury. We usually don't notice the important insulating function of fat tissue, because we wear clothes and add more as needed. A layer of insulating fat is important in animals living in cold climates. Polar bears, walruses, and whales all build a thick layer of fat tissue around themselves to insulate against cold-weather environments. The extra fat also provides energy storage for times when food is scarce.

Transporting Fat-Soluble Vitamins

Triglycerides and other fats in food carry fat-soluble vitamins to the small intestine and aid their absorption. People who absorb fat poorly, such as those with the disease cystic fibrosis, are at risk for deficiencies of fat-soluble vitamins, especially vitamin K. A similar risk comes from taking mineral oil as a laxative at mealtimes. The body cannot digest or absorb mineral oil, so the undigested oil carries the fat-soluble vitamins from the meal into the feces, where they are eliminated. Unabsorbed fatty acids can bind minerals, such as calcium and magnesium, and draw them into the stool for elimination. This can harm mineral status (see Chapter 9). Recall that the main problem with the fat replacer, olestra, is that it can bind the fat-soluble vitamins and reduce their absorption.

5.8 Phospholipids in the Body

Many types of phospholipids exist in the body, especially in the brain. They form important parts of cell membranes. Phospholipids are found in body cells, and they participate in fat digestion in the intestine. Recall that the various forms of lecithin (discussed earlier) are common examples of phospholipids (review Fig. 5-4b).

Cell membranes are composed primarily of phospholipids. A cell membrane looks much like a sea of phospholipids with protein "islands" (Fig. 5-15). The proteins

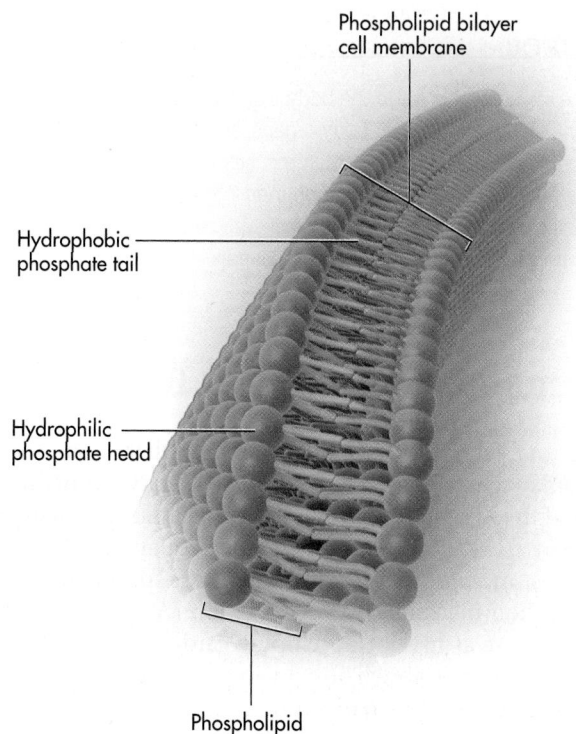

Phospholipid bilayer
cell membrane

Hydrophobic
phosphate tail

Hydrophilic
phosphate head

Phospholipid

FIGURE 5-15 ▶ Phospholipids are the main components of cell membranes, forming a double or bilayer of lipid.

form receptors for hormones, function as enzymes, and act as transporters for nutrients. The fatty acids on the phospholipids serve as a source of essential fatty acids for the cell. Some cholesterol is also present in the membrane.

In some foods, phospholipids function as emulsifiers (as covered earlier) allowing fat and water to mix. By breaking fat globules into small droplets, emulsifiers enable a fat to be suspended in water. They act as bridges between the oil and water that in turn lead to the formation of tiny oil droplets surrounded by thin shells of water. In an emulsified solution, such as salad dressing or mayonnaise, millions of tiny oil droplets are separated by shells of water (review Fig. 5-7).

The body's main emulsifiers are the lecithins and bile acids, produced by the liver and released into the small intestine via the gallbladder during digestion.

5.9 Cholesterol in the Body

Cholesterol plays many vital roles in the body. It forms part of some important hormones, such as estrogen, testosterone, and a form of the active vitamin D hormone. Cholesterol is also the building block of bile acids, needed for fat digestion. Finally, cholesterol is an essential structural component of cells and the outer layer of the lipoprotein particles that transport lipids in the blood. The cholesterol content of the heart, liver, kidney, and brain is high, reflecting its critical role in these organs.

About two-thirds of the cholesterol circulating through your body is made by body cells; the remaining one-third is consumed in the diet. Each day, our cells produce approximately 875 milligrams of cholesterol. Of the 875 milligrams of cholesterol made by the body, about 400 milligrams are used to make new bile acids to replenish those lost in the feces, and about 50 milligrams are used to make hormones. In addition to all the cholesterol cells make, we consume about 180 to 325 milligrams of cholesterol per day from animal-derived food products, with men consuming the higher amount compared to women. Absorption of cholesterol from food ranges from about 40% to 65%. The effect of blood cholesterol, especially LDL cholesterol, on cardiovascular disease risk will be discussed in the "Nutrition and Your Health" section.

See Nutrition and Your Health:
Lipids and Cardiovascular Disease
at the end of Chapter 5.

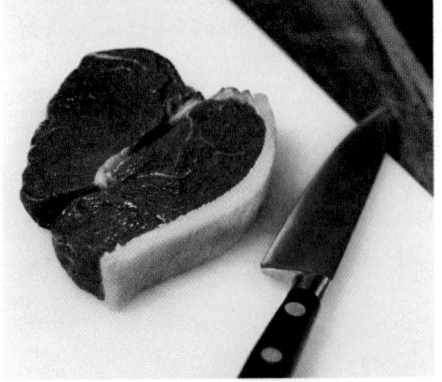

▲ Trimming the fat off meats can help reduce saturated fat intake. Limiting intake of meat that is highly marbled with fat (streaks of fat running through the lean) helps, too.

CONCEPT CHECK

Triglycerides are the major form of fat in the body. They are used for energy and stored in adipose tissue, they insulate and protect body organs, and they transport fat-soluble vitamins. Phospholipids are emulsifiers—compounds that can suspend fat in water. Phospholipids also form parts of cell membranes and various compounds in the body. Cholesterol, a sterol, forms part of cell membranes, hormones, and bile acids. If sufficient amounts are not consumed, the body makes what phospholipids and cholesterol it needs.

5.10 Recommendations for Fat Intake

There is no RDA for total fat intake for adults, although there is an Adequate Intake set for total fat for infants (see Chapter 15). The 2010 Dietary Guidelines for Americans recommendation and the Acceptable Macronutrient Distribution Range is that total fat intake should be 20% to 35% of total calories, which equates to 44 to 78 grams per day for a person who consumes 2000 kcal daily. The most specific recommendations for fat intake come from the American Heart Association (AHA) (see Further Reading 9). Many North Americans are at risk for developing cardiovascular disease, so AHA promotes dietary and lifestyle goals aimed at reducing this risk. The AHA diet and lifestyle goals for cardiovascular disease risk reduction for the general public are presented in Table 5-3. These goals include aiming for an overall healthy eating pattern; appropriate

TABLE 5-3 American Heart Association 2006 Diet and Lifestyle Goals for Cardiovascular Disease Risk Reduction

- Consume an overall healthy diet.
- Aim for a healthy body weight.
- Aim for recommended levels of low-density lipoprotein (LDL) cholesterol, high-density lipoprotein (HDL) cholesterol, and triglycerides.
- Aim for a normal blood pressure.
- Aim for a normal blood glucose level.
- Be physically active.
- Avoid use of and exposure to tobacco products.

From: Lichtenstein AH and others: Diet and lifestyle recommendations revision 2006. A scientific statement from the American Heart Association Nutrition Committee. *Circulation* 114:82, 2006.

body weight; and a desirable blood cholesterol profile, blood pressure, and blood glucose level. In Table 5-4, a more detailed list of recommendations is provided for those who currently are at high risk or have cardiovascular disease.

To reduce risk for cardiovascular disease, the AHA recommends that no more than 7% of total calories come from saturated fat and no more than 1% from *trans* fat. These are the primary fatty acids that raise LDL. In addition, cholesterol should amount to a maximum of 300 mg per day. Table 5-5 lists the cholesterol content of some foods. This often happens along with the reduction in saturated fat and *trans* fat intake. Table 5-6 is an example of a diet that adheres to 20% or 30% of calories as fat. Compare these recommendations to the actual dietary intake patterns of these fats by North Americans: 33% of calories from total fat, about 13% of calories from saturated fat, and 180 to 320 milligrams of cholesterol each day.

TABLE 5-4 American Heart Association 2006 Diet and Lifestyle Recommendations for Cardiovascular Disease Risk Reduction

- Balance calorie intake and physical activity to achieve or maintain a healthy body weight.
- Consume a diet rich in vegetables and fruits.
- Choose whole-grain, high-fiber foods.
- Consume fish, especially oily fish, at least twice a week.
- Limit your intake of saturated fat to less than 7% of energy, *trans* fat to less than 1% of energy, and cholesterol to less than 300 milligrams per day by
  — choosing lean meats and vegetable alternatives;
  — selecting fat-free (skim), 1%-fat, and low-fat dairy products; and
  — minimizing intake of partially-hydrogenated fats.
- Minimize your intake of beverages and foods with added sugars.
- Choose and prepare foods with little or no salt.
- If you consume alcohol, do so in moderation.
- When you eat food prepared outside of the home, follow the AHA Diet and Lifestyle Recommendations.

From: Lichtenstein AH and others: Diet and lifestyle recommendations revision 2006. A scientific statement from the American Heart Association Nutrition Committee. *Circulation* 114:82, 2006.

One goal of *Healthy People 2020* is to reduce consumption of saturated fat in the population ages 2 years and older to 9.5% of total calorie intake.

TABLE 5-5 Cholesterol Content of Foods

3 oz beef brains	2635 mg
3 oz beef liver	337 mg
1 large egg yolk*	209 mg
3 oz shrimp	166 mg
3 oz beef*	75 mg
3 oz pork	75 mg
3 oz chicken or turkey (white meat)*	75 mg
1 cup ice cream	63 mg
3 oz trout	60 mg
3 oz tuna	45 mg
3 oz hot dog	38 mg
1 oz cheddar cheese*	30 mg
1 cup whole milk*	24 mg
1 cup 1% milk	12 mg
1 cup fat-free milk	5 mg
1 large egg white	0 mg

*Leading dietary sources of cholesterol in American diets.

Some advice regarding fat intake from the 2010 Dietary Guidelines:

- Consume less than 10% of calories from saturated fatty acids by replacing them with monounsaturated and polyunsaturated fatty acids.
- Consume less than 300 mg per day of dietary cholesterol.
- Keep *trans* fatty acid consumption as low as possible by limiting foods that contain synthetic sources of *trans* fats, such as partially hydrogenated oils, and by limiting other solid fats.
- Reduce the intake of calories from solid fats and added sugars.

Continued

- Use oils to replace solid fats where possible.
- Limit the consumption of foods that contain refined grains, especially refined grain foods that contain solid fats, added sugars, and sodium.
- Replace protein foods that are higher in solid fats with choices that are lower in solid fats and calories and/or are sources of oils.
- Increase the amount and variety of seafood in place of same meat and poultry.
- Increase intake of fat-free or low-fat milk and milk products, such as milk, yogurt, cheese, or fortified soy beverages.

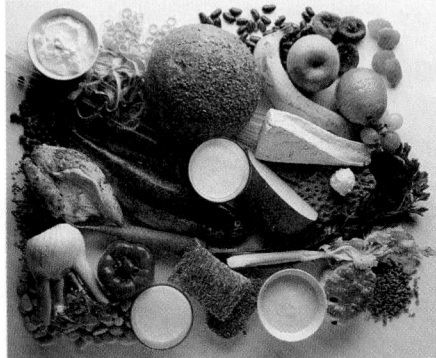

▲ **Whole grains** (shredded wheat, whole-wheat bread, oatmeal cookies, popcorn), **fruits** (orange juice, apple, banana, raisins), **vegetables** (carrots, lettuce, tomato), **lean meats** (roast beef, turkey, chicken), and **fat-free milk** are the primary components of the low-fat menus in Table 5-6.

The advice to consume 20% to 35% of calories as fat does not apply to infants and toddlers below the age of 2 years. These youngsters are forming new tissue that requires fat, especially in the brain, so their intake of fat and cholesterol should not be greatly restricted.

TABLE 5-6 Daily Menu Examples Containing 2000 kcal and 30% or 20% of Calories as Fat

30% of Calories as Fat		20% of Calories as Fat	
Food	Fat (grams)	Food	Fat (grams)
Breakfast			
Orange juice, 1 cup	0.5	Same	0.5
Shredded wheat, ¾ cup	0.5	Shredded wheat, 1 cup	0.7
Toasted bagel	1.1	Same	1.1
Tub margarine, 3 teaspoons	11.4	Tub margarine, 2 teaspoons	7.6
1% low-fat milk, 1 cup	2.5	Fat-free milk, 1 cup	0.6
Lunch			
Whole-wheat bread, 2 slices	2.4	Same	2.4
Roast beef, 2 ounces	4.9	Light turkey roll, 2 ounces	0.9
Mayonnaise, 3 teaspoons	11.0	Mayonnaise, 2 teaspoons	7.3
Lettuce	—	Same	—
Tomato	—	Same	—
Oatmeal cookie, 1	3.3	Oatmeal cookie, 2	6.6
Snack			
Apple	—	Same	—
Dinner			
Chicken tenders frozen meal	18.0	Fat-free chicken tenders	—
Carrots, ½ cup	—	Same	—
Dinner roll, 1	2.0	Same	2.0
Margarine, 1 teaspoon	3.8	Same	3.8
Banana	0.6	Same	0.6
1% low-fat milk, 1 cup	2.5	Fat-free milk, 1 cup	0.6
Snack			
Raisins, 2 teaspoons	—	Raisins, ½ cup	—
Air-popped popcorn, 3 cups	1.0	Air-popped popcorn, 6 cups	2.0
Margarine, 2 teaspoons	7.6	Same	7.6
Totals	**73.1**		**44.3**

The American Dietetic Association, the Dietitians of Canada (see Further Reading 1), the National Cholesterol Education Program (NCEP), and the Food and Nutrition Board are in agreement with the advice of the AHA. The 2010 Dietary Guidelines also support this advice. In addition to fat intake, controlling total calorie intake is also significant, as weight control is a vital component of cardiovascular disease prevention.

Regarding essential fatty acids, the Food and Nutrition Board has issued recommendations for both omega-6 and omega-3 fatty acids. The amounts listed in Table 5-7 work out to about 5% of calorie in-take for the total of both essential fatty acids. Infants and children have lower needs (again, see Chapter 15). Consumption of fish at least twice a week is one step toward meeting requirements for essential fatty acids.

The typical North American diet derives about 7% of calories from polyunsaturated fatty acids, and thus meets essential fatty acid needs. An upper limit of 10% of calorie intake as polyunsaturated fatty acids is often recommended, in part because the breakdown (oxidation) of those present in lipoproteins is linked to increased cholesterol deposition in the arteries (see the Nutrition and Your Health section in this chapter). Depression of immune function is also suspected to be caused by an excessive intake of polyunsaturated fatty acids.

TABLE 5-7 Food and Nutrition Board Recommendations for Omega-6 and Omega-3 Fatty Acids per Day

	Men (grams per day)	Women (grams per day)
Linoleic acid (omega-6)	17	12
Alpha-linolenic acid (omega-3)	1.6	1.1

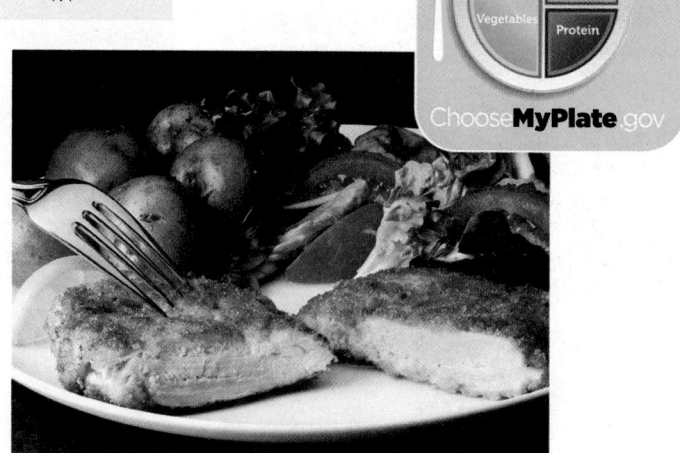

In recent years, the Mediterranean diet (see Newsworthy Nutrition in margin) has attracted a lot of attention as a result of lower rates of chronic diseases seen in people following such a diet plan. The major sources of fat in the Mediterranean diet include liberal amounts of olive oil compared to a small amount of animal fat (from animal flesh and dairy products). In contrast, major sources of fat in the typical North American diet include animal flesh, whole milk, pastries, cheese, margarine, and mayonnaise. While dietary fat sources definitely play a role in prevention of chronic disease, it is important to remember that other aspects of one's lifestyle also contribute to disease risk. People who follow a Mediterranean diet also tend to consume moderate alcohol (usually in the form of red wine, which contains many antioxidants), eat plenty of whole grains and few refined carbohydrates, and are also more physically active than typical North Americans.

An alternative plan for reduction of cardiovascular disease is Dr. Dean Ornish's purely vegetarian (**vegan**) diet plan (see Further Reading 12). This diet is very low in fat, including only a scant quantity of vegetable oil used in cooking and the small amount of oils present in plant foods. Individuals restricting fat intake to 20% of calories should be monitored by a physician, as the resulting increase in carbohydrate intake can increase blood triglycerides in some people, which is not a healthful change. Over time, however, the initial problem of high blood triglycerides on a low-fat diet may self-correct. Among people following the Ornish plan, blood triglycerides initially increased, but within a year, fell to normal values as long as they emphasized high-fiber carbohydrate sources, controlled (or improved) body weight, and followed a regular exercise program.

In summary, the general consensus among nutrition experts suggests that limitation of saturated fat, cholesterol, and *trans* fat intake should be the primary focus, and that the diet needs to contain some omega-3 and omega-6 fatty acids (Table 5-8). Furthermore, if fat intake exceeds 30% of total calories, the extra fat should come from monounsaturated fat.

▲ If you are looking to decrease the amount of saturated and *trans* fats in your diet, it is a good idea to opt for lower-fat substitutes for some of your current high-fat food choices. How do you think this meal compares with the fried meal on p. 179? How does it compare to MyPlate recommendations?

vegan A person who eats only plant foods.

NEWSWORTHY NUTRITION

Low-fat diet not necessary for weight loss

A low-fat; Mediterranean, or low-carbohydrate diet, was studied in moderately obese adults. Weight loss on the Mediterranean Diet (4.6 kg) and low-carbohydrate diet (5.5 kg) was greater than weight loss on the low-fat diet. This, along with the more favorable effects on lipids (low-carbohydrate diet) and on glycemic control (Mediterranean Diet), indicates they may be effective alternatives to low-fat diets.

Source: Shai I and others: Weight loss with a low-carbohydrate, Mediterranean, or low-fat diet. *New England Journal of Medicine* 359:229, 2008 (see Further Reading 14).

connect Check out the Connect site www.mcgrawhillconnect.com to further explore weight-loss diets.

CONCEPT CHECK

There is no RDA for fat. We need about 5% of total calorie intake from plant oils to obtain the needed essential fatty acids. Eating fatty fish at least twice a week is also advised to supply omega-3 fatty acids. Many health-related agencies recommend a diet containing no more than 35% of calorie intake as fat, with no more than 7% to 10% of calorie intake as a combination of saturated fat and *trans* fat for the general public. Cholesterol intake should be limited to 200 to 300 milligrams per day. These practices help maintain a normal LDL value in the blood. The North American diet contains about 33% of calories as fat, with about 13% of calories as saturated fat and about 3% as *trans* fatty acids. Cholesterol intake varies from about 200 to 400 milligrams per day.

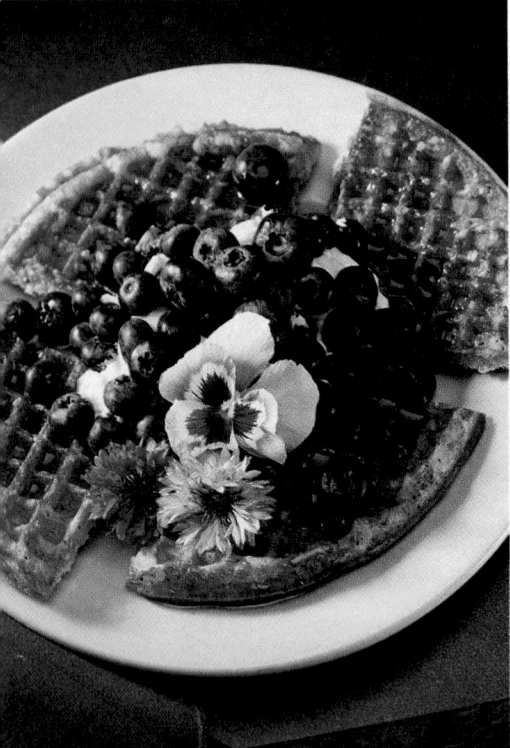

TABLE 5-8 Tips for Avoiding Too Much Fat, Saturated Fat, Cholesterol, and *Trans* Fat

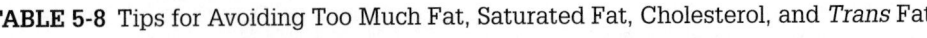

	Eat Less of These Foods	Eat More of These Foods
Grains	• Pasta dishes with cheese or cream sauces • Croissants • Pastries • Doughnuts • Pie crust	• Whole-grain breads • Whole-grain pasta • Brown rice • Angel food cake • Animal or graham crackers • Air-popped popcorn
Vegetables	• French fries • Potato chips • Vegetables cooked in butter, cheese, or cream sauces	• Fresh, frozen, baked, or steamed vegetables
Fruit	• Fruit pies	• Fresh, frozen, or canned fruits
Dairy	• Whole milk • Ice cream • High-fat cheese • Cheesecake	• Fat-free and reduced-fat milk • Low-fat frozen desserts (e.g., yogurt, sherbet, ice milk) • Reduced-fat/part-skim cheese
Protein	• Bacon • Sausage • Organ meats (e.g., liver) • Egg yolks	• Fish • Skinless poultry • Lean cuts of meat (with fat trimmed away) • Soy products • Egg whites/egg substitutes
Oils	• Butter and stick margarine	• Canola oil or olive oil • Tub or liquid margarine (in small amounts)

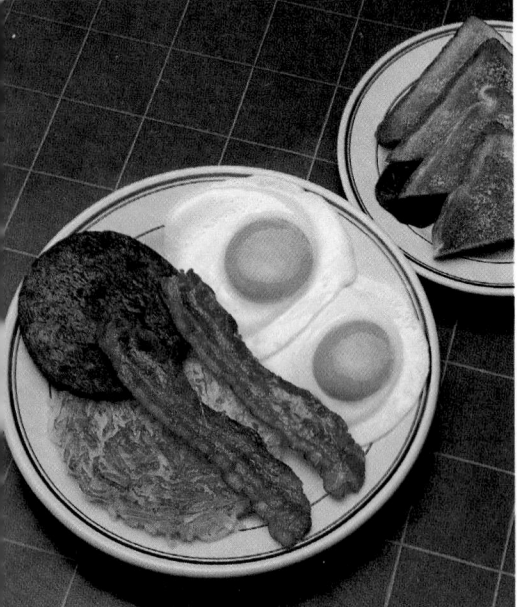

▲ To avoid too much saturated fat and cholesterol, for breakfast eat fewer foods like bacon, sausage, hash browns and whole eggs and more foods like whole-grain waffles and fresh fruit.

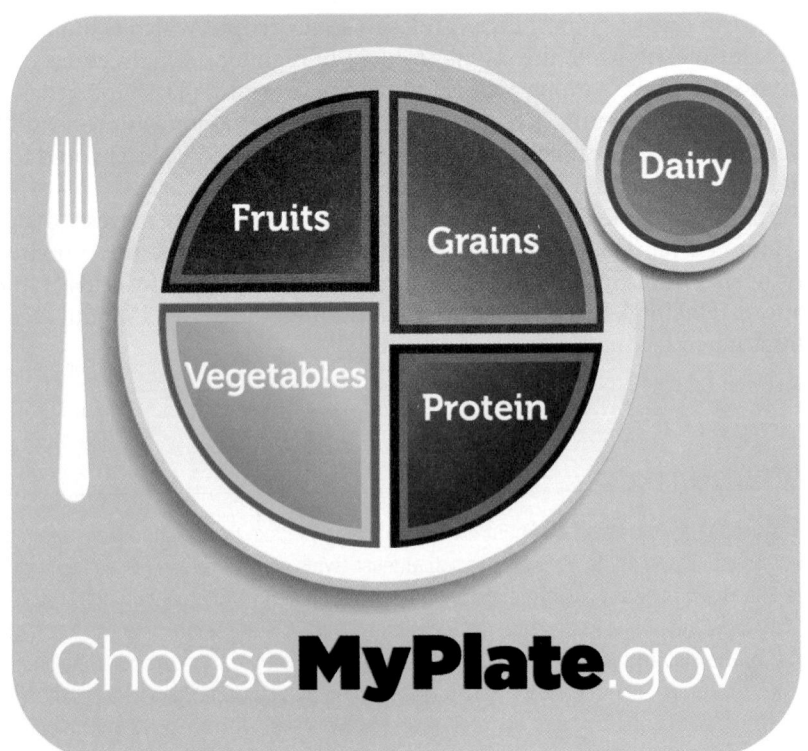

LIPIDS CONCEPT MAP

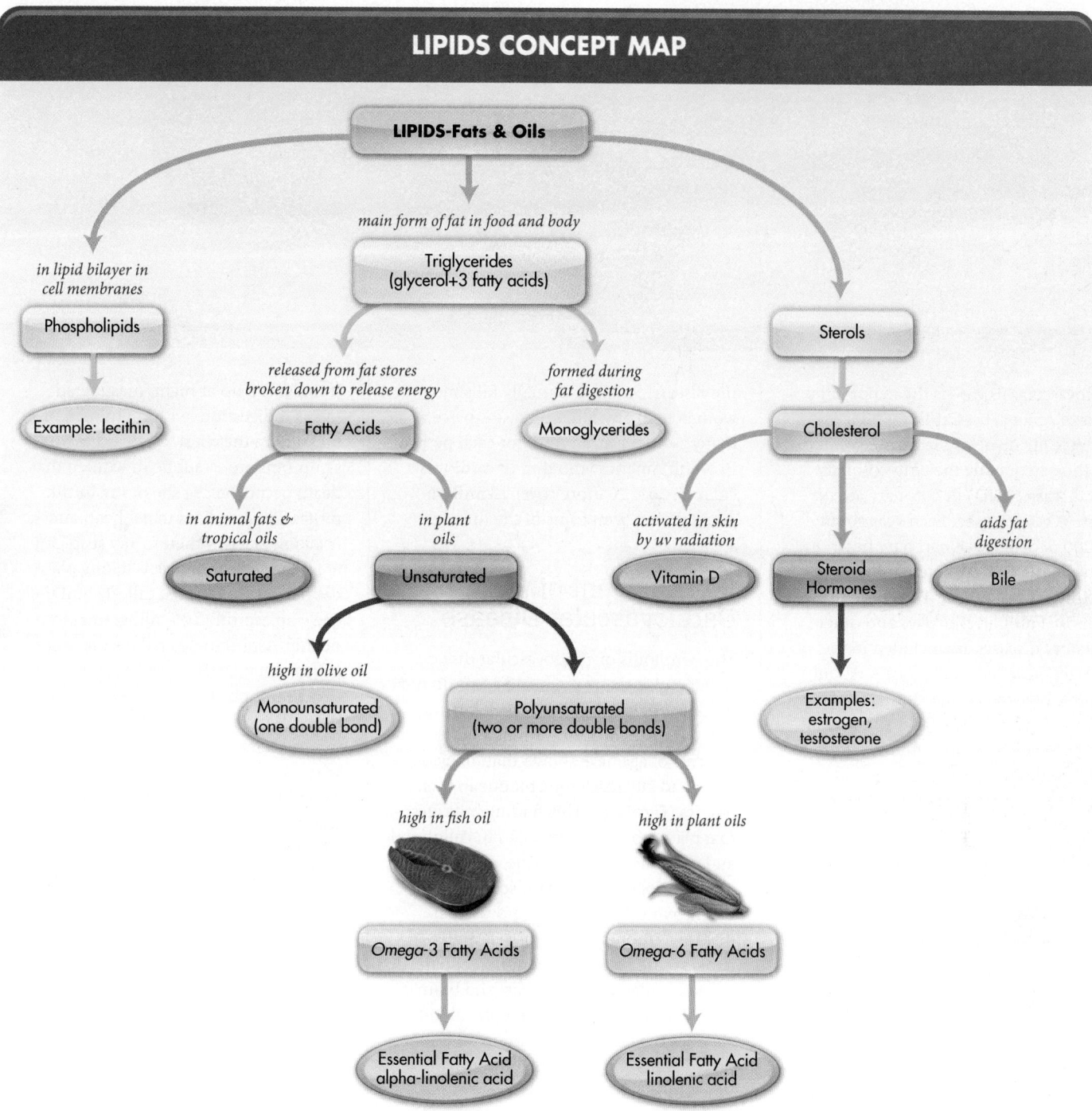

LIPIDS-Fats & Oils

main form of fat in food and body

Triglycerides
(glycerol+3 fatty acids)

in lipid bilayer in cell membranes

Phospholipids

Example: lecithin

released from fat stores broken down to release energy

Fatty Acids

formed during fat digestion

Monoglycerides

Sterols

Cholesterol

in animal fats & tropical oils

Saturated

in plant oils

Unsaturated

activated in skin by uv radiation

Vitamin D

Steroid Hormones

aids fat digestion

Bile

high in olive oil

Monounsaturated
(one double bond)

Polyunsaturated
(two or more double bonds)

Examples:
estrogen, testosterone

high in fish oil

high in plant oils

Omega-3 Fatty Acids

Omega-6 Fatty Acids

Essential Fatty Acid
alpha-linolenic acid

Essential Fatty Acid
linolenic acid

Lipids and Cardiovascular Disease

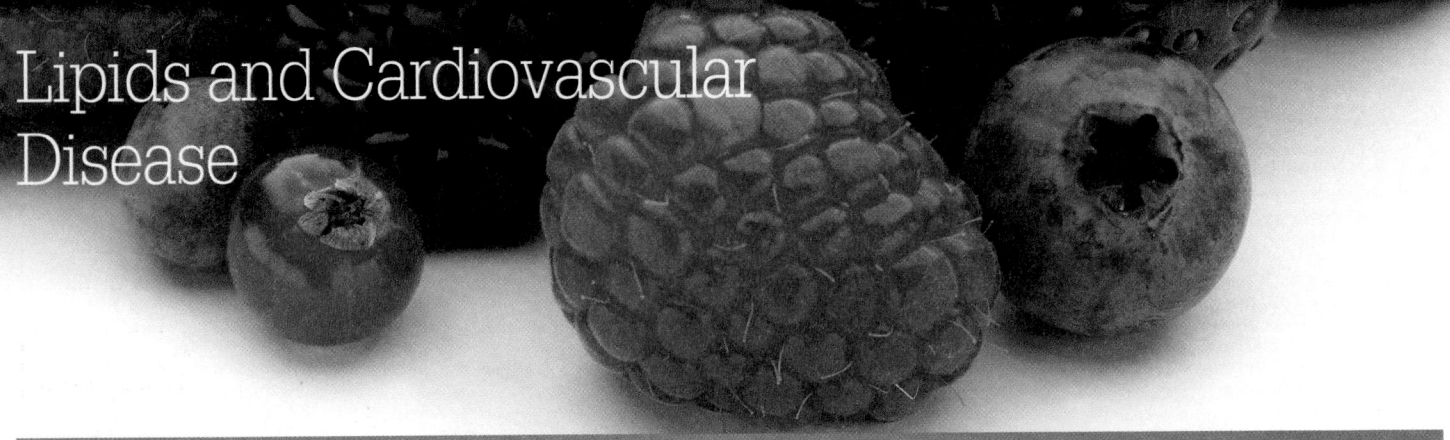

Cardiovascular disease is the major killer of North Americans. Cardiovascular disease typically involves the coronary arteries and, thus, frequently the term coronary heart disease (CHD) or coronary artery disease (CAD) is used. Each year about 500,000 people die of coronary heart disease in the United States, about 60% more than die of cancer. The figure rises to almost 1 million if strokes and other circulatory diseases are included in the global term *cardiovascular disease*. About 1.5 million people in the United States each year have a heart attack. The overall male-to-female ratio for cardiovascular disease is about 2:1. Women generally lag about 10 years behind men in developing

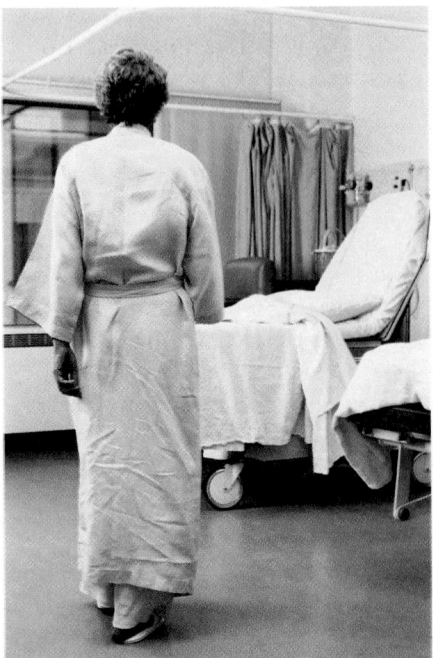

▲ Cardiovascular disease kills more women than any other disease—twice as many as does cancer.

the disease. Still, it eventually kills more women than any other disease—twice as many as does cancer. And, for each person in North America who dies of cardiovascular disease, 20 more (over 13 million people) have symptoms of the disease.

Development of Cardiovascular Disease

The symptoms of cardiovascular disease develop over many years and often do not become obvious until old age. Nonetheless, autopsies of young adults under 20 years of age have shown that many of them had atherosclerotic **plaque** in their arteries (Fig. 5-16). This finding indicates that plaque buildup can begin in childhood and continue throughout life, although it usually goes undetected for some time.

The typical forms of cardiovascular disease—coronary heart disease and strokes—are associated with inadequate blood circulation in the heart and brain related to buildup of this plaque. Blood supplies the heart muscle, brain, and other body organs with oxygen and nutrients. When blood flow via the coronary arteries surrounding the heart is interrupted, the heart muscle can be damaged. A heart attack, or **myocardial infarction,** may result (review Fig. 5-16). This may cause the heart to beat irregularly or to stop. About 25% of people do not survive their first heart attack. If blood flow to parts of the brain is interrupted long enough, part of the brain dies, causing a **cerebrovascular accident,** or stroke.

A heart attack can strike with the sudden force of a sledgehammer, with pain radiating up the neck or down the arm.

It can sneak up at night, masquerading as indigestion, with slight pain or pressure in the chest. Many times, the symptoms are so subtle in women that death occurs before she or the health professional realizes that a heart attack is taking place. If there is any suspicion at all that a heart attack is taking place, the person should first call 911 and then chew an aspirin (325 milligrams) thoroughly. Aspirin helps reduce the blood clotting that leads to a heart attack.

Continuous formation and breakdown of blood clots in the blood vessels is a normal process. However, in areas where plaques build up, blood clots are more likely to remain intact and then lead to a blockage, cutting off or diminishing the supply of blood to the heart (via the coronary arteries) or brain (via the carotid arteries). More than 95% of heart attacks are caused by such blood clots. Heart attacks generally are caused by total blockage of the coronary arteries due to a blood clot forming in an area of the artery already partially blocked by plaque. Disruption of the plaque may even lead to eventual clot formation.

plaque A cholesterol-rich substance deposited in the blood vessels; it contains various white blood cells, smooth muscle cells, various proteins, cholesterol and other lipids, and eventually calcium.

myocardial infarction Death of part of the heart muscle. Also termed a *heart attack.*

cerebrovascular accident (CVA) Death of part of the brain tissue due typically to a blood clot. Also termed a *stroke.*

▶ Typical warning signs of a heart attack are:

- Intense, prolonged chest pain or pressure, sometimes radiating to other parts of the upper body (men and women)
- Shortness of breath (men and women)
- Sweating (men and women)
- Nausea and vomiting (especially women)
- Dizziness (especially women)
- Weakness (men and women)
- Jaw, neck, and shoulder pain (especially women)
- Irregular heartbeat (men and women)

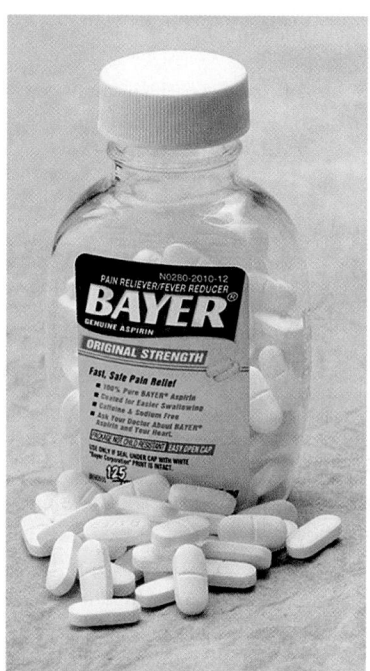

▲ At the first sign of a possible heart attack, the person should first call 911 and then thoroughly chew an aspirin.

▶ *Healthy People 2020* has set a goal of reducing death from coronary heart disease by 20%, compared with today's incidence.

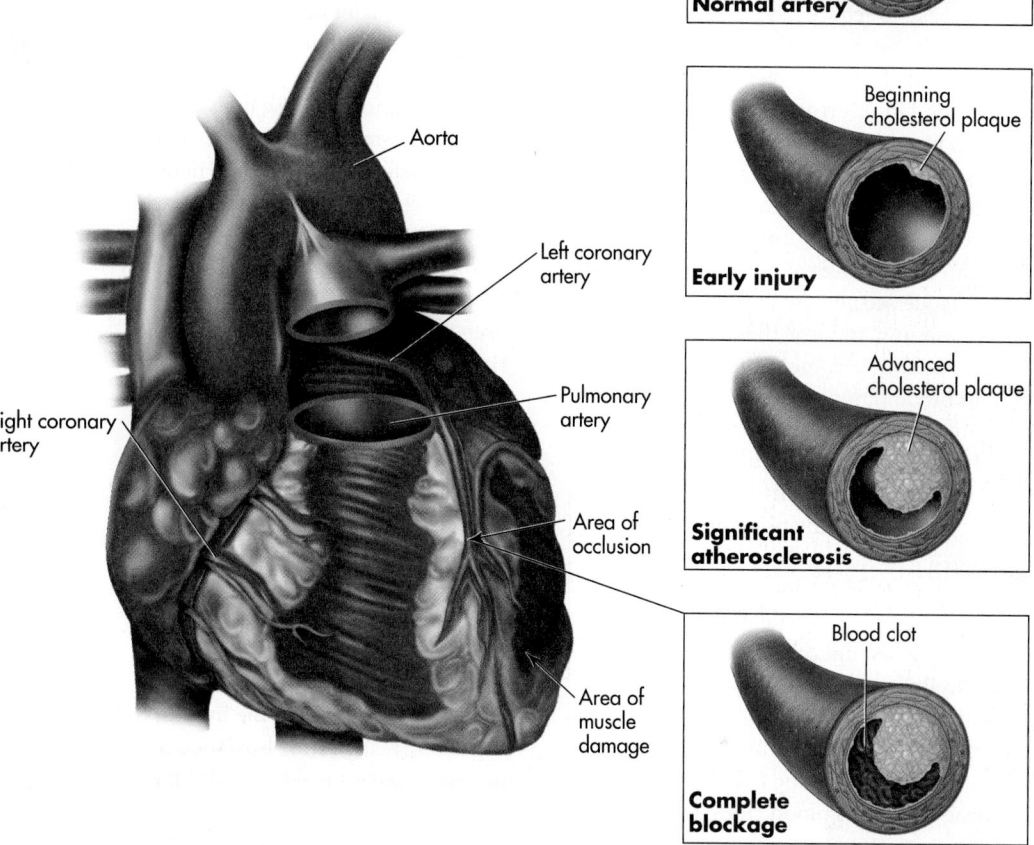

FIGURE 5-16 ▶ The road to a heart attack. Injury to an artery wall begins the process. This is followed by a progressive buildup of plaque in the artery walls. The heart attack represents the terminal phase of the process. Blockage of the left coronary artery by a blood clot is evident. The heart muscle served by the portion of the coronary artery beyond the point of blockage lacks oxygen and nutrients and is damaged and may die. This damage can lead to a significant drop in heart function and often total heart failure.

Atherosclerosis probably first develops to repair damage in a vessel lining. The damage that starts this process can be caused by smoking, diabetes, hypertension, LDL, and viral and bacterial infection. Ongoing inflammation in the blood vessel is also suspected to cause blood vessel damage. (A laboratory test for c-reactive protein in the blood is used to assess if inflammation is present.) (see Further Reading 3). Atherosclerosis can be seen in arteries throughout the body. The damage develops especially at points where an artery branches into two smaller vessels. A great deal of stress is placed on the vessel walls at these points due to changes in blood flow.

Once blood vessel damage has occurred, the next step in the development of atherosclerosis is the progression phase. This step is characterized by deposition of plaque at the site of initial damage. The rate of plaque buildup during the progression phase is directly related to the amount of LDL in the blood. The form of LDL that contributes to atherosclerosis is **oxidized** LDL (see Further Readings 6 and 10). This

oxidize In the most basic sense, the loss of an electron or gain of an oxygen by a chemical substance. This change typically alters the shape and/or function of the substance.

form is preferentially taken up by scavenger cells in the arterial wall. Nutrients and phytochemicals that have **antioxidant** properties may reduce LDL oxidation. Fruits and vegetables are particularly rich in these compounds. Eating fruits and vegetables regularly is one positive step we can make to reduce plaque buildup and slow the progression of cardiovascular disease. Some fruits and vegetables particularly helpful in this regard include legumes (beans), nuts, dried plums (prunes), raisins, berries, plums, apples, cherries, oranges, grapes, spinach, broccoli, red bell peppers, potatoes, and onions. Tea and coffee are also sources of antioxidants.

As plaque accumulates, arteries harden, narrow, and lose their elasticity. Affected arteries become further damaged as blood pumps through them and pressure increases. Finally, in the terminal phase, a clot or spasm in a plaque-clogged artery leads to a heart attack.

Factors that typically bring on a heart attack in a person already at risk include dehydration; acute emotional stress (such as firing an employee); strenuous physical activity when not otherwise physically fit (shoveling snow, for example); waking during the night or getting up in the morning (linked to an abrupt increase in stress); and consuming large, high-fat meals (increases blood clotting).

Risk Factors for Cardiovascular Disease

Many of us are free of the risk factors that contribute to rapid development of atherosclerosis. If so, the advice of health experts is to consume a balanced diet, perform regular physical activity, have a complete fasting lipoprotein analysis performed at age 20 or beyond, and reevaluate risk factors every 5 years.

For most people, however, the most likely risk factors are:

- **Total blood cholesterol over 200 milligrams per 100 milliliters of blood** (mg/dl; dl is short for deciliter or 100 milliliters). Risk is especially high when total cholesterol is at or over 240 mg/dl and LDL-cholesterol readings are over 130 to 160 mg/dl. (The terms LDL-cholesterol and HDL-cholesterol

are used when expressing the blood concentration because it is the cholesterol content of these lipoproteins that is measured.)

- **Smoking.** Smoking is the main cause of about 20% of cardiovascular disease deaths and generally negates the female advantage of later occurrence of the disease. A combination of smoking and oral contraceptive use increases the risk of cardiovascular disease in women even more. Smoking greatly increases the expression of a person's genetically linked risk for cardiovascular disease, even if one's blood lipids are low. Smoking also makes blood more likely to clot. Even secondhand smoke has been implicated as a risk factor.

- **Hypertension. Systolic blood pressure** over 139 (millimeters of mercury) and **diastolic blood pressure** over 89 indicate hypertension. Healthy blood pressure values are less than 120 and 80, respectively. (Treatment of hypertension is reviewed in Chapter 9.)

- **Diabetes.** Diabetes virtually guarantees development of cardiovascular disease and so puts a person with diabetes in the high-risk group. Insulin increases cholesterol synthesis in the liver, in turn increasing LDL in the bloodstream. This disease negates any female advantage.

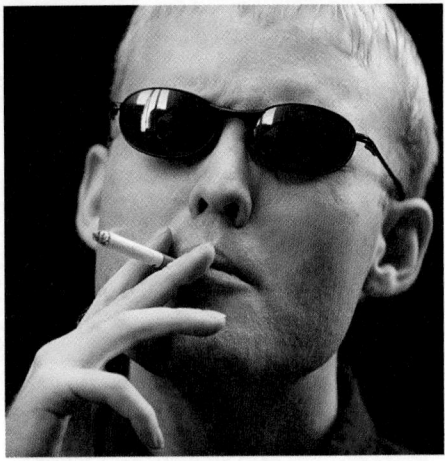

▲ Smoking is one of the four major risk factors for developing cardiovascular disease.

antioxidant Generally a compound that stops the damaging effects of reactive substances seeking an electron (i.e., oxidizing agents). This prevents breakdown (oxidizing) of substances in foods or the body, particularly lipids.

systolic blood pressure The pressure in the arterial blood vessels associated with the pumping of blood from the heart.

diastolic blood pressure The pressure in the arterial blood vessels when the heart is between beats.

MAKING **DECISIONS**

Antioxidant Supplements and Cardiovascular Disease

Are large doses of antioxidant vitamin supplements a reliable way to reduce LDL oxidation, and thereby prevent cardiovascular disease? Controversy about such dietary supplementation exists among the experts, as will be detailed in Chapter 8. The American Heart Association does not support use of antioxidant supplements (such as vitamin E) to reduce cardiovascular disease risk. This is because large-scale studies have shown no decrease in cardiovascular disease risk with use of antioxidant supplements. One study even showed a modest increase for heart failure in people with diabetes or otherwise at high risk for cardiovascular disease after taking antioxidant supplements. However, further trials of antioxidant supplementation (e.g., 600 IU of vitamin E every other day) for prevention of heart disease in men are ongoing. With regard to women, 600 IU of natural-source vitamin E taken every other day provided no overall benefit for major cardiovascular events (or cancer). More research is warranted, however, as a decrease in sudden cardiac death was seen in a subset of older women in this study. Some experts suggest daily vitamin E supplementation (100 IU to 400 IU) may be helpful for *preventing* cardiovascular disease, while other experts recommend against the practice. One thing is certain: any supplementation of vitamin E should be taken only under the guidance of a physician, because of interactions with vitamin K and anticlotting medications (and possibly high-dose aspirin use).

► For more information on cardiovascular disease, see the website of the American Heart Association at www.americanheart.org or the heart disease section of Healthfinder at www.healthfinder.gov/tours/heart.htm. This is a site created by the U.S. government for consumers. In addition, visit the website www.nhlbi.nih.gov/.

► *Healthy People 2020* has set a goal of reducing total blood cholesterol among adults from the average of 198 mg/dl to 178 mg/dl, as well as reducing the percentage of adults with high blood cholesterol from 15% to 13.5%.

► **Cardiovascular Disease Risk Factors**
- Total blood cholesterol > 200 mg/dl
- Smoking
- Hypertension
- Diabetes
- HDL cholesterol < 40 mg/dl
- Age: Men > 45 yr; Women > 55 yr
- Family history of cardiovascular disease
- Blood triglycerides > 200 mg/dl
- Obesity
- Inactivity

► Two approaches have been shown to cause reversal of atherosclerosis in the body. One employs a vegan diet and other lifestyle changes that are part of the Dr. Dean Ornish program. The other employs aggressive LDL lowering with medications.

► As noted earlier, aspirin in small doses reduces blood clotting. It is often used under a physician's guidance to treat people at risk for heart attack or stroke, especially if one has already occurred. About 80 to 160 milligrams per day is needed for such benefits. Individuals who may especially benefit from aspirin therapy are men over 40, smokers, postmenopausal women, and people with diabetes, hypertension, or a family history of cardiovascular disease.

Together, the previous four risk factors explain most cases of cardiovascular disease.

Other risk factors to consider:

- HDL-cholesterol under 40 mg/dl, especially when the ratio of total cholesterol to HDL-cholesterol is greater than 4:1 (3.5:1 or less is optimal). Women often have high values for HDL-cholesterol, and therefore it is important for this to be measured in women to establish cardiovascular disease risk. A value of 60 mg/dl or more is especially protective. Exercising for at least 45 minutes four times a week can increase HDL by about 5 mg/dl. Losing excess weight (especially around the waist) and avoiding smoking and overeating also help maintain or raise HDL, as does moderate alcohol consumption.
- Age. Men over 45 years and women over 55 years.
- Family history of cardiovascular disease, especially before age 50.
- Blood triglycerides 200 mg/dl or greater in the fasting state (less than 100 mg/dl is optimal).
- Obesity (especially fat accumulation in the waist). Typical weight gain seen in adults is a chief contributor to the increase in LDL seen with aging. Obesity also typically leads to insulin resistance, creating a diabetes-like state, and ultimately the disease itself. It also increases overall inflamation throughout the body.
- Inactivity. Exercise conditions the arteries to adapt to physical stress. Regular exercise also improves insulin action in the body. The corresponding reduction in insulin output leads to a reduction in lipoprotein synthesis in the liver. Both regular aerobic exercise and resistance exercise are recommended. A person with existing cardiovascular disease should seek physician approval before starting such a program, as should older adults.

Researchers are trying to unravel and quantify numerous other factors that may be linked to premature cardiovascular disease, such as the connection between inadequate intake of vitamin B-6, folate, and vitamin B-12, which can lead to increased homocysteine in the blood. As noted, homocysteine may damage the cells lining the blood vessels, in turn promoting atherosclerosis. Studies show that supplementation with folic acid and B vitamins does not reduce risk of recurrent cardiovascular disease in patients that had previous heart attacks or had existing vascular diseases.

The term *risk factor* is not equivalent to cause of disease; nevertheless, the more of these risk factors one has, the greater the chances of ultimately developing cardiovascular disease. A good example is the **metabolic syndrome** (also called *Syndrome X)* discussed in Chapter 4. A person with the metabolic syndrome would have abdominal obesity, high blood triglycerides, low HDL-cholesterol, hypertension, poor blood glucose regulation (i.e., high fasting blood glucose), and increased blood clotting. This profile raises the risk for cardiovascular disease considerably. On a positive note, cardiovascular disease is rare in populations who have low LDL-cholesterol, normal blood pressure, and do not smoke or have diabetes. By minimizing these risk factors, as well as following the dietary recommendations of the American Heart Association on page 193 and staying physically active, one will most likely reduce many of the other controllable risk factors listed. In other words, develop and follow a total lifestyle plan. Medications may also be added to lower blood lipids, as discussed next. Finally, if a person has a family history of cardiovascular disease but the usual risk factors aren't present, a rarer defect might be the cause. In this case, having a detailed physical examination for other potential causes is advised.

Medical Interventions to Lower Blood Lipids

Some people need even more aggressive therapy added to their regimen of a diet and lifestyle overhaul to treat elevated blood lipids. The clearest indication for this more aggressive approach is in people who already have had a heart attack or have cardiovascular disease symptoms or diabetes.

Medications are the cornerstone of this more aggressive therapy. The National

Cholesterol Education Program in the United States has developed a formula based on age, total blood cholesterol, HDL-cholesterol, smoking history, and blood pressure to determine who needs such medications. Check out this formula at http://hp2010.nhlbihin.net/atpiii/calculator.asp?usertype=pub. This formula provides an estimate for having a heart attack in the next 10 years.

Medications work to lower LDL in one of two ways. Some reduce cholesterol synthesis in the liver. Such medicines are known as "statins" (e.g., atorvistatin [Lipitor]). The cost of treatment with one of these drugs can be from $1,600 or more per year, depending on the dose needed. These medications lead to problems in some people, and so require physician monitoring, especially of liver function. Another group of medications binds bile acids or the cholesterol that is part of bile secreted into the small intestine. This binding leads to their elimination in the feces and so requires the liver to synthesize new bile acids and/or cholesterol. The liver removes LDL from the blood to do this. Some of these medications taste gritty and therefore are not popular.

The current therapeutic goal for people with (or at high risk for) cardiovascular disease (Table 5-9) is to drive LDL down to less than 70 mg/dl.

The statin drug simvastatin (Zocor) has been combined with another drug (ezetimibe) and is marketed as Vytorin, a drug that will treat the two sources of cholesterol, "food and family." While the statin reduces the cholesterol made by the liver, the ezetimibe helps block the absorption of cholesterol from food.

A third group of drugs can be used to lower blood triglycerides by decreasing the triglyceride production of the liver. These include gemfibrozil (Lopid) and megadoses of the vitamin nicotinic acid. The use of nicotinic acid does result in pesky side effects, however, but these are typically manageable.

Other Possible Medical Therapies for Cardiovascular Disease

FDA has approved two margarines that have positive effects on blood cholesterol levels—Benecol and Take Control. These margarines contain plant stanols/sterols.

The plant stanols/sterols, also called phytosterols, work by reducing cholesterol absorption in the small intestine and lowering its return to the liver. The liver responds by taking up more cholesterol from the blood so it can continue to make bile acids. The studies done on the cholesterol-lowering effect of these margarines have found that 2 to 5 grams of plant stanols/sterols per day reduces total blood cholesterol by 8% to 10% and LDL-cholesterol by 9% to 14% (similar to what is seen with some cholesterol-lowering drugs). (see Further Readings 7, 11, and 13.)

Benecol is made from plant stanols extracted from wood pulp. It is sold as margarine and has been added to salad dressings. Take Control is made from plant sterols isolated from soybeans. The recommended amount for both is about 2 to 3 grams per day as part of at least two meals; this works out to about 1 or 2 tablespoons per day. Use would cost about $1.00 per day, as these margarines are more expensive than regular margarines.

In people who have borderline high total blood cholesterol (between 200 and 239 mg/dl), these margarines can be helpful in avoiding future drug therapy. Plant stanols/sterols have been made available in pill form as well. Remember that plant sterols are naturally present in nuts in high concentrations. Wheat germ, sesame seeds, pistachios, and sunflower seeds are some of the richest sources.

The two most common surgical treatments for coronary artery blockage are percutaneous transluminal coronary angioplasty (PTCA) and coronary artery bypass graft (CABG). PTCA involves the insertion of a balloon catheter into an artery. Once it is advanced to the area of the lesion, the balloon is expanded to crush the lesion. This method works best when only one vessel is blocked, and it may be held open with metal mesh, called a stent. CABG involves the removal and use of a saphenous vein, a large vein in the leg, or use of a mammary artery. The relocated vein is sewn to the main heart vessel (aorta) and then used to bypass the blocked artery. The procedure can be performed on one or more blockages.

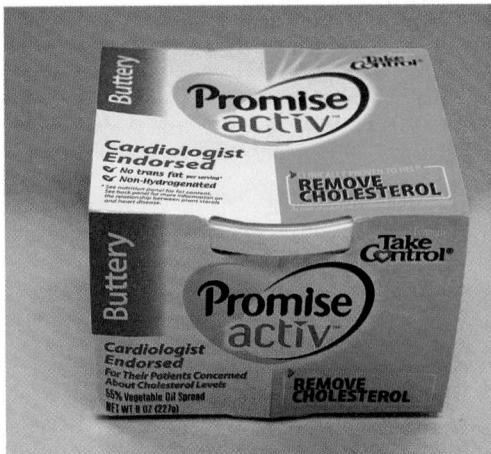

▲ Benecol and Take Control are margarines that are examples of "functional foods" because they contain added cholesterol-lowering plant stanols/sterols.

TABLE 5-9 Sorting Out One's Goals for Cardiovascular Disease Prevention/Treatment

Risk Class	This Is You If . . .	Your LDL (mg/dl) Goal
Very high	You have cardiovascular disease *and* other risk factors such as diabetes, obesity, smoking	Below 70
High	You have cardiovascular disease *or* diabetes *or* two or more risk factors for cardiovascular disease (e.g., smoking, hypertension)	Below 100
Moderately high	You have cardiovascular disease risks and an increased 10-year risk of developing a heart attack	100–130
Moderate	You have two or more risk factors and a marginal chance of developing cardiovascular disease in the next 10 years.	Below 130
Low	You have few or no cardiovascular disease risk factors	Below 160

Case Study Planning a Heart-Healthy Diet

Jackie is a 21-year-old health-conscious individual majoring in business. She recently learned that a diet high in saturated fat can contribute to high blood cholesterol and that exercise is beneficial for the heart. Jackie now takes a brisk 30-minute walk each morning before going to class, and she has started to cut as much fat out of her diet as she can, replacing it mostly with carbohydrates. A typical day for Jackie now begins with a bowl of Fruity Pebbles with 1 cup of skim milk and ½ cup of apple juice. For lunch, she might pack a turkey sandwich on white bread with lettuce, tomato, and mustard; a small package of fat-free pretzels; and a handful of reduced-fat vanilla wafers. Dinner could be a large portion of pasta with some olive oil and garlic mixed in, and a small iceberg lettuce salad with lemon juice squeezed over it. Her snacks are usually baked chips, low-fat cookies, fat-free frozen yogurt, or fat-free pretzels. She drinks diet soft drinks throughout the day as her main beverage.

Answer the following questions, and check your response in Appendix A.

1. Has Jackie made the best diet changes with regard to lowering blood cholesterol and maintaining heart health?
2. Is there much fat left in Jackie's new diet plan? Is it necessary for her to drastically lower her fat intake?
3. What types of fat should Jackie try to consume? Why are these types of fat the most desirable?
4. What types of foods has Jackie used to replace the fat in her diet?
5. What food groups are missing from her new diet plan? How many servings should she be including from these food groups?
6. Is Jackie's new exercise routine appropriate?

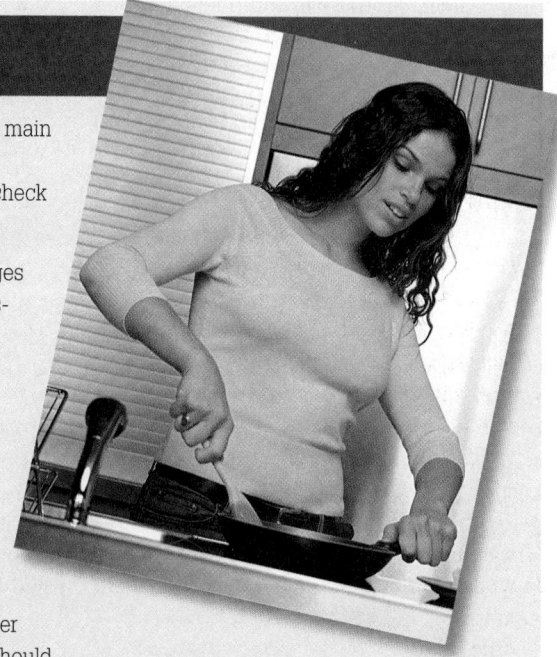

▲ Are there important food groups missing from Jackie's new diet plan?

Summary (Numbers refer to numbered sections in the chapter.)

5.1 Lipids are a group of compounds that do not dissolve in water. Fatty acids are the simplest form of lipid. There are three fatty acids on every triglyceride, the most common type of lipid found in the body and foods. Phospholipids and sterols are two other classes of lipids in food and our bodies.

5.2 Saturated fatty acids contain no carbon-carbon double bonds, monounsaturated fatty acids contain one carbon-carbon double bond, and polyunsaturated fatty acids contain two or more carbon-carbon double bonds in the carbon chain. In omega-3 polyunsaturated fatty acids, the first of the carbon-carbon double bonds is located three carbons from the methyl end of the carbon chain. In omega-6 polyunsaturated fatty acids, the first carbon-carbon double bond counting from the methyl end occurs at the sixth carbon. Both omega-3 and omega-6 fatty acids are essential fatty acids; these must be included in the diet to maintain health.

Triglycerides are formed from a glycerol backbone with three fatty acids.

Triglycerides rich in long-chain saturated fatty acids tend to be solid at room temperature, whereas those rich in monounsaturated and polyunsaturated fatty acids are liquid at room temperature. Triglyceride is the major form of fat in both food and the body. It allows for efficient energy storage, protects certain organs, transports fat-soluble vitamins, and helps insulate the body.

5.3 Foods rich in fat include salad oils, butter, margarine, and mayonnaise. Nuts, bologna, avocados, and bacon are also high in fat, as are peanut butter and cheddar cheese. Steak and hamburger are moderate in fat content, as is whole milk. Many grain products, and fruits and vegetables in general, are low in fat.

Fats and oils have several functions as components of foods. Fats add flavor and texture to foods and provide some satiety after meals. Some phospholipids are used in foods as emulsifiers, which suspend fat in water. When fatty acids break down, food becomes rancid, resulting in a foul odor and unpleasant flavor.

Hydrogenation is the process of converting carbon-carbon double bonds into single bonds by adding hydrogen at the point of unsaturation. The partial-hydrogenation of fatty acids in vegetable oils changes the oils to semisolid fats and helps in food formulation and reduces rancidity. Hydrogenation also increases *trans* fatty acid content. High amounts of *trans* fat in the diet are discouraged, as these increase LDL and reduce HDL.

5.4 Fat digestion takes place primarily in the small intestine. Lipase enzyme released from the pancreas digests long-chain triglycerides into smaller breakdown products—namely, monoglycerides (glycerol backbones with single fatty acids attached) and fatty acids. The breakdown products are then taken up by the absorptive cells of the small intestine. These products are mostly remade into triglycerides and eventually enter the lymphatic system, in turn passing into the bloodstream.

5.5 Lipids are carried in the bloodstream by various lipoproteins, which consist of a central triglyceride core encased in a shell of protein, cholesterol, and phospholipid. Chylomicrons are released from intestinal cells and carry lipids arising from dietary intake. Very-low-density lipoprotein (VLDL) and low-density lipoprotein (LDL) carry lipids both taken up by and synthesized in the liver. High-density lipoprotein (HDL) picks up cholesterol from cells and facilitates its transport back to the liver.

5.6 The essential fatty acids are linoleic acid (an omega-6 fatty acid) and alpha-linolenic acid (on omega-3 fatty acid). Body cells can synthesize hormone-like compounds from both omega-3 and omega-6 fatty acids.

5.7 The compounds produced from omega-3 fatty acids tend to reduce blood clotting, blood pressure, and inflammatory responses in the body. Those produced from omega-6 fatty acids tend to increase blood clotting.

5.8 Phospholipids are derivatives of triglycerides in which one or two of the fatty acids are replaced by phosphorus-containing compounds. Phospholipids are important parts of cell membranes, and some act as efficient emulsifiers.

5.9 Cholesterol forms vital biological compounds, such as hormones, components of cell membranes, and bile acids. Cells in the body make cholesterol whether we eat it or not. It is not a necessary part of an adult's diet.

5.10 There is currently no RDA for fat for adults. Plant oils should contribute about 5% of total calories to achieve the Adequate Intakes proposed for essential fatty acids (linoleic acid and alpha-linolenic acid). Fatty fish are a rich source of omega-3 fatty acids and should be consumed at least twice a week.

Many health agencies and scientific groups suggest a fat intake of no more than 30% to 35% of total calories. Some health experts advocate an even further reduction to 20% of calorie intake for some people to maintain a normal LDL value, but such a diet requires professional guidance. Medications such as "statins" may be added also to lower LDL. If fat intake exceeds 30% of total calories, the diet should emphasize monounsaturated fat. The typical North American diet contains about 33% of total calories as fat.

N&YH In the blood, elevated amounts of LDL and low amounts of HDL are strong predictors of the risk for cardiovascular disease. Additional risk factors for the disease are smoking, hypertension, diabetes, obesity, and inactivity.

Check Your Knowledge (Answers to the following questions are below.)

1. Margarine usually is made by a process called _____, in which hydrogen atoms are added to carbon-carbon double bonds in the polyunsaturated fatty acids found in vegetable oils.
   a. saturation
   b. esterification
   c. isomerization
   d. hydrogenation

2. Essential fatty acids that cause a decrease in blood clotting are
   a. omega-3.　　c. omega-9.
   b. omega-6.　　d. prostacyclins.

3. Cholesterol is
   a. a dietary essential; the human body cannot synthesize it.
   b. found in foods of plant origin.
   c. an important part of human cell membranes and necessary to make some hormones.
   d. All of the above.

4. Which of the following groups of foods would be important sources of saturated fatty acids?
   a. olive oil, peanut oil, canola oil
   b. palm oil, palm kernel oil, coconut oil

   c. safflower oil, corn oil, soybean oil
   d. All of the above.

5. Lipoproteins are important for
   a. transport of fats in the blood and lymphatic system.
   b. synthesis of triglycerides.
   c. synthesis of adipose tissue.
   d. enzyme production.

6. Which of the following foods is the best source of omega-3 fatty acids?
   a. fatty fish
   b. peanut butter and jelly
   c. lard and shortenings
   d. beef and other red meats

7. Immediately after a meal, newly digested and absorbed dietary fats appear in the lymph, and then blood, as part of which of the following?
   a. LDL
   b. HDL
   c. chylomicrons
   d. cholesterol

8. High blood concentrations of _____ decrease the risk for cardiovascular disease.

   a. low-density lipoproteins
   b. chylomicrons
   c. high-density lipoproteins
   d. cholesterol

9. Phospholipids such as lecithin are used extensively in food preparation because they
   a. provide the agreeable feel of fat melting on the tongue.
   b. are excellent emulsifiers.
   c. provide important textural features.
   d. impart delicate flavors.

10. The main form of lipid found in the food we eat is
    a. cholesterol.
    b. phospholipids.
    c. triglycerides.
    d. plant sterols

Answers: 1. d (LO 5.3), 2. a (LO 5.6), 3. c (LO 5.9), 4. b (LO 5.3), 5. a (LO 5.5), 6. a (LO 5.6), 7. c (LO 5.5), 8. c (LO 5.5), 9. b (LO 5.8), 10. c (LO 5.2)

Study Questions <small>(Numbers refer to Learning Outcomes)</small>

1. Describe the chemical structures of saturated and polyunsaturated fatty acids and their different effects in both food and the human body. (LO 5.3)

2. Relate the need for omega-3 fatty acids in the diet to the recommendation to consume fatty fish at least twice a week. (LO 5.7)

3. Describe the structures, origins, and roles of the four major blood lipoproteins. (LO 5.5)

4. What are the recommendations from various health-care organizations regarding fat intake? What does this mean in terms of food choices? (LO 5.10)

5. What are two important attributes of fat in food? How are these different from the general functions of lipids in the human body? (LO 5.3)

6. Describe the significance of and possible uses for reduced-fat foods. (LO 5.10)

7. Does the total cholesterol concentration in the bloodstream tell the whole story with respect to cardiovascular disease risk? (LO 5.9)

8. List the four main risk factors for the development of cardiovascular disease. (LO 5.11)

9. What three lifestyle factors decrease the risk of cardiovascular disease development? (LO 5.11)

10. When are medications most needed in cardiovascular disease therapy, and how in general do the various classes of medications operate to reduce risk? (LO 5.11)

What Would You Choose Recommendations

With heart health in mind you will want to choose the ground meat with the lowest fat, saturated fat, and cholesterol. Check the Nutrition Facts label to compare the lipid content of various products. Look for cuts of meat with "round " or "loin" in the name for lowest fat content.

The USDA allows up to 30% fat (by weight) in raw ground beef, so the cut of beef makes a difference. Regular ground beef typically contains the most fat (about 20% to 30% fat). Next comes ground chuck (about 15% fat), followed by ground round (about 10% fat), and ground sirloin (about 3% fat). Table 5-10 shows a further breakdown of the fat content of varieties of ground beef. Based on this information, you can see that the ground sirloin will give you the leanest burgers.

The ground sirloin, however, will also be the most expensive variety of ground beef. You may, therefore, want to take advantage of the fact that ground beef loses a lot of fat during cooking—as much as 50% for the highest fat products. Typically, regular ground beef is the least expensive product. As the % lean increases, so does price. You can purchase the higher-fat regular ground beef and reduce the amount of fat in the final product by draining, blotting with paper towels, or rinsing under warm water.

For foods in which the ground beef will be shaped then cooked (e.g., hamburger patties, meatballs, or meatloaf), bake, grill, or broil the ground meat on a rack so that fat will drain from the product as it cooks, then let the cooked product rest on paper

TABLE 5-10 Calorie, Fat and Cholesterol Content of Types of Ground Beef

	Energy (kcal)	Total Fat(g)	Saturated Fat (g)	Cholesterol (mg)
Regular ground beef, 3.5 oz cooked	273	18	7	82
Ground chuck, 3.5 oz cooked	232	14	5	86
Ground round, 3.5 oz cooked	204	11	4	82
Ground sirloin, 3.5 oz cooked	164	6	3	76

towels for 1 minute after cooking. For recipes that incorporate browned ground beef into a mixed dish (e.g., casseroles or spaghetti sauce), brown ground beef, crumbling as you cook, then blot with paper towels or rinse under warm water to achieve a final cooked product with nearly the same fat content as the ground round. Using the rinsing method, 100 grams (about 3.5 ounces) of ground beef yields a final product with just 4 grams of fat. Because a greater percentage of the starting product is lost during cooking, you will

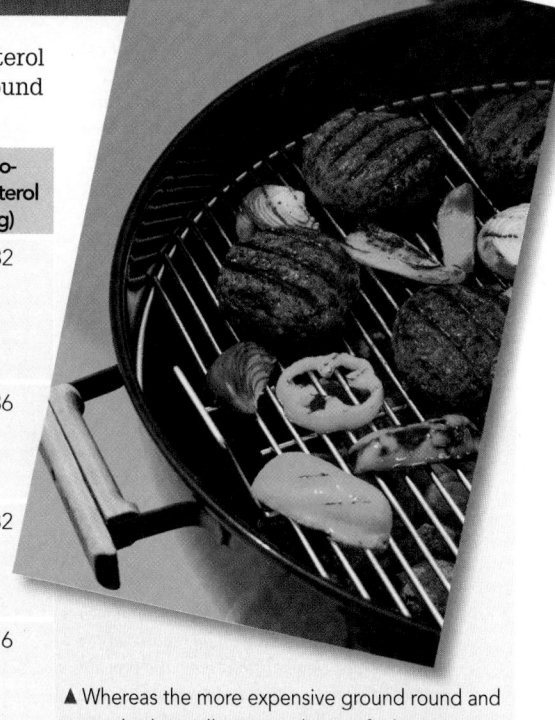

▲ Whereas the more expensive ground round and ground sirloin will give you lowest-fat burgers to start, the less expensive regular ground beef or ground chuck burgers will lose fat while cooking. You will therefore want to consider both fat content and cost when making your choice.

end up with less meat in the final product. However, this is not such a big deal because most Americans consume two to three times as much protein as they need. To further enhance the heart-healthiness of mixed dishes, replace some of that lost product with beans, Chili or tacos would be excellent recipes to try with this method.

Further Readings

1. ADA Reports: Position of the American Dietetic Association and Dietitians of Canada: Dietary fatty acids. *Journal of the American Dietetic Association* 107:1599, 2007.

   A diet is recommended that reduces fatty acids that increase risk of disease, while promoting fatty acids that benefit health. Dietary fat should provide 20% to 35% of energy and emphasize a reduction in saturated fatty acids and trans fatty acids and an increase in n-3 polyunsaturated fatty acids. A food-based approach should be used that includes fruits and vegetables, whole grains, legumes, nuts and seeds, lean protein, and fish. Nonhydrogenated margarines and oils are recommended such that unsaturated fatty acids are the predominant fat source in the diet.

2. Getz L: A burger and fries (hold the *trans* fats). *Today's Dietitian* 11(2):35, 2009.

   Several cities across the United States, including New York, Philadelphia, and Boston, have banned trans fat use in restaurants. Most eating establishments have willingly responded to the demand for healthier oils. It is important to remember that choosing trans fat-free foods does not necessarily make it a healthy choice.

3. Hansson GK: Inflammation, atherosclerosis, and coronary artery disease. *The New England Journal of Medicine* 352:1685, 2005.

   Excellent review of the role of inflammation in causing cardiovascular disease. Identifying atherosclerosis as an inflammatory disease offers new opportunities for the prevention and treatment of coronary artery disease.

4. He KA, Daviglus ML: A few more thoughts about fish and fish oil. *Journal of the American Dietetic Association* 105:428, 2005.

   Fish consumption has been shown to have beneficial effects on cardiovascular disease. Consuming whole fish is thought to have greater benefits and be safer than using fish oil supplements. Fish is not only a rich source of omega-3 fatty acids, but is also a valuable source of protein and trace elements that may also provide protective effects for the cardiovascular system. Broiled or baked fish is recommended rather than fried fish because frying may decrease the ratio of omega-3 to omega-6 fatty acids and may produce trans fatty acids and oxidized lipid products that may increase cardiovascular disease risk.

5. Kris-Etherton PM, Hill AM: n-3 fatty acids: Food or supplements? *Journal of the American Dietetic Association* 108:1125, 2008.

   A food-based approach is recommended for all fatty acids including the n-3 fatty acids. If an individual does not eat fish, the richest source of n-3 fatty acids, other options such as "designer" foods high in n-3 fatty acids, foods fortified with these fatty acids, or even supplements can be used. For vegans, algal supplements are an alternative source of DHA instead of fish or fish oil.

6. Kuller LH: Nutrition, lipids, and cardiovascular disease. *Nutrition Reviews* 64:S15, 2006.

   The development of coronary heart disease is discussed as an epidemic due to increased consumption of saturated fat and cholesterol, low intakes of polyunsaturated fat, and obesity. The risk of the disease is increased by hypertension, smoking, and diabetes. The careful monitoring and prevention of this disease beginning in young adults is important but expensive.

7. Lau VWY and others: Plant sterols are efficacious in lowering plasma LDL and non-HDL cholesterol in hypercholesterolemic type 2 diabetic and nondiabetic persons. *American Journal of Clinical Nutrition* 81:1351, 2005.

   Incorporation of plant sterols into a low-saturated-fat and low-cholesterol diet for persons at increased risk of CVD mortality could have a positive effect on reducing the mortality rate, including in those people with type 2 diabetes.

8. Lewis NM and others: The walnut: A nutritional nut case. *Today's Dietitian* 6(8):36, 2004.

   Compared to other nuts and seeds, walnuts are one of the richest sources of alpha-linolenic acid (2.6 grams per 1-ounce serving or 14 walnut halves). The DRI for alpha-linolenic acid is 1.6 grams/day for men and 1.1 grams/day for women. In addition, walnuts are a rich source of plant sterols known to inhibit intestinal absorption of cholesterol.

9. Lichtenstein AH and others: Diet and lifestyle recommendations revision 2006. A scientific statement from the American Heart Association Nutrition Committee. *Circulation* 114:82, 2006.

   The American Heart Association presents recommendations designed to reduce the risk of cardiovascular disease in the general population. Specific goals are presented and include consuming an overall healthy diet; to aim for a healthy body weight, recommended levels of low-density lipoprotein cholesterol, high-density lipoprotein cholesterol, and triglycerides; normal blood pressure; normal blood glucose level; being physically active; and avoiding the use of and exposure to tobacco products.

10. Meisinger C and others: Plasma oxidized low-density lipoprotein, a strong predictor for acute coronary heart disease events in apparently healthy, middle-aged men from the general population. *Circulation* 112:651, 2005.

    Elevated concentrations of oxidized low-density lipoprotein are predictive of future coronary heart disease events in apparently healthy men. Thus, oxidized LDL may represent a promising risk marker for clinical coronary heart disease complications and should be evaluated in further studies.

11. Micallef MA, Garg ML: The lipid-lowering effects of phytosterols and (n-3) polyunsaturated fatty acids are synergistic and complementary in hyperlipidemic men and women. *Journal of Nutrition* 138:1086, 2008.

    Phytosterols are plant compounds with structures similar to cholesterol. Some margarines and other products are enriched with phytosterols. Consuming phytosterols can reduce the intestinal absorption of cholesterol by 30% to 40%. Fish oils are rich in omega-3 polyunsaturated fatty acids (PUFA) and can reduce blood triglycerides and raise HDL-cholesterol. The combined effect of phytosterols and omega-3 PUFA on blood lipid profiles was studied in individuals with high blood lipids. The combined supplementation with phytosterols and omega-3 PUFA had synergistic and complementary lipid-lowering effects in men and women with high blood lipids, resulting in a reduction in plasma total and LDL-cholesterol concentrations, an increase in HDL-cholesterol concentration, and a decrease in plasma triglyceride concentration.

12. Palmer S: Fighting heart disease the Dean Ornish way. *Today's Dietitian* 2:48, 2009.

    The Ornish diet has been proven to prevent as well as reverse heart disease. Diet guidelines include eating no more than 10% of calories from fat from mostly a plant-based diet; consuming no more than 10 milligrams of cholesterol per day; and eating one serving of soy foods each day. Omega-3 fatty acids are recommended from supplements.

13. Phillips KM and others: Phytosterol composition of nuts and seeds commonly consumed in the United States. *Journal of Agriculture and Food Chemistry* 53:9436, 2005.

    This study set out to find the nuts and seeds that could provide the most heart-protective benefits. Of the 27 nuts and seeds analyzed, wheat germ and sesame seeds had the greatest concentration of phytosterols and Brazil nuts and walnuts ranked the lowest. Pistachio and sunflower seeds were the richest sources of phytosterols for products typically consumed as snack foods.

14. Shai I and others: Weight loss with a low-carbohydrate, Mediterranean, or low-fat diet. *The New England Journal of Medicine* 359:229, 2008.

Moderately obese adults (mean age, 52 years) were assigned to one of three diets: low-fat, restricted-calorie; Mediterranean, restricted-calorie; or low-carbohydrate, non-restricted-calorie, and studied for two years. The diet was monitored for various components, including amount and type of carbohydrates, fat, protein, and cholesterol. The mean weight loss among the 272 participants who remained on their diets was 3.3 kg for the low-fat group, 4.6 kg for the Mediterranean-diet group, and 5.5 kg for

the low-carbohydrate group. The results indicate that Mediterranean and low-carbohydrate diets may be effective alternatives to low-fat diets. The more favorable effects on lipids (with the low-carbohydrate diet) and on glycemic control (with the Mediterranean diet) suggest that personal preferences and metabolic considerations might inform individualized tailoring of dietary interventions.

15. Wang C and others: n-3 fatty acids from fish or fish oil supplements, but not alpha-linolenic acid, benefit cardiovascular disease outcomes in primary- and secondary-prevention studies: A systematic review. *American Journal of Clinical Nutrition* 84:5, 2006.

This review of previous studies found that consumption of omega-3 fatty acids from fish or fish oil but not alpha-linolenic acid, significantly reduced all-cause mortality, myocardial infarction, cardiac and sudden death, or stroke.

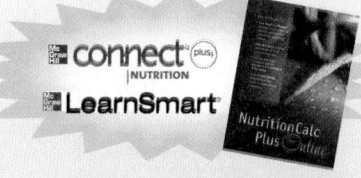

To get the most out of your study of nutrition, go to McGraw-Hill's online resources: Connect www.mcgrawhillconnect.com**, where you will find NutritionCalc Plus, LearnSmart, and many other dynamic tools.**

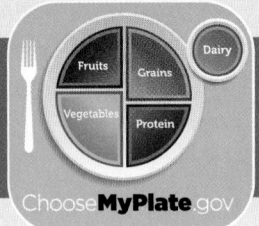
I. Is Your Diet High in Saturated and *Trans* Fat?

Instructions: In each row of the following list, circle your typical food selection from column A or B.

Column A		Column B
Bacon and eggs	or	Ready-to-eat whole-grain breakfast cereal
Doughnut or sweet roll	or	Whole-wheat roll, bagel, or bread
Breakfast sausage	or	Fruit
Whole milk	or	Reduced-fat, low-fat, or fat-free milk
Cheeseburger	or	Turkey sandwich, no cheese
French fries	or	Plain baked potato with salsa
Ground chuck	or	Ground round
Soup with cream base	or	Soup with broth base
Macaroni and cheese	or	Macaroni with marinara sauce
Cream/fruit pie	or	Graham crackers
Cream-filled cookies	or	Granola bar
Ice cream	or	Frozen yogurt, sherbet, or reduced-fat ice cream
Butter or stick margarine	or	Vegetable oils or soft margarine in a tub

Interpretation

The foods listed in column A tend to be high in saturated fat, *trans* fatty acids, cholesterol, and total fat. Those in column B generally are low in these dietary components. If you want to help reduce your risk of cardiovascular disease, choose more foods from column B and fewer from column A.

II. Applying the Nutrition Facts Label to Your Daily Food Choices

Imagine that you are at the supermarket looking for a quick snack to help you keep your energy up during afternoons. In the snack section, you settle on two choices (see labels a and b). Evaluate the products using the table on the left.

Compare the nutrients in each product by completing this list. For each serving, which product is lower in each of the following?

Calories	(a)	(b)	no difference
Calories from Fat	(a)	(b)	no difference
Total Fat	(a)	(b)	no difference
Saturated Fat	(a)	(b)	no difference
Trans Fat	(a)	(b)	no difference
Cholesterol	(a)	(b)	no difference
Sodium	(a)	(b)	no difference
Total Carbohydrates	(a)	(b)	no difference
Dietary Fiber	(a)	(b)	no difference
Sugars	(a)	(b)	no difference
Protein	(a)	(b)	no difference
Iron	(a)	(b)	no difference

Which package has more servings per container?

(a)　(b)　no difference

Which of the two brands would you choose?

(a)　(b)　no difference

What information on the Nutrition Facts labels contributed to your decision?

Nutrition Facts

Serving Size: 2 bars (42g)
Servings Per Container: 6

Amount Per Serving　　　　**2 bars**
Calories 180　　　Calories from Fat 50

	% Daily Value*
Total Fat 6g	**9**%
Saturated Fat 0.5g	**3**%
Trans fat 0g	**
Cholesterol 0mg	**0**%
Sodium 160mg	**7**%
Total Carbohydrates 29g	**10**%
Dietary Fiber 2g	**8**%
Sugars 11g	
Protein 4g	
Iron	6%

Not a significant source of Vitamin A, Vitamin C, and calcium.

** Intake of *trans* fat should be as low as possible.

* Daily values are based on a 2,000 calorie diet. Your daily values may be higher or lower depending on your calorie needs:

** Intake should be as low as possible.

		Calories	2,000	2,500
Total Fat	Less than		65g	80g
Saturated Fat	Less than		20g	25g
Cholesterol	Less than		300mg	300mg
Sodium	Less than		2,400mg	2,400mg
Total Carbohydrates			300g	375g
Dietary Fiber			25g	30g

INGREDIENTS: WHOLE GRAIN ROLLED OATS, SUGAR, CANOLA OIL, CRISP RICE WITH SOY PROTEIN (RICE FLOUR, SOY PROTEIN CONCENTRATE, SUGAR, MALT, SALT), HONEY, BROWN SUGAR SYRUP, HIGH FRUCTOSE CORN SYRUP, SALT, SOY LECITHIN, BAKING SODA, NATURAL FLAVOR, PEANUT FLOUR, ALMOND FLOUR, HAZELNUT FLOUR, WALNUT FLOUR, PECAN FLOUR.

(a)

Nutrition Facts

Serving Size: 2 cookies (38g)
Servings Per Container: about 12

Amount Per Serving
Calories 180　　　Calories from Fat 70

	% Daily Value*
Total Fat 7g	**11**%
Saturated Fat 2g	**10**%
Trans fat 2g	**
Cholesterol 0mg	**0**%
Sodium 100mg	**4**%
Total Carbohydrate 26g	**9**%
Dietary Fiber 1g	**4**%
Sugars 12g	
Protein 2g	

Vitamin A 0%	•	Vitamin C 0%	
Calcium 0%	•	Iron 2%	

** Intake of *trans* fat should be as low as possible.

* Daily values are based on a 2,000 calorie diet. Your daily values may be higher or lower depending on your calorie needs:

** Intake should be as low as possible.

		Calories	2,000	2,500
Total Fat	Less than		65g	80g
Saturated Fat	Less than		20g	25g
Cholesterol	Less than		300mg	300mg
Sodium	Less than		2,400mg	2,400mg
Total Carbohydrates			300g	375g
Dietary Fiber			25g	30g

Calories per gram: • Fat 9 • Carbohydrate 4
• Protein 4

INGREDIENTS: ENRICHED FLOUR (WHEAT FLOUR, NIACIN, REDUCED IRON, THIAMINE MONONITRATE, RIBOFLAVIN, FOLIC ACID), SUGAR, VEGETABLE OIL SHORTENING (PARTIALLY HYDROGENATED SOYBEAN, COCONUT, COTTONSEED, CORN AND/OR SAFFLOWER AND/OR CANOLA OIL), CORN SYRUP, HIGH FRUCTOSE CORN SYRUP, WHEY (A MILK INGREDIENT), CORN STARCH, SALT, SKIM MILK, LEAVENING (BAKING SODA, AMMONIUM BICARBONATE), ARTIFICIAL FLAVOR, SOYBEAN LECITHIN, COLOR (CONTAINING FD&C YELLOW #5 LAKE).

(b)

Chapter 6 Proteins

Student Learning Outcomes

Chapter 6 is designed to allow you to:

6.1 Distinguish between essential and nonessential amino acids and explain why adequate amounts of each of the essential amino acids are required for protein synthesis.

6.2 Describe how amino acids form proteins.

6.3 Distinguish between high-quality and lower-quality proteins, identify examples of each, and describe the concept of complementary proteins.

6.4 Describe how protein is digested and absorbed in the body.

6.5 List the primary functions of protein in the body.

6.6 Calculate the RDA for protein for an adult when a healthy weight is given.

6.7 Describe what is meant by positive protein balance, negative protein balance, and protein equilibrium.

6.8 Describe how protein-calorie malnutrition eventually can lead to disease in the body.

6.9 Develop vegetarian diet plans that meet the body's nutritional needs.

What Would You Choose?

About 3 weeks ago, you started lifting weights at the student recreation center. You are disappointed that you have not seen the results you were anticipating. You can lift more now than you could when you started, but you were hoping to tone and define the muscles in your arms, back, and abs. Perhaps you need more protein. Bodybuilding magazines have numerous advertisements for protein and amino-acid supplements, but they are expensive. What would you choose as optimal nutrition to support your weight-training regimen?

a Take whey protein supplements.

b Take individual amino-acid supplements.

c Increase your consumption of animal protein.

d Consume a diet that provides 10% to 35% of calories from a variety of sources of protein.

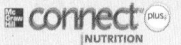 connect NUTRITION **Think about your choice as you read Chapter 6, then see our recommendations at the end of the chapter. To learn more about supplements and diet, check out the Connect site:** www.mcgrawhillconnect.com

Part Two
Energy Nutrients and Energy Balance

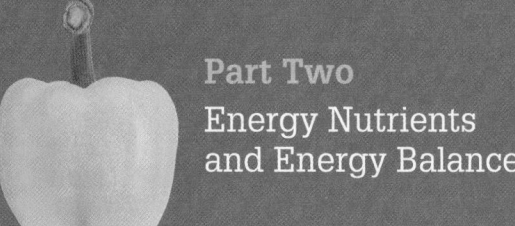

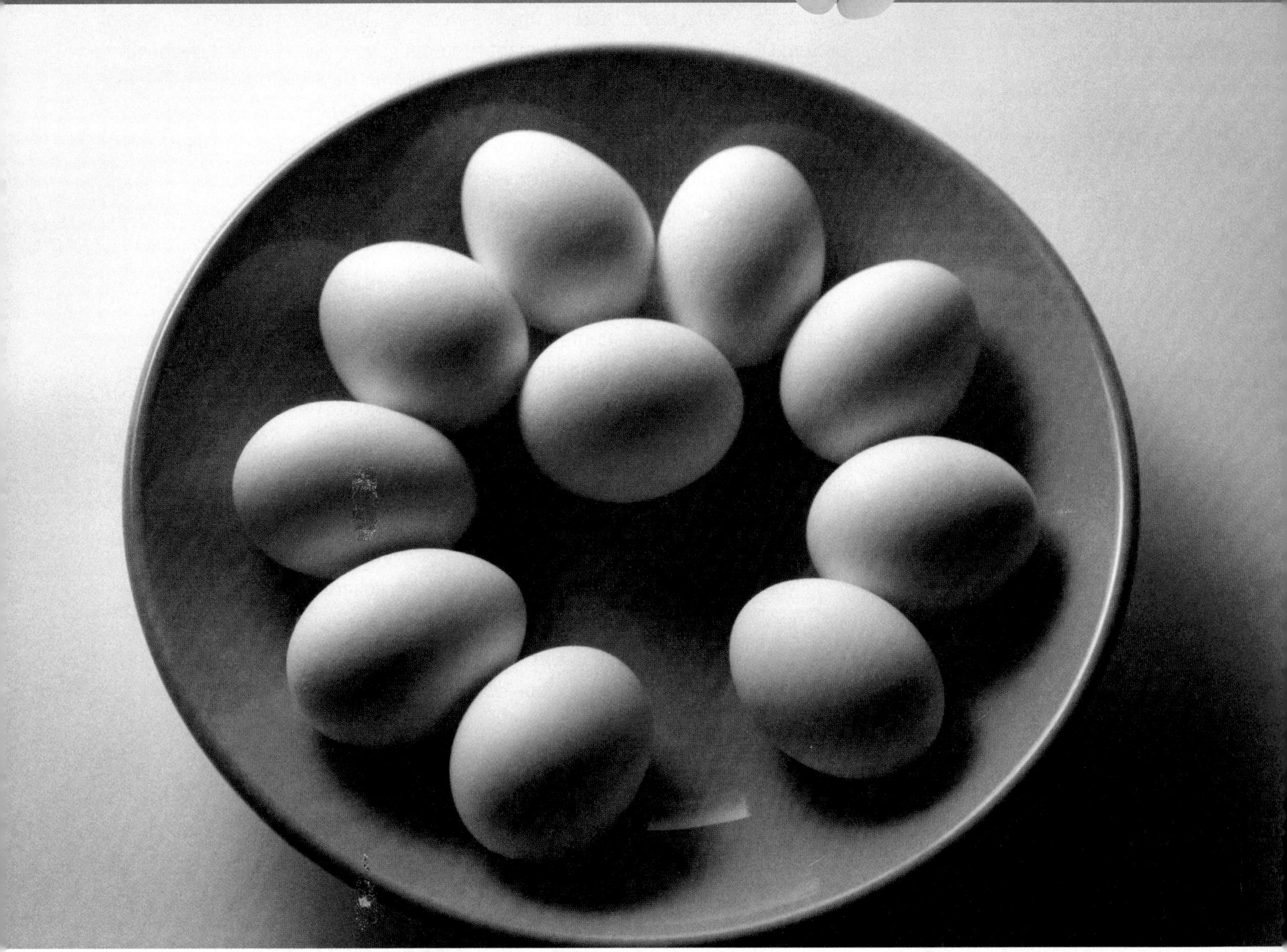

Consuming enough protein is vital for maintaining health. Proteins form important structures in the body, make up a key part of the blood, help regulate many body functions, and can fuel body cells.

North Americans generally eat more protein than is needed to maintain health. High-protein weight-loss diets have come and gone over the past 30 years. Our daily protein intake comes mostly from animal sources such as meat, poultry, fish, eggs, milk, and cheese. In contrast, in the developing world, diets can be deficient in protein.

Diets that are mostly vegetarian still predominate in much of Asia and areas of Africa, and, as suggested in the comic on the next page, some North Americans are currently adopting the practice. Plant sources of protein are worthy of more attention from North Americans. In the early 1900s, plant sources of proteins—nuts, seeds, and legumes—were consumed just as often as animal proteins. Over the years, though, plant proteins have been sidelined by meats. During this time, nuts have been viewed as high-fat foods, and beans have gotten the inferior reputation of "the poor man's meat." Contrary to these popular misconceptions, sources of plant proteins offer a wealth of nutritional benefits—from lowering blood cholesterol to preventing certain forms of cancer.

We could benefit from eating more plant sources of proteins. As shown in the comic in this chapter, it takes some knowledge to do so. It is possible—and desirable—to enjoy the benefits of animal and plant protein as we work toward the goal of meeting protein needs. This chapter takes a close look at protein, including the benefits of plant proteins in a diet. It will also examine vegetarian diets: their benefits and their risks, if not properly planned. Let's see why a detailed study of protein is worth your attention.

Refresh Your Memory

As you begin your study of proteins in Chapter 6, you may want to review:

- Organization of the cell in Chapter 3
- The processes of digestion and absorption in Chapter 3
- The nervous system and immune system in Chapter 3
- The role of carbohydrates in sparing protein for energy in Chapter 4

FRANK & ERNEST® by Bob Thaves

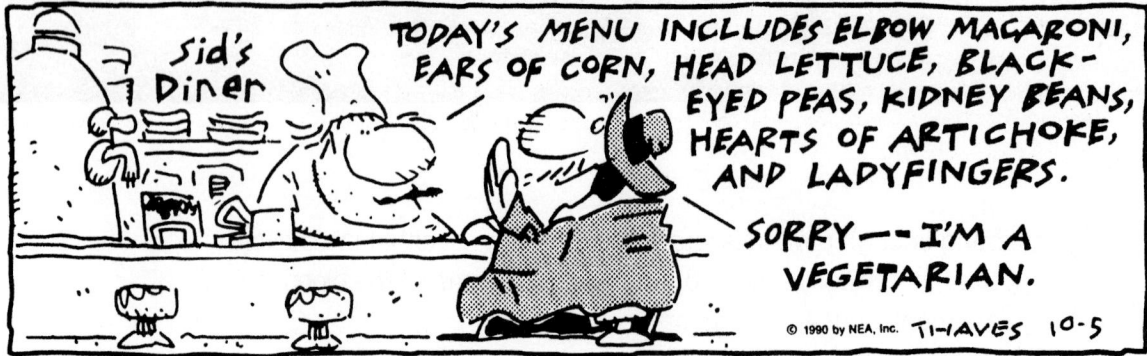

Can a vegetarian diet provide enough protein? What is prompting the growing interest in various forms of vegetarian diets? Why are plant protein sources, especially soy and nuts, gaining more attention? Should meat-eaters abandon that dietary practice? Chapter 6 provides some answers.

FRANK & ERNEST © United Features Syndicate. Reprinted by Permission.

6.1 Protein—An Introduction

Diets in the developed parts of the world, such as the United States and Canada, are typically rich in protein, and therefore a specific focus on eating enough protein is generally not needed. In the developing world, however, it is important to focus on protein in diet planning because diets in those areas of the world can be deficient in protein.

Thousands of substances in the body are made of proteins. Aside from water, proteins form the major part of lean body tissue, totaling about 17% of body weight. Amino acids—the building blocks for proteins—are unique in that they contain nitrogen along with carbon, oxygen, and hydrogen. Plants combine nitrogen from the soil with carbon and other elements to form amino acids. They then link these amino acids together to make proteins. We get the nitrogen we need by consuming dietary proteins. Proteins are thus an essential part of a diet because they supply nitrogen in a form we can readily use—namely, amino acids. Using simpler forms of nitrogen is, for the most part, impossible for humans.

Proteins are crucial to the regulation and maintenance of the body. Body functions such as blood clotting, fluid balance, hormone and enzyme production, visual processes, transport of many substances in the bloodstream, and cell repair require specific proteins. The body makes proteins in many configurations and sizes so that they can serve these greatly varied functions. Formation of these body proteins begins with amino acids from both the protein-containing foods we eat and those synthesized from other compounds within the body. Proteins can also be broken down to supply energy for the body—on average, 4 kcal per gram.

If you fail to consume an adequate amount of protein for weeks at a time, many metabolic processes slow down. This is because the body does not have enough amino acids available to build the proteins it needs. For example, the immune system no longer functions efficiently when it lacks key proteins, thereby increasing the risk of infections, disease, and death.

Amino Acids

Amino acids—the building blocks of proteins—are formed mostly of carbon, hydrogen, oxygen, and nitrogen. The following diagram shows the structure of a generic amino acid and also what one of the specific amino acids, glutamic acid, looks like. The amino acids have different chemical makeups, but all are slight variations of the generic amino acid pictured (see Appendix F). Each amino acid has an "acid" group; an "amino" group; and a "side" or R group specific to the amino acid.

The R group on some amino acids has a branched shape, like a tree. These so-called **branched-chain amino acids** are leucine, isoleucine, and valine (see Appendix F for the chemical structures of the amino acids). The branched-chain amino acids are the primary amino acids used by muscles for energy needs. This is one reason why proteins from milk (e.g., whey proteins) are popular with strength-training athletes (see Chapter 10 for details).

branched-chain amino acids Amino acids with a branching carbon backbone; these are leucine, isoleucine, and valine. All are essential amino acids.

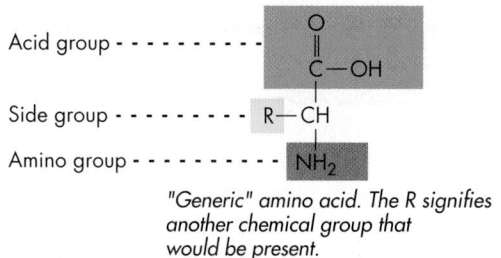

Acid group — — — — — — — —
Side group — — — — — — — —
Amino group — — — — — — — —

"Generic" amino acid. The R signifies another chemical group that would be present.

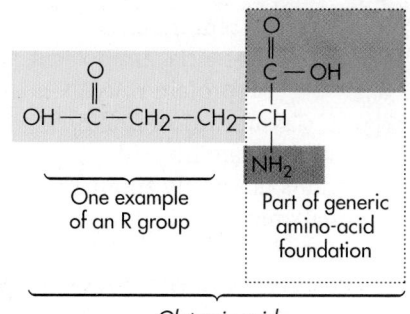

One example of an R group | Part of generic amino-acid foundation

Glutamic acid

nonessential amino acids Amino acids that can be synthesized by a healthy body in sufficient amounts; there are 11 nonessential amino acids. These are also called *dispensable amino acids.*

essential amino acids The amino acids that cannot be synthesized by humans in sufficient amounts or at all and therefore must be included in the diet; there are nine essential amino acids. These are also called *indispensable amino acids.*

limiting amino acid The essential amino acid in lowest concentration in a food or diet relative to body needs.

TABLE 6-1 Classification of Amino Acids

Essential Amino Acids	Nonessential Amino Acids
Histidine	Alanine
Isoleucine*	Arginine
Leucine*	Asparagine
Lysine	Aspartic acid
Methionine	Cysteine
Phenylalanine	Glutamic acid
Threonine	Glutamine
Tryptophan	Glycine
Valine*	Proline
	Serine
	Tyrosine

*A branched-chain amino acid.

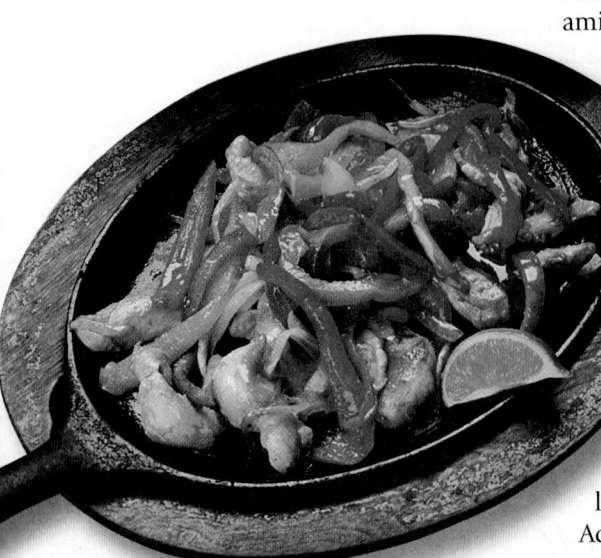

▲ When combined with vegetables, high-protein foods such as meats also help balance the amino-acid content of the diet.

Your body needs to use 20 different amino acids to function (Table 6-1). Although all these commonly found amino acids are important, 11 are considered **nonessential** (also called *dispensable*) with respect to our diets. Human cells can produce these certain amino acids as long as the right ingredients are present—the key factor being nitrogen that is already part of another amino acid. Therefore it is not essential that these amino acids be in our diet.

The nine amino acids the body cannot make in sufficient amounts or at all are known as **essential** (also called *indispensable*)—they must be obtained from foods. This is because body cells either cannot make the needed carbon-based foundation of the amino acid, cannot put a nitrogen group on the needed carbon-based foundation, or just cannot do the whole process fast enough to meet body needs.

Eating a balanced diet can supply us with both the essential and nonessential amino-acid building blocks needed to maintain good health. Both nonessential and essential amino acids are present in foods that contain protein. If you don't eat enough essential amino acids, your body first struggles to conserve what essential amino acids it can. However, eventually your body progressively slows production of new proteins until at some point you will break protein down faster than you can make it. When that happens, health deteriorates.

The essential amino acid in smallest supply in a food or diet in relation to body needs becomes the limiting factor (called the **limiting amino acid**) because it limits the amount of protein the body can synthesize. For example, assume the letters of the alphabet represent the 20 or so different amino acids we consume. If *A* represents an essential amino acid, we need three of these letters to spell the hypothetical protein *BANANA*. If the body had a *B*, two *N*s, but only two *A*s, the "synthesis" of *BANANA* would not be possible. *A* would then be seen as the limiting amino acid.

Adults need only about 11% of their total protein requirement to be supplied by essential amino acids. Typical diets supply an average of 50% of protein as essential amino acids.

The estimated needs for essential amino acids for infants and preschool children are 40% of total protein intake; however, in later childhood the need drops to 20%.

MAKING DECISIONS

Phenylketonuria

Some of the nonessential amino acids are also classed as conditionally essential. This means they must be made from essential amino acids if insufficient amounts are eaten. When that occurs, the body's supply of certain essential amino acids is depleted. Tyrosine is an example of a conditionally essential amino acid that can be made from the essential amino-acid phenylalanine.

The disease phenylketonuria (PKU) illustrates the importance of phenylalanine to make tyrosine. Recall from Chapter 4 that a person with PKU has a limited ability to metabolize the essential amino-acid phenylalanine. Normally, the body uses an enzyme to convert much of our dietary phenylalanine intake into tyrosine.

In PKU-diagnosed persons, the activity of the enzyme used in processing phenylalanine to tyrosine is insufficient. When the enzyme cannot synthesize enough tyrosine, both amino acids must be derived from foods. The point is that phenylalanine and tyrosine become *essential* in terms of dietary needs because the body can't produce enough tyrosine from phenylalanine. Phenylalanine levels in the blood increase because it is not converted to tyrosine. PKU is treated by limiting the consumption of phenylalanine with a special diet so that phenylalanine and its by-products do not rise to toxic concentrations in the body and cause the severe mental retardation seen in untreated PKU cases.

Rina is 7 months pregnant and has read about various tests that her baby will undergo when he or she is born. How can you explain to Rina the purpose and significance of one of those tests, the one that screens for PKU?

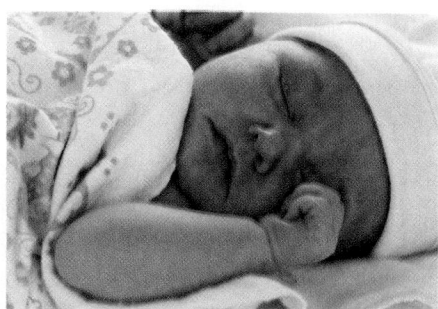

▲ Within the first few days of life all newborns are tested for phenylketonuria.

Diets designed for infants and young children need to take this into account to make sure enough proteins are present to yield a high-quality protein intake. Including some animal products in the diet, such as human milk or formula for infants, or cow's milk for children, helps ensure this. Otherwise, complementary amino acids from plant proteins should be consumed in each meal or within two subsequent meals. A major health risk for infants and children occurs in famine situations in which only one type of cereal grain is available, increasing the probability that one or more of the nine essential amino acids is lacking in the total diet. This is discussed further in a later section on protein-calorie malnutrition.

CONCEPT CHECK

The human body uses 20 different amino acids from protein-containing foods. A healthy body can synthesize 11 of the amino acids, so it is not necessary to obtain all amino acids from foods—only nine of these must come from the diet and are therefore termed *essential (indispensable) amino acids*. The essential amino acid in smallest supply in a food in relation to body needs is called the limiting amino acid because it limits the amount of protein the body can synthesize.

6.2 Proteins—Amino Acids Bonded Together

Amino acids are linked together by chemical bonds—technically called **peptide bonds**—to form proteins. Although these bonds are difficult to break, acids, enzymes, and other agents are able to do so—for example, during digestion.

The body can synthesize many different proteins by linking together the 20 common types of amino acids with peptide bonds.

peptide bond A chemical bond formed between amino acids in a protein.

polypeptide A group of amino acids bonded together, from 50 to 2000 or more.

Protein Synthesis

Our discussion of protein synthesis, begins with DNA. DNA is present in the nucleus of the cell and contains coded instructions for protein synthesis (i.e., which specific amino acids are to be placed in a protein and in which order). Recall from Chapter 3 that DNA is a double-stranded molecule.

Protein synthesis in a cell, however, takes place in the cytoplasm, not in the nucleus. Thus, the DNA code used for synthesis of a specific protein must be transferred from the nucleus to the cytoplasm to allow for protein synthesis. This transfer is the job of messenger RNA (mRNA). Enzymes in the nucleus read the code on one segment (a gene) of one strand of the DNA and *transcribe* that information into a single-stranded mRNA molecule (Fig. 6-1). This mRNA undergoes processing and then it is ready to leave the nucleus.

Once in the cytoplasm, mRNA travels to the ribosomes. The ribosomes read the mRNA code and *translate* those instructions to produce a specific protein. Amino acids are added one at a time to the growing **polypeptide** chain according to the instructions on the mRNA. Another key participant in protein synthesis, transfer RNA (tRNA), is responsible for bringing the specific amino acids to the ribosomes as needed during protein synthesis (review Fig. 6-1). Energy input is required to add each amino acid to the chain, making protein synthesis "costly" in terms of calorie use.

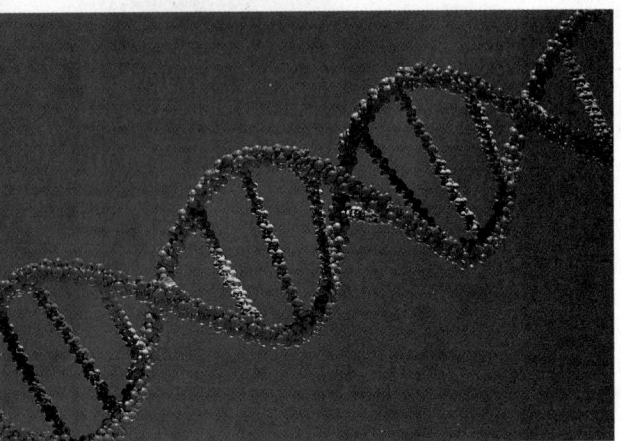

▲ Genes are present on DNA—a double-stranded helix. The cell nucleus contains most of the DNA in the body.

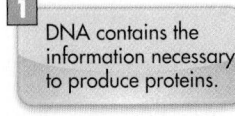

1 DNA contains the information necessary to produce proteins.

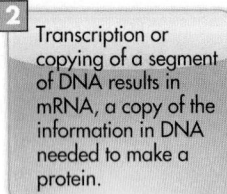

2 Transcription or copying of a segment of DNA results in mRNA, a copy of the information in DNA needed to make a protein.

3 The mRNA leaves the nucleus and goes to a ribosome.

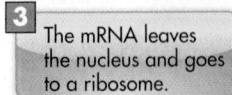

4 Amino acids, the building blocks of proteins, are carried to the ribosome by tRNAs containing the code that matches that on the mRNA.

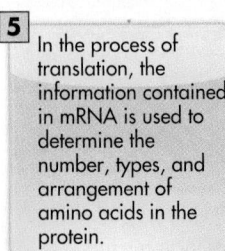

5 In the process of translation, the information contained in mRNA is used to determine the number, types, and arrangement of amino acids in the protein.

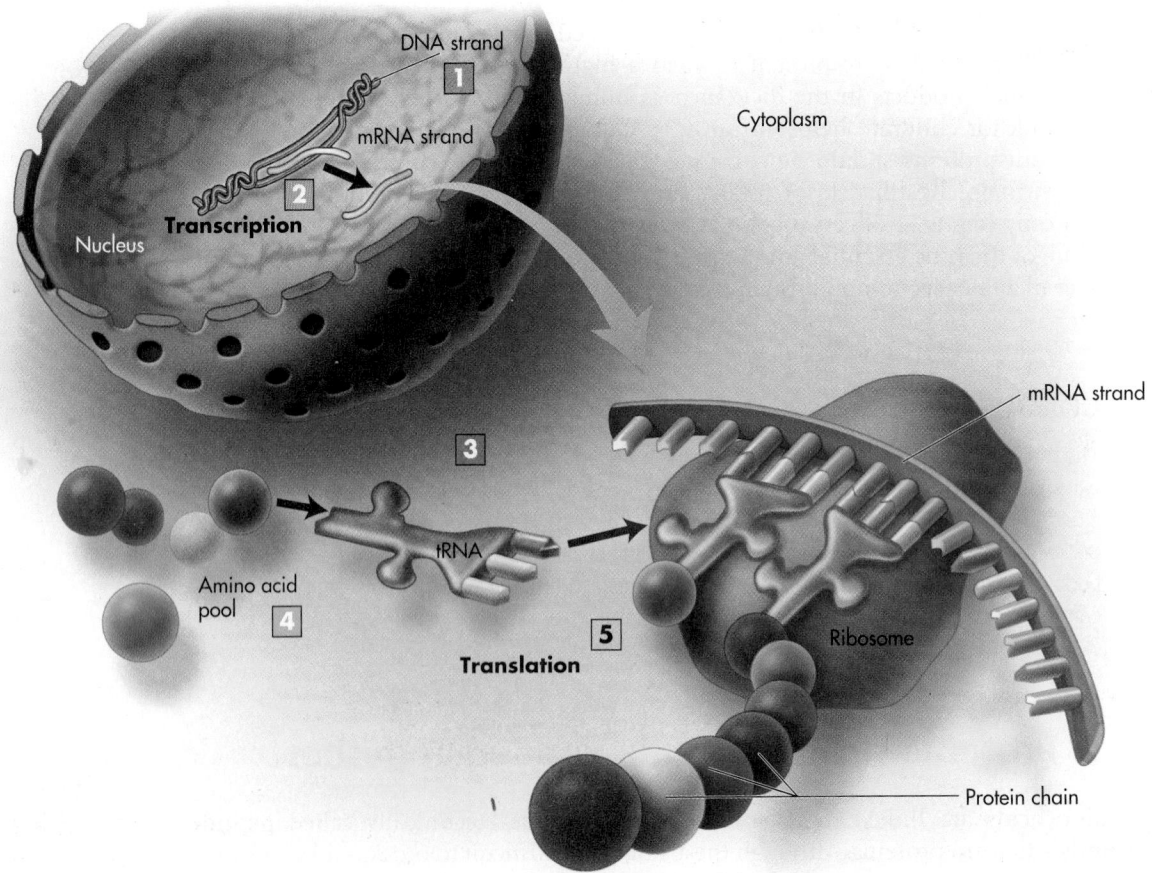

FIGURE 6-1 ▶ Protein synthesis (simplified). Once the mRNA is fully read, the amino acids have been connected into the polypeptide, which is released into the cytoplasm. It generally is then processed further to become a cell protein.

Once synthesis of a polypeptide is complete, it twists and folds into the appropriate three-dimensional structure of the intended protein. These structural changes occur based on specific interactions between the amino acids that make up the polypeptide chain (see the next section on protein organization for details). Some polypeptides, such as the hormone insulin, also undergo further changes in the cell before they are functional.

The important message in this discussion is the relationship between DNA and the proteins eventually produced by a cell. If the DNA code contains errors, an incorrect mRNA will be produced. The ribosomes will then read this incorrect message and an incorrect amino acid will be added and an incorrect polypeptide chain will be produced. As discussed in Chapter 3, genetic engineering may ultimately be able to correct many gene defects in humans, by placing the correct DNA code in the nucleus, so that the correct protein can be made by the ribosomes.

Protein Organization

As noted before, by bonding together various combinations of the 20 common types of amino acids, the body synthesizes thousands of different proteins. The sequential order of the amino acids then ultimately determines the protein's shape. The main point is that only correctly positioned amino acids can interact and fold properly to form the intended shape for the protein. The resulting unique, three-dimensional form goes on to dictate the function of each particular protein (Fig. 6-2). If it lacks the proper structure, a protein cannot function.

Sickle cell disease (also called **sickle cell anemia**) is one example of what happens when amino acids are out of order on a protein. North Americans of African descent are especially prone to this genetic disease. It occurs because of defects in the structure of the protein chains of hemoglobin, a protein that carries oxygen in red blood cells. In two of its four protein chains, an error in the amino-acid order occurs. This error produces a profound change in hemoglobin structure. It can no longer form the shape needed to carry oxygen efficiently inside the red blood cell. Instead of forming normal circular disks, the red blood cells collapse into crescent (or sickle) shapes (Fig. 6-3). Health deteriorates, and eventually episodes of severe pain in the bones and joints, abdominal pain, headaches, convulsions, and paralysis may occur.

These life-threatening symptoms are caused by a minute, but critical, error in the hemoglobin amino-acid order. Why does this error happen? It results from a defect in a person's genetic blueprint, DNA, inherited through one's parents. A defect in the DNA can dictate that a wrong amino acid will be built into the sequence of the body proteins. Many diseases, including cancer, stem from errors in the DNA code.

Denaturation of Proteins

Exposure to acid or alkaline substances, heat, or agitation can alter a protein's structure, leaving it uncoiled or otherwise deformed. This process of altering the three-dimensional structure of a protein is called **denaturation** (see Fig. 6-7 on p. 219). Changing a protein's shape often destroys its ability to function normally, such that it loses its biological activity.

Denaturation of proteins is useful for some body processes, especially digestion. The heat produced during cooking denatures some proteins. After food is ingested, the secretion of stomach acid denatures some bacterial proteins, plant hormones, many active enzymes, and other forms of proteins in foods, making it safer to eat. Digestion is also enhanced by denaturation because the unraveling increases exposure of the polypeptide chain to digestive enzymes. Denaturing proteins in some foods can also reduce their tendencies to cause allergic reactions.

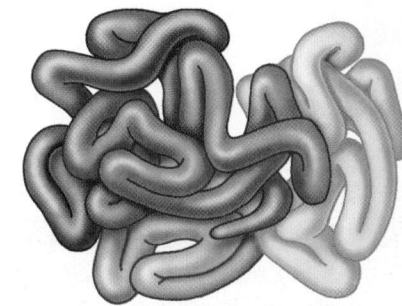

FIGURE 6-2 ▶ Protein organization. Proteins often form a coiled shape, as shown by this drawing of the blood protein hemoglobin. This shape is dictated by the order of the amino acids in the protein chain. To get an idea of its size, consider that each teaspoon (5 milliliters) of blood contains about 10^{18} hemoglobin molecules. One billion is 10^9.

sickle cell disease (sickle cell anemia) An illness that results from a malformation of the red blood cell because of an incorrect structure in part of its hemoglobin protein chains. The disease can lead to episodes of severe bone and joint pain, abdominal pain, headache, convulsions, paralysis, and even death.

denaturation Alteration of a protein's three-dimensional structure, usually because of treatment by heat, enzymes, acid or alkaline solutions, or agitation.

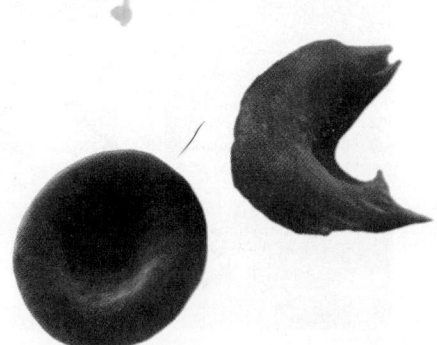

FIGURE 6-3 ▶ An example of the consequences of errors in DNA coding of proteins. (a) Normal red blood cell; (b) red blood cell from a person with sickle cell anemia—note its abnormal crescent (sicklelike) shape.

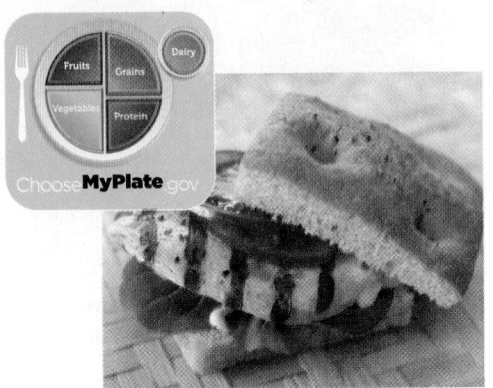

Recall that we need the essential amino acids that the proteins in the diet supply—not the proteins themselves. We dismantle ingested dietary proteins and use the amino-acid building blocks to assemble the proteins we need.

CONCEPT CHECK

Amino acids are bonded together in specific sequences to form distinct proteins. DNA provides the directions for synthesizing these new proteins. Specifically, DNA directs the order of the amino acids on the protein. The amino-acid order within a protein determines its ultimate shape and function. Destroying the shape of a protein denatures it. Stomach acid, heat, and other factors can denature proteins, causing them to lose their biological activity. Proteins must be denatured during digestion so that amino acids are available for absorption.

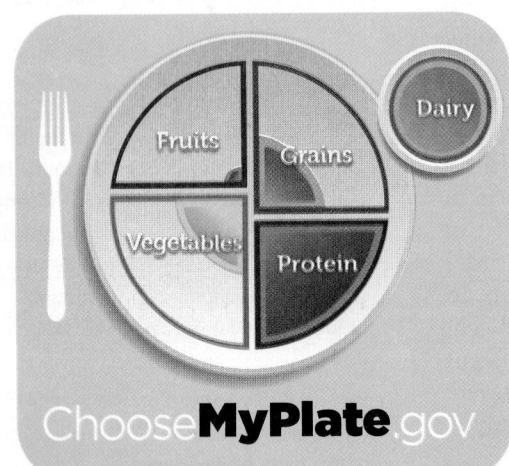

▲ This grilled chicken (protein) sandwich with lettuce and tomato (vegetables) on foccacia bread (grains) completes three section of MyPlate and provides a good source of protein. Which sections are missing?

6.3 Protein in Foods

Of the typical foods we eat, about 70% of our protein comes from animal sources (Fig. 6-4). The most nutrient-dense source of protein is water-packed tuna, which has 87% of calories as protein (Fig. 6-5). The top five contributors of protein to the North

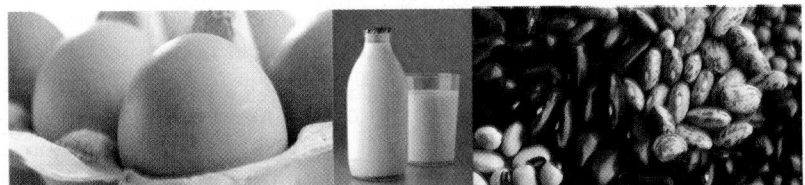

MyPlate:
Sources of Protein

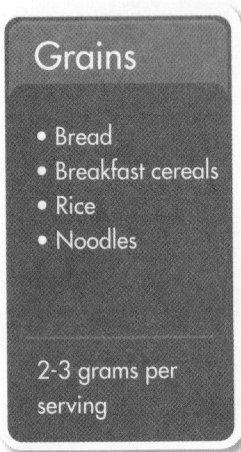
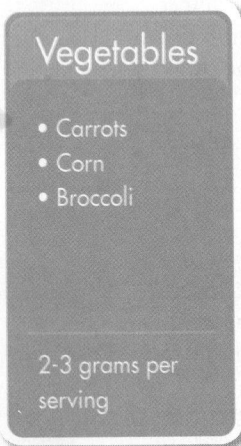
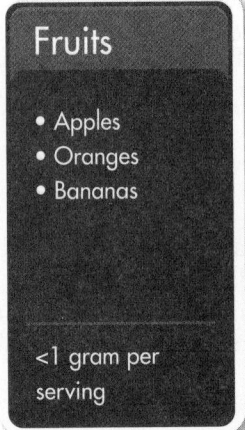
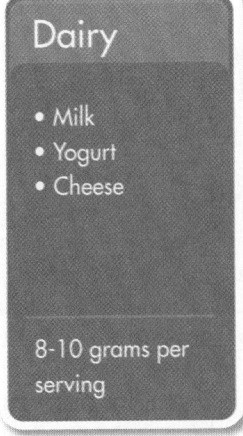
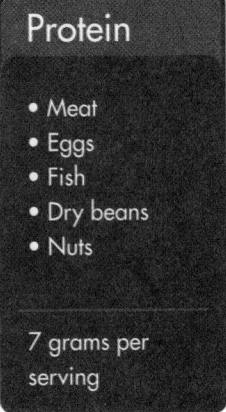

Grains
- Bread
- Breakfast cereals
- Rice
- Noodles

2-3 grams per serving

Vegetables
- Carrots
- Corn
- Broccoli

2-3 grams per serving

Fruits
- Apples
- Oranges
- Bananas

<1 gram per serving

Dairy
- Milk
- Yogurt
- Cheese

8-10 grams per serving

Protein
- Meat
- Eggs
- Fish
- Dry beans
- Nuts

7 grams per serving

FIGURE 6-4 ▶ Sources of protein from MyPlate. The fill of the background color (none, 1/3, 2/3, or completely covered) within each group on the plate indicates the average nutrient density for protein in that group. Overall, the dairy group and the protein group contain many foods that are nutrient-dense sources of protein. Based on serving sizes listed for MyPlate, the fruits group provides little or no protein (less than 1 gram per serving). Food choices from the vegetables group and grains group provide moderate amounts of protein (2 to 3 grams per serving). The dairy group provides much protein (8 to 10 grams per serving), as does the protein group (7 grams per serving).

leaches the indigestible carbohydrates into the water so they can be disposed. However, intestinal gas is not harmful. In fact, fermentation products of ingestible carbohydrates promote the health of your colon (review Chapter 3 for more information on probiotics and prebiotics).

The impact of plant proteins on health will be discussed in the Nutrition and Your Health section at the end of this chapter.

MAKING DECISIONS

Soy and Nut Allergies

For some of us, food allergies from soy, peanuts and tree nuts (e.g., almonds and walnuts), and wheat are a concern. Overall, food allergies occur in up to 8% of children 4 years of age or younger and in up to 2% of adults. Eight foods account for 90% of food-related allergies; soy, peanuts, tree nuts, and wheat are four of these foods (see Further Reading 11). (The other foods are milk, egg, fish, and shellfish.) The allergic reactions can range from a mild intolerance to fatal allergic reactions (see Nutrition and Your Health in Chapter 15 for details). For prevention of food allergies, exclusive breastfeeding for the first six months of life is the best strategy. Although experts no longer recommend delaying introduction of potentially allergenic foods past six months of age, for those people with allergies to specific proteins, such as wheat, soy, peanuts, and tree nuts, strict avoidance of these foods is the only proven treatment.

In sum, plant proteins are a nutritious alternative to animal proteins. They are inexpensive, versatile, tasty, add color to your plate, and benefit health beyond their contribution of protein to the diet. Simply adding these foods to your diet can lead to weight gain, but learning to substitute plant proteins in place of other less healthy foods is one way to reduce your risk for many diseases. Watch for news about additional research progress into this area.

6.4 Protein Digestion and Absorption

As with carbohydrate digestion, protein digestion begins with the cooking of food. Cooking unfolds (denatures) proteins (Fig. 6-7) and softens tough connective tissue in meat. Cooking also makes many protein-rich foods easier to chew and swallow and facilitates their breakdown during later digestion and absorption. As you will see in Chapter 13, cooking also makes many protein-rich foods, such as meats, eggs, fish, and poultry, much safer to eat.

Digestion

The enzymatic digestion of protein begins in the stomach (Fig. 6-8). Proteins are first denatured by stomach acid. **Pepsin,** a major stomach enzyme for digesting proteins, then goes to work on the unraveled polypeptide chains. Pepsin breaks the polypeptide into shorter chains of amino acids because it can break only a few of the many peptide bonds found in these large molecules. The release of pepsin is controlled by the hormone gastrin. Thinking about food or chewing food stimulates gastrin release in the stomach. Gastrin also strongly stimulates the stomach to produce acid.

The partially digested proteins move from the stomach into the small intestine along with the rest of the nutrients and other substances in a meal (chyme). Once in the small intestine, the partially digested proteins (and any fats accompanying them) trigger the release of the hormone cholecystokinin (CCK) from the walls of the small intestine. CCK, in turn, travels through the bloodstream to the pancreas where it causes the pancreas to release protein-splitting enzymes, such as **trypsin.** These digestive enzymes further divide the chains of amino acids into segments of two to three amino acids and some individual amino acids. Eventually, this mixture is digested

See Nutrition and Your Health: Vegetarian and Plant-Based Diets at the end of Chapter 6.

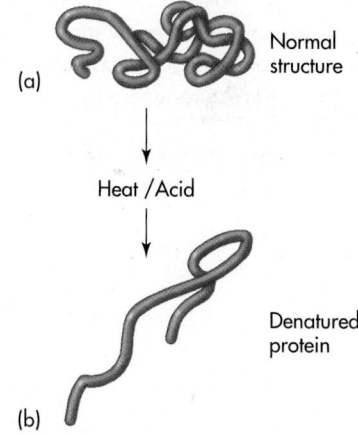

FIGURE 6-7 ▶ Denaturation. (a) Protein showing typical coiled state. (b) Protein is now partly uncoiled. This uncoiling can reduce biological activity and allow digestive enzymes to act on peptide bonds.

pepsin A protein-digesting enzyme produced by the stomach.

trypsin A protein-digesting enzyme secreted by the pancreas to act in the small intestine.

into amino acids, using other enzymes from the lining of the small intestine and enzymes present in the absorptive cells themselves.

Absorption

The short chains of amino acids and any individual amino acids in the small intestine are taken up by active transport into the absorptive cells lining the small intestine. Any remaining peptide bonds are broken down to yield individual amino acids inside the intestinal cells. They are water-soluble, so the amino acids travel to the liver via the portal vein, which drains absorbed nutrients from the intestinal tract. In the liver, individual amino acids can undergo several modifications, depending on the needs of the body. Individual amino acids may be combined into the proteins needed by the body; broken down for energy needs; released into the bloodstream; or converted to nonessential amino acids, glucose, or fat. With excess protein intake, amino acids are converted to fat as a last resort.

Except during infancy, it is uncommon for intact proteins to be absorbed from the digestive tract. In infants up to 4 to 5 months of age, the gastrointestinal tract is somewhat permeable to small proteins, so some whole proteins can be absorbed. Because proteins from some foods (e.g., cow's milk and egg whites) may predispose an infant to food allergies, pediatricians and registered dietitians recommend waiting until an infant is at least 6 to 12 months of age before introducing commonly allergenic foods (see Chapter 15 for details).

FIGURE 6-8 ▶ A summary of protein digestion and absorption. Enzymatic protein digestion begins in the stomach and ends in the absorptive cells of the small intestine, where any remaining short groupings of amino acids are broken down into single amino acids. Stomach acid and enzymes contribute to protein digestion. Absorption from the intestinal lumen into the absorptive cells requires energy input.

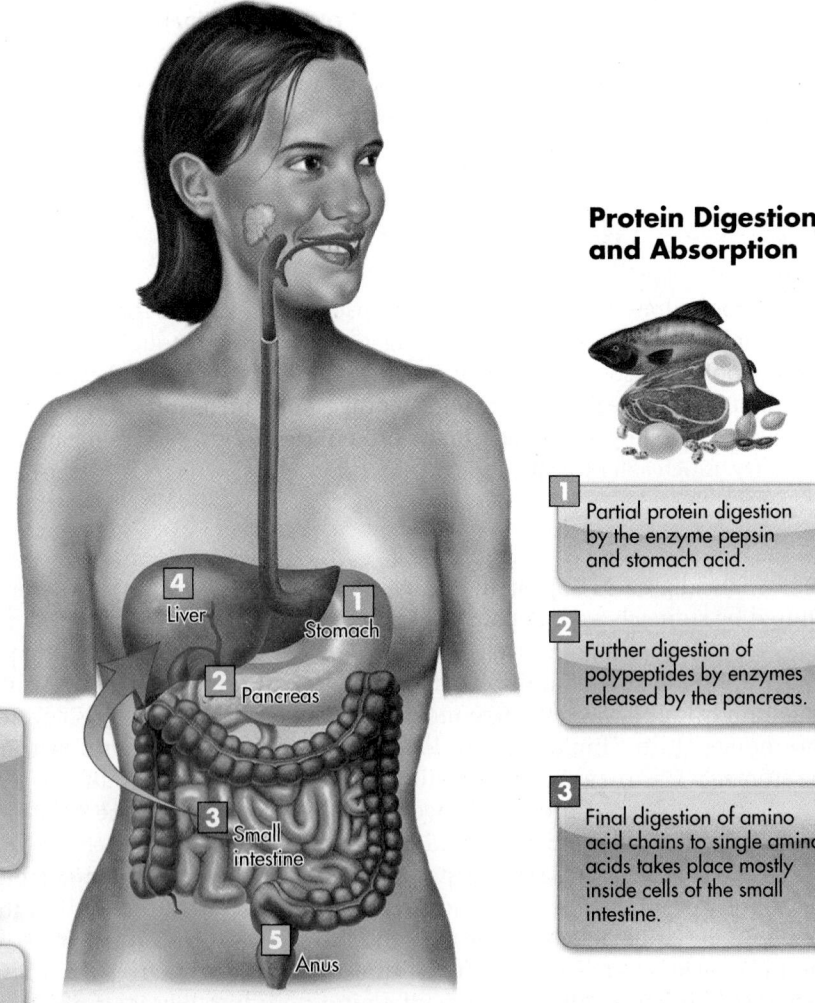

Protein Digestion and Absorption

1 Partial protein digestion by the enzyme pepsin and stomach acid.

2 Further digestion of polypeptides by enzymes released by the pancreas.

3 Final digestion of amino acid chains to single amino acids takes place mostly inside cells of the small intestine.

4 Liver 1 Stomach

2 Pancreas

4 Amino acids absorbed into the portal vein and transported to the liver. From there they enter the general bloodstream.

3 Small intestine

5 Anus

5 Little dietary protein is present in feces.

CONCEPT CHECK

Protein digestion begins with cooking, as proteins are denatured by heat. Once protein reaches the stomach, enzymes cleave proteins into smaller segments of amino acids. As food travels through the small intestine, protein breakdown products formed in the stomach are broken down further to individual amino acids or short segments of amino acids and taken up into the absorptive cells of the small intestine where final breakdown into amino acids occurs. The amino acids then travel to the liver via the portal vein.

6.5 Putting Proteins to Work in the Body

Proteins function in many crucial ways in human metabolism and in the formation of body structures. We rely on foods to supply the amino acids needed to form these proteins. However, only when we also eat enough carbohydrate and fat can food proteins be used most efficiently. If we don't consume enough calories to meet needs, some amino acids from proteins are broken down to produce energy, rendering them unavailable to build body proteins.

Producing Vital Body Structures

Every cell contains protein. Muscles, connective tissue, mucus, blood-clotting factors, transport proteins in the bloodstream, lipoproteins, enzymes, immune antibodies, some hormones, visual pigments, and the support structure inside bones are primarily made of protein. Excess protein in the diet doesn't enhance the synthesis of these body components, but eating too little protein can prevent it.

Most vital body proteins are in a constant state of breakdown, rebuilding, and repair. For example, the intestinal tract lining is constantly sloughed off. The digestive tract treats sloughed cells just like food particles, digesting them and absorbing their amino acids. In fact, most of the amino acids released throughout the body can be recycled to become part of the pool of amino acids available for synthesis of future proteins. Overall, **protein turnover** is a process by which a cell can respond to its changing environment by producing proteins that are needed and disassembling proteins that are not needed.

During any day, an adult makes and degrades about 250 grams of protein, recycling many of the amino acids. Relative to the 65 to 100 grams of protein typically consumed by adults in North America, recycled amino acids make an important contribution to total protein metabolism.

If a person's diet is low in protein for a long period, the processes of rebuilding and repairing body proteins will slow down. Over time, skeletal muscles; blood proteins; and vital organs, such as the heart and liver, will decrease in size or volume. Only the brain resists protein breakdown.

Maintaining Fluid Balance

Blood proteins help maintain body fluid balance. Normal blood pressure in the arteries forces blood into capillary beds. The blood fluid then moves from the **capillary beds** into the spaces between nearby cells (**extracellular spaces**) to provide nutrients to those cells (Fig. 6-9). Proteins in the bloodstream are too large however, to move out of the capillary beds into the tissues. The presence of these proteins in the capillary beds attracts the proper amount of fluid back to the blood, partially counteracting the force of blood pressure.

With an inadequate consumption of protein, the concentration of proteins in the bloodstream drops below normal. Excessive fluid then builds up in the surrounding tissues because the counteracting force produced by the smaller amount of blood proteins is too weak to pull enough of the fluid back from the tissues into the bloodstream. As

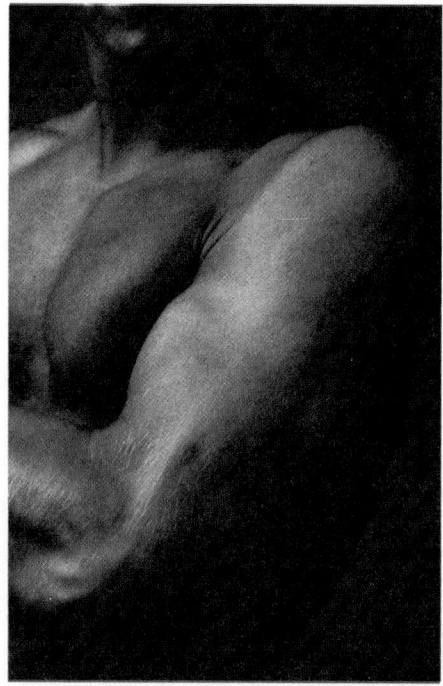

▲ Protein contributes to the structure and function of muscle.

protein turnover The process by which cells break down old proteins and resynthesize new proteins. In this way the cell will have the proteins it needs to function at that time.

capillary bed Network of one-cell-thick vessels that create a junction between arterial and venous circulation. It is here that gas and nutrient exchange occurs between body cells and the blood.

extracellular space The space outside cells; represents one-third of body fluid.

FIGURE 6-9 ▶ Blood proteins in relation to fluid balance. (a) Blood proteins are important for maintaining the body's fluid balance. (b) Without sufficient protein in the bloodstream, edema develops.

Arterial end of a capillary bed

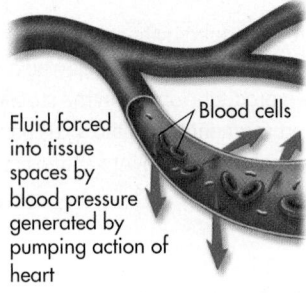

Fluid forced into tissue spaces by blood pressure generated by pumping action of heart

Blood cells

(a)

Venous end of a capillary bed

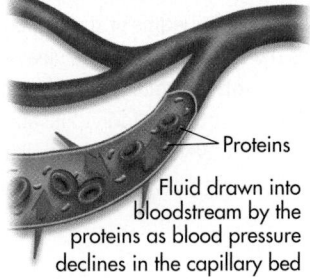

Proteins

Fluid drawn into bloodstream by the proteins as blood pressure declines in the capillary bed

Normal tissue

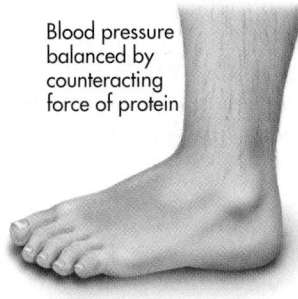

Blood pressure balanced by counteracting force of protein

Swollen tissue (edema)

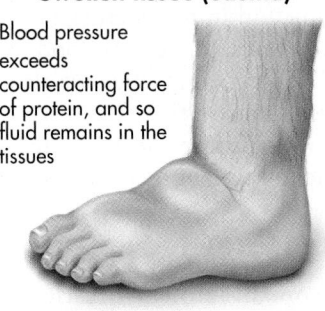

Blood pressure exceeds counteracting force of protein, and so fluid remains in the tissues

(b)

edema The buildup of excess fluid in extracellular spaces.

buffers Compounds that cause a solution to resist changes in acid-base conditions.

Neurotransmitters, released by nerve endings, are often derivatives of amino acids. This is true for dopamine and norepinephrine (both synthesized from the amino-acid tyrosine), and serotonin (synthesized from the amino-acid tryptophan).

The vitamin niacin can be made from the amino-acid tryptophan, illustrating another role of proteins.

fluids accumulate in the tissues, the tissues swell, causing **edema.** Edema may be a symptom of a variety of medical problems, so its cause must be identified. An important step in diagnosing the cause is to measure the concentration of blood proteins.

Contributing to Acid-Base Balance

Proteins help regulate acid-base balance in the blood. Proteins located in cell membranes pump chemical ions in and out of cells. The ion concentration that results from the pumping action, among other factors, keeps the blood slightly alkaline. In addition, some blood proteins are especially good **buffers** for the body. Buffers are compounds that maintain acid-base conditions within a narrow range.

Forming Hormones and Enzymes

Amino acids are required for the synthesis of many hormones—our internal body messengers. Some hormones, such as the thyroid hormones, are made from only one type of amino acid, tyrosine. Insulin, on the other hand, is a hormone composed of 51 total amino acids. Almost all enzymes are proteins or have a protein component.

Contributing to Immune Function

Proteins are a key component of the cells within the immune system. An example is the antibodies, proteins produced by one type of white blood cell. These antibodies can bind to foreign proteins in the body, an important step in removing invaders from the body. Without sufficient dietary protein, the immune system lacks the materials needed to function properly. For example, a low protein status can turn measles into a fatal disease for a malnourished child.

Forming Glucose

In Chapter 4 you learned that the body must maintain a fairly constant concentration of blood glucose to supply energy for the brain, red blood cells, and nervous tissue. At rest, the brain uses about 19% of the body's energy requirements, and it gets most

PROTEIN CONCEPT MAP

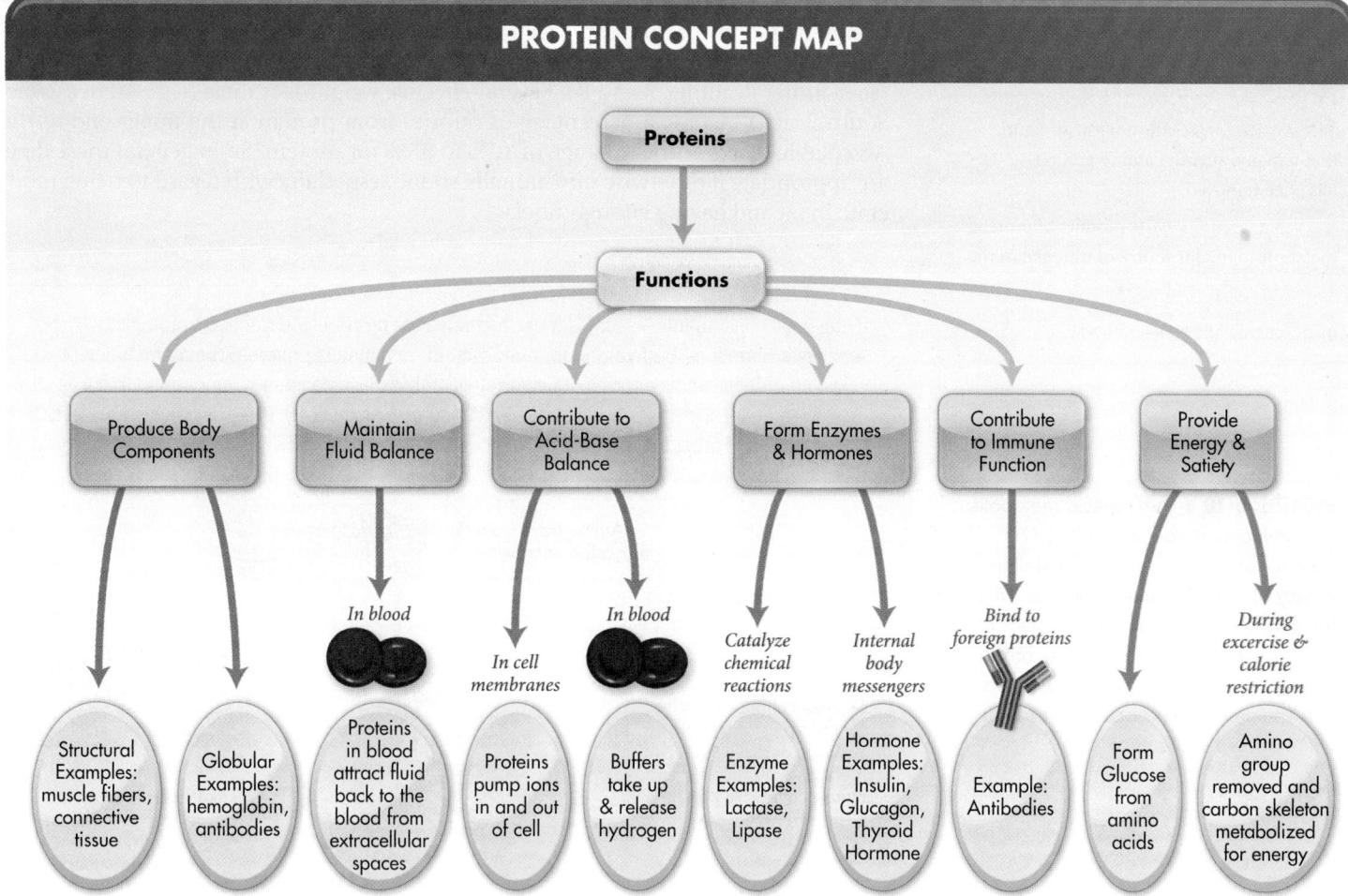

of that energy from glucose. If you don't consume enough carbohydrate to supply the glucose, your liver (and kidneys, to a lesser extent) will be forced to make glucose from amino acids present in body tissues (Fig. 6-10).

Making some glucose from amino acids is normal. For example, when you skip breakfast and haven't eaten since 7 P.M. the preceding evening, glucose must be manufactured. In an extreme situation, however, such as in starvation, amino acids from muscle tissue are converted into glucose, which wastes muscle tissue and can produce edema.

Providing Energy

Proteins supply little energy for a weight-stable person. Two situations in which a person does use protein to meet energy needs are during prolonged exercise (see Chapter 10 for information about the use of amino acids for energy needs during exercise) and during calorie restriction, as with a weight-loss diet. In these cases, the amino group ($-NH_2$) from the amino acid is removed and the remaining carbon skeleton is metabolized for energy needs (Fig. 6-10). Still, under most conditions, cells primarily use fats and carbohydrates for energy needs. Although proteins contain the same amount of calories (on average, 4 kcal per gram) as carbohydrates, proteins are a costly source of calories, considering the amount of processing the liver and kidneys must perform to use this calorie source.

Contributing to Satiety

Compared to the other macronutrients, proteins provide the highest feeling of **satiety** after a meal. Thus, including some protein with each meal helps control overall

satiety A state in which there is no longer a desire to eat; a feeling of satisfaction.

pool The amount of a nutrient stored within the body that can be mobilized when needed.

carbon skeleton Amino-acid structure that remains after the amino group (—NH$_2$) has been removed.

urea Nitrogenous waste product of protein metabolism; major source of nitrogen in the urine, chemically NH$_2$—C—NH$_2$.

food intake. Many experts warn against skimping on protein when trying to reduce energy intake to lose weight. Meeting protein needs is still important and exceeding needs somewhat may provide an additional benefit when dieting to lose weight (see Further Readings 7 and 8). Several effective weight-loss diets (e.g., Atkins, Zone, South Beach) include a percentage of calories from protein at the upper end of the Acceptable Macronutrient Range of 10% to 35% for protein. So in general these diets are appropriate if otherwise nutritionally sound, especially with regard to being moderate in fat and having enough fiber.

CONCEPT CHECK

Vital body constituents—such as muscle, connective tissue, blood transport proteins, enzymes, hormones, buffers, and immune factors—are mainly proteins. The degradation of existing proteins and synthesis of new proteins takes place constantly, amounting to a turnover rate of about 250 grams a day for the entire human body. Proteins can also be used for glucose and other fuel production and contributes to satiety.

FIGURE 6-10 ▶ Amino-acid metabolism. The amino-acid **pool** in a cell can be used to form body proteins, as well as a variety of other possible products. When the **carbon skeletons** of amino acids are metabolized to produce glucose or fat, ammonia (NH$_3$) is a resulting waste product. The ammonia is converted to **urea** and excreted in the urine.

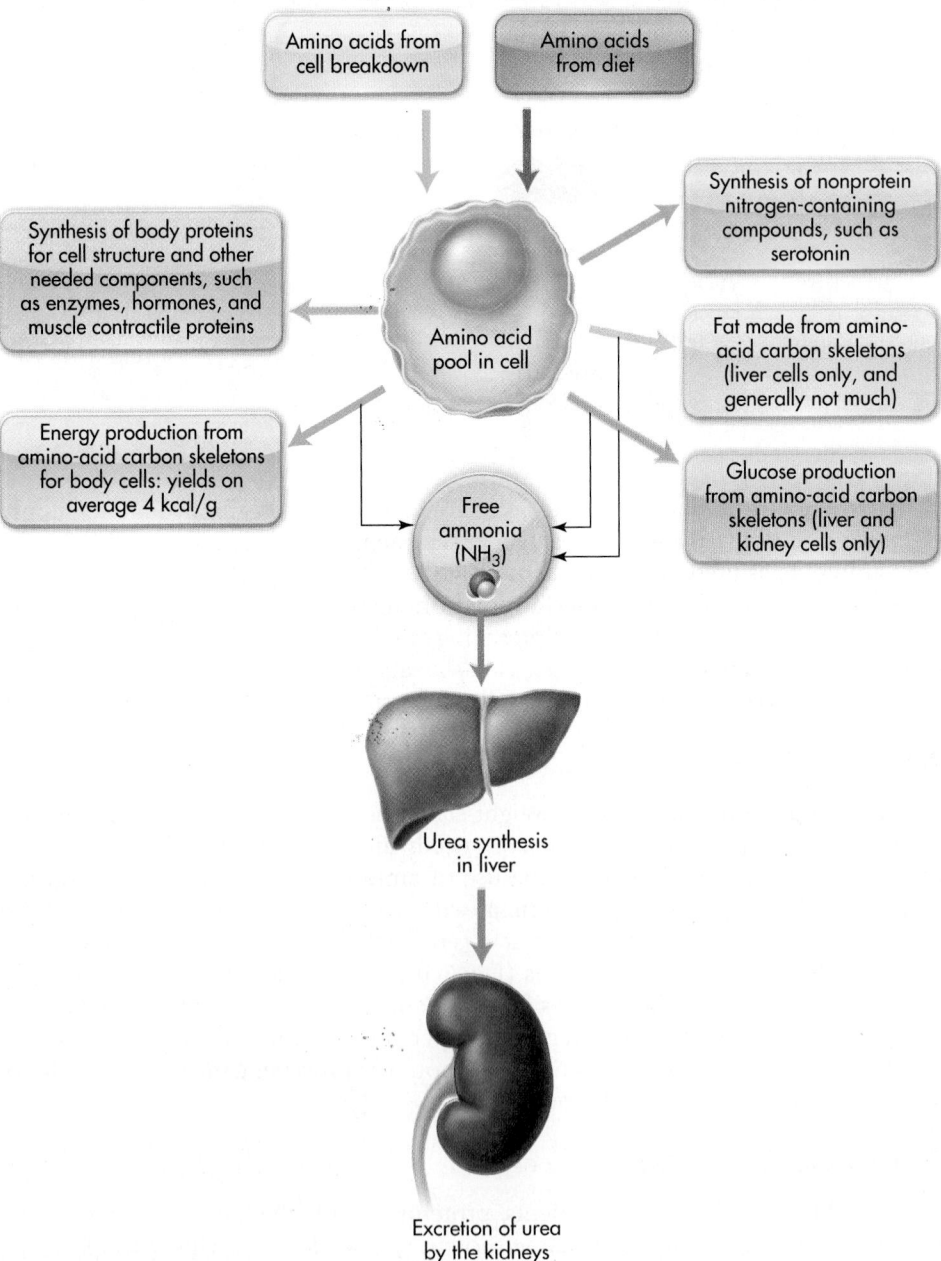

6.6 Protein Needs

How much protein (actually, amino acids) do we need to eat each day? People who aren't growing need to eat only enough protein to match whatever they lose daily from protein breakdown. The amount of breakdown can be determined by measuring the amount of urea and other nitrogen-containing compounds in the urine, as well as losses of protein from feces, skin, hair, nails, and so on. In short, people need to balance protein intake with such losses to maintain a state of **protein equilibrium,** also called *protein balance* (Fig. 6-11).

When a body is growing or recovering from an illness or injury, it needs a **positive protein balance** to supply the raw materials required to build new tissues. To achieve this, a person must eat more protein daily than he or she loses. In addition, the hormones insulin, growth hormone, and testosterone all stimulate positive protein balance. Resistance exercise (weight training) also enhances positive protein balance. Consuming less protein than needed leads to **negative protein balance,** such as when acute illness reduces the desire to eat and so one loses more protein than consumed.

For healthy people, the amount of dietary protein needed to maintain protein equilibrium (wherein intake equals losses) can be determined by increasing protein intake until it equals losses of protein and its related breakdown products (e.g., urea). Calorie needs must also be met so that amino acids are not diverted for such use.

Today, the best estimate for the amount of protein required for nearly all adults to maintain protein equilibrium is 0.8 grams of protein per kilogram of healthy

protein equilibrium A state in which protein intake is equal to related protein losses; the person is said to be in protein balance.

positive protein balance A state in which protein intake exceeds related protein losses, as is needed during times of growth.

negative protein balance A state in which protein intake is less than related protein losses, as is often seen during acute illness.

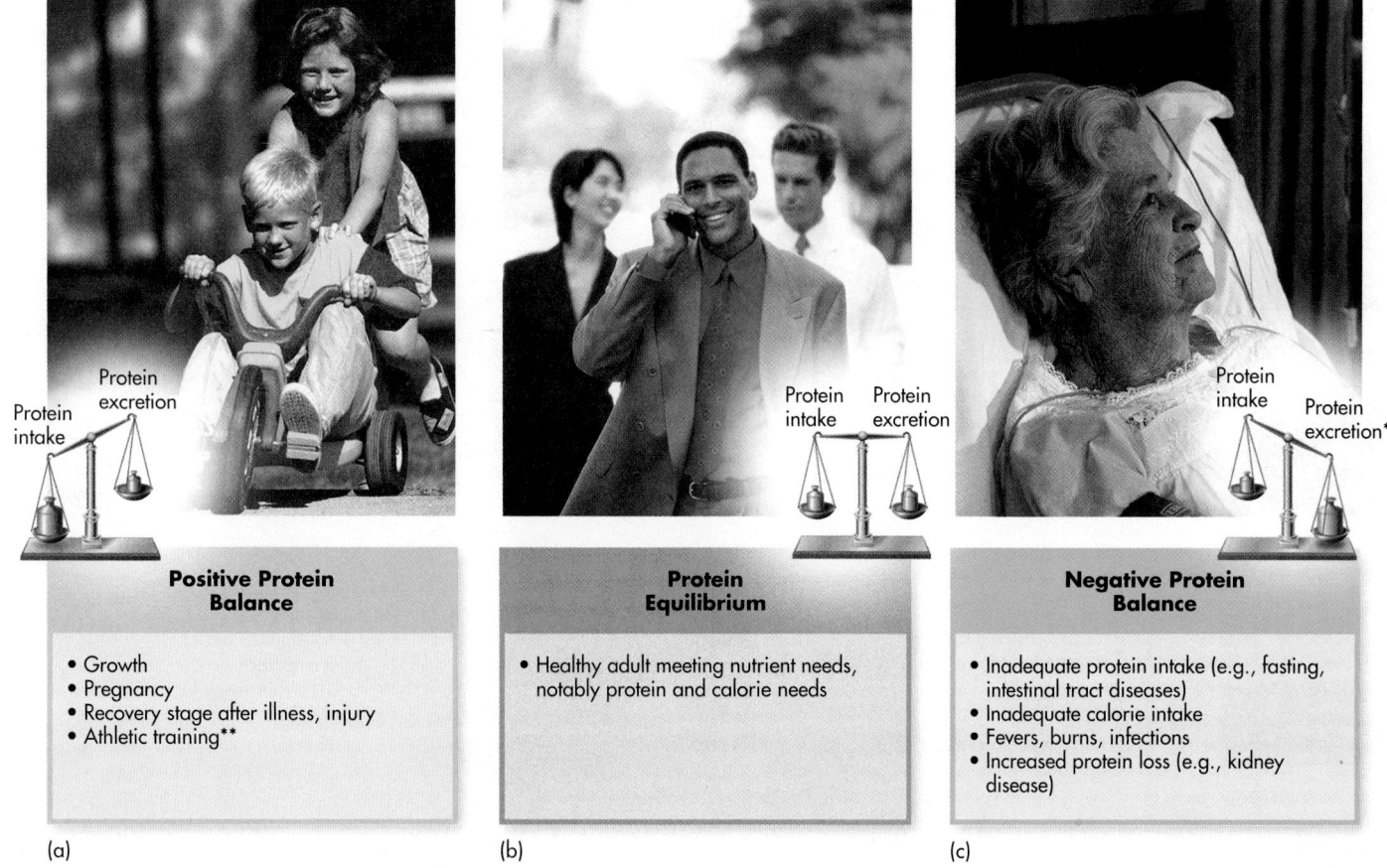

Positive Protein Balance
• Growth
• Pregnancy
• Recovery stage after illness, injury
• Athletic training**

Protein Equilibrium
• Healthy adult meeting nutrient needs, notably protein and calorie needs

Negative Protein Balance
• Inadequate protein intake (e.g., fasting, intestinal tract diseases)
• Inadequate calorie intake
• Fevers, burns, infections
• Increased protein loss (e.g., kidney disease)

(a) (b) (c)

*Based on losses of urea and other nitrogen-containing compounds in the urine, as well as protein lost from feces, skin, hair, nails, and other minor routes.
**Only when additional lean body mass is being gained. Nevertheless, the athlete is probably already eating enough protein to support this extra protein synthesis; protein supplements are not needed.

FIGURE 6-11 ▶ Protein balance in practical terms: (a) positive protein balance; (b) protein equilibrium; (c) negative protein balance.

The 2010 Dietary Guidlines for Americans in "**Food and Nutrients to Increase**," provide the following recommendatins regarding protein intake as part of healthy eating pattern and while staying within their calorie needs:

- Increase intake of fat-free or low-fat milk and milk product, such as milk, yogurt, cheese, or fortified soy beverages.
- Choose a variety of protein foods, which include seafood, lean meat and poultry, eggs, beans and peas, soy products, and unsalted nuts and seeds.
- Increase the amount and variety of seafood consumed by choosing seafood in place of some meat and poultry.
- Replace protein foods that are higher in solid fats with choices that are lower in solid fats and calories and/or are sources of oils.

body weight. This is the RDA for protein. Requirements are higher during periods of growth, such as pregnancy and infancy (see Chapters 14 and 15 for specific values for pregnant women, infants, and children). Healthy weight is used as a reference in the determination of protein needs because excess fat storage doesn't contribute much to protein needs (see Chapter 7 for insight into the concept of healthy weight). Calculations using this RDA are shown in the margin and estimate a requirement of about 56 grams of protein daily for a typical 70-kilogram (154-pound) man and about 46 grams of protein daily for a typical 57-kilogram (125-pound) woman.

The RDA for protein translates into about 10% of total calories. Many experts recommend up to 15% of total calories to provide more flexibility in diet planning, in turn allowing for the variety of protein-rich foods North Americans typically consume. Protein-rich foods are also part of the "Food and Nutrients to increase" in the 2010 Dietary Guidelines. As noted earlier, the Food and Nutrition Board has set an upper range for protein intake at 35% of calories consumed. It is easy to meet currently suggested daily protein needs (Table 6-2). On a daily basis, typical North American protein intakes are about 100 grams of protein for men and 65 grams for women. Thus, most of us consume much more protein than the RDA recommends because we like many high-protein foods and can afford to buy them. Our bodies cannot store excess protein once it is consumed, so the excess amino acids are converted to carbon skeletons that are turned into glucose or fat and then stored as fat or metabolized for energy needs (review Fig. 6-10).

TABLE 6-2 Protein Content of Sample Menus Containing 1600 kcal and 2000 kcal

Menu	1600 kcal		2000 kcal	
	Serving Size	Protein (g)	Serving Size	Protein (g)
Breakfast				
Low-fat granola	²⁄₃ cup	5	²⁄₃ cup	5
Blueberries	1 cup	1	1 cup	1
Fat-free (skim) milk	1 cup	8.5	1 cup	8.5
Coffee	1 cup	0	1 cup	0
Lunch				
Broiled chicken breast	3 oz	25	4 oz	33
Salad greens	3 cups	5	3 cups	5
Baked taco shell strips	½ cup	2	½ cup	2
Low-fat salad dressing	2 tbsp	0	2 tbsp	0
Fat-free (skim) milk	1 cup	8.5	1 cup	8.5
Dinner				
Yellow rice	1¼ cups	5	2½ cups	10
Shrimp	4 large	5	6 large	7
Mussels	4 medium	8	6 medium	12
Clams	5 small	12	10 small	24
Peas	¼ cup	4	½ cup	4
Sweet red pepper	¼ cup	0	½ cup	0
Snack				
Muffin	1 small	4	1 small	4
Swiss cheese	1 oz	7.5	1 oz	7.5
Banana	½ small	0.5	½ small	0.5
Total		101		132

Mental stress, physical labor, and recreational weekend sports activities do not require an increase in the protein RDA. For some highly trained athletes, such as those participating in endurance or strength training, protein consumption may need to exceed the RDA. This is an area of debate in sports nutrition: the Food and Nutrition Board does not support an increased need, but some experts suggest an increase to about 1.7 grams per kilogram. Many North Americans already consume that much protein, especially men.

6.7 Does Eating a High-Protein Diet Harm You?

People frequently ask about the potential harm of protein intakes in excess of the RDA. Problems with diets that are high in protein foods primarily stem from the fact that they typically rely on animal sources of protein. Diets rich in animal products will most likely be simultaneously low in the beneficial substances found in plant sources, including fiber, some vitamins (e.g., folate), some minerals (e.g., magnesium), as well as phytochemicals, and high in substances such as saturated fat and cholesterol. A high animal-protein diet, therefore, is unlikely to follow the recommendations of the Dietary Guidelines for Americans or the Food and Nutrition Board in terms of reducing risk for cardiovascular disease.

Some, but not all, studies show that high-protein diets can increase calcium losses in urine. For people with adequate calcium intakes, little concern about this relationship is warranted, but keep in mind that calcium is commonly deficient in North American diets.

Meat is one of the richest sources of protein. Excessive intake of red meat, however, especially processed forms, is linked to colon cancer in population studies (see Further Reading 3). This association is still being studied (see Newsworthy Nutrition in margin), and there are several possible explanations for this connection. The curing agents used to process meats such as ham and salami may cause cancer. Substances that form during cooking of red meat at high temperatures may also cause cancer. The excessive fat or low-fiber contents of diets rich in red meat may also be a contributing factor. Because of these concerns, some nutrition experts suggest we focus more on poultry, fish, nuts, legumes, and seeds to meet protein needs. In addition, any red or other type of meat should be trimmed of all visible fat before grilling.

Some researchers have expressed concern that a high-protein intake may overburden the kidneys by forcing them to excrete the extra nitrogen as urea. Additionally, animal proteins may contribute to kidney stone formation in certain individuals. There is some support for limiting protein intake for people in the early stages of kidney disease, because low-protein diets somewhat slow the decline in kidney function. Laboratory animal studies show that moderate protein intakes that just meet nutritional needs preserve kidney function over time better than high-protein diets. Preserving kidney function is especially important for those who have diabetes, early signs of kidney disease, or only one functioning kidney, so a high-protein diet is not recommended for these people. High-protein diets increase urine output, in turn posing a risk for dehydration. This is a special concern for athletes (see Chapter 10).

Convert weight from pounds to kilograms:	154 pounds
	2.2 pounds/kilogram
	= 70 kilograms
	125 pounds
	2.2 pounds/kilogram
	= 57 kilograms

Calculate protein RDA:

$$70 \text{ kilograms} \times \frac{0.8 \text{ grams protein}}{\text{kilogram body weight}}$$
$$= 56 \text{ grams}$$

$$57 \text{ kilograms} \times \frac{0.8 \text{ grams protein}}{\text{kilogram body weight}}$$
$$= 46 \text{ grams}$$

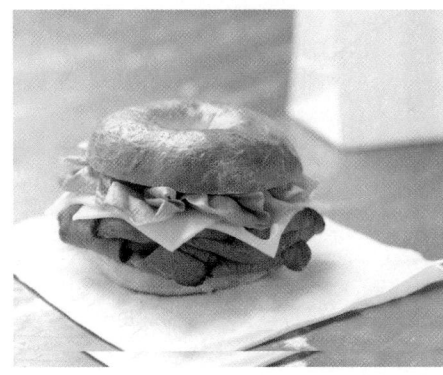

▲ Animal protein foods, such as the roast beef and swiss cheese on this bagel, are typically our main sources of protein in the North American diet.

NEWSWORTHY NUTRITION | Link between colon cancer and recent fat, protein, and red meat consumption not supported

The risk of distal colorectal cancer and the consumption of fat, protein, and red and processed meat was determined in whites and African-Americans. The diet was assessed for the previous 12 months in the 945 cases of colon cancer and 959 controls. No association was found between total, saturated, or monounsaturated fat intake and colon cancer risk; the percentages of calories from protein and red meat intake were both associated with a reduction (rather than increase) in risk of colon cancer, in whites. Although these results do not support the general hypotheses that fat, protein and red meat increase the risk of colon cancer, we must remember that the diet was only measured for 12 months prior to the study. A more long-term effect of these dietary factors, therefore, cannot be ruled out.

Source: Williams CD and others: Associations of red meat, fat, and protein intake with distal colorectal cancer risk. *Nutrition and Cancer* 62(6): 701, 2010 (see Further Reading 14).

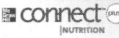 Check out the Connect site www.mcgrawhillconnect .com to further explore diet and colorectal cancer.

MAKING DECISIONS

Amino-Acid Supplements

Protein and amino-acid supplements are used primarily by athletes and dieters. Athletes use them hoping they will help build muscle. The branched-chain amino acids described earlier are especially popular with athletes looking to enhance their performance. Dieters have turned to these supplements hoping they will increase their weight loss. Although the right amount of protein in the diet will aid athletic performance and help in weight control, consuming this protein in the form of amino-acid supplements cannot be considered safe.

Earlier in this chapter, you learned that the body is designed to handle whole proteins as a dietary source of amino acids. When individual amino-acid supplements are taken, they can overwhelm the absorptive mechanisms in the small intestine, triggering amino-acid imbalances in the body. Imbalances occur because groups of chemically similar amino acids compete for absorption sites in the absorptive cells. For example, lysine and arginine are absorbed by the same transporter, so an excess of lysine can impair absorption of arginine. The amino acids most likely to cause toxicity when consumed in large amounts are methionine, cysteine, and histidine. Due to the potential for imbalances and toxicities of individual amino acids, the best advice to ensure adequacy is to stick to whole foods rather than supplements as sources of amino acids. Amino acids as such also have a disagreeable odor and flavor and are also much more expensive than food protein. In Canada the sale of individual amino acids to consumers is banned. Read more about this issue in the What Would You Choose Recommendations at the end of this chapter.

CONCEPT CHECK

The Recommended Dietary Allowance (RDA) for adults is 0.8 grams of protein per kilogram of healthy body weight. This is approximately 56 grams of protein daily for a 70-kilogram (156-pound) person. The average North American man consumes about 100 grams of protein daily, and a woman consumes about 65 grams. Thus, typically we eat more than enough protein to meet our needs. This even includes well-balanced vegetarian diets. Diets high in protein can compromise kidney health in people with diabetes and those with kidney disease, and animal protein sources likely increase cardiovascular disease and kidney stone risk when consumed in high amounts.

6.8 Protein-Calorie Malnutrition

protein-calorie malnutrition (PCM) A condition resulting from regularly consuming insufficient amounts of calories and protein. The deficiency eventually results in body wasting, primarily of lean tissue, and an increased susceptibility to infections.

kwashiorkor A disease occurring primarily in young children who have an existing disease and consume a marginal amount of calories and insufficient protein in relation to needs. The child generally suffers from infections and exhibits edema, poor growth, weakness, and an increased susceptibility to further illness.

marasmus A disease resulting from consuming a grossly insufficient amount of protein and calories; one of the diseases classed as protein-calorie malnutrition. Victims have little or no fat stores, little muscle mass, and poor strength. Death from infections is common.

Protein deficiency is rarely an isolated condition and usually accompanies a deficiency of calories and other nutrients resulting from insufficient food intake. In the developed world, alcoholism can lead to cases of protein deficiency because of the low protein content of alcoholic beverages. Protein and calorie malnutrition is a significant problem in hospitals worldwide, affecting patients of all ages from infants to geriatric patients. Malnutrition can be caused by the illnesses or injuries for which the patients are admitted to the hospital and by the hospitalization itself (see Further Reading 4). In developing areas of the world, people often have diets low in calories and also in protein. This state of undernutrition stunts the growth of children and makes them more susceptible to disease throughout life. (Undernutrition is a main focus of Chapter 12.) People who consume too little protein calories can eventually develop **protein-calorie malnutrition (PCM),** also referred to as *protein-energy malnutrition (PEM).* In its milder form, it is difficult to tell if a person with PCM is consuming too little calories or protein, or both. When an inadequate intake of nutrients, including protein, is combined with an already existing disease, especially an infection, a form of malnutrition called **kwashiorkor** can develop. But if the nutrient deficiency—especially for calories—becomes severe, a deficiency disease called **marasmus** can result. Both conditions are seen primarily in children but also may develop in adults, even in those hospitalized in North America. These two conditions form the tip of the iceberg with respect to states of undernutrition, and symptoms of these two conditions can even be present in the same person (Fig. 6-12).

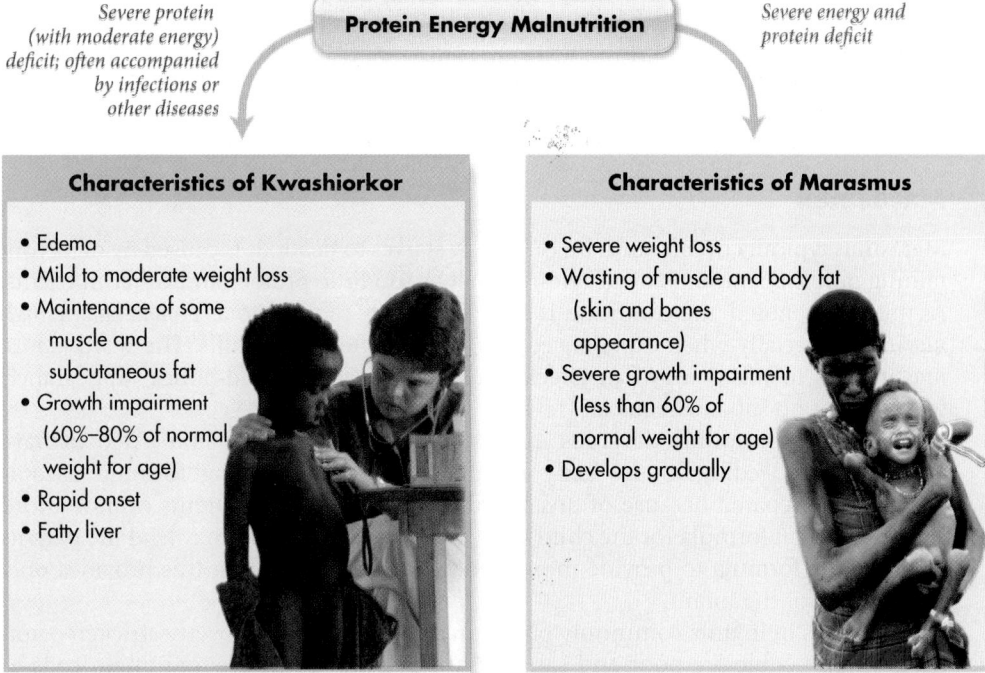

FIGURE 6-12 ▶ Classification of undernutrition in children.

Kwashiorkor

Kwashiorkor is a word from Ghana that means "the disease that the first child gets when the new child comes." From birth, an infant in developing areas of the world is usually breastfed. Often by the time the child reaches 1 to 1.5 years of age, the mother is pregnant or has already given birth again, and the new child gets preference for breastfeeding. The older child's diet then abruptly changes from nutritious human milk to starchy roots and **gruels.** These foods have low-protein densities, compared with total energy. Additionally, the foods are usually full of plant fibers, often bulky, making it difficult for the child to consume enough to meet calorie needs. The child generally also has infections, which acutely raise calorie and protein needs. For these reasons, calorie needs of these children are met just barely, at best, and their protein consumption is grossly inadequate, especially in view of the increased amount needed to combat infections. Many vitamin and mineral needs are also far from being fulfilled. Famine victims face similar problems.

The major symptoms of kwashiorkor are apathy, diarrhea, listlessness, failure to grow and gain weight, and withdrawal from the environment. These symptoms complicate other diseases present. For example, a condition such as measles, a disease that normally makes a healthy child ill for only a week or so, can become severely debilitating and even fatal. Further symptoms of kwashiorkor are changes in hair color, potassium deficiency, flaky skin, fatty liver, reduced muscle mass, and massive edema in the abdomen and legs. The presence of edema in a child who has some subcutaneous fat (i.e., directly under the skin) is the hallmark of kwashiorkor (review Fig. 6-12). In addition, these children seldom move. If you pick them up, they don't cry. When you hold them, you feel the plumpness of edema, not muscle and fat tissue.

Many symptoms of kwashiorkor can be explained based on what we know about proteins. Proteins play important roles in fluid balance, lipoprotein transport, immune function, and production of tissues, such as skin, cells lining the GI tract, and hair. Children with an insufficient protein intake do not grow and mature normally.

If children with kwashiorkor are helped in time—if infections are treated and a diet ample in protein, calories, and other essential nutrients is provided—the disease

gruels A thin mixture of grains or legumes in milk or water.

Toxic products in moldy grains may also contribute to kwashiorkor.

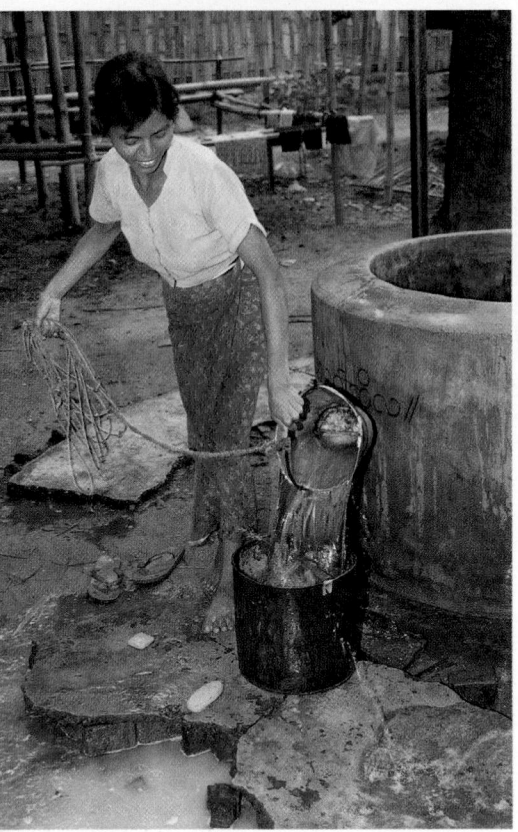

▲ Unsafe water supplies in developing countries contribute to the incidence of marasmus, particularly in bottle-fed infants.

preterm An infant born before 37 weeks of gestation; also referred to as premature.

process reverses. They begin to grow again and may even show no signs of their previous condition, except perhaps shortness of stature. Unfortunately, by the time many of these children reach a hospital or care center, they already have severe infections. Despite the best care, they still die. Or, if they survive, they return home only to become ill again.

Marasmus

Marasmus typically occurs as an infant slowly starves to death. It is caused by diets containing minimal amounts of calories, as well as too little protein and other nutrients. As previously noted, the condition is also commonly referred to as *protein-calorie malnutrition*, especially when experienced by older children and adults. The word *marasmus* means "to waste away," in Greek. Victims have a "skin-and-bones" appearance, with little or no subcutaneous fat (review Fig. 6-12).

Marasmus commonly develops in infants who either are not breastfed or have stopped breastfeeding in the early months. Often the weaning formula used is improperly prepared because of unsafe water and because the parents cannot afford sufficient infant formula for the child's needs. The latter problem may lead the parents to dilute the formula to provide more feedings, not realizing that this provides only more water for the infant.

Marasmus in infants commonly occurs in the large cities of poverty-stricken countries. When people are poor and sanitation is lacking, bottle feeding often leads to marasmus. In the cities, bottle feeding is often necessary because the infant must be cared for by others when the mother is working or away from home. An infant with marasmus requires large amounts of calories and protein—like a **preterm** infant—and, unless the child receives them, full recovery from the disease may never occur. The majority of brain growth occurs between conception and the child's first birthday. In fact, the brain is growing at its highest rate after birth. If the diet does not support brain growth during the first months of life, the brain may not grow to its full adult size. This reduced or retarded brain growth may lead to diminished intellectual function. Both kwashiorkor and marasmus plague infants and children; mortality rates in developing countries are often 10 to 20 times higher than in North America.

CONCEPT CHECK

Most undernutrition consists of mild deficits in calories, protein, and often other nutrients. If a person needs more nutrients because of disease and infection but does not consume enough calories and protein, a condition known as kwashiorkor can develop. The person suffers from edema and weakness. Children around age 2 are especially susceptible to kwashiorkor, particularly if they already have other diseases. Famine situations in which only starchy root products are available to eat contribute to this problem. Marasmus is a condition wherein people—infants, especially—starve to death. Symptoms include muscle wasting, absence of fat stores, and weakness. Both an adequate diet and the treatment of concurrent diseases must be promoted to regain and then maintain nutritional health.

Vegetarian and Plant-Based Diets

Vegetarianism has evolved over the centuries from a necessity into an option. Historically, vegetarianism was linked with specific philosophies and religions or with science. Today, about 1 in 40 adults in the United States (and about 1 in 25 in Canada) is a vegetarian. Vegetarian diets have evolved to include such new products as soy-based sloppy joes, chili, tacos, burgers, and more. In addition, cookbooks that feature the use of a variety of fruits, vegetables, and seasonings are enhancing food selection for vegetarians of all degrees.

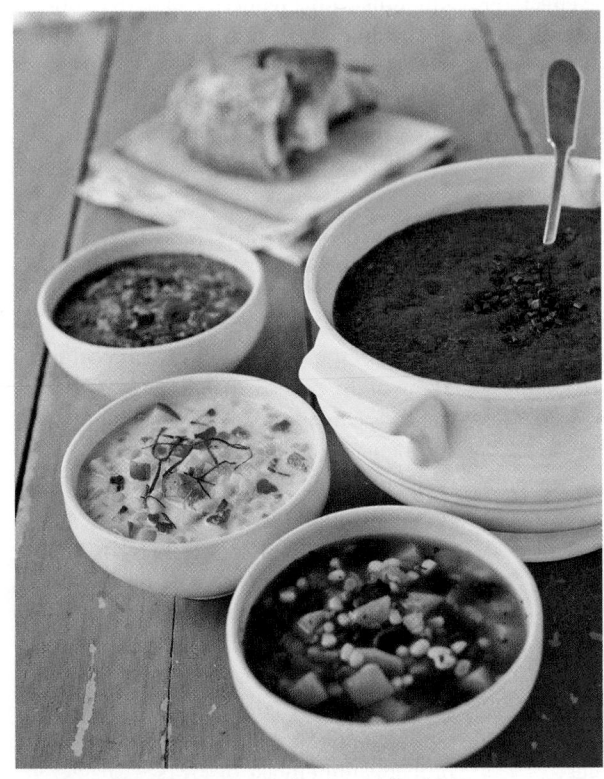

▲ Recipes for vegetarian and plant-based foods are widely available today. Soups are an excellent way to combine complementary plant proteins.

Vegetarianism is popular among college students. Fifteen percent of college students in one survey said they select vegetarian options at lunch or dinner on any given day. In response, dining services offer vegetarian options at every meal, such as pastas with meatless sauce and pizza. Many teenagers are also turning to vegetarianism. Many restaurants offer vegetarian meals in response to the growing number of its customers who want a vegetarian option when they eat out (see Further Reading 13). Many customers cite health and taste as reasons for choosing vegetarian meals.

As nutrition science has grown, new information has enabled the design of nutritionally adequate vegetarian diets. It is important for vegetarians to take advantage of this information because a diet of only plant-based foods has the potential to promote various nutrient deficiencies and substantial growth retardation in infants and children. People who choose a vegetarian diet can meet their nutritional needs by following a few basic rules and knowledgeably planning their diets.

Studies show that death rates from some chronic diseases, such as certain forms of cardiovascular disease, hypertention, many forms of cancer, type 2 diabetes, and obesity, are lower for vegetarians than for non-vegetarians. Vegetarians often live longer, as shown in

religious groups that practice vegetarianism. Other aspects of healthful lifestyles, such as not smoking, abstaining from alcohol and drugs, and regular physical activity often go along with vegetarianism and probably partially account for the lower risks of chronic disease and longer lives seen in this population.

As you learned in Chapter 2, MyPlate and the 2010 Dietary Guidelines for Americans emphasize a plant-based diet of whole-grain breads and cereals, fruits, and vegetables. In addition, the American Institute for Cancer Research promotes "The New American Plate," which includes plant-based foods covering two-thirds (or more) of the plate and meat, fish, poultry, or lowfat dairy covering only one-third (or less) of the plate. Although these recommendations do allow the inclusion of animal products, they are definitely more "vegetarian-like" than typical North American diets.

Why Do People Become Vegetarians?

People choose vegetarianism for a variety of reasons including ethics, religion, economics, and health. Some believe that killing animals for food is unethical. Hindus and Trappist monks eat vegetarian meals as a practice of their religion. In North America, many Seventh Day Adventists base their practice of vegetarianism on biblical texts and believe it is a more healthful way to live.

Some advocates of vegetarianism base their food preference upon the inefficient use of animals as a source of protein. Forty percent of the world's grain production is used to raise meat-producing animals.

The New American Plate

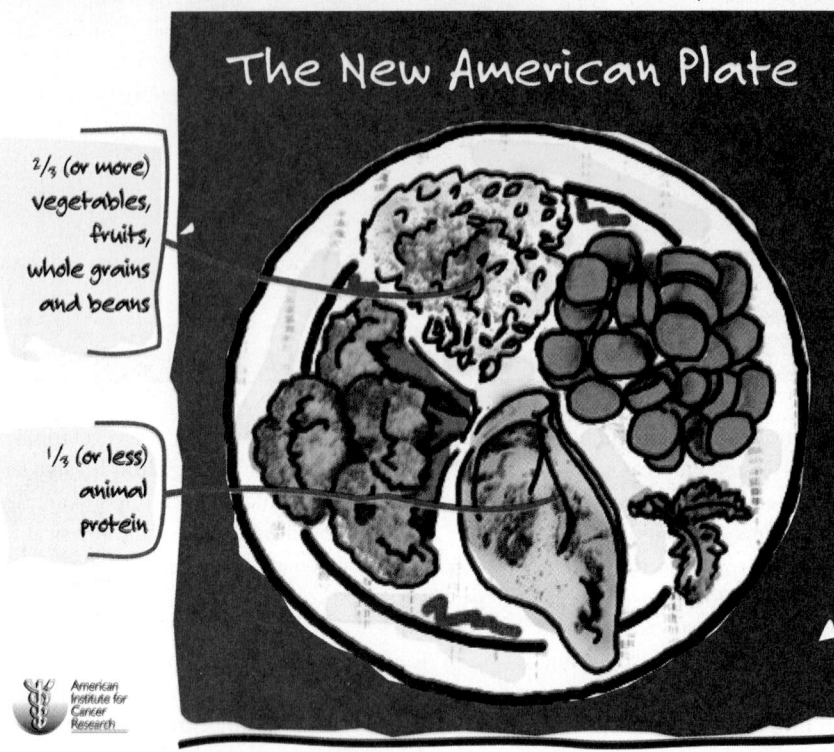

The New American Plate

2/3 (or more) vegetables, fruits, whole grains and beans

1/3 (or less) animal protein

American Institute for Cancer Research

▶ American Institute for Cancer Research Diet and Health Guidelines for Cancer Prevention

1. Choose a diet rich in a variety of plant-based foods.
2. Eat plenty of vegetables and fruit.
3. Maintain a healthy weight and be physically active
4. Drink alcohol only in moderation, if at all.
5. Select foods low in fat and salt.
6. Prepare and store food safely.

And always remember. . .

Do not use tobacco in any form.

▶ "The New American Plate" published by the Amercian Institute for Cancer Research, was a forerunner of and embodies the same concepts as the new ChooseMyPlate program.

Although animals that humans eat sometimes eat grasses that humans cannot digest, many also eat grains that humans can eat.

People might also practice vegetarianism because it limits saturated fat and cholesterol intake, while encouraging a high intake of complex carbohydrates, vitamins A, E, and C, carotenoids, magnesium, and fiber.

Good for Disease Prevention

Plant sources of proteins can positively impact heart health in several ways (see Further Readings 5, 6, 9, and 10). First, the plant foods we eat contain no cholesterol nor *trans* fat and little saturated fat. The major type of fats in plant foods are monounsaturated and polyunsaturated fats. Nuts in particular are high in monounsaturated fat, which helps to keep blood cholesterol low.

Beans and nuts contain soluble fiber, which binds to cholesterol in the small intestine and prevents it from being absorbed by the body. Also, due to the activity of some phytochemicals, foods

made from soybeans can lower production of cholesterol by the body. The effect is modest (about a 2% to 6% drop). In 1999, the Food and Drug Administration allowed health claims for the cholesterol-lowering properties of soy foods, and in 2000, the American Heart Association recommended inclusion of some soy protein in the diets of people with high blood cholesterol. As noted in Chapter 2, to list a health claim for soy on the label, a food product must have at least 6.25 grams of soy protein and less than 3 grams of fat, 1 gram of saturated fat, and 20 milligrams of cholesterol per serving.

There are several other compounds in plant foods under study for their heart-protective roles. Some of the phytochemicals may help to prevent blood clots and relax the blood vessels. Nuts are an especially good source of nutrients implicated in heart health, including vitamin E, folate, magnesium, and copper. Frequent consumption of nuts (about 1 ounce of nuts five times per week) is associated with a decreased risk of cardiovascular disease. Recall from Chapter 2 that FDA

also allows a provisional health claim to link nuts with a reduced risk of developing cardiovascular disease. As noted in Chapter 5, a vegan diet coupled with regular exercise and other lifestyle changes can lead to a reversal of atherosclerotic plaque in various arteries in the body.

Cancer-Fighting Agents

The numerous phytochemicals in plant foods are thought to aid in preventing cancers of the breast, prostate, and colon. Many of the proposed anticancer effects of foods containing plant protein are through antioxidant mechanisms.

Consumption of plant sources of proteins can aid in prevention of cardiovascular disease and cancer, but there are also other areas for future study. Some studies show that replacing animal proteins with plant proteins is beneficial for kidney health. However, because plant foods such as soy are high in oxalates, people with a history of kidney stones should probably limit intake of soy (see Chapter 9 for more about oxalates). Plants may be particularly good sources of protein for people with diabetes or impaired glucose tolerance because the high fiber content of plant foods leads to a slower increase in blood glucose (review Chapter 4 for a discussion of glycemic load). Frequent nut consumption may even reduce the risk of developing gallstones, obesity, and type 2 diabetes. A recent review of 18 studies concluded that soy consumption was associated with a 14% reduction in breast cancer risk, but several other studies have shown little benefit of soy in preventing many forms of cancer, in lowering blood cholesterol, contributing to bone maintenance in women after menopause, and in treating menopausal symptoms in women (see Further Readings 12 and 15).

Increasing Plant Proteins in Your Diet

Now that you've seen how much you can benefit from including plant proteins in your diet, here are some suggestions for putting the theory onto your plate:

- At your next cookout, try a veggie burger instead of a hamburger. These are usually made from beans and are available in the frozen foods section of the grocery store and come in a variety of delicious flavors. Many restaurants have added veggie burgers to their menus.
- Sprinkle sunflower seeds or chopped almonds on top of your salad to add taste and texture.
- Mix chopped walnuts into the batter of your banana bread to boost your intake of monounsaturated fats.
- Eat soy nuts (oil-roasted soybeans) as a great snack.
- Spread some peanut butter on your bagel instead of butter or cream cheese.
- Instead of having beef or chicken tacos for dinner, heat up a can of great northern beans in your skillet with one half of a packet of taco seasoning and chopped tomatoes. Use this as a filling in a tortilla shell.
- Consider using soy milk, especially if you have lactose malabsorption or lactose intolerance. Look for varieties fortified with calcium.

Food Planning for Vegetarians

There are a variety of vegetarian diet styles. **Vegans**, or "total vegetarians," eat only plant foods (and do not use animal products for other purposes, such as leather shoes or feather pillows). **Fruitarians** primarily eat fruits, nuts, honey, and vegetable oils. This plan is not recommended because it can lead to nutrient deficiencies in people of all ages. **Lactovegetarians** modify vegetarianism a bit—they include dairy products in their plant-based diet. **Lactoovovegetarians** modify the diet even further and eat dairy products and eggs, as well as plant foods. Including these animal products makes food planning easier because they are rich in some nutrients that are missing or minimal in plants, such as vitamin B-12 and calcium. The more variety in the diet, the easier it is to meet nutritional needs. Thus, the practice of eating no animal sources of food significantly separates the vegans and fruitarians from all other semivegetarian styles.

Most people who call themselves vegetarians consume at least some dairy products, if not all dairy products and eggs. A food-group plan has been developed for lactovegetarians and vegans (Table 6-3). This plan includes servings of nuts, grains, legumes, and seeds to help meet protein needs. There is also a vegetable group, a fruit group, and a milk group.

Vegan Diet Planning

Planning a vegan diet requires knowledge and creativity to yield high-quality protein and other key nutrients without animal products. Earlier in this chapter, you learned about complementing proteins, whereby the essential amino acids deficient in one protein source are supplied by those of another consumed at the same meal or the next (Fig. 6-13). Many legumes are deficient in the essential amino-acid methionine, while cereals are limited in lysine. Eating a combination of legumes and cereals, such as beans and rice, will supply the body with adequate amounts of all essential amino acids (Fig. 6-13). As for

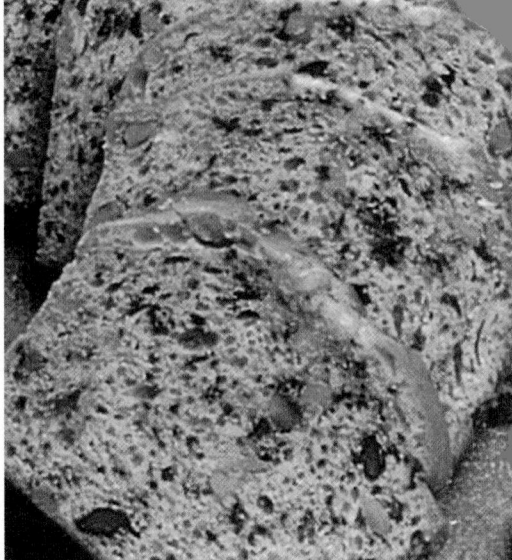

▲ Plant proteins, like those in walnuts, can be incorporated into one's diet in numerous ways, such as adding them to banana bread.

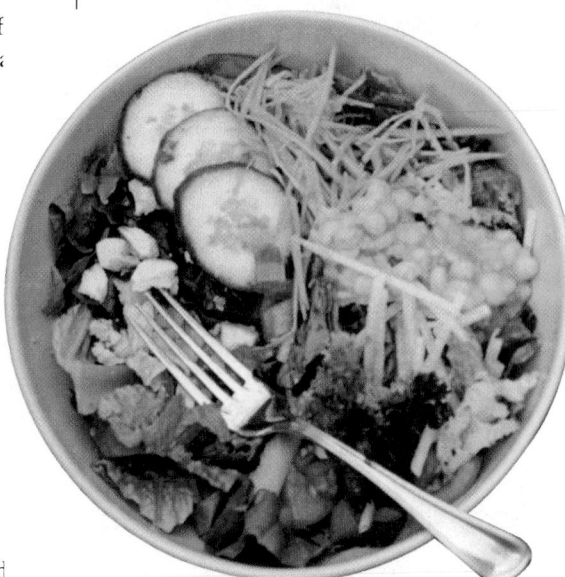

▲ A salad containing numerous types of vegetables and legumes is a healthy vegetarian choice.

vegan A person who eats only plant foods.

fruitarian A person who primarily eats fruits, nuts, honey, and vegetable oils.

lactovegetarian A person who consumes plant products and dairy products.

lactoovovegetarian A person who consumes plant products, dairy products, and eggs.

TABLE 6-3 Food Plan for Vegetarians Based on MyPlate

Food Group	MyPlate Servings Lactovegetarian[a]	Vegan[b]	Key Nutrients Supplied[c]
Grains	6–11	8–11	Protein, thiamin, niacin, folate, vitamin E, zinc, magnesium, iron, and fiber
Beans and other legumes	2–3	3	Protein, vitamin B-6, zinc, magnesium, and fiber
Nuts, seeds	2–3	3	Protein, vitamin E, and magnesium
Vegetables	3–5 (include 1 dark-green or leafy variety daily)	4–6 (include 1 dark-green or leafy variety daily)	Vitamin A, vitamin C, folate, vitamin K, potassium, and magnesium
Fruits	2–4	4	Vitamin A, vitamin C, and folate
Milk	3	_____	Protein, riboflavin, vitamin D, vitamin B-12, and calcium
Fortified soy milk	_____	3	Protein, riboflavin, vitamin D, vitamin B-12, and calcium

[a]This plan contains about 75 grams of protein in 1650 kcal.

[b]This plan contains about 79 grams of protein in 1800 kcal.

[c]One serving of vitamin- and mineral-enriched ready-to-eat breakfast cereal is recommended to meet possible nutrient gaps. Alternatively, a balanced multivitamin and mineral supplement can be used. Vegans also may benefit from the use of fortified soy milk to provide calcium, vitamin D, and vitamin B-12.

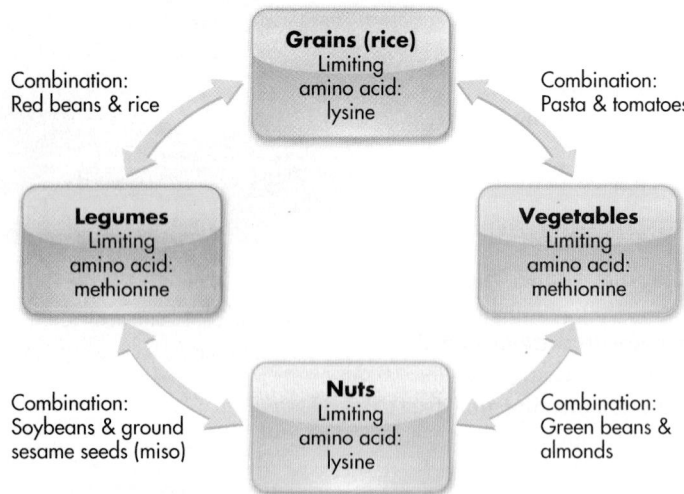

FIGURE 6-13 ▶ Plant group combinations in which the proteins complement each other in a meal based on their limiting amino acids.

any diet, variety is an especially important characteristic of a nutritious vegan diet.

Aside from amino acids, low intakes of certain micronutrients can be a problem for the vegan. At the forefront of nutritional concerns are riboflavin, vitamins D and B-12, iron, zinc, iodide, and calcium. The following dietary advice should be implemented. In addition, use of a balanced multivitamin and mineral supplement can help as well.

Riboflavin can be obtained from green leafy vegetables, whole grains, yeast, and legumes—components of most vegan diets. Alternate sources of vitamin D include fortified foods (e.g., margarine), as well as regular sun exposure (see Chapter 8).

Vitamin B-12 only occurs naturally in animal foods. Plants can contain soil or microbial contaminants that provide trace amounts of vitamin B-12, but these are negligible sources of the vitamin. Because the body can store vitamin B-12 for about 4 years, it may take a long time after removal of animal foods from the diet for a vitamin B-12 deficiency to surface. If dietary B-12 inadequacy persists, deficiency can lead to a form of anemia, nerve damage, and mental dysfunction. These deficiency consequences have been noted in the infants of vegetarian mothers whose breast milk was low in vitamin B-12. Vegans can prevent a vitamin B-12 deficiency by finding a reliable source of vitamin B-12,

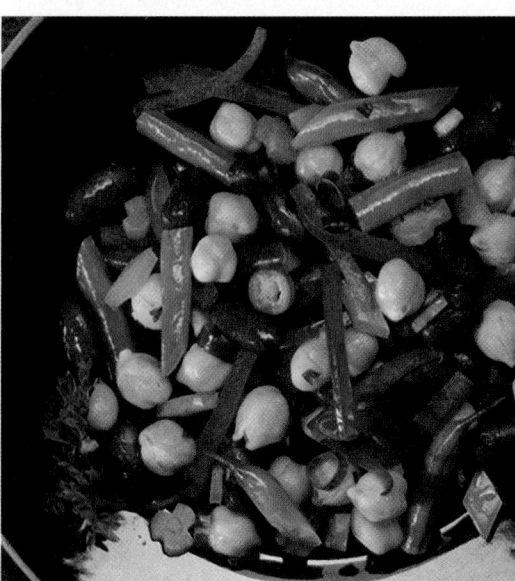

▲ Keep in mind that amino acids in vegetables are best used when a combination of sources is consumed.

such as fortified soybean milk, ready-to-eat breakfast cereals, and special yeast grown on media rich in vitamin B-12.

For iron, the vegan can consume whole grains (especially ready-to-eat breakfast cereals), dried fruits and nuts, and legumes. The iron in these foods is not absorbed as well as iron in animal foods. A good source of vitamin C helps with the absorption of iron so it is recommended that vitamin C be consumed with every meal that contains iron-rich plant foods. Cooking in iron pots and skillets can also add iron to the diet (see Chapter 9).

The vegan can find zinc in whole grains (especially ready-to-eat breakfast cereals), nuts, and legumes, but phytic acid and other substances in these foods limit zinc absorption. Breads are a good source of zinc because the leavening process (rising of the bread dough) reduces the influence of phytic acid. Iodized salt is a reliable source of iodide. It should be used instead of plain salt, both of which are found in U.S. supermarkets.

Of all nutrients, calcium is the most difficult to consume in sufficient quantities for vegans. Fortified foods including fortified soy milk, fortified orange juice, calcium-rich tofu (check the label), as well as certain ready-to-eat breakfast cereals and snacks are the vegan's best option for obtaining calcium. Green leafy vegetables and nuts also contain calcium, but the mineral is either not well absorbed or not very plentiful from these sources. Calcium supplements are another option (see Chapter 9). Special diet planning is always required, because even a multivitamin and mineral supplement will not supply enough calcium to meet the needs of the body.

Consuming adequate quantities of omega-3 fatty acids is yet another nutritional concern for vegetarians, especially vegans. Fish and fish oils, abundant sources of these

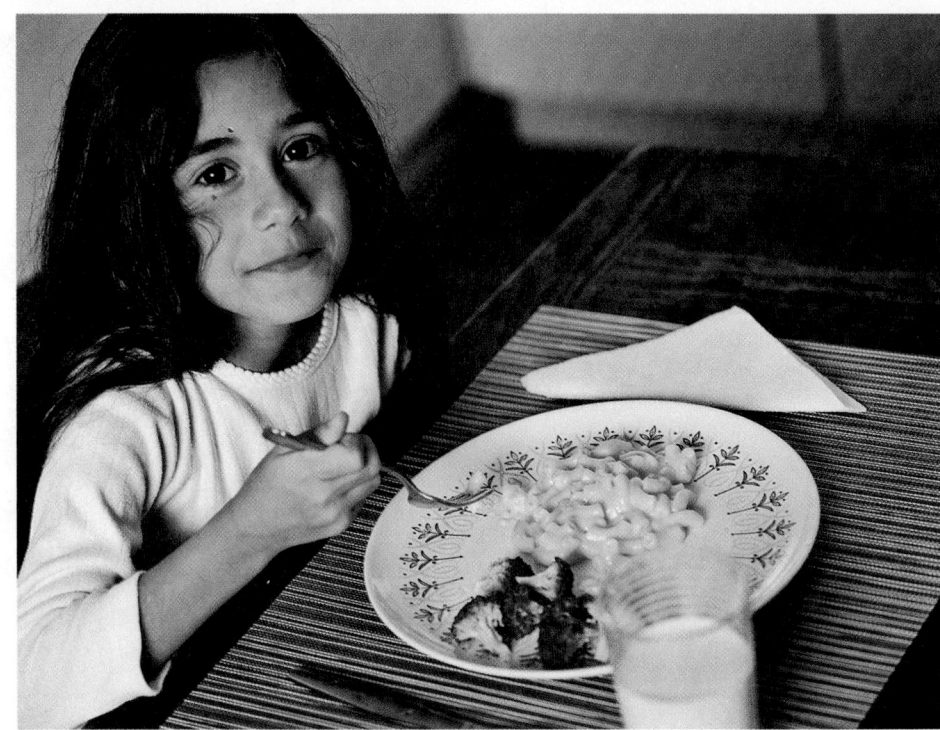

▲ Children can safely enjoy vegetarian and vegan diets as long as certain adjustments are made to meet their age-specific nutritional needs.

heart-healthy fats, are omitted from many types of vegetarian diets. Alternative plant sources of omega-3 fatty acids include canola oil, soybean oil, seaweed, microalgae, flax seeds, and walnuts.

Special Concerns for Infants and Children

Infants and children, notoriously picky eaters in the first place, are at highest risk for nutrient deficiencies as a result of improperly planned vegetarian and vegan diets. With the use of complementary proteins and good sources of problem nutrients just discussed, the calorie, protein, vitamin, and mineral needs of vegetarian and vegan infants and children can be met (see Further Reading 1). The most common nutritional concerns for infants and children following vegetarian and vegan diets are deficiencies of iron, vitamin B-12, vitamin D, and calcium.

Vegetarian and vegan diets tend to be high in bulky, high-fiber, low-calorie foods that cause a feeling of fullness. While this is a welcome advantage for adults, children have small stomach volume and relatively high nutrient needs compared to their size, and therefore may feel full before their calorie needs are met. For this reason, the fiber content of a child's diet may need to be decreased by replacing high-fiber sources with some refined grain products, fruit juices, and peeled fruit. Other concentrated sources of calories for vegetarian and vegan children include fortified soy milk, nuts, dried fruits, avocados, and cookies made with vegetable oils or tub margarine.

Case Study Planning a Vegetarian Diet

Jordan is a freshman in college. He lives in a campus residence hall and teaches martial arts in the afternoon. He eats two or three meals a day at the residence hall cafeteria and snacks between meals. Jordan and his roommate both decided to become vegetarians because they recently read a magazine article describing the health benefits of a vegetarian diet. Yesterday Jordan's vegetarian diet consisted of a Danish pastry for breakfast and a tomato-rice dish (no meat) with pretzels and a diet soft drink for lunch. In the afternoon, after his martial arts class, he had a milk shake and two cookies. At dinnertime he had a vegetarian sub sandwich consisting of lettuce, sprouts, tomatoes, cucumbers, and cheese, with two glasses of fruit punch. In the evening, he had a bowl of popcorn.

Answer the following questions, and check your response in Appendix A.

1. What type of health benefits can Jordan expect from following a well-planned vegetarian diet?
2. What is missing from Jordan's current diet plan in terms of foods that should be emphasized in a vegetarian diet?
3. Which nutrients are missing in this current diet plan?
4. Are there any food components in the current diet plan that should be minimized or avoided?
5. How could he improve his new diet at each meal and snack to meet his nutritional needs and avoid undesirable food components?

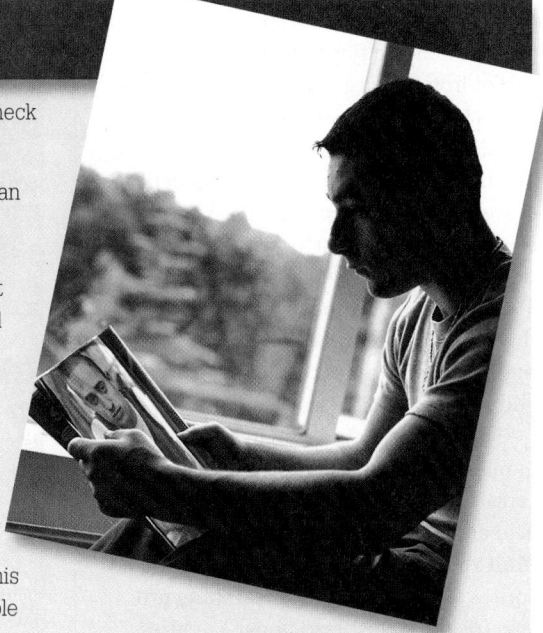

▲ Has Jordan planned a healthy and nutritious vegetarian diet?

Summary (Numbers refer to numbered sections in the chapter.)

6.1 Amino acids, the building blocks of proteins, contain a very usable form of nitrogen for humans. Of the 20 common types of amino acids found in food, nine must be consumed in food (essential) and the rest can be synthesized by the body (nonessential).

6.2 Individual amino acids are bonded together to form proteins. The sequential order of amino acids determines the protein's ultimate shape and function. This order is directed by DNA in the cell nucleus. Diseases such as sickle cell anemia can occur if the amino acids are incorrect on a polypeptide chain. When the three-dimensional shape of a protein is unfolded—denatured—by treatment with heat, acid or alkaline solutions, or other processes, the protein also loses its biological activity.

6.3 Almost all animal products are nutrient-dense sources of protein. The high quality of these proteins means that they can be easily converted into body proteins. Rich plant sources of protein, such as beans, are also available.

High-quality (complete) protein foods contain ample amounts of all nine essential amino acids. Furthermore, foods derived from animal sources provide high

biological value protein. Lower-quality (incomplete) protein foods lack sufficient amounts of one or more essential amino acids. This is typical of plant foods, especially cereal grains. Different types of plant foods eaten together often complement each other's amino-acid deficits, thereby providing high-quality protein in the diet.

6.4 Protein digestion begins in the stomach, dividing the proteins into breakdown products containing shorter polypeptide chains of amino acids. In the small intestine, these polypeptide chains eventually separate into amino acids in the absorptive cells. The free amino acids then travel via the portal vein that connects to the liver. Some then enter the bloodstream.

6.5 Important body components—such as muscles, connective tissue, transport proteins in the bloodstream, visual pigments, enzymes, some hormones, and immune cells—are made of proteins. These proteins are in a state of constant turnover. The carbon chains of proteins may be used to produce glucose (or fat) when necessary.

6.6 The protein RDA for adults is 0.8 grams per kilogram of healthy body weight. For a typical 70-kilogram (154-pound) person, this corresponds to 56 grams of

protein daily; for a 57-kilogram (125-pound) person, this corresponds to 46 grams per day. The North American diet generally supplies plenty of protein. Men typically consume about 100 grams of protein daily, and women consume closer to 65 grams. These usual protein intakes are also of sufficient quality to support body functions. This is even true for well-balanced vegetarian diets.

6.7 People need to balance protein intake with such losses to maintain a state of protein equilibrium, also called *protein balance.*

When a body is growing or recovering from an illness or injury, it needs a positive protein balance to supply the raw materials required to build new tissues. To achieve this, a person must eat more protein daily than he or she loses. Consuming less protein than needed leads to negative protein balance, such as when acute illness reduces the desire to eat and so one loses more protein than consumed.

6.8 Undernutrition can lead to protein-calorie malnutrition in the form of kwashiorkor or marasmus. Kwashiorkor results primarily from an inadequate calorie and protein intake in comparison with body needs, which often increase with concurrent disease and infection. Kwashiorkor often occurs when a child is weaned from human milk and fed mostly starchy gruels. Marasmus results from extreme starvation—a negligible intake of both protein and calories. Marasmus commonly occurs during famine, especially in infants.

N&YH Consumption of vegetarian and other plant-based diets provides many health benefits, including lower risks of chronic diseases including cardiovascular disease, diabetes, and certain cancers. The benefits associated with the plant-based diets appear to stem from the lower content of saturated fat and cholesterol and the higher amount of fiber, vitamins, minerals, and phytochemicals.

Check Your Knowledge (Answers to the following questions are below.)

1. The "instructions" for making proteins are located in the
   a. cell membrane.
   b. DNA and RNA genetic material.
   c. stomach.
   d. small intestine.

2. A nutrient that could easily be deficient in the diet of a vegan would be
   a. vitamin C.
   b. folic acid.
   c. calcium.
   d. All of the above.

3. If an essential amino acid is unavailable for protein synthesis, the
   a. cell will make the amino acid.
   b. synthesis of the protein will stop.
   c. cell will continue to attach amino acids to the protein.
   d. partially completed protein will be stored for later completion.

4. An example of protein complementation used in vegetarian diet planning would be the combination of
   a. cereal and milk.
   b. bacon and eggs.
   c. rice and beans.
   d. macaroni and cheese.

5. An individual who eats only plant food is referred to as a
   a. planetarium.
   b. vegan.
   c. lactovegetarian.
   d. ovovegetarian.

6. Which of the following groups accounts for the differences among amino acids?
   a. amine group
   b. side chain
   c. acid group
   d. keto group

7. Absorption of amino acids takes place in the
   a. stomach.
   b. liver.
   c. small intestine.
   d. large intestine.

8. Jack is not an athlete and weighs 176 pounds (80 kilograms). His RDA for protein would be _____ grams.
   a. 32
   b. 40
   c. 64
   d. 80

9. Which of the following is true about protein intake of people in the United States?
   a. Most do not consume enough protein.
   b. Most consume approximately the amount needed to balance losses.
   c. Athletes generally do not get enough protein without supplementation.
   d. Most consume more than is needed.

10. The basic building block of a protein is called a(n)
    a. fatty acid.
    b. monosaccharide.
    c. amino acid.
    d. gene.

Answers Key: 1. b (LO 6.2), 2. c (LO 6.3), 3. b (LO 6.2), 4. c (LO 6.9), 5. b (LO 6.9), 6. b (LO 6.1), 7. c (LO 6.4), 8. c (LO 6.6), 9. d (LO 6.7), 10. c (LO 6.1)

Study Questions (Numbers refer to Learning Outcomes)

1. Discuss the relative importance of essential and nonessential amino acids in the diet. Why is it important for essential amino acids lost from the body to be replaced in the diet? (LO 6.1)

2. Describe the concept of complementary proteins. (LO 6.3)

3. What is a limiting amino acid? Explain why this concept is a concern in a vegetarian diet. How can a vegetarian compensate for limiting amino acids in specific foods? (LO 6.9)

4. Briefly describe the organization of proteins. How can this organization be altered or damaged? What might be a result of damaged protein organization? (LO 6.2)

5. Describe four functions of proteins. Provide an example of how the structure of a protein relates to its function. (LO 6.5)

6. How are DNA and protein synthesis related? (LO 6.2)

7. What would be one health benefit of reducing high-protein intake(s) to RDA amounts for some people? (LO 6.6)

8. What characteristics of vegetable proteins could improve the North American diet? What foods would you include to provide a diet that has ample protein from both plant and animal sources but is moderate in fat? (LO 6.9)

9. Outline the major differences between kwashiorkor and marasmus. (LO 6.8)

10. What are the possible long-term effects of an inadequate intake of dietary protein among children between the ages of 6 months and 4 years? (LO 6.8)

What Would You Choose Recommendations

It is not a good idea to take individual amino-acid supplements. Your digestive tract is made to handle whole proteins—hydrochloric acid and enzymes break polypeptides into amino acids that can be absorbed by the cells of the small intestine. Taking large doses of one amino acid can impair the absorption and/or metabolism of other amino acids.

Whey protein, a by-product of cheese production from cow's milk, is considered to be a high-quality protein because it is easily digested and contains all of the essential amino acids. It is a source of the branched-chain amino acids, valine, leucine, and isoleucine. BCAAs can be used for fuel by exercising muscles and are particularly important for synthesizing muscle tissue. The rationale is that whey protein supports muscle recovery and anabolism after exercise.

Consuming adequate protein is important for muscle repair and synthesis, but consuming excessive protein from any source provides no advantage. Excess protein will be metabolized as fuel or stored as fat, not muscle. In fact, some excess subcutaneous fat is probably the reason you have not seen your toned muscles yet. Cutting back on calories or including more endurance exercise in your routine can help to reduce body weight and body fat as you tone your muscles. Animal protein, in particular, is often a source of excess total fat, saturated fat, and cholesterol. Not only will this hinder efforts at weight loss, but it is detrimental to heart health.

Americans typically consume two to three times as much protein as they actually need. The average American intake of 100 grams per day for men or 65 grams per day for women easily meets even the highest protein recommendations for resistance exercise (1.7 grams of protein per kilogram). Also, omnivorous diets and even appropriately planned vegan diets can supply ample amino acids to support muscle recovery and synthesis. Protein and amino

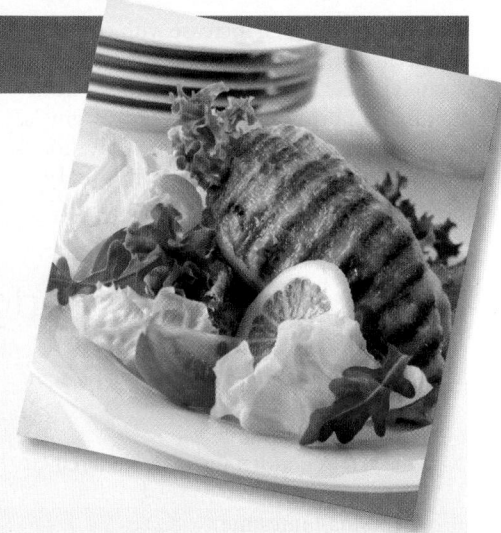

▲ This 4-ounce grilled chicken breast is an excellent choice, providing 38 grams of high-quality yet inexpensive lean protein.

acid supplements are expensive and may be detrimental to health. It is safer and more economical to focus on a diet that provides 10% to 35% of calories from a variety of lean sources of protein.

Further Readings

1. ADA Reports: Position of the American Dietetic Association and Dietitians of Canada: Vegetarian diets. *Journal of the American Dietetic Association* 109:1266, 2009.

   It is the position of the American Dietetic Association and Dietitians of Canada that appropriately planned vegetarian diets are healthful, nutritionally adequate, and provide health benefits in the prevention and treatment of certain diseases. Vegetarian diets are appropriate for all stages of the life cycle.

2. Barnard ND and others: A low-fat vegan diet improves glycemic control and cardiovascular risk factors in a randomized clinical trial in individuals with type 2 diabetes. *Diabetes Care* 29:1777, 2006.

   Improvements in glycemic (decreased hemoglobin A1C) and lipid (decreased LDL cholesterol) control were greater in type 2 diabetic patients that followed a low-fat vegan diet compared to a diet based on American Diabetes Association

   guidelines. In the vegan group, 43% of the subjects reduced their diabetes medications compared to 26% of the subjects on the ADA diet.

3. Chao A and others: Meat consumption and colorectal cancer. *Journal of the American Medical Association* 293:172, 2005.

   Diets rich in red meat, especially processed meat, increase the risk of colon cancer. Protein from poultry and fish, in contrast, does not pose the same risk.

4. Fessler TA: Malnutrition: A serious concern for hospitalized patients. *Today's Dietitian* 10(7): 44, 2008.

   Malnutrition continues to be a significant problem in hospitals worldwide, affecting patients of all ages from infants to geriatric patients. Malnutrition can be caused by the illnesses or injuries for which the patients are admitted to the hospital and by the hospitalization itself. This article outlines the need for prompt identification, treatment, and monitoring

   of malnourished patients among healthcare professionals.

5. Gardner CD and others: The effect of a plant-based diet on plasma lipids in hypercholesterolemic adults. *Annals of Internal Medicine* 142:725, 2005.

   Adding plant proteins to a diet already low in saturated fat and cholesterol provides additional benefits regarding lowering blood cholesterol. The authors emphasize the importance of including fruits, vegetables, legumes, and whole grains in a diet.

6. Key TJ and others: Health effects of vegetarian and vegan diets. *Proceedings of the Nutrition Society* 65:35, 2006.

   This study reviewed recent findings from large studies and summarizes the latest understanding of the health effects of vegetarian and vegan diets. Results indicated that vegetarians have a lower BMI and lower obesity rates than comparable nonvegetarians; total plasma cholesterol is lower in vegetarians that nonvegetarians; between vegetarians and nonvegetarians there is no significant differences in blood pressure; studies of vegetarians indicate a moderate reduction in mortality from ischemic heart disease; and studies showed no differences between vegetarians and nonvegetarians for colorectal cancer, breast cancer, prostate cancer, or total mortality.

7. Lejeune MP and others: Additional protein intake limits weight regain after weight loss in humans. *British Journal of Nutrition* 93:281, 2005.

Adding 30 grams of protein per day to their usual diets helped people in this study limit weight regain after weight loss. The diet ended up 18% of calorie intake as protein, compared to 15% in the control group. This protein intake in the experimental group would not be considered excessive given an upper limit of 35% of calorie intake set by the Food and Nutrition Board.

8. Mangels R: Weight control the vegan way. *Vegetarian Journal* XXV(1), 2006.

This article provides suggestions for vegans, or people interested in following a vegan diet, who want to lose weight. Two eating plans are included that were developed for people who are moderately active, spending 30 to 60 minutes daily in moderate physical activity. The first eating plan has approximately 1500 calories and is designed for women who want to lose 1 to 2 pounds per week. The second has about 1900 calories and is designed for men who want to lose 1 to 2 pounds per week. Protein foods include kidney beans, chickpeas, and other beans; tofu; lite or plain soymilk; nuts and nut butters; seitan (say-than, wheat meat); and meat analogs. Recipes are also included.

9. Newby PK: Risk of overweight and obesity among semivegetarian, lactovegetarian, and vegan women. *American Journal of Clinical Nutrition* 81:1267, 2005.

Semivegetarian women in this study were less likely to be overweight and obese compared to

omnivorous women. Consuming more plant foods and less animal products may help individuals control their weight.

10. Sacks FM and others: Soy protein, isoflavones, and cardiovascular health. An American Heart Association Science Advisory for Professionals From the Nutrition Committee. *Circulation* 113:1034, 2006.

This scientific advisory evaluates recent work published on soy protein and its component isoflavones and their potential role in improving risk factors for cardiovascular disease. In the majority of studies, soy protein with isoflavones, as compared with milk or other proteins, decreased LDL cholesterol concentrations; the average effect was ~ 3% and no significant effects on HDL cholesterol, triglycerides, lipoprotein(a), or blood pressure were evident. The authors conclude that soy products should be beneficial to cardiovascular and overall health because of their high content of polyunsaturated fats, fiber, vitamins, and minerals and low content of saturated fat.

11. Taylor SL: Estimating prevalence of soy protein allergy. *The Soy Connection* 14(2):1, 2006.

This article discusses the issue of soy protein allergy. Although soy protein has been designated one of the major allergens by the U.S. Food and Drug Administration, rigorous prevalence data for this allergy are not available, and indirect evidence suggests it occurs less frequently than other common allergens including shellfish, peanuts, tree nuts, and fish.

12. Trock BJ and others: Meta-analysis of soy intake and breast cancer risk. *Journal of the National Cancer Institute* 98(7):459, 2006.

This study analyzed data from 18 previously published studies and concludes that consumption of soy foods among healthy women was associated with a significant reduction (14%) in breast cancer risk.

13. Who's the veggie-friendliest of them all? *Vegetarian Journal* XXVII, p. 14, 2008.

The Vegetarian Resource Group evaluated the menus of the 400 largest restaurant chains in the United States. This article highlights the establishments that appeared to make the best effort at serving vegetarians of diverse needs. You can find more than 2000 veggie-friendly restaurants at their website *www.vrg.org*.

14. Williams CD and other: Associations of red meat, fat, and protein intake with distal colorectal cancer risk. *Nutrition and Cancer* 62(6):701, 2010.

Studies suggest that red and processed meat consumption increase the risk of colon cancer. The risk of distal colorectal cancer (CRC) associated with red and processed meat, fat, and protein intakes was determined in whites and African-Americans. Dietary intake was assessed in 945 cases of distal CRC and in 959 controls in the previous 12 months. The results did not support the hypothesis that fat, protein, and red meat increase the risk of distal CRC. There was no association between total, saturated, or monounsaturated fat and distal CRC risk, and the percentages of energy from protein and red meat consumption were associated with a risk reduction (rather than increase).

15. Xiao CW: Health effects of soy protein and isoflavones in humans. *Journal of Nutrition* 138:1244S, 2008.

The results of epidemiological and clinical studies have suggested that soy consumption may be associated with a lower incidence of certain chronic diseases and a reduction in the risk factors for cardiovascular disease. These results led to an FDA-approved food-labeling health claim for soy proteins in the prevention of coronary heart disease. This article reviews the evidence for health claims on the effects of soy protein and isoflavones in humans and concludes that the existing data are inconsistent or inadequate to support most of the suggested health benefits of consuming soy protein or ISF.

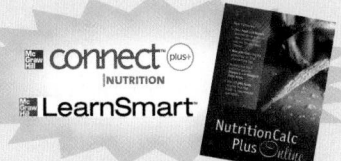

To get the most out of your study of nutrition, go to McGraw-Hill's online resources: Connect **www.mcgrawhillconnect.com**, where you will find NutritionCalc Plus, LearnSmart, and many other dynamic tools.

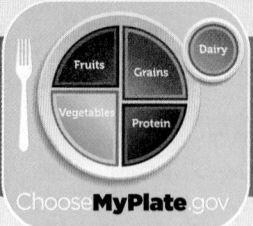

RATE YOUR PLATE

ChooseMyPlate.gov

I. Protein and the Vegetarian

Alana is excited about all the health benefits that might accompany a vegetarian diet. However, she is concerned that she will not consume enough protein to meet her needs. She is also concerned about possible vitamin and mineral deficiencies. Use NutritionCalc Plus or a food composition table to calculate her protein intake and see if her concerns are valid.

	Protein (g)
Breakfast Calcium fortified orange juice, 1 cup Soy milk, 1 cup Fortified bran flakes, 1 cup Banana, medium	
Snack Calcium-enriched granola bar	
Lunch GardenBurger, 4 oz Whole-wheat bun Mustard, 1 tbsp Soy cheese, 1 oz Apple, medium Green leaf lettuce, 1 ½ cups Peanuts, 1 oz Sunflower seeds, 1/4 cup Tomato slices, 2 Mushrooms, 3 Vinaigrette salad dressing, 2 tbsp Iced tea	
Dinner Kidney beans, ½ cup Brown rice, 3/4 cup Fortified margarine, 2 tbsp Mixed vegetables, 1/4 cup Hot tea	
Dessert Strawberries, ½ cup Angel food cake, 1 small slice Soy milk, ½ cup	
	TOTAL PROTEIN (grams) _____

Alana's diet contained 2150 kcal, with _____ grams (you fill in) of protein (Is this plenty for her?), 360 grams of carbohydrate, 57 grams of total dietary fat (only 9 grams of which came from saturated fat), and 50 grams of fiber. Her vitamin and mineral intake with respect to those of concern to vegetarians—vitamin B-12, vitamin D, calcium, iron, and zinc—met her needs.

II. Meeting Protein Needs When Dieting to Lose Weight

Your father has been steadily gaining weight for the last 30 years and now has developed hypertension and type 2 diabetes as a result. His physician recommends that he lose some weight by following an 1800 kcal diet. You know that it will be important for your father to meet protein needs as he tries to lose weight. Design a 1-day diet for him that contains about 20% of calorie intake as protein. Table 6-2 will provide some help. Will this diet meet his protein RDA? Does the diet look like a plan you could also follow?

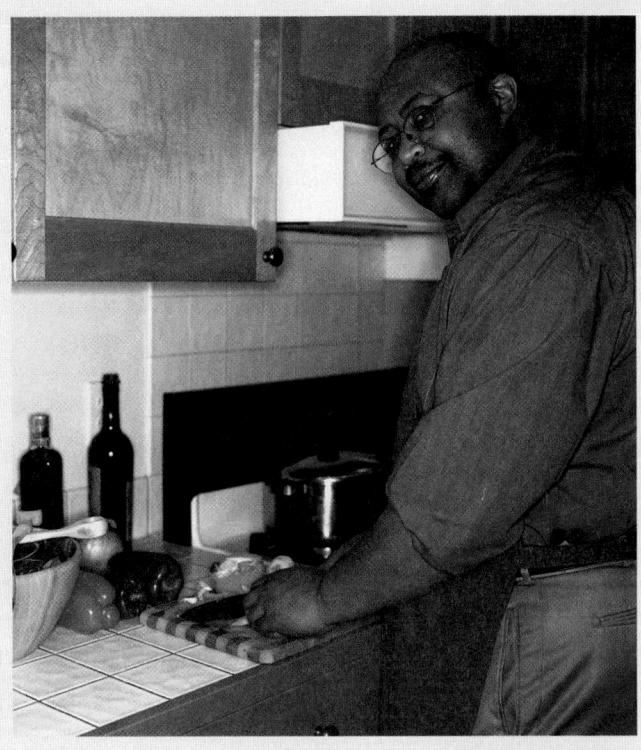

Chapter 7 Energy Balance and Weight Control

Student Learning Outcomes

Chapter 7 is designed to allow you to:

7.1 Describe energy balance and the uses of energy by the body.

7.2 Compare methods to determine energy use by the body.

7.3 Discuss methods for assessing body composition and determining whether body weight and composition are healthy.

7.4 Outline the risks to health posed by overweight and obesity.

7.5 Explain factors associated with the development of obesity.

7.6 List and discuss characteristics of a sound weight-loss program

7.7 Describe why reduced calorie intake is the main key to weight loss and maintenance.

7.8 Discuss why physical activity is a key to weight loss and especially important for later weight maintenance.

7.9 Describe why and how behavior modification fits into a weight-less program.

7.10 Outline the benefits and hazards of various weight-loss methods for severe obesity.

7.11 Discuss the causes and treatment of underweight.

7.12 Evaluate popular weight-reduction diets and determine which are unsafe, doomed to fail, or both.

What Would You Choose?

There are so many choices when it comes to controlling calorie intake. Is it possible to have dessert and still manage your weight? Consider the following frozen treats: regular ice cream, light ice cream, and frozen yogurt. Which of these desserts would you choose to cut back on calories? What information from the Nutrition Facts label is most helpful when it comes to weight management?

a Regular ice cream

b Light ice cream

c Frozen yogurt

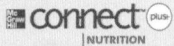 Think about your choice as you read Chapter 7, then see our recommendations at the end of the chapter. To learn more about controlling calorie intake, check out the Connect site: www.mcgrawhillconnect.com

Part Two
Energy Nutrients and Energy Balance

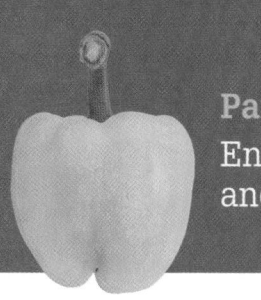

In the last 25 years (the years since most college students were born), there has been a dramatic increase in the percentage of individuals who are overweight or obese. The ranks of the obese are growing in North America and worldwide. Recall from Chapter 1 that an estimated 1 billion people in the world are overweight. This problem is increasing not only in the United States but also globally among affluent peoples and in developing countries where Westernized diets (high-fat, high-calorie) are increasing in popularity. Excess weight increases the likelihood of many health problems, such as cardiovascular disease, cancer, hypertension, strokes, certain bone and joint disorders, and type 2 diabetes, especially if a person performs minimal physical activity.

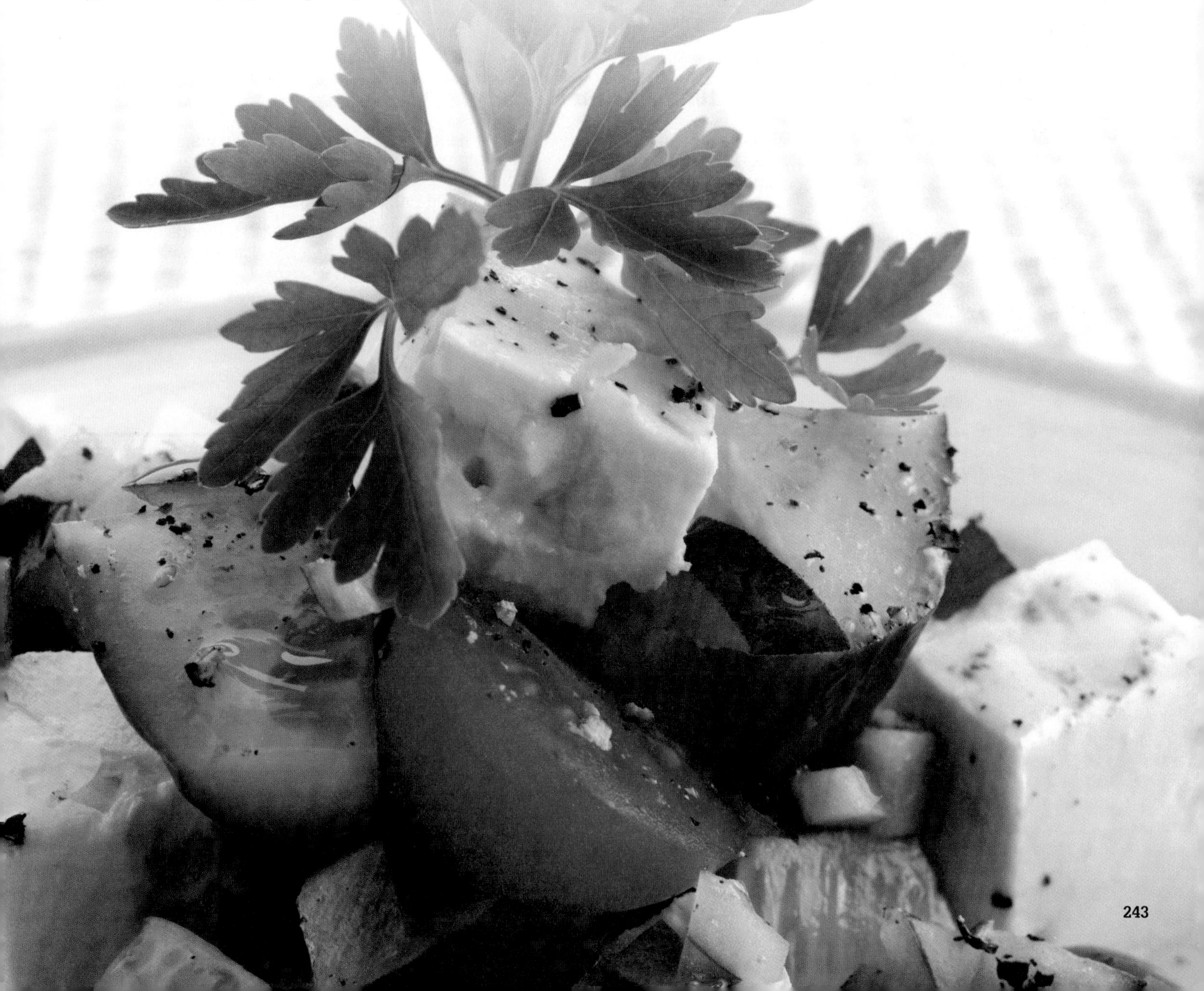

Currently, most weight-reduction efforts fizzle before bodies fall into a healthy weight range. As suggested in this chapter's comic, typical popular ("fad") diets are generally monotonous, ineffective, and confusing. They may even endanger some populations, such as children, teenagers, pregnant women, and people with various health disorders. A more logical approach to weight loss is straightforward: (1) eat less; (2) increase physical activity; and (3) change problematic eating behaviors.

A national commitment has begun from a variety of groups, including government agencies, the food industry, health professionals, and communities, to address the growing weight problem in North America. It has become obvious that, without this national effort to promote weight maintenance and effective new approaches to making our social environment more favorable to maintaining healthy weight, the current trends will not be reversed (Fig. 7-1) (see Futher Readings 3 and 9). Chapter 7 discusses these recommendations to help you understand obesity's causes, consequences, and potential treatments.

Refresh Your Memory

As you begin your study of weight control in Chapter 7, you may want to review:

- Biological and social influences of food intake in Chapter 1
- The concept of energy density and appropriate serving sizes for foods in Chapter 2
- The role of fiber in weight regulation in Chapter 4
- The fat content of various foods in Chapter 5
- The long-term risks of high-protein diets in Chapter 6

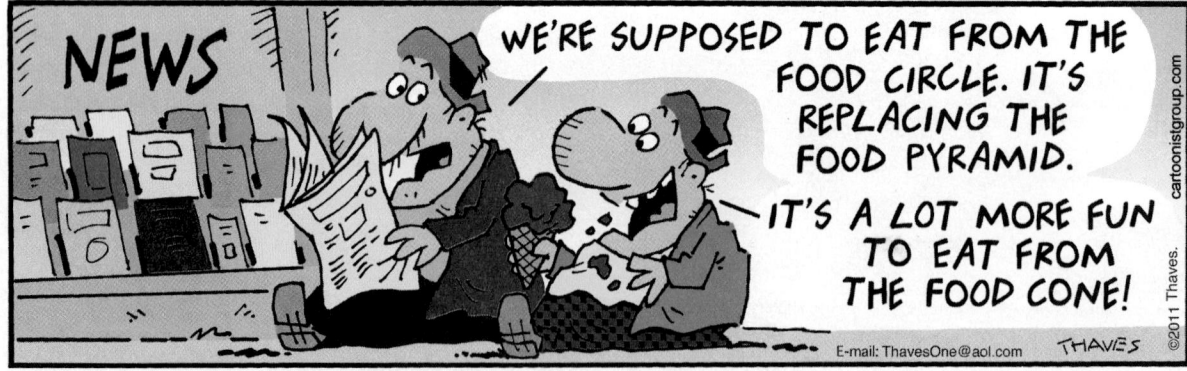

What components make up a successful diet plan? What constitutes a "fad" diet? Why are overweight and obesity growing problems worldwide? What might be the future consequences of this trend? Chapter 7 provides some answers.

"Frank and Ernest" used with the permission of the Thaves and the Cartoonist Group. All rights reserved. 2/28/1997

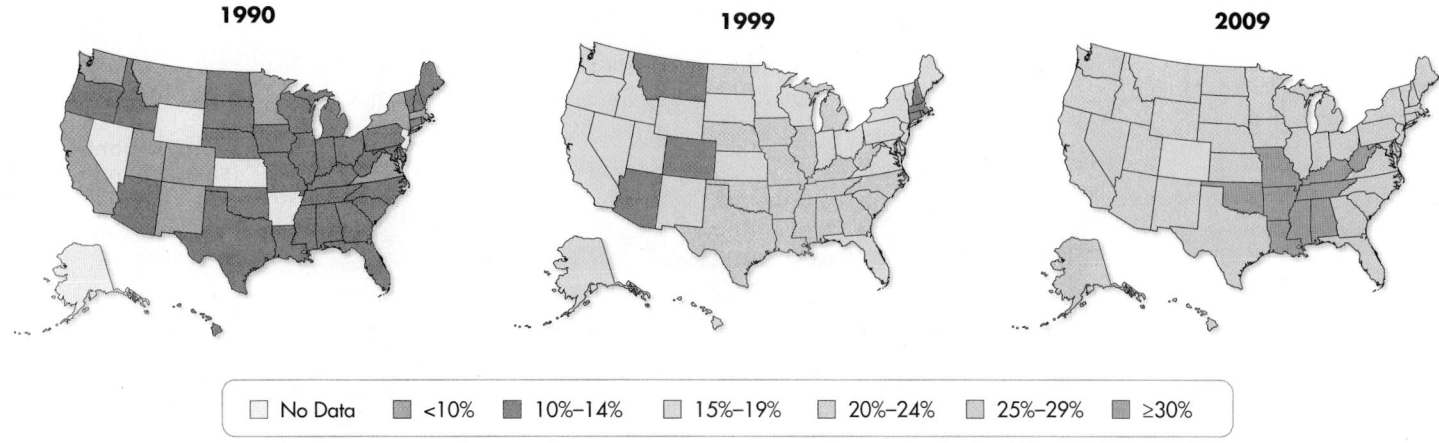

1990 **1999** **2009**

☐ No Data ▪ <10% ▪ 10%–14% ☐ 15%–19% ▪ 20%–24% ▪ 25%–29% ▪ ≥30%

FIGURE 7-1 ▶ Obesity trends among U.S. adults: 1990, 1999, 2009 (BMI ≥ 30, or about 30 pounds overweight for 5'4" person).

Source: CDC Behavioral Risk Factor Surveillance System.

7.1 Energy Balance

We begin this chapter with some good news and some bad news. The good news is that if you stay at a healthy body weight, you increase your chances of living a long and healthy life. The bad news is that currently 68% of all North American adults are overweight, significantly more than in the 1980s. Of those, about 50% (34% of the total population) are obese. There is a good chance that any of us could become part of those statistics if we do not pay attention to the prevention of significant weight gain in adulthood. Gaining more than 10 pounds or 2 inches in waist circumference are signals that a reevaluation of diet and lifestyle is in order.

There is no quick cure for overweight, despite what the advertisements claim. Successful weight loss comes from hard work and commitment. A combination of decreased calorie intake, increased physical activity, and behavior modification is considered to be the most reliable treatment for the overweight condition. And without a doubt, the prevention of the overweight condition in the first place is the most successful approach.

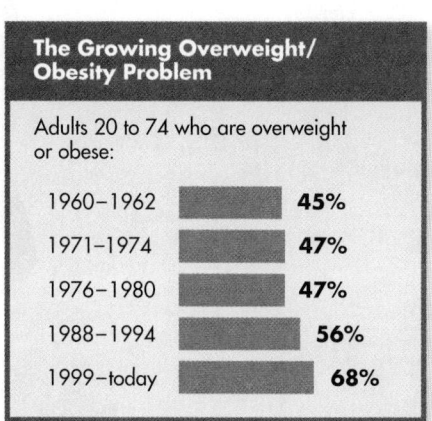

The Growing Overweight/ Obesity Problem

Adults 20 to 74 who are overweight or obese:

1960–1962 **45%**
1971–1974 **47%**
1976–1980 **47%**
1988–1994 **56%**
1999–today **68%**

Positive and Negative Energy Balance

A healthy weight can result from paying more attention to the important concept of **energy balance.** Think of energy balance as an equation:

Energy Input (calories from food intake) = Energy Output (metabolism; digestion, absorption, and transport of nutrients; physical activity)

The balance of calories (measured in kcals) on the two sides of this equation can influence energy stores, especially the amount of triglyceride stored in adipose tissue (Fig. 7-2). Fat tissue contains about 3500 calories per pound. Therefore to lose 1 pound of fat per week, calorie intake must be decreased by about 500 calories per day. When energy input is greater than energy output, the result is **positive energy balance.** The excess calories consumed are stored, which results in weight gain. There are some situations in which positive energy balance is normal and healthy. During pregnancy, a surplus of calories supports the developing fetus. Infants and children require a positive energy balance for growth and development. In adults, however, even a small positive energy balance is usually in the form of fat storage rather than muscle and bone and, over time, can cause body weight to climb.

energy balance The state in which energy intake, in the form of food and beverages, matches the energy expended, primarily through basal metabolism and physical activity.

positive energy balance The state in which energy intake is greater than energy expended, generally resulting in weight gain.

FIGURE 7-2 ▶ A model for energy balance—input versus output. This figure depicts energy balance in practical terms.

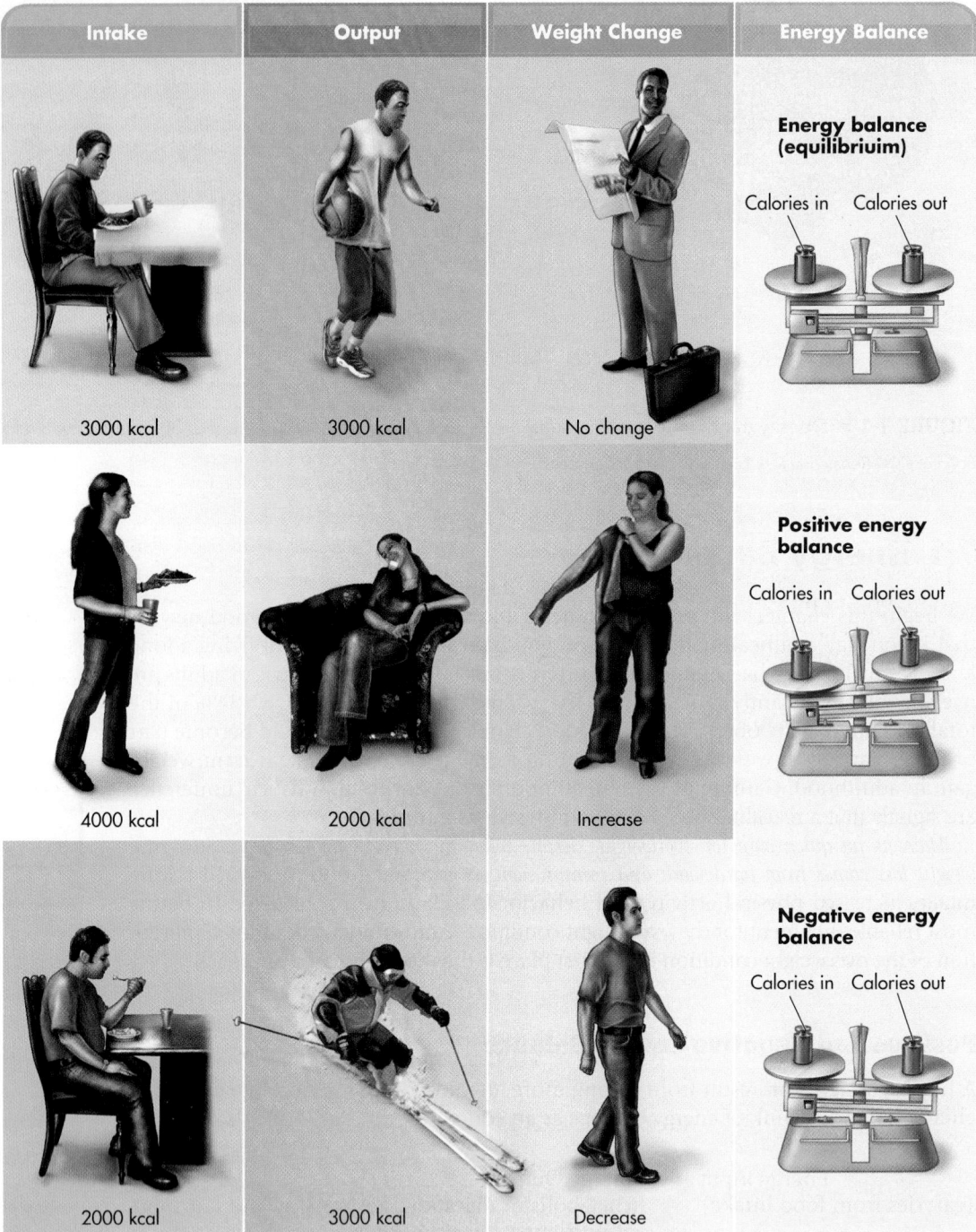

Intake	Output	Weight Change	Energy Balance
			Energy balance (equilibriuim) Calories in Calories out
3000 kcal	3000 kcal	No change	
			Positive energy balance Calories in Calories out
4000 kcal	2000 kcal	Increase	
			Negative energy balance Calories in Calories out
2000 kcal	3000 kcal	Decrease	

CRITICAL THINKING

As she gets closer to age 30, a 28-year-old classmate of yours has been thinking about the process of aging. One of the things she fears most as she gets older is gaining weight. How would you explain energy balance to her?

negative energy balance The state in which energy intake is less than energy expended, resulting in weight loss.

On the other hand, if energy input is less than energy output, there is a calorie deficit and **negative energy balance** results. A negative energy balance is necessary for successful weight loss. It is important to realize that during negative energy balance, weight loss involves a reduction in both lean and adipose tissue, not just "fat."

The maintenance of energy balance substantially contributes to health and well-being in adults by minimizing the risk of developing many common health problems. Adulthood is often a time of subtle increases in weight gain, which eventually turns into obesity if left unchecked. The process of aging does not cause weight gain; rather the problem stems from a pattern of excess food intake coupled with limited physical activity and slower metabolism. Let's look in detail at the factors that affect the energy balance equation.

Energy Intake

Energy needs are met by food intake, represented by the number of calories eaten each day. Determining the appropriate amount and type of food to match our energy needs is a challenge for many of us. Our desire to consume food and the ability of our bodies to use it efficiently are survival mechanisms that have evolved with humans. However, because of current North American food supplies and accessibility, many of us are now too successful in obtaining food energy. The abundant food supply has essentially replaced the need to store body fat. Given the wide availability of food in vending machines, drive-up windows, social gatherings, and fast-food restaurants—combined with *supersized* portions—it is no wonder that the average adult is 8 pounds heavier than just 10 years ago. In response to this cultural trend of food being widely available, "defensive eating" (i.e., making careful and conscious food choices, especially in regard to portion size) on a continual basis is important for many of us.

The number of calories in a food is determined with an instrument called a **bomb calorimeter.** This calorie determination is described in Figure 7-3. The bomb calorimeter measures the amount of calories coming from carbohydrate, fat, protein, and alcohol. Recall that carbohydrates yield about 4 kcal per gram, proteins yield about 4 kcal per gram, fats yield about 9 kcal per gram, and alcohol yields 7 kcal per gram. These energy figures have been adjusted for (1) our ability to digest the food and (2) substances in food, such as fibrous plant parts that burn in the bomb calorimeter but do not provide calories to the human body. The figures are then rounded to whole numbers. However, today it is also possible and more common to determine the calorie content of a food by quantifying its carbohydrate, protein, and fat (and possibly alcohol) content. Then the kcal per gram factors listed previously are used to calculate the total kcals. (Recall that Chapter 1 showed how to do this calculation.)

Energy Output

So far, some factors concerning energy intake have been discussed. Now let's look at the other side of the equation—energy output.

The body uses energy for three general purposes: basal metabolism; physical activity; and digestion, absorption, and processing of ingested nutrients. A fourth minor form of energy output, known as thermogenesis, refers to energy expended during fidgeting or shivering in response to cold (Fig. 7-4).

bomb calorimeter An instrument used to determine the calorie content of a food.

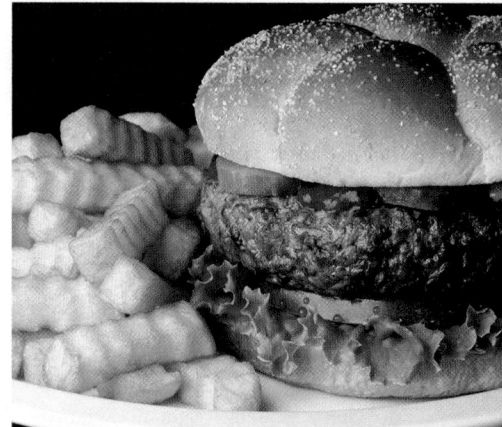

▲ The cultural trend of serving large quantities can easily lead to positive energy balance. Sharing your meal with another person is a good way to avoid overeating when served large portions.

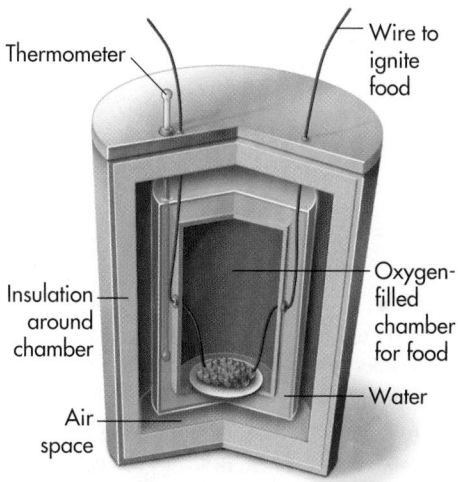

FIGURE 7-3 ▶ Bomb calorimeters measure calorie content by igniting and burning a dried portion of food. The burning food raises the temperature of the water surrounding the chamber holding the food. The increase in water temperature indicates the number of kilocalories in the food because 1 kilocalorie equals the amount of heat needed to raise the temperature of 1 kg of water by 1°C.

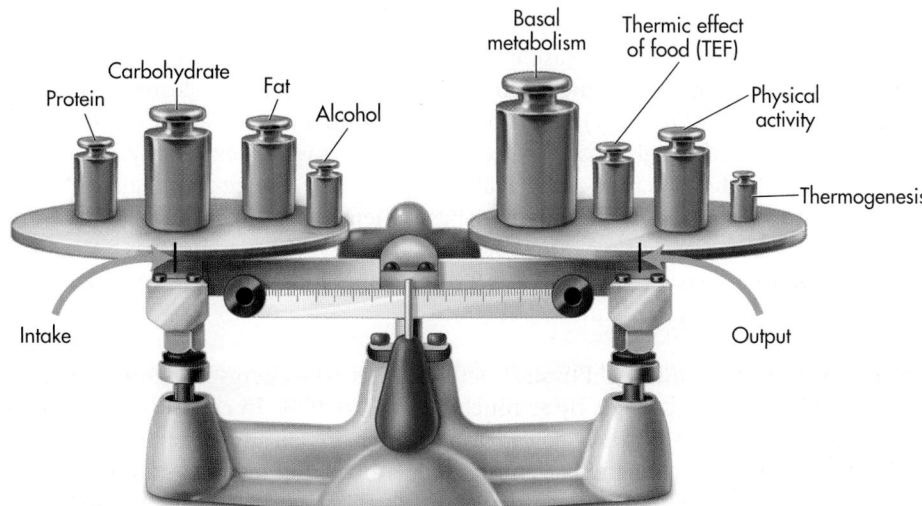

FIGURE 7-4 ▶ The components of energy intake and expenditure. This figure incorporates the major variables that influence energy balance. *Remember that alcohol is an additional source of energy for some of us.* The size of each component shows the relative contribution of that component to energy balance.

basal metabolism The minimal amount of calories the body uses to support itself in a fasting state when resting (e.g., 12 hours for both) and awake in a warm, quiet environment. It amounts to roughly 1 kcal per kilogram per hour for men and 0.9 kcal per kilogram per hour for women; these values are often referred to as *basal metabolic rate (BMR)*.

resting metabolism The amount of calories the body uses when the person has not eaten in 4 hours and is resting (e.g., 15 to 30 minutes) and awake in a warm, quiet environment. It is roughly 6% higher than basal metabolism due to the less strict criteria for the test; often referred to as *resting metabolic rate (RMR)*.

lean body mass Body weight minus fat storage weight equals lean body mass. This includes organs such as the brain, muscles, and liver, as well as bone and blood and other body fluids.

While a person is resting, the percentage of total energy use and corresponding energy use by various organs is approximately as follows:

Brain	19%	265 kcal/day
Skeletal muscle	18%	250 kcal/day
Liver	27%	380 kcal/day
Kidney	10%	140 kcal/day
Heart	7%	100 kcal/day
Other	19%	265 kcal/day

Basal Metabolism. **Basal metabolism** is expressed as basal metabolic rate (BMR) and represents the minimal amount of calories expended in a fasting state (for 12 hours or more) to keep a resting, awake body alive in a warm, quiet environment. For a sedentary person, basal metabolism accounts for about 60% to 70% of total energy use by the body. Some of the processes involved include the beating of the heart, respiration by the lungs, and the activity of other organs such as the liver, brain, and kidney. It does not include energy used for physical activity or digestion, absorption, and processing of recently consumed nutrients. If the person is not fasting or completely rested, the term **resting metabolism** is used and expressed as resting metabolic rate (RMR). An individual's RMR is typically 6% higher than his or her BMR.

To see how basal metabolism contributes to energy needs, consider a 130-pound woman. First, knowing that there are 2.2 pounds for every kilogram, convert her weight into metric units:

$$130 \text{ lbs} \div 2.2 \text{ lbs/kilograms} = 59 \text{ kilograms}$$

Then, using a rough estimate of basal metabolic rate of 0.9 kcal per kilogram per hour for an average female (1.0 kcal per kilogram per hour is used for an average male), calculate her basal metabolic rate:

$$59 \text{ kg} \times 0.9 \text{ kcal/kg} = 53 \text{ kcal per hour}$$

Finally, use this hourly basal metabolic rate to find her basal metabolic rate for an entire day:

$$53 \text{ kcal/hr} \times 24 \text{ hrs} = 1272 \text{ kcal}$$

These calculations give only an estimate of basal metabolism, as it can vary 25% to 30% among individuals. Factors that increase basal metabolism include:

- Greater **lean body mass**
- Larger body surface area per body volume
- Male gender (caused by greater lean body mass)
- Body temperature (fever or cold environmental conditions)
- Thyroid hormones
- Aspects of nervous system activity (release of norepinephrine)
- Pregnancy
- Caffeine and tobacco use (Using the practice of smoking to control body weight is not recommended as too many health risks are increased.)

Of those factors, the amount of lean body mass a person has is the most important one.

In contrast to factors that increase basal metabolism, a low calorie intake, such as that during an extreme diet regime, decreases basal metabolism by about 10% to 20% (about 150 to 300 kcal per day) as the body shifts into a conservation mode. This is a barrier to sustained weight loss during dieting that involves extremely low calorie diets. In addition, the effects of aging make weight maintenance a challenge. As lean body mass slowly and steadily decreases, basal metabolism declines 1% to 2% for each decade past the age of 30. However, because physical activity aids in maintenance of lean body mass, remaining active as one ages helps to preserve a high basal metabolism and, in turn, aids in weight control.

Energy for Physical Activity. Physical activity increases energy expenditure above and beyond basal energy needs by as much as 25% to 40%. In choosing to be active or inactive, we determine much of our total calorie expenditure for a day. Calorie expenditure from physical activity varies widely among people. For example, climbing stairs rather than riding the elevator, walking rather than driving to the store, and standing in a bus rather than sitting increase physical activity and, hence, energy use. The alarming incidence of and recent increase in obesity in North America are partially the result of our inactivity. Jobs demand less physical activity, and leisure time is often spent in front of a television or computer.

Thermic Effect of Food (TEF). In addition to basal metabolism and physical activity, the body uses energy to digest food, and absorb and further process the nutrients recently consumed. Energy used for these tasks is referred to as the **thermic effect of food (TEF).** TEF is similar to a sales tax—it is like being charged about 5% to 10% for the total amount of calories you eat to cover the cost of processing that food eaten. We may even recognize this increase in metabolism as a warming of the body during and right after a meal. Because of this "tax," you must eat between 105 and 110 kcal (5 to 10 kcal extra) for every 100 kcal needed for basal metabolism and physical activity. If your daily calorie intake was 3000 kcal, TEF would account for 150 to 300 kcal. As with other components of energy output, the total amount can vary somewhat among individuals.

Food composition influences TEF. For example, the TEF value for a protein-rich meal is 20% to 30% of the calories consumed and is higher than that of a carbohydrate-rich (5% to 10%) or fat-rich (0% to 3%) meal. This is because it takes more energy to metabolize amino acids into fat than to convert glucose into glycogen or transfer absorbed fat into adipose stores. In addition, large meals result in higher TEF values than the same amount of food eaten over many hours.

Thermogenesis. Thermogenesis represents the increase in nonvoluntary physical activity triggered by cold conditions or overeating. Some examples of nonvoluntary activities include shivering when cold, fidgeting, maintenance of muscle tone, and maintaining body posture when not lying down. Studies have shown that some people are able to resist weight gain from overfeeding by inducing thermogenesis, while others are not able to do so to a great extent.

The contribution of thermogenesis to overall calorie output is fairly small. The combination of basal metabolism and TEF accounts for 70% to 80% of energy used by a sedentary person. The remaining 20% to 30% is used mostly for physical activity, with a small amount used for thermogenesis.

Brown adipose tissue is a specialized form of adipose tissue that participates in thermogenesis. It is found in small amounts in infants. The brown appearance results from its rich blood flow. Brown adipose tissue contributes to thermogenesis by releasing some of the energy from energy-yielding nutrients into the environment as heat. In infants, brown adipose tissue contributes as much as 5% of body weight and is thought to be important for heat regulation. Hibernating animals also use brown adipose tissue to generate heat to withstand a long winter. Adults have very little brown adipose tissue, and its role in adulthood is unknown.

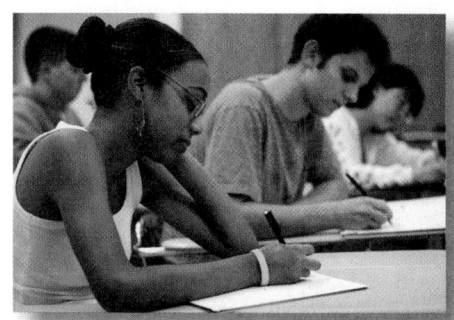
▲ Classwork leads to mental stress but puts little physical stress on the body. Hence, energy needs are only about 1.5 kcal per minute.

The TEF value for alcohol is 20%.

thermic effect of food (TEF) The increase in metabolism that occurs during the digestion, absorption, and metabolism of energy-yielding nutrients. This represents 5% to 10% of calories consumed.

thermogenesis This term encompasses the ability of humans to regulate body temperature within narrow limits (thermoregulation). Two visible examples of thermogenesis are fidgeting and shivering when cold.

brown adipose tissue A specialized form of adipose tissue that produces large amounts of heat by metabolizing energy-yielding nutrients without synthesizing much useful energy for the body. The unused energy is released as heat.

CONCEPT CHECK

Energy balance involves matching energy intake with energy output. Energy content of food is expressed in kcals and can be determined using a bomb calorimeter. This analysis yields the 4-9-4-7 estimates for the kcals in a gram of carbohydrate, fat, protein, and alcohol, respectively.

The body uses energy for four main purposes:

1. Basal metabolism (60% to 70% of total energy output) represents the minimal amount of calories needed to maintain the body at rest. Primary determinants of basal metabolic rate include quantity of lean body mass, amount of body surface, and thyroid hormone concentrations in the bloodstream.
2. Physical activity calorie expenditure (20% to 30% of total energy output) represents calorie use for total body cell metabolism above what is needed during rest.
3. Thermic effect of food (5% to 10% of total energy output) represents the calories needed to digest food and absorb and process nutrients recently consumed.
4. Thermogenesis (small, variable percentage of total energy output) includes nonvoluntary, heat-producing activities, such as fidgeting, as well as shivering when cold.

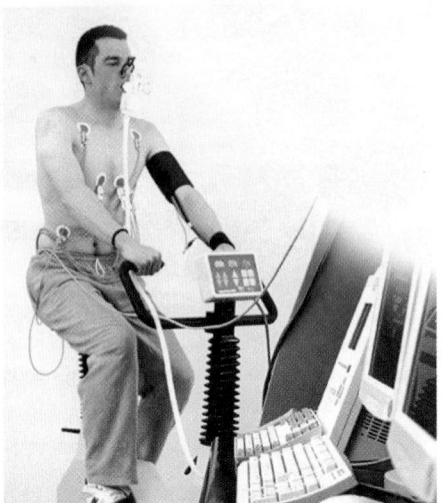

FIGURE 7-5 ▶ Indirect calorimetry measures oxygen intake and carbon dioxide output to determine energy expended during daily activities.

direct calorimetry A method of determining a body's energy use by measuring heat released from the body. An insulated chamber is usually used.

indirect calorimetry A method to measure energy use by the body by measuring oxygen uptake. Formulas are then used to convert this gas exchange value into energy use.

7.2 Determination of Energy Use by the Body

The amount of energy a body uses can be measured by both direct and indirect calorimetry or can be estimated based on height, weight, degree of physical activity, and age.

Direct and Indirect Calorimetry

Direct calorimetry measures the amount of body heat released by a person. The subject is put into an insulated chamber, often the size of a small bedroom, and body heat released raises the temperature of a layer of water surrounding the chamber. A kcal, as you recall, is related to the amount of heat required to raise the temperature of water. By measuring the water temperature in the direct calorimeter before and after the body releases heat, scientists can determine the energy expended.

Direct calorimetry works because almost all the energy used by the body eventually leaves as heat. However, few studies use direct calorimetry, mostly because of its expense and complexity.

The most commonly used method of **indirect calorimetry** measures the amount of oxygen a person consumes instead of measuring heat output (Fig. 7-5). A predictable relationship exists between the body's use of energy and oxygen. For example, when metabolizing a typical mixed diet of the energy-yielding nutrients, carbohydrate, fat, and protein, the human body uses 1 liter of oxygen to yield about 4.85 kcal of energy.

Instruments to measure oxygen consumption for indirect calorimetry are widely used. They can be mounted on carts and rolled up to a hospital bed or carried in backpacks while a person plays tennis or jogs. There are even newly developed handheld instruments (Body Gem). Tables showing energy costs of various forms of exercises rely on information gained from indirect calorimetry studies.

Estimates of Energy Needs

As covered in Chapter 2, the Food and Nutrition Board has published a number of formulas to estimate energy needs, called Estimated Energy Requirements (EERs). Those for adults are shown here (remember to do multiplication and division before addition and subtraction). (Formulas for pregnant women, lactating women, children, and teenagers, are listed in Chapters 14 and 15.) The calories used for basal metabolism are already factored into these formulas.

Estimated Energy Requirement Calculation for Men 19 Years and Older

$$EER = 662 - (9.53 \times AGE) + PA \times (15.91 \times WT + 539.6 \times HT)$$

Estimated Energy Requirement Calculation for Women 19 Years and Older

$$EER = 354 - (6.91 \times AGE) + PA \times (9.36 \times WT + 726 \times HT)$$

The variables in the formulas correspond to the following:

EER = Estimated Energy Requirement
AGE = age in years
PA = Physical Activity Estimate (see following table)
WT = weight in kilograms (pounds ÷ 2.2)
HT = height in meters (inches ÷ 39.4)

Physical Activity (PA) Estimates

Activity Level	PA (Men)	PA (Women)
Sedentary (e.g., no exercise)	1.00	1.00
Low activity (e.g., walks the equivalent of 2 miles per day at 3 to 4 mph)	1.11	1.12
Active (e.g., walks the equivalent of 7 miles per day at 3 to 4 mph)	1.25	1.27
Very active (e.g., walks the equivalent of 17 miles per day at 3 to 4 mph)	1.48	1.45

The following is a sample calculation for a man who is 25 years old, 5 feet, 9 inches (1.75 meters), 154 pounds (70 kilograms), and has an active lifestyle. His EER is:

$$EER = 662 - (9.53 \times 25) + 1.25 \times (15.91 \times 70 + 539.6 \times 1.75) = 2997 \text{ kcal}$$

The next equation is a sample calculation for a woman who is 25 years old, 5 feet, 4 inches (1.62 meters), 120 pounds (54.5 kilograms), and has an active lifestyle. Her EER is:

$$EER = 354 - (6.91 \times 25) + 1.27 \times (9.36 \times 54.5 + 726 \times 1.62) = 2323 \text{ kcal}$$

You have determined the man's EER to be about 3000 kcal and the woman's EER to be about 2300 kcal per day. Remember that this is only an estimate; many other factors, such as genetics and hormones, can affect actual energy needs.

A simple method of tracking your energy expenditure, and thus your energy needs, is to use the forms in Appendix E. Begin by taking an entire 24-hour period and listing all activities performed, including sleep. Record the number of minutes spent in each activity; the total should equal 1440 minutes (24 hours). Next record the energy cost for each activity in kcal per minute following the directions in Appendix E. Multiply the energy cost by the minutes. This gives the energy expended for each activity. Total all the kcal values. This gives your estimated energy expenditure for the day.

The www.ChooseMyPlate.gov website provides an interactive tool to estimate your calorie needs called Daily Food Plan. Figure 7-6 shows the range of activity levels and calorie recommendations for age and gender groups.

MyPlate Calorie Guidelines

Children	Sedentary →	Active
2–3 years	1000 →	1400

Females	Sedentary →	Active
4–8 years	1200 →	1800
9–13	1400 →	2200
14–18	1800 →	2400
19–30	1800 →	2400
31–50	1800 →	2200
51+	1600 →	2200

Males	Sedentary →	Active
4–8 years	1200 →	2000
9–13	1600 →	2600
14–18	2000 →	3200
19–30	2400 →	3000
31–50	2200 →	3000
51+	2000 →	2800

FIGURE 7-6 ▶ MyPlate Calorie Guidelines for age and gender groups.

CONCEPT CHECK

Energy use by the body can be measured as heat given off by direct calorimetry or as oxygen used by indirect calorimetry. A person's Estimated Energy Requirement can be calculated based on the following factors: gender, height, weight, age, and amount of physical activity.

7.3 Estimation of a Healthy Weight

Numerous methods are used to establish what body weight should be, typically called *healthy weight.* Healthy weight is currently the preferred term to use for weight recommendations. Older terms, such as *ideal weight* and *desirable weight*, are subjective and are no longer used in medical literature. Several tables exist, generally based on weight for height. These tables arise from studies of large population groups. When applied to a population, they provide good estimates of weight associated with health and longevity. However, they do not necessarily indicate the healthiest body weight

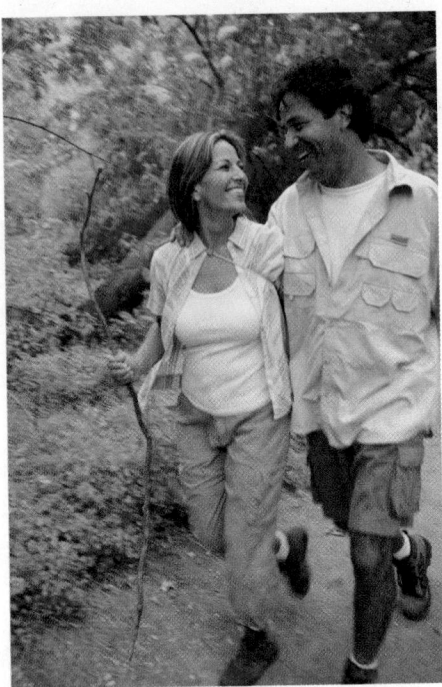

▲ Physical activity, such as walking, is an important component of our energy expenditure.

One BMI unit = 6 to 7 pounds

body mass index (BMI) Weight (in kilograms) divided by height (in meters) squared; a value of 25 and above indicates overweight and a value of 30 and above indicates obesity.

for each individual. For example, *athletes with large, lean body mass but low-fat content will have greater healthy weights than sedentary individuals.*

Overall, the individual, under a physician's guidance, should establish a "personal" healthy weight (or need for weight reduction) based on weight history, fat distribution patterns, family history of weight-related disease, and current health status. Indications that your weight is not healthy would include the following weight-related conditions:

- Hypertension
- Elevated LDL-cholesterol
- Family history of obesity, cardiovascular disease, or certain forms of cancer (e.g., uterus, colon)
- Pattern of fat distribution in the body
- Elevated blood glucose

This assessment points out how well the person is tolerating any existing excess weight. Thus, current height/weight standards are only a rough guide. On a more practical note, other questions can be pertinent: What is the least one has weighed as an adult for at least a year? What is the largest size clothing one would be happy with? What weight has one been able to maintain during previous diets without feeling constantly hungry? Furthermore, a healthy lifestyle may make a more important contribution to a person's health status than the number on the scale. Fit and overweight are not necessarily mutually exclusive (although not often seen together), and neither is thin synonymous with healthy if the person is not also physically active.

Body Mass Index (BMI)

For the past 50 years, weight-for-height tables issued by the Metropolitan Life Insurance Company have been the typical way healthy weight was established. These tables are organized by gender and frame size, predicting the weight range at a specific height that was associated with the greatest longevity. The latest table (issued in 1983) and methods for determining frame size can be found in Appendix G.

Currently, **body mass index (BMI)** is the preferred weight-for-height standard because it is the clinical measurement most closely related to body fat content (Fig. 7-7).

Body mass index is calculated as

$$\frac{\text{body weight (in kilograms)}}{\text{height}^2 \text{ (in meters)}}$$

An alternate method for calculating BMI is

$$\frac{\text{weight (pounds)} \times 703}{\text{height}^2 \text{ (inches)}}$$

Figure 7-8 lists the BMI for various heights and weights. A healthy weight for height is a BMI between 18.5 to 24.9. Health risks from excess weight may begin when the body mass index is 25 or more. What is your BMI? How much would your weight need to change to yield a BMI of 25? 30? These are general cutoff values for the presence of overweight and obesity, respectively. BMI offers another way to define obesity (Fig. 7-8).

| 30 to 39.9 | Obese | Increased health risk |
| 40 or greater | Severely obese | Major health risk (The number of North Americans falling into this category is increasing rapidly.) |

The concept of body mass index is convenient to use because the values apply to both men and women (i.e., gender neutral). However, any weight-for-height standard is a crude measure. Keep in mind, also, that a BMI of 25 to 29.9 is a marker of *overweight* (compared to a standard population) and not necessarily a marker of *overfat*. Many men (especially athletes) have a BMI greater than 25 because of extra muscle tissue. Also, very short adults (under 5 feet tall) may have high BMIs that may not reflect overweight or fatness. For this reason, BMI should be used only as a screening test for overweight or obesity. Even agreed upon weight standards for BMI are not for everyone. Adult BMIs should not be applied to children, still growing adolescents, frail older people, pregnant and lactating women, and highly muscular individuals. Pregnant women and children have unique BMI standards (see Chapters 14 and 15).

Still, overfat and overweight conditions generally appear together. The focus is on BMI in clinical settings mainly because this is easier to measure than total body fat.

Putting Healthy Weight into Perspective

Listening to the body for hunger cues, regularly eating a healthy diet, and remaining physically active (not to be overlooked) eventually helps one maintain an appropriate height/weight value. This concept will be further addressed in the upcoming discussion on treatment for obesity. Another school of thought is to let nature take its course with regard to body weight. Support for this proposal is that after weight is lost during dieting, people often regain their original weight plus more. The clearest idea regarding a healthy weight is that it is personal. Weight has to be considered in terms of health, not a mathematical calculation.

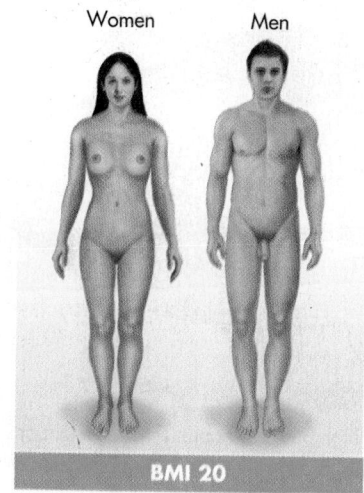

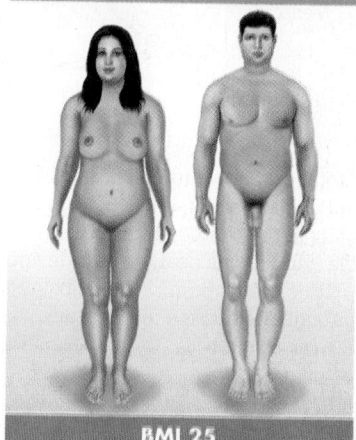

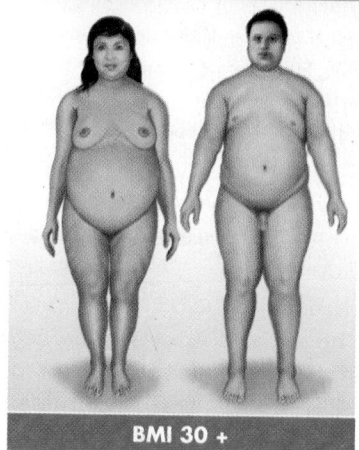

FIGURE 7-7 ▶ Estimates of body shapes at different BMI values.

Weight in pounds

	120	130	140	150	160	170	180	190	200	210	220	230	240	250
4'6"	29	31	34	36	39	41	43	46	48	51	53	56	58	60
4'8"	27	29	31	34	36	38	40	43	45	47	49	52	51	56
4'10"	25	27	29	31	34	36	38	40	42	44	46	48	50	52
5'0"	23	25	27	29	31	33	35	37	39	41	43	45	47	49
5'2"	22	24	26	27	29	31	33	35	37	38	40	42	44	46
5'4"	21	22	24	26	28	29	31	33	34	36	38	40	41	43
5'6"	19	21	23	24	26	27	29	31	32	34	36	37	39	40
5'8"	18	20	21	23	24	26	27	29	30	32	34	35	37	38
5'10"	17	19	20	22	23	24	26	27	29	30	32	33	35	36
6'0"	16	18	19	20	22	23	24	26	27	28	30	31	33	34
6'2"	15	17	18	19	21	22	23	24	26	27	28	30	31	32
6'4"	15	16	17	18	20	21	22	23	24	26	27	28	29	30
6'6"	14	15	16	17	19	20	21	22	23	24	25	27	28	29
6'8"	13	14	15	17	18	19	20	21	22	23	24	26	26	28

Height in feet and inches

◻ Healthy weight   ◻ Overweight   ◼ Obese

Developed by the National Center for Health Statistics in collaboration with the National Center for Chronic Disease Prevention and Health Promotion

FIGURE 7-8 ▶ Convenient height/weight table based on BMI. A healthy weight for height generally falls within a BMI range of 18.5 to 24.9 kilograms/meters².

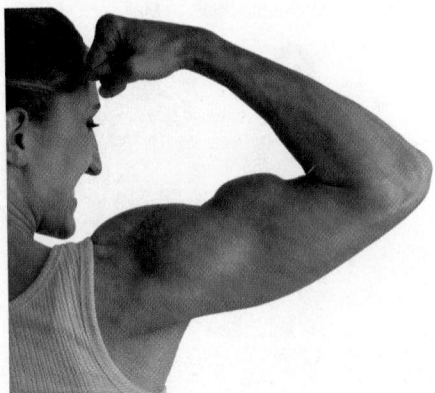

▲ A high BMI may not reflect overweight or fatness. Extra muscle tissue can result in a BMI greater than 25.

The total cost attributable to weight-related disease is about $147 billion annually in the United States. This is double what it was nearly a decade ago. Half of this cost is borne by the taxpayers through Medicare and Medicaid.

underwater weighing A method of estimating total body fat by weighing the individual on a standard scale and then weighing him or her again submerged in water. The difference between the two weights is used to estimate total body volume.

air displacement A method for estimating body composition that makes use of the volume of space taken up by a body inside a small chamber.

bioelectrical impedance The method to estimate total body fat that uses a low-energy electrical current. The more fat storage a person has, the more impedance (resistance) to electrical flow will be exhibited.

CONCEPT CHECK

Healthy body weight is generally determined in a clinical setting using a body mass index or another weight-for-height standard. The presence of existing weight-related diseases should be factored into the determination of healthy body weight. Total health history and lifestyle should be the major considerations when determining healthy weight.

7.4 Energy Imbalance

If calorie intake exceeds output over time, overweight (and often obesity) is a likely result. Often, health problems eventually follow (Table 7-1) (see Further Readings 1 and 12). As just discussed, BMI values can be used as a convenient clinical tool to estimate overweight (BMI ≥ 25), obesity (BMI ≥ 30), and severe obesity (BMI ≥ 40) in individuals greater than 20 years of age. Medical experts, however, recommend that an individual's diagnosis of obesity should not be based primarily on body weight but, rather, on the total amount of fat in the body, the location of body fat, and the presence or absence of weight-related medical problems.

Estimating Body Fat Content and Diagnosing Obesity

Body fat varies widely among individuals and can range from 2% to 70% of body weight. Desirable amounts of body fat are about 8% to 24% for men and 21% to 35% for women. Men with over 24% body fat and women with over about 35% body fat are considered obese. The higher range of body fat percentage for women is needed physiologically to maintain reproductive functions, including estrogen production.

To measure body fat content accurately using typical methods, both body weight and body volume of the person must be known. Body weight is easy to measure on a conventional scale. Of the typical methods used to estimate body volume, **underwater weighing** is the most accurate. This technique determines body volume using the difference between conventional body weight and body weight under water, along with the relative densities of fat tissue and lean tissue, and a specific mathematical formula. This procedure requires that an individual be totally submerged in a tank of water, with a trained technician directing the procedure (Fig. 7-9). **Air displacement** is another method of determining body volume. Body volume is quantified by measuring the space a person takes up inside a measurement chamber, such as the BodPod (Fig. 7-10). A less accurate method to measure body volume is to submerge a person in a tank and observe the level of the water before and after submersion. The volume of the displaced water is then calculated.

Once body volume is known, it can be used along with body weight in the following equation to calculate body density. Then using body density, body fat content finally can be determined.

$$\text{Body density} = \frac{\text{body weight}}{\text{body volume}}$$

$$\%\text{ body fat} = (495 \div \text{body density}) - 450$$

For example, assume that the individual in the underwater weighing tank in Figure 7-9 has a body density of 1.06 grams per centimeter³. We can use the second formula to calculate that he has 17% body fat ([495 ÷ 1.06] − 450 = 17).

Skinfold thickness is also a common anthropometric method to estimate total body fat content, although there are some limits to its accuracy. Clinicians use calipers to measure the fat layer directly under the skin at multiple sites and then plug these values into a mathematical formula (Fig. 7-11).

The technique of **bioelectrical impedance** is also used to estimate body fat content. The instrument sends a painless, low-energy electrical current to and from the

TABLE 7-1 Health Problems Associated with Excess Body Fat

Health Problem	Partially Attributable To
Surgical risk	Increased anesthesia needs, as well as greater risk of wound infections (the latter is linked to a decrease in immune function)
Pulmonary disease and sleep disorders	Excess weight over lungs and pharynx
Type 2 diabetes	Enlarged adipose cells, which poorly bind insulin and poorly respond to the message insulin sends to the cell; less synthesis of factors that aid insulin action, and greater synthesis of factors by adipose cells that lessen insulin action
Hypertension	Increased miles of blood vessels found in the adipose tissue, increased blood volume, and increased resistance to blood flow related to hormones made by adipose cells
Cardiovascular disease (e.g., coronary heart disease and stroke)	Increases in LDL-cholesterol and triglyceride values, low HDL-cholesterol, decreased physical activity, and increased synthesis of blood clotting and inflamatory factors by enlarged adipose cells. A greater risk for heart failure is also seen, due in part to altered heart rhythm.
Bone and joint disorders (including gout)	Excess pressure put on knee, ankle, and hip joints
Gallstones	Increased cholesterol content of bile
Skin disorders	Trapping of moisture and microorganisms in tissue folds
Various cancers, such as in the kidney, gall-bladder, colon and rectum, uterus (women), and prostate gland (men)	Estrogen production by adipose cells; animal studies suggest excess calorie intake encourages tumor development
Shorter stature (in some forms of obesity)	Earlier onset of puberty
Pregnancy risks	More difficult delivery, increased number of birth defects, and increased needs for anesthesia
Reduced physical agility and increased risk of accidents and falls	Excess weight that impairs movement
Menstrual irregularities and infertility	Hormones produced by adipose cells, such as estrogen
Vision problems	Cataracts and other eye disorders are more often present
Premature death	A variety of risk factors for disease listed in this table
Infections	Reduced immune system activity
Liver damage and eventual failure	Excess fat accumulation in the liver
Erectile dysfunction in men	Low-grade inflammation caused by excess fat mass and reduced function of the cells lining the blood vessels associated with being overweight

The greater the degree of obesity, the more likely and the more serious these health problems generally become. They are much more likely to appear in people who show an upper-body fat distribution pattern and/or are greater than twice healthy body weight.

body via wires and electrode patches to estimate body fat. This estimation is based on the assumption that adipose tissue resists electrical flow more than lean tissue because it has a lower electrolyte and water content than lean tissue. More adipose tissue therefore means proportionately greater electrical resistance. Within a few seconds, bioelectrical impedance analyzers convert body electrical resistance into an approximate estimate of total body fat, as long as body hydration status is normal (Fig. 7-12). Body composition monitors, better known as body fat calculators, that use bioelectric impedence are now available for home use. These machines are similar in shape and use to bathroom scales but their main purpose is to measure body fat. A current passes easily through conductive foot pads and/or handheld electrodes. These in-home devices will hopefully encourage people to be less concerned with what they weigh than whether their weight comes from fat or muscle.

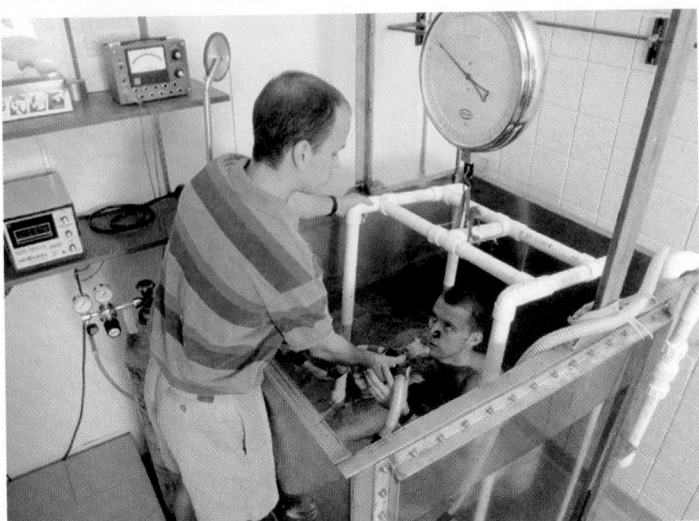

FIGURE 7-9 ▶ Underwater weighing. In this technique, the subject exhales as much air as possible and then holds his or her breath and bends over at the waist. Once the subject is totally submerged, the underwater weight is recorded. Using this value, body volume can be calculated.

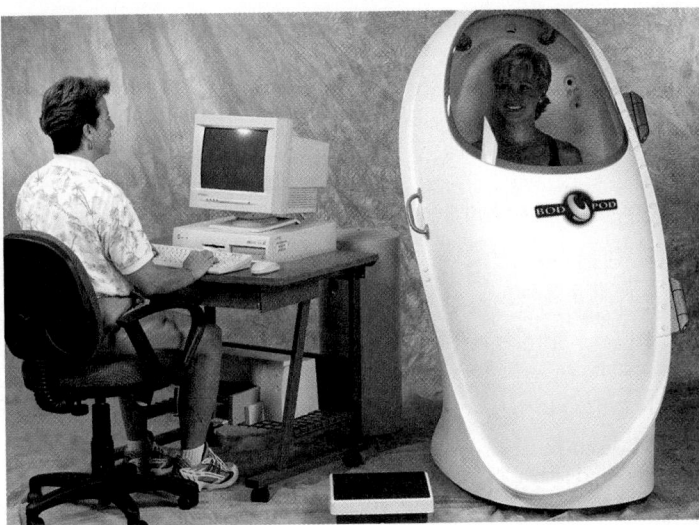

FIGURE 7-10 ▶ BodPod. This device determines body volume based on the volume of displaced air, measured as a person sits in a sealed chamber for a few minutes.

FIGURE 7-11 ▶ Skinfold measurements. Using proper technique and calibrated equipment, skinfold measurements around the body can be used to predict body fat content in about 10 minutes. Measurements are made at several locations including the triceps (photo and drawing) skinfolds.

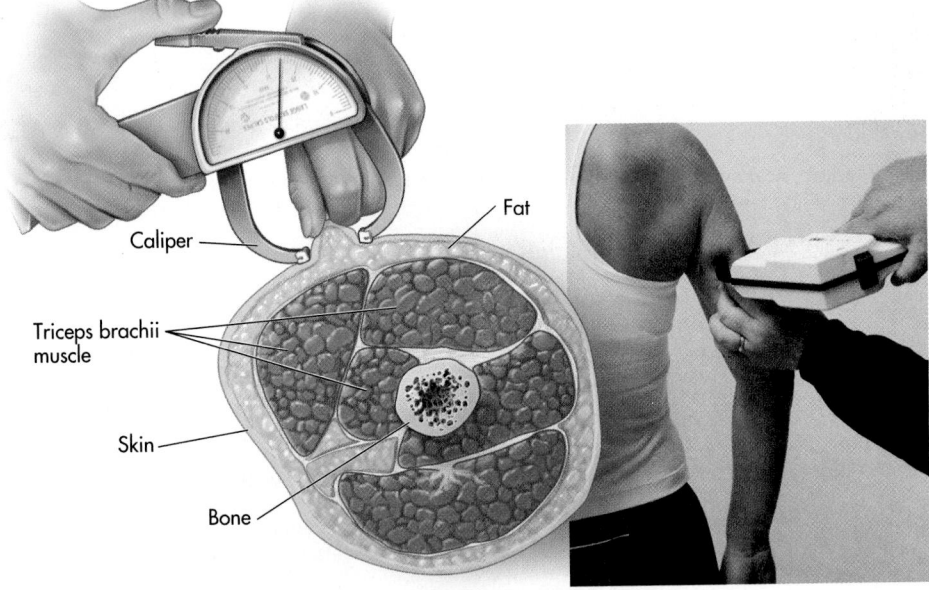

Caliper

Fat

Triceps brachii muscle

Skin

Bone

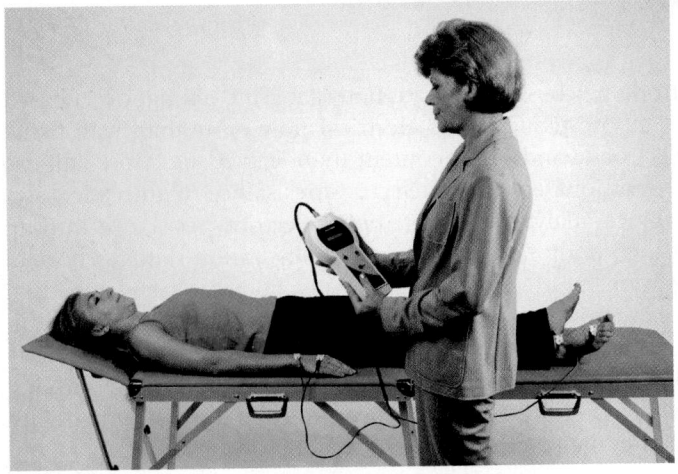

FIGURE 7-12 ▶ Bioelectrical impedance estimates total body fat in less than 5 minutes and is based on the principle that body fat resists the flow of electricity, since it is low in water and electrolytes. The degree of resistance to electrical flow is used to estimate body fatness.

A more advanced determination of body fat content can be made using **dual energy X-ray absorptiometry (DEXA).** DEXA is considered the most accurate way to determine body fat, but the equipment is expensive and not widely available for this use. This X-ray system allows the clinician to separate body weight into three separate components—fat, fat-free soft tissue, and bone mineral. The usual whole-body scan requires about 5 to 20 minutes and the dose of radiation is less than a chest X ray. An assessment of bone mineral density and the risk of osteoporosis also can be made using this method (Fig. 7-13).

Another method to assess body fat is to measure total-body electrical conductance (TOBEC) when placed in an electromagnetic field. Still another method, convenient and inexpensive, but not very accurate is **near-infrared reactance.** This method exposes the bicep muscle to a beam of near-infrared light and assesses the interactions of the light beam with fat and lean tissues in the upper arm after only 2 seconds.

In summary, although the DEXA is considered most accurate, the underwater weighing and air displacement methods of body fat estimation are also accurate because both body weight and body volume are measured. The adaptation of the bioelectrical impedence technology for in-home use is also a useful tool, providing valuable information about whether weight gain is coming from fat or muscle.

dual energy X-ray absorptiometry (DEXA) A highly accurate method of measuring body composition and bone mass and density using multiple low-energy X rays.

upper-body obesity The type of obesity in which fat is stored primarily in the abdominal area; defined as a waist circumference more than 40 inches (102 centimeters) in men and more than 35 inches (89 centimeters) in women; closely associated with a high risk for cardiovascular disease, hypertension, and type 2 diabetes. Also known as android obesity.

lower-body obesity The type of obesity in which fat storage is primarily located in the buttocks and thigh area. Also known as gynoid or gynecoid obesity.

Using Body Fat Distribution to Further Evaluate Obesity

In addition to the amount of fat we store, the location of that body fat is an important predictor of health risks. Some people store fat in upper-body areas, whereas others store fat lower on the body. Excess fat in either location generally spells trouble, but each storage space also has its unique risks. **Upper-body obesity,** characterized by a large abdomen, is more often related to cardiovascular disease, hypertension, and type 2 diabetes. Whereas other adipose cells empty fat into general blood circulation, the fat released from abdominal adipose cells goes directly to the liver, by way of the portal vein. This process likely interferes with the liver's ability to use insulin and negatively affects lipoprotein metabolism by the liver. These abdominal adipose cells also make substances that increase insulin resistance, blood clotting, blood vessel constriction, and inflammation in the body. These changes can lead to long-term health problems.

High blood testosterone (primarily a male hormone) levels apparently encourage upper-body obesity, as does a diet with a high glycemic load, alcohol intake, and smoking. This characteristic male pattern of fat storage is also called android obesity and is commonly known as the apple shape (large abdomen [pot belly] and small buttocks and thighs). Upper-body obesity is assessed by measuring the waist at the widest point just above the hips when relaxed. A waist circumference more than 40 inches (102 centimeters) in men and more than 35 inches (88 centimeters) in women indicates upper-body obesity (Fig. 7-14). If BMI is also 25 or more, health risks are significantly increased.

Estrogen and progesterone (primarily female hormones) encourage lower-body fat storage and **lower-body (gynecoid or gynoid) obesity**—the typical female pattern. The small abdomen and much larger buttocks and thighs give a pearlike appearance. Fat deposited in the lower body is not mobilized as easily as the other type and often resists being shed. After menopause, blood estrogen falls, encouraging upper-body fat distribution.

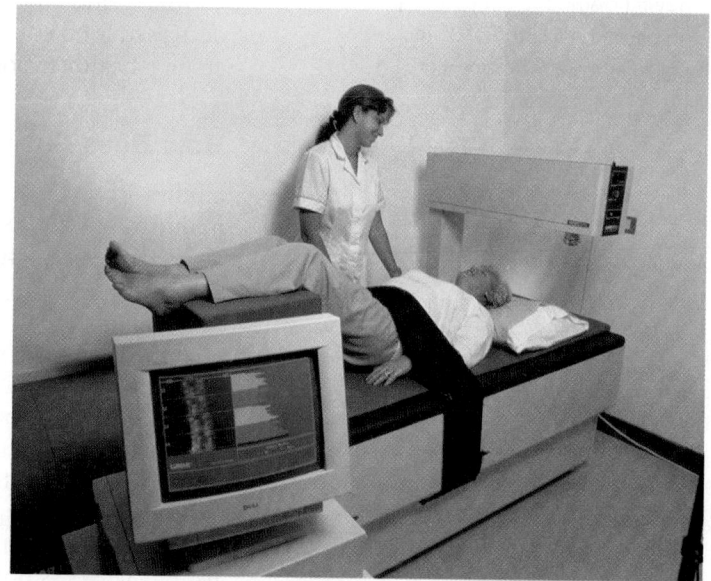

FIGURE 7-13 ▶ Dual energy X-ray absorptiometry (DEXA). This method measures body fat by passing small doses of radiation through the body. The radiation reacts differently with fat, lean tissue, or bone allowing these components to be quantified. The scanner arm moves from head to toe and in doing so can determine body fat as well as bone density. DEXA is currently considered the most accurate method for determining body fat (as long as the person can fit under the arm of the instrument). The radiation dose is minimal.

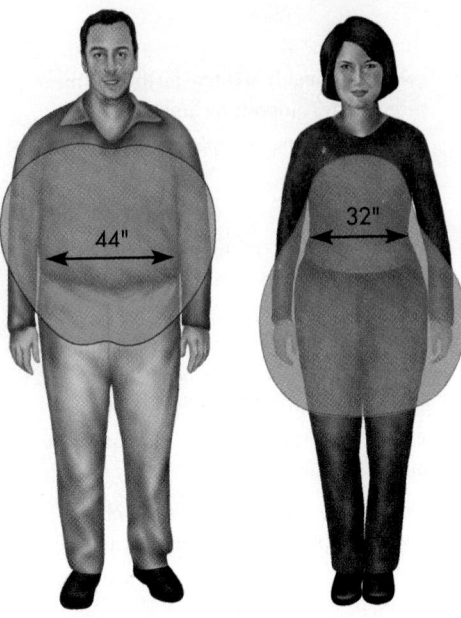

Upper-body fat
distribution
(android: apple shape)

Lower-body fat
distribution
(gynoid: pear shape)

FIGURE 7-14 ▶ Body fat stored primarily in the upper-body (android) form brings higher risks of ill health associated with obesity than does lower-body (gynoid) fat. The woman's waist circumference of 32 inches and the man's waist circumference of 44 inches indicate that the man has upper-body fat distribution but the woman does not, based on a cutoff of 35 inches for women and 40 inches for men.

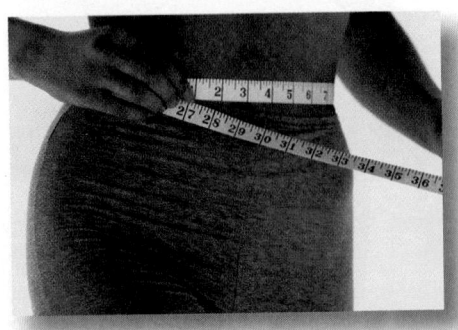

▲ Waist circumference is an important measure of weight-related health risk.

identical twins Two offspring that develop from a single ovum and sperm and, consequently, have the same genetic makeup.

CONCEPT CHECK

Overweight and obesity typically are associated with excessive body fat storage. The risk of health problems related to being overweight especially increases under the following conditions:

- A man's percentage of body fat exceeds 25%; a woman's exceeds about 35%.
- Excess fat is primarily stored in the upper-body region.
- Body mass index (BMI) is 30 or more (calculated as weight in kilograms divided by height squared in meters).

However, these are merely guidelines. A more individualized approach to assessment is warranted as long as a person is following a healthy lifestyle and has no existing health problems.

Body fat content can be estimated using a variety of methods such as underwater weighing, air displacement, skinfold thickness, bioelectrical impedance, and DEXA. Fat storage distribution further specifies an obese state as either upper-body or lower-body. Obesity leads to an increased risk for cardiovascular disease, some types of cancer, hypertension, type 2 diabetes, certain bone and joint disorders, and some digestive disorders. The risks for some of these diseases are greater with upper-body fat storage.

7.5 Why Some People Are Obese—Nature Versus Nurture

Both genetic (nature) and environmental (nurture) factors can increase the risk for obesity (Table 7-2). The eventual location of fat storage is strongly influenced by genetics. Consider the possibility that obesity is nurture allowing nature to express itself. Some obese people begin life with a slower basal metabolism; maintain an inactive lifestyle; and consume highly-refined, calorie-dense diets. These people in turn are nurtured into gaining weight, promoting their natural tendency toward obesity.

Still, genes do not fully control destiny. With increased physical activity and decreased food consumption, even those with a genetic tendency toward obesity can attain a healthier body weight.

How Does Nature Contribute to Obesity?

Studies in pairs of **identical twins** give us some insight into the contribution of nature to obesity. Even when identical twins are raised apart, they tend to show similar weight gain patterns, both in overall weight and body fat distribution. It appears that nurture—eating habits and nutrition, which varies between twins raised apart—has less to do with obesity than nature does. In fact, research suggests that genes account for up to 70% of weight differences between people. A child with no obese parent has only a 10% chance of becoming obese. When a child has one obese parent (common in our society), that risk advances up to 40%, and with two obese parents, it soars to 80%. Our genes help determine metabolic rate, fuel use, and differences in brain chemistry—all of which affect body weight.

We also inherit specific body types. Tall, thin people appear to have an inherently easier time maintaining healthy body weight. This is probably because basal metabolism increases as body surface increases, and therefore taller people use more calories than shorter people, even at rest.

Many of us probably have inherited a thrifty metabolism that enables us to store fat more readily than the typical human, so that we require fewer calories to get through the day. In earlier times, when food supplies were scarce, a thrifty metabolism would have been a built-in safeguard against starvation. Now, with a general abundance of food, people operating in this low gear require much physical activity and wise food choices to prevent obesity. If you think you are prone to weight gain, you likely have inherited a thrifty metabolism.

TABLE 7-2 What Encourages Excess Body Fat Stores and Obesity?

Factor	How Fat Storage is Affected
Age	Excess body fat is more common in adults and middle-age individuals.
Menopause	Increase in abdominal fat deposition is typical.
Gender	Females have more fat.
Positive energy balance	Over a long period promotes storage of fat.
Composition of diet	Excess calorie intake from fat, alcohol, and calorie dense (sugary, fat-rich) foods contributes to obesity.
Physical activity	Low physical activity ("couch potato") leads to positive energy balance and body fat storage.
Basal metabolism	A low BMR is linked to weight gain.
Thermic effect of food	Low for some obesity cases.
Increased hunger sensations	Some people have trouble resisting the abundant availability of food, which is likely linked to the activity of various brain chemicals.
Ratio of fat to lean tissue	A high ratio of fat mass to lean body mass is correlated with weight gain.
Fat uptake by adipose tissue	This is high in some obese individuals and remains high (perhaps even increases) with weight loss.
Variety of social and behavioral factors	Obesity is associated with socioeconomic status; familial conditions; network of friends; busy lifestyles that discourage balanced meals; binge eating; easy availability of inexpensive, "supersized" high-fat food; pattern of leisure activities; television time; smoking cessation; excessive alcohol intake; and number of meals eaten away from home.
Undetermined genetic characteristics	These affect components of energy balance, particularly energy expenditure, the deposition of the energy surplus as adipose tissue or as lean tissue, and the relative proportion of fat and carbohydrate used by the body.
Race	In some ethnic groups, higher body weight may be more socially acceptable.
Certain medications	Food intake increases.
Childbearing	Women may not lose all weight gained in pregnancy.
National region	Regional differences, such as high-fat diets and sedentary lifestyles in the Midwest and areas of the South, lead to geographically different rates of obesity.

Does the Body Have a Set Point for Weight?

The **set-point** theory of weight maintenance proposes that humans have a genetically predetermined body weight or body fat content, which the body closely regulates. Some research suggests that the **hypothalamus** region of the brain monitors the amount of body fat in humans and tries to keep that amount constant over time. The hypothalamus has two sites—the feeding center and the satiety center—that play a role in regulating hunger. The hormone **leptin** forms a communication link between adipose cells and the brain, which allows for some weight regulation.

Several physiological changes that occur during calorie reduction and weight loss also endorse the set-point theory (see Further Reading 2). For example, when calorie intake is reduced, the blood concentration of thyroid hormones falls, which slows basal metabolism. In addition, as weight is lost, the calorie cost of weight-bearing activity decreases, so that an activity that burned 100 kcal before weight loss may only burn 80 kcal after weight loss. Furthermore, with weight loss, the body becomes more efficient at storing fat by increasing the activity of the enzyme *lipoprotein lipase*, which takes fat into cells. All of these changes protect the body from losing weight.

If a person overeats, in the short run, basal metabolism tends to increase. This causes some resistance to weight gain. However, in the long run, resistance to weight

set point Often refers to the close regulation of body weight. It is not known what cells control this set point or how it functions in weight regulation. There is evidence, however, that mechanisms exist that help regulate weight.

hypothalamus A region at the base of the brain that contains cells that play a role in the regulation of hunger, respiration, body temperature, and other body functions.

leptin A hormone made by adipose tissue in proportion to total fat stores in the body that influences long-term regulation of fat mass. Leptin also influences reproductive functions, as well as other body processes, such as release of the hormone insulin.

▶ Studies in identical twins give us insight into the genetic contribution to obesity.

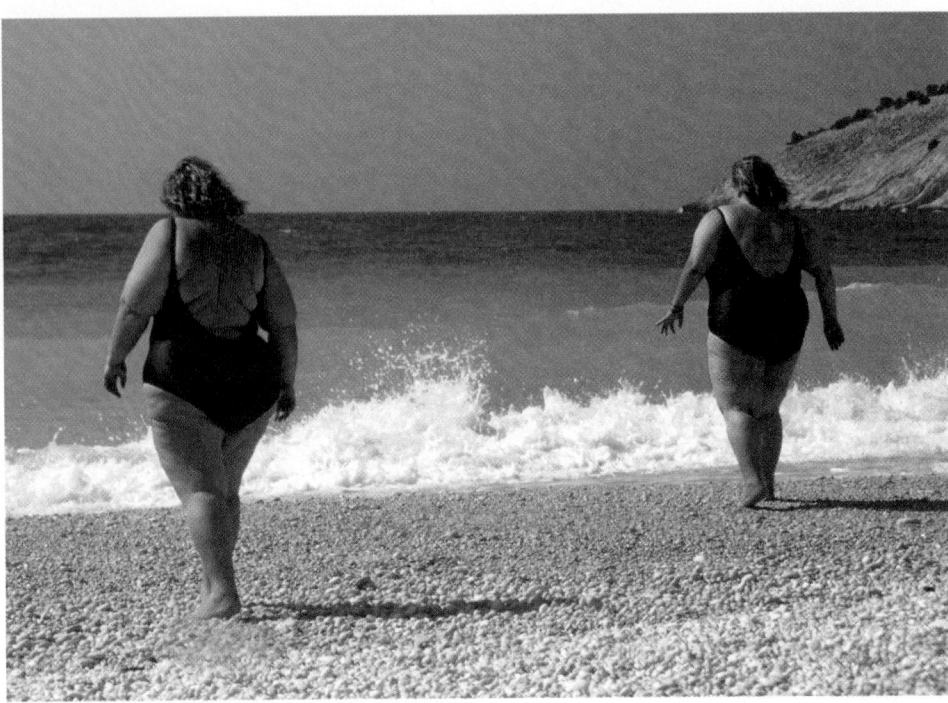

gain is much less than resistance to weight loss. When a person gains weight and stays at that weight for a while, the body tends to establish a new set point.

Opponents of the set-point theory argue that weight does not remain constant throughout adulthood—the average person gains weight slowly, at least until old age. Also, if an individual is placed in a different social, emotional, or physical environment, weight can be altered and maintained markedly higher or lower. These arguments suggest that humans, rather than having a set point determined by genetics or the number of adipose cells, settle into a particular stable weight based on their circumstances, often regarded as a "settling point."

The size-acceptance nondiet movement, "Health at Every Size," indirectly refers to a set point for weight by defining healthy weight as the natural weight the body adopts, given a healthy diet and meaningful levels of physical activity. Overall, the set point is weaker in preventing weight gain than in preventing weight loss. Even with a set point helping us, the odds are in favor of eventual weight gain unless we devote effort to a healthy lifestyle.

▼ Body weight is influenced by many factors related to both nature and nurture. We resemble our parents because of the genes we have inherited, as well as the lifestyle habits, including diet, that we have learned from them.

Does Nurture Have a Role?

Some would argue that body weight similarities between family members stem more from learned behaviors rather than genetic similarities. Even couples, who have no genetic link, may behave similarly toward food and eventually assume similar degrees of leanness or fatness. Proponents of nurture pose that environmental factors, such as high-fat diets and inactivity, literally shape us. This seems likely when we consider that our gene pool has not changed much in the past 50 years, whereas according to the U.S. Centers for Disease Control and Prevention the ranks of obese people have grown in epidemic proportions over the last 25 years.

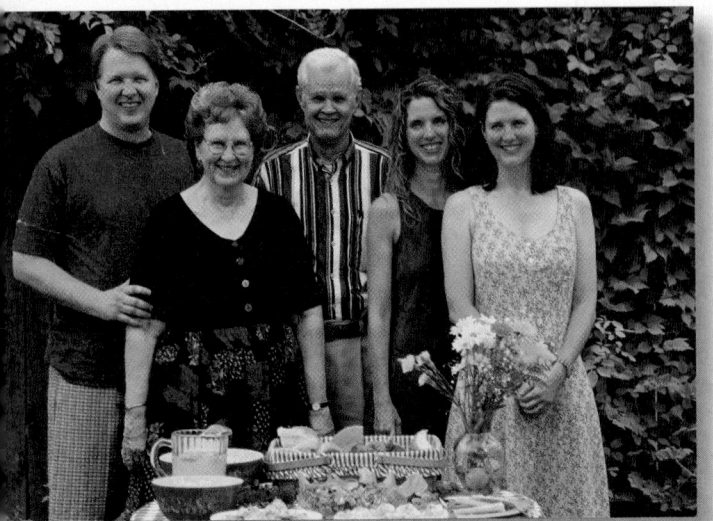

Adult obesity in women is often rooted in childhood obesity. In addition, relative inactivity and periods of stress or boredom, as well as excess weight gain during pregnancy, contribute to female obesity. (Chapter 14 notes that breastfeeding one's infant contributes to loss of some of the excess fat associated with pregnancy.) These patterns suggest both social and genetic links. Male obesity, however, is not strongly linked to childhood obesity and, instead, tends to appear after age 30. This powerful and prevalent pattern suggests a primary role of nurture in obesity, with less genetic influence.

Is poverty associated with obesity? Ironically, the answer is often yes. North Americans of lower socioeconomic status, especially females, are more likely to be obese than those in upper socioeconomic groups. Several social and behavioral factors promote fat storage. These factors include lower socioeconomic status, overweight friends and family, a cultural/ethnic group that prefers higher body weight, a lifestyle that discourages healthy meals and adequate exercise, easy availability of inexpensive high-calorie food, limited access to fresh fruits and vegetables, excessive television viewing, smoking cessation, lack of adequate sleep, emotional stress, and meals frequently eaten away from home.

7.6 Treatment of Overweight and Obesity

Treatment of overweight and obesity should be long-term, similar to that for any chronic disease. Treatments require long-term lifestyle changes, rather than a quick fix promoted by many popular (also called fad) diet books. We often view a "diet" as something one goes on temporarily, only to resume prior (typically poor) habits once satisfactory results have been achieved. This is a big reason that so many people regain lost weight. Instead, an emphasis on healthy, active living with acceptable dietary modifications will promote weight loss and later weight maintenance.

What to Look for in a Sound Weight-Loss Plan

A dieter can develop a plan of action by seeking advice from a health professional, such as a registered dietitian, or by using the interactive tools at www.ChooseMyPlate.gov. Either way, a sound weight-loss program (Fig. 7-15) should especially include these components:

1. Control of calorie intake. One recommendation is to decrease calorie intake by 100 kcal per day (and increase physical activity by 100 kcal per day). This should allow for slow and steady weight loss.
2. Increased physical activity.
3. Acknowledgment that maintenance of a healthy weight requires lifelong changes in habits, not a short-term weight-loss period.

A one-sided approach that focuses only on restricting calories is a difficult plan of action. Instead, adding physical activity and an appropriate psychological component

MAKING DECISIONS

Losing Body Fat

Rapid weight loss cannot consist primarily of fat loss because a high calorie deficit is needed to lose a large amount of adipose tissue. Adipose tissue, mostly fat, contains about 3500 kcal per pound. Weight loss, however, includes adipose tissue plus lean tissues that support it and represents approximately 3300 kcal per pound (about 7.2 kcal per gram). Therefore, to lose 1 pound of adipose tissue per week, calorie intake must be decreased by approximately 500 kcal per day, or physical activity must be increased by 500 kcal per day. Alternately, a combination of both strategies can be used. Diets that promise 10 to 15 pounds of weight loss per week cannot ensure that the weight loss is from adipose tissue stores alone. How many calories would need to be eliminated from the diet per day to lose 10 pounds per week? Is it possible to subtract enough calories from one's daily intake to lose that amount of adipose tissue? Lean tissue and water, rather than adipose tissue, account for the major part of the weight lost during these dramatic weight-loss programs.

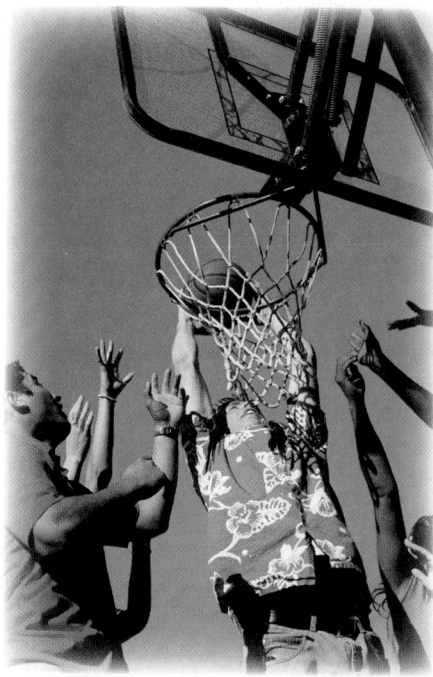

▲ Student life is often full of physical activity. This is not necessarily true for a person's later working life; hence, weight gain is a strong possibility.

▶ **Weight Status objectives from** *Healthy People 2020*

- Increase by 10% the proportion of adults who are at a healthy weight.
  - Target for 2020:   33.9%
  - Baseline in 2005–08: 30.8%
- Reduce by 10% the proportion of adults who are obese.
  - Target for 2020:   30.6%
  - Baseline in 2005–08: 34.0%
- Reduce by 10% the proportion of children and adolescents, 2 to 19 years, who are considered obese.
  - Target for 2020:   14.6%
  - Baseline in 2005–08: 16.2%
- Prevent inappropriate weight gain in youth and adults.

As you read brochures, articles, or research reports about specific diet plans, look beyond the weight loss promoted by the diet's advocate to see if the reported weight loss was maintained. If the weight-maintenance aspect was missing, then the program was not successful.

FIGURE 7-15 ▶ Characteristics of a sound weight-loss diet. Use this checklist to evaluate any new diet plan before putting it into practice.

RATE OF LOSS

☐ Encourages slow and steady weight loss, rather than rapid weight loss, to promote lasting weight
☐ Sets goal of 1 pound of fat loss per week
☐ Includes a period of weight maintenance for a few months after 10% of body weight is lost
☐ Evaluates need for further dieting before more weight loss begins

FLEXIBILITY

☐ Supports participation in normal activities (e.g., parties, restaurants)
☐ Adapts to individual habits and tastes

INTAKE

☐ Meets nutrient needs (except for energy needs)
☐ Includes common foods, with no foods being promoted as magical or special
☐ Recommends a fortified ready-to-eat breakfast cereal or balanced multivitamin/mineral supplement, especially when intake is less than 1600 kcal per day
☐ Uses MyPlate as a pattern for food choices

BEHAVIOR MODIFICATION

☐ Focuses on maintenance of healthy lifestyle (and weight) for a lifetime
☐ Promotes reasonable changes that can be maintained
☐ Encourages social support
☐ Includes plans for relapse, so that one does not quit after a setback
☐ Promotes changes that control problem eating behaviors

OVERALL HEALTH

☐ Requires screening by a physician for people with existing health problems, those over 40 (men) to 50 (women) years of age who plan to increase physical activity substantially, and those who plan to lose weight rapidly
☐ Encourages regular physical activity, sufficient sleep, stress reduction, and other healthy changes in lifestyle
☐ Addresses underlying psychological weight issues, such as depression or marital stress

The 2010 Dietary Guidelines for Americans provide the following recommendations regarding "Balancing Calories to Manage Weight" as part of healthy eating pattern and while staying within their calories need:

- Prevent and/or reduce overweight and obesity through improved eating and physical activity behaviors.

- Control total calorie intake to manage body weight. For people who are overweight or obese, this will mean consuming fewer calories from foods and beverages.

- Increase physical activity and reduce time spent in sedentary behaviors.

- Maintain appropriate calorie balance during each stage of life—childhood, adolescence, adulthood, pregnancy and breastfeeding, and older age.

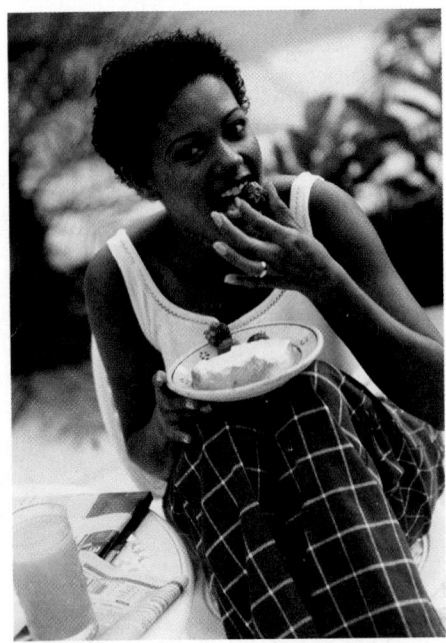

▲ Making a commitment to a healthier diet and lifestyle can be a challenge for many individuals. A sound weight-loss plan, however, does not require you to completely avoid certain favorite foods. Practical strategies include substituting lower-calorie choices, choosing high-calorie treats less often, and limiting portion sizes.

will contribute to success in weight loss and eventual weight maintenance (Fig. 7-16). From the 2010 Dietary Guidelines for Americans section on weight management, the key recommendations for those who need to lose weight is to aim for a slow, steady weight loss by decreasing calorie intake while maintaining an adequate nutrient intake and increasing physical activity.

Weight Loss in Perspective

These principles point to the importance of preventing obesity. This concept has wide support because conquering the disorder is so difficult. Public health strategies to address the current obesity problem must speak to all age groups. There is a particular need to focus on children and adolescents because patterns of excess weight and sedentary lifestyle developed during youth may form the basis for a lifetime

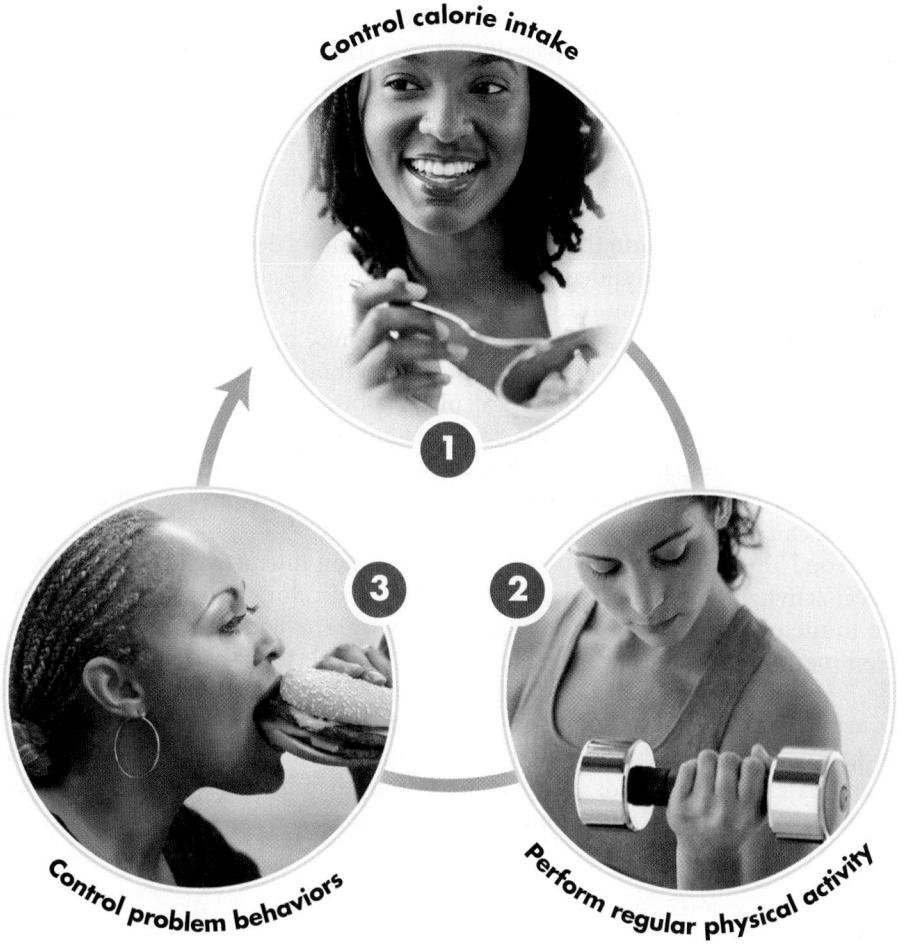

Control calorie intake

Control problem behaviors

Perform regular physical activity

FIGURE 7-16 ▶ Weight-loss triad. The key to weight loss and maintenance can be thought of as a triad, which consists of three parts: (1) controlling calorie intake, (2) performing regular physical activity, and (3) controlling problem behaviors. The three parts of the triad support each other in that without one part of the triad, weight loss and later maintenance become unlikely.

For more information on weight control, obesity, and nutrition, visit the Weight-Control Information Network (WIN) at http://win.niddk.nih.gov/index.htm or call 800-WIN-8098. Complete guidelines for weight management are available at www.nhlbi.nih.gov/guidelines/index .htm. Other websites include www .caloriecontrol.org, www.weight.com, www.obesity.org, and www.cyberdiet .com.

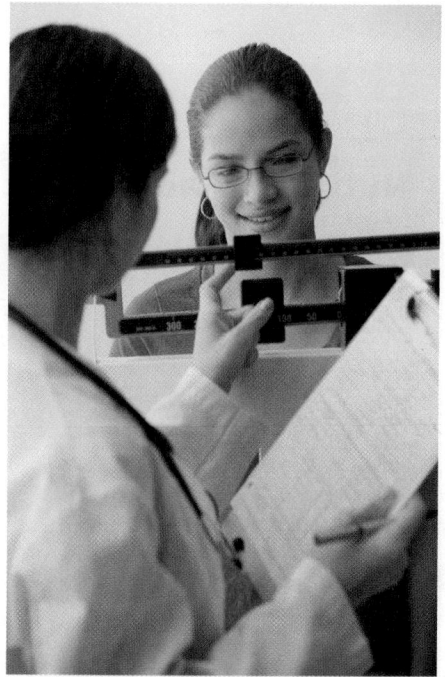

▲ Slow, steady weight loss is one of the characteristics of a sound weight-loss program.

CONCEPT CHECK

Obesity is a chronic disease that necessitates lifelong treatment. Emphasis should be placed especially on preventing obesity, because overcoming this disorder is difficult. Appropriate weight-loss programs have the following characteristics in common: (1) They meet nutritional needs; (2) they can adjust to accommodate habits and tastes; (3) they emphasize readily obtainable foods; (4) they promote changing habits that discourage overeating; (5) they encourage regular physical activity; and (6) they help change obesity-promoting beliefs and rally healthy social support.

of weight-related illness and increased mortality. In the adult population, attention should be directed toward weight maintenance and increased physical activity.

7.7 Control of Calorie Intake—The Main Key to Weight Loss and Weight Maintenance

A goal of losing 1 pound or so of stored fat per week may require limiting calorie intake to 1200 kcal per day for women and 1500 kcal for men. The calorie allowance could also be higher for very active people. Keep in mind that, in our sedentary society, decreasing calorie intake is vital because it is difficult to burn much energy without ample physical activity. With regard to consuming fewer calories, some experts

For interactive dietary and physical activity tools, check out the Food Tracker and Food Planner at www.ChooseMyPlate.gov.

NEWSWORTHY NUTRITION

Small changes result in large weight change over the years

Subjects in a large 20-year study of lifestyle factors and weight change gained an average of 20 pounds in 20 years. Less exercise led to weight gain but the kinds of foods people ate had a larger effect than changes in physical activity. Increased consumption of French fries alone led to an average weight gain of 3.4 pounds every 4 years. Greater intake of fruits, vegetables, whole grains, yogurt, and nuts resulted in weight loss or no gain. The result of this study show how small changes in eating, exercise, and other habits can result in large changes in body weight over the years.

Source: Mozaffarian D and others: Changes in diet and lifestyle and long-term weight gain in women and men. *New England Journal of Medicine* 364:2392 2011, (see Further Reading 8).

■ connect NUTRITION **Check out the Connect site** www.mcgrawhillconnect.com **to further explore long-term weight gain.**

suggest consuming less fat (especially saturated fat and *trans* fat), while others suggest consuming less carbohydrate, especially refined (high glycemic load) carbohydrate sources. Protein intakes in excess of what is typically needed by adults are also receiving attention. Using all these approaches simultaneously is fine. At this time, the low-fat, high-fiber approaches have been the most successful in long-term studies. A recent report (see Newsworthy Nutrition) confirms that the kinds of food we eat have a large effect on weight gain over the years. Finding what works for an individual is a process of trial and error. The notion that any type of diet promotes significantly greater calorie use by the body is unfounded (see Further Readings 13, 14, and 15).

One way for a dieter to monitor calorie intake at the start of a weight-loss program is by reading labels. Label reading is important, because many foods are more energy dense than people suppose (Fig. 7-17). Another method is to write down food intake for 24 hours (Appendix E) and then calculate calorie intake from the food table in the textbook supplement or by using your diet-analysis software. With knowledge of current calorie intake, future food choices can be adjusted as needed. People often underestimate portion size when recording food intake, so measuring cups and a food scale can help.

The Food Tracker at www.ChooseMyPlate.gov is an interactive online dietary and physical activity assessment tool that tracks the food calories you eat and compares them to the energy you expend in physical activity. The Food Planner is an interactive online tool for planning menus based on your personal ChooseMyPlate goals. Table 7-3 shows how to start reducing calorie intake. As you should realize, it is best to consider healthy eating a lifestyle change, rather than a weight-loss plan. Also, liquids deserve attention, because liquid calories do not stimulate satiety mechanisms to the same extent as solid foods. The corresponding advice from experts is to use beverages that have few or no calories and limit sugar-sweetened beverages.

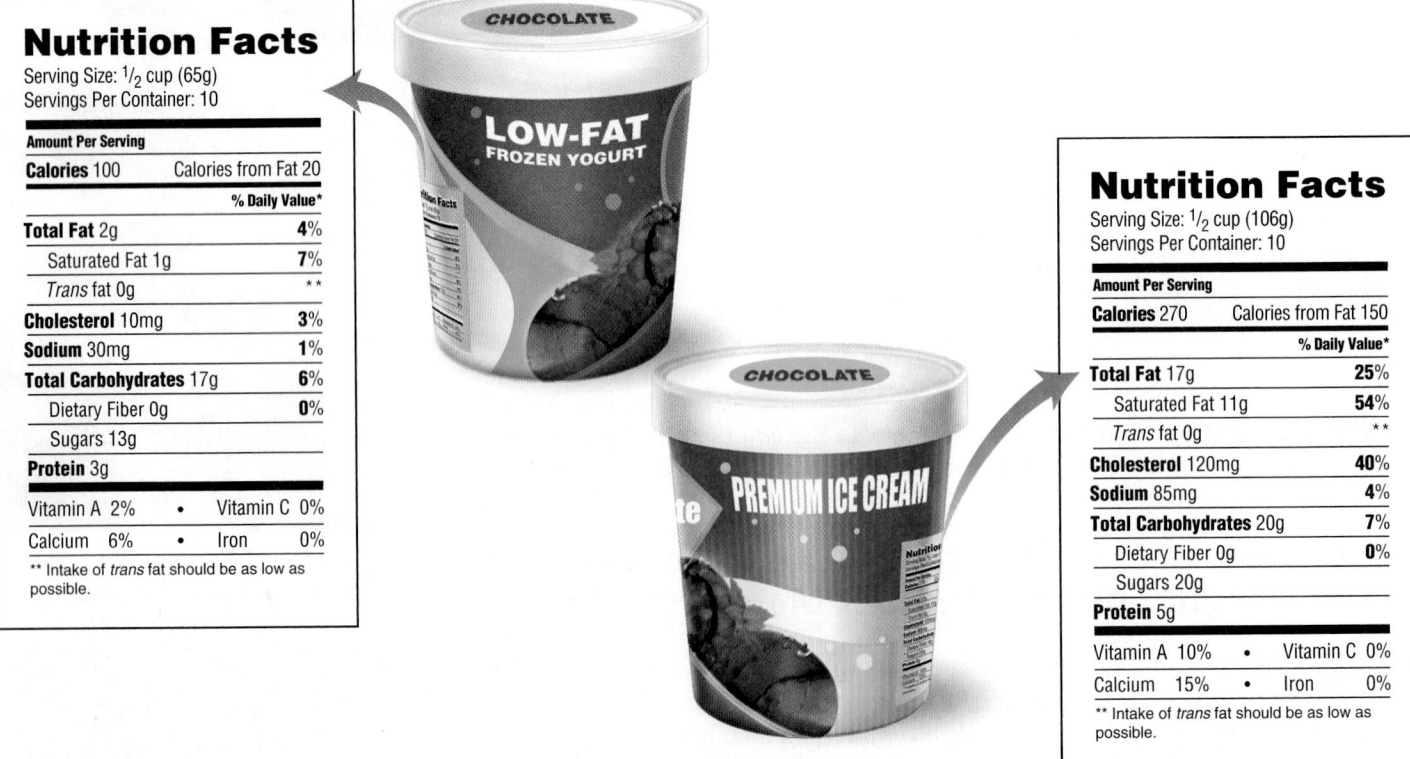

FIGURE 7-17 ▶ Reading labels helps you choose foods with fewer calories. Which of these frozen desserts is the best choice, per ½ cup serving, for a person on a weight-loss diet? The % Daily Values are based on a 2000 kcal diet. Read more about these dessert choices in What Would You Choose Recommendations.

TABLE 7-3 Lowering kcal: Point of Purchase and Consumption Decisions

Instead of	Try	Number of kcal Saved
3 oz well-marbled meat (prime rib)	3 oz lean meat (eye of round)	140
½ chicken breast, batter-fried	½ chicken breast, broiled with lemon	175
½ cup home-fried potatoes	1 medium baked potato	65
½ cup green bean-mushroom casserole	½ cup cooked green beans	50
½ cup potato salad	1 cup raw vegetable salad	140
½ cup pineapple chunks in heavy syrup	½ cup pineapple chunks canned in juice	25
2 tbsp bottled French dressing	2 tbsp low-calorie French dressing	150
$\frac{1}{8}$ 9-inch apple pie	1 baked apple, unsweetened	308
3 oatmeal-raisin cookies	1 oatmeal-raisin cookie	125
½ cup ice cream	½ cup ice milk	45
1 danish pastry	½ English muffin	150
1 cup sugar-coated corn flakes	1 cup plain corn flakes	60
1 cup whole milk	1 cup 1% low-fat milk	45
1 oz bag potato chips	1 cup plain popcorn	120
$\frac{1}{12}$ 8-inch white layer cake with chocolate frosting	$\frac{1}{12}$ angel food cake, 10-inch tube	185
12-fluid-ounce cola	12-fluid-ounce diet cola	150

7.8 Regular Physical Activity—A Second Key to Weight Loss and Especially Important for Later Weight Maintenance

Regular physical activity is important for everyone, especially those trying to lose weight or maintain a lower body weight. Calorie burning is enhanced both during and after physical activity. Therefore, activity greatly complements a reduction in calorie intake for weight loss. Many of us rarely do more than sit, stand, and sleep. More calories are used during physical activity than at rest. Expending only 100 to 300 extra kcal per day above and beyond normal daily activity, while controlling calorie intake, can lead to a steady weight loss. Furthermore, physical activity has so many other benefits, including a boost for overall self-esteem. A Key Recommendation from the 2010 Dietary Guidelines is to increase physical activity and reduce time spent in sedentary behaviors. The Dietary Guidelines point to the 2008 Physical Activity Guidelines for Americans for specific recommendations. Weight management, as well as other health outcomes including diseases and risk factors for disease, was considered in developing the Physical Activity Guidelines. Although some adults will need a higher level of physical activity than others, it is recommended that adults should do the equivalent of 150 minutes of moderate-intensity aerobic activity each week to achieve and maintain a healthy body weight. Some may need more than the equivalent of 300 minutes per week of moderate-intensity activity.

Adding any of the activities in Table 7-4 to one's lifestyle can increase calorie use. Duration and regular performance, rather than intensity, are the keys to success with this approach to weight loss. One should search for activities that can be continued over time. In this regard, walking vigorously 3 miles per day can be as helpful as

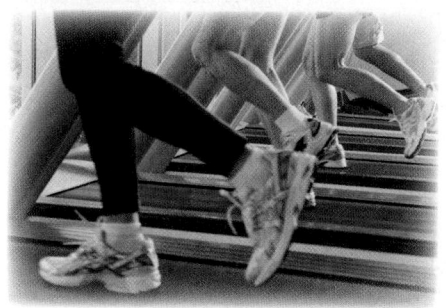

▲ Physical activity complements any diet plan.

TABLE 7-4 Approximate Calorie Costs of Various Activities and Specific Calorie Costs Projected for a 150-Pound (68-Kilogram) Person

Activity	kcal per kilogram per Hour	Total kcal per Hour	Activity	kcal per kilogram per Hour	Total kcal per Hour
Aerobics—heavy	8.0	544	Horseback riding	5.1	346
Aerobics—medium	5.0	340	Ice skating (10 mph)	5.8	394
Aerobics—light	3.0	204	Jogging—medium	9.0	612
Backpacking	9.0	612	Jogging—slow	7.0	476
Basketball—vigorous	10.0	680	Lying—at ease	1.3	89
Bowling	3.9	265	Racquetball—social	8.0	544
Calisthenics—heavy	8.0	544	Roller skating	5.1	346
Calisthenics—light	4.0	272	Running or jogging (10 mph)	13.2	897
Canoeing (2.5 mph)	3.3	224	Skiing downhill (10 mph)	8.8	598
Cleaning (female)	3.7	253	Sleeping	1.2	80
Cleaning (male)	3.5	236	Swimming (.25 mph)	4.4	299
Cooking	2.8	190	Tennis	6.1	414
Cycling (13 mph)	9.7	659	Volleyball	5.1	346
Cycling (5.5 mph)	3.0	204	Walking (3.75 mph)	4.4	299
Dressing/showering	1.6	106	Walking (2.5 mph)	3.0	204
Driving	1.7	117	Water skiing	7.0	476
Eating (sitting)	1.4	93	Weight lifting—heavy	9.0	612
Food shopping	3.6	245	Weight lifting—light	4.0	272
Football—touch	7.0	476	Window cleaning	3.5	240
Golf (using power cart)	3.6	244	Writing (sitting)	1.7	118

The values in Table 7-4 refer to total energy expenditure, including that needed to perform the physical activity, plus that needed for basal metabolism, the thermic effect of food, and thermogenesis. Use your diet-analysis software for your personal estimate.

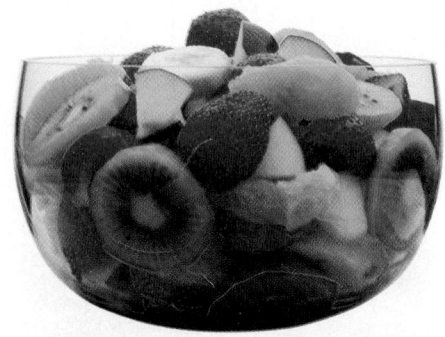

▲ Fruit is a great low-cal snack—high in nutrient density and low in calories.

aerobic dancing or jogging, if it is maintained. Moreover, activities of lighter intensity are less likely to lead to injuries. Some resistance exercises (weight training) also should be added to increase lean body mass and, in turn, fat use (see Chapter 10). As lean muscle mass increases, so will one's overall metabolic rate. An added benefit of including exercise in a weight-reduction program is maintenance of bone health.

Unfortunately, opportunities to expend calories in our daily lives are diminishing as technology systematically eliminates almost every reason to move our muscles. The easiest way to increase physical activity is to make it an enjoyable part of a daily routine. To start, one might pack a pair of athletic shoes and walk around the parking lot before coming home after school or work every day. Other ideas are avoiding elevators in favor of stairs and parking the car farther away from the shopping mall.

A pedometer is an inexpensive device that monitors activity as steps. A recommended goal for activity is to take at least 10,000 steps per day—typically we take half that many or less. A pedometer tracks this activity. Calorie counters, such as the Body-bugg, are new devices that track calorie expenditures throughout the day. The counters calculate calories by measuring heart rate, sweat rate, or heat loss and production. Like pedometers, calorie counters can motivate users to do more activity.

7.9 Behavior Modification—A Third Strategy for Weight Loss and Management

Controlling calorie intake also means modifying *problem* behaviors. Only the dieter can decide what behaviors are preventing calorie control. What events cause us to start (or stop) eating? What factors influence food choices?

The 2010 Dietary Guidelines identify the following behaviors as having the strongest evidence related to body weight:

- Focus on the total number of calories consumed.
- Monitor food intake.
- When eating out, choose smaller portions or lower-calorie options.
- Prepare, serve, and consume smaller portions of foods and beverages, especially those high in calories.
- Eat a nutrient-dense breakfast.
- Limit screen time.

Chain-breaking, stimulus control, cognitive restructuring, contingency management, and *self-monitoring* are behavior modification strategies used by psychologists that (Table 7-5) help place the problem in perspective and organize the intervention into manageable steps.

Chain-breaking separates behaviors that tend to occur together—for example, snacking on chips while watching television. Although these activities do not have to occur together, they often do. Dieters may need to break the chain reaction (see Rate Your Plate at the end of this chapter for more details).

Stimulus control puts us in charge of temptations. Options include pushing tempting food to the back of the refrigerator, removing fat-laden snacks from the kitchen counter, and avoiding the path by the vending machines. Provide a positive stimulus by keeping low-fat snacks available to satisfy hunger/appetite.

Cognitive restructuring changes our frame of mind. For example, after a hard day, avoid using alcohol or comfort foods as quick relief for stress. Instead, plan for healthful, relaxing activities for stress reduction. For example, take a walk around the neighborhood or have a satisfying talk with a friend.

Labeling some foods as "off limits" sets up an internal struggle to resist the urge to eat that food. This hopeless battle can keep us feeling deprived. We lose the fight. Managing food choices with the principle of moderation is best. If a favorite food becomes troublesome, place it off limits only temporarily, until it can be enjoyed in moderation.

Contingency management prepares one for situations that may trigger overeating (e.g., when snacks are served at a party) or hinder physical activity (e.g., rain).

A **self-monitoring** record can reveal patterns—such as unconscious overeating—that may explain problem eating habits. This record can encourage new habits that will counteract unwanted behaviors. Obesity experts note that this is the key behavioral tool to use in any weight-loss program (see Further Readings 4 and 6). See the margin for a list of free online tools available for self-monitoring.

Overall, it's important to address specific problems, such as snacking, compulsive eating, and mealtime overeating. Behavior Modification principles (review Table 7-5) are critical components of weight reduction and maintenance. Without them it is difficult to make lifelong lifestyle changes needed to meet weight-control goals.

Relapse Prevention Is Important

Preventing relapse is thought to be the hardest part of weight control—even harder than losing weight. A dieter needs to plan for lapses, not overreact, and take charge immediately. Change responses such as "I ate that cookie; I'm a failure" to "I ate that cookie, but I did well to stop after only one!" When dieters lapse from their diet plan, newly learned food habits should steer them back toward the plan. Without a strong behavioral program for **relapse prevention** in place, a lapse frequently turns into a relapse and a potential collapse. Once a pattern of poor food choices begins, dieters may feel

---

The motivation to lose weight and keep it off generally comes with a proverbial "flip of the switch," in which the desire to lose weight finally becomes more important than the desire to overeat.

chain-breaking Breaking the link between two or more behaviors that encourage overeating, such as snacking while watching television.

stimulus control Altering the environment to minimize the stimuli for eating—for example, removing foods from sight and storing them in kitchen cabinets.

cognitive restructuring Changing one's frame of mind regarding eating—for example, instead of using a difficult day as an excuse to overeat, substituting other pleasures for rewards, such as a relaxing walk with a friend.

contingency management Forming a plan of action to respond to a situation in which overeating is likely, such as when snacks are within arm's reach at a party.

self-monitoring Tracking foods eaten and conditions affecting eating; actions are usually recorded in a diary, along with location, time, and state of mind. This is a tool to help people understand more about their eating habits.

relapse prevention A series of strategies used to help prevent and cope with weight-control lapses, such as recognizing high-risk situations and deciding beforehand on appropriate responses.

Food and Activity Tracking
Here are some websites where you can record your food and physical activity online for free:

www.fitday.com
http://www.livestrong.com
www.mypyramidtracker.gov
http://nutritiondata.self.com
www.sparkpeople.com

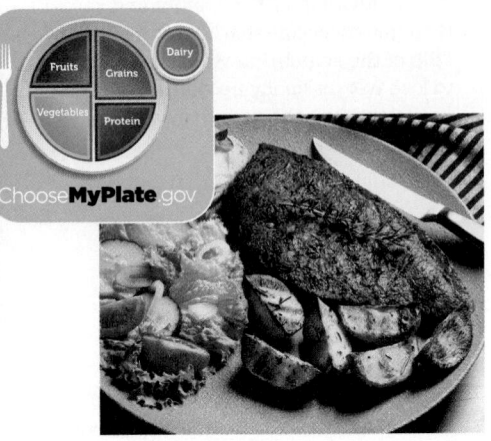

ChooseMyPlate.gov

▲ Large portions of food, such as this steak, provide us with many opportunities to overeat. It takes much perseverance to eat sensibly. How do the portion sizes shown here compare to those recommended on MyPlate?

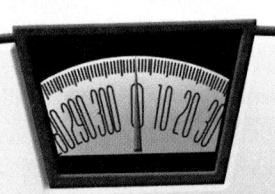

Successful weight losers and maintainers from the National Weight Control Registry:

- Eat a low-fat, high-carbohydrate diet (on average 25% of calorie intake as fat).
- Eat breakfast almost every day.
- Self-monitor by regularly weighing oneself and keeping a food journal.
- Exercise for about 1 hour per day.
- Eat at restaurants only once or twice per week.

Other recent studies support this approach, especially the last four characteristics.

TABLE 7-5 Behavior Modification Principles for Weight Loss

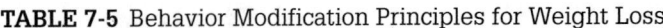

Shopping
1. Shop for food after eating—buy nutritious foods.
2. Shop from a list; limit purchases of irresistible "problem" foods. Shopping for fresh foods around the perimeter of the store first helps.
3. Avoid ready-to-eat foods.
4. Put off food shopping until absolutely necessary.

Plans
1. Plan to limit food intake as needed.
2. Substitute periods of physical activity for snacking.
3. Eat meals and snacks at scheduled times; don't skip meals.

Activities
1. Store food out of sight, preferably in the freezer, to discourage impulsive eating.
2. Eat all food in a "dining" area.
3. Keep serving dishes off the table, especially dishes of sauces and gravies.
4. Use smaller dishes and utensils.

Holidays and Parties
1. Drink fewer alcoholic beverages.
2. Plan eating behavior before parties.
3. Eat a low-calorie snack before parties.
4. Practice polite ways to decline food.
5. Don't get discouraged by an occasional setback.

Eating Behavior
1. Put fork down between mouthfuls.
2. Chew thoroughly before taking the next bite.
3. Leave some food on the plate.
4. Pause in the middle of the meal.
5. Do nothing else while eating (for example, reading, watching television).

Reward
1. Plan specific rewards for specific behavior (behavioral contracts).
2. Solicit help from family and friends and suggest how they can help you. Encourage family and friends to provide this help in the form of praise and material rewards.
3. Use self-monitoring records as basis for rewards.

Self-Monitoring
1. Note the time and place of eating.
2. List the type and amount of food eaten.
3. Record who is present and how you feel.
4. Use the diet diary to identify problem areas.

Cognitive Restructuring
1. Avoid setting unreasonable goals.
2. Think about progress, not shortcomings.
3. Avoid imperatives such as *always* and *never*.
4. Counter negative thoughts with positive restatements.

Portion Control
1. Make substitutions, such as a regular hamburger instead of a "quarter pounder" or cucumbers instead of croutons in salads.
2. Think small. Order the entrée and share it with another person. Order a cup of soup instead of a bowl or an appetizer in place of an entrée.
3. Use a doggie bag. Ask your server to put half the entrée in a doggie bag before bringing it to the table.

As we said at the start of this chapter, many of us need to become "defensive eaters." Know when to refuse food after satiety registers, and reduce portion sizes.

failure and stray farther from the plan. As the relapse lengthens, the diet plan collapses, and falls short of the weight-loss goal. Losing weight is difficult. Overall, maintenance of weight loss is fostered by the "3 *Ms*": motivation, movement, and monitoring.

Social Support Aids Behavioral Change

Healthy social support is helpful in weight control. Helping others understand how they can be supportive can make weight control easier. Family and friends can provide praise and encouragement. A registered dietitian or other weight-control professional can keep dieters accountable and help them learn from difficult situations. Long-term contact with a professional can be helpful for later weight maintenance. Groups of individuals attempting to lose weight or maintain losses can provide empathetic support.

Societal Efforts to Reduce Obesity

The incidence of obesity in the United States is now considered an epidemic. Improvement in the health of our nation requires an approach that includes many sectors. Although we ultimately make our own choices at an individual level, partnerships, programs, and policies that support healthy eating and active living must be coordinated. The 2010 Dietary Guidelines' Call to Action includes three guiding principles:

1. Ensure that all Americans have access to nutritious foods and opportunities for physical activity.
2. Facilitate individual behavior change through environmental strategies.
3. Set the stage for lifelong healthy eating, physical activity, and weight-management behaviors.

Public, private, and nonprofit organizations have begun to work together to address and reverse this public health crisis. For example, the U.S. Food and Drug Administration has brought together leaders from industry, government, academia, and the public health community to seek solutions to the obesity epidemic by making changes in foods eaten outside the home (restaurant and carry-out foods). These groups have collaborated and made recommendations to support the consumer's ability to manage calorie intake. Recommendations include "social marketing" programs that promote healthy eating and active living.

CRITICAL THINKING

With regard to readiness to lose weight, what would you say to a young woman who has just had a baby, needs to find a new job, and recently has gone back to school part-time?

CONCEPT CHECK

Increasing physical activity in daily life should be part of any weight-loss plan. Daily activity, such as walking and stair climbing, is recommended. Behavior Modification can improve conditions for losing weight. One key step is to break behavior chains that encourage overeating, such as snacking while watching television. Another tactic is to modify the environment to reduce temptation; for example, put foods into cupboards to keep them out of sight. In addition, rethinking attitudes about eating—for example, substituting pleasures other than food as a reward for coping with a stressful day—can be important for altering undesirable behavior. Advanced planning to prevent and deal with lapses is vital, as is rallying healthy social support. Finally, careful observation and recording of eating habits can reveal subtle cues that lead to overeating. Overall, weight loss and maintenance are fostered by controlling calorie intake, performing regular physical activity, and modifying "problem" behaviors.

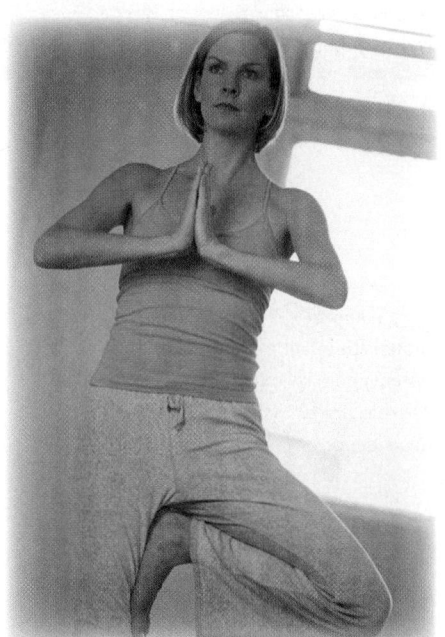

▲ Individuals who successfully maintain their weight loss employ a variety of strategies to cope with the stresses and challenges of changing problem behaviors.

7.10 Professional Help for Weight Loss

The first professional to see for advice about a weight-loss program is one's family physician. Doctors are best equipped to assess overall health and the appropriateness of weight loss. The physician may then recommend a registered dietitian for a specific weight-loss plan and answers to diet-related questions. Registered dietitians are uniquely qualified to help design a weight-loss plan because they understand both food composition and the psychological importance of food. Exercise physiologists can provide advice about programs to increase physical activity. The expense for such

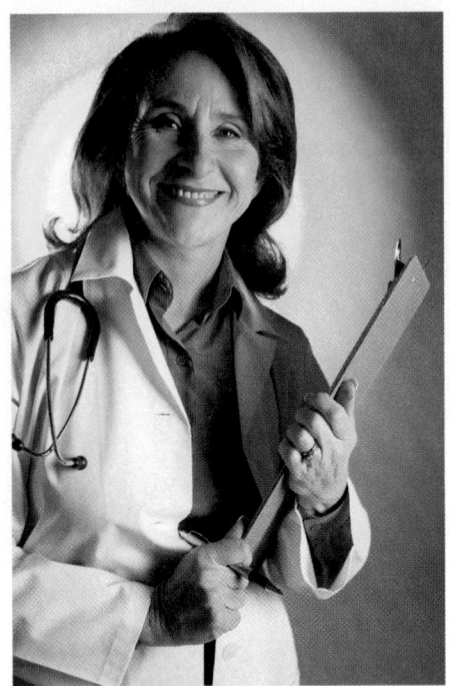

▲ All weight loss programs should begin with a visit to your family physician.

amphetamine A group of medications that induce stimulation of the central nervous system and have other effects in the body. Abuse is linked to physical and psychological dependence.

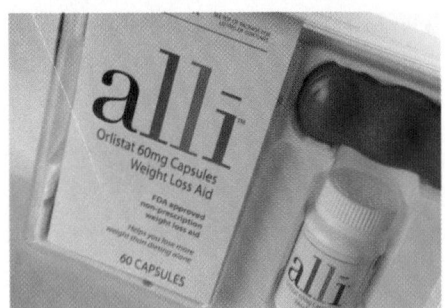

professional interventions is tax deductible in the United States in some cases (see a tax advisor) and often covered by health insurance plans if prescribed by a physician.

Many communities have a variety of weight-loss organizations. These include self-help groups, such as Take Off Pounds Sensibly and Weight Watchers. Other programs, such as Jenny Craig and Physicians' Weight Loss Center, are less desirable for the average dieter. Often, the employees are not registered dietitians or other appropriately trained health professionals. These programs also tend to be expensive because of their requirements for intense counseling or mandatory diet foods and supplements. In addition, the Federal Trade Commission has charged these and other commercial diet-program companies with misleading consumers through unsubstantiated weight-loss claims and deceptive testimonials.

North Americans are willing to try almost anything to shed unwanted pounds. Operation Waistline is a program designed by the U.S. Federal Trade Commission to terminate fraudulent claims being made by weight-loss charlatans with regard to diet products. The program hopes to put an end to the $6 billion spent annually in the United States on counterfeit products. The Enforma Natural Products Corporation had to pay $10 million in response to false claims for its "Fat Trapper" product.

Medications for Weight Loss

Candidates for medications for obesity include those with a BMI of 30 or more, or a BMI of 27 to 29.9 with weight-related health conditions, such as type 2 diabetes, cardiovascular disease, hypertension, or excess waist circumference; those with no contraindications to use the medication; and those ready to undertake lifestyle change. Drug therapy alone has not been found to be successful. Success with medications has been shown only in those who also modify their behavior, decrease calorie intake, and increase physical activity. In addition, if a person has not lost at least 4.4 pounds (2 kilograms) after 4 weeks, it is not likely that the person will benefit from further use of the medication.

Three main classes of medications have been used. An **amphetamine**-like medication (phenteramine [Fastin or Ionamin]) prolongs the activity of epinephrine and norepinephrine in the brain. This therapy is effective for some people in the short run but has not yet been proven effective in the long run. Most state medical boards limit use of this drug to 12 weeks unless the person is participating in a medical study using the product. The medication should not be used in pregnant or nursing women or those under 18 years of age.

The second class of medication approved by FDA for weight loss and the only weight-loss medication approved for long-term use is orlistat (Xenical). This medication reduces fat digestion by about 30% by inhibiting lipase enzyme action in the small intestine (Fig. 7-18). This cuts absorption of dietary fat by one-third for about 2 hours when taken along with a meal containing fat. This malabsorbed fat is deposited in the feces. *Fat intake has to be controlled*, however, because large amounts of fat in the feces cause numerous side effects, such as gas, bloating, and oily discharge. Interestingly, orlistat use can remind the person to follow a fat-controlled diet, as the symptoms resulting from consuming a high-fat meal are unpleasant and develop quickly. Orlistat is taken with each meal containing fat. The malabsorbed fat also carries fat-soluble vitamins into the feces, so the person taking orlistat must take a multivitamin and mineral supplement at bedtime. In this way, any micronutrients not absorbed during the day can be replaced; fat malabsorption from the dinner meal will not greatly influence micronutrient absorption in the late evening. A low-dose form of orlistat (alli™) is now available over the counter without a prescription.

Sibutramine (Meridia) is a third class of medication that was approved by FDA for weight loss and was available until October 2010. It enhances both norepinephrine and serotonin activity in the brain by reducing reuptake of these neurotransmitters by nerve cells. The neurotransmitters then remain active in the brain for

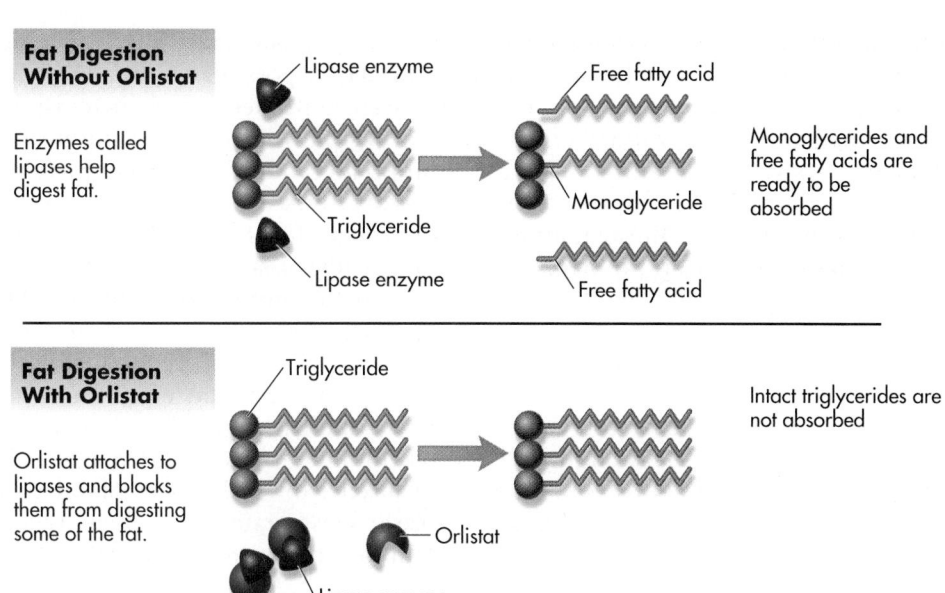

Fat Digestion Without Orlistat

Enzymes called lipases help digest fat.

Lipase enzyme

Free fatty acid

Triglyceride

Lipase enzyme

Monoglycerides and free fatty acids are ready to be absorbed

Monoglyceride

Free fatty acid

Fat Digestion With Orlistat

Orlistat attaches to lipases and blocks them from digesting some of the fat.

Triglyceride

Intact triglycerides are not absorbed

Orlistat

Lipase enzyme

FIGURE 7-18 ▶ Orlistat is a weight-loss drug that works in the digestive system to block digestion of about one-third of the fat in the food we eat. A low-dose form of this drug (alli™) is now available without a prescription.

a longer time and so prolong a sense of reduced hunger. The main effect is to moderately reduce appetite so that people eat less. Production of subutramine was voluntarily stopped at the request of FDA and based on increased risk of heart attacks and strokes observed in people taking sibutramine. Read more about this study in Newsworthy Nutrition.

Drug companies are working on many other types of medications and hopes that some of these will prove to be safe and effective for weight loss. In addition, physicians may prescribe medications not approved for weight loss but that have weight loss as a side effect. Certain antidepressants are an example. Such an application is termed *off-label*, because the product label does not include weight loss as an FDA-approved use. Over-the-counter medications and supplements are widely marketed as miracle cures for obesity, but in some cases, they do more harm than good (see Further Reading 11). Today more than ever, let the buyer beware concerning any purported weight-loss aid not prescribed by a physician.

Overall, in skilled hands, prescription medications can aid weight loss in some instances. However, they do not replace the need for reducing calorie intake, modifying "problem" behaviors, and increasing physical activity, both during and after therapy. Often, any weight loss during drug treatment can be attributed mostly to the individual's hard work at balancing calorie intake with calorie output.

Treatment of Severe Obesity

Severe (morbid) obesity, having a BMI greater than or equal to 40 or weighing at least 100 pounds over healthy body weight (or twice one's healthy body weight), requires professional treatment. Because of the serious health implications of severe obesity, drastic measures may be necessary. Such treatments are recommended only when traditional diets and medications fail. Drastic weight-loss procedures are not without side effects, both physical and psychological, making careful monitoring by a physician a necessity.

NEWSWORTHY NUTRITION | Popular weight-loss drug withdrawn from the market

In October 2010, the FDA withdrew the obesity drug sibutramine (Meridia) from the market based on the results of the Sibutramine Cardiovascular OUTcomes Trial. This study evaluated the cardiovascular safety of the drug in patients at high risk for cardiovascular events. Subjects receiving sibutramine long-term (~3.4 years) had 16% increased risk of nonfatal heart attacks and strokes. Based on these results and the small difference in weight loss among those taking the drug and those receiving a placebo, sibutramine should not be used in patients with preexisting cardiovascular disease. At the time of its withdrawal from the market in the United States and several other countries, about 100,000 people in the United States were taking Meridia.

Source: James WPT and others: Effect of sibutramine on cardiovascular outcomes in overweight and obese subjects. *New England Journal of Medicine* 363(10):905, 2010 (see Further Reading 5).

connect NUTRITION   **Check out the connect site** www.mcgrawhillconnect.com **to further explore long-term weight-loss medications.**

very-low-calorie diet (VLCD) Known also as *protein-sparing modified fast (PSMF)*, this diet allows a person 400 to 800 kcal per day, often in liquid form. Of this, 120 to 480 kcal is carbohydrate, and the rest is mostly high-quality protein.

bariatrics The medical specialty focusing on the treatment of obesity.

adjustable gastric banding A restrictive procedure in which the opening from the esophagus to the stomach is reduced by a hollow gastric band.

gastroplasty Gastric bypass surgery performed on the stomach to limit its volume to approximately 30 milliliters. Also referred to as stomach stapling.

Very-Low-Calorie Diets. If more traditional diet changes have failed, treating severe obesity with a **very-low-calorie diet (VLCD)** is possible, especially if the person has obesity-related diseases that are not well controlled (e.g., hypertension, type 2 diabetes). Some researchers believe that people with body weight greater than 30% above their healthy weight are appropriate candidates. VLCD programs are offered almost exclusively by medical centers or clinics since careful monitoring by a physician is crucial throughout this very restrictive form of weight loss. Major health risks include heart problems and gallstones. Optifast is one such commercial program. In general, the diet allows a person to consume only 400 to 800 kcal per day, often in liquid form. (These diets were previously known as protein-sparing modified fasts.) Of this amount, about 30 to 120 grams (120 to 480 kcal) is carbohydrate. The rest is high-quality protein, in the amount of about 70 to 100 grams per day (280 to 400 kcal). This low carbohydrate intake often causes ketosis, which may decrease hunger. However, the main reasons for weight loss are the minimal energy consumption and the absence of food choice. About 3 to 4 pounds can be lost per week; men tend to lose at a faster rate than women. When physical activity and resistance training augment this diet, a greater loss of adipose tissue occurs.

Weight regain remains a nagging problem, especially without a behavioral and physical activity component. If behavioral therapy and physical activity supplement a long-term support program, maintenance of the weight loss is more likely but still difficult. Any program under consideration should include a maintenance plan. Today, antiobesity medications also may be included in this phase of the program.

Bariatric Surgery. Bariatrics is the medical specialty focusing on the treatment of obesity. Bariatric surgery is only considered for people with severe obesity and includes operations aimed at promoting weight loss. Two types of bariatric operations are now common and effective (see Further Readings 7 and 10). Both procedures can be performed using an open (8- to 10-inch) incision in the middle of the abdomen or a laparoscopic approach in which several smaller (½- to 2-inch) incisions are used that allow cameras and instruments to enter the abdomen. **Adjustable gastric banding** (also known as the lap-band procedure) is a restrictive procedure in which the opening from the esophagus to the stomach is reduced by a hollow gastric band. This creates a small pouch and a narrow passage into the rest of the stomach and thus decreases the amount of food that can be eaten comfortably. The band can be inflated or deflated via an access port placed just under the skin. Studies have demonstrated that adjustable gastric banding is more effective long term than a very low-calorie diet (500 kcal) for people who are about 50 pounds overweight.

Gastric bypass (also called **gastroplasty** or stomach stapling) is another bariatric surgical procedure used for treating severe obesity. The most common and effective approach (the Roux-en-Y gastric bypass procedure) works by reducing the stomach capacity to about 30 milliliters (the volume of one egg or shot glass) and bypassing a short segment of the upper small intestine (Fig. 7-19). Weight loss is promoted mainly because overeating of solid foods is now less likely due to rapid satiety and discomfort or vomiting after overeating. About 75% of people with severe obesity eventually lose 50% or more of excess body weight with this method. In addition, the surgery's success at long-term maintenance often leads to dramatic health improvements, such as reduced blood pressure and elimination of type 2 diabetes. Risks of the surgery include bleeding, blood clots, hernias, and severe infections. In the long run, nutrient deficiencies can develop if the person is not adequately treated in the years following the surgery. Anemia and bone loss might then be the result. Risk of death from this demanding surgery can be as high as 2% (less risk with experienced surgeons).

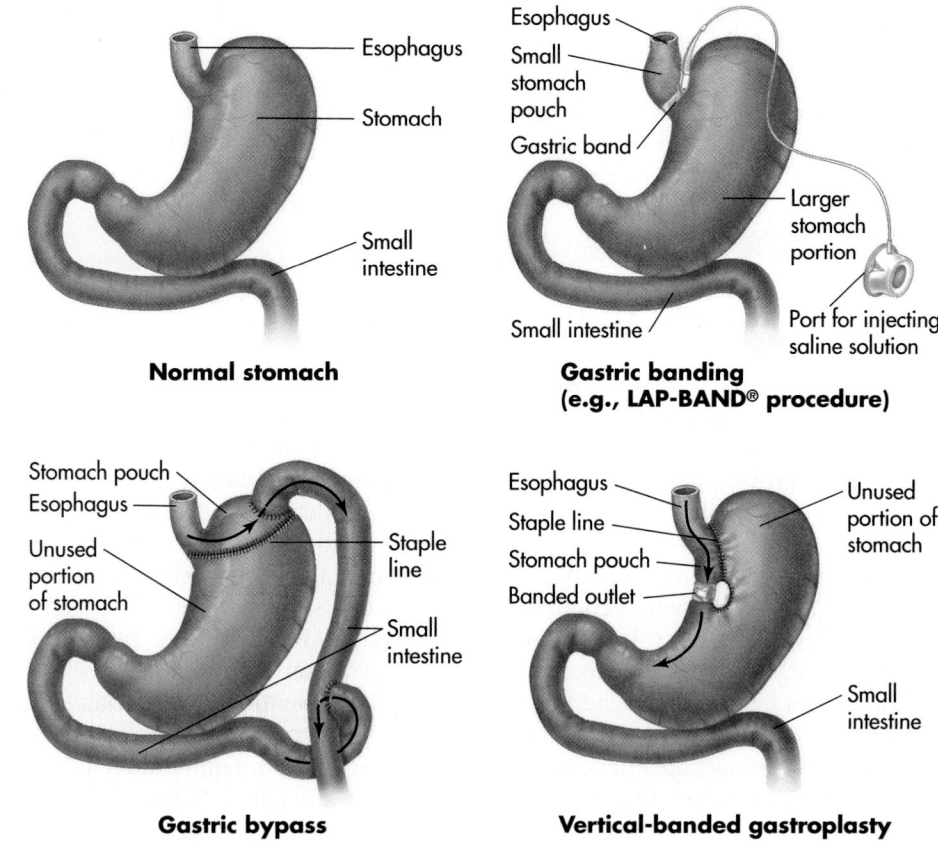

Normal stomach

Gastric banding (e.g., LAP-BAND® procedure)

Gastric bypass

Vertical-banded gastroplasty

FIGURE 7-19 ▶ The most common forms of gastroplasty for treating severe obesity. The gastric bypass is the most effective method. In banded gastroplasty, the band prevents expansion of the outlet for the stomach pouch.

Patient selection criteria for bariatric surgery include:

- BMI should be greater than 40.
- BMI between 35 and 40 is considered when there are serious obesity-related health concerns.
- Obesity must be present for a minimum of 5 years, with several nonsurgical attempts to lose weight.
- There should be no history of alcoholism or major untreated psychiatric disorders.

The person also must consider that the surgery is costly and may not be covered by medical insurance. The average cost for gastric bypass produres is $18,000 to $35,000 and for adjustable gastric banding is $17,000 to $30,000. In addition, follow-up surgery is often needed after weight loss to correct stretched skin, previously filled with fat. Furthermore, the surgery necessitates major lifestyle changes, such as the need to plan frequent, small meals. Therefore, the dieter who has chosen this drastic approach to weight loss faces months of difficult adjustments.

MAKING DECISIONS

Lipectomy

Spot-reducing by using diet and physical activity is not possible. "Problem" local fat deposits can be reduced in size, however, using suction lipectomy. Lipectomy or liposuction means surgical removal of fat. A pencil-thin tube is inserted into an incision in the skin, and the fat tissue, such as that in the buttocks and thigh area, is suctioned. This procedure carries some risks, such as infection; lasting depressions in the skin; and blood clots, which can lead to kidney failure and sometimes death. The procedure is designed to help a person lose about 4 to 8 pounds per treatment. Cost is about $1800 per site; total costs range as high as $2600 to $9000.

CONCEPT CHECK

Severely obese people who have failed to lose weight with conservative weight-loss strategies may consider other options. Their doctors may recommend undergoing surgery such as reducing the volume of the stomach to approximately 30 milliliters or following a very-low-calorie diet plan containing 400 to 800 kcal per day. Careful monitoring by a physician is crucial in both cases.

7.11 Treatment of Underweight

underweight A body mass index below 18.5. The cutoff is less precise than for obesity because this condition has been less studied.

Underweight is defined by a BMI less than 18.5 and can be caused by a variety of factors, such as cancer, infectious disease (e.g., tuberculosis), digestive tract disorders (e.g., chronic inflammatory bowel disease), and excessive dieting or physical activity. Genetic background may also lead to a higher resting metabolic rate, a slight body frame, or both. Health problems associated with underweight include the loss of menstrual function, low bone mass, complications with pregnancy and surgery, and slow recovery after illness. Significant underweight is also associated with increased death rates, especially when combined with cigarette smoking. We frequently hear about the risks of obesity, but seldom of underweight. In our culture, being underweight is much more socially acceptable than being obese.

Sometimes being underweight requires medical intervention. A physician should be consulted first to rule out hormonal imbalances; depression; cancer; infectious disease; digestive tract disorders; excessive physical activity; and other hidden disease, such as a serious eating disorder (see Chapter 11 for a detailed discussion of eating disorders).

The causes of underweight are not altogether different from the causes of obesity. Internal and external satiety-signal irregularities, the rate of metabolism, hereditary tendencies, and psychological traits can all contribute to underweight.

In growing children, the high demand for calories to support physical activity and growth can cause underweight. During growth spurts in adolescence, active children may not take the time to consume enough calories to support their needs. Moreover, gaining weight can be a formidable task for an underweight person. An extra 500 kcal per day may be required to gain weight, even at a slow pace, in part because of the increased expenditure of energy in thermogenesis. In contrast to the weight loser, the weight gainer may need to increase portion sizes.

When underweight requires a specific intervention, one approach for treating adults is to gradually increase their consumption of calorie-dense foods, especially those high in vegetable fat. Italian cheeses, nuts, and granola can be good calorie sources with low saturated-fat content. Dried fruit and bananas are good fruit choices. If eaten at the end of a meal, they don't cause early satiety. The same advice applies to salads and soups. Underweight people should replace such foods as diet soft drinks with good calorie sources, such as fruit juices and smoothies.

Encouraging a regular meal and snack schedule also aids in weight gain and maintenance. Sometimes underweight people have experienced stress at work or have been too busy to eat. Making regular meals a priority may not only help them attain an appropriate weight but also help with digestive disorders, such as constipation, sometimes associated with irregular eating times.

Excessively physically active people can reduce activity. If their weight remains low, they can add muscle mass through a resistance training (weight-lifting) program, but they must also increase their calorie intake to support that physical activity. Otherwise, weight gain will be hindered.

If these efforts fail to help a person achieve a healthy weight, they should at least prevent the health problems associated with being underweight. After achieving that, they may have to accept their lean frames.

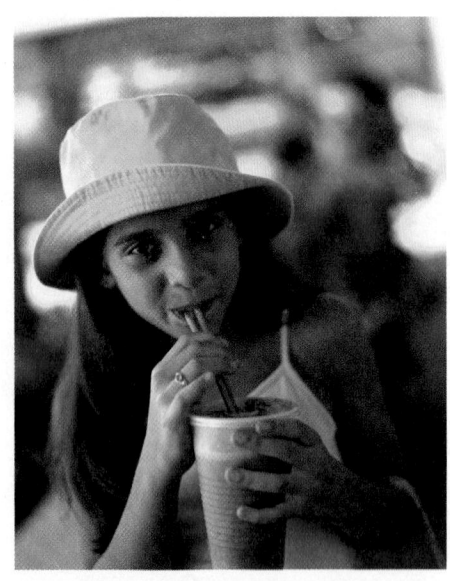

▲ Underweight people should increase their consumption of calorie-dense foods, such as smoothies, that are also loaded with nutrients.

Popular Diets—Cause for Concern

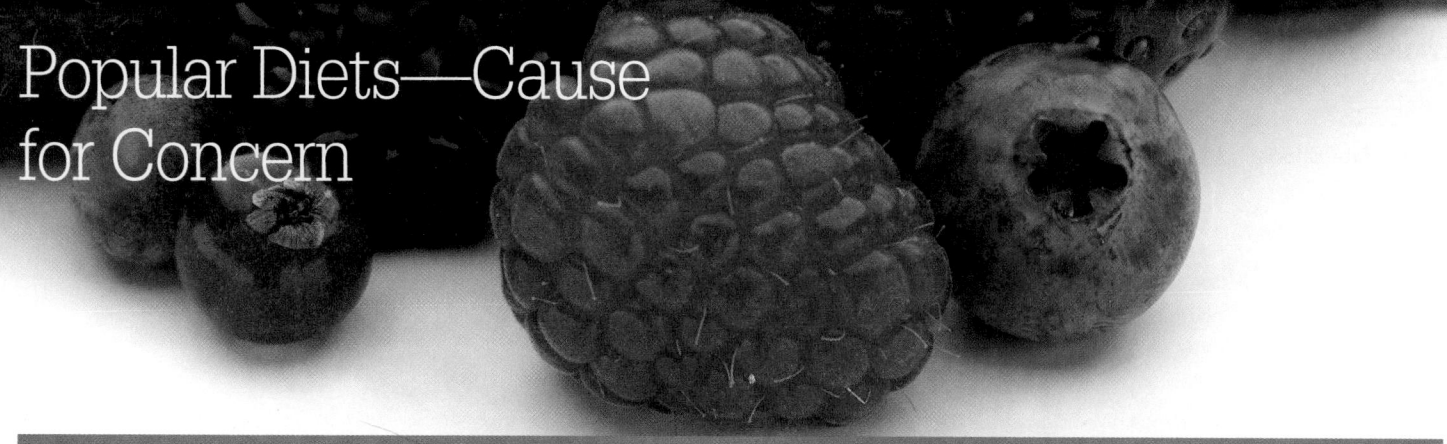

Many overweight people try to help themselves by using the latest popular (also called fad) diet book. But, as you will see, most of these diets do not help, and some can actually harm those who follow them (Table 7-6). Research has shown that early dieting and other unhealthful weight control practices in adolescents lead to an increased risk of weight gain, overweight, and eating disorders.

Recently, weight-loss experts came together at the request of the USDA to evaluate weight-loss diets. They came to this conclusion: Forget these fads when it comes to dieting. Most of the popular diets are nutritionally inadequate and include certain foods that people would not normally choose to consume in large amounts. The experts stated that eating less of one's favorite foods and becoming more physically active can be much more effective when trying to implement a weight-loss diet. People need a plan they can live with in the long run so that weight control becomes permanent. The goal should be weight control over a lifetime, not immediate weight loss. Every popular diet leads to some immediate weight loss simply because daily in-take is monitored and monotonous food choices are typically part of the plan. A well-known example of the effectiveness of monotony contributing to weight loss is the experience of Jared Fogle. He ate primarily Subway sandwiches for 11 months and lost 245 pounds. He notes however that this is not a miracle diet—it takes a lot of hard work to lead to the success he experienced. There are also many other examples where diet monotony has led to weight loss. Overall, a traditional moderate diet coupled with regular physical activity is adequate for weight loss.

People on diets often fall within a healthy BMI of 18.5 to 25. Rather than worrying about weight loss, these individuals should be focusing on a healthy lifestyle that allows for weight maintenance. Incorporating necessary lifestyle changes and learning to accept one's particular body characteristics should be the overriding goals.

The dieting mania can be viewed as mostly a social problem, stemming from unrealistic weight expectations (especially for women) and lack of appreciation for the natural variety in body shape and weight. Not every woman can look like a fashion model, nor can every man look like a Greek god, but all of us can strive for good health and, if physically possible, an active lifestyle.

The size-acceptance nondiet movement, "Health at Every Size," has attempted to shift the paradigm away from the use of "popular" weight loss diets. The goals of the movement are all independent of body weight and include improvement of self-image, normalization of eating behavior, and increase in physical activity.

How to Recognize an Unreliable Diet

The criteria for evaluating weight-loss programs with regard to their safety and effectiveness were discussed previously (review Fig. 7-15). In contrast, unreliable diets typically share some common characteristics:

1. They promote quick weight loss. This is the primary temptation that the dieter falls for. As mentioned, this initial weight loss primarily results from water loss and lean muscle mass depletion.

2. They limit food selections and dictate specific rituals, such as eating only fruit for breakfast or cabbage soup every day.

3. They use testimonials from famous people and tie the diet to well-known cities, such as Beverly Hills and South Beach.

4. They bill themselves as cure-alls. These diets claim to work for everyone, whatever the type of obesity or the person's specific strengths and weaknesses.

5. They often recommend expensive supplements.

6. No attempts are made to change eating habits permanently. Dieters follow the diet until the desired weight is reached and then revert to old eating habits—they are told, for example, to eat rice for a month, lose weight, and then return to old habits.

7. They are generally critical of and skeptical about the scientific community. The lack of a quick fix from medical and dietetic professionals has led some of the public to seek advice from those who appear to have the answer.

8. They claim that there is no need to exercise.

Probably the cruelest characteristic of these diets is that they essentially guarantee failure for the dieter. The diets are not designed for permanent weight loss. Habits are not changed, and the food selection is so limited that the person cannot follow the diet in the long run. Although dieters assume they have lost fat, they have lost mostly muscle and other lean tissue mass. As soon as they begin

TABLE 7-6 Summary of Popular Diet Approaches to Weight Control

Approach	Examples*	Characteristics	Dietitian's Review
Moderate calorie restriction	• *Dieting for Dummies* (2003) • *Dieting with the Duchess* (2000) • *Dr. Phil's Ultimate Weight Solution* (2003, 2005) • Flat Belly Diet (2008) • *Jenny Craig* (1980s) • *Picture Perfect Weight Loss* (2003) • Slim-fast (1980s) • *Sonoma Diet* (2005) • *Volumetrics* (2000) • *Wedding Dress Diet* (2000) • Weight Watchers (1960s) • You on a Diet (2006)	• Generally 1200 to 1800 kcal per day • Moderate fat intake • Reasonable balance of macronutrients • Encourage exercise • May use behavioral approach	These diets are acceptable if a multivitamin and mineral supplement is used and permission of family physician is granted.
Carbohydrate focused	• *Carbohydrate Addicts Diet* (1993, 2001) • *Dr. Atkin's Diet Revolution* (1973, 2002) • *Dr. Gott's No Flour, No Sugar Diet* (2006) • *Eat, Drink & Weigh Less* (2006) • *G.I. (Glycemic Index) Diet* (2003) • *Healthy for Life* (2005) • *New Glucose Revolution* (2002) • Nutrisystem (2003) • *South Beach Diet* (especially initial phases) (2003) • *Sugar Busters Diet* (1998, 2003) • *Zone Diet* (1995)	• Restricted carbohydrate diets generally advise consumption of less than 100 grams of carbohydrate per day • Some plans focus on carbohydrate choices (e.g., choosing low rather than high glycemic index foods)	Selecting high-fiber, whole-grain sources of carbohydrates is an advisable practice for weight control and prevention of several chronic diseases. However, severe carbohydrate restriction may lead to ketosis, reduced exercise capacity (due to poor glycogen stores in the muscles), excessive animal fat intake, constipation, headaches, halitosis (bad breath), and muscle cramps. Severe carbohydrate restriction is not a nutritionally sound, long-term, weight-loss solution.
Low fat	• *20/30 Fat and Fiber Diet Plan* (2000) • *Complete Hip and Thigh Diet* (1989, 1999) • *Eat More, Weigh Less* (1993, 2001) • *Fit or Fat* (1977, 2005) • *Foods That Cause You to Lose Weight* (1992, 2003) • *McDougall Program* (1983, 1995) • *Pritikin Diet* (1984, 1995) • *Rice Diet Solution* (2005) • *T-Factor Diet* (1989, 2001) • *Okinawa Program* (2002)	• Generally less than 20% of calories from fat • Limited (or elimination of) animal protein sources; also limited plant oils, nuts, seeds	Low-fat diet plans are not necessarily to be avoided, but certain aspects may be unacceptable. Some potentially negative outcomes include flatulence, poor mineral absorption (from excess fiber intake), and a sense of deprivation (due to limited food choices).
Novelty diets	• *17-Day Diet* (2011) • *3-Hour Diet* (2005) • *Beverly Hills Diet* (1981, 1996) • *Cabbage-Soup Diet* (2004) • *Eat Right 4 Your Type* (1996) • *Fat Smash Diet* (2006) • *Fit for Life* (1987, 2001) • *Metabolic Typing Diet* (2002) • *New Hilton Head Metabolism Diet* (1983, 1996) • *Ultrametabolism* (2006) • *Weigh Down Diet* (2002)	• Promote certain nutrients, foods, or combinations of foods as having unique, magical, or previously undiscovered qualities	Novelty diets are usually not nutritionally balanced, thus malnutrition is a possible result. Also, failure to make long-term changes may lead to relapse, and unrealistic food choices lead to possible bingeing.

*Dates listed are original release date followed by most recent release date, if applicable.

eating normally again, much of the lost tissue is replaced. In a matter of weeks, most of the lost weight is back. The dieter appears to have failed, when actually the diet has failed. The gain and loss cycle is called weight cycling or "yo-yo" dieting. This whole scenario can add more blame and guilt, challenging the self-worth of the dieter. It can also come with some health costs, such as increased upper-body fat deposition. If someone needs help losing weight, professional help is advised. It is unfortunate that current trends suggest that people are spending more time and money on "quick fixes" rather than on such professional help.

Types of Popular Diets

Low- or Restricted-Carbohydrate Approaches

Low-carbohydrate diets have recently been the most popular diets. The low-carbohydrate intake leads to less glycogen synthesis, and therefore less water in the body (about 3 grams of water are stored per gram of glycogen). As discussed in Chapter 4, a very-low-carbohydrate intake also forces the liver to produce needed glucose. The source of carbons for this glucose is mostly proteins from tissues such as muscle resulting in loss of protein tissue, about 72% water. Essential ions, such as potassium are also lost in the urine. With the loss of glycogen stores, lean tissue and water, the dieter loses weight very rapidly. When a normal diet is resumed, the protein tissue is rebuilt and the weight is regained.

Although low-carbohydrate diets work in the short run primarily because they limit total food intake, recent results indicate that low-carbohydrate diets may be effective alternatives to low-fat diets. In a recent 2-year study published in the New England Journal of Medicine, moderately obese adults on a low-carbohydrate diet lost and kept off about 12 pounds, compared to 10 pounds for those following the traditional Mediterranean diet, and 7 pounds for those on a restricted-fat plan.

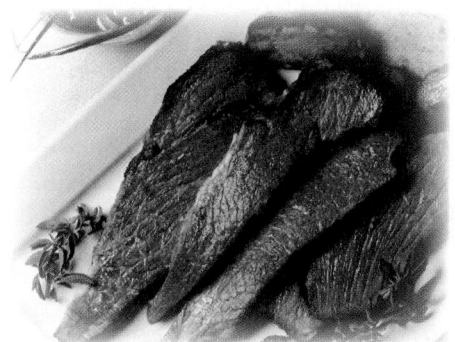

▲ In time, the very-low-carbohydrate, high-protein diets typically leave a person wanting more variety in meals, and so the diets are abandoned. Dropout rates are high on these diets.

The most popular diet using a low-carbohydrate approach is the Dr. Atkins' New Diet Revolution. More moderate approaches are found in the various Zone diets (40% of calorie intake as carbohydrate), Sugar Busters diet, and the South Beach diet (especially initial phases).

Carbohydrate-Focused Diets

Several recent diets, including Sugar Busters the Glucose Revolution, and Eat, Drink and Weigh Less, do not restrict carbohydrates, but rather emphasize the "good" carbohydrates in place of the "bad" or "harmful" ones. These diets recommend eating plenty of fruits, vegetables, whole grains, and cutting out simple sugars and processed grains. The carbohydrate-focused diets rely largely on low glycemic index and low glycemic load foods. In theory, these foods will cause a slow, steady rise in blood sugar, which will help control hunger.

Low-Fat Approaches

The very-low-fat diets contain approximately 5% to 10% of calories as fat and are very high in carbohydrates. The most notable are the Pritikin Diet and the Dr. Dean Ornish "Eat More, Weigh Less" diet plans. This approach is not harmful for healthy adults, but it is difficult to follow. People are quickly bored with this type of diet because they cannot eat many of their favorite foods. These dieters eat primarily grains, fruits, and vegetables, which most people cannot do for very long. Eventually, the person wants some foods higher in fat or protein. These diets are just too different from the typical North American diet for many adults to follow consistently, but may be acceptable for some people.

Novelty Diets

A variety of diets are built on gimmicks. Some novelty diets emphasize one food or food group and exclude almost all others. A rice diet was designed in the 1940s to lower blood pressure; now it has resurfaced as a weight-loss diet. The first phase consists of eating only rice and fruit. On the Beverly Hills Diet, you eat mostly fruit.

The rationale behind these diets is that you can eat only rice or fruit for just so long before becoming bored and, in theory, reducing your calorie intake. However,

chances are that you will abandon the diet entirely before losing much weight.

The most questionable of the novelty diets propose that "food gets stuck in your body." Fit for Life, the Beverly Hills Diet, and Eat Great, Lose Weight are examples. The supposition is that food gets stuck in the intestine, putrefies, and creates toxins, which invade the blood and cause disease. In response, recommendations are to not consume meat with potatoes or to consume fruits only after noon. These recommendations make no physiological sense.

Meal Replacements

Meal replacements come in many forms, including beverages or formulas, frozen or shelf-stable entrees, and meal or snack bars. Most meal replacements are fortified with vitamins and minerals and are appropriate to replace one or two regular meals or snacks per day. Although they are not a "magic bullet" for weight loss, they have been shown to help some people lose weight. Advantages of these convenient products are that they provide portion- and calorie-controlled foods that can serve as a visual education on appropriate portion sizes.

Quackery Is Characteristic of Many Popular Diets

Many popular diets fall under the category of quackery—people taking advantage of others. They usually involve a product or service that costs a considerable amount of money. Often, those offering the product or service don't realize that they are promoting quackery, because they were victims themselves. For example, they tried the product and by pure coincidence it worked for them, so they wish to sell it to all their friends and relatives.

Numerous other gimmicks for weight loss have come and gone and are likely to resurface. If in the future an important aid for weight loss is discovered, you can feel confident that major journals, such as the *Journal of the American Dietetic Association,* the *Journal of the American Medical Association,* or *The New England Journal of Medicine,* will report it. You don't need to rely on paperback books, infomercials, billboards, or newspaper advertisements for information about weight loss.

Case Study Choosing a Weight-Loss Program

Joe has a hectic schedule. During the day he works full-time at a warehouse distribution center filling orders. At night, three times a week, he attends class at the local community college in pursuit of computer certification. On weekends he likes to watch sports on TV, spend time with family and friends, and study. Joe has little time to think about what he eats—convenience rules. He stops for coffee and a pastry on his way to work, has a burger or pizza for lunch at a quick service restaurant, and for dinner picks up fried chicken or fish at the drive-through on his way to class. Unfortunately, over the past few years Joe's weight has been climbing. Watching a game on television a few nights ago, he saw an infomercial for a product that promises he can eat large portions of tasty foods but not gain weight. A famous actor supports the claim that this product allows one to eat at will and not gain weight. This claim is tempting to Joe.

Answer the following questions, and check your response in Appendix A.

1. Has Joe been experiencing positive or negative energy balance over the past few years?
2. What aspects of Joe's lifestyle (other than diet) are causing this effect on his energy balance? What changes could Joe make in his habits to promote weight loss or maintenance?
3. What changes could Joe make in his diet that would promote weight loss or maintenance?
4. Why should Joe be skeptical of the claims he heard about the weight-loss product in the infomercial?
5. What advice can you offer Joe for evaluation of weight-loss programs?

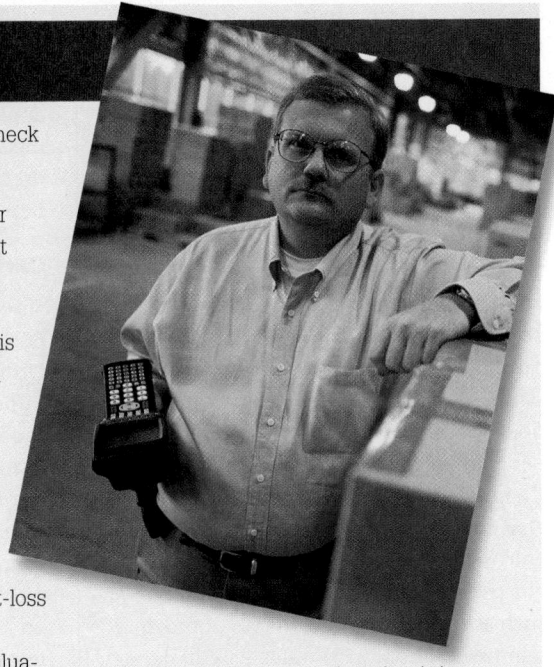

▲ What changes can Joe make in his daily routine and diet to stop his weight gain?

Summary (Numbers refer to numbered sections in the chapter.)

7.1 Energy balance considers energy intake and energy output. Negative energy balance occurs when energy output surpasses energy intake, resulting in weight loss. Positive energy balance occurs when calorie intake is greater than output, resulting in weight gain.

Basal metabolism, the thermic effect of food, physical activity, and thermogenesis account for total energy use by the body. Basal metabolism, which represents the minimum amount of calories required to keep the resting, awake body alive, is primarily affected by lean body mass, surface area, and thyroid hormone concentrations. Physical activity is energy use above that expended at rest. The thermic effect of food describes the increase in metabolism that facilitates digestion, absorption, and processing of the nutrients recently consumed. Thermogenesis is heat production caused by shivering when cold, fidgeting, and other stimuli. In a sedentary person, about 70% to 80% of energy use is accounted for by basal metabolism and the thermic effect of food.

7.2 Energy use by the body can be measured as heat given off by direct calorimetry or as oxygen used by indirect calorimetry. A person's Estimated Energy Requirement can be calculated based on the following factors: gender, height, weight, age, and amount physical activity.

7.3 A person of healthy weight shows good health and performs daily activities without weight-related problems. A body mass index (weight in kilograms ÷ height² in meters) of 18.5 to 25 is one measure of healthy weight. A healthy weight is best determined in conjunction with a thorough health evaluation by a physician. A body mass index of 25 to 29.9 represents overweight. Obesity is defined as a total body fat percentage over 25% (men) or 35% (women) or a body mass index of 30 or more.

7.4 If calorie intake exceeds output, an energy imbalance occurs that results in overweight. Fat distribution greatly determines health risks from obesity. Upper-body fat storage, as measured by a waist circumference greater than 40 inches (102 centimeters) for men or 35 inches (88 centimeters) for women typically results in higher risks of hypertension, cardiovascular disease, and type 2 diabetes than does lower-body fat storage.

7.5 Both genetic (nature) and environmental (nurture) factors can increase the risk of obesity. The set-point theory proposes that we have a genetically predetermined body weight or body fat content, which the body regulates.

7.6 A sound weight-loss program meets the dieter's nutritional needs by emphasizing a wide variety of low-calorie, bulky foods; adapts to the dieter's habits; consists of readily obtainable foods; strives to change poor eating habits; stresses regular physical activity; and stipulates the supervision by a physician if weight is to be lost rapidly or if the person is over the age of 40 (men) or 50 (women) and plans to perform substantially greater physical activity than usual.

7.7 A pound of adipose tissue contains about 3500 kcal. Loss or gain of a pound of adipose tissue—the fat itself plus lean support tissue—represents approximately 3300 kcal. Thus, if energy output exceeds calorie intake by about 500 kcal per day, a pound of adipose tissue can be lost per week.

7.8 Physical activity as part of a weight-loss program should be focused on duration rather than intensity. Ideally, vigorous activity for 60 minutes should be part of each day to prevent adult weight gain.

7.9 Behavior modification is a vital part of a weight-loss program because the dieter may have many habits that discourage weight maintenance. Specific behavior modification techniques, such as stimulus control and self-monitoring, can be used to help change problem behavior.

7.10 Medications to blunt appetite, such as phenteramine (Fastin), can aid weight-reduction strategies. Orlistat (Xenical) reduces fat absorption from a meal when taken with the meal. Weight-loss drugs are reserved for those who are obese or have weight-related problems, and they must be administered under close physician supervision.

The treatment of severe obesity may include surgery to reduce stomach volume to approximately 30 milliliters (1 ounce) or very-low-calorie diets containing 400 to 800 kcal per day. Both of these measures should be reserved for people who have failed at more conservative approaches to weight loss. They also require close medical supervision.

7.11 Underweight can be caused by a variety of factors, such as excessive physical activity and genetic background. Sometimes being underweight requires medical attention. A physician should be consulted first to rule out underlying disease. The underweight person may need to increase portion sizes and learn to like calorie-dense foods. In addition, encouraging a regular meal and snack schedule aids in weight gain, as well as weight maintenance.

N&YH Many overweight people try popular diets that most often are not helpful and may actually be harmful. Unreliable diets typically share some common characteristics, including promoting quick weight loss, limiting food selections, using testimonials as proof, and requiring no exercise.

Check Your Knowledge (Answers to the following questions are below.)

1. Decreasing energy intake by about 500 kcal per day would mean a loss of 1 pound of body fat stores in _____ days.
   a. 2   c. 10
   b. 7   d. 14

2. Thermic effect of food represents the energy cost of
   a. chewing food.
   b. peristalsis
   c. basal metabolism.
   d. digesting, absorbing, and packaging nutrients.

3. A well-designed diet should
   a. increase physical activity.
   b. alter problem behaviors.
   c. reduce energy intake.
   d. All of the above.

4. All of the following factors are associated with a higher basal metabolic rate *except*
   a. stress.   c. fever.
   b. starvation.   d. pregnancy.

5. The intent of bariatric surgery is to
   a. limit stomach volume.
   b. speed transit time.
   c. surgically remove adipose tissue.
   d. prevent snacking.

6. Basal metabolism
   a. represents about 30% of total energy expenditure.
   b. is energy used to maintain heartbeat, respiration, and other basic functions and daily activities.
   c. represents about 60% to 70% of total calories used by the body during a day.
   d. includes energy to digest food.

7. Dr. Atkins' New Diet Revolution, The Zone, and the South Beach Diet are all examples of low- _____ diets.
   a. fat
   b. carbohydrate
   c. protein
   d. fiber

8. Probably the most important reason for obesity today in the United States is
   a. watching TV.
   b. snacking practices.
   c. inactivity.
   d. eating French fries.

9. The major goal for weight reduction in the treatment of obesity is the loss of
   a. weight.   c. body water.
   b. body fat.   d. body protein.

10. For most adults, the greatest portion of their energy expenditure is for
    a. physical activity.
    b. sleeping.
    c. basal metabolism.
    d. the thermic effect of food.

Answers: 1. b (LO 7.6), 2. d (LO 7.2), 3. d (LO 7.6), 4. b (LO 7.1), 5. a (LO 7.10), 6. c (LO 7.1), 7. b (LO 7.12), 8. c (LO 7.5), 9. b (LO 7.6), 10. c (LO 7.1)

Study Questions (Numbers refer to Learning Outcomes)

1. After reexamining the nature and nurture aspects of weight control, propose two hypotheses for the development of obesity. **(LO 7.5)**

2. Propose two hypotheses for the development of obesity, based on the four contributors to energy expenditure. **(LO 7.1)**

3. Define a healthy weight in a way that makes the most sense to you. **(LO 7.3)**

4. Describe a practical method to define obesity in a clinical setting. **(LO 7.3)**

5. What are the two most convincing pieces of evidence that both genetic and environmental factors play significant roles in the development of obesity? **(LO 7.5)**

6. List three health problems that obese people typically face and a reason that each problem arises. **(LO 7.4)**

7. What are three key characteristics of a sound weight-loss program? **(LO 7.6)**

8. Why is the claim for quick, effortless weight loss by any method always misleading? **(LO 7.6)**

9. Define the term *behavior modification*. Relate it to the terms *stimulus control*, *self-monitoring*, *chain-breaking*, *relapse prevention*, and *cognitive restructuring*. Give examples of each. **(LO 7.9)**

10. Why should obesity treatment be viewed as a lifelong commitment rather than a short episode of weight loss? **(LO 7.12)**

What Would You Choose Recommendations

Regular varieties of ice cream contain at least 10% milk fat by weight and are therefore a source of fat, saturated fat, and cholesterol. The milk fat gives the product the smooth, creamy texture for which ice cream is famous. You can see that the regular ice cream in the choices provided has 180 kcal, 10 grams of fat, 6 grams of saturated fat, and 65 mg of cholesterol. The sugar content is 19 grams—some of this comes from natural milk sugar (lactose), and some sugar is added for flavor.

Premium ice cream varieties, such as those you would find in an ice cream shop, may have up 300 kcal, 18 grams of fat, and 30 grams of sugar per ½-cup serving! That's equivalent to 4 teaspoons of butter and 7 teaspoons of sugar. Such decadent treats can be enjoyed in moderation, but are best reserved for special occasions.

Reduced-fat, low-fat, light, or fat-free varieties of ice cream have less than 10% milk fat. This can be accomplished by starting with lower-fat milk, using gelatin instead of eggs, using fat replacers incorporating more air into the product (e.g., "churned"), or any combination thereof. "Reduced fat" means the product has at least 25% less fat than the original product. "Low fat" sets the standard at 3 grams of fat or less per ½-cup serving. "Light" ice cream has at least 50% less fat than the original product. "Fat free" signifies 0.5 grams of fat or less per ½-cup serving. The brand shown here is "light"—it contains lower fat and sugar than the regular ice cream. It has 110 kcal, 3 grams of fat, 2 grams of saturated fat, 10 mg cholesterol, and 14 grams of sugar per serving. For weight-management purposes, this saves you 70 kcals, 7 grams of fat, and 5 grams of sugar per serving compared to regular ice cream. Reducing the fat content of ice cream might also reduce the creamy texture, but for most reduced-fat, low-fat, and light products, the change is barely noticeable.

Frozen yogurt is not always a lower-calorie option than ice cream. It does not have to comply with the same 10% milk fat standard as ice cream does, so there may be a wide range of fat and sugar content. This brand of frozen yogurt has 180 kcal, 3 grams of fat, 1 gram of saturated fat, and 45 mg cholesterol—very similar to the regular ice cream. The product is marketed as "low fat"— and it does only contain 3 grams of fat per ½-cup serving—but there are still 22 grams of sugar. This is a great example of how low fat does not necessarily mean low calorie.

Serving size is the most important part of the Nutrition Facts panel when it comes to calorie control. No matter how low the calorie, fat, and sugar content are, if you consume multiple servings of any product, you are likely to take in too many calories.

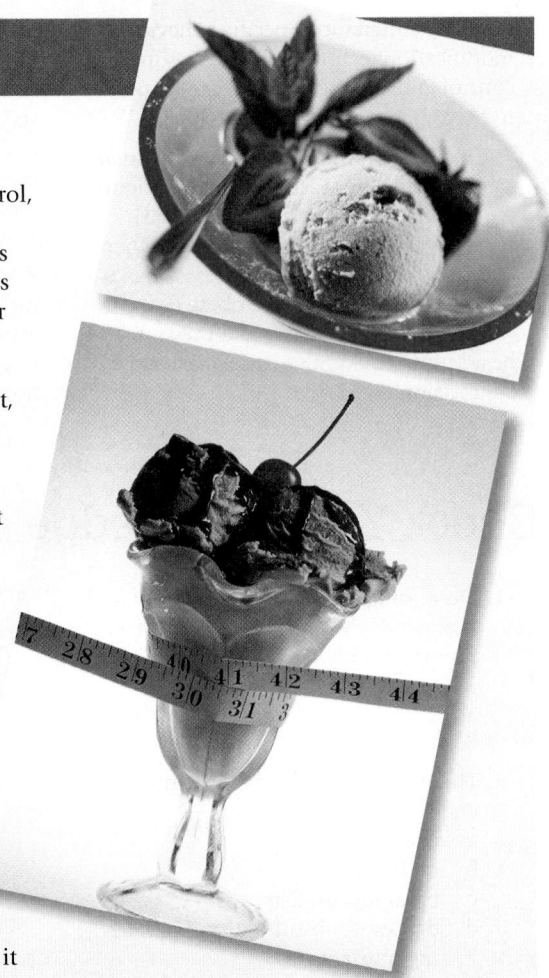

▲ One serving (one scoop) of ice cream with berries is a lower-calorie choice than several scoops with chocolate sauce and cherry.

NUTRITION FACTS			
Kroger Private Selection—Country Made Vanilla Ice Cream			
Serving: 1/2 cup			
Calories	180	Sodium	45 mg
Total Fat	10 g	Potassium	0 g
Saturated	6 g	Total Carbs	19 g
Polyunsaturated	0 g	Dietary Fiber	0 g
Monounsaturated	0 g	Sugars	19 g
Trans	0 g	Protein	6 g
Cholesterol	65 mg		
Vitamin A	8%	Calcium	10%
Vitamin C	2%	Iron	2%
*Percent Daily Values are based on a 2000 calorie diet. Your daily values may be higher or lower depending on your calories needs.			

NUTRITION FACTS			
Kroger Deluxe—Vanilla Bean Light Ice Cream			
Serving: 1/2 cup			
Calories	110	Sodium	50 mg
Total Fat	3 g	Potassium	0 g
Saturated	2 g	Total Carbs	17 g
Polyunsaturated	0 g	Dietary Fiber	0 g
Monounsaturated	0 g	Sugars	14 g
Trans	0 g	Protein	3 g
Cholesterol	10 mg		
Vitamin A	6%	Calcium	10%
Vitamin C	2%	Iron	0%
*Percent Daily Values are based on a 2000 calorie diet. Your daily values may be higher or lower depending on your calories needs.			

NUTRITION FACTS			
Haagen-Dazs—Yogurt Frozen Low Fat Vanilla			
Serving: 1/2 cup			
Calories	180	Sodium	45 mg
Total Fat	3 g	Potassium	0 g
Saturated	1 g	Total Carbs	30 g
Polyunsaturated	0 g	Dietary Fiber	0 g
Monounsaturated	0 g	Sugars	22 g
Trans	0 g	Protein	9 g
Cholesterol	45 mg		
Vitamin A	2%	Calcium	20%
Vitamin C	0%	Iron	0%
*Percent Daily Values are based on a 2000 calorie diet. Your daily values may be higher or lower depending on your calories needs.			

Further Readings

1. Adams KF and others: Overweight, obesity, and mortality in a large prospective cohort of persons 50 to 71 years old. *The New England Journal of Medicine* 355:763, 2006.

   Excess body weight during midlife was associated with an increased risk of death. Risk of death increased by 20% to 40% among overweight persons and by two to three times among obese persons.

2. Blackburn GL, Corliss J: *Break Through Your Set Point.* New York: Harper Collins, 2007.

   This book outlines strategies for "breaking through" weight-loss plateaus by working with the body's natural tendency to stay at a fixed weight. The key is slow, gradual weight loss, followed by a 6-month period of holding steady at your new weight.

3. Flegal KM and others: Prevalence and trends in obesity among U.S. adults, 1999–2008. *Journals of the American Medical Association* 303(3):235, 2010.

   In the United States adult obesity rates have increased significantly. In the late 1970s, 15% of adults were obese compared to 34% in 2008.

4. Hollis JF and others: Weight loss during the intensive intervention phase of the weight-loss maintenance trial. *American Journal of Preventive Medicine* 35:118, 2008.

   Overweight or obese participants lost an average of 12 pounds. Keeping a daily record of food and physical activity helped them succeed suggesting that the willingness to record your eating habits could lead to a healthier weight.

5. James WPT and others: Effect of sibutramine on cardiovascular outcomes in overweight and obese subjects. *New England Journal of Medicine* 363(10):905, 2010.

   Sibutramine (Meridia) was withdrawn from the market in October 2010 based primarily on results from the SCOUT study (Sibutramine Cardiovascular OUTcomes Trial). Among subjects who were receiving long-term sibutramine treatment (~3.4 years), those with preexisting cardiovascular conditions had an increased risk of nonfatal heart attacks and stroke. More than 90% of the 10,000 patients in the study had underlying cardiovascular disease and therefore should not have received sibutramine. It was concluded that sibutramine should not be used in patients with preexisting cardiovascular disease.

6. Kruger J and others: Dietary and physical activity behaviors among adults successful at weight-loss maintenance. *International Journal of Behavioral Nutrition and Physical Activity* 3:17, 2006.

   Strategies practiced more frequently by successful weight losers included weighing oneself, planning meals, tracking fat and calories, exercising 30 or more minutes daily, and adding physical activity to their daily routines.

7. Madan AT, Orth WD: Vitamin and trace mineral levels after laparoscopic gastric bypass. *Obesity Surgery* 16:603, 2006.

   Vitamin and mineral deficiencies are thought to be a common long-term outcome of bariatric surgery. In this study, of 100 patients who underwent laparoscopic Roux-en-Y gastric bypass, most vitamins and minerals were slightly lower at 1-year postoperative. Significant decreases were observed only for vitamin D and selenium.

8. Mozaffarian D and others: Changes in diet and lifestyle and long-term weight gain in women and men. *New England Journal of Medicine* 364:2392, 2011.

   Relationships between lifestyle factors and weight change were evaluated. Subjects gained an average of 3.35 pounds every 4 years, adding up to 20 pounds in 20 years. Those with the greatest increase in physical activity gained 1.76 fewer pounds. The kind of foods eaten had a larger effect than changes in physical activity. Weight gained was associated with greater intake of French fries, potato chips, potatoes, sugar-sweetened beverages, unprocessed red meats, and processed meats. Foods that resulted in weight loss or no gain were fruits, vegetables, whole grains, yogurt, and nuts. Results show how small changes in eating, exercise, and other habits can result in large changes in body weight over the years.

9. National Center for Chronic Disease Prevention and Health Promotion: *Obesity: Halting the Epidemic by Making Health Easier.* Center for Disease Control and Prevention, Department of Health and Human Services, 2009. www.cdc.gov/nccdphp/dnpa.

   In the United States, obesity rates did not increase significantly between 2003–2004 and 2005–2006. Increased awareness of obesity as a national health problem, innovative policy and environmental changes in communities, work sites, and schools, and increased exercise and reduced consumption of high-calorie and fatty foods have likely led to this leveling of rates.

10. O'Brien PE and others: Treatment of mild to moderate obesity with laparoscopic adjustable gastric banding or an intensive medical program: A randomized trial. *Annals of Internal Medicine* 144:625, 2006.

    Surgical patients lost weight more rapidly and also had greater improvement in the metabolic syndrome and quality of life.

11. Robb M, Robb N: Tiny pills, big promises. *Today's Diet & Nutrition* 4(4):58, 2008.

    Information is provided about the latest dietary aids/diet pills for weight loss. Diet pills rely on one of three strategies: suppressing appetite, boosting metabolism, or blocking absorption of fats or carbohydrates. Each strategy is reviewed.

12. See R and others: The association of differing measures of overweight and obesity with prevalent atherosclerosis: the Dallas Heart Study. *Journal of American College of Cardiologists* 50:752, 2007.

    A study of associations between different measures of obesity (body mass index, waist circumference, and waist-to-hip ratio) and atherosclerosis found that waist-to-hip ratio was more strongly associated with atherosclerosis than body mass index or waist circumference. These results indicate that apple-shaped people are at greater risk for obesity-related diseases and heart attack than pear-shaped ones.

13. Shai I and others: Weight loss with a low-carbohydrate, Mediterranean, or low-fat diet. *New England Journal of Medicine* 359:229, 2008.

    Moderately obese adults were assigned to either a low-fat Mediterranean or low-carbohydrate diet, and studied for 2 years. Participants on the low-carbohydrate diet lost and kept off about 12 pounds; those on the Mediterranean Diet, kept off a 10-pounds weight loss; and those on the restricted-fat plan kept off 7 pounds. The results indicate that Mediterranean and low-carbohydrate diets may be effective alternatives to low-fat diets.

14. Slavin J and others: How fiber affects weight regulation. *Food Technology,* p. 34, February 2008.

    Dietary fiber has intrinsic, hormonal, and intestinal effects that decrease food intake by promoting satiety. Effects include decreased gastric emptying and/or slowed energy and nutrient absorption.

15. Svetkey LP and others: Comparison of strategies for sustaining weight loss: The weight-loss maintenance randomized controlled trial. *Journal of the American Medical Association* 299:1139, 2008.

    Participants weighed an average of 213 pounds, followed the Dietary Approaches to Stop Hypertension (DASH) diet for 6 months, and were encouraged to do 180 minutes of moderate exercise a week. Average weight loss was 19 pounds. After 2 ½ years, dieters kept more weight off if they reported to a nutrition counselor every month.

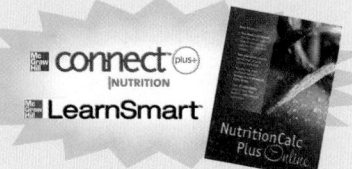

To get the most out of your study of nutrition, go to McGraw-Hill's online resources: Connect www.mcgrawhillconnect.com, **where you will find NutritionCalc Plus, LearnSmart, and many other dynamic tools.**

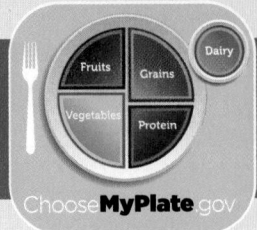

I. A Close Look at Your Weight Status

Determine the following two indices of your body status: body mass index and waist circumference.

Body Mass Index (BMI)

Record your weight in pounds: _____ pounds
Divide your weight in pounds by 2.2 to determine your weight in kilograms: _____ kilograms
Record your height in inches: _____ in
Divide your height in inches by 39.4 to determine your height in meters: _____ meters
Calculate your BMI using the following formula:
BMI = weight (kilograms)/height^2 (meters)
BMI = _____ kg/ _____ m^2 = _____

Waist Circumference

Use a tape measure to measure the circumference of your waist (at the umbilicus with stomach muscles relaxed). Circumference of waist (umbilicus) = _____ in

Interpretation

1. When BMI is greater than 25, health risks from obesity often begin. It is especially advisable to consider weight loss if your BMI exceeds 30. Does yours exceed 25 (or 30)?

   Yes _____ No _____

2. When a person has a BMI greater than 25 and a waist circumference of more than 40 inches (102 centimeters) in men or 35 inches (88 centimeters) in women, there is an increased risk of cardiovascular disease, hypertension, and type 2 diabetes. Does your waist circumference exceed the standard for your gender?

   Yes _____ No _____

3. Do you feel you need to pursue a program of weight loss?

   Yes _____ No _____

Application

From what you have learned in Chapter 7, what can you do to change your patterns of eating and physical activity to lose weight and help ensure maintenance of any loss?

_____

_____

_____

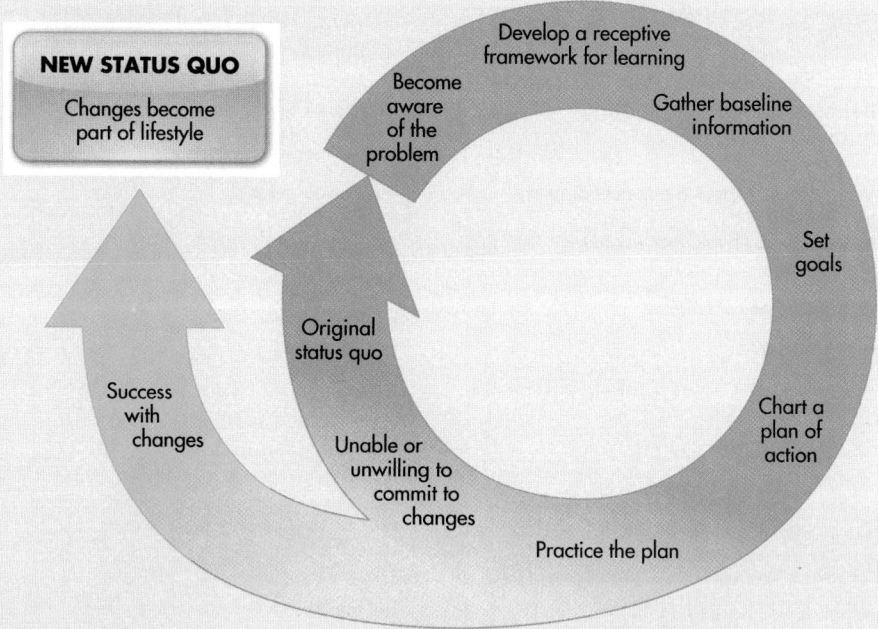

FIGURE 7-20 ▶ A model for behavior change. It starts with awareness of the problem and ends with the incorporation of new behaviors intended to address the problem.

II. An Action Plan to Change or Maintain Weight Status

Now that you have assessed your current weight status, do you feel that you would like to make some changes? Following is a step-by-step guide to behavioral change. This process can be useful even for those satisfied with their current weight, as it can be applied to changing exercise habits, self-esteem, and a variety of other behaviors (Fig. 7-20).

Becoming Aware of the Problem

By calculating your current weight status, you have already become aware of the problem, if one exists. From here, it is important to find out more information about the cause of the problem and whether it is worth working toward a change.

1. What are the factors that most influence your eating habits? Do you eat due to stress, boredom, or depression? Is volume of food your problem, or do you eat mainly the wrong foods for you? Take some time to assess the root causes of your eating habits.

2. Once you have more information about your specific eating practices, you must decide if it is worth changing these practices. A benefits and costs analysis can be a useful tool in evaluating whether it is worth your effort to make life changes. Use the following example as a guide for listing benefits and costs pertinent to your situation (Fig. 7-21).

Setting Goals

What can we accomplish, and how long will it take? Setting a realistic, achievable goal and allowing a reasonable amount of time to pursue it increase the likelihood of success.

1. Begin by determining the outcome you would like to achieve. If you are trying to change your eating behaviors to be more healthy, list your reasons for doing so (e.g., overall health, weight loss, self-esteem).

Overall goal:

_____

_____

FIGURE 7-21 ▶ Benefits and costs analysis applied to increasing physical activity. This process helps put behavior change into the context of total lifestyle.

Benefits and Costs Analysis

1 Benefits of changing eating habits?

What do you expect to get, now or later, that you want?
What may you avoid that would be unpleasant?

feel better physically and psychologically
look better

2 Benefits of not changing eating habits?

What do you get to do that you enjoy doing?
What do you avoid having to do?

no need for planning
can eat without feeling guilty

3 Costs involved in changing eating habits?

What do you have to do that you don't want to do?
What do you have to stop doing that you would rather continue doing?

take time to plan meals and shop
must give up some food volume

4 Costs of not changing eating habits?

What unpleasant or undesirable effects are you likely to experience now or in the future?
What are you likely to lose?

creeping weight gain
low self-esteem and poor health

Reasons to pursue goal:

_____

_____

_____

2. Now list several steps that will be necessary to achieve your goal. Keep in mind, however, that it is generally best to change only a few specific behaviors at first—walking briskly for 60 minutes each day, reducing fat intake, using more whole-grain products, and not eating after 7 P.M. Attempting small and perhaps easier dietary changes first reduces the scope of the problem and increases the likelihood of success.

Steps toward achieving goal:

1. _____

2. _____

3. _____

If you are having trouble deciphering the steps needed to achieve your goal, health professionals are an excellent resource for aid in planning.

Measuring Commitment

Now that you have collected information and know what is required to reach your goal, you must ask yourself, "Can I do this?" Commitment is an essential component in the success of behavioral change. Be honest with yourself. Permanent change is not quick or easy. Once you have decided that you have the commitment required to see this through, continue on to the following sections.

Making It Official with a Contract

Drawing up a behavioral contract often adds incentive to follow through with a plan. The contract could list goal behaviors and objectives, milestones for measuring progress, and regular rewards for meeting the terms of the contract. After finishing a contract, you should sign it in the presence of some friends. This encourages commitment.

Initially, plans should reward positive behaviors, and then they should focus on positive results. Positive behaviors, such as regular physical activity, eventually lead to positive outcomes, such as increased stamina.

Figure 7-22 is a sample contract for increasing physical activity. Keep in mind that this sample contract is only a suggestion; you can add your ideas as well.

Psyching Yourself Up

Once your contract is in place, you need to psych yourself up. Discouragement from peers and your temptations to stray from your plan need to be anticipated. Psyching yourself up can enable you to progress toward your goals in spite of others' attitudes and

Name _Alan Young_

Goal

I agree to _ride my exercise bike_
             (specify behavior)

under the following circumstances _for 30 minutes, 4 times per week in the evening_
                                   (specify where, when, how much, etc.)

Substitute behavior and/or reinforcement schedule _I will reinforce myself if I've achieved my goal after a month with a weekend off campus with my roommate._

Environmental planning

In order to help me do this, I am going to (1) arrange my physical and social environment by _buying a new portable CD player_

and (2) control my internal environment (thoughts, images) by _coordinating riding the bike with the first T.V. watching I do in the evening_

Reinforcements

Reinforcements provided by me daily or weekly (if contract is kept):
I will buy myself a new piece of clothing for off campus trip

Reinforcements provided by others daily or weekly (if contract is kept):
at the end of a month if I've completed my goal my parents will buy me a fitness club membership for winter.

Social support

Behavior change is more likely to take place when other people support you. During the quarter/semester please meet with the other person at least three times to discuss your progress.

The name of my "significant helper" is: _Mr. and Mrs. Young_

This contract should include:

1. Baseline data (one week)
2. Well-defined goal
3. Simple method for charting progress (diary, counter, charts, etc.)
4. Reinforcements (immediate and long-term)
5. Evaluation method (summary of experiences, success, and/or new learnings about self).

FIGURE 7-22 ▶ Alan's behavior contract. Completing such a contract can help generate commitment to behavior change. What would your contract look like?

opinions. Almost everyone benefits from some assertiveness training when it comes to changing behaviors. The following are a few suggestions. Can you think of any others?

- No one's feelings should be hurt if you say, "No, thank you," firmly and repeatedly when others try to dissuade you from a plan. Tell them you have new diet behavior and your needs are important.

- You don't have to eat a lot to accommodate anyone—your mother, business clients, or the chef. For example, at a party with friends, you may feel you have to eat a lot to participate, but you don't. Another trap is ordering a lot just because someone else is paying for the meal.

- Learn ways to handle put-downs—inadvertent or conscious. An effective response can be to communicate feelings honestly, without hostility. Tell criticizers that they have annoyed or offended you, that you are working to change your habits and would really like understanding and support from them.

Practicing the Plan

Once you've set up a plan, the next step is to implement it. Start with a trial of at least 6 to 8 weeks. Thinking of a lifetime commitment can be overwhelming. Aim for a total duration of 6 months of new activities before giving up. We may have to persuade ourselves more than once of the value of continuing the program. The following are some suggestions to help keep a plan on track:

- *Focus on reducing but not necessarily extinguishing undesirable behaviors.* For example, it's usually unrealistic to say, "I'll never eat a certain food again." It's better to say, "I won't eat that *problem* food as often as before."

- *Monitor progress.* Note your progress in a diary and reward yourself according to your contract. While conquering some habits and seeing improvement, you may find yourself quite encouraged, even enthusiastic, about your plan of action. That can give you the impetus to move ahead with the program.

- *Control environments.* In the early phases of behavioral change, try to avoid problem situations, such as parties, coffee breaks, and favorite restaurants. Once new habits are firmly established, you can probably more successfully resist the temptations of these environments.

Reevaluating and Preventing Relapse

After practicing a program for several weeks to months, it is important to reassess the original plan. In addition, you may now be able to pinpoint other problem areas for which you need to plan appropriately.

1. Begin by taking a close and critical look at your original plan. Does it lead to the goals you set? Are there any new steps toward your goal that you feel capable of adding to your contract? Do you need new reinforcements? It may even be necessary to make a new contract. For permanent change, it is worth this time of reassessment.

2. In practicing your plan over the past weeks or months, you have likely experienced relapses. What triggered these relapses? To prevent a total retreat to your old habits, it is important to set up a plan for such relapses. You can do this by identifying high-risk situations, rehearsing a response, and remembering your goals.

You may have noticed a behavior chain in some of your relapses. That is, the relapse may stem from a series of interconnected habitual activities. The way to break the chain is to first identify the activities, pinpoint the weak links, break those links, and substitute other behaviors. Figure 7-23 illustrates a sample behavior chain and a substitute activities list. Consider compiling a list based on your behavior chains.

Epilogue

If you have used the activities in this section, you are well on your way to permanent behavioral change. Recall that this exercise can be used for a variety of desired changes, including quitting smoking, increasing physical activity, and improving study habits. It is by no means an easy process, but the results can be well worth the effort. Overall, the keys to success are motivation (keeping the problem in the forefront of your mind), having a plan of action, securing the resources and skills needed for success, and looking for help from family, friends, or a group.

SUBSTITUTE ACTIVITIES

Pleasant activities
1. _Singing / washing hair_
2. _Reading comics / biking_
3. _Sewing / calling a friend_

Necessary activities
1. _Ironing_
2. _Vacuuming_
3. _Straightening apartment_

Situations when used
1. _Wanted ice cream – delayed with bath_
2. _Wanted wheat thins – cleaned up apt._
3. _Wanted snack – went for walk_
4. _Wanted cookies – did dishes first_
5. _Saw leftovers – went for bike ride_
6. _Tempted by cookies – set timer_
7. _Wanted snack – read comics_

BEHAVIOR CHAIN

Identify the links in your eating response chain on the following diagram. Draw a line through the chain where it was interrupted. Add the link you substituted and the new chain of behavior this substitution started.

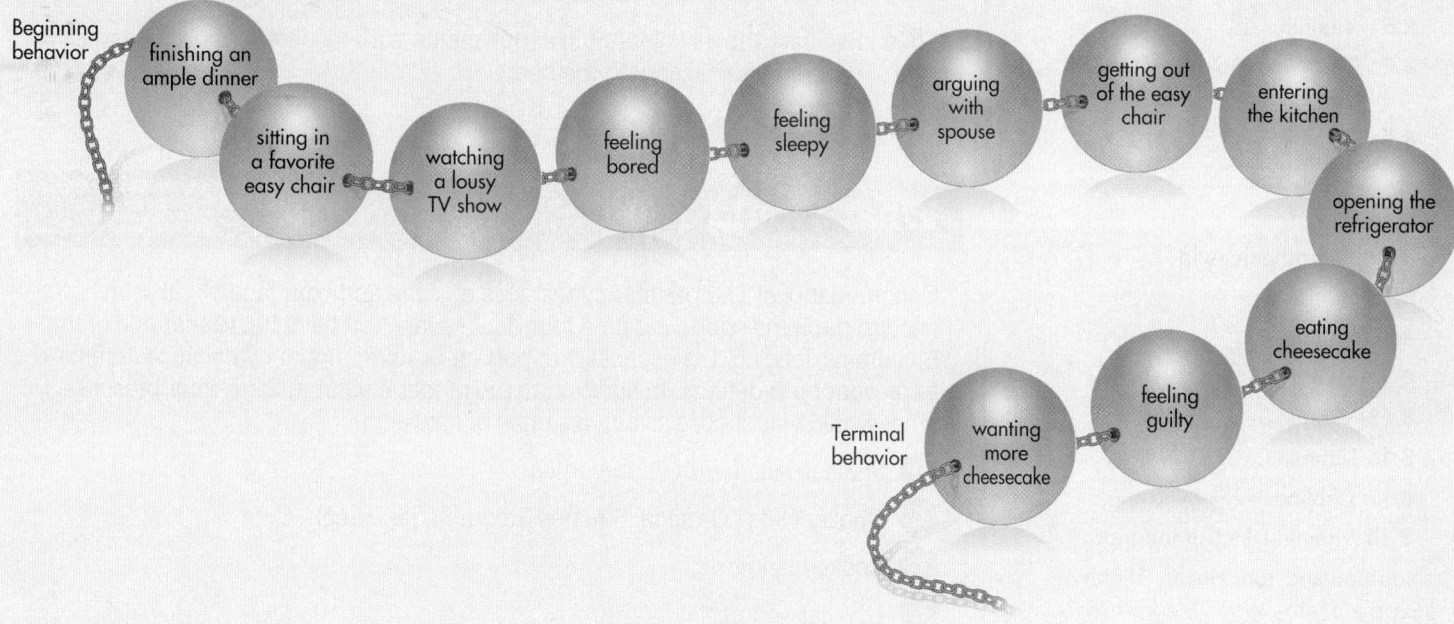

FIGURE 7-23 ▶ Identifying behavior chains. This is a good tool for understanding more about your habits and pinpointing ways to change unwanted habits. The earlier in the chain you substitute a nonfood link, the easier it is to intervene. Four types of behaviors can be substituted in an ongoing behavior chain.

1. Fun activities (taking a walk, reading a book)
2. Necessary activities (cleaning a room, balancing your checkbook)
3. Incompatible activities (taking a shower)
4. Urge-delaying activities (setting a kitchen timer for 20 minutes before allowing yourself to eat)

Using activities to interrupt behavior patterns that lead to inappropriate eating (or inactivity) can be a powerful means of changing habits.

Chapter 8 Vitamins

Student Learning Outcomes

Chapter 8 is designed to allow you to:

8.1 Define the term *vitamin* and list three characteristics of vitamins as a group.

8.2 Classify the vitamins according to whether they are fat soluble or water soluble.

8.3 List the major functions and deficiency symptoms for each vitamin.

8.4 List three important food sources for each vitamin.

8.5 Describe toxicity symptoms from excess consumption of certain vitamins.

8.6 Evaluate the use of vitamin supplements with respect to their potential benefits and hazards to the body.

What Would You Choose?

Congratulations! The pregnancy test was positive and your family will soon need to ditch the sports car for a four-door sedan! You have heard that one of the B vitamins, folic acid, is especially important during pregnancy because it helps to prevent birth defects. In addition to the prenatal vitamin the doctor prescribed, what would you choose as a rich source of folic acid?

a Spinach salad with strawberries

b Quaker Oats® Oatmeal Squares Brown Sugar cereal

c Cooked lentils

d Low-fat yogurt

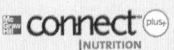 **Think about your choice as you read Chapter 8, then see our recommendations at the end of the chapter. To learn more about nutrient needs during pregnancy, check out the Connect site:** www.mcgrawhillconnect.com

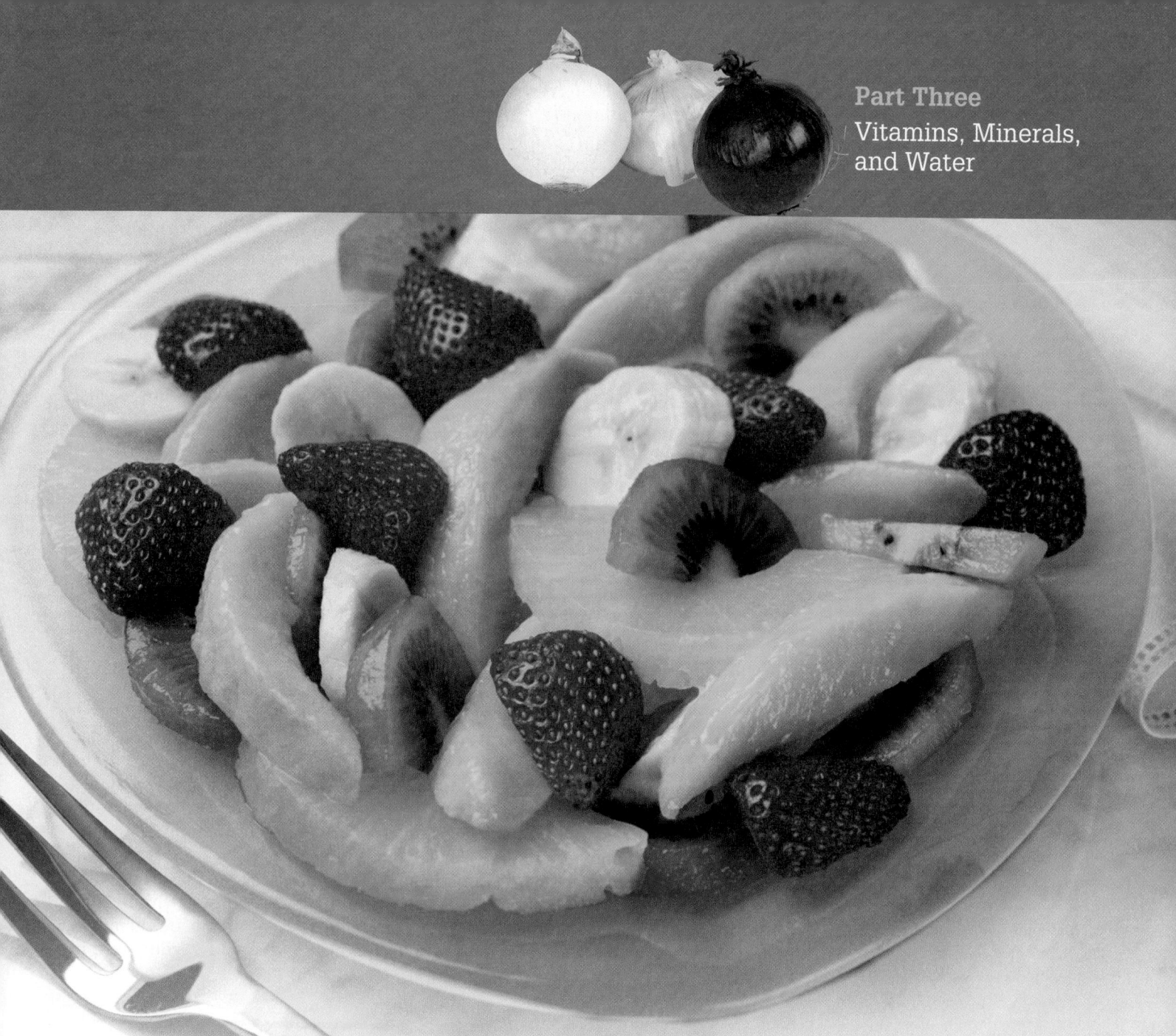

Although the vitamins are essential nutrients, the amount of vitamins we need to prevent deficiency is small. In general, humans require a total of about 1 ounce (28 grams) of vitamins for every 150 pounds (70 kilograms) of food consumed. Some people believe that consuming vitamins far in excess of their needs provides them with extra energy, protection from disease, and prolonged youth. They seem to think that if a little is good, then more must be better. More than half of the U.S. adult population have taken vitamin and/or mineral supplements on a regular basis, some at unsafe levels. In 2010, we spent $28.7 billion on dietary supplements. Sales for vitamin D at $550 million were up 30% over 2009. The health-related value of this practice is hotly debated.

Vitamins are found in plants and animals. Plants synthesize all the vitamins they need and, as the chapter comic suggests, are a healthy source of vitamins for animals. Animals vary in their ability to synthesize vitamins. For example, guinea pigs and humans are two of the few organisms unable to make their own supply of vitamin C.

Chapter 8 reviews some general properties of vitamins. These vital nutrients are divided into two groups: the fat-soluble vitamins and the water-soluble vitamins. The chapter focuses on the functions and sources of each vitamin and human needs for them. The current controversy over vitamin and mineral supplement use is also explored.

Refresh Your Memory

As you begin your study of vitamins in Chapter 8, you may want to review:

- Implications of the Dietary Supplement Health and Education Act (DSHEA) in Chapter 2
- The gastrointestinal system for the digestion and absorption of nutrients and the urinary system for vitamin D activation in Chapter 3
- The digestion and absorption of dietary lipids, the formation of lipoproteins, and the definition of antioxidants in Chapter 5
- Amino-acid metabolism, protein synthesis, and protein-calorie malnutrition in Chapter 6

8.1 Vitamins: Vital Dietary Components

By definition, **vitamins** are essential organic (carbon-containing) substances needed in small amounts in the diet for normal function, growth, and maintenance of the body. Although vitamins yield no energy to the body, they often participate in energy-yielding reactions. Vitamins A, D, E, and K are **fat soluble,** whereas the B vitamins and vitamin C are **water soluble.** In addition, the B vitamins and vitamin K function as parts of **coenzymes** (compounds that help enzymes function).

Vitamins are generally essential in human diets because they can't be synthesized in the human body or because their synthesis can be decreased by environmental factors. Notable exceptions to having a strict dietary need for a vitamin are vitamin A, which we can synthesize from certain pigments in plants; vitamin D, synthesized in

vitamin Compound needed in small amounts in the diet to help regulate and support chemical reactions and processes in the body.

fat-soluble vitamins Vitamins that dissolve in fat and such substances as ether and benzene but not readily in water. These vitamins are A, D, E, and K.

water-soluble vitamins Vitamins that dissolve in water. These vitamins are the B vitamins and vitamin C.

coenzyme A compound that combines with an inactive enzyme to form a catalytically active form. In this manner, coenzymes aid in enzyme function.

Increasing our intake of fruits and vegetables is one of the recurring Dietary Guidelines. Which vitamins are especially found in fruits and vegetables? What are some other health-related attributes of fruits and vegetables in general? Which chronic diseases are associated with a poor intake of fruits and vegetables? Should we take a daily vitamin supplement if we do not include fruits and vegetables in our diet? Chapter 8 provides some answers.

ZIGGY

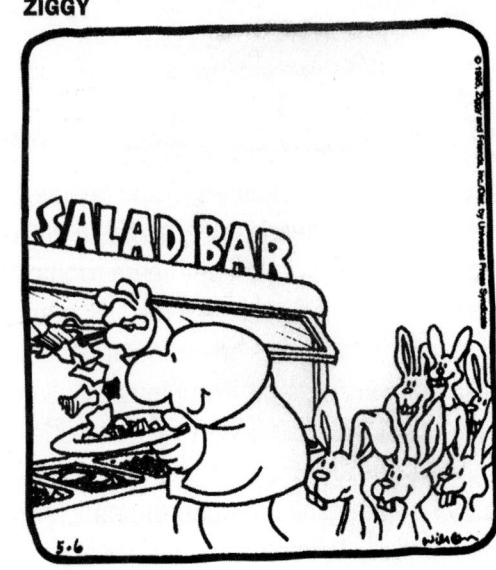

ZIGGY © ZIGGY AND FRIENDS, INC. Reprinted with permission of UNIVERSAL PRESS SYNDICATE. All rights reserved.

the body if the skin is exposed to adequate sunlight; niacin, synthesized from the amino acid tryptophan; and vitamin K and biotin, synthesized to some extent by bacteria in the intestinal tract.

To be classified as a vitamin, a compound must meet the following criteria to be an essential nutrient: (1) the body is unable to synthesize enough of the compound to maintain health; and (2) absence of the compound from the diet for a defined period produces deficiency symptoms that, if caught in time, are quickly cured when the substance is resupplied. A substance does not qualify as a vitamin merely because the body can't make it. Evidence must suggest that health declines when the substance is not consumed.

As scientists began to identify various vitamins, related deficiency diseases such as scurvy, beriberi, pellagra, and rickets were dramatically cured. For the most part, as the vitamins were discovered, they were named alphabetically: A, B, C, D, E, and so on. Later, many substances originally classified as vitamins were found not to be essential for humans and were dropped from the list. Other vitamins, thought at first to be only one chemical turned out to be several chemicals, so the alphabetical names had to be broken down by numbers (B-6, B-12, and so on).

In addition to their use in correcting deficiency diseases, a few vitamins have also proved useful in treating several nondeficiency diseases. These medical applications require administration of pharmacological amounts or **megadoses,** well above typical human needs for the vitamins. For example, megadoses of a form of niacin can be used as part of blood cholesterol–lowering treatment for certain individuals. This chapter will mention others as well. Still, any claimed benefits from use of vitamin supplements, especially intakes in excess of the Upper Level (if set), should be viewed critically because unproven claims are common.

Both plant and animal foods supply vitamins in the human diet. Vitamins isolated from foods or synthesized in the laboratory are the same chemical compounds and generally work equally well in the body. Contrary to claims in the health-food literature, "natural" vitamins isolated from foods are, for the most part, no more healthful than those synthesized in a laboratory, but there are exceptions. Vitamin E is much more potent in its natural form than in its synthetic form. In contrast, synthetic folic acid, the form of the vitamin added to ready-to-eat breakfast cereals and flour, is 1.7 times more potent than the natural vitamin form.

Have Scientists Found All the Vitamins?

You may wonder whether there are vitamins in foods that have yet to be discovered. After all, the first chemical formula of a vitamin (thiamin) was not determined until 1937, and the last structure was characterized in 1948 (vitamin B-12). Although some optimistic researchers hope to discover that one or more additional compounds (e.g., choline; see p. 330) are vitamins, most scientists are confident that all compounds that meet the criteria for classification as a vitamin have been discovered. Evidence supports this assumption. For example, people have lived well for years when receiving only intravenous administration of solutions that consist of protein, carbohydrate, fat, all the known vitamins, and the essential minerals. With appropriate medical monitoring, these people not only continue to live, but also build new body tissues, heal wounds, fight existing diseases, and even have babies.

Storage of Vitamins in the Body

Except for vitamin K, the fat-soluble vitamins are not readily excreted from the body. In contrast, excess amounts of the water-soluble vitamins are generally lost from the body rapidly, partly because the water in cells dissolves these vitamins and excretes them out of the body via the kidneys. Water-soluble vitamin B-6 and vitamin B-12 are exceptions; these are stored much more readily than the other water-soluble vitamins.

megadose Intake of a nutrient beyond estimates of needs to prevent a deficiency or what would be found in a balanced diet; 2 to 10 times human needs is a starting point for such a pharmacological dosage.

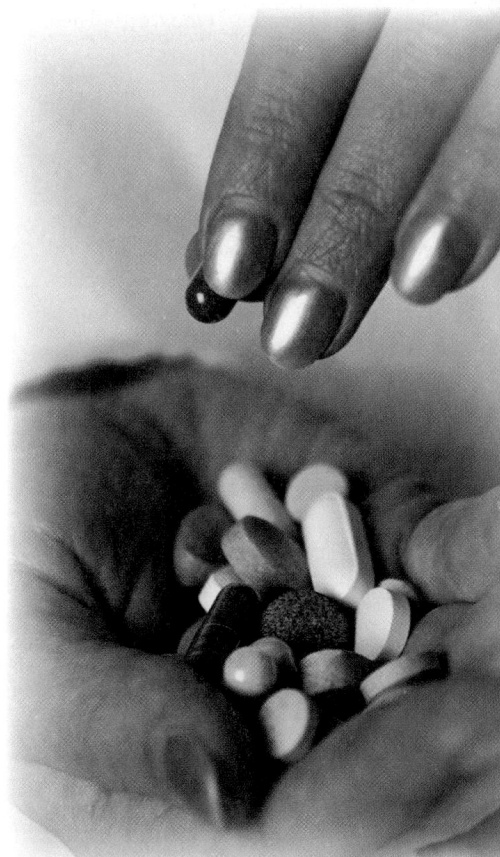

▲ Vitamins are not likely to be toxic unless taken in large amounts as supplements.

Because of the limited storage of many vitamins, they should be consumed in the diet daily, although an occasional lapse in the intake of even water-soluble vitamins generally causes no harm. Symptoms of a vitamin deficiency occur only when that vitamin is lacking in the diet and body stores are essentially exhausted. For example, an average person must consume no thiamin for 10 days or no vitamin C for 20 to 40 days before developing the first symptoms of deficiency of these vitamins.

Vitamin Toxicity

Fat-soluble vitamins are not readily excreted, so some can easily accumulate in the body and cause toxic effects. And, although a toxic effect from an excessive intake of any vitamin is theoretically possible, toxicity of the fat-soluble vitamin A is the most frequently observed. Vitamin E and the water-soluble vitamins niacin, vitamin B-6, and vitamin C can also cause toxic effects, but only when consumed in large amounts (15 to 100 times human needs or more). These five vitamins are unlikely to cause toxic effects unless taken in supplement (pill) form. Vitamin A even causes toxicity with long-term intake as little as two times human needs.

A "one-a-day" type of multivitamin and mineral supplement usually contains less than two times the Daily Values of the components, so daily use of these products is unlikely to cause toxic effects in men and nonpregnant women. But consuming many vitamin pills, especially highly potent sources of vitamin A, can cause problems. Today, concentrated vitamin A supplements are widely available in grocery, drug, and health-food stores and pose risks for toxicity when used inappropriately. See the later Nutrition and Your Health section to find out more about whether you should take a multivitamin and mineral supplement and, if so, how to do it safely.

Preservation of Vitamins in Foods

Substantial amounts of vitamins can be lost from the time a fruit or vegetable is picked until it is eaten. The water-soluble vitamins—particularly thiamin, vitamin C, and folate—can be destroyed with improper storage and excessive cooking. Heat, light, exposure to the air, cooking in water, and alkalinity are all factors that can destroy vitamins. The sooner a food is eaten after harvest, the less chance of nutrient loss. Food cooperatives, **community-supported agriculture (CSA)** and farmers' markets are great sources of freshly harvested fruits and vegetables.

In general, if the food is not eaten within a few days, freezing is the best preservation method to retain nutrients. Fruits and vegetables are often frozen immediately after harvesting, so frozen vegetables and fruits are often as nutrient-rich as freshly picked ones. As part of the freezing process, vegetables are quickly blanched in boiling water. This destroys the enzymes that would otherwise degrade the vitamins. Table 8-1 provides some tips to aid in preserving the vitamins in food.

See Nutrition and Your Health: Dietary Supplements—Who Needs Them? at the end of Chapter 8.

Community-supported agriculture (CSA) Farms that are supported by a community of growers and consumers who provide mutual support and share the risks and benefits of food production, usually including a system of weekly delivery or pick-up of vegetables and fruit, sometimes dairy products and meat.

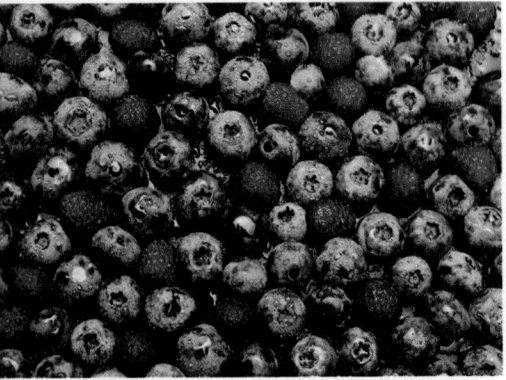

▲ Frozen fruits and vegetables are often as nutrient rich as freshly picked ones.

CONCEPT CHECK

In general, the fat-soluble vitamins—A, D, E, and K—are less readily excreted than the water-soluble B vitamins and vitamin C. Regular consumption of foods rich in both water-soluble and fat-soluble vitamins is important for health. However, the occasional inadequate consumption of any one vitamin is of little health concern, because even water-soluble vitamins persist in the body to some extent. For example, when a person ingests a vitamin-free diet, the first deficiency signs (due to lack of thiamin) will not appear for about 10 days. When taken in supplement form, the fat-soluble vitamin A poses the greatest risk of toxicity. For the most part, there is little risk of toxicity when vitamins are obtained from a variety of foods.

TABLE 8-1 Tips for Preserving the Vitamin Content of Foods

What to Do	Why
Keep fruits and vegetables cool.	Enzymes in food begin to degrade vitamins once the fruit or vegetable is picked. Chilling reduces this process. Refrigerate fresh produce (except for potatoes, tomatoes, onions, and bananas) until they are consumed.
Refrigerate foods in moisture-proof, air-tight containers.	Nutrients keep best at temperatures near freezing, at high humidity, and away from air.
Trim, peel, and cut fruits and vegetables minimally—just enough to remove rotten or inedible parts.	Oxygen breaks down vitamins faster when more surface is exposed. Outer leaves of lettuce and other greens have higher values of vitamins and minerals than the inner, tender leaves or stems. Potato skins and apple skins are higher in vitamins and minerals than the inner parts.
Microwave, steam, or use a pan or wok with very small amounts of fat and a tight-fitting lid to cook vegetables.	More nutrients are retained when there is less contact with water and shorter cooking time. Whenever possible, cook fruits or vegetables in their skins.
Minimize reheating food.	Prolonged reheating reduces vitamin content.
Do not add fats to vegetables during cooking if you plan to discard the liquid.	Fat-soluble vitamins will be lost in discarded fat. Add fats to vegetables after they are fully cooked and drained.
Do not add baking soda to vegetables to enhance the green color.	Alkalinity destroys much thiamin, and other vitamins.
Store canned foods in a cool place.	Canned foods vary in the amount of nutrients lost, largely because of differences in storage time and temperatures. To get maximal nutritive value from canned goods, serve any liquid packed with the food whenever possible.

▲ Rapid cooking of vegetables in minimal fluids aids in preserving vitamin content. Steaming is one effective method.

8.2 The Fat-Soluble Vitamins—A, D, E, and K

Let's look at what we know about the fat-soluble vitamins—vitamins A, D, E, and K.

Absorption of Fat-Soluble Vitamins

Vitamins A, D, E, and K are absorbed along with dietary fat, because they are fat-soluble. These vitamins then travel with dietary fats through the bloodstream to reach body cells. Special carriers in the bloodstream help distribute some of these vitamins. Fat-soluble vitamins are stored mostly in the liver and fatty tissues.

When fat absorption is efficient, about 40% to 90% of the fat-soluble vitamins are absorbed. Anything that interferes with normal digestion and absorption of fats, however, also interferes with fat-soluble vitamin absorption. For example, people with cystic fibrosis, a disease that often inhibits fat absorption, may develop deficiencies of fat-soluble vitamins. Some medications, such as the weight-loss drug orlistat (Xenical), that we discussed in Chapter 7, also interfere with fat absorption. Unabsorbed fat carries these vitamins to the large intestine, where they are excreted in the feces. People with such conditions are especially susceptible to vitamin K deficiency because body stores of vitamin K are lower than those of the other fat-soluble vitamins. Vitamin supplements, taken under a physician's guidance, are part of the treatment for preventing a vitamin deficiency associated with fat malabsorption. Finally, people who use mineral oil as a laxative at mealtimes risk fat-soluble vitamin deficiencies. The intestine does not absorb mineral oil, so fat-soluble vitamins are eliminated with the mineral oil in the feces.

8.3 Vitamin A

The amount of vitamin A you consume is important, as both deficiency and toxicity of this vitamin can cause severe problems. In addition, there is a narrow range of optimal intakes between these two states. Vitamin A is found in foods in a variety of forms. **Retinoids,** or preformed vitamin A, are only found in foods of animal origin, such as fish and organ meats. However, plants contain pigments called **carotenoids,** which can be turned into vitamin A in the body as needed. They can be termed **provitamin A.** Only three of the more than 600 carotenoids found in nature are known to serve as provitamin A in humans, but there may be more. Beta-carotene, the orange-yellow pigment in carrots, is the most potent form of provitamin A. The other known provitamin A carotenoids are lutein and zeaxanthin. Together, preformed vitamin A from animal sources and provitamin A carotenoids make up what is generally called vitamin A.

Functions of Vitamin A and Carotenoids

Vitamin A plays many important roles in the body. The best known and most clearly understood of its roles is in vision. Body changes that occur when vitamin A is lacking provide insight to this and other actions of this fat-soluble nutrient.

Vision. Vitamin A performs important functions in light-dark vision, and to a lesser extent, color vision. One form of vitamin A (retinal) allows certain cells in the eye to adjust from bright to dim light (such as after seeing the headlights of an oncoming car). Without sufficient dietary vitamin A, the cells in the eye cannot quickly readjust to dim light. This condition, known as **night blindness,** is an early sign of vitamin A deficiency.

If vitamin A deficiency progresses, the cells that line the cornea of the eye (the clear window of the eye) also lose their ability to produce **mucus.** The eye then becomes dry. Eventually, when dirt particles scratch the dry surface of the eye, bacteria infect it. The infection soon spreads to the entire surface of the eye and leads to blindness. This disease process is called **xerophthalmia,** which means *dry eye* (Fig. 8-1).

Vitamin A deficiency is second only to accidents as a worldwide cause of blindness. North Americans are at little risk because of generally good diets. However, people—especially children—in less-developed nations are susceptible to vitamin A deficiency. Poor vitamin A intakes, low fat intakes that do not allow for sufficient vitamin A absorption, and low stores of vitamin A lessen the ability of the children to meet high needs during rapid childhood growth. Hundreds of thousands of children in developing nations, especially Asia, become blind each year because of vitamin A deficiency and ultimately die from infections. In North America, the leading cause of blindness in adults is diabetes; in children, it is accidents. As covered in more detail in Chapter 12, worldwide attempts to reduce this problem have included giving large doses of vitamin A twice yearly and fortifying sugar, margarine, and monosodium glutamate with vitamin A. These food vehicles are used because they are commonly consumed by the populations of less-developed nations. This effort has proven effective in some countries.

Age-related **macular degeneration** is a leading cause of legal blindness among North American adults over the age of 65 (Fig. 8-2). The disease is associated with changes in the macular area of the eye, which provides the most detailed vision. Age, smoking, and genetics are risk factors. The macula contains the carotenoids lutein and zeaxanthin in high enough concentrations to impart a yellow color. In one study, the higher the total number of carotenoids (beta-carotene, lutein, and zeaxanthin) consumed in the diet, the lower was the risk for age-related macular degeneration. These carotenoids may also decrease the risk of cataracts in the eyes. Consumption of fruits and vegetables high in carotenoids, rather than the intake of these specific carotenoids in supplements, may reduce the risk for these eye disorders. Multivitamin and mineral supplements formulated for older adults (e.g., Centrum Silver™) are being marketed as a source of lutein.

retinoids Chemical forms of preformed vitamin A; one source is animal foods.

carotenoids Pigment materials in fruits and vegetables that range in color from yellow to orange to red; three of the various carotenoids yield vitamin A. Many are antioxidants.

provitamin/precursor A substance that can be made into a vitamin if the body needs it.

night blindness A vitamin A deficiency condition in which the retina (in the eye) cannot adjust to low amounts of light.

mucus A thick fluid secreted by many cells throughout the body. It contains a compound that has both carbohydrate and protein parts. It acts as a lubricant and means of protection for cells.

xerophthalmia Literally "dry eye." This is a cause of blindness that results from a vitamin A deficiency. A lack of mucus production by the eye, which leaves it at a greater risk of damage from surface dirt and bacteria.

macular degeneration A painless condition leading to disruption of the central part of the retina (in the eye) and, in turn, blurred vision.

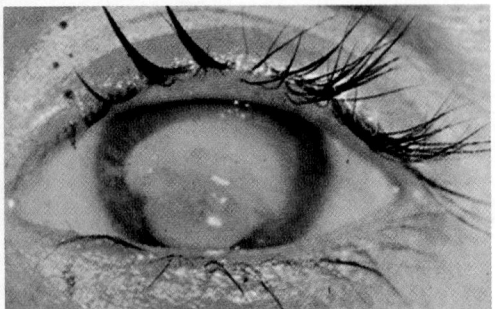

FIGURE 8-1 ▶ Vitamin A deficiency that eventually led to blindness. Note the severe effects on this eye. This problem is commonly seen today in southeast Asia.

Health of Other Cells. Vitamin A also maintains the health of cells that line internal and external surfaces of the lungs, intestines, stomach, vagina, urinary tract, and bladder, as well as those of the eyes and skin. These cells (called **epithelial cells**) serve as important barriers to bacterial infection. As just noted for the eye, some epithelial cells secrete mucus, a needed lubricant. Without vitamin A, mucus-forming cells deteriorate and no longer synthesize mucus. Vitamin A deficiency also causes insufficient mucus production in the intestines and lung cells, and poor health of cells in general. Vitamin A deficiency also reduces the activity of certain immune system cells. Together, these effects leave the vitamin A–deficient person at great risk for infections. For many years, vitamin A has been dubbed the "anti-infection" vitamin.

Growth, Development, and Reproduction. Vitamin A participates in the processes of growth, development, and reproduction in several ways. This role has been demonstrated in vitamin A deficient children experiencing growth retardation when vitamin A supplementation increased their growth. At the genetic level, vitamin A (as retinoic acid) binds to receptors on DNA to increase synthesis of a variety of proteins (review Fig. 6-1 regarding the role of DNA in protein synthesis). In doing so, vitamin A is said to be affecting **gene expression.** Some of these proteins are required for growth, such as bone growth. In laboratory animals, another consequence of vitamin A deficiency is an inability to reproduce.

Cardiovascular Disease Prevention. Carotenoids may play a role in preventing cardiovascular disease in persons at high risk, possibly linked to carotenoids' antioxidant capability. Until definitive studies are complete, many scientists recommend that we increase our intake of carotenoids and other nutrients and compounds by consuming at least 5 servings of fruits and vegetables per day as part of an effort to reduce the risk of cardiovascular disease (see Further Reading 13).

Cancer Prevention. Most forms of cancer arise from cells influenced by vitamin A. Coupled with its ability to aid immune system activity, vitamin A may be a valuable tool in the fight against cancer. This is especially true for skin, lung, bladder, and breast cancers. Still, because of the potential for toxicity, unsupervised use of megadose vitamin A supplements to reduce cancer risk is not advised.

Carotenoids by themselves also may help prevent cancer, acting again as antioxidants. Population studies show that regular consumption of foods rich in carotenoids decreases the risk of lung and oral cancers. Cancer of the **prostate gland** is one of the most common cancers among North American men. The dietary carotenoid found in tomatoes, (the red pigment lycopene) seems to protect against this type of cancer and may also decrease skin cancer risk.

In contrast to the potential benefits of carotenoids in food, recall from Chapter 1 that recent studies from the United States and Finland failed to show a reduction in lung cancer in male smokers and nonsmokers given supplements of the carotenoid beta-carotene for 5 or more years. In fact, beta-carotene use in male smokers increased the number of lung cancer cases compared with the control groups. No comparable studies have been done with women. Although further research continues, most researchers are now convinced that beta-carotene supplementation offers no protection against cancer. Thus, overwhelming advice is to rely on food sources of this or any other carotenoids.

Vitamin A Analogs for Acne. The acne medication tretinoin (Retin-A) is made of one **analog** form of vitamin A. It is used as a topical treatment (applied to the skin) for acne. It appears to work by irritating the skin, which leads to opening of pores and a generalized peeling of the skin layer. It also can block the deleterious effects that skin bacteria have on acne lesions. Similar vitamin A derivatives are also used in antiaging creams because they increase cell turnover and interrupt the path-

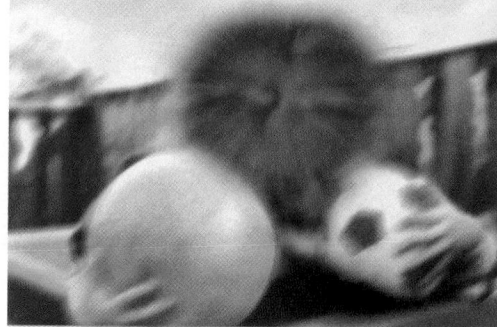

FIGURE 8-2 ▶ Age-related macular degeneration causing a blind spot in the center of the visual field. Increased dietary lutein and zeaxanthin are associated with decreased risk of macular degeneration. Further research is needed to better understand the relationship between macular degeneration and carotenoids.

epithelial cells The cells that line the outside of the body and the inside of all external passages within it, such as the GI tract.

gene expression Use of DNA information on a gene to produce a protein. This is a major determinant of cell development.

prostate gland A solid, chestnut-shaped organ surrounding the first part of the urinary tract in the male. The prostate gland secretes substances into the semen.

analog A chemical compound that differs slightly from another, usually natural, compound. Analogs generally contain extra or altered chemical groups and may have similar or opposite metabolic effects compared with the native compound. Also spelled *analogue.*

▼ Many vegetables are rich in provitamin A carotenoids.

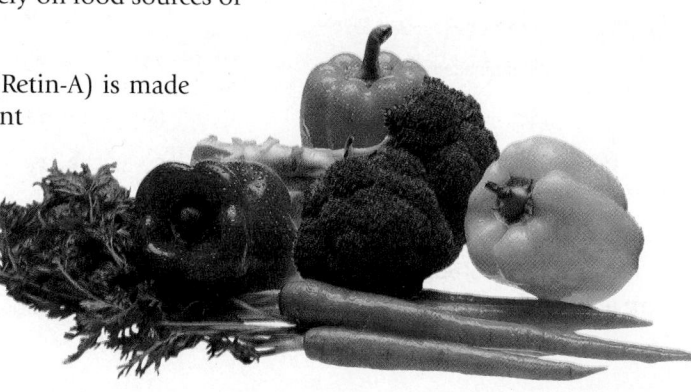

ways of UV skin damage. Another derivative of vitamin A, isotretinoin (Accutane), is an oral drug used to treat serious acne. It acts in part to regulate development of cells in the skin (the gene expression role discussed earlier). Taking high doses of vitamin A itself would not be safe. The use of isotretinoin (Accutane) is strictly monitored by the U.S. Food and Drug Administration (FDA) in order to prevent the use of the drug during pregnancy due to the high risk of birth defects. iPLEDGE is a mandatory distribution program required since March 2006 by the FDA. In order for women to receive this medication, they must have two negative pregnancy tests; sign a patient information/consent form; agree to use two effective forms of birth control; register, along with their doctors and pharmacists, with iPLEDGE by phone or on the Internet, and agree to follow all instructions in the iPLEDGE program.

Vitamin A Sources and Needs

Preformed vitamin A is found in liver, fish, fish oils, fortified milk and yogurt, and eggs (Fig. 8-3). Although liver is a rich food source of vitamin A and other nutrients that are stored in the liver. Focusing on liver to meet nutrient needs is not a good idea because it also provides a high concentration of cholesterol and other fats. Margarine is also fortified with vitamin A. The provitamin A carotenoids mentioned before are mainly found in dark green and yellow-orange vegetables and some fruits. Carrots, spinach and other greens, winter squash, sweet potatoes, broccoli, mangoes, cantaloupe, peaches, and apricots are examples of such sources. About 65% of the vitamin A in the typical North American diet comes from preformed vitamin A sources, whereas provitamin A dominates in the diet among poor people in other parts of the world.

Food Sources of Vitamin A

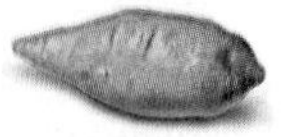

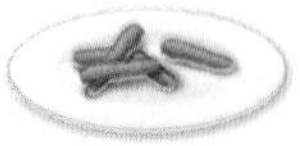

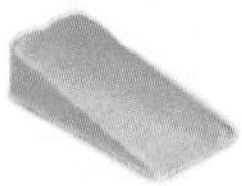

Food Item and Amount	Vitamin A (micrograms RAE*)	Adult Male RDA = 900 micrograms %RDA	Adult Female RDA = 700 micrograms %RDA
RDA	700-900 micrograms	100%	100%
Sweet potato, ½ cup	958	106%	137%
Spinach, ⅔ cup	494	55%	71%
Mango, 1	402	45%	57%
Baby carrots, 5	375	42%	54%
Acorn squash, ⅔ cup	244	27%	35%
Cooked kale, ½ cup	206	23%	29%
Nonfat milk, 1 cup	150	17%	21%
Broccoli, 1 cup	138	15%	20%
Apricot, 3	137	15%	20%
Cheddar cheese, 1 ounce	78	9%	11%
Romaine lettuce, 1 cup	72	8%	10%
Soft margarine, 1 tsp	50	6%	7%
Scallions, 1 tablespoon	32	4%	5%
Peach, 1	26	3%	4%

Daily Value = 1000 micrograms

Key:
- Grains
- Vegetables
- Fruits
- Dairy
- Protein
- Oils

ChooseMyPlate.gov

* Retinol activity equivalents.

FIGURE 8-3 ▶ Food sources of vitamin A compared to the RDA for adult males and females.

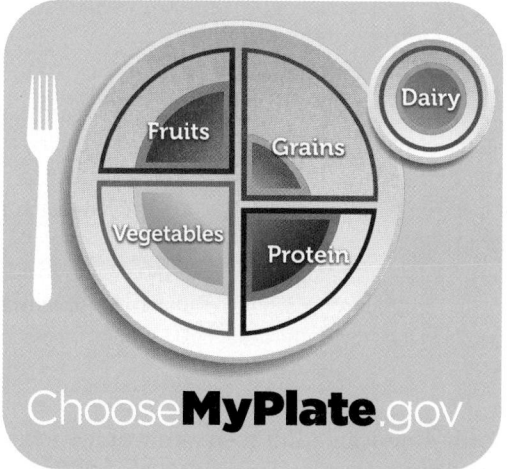

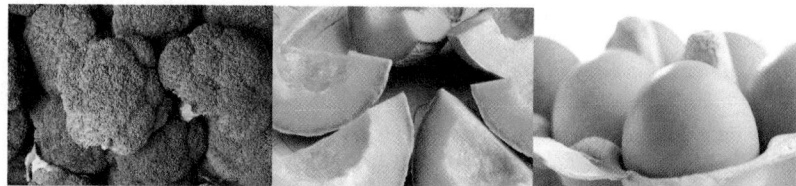

MyPlate:
Sources of Vitamin A

Grains	Vegetables	Fruits	Dairy	Protein
• Fortified break-fast cereals • Fortified meal replacement bars	• Carrots • Broccoli • Spinach • Squash • Sweet potatoes	• Peaches • Apricots • Cantaloupes • Mangoes • Papayas	• Fortified milk • Fortified yogurt • Cheese	• Liver • Eggs

FIGURE 8-4 ▶ Sources of vitamin A from MyPlate. The fill of the background color (none, 1/3, 2/3, or completely covered) within each group on the plate indicates the average nutrient density for vitamin A in that group. Overall, the vegetables group, fruits group, and certain choices in the protein group provide the richest sources. The grains group contains some foods that are nutrient-dense sources of vitamin A because they are fortified with the vitamin. With regard to physical activity, vitamin A plays no specific role *per se* in such endeavors.

Among common foods, those especially rich in vitamin A are carrots, spinach and other greens, sweet potatoes, winter squash, romaine lettuce, broccoli, apricots, and fat-free and low-fat milk. Many of the vegetables listed in Figs. 8-3 and 8-4 are good sources of beta-carotene and the other two provitamin A carotenoids. Marine oils are rich in vitamin A, and consumption of large amounts of such oils can lead to symptoms of vitamin A toxicity.

Beta-carotene accounts for some of the orange color of carrots. In vegetables such as broccoli, this yellow-orange color is masked by dark-green chlorophyll pigments. Still, green vegetables contain provitamin A. Green, leafy vegetables, such as spinach and kale, have a high concentration of lutein and zeaxanthin. Tomato juice and other tomato products, such as pizza sauce, contain significant amounts of lycopene.

The RDA for vitamin A is 700 to 900 micrograms of retinol activity equivalents (RAEs). These RAE units take into account the activity of both preformed vitamin A and the three carotenoids that also are known to yield vitamin A in humans. The total RAE value for a food is calculated by adding the concentration of preformed vitamin A to the amount of provitamin A carotenoids in the food that will be converted to vitamin A. The retinol equivalent (RE) is an older unit for vitamin A. This RE is similar to the RAE but assumed that there was a greater contribution to vitamin A needs from carotenoids than we assume today. Food composition tables and nutrient databases still contain some values based on this older RE standard. It will take some time to update these resources. The Daily Value used on food and supplement labels is 1000 micrograms (5000 IU).

▲ Provitamin A carotenoids are the safest way to meet vitamin A needs. A serving of these carrots would be an excellent addition to the vegetable section of MyPlate.

international unit (IU) A crude measure of vitamin activity, often based on the growth rate of animals in response to the vitamin. Today IUs have largely been replaced by more precise milligram or microgram measures.

fetus The developing human life form from 8 weeks after conception until birth.

MAKING DECISIONS

Expressing Vitamin A Content

In the past, most nutrient amounts in foods, including vitamin A, were formerly expressed in less precise **international units (IUs).** Some food and supplement labels still show the IU value for vitamin A. To compare the older IU standards to current RAE recommendations, assume that for any preformed vitamin A in a food or added to food, 3.3 IU = RAE. The same is true for any beta-carotene added to foods.

There is no easy way to convert IU units to RAE units for foods that naturally contain provitamin A carotenoids, such as carrots, spinach, and apricots. A general rule of thumb is to divide the IU units for foods containing carotenoids by 2, and then divide the result by 3.3 as just discussed.

Average intakes of vitamin A for North American adult men and women meet the RDA. Most adults in North America have liver reserves of vitamin A three to five times greater than needed to provide good health. Thus, the use of vitamin A supplements by most people is unnecessary. At present, there is no separate RDA for beta-carotene or any of the other provitamin A carotenoids.

Deficient vitamin A status in North America may be seen in preschool children who do not eat enough vegetables. The urban poor, older adults, and people with alcoholism or liver disease (which limits vitamin A storage) can also show diminished vitamin A status, especially with respect to stores. Finally, children and adults with severe fat-malabsorption may also experience vitamin A deficiency.

Upper Level for Vitamin A

The Upper Level for vitamin A intake is established at 3000 micrograms of preformed vitamin A (3000 RAE or 10,000 IU) per day for adult men and women. This is based on the increases in birth defects and liver toxicity that accompany intakes in excess of 3000 micrograms of vitamin A per day. Above the Upper Level, other possible side effects include an increased risk of hip fracture and poor pregnancy outcomes.

During the early months of pregnancy, a high intake of preformed vitamin A is especially dangerous because it may cause **fetal** malformations and spontaneous abortions. This is because vitamin A binds to DNA and so influences cell development. FDA recommends that women of childbearing age limit their overall intake of preformed vitamin A to a total of about 100% of the Daily Value (1000 micrograms RAE or 5000 IU). Therefore, it is important to limit consumption of rich food sources, such as liver. These precautions also apply to women who may possibly become pregnant. Vitamin A is stored in the body for long periods, so women who take large amounts during the months before pregnancy place their fetuses at risk.

The consumption of large amounts of vitamin A–yielding carotenoids does not cause toxic effects. A high carotenoid concentration in the blood can occur if someone consumes large amounts of carrots or takes pills containing beta-carotene (more than 30 milligrams daily) or if infants eat a great deal of squash. This can turn the skin yellow-orange. The palms of the hands and soles of the feet in particular become colored. This condition does not appear to cause harm and disappears when carotenoid intake decreases. Dietary carotenoids do not produce toxic effects because (1) their rate of conversion into vitamin A is relatively slow and regulated, and (2) the efficiency of carotenoid absorption from the small intestine decreases markedly as oral intake increases.

8.4 Vitamin D

Vitamin D is not just a vitamin. It is primarily considered a hormone. A cholesterol-like substance in the skin cells is converted to the prohormone vitamin D when exposed to ultraviolet B (UVB) rays from sunlight or tanning beds (Fig. 8-5). Liver and kidney cells then convert the prohormone to its active hormone form. The skin,

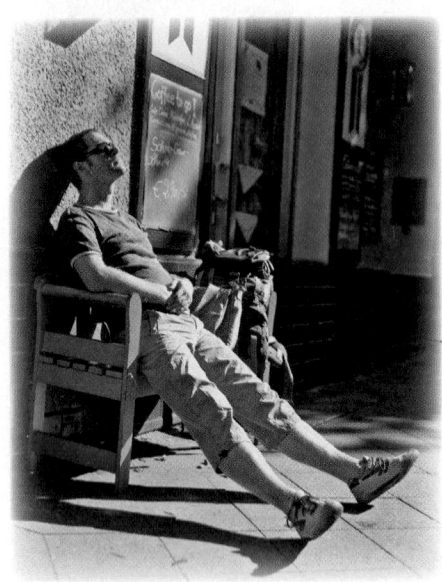

▲ Solar radiation on the skin provides about 80% to 100% of the vitamin D humans use. This is also the most reliable way to maintain vitamin D status. Dietary vitamin D is also effective, but less so.

8-4

liver, and kidney cells that participate in vitamin D synthesis are different from the bone and intestinal cells that are responsive to vitamin D. Having a site of synthesis different from the location of action is characteristic of hormones.

For many individuals, UVB exposure provides about 80% to 100% of our vitamin D needs. The amount of sun exposure needed by individuals to produce vitamin D depends on their skin color, age, time of day, season, and location. Experts recommend that people should expose their hands, face, and arms at least two to three times a week for 25% of the time it takes to turn one's skin pink (e.g., 5 to 10 minutes) to make enough vitamin D. Persons with dark skin would need additional exposure, about three to five times the amount just recommended (or maybe even more). The large amount of melanin pigment in dark-skinned people is a potent natural sunscreen.

Sun exposure is only effective for vitamin D synthesis between about 8:00 A.M. and 4:00 P.M. and without sunscreen over SPF 8. Although excessive exposure to the sun can increase the risk of skin cancer, the minimal amount of UVB exposure needed for vitamin D synthesis is encouraged. Still, this practice is not effective at all when there is little skin exposed to sun in the winter in northern climates. Although some people may have enough vitamin D stored in their adipose cells from summer months, most people in northern climates should find alternate vitamin D sources in the winter months. Overall, anyone who does not receive enough sunshine to synthesize an adequate amount of vitamin D must have a dietary source of the vitamin. About 80% of dietary vitamin D is absorbed.

Functions of Vitamin D

The main function of the vitamin D hormone (1,25-dihydroxyvitamin D) is to help regulate calcium and bone metabolism. Working with other hormones, especially **parathyroid hormone (PTH)**, the vitamin D hormone closely regulates blood calcium so that appropriate amounts of it will be supplied to all cells. This regulation involves two main processes: the vitamin D hormone helps regulate absorption of calcium and phosphorus from the intestine and the deposition of calcium in the bones.

More interestingly, the vitamin D hormone is also capable of ensuring normal development of some cells, such as skin, colon, prostate, ovary, and breast cells, in turn reducing cancer risk in these sites (see Further Readings 4 and 7). The vitamin D hormone controls the growth of the parathyroid gland; aids in the function of the immune system; and contributes to skin cell development, muscle and gum health, and blood pressure regulation.

The most obvious result of the vitamin D hormone action is increased calcium and phosphorus deposition in bones. Without adequate calcium and phosphorus deposition during bone synthesis, bones weaken and bow under pressure. A child with these symptoms has the disease **rickets.** Symptoms also include enlarged head, joints, and rib cage and a deformed pelvis (Fig. 8-6) (see Further Readings 6, 7, and 11).

Studies have shown rickets to be a problem in breastfed infants who receive little sun exposure. For the prevention of rickets, breastfed infants should be provided supplemental vitamin D (under a physician's guidance). Keep in mind that supplements need to be used very carefully to avoid vitamin D toxicity in the infant. Rickets in children is also associated with fat malabsorption, such as that occurring in children with cystic fibrosis.

Osteomalacia, which means *soft bones,* is an adult disease comparable to rickets. It results from inefficient calcium absorption in the intestine or poor conservation of calcium by the kidneys. Both of these calcium-related problems can be caused by vitamin D deficiency. Bones then lose their minerals and become porous and weak and break easily. This leads to fractures in the hip and other bones. The risk of vitamin D deficiency increases in older adults. Adults with limited sun exposure may also develop the disease as may many African-American individuals. Combinations of sun exposure, vitamin D intake, or both can prevent this problem. Older people are advised to get sun exposure during early morning and late afternoon to receive the benefit of vitamin D synthesis without also increasing skin cancer risk. Aging decreases production of vitamin D in the skin by about 70% by the time one reaches the age of 70. One study showed that treatment with 10 to 20 micrograms per day

FIGURE 8-5 ▶ The synthesis of vitamin D can take place in the body.

parathyroid hormone (PTH) A hormone made by the parathyroid glands that increases synthesis of the vitamin D hormone and aids calcium release from bone and calcium conservation by the kidneys, among other functions.

rickets A disease characterized by poor mineralization of newly synthesized bones because of low calcium content. This deficiency disease arises in infants and children from insufficient amounts of the vitamin D hormone in the body.

osteomalacia Adult form of rickets. The weakening of the bones seen in this disease is caused by low calcium content. A reduction in the amount of the vitamin D hormone in the body is one cause.

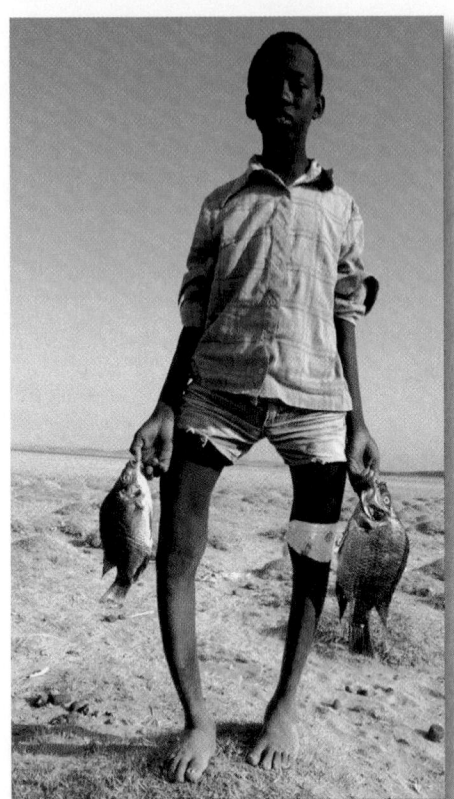

FIGURE 8-6 ▶ Vitamin D deficiency causes rickets, in which the bones and teeth do not develop normally.

Be careful not to confuse osteomalacia with osteoporosis, another type of bone disorder discussed in Chapter 9.

(400 to 800 IU per day) of vitamin D (in conjunction with adequate dietary calcium) greatly decreased fracture risk in older people in nursing homes. Follow-up studies support this role of vitamin D in reducing hip fracture risk (see Further Reading 16).

MAKING DECISIONS

New Benefits and Concerns about Vitamin D

Physicians are increasing the testing of blood levels of vitamin D. The jump in vitamin D testing stems from an abundance of emerging research linking vitamin D deficiency not only with osteoporosis and osteomalacia but also with some infectious diseases, cancers, autoimmune disorders, and cardiovascular disease. A recent study found that individuals with low vitamin D levels had a 60% greater risk of cardiac events such as heart attacks and stroke, and when both a vitamin D deficiency and high blood pressure were present, the risk for a serious cardiovascular event was doubled (see Further Readings 5 and 14). These results are of concern because vitamin D deficiency is becoming more common than previously believed in the United States, especially in people living at higher latitudes where vitamin D is less available from exposure to sunlight. Statistics indicate that 36% of Americans are vitamin D deficient and 40% of infants and toddlers have tested below the optimal blood threshold for vitamin D. A normal vitamin D test result is 30 nanograms/milliliter (ng/ml) or above, whereas under 20 ng/ml is considered deficient. Children are at risk of vitamin D insufficiency as a result of too little exposure to the sun stemming from concerns about skin cancer and increasing playtime indoors.

Vitamin D Sources and Needs

Few foods contain significant amounts of vitamin D. Rich sources are fatty fish (e.g., sardines and salmon), fortified milk and yogurt, and some ready-to-eat breakfast cereals (Fig. 8-7). In the United States and Canada, milk usually is fortified with 10 micrograms (400 IU) per quart. Although eggs, butter, liver, and a few brands of margarine contain some vitamin D, large servings must be eaten to obtain an adequate amount of the vitamin from these sources.

The Food and Nutrition Board established the first RDA for vitamin D in 2010. The RDA for healthy people ages 1 to 70 is 15 micrograms (600 IU) based on a daily intake that is sufficient to maintain bone health and normal calcium metabolism and on the basis of minimal sun exposure. The Daily Value used on food and supplement labels is 10 micrograms (400 IU). As mentioned, young, light-skinned people can synthesize all the vitamin D needed from casual sun exposure. For adults age 70 and over who have limited sun exposure, the RDA is set at 20 micrograms (800 IU) and can be obtained from a combination of vitamin D-fortified foods and a multivitamin and mineral supplement. Within the 2010 Dietary Guidelines for Americans, a key recommendation is to choose foods that provide more vitamin D, which is a nutrient of concern in American diets.

Upper Level for Vitamin D

The Upper Level for vitamin D is 100 micrograms per day (4000 IU per day) for children over age 9 and adults. Too much vitamin D taken regularly can create problems, especially in some infants and young children. For adults, intakes somewhat above the Upper Level appear to be safe. The Upper Level is based on the risk of too much vitamin D causing the overabsorption of calcium, which eventually leads to calcium deposits in the kidneys and other organs. These high intakes of vitamin D would also cause the typical symptoms of high blood calcium: weakness, loss of appetite, diarrhea, vomiting, mental confusion, and increased urine output. Calcium deposits in organs cause metabolic disturbances and cell death. However, vitamin D toxicity does not result from tanning in the sun too long because the body regulates the amount made in the skin.

Food Sources of Vitamin D

Food Item and Amount	Vitamin D (micrograms) Daily Value = 15 micrograms	Vitamin D (IU)	Adult Male and Female RDA = 15 micrograms %RDA
RDA	15	600	100%
Baked Salmon, 3 ounces	11.0	438	73%
Sardines, 1 ounce	3.4	136	23%
Canned tuna, 3 ounces	3.4	136	23%
1% milk, 1 cup	2.5	99	17%
Nonfat milk, 1 cup	2.5	98	17%
Soft margarine, 1 teaspoon	1.5	60	10%
Italian pork sausage, 3 ounces	1.1	44	7%
Soy milk, 1 cup	1.0	40	7%
Raisin Bran cereal, ¾ cup	1.0	38	7%
Baked bluefish, 3 ounces	0.9	34	6%
Special K cereal, ¾ cup	0.8	30	5%
Cooked egg yolk, 1	0.6	25	4%

Key:
- Grains
- Vegetables
- Fruits
- Dairy
- Protein
- Oils

ChooseMyPlate.gov

FIGURE 8-7 ▶ Food sources of vitamin D compared to the Adequate Intake for adults.

CONCEPT CHECK

Vitamin A is found in foods as preformed vitamin A and as provitamin A carotenoids. The most fully understood function of vitamin A is its importance in vision. Blindness caused by vitamin A deficiency is a major problem in many parts of the world. Vitamin A is also needed to maintain the health of many types of cells, support the immune system, and promote proper growth and development. Vitamin A and some carotenoids may be important in preventing cancer. However, because taking supplements of preformed vitamin A can be toxic, especially in pregnancy, the best recommendation is to focus primarily on eating plenty of provitamin A–rich foods, such as fruits and vegetables.

Vitamin D is a true vitamin only for people who fail to produce enough from sunlight, such as some older people and those with dark skin. Humans synthesize vitamin D from a cholesterol-like substance by the action of sunlight on their skin. The vitamin D is later acted on by the liver and kidneys to form the hormone 1,25-dihydroxyvitamin D. This hormone increases calcium absorption in the intestine and works with another hormone (parathyroid hormone) to maintain calcium in bones. Statistics indicating that 36% of Americans are vitamin D deficient have led to an increase in the recommended vitamin D intake and the first RDA for vitamin D. Rich food sources of vitamin D are fish oils and fortified milk. Megadose vitamin D intake can be toxic, especially in infancy and early childhood.

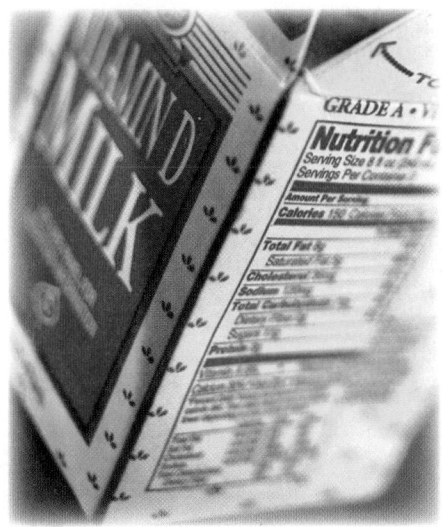

▲ Milk is usually fortified with vitamin D as well as vitamin A.

8.5 Vitamin E

In the past North Americans have spent more than $1 billion on vitamin E supplements each year. Sales of vitamin E supplements have declined in recent years, however, after studies raised concerns about higher deaths in those taking more than 800 IU of vitamin E per day. The following section attempts to sort out fact from fiction in the debate over this high-profile vitamin.

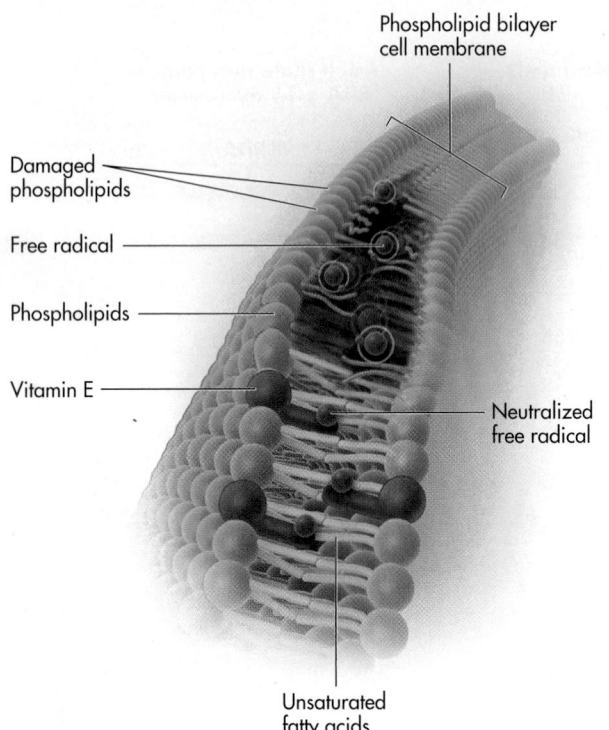

Phospholipid bilayer
cell membrane

Damaged
phospholipids

Free radical

Phospholipids

Vitamin E

Neutralized
free radical

Unsaturated
fatty acids

FIGURE 8-8 ▶ Fat-soluble vitamin E can
donate an electron to stop free radical reactions. If not interrupted, these reactions cause
extensive oxidative damage to cell membranes.

hemolysis Destruction of red blood cells.
The red blood cell membrane breaks down,
allowing cell contents to leak into the fluid
portion of the blood.

Functions of Vitamin E

Acting as a fat-soluble antioxidant, vitamin E resides mostly in cell membranes. As discussed in Chapter 5, an antioxidant can form a barrier between a target molecule—an unsaturated fatty acid in a cell membrane, for example—and a compound seeking its electrons (Fig. 8-8). The antioxidant donates electrons or hydrogens to the electron-seeking compound. This protects other molecules or parts of a cell from having electrons stolen (such as from double bonds of unsaturated fatty acids).

Free radicals are highly reactive compounds containing an unpaired electron. Production of free-radicals is a normal result of cell metabolism and immune system function. For example, white blood cells generate free radicals as part of their action to stop infection. Some exposure to free radicals, then, is an important part of life. If vitamin E is not available to do its job, the electron-seeking free radicals can pull electrons from cell membranes, DNA, and other electron-dense cell components. This either alters the cell's DNA, which may increase the risk for cancer, or injures cell membranes, possibly causing the cell to die. Overall, the body needs antioxidants like vitamin E to carefully regulate exposure to free radicals and thereby prevent cellular damage.

Cells do not rely exclusively on vitamin E for protection from free radicals. Many other antioxidant systems exist in cells, some of which use minerals, such as copper, selenium, and manganese (see Chapter 9 for details). As discussed earlier in this chapter, carotenoids in fruits and vegetables also act as antioxidants. In addition, cells have mechanisms other than antioxidants to repair molecules (such as DNA) that have been damaged by free radicals.

Thus, vitamin E is just one component of the antioxidant system. There is evidence that vitamin E helps prevent or delay heart diseases and certain cancers. Consuming vitamin E as a dietary supplement, however, may not be the most effective way to produce these effects. Two large recent studies have shown no benefit from vitamin E supplements on the prevention of certain diseases in males (see Further Readings 8 and 12). In the Physician's Health Study II, neither vitamin E nor C had an effect on major cardiovascular events including heart attacks, stroke, or death. The major prostate cancer SELECT trial also found no benefit of vitamin E or selenium supplements on prostate cancer. These results suggest that pulling a nutrient out of the whole diet, may not produce the same effects. Furthermore, there is far stronger evidence to support the benefits of lifestyle changes such as improving diet (especially fruit, vegetable, and whole-grain bread and cereal intake), performing regular physical activity, not smoking, and maintaining a healthy body weight than there is for the postulated benefits of supplemental antioxidants, including vitamin E. Thus, as reviewed in Chapter 5, even if antioxidant supplements are eventually determined to be effective in preventing cardiovascular disease or cancer, they should be used only as an adjunct—not as an alternative—to a healthful lifestyle. In fact, the American Heart Association and a group of leading cardiologists stated that it is premature to recommend vitamin E supplements to the general population, based on current knowledge and the failure of major clinical trials to show any benefit (review Chapter 5). This conclusion is in agreement with the latest report on vitamin E by the Food and Nutrition Board of the National Academy of Sciences. In addition, FDA has denied the request of the supplement industry to make a health claim that vitamin E supplements reduce the risk of cardiovascular disease and cancer. Still, some experts recommend vitamin E supplements (50 IU to 400 IU per day), while at the same time noting that evidence supporting this recommendation is sketchy.

A deficiency of vitamin E causes cell membranes to break down. The double bonds in the unsaturated fatty acids in cell membranes are sensitive to attack by oxidizing compounds. Vitamin E neutralizes these compounds, so it protects cell membranes from damage. When oxidative damage causes the cell membranes of red blood cells to break down, it is called **hemolysis.**

3000 micro

Vitamin E Sources and Needs

Vitamin E is a family of four **tocopherols**, called alpha, beta, gamma, and delta. Alpha-tocopherol is the main form in the human body, whereas gamma-tocopherol is the main form in foods. Major sources of vitamin E include plant oils, the main components of products such as salad dressings and mayonnaise, ready-to-eat breakfast cereals, some fruits and vegetables (e.g., asparagus, tomatoes, and green leafy vegetables), eggs, and margarine. Also, whole grains, nuts (e.g., almonds), and seeds (e.g., sunflower seeds) are good sources of vitamin E (Fig. 8-9). Plant oils are made up of mainly unsaturated fatty acids, and the vitamin E in plant oils protects these unsaturated fats from oxidation. Animal fats and fish oils, on the other hand, have practically no vitamin E (Fig. 8-10). The actual vitamin E content of a food depends on how it was harvested, processed, stored, and cooked because vitamin E is susceptible to destruction by oxygen, metals, light, and especially repeated use in deep-fat frying.

The RDA of vitamin E for adults is 15 milligrams per day of alpha-tocopherol, the most active form of vitamin E. The 15-milligram allotment is equivalent to 22 IU of a natural source and 33 IU of a synthetic source. Typically, North American adults consume about two-thirds of the RDA for vitamin E from food sources. Daily intake of nuts and seeds, ready-to-eat breakfast cereals containing vitamin E, or use of a multivitamin and mineral supplement would close this gap between needs and actual intakes. A Daily Value of 30 IU is used to express the vitamin E content on food and supplement labels.

The chemical structure of vitamin E varies depending on its source. The dl form or isomer is found in synthetic vitamin E and the d isomer is found in natural sources of vitamin E. Within the older IU system, 1 IU equals about 0.45 milligrams vitamin E,

tocopherols The chemical name for some forms of vitamin E. The alpha form is the most potent.

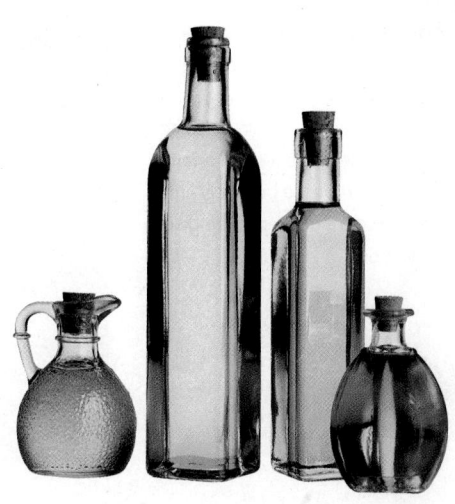

▲ Plant oils are rich sources of vitamin E.

Food Sources of Vitamin E

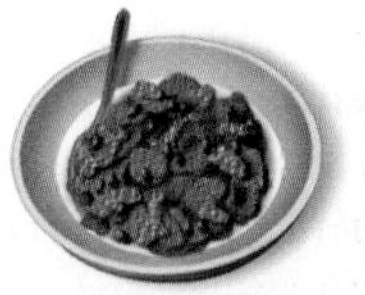

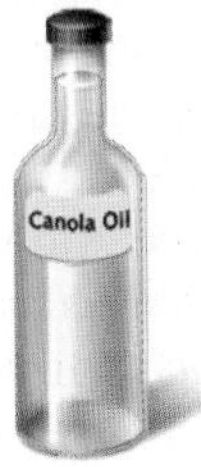

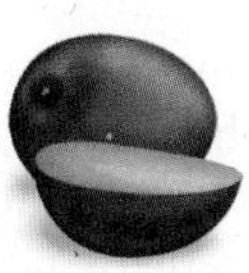

Food Item and Amount	Vitamin E (milligrams)	Vitamin E (IU)	Adult Male and Female RDA = 15 milligrams
	Daily Value = 30 IU		%RDA
RDA	15	22-33	100%
Fortified Bran cereal, ¾ cup	22.5	33.5	150%
Sunflower oil, 2 tablespoons	16.3	24.3	109%
Dry-roasted sunflower seeds, 1 ounce	14.3	21.2	95%
Dry-roasted almonds, 1 ounce	7.5	11.1	50%
Safflower oil, 1 tablespoon	5.9	8.7	39%
Canola oil, 2 tablespoons	5.7	8.5	38%
Wheat germ, ¼ cup	5.2	7.7	35%
Almonds, 1 ounce	4.5	6.8	30%
Oil-roasted sunflower seeds, 1 tablespoon	3.4	5.0	23%
Italian dressing, 2 tablespoons	3.1	4.5	21%
Mayonnaise, 1 tablespoon	3.0	4.5	20%
Avocado, 1	2.7	4.0	18%
Chunky peanut butter, 2 tablespoons	2.4	3.6	16%
Mango, 1	2.3	3.5	15%
Peanuts, 1 ounce	2.1	3.1	14%

Key:
- Grains
- Vegetables
- Fruits
- Dairy
- Protein
- Oils

ChooseMyPlate.gov

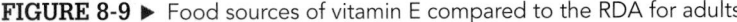

FIGURE 8-9 ▶ Food sources of vitamin E compared to the RDA for adults.

FIGURE 8-10 ▶ Sources of vitamin E from MyPlate. The fill of the background color (none, 1/3, 2/3, or completely covered) within each group on the plate indicates the average nutrient density for vitamin E in that group. Overall, plant oils are the richest source, followed by nuts and seeds in the protein group. With regard to physical activity, vitamin E has no primary role in the related energy metabolism *per se* but likely limits some oxidant damage during such endeavors.

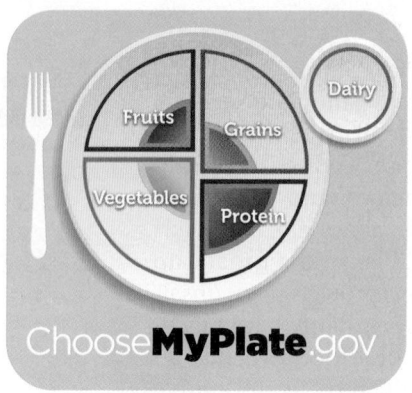

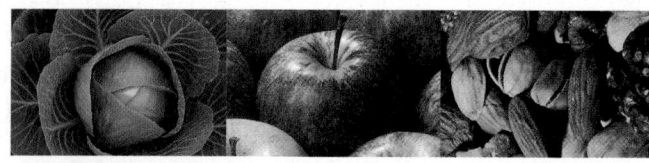

MyPlate: Sources of Vitamin E

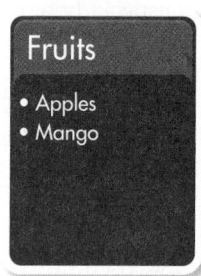
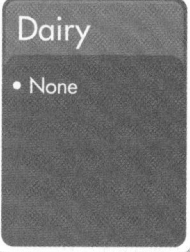
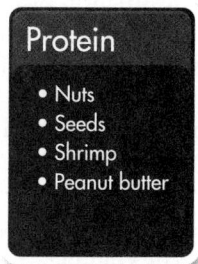

Grains
• Wheat germ (whole grains)
• Some fortified breakfast cereals

Vegetables
• Cabbage
• Asparagus
• Avocados
• Sweet potatoes
• Tomatoes

Fruits
• Apples
• Mango

Dairy
• None

Protein
• Nuts
• Seeds
• Shrimp
• Peanut butter

isomers Different chemical structures for compounds that share the same chemical formula.

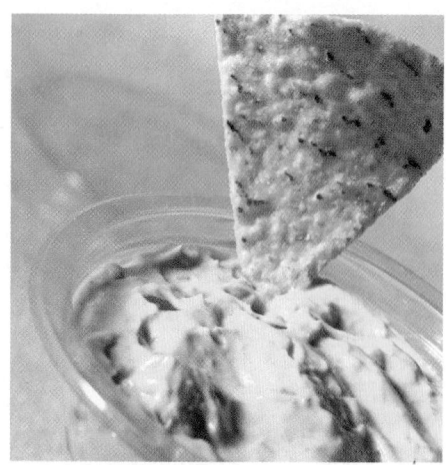

▲ The avocado in guacamole and the oil in the tortilla chip are good sources of vitamin E.

hemorrhage An escape of blood from blood vessels.

based on the synthetic form (dl **isomer**) of vitamin E found in most supplements. If vitamin E is from a natural source (d isomer), 1 IU equals 0.67 milligrams, because the natural form of vitamin E is more potent than the synthetic form.

The maximum dose the body can retain on a daily basis is thought to be 200 milligrams. This would represent 300 IU of the d isomer (200/0.67 = 300) to 450 IU of the dl isomer (200/0.45 = 450).

Cell damage by free radicals occurs over an extended period. Therefore, the beneficial effects of vitamin E and other antioxidants in counteracting this damage is most apparent when viewed over the long term. Research on a possible benefit of intakes of vitamin E in excess of the RDA for healthy adults is currently underway.

Several populations are especially susceptible to developing marginal vitamin E status. Preterm infants are born with low vitamin E stores, because this vitamin is transferred from mother to baby during late stages of pregnancy. Hemolysis (described on page 302) is of particular concern for preterm infants, due to red blood cell damage that occurs in the absence of adequate vitamin E. The rapid growth of preterm infants, coupled with the high oxygen needs of their immature lungs, greatly increases the stress on red blood cells. Special formulas and supplements designed for preterm infants can help compensate for their low vitamin E status. Smokers are another group at high risk for vitamin E deficiency, as smoking readily destroys vitamin E in the lungs. Still, one study showed that even using megadoses of vitamin E was ineffective in preventing this damage in smokers. Others at considerable risk of vitamin E deficiency include adults on very low-fat diets or those with fat malabsorption.

Upper Level for Vitamin E

The Upper Level for vitamin E for a healthy population is 1000 milligrams per day of supplemental alpha-tocopherol. The upper level has been established because excessive amounts of vitamin E can interfere with vitamin K's role in the clotting mechanism, leading to **hemorrhage.** Individuals who are vitamin K deficient or taking anticoagulants (e.g., Coumadin) or heavy doses of aspirin are especially at risk for hemorrhage from megadose vitamin E use. In international units, the Upper Level is 1500 IU for vitamin E isolated from natural sources (d isomer; 1000/0.67 = 1500) and 1100 IU for synthetic vitamin E (dl isomer; 1000/0.45/2 = 1100). The lower IU value for the synthetic form reflects the greater number of forms present in the synthetic product, only half or less of which contribute to vitamin E activity in cells, but are still absorbed. This Upper Level is set for a healthy population.

8.6 Vitamin K

A family of compounds known collectively as vitamin K is found in plants, plant oils, fish oils, and meats. While most vitamin K comes from our diet, another form is also synthesized by bacteria in the human intestine. This form supplies us with about 10% of the vitamin K we need.

Functions of Vitamin K

Vitamin K is vital for blood clotting, working along with various proteins and calcium. The *K* stems from the Danish spelling of **coagulation** because a Danish researcher first noted the relationship between vitamin K and blood clotting. Vitamin K is needed for the activation of several blood-clotting factors (Fig. 8-11). Vitamin K

coagulation Blood clotting; essentially a transition of blood from a liquid cell suspension into a solid, gel-like form.

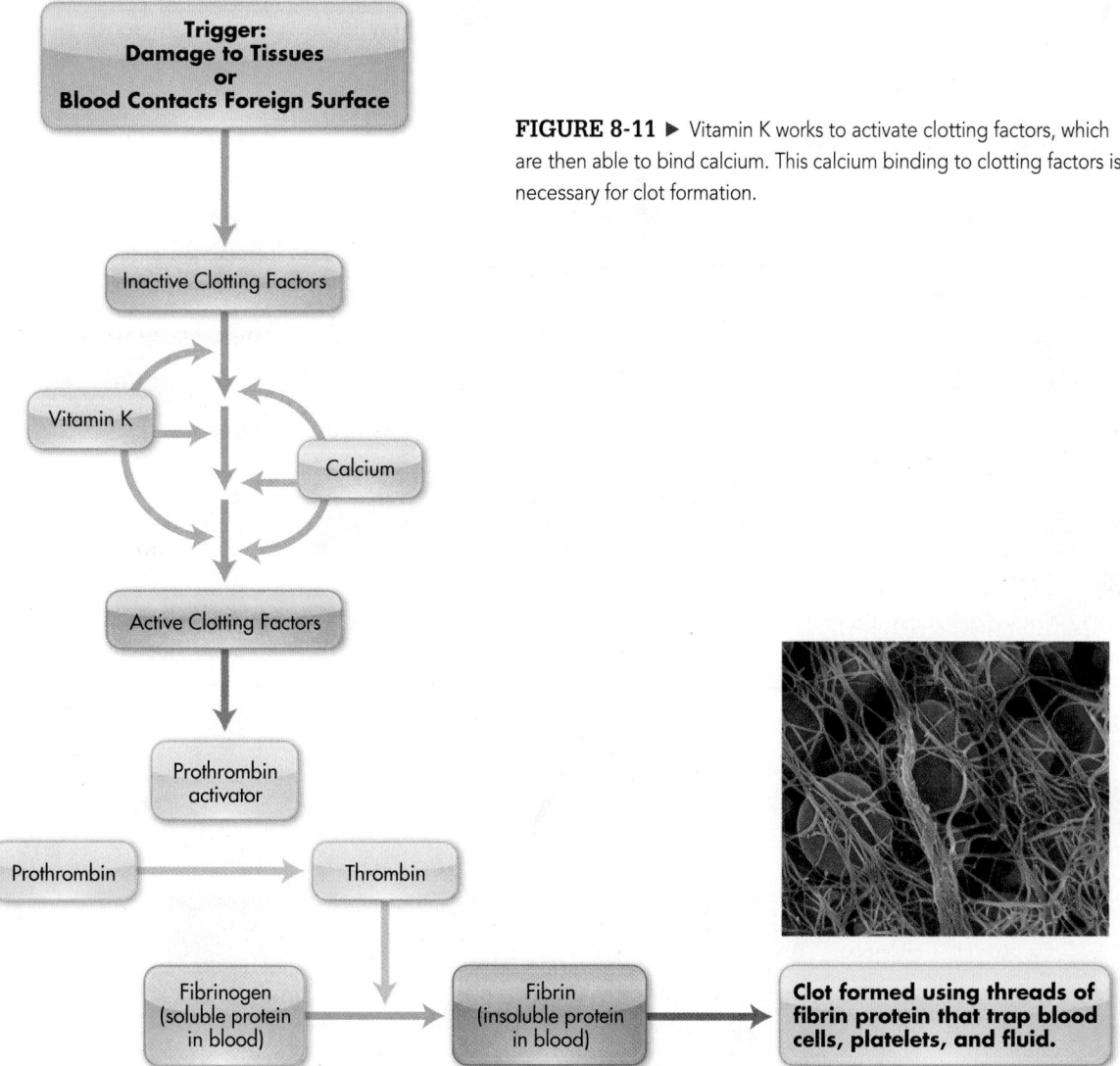

FIGURE 8-11 ▶ Vitamin K works to activate clotting factors, which are then able to bind calcium. This calcium binding to clotting factors is necessary for clot formation.

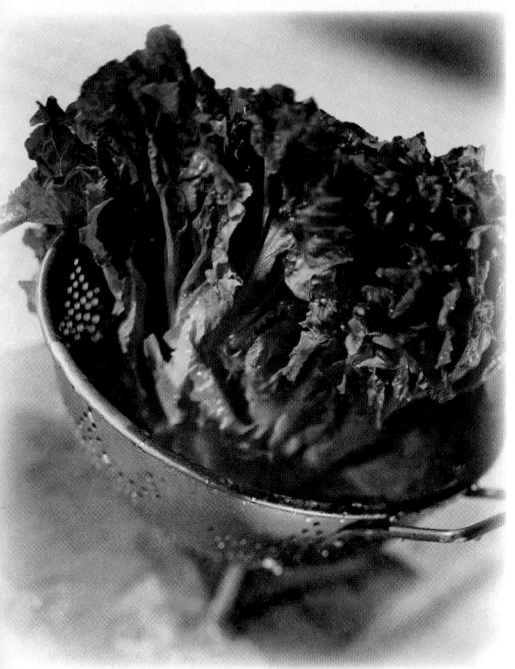

▲ A salad containing dark greens (or other green vegetables) each day provides abundant vitamin K for a diet.

also activates proteins present in bone, muscle, and kidneys, to give calcium-binding ability to these organs. A poor vitamin K intake has been linked to an increase in hip fractures because of its effect on various proteins in bone (see Further Reading 16).

At birth, a newborn's intestinal tract lacks a sufficient amount of bacteria to produce enough vitamin K to allow for effective blood clotting. Therefore, vitamin K also is routinely given by injection shortly after birth to insure blood clotting if the infant is injured or needs surgery. In adults, deficiencies of vitamin K have occurred in the presence of severe, long-standing fat malabsorption or when a person takes long-term antibiotics that destroy many of the intestinal bacteria that produce vitamin K.

Vitamin K Sources and Needs

Major food sources of vitamin K are liver, green leafy vegetables (e.g., kale, turnip greens, dark-green lettuce, and spinach), broccoli, peas, and green beans (Fig. 8-12). Other sources are soybean and canola oils and certain fortified chocolate confections (these also contain extra calcium). Thus, another reason to consume a diet rich in green vegetables is to obtain sufficient vitamin K. Most vitamin K consumed in a day disappears from the body by the next day. Nevertheless, vitamin K is abundant in a balanced diet, and a deficiency is uncommon. Vitamin K is resistant to cooking losses.

The Adequate Intake for vitamin K is 90 and 120 micrograms per day for adult women and men, respectively. Most North Americans consume at least this much. A Daily Value of 80 micrograms is used to express vitamin K content on food and supplement labels. Older adults may be at risk of a deficiency because of low consumption of green vegetables.

Food Sources of Vitamin K

Food Item and Amount	Vitamin K (micrograms)	Adult Male AI = 120 micrograms %AI	Adult Female AI = 90 micrograms %AI
RDA	90-120	100%	100%
Cooked kale, ½ cup	530	442%	589%
Cooked turnip greens, 1 cup	520	433%	578%
Cooked spinach, 1 cup	480	400%	533%
Cooked Brussel sprouts, ½ cup	150	125%	167%
Raw spinach, 1 cup	144	120%	160%
Cooked asparagus, 1 cup	144	120%	160%
Cooked broccoli, ½ cup	110	92%	122%
Looseleaf lettuce, 1 cup	97	81%	108%
Cooked green beans, ½ cup	49	41%	54%
Raw cabbage, 1 cup	42	35%	47%
Sauerkraut, ½ cup	30	25%	33%
Green peas, ½ cup	26	22%	29%
Soybean oil, 1 tablespoon	25	21%	28%
Cooked cauliflower, 1 cup	20	17%	22%
Canola oil, 1 tablespoon	17	14%	19%

Daily Value = 80 micrograms

Key:
■ Grains
■ Vegetables
■ Fruits
□ Dairy
■ Protein
□ Oils

ChooseMyPlate.gov

FIGURE 8-12 ▶ Food sources of vitamin K compared to the Adequate Intake for adult males and females.

Oral vitamin K generally poses no risk of toxicity, so no Upper Level has been set. The main problem with megadose use is reduced effectiveness of oral medications used to reduce blood clotting (e.g., Coumadin). These medications are used to lessen blood clotting especially in those who have undergone recent cardiovascular surgery.

Table 8-2 reviews what we have covered so far regarding the fat-soluble vitamins.

TABLE 8-2 Summary of the Fat-Soluble Vitamins

Vitamin	Major Functions	RDA or Adequate Intake	Dietary Sources	Deficiency Symptoms	Toxicity Symptoms
Vitamin A (preformed vitamin A and provitamin A)	• Promote vision: night and color • Promote growth • Prevent drying of skin and eyes • Promote resistance to bacterial infection and overall immune system function	Females: 700 micrograms RAE Males: 900 micrograms RAE 2300–3000 IU if as preformed (vitamin A)	Preformed Vitamin A: • Liver • Fortified milk • Fortified breakfast cereals Provitamin A: • Sweet potatoes • Spinach • Greens • Carrots • Cantaloupe • Apricots • Broccoli	• Night blindness • Xerophthalmia • Poor growth • Dry skin	• Fetal malformations • Hair loss • Skin changes • Bone pain • Fractures Upper Level is 3000 micrograms of preformed vitamin A (10,000 IU) based on the risk of birth defects and liver toxicity
Vitamin D	• Increase absorption of calcium and phosphorus • Maintain optimal blood calcium and calcification of bone	15 micrograms (600 IU)	• Vitamin D fortified milk • Fortified breakfast cereals • Fish oils • Sardines • Salmon	• Rickets in children • Osteomalacia in adults	• Growth retardation • Kidney damage • Calcium deposits in soft tissue Upper Level is 100 micrograms (4000 IU) based on the risk of elevated blood calcium
Vitamin E	• Antioxidant prevents breakdown of vitamin A and unsaturated fatty acids	15 milligrams alpha-tocopherol 22 IU natural form, 33 IU (synthetic form)	• Plant oils • Products made from plant oils • Some greens • Some fruits • Nuts and seeds • Fortified breakfast cereals	• Hemolysis of red blood cells • Nerve degeneration	• Muscle weakness • Headaches • Nausea • Inhibition of vitamin K metabolism Upper Level is 1000 milligrams (1100 IU synthetic form, 1500 IU natural form) based on the risk of hemorrhage
Vitamin K	• Activation of blood-clotting factors • Activation of proteins involved in bone metabolism	Females: 90 micrograms Males: 120 micrograms	• Green vegetables • Liver • Some plant oils • Some calcium supplements	• Hemorrhage • Fractures	No Upper Level has been set

Abbreviations: RAE = retinol activity equivalents; IU = international units

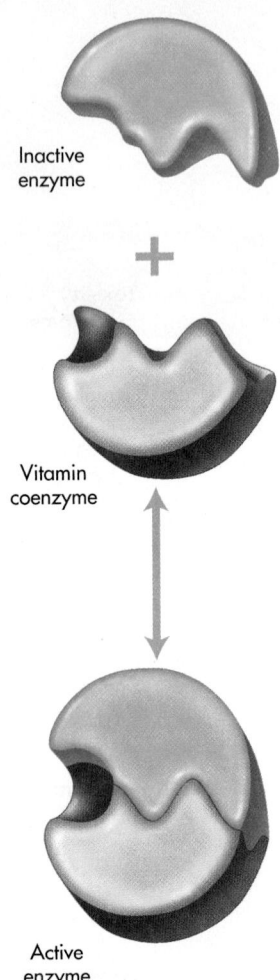

Inactive
enzyme

+

Vitamin
coenzyme

Active
enzyme

FIGURE 8-13 ▶ Coenzymes, such as those formed from B vitamins, aid in the function of various enzymes. Without the coenzyme, the enzyme cannot function, and deficiency symptoms associated with the missing vitamin eventually appear. Health-food stores sell the coenzyme forms of some vitamins. These more expensive forms of vitamins are unnecessary. The body makes all the coenzymes it needs from vitamin precursors.

bioavailability The degree to which an ingested nutrient is absorbed and thus is available to the body.

CONCEPT CHECK

Vitamin E functions primarily as an antioxidant. It can donate electrons to electron-seeking free radical (oxidizing) compounds. By neutralizing these compounds, vitamin E helps prevent cell destruction, especially the destruction of red blood cell membranes. Vitamin E occurs in a wide variety of foods, but its richest sources are plant oils, foods rich in these oils, and nuts. Studies using dietary supplements of vitamin E have not shown beneficial effects on the risk of diseases including heart disease and cancer.

Vitamin K plays a key role in efficient blood clotting; it contributes to the activation of certain blood-clotting proteins. In addition, vitamin K contributes to the synthesis of the calcium-binding proteins in some organs, such as bones. About 10% of the vitamin K we absorb every day is synthesized by our intestinal bacteria; the rest comes from our diets. The amount in the diet alone generally meets our daily needs. Thus, except for newborns and possibly older adults, a deficiency of vitamin K is unlikely.

8.7 The Water-Soluble Vitamins and Choline

Regular consumption of good sources of the water-soluble vitamins is important. Most water-soluble vitamins are readily excreted from the body with any excess generally ending up in the urine or stool and very little being stored. They dissolve in water, so large amounts of these vitamins can be lost during food processing and preparation. Vitamin content is best preserved by light cooking methods, such as stir-frying, steaming, and microwaving (review Table 8-1).

The B vitamins are thiamin, riboflavin, niacin, pantothenic acid, biotin, vitamin B-6, folate, and vitamin B-12. Choline is a related nutrient, but currently is not classified as a vitamin. Vitamin C is also a water-soluble vitamin.

The B vitamins often occur together in the same foods, so a lack of one B vitamin may mean other B vitamins are also low in a diet. The B vitamins function as coenzymes, small molecules that interact with enzymes to enable the enzymes to function. In essence, the coenzymes contribute to enzyme activity (Fig. 8-13).

As coenzymes, the B vitamins play many key roles in metabolism. The metabolic pathways used by carbohydrates, fats, and amino acids all require input from B vitamins. Because of their role in energy metabolism, needs for many B vitamins increase somewhat as energy expenditure increases. Still, this is not a major concern because this increase in energy expenditure usually results in a corresponding increase in food intake, which contributes more B vitamins to a diet. Many B vitamins are interdependent because they participate in the same processes (Fig. 8-14). B vitamin deficiency symptoms typically occur in the brain and nervous system, skin, and GI tract. Cells in these tissues are metabolically active, and those in the skin and GI tract are also constantly being replaced.

After being ingested, the B vitamins are first broken down from their active coenzyme forms into free vitamins in the stomach and small intestine. The vitamins are then absorbed, primarily in the small intestine. Typically, about 50% to 90% of the B vitamins in the diet are absorbed, which means they have relatively high **bioavailability**. Once inside cells, the active coenzyme forms are resynthesized. There is no need to consume the coenzyme forms themselves. Some vitamins are sold in their coenzyme forms but these are broken down during digestion and we activate them when needed.

B Vitamin Intakes of North Americans

The nutritional health of most North Americans with regard to the B vitamins is generally good. Typical diets contain a good amount and variety of natural sources of

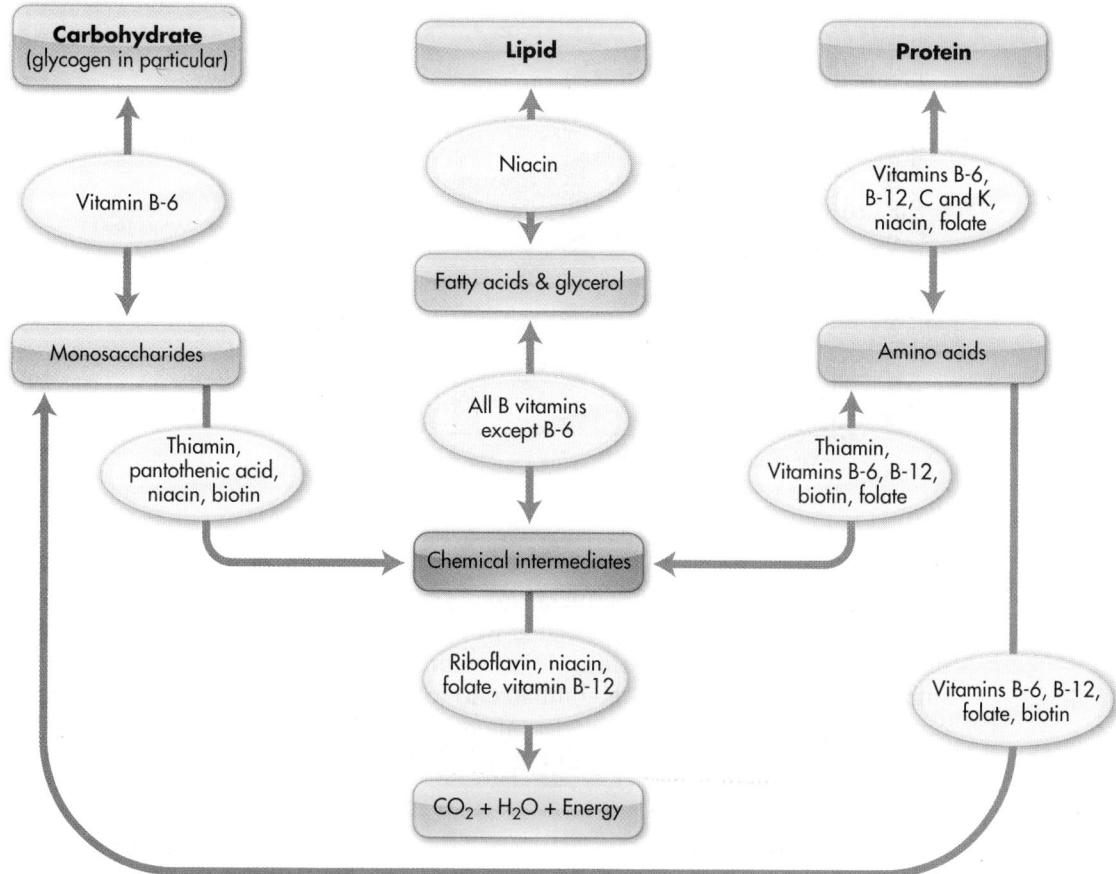

FIGURE 8-14 ▶ Examples of metabolic pathways for which water soluble vitamins are essential. The metabolism of energy-yielding nutrients requires vitamin input.

these vitamins. In addition, many common foods, such as ready-to-eat breakfast cereals, are fortified with one or more of the water-soluble vitamins. In some developing countries, however, deficiencies of the water-soluble vitamins are more common, and the resulting deficiency diseases pose significant public health problems. (A detailed discussion of nutritional deficiencies worldwide is presented in Chapter 12.)

Despite the generally good B vitamin status of North Americans, marginal deficiencies of the water-soluble vitamins may occur in some cases, especially in older people who eat little food and in people who follow poor dietary patterns. The long-term effects of such marginal deficiencies are unknown, but increased risk of cardiovascular disease, cancer, and cataracts of the eye is suspected. However, in the short run, such a marginal deficiency in most people likely leads only to fatigue or other bothersome and unspecific physical effects. With rare exceptions, healthy adults do not develop the more serious B vitamin deficiency diseases from dietary inadequacies alone. The main exceptions are people with alcoholism. The combination of extremely unbalanced diets and alcohol-induced alterations of vitamin absorption and metabolism creates significant risks for serious nutrient deficiencies among people with alcoholism (see Chapter 16).

Grains: One Important Source of B Vitamins The milling of grains leads to losses of vitamins and minerals. In the milling process, seeds are crushed and the germ, bran, and husk layers are discarded, leaving just the starch-containing endosperm in the refined grains. The starch is used to make flour, bread, and cereal products. Unfortunately, many nutrients are lost along with the discarded germ, bran, and husk materials. To counteract these losses, in the United States, bread and cereal products made from milled grains are enriched with four B vitamins (thiamin, riboflavin, niacin,

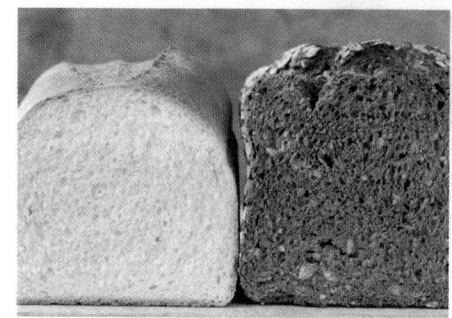

▲ The white bread on the left is made from refined flour that has been enriched with four B vitamins and iron to achieve the nutrient level in the whole-grain bread on the right.

FIGURE 8-15 ▶ Compare the relative nutrient contents of refined versus whole grains. Nutrients are expressed as a percentage of the nutrient contribution of the whole grain product.

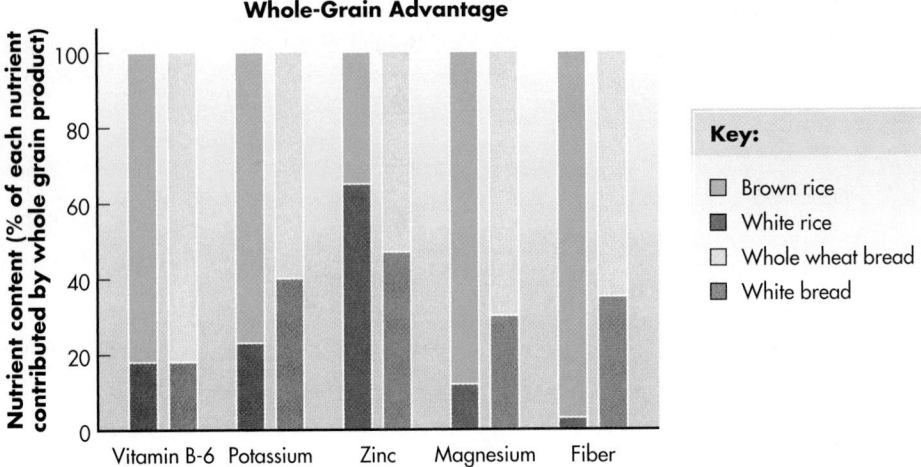

Whole-Grain Advantage

Key:
- Brown rice
- White rice
- Whole wheat bread
- White bread

Nutrient content (% of each nutrient contributed by whole grain product)

Vitamin B-6   Potassium   Zinc   Magnesium   Fiber

and folic acid) and with the mineral iron. This addition helps protect us from the common deficiency diseases associated with a dietary lack of these nutrients. Unfortunately, these products remain lower in vitamin E, vitamin B-6, potassium, magnesium, fiber, and other nutrients compared to whole-grain products (Fig. 8-15). This is one reason why nutrient experts advocate regular consumption of whole-grain products, such as whole-wheat bread and brown rice, rather than refined grain products.

8.8 Thiamin

beriberi The thiamin deficiency disorder characterized by muscle weakness, loss of appetite, nerve degeneration, and sometimes edema.

Thiamin (formerly called *vitamin B-1*) is used, among other purposes, to help release energy from carbohydrate. Its coenzyme form participates in reactions in which a carbon dioxide (CO_2) is lost from a larger molecule. This reaction is particularly important in the breakdown of carbohydrates and certain amino acids for energy needs (review Fig. 8-14).

The thiamin deficiency disease is called **beriberi,** a word that means "I can't, I can't" in the Sri Lanka language of Sinhalese. The symptoms include weakness, loss of appetite, irritability, nervous tingling throughout the body, poor arm and leg coordination, and deep muscle pain in the calves. A person with beriberi often develops an enlarged heart and sometimes severe edema.

Beriberi results when glucose, the primary fuel for brain and nerve cells, cannot be metabolized to release energy. The thiamin coenzyme participates in glucose metabolism, so problems with body functions associated with brain and nerve action are the first signs of a thiamin deficiency, some after only 10 days on a thiamin-free diet.

Beriberi is seen in areas where rice is a staple and polished (white) rice is consumed rather than brown (whole-grain) rice. In most parts of the world, brown rice has had its bran and germ layer removed to make white rice, a poor source of thiamin, unless it is enriched.

Thiamin Sources and Needs

Major sources of thiamin include pork products, whole grains (wheat germ), ready-to-eat breakfast cereals, enriched grains, green beans, milk, orange juice, organ meats, peanuts, dried beans, and seeds (Figs. 8-16 and 8-17).

The adult RDA for thiamin is 1.1 to 1.2 milligrams per day. The Daily Value of 1.5 milligrams is used to express the thiamin content on food and supplement labels. Average daily intakes for men exceed this by 50% or more, and women generally meet the RDA. Some groups, such as low-income and older people, may barely meet

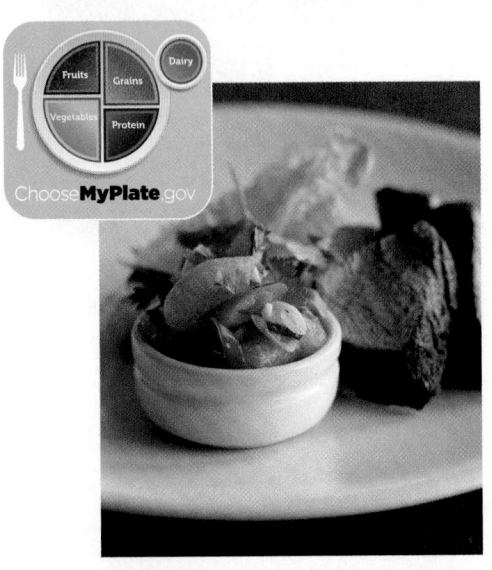

▲ The roasted pork filet and mandarin orange and chili pepper salad are good sources of thiamin from the protein, fruit, and vegetable sections of MyPlate. Which sections are missing?

Food Sources of Thiamin

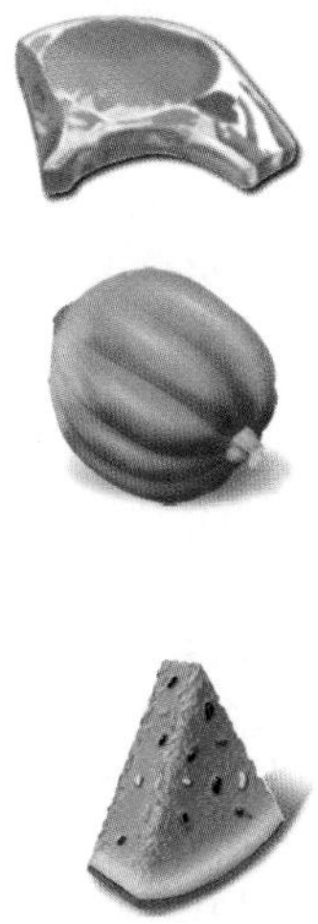

Food Item and Amount	Thiamin (milligrams)	Adult Male RDA = 1.2 milligrams %RDA	Adult Female RDA = 1.1 milligrams %RDA
RDA	1.1-1.2	100%	100%
Canned lean ham, 3 ounces	0.9	75%	82%
Pork chops, 4 ounces	0.6	50%	55%
Wheat germ, ¼ cup	0.5	42%	45%
Canadian bacon, 2 ounces	0.5	42%	45%
Acorn squash, 1 cup	0.4	33%	36%
Soy milk, 1 cup	0.4	33%	36%
Flour tortilla, 1	0.4	33%	36%
Ham lunch meat, 2 pieces	0.3	25%	27%
Watermelon, 1 slice	0.2	17%	18%
Fresh orange juice, 1 cup	0.2	17%	18%
Cooked green peas, ½ cup	0.2	17%	18%
Baked beans, ½ cup	0.2	17%	18%
Navy beans, ½ cup	0.2	17%	18%
Corn, ½ cup	0.2	17%	18%

Daily Value = 1.5 mg

Key:
- Grains
- Vegetables
- Fruits
- Dairy
- Protein

FIGURE 8-16 ▶ Food sources of thiamin compared to the RDA for adult males and females.

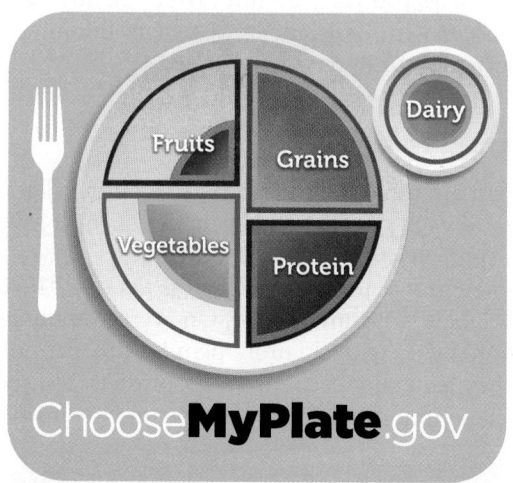

MyPlate: Sources of Thiamin, Riboflavin, and Niacin

Grains Vegetables Fruits Dairy Protein

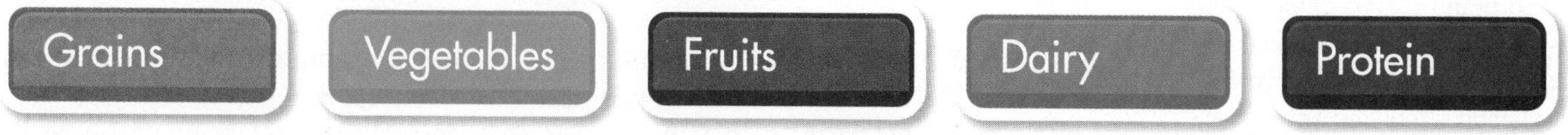

FIGURE 8-17 ▶ Sources of thiamin, riboflavin, and niacin from MyPlate. The fill of the background color (none, 1/3, 2/3, or completely covered) within each group in the plate indicates the average nutrient density for these vitamins in that group. Overall, the protein group and the grains group contain many foods that are nutrient-dense sources of thiamin, riboflavin, and niacin. As well, foods from the dairy group are especially rich sources of riboflavin.

their needs for thiamin. A diet dominated by highly processed and unenriched foods, sugar, fat, and alcohol also creates a potential for thiamin deficiency. Oral thiamin supplements are typically nontoxic because excess thiamin is rapidly lost in the urine. Thus, no Upper Level has been set for thiamin.

MAKING DECISIONS

Thiamin and Alcohol

People with alcoholism are at the greatest risk for thiamin deficiency because absorption and use of thiamin are profoundly diminished and excretion is increased by consumption of alcohol. Furthermore, the low-quality diet that often accompanies severe alcoholism makes matters worse. There is limited thiamin storage in the body, so an alcoholic binge lasting 1 to 2 weeks may quickly deplete already diminished amounts of the vitamin and result in deficiency symptoms.

8.9 Riboflavin

The name *riboflavin* comes from its yellow color (*flavus* means yellow in Latin). Riboflavin was formerly referred to as *vitamin B-2*.

The coenzyme forms of riboflavin participate in many energy-yielding metabolic pathways. When cells generate energy using oxygen-requiring pathways, such as when fatty acids are broken down and burned for energy, the coenzymes of riboflavin are used (review Fig. 8-14). Some vitamin and mineral metabolism also requires riboflavin. In addition, because of its link to the activity of certain enzymes, riboflavin has an antioxidant role in the body.

The symptoms associated with riboflavin deficiency include inflammation of the mouth and tongue, dermatitis, cracking of tissue around the corners of the mouth (called *cheilosis*), various eye disorders, sensitivity to the sun, and confusion (Fig. 8-18). Such symptoms develop after approximately 2 months on a riboflavin-poor diet. In addition, riboflavin deficiencies probably do not exist by themselves. Instead, a riboflavin deficiency would occur with deficiencies of niacin, thiamin, and vitamin B-6 because these nutrients often occur in the same foods.

Riboflavin Sources and Needs

Major sources of riboflavin are milk and milk products, enriched grains, ready-to-eat breakfast cereals, meat, and eggs (Fig. 8-19). Vegetables such as asparagus, broccoli, and various greens (e.g., spinach) are also good sources.

The adult RDA of riboflavin is 1.1 to 1.3 milligrams per day. The Daily Value used on food and supplement labels is 1.7 milligrams. On average, daily intakes of riboflavin are slightly above the RDA. As with thiamin, people with alcoholism risk riboflavin deficiency because they generally eat nutrient-poor diets. No specific symptoms indicate that riboflavin taken in megadoses is toxic, so no Upper Level has been set.

8.10 Niacin

Niacin functions in the body as one of two related compounds: nicotinic acid and nicotinamide. Niacin was formerly referred to as *vitamin B-3.*

The coenzyme forms of niacin function in many cellular metabolic pathways. In general, when energy is being released from the energy nutrients and used by cells, a niacin coenzyme is used. Synthetic pathways in the cell—those that make new compounds—also often use a niacin coenzyme. This is especially true for fatty acid synthesis (review Fig. 8-14).

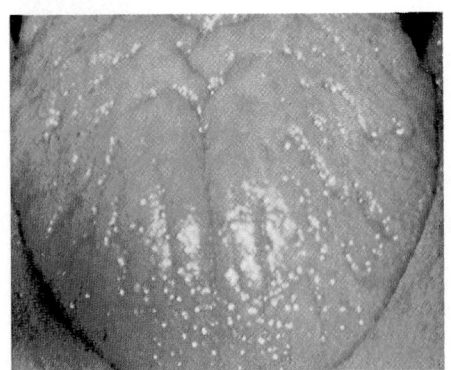
(a)

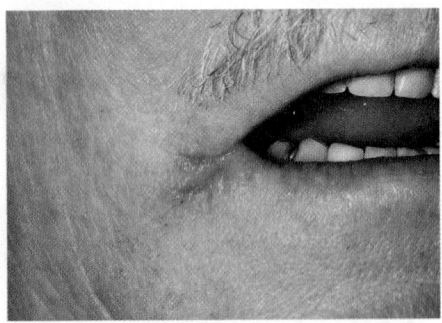
(b)

FIGURE 8-18 ▶ (a) Glossitis is a painful, inflamed tongue that can signal a deficiency of riboflavin, niacin, vitamin B-6, folate, or vitamin B-12. (b) Angular cheilitis, also called cheilosis or angular stomatitis, is another result of a riboflavin deficiency. It causes painful cracks at the corners of the mouth. Both glossitis and angular cheilitis can be caused by other medical conditions; thus, further evaluation is required before diagnosing a nutrient deficiency.

Food Sources of Riboflavin

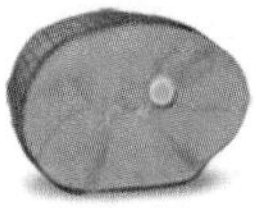

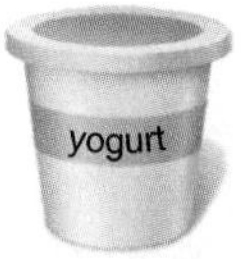

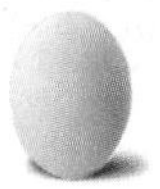

Food Item and Amount	Riboflavin (milligrams)	Adult Male RDA = 1.3 milligrams %RDA	Adult Female RDA = 1.1 milligrams %RDA
RDA	1.1-1.3	100%	100%
Multigrain oat cereal, ¾ cup	1.3	100%	110%
Fried beef liver, 1 ounce	1.2	92%	109%
Steamed oysters, 10	1.1	85%	100%
Plain yogurt, 1 cup	0.5	38%	45%
Raw mushrooms, 5	0.5	38%	45%
Braunschweiger sausage, 1	0.4	31%	36%
Cooked spinach, 1 cup	0.4	31%	36%
1% milk, 1 cup	0.4	31%	36%
Buttermilk, 1 cup	0.4	31%	36%
Boiled egg, 1	0.3	23%	27%
Sirloin steak, 3 ounces	0.3	23%	27%
Feta cheese, 1 ounce	0.2	15%	18%
Tortilla, 1	0.2	15%	18%
Lean ham, 3 ounces	0.2	15%	18%

Daily Value = 1.7 milligrams

Key: Grains, Vegetables, Fruits, Dairy, Protein — ChooseMyPlate.gov

FIGURE 8-19 ▶ Food sources of riboflavin compared to the RDA for adult males and females.

Almost every cellular metabolic pathway uses a niacin coenzyme, so a deficiency causes widespread changes in the body. The group of niacin deficiency symptoms is known as *pellagra,* which means rough or painful skin. The symptoms of the disease are **dementia,** diarrhea, and dermatitis (especially on areas of skin exposed to the sun) (Fig. 8-20). Later, death often results. Early symptoms include poor appetite, weight loss, and weakness.

Pellagra is the only dietary deficiency disease ever to reach epidemic proportions in the United States. It became a major problem in the southeastern United States in the late 1800s and persisted until the late 1930s when standards of living and diets improved. Today, pellagra is rare in Western societies, but can be seen in the developing world.

High does of niacin, beyond what is available from food, are also prescribed as a treatment to increase HDL-cholesterol (good). Niacin can raise HDL-cholesterol by 15% to 35%, making niacin the most effective drug available for raising HDL-cholesterol.

dementia A general loss or decrease in mental function.

MAKING DECISIONS

Niacin in Corn

Do you enjoy corn tortillas? Niacin in corn is bound by a protein that hampers its absorption. Soaking corn in an alkaline solution, such as lime water (water with calcium hydroxide), releases bound niacin and renders it more usable. Hispanic people in North America traditionally soak corn in lime water before making tortillas. This treatment is one reason this Hispanic population never experienced much pellagra.

FIGURE 8-20 ▶ The dermatitis of pellagra. (a) Dermatitis on both sides (bilateral) of the body is a typical symptom of pellagra. Sun exposure worsens the condition. (b) The rough skin around the neck is referred to as Casal's necklace.

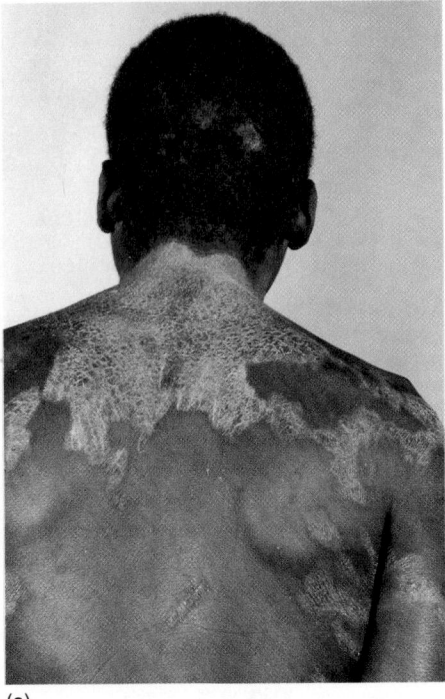 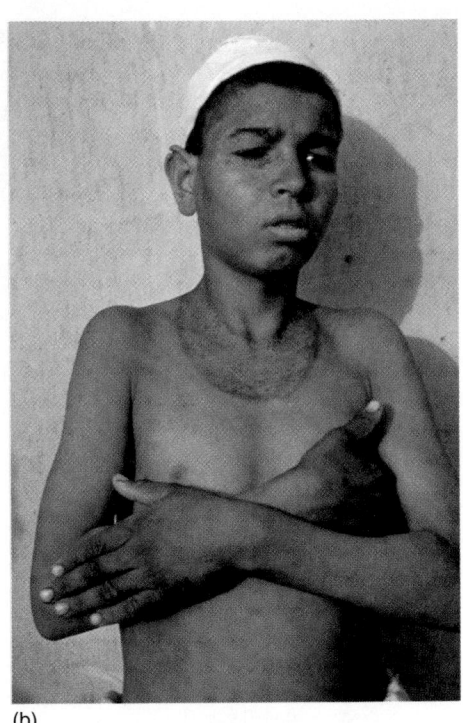

(a)   (b)

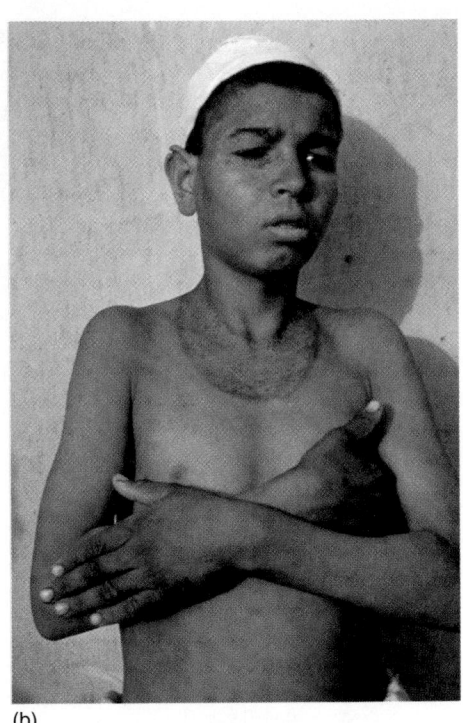

▲ Chicken is a good source of niacin. The tryptophan present can also be metabolized to niacin. How does this dish compare to ChooseMyPlate recommendations?

Niacin Sources and Needs

Major sources of niacin are poultry, ready-to-eat breakfast cereals, beef, wheat bran, tuna and other fish, asparagus, and peanuts (Fig. 8-21). Coffee and tea also contribute some niacin to the diet. Niacin is heat stable; little is lost in cooking.

Besides the preformed niacin found in protein foods, we can synthesize niacin from the amino acid tryptophan: 60 milligrams of tryptophan in a diet yield about 1 milligram of niacin. In this manner, we synthesize about 50% of the niacin we need.

The adult RDA of niacin is 14 to 16 milligrams per day. The RDA is expressed as niacin equivalents (NE) to account for niacin received intact from the diet, as well as that made from tryptophan. A Daily Value of 20 milligrams is used to express niacin content on food and supplement labels. Intakes of niacin by adults are about double the RDA, without considering the contribution from tryptophan. (Tables of food composition values also ignore this contribution.) People with alcoholism and those with rare disorders of tryptophan metabolism are generally the only groups to show a niacin deficiency.

Upper Level for Niacin

The Upper Level for niacin is 35 milligrams per day of the nicotinic acid form. Effects of high intakes include headache, itching, and increased blood flow to the skin, causing a general blood vessel dilation or flushing in various parts of the body, especially when intakes are above 100 milligrams per day. In the long run, GI tract and liver damage is possible, so any use of megadoses, including large doses recommended for treatment of cardiovascular disease, requires close physician scrutiny (review Chapter 5).

Food Sources of Niacin

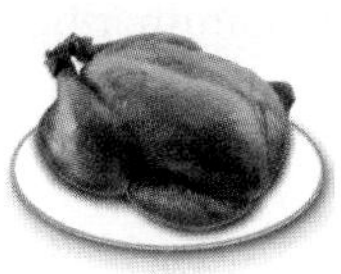

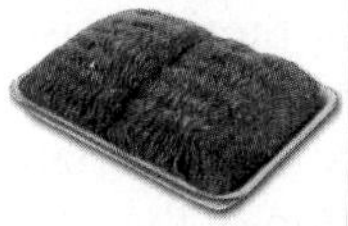

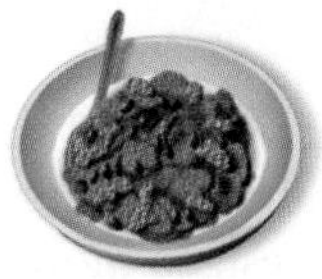

Food Item and Amount	Niacin (milligrams)	Adult Male RDA = 16 milligrams	Adult Female RDA = 14 milligrams
		Daily Value = 20 milligrams	
		%RDA	%RDA
RDA	14-16	100%	100%
Tuna, 3 ounces	11.3	71%	81%
Roasted chicken, 3 ounces	10.1	63%	72%
Peanuts, ½ cup	9.9	62%	71%
Baked salmon, 3 ounces	8.6	54%	61%
Turkey lunch meat, 3 ounces	5.4	34%	39%
Ground beef, 3 ounces	5.0	31%	36%
Raw mushrooms, 5	4.7	29%	34%
Lean steak, 4 ounces	4.5	28%	32%
Chunky peanut butter, 2 tablespoons	4.4	28%	31%
Fried beef liver, 1 ounce	4.1	26%	29%
Raisin Nut Bran cereal, ¾ cup	3.8	24%	27%
Tortilla, 1	2.6	16%	19%
Baked cod, 3 ounces	2.1	13%	15%
Potato, 1	2.1	13%	15%
Broiled halibut, 3 ounces	1.6	10%	11%

Key:
- Grains
- Vegetables
- Fruits
- Dairy
- Protein

ChooseMyPlate.gov

FIGURE 8-21 ▶ Food sources of niacin compared to the RDA for adult males and females.

CONCEPT CHECK

The B vitamins thiamin, riboflavin, and niacin are important in the metabolism of carbohydrates, proteins, and fats. Energy metabolism in particular requires adequate amounts of the coenzyme forms of these three vitamins. Deficiency symptoms typically occur in the brain and nervous system, skin, and GI tract. Cells in these tissues are metabolically active, and those in the skin and GI tract are also constantly being replaced. Enriched grains and ready-to-eat breakfast cereals are adequate sources of all three vitamins. Additionally, pork is an excellent source of thiamin, milk is an excellent source of riboflavin, and protein foods in general—such as chicken—are excellent sources of niacin. Deficiencies of all three vitamins can occur with alcoholism; a thiamin deficiency is the most likely of the three.

8.11 Pantothenic Acid

Like the other B vitamins, pantothenic acid helps release energy from carbohydrates, fats, and protein. By forming its coenzyme (coenzyme A or CoA) pantothenic acid allows many energy-yielding metabolic reactions to occur (review Fig. 8-14). This coenzyme also activates fatty acids so they can yield energy. It is also used in the beginning steps of fatty acid synthesis. Pantothenic acid is so widespread in foods that a nutritional deficiency among healthy people who eat varied diets is unlikely.

Pantothenic Acid Sources and Needs

Rich sources of pantothenic acid are sunflower seeds, mushrooms, peanuts, and eggs. Other sources are meat, milk, and many vegetables (Fig. 8-22).

The Adequate Intake set for pantothenic acid is 5 milligrams per day for adults, and we generally consume that amount or more. A Daily Value of 10 milligrams is used to express pantothenic acid content on food and supplement labels. A deficiency of pantothenic acid might occur when alcoholism is accompanied by a nutrient-deficient diet. However, the symptoms would probably be hidden among deficiencies of thiamin, riboflavin, vitamin B-6, and folate, so the pantothenic acid deficiency might be unrecognizable. No toxicity is known for pantothenic acid, therefore no Upper Level has been set.

8.12 Biotin

In its coenzyme form, biotin aids in fat and carbohydrate metabolism. Biotin assists in the addition of carbon dioxide to other compounds. By doing so, it promotes the synthesis of glucose and fatty acids, while also helping to break down certain amino acids. Symptoms of biotin deficiency include a scaly inflammation of the skin, changes in the tongue and lips, decreased appetite, nausea, vomiting, a form of anemia, depression, muscle pain and weakness, and poor growth.

Biotin Sources and Needs

Cauliflower, egg yolks, peanuts, and cheese are good sources of biotin (Fig. 8-23). Intestinal bacteria synthesize and supply some biotin, making a biotin deficiency unlikely. However, scientists are not sure how much of the bacteria-synthesized biotin

FIGURE 8-22 ▶ Food sources of pantothenic acid compared to the Adequate Intake for adults.

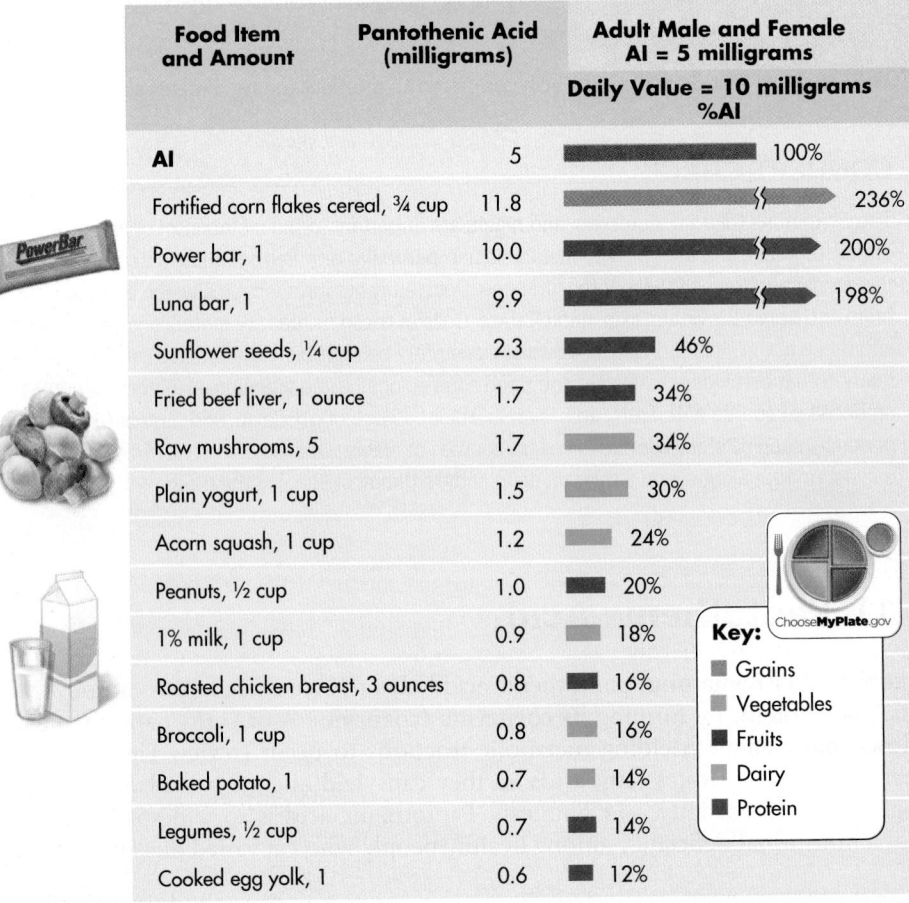

Food Sources of Pantothenic Acid

Food Item and Amount	Pantothenic Acid (milligrams)	Adult Male and Female AI = 5 milligrams / Daily Value = 10 milligrams %AI
AI	5	100%
Fortified corn flakes cereal, ¾ cup	11.8	236%
Power bar, 1	10.0	200%
Luna bar, 1	9.9	198%
Sunflower seeds, ¼ cup	2.3	46%
Fried beef liver, 1 ounce	1.7	34%
Raw mushrooms, 5	1.7	34%
Plain yogurt, 1 cup	1.5	30%
Acorn squash, 1 cup	1.2	24%
Peanuts, ½ cup	1.0	20%
1% milk, 1 cup	0.9	18%
Roasted chicken breast, 3 ounces	0.8	16%
Broccoli, 1 cup	0.8	16%
Baked potato, 1	0.7	14%
Legumes, ½ cup	0.7	14%
Cooked egg yolk, 1	0.6	12%

Key:
■ Grains
■ Vegetables
■ Fruits
■ Dairy
■ Protein

Food Sources of Biotin

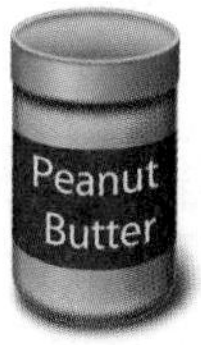

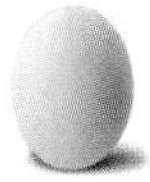

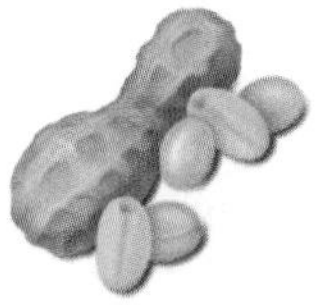

Food Item and Amount	Biotin (micrograms)	Adult Male and Female AI = 30 micrograms Daily Value = 30 micrograms %AI
AI	30.0	100%
Smooth peanut butter, 2 tablespoons	30.1	100%
Cooked lamb liver, 1 ounce	11.6	39%
Boiled egg, 1	9.3	31%
Cooked egg yolk, 1	8.1	27%
Yogurt, 1 cup	7.4	25%
Wheat germ, ¼ cup	7.2	24%
Roasted peanuts, 5	6.5	22%
Wheat bran, ¼ cup	6.4	21%
Nonfat milk, 1 cup	4.9	16%
Salmon, 3 ounces	4.3	14%
Egg noodles, 1 cup	4.0	13%
Swiss cheese, 2 ounces	2.2	7%
Cheddar cheese, 2 ounces	1.7	6%
Raw cauliflower, 1 cup	1.5	5%
American cheese, 2 ounces	1.4	5%

Key: Grains, Vegetables, Fruits, Dairy, Protein

FIGURE 8-23 ▶ Food sources of biotin compared to the Adequate Intake for adults.

in our intestines is absorbed. If intestinal bacterial synthesis is not sufficient, as in people missing a large part of the small intestine or who take antibiotics for many months, special attention should be paid to meeting biotin needs. A protein called *avidin* in raw egg whites binds biotin and inhibits its absorption. Consuming many raw egg whites eventually leads to the deficiency disease. Cooking denatures avidin in eggs such that it cannot bind biotin.

The Adequate Intake set for biotin is 30 micrograms per day for adults. Our food supply is thought to provide 40 to 60 micrograms per person per day. A Daily Value of 30 micrograms is used to express biotin content on food and supplement labels and is 10 times our current estimate of needs. Biotin is relatively nontoxic. Large doses have been given over an extended period without harmful side effects to children who exhibit defects in biotin metabolism. Thus, no Upper Level for biotin has been set.

8.13 Vitamin B-6

Vitamin B-6 can exist in three chemical forms, all of which can be changed to the active vitamin B-6 coenzyme. Pyridoxine is the general vitamin name and form added to foods.

Functions of Vitamin B-6

The coenzymes of vitamin B-6 are needed for the activity of many enzymes involved in carbohydrate, protein, and fat metabolism. Vitamin B-6 is needed in many areas of metabolism, so a deficiency results in widespread symptoms, such as depression, vomiting, skin disorders, irritation of the nerves, and impaired immune response.

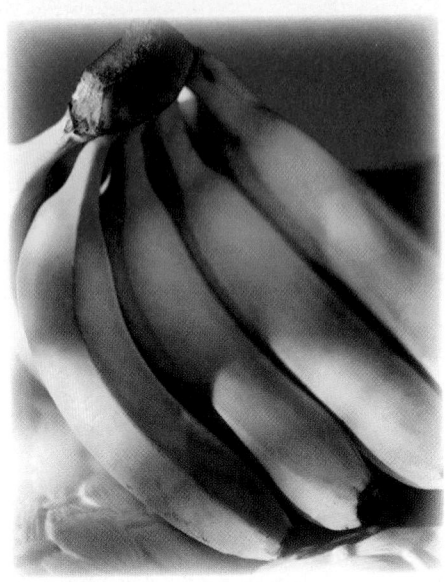

▲ Bananas are a plant source of vitamin B-6.

Vitamin B-6 plays a particularly important role in protein and amino acid metabolism (review Fig. 8-14). The coenzyme helps to remove the nitrogen group (–NH$_2$) from certain amino acids, making nitrogen available to another amino acid. These amino acid reactions allow a cell to synthesize nonessential (dispensable) amino acids. In a related function, vitamin B-6 plays a role in homocysteine metabolism.

Another important role of vitamin B-6 is the synthesis of many neurotransmitters. Recall from Chapter 3 that neurotransmitters allow nerve cells to communicate with each other and with other body cells. A vitamin B-6 deficiency can cause a decrease in these neurotransmitters and lead to symptoms, especially convulsions. This problem occurred in the 1950s when heat destroyed vitamin B-6 in formulas fed to infants.

The vitamin B-6 coenzyme is important for the synthesis of hemoglobin and its function as the oxygen-carrying part of the red blood cell. Vitamin B-6 is also necessary for the synthesis of white blood cells, which perform a major role in the immune system.

Vitamin B-6 Sources and Needs

Major sources of vitamin B-6 are animal products, ready-to-eat breakfast cereals, potatoes, and milk. Other sources are fruits and vegetables such as bananas, cantaloupes, broccoli, and spinach (Figs. 8-24 and 8-25). Overall, animal sources and fortified products are the most reliable because the vitamin B-6 they contain is more absorbable than that in plant foods.

The adult RDA of vitamin B-6 is 1.3 to 1.7 milligrams per day. A Daily Value of 2 milligrams is used to express vitamin B-6 content on food and supplement labels. Average daily consumption of vitamin B-6 for men and women is somewhat above the RDA.

FIGURE 8-24 ▶ Food sources of vitamin B-6 compared to the RDA for adults.

Food Sources of Vitamin B-6

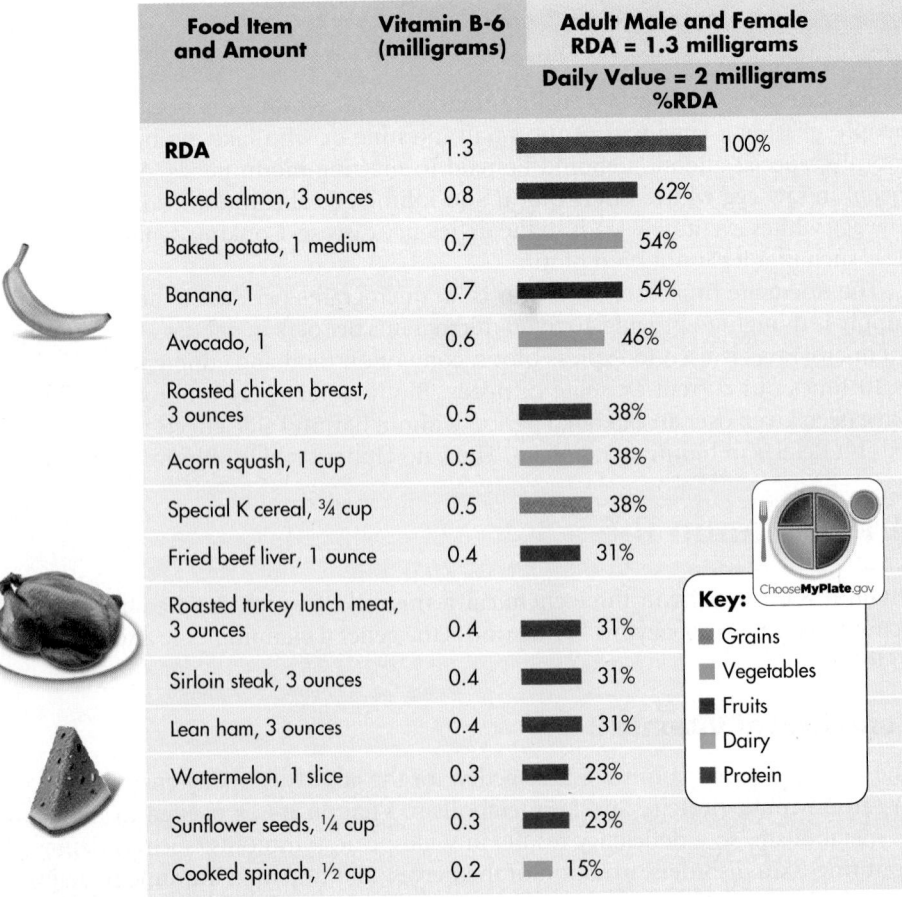

Food Item and Amount	Vitamin B-6 (milligrams)	Adult Male and Female RDA = 1.3 milligrams / Daily Value = 2 milligrams %RDA
RDA	1.3	100%
Baked salmon, 3 ounces	0.8	62%
Baked potato, 1 medium	0.7	54%
Banana, 1	0.7	54%
Avocado, 1	0.6	46%
Roasted chicken breast, 3 ounces	0.5	38%
Acorn squash, 1 cup	0.5	38%
Special K cereal, ¾ cup	0.5	38%
Fried beef liver, 1 ounce	0.4	31%
Roasted turkey lunch meat, 3 ounces	0.4	31%
Sirloin steak, 3 ounces	0.4	31%
Lean ham, 3 ounces	0.4	31%
Watermelon, 1 slice	0.3	23%
Sunflower seeds, ¼ cup	0.3	23%
Cooked spinach, ½ cup	0.2	15%

Key: Grains, Vegetables, Fruits, Dairy, Protein

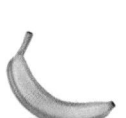
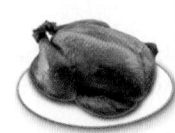

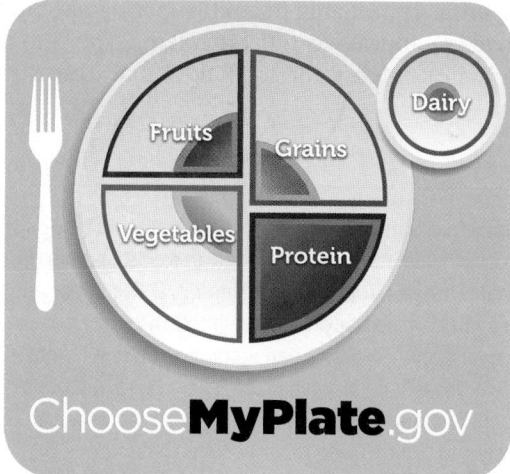

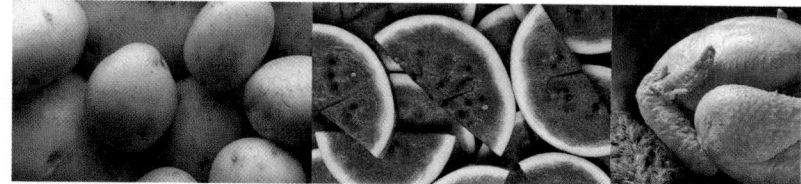

MyPlate:
Sources of Vitamin B-6

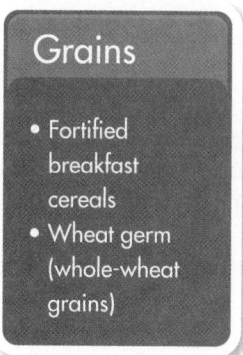
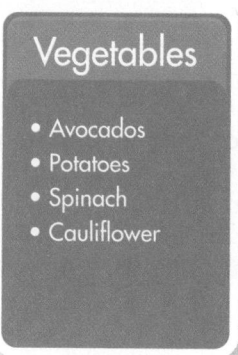
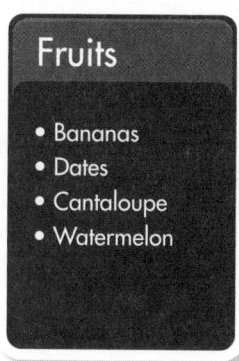
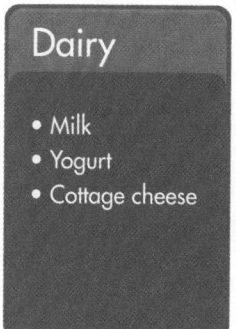
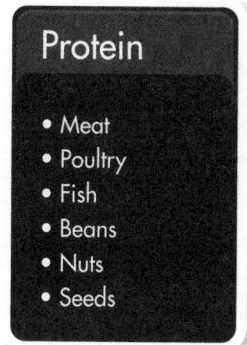

Grains
- Fortified breakfast cereals
- Wheat germ (whole-wheat grains)

Vegetables
- Avocados
- Potatoes
- Spinach
- Cauliflower

Fruits
- Bananas
- Dates
- Cantaloupe
- Watermelon

Dairy
- Milk
- Yogurt
- Cottage cheese

Protein
- Meat
- Poultry
- Fish
- Beans
- Nuts
- Seeds

FIGURE 8-25 ▶ Sources of vitamin B-6 from MyPlate. The fill of the background color (none, 1/3, 2/3, or completely covered) within each group in the plate indicates the average nutrient density for vitamin B-6 in that group. Overall, the protein group especially contains many foods that are nutrient-dense sources of vitamin B-6. With regard to physical activity, vitamin B-6 participates in the related energy metabolism during such endeavors.

Athletes may need slightly more vitamin B-6 than sedentary adults. The athlete's body processes a great deal of glycogen and ingested protein (in the form of amino acids) for fuel, and the metabolism of these compounds requires vitamin B-6. However, athletes are likely to consume plenty of protein-rich foods—enough to supply needed amounts of vitamin B-6.

People with alcoholism are susceptible to a vitamin B-6 deficiency because a metabolite formed in alcohol metabolism can displace the coenzyme form from enzymes, increasing its tendency to be destroyed. In addition, alcohol decreases the absorption of vitamin B-6 and the synthesis of its coenzyme form. Cirrhosis and hepatitis (both of which may accompany alcoholism) also disable liver tissue from metabolizing vitamin B-6, which decreases synthesis of its coenzyme form.

Nausea is experienced by 70% to 85% of women during the first trimester of pregnancy (see Chapter 14). Sometimes physicians recommend vitamin B-6 supplementation, typically 30 to 75 milligrams per day, to reduce nausea. A review of the research on treating nausea during pregnancy suggests that this therapy is both safe and likely to help reduce nausea. Even though vitamin B-6 supplements to treat nausea are available over-the-counter without a prescription, pregnant women should first discuss this treatment option with their physicians.

▲ This grilled salmon with red onion, potatoes, and lemon provides good sources of vitamin B-6 from the protein and vegetable sections of MyPlate. Which sections of MyPlate are missing?

Upper Level for Vitamin B-6

The Upper Level for vitamin B-6 is 100 milligrams per day, based on the risk of developing nerve damage. Studies have shown that intakes of 2 to 6 grams of vitamin B-6 per day for 2 or more months especially can lead to irreversible nerve damage. Symptoms of vitamin B-6 toxicity include walking difficulties and hand and foot numbness. Some nerve damage in individual sensory neurons is probably reversible, but damage to the ganglia (where many nerve fibers converge) appears to be permanent. With 500 milligram tablets of vitamin B-6 available in health-food stores, taking a toxic dose is easy.

CONCEPT CHECK

Pantothenic acid and biotin both participate in the metabolism of carbohydrate and fat. A deficiency of either vitamin is unlikely; pantothenic acid is found widely in foods, and our need for biotin is partially met by intestinal synthesis from bacteria. Vitamin B-6 is important for protein metabolism, neurotransmitter synthesis, homocysteine metabolism, and other key metabolic functions. Headache, a form of anemia, nausea, and vomiting can result from a vitamin B-6 deficiency. Increased risk of cardiovascular disease is also likely. Animal protein foods, ready-to-eat breakfast cereals, broccoli, spinach, and bananas are some food sources of vitamin B-6. Megadose supplements of vitamin B-6 can lead to nerve damage.

8.14 Folate

The term *folate* encompasses a variety of food forms of the vitamin. Folic acid is the synthetic chemical form added to foods and present in supplements. Folic acid is more readily absorbed (1.7 times greater) than natural forms of folate. The structure of natural food folate differs from folic acid by containing extra units of the amino acid, glutamic acid. These extra units must be removed before absorption, yielding free folic acid.

Functions of Folate

A key role of the folate coenzymes is to supply or accept single carbon compounds. In this role, the coenzymes help form DNA and also metabolize various amino acids and their derivatives, such as homocysteine.

One major result of a folate deficiency is decreased red blood cell synthesis. Without folate, the immature cells cannot divide because they cannot form new DNA. The cells grow progressively larger because they can still synthesize enough protein and other cell parts to make new cells. When the time comes for the cells to divide, however, the amount of DNA is insufficient to form two nuclei. The cells then remain in a large immature form, known as a **megaloblast** (Fig. 8-26).

The bone marrow of a folate-deficient person, therefore, produces mostly immature megaloblast cells, and very few mature red blood cells (called **erythrocytes**). With fewer mature red blood cells in the bloodstream, the blood's capacity to carry oxygen decreases, causing folate deficiency anemia called **megaloblastic anemia** (also called macrocytic anemia).

The changes in red blood cell formation occur after 7 to 16 weeks on a folate-free diet, depending on the person's folate stores. White blood cell formation is also affected, but to a lesser degree. In addition, cell division throughout the entire body is disrupted. Clinicians focus primarily on red blood cells because they are easy to collect and examine. Other symptoms of folate deficiency are inflammation of the tongue, diarrhea, poor growth, mental confusion, depression, and problems in nerve function.

About 10% of the North American population has a genetic defect in an important aspect of folate metabolism. They may need up to twice the RDA to compensate for the defect. Genetic testing for this defect is not routine in medical practice, but one day it may be.

A maternal deficiency of folate along with this genetic abnormality related to folate metabolism has been linked to development of **neural tube defects** in the fetus (Fig. 8-27). These defects include spina bifida (spinal cord or spinal fluid bulge

megaloblast A large, immature red blood cell that results from the particular cell's inability to divide normally.

erythrocytes Mature red blood cells. These have no nucleus and a life span of about 120 days; they contain hemoglobin, which transports oxygen and carbon dioxide.

megaloblastic anemia Anemia characterized by the presence of abnormally large red blood cells.

neural tube defect A defect in the formation of the neural tube occurring during early fetal development. This type of defect results in various nervous system disorders, such as spina bifida. Folate deficiency in the pregnant woman increases the risk that the fetus will develop this disorder.

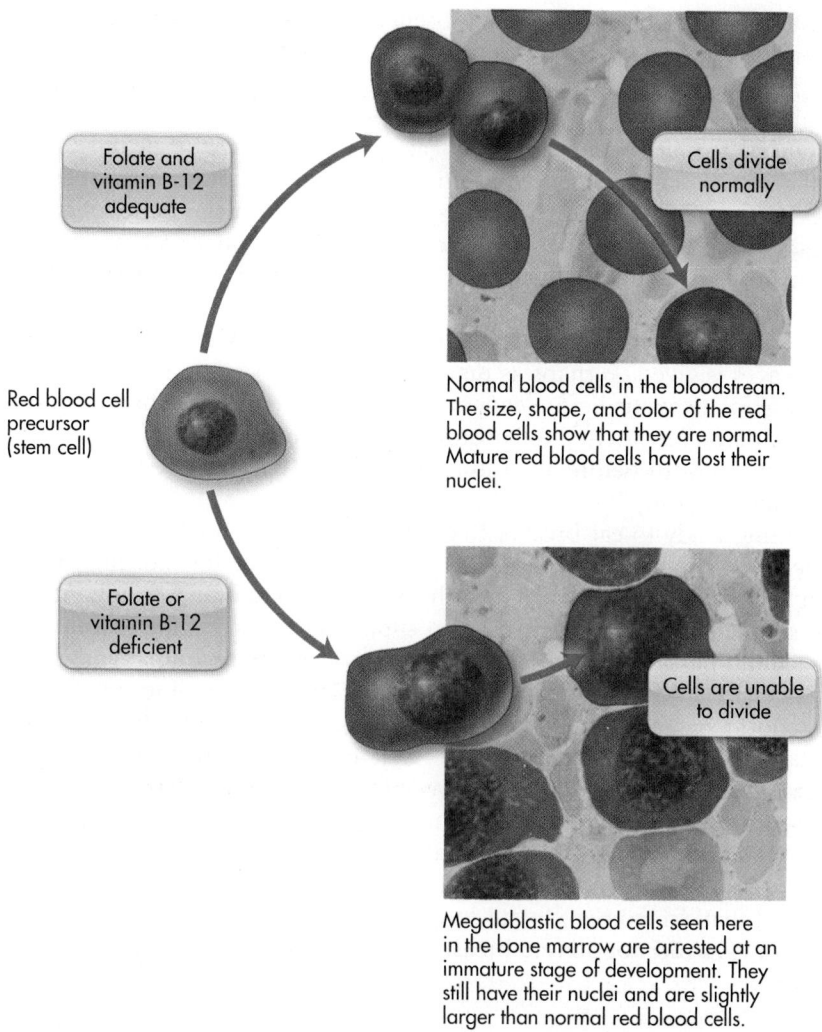

Folate and vitamin B-12 adequate

Cells divide normally

Red blood cell precursor (stem cell)

Normal blood cells in the bloodstream. The size, shape, and color of the red blood cells show that they are normal. Mature red blood cells have lost their nuclei.

Folate or vitamin B-12 deficient

Cells are unable to divide

Megaloblastic blood cells seen here in the bone marrow are arrested at an immature stage of development. They still have their nuclei and are slightly larger than normal red blood cells.

FIGURE 8-26 ▶ Megaloblastic anemia occurs when blood cells are unable to divide, leaving large, immature red blood cells. Either a folate or vitamin B-12 deficiency may cause this condition. Measurements of blood concentrations of both vitamins are taken to help determine the cause of the anemia.

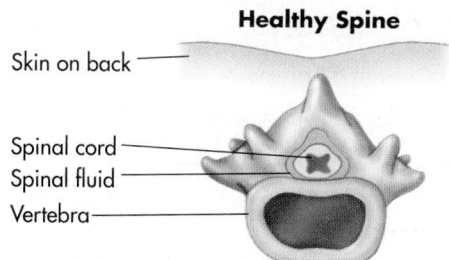

Healthy Spine

Skin on back

Spinal cord
Spinal fluid
Vertebra

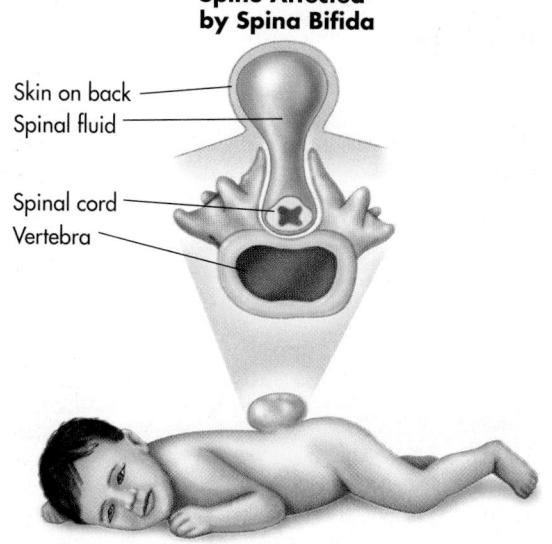

Spine Affected by Spina Bifida

Skin on back
Spinal fluid

Spinal cord
Vertebra

FIGURE 8-27 ▶ Neural tube defects result from a developmental failure affecting the spinal cord or brain in the embryo. Very early in fetal development, a ridge of neural-like tissue forms along the back of the embryo. As the fetus develops, this material develops into both the spinal cord and nerves at the lower end and into the brain at the upper end. At the same time, the bones that make up the back gradually surround the spinal cord on all sides. If any part of this sequence goes awry, many defects can appear. The worst case is total lack of a brain (anencephaly). Spina bifida, in which the back bones do not form a complete ring to protect the spinal cord, is much more common. Deficient folate status in the mother during the beginning of pregnancy, especially in combination with a genetic abnormality in folate metabolism, greatly increases the risk of neural tube defects.

NEWSWORTHY
NUTRITION

Folic acid added to cereal reduces number of neural tube defects

Fortification of cereal products with folic acid became mandatory in Canada and the United States in 1998. As a result of the fortification, the prevalence of neural tube defects decreased 46% in Canada from 1.58 per 1000 births before fortification to 0.86 per 1000 births after fortification. The reduction rate was greatest for spina bifida (a decrease of 53%). Declines have also been observed in the United States.

Source: DeWals P and others: Reduction in neural tube defects after folic acid fortification in Canada. *New England Journal of Medicine* 357:135, 2007 (see Further Reading 3).

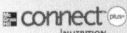 **connect** NUTRITION   **Check out the Connect site** www.mcgrawhillconnect.com **to further explore vitamin-fortified foods.**

through the back) and anencephaly (absence of a brain). About 2000 infants are affected with neural tube defects annually in the United States. Victims of spina bifida exhibit paralysis, incontinence, learning disabilities, and other health problems. Children born with anencephaly die shortly after birth. Adequate folate nurture is crucial for all women of childbearing age because the neural tube closes within the first 28 days of pregnancy, a time when many women are not even aware that they are pregnant. Research that has been done with synthetic folic acid supplementation has resulted in a recommendation that ample folate, specifically 400 micrograms of synthetic folic acid per day, be consumed at least 6 weeks before conception. It appears that even those women with varied diets may not consume adequate synthetic folic acid to prevent neural tube defects unless specific attention to rich sources is given. Perhaps as many as 70% of these defects could be avoided by adequate folate status before conception. (Women who have had a child with a neural tube defect are advised to consume 4 milligrams per day of folic acid, beginning at least 1 month before any future pregnancy. This must be done under strict physician supervision.)

Consuming ready-to-eat breakfast cereals that contain 100% of the Daily Value for folate (this is the same as the RDA) is a good practice for meeting the goal for synthetic folic acid intake (see Newsworthy Nutrition in margin). A multivitamin and mineral supplement can also be used to supply adequate synthetic folic acid, but women should be careful to monitor the amount of any accompanying preformed vitamin A content (do not exceed 100% of the Daily Value). Since 1992, there has been an effort to get all women of childbearing age to take daily vitamins containing folic acid. A March of Dimes survey found that 40% of these women did so in 2007.

Research is underway on the link between folate and cancer protection. Folate aids in DNA synthesis, so it is hypothesized that even mild folate deficiency contributes to abnormal DNA integrity, which in turn affects certain cancer-protecting genes. Meeting the RDA for folate is thought to be one way to reduce cancer risk. A recent 7-year study found that, in women, folate supplements in combination with vitamin B-6 and vitamin B-12 did not prevent breast cancer or other invasive cancers (see Further Reading 15).

MAKING DECISIONS

Folate and Cancer Therapy

Some forms of cancer therapy provide a vivid example of the effects of a folate deficiency on DNA metabolism. A cancer drug, methotrexate, closely resembles a form of folate but cannot act in its place. Because of this resemblance, when methotrexate is taken in high doses, it hampers folate metabolism. In essence, methotrexate crowds out folate in the metabolic pathways. DNA synthesis and, consequently, cell division, then decrease. Cancer cells are among the most rapidly dividing cells in the body, so they are among those first affected. However, other rapidly dividing cells, such as intestinal cells and skin cells, are also affected. Not surprisingly, typical side effects of methotrexate therapy are diarrhea, vomiting, and hair loss. These are also typical symptoms of folate deficiency. Today when patients are given methotrexate, they need to follow a high-folate diet and/or take folic acid supplements because this reduces the toxic side effects of the drug. High supplemental doses generally have little or no influence on methotrexate's effectiveness as a cancer therapy.

Folate Sources and Needs

Green, leafy vegetables (*folate* is derived from the Latin word *folium*, which means *foliage* or *leaves*), organ meats, sprouts, other vegetables, dried beans, and orange juice are the richest sources of folate (Figs. 8-28 and 8-29). The vitamin C in orange juice also reduces folate destruction. Ready-to-eat breakfast cereals, milk, and bread also are important sources of folate for many adults.

Folate is susceptible to destruction by heat. Food processing and preparation destroy 50% to 90% of the folate in food. This underscores the importance of regularly eating fresh fruits and raw or lightly cooked vegetables. As mentioned, vegetables retain their nutrients best when cooked quickly in minimal water—steaming, stir-frying, or microwaving (review Table 8-1).

The RDA of folate for adults is 400 micrograms per day, as is the Daily Value used to express folate content on food and supplement labels. Folate recommendations for all but women of childbearing age (these women should meet such recommendations with synthetic folic acid), are based on dietary folate equivalents (DFE). To compute folate intake in DFE units, one has to determine how much of a day's folate intake comes from food folate and how much comes from synthetic folic acid added to foods. When in doubt, assume all folate in a diet is in the food form, except that coming from ready-to-eat breakfast cereals and refined grain products. Also included in this second category is any folic acid in supplements. To calculate the DFE, multiply total synthetic folic acid intake by 1.7, and add that value to the food folate consumed. For example, if a person consumed 300 micrograms as food folate and 200 micrograms from a ready-to-eat breakfast cereal, total DFE would be 640 micrograms (300 + [200 × 1.7] = 640). Compared to the RDA of 400 micrograms, this intake would be sufficient.

Prior to 1998, average daily folate intakes in the United States were approximately 320 micrograms for men and 220 micrograms for women. In 1998, the fortification of grain products with folate was mandated in the United States and Canada, with the aim of reducing birth defects of the spine. With this mandate, average intakes have increased by about 200 micrograms per day. Studies have shown this practice has decreased rates of neural tube defects in infants (see Further Reading 3).

CRITICAL THINKING

Suzanne and Ted are planning to start a family. They are especially concerned because Suzanne's sister gave birth last year to a baby with spina bifida. In preparation for her pregnancy, Suzanne takes a multivitamin supplement and eats fortified breakfast cereal most days. She also tries to include oranges, orange juice, broccoli, and spinach salads in her diet. What is spina bifida? How do Suzanne's diet and multivitamin supplement help prevent this serious disorder? Read more about this issue in What Would You Do Recommendations at the end of Chapter 8.

Food Sources of Folate

Food Item and Amount	Folate (micrograms)	Adult Male and Female RDA = 400 micrograms Daily Value = 400 micrograms %RDA
RDA	400	100%
Asparagus, 1 cup	263	66%
Cooked spinach, 1 cup	262	66%
Cooked lentils, ½ cup	179	45%
Black-eyed peas, ½ cup	179	45%
Romaine lettuce, 1½ cups	114	29%
Great Grains cereal, ¾ cup	114	29%
Tortilla, 1	89	22%
Cooked turnips, ½ cup	85	21%
Cooked broccoli, 1 cup	78	20%
Sunflower seeds, ¼ cup	76	19%
Fresh orange juice, 1 cup	75	19%
Cooked beets, ½ cup	68	17%
Kidney beans, ½ cup	65	16%

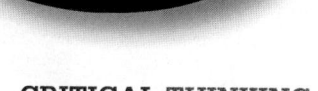

Key:
- Grains
- Vegetables
- Fruits
- Dairy
- Protein

FIGURE 8-28 ▶ Food sources of folate compared to the RDA for adults.

FIGURE 8-29 ▶ Sources of folate from MyPlate. The fill of the background color (none, 1/3, 2/3, or completely covered) within each group in the plate indicates the average nutrient density for folate in that group. Overall, the vegetables group provides the richest sources, but the fruits group and the grains group contain some foods that are nutrient-dense sources of folate.

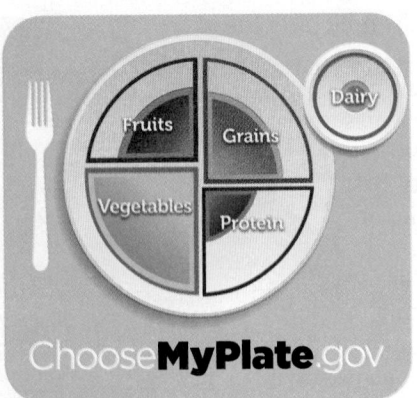

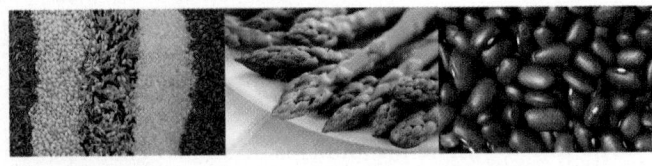

MyPlate: Sources of Folate

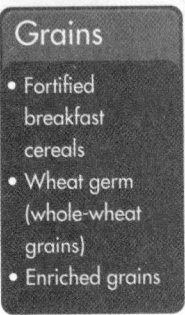
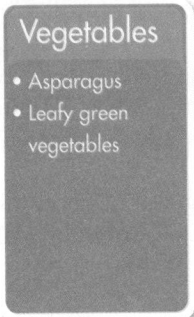
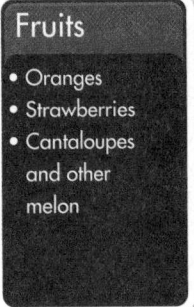
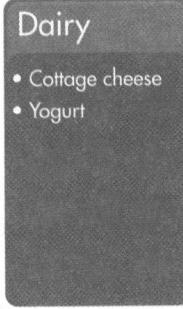
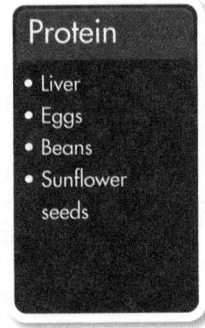

Grains
- Fortified breakfast cereals
- Wheat germ (whole-wheat grains)
- Enriched grains

Vegetables
- Asparagus
- Leafy green vegetables

Fruits
- Oranges
- Strawberries
- Cantaloupes and other melon

Dairy
- Cottage cheese
- Yogurt

Protein
- Liver
- Eggs
- Beans
- Sunflower seeds

See Nutrition and Your Health: Dietary Supplements—Who Needs Them? at the end of Chapter 8.

Pregnant women need extra folate (a total of 600 micrograms DFE) to accommodate the increased rates of cell division and DNA synthesis in their own bodies and in the developing fetus. A healthy diet easily supplies this much. Although most vitamin supplements have no proven health benefits in most people (See the Nutrition and Your Health section at the end of this chapter), supplemental folic acid is effective at preventing birth defects. Prenatal care often includes a specially formulated multivitamin and mineral supplement enriched with synthetic folic acid to help compensate for the extra needs associated with pregnancy. Within the 2010 Dietary Guidelines for Americans, a key recommendation for women of childbearing age who may become pregnant and those in the first trimester of pregnancy is to consume 400 micrograms per day of synthetic folic acid daily (from fortified foods or supplements) in addition to food forms of folate from a varied diet.

Older people are also at risk for folate deficiency, possibly due to a combination of inadequate folate intake and decreased absorption. Perhaps these people fail to consume sufficient amounts of fruits and vegetables because of poverty or physical problems, such as poor dental health. In addition, folate deficiencies often occur with alcoholism, due mostly to poor intake and absorption. Symptoms of a folate-related anemia can alert a physician to the possibility of alcoholism.

MAKING DECISIONS

Dietary Folate Equivalents

The use of dietary folate equivalents (DFEs) instead of the actual amount of folate in a food has some important implications. Typically, many foods will be richer in folate than the Nutrition Facts label suggests because folate content is due primarily to synthetic folic acid added to the foods, such as in enriched grains and ready-to-eat breakfast cereals. This contributes substantially to the DFE calculation. Another implication is that food composition tables and diet-analysis software programs (such as that supplied with this book) also underestimate the true folate contribution of a diet compared to folate needs because these have not been updated to DFE units.

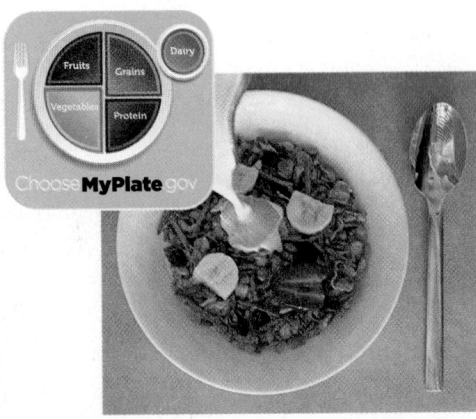

▲ Enriched grains and ready-to-eat breakfast cereals are good sources of synthetic folic acid. The cereal, fruit, and milk provide good sources of vitamins from the grains, fruit, and dairy sections of MyPlate.

Upper Level for Folate

The Upper Level for folate is 1 milligram (1000 micrograms) per day but only refers to the synthetic source. This is because folate naturally present in foods has limited absorption. Large doses of folate can hide the signs of vitamin B-12 deficiency and therefore complicate its diagnosis. Specifically, regular consumption of large amounts of folate can prevent the appearance of an early warning sign of vitamin B-12 deficiency—enlarged red blood cell size. To prevent such masking of vitamin B-12 deficiency, the goal of the folate fortification of grains program is, to increase the folate status of women of childbearing age without causing excessive intake (over 1 milligram of synthetic folic acid per day) by other individuals. Also, because of risk of masking a vitamin B-12 deficiency, FDA limits supplements for nonpregnant adults and food fortification to 400 microgram amounts.

8.15 Vitamin B-12

Vitamin B-12 represents a family of compounds that contain the mineral cobalt. All vitamin B-12 compounds are synthesized by bacteria, fungi, and other lower organisms.

The body has a complex means of absorbing vitamin B-12. Vitamin B-12 in food enters the stomach and is digested from other materials, especially by stomach acid. The free vitamin B-12 in the stomach binds with a protein produced by the salivary glands in the mouth, and that protects vitamin B-12 from stomach acid. Vitamin B-12 is later freed from this protein in the small intestine. Finally, vitamin B-12 binds in the small intestine with a compound made in the stomach called **intrinsic factor.** The resulting intrinsic factor/vitamin B-12 complex travels to the last portion of the small intestine for absorption. After these digestion steps, approximately 50% of dietary vitamin B-12 is absorbed, depending on the body's need for it.

If a person has a defect in the digestion and absorption of vitamin B-12, the body may only be able to use 1% to 2% of dietary vitamin B-12. Monthly injections of vitamin B-12 or vitamin B-12 nasal gels are used to bypass the need for absorption or megadoses of a supplemental form (300 times the RDA) are needed to overcome the absorption defect by providing enough of the vitamin via simple diffusion across the intestinal tract.

About 95% of all cases of vitamin B-12 deficiencies in healthy people result from defective vitamin B-12 absorption, rather than from inadequate intakes. This is especially true for older people. As we age, our stomachs have a decreased ability to synthesize the intrinsic factor needed for vitamin B-12 absorption.

intrinsic factor A proteinlike compound produced by the stomach that enhances vitamin B-12 absorption.

Functions of Vitamin B-12

Vitamin B-12 participates in a variety of cellular processes. The most important function is in folate metabolism. Vitamin B-12 is required to convert folate coenzymes to the active forms needed for metabolic reactions, such as DNA synthesis. Without vitamin B-12, reactions that require certain active forms of folate do not take place in the cell. Thus, a vitamin B-12 deficiency can result in symptoms of a folate deficiency. Another vital function of vitamin B-12 is maintaining the myelin sheaths that insulate neurons from each other. People with vitamin B-12 deficiencies have destruction of segments of the myelin sheaths. This destruction eventually causes paralysis and, perhaps, death. Vitamin B-12 also participates in homocysteine metabolism and certain minor metabolic pathways.

In the past, the inability to absorb enough vitamin B-12 eventually led to death, mainly because it destroyed nerves. This phenomenon was

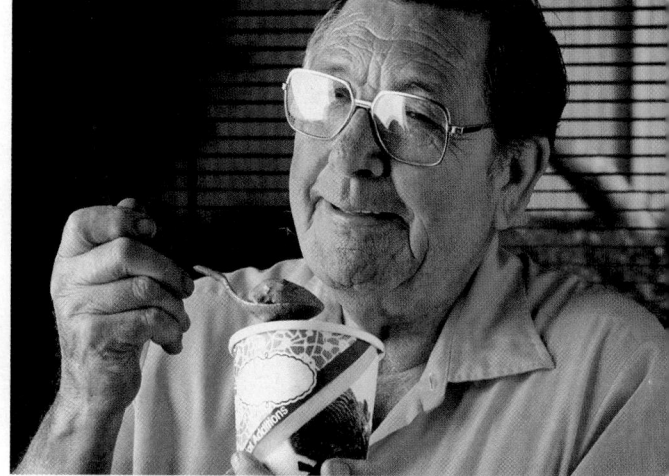

▼ As we age, our digestive system absorbs vitamin B-12 from food less efficiently.

pernicious anemia The anemia that results from a lack of vitamin B-12 absorption; it is pernicious because of associated nerve degeneration that can result in eventual paralysis and death.

called **pernicious anemia** (*pernicious* literally means "leading to death"). Clinically, the anemia looks much like a folate-deficiency anemia, characterized by the appearance of many large red blood cells in the bloodstream. However, the true cause of pernicious anemia is poor vitamin B-12 absorption rather than inadequate folate intakes.

Symptoms of pernicious anemia include weakness, sore tongue, back pain, apathy, and tingling in the extremities. We store significant amounts of vitamin B-12, so symptoms of nerve destruction generally do not develop until at least 3 years after the onset of the deficiency. Unfortunately, significant nerve destruction often occurs before the anemia is detected, and this destruction is irreversible. Pernicious anemia and its accompanying nerve destruction generally start after middle age, affecting up to 10% to 20% of older adults. The explanation for this age-associated pernicious anemia is twofold. First, aging is often associated with low production of stomach acid. Thus, vitamin B-12 is not properly cleaved from other food components during digestion. Second, aging may be accompanied by reduced output of intrinsic factor, resulting in decreased absorption of the vitamin (see Further Reading 2).

Infants who are breastfed by vegetarian or vegan mothers are at risk for vitamin B-12 deficiency accompanied by anemia and long-term nervous system problems, such as diminished brain growth, degeneration of the spinal cord, and poor intellectual development. The problems may have their origins during pregnancy, when the mother is deficient in vitamin B-12. Vegan diets supply little vitamin B-12 unless they include vitamin B-12–enriched food or supplements, so achieving an adequate vitamin B-12 intake is a key diet-planning goal for vegans (review Chapter 6).

Vitamin B-12 Sources and Needs

Major sources of vitamin B-12 include meat, milk, ready-to-eat breakfast cereals, poultry, seafood, and eggs (Fig. 8-30). Organ meats (especially liver, kidneys, and heart) are especially rich sources of vitamin B-12. Adults over age 50 are encouraged

FIGURE 8-30 ▶ Food sources of vitamin B-12 compared to the RDA for adults.

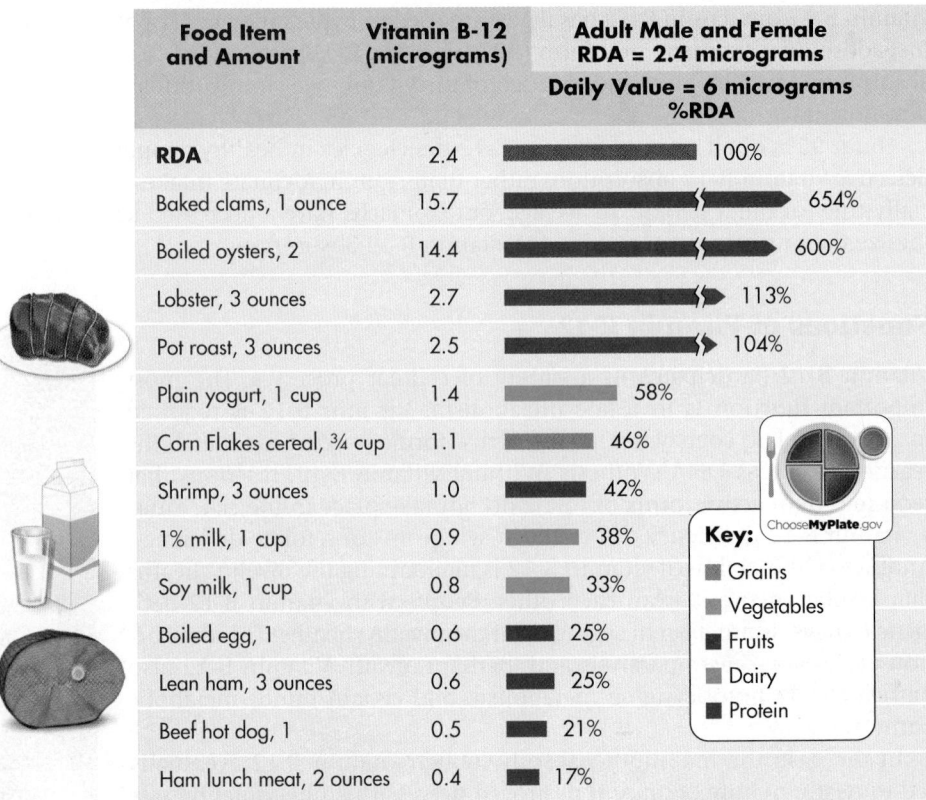

Food Sources of Vitamin B-12

Food Item and Amount	Vitamin B-12 (micrograms)	Adult Male and Female RDA = 2.4 micrograms Daily Value = 6 micrograms %RDA
RDA	2.4	100%
Baked clams, 1 ounce	15.7	654%
Boiled oysters, 2	14.4	600%
Lobster, 3 ounces	2.7	113%
Pot roast, 3 ounces	2.5	104%
Plain yogurt, 1 cup	1.4	58%
Corn Flakes cereal, ¾ cup	1.1	46%
Shrimp, 3 ounces	1.0	42%
1% milk, 1 cup	0.9	38%
Soy milk, 1 cup	0.8	33%
Boiled egg, 1	0.6	25%
Lean ham, 3 ounces	0.6	25%
Beef hot dog, 1	0.5	21%
Ham lunch meat, 2 ounces	0.4	17%

Key:
- Grains
- Vegetables
- Fruits
- Dairy
- Protein

to seek a synthetic vitamin B-12 source to aid absorption, which can be limited due to reduced intrinsic factor and stomach acid output seen in aging, as mentioned. Synthetic vitamin B-12 is not food bound, so it doesn't need stomach acid to release it from foods. Thus, it will be more readily absorbed than the food form. Ready-to-eat breakfast cereals and a multivitamin and mineral supplement are two possible synthetic sources.

The RDA of vitamin B-12 for adults is 2.4 micrograms per day. The Daily Value of 6 micrograms is used on food and supplement labels. On average, adults consume 2 times the RDA or more. This high intake provides the average meat-eating person with storage of vitamin B-12 in the liver for about 2 to 3 years.

It takes a person approximately 20 years of consuming a diet essentially free of vitamin B-12 to exhibit nerve destruction caused by a diet deficiency. Still, vegans, who eat no animal products, should find a reliable source of vitamin B-12, such as fortified soybean milk, ready-to-eat breakfast cereals, and a supplemental form of vitamin B-12 enriched yeast. Use of a multivitamin and mineral supplement containing vitamin B-12 is another option. As noted earlier, older persons are at significant risk for developing pernicious anemia due to the loss of vitamin B-12 absorption capacity. Within the 2010 Dietary Guidelines for Americans, a key recommendation for people over age 50 is to consume foods fortified with vitamin B-12, such as fortified cereals, or dietery supplements. Regular physical examinations should test for pernicious anemia in older adults. Vitamin B-12 supplements are essentially non-toxic, so no Upper Level has been set.

People with HIV/AIDS also are at risk of vitamin B-12 deficiency, linked to long-standing malabsorption that they often experience. In a few studies, adequate vitamin B-12 status has been shown to lessen the decline in health experienced by those with HIV/AIDS.

CONCEPT CHECK

Folate is needed for cell division because it influences DNA synthesis. A folate deficiency results in megaloblastic (macrocytic) anemia, as well as elevated blood homocysteine, inflammation of the tongue, diarrhea, and poor growth. Excess folate intake can mask a vitamin B-12 deficiency because these vitamins work together in metabolism. Folate is found in fruits and vegetables, beans, and organ meats. Emphasizing fresh and lightly cooked vegetables in the diet is important because much folate is lost during cooking. Women of childbearing age should meet needs by consuming a source of synthetic folic acid. Folate needs during pregnancy are especially high; a deficiency around the time of conception and in the first month of pregnancy may lead to neural tube defects in the fetus.

Vitamin B-12 is necessary for folate metabolism. Without dietary vitamin B-12, folate deficiency symptoms, such as macrocytic anemia, develop. In addition, vitamin B-12 is necessary for maintaining the nervous system. Paralysis can develop from a vitamin B-12 deficiency. Vitamin B-12 also participates in homocysteine metabolism. The absorption of vitamin B-12 requires a number of specific factors. If absorption is inhibited, the resulting deficiency can lead to pernicious anemia and its associated nerve destruction. Concentrated amounts of vitamin B-12 are found only in animal foods; meat-eaters generally have a 2- to 3-year supply stored in the liver. Vegans need to find an alternate source. Vitamin B-12 absorption may decline as we age. Monthly injections, nasal gels, or megadoses can make up for this.

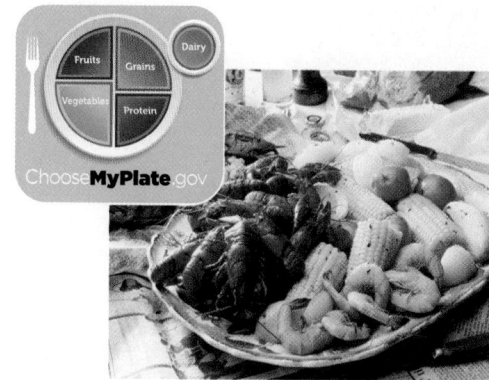

▲ Seafood, is a good source of vitamin B-12. Servings of seafood, corn, and potatoes can fill the protein and vegetables sections of MyPlate.

8.16 Vitamin C

Vitamin C (ascorbic acid) is found in all living tissues, and most animals (but not humans) synthesize it from the simple sugar glucose. Vitamin C is absorbed in the small intestine. About 70% to 90% of vitamin C is absorbed when a person eats between 30 and 180 milligrams of it per day. If someone ingests 1 gram (1000 milligrams) per day, absorption efficiency drops to about 50%. A common side effect of megadose vitamin C use is diarrhea. The unabsorbed vitamin C stays in the small intestine and attracts water, resulting in diarrhea (see the section on toxicity of vitamin C).

CRITICAL THINKING

Carlos just returned from a local mall and is excited because he saw an advertisement claiming that vitamin C will cure just about everything, from colds to heart disease. How would you explain vitamin C's main functions in the human body to Carlos?

Functions of Vitamin C

Collagen Synthesis The best understood function of vitamin C is its role in synthesizing the protein collagen. This protein is highly concentrated in connective tissue, bone, teeth, tendons, and blood vessels. It is important for wound healing. Vitamin C increases the cross-connections between amino acids in collagen, greatly strengthening the structural tissues it helps form.

On long sea voyages, captains often lost half or more of their crews to scurvy, the vitamin C deficiency disease. Its symptoms include weakness, slow wound healing, opening of previously healed wounds, bone pain, fractures, bleeding gums, diarrhea, and pinpoint hemorrhages around hair follicles on the back of the arms and legs. In 1740, the Englishman Dr. James Lind first showed that citrus fruits—two oranges and one lemon a day—could cure scurvy. Fifty years after Lind's discovery, rations for British sailors included limes to prevent scurvy (thus their nickname, limeys).

A vitamin C deficiency can cause widespread changes in tissue metabolism. Most symptoms of scurvy are linked to a decrease in collagen synthesis, such as in the skin. About 20 to 40 days with no vitamin C intake are required for the first symptoms of scurvy to appear (Fig. 8-31).

Antioxidant Activity Vitamin C has antioxidant properties. This may allow vitamin C to reduce the formation of cancer-causing nitrosamines in the stomach and also keep the folate coenzymes intact, preventing their destruction. Vitamin C may work as a free radical scavenger. Vitamin C also may aid in reactivating oxidized vitamin E so that it can be reused. The extent to which all this antioxidant activity happens in the body, however, is debatable and not proven as of now. Population studies suggest that vitamin C is effective in helping prevent certain cancers (of the esophagus, mouth, and stomach) and cataracts in the eye, probably because of its antioxidant properties.

Iron Absorption Vitamin C enhances iron absorption by keeping iron in its most absorbable form, especially as the mineral travels through the small intestine's alkaline environment. This is seen with a vitamin C intake of 75 milligrams or more at a meal. Increasing intake of vitamin C-rich foods is beneficial for those with poor iron stores. Within the 2010 Dietary Guidelines for Americans, a key recommendation for women of childbearing age who may become pregnant is to choose foods that supply heme iron, which is more readily absorbed by the body, additional iron sources, and enhancers of iron absorption, such as vitamin C-rich foods.

Immune Function Finally, vitamin C is vital for the function of the immune system, especially for the activity of certain immune cells. Thus, disease states that increase the need for immune function can increase the need for vitamin C, possibly above the RDA. Partly on the basis of this observation, Dr. Linus Pauling gained great notoriety by claiming that vitamin C could combat the common cold. He claimed that 1000 milligrams (1 gram) or more of vitamin C daily could reduce the number of colds for most people by nearly half. As a result of the popularity of his books and the respectability of his scientific credentials, millions of North Americans supplement their diets with vitamin C.

But does vitamin C reliably and effectively work against colds and other infections? Most medical and nutrition scientists disagree with Pauling's views of vitamin C. Numerous well-designed, double-blind studies have not shown megadoses of vitamin C to reliably prevent colds, though it seems to reduce the duration of symptoms by a day or so.

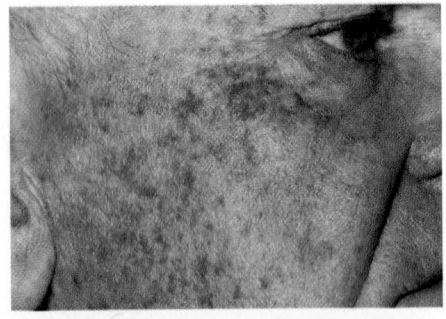

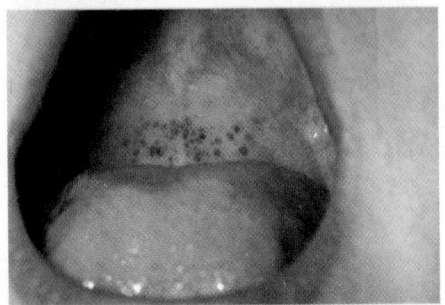

FIGURE 8-31 ▶ Pinpoint hemorrhages of the skin—an early symptom of scurvy. The spots on the skin are caused by slight bleeding. The person may experience poor wound healing. These are all signs of defective collagen synthesis.

Vitamin C Sources and Needs

Major sources of vitamin C are citrus fruits, green peppers, cauliflower, broccoli, cabbage, strawberries, papayas, and romaine lettuce. Potatoes, ready-to-eat breakfast cereals, and fortified fruit drinks are also good sources of vitamin C (Figs. 8-32 and 8-33).

Food Sources of Vitamin C

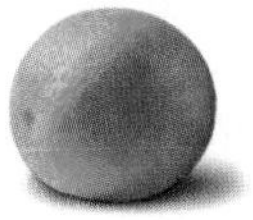

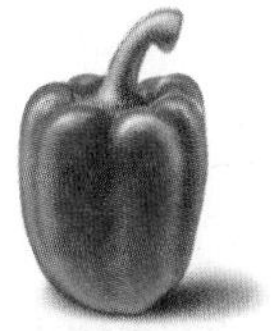

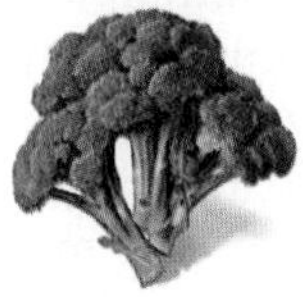

Food Item and Amount	Vitamin C (milligrams)	Adult Male RDA = 90 milligrams	Adult Female RDA = 75 milligrams
		Daily Value = 60 milligrams %RDA	%RDA
RDA	75-90	100%	100%
Orange, 1	98	109%	131%
Cooked Brussels sprouts, 1 cup	97	108%	129%
Strawberries, 1 cup	94	104%	125%
Grapefruit juice, 1 cup	80	89%	107%
Red peppers, ¼ cup	71	79%	95%
Kiwi fruit, 1	57	63%	76%
Green pepper rings, 5	45	50%	60%
Tomato juice, 1 cup	45	50%	60%
Cooked broccoli, ½ cup	33	37%	44%
Kale, ½ cup	27	30%	36%
Raw cauliflower, ½ cup	23	26%	31%
Sweet potato, 1	17	19%	23%
Baked potato, 1 medium	16	18%	21%
Pineapple chunks, ½ cup	12	13%	16%
Cooked spinach, ½ cup	9	10%	12%

Key:
- Grains
- Vegetables
- Fruits
- Dairy
- Protein

FIGURE 8-32 ▶ Food sources of vitamin C compared to the RDA for adult males and females.

FIGURE 8-33 ▶ Sources of vitamin C from MyPlate. The fill of the background color (none, 1/3, 2/3, or completely covered) within each group on the plate indicates the average nutrient density for vitamin C in that group. Overall, the vegetables group and the fruits group contain many foods that are nutrient-dense sources of vitamin C. With regard to physical activity, vitamin C has no primary role in the related energy metabolism *per se*, but likely limits some oxidant damage during such endeavors.

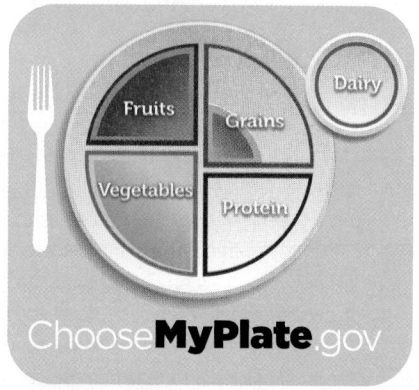

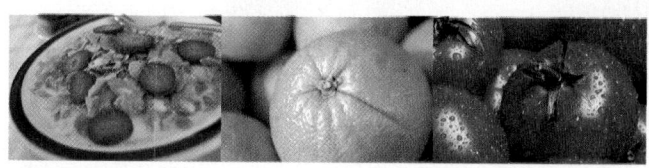

MyPlate: Sources of Vitamin C

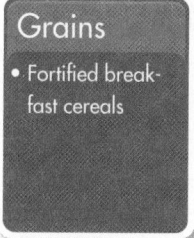

Grains
- Fortified breakfast cereals

Vegetables
- Tomatoes
- Potatoes
- Cauliflower
- Green vegetables

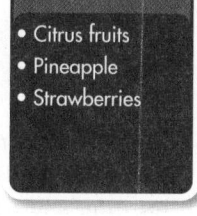

Fruits
- Citrus fruits
- Pineapple
- Strawberries

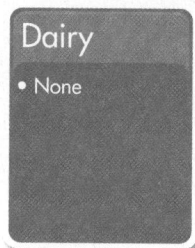

Dairy
- None

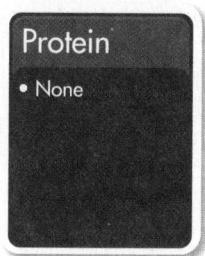

Protein
- None

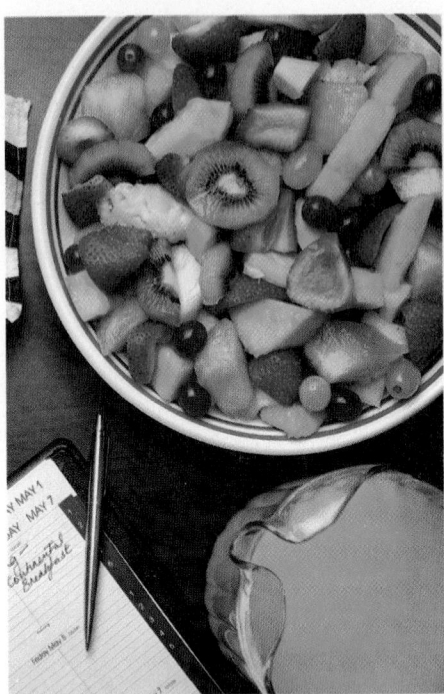

▲ In addition to orange juice, fruits such as strawberries and kiwis are excellent sources of vitamin C.

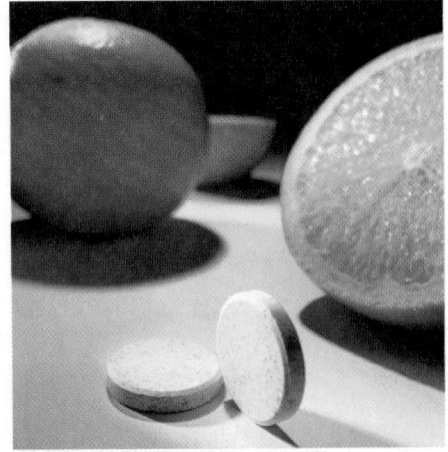

▲ Oranges are a rich source of vitamin C. The many phytochemicals they provide are an additional benefit and are not found in vitamin C supplements.

Meeting the servings for fruits and vegetables recommended by MyPyramid can easily provide enough vitamin C. Vitamin C is rapidly lost in processing and cooking as it is unstable in the presence of heat, iron, copper, or oxygen and is water soluble.

The adult RDA of vitamin C is 75 to 90 milligrams per day. The Daily Value of 60 milligrams is used to express vitamin C content on food and supplement labels. Cigarette smokers need to add an extra 35 milligrams per day to the RDA because of the great stress on their lungs from oxygen and toxic by-products of cigarette smoke. Nearly all North Americans likely meet their daily needs for vitamin C. We consume an average 70 to 100 milligrams per day. Respected nutrition experts who advocate increased use of vitamin C often recommend intakes of about 200 milligrams per day. Still, this amount can be obtained by sufficient fruit and vegetable intake. Today, vitamin C deficiency appears mostly in alcoholic people who eat nutrient-poor diets and in some older persons with inadequate food intakes.

Upper Level for Vitamin C

Most vitamin C consumed in large doses in supplements ends up in the feces or the urine. Only a small fraction of such large doses can be used. The kidneys start rapidly excreting excess vitamin C, beginning at intakes of about 100 milligrams per day. This means that if more than that is ingested, much is quickly excreted. At dosages of 500 milligrams per day, almost all of consumed vitamin C is excreted. The Upper Level for vitamin C is 2 grams per day. Regularly consuming more than that may cause stomach inflammation and diarrhea. Other suggested toxicity symptoms have been discounted in healthy people.

MAKING DECISIONS

High Doses of Vitamin C

If people want to experiment with large doses of vitamin C, they should alert their physician. High doses of vitamin C can change reactions to medical tests for blood in the feces and glucose in the urine (test for diabetes). Vitamin C can interact with the testing procedures because much of a high dose of vitamin C will not be absorbed and end up in the feces, or if absorbed, will be rapidly excreted in the urine. Physicians may misdiagnose conditions when large doses of vitamin C are consumed without their knowledge.

CONCEPT CHECK

Vitamin C is important in the synthesis of collagen, a major connective tissue protein. A vitamin C deficiency, known as scurvy, causes many changes in the skin and gums, such as small hemorrhages. This is mainly because of poor collagen synthesis. Vitamin C also modestly improves iron absorption, is involved in synthesizing certain hormones and neurotransmitters, and likely acts as a general body antioxidant. Citrus fruits, green peppers, cauliflower, broccoli, strawberries, and ready-to-eat breakfast cereals are good sources of vitamin C. As with folate, eating fresh or lightly cooked foods is important because vitamin C loses a lot of its potency in cooking. High doses of vitamin C can lead to diarrhea and foil various medical tests.

8.17 Choline

The dietary component choline is the latest addition to the list of essential nutrients. Choline is part of acetylcholine, a neurotransmitter associated with attention, learning and memory, muscle control, and many other functions. It is also part of phospholipids, such as **lecithin,** the major component of the cell membrane. Finally, choline participates in some aspects of homocysteine metabolism.

There has been only one published study examining the effect of inadequate dietary intake of choline in healthy humans. The study of male volunteers showed decreased choline stores and liver damage when humans were fed choline-deficient total parental (intravenous) nutrition solutions. Based on this human study and several laboratory animal studies, choline has been deemed essential, but is not yet classified as a vitamin.

lecithin A group of phospholipid compounds that are major components of cell membranes.

Choline Sources and Needs

Choline is widely distributed in foods (Fig. 8-34). Milk, liver, and peanuts are sources. Lecithins often are added to food during processing, so this is yet another source. There is so much choline available in ordinary foods that it is unlikely that a dietary deficiency exists naturally. Choline also can be synthesized from the nonessential (dispensable) amino-acid serine.

The Adequate Intake for choline for adults is 425 to 550 milligrams per day. We do not know if a dietary supply is needed at all life stages. Although Adequate Intakes are set for choline, it may be that the choline requirement can be met by body synthesis at some or all stages of life. We consume ample choline from food, at least 700 to 1000 milligrams per day.

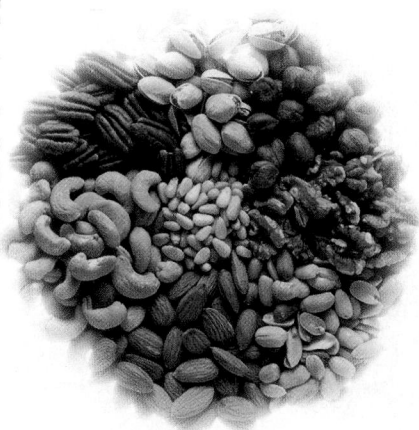

▲ Nuts, such as peanuts, are a good source of choline. Body cells also produce choline.

Upper Level for Choline

The Upper Level for adults is 3.5 grams per day. This is based on development of a fishy body odor and low blood pressure at excessive intakes.

8.18 Vitamin-Like Compounds

A variety of vitamin-like compounds are found in the body. These include the following:

- Carnitine, needed to transport fatty acids into cell mitochondria
- Inositol, part of cell membranes

Food Sources of Choline

Food Item and Amount	Choline (milligrams)	Adult Male AI=550 milligrams %AI	Adult Female AI=425 milligrams %AI
AI	425-550	100%	100%
Egg, 1 each	126	23%	30%
Cod, 3 ounces	70	13%	16%
Chicken, 3 ounces	56	10%	13%
Fat-free milk, 1 cup	37	7%	9%
Beef, 3 ounces	36	7%	8%
Yogurt, 1 cup	31	6%	7%
Wheat germ, 2 tablespoons	21	4%	5%
Peanut butter, 2 tablespoons	20	4%	5%
Cottage cheese, ½ cup	20	4%	5%

Key:
■ Grains
■ Vegetables
■ Fruits
■ Dairy
■ Protein

FIGURE 8-34 ▶ Food sources of choline compared to the Adequate Intake for adult males and females.

- Taurine, part of bile acids
- Lipoic acid, which participates in carbohydrate metabolism and acts as an antioxidant

These vitamin-like compounds can be synthesized by cells using common building blocks, such as amino acids and glucose. Our diets are also a source. In disease states or periods of active growth, synthesis of vitamin-like compounds may not meet needs, so dietary intake can be crucial. The needs for vitamin-like compounds in certain groups of individuals, such as for preterm infants, are being investigated. Although promoted and sold by health-food stores, these vitamin-like compounds need not be included in the diet of the average healthy adult.

Table 8-3 summarizes much of what we know about the water-soluble vitamins. Now that you have studied the vitamins, review MyPlate and note how each food group can make an important vitamin contribution (Fig. 8-35).

Figure 8-36 summarizes much of what we have covered about the functions of the fat-soluble and water-soluble vitamins. Many vitamins work together for a common purpose.

TABLE 8-3 Summary of the Water-Soluble Vitamins and Choline

Vitamin	Major Functions	RDA or Adequate Intake	Dietary Sources*	Deficiency Symptoms	Toxicity Symptoms
Thiamin	• Coenzyme of carbohydrate metabolism • Nerve function	1.1–1.2 milligrams	• Sunflower seeds • Pork • Whole and enriched grains • Dried beans • Peas	*Beriberi* • Nervous tingling • Poor coordination • Edema • Heart changes • Weakness	None
Riboflavin†	• Coenzyme of carbohydrate metabolism	1.1–1.3 milligrams	• Milk • Mushrooms • Spinach • Liver • Enriched grains	• Inflammation of the mouth and tongue • Cracks at the corners of the mouth • Eye disorders	None
Niacin	• Coenzyme of energy metabolism • Coenzyme of fat synthesis • Coenzyme of fat breakdown	14–16 milligrams (niacin equivalents)	• Mushrooms • Bran • Tuna • Salmon • Chicken • Beef • Liver • Peanuts • Enriched grains	*Pellagra* • Diarrhea • Dermatitis • Dementia • Death	Upper Level is 35 milligrams from supplements, based on flushing of skin
Pantothenic acid	• Coenzyme of energy metabolism • Coenzyme of fat synthesis • Coenzyme of fat breakdown	5 milligrams	• Mushrooms • Liver • Broccoli • Eggs *Most foods have some*	• No natural deficiency disease or symptoms	None
Biotin	• Coenzyme of glucose production • Coenzyme of fat synthesis	30 micrograms	• Cheese • Egg yolks • Cauliflower • Peanut butter • Liver	• Dermatitis • Tongue soreness • Anemia • Depression	Unknown

Vitamin	Major Functions	RDA or Adequate Intake	Dietary Sources*	Deficiency Symptoms	Toxicity Symptoms
Vitamin B-6†	• Coenzyme of protein metabolism • Neurotransmitter synthesis • Hemogloblin synthesis *Many other functions*	1.3–1.7 milligrams	• Animal protein foods • Spinach • Broccoli • Bananas • Salmon • Sunflower seeds	• Headache • Anemia • Convulsions • Nausea • Vomiting • Flaky skin • Sore tongue	Upper Level is 100 milligrams, based on nerve destruction
Folate (folic acid)†	• Coenzyme involved in DNA synthesis *Many other functions*	400 micrograms (dietary folate equivalents)	• Green leafy vegetables • Orange juice • Organ meats • Sprouts • Sunflower seeds	• Megaloblastic anemia • Inflammation of tongue • Diarrhea • Poor growth • Depression	None likely Upper Level for adults set at 1000 micrograms for synthetic folic acid (exclusive of food folate), based on masking of B-12 deficiency
Vitamin B-12†	• Coenzyme of folate metabolism • Nerve function *Many other functions*	2.4 micrograms *Older adults and vegans should use fortified foods or supplements.*	• Animal foods (not natural in plants) • Organ meats • Oysters • Clams • Fortified, ready-to-eat breakfast cereals	• Macrocytic anemia • Poor nerve function	None
Vitamin C	• Connective tissue synthesis • Hormone synthesis • Neurotransmitter synthesis • Possible antioxidant activity	75–90 milligrams *Smokers should add 35 milligrams*	• Citrus fruits • Strawberries • Broccoli • Greens	• Scurvy • Poor wound healing • Pinpoint hemorrhages • Bleeding gums	Upper Level is 2 grams, based on development of diarrhea Can also alter some diagnostic tests
Choline†	• Neurotransmitter synthesis • Phospholipid synthesis	425–550 milligrams	Widely distributed in foods and synthesized by the body	No natural deficiency	Upper Level is 3.5 grams per day based on development of fishy body odor and reduced blood pressure

*Fortified ready-to-eat breakfast cereals are good sources for most of these vitamins and a common source of B vitamins for many of us.

†These nutrients also participate in homocysteine metabolism, which in turn may reduce the risk of developing cardiovascular disease.

FIGURE 8-35 ▶ Certain groups of MyPlate are especially rich sources of various vitamins and choline. This is true for those listed. Each may be also found in other groups on the plate but in lower amounts. Pantothenic acid is also present in moderate amounts in many groups.

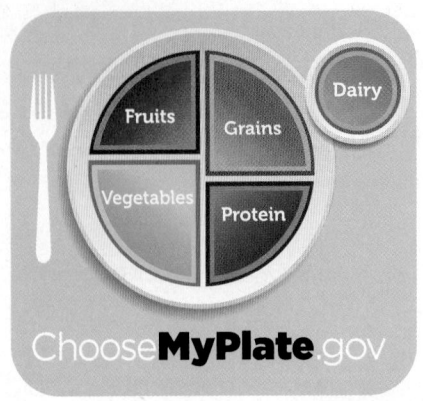

MyPlate: Sources of Vitamins and Choline

Grains	Vegetables	Fruits	Dairy	Protein
• Thiamin	• Vitamin A	• Vitamin A	• Vitamin D	• Thiamin
• Riboflavin	• Vitamin K	• Vitamin C	• Riboflavin	• Riboflavin
• Niacin	• Folate		• Vitamin B12	• Niacin
• Folic acid	• Vitamin C		• Choline	• Biotin
				• Vitamin B6
				• Vitamin B12
				• Choline

FIGURE 8-36 ▶ Vitamins and related compounds (e.g., choline) work together to maintain health.

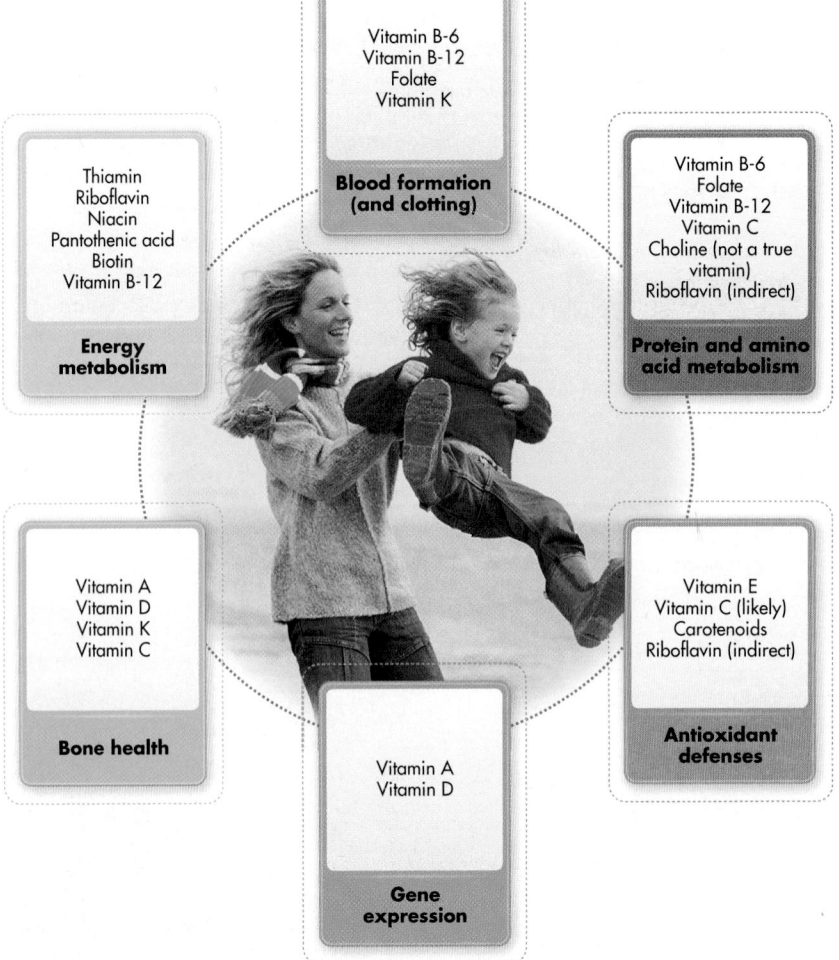

Vitamin B-6
Vitamin B-12
Folate
Vitamin K

Blood formation (and clotting)

Thiamin
Riboflavin
Niacin
Pantothenic acid
Biotin
Vitamin B-12

Energy metabolism

Vitamin B-6
Folate
Vitamin B-12
Vitamin C
Choline (not a true vitamin)
Riboflavin (indirect)

Protein and amino acid metabolism

Vitamin A
Vitamin D
Vitamin K
Vitamin C

Bone health

Vitamin A
Vitamin D

Gene expression

Vitamin E
Vitamin C (likely)
Carotenoids
Riboflavin (indirect)

Antioxidant defenses

Dietary Supplements—
Who Needs Them?

The term *multivitamin and mineral supplement* has been mentioned many times so far in this textbook. Often, these and other supplements are marketed as cures for anything and everything. This cure-all approach is promoted by the supplement industry and countless health-food stores, pharmacies, and supermarkets.

According to the Dietary Supplement Health and Education Act of 1994 (discussed in Chapter 1), a supplement in the United States is a product intended to supplement the diet that contains one or more of the following ingredients:

- A vitamin
- A mineral
- An herb or another botanical
- An amino acid
- A dietary substance to supplement the diet, which could be an extract or a combination of the first four ingredients in this list

The definition is broad and covers a wide variety of nutritional substances. The use of dietary supplements is a common practice among North Americans and generates about $28–29 billion annually for the industry in the United States (Fig. 8-37). Supplements can be sold without proof that they are safe and effective. Unless FDA has evidence that a supplement is inherently dangerous or marketed with an illegal claim, it will not regulate such products closely. (The vitamin folate is an exception.) FDA has limited resources to police supplement manufacturers and has to act against these manufacturers one at a time. Thus, we cannot rely on FDA to protect us from vitamin and mineral supplement overuse and misuse. We bear that responsibility ourselves, with the help of professional advice from a physician or registered dietitian.

The supplement makers can make broad claims about their products under the "structure or function" provision of the law. The products, however, cannot claim to prevent, treat, or cure a disease. Menopause in women and aging are not diseases *per se*, so products alleging to treat symptoms of these conditions can be marketed without FDA approval. For example, a product that claims to treat hot flashes arising during menopause can be sold without any evidence to prove that the product works, but a product that claims to decrease the risk of cardiovascular disease by reducing blood cholesterol must have results from scientific studies that justify the claim.

Why do people take supplements? Frequently given reasons include to:

- Reduce susceptibility to health problems (e.g., colds)
- Prevent heart attacks
- Prevent cancer
- Reduce stress
- Increase "energy"

FIGURE 8-37 ▶
The dietary supplement industry is a growing multibillion dollar business.

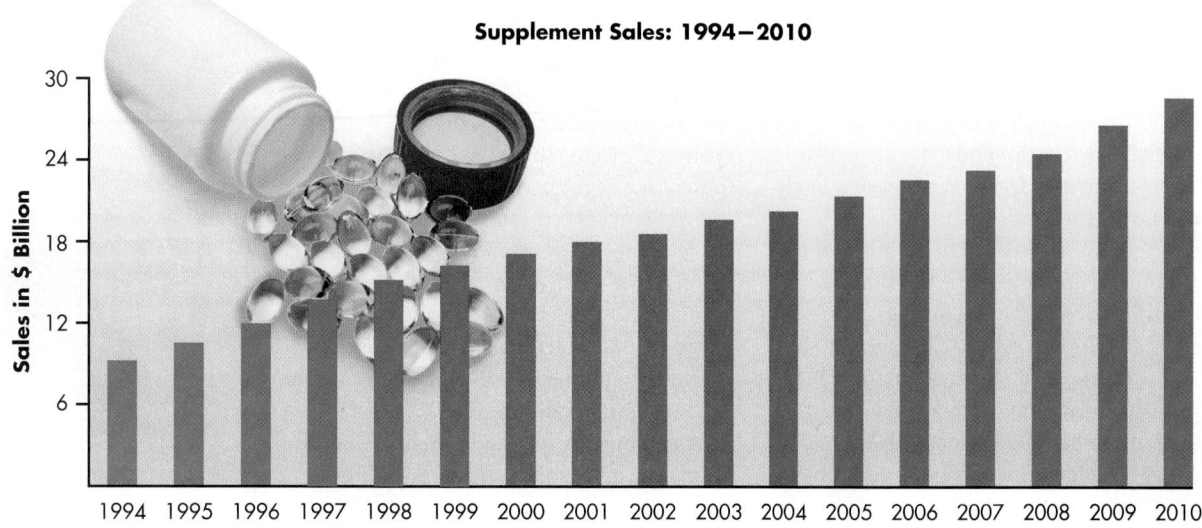

Supplement Sales: 1994–2010

Sales in $ Billion (y-axis: 6, 12, 18, 24, 30)

1994 1995 1996 1997 1998 1999 2000 2001 2002 2003 2004 2005 2006 2007 2008 2009 2010

Should You Take a Supplement?

Opinions vary about the wisdom and safety of supplement use even among knowledgeable scientists. Typically, nutrition scientists have recommended that supplement use is needed only by a few groups (see Further Reading 9). The National Institutes of Health came to the same conclusion, noting there is insufficient evidence to support the recommendation of use of a multivitamin and mineral supplement by the general population. The experts found that only a few studies of vitamins and minerals demonstrate beneficial effects for the prevention of chronic disease, including increased bone mineral density and decreased fractures in postmenopausal women who use calcium and vitamin D supplements. (See the next section in this feature for more specific examples.) In contrast, several other studies provide disturbing evidence of risk, such as increased lung cancer risk with beta-carotene use among smokers. The NIH State-of-the-Science report (see Further Reading 10) concludes that the present evidence is insufficient to recommend either for or against the use of multivitamin/mineral supplements by Americans to prevent chronic disease.

The rationale for widespread use of a multivitamin and mineral supplement is primarily because many North Americans have been unwilling to change their food habits to include the recommended servings of fruits, vegetables, and whole grains. As for individual vitamins, there are specific cases in which supplements are advised. As discussed in Chapter 8, adequate folate status when a woman becomes pregnant helps reduce the risk of certain birth defects in her offspring (400 micrograms per day of synthetic folic acid is recommended). Folate also limits homocysteine in the blood, a likely risk factor for cardiovascular disease that can affect all of us. In addition, the committee appointed by the Food and Nutrition Board that set current nutrient standards for vitamin B-12 suggested that adults over age 50 consume vitamin B-12 in a synthetic form, such as that added to ready-to-eat breakfast cereals or present in supplements. Synthetic vitamin B-12 is more easily absorbed than that found in food; this helps compensate for the fall in vitamin B-12 absorption often seen in one's older years.

Whether experts support use of a multivitamin and mineral supplement or not, they all emphasize that many of the health-promoting effects of foods cannot be found in a bottle. Recall the discussions of phytochemicals in Chapter 2 and the benefits of fiber in Chapter 4. Few or no phytochemicals and no fiber are present in supplements. Multivitamin and mineral supplements also contain little calcium to keep the pill size small, and the oxide forms of magnesium, zinc, and copper used in many supplements are not as well absorbed as forms found in foods.

Overall, supplement use cannot fix a poor diet in all respects. Uninformed megadose supplement use also can lead to harm—most cases of nutrient toxicity are a result of supplement use. Thus, we are advised to first take a good look at our dietary habits and then improve them, as outlined in Chapter 2 (Fig. 8-38). Then we should find out which nutrient gaps remain, and identify food sources that can help. Such a source could be ready-to-eat breakfast cereals to increase vitamin E, folic acid, and vitamin B-6 intake, and as well provide highly absorbable forms of vitamin B-12. Calcium-fortified orange juice could be used to increase calcium intake, or milk and yogurt to increase vitamin D and calcium intake. You need to be careful of highly fortified foods, however, as these products may provide the appropriate amount of nutrients in 1 serving, but the typical consumer may eat more than 1 serving. This can lead to an excessive intake of some nutrients, such as vitamin A, iron, and synthetic folic acid.

If supplement use is desired, you should discuss this practice with a physician or registered dietitian, as some supplements can interfere with certain medicines. For example, high intakes of vitamin K or vitamin E alter the action of anticlotting medications. Vitamin B-6 can offset the action of L-dopa (used in treating Parkinson's disease). Large doses of vitamin C can interfere with certain cancer therapy regimens, excessive zinc intake can inhibit copper absorption.

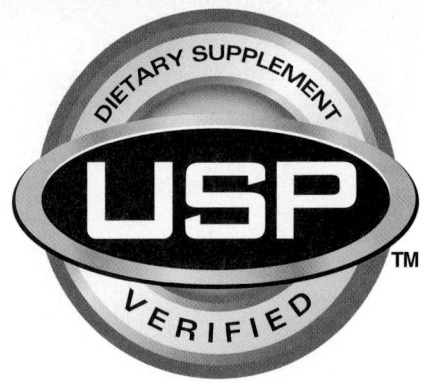

▲ The USP (United States Pharmacopeia) label indicates the product meets USP standards.

▶ Because research on a variety of nutrient supplements has revealed a lack of product quality, FDA now requires supplement makers to test the purity, strength, and composition of all their products. The USP (United States Pharmacopeia) designation, which has been extended to an increasing number of nutrient supplements, establishes professionally accepted standards for these products and can be used to evaluate supplements. The USP standards designate strength, quality, purity, packaging, labeling, speed of dissolution, and acceptable length of storage of ingredients for drugs.

Top Five Dietary Supplements in 2010:

1. Fish/Oil
2. Multivitamins
3. Vitamin D
4. Calcium
5. Coenzyme Q

Source: www.Consumerlab.com

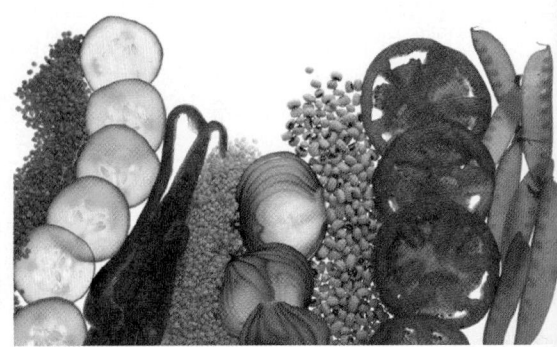

▲ Focus first on foods that meet nutrient needs.

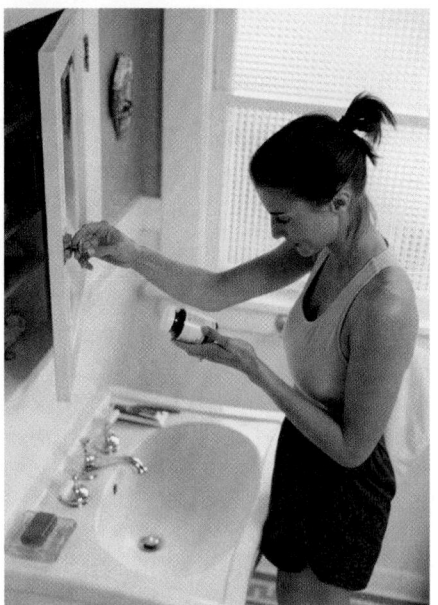

▲ Long-term intake of just three times the Daily Value for some fat-soluble vitamins—particularly preformed vitamin A—can cause toxic effects. Know what you are taking if you use supplements.

Healthy Diet Rich in Vitamins and Minerals

↓

Fortified Foods

↓

Possible Multivitamin and Mineral Supplement Use

↓

Individual Supplements in Some Cases

FIGURE 8-38 ▶ Supplement savvy—an approach to the use of nutrient supplementation. Emphasizing a healthy diet rich in vitamins and minerals is always the first option.

CRITICAL THINKING

Believing that supplements provide the nutrition her body needs, Janice regularly takes numerous supplements while paying relatively little attention to daily food choices. How would you explain to her that this practice may lead to health problems?

Large amounts of folate can mask signs and symptoms of a vitamin B-12 deficiency (review the section on toxicity of folate in this chapter). Remember, you *can* get too much of a good thing.

People Most Likely to Need Supplements

As you might guess, generally the people who take supplements in our society are already healthy. Various medical and health-related organizations suggest that the following vitamin and mineral supplements can be important for certain groups of healthy people:

- Women of childbearing age may need extra synthetic folic acid if their dietary patterns do not supply the recommended amount (400 micrograms).
- Women with excessive bleeding during menstruation may need extra iron.
- Women who are pregnant or breast-feeding may need extra iron, folate, and calcium.
- People with low calorie intakes (less than about 1200 kcal per day) may need a range of vitamins and minerals. This is true of some women and many older people.
- Strict vegans may need extra calcium, iron, zinc, and vitamin B-12.
- Newborns need a single dose of vitamin K, as directed by a physician.
- Some older infants may need fluoride supplements, as directed by a dentist.
- People with limited milk intake and sunlight exposure may need extra vitamin D. This includes breastfed infants and many African-American and older people.
- People with lactose maldigestion or lactose intolerance, and those with allergies to dairy products, may need extra calcium.
- Adults over age 50 may need a synthetic source of vitamin B-12.
- People on low-fat diets or diets low in plant oils and nuts may need some extra vitamin E.
- People who consume a large part of their diet as refined foods rather than as fruits, vegetables, or whole grains may need a range of vitamins and minerals.

Individuals with certain medical conditions (e.g., vitamin-resistant diseases or longstanding fat malabsorption) and those who use certain medications also may require supplementation with specific vitamins and minerals. Children who are "picky eaters" may require supplementation as well (see Chapter 15). Finally, smokers and alcohol abusers may benefit from supplementation, but cessation of these two activities is far more beneficial than any supplementation.

Which Supplement Should You Choose?

If you decide to take a multivitamin and mineral supplement, which one should you choose? As a start, choose a nationally recognized brand (from a supermarket or pharmacy) that contains about 100% of the Daily Values for the nutrients present. A multivitamin and mineral supplement should generally be taken with or just after meals to maximize absorption. Make sure also that intake from the total of this supplement, any other supplements used, and highly fortified foods (such as ready-to-eat breakfast cereals) provide no more than the Upper Level for each vitamin and mineral. (See the inside cover of this text book for Upper Levels.) This is especially important with regard to preformed vitamin A intake. Two exceptions are (1) both men and older women should make sure any product used is low in iron or iron-free to avoid possible iron overload (see Chapter 9 for details), and (2) somewhat exceeding the Upper Level for vitamin D is likely a safe practice for adults. One should read the labels carefully to be sure of what is being taken (Fig. 8-39).

Another consideration in choosing a supplement is avoiding superfluous ingredients, such as para-aminobenzoic acid (PABA), hesperidin complex, inositol, bee pollen, and lecithins. These are not needed in our diets. They are especially common in expensive supplements sold in health-food stores and by mail. In addition, use of l-tryptophan and high doses of beta-carotene or fish oils is discouraged.

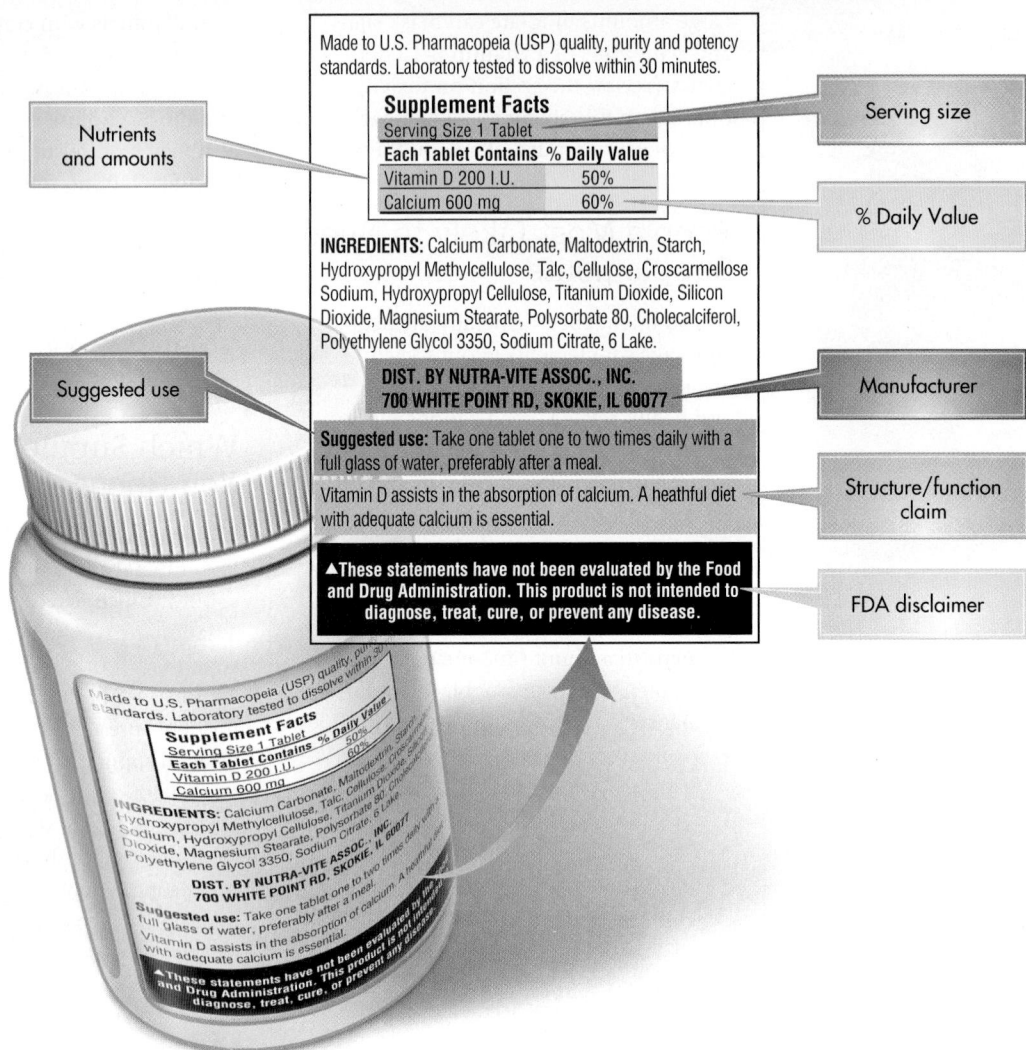

Made to U.S. Pharmacopeia (USP) quality, purity and potency standards. Laboratory tested to dissolve within 30 minutes.

Supplement Facts
Serving Size 1 Tablet

Each Tablet Contains	% Daily Value
Vitamin D 200 I.U.	50%
Calcium 600 mg	60%

INGREDIENTS: Calcium Carbonate, Maltodextrin, Starch, Hydroxypropyl Methylcellulose, Talc, Cellulose, Croscarmellose Sodium, Hydroxypropyl Cellulose, Titanium Dioxide, Silicon Dioxide, Magnesium Stearate, Polysorbate 80, Cholecalciferol, Polyethylene Glycol 3350, Sodium Citrate, 6 Lake.

DIST. BY NUTRA-VITE ASSOC., INC.
700 WHITE POINT RD, SKOKIE, IL 60077

Suggested use: Take one tablet one to two times daily with a full glass of water, preferably after a meal.

Vitamin D assists in the absorption of calcium. A heathful diet with adequate calcium is essential.

▲**These statements have not been evaluated by the Food and Drug Administration. This product is not intended to diagnose, treat, cure, or prevent any disease.**

Nutrients and amounts

Suggested use

Serving size

% Daily Value

Manufacturer

Structure/function claim

FDA disclaimer

FIGURE 8-39 ▶ Nutrient supplements display a nutrition label different from that of foods. This Supplement Facts label must list the ingredient(s), amount(s) per serving, serving size, suggested use, and % Daily Value if one has been established. This label also includes structure/function claims. Thus, it also must include the FDA warning that these claims have not been evaluated by the agency.

Six websites to help you evaluate ongoing claims and evaluate safety of supplements are:

www.acsh.org
www.quackwatch.com
www.ncahf.org
http://ods.od.nih.gov
www.eatright.org
www.usp.org/USPVerified/dietarySupplements/

These sites are maintained by groups or individuals committed to providing reasoned and authoritative nutrition and health advice to consumers. See Further Reading 1 for more advice on nutrient supplementation.

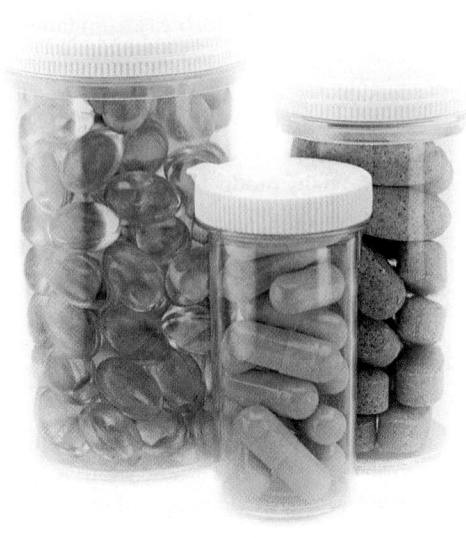

◀ The regular use of individual nutrient supplements could lead to health risks. These should be used with caution.

Food source — Choline
Function — dofi Biotin   Summary, Concept Check, 1st para lin!

Chapter 8: Vitamins   **339**

Case Study Choosing a Dietary Supplement

Amy works the "pre-dawn" shift as a baker at a popular bistro. Amy is also a full-time student, and the combination of taking a full course load at college and working early hours while her friends are sleeping has created a lot of stress for her. Amy's many commitments also make it important that she not become ill. Recently one of her coworkers suggested that she take *Nutramega* supplements to help prevent colds, flu, and other illnesses. The product's label suggests that *Nutramega* helps prevent such problems, especially those associated with the changing of seasons. The label recommends taking two to three tablets daily for health maintenance and two to three tablets every 3 hours at the first sign of feeling ill. Amy looks at the Supplement Facts label on the bottle and finds that each tablet contains (as percent of the Daily Value): 33% for vitamin A (three-quarters is preformed vitamin A), 700% for vitamin C, 200% for niacin, and 100% for vitamin B-6. A month's supply costs about $50.

Answer the following questions, and check your response in Appendix A.

1. Are there any health risks associated with taking the "maintenance" dose of two to three tablets per day? How does this dose compare with the Upper Tolerable Intake Levels for the four nutrients?

2. How many tablets would be taken per day if Amy was feeling ill?
   a. For vitamin A, use the % Daily Value to calculate the micrograms RAE that would be in this larger dose. How does this compare to the Upper Level for Vitamin A?
   b. Use the % Daily Value to calculate the milligrams of vitamin C in this larger dose. How does this compare to the Upper Level for vitamin C?
   c. Use the % Daily Value to calculate the milligrams of niacin in this larger dose. How does this compare to the Upper Level for niacin?
   d. Use the % Daily Value to calculate the micrograms of vitamin B-6 in this larger dose. How does this compare to the Upper Level for vitamin B-6?
   e. Does the recommended dosage of any of these nutrients pose any health risks?

3. Does the cost of this supplement seem reasonable? How does it compare to the

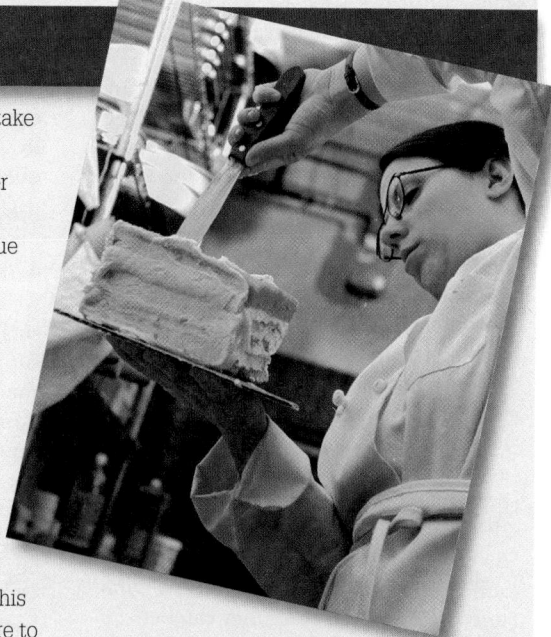

▲ Is a dietary supplement a safe way for Amy to prevent colds and the flu?

cost of a typical multivitamin supplement available at your local drug store?

4. Should Amy be concerned about meeting her nutrient needs? Does the type of stress she is under increase her nutrient needs?

5. After studying Chapter 8, what diet and supplement advice would you offer to Amy?

Summary (Numbers refer to numbered learning outcomes.)

8.1 Vitamins are carbon-containing compounds we generally need daily in small amounts from foods. They yield no energy directly, but many contribute to energy-yielding chemical reactions in the body and promote growth and development. Many vitamins act as coenzymes, which help enzymes function.

8.2 Vitamins A, D, E, and K are fat soluble, whereas the B vitamins, vitamin C and choline are water soluble.

8.3 Vitamin A is a family of compounds that includes several forms of preformed vitamin A. Three forms of carotenoids can also yield vitamin A; some also function as antioxidants. Vitamin A contributes to vision, immune function, and cell development. Vitamin D is both a hormone and a vitamin. It can be synthesized in the human body using sunshine and a cholesterol-like substance in the skin. The active hormone form of vitamin D helps regulate blood calcium in part by increasing calcium absorption from the intestine. Infants and children who don't get enough vitamin D may develop rickets, and adults develop osteomalacia. Vitamin E functions primarily as an antioxidant. By donating electrons to electron-seeking, free-radical (oxidizing) compounds, it neutralizes them. This effect shields cell membranes and red blood cells from breakdown. Vitamin K helps blood clot and increases the calcium-binding potential of some organs. Vitamin K is poorly stored in the body, but our dietary intake alone is usually sufficient to meet needs. People who can't

absorb fat well or who are on antibiotics for long periods may need extra vitamin K. Thiamin, riboflavin, and niacin play key roles as coenzymes in energy-yielding reactions. They help metabolize carbohydrates, fats, and proteins. Alcoholism and a poor diet can create deficiencies of these three nutrients, which often show up as symptoms in the brain and nervous system, skin, and GI tract. Pantothenic acid, which participates in many aspects of cell metabolism. Biotin, which participates in glucose production, fatty acid synthesis, and DNA synthesis, can be synthesized by bacteria in the intestine. Vitamin B-6 performs a vital role in protein metabolism, especially in synthesizing nonessential amino acids. It also helps synthesize neurotransmitters and performs other metabolic roles, such as metabolism of homocysteine. Headaches, a form of anemia, nausea, and vomiting result from a B-6 deficiency. Folate plays an important role in DNA synthesis and homocysteine metabolism. Symptoms of a deficiency include generally poor cell division in various areas of the body, megaloblastic anemia, tongue inflammation, diarrhea, and poor growth. Pregnancy puts high demands for folate on the body; deficiency during the first month of pregnancy can result in neural tube defects in offspring. A deficiency can also occur in people with alcoholism. Vitamin B-12 is needed to metabolize folate and homocysteine, and maintain the insulation surrounding nerves. A deficiency results in anemia (because of its relationship to folate) and nerve degeneration. Older people often suffer from inefficient absorption of vitamin B-12, in which case they can benefit from monthly injections or megadoses of the vitamin. Vitamin C is mainly used to synthesize collagen, a major protein for building connective tissue. A vitamin C deficiency results in scurvy, evidenced by poor wound healing, pinpoint hemorrhages in the skin, and bleeding gums. Vitamin C also modestly enhances iron absorption, is likely a general antioxidant, and is needed for synthesizing some hormones and neurotransmitters. Deficiencies can occur in people with alcoholism and those whose diets lack sufficient fruits and vegetables. Smoking makes matters worse for people already at risk. Choline is used to form a neurotransmitter, and has other functions, including a role in homocysteine metabolism. Nutritional needs have recently been set. No natural deficiency of choline has been reported. The vitamin-like compounds carnitine, inositol, taurine, and lipoic acid, while participating in many important chemical reactions in the body, are not true vitamins because they can be synthesized in the body from readily available building blocks; they are also obtained from the diet.

8.4 Vitamin A is found in liver and fish oils; carotenoids are especially plentiful in dark green and orange vegetables. If we don't spend enough time in the sun, such foods as fish and fortified milk can supply vitamin D. Older people, African-Americans, and breastfed infants often need a supplemental source. Vitamin E is found in plant oils. Claims are made about the curative powers of vitamin E, but more information is needed before megadose vitamin E recommendations for healthy adults can be made with certainty. Some vitamin K absorbed each day comes from bacterial synthesis in the intestine, but most comes from foods, primarily green, leafy vegetables. Enriched grain products are common sources of thiamin, riboflavin, and niacin. Pantothenic acid is widely distributed among foods. Biotin comes from foods such as eggs, peanuts, and cheese. Regular consumption of animal protein foods and rich plant sources such as broccoli provide needed vitamin B-6. Food sources of folate are leafy vegetables, organ meats, and orange juice. Women of child-bearing age need to meet the RDA with synthetic folic acid. Great amounts of folate can be lost in prolonged cooking. Generally, a dietary deficiency is unlikely because vitamin B-12 is highly concentrated in animal foods, which constitute a major part of the North American diet. Vitamin B-12 does not occur naturally in plant foods. Vegans need a supplemental source, and adults over age 50 should consume a synthetic source, such as that in ready-to-eat breakfast cereals. Fresh fruits and vegetables, especially citrus fruits, are generally good sources. A great amount of vitamin C is lost in cooking, so a diet should emphasize fresh or lightly cooked vegetables. Choline is a dietary component available from a wide variety of foods and is synthesized in the body.

8.5 Vitamin A can be toxic, even when taken at just 3 times the RDA for preformed vitamin A (the Upper Level). High vitamin A intakes are especially dangerous during pregnancy. Vitamin D is potentially a toxic substance in infancy and early childhood. The Upper Level for vitamin E is set at about 50 times adult needs. Niacin has an Upper Level (2.5 times adult needs). Taking high doses of vitamin B-6 causes damage to the nervous system. The Upper Level is about 60 times adult needs. Excess folate in the diet can mask a vitamin B-12 deficiency, so an Upper Level has been set at 2½ times adult needs (refers to synthetic folic acid only). The Upper Level of vitamin C is set at about 20 times adult needs. The Upper Level of choline is set at about eight times adult needs.

N&YH Taking a multivitamin and mineral supplement to help meet nutrient needs is recommended by some experts, while other experts suggest that only some in the population need such supplementation. Taking many nutrient supplements can lead to nutrient-related toxicity, so any such use should be carefully considered. The clearest evidence is for a diet rich in fruits and vegetables and whole-grain breads and cereals, not reliance on supplements.

Check Your Knowledge (Answers to the following questions are below.)

1. Vitamins are classified as
   a. organic and inorganic.
   b. fat-soluble and water-soluble.
   c. essential and nonessential.
   d. elements and compounds.

2. Vitamin D is called the sunshine vitamin because
   a. it is available in orange juice.
   b. exposure to sunlight converts a precursor to vitamin D.
   c. it can be destroyed by exposure to sunlight.
   d. All of the above.

3. Vitamin E functions as
   a. a coenzyme.
   b. an antioxidant.
   c. a hormone.
   d. a peroxide.

4. A deficiency of vitamin A can lead to the disease called
   a. xerophthalmia.
   b. osteomalacia.
   c. scurvy.
   d. pellagra.

5. A high intake of vitamin E can
   a. inhibit vitamin K metabolism.
   b. lead to lead poisoning.
   c. inhibit copper absorption.
   d. cause baldness.

6. A vitamin synthesized by bacteria in the intestine is
   a. A.
   b. D.
   c. E.
   d. K.

7. Bowed legs, an enlarged and misshapen head, and enlarged knee joints in children are all symptoms of
   a. rickets.
   b. xerophthalmia.
   c. osteoporosis.
   d. vitamin D toxicity.

8. Thiamin, riboflavin, and niacin are called the "energy" vitamins because they
   a. can be broken down to provide energy.

   b. are coenzymes needed for release of energy from carbohydrates, fats, and proteins.
   c. are ingredients in energy drinks such as Powerade.
   d. are needed in large amounts by competitive athletes.

9. A deficient intake of _____ has been shown to increase the risk of having a baby with a neural tube defect such as spina bifida.
   a. vitamin A
   b. vitamin C
   c. vitamin E
   d. folic acid

10. Vitamin C is necessary for the production of
    a. stomach acid.
    b. collagen.
    c. hormones.
    d. clotting factors.

Answers: 1.b (LO 8.1), 2.b (LO 8.4), 3.b (LO 8.3), 4.a (LO 8.3), 5.a (LO 8.5), 6.d (LO 8.4), 7.a (LO 8.3), 8.b (LO 8.3), 9.d (LO 8.3), 10.b (LO 8.3)

Study Questions (Numbers refer to Learning Outcomes)

1. Why is the risk of toxicity greater with the fat-soluble vitamins A and D than with water-soluble vitamins in general? **(LO 8.2)**

2. How would you determine which fruits and vegetables displayed in the produce section of your supermarket are likely to provide plenty of carotenoids? **(LO 8.4)**

3. What is the primary function of the vitamin D hormone? Which groups of people likely need to supplement their diets with vitamin D, and on what do you base your answer? **(LO 8.3)**

4. Describe how vitamin E functions as an antioxidant. Use the term *free radical* **(LO 8.3)**

5. Describe how the RDA, Daily Value, and Upper Level for vitamin B-6 should be used in everyday life. How do the RDA and Daily Value for vitamin B-6 differ? **(LO 8.4)**

6. The need for certain vitamins increases as energy expenditure increases. Name two such vitamins and explain why this is the case. **(LO 8.3)**

7. Take one of the B vitamins that might be low in the North American diet and explain why a deficiency might occur. **(LO 8.3)**

8. Which vitamins are lost from cereal grains as a result of the "refining" process? Which vitamins must be replaced

by law in the subsequent enrichment process? **(LO 8.4)**

9. Why does FDA limit the amount of folate that may be included in supplements and fortified foods? **(LO 8.4)**

10. Is it necessary for North Americans to consume a great excess of vitamin C to avoid the possibility of a deficiency? Do vitamin C intakes well above the RDA have any negative consequences? **(LO 8.5)**

What Would You Choose Recommendations

Folate is especially important during pregnancy because it is required for DNA synthesis. During pregnancy, folate needs increase from 400 to 600 micrograms per day. Obstetricians typically prescribe prenatal vitamins that contain 800 micrograms of folic acid, but good food sources of folate have benefits besides the nutrient itself, such as phytochemicals and fiber.

Meats and other animal products are not particularly good sources of folate. Dairy foods do contribute some—your low-fat yogurt supplies about 27 micrograms of folate per 1-cup container. Other dairy products, such as skim milk, provide about 12 micrograms of folate. To find more folate, seek out plant sources.

Lentils and other dried beans are among the richest sources of folate. A 1/2-cup serving of cooked lentils provides about 179 micrograms of folate. Beans are also great sources of other nutrients that are typically low in American diets, such as fiber, potassium, magnesium. Plus, they are low in fat and cholesterol-free.

Spinach and other leafy green vegetables are excellent sources of folate. Two cups of fresh, chopped spinach provide 116 micrograms of folate. Half a cup of sliced strawberries adds an additional 20 micrograms, so this delicious spinach salad supplies almost 25% of the RDA for folate during pregnancy. Even with 1 tablespoon of low-fat vinaigrette, this salad is a very nutrient-dense source of folate (recall Chapter 2): 136 micrograms folate compared to only 50 kcal. Cooked spinach (as presented in Figure 8-28) is an even more concentrated source of folate because greens cook down to a smaller volume, so you are actually consuming more vegetables per cup.

Recall that grain products, such as the whole-wheat bread in your turkey sandwich, are fortified with folic acid. Fortified breakfast cereals are a fabulous source of synthetic folic acid. One cup of Oatmeal Squares cereal contains 400 micrograms (100% of the DV) of folic acid in one serving! Also, the synthetic folic acid incorporated into fortified foods is more bioavailable than natural sources of folate. During pregnancy—or any life stage—a fortified, whole-grain, ready-to-eat breakfast cereal is an excellent way to start the day.

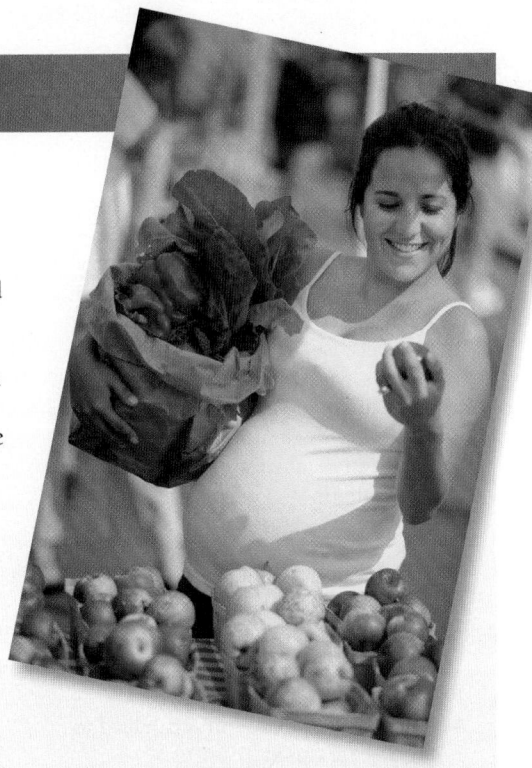

▲ Spinach and other leafy green vegetables are excellent sources of folate. Your next choice—should you decorate the nursery pink or blue?

Further Readings

1. ADA Reports: Position of the American Dietetic Association: Nutrient supplementation. *Journal of the American Dietetic Association* 109:2073, 2009.
   The best nutrition-based strategy for promoting optimal health and reducing the risk of chronic disease is to wisely choose a wide variety of foods. Additional nutrients and/or supplements can help some people meet their nutritional needs as set by science-based nutrition standards (e.g., the Dietary Reference Intakes).

2. Andres E and others: Food-cobalamin malabsorption in elderly patients: Clinical manifestations and treatments. *American Journal of Medicine* 118:1154, 2005.
   About 15% of older adults show defective vitamin B-12 absorption. This condition especially affects absorption of the vitamin B-12 found naturally in foods. Consumption of crystalline vitamin B-12 in contrast is not so affected and was found to be a useful form of therapy for the older adults in this study.

3. DeWals P and others: Reduction in neural tube defects after folic acid fortification in Canada. *New England Journal of Medicine* 357:135, 2007.
   Changes in the prevalence of neural tube defects were assessed in Canada before and after food fortification of cereal products with folic acid became mandatory in 1998. A 46% reduction in the prevalence of neural tube defects occurred during the full-fortification period, with a decrease from 1.58 per 1000 births before fortification to 0.86 per 1000 births after fortification. The reduction rate was greater for spina bifida (a decrease of 53%) than for anencephaly and encephalocele (decreases of 38% and 31%, respectively).

4. Garland CF and others: Vitamin D and prevention of breast cancer: Pooled analysis. *Journal of Steroid Biochemistry & Molecular Biology* 103:708, 2007.
   This review of all studies reported risk of breast cancer and assessed the dose-response association between serum 25(OH)D and risk of breast cancer. The conclusion of this review is that daily intake of 2000 IU of Vitamin D3, and, when possible, very moderate exposure to sunlight, could raise serum 25(OH)D to 52 ng/ml, a level associated with reduction by 50% in incidence of breast cancer, according to observational studies.

5. Giovannucci E and others: 25-Hydroxyvitamin D and risk of myocardial infarction in men: A prospective study. *Archives Internal Medicine* 168:1174, 2008.
   Vitamin D deficiency is thought to be involved in the development of atherosclerosis and coronary heart disease in humans. This study found men 40 to 75 years of age with vitamin D levels

below normal had a higher risk of heart attack even after controlling for factors known to be associated with coronary artery disease. Even men with intermediate vitamin D levels were at elevated risk of heart disease relative to those with sufficient vitamin D levels.

6. Gordon CM and others: Prevalence of vitamin D deficiency among healthy infants and toddlers. *Archives of Pediatric and Adolescent Medicine* 162:505, 2008.

   The prevalence of vitamin D deficiency was determined and 25-hydroxyvitamin D concentration was examined as a function of skin pigmentation, season, sun exposure, breastfeeding, and vitamin D supplementation. Suboptimal vitamin D status was common among otherwise healthy young children with 40% of infants and toddlers testing below average for vitamin D. One-third of the vitamin D deficient infant and toddlers exhibited demineralization a hallmark of the deleterious skeletal effects of this condition.

7. Holick MF: Vitamin D deficiency. *New England Journal of Medicine* 357:266, 2007.

   This is a review of numerous studies that have shown that vitamin D does more than just enhance bone health in children and adults. Studies show that vitamin D deficiency in adults has been linked to an increased risk for osteoporosis and osteomalacia but also certain cancers.

8. Lee I and others: Vitamin E in the primary prevention of cardiovascular disease and cancer: The women's health study: A randomized controlled trial. *Journal of the American Medical Association* 294:56, 2005.

   The data from this large trial indicated that 600 IU of natural-source vitamin E taken every other day provided no overall benefit for major cardiovascular events or cancer. These data do not support recommending vitamin E supplementation for cardiovascular disease or cancer prevention among healthy women, but more research is warranted, because a decrease in sudden cardiac death was seen in a subset of older women in this study.

9. Lichtenstein AH, Russell RM: Essential nutrients: Food or supplements? Where should the emphasis be? *Journal of the American Medical Association* 294:351, 2005.

   There is insufficient evidence to justify a shift in public health policy from one that emphasizes a food-based diet to fulfill nutrient requirements and promote optimal health to one that emphasizes dietary supplementation. Targeted nutrient supplementation is appropriate in some cases, however, as reviewed by these authors.

10. NIH State-of-the-Science Conference Statement on Multivitamin/Mineral Supplements and Chronic Disease Prevention. *NIH consensus State-of-the-Science Statements* 23(2):1, 2006.

    Use of multivitamins/minerals (MVMs) has grown rapidly over the past several decades. Due in part to the fortification of foods, there is still insufficient knowledge about the actual amount of total nutrients that Americans consume from diet and supplements. The cumulative effects of supplementation and fortification have raised safety concerns about exceeding upper levels. Most studies do not provide strong evidence for beneficial health-related effects of supplements taken singly, in pairs, or in combinations of three or more. Although there is encouraging evidence of increased bone mineral density and decreased fractures in postmenopausal women who use calcium and vitamin D supplements, several other studies provide disturbing evidence of risk, such as increased lung cancer risk with beta-carotene use among smokers. The present evidence is insufficient to recommend either for or against the use of MVMs by the American public to prevent chronic disease.

11. Nield LS and others: Rickets: Not a disease of the past. *American Family Physician* 74(4), 200:619, 2006.

    This review article emphasizes the current need to screen for rickets even in developed countries. Background and support is given for the recent recommendation by the American Academy of Pediatrics (AAP) to provide a daily vitamin D supplement for all solely breastfed babies beginning in the first 2 months of life. Until recently, vitamin D supplementation was not advised for breastfed infants. Multiple case reports of nutritional rickets in the United States have promoted the AAP recommendation.

12. Sesso HD and others: Vitamins E and C in the prevention of cardiovascular disease in men. The Physicians' Health Study II Randomized Controlled Trial. *Journal of American Medical Association* 300:2123, 2008.

    Men enrolled in the Physician's Health Study II were placed into four groups, which were given vitamin C and a placebo, vitamin E and a placebo, C and E together, and placebo only. Neither C nor E had an effect on major cardiovascular events, which include heart attacks, stroke, or death. The results suggest that when you pull a nutrient out of the whole diet, you do not see the same effects.

13. Voutilainen S and others: Carotenoids and cardiovascular health. *American Journal of Clinical Nutrition* 83:1265, 2006.

    This report reviews the role of carotenoids in the prevention of heart disease. Although fruit and vegetables are recognized as having protective effects against cardiovascular disease, the role of a single group of compounds such as carotenoids cannot be ascertained. Therefore, the consumption of carotenoids in supplemental forms cannot be recommended.

14. Wang TJ and others: Vitamin D deficiency and risk of cardiovascular disease. *Circulation* 117:503, 2008.

    This study was conducted over 5 years and examined the vitamin D levels in the blood of 1739 people with an average age of 59 years and no prior history of cardiovascular disease. Individuals with low vitamin D levels had a 60% greater risk of cardiac events such as heart attacks and stroke. For people with both a vitamin D deficiency and high blood pressure, the risk for a serious cardiovascular event was doubled. These results are of concern because vitamin D is becoming more common, especially in people living at higher latitudes where vitamin D is less available from exposure to sunlight.

15. Zhang SM and others: Effect of combined folic acid, vitamin B-6, and vitamin B-12 on cancer risk in women: A randomized trial. *Journal of the American Medical Association* 300(17):2012, 2008.

    Use of a combined supplement of folic acid, vitamin B-6, and vitamin B-12 had no significant effect on overall risk of total invasive cancer or breast cancer in a 7-year study of 5442 women. This was the longest-running trial of its kind and occurred at the time that background fortification of the food supply with folic acid had begun.

16. Yaegashi Y and others: Association of hip fracture incidence and intake of calcium, magnesium, vitamin D, and vitamin K. *European Journal of Epidemiology* 23(3):219, 2008.

    An association was found between the dietary intakes of magnesium, vitamin D, and vitamin K and the incidence of hip fractures and osteoporosis in Japanese men and women. The strongest inverse correlation was found between hip fracture incidence and vitamin K intake. It was concluded that vitamin K-2 consumption can aid recovery from hip fracture as well as have potential osteoporosis benefits.

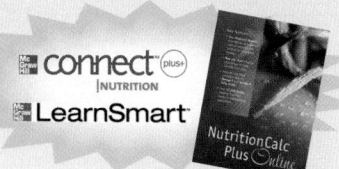

To get the most out of your study of nutrition, go to McGraw-Hill's online resources: Connect www.mcgrawhillconnect.com, **where you will find NutritionCalc Plus, LearnSmart, and many other dynamic tools.**

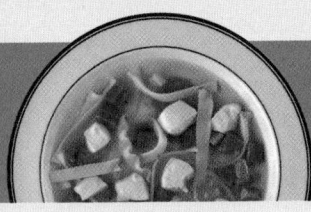

RATE YOUR PLATE

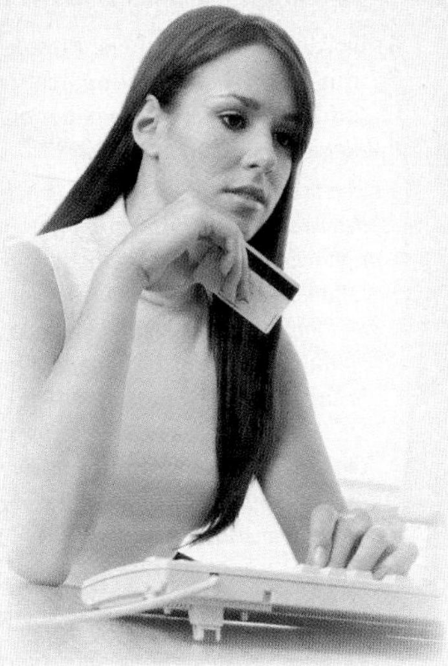

I. Spotting Fraudulent Claims on the Internet

Search for vitamins and vitamin-like substances sold over the Internet. Then write a report concerning any claims made on behalf of these products that you consider fraudulent or misleading. Are the websites selling vitamins, or are they a cover for selling something else? Compare the price of the vitamins from these sites with the price you would pay at the local supermarket or drugstore. Do any of these sites display any disclaimers or warnings about the products?

II. A Closer Look at Supplement Use

With the current popularity of vitamin and mineral supplements, it is more important than ever to understand how to evaluate a supplement. Study the label of a supplement you use or one readily available from a friend or the supermarket. Then answer the following questions.

1. What is the recommended dosage of this supplement?

   _____

   _____

2. Based on the recommended dosage, are there any individual vitamins for which the intake would be greater than 100% of the Daily Value? List these vitamins.

   _____

   _____

3. Are any suggested intakes above the Upper Level for the nutrient?

   _____

   _____

4. Are there any superfluous ingredients, such as herbs or flavors, in the supplement? You can often determine these by looking for ingredients that do not have a percent of Daily Value.

   _____

   _____

5. Does at least 50% of the vitamin A in the product come from beta-carotene or other provitamin A carotenoids (to reduce risk of preformed vitamin A toxicity)?

   _____

   _____

   _____

6. Are there any warnings on the label as to populations who should not consume this product?

   _____

   _____

7. Are there any other signs that tip you off that this product may not be safe?

   _____

   _____

344

Chapter 9 Water and Minerals

Student Learning Outcomes

Chapter 9 is designed to allow you to:

9.1 List and briefly explain the functions of water in the body.

9.2 Discuss healthy water intake and output levels to maintain water balance.

9.3 List safety concerns about our water supply.

9.4 Classify the minerals as major or trace minerals.

9.5 List conditions of the body, dietary factors, and other pertinent relationships that influence the absorption, retention, and availability of specific minerals.

9.6 List key functions and at least two food sources of the major and trace minerals. Identify possible deficiency and toxicity symptoms associated with the major and trace minerals.

9.7 Explain the role of nutrition in maintaining a healthy blood pressure.

9.8 Describe the processes involving minerals that aid in maintaining bone health and preventing osteoporosis.

What Would You Choose?

Water is the best choice for everyday hydration—it quenches thirst without calories. There are currently many "water" choices available. Do you need water that contains vitamins and minerals? What's the difference between spring water and mineral water? Is bottled water safer to drink than tap water? As you peruse the convenience store shelves, which is the healthiest choice to take along to the student recreation center for your workout?

a 20-ounce reusable bottle filled with tap water

b 16.9-ounce bottle of Aquafina® Pure Water

c 16.9-ounce bottle of San Pellegrino Mineral Water

d 20-ounce bottle of vitaminwater®

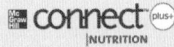 **Think about your choice as you read Chapter 9, then see our recommendations at the end of the chapter. To learn more about water choices, check out the Connect site:** www.mcgrawhillconnect.com

Part Three
Vitamins, Minerals, and Water

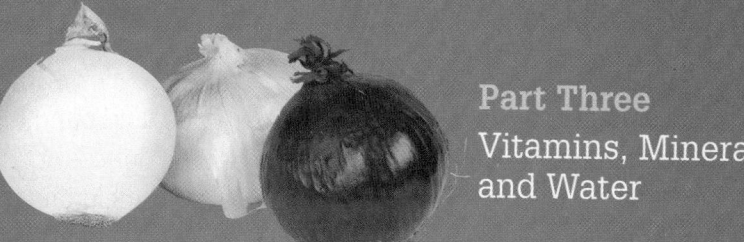

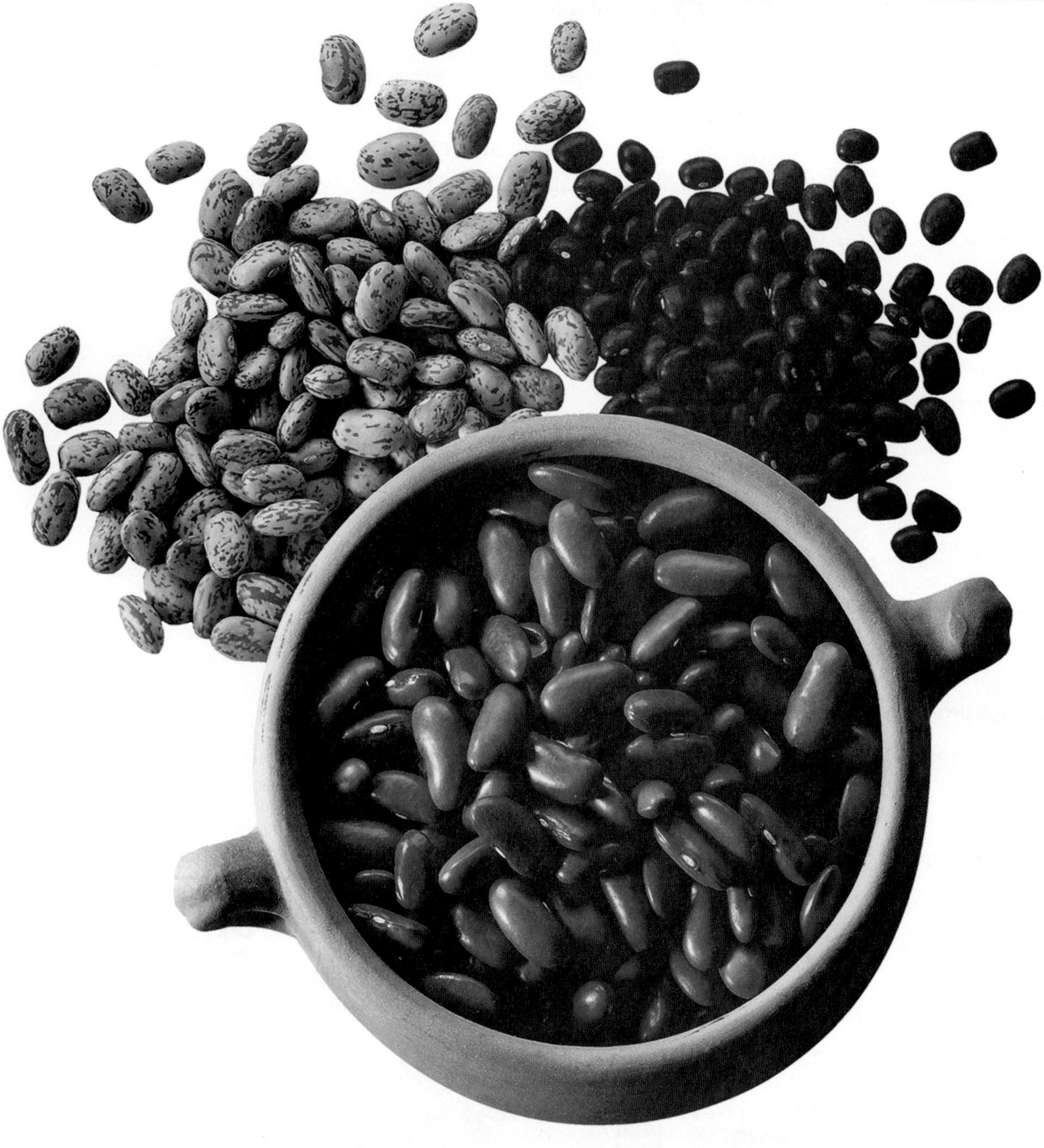

Water—the most versatile medium for a variety of chemical reactions—constitutes the major portion of the human body. Without water, biological processes necessary to life would cease in a matter of days. We must replenish water regularly, as the comic in the chapter suggests, because the body does not store it *per se*. We recognize this constant demand for water as thirst. Recent beverage guidelines recommend a water intake of approximately 50 fluid ounces (1.7 liters) per day, with other beverages totaling about 48 fluid ounces (1.4 liters).

Many nutrients, including minerals, exist in the body dissolved in water. The functions of several minerals are related to the characteristics of water, so water and its roles in the body are explored first in Chapter 9.

Many minerals, like water, are vital to health. They are considered inorganic because they are typically not bonded to carbon atoms. Minerals are key participants in body metabolism, muscle movement, body growth, water balance, and other wide-ranging processes. We also know that some mineral deficiencies can cause severe health problems. For this reason, the study of minerals in Chapter 9 also is critical to understanding human nutrition.

 Refresh Your Memory

As you begin your study of water and minerals in Chapter 9, you may want to review:

- Cell structure and function, digestion and absorption of nutrients, cardiovascular function, immunity, and endocrine function in Chapter 3
- The functions of vitamin D and vitamin K related to calcium and bone health in Chapter 8
- The role of vitamin C in collagen synthesis in Chapter 8

9.1 Water

solvent A liquid substance in which other substances dissolve.

Life as we know it could not exist without water. Acting as a **solvent,** it dissolves many body compounds such as sodium chloride (table salt). Water is the perfect medium for body processes because it enables chemical reactions to occur. Water even participates directly in many of these reactions. It forms the greatest component

FRANK & ERNEST by Bob Thaves

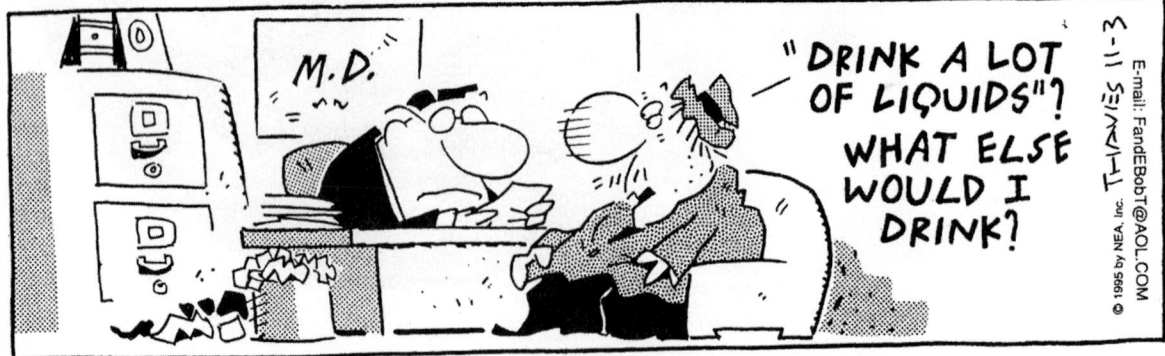

As suggested in the comic, replacing fluids—water as part of foods, beverages, and water itself—is an important daily task. Why is this so critical for maintaining health? And why are infants, athletes, and older adults particularly at risk for dehydration? In addition, how does water interact with some of the minerals used by the body? Chapter 9 provides some answers.

FRANK & ERNEST © Reprinted by permission of Newspaper Enterprise Association, Inc.

of the human body, making up 50% to 70% of the body's weight (about 10 gallons or 40 liters). Lean muscle tissue contains about 73% water. Adipose tissue is about 20% water. Thus, as fat content increases (and the percentage of lean tissue decreases) in the body, total body water content drifts downward toward 50%.

Depending on the amount of fat stores present, an adult can survive for about 8 weeks without eating food but only a few days without drinking water. This occurs not because water is more important than carbohydrate, fat, protein, vitamins, or minerals, but rather because we cannot conserve or store water as well as we can the other components of our diet.

Water in the Body—Intracellular and Extracellular Fluid

Water flows in and out of body cells through cell membranes. Water inside cells forms part of the **intracellular fluid.** When water is outside cells or in the bloodstream, it is part of the **extracellular fluid** (Fig. 9-1). Cell membranes are permeable to water, so water shifts freely in and out of cells. For example, if blood volume decreases, water can move into the bloodstream from the areas inside and around cells to increase blood volume. On the other hand, if blood volume increases, water can shift out of the bloodstream into cells and the surrounding areas, leading to edema (review Fig. 6-8 in Chapter 6).

The body controls the amount of water in the intracellular and extracellular compartments mainly by controlling *ion* movement and concentrations. Ions are minerals that have electrical charges and so are called **electrolytes.** Water is attracted to ions, such as sodium, potassium, chloride, phosphate, magnesium, and calcium. By controlling the movements of ions in and out of the cellular compartments, the body maintains the appropriate amount of water in each compartment using a process called **osmosis.** Overall, where ions go, water follows (Fig. 9-2).

intracellular fluid Fluid contained within a cell; it represents about two-thirds of body fluid.

extracellular fluid Fluid present outside the cells; represents about one-third of body fluid.

electrolytes Substances that separate into ions in water and, in turn, are able to conduct an electrical current. These include sodium, chloride, and potassium.

osmosis The passage of a solvent such as water through a semipermeable membrane from a less concentrated compartment to a more concentrated compartment.

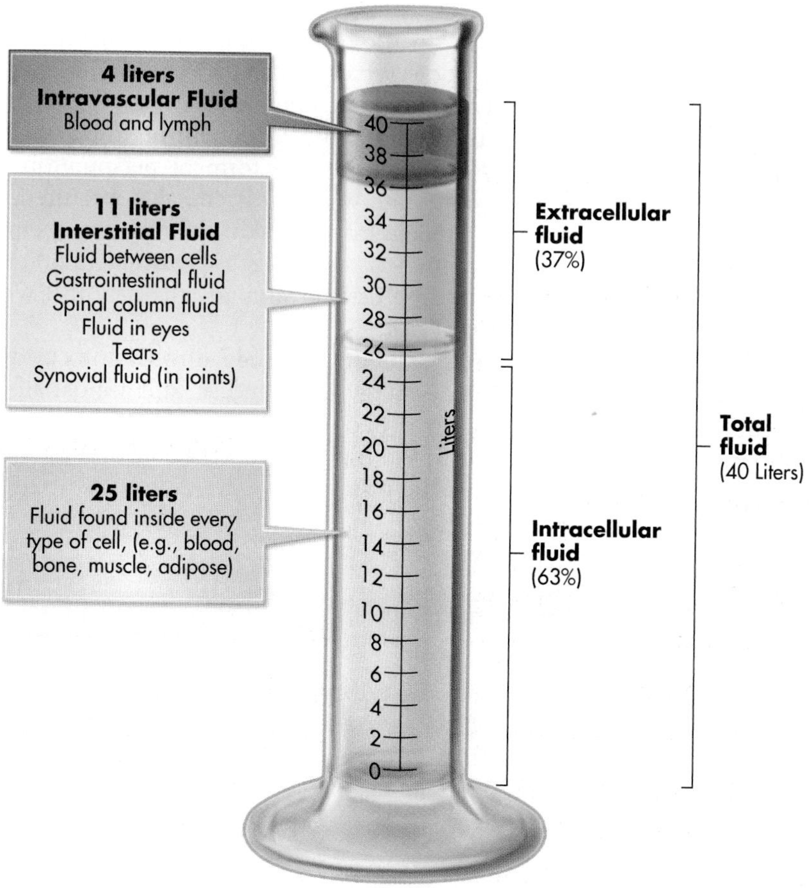

FIGURE 9-1 ▶ Fluid compartments in the body. Total fluid volume is about 10 gallons (40 liters).

FIGURE 9-2 ▶ Effects of various ion concentrations in a fluid on red blood cells. This shows the process of osmosis. Fluid is shifting in and out of the red blood cells in response to changing ion concentrations in the flasks.

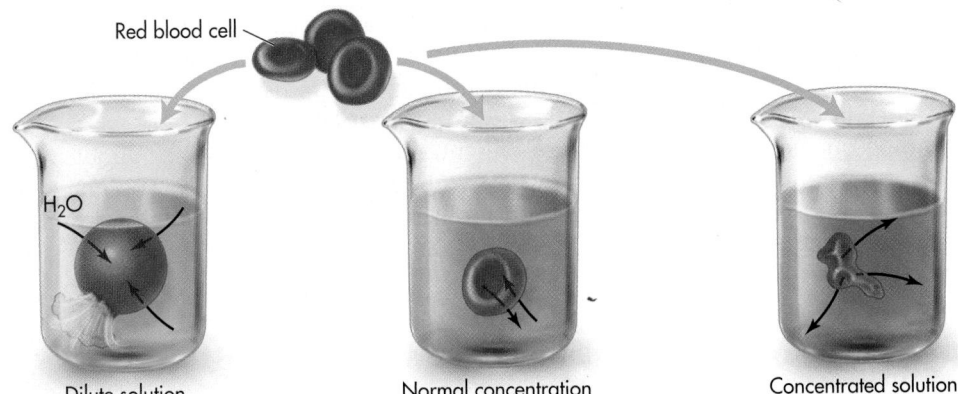

Red blood cell

H₂O

Dilute solution

Normal concentration

Concentrated solution

(a) A dilute solution with a low ion concentration results in swelling (*black arrows*) and subsequent rupture (*puff of red in the lower left part of the cell*) of a red blood cell placed into the solution.

(b) A normal concentration (a concentration of ions outside the cell equal to that inside the cell) results in a typically shaped red blood cell. Water moves into and out of the cell in equilibrium (*black arrows*), but there is no net water movement.

(c) A concentrated solution, with a high ion concentration, causes shrinkage of the red blood cell as water moves out of the cell and into the concentrated solution (*black arrows*).

Positive ions, such as sodium and potassium, end up pairing with negative ions, such as chloride and phosphate. Maintenance of intracellular water volume depends primarily on intracellular potassium and phosphate concentrations. Extracellular water volume depends primarily on the extracellular sodium and chloride concentrations.

Water Contributes to Body Temperature Regulation

Water temperature changes slowly because it has a great ability to hold heat. It takes much more energy to heat water than it does to heat fat. Water molecules are attracted to each other, and it takes much energy to separate them. Because water requires so much energy to change states—for example, from a liquid to a gas in the evaporation of perspiration—it forms an ideal medium for removing heat from the body.

When overheated, the body secretes fluids in the form of perspiration, which evaporates through skin pores. To evaporate water, heat energy is required. So, as perspiration evaporates, heat energy is taken from the skin, cooling it in the process. Each quart (liter) of perspiration evaporated represents approximately 600 kcal of energy lost from the skin and surrounding tissues. Similarly the heat lost when we have a fever increases one's need for calories.

About 60% of the chemical energy in food is turned directly into body heat; the other 40% is converted to forms of energy cells can use, and almost all of that energy eventually leaves the body in the form of heat. If this heat could not be dissipated, the body temperature would rise too high, preventing enzyme systems from functioning efficiently. Perspiration is the primary way to prevent this rise in body temperature.

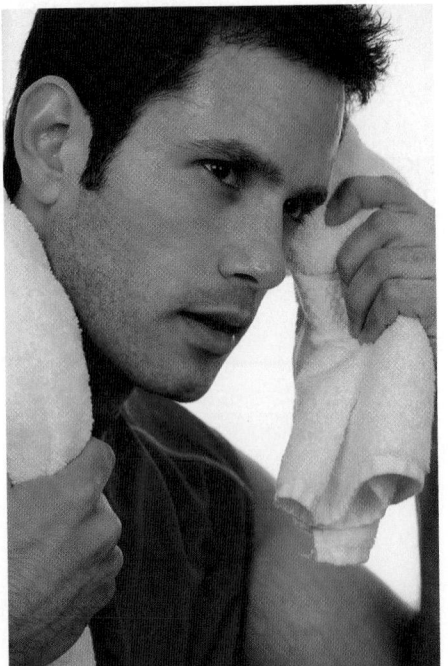

▲ The evaporation of sweat is an important part of temperature regulation.

MAKING DECISIONS

Importance of Perspiration

To cool efficiently, perspiration must be allowed to evaporate. If it simply rolls off the skin or soaks into clothing, perspiration doesn't cool the body as much. Evaporation of perspiration occurs quickly when humidity is low. This is why humans can cool off and therefore tolerate hot, dry climates far better than they do hot, humid climates. This is also why increasing air circulation with a fan cools the body during an exercise workout.

Water Helps Remove Waste Products

Water is an important vehicle for transporting substances throughout the body and for removing waste products from the body. Most unusable substances in the body can dissolve in water and exit the body through the urine.

Urea is a major body waste product. This by-product of protein metabolism contains nitrogen. The more protein we eat in excess of needs, the more nitrogen we remove from amino acids and excrete—in the form of urea—in the urine. Likewise, the more sodium we consume, the more sodium we excrete in the urine. Overall, the amount of urine a person needs to produce is determined primarily by excess protein and salt intake. By limiting excess protein and salt intakes, it is possible to limit urine output—a useful practice, for example, in space flights and in the treatment of some kidney diseases wherein the ability to produce urine is hampered.

A typical volume of urine produced per day is about 1 liter (1 quart) or more, depending mostly on the intake of fluid, protein, and sodium. A somewhat greater urine output than that is fine, but less—especially less than 500 milliliters (2 cups)—forces the kidneys to form concentrated urine. The simplest way to determine if water intake is adequate is to observe the color of one's urine. Whereas urine should be clear or pale yellow, concentrated urine is very dark yellow. The heavy ion content of concentrated urine in turn increases the risk of kidney stone formation in susceptible people (generally men). Kidney stones are formed from minerals and other substances that have precipitated out of the urine and accumulate in kidney tissues.

Other Functions of Water

Water helps form the lubricants found in knees and other joints of the body. It is the basis for saliva, bile, and **amniotic fluid.** Amniotic fluid acts as a shock absorber surrounding the growing fetus in the mother's womb. Ion concentrations vary in each fluid compartment to accommodate Specific needs, such as the ability to transfer nerve impulses.

How Much Water Do We Need per Day?

The Adequate Intake for total water intake per day is 2.7 liters (11 cups) for adult women and 3.7 liters (15 cups) for adult men. This is based primarily on our typical total water intakes from a combination of fluids and foods. For fluid alone this corresponds to about 2.2 liters (9 cups) for women and about 3 liters (13 cups) for men. (Keep in mind also that it does not indicate that water *per se* must be used to meet fluid needs.) At minimum, adults need 1 to 3 liters of fluid to replace daily water losses.

We consume water in various liquids, such as fruit juice, coffee, tea, soft drinks, and water itself. Note that coffee, tea, and soft drinks often contain caffeine, which increases urine output. However, the fluid consumed from these beverages is not completely lost in urine, so these fluids still help to meet water needs. Foods also supply water; many fruits and vegetables are more than 80% water (Fig. 9.3). Water as a by product of metabolism provides approximately 250 to 350 milliliters (1 to 1½ cups) of additional water.

Much of the water needed is used to produce urine (500 to 1000 milliliters or more). The rest compensates for typical water losses through the lungs (250 to 350 milliliters), feces (100 to 200 milliliters), and skin (450 to 1900 milliliters) (Fig. 9.4). These are just estimates: altitude, caffeine intake, alcohol intake, and humidity can affect these individual losses.

When we consider the large amount of water used to lubricate the gastrointestinal (GI) tract, the loss of only 100 to 200 milliliters of water each day through the feces is remarkable. About 8000 milliliters of water enter the GI tract daily through secretions from the mouth, stomach, intestine, pancreas, and other organs, while the diet

urea Nitrogen-containing waste product of protein metabolism; major source of nitrogen in the urine.

Functions of water:
- Chemical processes
- Temperature regulation
- Removal of waste products
- Primary component of body fluids, such as in joints

amniotic fluid Fluid contained in a sac within the uterus. This fluid surrounds and protects the fetus during development.

FIGURE 9-3 ▶ Water content of foods by weight. In addition to the MyPlate food groups, pink is used for substances that do not fit easily into food groups (e.g., honey, candy, coffee, alcohol, and table salt).

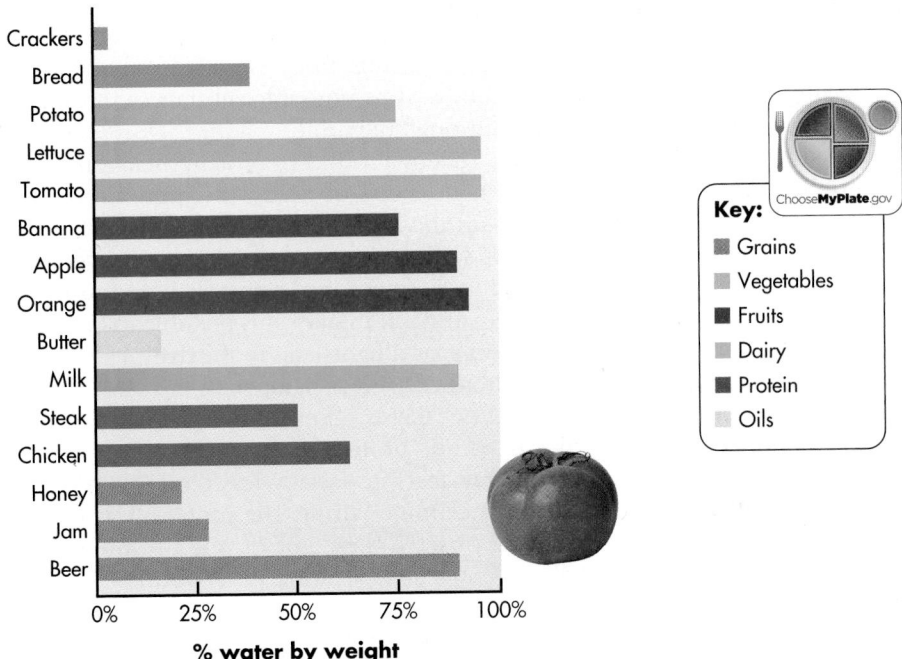

Key:
- Grains
- Vegetables
- Fruits
- Dairy
- Protein
- Oils

% water by weight

supplies an additional 30% to 50% or more. The small intestine reabsorbs most of this water, while the large intestine takes up a lesser—but still important—amount. The kidneys also greatly conserve water. They reabsorb about 97% of the water filtered from waste products.

MAKING DECISIONS

Hard Water or Soft Water?

Water can be classified by whether it is hard or soft. Hard water generally comes from underground wells and usually contains calcium, magnesium, and iron. The more minerals the water contains, the harder it is. Soft water has a low content of these minerals and is often produced by replacing other minerals with sodium.

▶ Regular intake of water and water-rich fluids are essential to replace daily fluid losses. One trend in North America is to carry bottles of water with us.

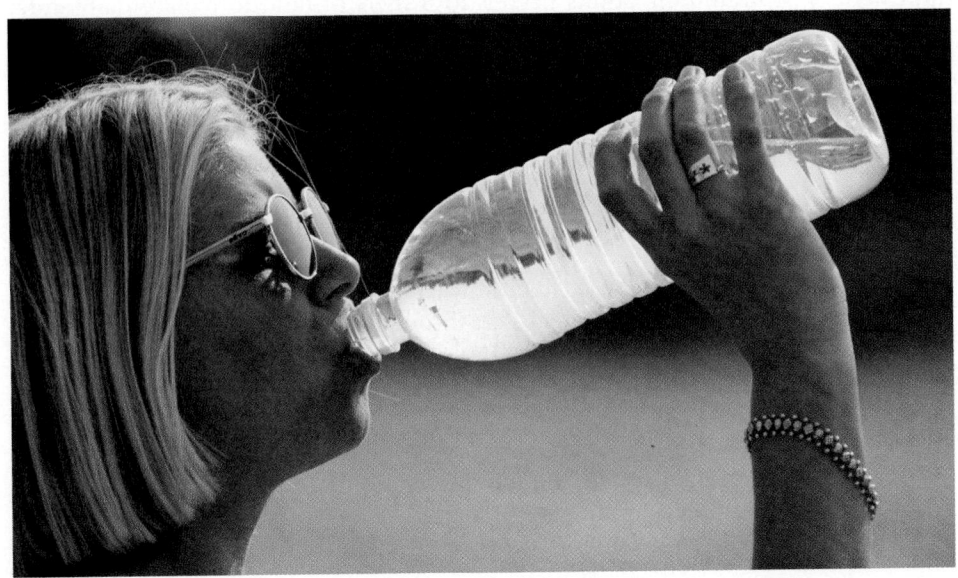

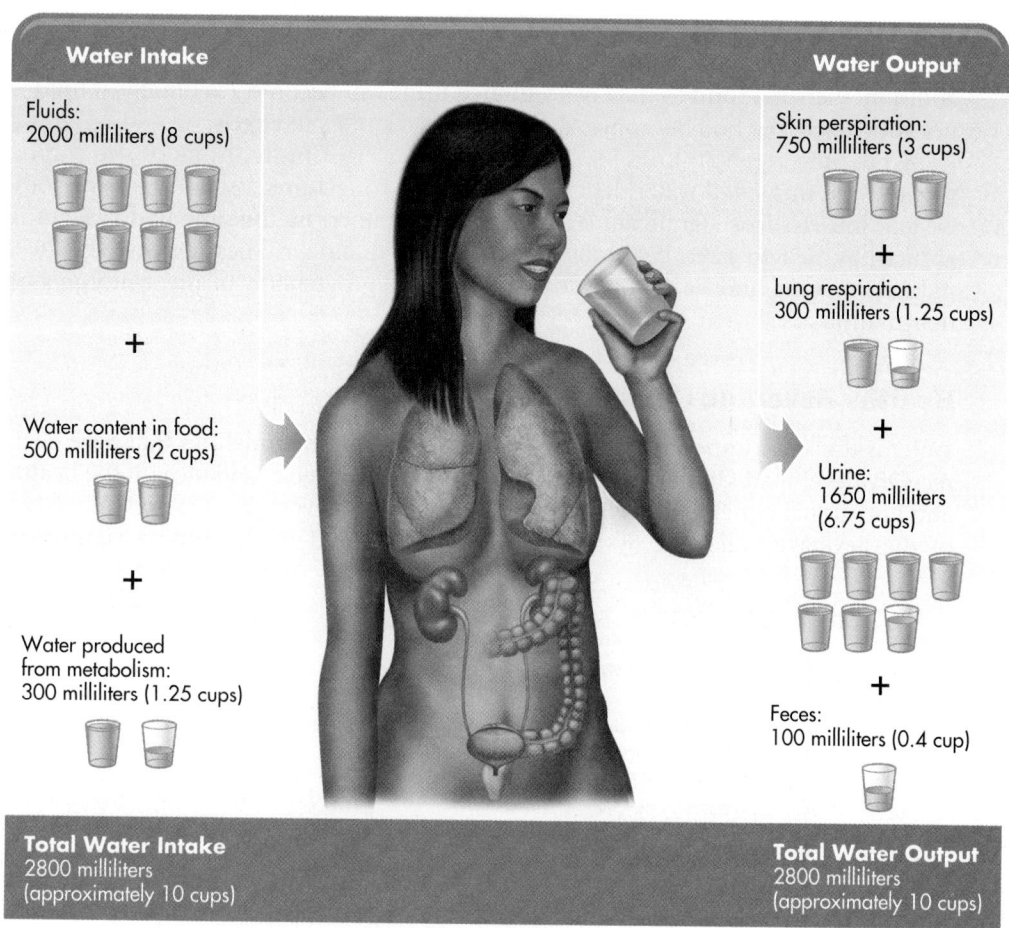

FIGURE 9-4 ▶ Estimate of water balance—intake versus output—in a woman. We primarily maintain body fluids at an optimum amount by adjusting water output to intake. As you can see for this woman, most water comes from the liquids we consume. Some comes from the moisture in more solid foods, and the remainder is manufactured during metabolism. Water output includes that lost via lungs, urine, skin, and feces.

Thirst

If you don't drink enough water, your body eventually lets you know by signaling thirst. Your brain is communicating the need to drink. This thirst mechanism can lag behind actual water loss, however, during prolonged exercise and illness, as well as in one's older years. For this reason, athletes should carefully monitor fluid status—they should weigh themselves before and after training sessions to determine their rate of water loss and, thus, their water needs. The current goal for athletes is to consume 2 to 3 cups of fluid for every pound lost (see Chapter 10 for details). Sick children—especially those with fever, vomiting, diarrhea, and increased perspiration—and older persons often need to be reminded to drink plenty of fluids (see Chapters 15 and 16 for details). As Chapter 15 discusses in further detail, infants can easily become dehydrated.

What If the Thirst Message Is Ignored?

Once the body registers a shortage of available water, it increases fluid conservation. Two hormones that participate in this process are **antidiuretic hormone** and **aldosterone**. The pituitary gland releases antidiuretic hormone to force the kidneys to conserve water. The kidneys respond by reducing urine flow. At the same time, as fluid volume decreases in the bloodstream, blood pressure falls. This eventually triggers the release of the hormone aldosterone, which signals the kidneys to retain more sodium and, in turn, more water.

Alcohol inhibits the action of antidiuretic hormone. One reason people feel so weak the day after heavy drinking is that they are dehydrated. Even though they may have consumed a lot of liquid in their drinks, they have lost even more liquid because alcohol has inhibited antidiuretic hormone.

antidiuretic hormone A hormone that is secreted by the pituitary gland and that acts on the kidneys to decrease water excretion.

aldosterone A hormone produced by the adrenal glands that acts on the kidneys to conserve sodium (and therefore water).

However, despite mechanisms that work to reduce water loss via the kidneys, fluid continues to be lost via the feces, skin, and lungs. Those losses must be replaced. In addition, there is a limit to how concentrated urine can become. Eventually, if fluid is not consumed, the body becomes dehydrated and suffers ill effects.

By the time a person loses 1% to 2% of body weight in fluids, he or she will be thirsty. Even this small water deficit can cause one to feel tired. At a 4% loss of body weight, muscles lose significant strength and endurance. By the time body weight is reduced by 10% to 12%, heat tolerance is decreased and weakness results. At a 20% reduction, coma and death may soon follow. The progression of the symptoms of dehydration are shown in Figure 9-5.

Healthy Beverage Consumption Guidelines

Water is the key component in the beverage consumption guidelines that have been recently developed (Table 9-1). These recommendations give guidance on the health and nutritional benefits as well as the risks of various beverage categories. The basis of the Beverage Guidance System is that fluids should not provide a significant

FIGURE 9-5 ▶ The effects of dehydration can range from thirst to death, depending on the extent of water weight lost.

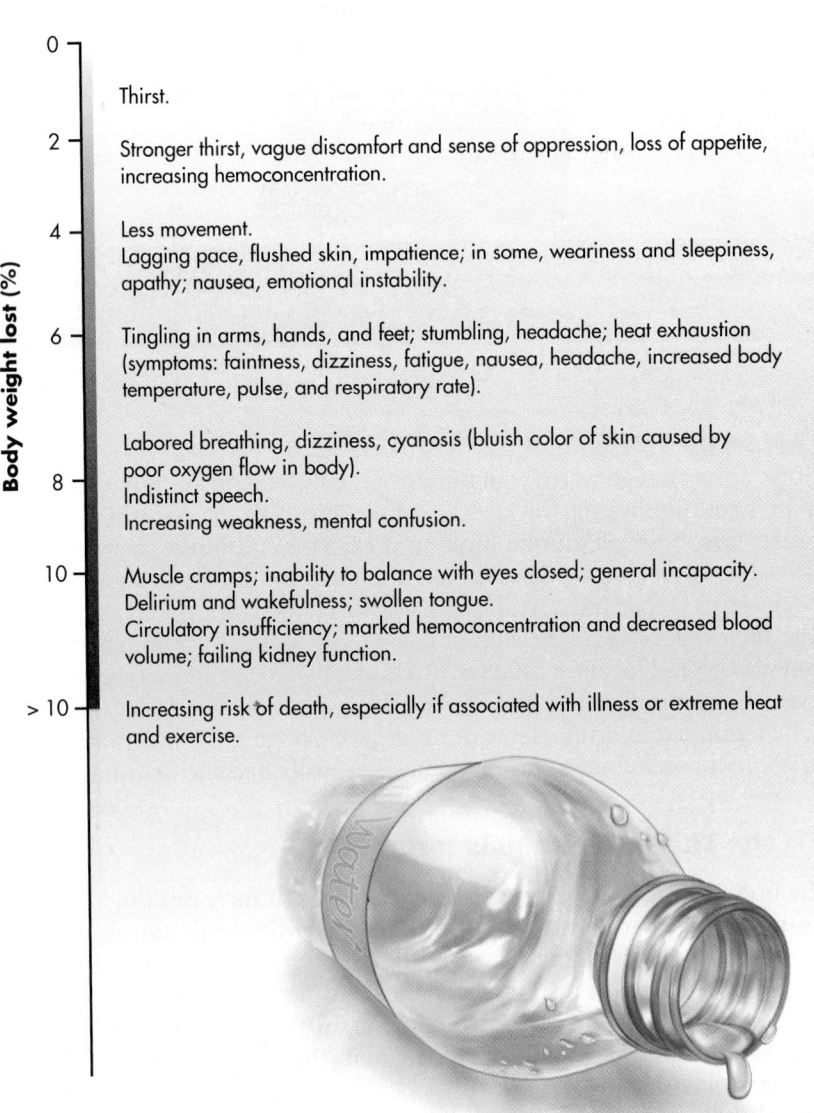

Body weight lost (%)

0 —

Thirst.

2 —
Stronger thirst, vague discomfort and sense of oppression, loss of appetite, increasing hemoconcentration.

4 —
Less movement.
Lagging pace, flushed skin, impatience; in some, weariness and sleepiness, apathy; nausea, emotional instability.

6 —
Tingling in arms, hands, and feet; stumbling, headache; heat exhaustion (symptoms: faintness, dizziness, fatigue, nausea, headache, increased body temperature, pulse, and respiratory rate).

Labored breathing, dizziness, cyanosis (bluish color of skin caused by poor oxygen flow in body).
Indistinct speech.
8 —
Increasing weakness, mental confusion.

10 —
Muscle cramps; inability to balance with eyes closed; general incapacity.
Delirium and wakefulness; swollen tongue.
Circulatory insufficiency; marked hemoconcentration and decreased blood volume; failing kidney function.

> 10 —
Increasing risk of death, especially if associated with illness or extreme heat and exercise.

TABLE 9-1 The Beverage Guidance System

Level	Category*	Recommended Servings per day
1	Water	50 fluid ounces (1.7 liters)
2	Tea or coffee, unsweetened	0 to 40 fluid ounces (0 to 1.4 liters)
3	Low-fat and skim milk and soy beverages	0 to 16 fluid ounces (0 to 0.5 liter)
4	Non-calorically sweetened beverages (diet drinks)	0 to 32 fluid ounces (0 to 1 liter)
5	Calorie beverages with some nutrients (100% fruit juices, alcoholic beverages, whole milk, sports drinks)	0 to 8 fluid ounces (0 to 0.25 liter) 0 to 2 alcoholic drinks for men 0 to 8 fluid ounces (0 to 0.25 liter)
6	Calorically sweetened beverages (regular soft drinks)	0 to 1 alcoholic drinks for women,

*Categories established based on their possible health benefits or risks.

Adapted from Popkin and others: *Am J Clin Nutr* 83:529, 2006.

amount of the energy or nutrients in a healthy diet. More specifically, the system recommends that beverages provide less than 10% of total calories consumed for a 2200 kcal diet (see Further Reading 14).

Is There Such a Thing as Too Much Water?

Consuming too much water—whatever amount the kidneys are unable to excrete—can also lead to ill health, especially if concentrations of blood electrolytes, notably sodium, become too low. However, an excessive amount would have to approach many quarts (liters) each day. When excessive water intake overwhelms the kidneys' capacity to excrete fluid, blurred vision is one resulting symptom. Such water toxicity risks during athletic events are covered in Chapter 10.

CONCEPT CHECK

The body can neither readily store nor conserve water, so we can survive only a few days without it. Water transports nutrients and waste products, serves as a medium for chemical reactions and as a lubricant, and aids in temperature regulation. Water accounts for 50% to 70% of body weight and distributes itself all over the body—among lean and other tissues (in both intracellular and extracellular fluids) and in urine and other body fluids. The Adequate Intake for total water intake is 2.7 liters (11 cups) for women and 3.7 liters (15 cups) for men per day. Thirst is the body's first sign of dehydration. If this thirst mechanism is faulty, as it may be during illness or vigorous exercise, hormonal mechanisms also help conserve water by reducing urine output. Excess fluid intake can be hazardous to a person's health. Overall, the United States enjoys a safe water supply. However, people with poor immune status should boil water used for drinking and cooking to avoid waterborne illness. Bottled water can also be used if desired.

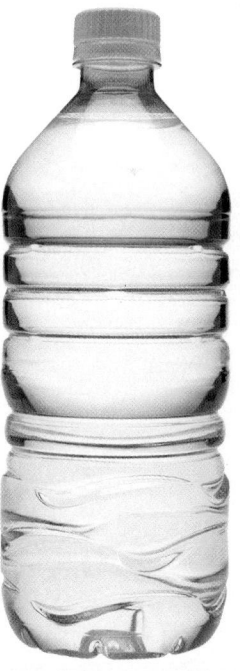

▲ Bottled water is a convenient but relatively expensive source of water. In most cases, tap water is just as healthy a choice to meet our water needs.

Our Water Supply: Safety Issues

Many people choose bottled water over tap water because they doubt the safety of their public drinking water. Some concern over municipal water supplies is warranted. For example, contamination of the public water supply by the parasite *Cryptosporidium* is possible. This parasite is usually found in lakes and rivers; the typical chlorination procedures used to treat public water supplies do not kill *Cryptosporidium*.

This parasite poses little risk to healthy people—other than a case of diarrhea—but it can harm people who have AIDS or other diseases that compromise function of the immune system (such as some forms of cancer therapy or organ transplant therapy). High-risk people have been advised to boil for at least 1 minute any tap water they use for cooking or drinking to ensure that the parasite is destroyed. Alternatively, individuals can purchase a water filter that screens out *Cryptosporidium* (the National Sanitation Foundation at (800) 673-8010 can provide a list of manufacturers) or use bottled water certified to be free of the parasite (contact the supplier if in doubt). Generally, distilled water or that which has undergone reverse osmosis is parasite free.

Monitoring the Safety of Your Water

Under the Safe Water Drinking Act, all public drinking water supplies are monitored for contaminants such as bacteria, various chemicals, and toxic metals (such as lead and mercury). The local municipal water department must mail the results of these tests each year to its consumers. According to the Environmental Protection Agency (EPA), the U.S. water supply ranks among the safest in the world. However, this water does sometimes fail to meet the agency's standards for contaminants such as lead and nitrates. Generally, the public will be warned about the latter, because it is dangerous to use nitrate-rich water for mixing infant formulas (Chapter 15). Some studies indicate that in 1 year, about one in five Americans consumes water not up to standards, especially in rural areas. These people could consider using a home water filter or bottled water. The local water department can help a person evaluate whether health risks are worth the cost of home water filters or bottled water.

As a safeguard against contamination, chlorine and ammonia are added to kill bacteria. The addition of such chemicals has raised concern that drinking water may increase rectal and bladder cancer risk, though there is no conclusive proof of such risk. If chlorine in tap water does increase cancer risk, the risk is likely extremely small (perhaps two cases of cancer in 1 million people).

If you find the taste of chlorinated tap water unpleasant or are concerned about the possible cancer risk, you can remove the chlorine from tap water by boiling it or by letting a large container filled with water stand uncovered overnight. In both cases, the chlorine will evaporate, taking its characteristic flavor with it. Alternatively, you can install a filter on the household spigot from which you obtain your water. It should be designed to remove trihalomethanes, common chlorine by-products.

Options Regarding Your Water Source

Keep in mind that by most standards, bottled water ranges from moderately expensive to expensive. In many cases, you are paying for water not much different from the water you get from your tap. If you are concerned about the safety of your tap water, you can ask the municipal water department for its most recent test results, or you can have the water tested. A local testing laboratory or state health department can be of service, as can the EPA at (800) 426-4791, if local information is not available (for example, if you have a well). This testing can point out whether there are health risks associated with your water supply. Compared with the cost of bottled water, the testing fee will be insignificant. Letting cold water run for a minute or so before taking a drink or before using it in meal preparation is a good way to limit possible lead exposure, especially if the water has been off for more than two hours. In addition, do not use hot tap water for food preparation. For more information, see the website www.epa.gov/safewater.

9.2 Minerals—An Overview

cofactor A mineral or other substance that binds to a specific region on a protein, such as an enzyme, and is necessary for the protein's function.

The metabolic roles of minerals and the amounts of them in the body vary considerably (Fig. 9-6). Some minerals, such as copper and selenium, work as **cofactors,** enabling various proteins, such as enzymes, to function. Minerals also contribute

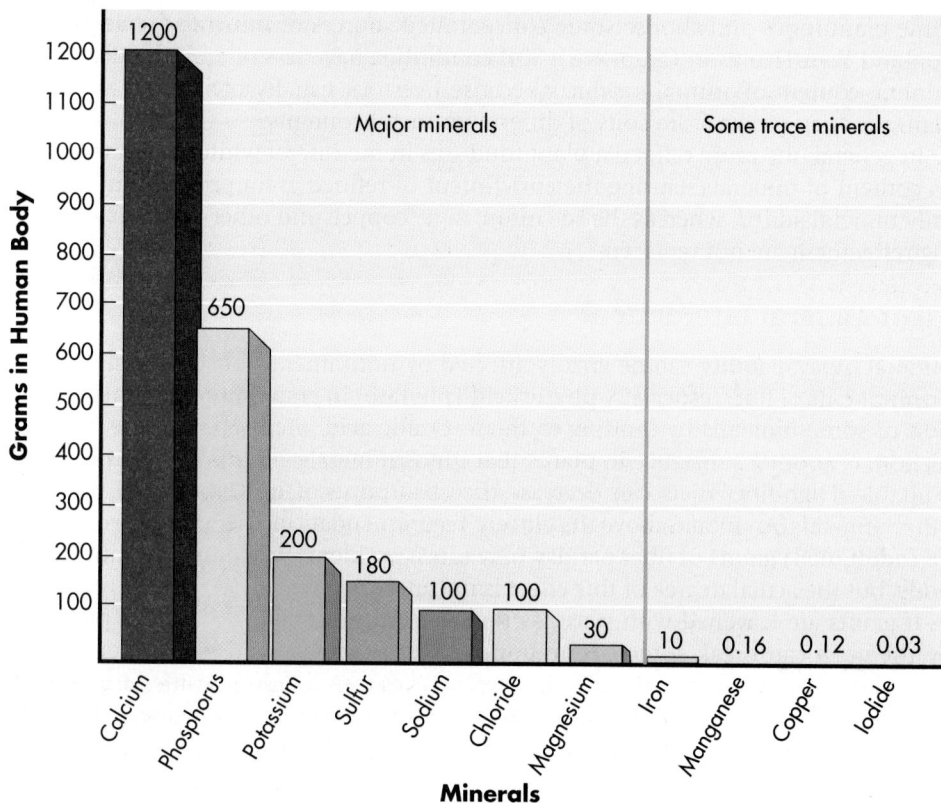

FIGURE 9-6 ▶ Approximate amounts of various minerals present in the average human body. Other trace minerals of nutritional importance not listed include chromium, fluoride, molybdenum, selenium, and zinc.

to many body compounds. For example, iron is a component of red blood cells. Sodium, potassium, and calcium aid in the transfer of nerve impulses throughout the body. Body growth and development also depend on certain minerals, such as calcium and phosphorus. Water balance requires sodium, potassium, calcium, and phosphorus. At all levels—cellular, tissue, organ, and whole body—minerals clearly play important roles in maintaining body functions.

Minerals are categorized based on the amount we need per day. Recall from Chapter 1 that if we require greater than 100 milligrams (1/50 of a teaspoon) of a mineral per day, it is considered a **major mineral;** otherwise, it is considered a **trace mineral.** For example, calcium and phosphorus are major minerals and iron and zinc are trace minerals.

The roles and nutritional significance of both the major and the trace minerals are discussed in this chapter. But before examining the properties of the individual minerals, let's consider some topics that apply to all these nutrients.

Mineral Bioavailability

Foods offer us a plentiful supply of many minerals, but the ability of our bodies to absorb and use them varies. The degree to which an ingested nutrient is absorbed from food sources and is available to the body is called **bioavailability.** The bioavailability of minerals depends on many factors. The mineral content listed in a food composition table for the amount of a mineral in a food is just a starting point for estimating the actual contribution the food will make to our mineral needs. Spinach, for example, contains plenty of calcium, but only about 5% of it can be absorbed because of the vegetable's high concentration of **oxalic acid (oxalate),** a calcium-binder. Usually, about 25% of dietary calcium is absorbed by adults.

The average North American diet derives minerals from both plant and animal sources. Overall, minerals from animal products are better absorbed than those from plants because binders such as fiber are not present to hinder absorption. The mineral content of plants greatly depends on mineral concentrations of the soil in which they are grown. Vegans must be aware of the potentially poor mineral content of

major mineral A mineral vital to health that is required in the diet in amounts greater than 100 milligrams per day.

trace mineral A mineral vital to health that is required in the diet in amounts less than 100 milligrams per day.

bioavailability The degree to which an ingested nutrient is absorbed and available to the body.

oxalic acid (oxalate) An organic acid found in spinach, rhubarb, and other leafy green vegetables that can depress the absorption of certain minerals present in the food, such as calcium.

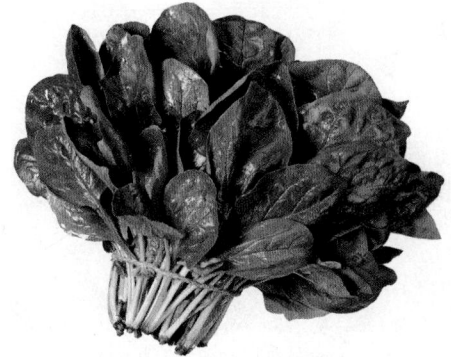

▲ Spinach is often touted as a rich source of calcium, but little of the calcium present is available to the body.

some plant foods and choose some concentrated sources of minerals (review Nutrition and Your Health in Chapter 6). Soil conditions have less of an influence on the mineral content of animal products because livestock usually consume a variety of plant products grown from soils of differing mineral contents.

In general, the more refined a plant food—as in the case of white flour—the lower its content of minerals. During the enrichment of refined grain products, iron is the only mineral added, whereas the selenium, zinc, copper, and other minerals lost during refinement are not replaced.

Fiber-Mineral Interactions

phytic acid (phytate) A constituent of plant fibers that binds positive ions to its multiple phosphate groups.

Mineral bioavailability can be greatly affected by nonmineral substances in the diet. Components of fiber, especially **phytic acid (phytate)** in grain fiber, can limit absorption of some minerals by binding to them. Oxalic acid, mentioned in the previous section, is another substance in plants that binds minerals and makes them less bioavailable. High-fiber diets can decrease the absorption of iron, zinc, and probably other minerals. An intake above the current recommendation of 25 (adult women) to 38 (adult men) grams of fiber per day may cause problems with mineral status of the body, but the actual degree of this effect is uncertain.

If grains are leavened with yeast, as they are in breadmaking, enzymes produced by the yeast can break some of the bonds between phytic acid and minerals. This increases mineral absorption. The zinc deficiencies found among some Middle Eastern populations are attributed partly to their consumption of unleavened breads, resulting in low bioavailability of dietary zinc. Zinc bioavailability is discussed in greater detail in a later section.

Mineral-Mineral Interactions

Many minerals, such as magnesium, calcium, iron, and copper, are of similar sizes and electrical charges. Having similar sizes and the same electrical charge causes these minerals to compete with each other for absorption, and therefore they affect each other's bioavailability. Simply stated, an excess of one mineral decreases the absorption and metabolism of other minerals. For example, a large intake of zinc decreases copper absorption. Because of this, people should avoid taking individual mineral supplements unless a dietary deficiency or medical condition specifically warrants it. Food sources, however, pose little risk for these mineral interactions, giving us another reason to emphasize foods in meeting nutrient needs.

Vitamin-Mineral Interactions

Several beneficial vitamin-mineral interactions occur during nutrient absorption and metabolism. When consumed in conjunction with vitamin C, absorption of certain forms of iron—such as that in plant products—improves. The active vitamin D hormone improves calcium absorption. Many vitamins require specific minerals to act as components in their structure and function. For example, the thiamin coenzyme requires magnesium or manganese to function efficiently.

Mineral Toxicities

An excessive mineral intake, especially of trace minerals, such as iron and copper, can have toxic results. For many trace minerals, the gap between just enough and too much is small. Taking minerals as supplements poses the biggest threat for mineral toxicity, whereas food sources are unlikely culprits. Mineral supplements exceeding current standards for mineral needs—especially those that supply more than 100% of the Daily Values on supplement labels—should be taken only under a physician's supervision. The Daily Values are for the most part higher than our current standards (e.g., RDA) for mineral needs. Without close monitoring, doses of minerals should not exceed any Upper Level set on a long-term basis.

▲ Mineral supplements pose a high risk for toxicity. Generally, mineral intake from a supplement should not exceed 100% of the Daily Value, unless otherwise specified by a physician.

The potential for toxicity is not the only reason to carefully consider the use of mineral supplements. Harmful interactions with other nutrients are possible. Also, contamination of mineral supplements—with lead, for example—is a possibility. Use of brands approved by the United States Pharmacopeia (USP) lessens this risk (review Nutrition and Your Health in Chapter 8). In summary, even with the best intentions, people may harm themselves using mineral supplements.

CONCEPT CHECK

Minerals are vital to the functioning of many body processes. Their bioavailability depends on many factors, including a mineral's interaction with fiber, vitamins, and other minerals. Animal products often yield better mineral absorption than do plants. Still, both animal and plant sources help us meet our mineral needs. Taking megadoses of an individual mineral supplement can greatly diminish the absorption and metabolism of other minerals. In addition, some minerals are potentially toxic in amounts not much in excess of body needs. These are two good reasons to carefully consider any use of mineral supplements exceeding the Daily Value on the label, particularly long-term use of supplements that lead to intakes in excess of the Upper Level set for any mineral.

9.3 Major Minerals

Up to now, some general characteristics of minerals and how some of them interact with water in the body have been covered. Now let us review the individual properties of the major minerals (also called macrominerals) in the context of the North American diet.

9.4 Sodium (Na)

Our primary dietary source of sodium is table salt, chemically known as sodium chloride, added during food processing. This mineral is an essential part of our diets and adds flavor to our foods, but there is concern that an overabundance of sodium in the diet may cause harm. Table salt is 40% sodium and 60% chloride. For example, dietary intake of 10 grams of salt translates into about 4 grams of sodium. A teaspoon of salt contains about 2 grams of sodium (2000 milligrams).

The human body absorbs almost all sodium that gets eaten. Once absorbed, sodium becomes the major positive ion outside of cells in extracellular fluid and a key factor for retaining body water. Fluid balance throughout the body depends partly on the variation in the sodium and other ion concentrations among the water-containing compartments in the body. Sodium ions also function in nerve impulse conduction and absorption of some nutrients (e.g., glucose).

A dietary deficiency of sodium is rare. However, a diet low in sodium—coupled with excessive perspiration, persistent vomiting, or diarrhea—has the ability to deplete the body of sodium. This state can lead to muscle cramps, nausea, vomiting, dizziness, and later, shock and coma. The likelihood of this happening, however, is low because the kidney responds early to low sodium status, eventually triggering the body to conserve sodium. This conservation of sodium by the body demonstrates how important small amounts of sodium are to body functions.

Only when perspiration leads to weight loss exceeding 2% to 3% of total body weight (or about 5 to 6 pounds) should sodium losses raise concern. Even then, merely salting foods is sufficient to restore body sodium for most people. Certain endurance athletes, however, may need to consume sports drinks during competition to replace sodium losses from perspiration in order to avoid depletion of sodium (see Chapter 10). Although perspiration tastes salty on the skin, sodium is not highly concentrated in perspiration. Rather, water evaporating from the skin leaves concentrated

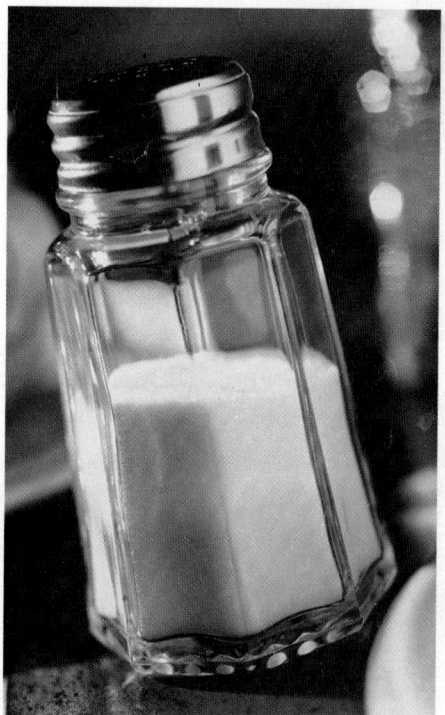

For your information, the chemical symbols for the minerals discussed are given next to each mineral heading.

▲ Table salt is our primary source of the minerals sodium and chloride.

sodium behind. Perspiration contains about two-thirds the sodium concentration found in blood.

Sodium Sources and Needs

About 80% of the sodium we consume is added to foods during manufacturing and preparation at restaurants (Fig. 9-7). Sodium added in cooking provides about 10% of our intakes, and sodium naturally present in foods provides the rest, about another 10%. Almost all foods naturally contain a little sodium; the higher amount found in milk (about 120 milligrams per cup) is one exception.

The more processed and restaurant food one consumes, generally the higher one's sodium intake. Conversely, the more home cooking one does, the more sodium control that person has. The foods that contribute most of the sodium in the adult diet (white bread and rolls, hot dogs and lunch meats, cheese, soups, and foods with tomato sauce) do so partly because they are eaten so often. Other foods that generally are especially high in sodium include salted snack foods, French fries and potato chips, and sauces and gravies (Fig. 9-8).

If we ate only unprocessed foods and added no salt, we would consume about 500 milligrams of sodium per day. In comparison, the Adequate Intake for sodium for adults under age 51 is 1500 milligrams, a generous amount; this is reduced by 100 to 200 milligrams for older adults. (See the inside back cover for references to mineral needs for various age groups.) The 2010 Dietary Guidelines for Americans recommends that the general population consume less than 2300 milligrams (approximately 1 teaspoon of salt) of sodium per day. The Dietary Guidelines for individuals with hypertension, diabetes, or chronic kidney disease; blacks; and middle-aged and older adults are to aim to consume no more than 1500 milligrams of sodium per day. We really need only about 200 milligrams per day to maintain physiological functions. (Additional sodium above needs was added to establish the Adequate Intake to allow for a more varied diet where not all foods are low in sodium.)

If we compare 500 milligrams of sodium from unprocessed food with the amount typically eaten by adults (2300 to 4700 milligrams or more), it is clear that food processing and cooking contribute most of our dietary sodium. As discussed in Chapter 2, nutrition labels list a food's sodium content. When dietary sodium must be severely restricted, attention to food labels is of utmost importance. Under FDA food and supplement labeling rules, the Daily Value for sodium is 2400 milligrams (2.4 grams).

Most humans can adapt somewhat to various dietary salt intakes, though very high intakes can be toxic. For most people, today's sodium intake simply will be in tomorrow's urine output. However, approximately 10% to 15% of adults, such as African-Americans and people who have diabetes and/or are overweight, are especially *sodium sensitive.* For these people, high sodium intakes can increase blood pressure, whereas lower-sodium diets (about 2000 milligrams daily) often help correct the problem (see the Nutrition and Your Health section on minerals and hypertension at the end

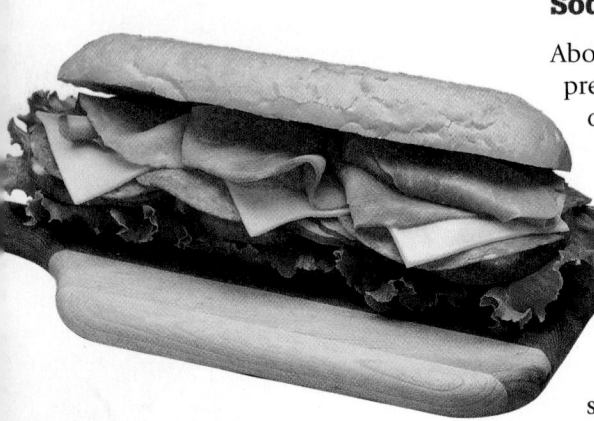

▲ Deli meats, such as ham, are high in sodium (salt).

FIGURE 9-7 ▶ Salt arrives in the American diet largely as a result of food processing.

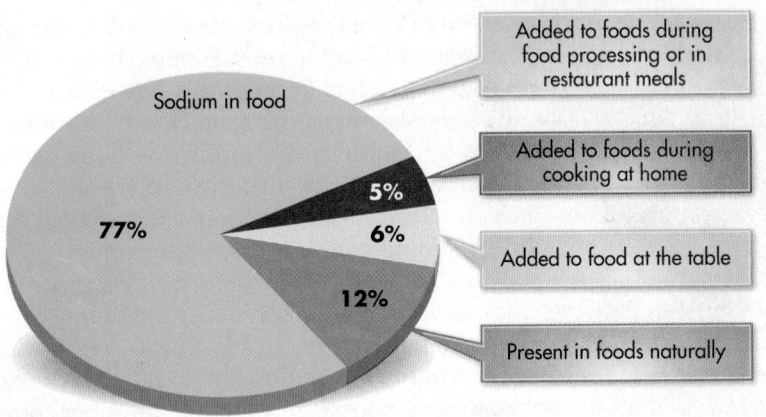

Sodium in food

77%

5% — Added to foods during food processing or in restaurant meals

6% — Added to foods during cooking at home

12% — Added to food at the table

Present in foods naturally

Food Sources of Sodium

Food Item and Amount	Sodium Content (milligrams)	Adult Male and Female AI = 1500 milligrams Daily Value = 2400 milligrams %AI
AI*	1500	100%
Pepperoni pizza, 2 slices	2045	136%
Ham, sliced, 1 ounce	1215	81%
Chicken noodle soup, canned, 1 cup	1106	74%
V8 vegetable juice, 8 ounces	620	41%
Macaroni salad, ½ cup	561	37%
Hard pretzels, 1 ounce	486	32%
Hamburger with bun, 1 each	474	32%
Green beans, canned, ½ cup	390	26%
Saltine crackers, 6 each	234	16%
Cheddar cheese, 1 ounce	176	12%
Peanut butter, 2 tablespoons	156	10%
Nonfat milk, 1 cup	127	8%
Seven grain bread, 1 slice	126	8%
Animal crackers, 1 ounce	112	7%
Grape juice, 1 cup	10	1%

Key:
- ▪ Grains
- ▪ Vegetables
- ▪ Fruits
- ▪ Dairy
- ▪ Protein

* For adults; see the DRI table in the back of this book for age-specific recommendations.

FIGURE 9-8 ▶ Food sources of sodium compared to the Adequate Intake.

of the chapter and the Newsworthy Nutrition in the margin). Still, keep in mind that other lifestyle factors, such as being overweight and inactive, are more likely to contribute to hypertension.

Scientific groups typically suggest that adults in general reduce sodium intake, mostly to limit the risk of developing hypertension later. It is also a good idea to have your blood pressure checked regularly. If you have hypertension, you should try to reduce your sodium intake as you follow a comprehensive plan to treat this disease. Reducing sodium intake also helps to maintain healthy calcium status, because urinary calcium loss is increased along with sodium when sodium intake is greater than about 2000 milligrams per day (see Further Reading 5).

It is not that hard to follow a low-sodium diet, but many typical food choices such as processed meats and salty snacks will have to be limited (see the first Rate Your Plate activity at the end of this chapter). At first, foods may also taste bland, but eventually you will perceive more flavor as the tongue becomes more sensitive to the salt content of foods. By slowly reducing dietary sodium and substituting lemon juice, herbs and spices, you can eventually become accustomed to a diet that contains minimal sodium but does not result in much of a flavor trade-off. Many new cookbooks offer excellent recipes for flavorful low-sodium foods.

Upper Level for Sodium

The Upper Level for sodium for adults is 2300 milligrams (2.3 grams). Intakes exceeding this amount are common but are not recommended because they typically

NEWSWORTHY NUTRITION

Lower sodium and higher potassium intakes reduce risk of cardiovascular disease

Increasing potassium intakes appears effective in lowering blood pressure and is most effective at reducing risk of cardiovascular disease when combined with lower intake of sodium. The sodium-to-potassium ratio in urine is a good predictor of cardiovascular disease.

Source: Cook NR and others: Joint effects of sodium and potassium intake on subsequent cardiovascular disease. *Archives of Internal Medicine* 169:32, 2009 (see Further Reading 3).

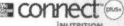 **Check out the Connect site** www.mcgrawhillconnect.com to further explore the roles of sodium and potassium.

increase blood pressure. About 95% of North American adults have sodium intakes that exceed the Upper Level.

CRITICAL THINKING

Mrs. Massa has recently seen and heard a lot about the amount of salt (sodium) in foods. She has been surprised by the number of articles that advise the public to decrease the amount of salt in their food. If sodium is such a bad thing, Mrs. Massa wonders, why do you need to have any at all? How would you respond to her question?

CONCEPT CHECK

Sodium is the major positive ion in the extracellular fluid. It is important for maintaining fluid balance and conducting nerve impulses. Sodium depletion is unlikely, because the typical North American's diet has abundant sources of sodium and most of it gets absorbed. Compared to dining out or buying commercially prepared foods, preparation of foods in the home allows greater control over sodium intake. The Adequate Intake for sodium for adults is 1500 milligrams per day. The average adult consumes 2300 to 4700 milligrams or more daily. About 10% to 15% of the population is especially sensitive to sodium, such as overweight individuals and African-Americans. In these people, hypertension can develop as a result of high-sodium diets, but many other lifestyle habits also contribute to hypertension. Nutrition experts suggest that for young adults, sodium intake should be about 1500 milligrams (1.5 grams) and not exceed 2300 milligrams (2.3 grams) on a regular basis. Sodium in the North American diet is provided predominantly through processed and restaurant foods.

9.5 Potassium (K)

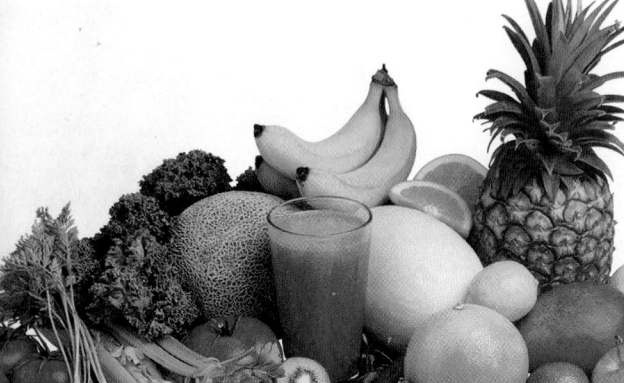

▲ Vegetables in general are a rich source of potassium, as are fruits.

Potassium performs many of the same functions as sodium, such as fluid balance and nerve impulse transmission. However, it operates inside, rather than outside cells. Intracellular fluids—those inside cells—contain 95% of the potassium in the body. Also, unlike sodium, increasing potassium intake is associated with lower rather than higher blood pressure values. We absorb about 90% of the potassium we eat.

Low blood potassium is a life-threatening problem. Symptoms often include a loss of appetite, muscle cramps, confusion, and constipation. Eventually, the heart beats irregularly, which decreases its capacity to pump blood.

Potassium Sources and Needs

Generally, unprocessed foods are rich sources of potassium. This includes fruits, vegetables, milk, whole grains, dried beans, and meats (Fig. 9-9). Major contributors of potassium to the adult diet include milk, potatoes, beef, coffee, tomatoes, and orange juice (Fig. 9-10).

The Adequate Intake for potassium for adults is 4700 milligrams (4.7 grams) per day. The Daily Value used to express potassium content on food and supplement labels is 3500 milligrams. On average, North Americans consume 2000 to 3000 milligrams per day. Thus, many of us need to increase our potassium intakes, preferably by increasing fruit and vegetable intake.

diuretic A substance that increases the volume of urine.

Diets are more likely to be lower in potassium than sodium because we generally do not add potassium to foods. Some **diuretics** used to treat high blood pressure also deplete the body's potassium. Thus, people who take potassium-wasting diuretics need to monitor their potassium intakes carefully. For these people, high-potassium foods are good additions to the diet, as are potassium chloride supplements if prescribed by a physician.

A chronically deficient food intake, as may be the case in alcoholism, can result in a severe potassium deficiency that requires medical attention. People with certain eating disorders, whose diets are poor and whose bodies can be depleted of nutrients because of vomiting, are also at risk for severe potassium deficiency (see Chapter 11).

Food Sources of Potassium

Food Item and Amount	Potassium (milligrams)	Adult Male and Female AI = 4700 milligrams
		Daily Value = 3500 milligrams %AI
AI*	4700	100%
Kidney beans, 1 cup	715	15%
Winter squash, ¾ cup	670	14%
Plain yogurt, 1 cup	570	12%
Orange juice, 1 cup	495	11%
Cantaloupe, 1 cup	495	11%
Lima beans, ½ cup	480	10%
Banana, 1 medium	470	10%
Zucchini, 1 cup	450	10%
Soybeans, ½ cup	440	9%
Artichoke, 1 medium	425	9%
Tomato juice, ¾ cup	400	9%
Pinto beans, ½ cup	400	9%
Baked potato, 1 small	385	8%
Buttermilk, 1 cup	370	8%
Sirloin steak, 3 ounces	345	7%

Key:
- Grains
- Vegetables
- Fruits
- Dairy
- Protein

* For adults; see the DRI table in the back of this book for age-specific recommendations.

FIGURE 9-9 ► Food sources of potassium compared to the Adequate Intake.

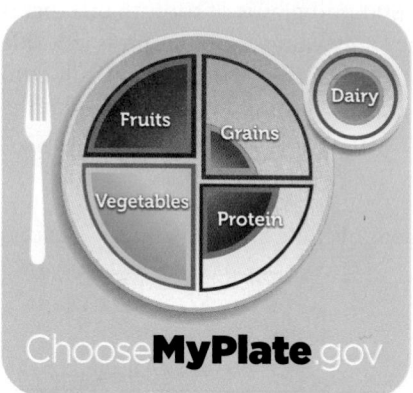
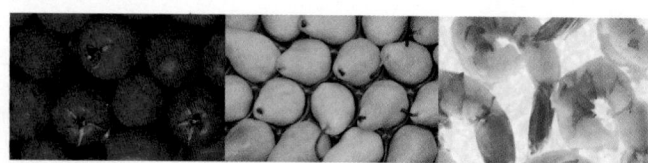

MyPlate: Sources of Potassium

Grains	Vegetables	Fruits	Dairy	Protein
• Whole-wheat bread • Whole-grain products	• Avocados • Spinach • Squash • Potatoes • Tomatoes • Lettuce • Lima beans	• Pears • Prunes • Peaches • Cantaloupes • Bananas	• Milk • Yogurt • Cottage cheese • Ricotta cheese	• Meat • Chicken • Fish • Shrimp • Beans

FIGURE 9-10 ► Sources of potassium from MyPlate. The fill of the background color (none, 1/3, 2/3, or completely covered) within each group on the plate indicates the average nutrient density for potassium in that group. Overall, the vegetables group and the fruits group contain many foods that are nutrient-dense sources of potassium, with the dairy group and protein group following close behind.

Other populations especially at risk for a severe potassium deficiency include people on very low-calorie diets and athletes who exercise heavily. As covered in Chapters 7 and 10, all of these people should compensate for potentially low body potassium by consuming potassium-rich foods.

If the kidneys function normally, typical food intakes will not lead to potassium toxicity. Thus, no Upper Level for potassium has been set. When the kidneys function poorly, potassium builds up in the blood. This inhibits heart function, causing slowed heartbeat. If untreated, this can be fatal, as the heart eventually stops beating. Consequently, in cases of reduced kidney function, close control of potassium intake becomes critical.

9.6 Chloride (Cl)

In our bodies, chloride—an ion form of chlorine—is an important negative ion for the extracellular fluid. Chlorine, on the other hand, is a poisonous gas. Chloride ions are a component of the acid produced in the stomach and are also used during immune responses as white blood cells attack foreign cells. In addition, nerve function relies on the presence of chloride. As is the case with sodium, most of the body's chloride is excreted by the kidneys; some is lost in perspiration. It is also thought to contribute to the blood pressure-raising ability of sodium chloride.

A chloride deficiency is unlikely because our dietary sodium chloride (salt) intake is so high. Frequent and lengthy bouts of vomiting—if coupled with a nutrient-poor diet—can, however, contribute to a deficiency because stomach secretions contain much chloride.

Chloride Sources and Needs

A few fruits and some vegetables are naturally good sources of chloride. Chlorinated water is also a source. However, the chloride we consume is mostly in the salt added to foods. Knowing a food's salt content allows for a close prediction of its chloride content; recall salt is 60% chloride.

The Adequate Intake for chloride for adults is 2300 milligrams per day. This is based on the 40:60 ratio of sodium to chloride in salt (1500 milligrams of sodium in a diet is accompanied by 2300 milligrams of chloride). The Daily Value used to express chloride content on food and supplement labels is 3400 milligrams. If the average adult consumes about 9 grams of salt daily, that yields 5.4 grams (5400 milligrams) of chloride.

Upper Level for Chloride

The Upper Level is 3600 milligrams. The average adult typically consumes an excess amount of this ion.

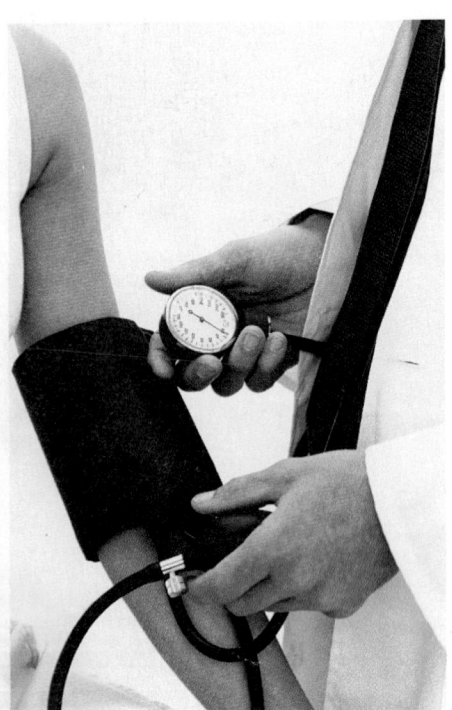

▲ Chloride is likely part of the blood pressure-raising property of sodium chloride (salt).

CONCEPT CHECK

The functions of potassium closely parallel those of sodium, but whereas sodium is found outside cells, potassium is the main positive ion found inside cells. Potassium is vital to fluid balance and nerve transmission. A potassium deficiency—caused by an inadequate intake of potassium, persistent vomiting, or use of some diuretics—can eventually lead to loss of appetite, muscle cramps, confusion, and heartbeat irregularities. Fruits and vegetables are generally rich sources of potassium. Potassium intake can be toxic if a person's kidneys do not function properly. Chloride is the major negative ion of extracellular fluid. Chloride also functions in digestion as part of stomach acid and in immune and nervous system responses. Deficiencies of chloride are highly unlikely because we eat so much sodium chloride (salt).

9.7 Calcium (Ca)

All cells need calcium, but more than 99% of the calcium in the body is used to strengthen bones and teeth. This calcium represents 40% of all the minerals present in the body and equals about 2.5 pounds (1200 grams). The calcium circulating in the bloodstream supplies the calcium needs of body cells. Growth and bone development require an adequate calcium intake.

Unlike sodium, potassium, and chloride, the amount of calcium in the body depends greatly on its absorption from the diet. Calcium requires an acidic environment in the GI tract to be absorbed efficiently. Absorption occurs primarily in the upper part of the small intestine. This area tends to be the most acidic portion of the small intestine because it receives the acidic stomach contents. Calcium absorption in the upper small intestine also depends on the active vitamin D hormone.

Adults absorb about 25% of the calcium in the foods eaten, but during times when the body needs extra calcium—such as in infancy and pregnancy—absorption increases to as high as 60%. Young people tend to absorb calcium better than do older people, especially those older than 70.

Many factors enhance calcium absorption, including:

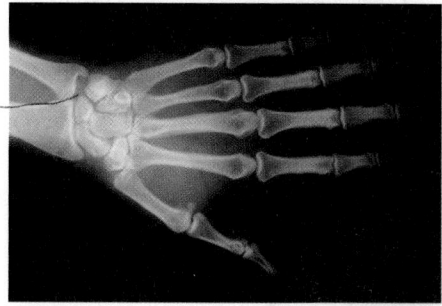

▲ Ninety-nine percent of calcium in the body is in bones.

- Blood levels of parathyroid hormone
- The presence of glucose and lactose in the diet
- The gradual flow (motility) of digestive contents through the intestine

On the other hand, several factors limit calcium absorption, such as:

- Large amounts of phytic acid in fiber from grains
- Great excess of phosphorus (and possibly magnesium) in the diet
- Polyphenols (tannins) in tea
- Vitamin D deficiency
- Diarrhea
- Old age

We have excellent hormonal systems to control blood calcium, so a normal blood calcium value can be maintained despite an inadequate calcium intake. The bones, however, pay the price. Bones can be seen as a calcium bank to which calcium can be added or withdrawn. Bone loss caused by a net calcium loss from this bank proceeds slowly. Only after many years of calcium loss are clinical symptoms apparent. By not meeting calcium needs, some people—especially women—are most likely setting the stage for future bone fractures.

Functions of Calcium

Forming and maintaining bones are calcium's major roles in the body. This is discussed in detail in the second Nutrition and Your Health section on minerals and **osteoporosis** found at the end of this chapter. However, calcium is important in many other processes as well. Calcium is essential for blood clotting and for muscle contraction. If blood calcium falls below a critical point, muscles cannot relax after contraction; the body stiffens and shows involuntary twitching, called **tetany**. In nerve transmission, calcium assists in the release of neurotransmitters and permits the flow of ions in and out of nerve cells. Without sufficient calcium, nerve function fails, which can also cause tetany. Finally, calcium helps regulate cellular metabolism by influencing the activities of various enzymes and hormonal responses. It is the hormonal regulation of blood calcium that keeps all of these processes going, even if a person fails to consume enough calcium on a daily basis.

osteoporosis Decreased bone mass related to the effects of aging, genetic background, and poor diet in both genders, and hormonal changes at menopause in women.

tetany A body condition marked by sharp contraction of muscles and failure to relax afterward; usually caused by abnormal calcium metabolism.

Other Possible Health Benefits of Calcium

Researchers have been examining links between calcium intake and risks for a variety of diseases including certain cancers, kidney stones, hypertension, high blood

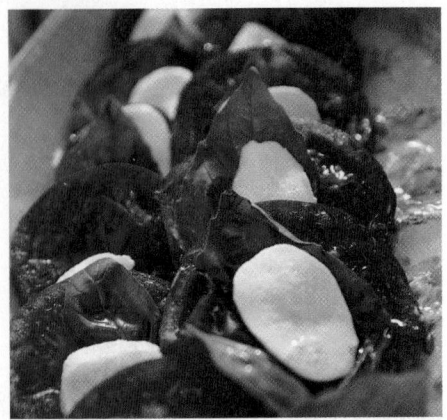

▲ To enhance intake of calcium and other nutrients, the 2010 Dietary Guidelines recommend an increased intake of fat-free or low-fat milk and milk products such as the mozzarella cheese on this tomato-basil salad.

cholesterol, and most recently, obesity. An adequate calcium intake can reduce the risk of colon cancer, especially in people who consume a high-fat diet (see Further Reading 13). A decreased risk of some forms of kidney stones and reduced lead absorption are other possible benefits when calcium is part of a meal. Calcium intakes of 800 to 1200 milligrams per day can also decrease blood pressure, compared with intakes of 400 milligrams per day or less. As covered in Chapter 5, calcium intakes of 1200 milligrams per day in combination with a low-fat, low-cholesterol diet can help people with elevated LDL cholesterol improve their blood lipid profiles. A link between a low calcium intake and overweight/obesity is also under study. Although the true benefit in this regard is not clear, studies suggest that an adequate calcium intake (compared to a very low intake [e.g., 400 milligrams per day]), coupled with a low calorie intake, may promote even more weight loss than the low calorie diet alone. Focusing on dairy sources of calcium is recommended because other components in dairy foods, such as some of the specific dairy proteins, contribute to this potential weight loss benefit. For women, an adequate calcium in-take might also reduce the risk of premenstrual syndrome and high blood pressure that can develop during pregnancy. Overall, the benefits of a diet providing adequate calcium extend beyond bone health.

Calcium Sources and Needs

Dairy products, such as milk and cheese, provide about 75% of the calcium in North American diets. The exception is cottage cheese, because most calcium is lost during production. Bread, rolls, crackers, and other foods made with milk products are secondary contributors. Other calcium sources are leafy greens (such as spinach), broccoli, sardines, and canned salmon (Fig. 9-11). It is important to remember that much of the calcium in some leafy green vegetables, notably spinach, is not absorbed because of the presence of oxalic acid. This effect is not as strong, however, in kale,

FIGURE 9-11 ▶ Food sources of calcium compared to the Adequate Intake.

Food Sources of Calcium

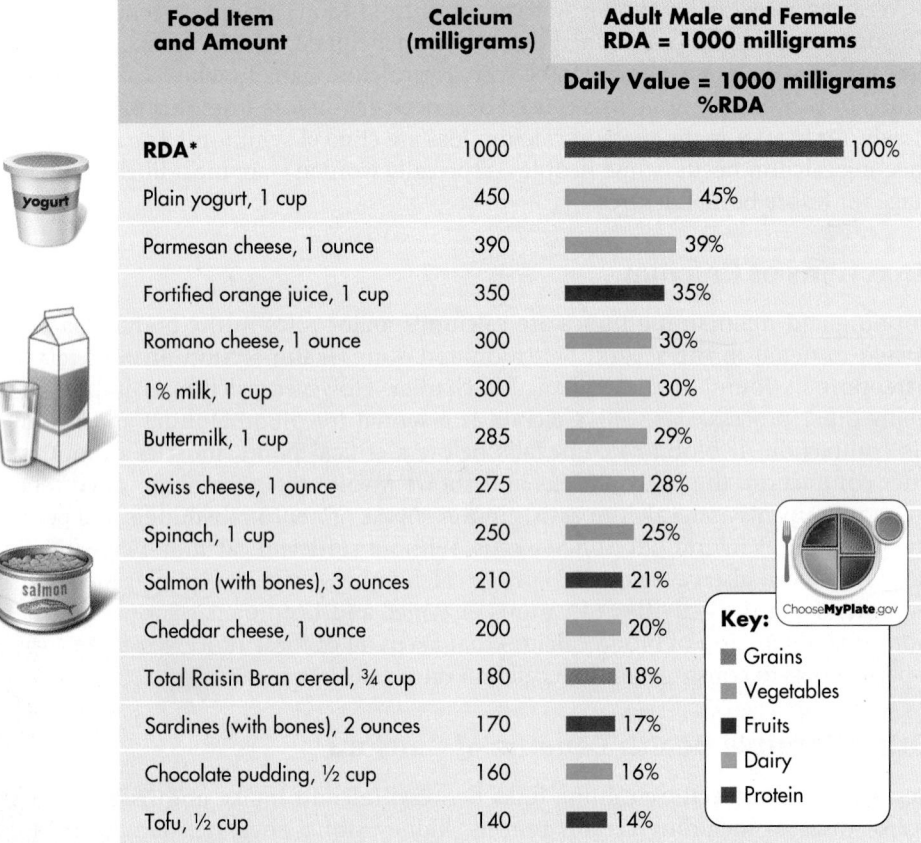

Food Item and Amount	Calcium (milligrams)	Adult Male and Female RDA = 1000 milligrams Daily Value = 1000 milligrams %RDA
RDA*	1000	100%
Plain yogurt, 1 cup	450	45%
Parmesan cheese, 1 ounce	390	39%
Fortified orange juice, 1 cup	350	35%
Romano cheese, 1 ounce	300	30%
1% milk, 1 cup	300	30%
Buttermilk, 1 cup	285	29%
Swiss cheese, 1 ounce	275	28%
Spinach, 1 cup	250	25%
Salmon (with bones), 3 ounces	210	21%
Cheddar cheese, 1 ounce	200	20%
Total Raisin Bran cereal, ¾ cup	180	18%
Sardines (with bones), 2 ounces	170	17%
Chocolate pudding, ½ cup	160	16%
Tofu, ½ cup	140	14%

Key:
■ Grains
■ Vegetables
■ Fruits
■ Dairy
■ Protein

*For adults; see the DRI table in the back of this book for age-specific recommendations.

collard, turnip, and mustard greens. Overall, fat-free milk is the most nutrient-dense (milligrams per kcal) source of calcium because of its high bioavailability and low calorie content, with some of the vegetables just noted following close behind (Fig. 9-12). The new calcium-fortified versions of orange juice and other beverages (e.g., soy milk), as well as calcium-fortified cottage cheese, breakfast cereals, breakfast bars, snacks, and certain chewable candies, also follow as close competitors. Another source of calcium is soybean curd (tofu) if it is made with calcium carbonate (check the label). Also, the bones in canned fish, such as salmon and sardines, supply calcium. High-calcium mineral waters appear to provide useful quantities of bioavailable calcium. Read more about these mineral waters in Further Reading 6 and in the What Would You Choose Recommendations at the end of this chapter.

Information about calcium is mandatory on food labels. The Daily Value used to express the calcium content on food and supplement labels is 1000 milligrams.

The Recommended Dietary Allowance for calcium for adults ranges from 1000 to 1200 milligrams per day for adults and is based on the amount of calcium needed each day to offset calcium losses in urine, feces, and other routes. The RDA for adolescents and teens is 1300 milligrams to allow for increases in bone mass during growth and development. In the United States, average calcium intakes are approximately 800 milligrams for women and 1000 milligrams for men. Thus, dietary intakes of calcium by many women, especially young women, are below the RDA, whereas intakes by most men are roughly equivalent to the RDA. It is also important for vegans to focus on eating good plant sources of calcium as well as on the total amount of calcium ingested.

To estimate your calcium intake, use the rule of 300s. Count 300 milligrams for the calcium provided by foods scattered throughout the diet. Add to that another 300 milligrams for every cup of milk or yogurt or 1.5 ounces of cheese. If you eat a lot of tofu, almonds, or sardines, or drink calcium-fortified beverages, use the second "Rate Your Plate" activity at the end of this chapter or your diet-analysis software to get a more accurate calculation of your calcium intake.

▲ Milk is a rich as well as convenient source of calcium.

Calcium Supplements

Calcium supplements can be used by people who do not like milk or who cannot incorporate enough calcium-containing foods into their diets. Calcium carbonate, the

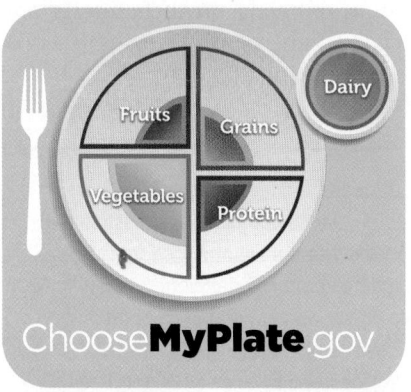

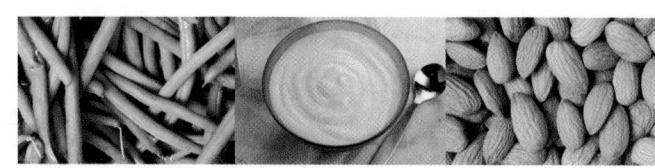

MyPlate:
Sources of Calcium

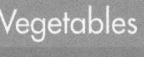

FIGURE 9-12 ▶ Sources of calcium from MyPlate. The height of the background color (none, 1/3, 2/3, or completely covered) within each group on the plate indicates the average nutrient density for calcium in that group. Overall, foods from the dairy group and many fortified foods are nutrient-dense and bioavailable sources of calcium. Additional calcium-fortified foods appear in stores each year and thus will add to the food sources listed for various groups.

Grains	Vegetables	Fruits	Dairy	Protein
• Calcium-fortified snack foods • Calcium-fortified flour tortillas • Calcium-fortified breakfast cereals	• Greens • Spinach • Broccoli • Green beans	• Calcium-fortified orange juice	• Milk • Yogurt • Cheese	• Tofu • Almonds • Shrimp • Sardines • Canned salmon

MAKING DECISIONS

Choosing a Calcium Supplement

Here is how to determine the calcium content of typical supplements based on the form of calcium, as listed on the supplement label and the percentage of calcium per unit of weight.

- Calcium carbonate: 40%
- Calcium phosphate (tribasic): 38%
- Calcium citrate: 21%
- Calcium lactate: 13%
- Calcium gluconate: 9%

To calculate the amount of calcium in a supplement, multiply the weight of the capsule by the percentage listed above. For example, if 1 tablet of calcium citrate weighs 500 milligrams, it contains 105 milligrams of calcium.

500 milligrams × 0.21 = 105 milligrams

Some calcium supplements are poorly digested because they do not readily dissolve. To test for this, put a supplement in ¾ cup of cider vinegar. Stir every 5 minutes. It should dissolve within 30 minutes. You now see that the type of calcium supplement chosen can make a big difference in how much calcium is in each pill.

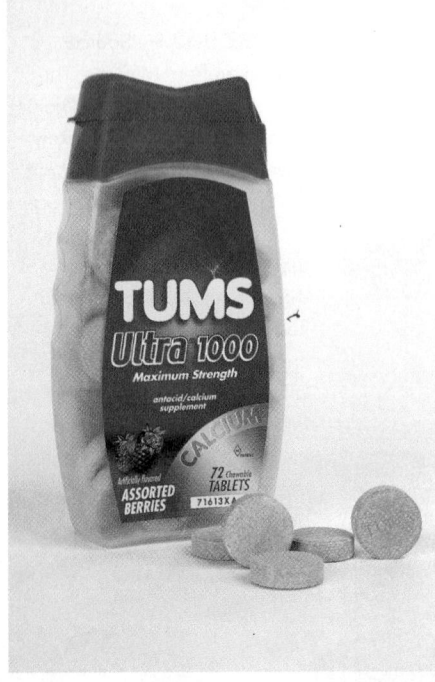

▲ Tums is an antacid that is also a good source of calcium carbonate.

form found in calcium-based antacid tablets, is the most common supplement used. People should take this supplement with or just after meals in doses of about 500 milligrams so that stomach acid produced during digestion can aid with absorption of this mineral. On the other hand, a supplement containing calcium citrate, which is acidic itself, can be taken without regard to meals. Studies have shown that supplements containing calcium citrate reduce bone loss and height loss in postmenopause women (see Further Reading 15).

With calcium supplements, interactions with other minerals are a valid concern. Perhaps most importantly, there is some evidence that calcium supplements may decrease zinc absorption. Therefore, calcium supplements should not be taken with meals rich in zinc. An effect of calcium supplementation on iron absorption is possible; however, this appears to be small over the long term. To be safe, people should notify their physician if using a calcium supplement on a regular basis.

Some calcium supplements also contain lead. FDA has no standards for lead content in food supplements, but does plan to regulate the lead content of supplements, including calcium, in the future. Until then, it is important to avoid supplements made from bonemeal, the worst offender when it comes to lead. Tablet or liquid calcium supplements with the USP seal of approval are less likely than others to contain high concentrations of contaminants.

No form of natural calcium, such as coral calcium, is superior to typical supplement forms. People making such claims of superiority have been prosecuted by the U.S. Federal Trade Commission for false advertising.

Upper Level for Calcium

The Upper Level for calcium intake is 2500 milligrams per day, based on the observation that greater intakes increase the risk for some forms of kidney stones. Excessive calcium intakes by some people also can cause high blood and urinary calcium concentrations, irritability, headache, kidney failure, soft tissue calcification, and decreased absorption of other minerals, as noted above.

So, which is better: calcium from food or supplements? Taking 1000 milligrams of calcium carbonate or calcium citrate daily in divided doses (about 500 milligrams per tablet) is probably safe in many instances. However, people often have difficulty adhering to a supplement regimen. If possible, modification of eating habits to include foods that are good sources of calcium is a better plan. In addition to this important mineral, foods that contain calcium also supply other vitamins, minerals, phytochemicals, and fats needed to support health. Plus, problems associated with excessive consumption of calcium are not likely when foods are one's sources of calcium.

CONCEPT CHECK

About 99% of calcium in the body is found in the bones. Aside from its critical role in bone, calcium also functions in blood clotting, muscle contraction, nerve-impulse transmission, and cell metabolism. Calcium requires a slightly acid pH and the vitamin D hormone for efficient absorption. Factors that reduce calcium absorption include a vitamin D deficiency, large amounts of fiber (especially excess wheat bran), and old age in general. Blood calcium is regulated primarily by hormones and does not closely reflect daily intake.

Dairy products are rich food sources of calcium. Other foods, such as calcium-fortified beverages, are rich sources as well. Supplemental forms, such as calcium carbonate, are well-absorbed by most people. However, overzealous supplementation can also result in the development of kidney stones and other health problems.

9.8 Phosphorus (P)

Although no disease is currently associated with an inadequate phosphorus intake, a deficiency may contribute to bone loss in older women. The body efficiently absorbs phosphorus, at about 70% of dietary intake. This high absorption, plus the wide availability of phosphorus in foods, makes this mineral less important than is calcium in diet planning. The active vitamin D hormone enhances phosphorus absorption, as it does for calcium. Blood phosphorus concentration is regulated primarily by kidney excretion and also by changes in the degree of absorption.

Phosphorus is a component of enzymes, other key compounds, DNA (genetic material), cell membranes, and bone. About 85% of the body's phosphorus is inside bone. The remaining phosphorus circulates freely in the bloodstream and functions inside cells.

Phosphorus Sources and Needs

Milk, cheese, meat, and bread provide most of the phosphorus in the adult diet. Breakfast cereals, bran, eggs, nuts, and fish are also good sources (Fig. 9-13). About 20% to 30% of dietary phosphorus comes from food additives, especially in baked goods, cheeses, processed meats, and many soft drinks with about 75 milligrams per 12-ounce (⅓-liter) serving of soft drinks. Next time you have a soft drink, look for a listing of phosphoric acid on the label.

The RDA for phosphorus for adults over age 18 is 700 milligrams daily, based on the amount needed to maintain normal blood concentrations of phosphorus. The Daily Value used to express phosphorus content on food and supplement labels is 1000 milligrams. Adults consume about 1000 to 1600 milligrams of phosphorus per day. Thus, deficiencies of phosphorus are unlikely in healthy adults, especially because it is so efficiently absorbed.

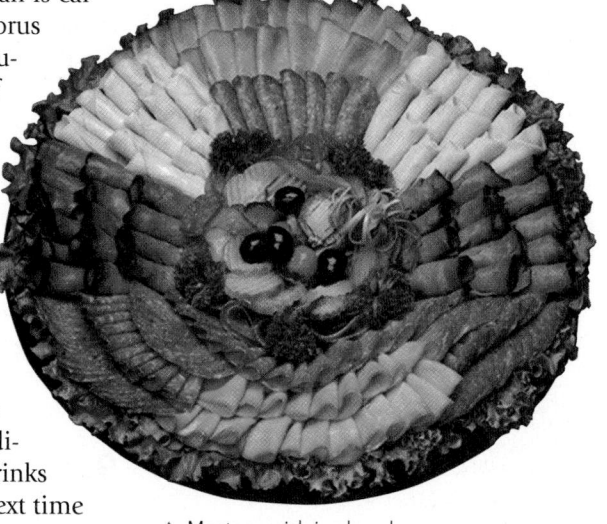
▲ Meats are rich in phosphorus.

Food Sources of Phosphorus

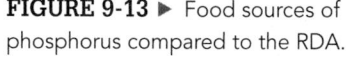

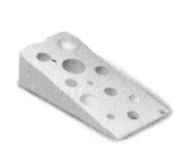
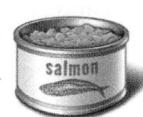
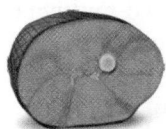

Food Item and Amount	Phosphorus (milligrams)	Adult Male and Female RDA = 700 milligrams / Daily Value = 1000 milligrams %RDA
RDA*	700	100%
Plain yogurt, 1 cup	350	50%
Swiss cheese, 2 ounces	345	49%
Almonds, ½ cup	340	49%
Sunflower seeds, 1 ounce	330	47%
1% milk, 1 cup	235	34%
Cheddar cheese, 1.5 ounces	220	31%
Salmon, 3 ounces	220	31%
Raisin Bran cereal, 1 cup	215	31%
Sirloin steak, 3 ounces	210	30%
Egg, 2 hard boiled	200	29%
Chicken breast, 3 ounces	180	26%
Roasted turkey, 3 ounces	180	26%
Pot roast, 3 ounces	170	24%
Lean ham, 3 ounces	165	24%
American cheese, 1 slice	155	22%

Key:
▪ Grains
▪ Vegetables
▪ Fruits
▪ Dairy
▪ Protein

*For adults; see the DRI table in the back of this book for age-specific recommendations.

FIGURE 9-13 ▶ Food sources of phosphorus compared to the RDA.

Marginal phosphorus status can be found in preterm infants, vegans, people with alcoholism, older people on nutrient-poor diets, and people with long-term bouts of diarrhea.

Upper Level for Phosphorus

The Upper Level for phosphorus intake is 3 to 4 grams per day. Intakes greater than this impair kidney function. High intakes are especially a problem in people with certain kidney diseases. In addition, a chronically high phosphorus intake coupled with a low calcium intake can cause an imbalance in the calcium-to-phosphorus ratio in the diet, which can contribute to bone loss. This situation most likely arises when the Adequate Intake for calcium is not met, as can occur in adolescents and adults who regularly substitute soft drinks for milk or otherwise underconsume calcium.

9.9 Magnesium (Mg)

Magnesium is important for nerve and heart function and aids many enzyme reactions. It is found mostly in the plant pigment chlorophyll, where it functions in respiration. We normally absorb about 40% to 60% of the magnesium in our diets, but absorption efficiency can increase up to about 80% if intakes are low.

Bone contains 60% of the body's magnesium. The rest circulates in the blood and operates inside cells. Over 300 enzymes use magnesium, and many energy-yielding compounds in cells require magnesium to function properly, as does the hormone insulin.

In humans, a magnesium deficiency causes an irregular heartbeat, sometimes accompanied by weakness, muscle pain, disorientation, and seizures. Adequate magnesium intakes decrease cardiovascular disease risk by decreasing blood pressure by dilating arteries and preventing heart rhythm abnormalities. People with cardiovascular disease should closely monitor magnesium intake, especially because they are often on medications such as diuretics that reduce magnesium status. Keep in mind that a magnesium deficiency develops slowly because our bodies store it readily.

Magnesium Sources and Needs

Rich sources for magnesium are plant products, such as whole grains (like wheat bran), broccoli, potatoes, squash, beans, nuts, and seeds (Fig. 9-14). Animal products, such as milk and meats, and even chocolate supply some magnesium, although less than the foods in the magnesium plate (Fig. 9-15). Two other sources of magnesium are hard tap water, which contains a high mineral content, and coffee.

The adult RDA for magnesium is about 400 milligrams per day for men and about 310 milligrams per day for women. This is based on the amount needed to offset daily losses. The Daily Value used to express magnesium content on food and supplement labels is 400 milligrams. Adult men consume an average of 320 milligrams daily, whereas women consume closer to 220 milligrams daily. A study has shown that a diet high in magnesium-rich foods, especially whole grains, decreases the risk of type 2 diabetes in U.S. black women (see Further Reading 16). This suggests that many of us should improve our intakes of magnesium-rich foods, such as whole-grain breads and cereals.

The refined grain products that dominate the diets of many North Americans are poor sources of this mineral. If dietary means are not enough, a balanced multivitamin and mineral supplement containing approximately 100 milligrams of magnesium can help to close the gap between intake and needs. The typical form used in supplements (magnesium oxide) is not as well absorbed as the forms of magnesium found in foods but still contributes to meeting magnesium needs.

Poor magnesium status is found especially among users of certain diuretics. In addition, heavy perspiration for weeks in hot climates and bouts of long-standing

Diabetes and hypertension have both been linked with low levels of magnesium in the blood. However, the cause for low magnesium in people with these diseases is unclear. Research is underway to uncover the potential role of magnesium in treatment and/or prevention of these chronic diseases.

Food Sources of Magnesium

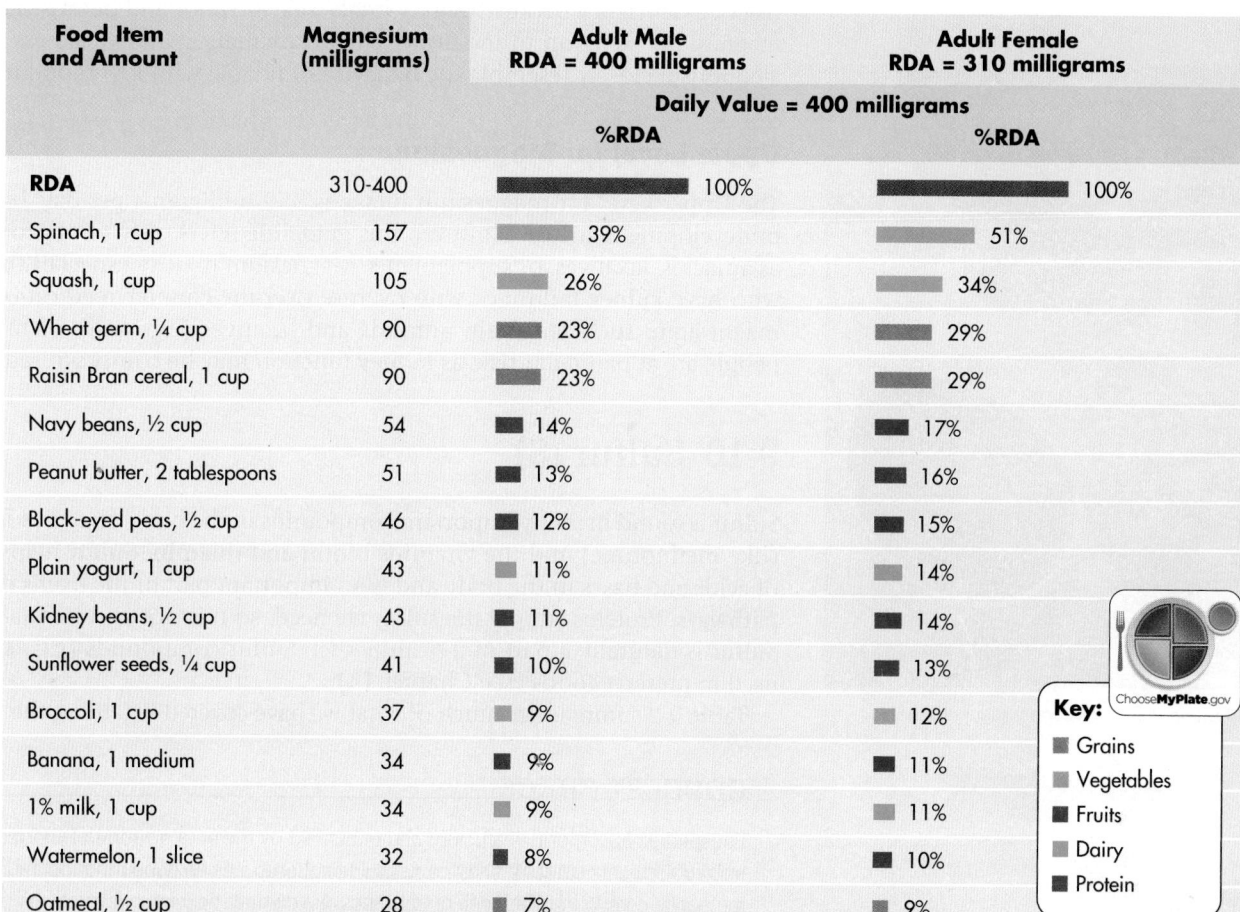

Food Item and Amount	Magnesium (milligrams)	Adult Male RDA = 400 milligrams	Adult Female RDA = 310 milligrams
		Daily Value = 400 milligrams	
		%RDA	%RDA
RDA	310-400	100%	100%
Spinach, 1 cup	157	39%	51%
Squash, 1 cup	105	26%	34%
Wheat germ, ¼ cup	90	23%	29%
Raisin Bran cereal, 1 cup	90	23%	29%
Navy beans, ½ cup	54	14%	17%
Peanut butter, 2 tablespoons	51	13%	16%
Black-eyed peas, ½ cup	46	12%	15%
Plain yogurt, 1 cup	43	11%	14%
Kidney beans, ½ cup	43	11%	14%
Sunflower seeds, ¼ cup	41	10%	13%
Broccoli, 1 cup	37	9%	12%
Banana, 1 medium	34	9%	11%
1% milk, 1 cup	34	9%	11%
Watermelon, 1 slice	32	8%	10%
Oatmeal, ½ cup	28	7%	9%
Whole-wheat bread, 1 slice	25	6%	8%

Key:
- Grains
- Vegetables
- Fruits
- Dairy
- Protein

FIGURE 9-14 ▶ Food sources of magnesium compared to the RDA for adult males and females.

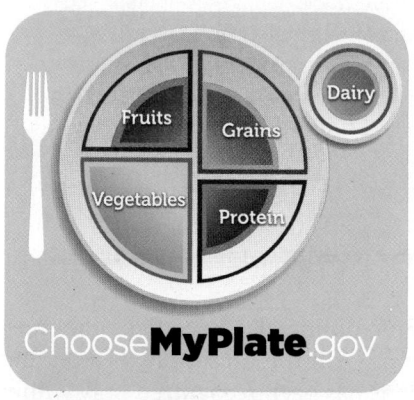

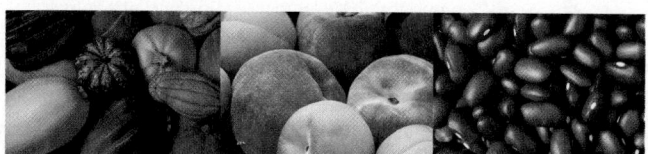

**MyPlate:
Sources of Magnesium**

FIGURE 9-15 ▶ Sources of magnesium from MyPlate. The fill of the background color (none, 1/3, 2/3, or completely covered) within each group on the plate indicates the average nutrient density for magnesium in that group. Overall, the vegetables group provides the richest sources. Whole-grain choices in the grains group are also rich sources.

Grains
- Wheat bran
- Wheat germ
- Whole-grain products

Vegetables
- Avocados
- Spinach
- Greens
- Broccoli
- Lima beans
- Potatoes
- Squash

Fruits
- Figs
- Peaches
- Bananas
- Berries

Dairy
- Milk
- Yogurt

Protein
- Tofu
- Nuts
- Shrimp
- Kidney beans
- Sunflower seeds

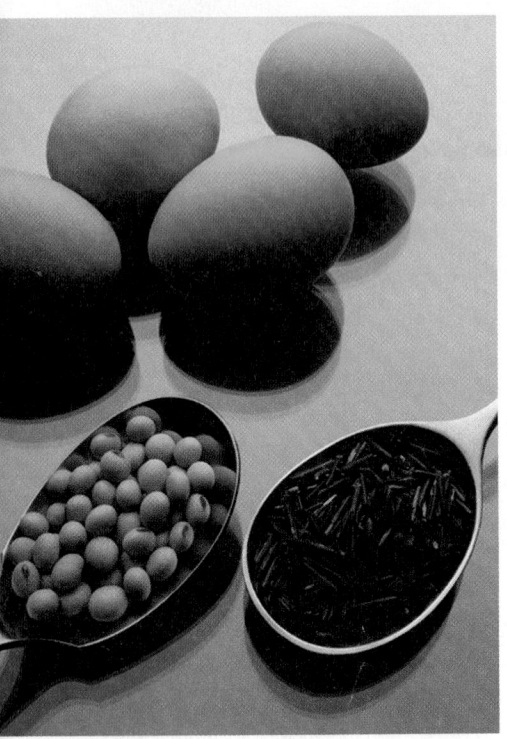

▲ Protein-rich foods supply sulfur in the diet.

diarrhea or vomiting cause significant magnesium loss. Alcoholism also increases the risk of a deficiency because dietary intake may be poor and because alcohol increases magnesium excretion in the urine. The disorientation and weakness associated with alcoholism closely resemble the behavior of people with low blood magnesium.

Upper Level for Magnesium

The Upper Level for magnesium intake is 350 milligrams per day, based on the risk of developing diarrhea. However, this guideline refers only to nonfood sources such as antacids, laxatives, or supplements. Magnesium toxicity especially occurs in people who have kidney failure or who overuse over-the-counter medications that contain magnesium, such as certain antacids and laxatives (e.g., milk of magnesia). Older people are at particular risk, as kidney function may be compromised.

9.10 Sulfur (S)

Sulfur is found in many important compounds in the body, such as some amino acids (like methionine) and the vitamins biotin and thiamin. Sulfur helps in the balance of acids and bases in the body and is an important part of the liver's drug-detoxifying pathways. Proteins supply the sulfur we need, so it is not an essential nutrient *per se.* Sulfur is naturally a part of a healthy diet. Sulfur compounds (e.g., sulfites) are also used to preserve foods (see Chapter 13).

Table 9-2 summarizes much of what we have covered regarding the major minerals.

CONCEPT CHECK

Phosphorus absorption is efficient and enhanced by the active vitamin D hormone. Urinary excretion mainly controls body content. Phosphorus aids enzyme function and is part of key metabolic compounds and cell membranes. No distinct deficiency symptoms caused by an inadequate phosphorus intake have been reported. Food sources for phosphorus include dairy products, baked goods, and meat. The RDA is met by most North Americans. An excess intake of phosphorus can compromise bone health, if sufficient calcium is not consumed, and can impair kidney function. Magnesium is required for nerve and heart function; it also aids activity for many enzymes. Food sources of magnesium are whole grains (wheat bran), vegetables, beef, coffee, beans, nuts, and seeds. People using certain diuretics and people with alcoholism are at greatest risk of developing a deficiency. Magnesium toxicity is most likely in people with kidney failure or people using certain forms of laxatives and antacids. Sulfur is a component of certain vitamins and amino acids. The protein we consume supplies sufficient sulfur for the body's needs.

9.11 Trace Minerals—An Overview

Information about trace minerals (also called microminerals) is perhaps the most rapidly expanding area of knowledge in nutrition. With the exceptions of iron and iodide, the importance of trace minerals to humans has been recognized only within the last 40 years. Although we need 100 milligrams or less of each trace mineral daily, they are as essential to good health as major minerals.

In some cases, discovering the importance of a trace mineral reads like a detective story, and the evidence is still unfolding. In 1961, researchers linked dwarfism among Middle Eastern villagers to a zinc deficiency. Other scientists recognized that a rare form of heart disease in an isolated area of China was linked to a selenium deficiency. In North America, some trace mineral deficiencies were first observed in the late 1960s and early 1970s when the minerals were not added to newly developed synthetic formulas used for intravenous feeding.

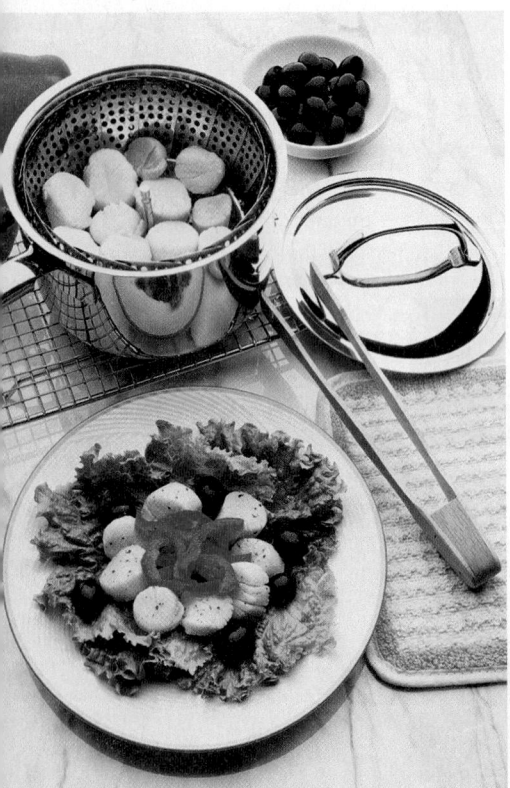

▲ Seafood, such as scallops, is a good source of many trace minerals.

TABLE 9-2 Summary of the Major Minerals

Mineral	Major Functions	RDA, or Adequate Intake	Dietary Sources	Deficiency Symptoms	Toxicity Symptoms
Sodium	• Major positive ion of the extracellular fluid • Aids nerve impulse transmission • Water balance	*Age 19–50 years:* 1500 milligrams *Age 51–70 years:* 1300 milligrams *Age > 70 years* 1200 milligrams	• Table salt • Processed foods • Condiments • Sauces • Soups • Chips	• Muscle cramps	• Contributes to hypertension in susceptible individuals • Increases calcium loss in urine • Upper Level is 2300 milligrams
Potassium	• Major positive ion of intracellular fluid • Aids nerve impulse transmission • Water balance	4700 milligrams	• Spinach • Squash • Bananas • Orange juice • Milk • Meat • Legumes • Whole grains	• Irregular heart beat • Loss of appetite • Muscle cramps	• Slowing of the heartbeat, as seen in kidney failure
Chloride	• Major negative ion of extracellular fluid • Participates in acid production in stomach • Aids nerve impulse transmission • Water balance	2300 milligrams	• Table salt • Some vegetables • Processed foods	• Convulsions in infants	• Linked to hypertension in susceptible people when combined with sodium • Upper Level is 3600 milligrams
Calcium	• Bone and tooth structure • Blood clotting • Aids in nerve impulse transmission • Muscle contractions • Other cell functions	*Age 9–18 years:* 1300 milligrams *Age > 18 years:* 1000–1200 milligrams	• Dairy products • Canned fish • Leafy vegetables • Tofu • Fortified orange juice (and other fortified foods)	• Increased risk of osteoporosis	• May cause kidney stones and other problems in susceptible people • Upper Level is 2500 milligrams
Phosphorus	• Major ion of intracellular fluid • Bone and tooth strength • Part of various metabolic compounds • Acid/base balance	*Age 9–18 years:* 1250 milligrams *Age > 18 years:* 700 milligrams	• Dairy products • Processed foods • Fish • Soft drinks • Bakery products • Meats	• Possibility of poor bone maintenance	• Impairs bone health in people with kidney failure • Poor bone mineralization if calcium intakes are low • Upper Level is 3 to 4 grams
Magnesium	• Bone formation • Aids enzyme function • Aids nerve and heart function	*Men:* 400–420 milligrams *Women:* 310–320 milligrams	• Wheat bran • Green vegetables • Nuts • Chocolate • Legumes	• Weakness • Muscle pain • Poor heart function	• Causes diarrhea and weakness in people with kidney failure • Upper Level is 350 milligrams, but refers to nonfood sources (e.g., supplements) only
Sulfur	• Part of vitamins and amino acids • Aids in drug detoxification • Acid/base balance	None	• Protein foods	• None observed	• None likely

It is difficult to precisely define our trace mineral needs because we need only minute amounts. Highly sophisticated technology is required to measure such small amounts in both food and body tissues.

9.12 Iron (Fe)

Although the importance of dietary iron has been recognized for centuries, today, iron deficiency is still one of the most common nutrient deficiencies worldwide. Iron is the only nutrient for which young women have a greater RDA than do adult men. Iron is found in every living cell, adding up to about 5 grams (1 teaspoon) for the entire body.

Absorption and Distribution of Iron

Controlling absorption is important because our bodies cannot easily eliminate excess iron once it is absorbed. The body uses several mechanisms to regulate iron absorption. Overall, iron absorption depends on its form in the food, the body's need for it, and a variety of other factors. Healthy people absorb about 18% of that present in food, whereas people with iron deficiency absorb somewhat more.

The form of iron in foods especially influences how much is absorbed. About 40% of the total iron in animal flesh is in the form of **hemoglobin** (the same form as in red blood cells) and **myoglobin** (pigment found in muscle cells). This type of iron, called **heme iron,** is absorbed about two to three times more efficiently than the simple elemental iron, called **nonheme iron.** Nonheme iron is added to grain products during the enrichment process and is also present in animal flesh, as well as in eggs, milk, vegetables, grains, and other plant foods.

Consuming heme iron and nonheme iron together increases nonheme iron absorption. A protein factor in meats may also aid nonheme absorption. Overall, eating meat with vegetables and grain products enhances the absorption of all nonheme iron present.

Vitamin C in amounts of about 75 milligrams can also increase nonheme iron absorption. Drinking a glass of orange juice when taking an iron supplement, therefore, will enhance the iron absorbed from the supplement. Consuming more foods rich in vitamin C is particularly desirable if dietary iron is inadequate or if blood iron is low. Iron use in the body is also aided by copper, as explained in the later section on copper.

In contrast, several dietary factors interfere with our ability to absorb nonheme iron. Phytic acid and other factors in grain fibers and oxalic acid in vegetables can all bind this iron and reduce its absorption. Polyphenols (tannins) found in tea also reduce nonheme iron absorption. It is a good idea to moderate intake of tannins if one has iron deficiency and keep fiber intake within current recommendations. Taking zinc supplements will also interfere with nonheme iron because zinc will compete with iron for absorption.

Overall, the most important factor influencing nonheme iron absorption is the body's need for it. Iron needs are increased during pregnancy and growth. At high altitudes, the need for iron is also increased because the lower oxygen concentration of the air causes an increase in the hemoglobin concentration of blood. During an iron deficiency state, nonheme iron absorption can increase. When iron stores are inadequate, the main protein that carries iron in blood readily binds more iron from intestinal cells and shifts it into the bloodstream. When iron stores are adequate and the iron-binding protein in the blood is fully saturated with iron, iron stays bound in the intestinal cells and little will be absorbed.

By this mechanism, under normal circumstances, iron, especially the nonheme form, is absorbed as needed. If not needed, iron stored in intestinal cells will be excreted when intestinal cells are shed at the end of their 2- to 5-day life cycle. High doses of iron can still be toxic, but absorption is carefully regulated under typical dietary conditions in most people.

hemoglobin The iron-containing part of the red blood cell that carries oxygen to the cells and some carbon dioxide away from the cells. The heme iron portion is also responsible for the red color of blood.

myoglobin Iron-containing protein that binds oxygen in muscle tissue.

heme iron Iron provided from animal tissues in the form of hemoglobin and myoglobin. Approximately 40% of the iron in meat is heme iron; it is readily absorbed.

nonheme iron Iron provided from plant sources and animal tissues other than in the forms of hemoglobin and myoglobin. Nonheme iron is less efficiently absorbed than heme iron; absorption is closely dependent on body needs.

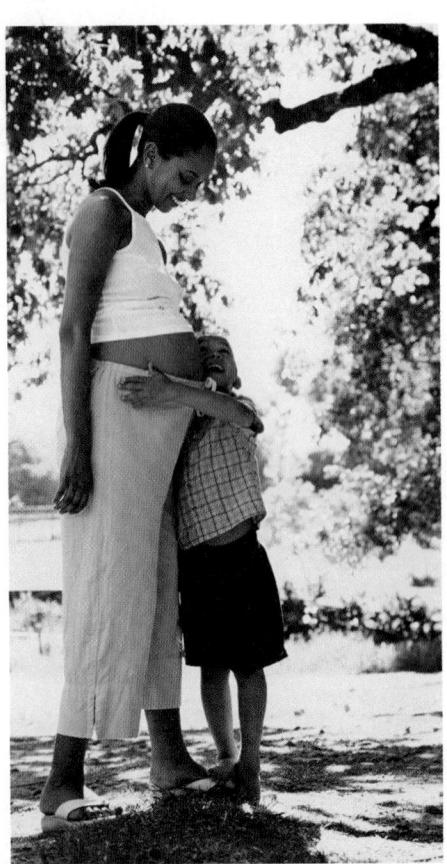

▲ Pregnancy greatly increases iron needs, as does growth in childhood.

Most iron in the body is contained in the hemoglobin molecules of the red blood cells. Some iron is stored in the bone marrow, and a small portion goes to other body cells, such as the liver, for storage. As iron is needed, it can be mobilized from these body stores. If dietary intake is chronically inadequate, these iron stores become depleted. Only then do signs of an iron deficiency appear.

Functions of Iron

Iron is part of the hemoglobin in red blood cells and myoglobin in muscle cells. Hemoglobin molecules in red blood cells transport oxygen (O_2) from the lungs to cells and assist in the return of some carbon dioxide (CO_2) from cells to the lungs for excretion. In addition, iron is used as part of many enzymes, some proteins, and compounds that cells use in energy production. Iron is also needed for brain and immune function and contributes to drug detoxification in the liver and to bone health.

If neither the diet nor body stores can supply the iron needed for hemoglobin synthesis, the number of red blood cells decreases in the bloodstream. The blood hemoglobin concentration also falls. Physicians use both the percentage of red blood cells (called the **hematocrit**) and the hemoglobin concentration in blood to assess iron status, along with the amount of iron and iron-containing proteins in the bloodstream. When hematocrit and hemoglobin fall, an iron deficiency is suspected. In severe deficiency, hemoglobin and hematocrit fall so low that the amount of oxygen carried in the bloodstream is decreased. Such a person has **anemia,** defined as a decreased oxygen-carrying capacity of the blood.

While there are many types of anemia, iron-deficiency anemia is the major type worldwide. About 30% of the world's population is anemic, and about half of those cases are caused by an iron deficiency. Probably about 10% of North Americans in high-risk categories have iron-deficiency anemia. This appears most often in infancy, the preschool years, and at puberty for both males and females. Growth, with accompanying expansion of blood volume and muscle mass, increases iron needs, making it difficult to consume enough iron. Women are also vulnerable during childbearing years from blood loss during menstruation. In addition, anemia is often found in pregnant women, as discussed in Chapter 14. Iron-deficiency anemia in adult men is usually caused by blood loss from ulcers, colon cancer, or hemorrhoids. Finally, athletes can develop iron-deficiency anemia, as discussed in Chapter 10.

Clinical symptoms of iron-deficiency anemia primarily include pale skin, fatigue upon exertion, poor temperature regulation, loss of appetite, and apathy. Insufficient iron for the synthesis of red blood cells and key cell compounds may cause the fatigue. Poor iron stores may also decrease learning ability, attention span, work performance, and immune status even before a person is anemic.

More North Americans have an iron deficiency without anemia than have iron-deficiency anemia. Their blood hemoglobin values are still normal, but they have no stores to draw from in times of pregnancy or illness, and basic functioning may be at decreased levels. These effects could range from having too little energy to perform everyday tasks in an efficient manner to difficulties staying alert in school or on the job.

To speed the cure of iron-deficiency anemia, a person needs to take iron supplements. A physician should determine the cause of the anemia, be it an inadequate diet or a bleeding ulcer, for example, so that the anemia does not recur. Changes in diet may prevent iron-deficiency anemia, but supplemental iron is the only reliable cure once it has developed.

Iron Sources and Needs

Because animal sources contain some heme iron, the most bioavailable form, they are our best iron sources. The major iron sources in the adult diet are ready-to-eat breakfast cereals, animal products, and bakery items, such as bread (Figs. 9-16 and 9-17). Most of the iron in bakery items has been added to refined flour in the

hematocrit The percentage of blood made up of red blood cells.

anemia Generally refers to a decreased oxygen-carrying capacity of the blood. This can be caused by many factors, such as iron deficiency or blood loss.

Food Sources of Iron

Food Item and Amount	Iron (milligrams)	Adult Male RDA = 8 milligrams		Adult Female RDA =18 milligrams	
		Daily Value = 18 milligrams			
		%RDA		%RDA	
RDA			100%		100%
Oat bran cereal, 1 cup	15		188%		83%
Baked clams, 3 ounces	14		175%		78%
Spinach, 1 cup	6.4		80%		36%
Kidney beans, 1 cup	5.3		66%		29%
Pot roast, 4 ounces	3.9		49%		22%
Sirloin steak, 4 ounces	3.8		48%		21%
Parsley, 1 cup	3.7		46%		21%
Fried beef liver, 2 ounces	3.6		45%		20%
Shrimp, 3 ounces	2.7		34%		15%
Braunschweiger sausage, 1 piece	2.7		34%		15%
Flour tortilla, 1	2.4		30%		13%
Garbanzo beans, ½ cup	2.4		30%		13%
Navy beans, ½ cup	2.3		29%		13%
Baked potato, 1	1.7		21%		9%
Artichoke, 1	1.6		20%		9%

Key:
- Grains
- Vegetables
- Fruits
- Dairy
- Protein

ChooseMyPlate.gov

FIGURE 9-16 ▶ Food sources of iron compared to the RDA for adult males and females.

FIGURE 9-17 ▶ Sources of iron from MyPlate. The fill of the background color (none, 1/3, 2/3, or completely covered) within each group on the plate indicates the average nutrient density for iron in that group. Overall, the protein group and the grains group contain many foods that are nutrient-dense sources of iron. Still, the iron content of a food containing mostly nonheme iron is only an approximate measure of the amount delivered to body cells, as body need greatly influences the absorption of nonheme iron.

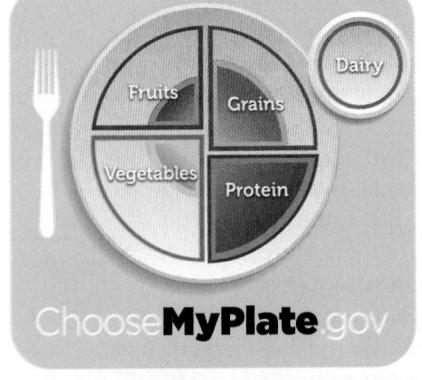

Choose**MyPlate**.gov

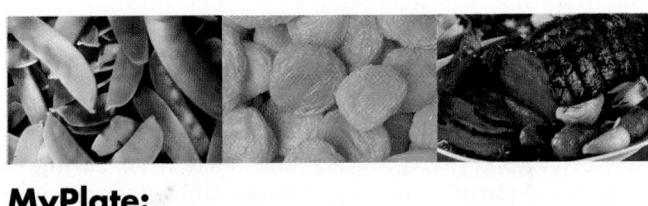

MyPlate: Sources of Iron

Grains	Vegetables	Fruits	Dairy	Protein
• Whole grains	• Spinach	• Peaches	• None	• Beef
• Enriched grains	• Peas	• Prune juice		• Tofu
• Wheat germ	• Potatoes	• Dried apricots		• Beans
• Oatmeal	• Green beans			• Seafood
	• Broccoli			• Organ meats

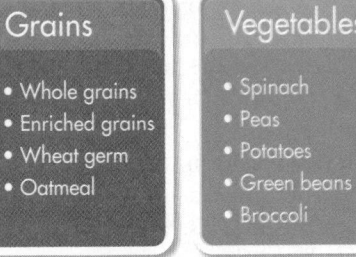
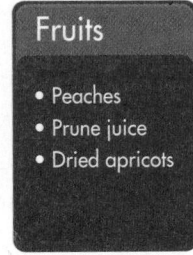
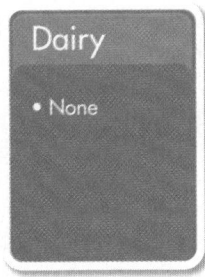

enrichment process. Other iron sources are spinach, peas, and legumes, but the iron is less available from these foods than from animal products.

Milk is a poor source of iron. A common cause of iron-deficiency anemia in children is an overreliance on milk, coupled with an insufficient meat intake. Total vegetarians (vegans) are particularly susceptible to iron-deficiency anemia because of their lack of dietary heme iron.

The daily adult RDA for iron for men, and for women over 50 years, is 8 milligrams. For women ages 19 to 50 years the RDA is 18 milligrams. The higher RDA for young and middle-age women is primarily because of menstrual blood loss. The variation in menstrual blood loss, and hence, loss of iron, makes it difficult to set an RDA for iron for women. Women who menstruate more heavily and longer than average may need even more dietary iron than those who have lighter and shorter flows. The Daily Value used to express iron content on food and supplement labels is 18 milligrams.

Most women do not consume 18 milligrams of iron daily. The average daily intake is closer to 13 milligrams, while in men it is about 18 milligrams per day. Women can close this gap between average daily intakes and needs by seeking out iron-fortified foods, such as ready-to-eat breakfast cereals that contain at least 50% of the Daily Value. Use of a balanced multivitamin and mineral supplement containing up to 100% of the Daily Value for iron is another option. Consuming more than that much iron is not advised unless a physician suggests otherwise (e.g., compensating for heavy menstrual loss).

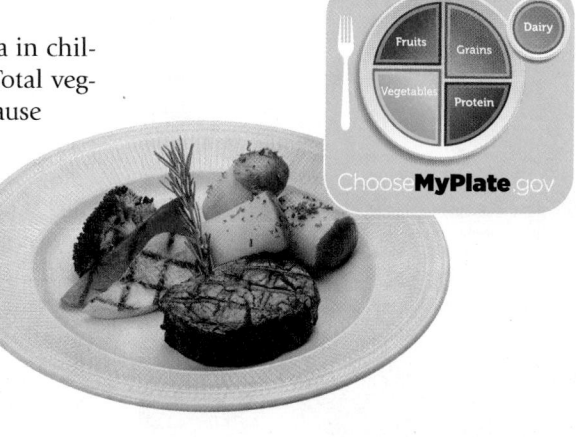

▲ Red meat is a major source of iron in the North American diet. The heme iron present is better absorbed than the nonheme iron found in meats and plants. The filet mignon, potatoes, and broccoli on this plate are good sources of iron from the protein and vegetable groups.

MAKING DECISIONS

Blood Donation

The adult human body contains about 21 cups (5 liters) of blood. Blood donations are generally 2 cups (500 milliliters). Thus, a blood donor gives about a tenth of his or her total supply with each donation. Healthy people generally can donate blood two to four times a year without harmful consequences. As a precaution, blood banks first screen potential donors' blood for the presence of anemia.

Upper Level for Iron

The Upper Level for iron is 45 milligrams per day. Higher amounts can lead to stomach irritation. Although iron overload is not as common as iron deficiency, it can be a serious result of misuse because iron can easily build up in the body and lead to toxic symptoms. Even a large single dose of 60 milligrams of iron can be life-threatening to a 1-year-old. Children are frequently victims of iron poisoning because iron pills and nutrient supplements containing iron are tempting when accessible on kitchen tables and even from cabinets.

FDA has ruled that all iron supplements must carry a warning about toxicity and that tablets with 30 milligrams of iron or more must be individually wrapped. Smaller doses of iron (but still greater than what is needed) over a long period can also cause problems. Repeated blood transfusions can also lead to iron toxicity.

Hemochromatosis. Iron toxicity can occur as a result of the genetic disease called hereditary **hemochromatosis.** The disease is associated with a substantial increase in iron absorption. Heme iron poses the greatest risk as body needs do not influence its absorption to a great extent. For people with this disease, iron in the body eventually builds up to dangerous amounts, especially in the blood and liver. Some iron is deposited in the muscles, pancreas, and heart. If not treated, the excess iron deposits contribute to severe organ damage, especially in the liver and heart.

Development of hereditary hemochromatosis requires that a person carry two defective copies of a particular gene. People with one defective gene and one normal

Chapter 8 noted that if men, in general, and older women take a multivitamin and mineral supplement, it should be low in iron or iron-free because of their increased risk for iron toxicity.

hemochromatosis A disorder of iron metabolism characterized by increased iron absorption and deposition in the liver and heart tissue. This eventually poisons the cells in those organs.

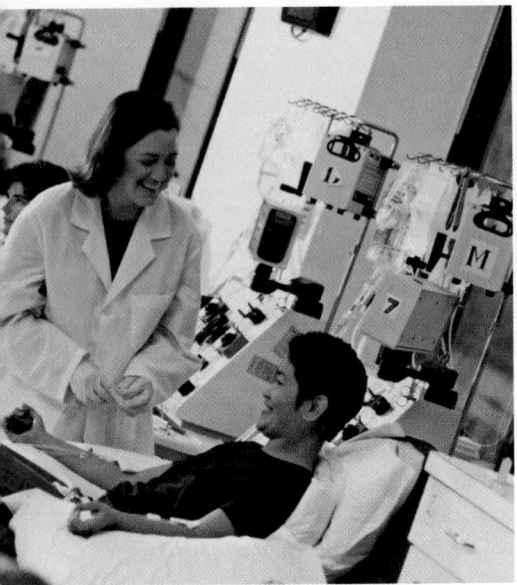

▲ Young adult women should avoid frequent blood donations because a significant amount of iron is lost in each donation. Blood donation, however, is an effective treatment for hemochromatosis.

gene, called carriers, may also absorb too much dietary iron but not to the same extent as those with two defective genes. About 5% to 10% of North Americans of Northern European descent are carriers of hemochromatosis. Approximately 1 in 250 North Americans has both hemochromatosis genes. These numbers are high considering that many physicians regard hemochromatosis as a rare disease and thus do not routinely test for it.

A reasonable approach is for you to ask to be screened for iron overload at your next visit to a physician (ask for a transferrin saturation test or a ferritin test to assess iron stores). Hemochromatosis can go undetected until a person is in their fifties or sixties, so some experts recommend screening for anyone over the age of 20. If the disease goes untreated, many organs will have become irreversibly damaged by one's middle years. If you show evidence of hemochromatosis, it would be wise to undergo therapy. This includes regular blood donations and avoidance of iron-rich foods and iron supplements (see the website www.americanhs.org).

Ideally, consent of a physician should precede any intake of iron from supplements, especially by men. When iron supplements are advised, there should be adequate follow-up so that supplementation does not exceed what is necessary. Probably the only factor keeping many people with hemochromatosis and carriers of one gene from experiencing serious effects of the disease is that they consume only a moderate amount of iron.

CONCEPT CHECK

Iron is absorbed depending mostly on its form and the body's need for it. Absorption is affected by iron needs but excess iron intake can override the system, leading to toxicity. Nonheme iron absorption increases somewhat in the presence of vitamin C and meat protein and decreases in the presence of large amounts of some components of grain fiber, such as phytic acid. Iron is used in synthesizing hemoglobin and myoglobin, in supporting immune function, and in energy metabolism. An iron deficiency can cause decreased red blood cell synthesis, which can lead to anemia. It is particularly important for women of childbearing age to consume adequate iron, primarily to replace that lost in menstrual blood. Sources include red meat, pork, liver, enriched grains and cereals, and oysters. Iron toxicity usually results from a genetic disorder called hemochromatosis. This disease causes overabsorption and accumulation of iron, which can result in severe liver and heart damage. Any use of iron supplements should be supervised by a physician because of the risk of toxicity.

9.13 Zinc (Zn)

Zinc deficiency was first recognized in humans in the early 1960s in Egypt and Iran. Zinc deficiencies were determined to cause growth retardation and poor sexual development in some groups of people, even though the zinc content of their diets was fairly high. The zinc bioavailability of the customary diet however, was decreased by the lack of animal protein and almost exclusive use of unleavened bread. Unleavened bread is very high in phytic acid and other factors that decrease zinc bioavailability.

In North America, zinc deficiencies were first observed in the early 1970s in hospitalized patients who were fed only intravenously via total parenteral nutrition containing individual amino acids as the protein source. Zinc deficiency symptoms quickly developed because amino-acid formulas are low in trace minerals compared to whole proteins.

Like iron, zinc absorption is influenced by the foods a person ingests. About 40% of dietary zinc is absorbed, especially when animal protein sources are used and when the body needs more zinc. Most people worldwide rely on cereal grains (low in zinc) for their sources of protein and calories. This makes consuming adequate zinc

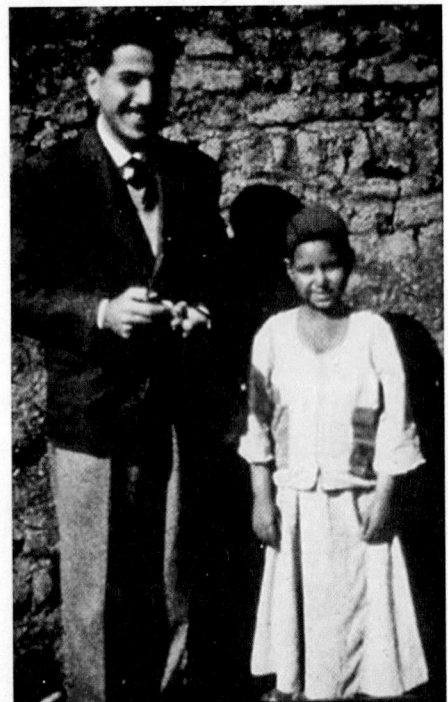

▲ Low intakes of zinc limit growth in people worldwide. On the right, an Egyptian farm boy, age 16 years old and 49 inches tall, with limited growth and sexual development associated with zinc deficiency.

a problem. In addition, high-dose calcium supplementation with meals decreases zinc absorption. Finally, zinc competes with copper and iron for absorption, and vice versa, when supplemental sources are taken.

Functions of Zinc

Up to 200 or so enzymes, such as alcohol dehydrogenase, require zinc as a cofactor for optimal activity. Adequate zinc intake is necessary to support many bodily functions, such as:

- DNA synthesis and function
- Protein metabolism, wound healing, and growth
- Immune function (intakes in excess of the RDA do not provide any extra benefit to immune function)
- Development of sexual organs and bones
- Storage, release, and function of insulin
- Cell membrane structure and function
- Indirect antioxidant as a component of two forms of superoxide dismutase, an enzyme that aids in the prevention of oxidative damage to cells.

Other possible functions of zinc are slowing the progression of macular degeneration of the eye and reducing the risk for developing certain forms of cancer. One study has shown that megadose zinc supplements (80 milligrams per day of zinc oxide) reduces the progression of macular degeneration by 25% in people who had a moderate case of the disease. The zinc supplements worked even better when provided in combination with 400 IU of vitamin E, 500 milligrams of vitamin C, and 15 milligrams of beta-carotene. (Copper oxide [2 milligrams] was also included because zinc decreases copper absorption.) Experts suggest that adults who have evidence of moderate macular degeneration talk to their physicians and eyecare specialists about the possibility of following such a protocol.

Symptoms of adult zinc deficiency include an acnelike rash, diarrhea, lack of appetite, reduced sense of taste and smell, and hair loss. In children and adolescents with zinc deficiency, growth, sexual development, and learning ability may also be hampered.

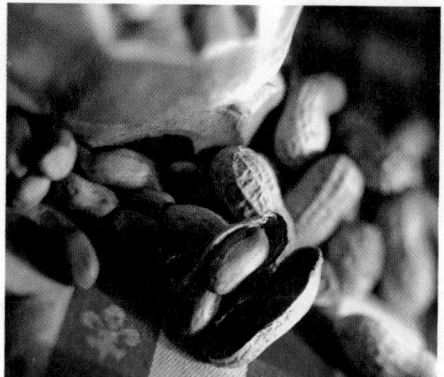

▲ Peanuts are a plant source of zinc.

Zinc Sources and Needs

In general, protein-rich diets are also rich in zinc. Animal foods supply almost half of an individual's zinc intake. Major sources of zinc are beef, fortified breakfast cereals, milk, poultry, and bread. As with iron, bioavailability is also important to consider for zinc. Animal foods are again our prime sources because zinc from animal sources is not bound by phytic acid. However, good plant sources of zinc—such as whole grains, peanuts, and legumes (beans)—should not be discounted. They can deliver substantial amounts of zinc to body cells (Figs. 9-18 and 9-19). Also, the form generally used in multivitamin and mineral supplements (zinc oxide) is not as well absorbed as zinc found naturally in foods, but still contributes to meeting zinc needs.

The adult RDA for zinc is 11 milligrams for men and 8 milligrams for women, based on the amount to cover daily losses of zinc. The Daily Value used to express zinc content on food and supplement labels is 15 milligrams. The average North American takes in 10 to 14 milligrams of zinc per day, with men consuming the higher values. There are no indications of moderate or severe zinc deficiencies in an otherwise healthy adult population. It is likely, however, that some North Americans—especially some women, poor children, vegans, older people, and people with alcoholism—have a marginal zinc status. These and other people who show deterioration in taste sensation, recurring infections, poor growth, or depressed wound healing should have zinc status checked. Unfortunately, it is difficult to detect early signs of a zinc deficiency (see Further Reading 9).

FIGURE 9-18 ▶ Sources of zinc from MyPlate. The fill of the background color (none, 1/3, 2/3, or completely covered) within each group on the plate indicates the average nutrient density for zinc in that group. Overall, the protein group and the grains group contain many foods that are nutrient-dense sources of zinc.

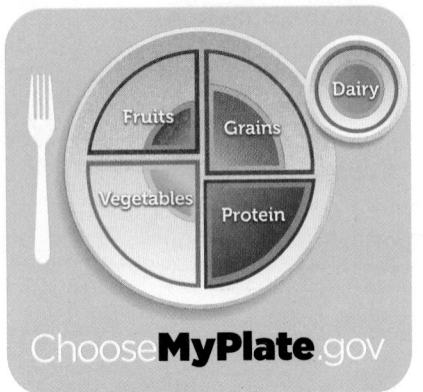

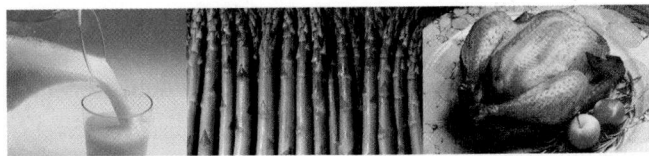

MyPlate: Sources of Zinc

Grains
- Whole-grain bread and cereals
- Fortified breakfast cereals

Vegetables
- Spinach
- Peas
- Asparagus

Fruits
- Avocados
- Dried Fruit

Dairy
- Milk
- Yogurt
- Cheese

Protein
- Beef
- Eggs
- Beans
- Nuts
- Shellfish
- Poultry

Food Sources of Zinc

Food Item and Amount	Zinc (milligrams)	Adult Male RDA = 11 milligrams %RDA	Adult Female RDA = 8 milligrams %RDA
RDA		100%	100%
Steamed oysters, 3	24.9	226%	311%
Sirloin steak, 4 ounces	7.4	67%	93%
Pot roast, 3 ounces	4.6	42%	58%
Special K cereal, 1 cup	3.8	35%	48%
Wheat germ, ¼ cup	3.5	32%	44%
Lamb chops, 3 ounces	2.7	25%	34%
Peanuts, ½ cup	2.4	22%	30%
Black-eyed peas, 1 cup	2.2	20%	28%
Plain yogurt, 1 cup	2.2	20%	28%
Lean ham, 3 ounces	1.9	17%	24%
Swiss cheese, 1.5 ounces	1.7	15%	21%
Ricotta cheese, ½ cup	1.7	15%	21%
Sunflower seeds, 1 ounce	1.5	14%	19%
Cheddar cheese, 1.5 ounces	1.3	12%	16%
Enriched white rice, ½ cup	1.1	10%	14%

Daily Value = 15 milligrams

Key:
- Grains
- Vegetables
- Fruits
- Dairy
- Protein

FIGURE 9-19 ▶ Food sources of zinc compared to the RDA for adult males and females.

Upper Level for Zinc

The Upper Level for zinc is 40 milligrams per day based on the potential interference with copper metabolism. Excessive zinc intakes over time can lead to problems by interfering with copper metabolism. An increased risk for prostate cancer with high intakes of zinc is also under study. Overall, if a person uses megadose zinc supplements (e.g., to try to slow macular degeneration), he or she should be under close medical supervision and also take a supplement containing copper (2 milligrams per day). Zinc intakes over 100 milligrams per day also result in diarrhea, cramps, nausea, vomiting, and depressed immune system function, especially if intake exceeds 2 grams per day.

MAKING DECISIONS

Zinc and the Common Cold

Many companies are singing the praises of zinc as a cold remedy. Products such as Cold-EEZE are lozenges that contain zinc, and their claims are based largely on one study done with 100 participants. The 50 individuals in the experimental group took 13 milligrams of zinc via the lozenges every 2 hours for the duration of their symptoms. Cold symptoms subsided after 4 days in the experimental group and 7 days in the control group. Nausea was a common side effect of the zinc lozenges. Of 10 other follow-up studies, however, only half have shown beneficial results from zinc. This may be due to differences in the bioavailability of various forms of zinc. Experts also note that we also have no idea of how the zinc would treat a cold, if it did. Adults can determine if the benefits outweigh the taste. Zinc expert Dr. Ananda Prasad recommends discontinuing use of zinc lozenges after 3 to 4 days unless they are showing evidence of effectiveness. Any use of such amounts beyond a week or so is potentially dangerous.

9.14 Selenium (Se)

Selenium exists in many readily absorbed forms. Like zinc, selenium has an indirect antioxidant function. Selenium's best understood role is as part of the enzyme (glutathione peroxidase) that works to reduce damage to cell membranes from electron-seeking, free-radical (oxidizing) compounds. Selenium also contributes to thyroid hormone metabolism and other functions.

In Chapter 8 you saw that vitamin E helps prevent attacks on cell membranes by donating electrons to electron-seeking compounds. Thus, vitamin E and selenium work together toward the same goal. The potential for free-radical compounds to cause cancer was also discussed in Chapter 8. Although selenium could prove to have a role in prevention of cancers, such as prostate cancer, it is premature to recommend megadose selenium supplementation for this purpose. Animal studies in this area are conflicting; recent studies with humans using supplemental intakes of 200 micrograms per day have shown no benefit of selenium in cancer prevention (see Further Reading 11).

Selenium deficiency symptoms in humans include muscle pain and wasting and a certain form of heart damage. In some areas of China, people develop characteristic muscle and heart disorders associated with inadequate selenium intake. Other factors probably also contribute.

Selenium Sources and Needs

Fish, meats (especially organ meats), eggs, and shellfish are good animal sources of selenium (Fig. 9-20). Grains and seeds grown in soils containing selenium are good plant sources. Major selenium contributors to the adult diet are animal and grain products.

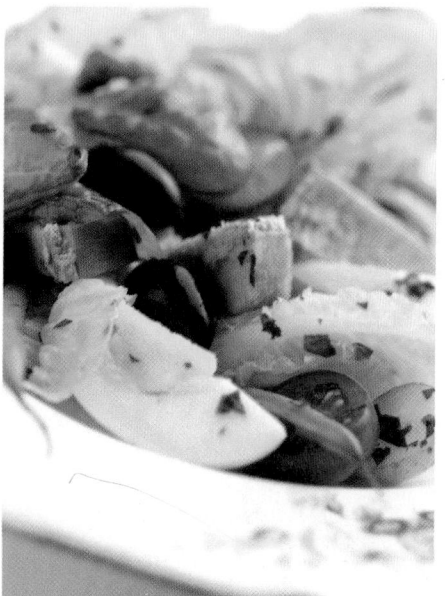

▲ The tuna and egg in this Salade Niçoise are excellent sources of selenium.

CRITICAL THINKING

Tammy read an article about antioxidants and their role in preventing free-radical damage to cells. When Tammy went to the drugstore to take a closer look at such supplements, she saw that selenium was one of the antioxidants in the supplements. Why does selenium deserve consideration as an antioxidant?

FIGURE 9-20 ▶ Food sources of selenium compared to the RDA.

Food Sources of Selenium

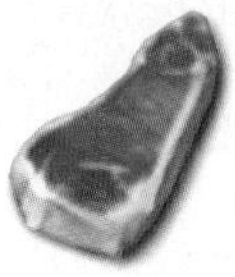

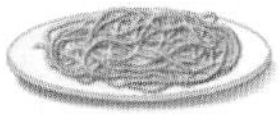

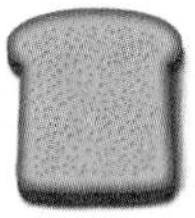

Food Item and Amount	Selenium (micrograms)	Adult Male and Female RDA = 55 micrograms
		Daily Value = 70 micrograms %RDA
RDA*	55	100%
Tuna, 3 ounces	68	124%
Sirloin steak, 5 ounces	47	85%
Lean ham, 3 ounces	42	76%
Clams, 3 ounces	41	75%
Salmon, 3 ounces	40	73%
Egg noodles, 1 cup	35	64%
Chicken breast, 3 ounces	20	36%
Special K cereal, 1 cup	17	31%
Oat bran cereal, 1 cup	14	25%
Whole-wheat bread, 1 slice	10	18%
Cooked oatmeal, 1 cup	10	18%
White bread, 1 slice	9	16%
Raisin bran cereal, 1 cup	4	7%

Key:
■ Grains
■ Vegetables
■ Fruits
■ Dairy
■ Protein

*For adults; see DRI table in the back of this book for gender- and age-specific recommendations.

We eat a varied diet of foods supplied from many geographic areas, so it is unlikely that low soil selenium in a few locations will mean inadequate selenium in our diets.

The RDA for selenium is 55 micrograms per day for adults. This intake maximizes the activity of selenium-dependent enzymes. The Daily Value used to express selenium content on food and supplement labels is 70 micrograms. In general, adults meet the RDA, consuming on average 105 micrograms of selenium each day.

Upper Level for Selenium

The Upper Level for selenium is 400 micrograms per day for adults. This is based on overt signs of selenium toxicity, such as hair loss.

CONCEPT CHECK

Zinc functions as a cofactor for many enzymes (including those that act as antioxidants) and is important for growth, cell membrane structure and function, immune function, and sense of taste. Beef, seafood, and whole grains are good food sources. As in the case of iron, zinc absorption is regulated according to the body's needs for the mineral. If taken in excess amounts, zinc competes with copper for absorption. Selenium activates an enzyme that helps change electron-seeking, free-radical (oxidizing) compounds into less toxic compounds so these do not attack and break down cell membranes. By helping to dismantle the free-radical compounds, selenium works toward the same goal as vitamin E in providing antioxidant protection to the body. A selenium deficiency results in muscle and heart disorders. Animal products and grains are good selenium sources; however, the selenium content in plants depends on the selenium concentration in the soil. The misuse of both selenium and zinc supplements can readily lead to toxic results.

9.15 Iodide (I)

Iodine in foods is found in an ion form, called iodide. During World War I, a link was discovered between a deficiency of iodide and the production of a **goiter,** an enlarged thyroid gland. Men drafted from areas such as the Great Lakes Region of the United States had a much higher rate of goiter than did men from some other areas of the country. The soils in these areas have low iodide contents. In the 1920s, researchers in Ohio found that low doses of iodide given to children over a 4-year period could prevent goiter. That finding led to the addition of iodide to salt beginning in the 1920s.

Today, many nations such as Canada require iodide fortification of salt. In the United States, salt can be purchased either iodized or plain. Iodized salt is clearly marked on the label of a package of salt. Some areas of Europe, such as northern Italy, have low levels of iodide in soil, but have yet to adopt an iodide fortification program. People in these areas, especially women, still suffer from goiter, as do people in areas of Latin America, the Indian subcontinent, Southeast Asia, and Africa. About 2 billion people worldwide are at risk of iodide deficiency, and approximately 800 million of these people have suffered the widespread effects of the deficiency. Eradication of iodide deficiency is a goal of many health-related organizations worldwide.

Function of Iodide

The thyroid gland actively accumulates and traps iodide from the bloodstream to support thyroid hormone synthesis. Thyroid hormones are synthesized using iodide and the amino acid tyrosine. These hormones help regulate metabolic rate and promote growth and development throughout the body, including the brain.

If a person's iodide intake is insufficient, the thyroid gland enlarges as it attempts to take up more iodide from the bloodstream. This eventually leads to goiter. Simple goiter is a painless condition, but if uncorrected can lead to pressure on the trachea (windpipe), which may cause difficulty in breathing. Although iodide can prevent goiter formation, it does not significantly shrink a goiter once it has formed. Surgical removal may be required in severe cases.

If a woman has an iodide-deficient diet during the early months of her pregnancy, the fetus suffers iodide deficiency because the mother's body uses up the available iodide. The infant then may be born with short length and develop mental retardation. The stunted growth and mental retardation that results is known as **cretinism.** Cretinism appeared in North America before iodide fortification of table salt began. Today, cretinism still appears in Europe, Africa, Latin America, and Asia.

Iodide Sources and Needs

Saltwater fish, seafood, iodized salt, dairy products, and grain products contain various forms of iodide (Fig. 9-21). Sea salt found in health-food stores, however, is not a good source because the iodide is lost during processing.

The RDA for iodide for adults is 150 micrograms to support thyroid gland function. This is the same as the Daily Value used to express iodide content on food and supplement labels. A half teaspoon of iodide-fortified salt (about 2 grams) supplies that amount. Most adults consume more iodide than the RDA—an estimated 190 to 300 micrograms daily, not including that from use of iodized salt at the table. The iodide in our diets adds up because dairies and fast-food restaurants use it as a sterilizing agent, bakeries use it as a dough conditioner, food producers use it as part of food colorants, and it is added to salt. There is concern, however, that vegans may not consume enough unless iodized salt is used.

Upper Level for Iodide

The Upper Level for iodide is 1.1 milligrams per day. When high amounts of iodide are consumed, thyroid hormone synthesis is inhibited, as in a deficiency. This can

goiter An enlargement of the thyroid gland; this is often caused by insufficient iodide in the diet.

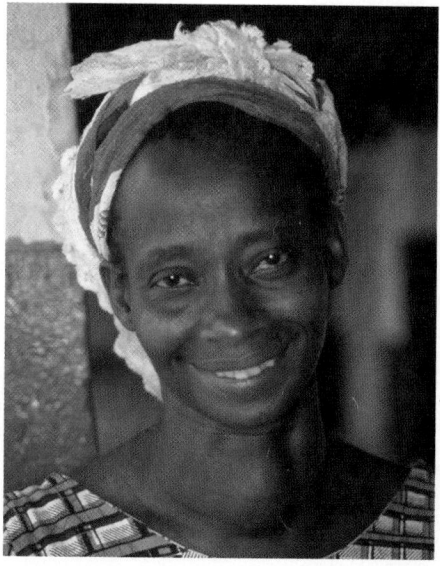

▲ This woman has an enlargement of the thyroid gland also known as a goiter caused by insufficient iodide in the diet.

cretinism The stunting of body growth and poor mental development in the offspring that results from inadequate maternal intake of iodide during pregnancy.

FIGURE 9-21 ▶ Food sources of Iodide compared to the RDA.

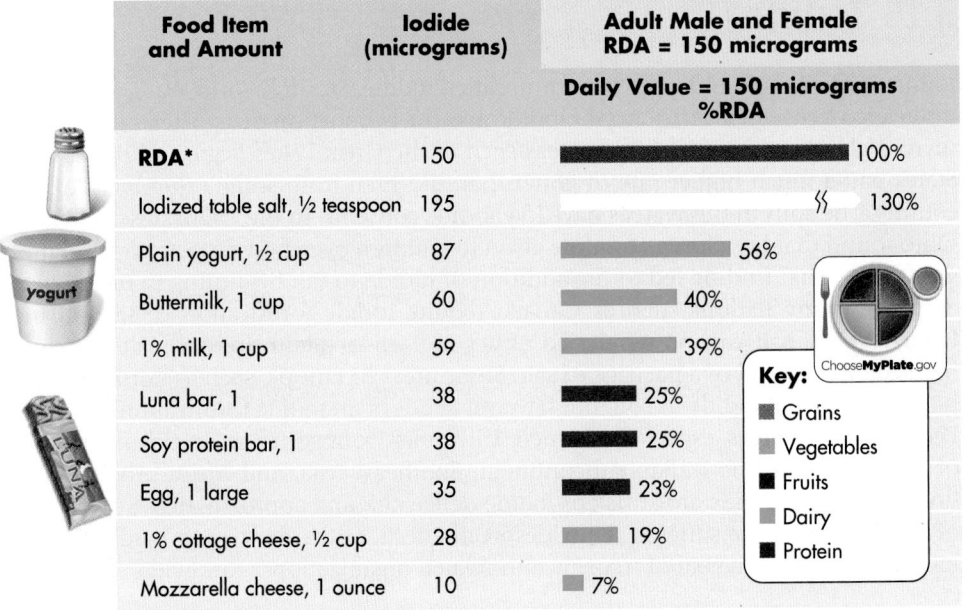

Food Item and Amount	Iodide (micrograms)	Adult Male and Female RDA = 150 micrograms
		Daily Value = 150 micrograms %RDA
RDA*	150	100%
Iodized table salt, ½ teaspoon	195	130%
Plain yogurt, ½ cup	87	56%
Buttermilk, 1 cup	60	40%
1% milk, 1 cup	59	39%
Luna bar, 1	38	25%
Soy protein bar, 1	38	25%
Egg, 1 large	35	23%
1% cottage cheese, ½ cup	28	19%
Mozzarella cheese, 1 ounce	10	7%

Key:
- Grains
- Vegetables
- Fruits
- Dairy
- Protein

ChooseMyPlate.gov

*For adults; see the DRI table in the back of this book for gender- and age-specific recommendations.

appear in people who eat a lot of seaweed, because some seaweeds contain as much as 1% iodide by weight. Total iodide intake then can add up to 60 to 130 times the RDA.

9.16 Copper (Cu)

Copper is involved in the metabolism of iron by functioning in the formation of hemoglobin and transport of iron. A copper-containing enzyme aids in the release of iron from storage. Copper is needed by enzymes that create cross-links in connective tissue proteins. Copper is also needed by other enzymes, such as those that defend the body against free-radical (oxidizing) compounds (e.g., a form of superoxide dismutase) and those that act in the brain and nervous system. Finally, copper performs in immune system function, blood clotting, and blood lipoprotein metabolism. About 12% to 75% of dietary copper is absorbed, with higher intakes associated with lower absorption. Absorption takes place primarily in the stomach and upper small intestine. Copper is excreted in the bile made by the liver and released by the gallbladder. Phytates, fiber, as well as zinc and iron supplements, may all interfere with copper absorption. Symptoms of copper deficiency include a form of anemia, low white blood cell count, bone loss, poor growth, and some forms of cardiovascular disease.

Copper Sources and Needs

Copper is found primarily in liver, seafood, cocoa, legumes, nuts, seeds, and whole-grain breads and cereals (Fig. 9-22).

The RDA for copper is 900 micrograms daily for adults, based on the amount needed for activity of copper-containing proteins and enzymes in the body. The Daily Value used to express copper content on food and supplement labels is 2 milligrams. The average adult intake is about 1 to 1.6 milligrams per day. Women generally consume the smaller amount. The form of copper typically found in multivitamin and mineral supplements (copper oxide) is not readily absorbed. It is best to rely on food sources to meet copper needs. The copper status of adults appears to be good, though we lack sensitive measures to determine copper status.

The groups most likely to develop copper deficiencies are preterm infants, infants recovering from semistarvation on a milk-dominated diet (a poor source of copper),

▲ Seafood is one source of copper in the diet

Food Sources of Copper

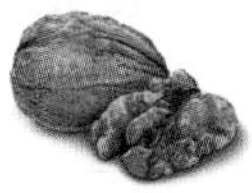

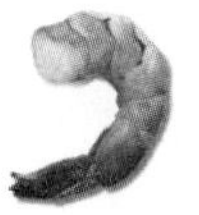

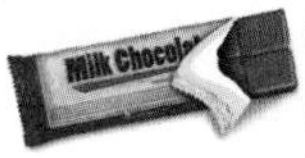

Food Item and Amount	Copper (milligrams)	Adult Male and Female RDA = 900 milligrams Daily Value = 2 milligrams %RDA
RDA*	900	100%
Fried beef liver, 3 ounces	3800	422%
Power bar, 1	700	78%
Walnuts, ½ cup	600	67%
Kidney beans, ½ cup	500	56%
Lobster, 3 ounces	400	44%
Molasses, 3 tablespoons	300	33%
Sunflower seeds, 2 tablespoons	300	33%
Shrimp, 3 ounces	300	33%
Raisin Bran cereal, 1 cup	300	33%
Great Grains cereal, 1 cup	300	33%
Black-eyed peas, ½ cup cooked	200	22%
Wheat germ, ¼ cup	200	22%
Milk chocolate, 1 ounce	110	12%
Whole-wheat bread, 1 slice	80	9%

Key:
- Grains
- Vegetables
- Fruits
- Dairy
- Protein
- Discretionary calories

ChooseMyPlate.gov

*For adults; see the DRI table in the back of this book for gender- and age-specific recommendations.

FIGURE 9-22 ▶ Food sources of copper compared to the RDA.

and people recovering from intestinal surgery (during which time copper absorption decreases). Recall that a copper deficiency can also result from overzealous supplementation of zinc, because zinc and copper compete with each other for absorption.

Upper Level for Copper

The Upper Limit for copper is 10 milligrams per day. High doses of copper can cause toxicity, including vomiting, at single doses of greater than 10 milligrams. Other effects, such as liver toxicity, are also possible with megadose uses.

9.17 Fluoride (F)

The fluoride ion (F^-) is the form of this trace mineral essential for human health. Like chlorine, fluorine (F_2) is a poisonous gas. This link was found as dentists in the early 1900s noticed a lower rate of dental caries (cavities) in the southwestern United States. These areas contained high amounts of fluoride in the water. The amounts of fluoride were sometimes so high that small spots on the teeth, called **mottling**, appeared. Even though mottled teeth were quite discolored, they contained very few dental caries. After experiments showed that fluoride in the water did indeed decrease the rate of dental caries, controlled fluoridation of water in parts of the United States began in 1945.

Those who grew up drinking fluoridated water generally have 40% to 60% fewer dental caries than people who did not drink fluoridated water as children. Dentists can provide topical fluoride treatments, and schools can provide fluoride tablets, but it is much less expensive and more reliable to add fluoride to a community's drinking

mottling The discoloration or marking of the surface of teeth from fluorosis.

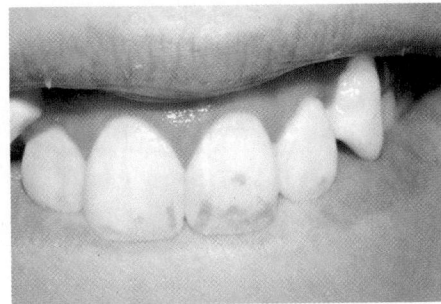

▲ Example of mottling in a tooth caused by overexposure to fluoride.

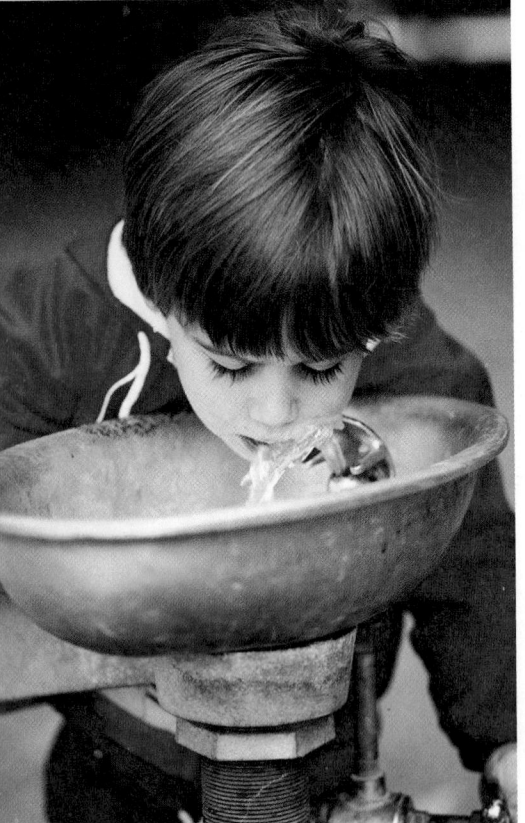

▲ Fluoridated water is responsible for much of the decrease in dental caries throughout North America.

water. State and private water sources do not always contain enough fluoride, however. When in doubt, contact your local water plant or have the water in your home analyzed for fluoride content. If it is less than 1 part fluoride per million parts of water (e.g., 1 milligram per kilogram or liter of water), talk to your dentist about the best means to obtain the fluoride.

Functions of Fluoride

Dietary fluoride consumed during childhood, when bones and teeth are developing, aids the synthesis of a form of tooth enamel that strongly resists acid. Therefore, teeth become resistant to dental caries. Fluoride also inhibits metabolism and growth of the bacteria that cause dental caries, and fluoride present in saliva directly inhibits tooth demineralization and enhances tooth remineralization.

Fluoride applied to the surface of the teeth by dentists or from toothpaste or rinses adds additional protection against dental caries. Thus, people of all ages benefit from the topical effects of fluoride, whether they consumed fluoridated water or fluoride supplements as children (see Further Reading 1).

Fluoride Sources and Needs

Tea, seafood, seaweed, and some natural water sources are the only good food sources of fluoride. Most of our fluoride intake comes from fluoride added to drinking water and toothpaste and from fluoride treatments performed by dentists. Fluoride is not added to bottled water. Therefore, if people such as children consume bottled water, they won't receive fluoride from such water intake.

The Adequate Intake for fluoride for adults is 3.1 to 3.8 milligrams per day. This range of intake provides the benefits of resistance to dental caries without causing ill effects. Typical fluoridated water contains about 1 milligram per liter, which works out to about 0.25 milligrams per cup.

Upper Level for Fluoride

The Upper Level for fluoride is set at 1.3 to 2.2 milligrams per day for young children, and 10 milligrams per day for children over 9 years of age and adults, based on skeletal and tooth damage seen with higher doses. If children swallow large amounts of fluoridated toothpaste as part of daily tooth care, tooth mottling may develop. Not swallowing toothpaste and limiting the amount used to "pea" size are the best ways to prevent this problem. In addition, children under 6 years should have toothbrushing supervised by an adult. Fluoride-related mottling only occurs during tooth development, so adults do not develop mottling from their fluoride exposure.

CONCEPT CHECK

Iodide is vital for the synthesis of thyroid hormones. A prolonged insufficient intake causes the thyroid gland to enlarge, resulting in a goiter. The use of iodized salt in North America has virtually eliminated this condition. Copper functions mainly in iron and free-radical metabolism, and in the cross-bonding of connective tissue. A deficiency can result in a type of anemia. Good food sources of copper are seafoods, legumes, nuts, dried fruits, and whole grains. Fluoride becomes incorporated into teeth during development and is present in salivary secretions. The presence of this trace mineral makes teeth resistant to acid and bacterial growth, in turn reducing development of dental caries. Fluoride also aids in remineralization of teeth once decay begins. Most of us receive adequate amounts of fluoride from that added to drinking water and toothpaste. An excessive fluoride intake during tooth development can lead to spotted (i.e., mottled) teeth and possibly bone damage.

9.18 Chromium (Cr)

The importance of chromium in human diets has been recognized only in the past 40 years. The most-studied function of chromium is the maintenance of glucose uptake into cells. Our current understanding is that chromium enters the cell and acts to enhance the transport of glucose across the cell membrane by aiding insulin function. Marginal to low chromium intakes may contribute to an increased risk for developing type 2 diabetes, but opinions are mixed on the true degree of this effect.

A chromium deficiency is characterized by impaired blood glucose control and elevated blood cholesterol and triglycerides. The mechanism by which chromium influences cholesterol metabolism is not known but may involve enzymes that control cholesterol synthesis. Chromium deficiency originally appeared in people maintained on intravenous total parenteral nutrition solutions not supplemented with chromium and in children with malnutrition. Sensitive measures of chromium status are not available, so marginal chromium deficiencies may go undetected.

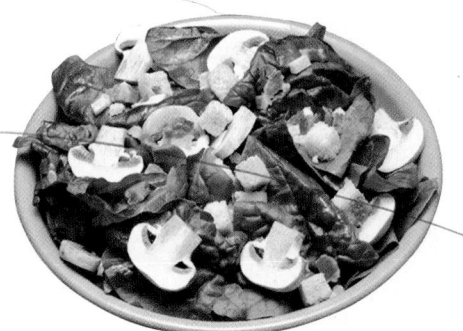

▲ The mushrooms in this spinach salad are a good source of chromium.

Chromium Sources and Needs

Specific data regarding the chromium content of various foods are limited, and most food composition tables do not include values for this trace mineral. Egg yolks, whole grains (bran), organ meats, other meats, mushrooms, nuts, and beer are good sources. Yeast is also a source. The amount of chromium in foods is closely tied to the local soil content of chromium. To provide yourself with a good chromium intake, regularly choose whole grains in place of mostly refined grains.

The Adequate Intake for chromium is 25 to 35 micrograms per day, based on the amount present in a balanced diet. The Daily Value used to express chromium content on food and supplement labels is about 4 times greater at 120 micrograms. Average adult intakes in North America are estimated at about 30 micrograms per day, but could be somewhat higher.

No Upper Level for chromium has been set because toxicity for that present in foods has not been observed. Chromium toxicity, however, has been reported in people exposed to industrial waste and in painters who use art supplies with a high chromium content. Liver damage and lung cancer can result. Use of any supplement should normally not exceed the Daily Value set unless supervised by a physician, because of the risk of toxicity.

Chromium supplements have been touted to help with exercise-induced increases in muscle mass and weight loss. Careful research, however, does not support this assertion.

9.19 Manganese (Mn)

The mineral manganese is easily confused with magnesium. Not only are their names similar, but they also often substitute for each other in metabolic processes. Manganese is needed by enzymes used in carbohydrate metabolism and by a form of superoxide dismutase used in free-radical metabolism. Manganese is also important in bone formation.

No human deficiency symptom is associated with a low manganese intake. Our need for manganese is low, and our diets tend to be adequate in this trace mineral.

Good food sources of manganese are nuts, rice, oats and other whole grains, beans, and leafy vegetables. The Adequate Intake for manganese is 1.8 to 2.3 milligrams to offset daily losses. Average intakes generally fall within this range. The Daily Value used to express manganese content on food and supplement labels is 2 milligrams.

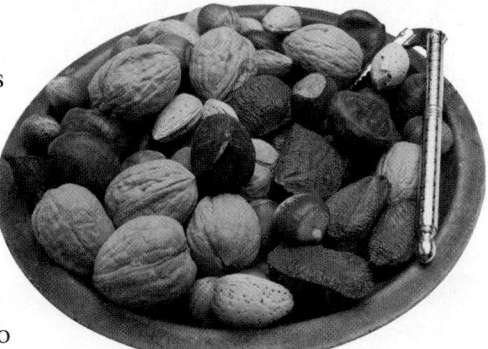

▲ Nuts are rich in manganese.

Upper Level for Manganese

Manganese is toxic at high doses. The Upper Level is 11 milligrams per day and is based on the development of nerve damage.

9.20 Molybdenum (Mo)

Several human enzymes use molybdenum. No molybdenum deficiency has been noted in people who consume normal diets, though deficiency symptoms have appeared in people maintained on intravenous total parenteral nutrition feedings. These symptoms include increased heart and respiration rates, night blindness, mental confusion, edema, and weakness.

Good food sources of molybdenum include milk and milk products, beans, whole grains, and nuts. The RDA for molybdenum is 45 micrograms to offset daily losses. The Daily Value used to express molybdenum content on food and supplement labels is 75 micrograms. Our daily intakes average 75 to 110 micrograms.

Upper Level for Molybdenum

The Upper Level for molybdenum is 2 milligrams per day. When consumed in high doses, molybdenum causes toxicity in laboratory animals, resulting in weight loss and decreased growth.

Table 9-3 summarizes what we have covered regarding the trace minerals, as does Figure 9-23. Figure 9-24 summarizes the various contributions of groups in MyPlate to mineral needs.

FIGURE 9-23 ▶ Water and minerals are involved in many processes in the body.

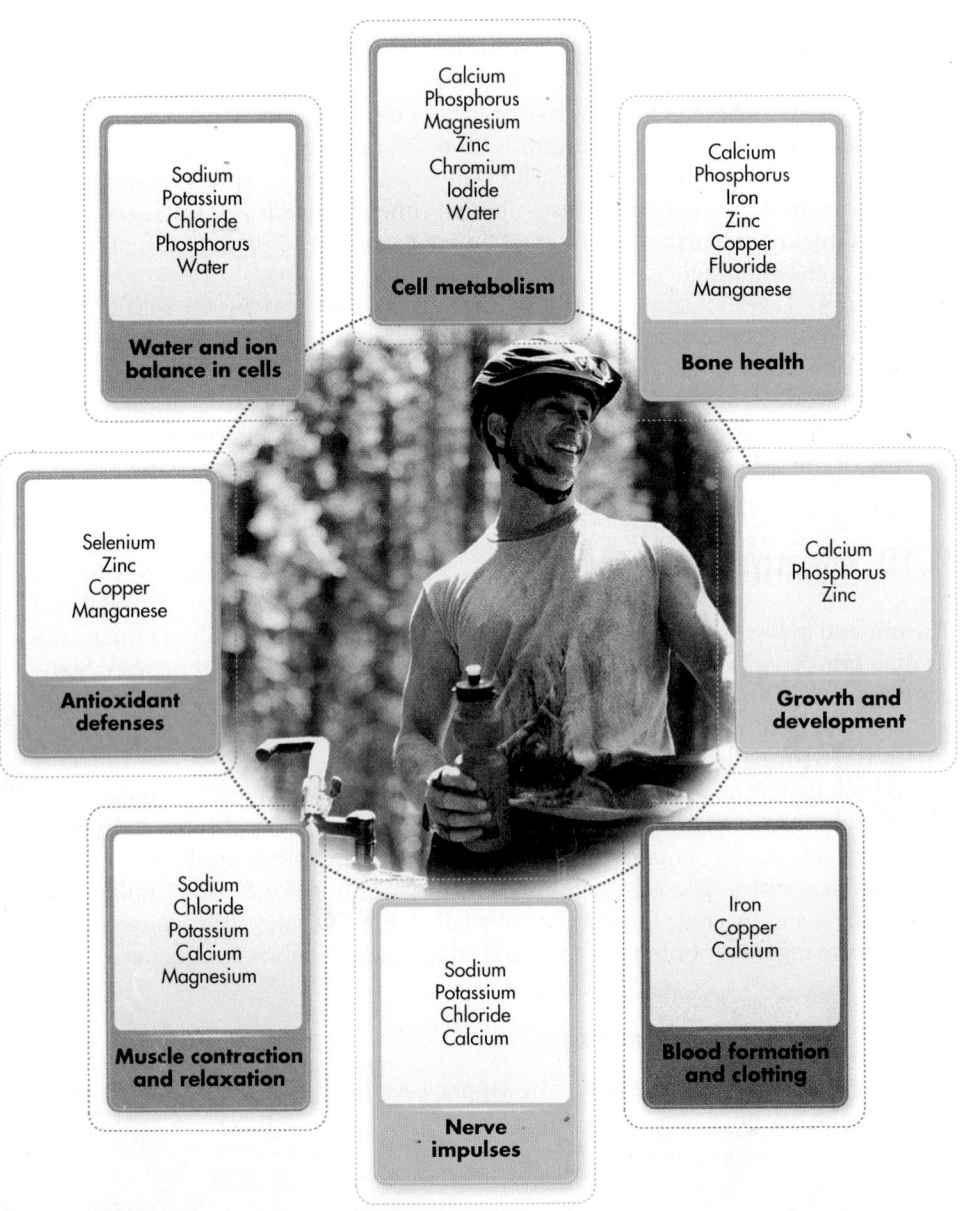

- Sodium
  Potassium
  Chloride
  Phosphorus
  Water
  Water and ion balance in cells

- Calcium
  Phosphorus
  Magnesium
  Zinc
  Chromium
  Iodide
  Water
  Cell metabolism

- Calcium
  Phosphorus
  Iron
  Zinc
  Copper
  Fluoride
  Manganese
  Bone health

- Selenium
  Zinc
  Copper
  Manganese
  Antioxidant defenses

- Calcium
  Phosphorus
  Zinc
  Growth and development

- Sodium
  Chloride
  Potassium
  Calcium
  Magnesium
  Muscle contraction and relaxation

- Sodium
  Potassium
  Chloride
  Calcium
  Nerve impulses

- Iron
  Copper
  Calcium
  Blood formation and clotting

TABLE 9-3 A Summary of Key Trace Minerals

Mineral	Major Functions	RDA, or Adequate Intake	Dietary Sources	Deficiency Symptoms	Toxicity Symptoms
Iron	• Components of hemoglobin and other key compounds used in respiration • Immune function • Cognitive development	*Men:* 8 milligrams *Premenopausal Women:* 18 milligrams	• Meats • Seafood • Broccoli • Peas • Bran • Enriched breads	• Fatigue • Anemia • Low blood hemoglobin values	• Liver and heart damage (extreme cases) • GI upset • Upper Level is 45 milligrams
Zinc	• Required for nearly 200 enzymes • Growth • Immunity • Alcohol metabolism • Sexual development • Reproduction • Antioxidant protection	*Men:* 11 milligrams *Women:* 8 milligrams	• Seafood • Meats • Greens • Whole grains	• Skin rash • Diarrhea • Decreased appetite and sense of taste • Hair loss • Poor growth and development • Poor wound healing	• Reduced copper absorption • Diarrhea • Cramps • Depressed immune function • Upper Level is 40 milligrams
Selenium	• Part of an antioxidant system	55 micrograms	• Meats • Eggs • Fish • Seafood • Whole grains	• Muscle pain • Weakness • Form of heart disease	• Nausea • Vomiting • Hair loss • Weakness • Liver disease • Upper Level is 400 micrograms
Iodide	• Component of thyroid hormones	150 micrograms	• Iodized salt • White bread • Saltwater fish • Dairy products	• Goiter • Mental retardation • Poor growth in infancy when mother is iodide deficient during pregnancy	• Inhibition of thyroid gland function • Upper Level is 1.1 milligrams
Copper	• Aids in iron metabolism • Works with many antioxidant enzymes • Involved with enzymes of protein metabolism and hormone synthesis	900 micrograms	• Liver • Cocoa • Beans • Nuts • Whole grains • Dried fruits	• Anemia • Low white blood cell count • Poor growth	• Vomiting • Nervous system disorders • Upper Level is 8–10 milligrams
Fluoride	• Increases resistance of tooth enamel to dental caries	*Men:* 3.8 milligrams *Women:* 3.1 milligrams	• Fluoridated water • Toothpaste • Tea • Seaweed • Dental treatments	• Increased risk of dental caries	• Stomach upset • Mottling (staining) of teeth during development • Bone pain • Upper Level is 10 milligrams for adults
Chromium	• Enhances insulin action	25–35 micrograms	• Egg yolks • Whole grains • Pork • Nuts • Mushrooms • Beer	• High blood glucose after eating	Caused by industrial contamination, not dietary excesses, so no Upper Level has been set
Manganese	• Cofactor of some enzymes, such as those involved in carbohydrate metabolism • Works with some antioxidant systems	1.8–2.3 milligrams	• Nuts • Oats • Beans • Tea	None observed in humans	• Nervous system disorders • Upper Level is 11 milligrams
Molybdenum	• Aids in action of some enzymes	45 micrograms	• Beans • Grains • Nuts	None observed in healthy humans	• Poor growth in laboratory animals • Upper Level is 2 milligrams

FIGURE 9-24 ▶ Certain groups of MyPlate are especially rich sources of various minerals. This is true for the minerals listed. Each mineral may also be found in other groups, but in lower amounts. Other trace minerals are also present in moderate amounts in many groups. With regard to the grains group, whole-grain varieties are the richest sources of most trace minerals listed.

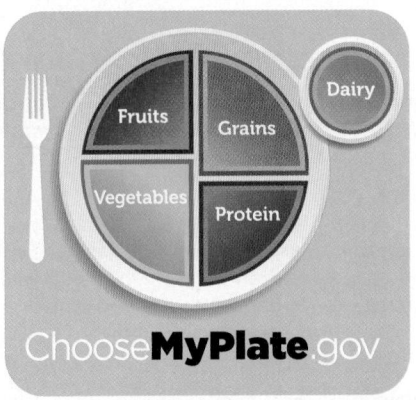

**MyPlate:
Sources of Minerals**

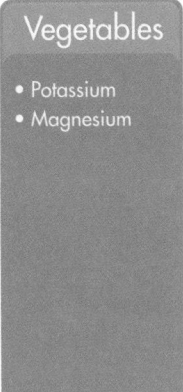
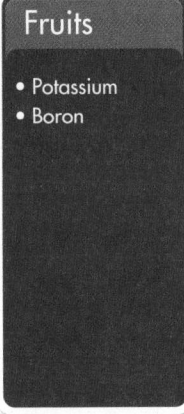
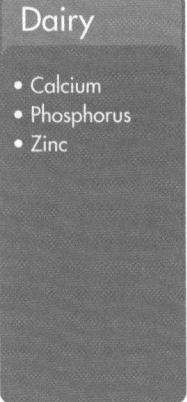

Grains	Vegetables	Fruits	Dairy	Protein
• Sodium chloride • Calcium (fortified products) • Phosphorus • Magnesium • Iron • Zinc • Copper • Selenium • Chromium	• Potassium • Magnesium	• Potassium • Boron	• Calcium • Phosphorus • Zinc	• Sodium chloride (processed foods) • Potassium • Phosphorus • Magnesium • Selenium • Iron • Zinc • Copper

9.21 Other Trace Minerals

Although a variety of other trace minerals is found in humans, many of them have not yet been shown to be required. The list of minerals in this category includes boron, nickel, vanadium, arsenic, and silicon. Widespread deficiency symptoms in humans have never been noted, probably because typical diets provide adequate amounts of these minerals and they are needed by very few enzymes and metabolic systems. Their potential for toxicity should make one question any supplementation not supervised by a physician. These trace minerals may achieve more importance as more research is reported.

CONCEPT CHECK

Chromium contributes to insulin function. The amount of chromium found in food depends on chromium content of the soil on which it was grown. Meats, whole grains, and egg yolks are good sources. Manganese is a component of bone and is used by many enzymes, including those involved in glucose production. Our need for manganese is low, so deficiencies are rare. Nuts, rice, oats, and beans are good food sources. Molybdenum is another trace mineral required by a few enzymes. Good sources include milk, beans, whole grains, and nuts. Deficiencies have appeared only in people nourished by unsupplemented total parenteral nutrition. The needs for some other trace minerals—such as boron, nickel, arsenic, and vanadium—have not been fully established in humans. If required, these minerals are needed in such small amounts that our current diets are probably adequate sources of them.

Maintaining a Healthy Blood Pressure

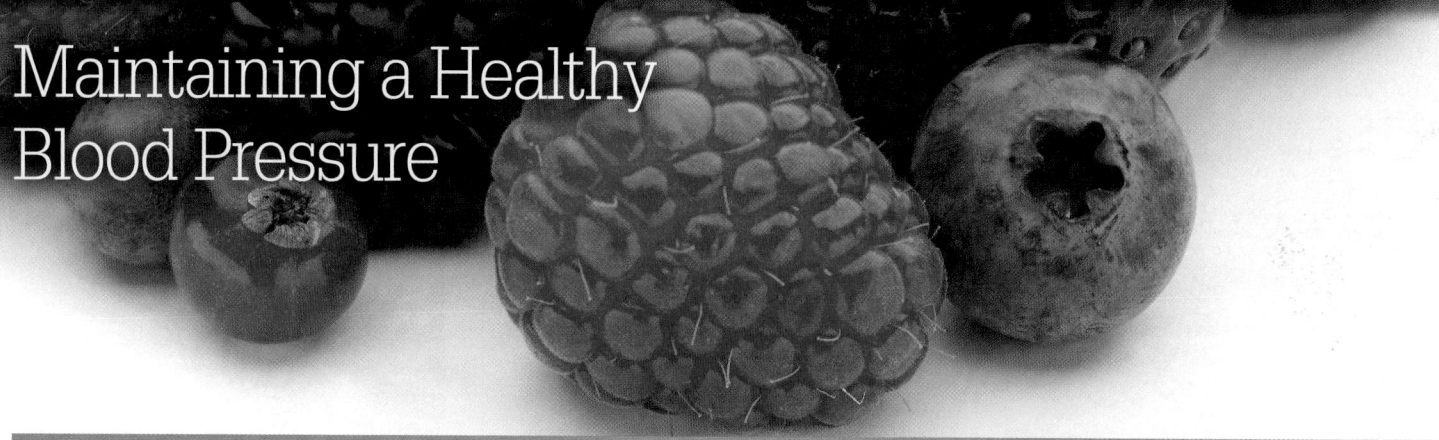

Among North Americans, an estimated 1 in 5 adults has hypertension. Over the age of 65, the number rises to 1 in every 2 adults. Only about half of cases are being treated. Blood pressure is expressed by two numbers. The higher number represents systolic blood pressure, the pressure in the arteries when the heart muscle is contracting and pumping blood into the arteries. Optimal systolic blood pressure is 120 millimeters of mercury (mm Hg) or less. The second value is diastolic blood pressure, the artery pressure when the heart is relaxed. Optimal diastolic blood pressure is 80 mm Hg or less. Elevations in both systolic and diastolic blood pressure are strong predictors of disease (Fig. 9-25).

Hypertension is defined as sustained systolic pressure exceeding 139 mm Hg or diastolic blood pressure exceeding 89 mm Hg. Most cases of hypertension (about 95% of cases) have no clear-cut cause. It is described as primary, or essential (i.e., essential hypertension). Kidney disease, sleep-disordered breathing (sleep apnea), and other causes often lead to the other 5% of cases, known as secondary hypertension. African-Americans are more likely than Caucasians to develop hypertension and to do so earlier in life.

Unless blood pressure is periodically measured, the development of hypertension is easily overlooked. Thus, it's described as a silent disorder, because it usually does not cause symptoms.

Why Control Blood Pressure?

Blood pressure needs to be controlled mainly to prevent cardiovascular disease, kidney disease, strokes and related declines in brain function, poor blood circulation in the legs, problems with vision, and sudden death. These conditions are much more likely to be found in individuals with hypertension than in people with normal blood pressure. Smoking and elevated blood lipoproteins make these diseases even more likely. Individuals with hypertension need to be diagnosed and treated as soon as possible, as the condition generally progresses to a more serious stage over time and even resists therapy if it persists for years.

Causes of Hypertension

A family history of hypertension is a risk factor, especially if both parents have (or had) the problem. In addition, blood pressure usually increases as a person ages. Some increase is caused by atherosclerosis. As plaque builds up in the arteries, the arteries become less flexible and cannot expand. When vessels remain rigid, blood pressure remains high. Eventually, the plaque begins to decrease the blood supply to the kidneys, decreasing their ability to control blood volume and, in turn, blood pressure.

An enzyme secreted by the kidneys and some hormonelike compounds are designed to maintain a healthy blood pressure. When blood pressure is elevated, the effect of these compounds can be reduced by anti-hypertension medications.

Overweight people have six times greater risk of having hypertension than lean people. Overall, obesity is considered the number one lifestyle factor related to hypertension.

This is especially the case in minority populations. Additional blood vessels

How High Is High?

If your systolic and diastolic pressures fall into different categories, your risk depends on the higher category

SYSTOLIC	DIASTOLIC
Hypertension (High)	
140	90
Pre-hypertension	
120	80
Normal	

Numbers (in millimeters of mercury) apply to adults who aren't taking drugs to lower their blood pressure.

FIGURE 9-25 ▶ The cutoff for hypertension is 140/90 mm Hg, but the risk of heart attacks and stroke precedes the rise in blood pressure.

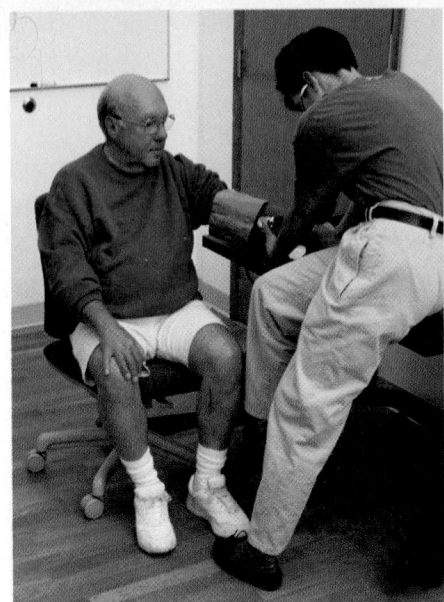

▲ Older adults are particularly at risk of hypertension.

develop to support excess tissue in overweight and obese individuals, and these extra miles of associated blood vessels increase work by the heart and also blood pressure. Hypertension is linked to obesity if elevated blood insulin levels result from insulin-resistant adipose cells. This increased insulin level increases sodium retention in the body and accelerates atherosclerosis. A weight loss of as little as 10 to 15 pounds often can help treat hypertension.

Inactivity is considered the number two lifestyle factor related to hypertension. If an obese person can engage in regular physical activity (at least 5 days per week for 30 to 60 minutes) and lose weight, blood pressure often returns to normal.

Third, excess alcohol intake is responsible for about 10% of all cases of hypertension, especially in middle-aged males and among African-Americans in general. When hypertension is caused by excessive alcohol intake, it is usually reversible. A sensible alcohol intake for people with hypertension is two or fewer drinks per day for men and one or no drinks per day for women and all older adults. Did you recognize that this is the same recommendation given in the 2010 Dietary Guidelines for Americans? Some studies suggest that such a minimal alcohol

intake may reduce the risk of ischemic stroke. These data, however, should not be used to encourage alcohol use.

In some people, particularly African-Americans and older overweight persons, blood pressure is especially sensitive to sodium. In these people, excess salt leads to fluid retention by the kidney and a corresponding increase in blood volume, which therefore increases blood pressure. It is not clear whether the sodium ion or the chloride ion is most responsible for the effect. Still, as reviewed in this chapter, if one reduces sodium intake, chloride intake naturally falls; the opposite is also true. For the most part, a recommendation to consume less sodium is equivalent to a call for less salt in the diet. Only some North Americans are very susceptible to increases in blood pressure from salt intake, so it is only the number four lifestyle factor related to hypertension. It is unfortunate that salt intake receives the major portion of public attention with regard to hypertension. Efforts to prevent hypertension should also focus on obesity, inactivity, and alcohol abuse.

Other Minerals and Blood Pressure

Minerals such as calcium, potassium, and magnesium also deserve attention when it comes to prevention and treatment of hypertension. Studies show that a diet rich in these minerals and low in salt can decrease blood pressure within days of beginning this type of diet, especially among African-Americans. The response is even similar to that seen with

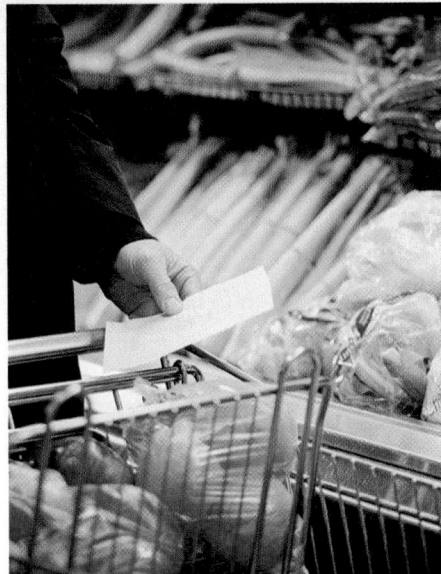

▲ Opting for the fruits, vegetables, and low-fat foods recommended by the DASH diet represents a sound approach to nutrition for most people regardless of hypertension risk.

commonly used medications. The diet is called the Dietary Approaches to Stop Hypertension (DASH) diet (Table 9-4). The diet, rich in calcium, phosphorus, and magnesium and low in salt, takes a standard MyPlate food plan and adds 1 to 2 extra vegetables and fruits servings and a serving of nuts, seeds, or legumes (beans) 4 to 5 days of the week. In DASH studies, participants also consumed no more than 3 grams of sodium and no more than one to two alcoholic drinks per day. A DASH 2 diet trial tested three daily sodium intakes (3300 milligrams, 2400 milligrams, and 1500 milligrams). People showed a steady decline in blood

TABLE 9-4 What Is the DASH Diet?

The DASH diet is characterized as low in fat and sodium and rich in fruits, vegetables, and low-fat dairy products. Here is the breakdown:

Per Day	Per Week
6–8 servings of grains and grain products	4–5 servings of nuts, seeds, or legumes
4–5 servings of fruit	5 servings of sweets and added sugars
4–5 servings of vegetables	
2–3 servings of low-fat or fat-free dairy products	
2 or less servings of meats, poultry, and fish	
2–3 servings of fats/oils	

pressure on the DASH diet as sodium intake declined. Over all, the DASH diet is seen as a total dietary approach to treating hypertension. It is not clear which of the many healthful practices of this diet are responsible for the fall in blood pressure (see Further Readings 2 and 4).

Other studies also show a reduction in stroke risk among people who consume a diet rich in fruits, vegetables, and vitamin C (recall that fruits and vegetables are rich vitamin C sources). Overall, a diet low in salt and rich in low-fat and fat-free dairy products, fruits, vegetables, whole grains, and some nuts can substantially reduce hypertension and stroke risk in many people, especially those with hypertension.

Medications to Treat Hypertension

Diuretic medications are one class of drugs used to treat hypertension. These "water pills" work to reduce blood volume (and therefore blood pressure) by increasing fluid output in the urine. Other medications act by slowing heart rate or by causing relaxation of blood vessels. A combination of two or more medications is commonly required to treat hypertension that does not respond to diet and lifestyle therapy. Read more about the importance of antihypertensive drugs compared to the reduction in salt intake in Further Reading 7.

Prevention of Hypertension

Many of the risk factors for hypertension and stroke are controllable, and appropriate lifestyle changes can reduce a person's risk (Fig. 9-26). Experts also recommend that those with hypertension lower blood pressure through diet and lifestyle changes before resorting to blood pressure medications.

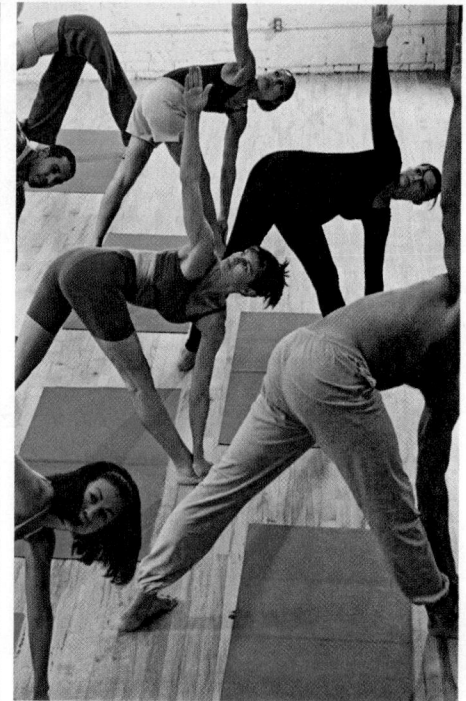

▲ Regular, moderate physical activity contributes to better blood pressure control.

FIGURE 9-26 ▶ What works? If your blood pressure is high, here's how much lifestyle changes should lower it.

Advice	Details	Drop in Systolic Blood Pressure
Lose excess weight	For every 20 pounds you lose	5 to 20 points
Follow a DASH diet	Eat a lower-fat diet rich in vegetables, fruits, and low-fat dairy foods	8 to 14 points
Exercise daily	Get 30 minutes a day of aerobic activity (such as brisk walking)	4 to 9 points
Limit sodium	Eat no more than 2400 mg per day (1500 mg per day is better)	2 to 8 points
Limit alcohol	Have no more than 2 drinks per day for men, 1 drink per day for women (1 drink = 12 oz. beer, 5 oz. wine, or 1.5 oz. 80-proof whiskey)	2 to 4 points

Source: *The Seventh Report of the Joint National Committee on Prevention, Detection, Evaluation, and Treatment of High Blood Pressure, May 2003* (www.nhibl.hih.gov/guidelines/hypertension).

Preventing Osteoporosis

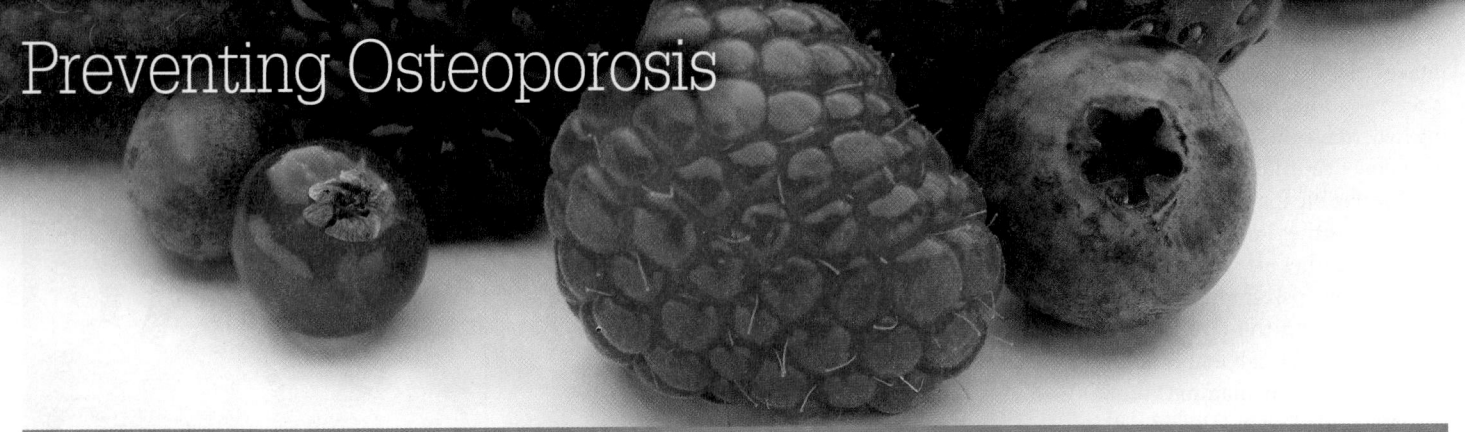

Widespread media attention has made it almost impossible for women to ignore osteoporosis. The crippling effect this disease has on older persons is now recognized as a major medical problem. Osteoporosis leads to approximately 1.5 million bone fractures per year in the United States, usually in the hip, spine, or wrist, leading to about $18 billion per year in health-care costs. Many older women in North America experience osteoporosis-related fractures in their lifetimes.

The slender, inactive woman who smokes is most susceptible to osteoporosis, but any person who lives long enough can suffer from the disease, including men. About 25% of women older than age 50 develop osteoporosis. Among people older than age 80, osteoporosis becomes the rule—not the exception. The spine fractures commonly found in women with osteoporosis cause considerable pain and deformity and decrease physical ability (Fig. 9-27); hip fractures are seen in both men and women with osteoporosis. Not only is this disease debilitating, it also can be fatal. Almost one-quarter of older persons who suffer hip fractures die within the first year from fracture-related complications.

Bone Structure and Strength

To better understand the role calcium plays in bone health and osteoporosis, it is important to understand how bone is constructed. Visual observation of the cross-sections of a bone reveals two primary bone structural types: **cortical**

bone and **trabecular bone.** These interact within each bone to form an engineering marvel of strength (Fig. 9-28).

The entire outer surface of all bones is composed of cortical bone, also known as compact bone, which is very dense. The shafts of long bones, such as those of the arm, are almost entirely cortical bone. Trabecular bone, also known as spongy bone, is found in the ends of the long bones, inside the spinal vertebrae,

cortical bone Dense, compact bone that comprises the outer surface and shafts of bone; also called compact bone.

trabecular bone The spongy, inner matrix of bone, found primarily in the spine, pelvis, and ends of bones; also called spongy or cancellous bone.

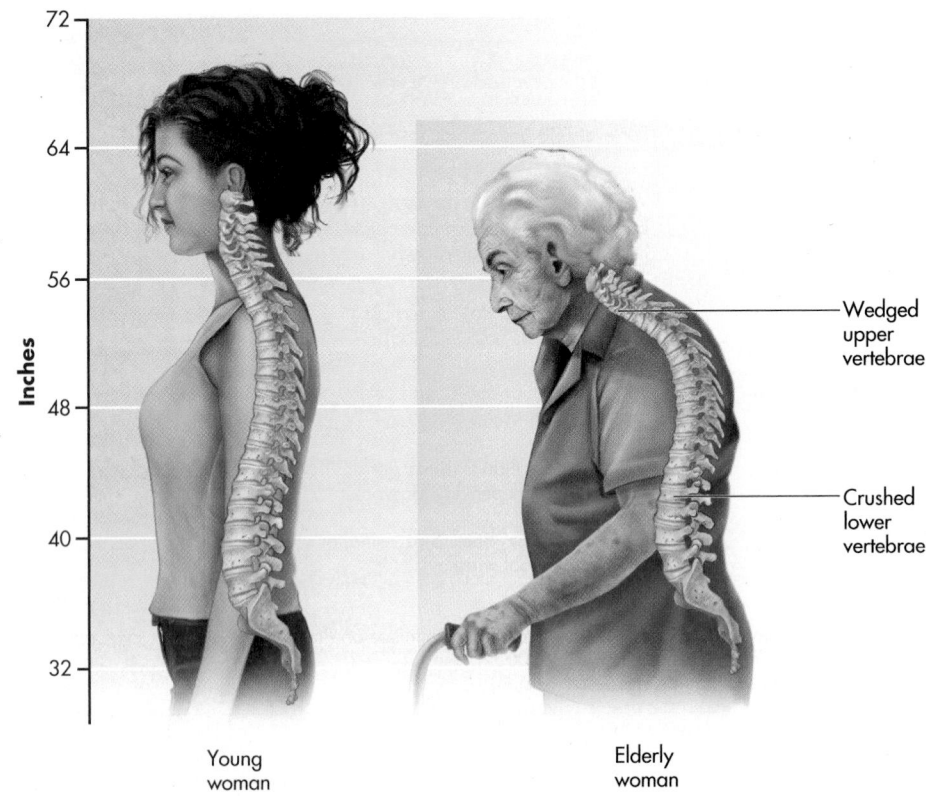

FIGURE 9-27 ▶ Normal and osteoporotic woman. Osteoporotic bones have less substance, so osteoporosis generally leads to loss of height, distorted body shape, fractures, and loss of teeth. Monitoring changes in adult height is one way to detect early evidence of osteoporosis.

and inside the flat bones of the pelvis. Trabecular bone is porous and forms an internal scaffolding-like network for a bone. It supports the outer cortical shell of the bone, especially in heavily stressed areas, such as joints. Like the beams of a building, the trabecular bone adds strength to the bone without the added weight of a more solid matrix. It is especially critical for the horizontal and vertical trabecular beams to extend continuously—without breaks. Any break in the trabecular beams weakens the support system of a bone and increases the risk for bone fracture. Once these beams are broken, there is no way to rebuild them. This is why it is so important to limit bone loss as people age.

Bone Mass Is Related to Age and Gender

Bone strength depends on a person's **bone mass** and **bone mineral density**. The more bone there is, and especially

the more densely packed bone crystals are in the bone, the stronger the bone structure. Rapid and continual bone growth and calcification occur throughout the adolescent years, ultimately resulting in what is called *peak bone mass*. In the adolescent growth spurt, bone mass is increasing at the rate of about 8.5% per year. Small increases in bone mass then continue between 20 and 30 years of age.

The ultimate amount of bone built by a person is clearly dependent on gender; race; familial patterns seen in the mother and father; and probably other genetically determined factors, such as the degree of calcium absorption. In addition, men have higher bone mass than women, and African-Americans have heavier skeletons than Caucasians. As a direct consequence, men and African-Americans in general have a somewhat lower risk of osteoporosis-related fractures than do other populations. Slender, small-framed Caucasian and Asian women show the

bone mass Total mineral substance (such as calcium or phosphorus) in a cross section of bone, generally expressed as grams per centimeter of length.

bone mineral density Total mineral content of bone at a specific bone site divided by the width of the bone at that site, generally expressed as grams per cubic centimeter.

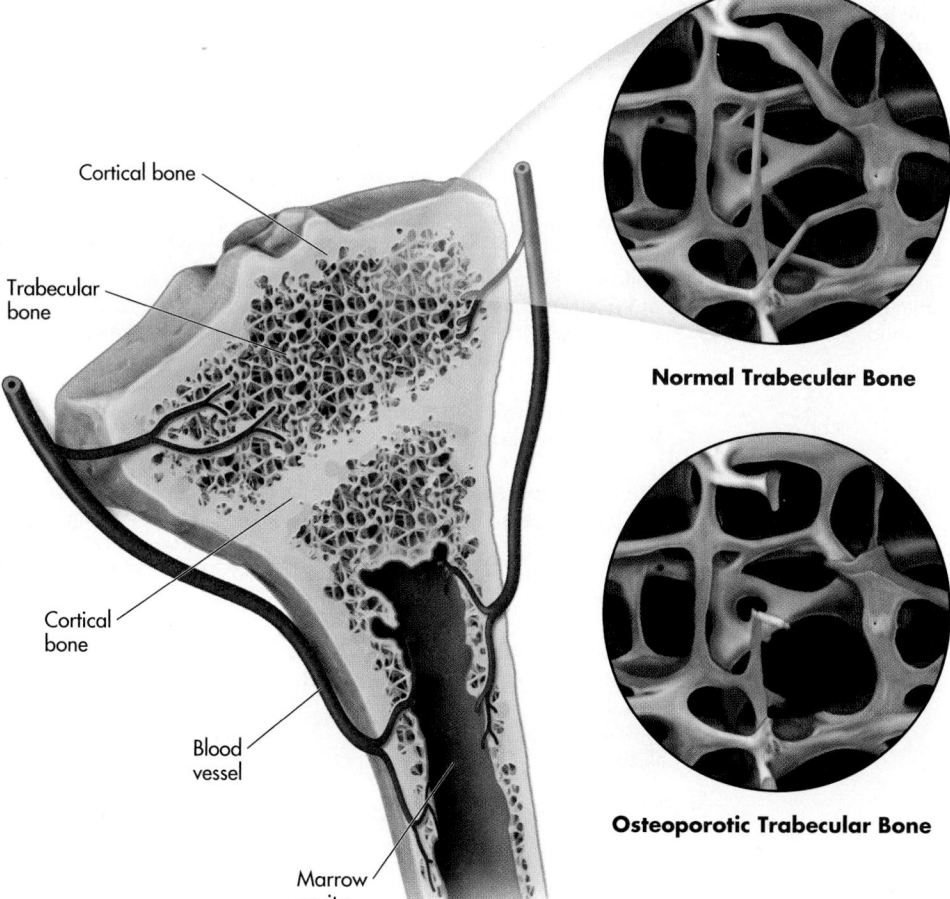

Normal Trabecular Bone

Osteoporotic Trabecular Bone

Cortical bone

Trabecular bone

Cortical bone

Blood vessel

Marrow cavity

FIGURE 9-28 ▶ Cortical and trabecular bone. Cortical bone forms the shafts of bones and their outer mineral covering. Trabecular bone supports the outer shell of cortical bone in various bones of the body, as in the illustration. Note how the osteoporotic bone has much less trabecular bone. This leads to a more fragile bone and is not reversible to any major extent with current therapies.

lowest bone mass values. Peak bone mass is also related to dietary intake of calcium and other nutrients, such as protein, phosphorus, vitamin A, vitamin D, vitamin K, magnesium, iron, zinc, and copper (Table 9-5). Recent studies also link a potassium-rich diet high in fruits and vegetables to osteoporosis prevention (see Further Reading 10). Thus, osteoporosis is not just a calcium story—many minerals and other nutrients play a part.

Bone mass varies among young adults; some have much denser bone than others, perhaps because they built more bone when they were young. Some people also may adapt more easily to lower-calcium diets. People who have developed more bone by early adulthood can sustain greater age-related bone loss with less risk of osteoporosis compared with those who reach adulthood with less bone. Thus, osteoporosis is considered to be a "pediatric disease" with geriatric (old age) consequences (Fig. 9-29).

For women, bone loss begins at age 30 and proceeds slowly and continuously to menopause (approximately age 50). It often speeds up at menopause with the decline in estrogen output and

continues at a high rate of loss for the next 10 years. By age 65 to 70, the rate of bone loss falls to about the same rate as before menopause. In men, bone loss is slow and steady from around age 30. Overall, this bone loss in both males and females progresses without noticeable short-term symptoms.

Osteoporosis

Failure to maintain enough bone mass in the body is generally diagnosed as osteoporosis. Bone loss can also be caused by the vitamin D deficiency disease osteomalacia, the use of certain medications (such as cortisol and antiseizure drugs), and cancer.

All women age 65 and older should be screened for this disease. The most accurate screening involves a **dual energy X-ray absorptiometry (DEXA) bone scan** of the whole body. (Somewhat less accurate instruments measure bone mineral density at a single site, such as the heel.) Younger women with associated risk factors are advised to do the same at menopause, because the results of the screening would help them decide

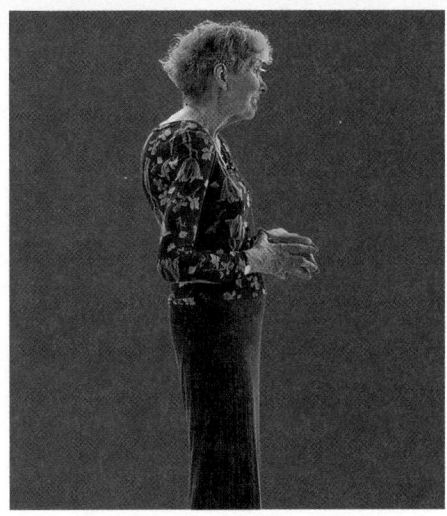

▲ Women with osteoporosis typically develop abnormal curvature of the upper spine. This results from fractures of the weakened vertebrae. This can lead to both physical and emotional pain.

Dual energy X-ray absorptiometry (DEXA) bone scan Method to measure bone density that uses small amounts of X-ray radiation. The ability of a bone to block the path of the radiation is used as a measure of bone density at that bone site.

TABLE 9-5 Diet and Lifestyle Factors Associated with Bone Status

Positive Diet and Lifestyle Factors	Call to Action
Adequate diet containing a sufficient amount of protein, calcium, phosphorus, magnesium, potassium, vitamin A, vitamin C, vitamin D, vitamin K, iron, zinc, copper, fluoride, and manganese and possibly boron.	• Follow MyPlate with special emphasis on adequate amounts of fruits, vegetables, and low-fat and fat-free dairy products. • Consider use of fortified foods (or supplements) to make up for specific nutrient shortfalls, such as vitamin D and calcium.
Healthy body weight	• Be aware that low body weight (slender figure) increases the risk for low bone mass.
Normal menses	• During childbearing years, seek medical advice if menses cease (such as in cases of anorexia nervosa or extreme athletic training). • Women at menopause and beyond should consider use of current medical therapies to reduce bone loss linked to the fall in estrogen output.
Weight-bearing physical activity	• Perform weight-bearing activity as this contributes to bone maintenance, whereas bed rest and a sedentary lifestyle lead to bone loss. Strength training is especially helpful for bone maintenance.
Negative Diet and Lifestyle Factors	**Call to Action**
Excessive intake of protein, phosphorus, sodium, caffeine, wheat bran, and alcohol	• Moderate intake of these dietary constituents is recommended. Problems primarily arise if adequate calcium is not consumed. • Excessive soft drink consumption is especially discouraged.
Smoking	• Smoking lowers estrogen output in women, so smoking cessation is advised.

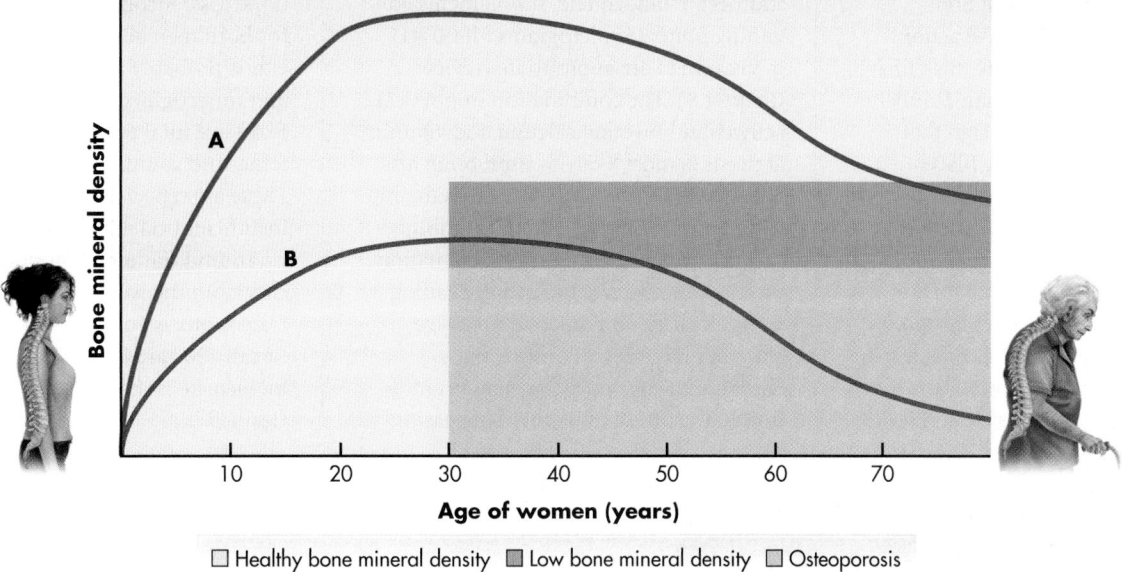

FIGURE 9-29 ▶ The relationship between peak bone mass and the ultimate risk of developing osteoporosis and related bone fractures
• **Woman A** had developed a high peak bone mass by age 30. Her bone loss was slow and steady between ages 30 and 50 and sped up somewhat after age 50 because of the effects of menopause. At age 75, the woman had a healthy bone mineral density value and did not show evidence of osteoporosis.
• **Woman B** with low peak bone mass experienced the same rate of bone loss as woman A. By age 50, she already had low mineral density and by age 70 kyphosis and spinal fractures had occurred.
Given the low calcium intakes that are common among young women today, line B is a sobering reality. Following a diet and lifestyle pattern that contributes to maximal bone mineral density can help women follow line A and significantly reduce their risk of developing osteoporosis.

whether medical therapy for bone loss is an appropriate plan for menopause.

For the DEXA test, a person will lie down on his or her back on a padded table while a movable imaging arm moves over the length of the body. The procedure usually takes about 20 to 30 minutes. The ability of a bone to block the path of radiation is used as a measure of bone mineral density at that bone site. A low dose of radiation is used for the DEXA—about one-tenth of the exposure from a chest X ray.

From the DEXA measurement of bone density, a T score is generated, which compares the observed bone density to that of a person at peak bone strength (e.g., age 30). Such a T score is interpreted as follows:

0 to −1	Normal
−1 to −2.4	Low bone mineral density
−2.5 or lower	Osteoporosis

Preventing Osteoporosis

Once osteoporosis is present, there is no way to repair the bone damage. This makes prevention important. Strategies for prevention of osteoporosis vary based on age and individual risk factors.

For young women, osteoporosis prevention involves three main elements. First, young women should focus on meeting calcium, vitamin D, protein, and other nutrient needs. Second, because the hormones of regular menstruation contribute to bone maintenance in young women, any sign of menstrual irregularities is reason to see a physician. Some nonmenstruating female athletes and other women with irregular menstrual cycles (e.g., women with anorexia nervosa) already exhibit low bone mineral density. Third, an active lifestyle that includes weight-bearing physical activity is also important. The increased muscle mass that stems from weight-bearing physical activity is associated with greater bone mineral density, as muscle keeps tension on bone. However, physical activity cannot prevent the bone loss associated with irregular menstruation. Even though female athletes may do plenty of weight-bearing physical activity, they should

be closely monitored by a physician if they have irregular menstrual cycles.

Once they have reached menopause, women should discuss approved osteoporosis-related therapies with a physician. The most common medications are **bisphosphonates.** These lessen bone breakdown. Estrogen replacement previously was the most common therapy for bone protection, but it has been shown to increase the risks in some women for cardiovascular disease and strokes, as well as cancers of the breast and ovaries. Estrogen replacement is now reserved for short-term use to control menopausal symptoms in most cases.

bisphosphonates Compounds primarily composed of carbon and phosphorus that bind to bone mineral and in turn reduce bone breakdown. Examples are alendronate (Fosamax), risedronate (Actonel), and ibandronate (Boniva).

As age advances, both men and women need to take preventive action. First, adults need to accurately track their height. A decrease of more than 1½ inches from young adult height is a sign that significant bone loss is taking place.

Older adults especially need to stay physically active—including some weight-bearing and resistance activities—and they should meet the Adequate Intake for calcium set for their particular age. Regular sun exposure and the consumption of food sources of vitamin D are also important. If sun exposure and food sources are inadequate, supplements containing up to 25 micrograms (1000 IU) of vitamin D are appropriate (review Chapter 8). The combination of physical activity and meeting calcium and vitamin D needs is most likely to limit bone loss in some areas of the body, such as the hip. Read more about the effect of combined calcium and vitamin D supplementation on hip bone density in Further Reading 8.

At any age, smoking and excessive alcohol intake decrease bone mass. Smoking lowers the estrogen concentration in the blood in women, increasing bone loss. Alcohol is toxic to bone cells for both men and women, and alcoholism is probably a major undiagnosed and unrecognized cause of osteoporosis. Excessive intakes of phosphorus, caffeine, and sodium are also discouraged. These are especially problematic when insufficient calcium is consumed.

To find out more about osteoporosis, check out the website of the National Osteoporosis Foundation (www.nof.org) or call (800)464-6700. Another helpful website is that of the National Dairy Council (www.nationaldairycouncil.org).

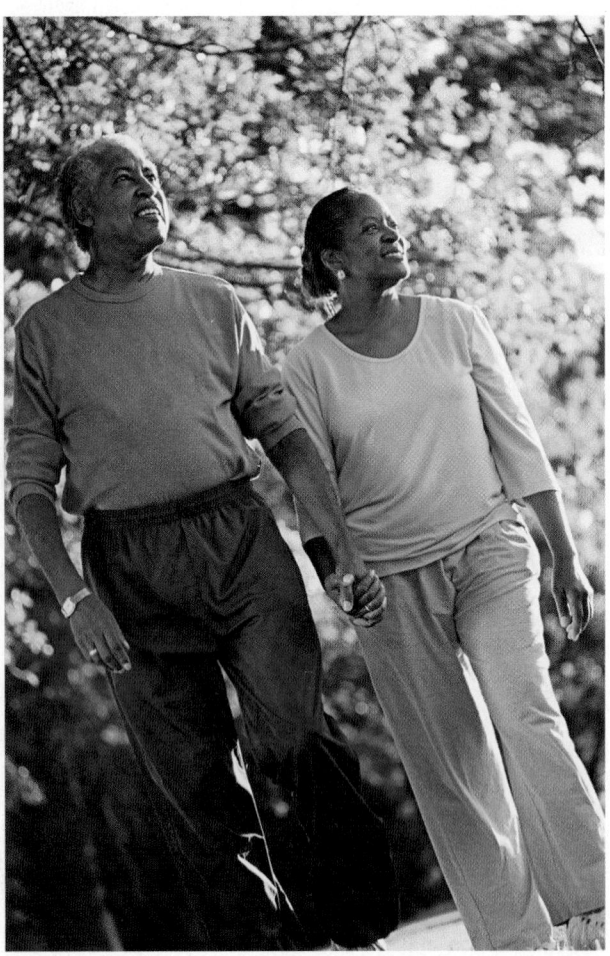

◀ Regular, moderate, weight-bearing physical activity contributes to bone health in both men and women. Note that men can also develop osteoporosis as they age.

Case Study Giving Up Milk

Ashley, a 19-year-old sophomore in college, recently gave up drinking milk. She thought this would help her stay slim by avoiding the calories in milk. Ashley's mother is concerned about her diet change. One of her primary concerns is the future risk of osteoporosis. Ashley also started smoking, and her only physical activity is practice for Women's Glee Club.

Ashley's typical diet consists of oatmeal made with water, a banana and a cup of fruit juice for breakfast. At midmorning, she buys a snack cake or candy bar from the vending machine. At lunch, she has pasta with vegetables, bread with olive oil, a side salad, 1 ounce of mixed nuts, and a soft drink. For dinner, she has a chicken or hamburger sandwich along with mixed vegetables and another soft drink. As an evening snack, she has some cookies and hot tea.

Answer the following questions about Ashley's situation and check your responses in Appendix A.

1. What nutrients are low in Ashley's typical diet that put her at risk of osteoporosis in the future?
2. Which of Ashley's lifestyle factors contribute to this increased risk of osteoporosis?
3. Is there any evidence that consumption of milk or other dairy products leads to weight gain?
4. What changes to her current diet could reduce the risk of osteoporosis and also help Ashley maintain her weight?
5. What lifestyle changes (other than the dietary changes) could Ashley make to decrease her risk of osteoporosis and maintain a healthy weight?

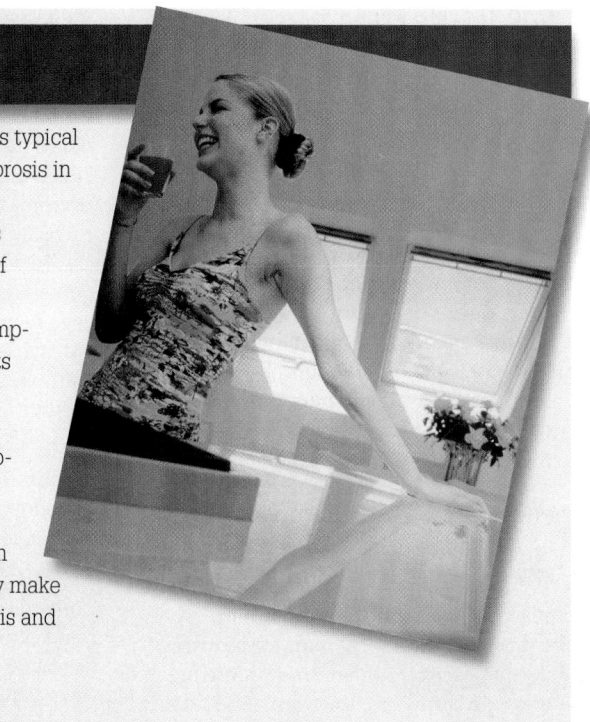

Summary (Numbers refer to numbered sections in the chapter.)

9.1 Water constitutes 50% to 70% of the human body. Its unique chemical properties enable it to dissolve substances as well as serve as a medium for chemical reactions, temperature regulation, and lubrication. Water also helps regulate the acid-base balance in the body.

For adults, daily water needs are estimated at 9 cups (women) to 13 cups (men) per day; fluid intake contributes to meeting this need.

Overall, the United States enjoys a safe water supply. However, people with poor immune status should boil water used for drinking and cooking to avoid waterborne illness. Bottled water can be used, but reliance on it to meet fluid needs is costly to the environment and our personal budgets.

9.2 Minerals are categorized based on the amount we need per day. If we require greater than 100 milligrams of a mineral per day, it is considered a major mineral; otherwise it is considered a trace mineral.

9.3 Many minerals are vital for sustaining life. For humans, animal products are the most bioavailable sources of most minerals. Supplements of minerals exceeding 100%

of the Daily Values listed on the label should be taken only under a physician's supervision. Toxicity and nutrient interactions are especially likely if the Upper Level (when set) is exceeded on a long-term basis.

9.4 Sodium, the major positive ion found outside cells, is vital in fluid balance and nerve impulse transmission. The North American diet provides abundant sodium through processed foods and table salt. About 10% to 15% of the adult population, such as overweight people, is especially sodium-sensitive and at risk for developing hypertension from consuming excessive sodium.

9.5 Potassium, the major positive ion found inside cells, has a similar function to sodium. Milk, fruits, and vegetables are good sources.

9.6 Chloride is the major negative ion found outside cells. It is important in digestion as part of stomach acid and in immune and nerve functions. Table salt supplies most of the chloride in our diets.

9.7 Calcium forms a part of bone structure and plays a role in blood clotting,

muscle contraction, nerve transmission, and cell metabolism. Calcium absorption is enhanced by stomach acid and the active vitamin D hormone. Dairy products are important calcium sources. Women are particularly at risk for not meeting calcium needs.

9.8 Phosphorus aids enzyme function and forms part of key metabolic compounds, cell membranes, and bone. It is efficiently absorbed, and deficiencies are rare, although there is concern about possible poor intake by some older women. Good food sources are dairy products, bakery products, and meats.

9.9 Magnesium is a mineral found mostly in plant food sources. It is important for nerve and heart function and as an activator for many enzymes. Whole-grain breads and cereals (bran portion), vegetables, nuts, seeds, milk, and meats are good food sources.

9.10 Sulfur is incorporated into certain vitamins and amino acids.

9.11 Trace minerals are essential to good health even though we only need 100 milligrams or less of each daily.

9.12 Iron absorption depends mainly on the form of iron present and the body's need for it. Heme iron from animal sources is better absorbed than the nonheme iron obtained primarily from plant sources. Consuming vitamin C or meat simultaneously with nonheme iron increases absorption. Iron operates mainly in synthesizing hemoglobin and myoglobin and in the action of the immune system. Women are at great risk for developing iron deficiency, which decreases blood hemoglobin and hematocrit. When this condition is severe, iron-deficiency anemia develops. This decreases the amount of oxygen carried in the blood. Iron toxicity usually results from a genetic disorder called hemochromatosis. This disease causes overabsorption and accumulation of iron, which can result in severe liver and heart damage.

9.13 Zinc aids in the action of up to 200 enzymes important for growth, development, cell membrane structure and function, immune function, antioxidant protection, wound healing, and taste. A zinc deficiency results in poor growth, loss of appetite, reduced sense of taste and smell, hair loss, and a persistent rash. Zinc is best absorbed from animal sources. The richest sources of zinc are oysters, shrimp, crab, and beef. Good plant sources are whole grains, peanuts, and beans.

9.14 An important role of selenium is decreasing the action of free-radical (oxidizing) compounds. In this way, selenium acts along with vitamin E in providing antioxidant protection. Muscle pain, muscle wasting, and a form of heart damage may result from a selenium deficiency. Meats, eggs, fish, and shellfish are good animal sources of selenium. Good plant sources include grains and seeds.

9.15 Iodide forms part of the thyroid hormones. A lack of dietary iodide results in the development of an enlarged thyroid gland or goiter. Iodized salt is a major food source.

9.16 Copper is important for iron metabolism, cross-linking of connective tissue, and other functions, such as enzymes that provide antioxidant protection. A copper deficiency can result in a form of anemia. Copper is found mainly in liver, seafood, cocoa, legumes, and whole grains.

9.17 Fluoride as part of regular dietary intake or toothpaste use makes teeth resistant to dental caries. Most North Americans receive the bulk of their fluoride from fluoridated water and toothpaste.

9.18–9.21 Chromium aids in the action of the hormone insulin. Egg yolks, meats, and whole grains are good sources of chromium. Manganese and molybdenum are used by various enzymes. One enzyme that uses manganese provides antioxidant protection. Clear deficiencies in otherwise healthy people are rarely seen for any of these three nutrients. Human needs for other trace minerals are so low that deficiencies are uncommon

N&YH Controlling weight and alcohol intake; exercising regularly; decreasing salt intake; and ensuring adequate potassium, magnesium, and calcium in the diet all can play a part in controlling high blood pressure.

Women are particularly at risk for developing osteoporosis as they age. Numerous lifestyle and medical options can help reduce this risk, including an adequate intake of calcium and many other minerals.

Check Your Knowledge (Answers to the following questions are below.)

1. Dietary heme iron is derived from
   a. elemental iron in food.
   b. animal flesh.
   c. breakfast cereal.
   d. vegetables.

2. Chloride is
   a. a component of hydrochloric acid.
   b. an intracellular fluid ion.
   c. a positively charged ion.
   d. converted to chlorine in the intestinal tract.

3. Minerals involved in fluid balance are
   a. calcium and magnesium.
   b. copper and iron.
   c. calcium and phosphorus.
   d. sodium and potassium.

4. In a situation where there is an insufficient intake of dietary iodide, the thyroid-stimulating hormone promotes the enlargement of the thyroid gland. This condition is called
   a. Graves' disease.
   b. goiter.
   c. hyperparathyroidism.
   d. cretinism.

5. Ninety-nine percent of the calcium in the body is found in
   a. intracellular fluid.
   b. bones and teeth.
   c. nerve cells.
   d. the liver.

6. At the end of long bones, inside the spinal vertebrae, and inside the flat bones of the pelvis, is a spongy type of bone known as _____ bone.
   a. osteoclastic
   b. osteoblastic
   c. trabecular
   d. compact

7. Which compartment contains the greatest amount of body fluid?
   a. intracellular
   b. extracellular
   c. They contain the same amount.

8. The primary function of sodium is to maintain

   a. bone mineral content.
   b. hemoglobin concentration.
   c. immune function.
   d. fluid distribution.

9. Hypertension is defined as a blood pressure greater than
   a. 110/60.
   b. 120/65.
   c. 140/90.
   d. 190/80.

10. Which of the following individuals are most likely to develop osteoporosis?
    a. premenopausal women athletes
    b. women taking estrogen replacement therapy
    c. slender, inactive women who smoke
    d. women who eat a lot of high-fat dairy products

Study Questions (Numbers refer to Learning Outcomes)

1. Approximately how much water do you need each day to stay healthy? Identify at least two situations that increase the need for water. Then list three sources of water in the average person's diet. **(LO 9.2)**

2. What is the relationship between sodium and water balance, and how is that relationship monitored as well as maintained in the body? **(LO 9.6)**

3. Identify four factors that influence the bioavailability of minerals from food. **(LO 9.5)**

4. What are two similarities and differences between sodium and potassium? Sodium and chloride? **(LO 9.6)**

5. In terms of total amounts in the body, calcium and phosphorus are the first and second most abundant minerals, respectively. What function do these minerals have in common? **(LO 9.6)**

6. What are the best food sources for zinc and copper? **(LO 9.6)**

7. Describe the symptoms of iron-deficiency anemia and explain possible reasons they occur. **(LO 9.6)**

8. Which trace minerals are lost from cereal grains when they are refined? Are any of these nutrients replaced by enrichment? **(LO 9.6)**

9. Describe the chief functions of fluoride, copper, and chromium in the body. **(LO 9.6)**

10. What are the practical consequences of the Daily Values on food and supplement labels exceeding the RDA or Adequate Intake for many trace minerals? **(LO 9.6)**

What Would You Choose Recommendations

Bottled water has become very popular. In 2009, each American consumed almost 28 gallons of bottled water, adding up to about 8.5 billion gallons for the nation. The public perception that bottled water is safer and healthier than tap water has stimulated the current bottle-toting habit. The truth is that bottled and tap water are both regulated: bottled water by the FDA and tap water by the Environmental Protection Agency (EPA). The FDA requirements for bottled water mimic those of the EPA for water quality, but neither has to be contaminant-free.

"Pure" is an advertising term and means nothing about the quality of the water. Recent controversy over misleading advertising by major companies such as Pepsico and Coca-Cola that use public source water in their respective products, Aquafina and Dasani, has led to the printing of "Public Source Water" or "PSW" on labels (see Further Reading 12).

Mineral water must contain consistent levels of natural elements from an underground source; no minerals may be added to the water. The precise mineral content varies by source, but some common minerals found in water include calcium, magnesium, potassium, sodium, sulfur, iron, fluoride, zinc, and some ultratrace

minerals. The minerals impart some taste to the water but are typically a minor contributor to overall mineral intake.

There is no legal definition for "vitamin water." Manufacturers of vitamin water (i.e., soft-drink companies) usually use filtered or distilled water and add sweeteners (e.g., high-fructose corn syrup) and citric acid as flavoring agents, plus several vitamins (mostly vitamin C and an assortment of B vitamins). In 2010, the Coca-Cola Bottling Company was sued by the Center for Science in the Public Interest for false marketing of its popular vitaminwater® brand as "nutritious." These products are marketed as healthy because they contain added vitamins, but most of them also supply a surprising amount of sugar. Recall that the American Heart Association recommends that men and women get no more than 150 or 100 kcal per day, respectively, from added sugars. A 20-ounce bottle of vitaminwater® has 33 grams of sugar, providing 132 kcal from added sugar. This is about half the sugar in a regular soft drink, but you can see how this can add up to excess. Furthermore, most North

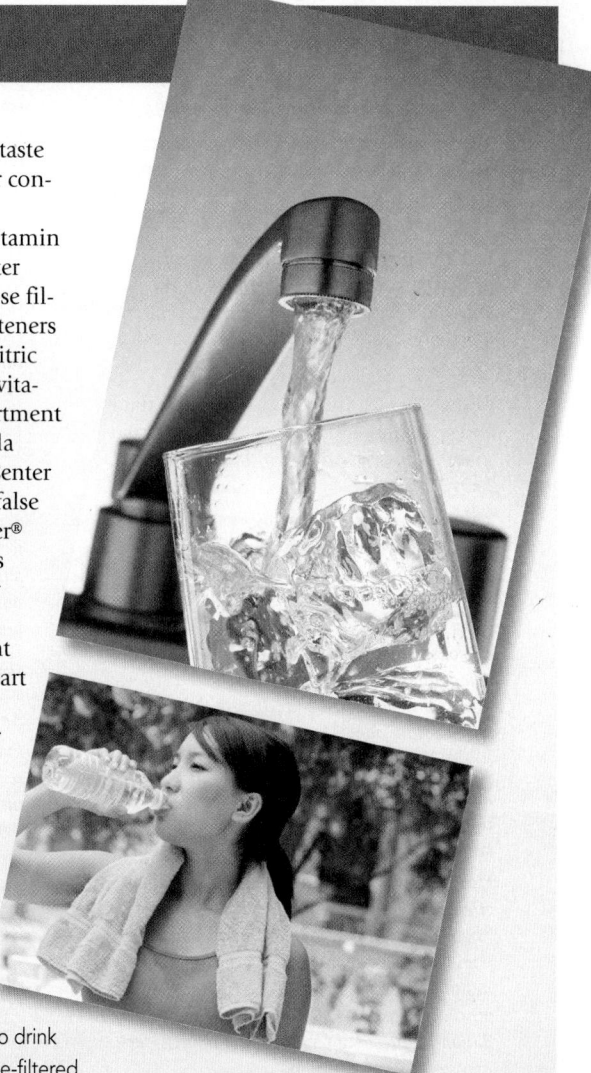

▲ While following the recommendations to drink more water, hydrate with tap water or home-filtered water in a reusable container.

Americans consume adequate amounts of vitamin C and the B vitamins without the aid of these beverages.

Consumers should also be aware of the FDA definitions for other types of bottled water.

- Artesian water must come from a confined aquifer.
- Springwater must flow naturally to the surface.

- Purified water is produced through an approved process such as distillation or reverse osmosis.

Relying on bottled water is an expensive habit, personally and environmentally. If you use bottled water to meet your recommended fluid needs, you will spend close to $1500 per year compared with about 50 cents for the same volume of tap water. On a larger scale, it is estimated that close to 90% of water bottles end up in the trash, clogging our landfills or being shipped to other countries for recycling. It is well known that America has some of the cleanest, safest tap water in the world.

Further Readings

1. ADA Reports: Position of the American Dietetic Association: The impact of fluoride on health. *Journal of the American Dietetic Association* 105:1620, 2005.

   The American Dietetic Association reaffirms that fluoride is an important element for all mineralized tissues in the body. Appropriate fluoride intake is beneficial to bone and tooth health.

2. Appel LJ and others: Dietary approaches to prevent and treat hypertension: A scientific statement from the American Heart Association. *Hypertension* 47:296, 2006.

   Latest advice from the American Heart Association on diet and hypertension. Key preventive factors are to avoid overweight and inactivity and to moderate alcohol and salt intake.

3. Cook NR and others: Joint effects of sodium and potassium intake on subsequent cardiovascular disease. *Archives of Internal Medicine* 169: 32, 2009.

   This study suggests that potassium is effective in lowering blood pressure. Furthermore, the combination of a higher intake of potassium and a lower intake of sodium seems to be more effective than either on its own in reducing the risk of cardiovascular disease. The sodium-to-potassium ratio in subjects' urine was a stronger predictor of cardiovascular disease than sodium or potassium alone.

4. Elliott P and others: Dietary phosphorus and blood pressure: International study of macro- and micro-nutrients and blood pressure. *Hypertension* 51:669, 2008.

   Little attention has been given to the possible effects of phosphorus intake on blood pressure. The results of this study indicate that increased phosphorus intake, as well as calcium and magnesium intake, have the potential to lower blood pressure. This may be an important recommendation for prevention and control of prehypertension and hypertension.

5. Havas S and others: The urgent need to reduce sodium consumption. *Journal of the American Medical Association* 298:1439, 2007.

   In the United States, 77% of sodium comes from processed and restaurant foods, with many processed foods containing 1000 mg or more per serving. There is a general consensus that sodium levels should be reduced substantially in processed and restaurant foods. Policy developments and possible solutions to address this problem are presented in this article.

6. Heaney RP: Absorbability and utility of calcium in mineral waters. *American Journal of Clinical Nutrition* 84(2):371, 2006.

   Published absorbability and utility of high-calcium mineral waters are summarized and integrated in this article. The absorbability of all the high-calcium mineral waters was equal to or slightly better than milk calcium. The utility of calcium as measured by increased urinary calcium, decreased serum parathyroid hormone, decreased bone resorption biomarkers, and protection of bone mass indicated that a significant quantity of calcium was absorbed. High-calcium mineral waters, therefore, appear to provide useful quantities of bioavailable calcium.

7. Hollenberg NK: The influence of dietary sodium on blood pressure. *Journal of the American College of Nutrition* 25:240S, 2006.

   Evidence relating salt intake to blood pressure is reviewed. The merit of mandating a reduction in salt intake is discussed. The author indicates that the evidence supporting such a policy is inconsistent and small. The importance of anti-hypertensive drugs is emphasized.

8. Jackson RD and others: Calcium plus vitamin D supplementation and the risk of fractures. *New England Journal of Medicine* 354 (7):669, 2006.

   Postmenopausal women, 50 to 79 years of age, who were enrolled in a Women's Health Initiative (WHI) clinical trial were assigned to receive 1000 mg of elemental calcium as calcium carbonate with 400 IU of vitamin D_3 daily or a placebo. The occurrence of fractures and bone density was determined for 7 years. Calcium with vitamin D supplementation resulted in a small but significant increase in hip bone density, but did not significantly reduce hip fracture and increased the risk of kidney stones.

9. King JC: Zinc: An essential but elusive nutrient. *American Journal of Clinical Nutrition* 94:679S, 2011.

   Zinc is essential for many biochemical functions. When zinc is insufficient in the diet, body stores give up zinc immediately to conserve the nutrient. There is probably a small zinc reserve in all cells in addition to the zinc in blood. Zinc concentrations in blood decline quickly with severe deficiencies and more slowly with marginal depletion. Blood zinc concentrations also decrease with conditions such as infection, trauma, stress, and steroid use due to redistribution of zinc from blood to tissues. This redistribution confuses the interpretation of low blood zinc concentrations and determining whether this redistribution is the cause of low blood zinc rather than poor nutrition.

10. Lanham-New SA. The balance of bone health: Tipping the scales in favor of potassium-rich, bicarbonate-rich foods. *Journal of Nutrition* 137:1725, 2008.

    About 10 million Americans have osteoporosis. This review article summarizes the current evidence linking potassium-rich, bicarbonate-rich foods (e.g., fruits and vegetables) to osteoporosis prevention.

11. Lippman SM and others: Effect of selenium and vitamin E on risk of prostate cancer and other cancers: The selenium and vitamin E cancer prevention trial (SELECT). *Journal of the American Medical Association* 301:39, 2009.

The results of this study showed no benefit to taking a supplement of selenium or vitamin E alone or in combination for the prevention of prostate cancer, colon cancer, lung cancer, all cancers, and cardiovascular disease and for overall survival.

12. Palmer S: Busting bottled water. *Today's Dietitian* 9(12):60, 2007.

    This article highlights several reasons why consumers have been wrong in assuming that bottled water is always better than tap water. The ecological, environmental, and economic problems with relying on bottled water for our fluids needs. The laws regulating bottled and tap water are also compared, suggesting that bottled water is generally not safer and healthier than tap water. The author recommends that we drink more water, but do it from the tap.

13. Park Y and others: Dairy food, calcium, and risk of cancer in the NIH-AARP diet and health study. *Archives of Internal Medicine* 169:391, 2009.

    The 7-year study of 493,000 older men and women provides evidence that diets rich in calcium may lower risk of total cancer and cancers of the digestive system, especially colorectal cancer. Benefits were mostly associated with foods high in calcium, rather than calcium supplements. Getting more than the recommended 1200 milligrams of calcium for older people did not result in greater cancer protection.

14. Popkin BM and others: A new proposed guidance system for beverage consumption in the United States. *American Journal of Clinical Nutrition* 83:529, 2006.

    Drinking water is recommended as the preferred beverage to fulfill water needs, with tea, coffee, and low-fat and skim milk also ranked high. The Beverage Guidance Panel suggests that beverages with no or few calories should be consumed more often than calorie-containing beverages. An intake of 98 fluid ounces is recommended daily for a person consuming 2200 calories.

15. Reid IR and others: Randomized controlled trial of calcium in healthy older women. *American Journal of Medicine* 119(9):777, 2006.

    In this study of postmenopausal women receiving 1 g/day as calcium citrate over 5 years, height loss was reduced by calcium but constipation was more common. The authors conclude that calcium results in a sustained reduction in bone loss and turnover, but its effect on fracture is uncertain.

16. Van Dam RM and others: Dietary calcium and magnesium, major food sources, and risk of type 2 diabetes in U.S. black women. *Diabetes Care* 29:2238, 2006.

    Magnesium and calcium intakes have been inversely associated with risk of type 2 diabetes in predominantly white populations. The results of this study of 41,186 participants of the Black Women's Health Study indicated that a diet high in magnesium-rich foods, particularly whole grains, is associated with a significantly lower risk of type 2 diabetes in U.S. black women.

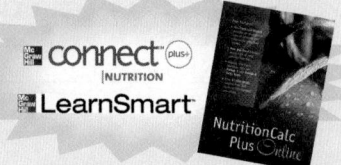

To get the most out of your study of nutrition, go to McGraw-Hill's online resources: Connect www.mcgrawhillconnect.com, **where you will find NutritionCalc Plus, LearnSmart, and many other dynamic tools.**

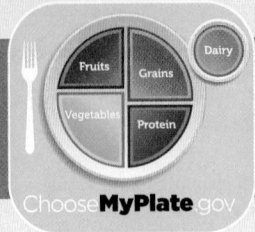

I. How High Is Your Sodium Intake?

Complete this questionnarie to evaluate your sodium habits with respect to typically rich sources.

How Often Do You...	Rarely	Occasionally	Often	Regularly (Daily)
1. Eat cured or processed meats, such as ham, bacon, sausage, frankfurters, and other luncheon meats?	☐	☐	☐	☐
2. Choose canned or frozen vegetables with sauce?	☐	☐	☐	☐
3. Use commercially prepared meals, main dishes, or canned or dehydrated soups?	☐	☐	☐	☐
4. Eat cheese, especially processed cheese?	☐	☐	☐	☐
5. Eat salted nuts, popcorn, pretzels, corn chips, or potato chips?	☐	☐	☐	☐
6. Add salt to cooking water for vegetables, rice, or pasta?	☐	☐	☐	☐
7. Add salt, seasoning mixes, salad dressings, or condiments—such as soy sauce, steak sauce, catsup, and mustard—to foods during preparation or at the table?	☐	☐	☐	☐
8. Salt your food before tasting it?	☐	☐	☐	☐
9. Ignore labels for sodium content when buying foods?	☐	☐	☐	☐
10. When dining out, choose obviously salty sauces or foods?	☐	☐	☐	☐

The more checks you put in the "often" or "regularly" columns, the higher your dietary sodium intake is. However, not all the habits in the table contribute the same amount of sodium. For example, many natural cheeses such as cheddar are relatively moderate in sodium, whereas processed cheeses and cottage cheese are much higher. To moderate sodium intake, choose lower-sodium foods from each food group more often and balance high-sodium food choices with low-sodium ones.

Adapted from *USDA Home and Garden Bulletin* No. 232–6, April 1986.

II. Working for Denser Bones

Osteoporosis and related low bone mass affect many adults in North America, especially older women. One-third of all women experience fractures because of this disease, amounting to about 2 million bone fractures per year.

Osteoporosis is a disease you can do something about. Some risk factors can't be changed, but others, such as a poor calcium intake, can. Is this true for you? To find out, complete this tool for estimating your current calcium intake. For all the following foods, write the number of servings you eat in a day. Total the number of servings in each category and then multiply the total number of servings by the amount of calcium for each category. Finally, add the total amount for each food category to estimate your calcium intake for that day.

Does your intake meet your RDA set for calcium?

Food	Serving Size	Number of Servings	Calcium (mg)	Total Calcium (mg)
Plain low-fat yogurt	1 cup	_____		
Fat-free dry milk powder	1/2 cup	_____		
Total servings		_____	× 400	= _____ mg
Canned sardines (with bones)	3 ounces	_____		
Fruit-flavored yogurt	1 cup	_____		
Milk: fat-free, reduced-fat, whole, chocolate, buttermilk	1 cup	_____		
Calcium-fortified soy milk (e.g., Silk)	1 cup	_____		
Parmesan cheese (grated)	1/4 cup	_____		
Swiss cheese	1 ounce	_____		
Total servings		_____	× 300	= _____ mg
Cheese (all other hard cheese)	1 ounce	_____		
Pancakes	3	_____		
Total servings		_____	× 200	= _____ mg
Canned pink salmon	3 ounces	_____		
Tofu (processed with calcium)	4 ounces	_____		
Total servings		_____	× 150	= _____ mg
Collards or turnip greens, cooked	1/2 cup	_____		
Ice cream or ice milk	1/2 cup	_____		
Almonds	1 ounce	_____		
Total servings		_____	× 75	= _____ mg
Chard, cooked	1/2 cup	_____		
Cottage cheese	1/2 cup	_____		
Corn tortilla	1 medium	_____		
Orange	1 medium	_____		
Total servings		_____	× 50	= _____ mg
Kidney, lima, or navy beans, cooked	1/2 cup	_____		
Broccoli	1/2 cup	_____		
Carrot, raw	1 medium	_____		
Dates or raisins	1/4 cup	_____		
Egg	1 large	_____		
Whole-wheat bread	1 slice	_____		
Peanut butter	2 tablespoons	_____		
Total servings		_____	× 25	= _____ mg
Calcium-fortified orange juice	6 ounces	_____		
Calcium-fortified snack bars	1 each	_____		
Calcium-fortified breakfast bars	1/2 bar	_____		
Total servings		_____	× 200	= _____ mg
Calcium-fortified chocolate candies	1 each	_____		
Calcium supplements*	1 each	_____	× 500	= _____ mg
Total servings		_____	Total calcium intake	= _____ mg

Other calcium sources to consider include many breakfast cereals (100 to 250 mg per cup) and some vitamin/mineral supplements (200 to 500 mg or more per tablet).

*Amount varies, so check the label for the amount in a specific product and then adjust the calculation as needed.

Reprinted with permission from *Topics in Clinical Nutrition*, "Putting Calcium into Perspective for Your Clients," G. Wardlaw and N. Weese, 11:1, p. 29. © 1995 Aspen Publishers, Inc.

Chapter 10 Nutrition: Fitness and Sports

Student Learning Outcomes

Chapter 10 is designed to allow you to:

10.1 List five positive health-related outcomes of a physically active lifestyle.

10.2 Design a fitness regimen.

10.3 Describe when and how glycogen, blood glucose, fat, and protein are used to meet energy needs during different types of physical activity.

10.4 Differentiate between anaerobic and aerobic use of glucose, and identify advantages and disadvantages of each.

10.5 Show how muscles and related organs adapt to an increase in physical activity.

10.6 Outline how to estimate an athlete's calorie needs and discuss the general principles for meeting overall nutrient requirements in the training diet.

10.7 Examine the problems associated with rapid weight loss by dehydration and outline the importance of water and/or sports drinks during exercise.

10.8 Understand how athletes can optimize performance by consuming foods and fluids before, during, and after exercise.

10.9 List several ergogenic aids and describe their effects, if any, on an athlete's performance.

What Would You Choose?

You are gearing up to run your first half-marathon in a few weeks. When your race packet arrived in the mail, it included your T-shirt, race number, and a bunch of free samples and coupons for sports nutrition products. From your long training runs, you know that you tend to lose your speed and motivation around mile nine. What would you choose to take along during the race to help you make it to the finish line?

a Clif Shot Turbo energy gel with 100 milligrams caffeine, 22 grams of carbohydrate, and electrolytes

b PowerBar ProteinPlus energy bar with 23 grams of protein

c Powerade sports drink with electrolytes, vitamins, and 14 grams of carbohydrate

d Essential Amino Energy drink with branched-chain amino acids

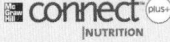 **connect** | NUTRITION

Think about your choice as you read Chapter 10, then see our recommendations at the end of the chapter. To learn more about store-bought and homemade sports nutrition products, check out the Connect site:
www.mcgrawhillconnect.com

Part Four
Nutrition: Beyond the Nutrients

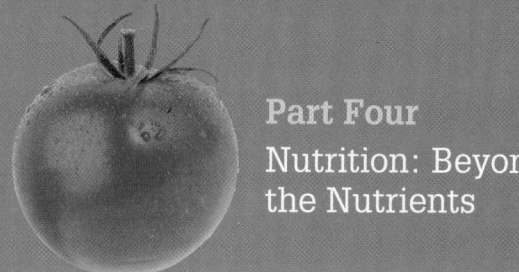

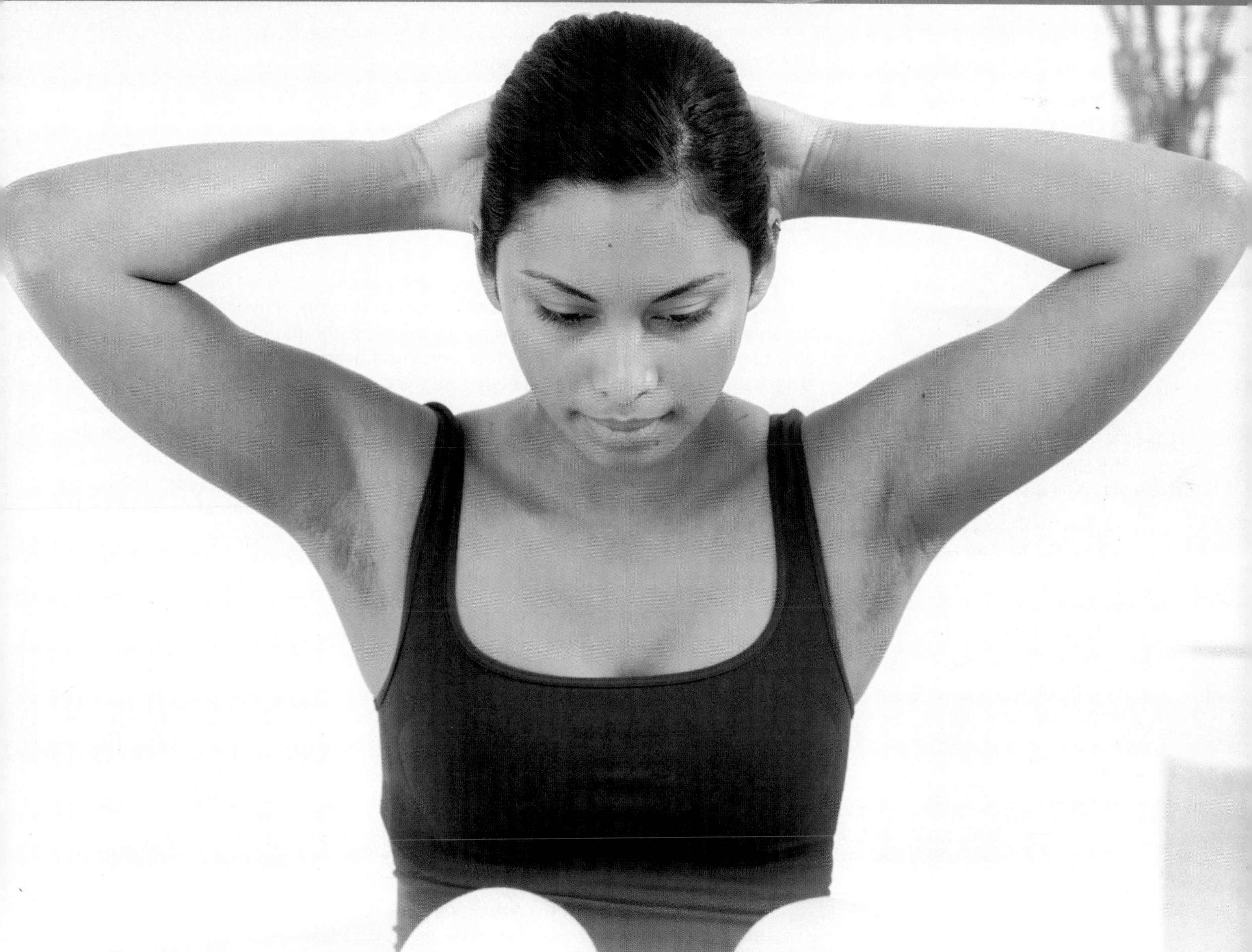

Athletes invest a lot of time and effort in training. Most athletes don't want to miss out on any advantage, whether real or perceived, that might give them the winning edge. Athletes often seek ways to enhance their diets to improve performance, so they make easy targets for purveyors of nutrition misinformation.

Although good eating habits can't substitute for physical training and genetic endowment, proper food and beverage choices are crucial for top-notch performance, contributing to endurance and helping to speed the repair of injured tissues.

Although experts might disagree on how much carbohydrate, protein, and fat we should consume, there is no argument over the health benefits of regular physical activity. It is even beneficial for overweight people who remain at that excess weight. As the comic in this chapter suggests, it takes a strong commitment to reap the benefits.

In Chapter 10, you will discover how physical fitness benefits the entire body and how nutrition relates to fitness and sports performance.

Refresh Your Memory

As you begin your study of nutrition for fitness and sports in Chapter 10, you may want to review:

- The current trend of consuming "energy bars" in Chapter 1
- Components of the cell in Chapter 3
- Concept of glycemic load in Chapter 4
- Various food sources of carbohydrates, proteins, and lipids in Chapters 4–7
- Food sources of calcium and iron in Chapter 9

10.1 The Close Relationship Between Nutrition and Fitness

Healthy people 2020 objectives focus on reducing the proportion of adults who engage in no leisure time physical activity and increasing the proportion of adults who meet the 2008 Physical Activity Guidelines for aerobic and muscle-strengthening physical activity.

Without a doubt, physical fitness has many health benefits. Physical fitness refers to the ability to perform moderate to vigorous activity without undue fatigue. The benefits of regular physical activity include enhanced heart function, less injury, better sleep habits, and improvement in body composition. Physical activity also can reduce stress and positively affect blood pressure, blood cholesterol, blood glucose regulation, and immune function. In addition, physical activity aids in weight control, both by raising resting energy expenditure for a short time after exercise and by increasing overall energy expenditure. In fact, as physical fitness improves, so does your ability to mobilize fat as a source of energy. See Figure 10-1 and Further Readings 8 and 11 for a further look at these and other benefits of a physically active lifestyle.

Unfortunately, as noted in Chapter 7, many North American adults lead sedentary lives. Most adults do not regularly practice moderate to vigorous physical activity and about half of all adults quit an exercise program within 3 months of initiation.

To help yourself stay with an exercise program, experts recommend the following:

- Start slowly.
- Vary your activities; make it fun.

Sherman's Lagoon by J.P. Toomey

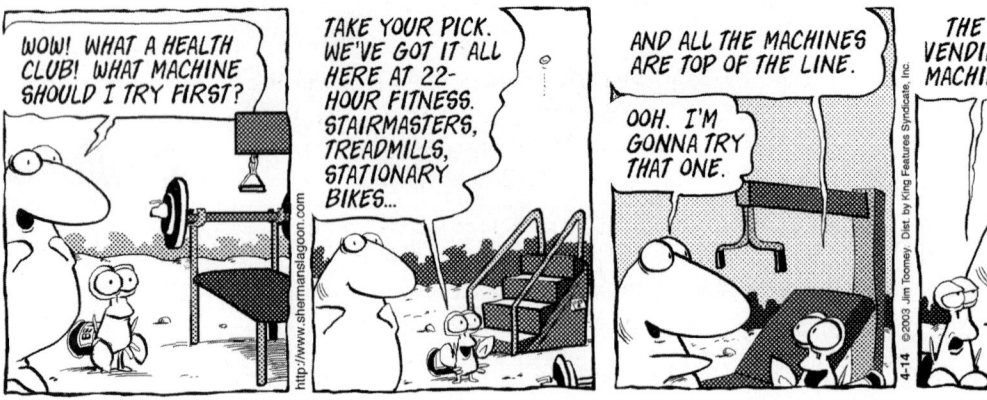

Why is regular physical activity—including some strength-building activities—generally advocated for all of us? What benefits accrue from this practice? How do strength-training and endurance athletes need to tailor their diets to support their vigorous physical activities? Chapter 10 provides some answers.

© Jim Toomey. Reprinted with special permission of King Features Syndicate.

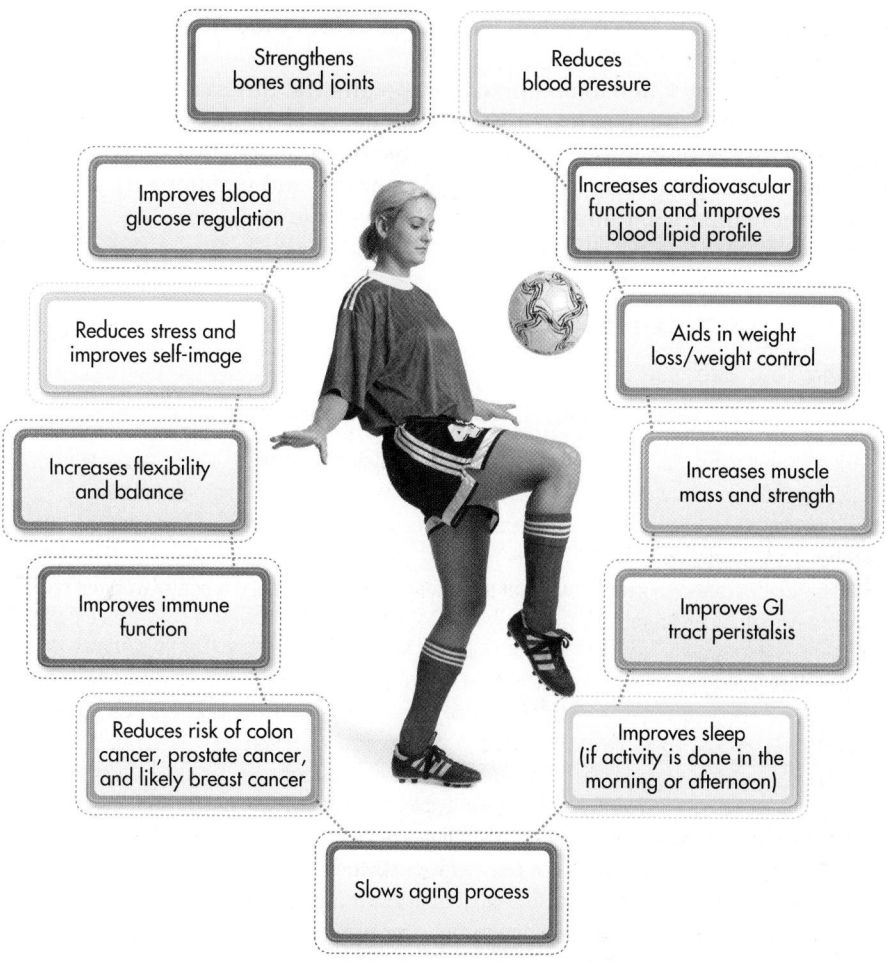

- Include friends and family members.
- Set specific, attainable goals and monitor progress.
- Set aside a specific time each day for exercise; build it into your routine, but make it convenient.
- Reward yourself for being successful in keeping up with your goals.
- Don't worry about occasional setbacks; focus on the long-term benefits to your health.

The 2008 Physical Activity Guidelines for Americans recommend that all adults should avoid inactivity. Some physical activity is better than none, and adults who participate in any amount of physical activity gain some health benefits. The Physical Activity Guidelines set specific time goals for adults (review Chapter 2):

- For substantial health benefits, adults should do at least 150 minutes (2 hours and 30 minutes) a week of **moderate-intensity,** or 75 minutes (1 hour and 15 minutes) a week of **vigorous-intensity aerobic physical activity**, or an equivalent combination of moderate- and vigorous-intensity aerobic activity. Aerobic activity should be performed in episodes of at least 10 minutes, and preferably, it should be spread throughout the week.
- For additional and more extensive health benefits, adults should increase their aerobic physical activity to 300 minutes (5 hours) a week of moderate-intensity, or 150 minutes a week of vigorous-intensity aerobic physical activity, or an equivalent combination of moderate- and vigorous-intensity activity. Additional health benefits are gained by engaging in physical activity beyond this amount.
- Adults should also include **muscle-strengthening activities** that involve all major muscle groups on 2 or more days a week.

moderate-intensity aerobic physical activity Aerobic activity that increases a person's heart rate and breathing to some extent (5–6 on RPE scale). Examples include brisk walking, dancing, swimming, or bicycling on level terrain.

vigorous-intensity aerobic physical activity Aerobic activity that greatly increases a person's heart rate and breathing (7–8 on RPE scale). Examples include jogging, singles tennis, swimming continuous laps, or bicycling uphill.

muscle-strengthening activity Physical activity, including exercise, that increases skeletal muscle strength, power, endurance, and mass. Examples include strength training, resistance training, and muscle strength and endurance exercises.

These recommendations are consistent with guidance from the American College of Sports Medicine (see Further Reading 3).

The Physical Activity Guidelines aim to develop physical fitness and reduce risk of chronic diseases. Performing at least 150 minutes per week of moderate-intensity or 75 minutes per week of vigorous-intensity aerobic physical activity can assist efforts at preventing weight gain during adulthood. Weight loss and maintenance of weight loss require more than 150 minutes of physical activity per week.

▶ To earn yourself a place in the *Guinness Book of World Records* for the Physical Fitness Challenge, you'll need to complete:

2 miles swimming,

12 miles running,

12 miles hiking with a 25-pound backpack,

1250 push-ups,

1250 leg lifts,

1250 jumping jacks,

110 miles cycling,

20 miles rowing,

20 miles cross-training on elliptical equipment,

3250 abdominal crunches, and

300,000 pounds lifting through various upper-body repetitions.

Oh, and by the way, this will all need to be accomplished (on videotape and with at least three official witnesses) within 18 hours, 25 minutes, and 40 seconds!

MAKING DECISIONS

Planning Your Exercise

Consider applying the dietary principles of variety, balance, and moderation to your exercise plan:

- Variety: Enjoy many different activities to exercise different muscles.
- Balance: Different activities have different benefits, so balance your exercise pattern. For overall fitness, you need exercises that build cardiovascular endurance, muscular strength, and flexibility.
- Moderation: Exercise to keep fit without overdoing it. You don't need a heavy workout every day to achieve fitness.

CONCEPT CHECK

Regular physical activity is a vital part of a healthy lifestyle, ideally consisting of a total of at least 150 minutes of moderate-intensity or 75 minutes of vigorous-intensity aerobic physical activity per week. In addition, muscle-strengthening activities should be included at least twice per week. Physically active people benefit from lower risks of cardiovascular disease, type 2 diabetes, obesity, and other common chronic diseases.

10.2 Guidelines for Achieving and Maintaining Physical Fitness

For healthy people, a gradual increase to a goal of regular physical activity is recommended. Men 40 years of age or older and women 50 years of age or older who have been inactive for many years, or who have an existing health problem, should discuss their fitness goals with their physician before increasing activity. Health problems that require medical evaluation before beginning an exercise program are obesity, cardiovascular disease (or family history of it), hypertension, diabetes (or family history), shortness of breath after mild exertion, and arthritis.

During the first phase of a fitness program to promote health, you should begin to incorporate short periods of physical activity into your daily routine. This includes walking, taking the stairs instead of the elevator, house cleaning, gardening, and other activities that cause you to "huff and puff" a bit. The goal is a total of 30 minutes of this moderate type of physical activity on most (and preferably all) days. If necessary, this can be broken up into increments lasting at least 10 minutes. Experts suggest starting with short intervals, building up to a total of 30 minutes of activity incorporated into each day's tasks. If there is not much time for activity, you can even go for more intensity in the activities over shorter periods to get the same benefits. Clearly, many of the activities just recommended are not very vigorous.

Once you can perform physical activity for 30 minutes per day, turn your attention to more specific goals, such as increasing muscle mass and strength, to reap even more benefits. Guidelines for designing a fitness program are listed in Table 10-1.

Aerobic, strength, and stretching activities are included, as well as considerations for duration, frequency, intensity, and progression.

Begin by warming up with 5 to 10 minutes of low-intensity exercises, such as walking, slow jogging, or any slow version of the anticipated activity. This warms up your muscles so that muscle filaments more easily slide over one another to increase range of motion and decrease the risk of injury.

Aerobic Workout

Daily aerobic activity is recommended. As you learned in Chapter 3, "aerobic" means "with oxygen." Aerobic exercises use large muscle groups in a rhythmic fashion. They are usually of low or moderate intensity and long duration (i.e., 30 minutes of brisk walking). Health benefits from regular physical activity are especially seen when you can achieve a moderate level of intensity of exercise.

There are a few ways to determine the intensity of exercise. A popular and simple method is to use a percentage of your age-predicted maximum heart rate (Fig. 10-2). To find maximum heart rate, subtract your age from 220. Multiplying maximum heart rate by 0.60 and 0.90 will result in a range of heart rates, sometimes called the *target zone*. For a 20-year-old person beginning an exercise program, maximum heart rate equals 200 beats per minute ($220 - 20 = 200$). Then, (200×0.6) and (200×0.9) yields a target zone of 120 to 180 beats per minute. Measuring heart rate (pulse) is easy: Stop and count your pulse for 10 seconds and then multiply that number by 6 to determine your heart rate for one minute. Some exercise equipment and high-tech watches contain heart rate monitors.

At the initiation of an exercise program, aim for the lower end of the target zone. As you progress and become more physically fit, you can work up to a higher heart rate. As with many of the prediction formulas, calculation of maximum heart rate is just an estimate. Medications, such as those for hypertension and other health conditions, may impact heart rate. If you have health concerns, a physician can help to personalize your target zone.

▲ What is the best exercise? One you want to continue to do.

TABLE 10-1 Designing a Fitness Program

Type of Activity	Aerobic (uses large muscle groups in rhythmic fashion)	Strength (resistance activity)	Stretching (uses major muscle groups; most beneficial when muscles are warm, such as during cooldown.)
Examples	Brisk walking, running, cycling, swimming, basketball, tennis, soccer	Weight lifting, pilates, push-ups, pull-ups	Yoga
Duration (time spent in exercise session)	20 to 60 minutes	8 to 12 repetitions of 8 to 10 different exercises	4 repetitions of 10 to 30 seconds per muscle group
Frequency (times activity is performed)	5 days per week	2 to 3 days per week	2 to 3 days per week and during warm-up and cooldown
Intensity (level of exertion)	55% to 90% maximum heart rate or RPE of 4 or above (see Figure 10-3)	Enough to condition major muscle groups of the upper and lower body	5 to 10 minutes during warm-up and cooldown
Progression (increase in frequency, intensity, and duration over time)	**Initiation phase:** 3 to 6 weeks **Improvement phase:** 5 to 6 months **Maintenance phase:** plateau in gains in fitness		Start with smaller muscle groups (e.g., arms) and work toward large muscle groups (e.g., legs and abdomen)

FIGURE 10-2 ▶ Heart rate training chart. This chart shows the number of heart beats per minute that corresponds to various exercise intensities.

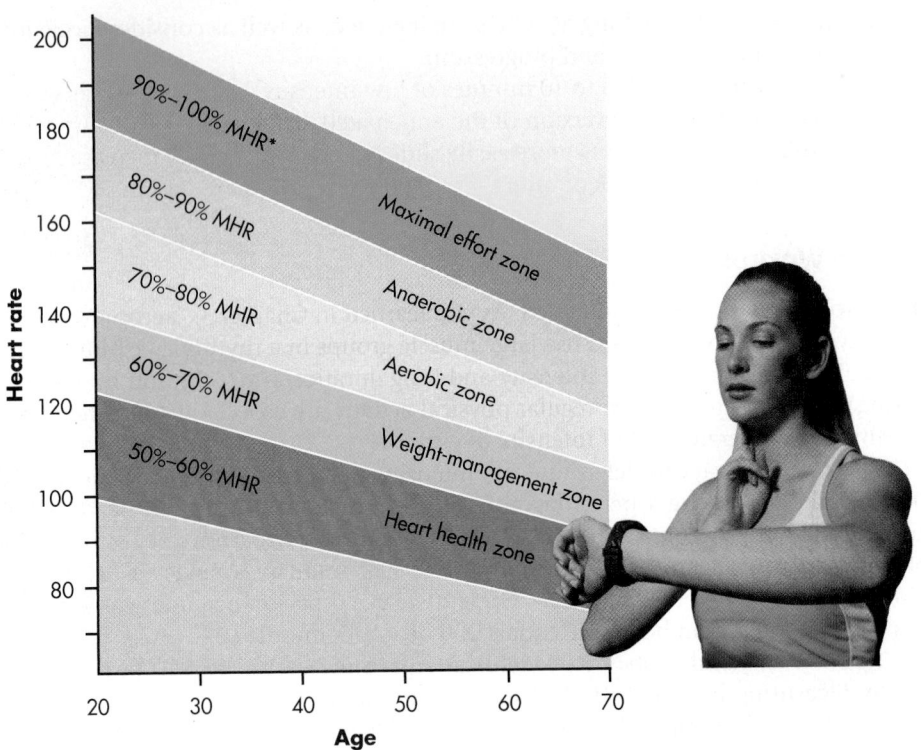

*MHR (maximum heart rate) = 220 - Age in years

Another way of determining the intensity of exercise is the Rating of Perceived Exertion scale (RPE). One version includes a range of 1 to 10, with each number corresponding to a subjective feeling of exertion. For example, the number 0 is "nothing at all" (sitting at a table) and the number 10 is considered close to maximal effort or "very, very strong" (all-out sprint) (Fig. 10-3).

When using the RPE scale, the goal is to aim for the number 4, which corresponds to the beginning of "somewhat strong." This is the point at which you begin to see significant fitness results. You should be working hard, but still be able to talk to an exercise partner (sometimes called the "talk test").

During cooldown, follow a reverse pattern of the warm-up: 5 to 10 minutes of low-intensity activity and add 5 to 10 minutes of stretching. The same exercises performed during warm-up are appropriate. The cooldown is essential to the prevention of injury and soreness.

10.3 Energy Sources for Exercising Muscles

Like other cells, muscle cells cannot directly use the energy released from breaking down glucose or triglycerides. Muscle cells need a specific form of energy for contraction. Body cells must first convert food energy (i.e., calories) to **adenosine triphosphate (ATP)**.

The chemical bonds between phosphates in ATP and related molecules are high-energy bonds. Using the energy obtained from foodstuffs, cells make ATP from its breakdown product **adenosine diphosphate (ADP)** and a phosphate group (abbreviated P_i).

$$ADP + Energy\ from\ food + P_i \rightarrow ATP$$

Conversely, to release energy from ATP, cells partially break the compound down into ADP and P_i. The released energy is used for many cell functions.

$$ATP \rightarrow Energy\ to\ do\ work + ADP + P_i$$

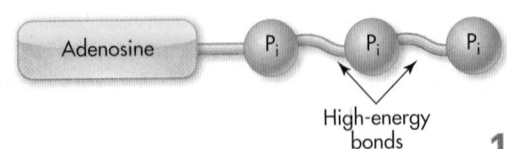

Structure of ATP

adenosine triphosphate (ATP) The main energy currency for cells. ATP energy is used to promote ion pumping, enzyme activity, and muscular contraction.

adenosine diphosphate (ADP) A breakdown product of ATP. ADP is synthesized into ATP using energy from foodstuffs and a phosphate group (abbreviated P_i).

RPE Scale*

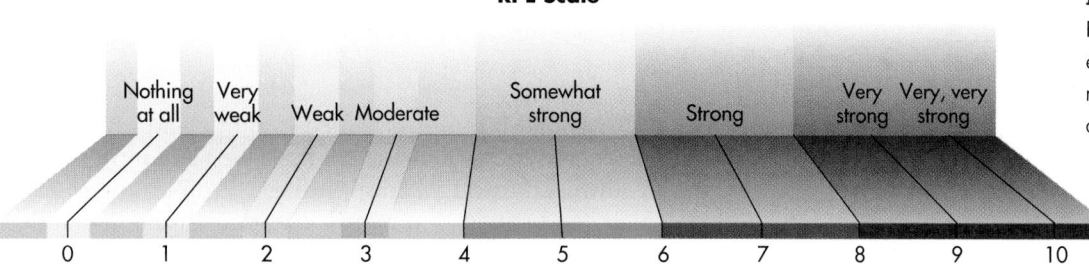

Nothing at all — Very weak — Weak — Moderate — Somewhat strong — Strong — Very strong — Very, very strong

0 1 2 3 4 5 6 7 8 9 10

* Rating of Perceived Exertion (RPE) beyond 10 is considered maximal.

FIGURE 10-3 ▶ Rating of Perceived Exertion scale. When exercising, aim for 4 for light/moderate activity or up to 8 for cardiorespiratory fitness.

Essentially, ATP is the immediate source of energy for body functions (Table 10-2). The primary goal in the use of any fuel, whether carbohydrate, fat, or protein, is to make ATP. A resting muscle cell contains only a small amount of ATP that can be used immediately. This amount of ATP could keep the muscle working maximally for only about 2 to 4 seconds if no resupply of ATP were possible. Fortunately, another type of high-energy compound—**phosphocreatine (PCr)**—is also present in muscle cells and can be quickly broken down to release enough energy to make more ATP. This supports the working muscle cells until metabolism of carbohydrate and fat for fuel begins in earnest. Overall, cells must constantly and repeatedly use and then re-form ATP, using a variety of energy sources.

Phosphocreatine Is the First Line of Defense for Resupplying ATP in Muscles

As soon as ATP stored in muscle cells begins to be used, another source of energy just mentioned, PCr, is used to produce ATP. An enzyme in the muscle cell is activated to split PCr into phosphate and **creatine**. This releases energy that can be used to re-form ATP from its breakdown products. If no other source of energy for ATP resupply were available, PCr could probably maintain maximal muscle contractions

phosphocreatine (PCr) A high-energy compound that can be used to re-form ATP. It is used primarily during bursts of activity, such as lifting and jumping.

creatine An organic (i.e., carbon-containing) molecule in muscle cells that serves as a part of a high-energy compound (termed creatine phosphate or phosphocreatine) capable of synthesizing ATP from ADP.

TABLE 10-2 Energy Sources Used by Resting and Working Muscle Cells

Energy Source*	When in Use	Activity
ATP	At all times	All types
Phosphocreatine (PCr)	All exercise initially; short bursts of exercise thereafter	Shotput, high jump, bench press
Carbohydrate (anaerobic)	High-intensity exercise, especially lasting 30 seconds to 2 minutes	200-yard (about 200 meters) sprint
Carbohydrate (aerobic)	Exercise lasting 2 minutes to 3 hours or more; the higher the intensity (for example, running a 6-minute mile), the greater the use	Basketball, swimming, jogging, power walking, soccer, tennis
Fat (aerobic)	Exercise lasting more than a few minutes; greater amounts are used at lower exercise intensities	Long-distance running, long-distance cycling; much of the fuel used in a 30-minute brisk walk is fat
Protein (aerobic)	Low amount during all exercise; slightly more in endurance exercise, especially when carbohydrate fuel is depleted	Long-distance running

*At any given time, more than one source is used. The relative amount of use differs during various activities.

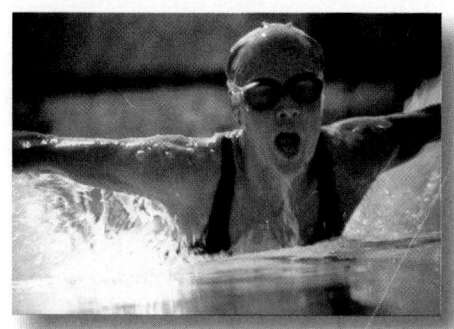

▲ Bursts of muscle activity use a variety of energy sources, including PCr and ATP.

See the Nutrition and Your Health Section: Ergogenic Aids and Athletic Performance at the end of Chapter 10.

aerobic Requiring oxygen.

anaerobic Not requiring oxygen.

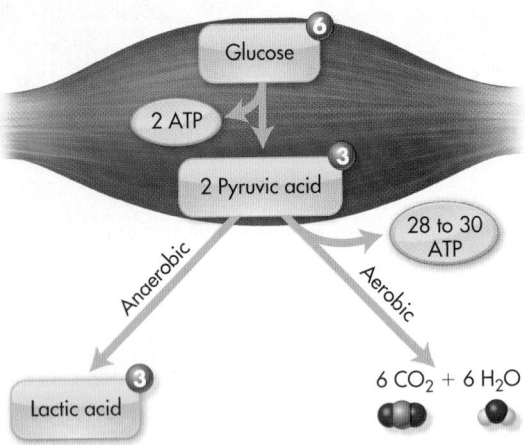

FIGURE 10-4 ▶ ATP yield from aerobic versus anaerobic glucose use. Encircled numbers indicate the number of carbons in each molecule.

pyruvic acid A three-carbon compound formed during glucose metabolism; also called *pyruvate*.

lactic acid A three-carbon acid formed during anaerobic cell metabolism; a partial breakdown product of glucose; also called *lactate*.

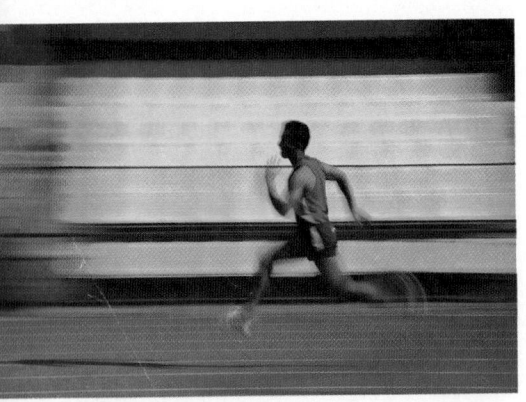

▲ Sprinting relies primarily on anaerobic glucose breakdown.

for about 10 seconds. Other sources of ATP resupply kick in, however, so PCr ends up as a source of energy for events lasting about 1 minute or less.

$$PCr + ADP \rightarrow ATP + Cr$$

The main advantage of PCr is that it can be activated instantly and can replenish ATP at rates fast enough to meet the energy demands of the fastest and most powerful actions, including jumping, lifting, throwing, and sprinting. The disadvantage of PCr is that not much of it is made and stored in the muscles. Strength-training athletes have begun to use creatine supplements in an effort to increase PCr in muscles.

Carbohydrate Fuel for Muscles

Carbohydrates are an important fuel for muscles. The most useful form of carbohydrate fuel is the simple sugar glucose, available to all cells from the bloodstream. As you will recall from Chapter 4, glucose is stored as glycogen in the liver and muscle cells. Blood glucose is maintained by the breakdown of liver glycogen. Breakdown of glycogen stored in a specific muscle also helps meet the carbohydrate demand of that muscle, but the actual amount of glycogen stored in muscle is limited (about 350 grams for all the muscles in the body, which would yield about 1400 kcal).

Depending on whether oxygen is available to exercising muscles, use of glucose to make ATP can be either **anaerobic** or **aerobic**.

Anaerobic Glucose Breakdown Yields Energy Fast. When oxygen supply in the muscle is limited (anaerobic conditions), glucose is broken down into a three-carbon compound called **pyruvic acid.** The pyruvic acid accumulates in the muscle and is then converted to **lactic acid.** Only about 5% of the total amount of ATP that could be formed from complete breakdown of glucose, is released through this anaerobic process (glucose → → lactic acid).

The advantage of anaerobic glucose breakdown is that it is the fastest way to resupply ATP, other than PCr breakdown. It therefore provides most of the energy needed for events that require a quick burst of energy, ranging from about 30 seconds to 2 minutes. Examples of activities that primarily rely on anaerobic glucose breakdown include sprinting 400 meters or swimming 100 meters.

The two major disadvantages of the anaerobic process are that (1) the high rate of ATP production cannot be sustained for long periods, and (2) the rapid accumulation of lactic acid greatly increases the acidity of the muscle. Acidity inhibits the activities of key enzymes in the muscle cells, slowing anaerobic ATP production and causing short-term fatigue. The acidity also leads to a net potassium loss from muscle cells, providing another cause of fatigue. We learn by trial-and-error a pace that will control muscle lactic acid concentrations during these anaerobic events.

For the most part, lactic acid builds up in active muscle cells until it is released into the bloodstream. The liver (and the kidneys, to some extent) takes up the lactic acid and resynthesizes it into glucose. Glucose can then reenter the bloodstream, where it is available for cell uptake and breakdown.

Aerobic Glucose Breakdown Is a Sustained Energy Source. If plenty of oxygen is available in the muscle (aerobic conditions), such as when the exercise is of low to moderate intensity, the bulk of the three-carbon pyruvic acid is shuttled to the mitochondria of the cell, where it is fully metabolized into carbon dioxide (CO_2) and water (H_2O) (Fig. 10-5). This aerobic breakdown of glucose yields approximately 95% of the ATP made from complete glucose metabolism (glucose → → CO_2 + H_2O).

Aerobic glucose breakdown supplies more ATP than does the anaerobic process, but it releases the energy more slowly. This slower rate of aerobic energy supply can be sustained for hours. One reason is that the products are carbon dioxide and water, not lactic acid. Aerobic glucose breakdown makes a major energy contribution to activities that last anywhere from 2 minutes to 3 hours or more. Examples of such activities include jogging or distance swimming (review Table 10-2).

Many researchers have studied the ability of various types of carbohydrate feeding regimens to maximize glucose supply to muscles during prolonged exercise. Overall, the techniques have succeeded. Consuming about 30 to 60 grams of carbohydrate per hour during strenuous endurance exercise that lasts 1 hour or more, such as cycling, can aid in maintaining adequate blood glucose, resulting in a delay of fatigue by 30 to 60 minutes. This attention to carbohydrate intake also helps one tolerate vigorous training on a daily basis.

As blood glucose declines during exercise, so does mental function. Cyclists refer to this diminished mental ability as "bonking." The fall in blood glucose is related to depletion of liver glycogen, not muscle glycogen, because liver glycogen is used to maintain blood glucose. See the later section, "Sports Drinks," to learn more about carbohydrate replacement during exercise.

CRITICAL THINKING

Marty started going to the gym about 8 weeks ago. At first, he noticed that he began "huffing and puffing" about 7 minutes into his aerobic workout. Now, however, he can work out for about 25 minutes without tiring. What is a possible explanation for this ability to work out longer?

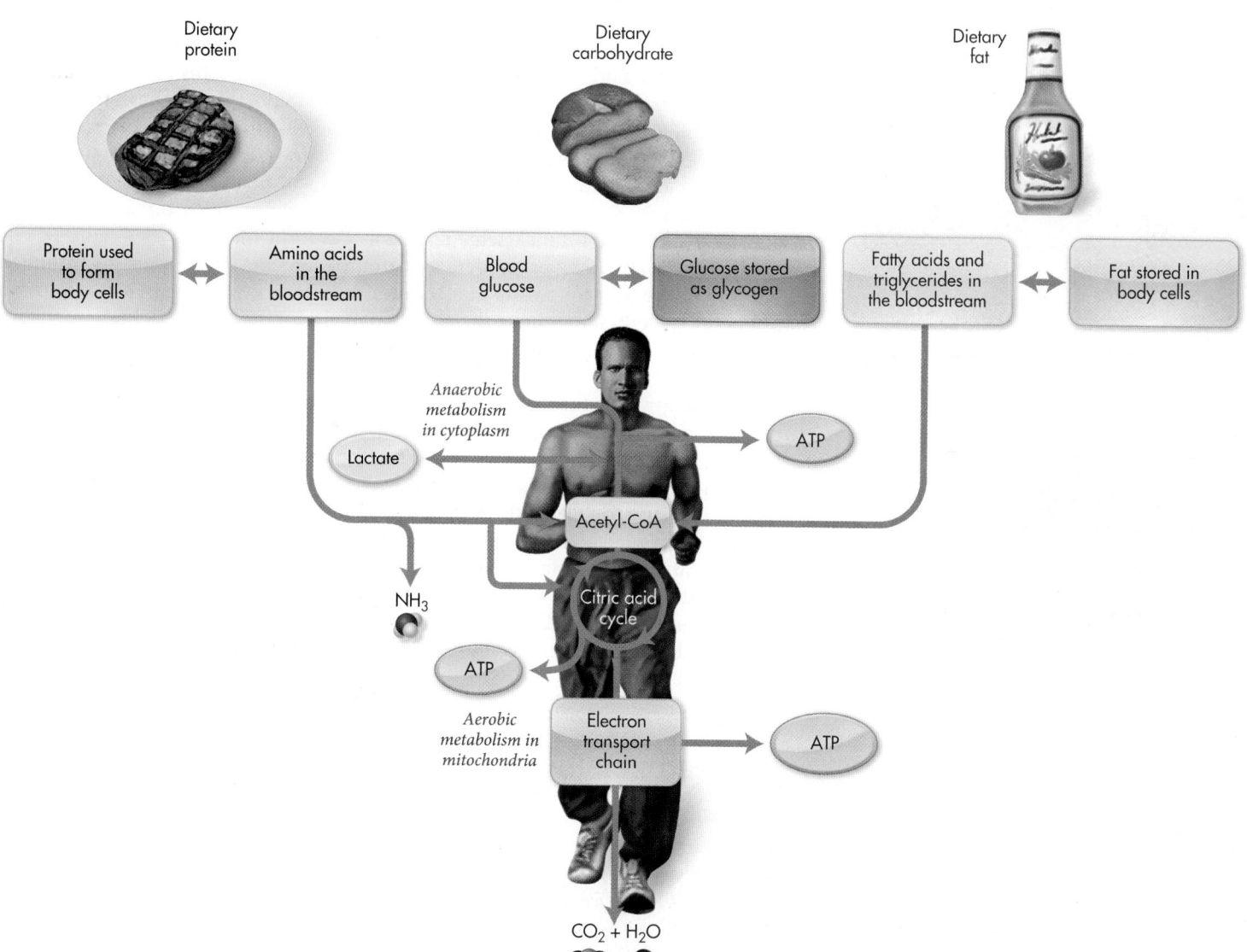

FIGURE 10-5 ▶ Simplified view of ATP formation from carbohydrate, fat, and protein. Along with phosphocreatine (PCr), all three macronutrients may be used for ATP synthesis, but glucose and fatty acids are primary sources. Glucose may be broken down anaerobically or may undergo complete aerobic metabolism. The products of fatty acid breakdown are channeled into aerobic metabolism. Although limited, products of amino-acid breakdown are channeled into the aerobic pathway as well. Recall also from Chapters 8 and 9 that many vitamins and minerals participate in these metabolic pathways.

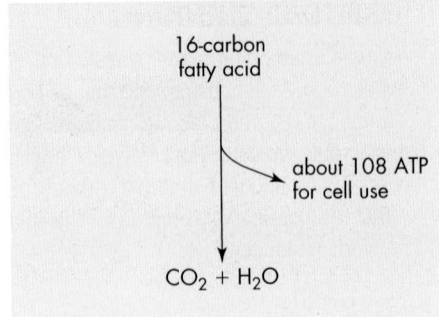

▲ ATP yield from aerobic fatty acid utilization.

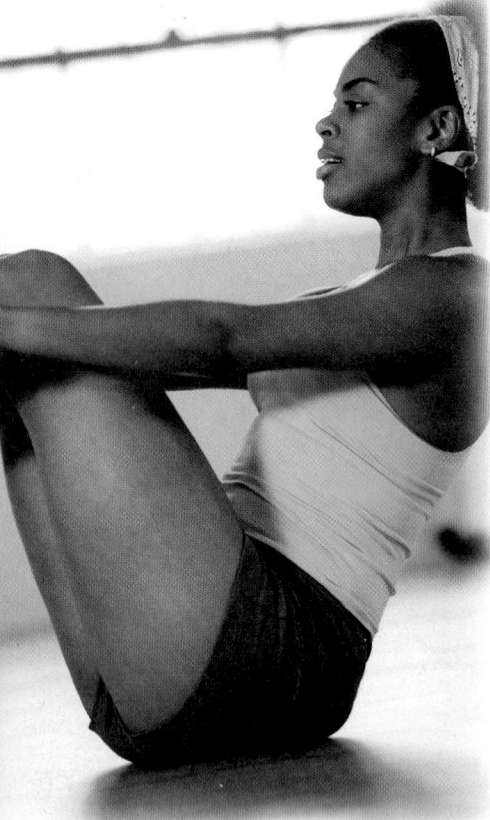

▲ Fatty acids can come from all over the body, not necessarily from fat stored near the active muscles. *This is why spot reducing does not work.* Exercise can tone the muscles near adipose tissue but does not preferentially use those stores.

Carbohydrate intake during exercise is not as important in shorter events (e.g., 30 minutes or so) because the muscles do not take up much blood glucose during short-term exercise, relying instead primarily on their glycogen stores for fuel.

Fat: The Main Fuel for Prolonged Low-Intensity Activity

When fat stores in body tissues begin to be broken down for energy, each triglyceride first yields three fatty acids and a glycerol. The majority of the stored energy is found in the fatty acids. During physical activity, fatty acids are released from various adipose tissue depots into the bloodstream and travel to the muscles, where they are taken into each cell and broken down aerobically to carbon dioxide and water. Some of the fat stored in muscles also is used, especially as activity increases from a low to a moderate pace (see Further Reading 2).

The rate at which muscles use fatty acids partly depends on the concentration of fatty acids in the bloodstream. In other words, the more fatty acids released from adipose tissue stores into the bloodstream, the more fat will be used by the muscles. Some cyclists and other endurance athletes have attempted to raise their blood concentrations of fatty acids by consuming caffeinated beverages. This practice can actually increase fatty acid release from the adipose tissue depots and is therefore helpful to certain athletes, but it is illegal under NCAA rules if the amount of caffeine in the body exceeds the equivalent of 6 to 8 cups of coffee (see the Nutrition and Your Health section at the end of this chapter).

Fat is not a very useful muscle fuel for intense, brief exercise, but it becomes a progressively more important energy source as duration increases, especially when exercise remains at a low or moderate (aerobic) rate for more than 20 minutes (Fig. 10-6). The reason for this is that some of the steps involved in fat breakdown cannot occur fast enough to meet the ATP demands of short-duration, high-intensity exercise. If fat were the only available fuel, we would be unable to exercise beyond a fast walk or jog.

The advantage of fat fuel is that it provides stores of energy in a relatively concentrated form, and we generally have a lot of it stored. For a given weight of fuel, fat supplies more than twice as much energy as carbohydrate does. For lengthy activities at a moderate pace (for example, hiking) or even sitting at a desk for 8 hours a day, fat supplies about 70% to 90% of the energy required. Carbohydrate use is much less. As intensity increases, such as in a 3-hour marathon run at a competitive pace, muscles use about a 50:50 ratio of fat to carbohydrate. In comparison, for short events, such as a 100-meter sprint or even a 1500-meter race, the contribution of fat to resupply ATP is minimal. To summarize, remember that the only fast-paced (anaerobic) fuel we eat is carbohydrate; slow and steady (aerobic) activity uses fat in addition to carbohydrate.

MAKING DECISIONS

Training Effect

As people start exercising regularly four or five times per week, they experience a "training effect." Initially, these individuals might be able to exercise for 20 minutes before tiring. Months later, exercise can be extended to an hour before they feel tired. During the months of training, muscle cells have produced more mitochondria and thus can burn more fat. Training also increases the number of capillaries in muscles, which increases oxygen supply to the muscles. As a result, lactic acid production from anaerobic glucose metabolism decreases. Lactic acid contributes to short-term muscle fatigue, so the less lactic acid produced, the longer the exercise can be sustained. Other contributors to the training effect include increased aerobic efficiency of the heart and muscles and elevations in muscle triglyceride content, with an enhanced ability of muscles to use triglycerides for energy needs.

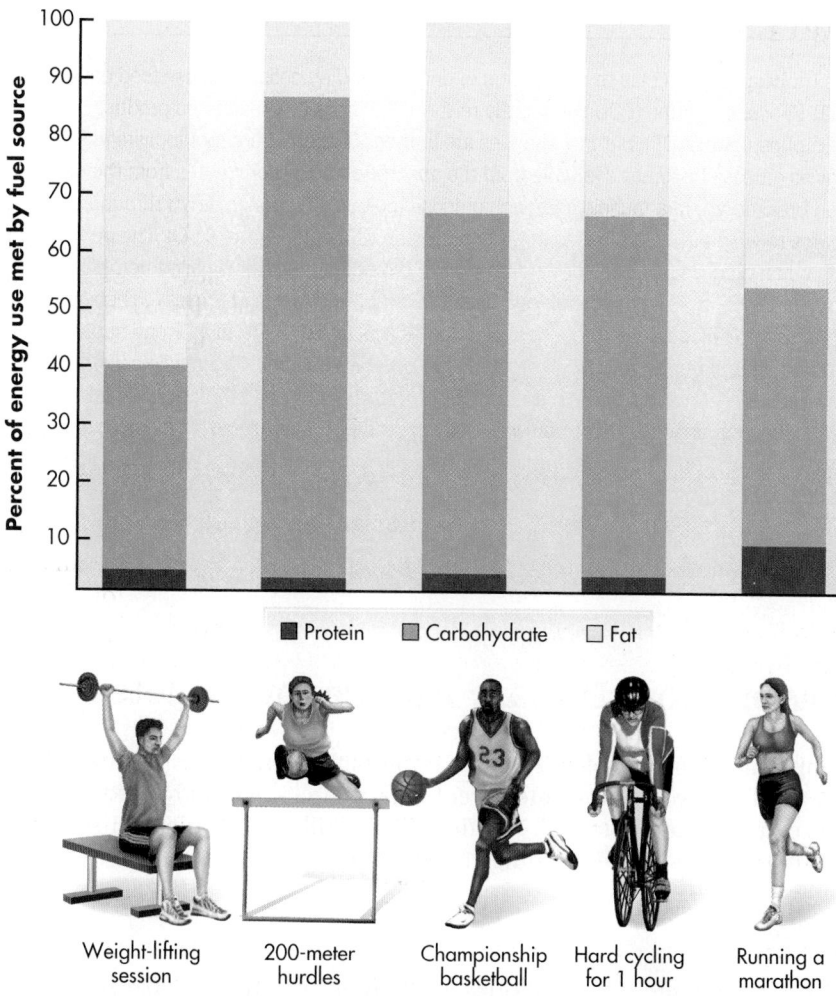

Weight-lifting session   200-meter hurdles   Championship basketball   Hard cycling for 1 hour   Running a marathon

■ Protein   ■ Carbohydrate   □ Fat

FIGURE 10-6 ▶ Rough estimates of fuel use during various forms of physical activity. With regard to the weight-lifting session, carbohydrate use could be somewhat greater and fat use somewhat less if the session is intense and fast-paced (e.g., circuit training). Fat use generally is higher because much of the time spent weight lifting is for rest periods and equipment-related activities.

Protein: A Minor Fuel Source, Primarily for Endurance Exercise

Although amino acids derived from protein can be used to fuel muscles, their contribution is relatively small, compared with that of carbohydrate and fat. As a rough guide, only about 5% of the body's general energy needs, as well as the typical energy needs of exercising muscles, is supplied by the metabolism of amino acids.

During endurance exercise, proteins can contribute importantly to energy needs, perhaps as much as 10% to 15%, especially as glycogen stores in the muscle are exhausted. Most of the energy supplied from protein comes from metabolism of the branched-chain amino acids—leucine, isoleucine, and valine. A normal diet provides ample branched-chain amino acids to supply this amount of fuel, so protein or amino-acid supplements are not needed. Contrary to what many athletes believe, protein is used for fuel less in resistance types of exercise (e.g., weight lifting) than in endurance exercise (e.g., running) (review Fig. 10-6). The primary muscle fuels for weight lifting are phosphocreatine (PCr) and carbohydrate for the brief bursts of activity, with fat providing energy during the resting stages, and with little use of protein overall. Despite this, high-protein products such as Pro-Complex, Amino Fuel 2000, High Voltage Protein Drink, and Instant Egg Protein are marketed specifically to weight lifters and bodybuilders in nearly every health-food and fitness store. Consuming high-carbohydrate, moderate-protein foods immediately after a weight-training workout enhances the muscle-building effect of the activity, most likely by increasing the concentrations of insulin and growth hormone released into the blood and contributing to protein synthesis. Still, it is impossible to increase muscle mass simply by eating protein. Overloading muscle through strength training or other physical activity is needed.

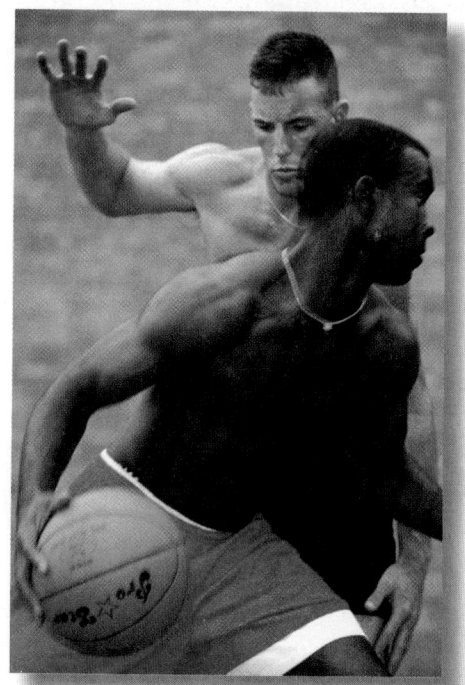

▲ The calories needed to perform come from carbohydrate, fat, and protein. The relative mix depends on the pace.

CONCEPT CHECK

Adenosine triphosphate (ATP) is the main form of energy used by cells. Cells use food energy to form ATP. Phosphocreatine (PCr) can rapidly re-form ATP from its breakdown product adenosine diphosphate (ADP), but PCr supplies are limited. Carbohydrate metabolism to form ATP begins as glucose becomes available from the absorption of carbohydrates from the diet or glycogen breakdown. In a muscle cell, each glucose molecule is broken down through a series of steps to yield either lactic acid or carbon dioxide (CO_2) plus water (H_2O). The process that occurs when glucose is broken down into carbon dioxide and water is called *aerobic* because oxygen is used. The conversion of glucose to lactic acid is called *anaerobic* because no oxygen is used. The anaerobic process allows the cell to quickly re-form ATP and supports the demand for energy during intense exercise. Fat is a key aerobic fuel for muscle cells, especially at low exercise outputs. At rest and during light activity, muscles burn primarily fat for energy needs. In comparison, little protein generally is used to fuel muscles. At most, protein supplies 10% to 15% of energy needs during endurance activities, especially when glycogen stores are depleted.

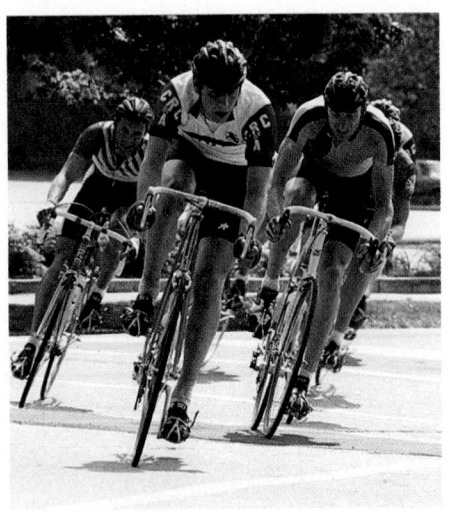

▲ Intense athletic training may require thousands of additional calories. This increased food intake should easily provide ample protein and other nutrients to support activity.

Review Table 7-4 in Chapter 7, which listed the energy costs of typical forms of physical activity.

10.4 Power Food: Dietary Advice for Athletes

Athletic training and genetic makeup are two important determinants of athletic performance. A good diet won't substitute for either factor, but diet can help to enhance and maximize an athlete's potential. On the other hand, a poor diet can seriously reduce performance (see Further Readings 12 and 15).

Calorie Needs

Athletes need varying amounts of calories, depending on each athlete's body size, body composition, and the type of training or competition being considered. A small person may need only 1700 kcal daily to sustain normal daily activities without losing body weight; a large, muscular man may need 4000 kcal. Review Chapter 7 or visit www.ChooseMyPlate.gov to calculate Estimated Energy Requirements (EERs) at various activity levels. These rough estimates can be viewed as starting points that need to be individualized by trial and error for each athlete.

An estimate of the calories required to sustain moderate activity is 5 to 8 kcal per minute. The calories required for sports training or competition then have to be added to those used to carry on normal activities. For example, an hour of bowling requires few calories in addition to that required to sustain normal daily living. At the other extreme, a 12-hour endurance bicycle race over mountains can require an additional 4000 kcal per day. Therefore, some athletes may need as much as 7000 kcal or more daily to maintain body weight while training, whereas others may need 1700 kcal or less. If an athlete experiences daily fatigue, the first consideration should be whether he or she is consuming enough food. Up to six meals per day may be needed, including one before each workout.

How can we know if an athlete is getting enough calories? Estimating daily intake from a food diary kept by the athlete is one way. Another step is to estimate the athlete's body fat percentage via skinfold measurements, bioelectrical impedance, or underwater weighing (review Chapter 7). Body fat should be the typical amount found for athletes in the specific sport practiced. This corresponds to 5% to 18% for most male athletes and 17% to 28% for most female athletes. The next step is to monitor body weight changes on a daily or weekly basis. If body weight starts to fall, calories should be increased; if weight rises and it is because of increases in body fat, the athlete should eat less.

MAKING DECISIONS

Making Weight

Wrestlers, boxers, judoists, jockeys, and oarsmen often try to lose weight before a competition, so that they can be certified to compete in a lower weight class. This helps them gain a mechanical advantage over an opponent of smaller stature. They usually lose this weight before stepping on the scale for weight certification. Athletes can lose up to 22 pounds (10 kilograms) of body weight as water in 1 day by sitting in a sauna, exercising in a plastic sweat suit, or taking diuretic drugs, which speed water loss from the kidneys. Losing as little as 2% of body weight by dehydration, however, can adversely affect endurance and performance, especially in hot weather. A pattern of repeated weight loss or gain of more than 5% of body weight by dehydration carries risk of kidney malfunction and heat-related illness. Death is also a possibility.

To prevent future deaths from such weight loss in athletes, the National Collegiate Athletic Association and many states have authorized physicians or athletic trainers to set safe weight and body fat content minimums (e.g., 7% or more of total body weight for male athletes and 12% or more for females) in weight-class sports. Under new guidelines, athletes are assigned to weight classes at the beginning of the season and are not allowed to "cut weight" to gain a competitive advantage. Weight gain in the days after a competition (reflecting regain of body water) can now be no greater than 2 pounds. If athletes, such as wrestlers, wish to compete in a lower-bodyweight class and have enough extra fat stores, they should begin a gradual, sustained reduction in calorie intake long before the competitive season starts.

If the body composition test shows that an athlete has too much body fat, the athlete should lower food intake by about 200 to 500 kcal per day, while maintaining a regular exercise program, until the desirable fat percentage is achieved. Reducing fat intake is the best nutrient-related approach. On the other hand, if an athlete needs to gain weight, increasing food intake by 500 to 700 kcal per day will eventually lead to the needed weight gain. A mix of carbohydrate, fat, and protein is advised, coupled with exercise to make sure this gain is mostly in the form of lean tissue and not fat stores.

Carbohydrate Needs

Anyone who exercises vigorously, especially for more than 1 hour per day on a regular basis, needs to consume a diet that includes moderate to high amounts of carbohydrates. The diet should provide a variety of foods, such as those portrayed by MyPlate. Numerous servings of grains, starchy vegetables, and fruits provide enough carbohydrate to maintain adequate liver and muscle glycogen stores, especially for replacing glycogen losses from workouts on the previous day. Relatively low-carbohydrate/high-protein diets, such as the Zone Diet, are not recommended. Recall that Chapter 7 discussed the Zone Diet. The carbohydrate content of this diet is only 40% of calories, rather than the 60% or more typically recommended for athletes.

Carbohydrate intake should be at least 5 grams per kilogram body weight. People engaged in aerobic training and endurance activities (60 minutes or more per day) may need as much as 7 grams per kilogram body weight. When exercise duration approaches several hours per day, the carbohydrate recommendation increases to up to 10 grams per kilogram of body weight. In other words, triathletes and marathoners should consider eating close to 500 to 600 grams of carbohydrates daily, and even more if necessary, to (1) prevent chronic fatigue and (2) load the muscles and liver with glycogen. Attention to carbohydrate intake is especially important when performing multiple training bouts in a day, such as swim practices, or heavy training on successive days, as in cross-country running. Depletion of carbohydrate ranks just behind depletion of fluid and electrolytes as a major cause of fatigue. Table 10-3 shows sample menus, based on MyPlate's Daily Food Plan recommendations, for

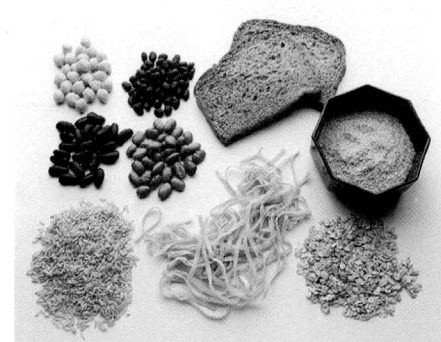

▲ High-carbohydrate foods should form the basis of the diet for athletes.

TABLE 10-3 Sample Daily Menus Based on MyPlate's Daily Food Plan* Recommendations That Provide Various Total Calorie Intakes

1500 kcal	2000 kcal	3000 kcal	4000 kcal	5000 kcal
Breakfast Fat-free milk, 1 cup Cheerios, 1/2 cup Bagel, 1/2 Cherry jam, 2 tsp Margarine, 1 tsp	**Breakfast** Fat-free milk, 1 cup Cheerios, 1 cup Bagel, 1/2 Cherry jam, 1 tbsp Margarine, 1 tsp	**Breakfast** Fat-free milk, 1 cup Cheerios, 2 cups Bagel, 1 Cherry jam, 2 tsp Margarine, 1 tsp Bran muffins, 2	**Breakfast** Fat-free milk, 1 cup Cheerios, 2 cups Orange, 1 Bran muffins, 2	**Breakfast** Fat-reduced milk, 1 cup Cheerios, 2 cups Bran muffins, 2 Orange, 1
			Snack Chopped dates, 3/4 cup	**Snack** Low-fat yogurt, 1 cup Chopped dates, 1 cup
Lunch Chicken breast (roasted), 2 oz Figs, 1 Fat-free milk, 1/2 cup Banana, 1	**Lunch** Chicken breast (roasted), 2 oz Wheat bread, 2 slices Mayonnaise, 1 tsp Raisins, 1/4 cup Cranberry juice, 1 1/2 cups Banana, 1	**Lunch** Chicken breast (roasted), 2 oz Wheat bread, 2 slices Provolone cheese, 1 oz Mayonnaise, 1 tsp Raisins, 1/3 cup Cranberry juice, 1 1/2 cups Low-fat fruit yogurt, 1 cup	**Lunch** Romaine lettuce, 1 cup Garbanzo beans, 1 cup Grated carrots, 1/2 cup French dressing, 2 tbsp Macaroni and cheese, 3 cups Apple juice, 1 cup	**Lunch** Chicken enchilada, 1 Romaine lettuce, 1 cup Garbanzo beans, 1 cup Shredded carrots, 3/4 cup Chopped celery, 1/2 cup Seasoned croutons, 1 oz French dressing, 2 tbsp Wheat bread, 2 slices Margarine, 1 tbsp Apple juice, 1 cup
Snack Oatmeal-raisin cookie, 1 Low-fat fruit yogurt, 1 cup	**Snack** Oatmeal-raisin cookies, 3 Low-fat fruit yogurt, 1 cup	**Snack** Banana, 1 Oatmeal-raisin cookies, 3	**Snack** Wheat bread, 2 slices Margarine, 1 tsp Jam, 2 tbsp	**Snack** Banana, 1 Bagel, 1 Cream cheese, 1 tbsp
Dinner Spaghetti w/meatballs, 1 cup Romaine lettuce, 1 cup Italian dressing, 2 tsp Green beans, 1/2 cup Cranberry juice, 1 1/2 cups	**Dinner** Broiled beef sirloin, 3 oz Romaine lettuce, 1 cup Italian dressing, 2 tsp Green beans, 1 cup Fat-free milk, 1/2 cup	**Dinner** Broiled beef sirloin, 3 oz Romaine lettuce, 1 cup Garbanzo beans, 1 cup Italian dressing, 2 tsp Spinach pasta noodles, 1 1/2 cups Margarine, 1 tsp Green beans, 1 cup Fat-free milk, 1/2 cup	**Dinner** Skinless turkey breast, 2 oz Mashed potatoes, 2 cups Peas and onions, 1 cup Banana, 1 Fat-free milk, 1 cup	**Dinner** Beef sirloin, 5 oz Mashed potatoes, 2 cups Spinach pasta noodles, 1 1/2 cups Grated parmesan cheese, 2 tbsp Green beans, 1 cup Oatmeal-raisin cookies, 3 Fat-reduced milk, 1 cup
			Snack Pasta, 1 cup cooked Margarine, 2 tsp Parmesan cheese, 2 tbsp Cranberry juice, 1 cup	**Snack** Air-popped popcorn, 4 cups Raisins, 1/3 cup Cranberry juice, 2 cups
18% protein (68 grams) 64% carbohydrate (240 grams) 19% fat (32 grams)	17% protein (85 grams) 63% carbohydrate (315 grams) 20% fat (44 grams)	17% protein (128 grams) 62% carbohydrate (465 grams) 21% fat (70 grams)	14% protein (140 grams) 61% carbohydrate (610 grams) 26% fat (116 grams)	14% protein (175 grams) 63% carbohydrate (813 grams) 24% fat (136 grams)

* Daily Food Plans are available online for diets supplying 1000 to 3200 kcal/day (see www.ChooseMyPlate.gov). Additional servings from each food group have been added to supply increased calories while maintaining healthy proportions of protein, carbohydrate and fat.

diets providing food energy ranging from 1500 to 5000 kcal per day. In addition, the Exchange System described in Appendix D is a very useful tool for planning all types of diets, including high-carbohydrate diets for athletes.

As noted, athletes should obtain at least 60% of their total energy needs from carbohydrate (rather than the 50% typical of most North American diets), especially if exercise duration is expected to exceed 2 hours and total caloric intake is about 3000 kcal per day or less. Diets providing 4000 to 5000 kcal per day can be as low as 50% carbohydrate, as these will still provide sufficient carbohydrate (e.g., 500 to 600 grams or so per day).

One does not have to give up any specific food when planning a high-carbohydrate diet. The focus is to include more high-carbohydrate foods while moderating concentrated fat sources. Sports nutritionists emphasize the difference between a high-carbohydrate meal and a high-carbohydrate/high-fat meal. Before endurance events, such as marathons or triathlons, some athletes seek to increase their carbohydrate reserves by eating foods such as potato chips, French fries, banana cream pie, and pastries. Although such foods provide carbohydrate, they also contain a lot of fat. Better high-carbohydrate food choices include pasta, rice, potatoes, bread, fruit and fruit juices, and many breakfast cereals (check the label for carbohydrate content) (Table 10-4). Sports drinks appropriate for carbohydrate loading, such as GatorLode and UltraFuel, can also help. Consuming a moderate rather than a high amount of fiber during the final day of training is a good precaution to reduce the chances of bloating and intestinal gas during the next day's event.

Carbohydrate Loading

For athletes who compete in continuous, intense aerobic events lasting more than 60 to 90 minutes (or in shorter events taking place more than once within a 24-hour period), a **carbohydrate-loading** regimen can help to maximize the amount of energy stored in the form of muscle glycogen for the event. (However, this amount of activity applies to few athletes.) In one possible regimen, during the week prior to the event, the athlete gradually reduces the intensity and duration of exercise ("tapering") while simultaneously increasing the percentage of total calories supplied by carbohydrate.

For example, consider the carbohydrate-loading schedule of a 25-year-old man preparing for a marathon. His typical calorie needs are about 3500 kcal per day. Six days before competition, he completes a final hard workout of 60 minutes. On that day, carbohydrates contribute 45% to 50% of his total calorie intake. As he goes through the rest of the week, the duration of his workouts decreases to 40 minutes, and then to about 20 minutes by the end of the week. Meanwhile, he increases the amount of carbohydrate in his diet to reach 70% to 80% of total calorie intake as the week continues. Total calorie intake should decrease as exercise time decreases throughout the week. On the final day before competition, he rests while maintaining the high-carbohydrate intake.

Carbohydrate Loading Regimen

Days Before Competition	6	5	4	3	2	1
Exercise time (minutes)	60	40	40	20	20	Rest
Carbohydrate (grams)	450	450	450	600	600	600

This carbohydrate-loading technique usually increases muscle glycogen stores by 50% to 85% over typical conditions (that is, when dietary carbohydrate constitutes only about 50% of total calorie intake).

A potential disadvantage of carbohydrate loading is that additional water (about 3 grams) is incorporated into the muscles along with each gram of glycogen. Although the additional water aids in maintaining hydration, for some individuals this additional water weight and related muscle stiffness detract from their sports performance, making carbohydrate loading inappropriate. Athletes considering a carbohydrate-loading regimen should try it during training (and well before an important competition) to experience its effects on performance. They can then determine whether it is worth the effort. Also, consuming carbohydrates during a competition provides about the same advantage as carbohydrate loading prior to the event. Expert advice is shifting away from carbohydrate loading and more toward this second method, coupled with a daily diet high in carbohydrate. In addition, remember the importance of the "training effect" discussed in " Making Decisions: Training Effect " on page 415.

CRITICAL THINKING

Joe is a wrestler who qualified for the 125-pound weight classification in the annual state high school competition. After a few matches, Joe began to feel dizzy and faint. He was disqualified because he was unable to continue the match. Later, the coach found out that Joe had spent 2 hours in the sauna before weighing in, which had made him dehydrated. What are the consequences of dehydration? What can you suggest as a safer alternative for weight loss?

carbohydrate loading A process in which a high carbohydrate intake is consumed for 6 days before an athletic event while tapering exercise duration in an attempt to increase muscle glycogen stores.

▶ **Carbohydrate Loading May Be Beneficial for These activities**

Marathons

Long-distance swimming

Cross-country skiing

30-kilometer runs

Triathlons

Tournament-play basketball

Soccer

Cycling time trials

Long-distance canoe racing

Carbohydrate Loading Is Not Beneficial for These Activities

American football games

10-kilometer or shorter runs

Walking and hiking

Most swimming events

Single basketball games

Weight lifting

Most track and field events

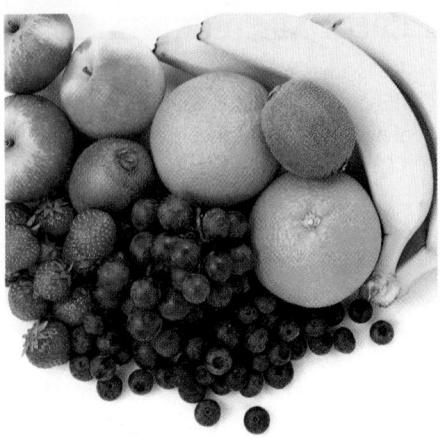

▲ Fruits provide a good source of carbohydrate, especially starch and natural sugars, for athletes.

TABLE 10-4 Grams of Carbohydrate Based on Serving Size of Typical Carbohydrate-Rich Foods

Starches—15 grams Carbohydrate per Serving (80 kcal)

One Serving

dry breakfast cereal*, 1/2–3/4 cup	baked potato, 1/4 large
cooked breakfast cereal, 1/2 cup	bagel, 1/4 (4 ounces)
cooked grits, 1/2 cup	English muffin, 1/2
cooked rice, 1/3 cup	bread, 1 slice
cooked pasta, 1/3 cup	pretzels, 3/4 ounces
baked beans, 1/3 cup	saltine crackers, 6
cooked corn, 1/2 cup	pancake, 4 inches in diameter, 1
cooked dry beans, 1/2 cup	taco shells, 2 (add 45 kcal)

Vegetables—5 grams Carbohydrate per Serving (25 kcal)

One Serving
cooked vegetables, 1/2 cup
raw vegetables, 1 cup
vegetable juice, 1/2 cup
Examples: carrots, green beans, broccoli, cauliflower, onions, spinach, tomatoes, vegetable juice

Fruits—15 grams Carbohydrate per Serving (60 kcal)

One Serving

canned fruit or berries, 1/2 cup	grapes (small), 17
fruit juice, 1/2 cup	grapefruit, 1/2
figs (dried), 1 1/2	dates, 3
apple or orange, 1 small	peach, 1
apricots (dried), 8	watermelon cubes, 1 1/4 cups
banana, 1 small	

Milk—12 grams Carbohydrate per Serving

One Serving
milk, 1 cup
plain low-fat yogurt, 2/3 cup

soymilk, 1 cup

Sweets—15 grams Carbohydrate per Serving (variable calories)

One Serving

cake, 2-inch square	ice cream, 1/2 cup
cookies, 2 small	sherbet, 1/2 cup

*The carbohydrate content of dry cereal varies widely. Check the labels of the ones you choose and adjust the serving size accordingly.

Modified from *Choose Your Foods: Exchange Lists for Diabetes* by the American Diabetes Association and American Dietetic Association, 2008, Chicago, American Dietetic Association.

Fat Needs

A diet containing up to 35% of calories from fat is generally recommended for athletes. Rich sources of monounsaturated fat, such as canola oil, should be emphasized, and saturated fat and *trans* fat intake should be limited.

Protein Needs

For athletes, the American College of Sports Medicine, American Dietetic Association, and Dietitians of Canada recommend protein intake within the range of 0.8 to 1.7 grams of protein per kilogram of body weight. The International Society of Sports Nutrition recommends up to 2.0 grams of protein per-kilogram (see Further Reading 7). This advice is considerably higher than the RDA of 0.8 grams per kilogram body weight for nonathletes recommended by the Food and Nutrition Board for all adults, including athletes. Estimates of protein needs vary by the type of physical activity (Table 10-5).

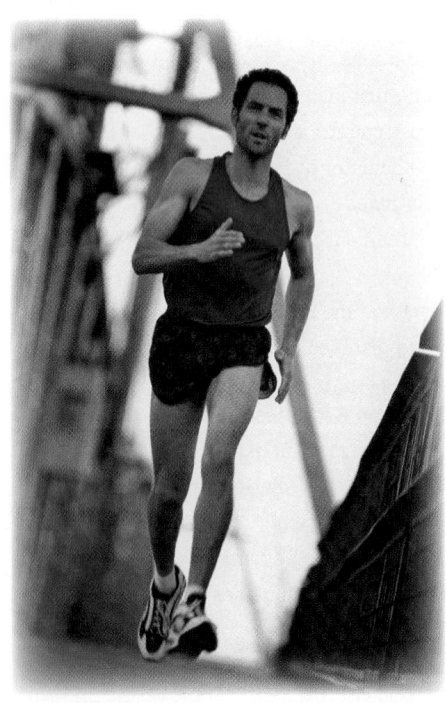

▲ Carbohydrate loading is appropriate only for endurance activities such as a long-distance race.

TABLE 10-5 Estimated Protein Needs of Athletes Based on Kilograms Body Weight[1]

Activity Level	Males	Females	Amount for a 70-kilogram (154-pound) Man
Sedentary adults[2]	0.8 g/kg	0.8 g/kg	56 g/d
Recreational endurance athletes[3]	0.8–1.0 g/kg	0.8–0.9 g/kg	56–70 g/d
Moderate-intensity endurance athletes[4]	1.2 g/kg	1.0–1.1 g/kg	84 g/d
Elite endurance athletes	1.6 g/kg	1.3–1.4 g/kg	112 g/d
Football, power sports	1.4–1.7 g/kg	1.1–1.5 g/kg	98–119 g/d
Resistance athletes (early training)	1.5–1.7 g/kg	1.2–1.5 g/kg	105–119 g/d
Resistance athletes (steady state)	1.0–1.2 g/kg	0.8–1.1 g/kg	70–84 g/d

Source: Adapted from Burke L, Deakin V: *Clinical Sports Nutrition*, 4th ed., McGraw-Hill, Australia, 2009.

[1]Calculate kilograms by dividing pounds by 2.2.

[2]RDA, as recommended by the Food and Nutrition Board.

[3]Exercising four to five times per week for 30 minutes.

[4]Exercising four to five times per week for 45–60 minutes.

For athletes beginning a strength-training program, some experts recommend up to 2.0 grams of protein per kilogram of body weight. That is more than twice the RDA for protein. To date, the value of such an excessive protein intake during the initial phases of strength training has not been supported by sufficient research. In addition, protein intakes above this amount result in an increased use of amino acids for energy needs; no further increase in muscle protein synthesis is seen. Recall from earlier in this chapter that phosphocreatine and carbohydrate (not extra protein) primarily fuel the body during strength-training activities. The extra protein, theoretically, is required for the synthesis of new muscle tissue brought on by the loading effect of strength training. Once the desired muscle mass is achieved, protein intake need not exceed 1.2 grams per kilogram of body weight.

Table 10-5 summarizes recommended ranges of protein intakes for various types of activity. Any athlete not specifically on a low-calorie regimen can easily meet these protein recommendations by eating a variety of foods (review Table 10-3). To illustrate, a 123-pound (53-kilogram) woman performing moderate-intensity endurance activity can consume 58 grams of protein (53 × 1.1) during a single day by including 3 ounces of chicken (one chicken breast), 3 ounces of beef (a small, lean hamburger), and two glasses of milk in her diet. Similarly, a 180-pound (77-kilogram) man who aims to gain muscle mass through strength training needs to consume only 6 ounces of chicken (a large chicken breast), ½ cup of cooked beans, a 6-ounce can of tuna, and three glasses of milk to achieve an intake of 130 grams of protein (77 × 1.7) in a day. And, for both athletes, these calculations do not even include the protein present in grains or vegetables they will also eat. As you can see, by meeting their calorie needs, many athletes consume much more protein than is required. Despite marketing claims, protein supplements are an expensive and unnecessary part of a fitness plan.

Consuming excessive amounts of protein has drawbacks. As noted in Chapter 6, it increases calcium loss somewhat in the urine. It also leads to increased urine production, possibly compromising body hydration. It also may lead to kidney stones in people with a history of this or other kidney problems. Finally, enough carbohydrate fuel may not be consumed on such a diet, leading to fatigue. Athletes who either feel they must significantly limit their calorie intake or are vegetarians should specifically determine how much protein they eat. They should make sure to follow a diet that provides at least 1.2 grams of protein per kilogram of body weight per day, the upper recommendation for most athletes.

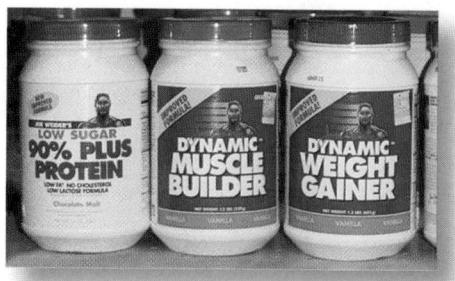

▲ High-protein products, often marketed to athletes, are unnecessary. The same holds true for high-protein bars, a trend in marketing products to athletes.

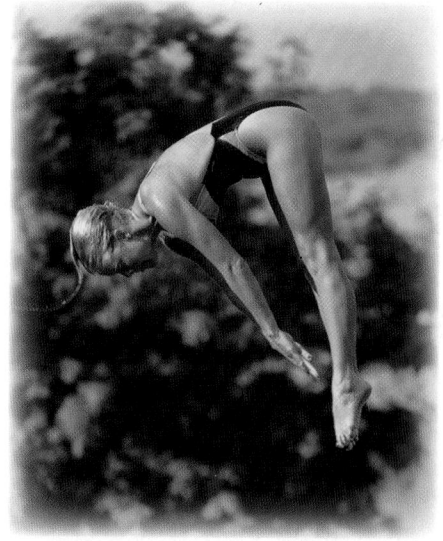

▲ Weight-restricted athletes especially should make sure they are consuming enough protein as well as other essential nutrients.

Vitamin and Mineral Needs

Vitamin and mineral needs are the same or slightly higher for athletes, compared with those of sedentary adults. Athletes usually have high calorie intakes, so they tend to consume plenty of vitamins and minerals. An exception is athletes consuming low-calorie diets (about 1200 kcal or less), such as seen with some female athletes participating in events in which maintaining a low body weight is crucial. These diets may not meet B-vitamin and other micronutrient needs. Vegetarian athletes are also a concern. In these cases, consuming fortified foods, such as ready-to-eat breakfast cereals or a balanced multivitamin and mineral supplement is recommended.

Athletes' needs for antioxidants such as vitamin E and vitamin C may be somewhat greater because of the potential protection these nutrients provide; this effect could be especially important in the face of high oxygen use by muscles. The use of large doses of vitamin E and vitamin C, however, requires more study and is not currently an accepted part of the dietary guidance for athletes. Experts suggest consuming a diet containing foods rich in antioxidants, such as fruits, vegetables, whole-grain breads and cereals, and vegetable oils. In addition, there is evidence that antioxidant systems in the body increase in activity as exercise training progresses. There is also speculation that the "oxidative stress" produced during exercise might have benefits, such as for muscle adaptation to exercise, and so trying to block this process may not be advantageous (see Further Reading 9).

Iron Deficiency Impairs Performance. Iron is involved in red blood cell production, oxygen transport, and energy production, so a deficiency of this mineral can noticeably detract from optimal athletic performance. The potential causes for iron deficiency in athletes vary (see Further Reading 1). As in the general population, female athletes are most susceptible to low iron status due to monthly menstrual losses. Special diets followed by athletes, such as low-calorie and vegetarian (especially vegan) diets are likely to be low in iron. Distance runners should pay special attention to iron intake, because their intense workouts may lead to gastrointestinal bleeding. Another concern is *sports anemia*—which occurs because exercise causes blood plasma volume to expand, particularly at the start of a training regimen before the synthesis of red blood cells increases. This results in dilution of the blood. In this case, even if iron stores are adequate, blood iron tests may appear low.

Sports anemia is not detrimental to performance, but it is hard to differentiate between sports anemia and true anemia. If iron status is low and not replenished, iron-deficiency anemia and markedly impaired endurance performance can eventually result. Although true anemia (a depressed blood hemoglobin level) is not that common among athletes, it is a good idea for athletes (especially adult women), to have their iron status checked at the beginning of a training season and at least once during midseason to monitor dietary iron intake.

Any blood test indicating low iron status—sports anemia or not—is cause for follow-up. For some, the use of iron supplements may be advisable. However, indiscriminate use of iron supplements is not advised because toxic effects are possible. It is important that physicians investigate the cause of the deficiency because iron deficiency can be caused by blood loss. If caught early, some serious medical conditions such as this can be treated or prevented.

Some studies have suggested that iron deficiency without anemia may also have a negative effect on physical activity and performance. Also, once depleted, iron stores can take months to replenish. For this reason, athletes must be especially careful to meet iron needs.

Calcium Intake Is Important, Especially in Women. Athletes, especially women trying to lose weight by restricting their intake of dairy products, can have marginal or low dietary intakes of calcium. This practice compromises optimal bone health. Of still greater concern are women athletes who have stopped menstruating because their arduous training and low body fat content interferes with the normal secretion of reproductive hormones. Disturbing reports show that female athletes who do not menstruate regularly have spinal bones far less dense than those of both nonathletes

R̲ecall from Chapter 8 that nutrients in dietary supplements should not exceed any Upper Levels set over the long term. As well, men should be cautious about any use of supplements containing iron.

"B̲lood doping" is the injection of red blood cells, naturally containing iron, to enhance aerobic capacity. This is an illegal practice under Olympic guidelines.

See the Nutrition and Your Health: Ergogenic Aids and Athletic Performance at the end of Chapter 10.

and female athletes who menstruate regularly. This places them at increased risk for bone fractures during training and competition and osteoporosis in later life. The negative impacts of low dietary calcium intake and irregular menses in female athletes outweigh the benefits of weight-bearing exercise on bone density. Increasing energy intake to restore body weight and body fat stores is important to correct hormonal imbalances and prevent further bone loss. This topic is discussed further in Chapter 11, with respect to the female athlete triad, and in Chapter 9, where osteoporosis was reviewed in detail (also see Further Readings 5 and 11).

Research has clearly documented the importance of regular menstruation to maintain bone mineral density. Studies show that a woman runner who does not menstruate regularly may also have a higher risk for the development of a **stress fracture.** Thus, female athletes whose menstrual cycles become irregular should consult a physician to determine the cause. Decreasing the amount of training or increasing energy intake and body weight often restores regular menstrual cycles. If irregular menstrual cycles persist, severe bone loss (much of which is not reversible) and osteoporosis can result. Extra calcium in the diet does not necessarily compensate for these damaging effects of menstrual irregularities, but inadequate dietary calcium can make matters worse.

stress fracture A fracture that occurs from repeated jarring of a bone. Common sites include bones of the foot.

10.5 A Focus on Fluid Needs

Fluid needs for an average adult are about 9 cups per day for women and 13 cups per day for men. Athletes generally need even more water to regulate internal temperature and keep cool. Heat production in contracting muscles can rise 15 to 20 times above that of resting muscles. Unless this heat is quickly dissipated, heat exhaustion, heat cramps, and potentially fatal heatstroke may ensue.

Fluid intake during exercise, when possible, should be adequate to minimize body weight loss; following this practice is a good idea even when sweating can go unnoticed, such as when swimming or during the winter. Fluid and electrolyte needs vary widely, based on differences in body mass, environmental conditions, level of training, event duration, and even genetics. Because fluid needs are highly individualized and dynamic, it is not appropriate to make general recommendations for fluid replacement (see Further Reading 14). Rather, an athlete should aim to replace the total amount of fluid lost during exercise. This can be accomplished by knowing the body's hourly sweat rate, which can be calculated from the weight lost during exercise per hour plus the fluid consumed during exercise per hour.

The American College of Sports Medicine recommends losing no more than 2% of body weight during exercise, especially in hot weather. Athletes should first calculate 2% of their body weight and then by trial and error determine how much fluid they must take in to avoid excessive losses. Monitoring pre- and post-workout body weight is the most straightforward method of determining fluid losses. Much of this fluid replacement will have to take place after exercise because it is difficult to consume enough fluid during exercise to prevent weight loss. If weight change can't be monitored, urine color is another measure of hydration status. Urine color should be no more yellow than lemonade.

Thirst is a late sign of dehydration. An athlete who drinks only when thirsty may take 48 hours to replenish fluid losses. After several days of training, an athlete relying on thirst can build up a fluid debt that will impair performance. The following fluid-replacement approach can meet athletes' fluid needs in most cases:

- Freely drink beverages (e.g., water, diluted fruit juice, sports drinks) during the 24-hour period before an event, even if not particularly thirsty.
- Drink 5 to 7 milliliters per kilogram of body weight (about 1.5 to 2 cups for a 150-pound male) of water or sports drink at least 4 hours before exercise. This allows time for both adequate hydration and excretion of excess fluid.
- During events lasting more than 30 minutes, athletes should consume fluid to prevent dehydration (i.e., losses of >2% body weight). Research in marathon runners suggests about 1 ½ to 3 ½ cups (400 to 800 milliliters) per hour to prevent

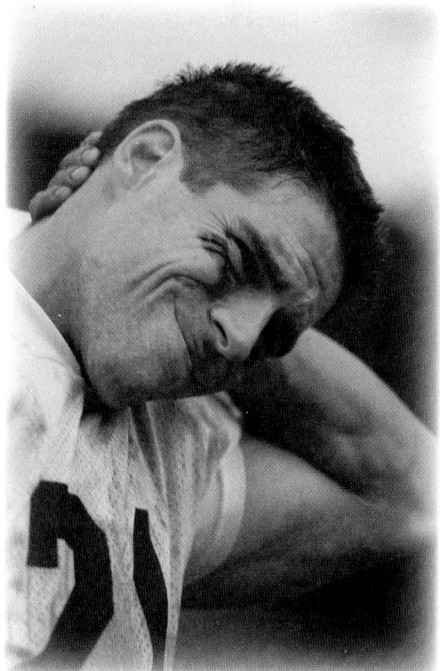

▲ Dehydration, which can lead to illness and death, is a problem that must be avoided during physical activity in hot, humid environments.

NEWSWORTHY NUTRITION

Sports drinks and energy drinks are not interchangeable

The value of electrolyte- and carbohydrate-containing *sports* drinks (e.g., Gatorade) is well documented for replenishing fluids during physical activity lasting more than 1 hour. However, an assortment of *energy* drinks are now marketed alongside sports drinks to young people, especially male athletes. Experts caution athletes against using energy drinks, such as the top-selling Red Bull, Rockstar, Monster, and Throttle, to meet fluid needs during exercise. The sugar content is too high, and a multitude of additives, including caffeine, taurine, ginseng, guarana, and others, have limited if any documented benefits for athletes. In fact, binge consumption of energy drinks with stimulants has led to illness and at least four deaths. Combining energy drinks with alcohol can mask the symptoms of intoxication and result in hazardous behavior and accidents. Experts recommend limiting use of energy beverages to 1 serving (500 milliliters) per day, avoiding combinations with alcohol, and, for people with cardiac problems, consulting a physician before use. Athletes should use a sports drink rather than an energy drink for the purpose of rehydration during physical activity.

Source: Higgins JP and others: Energy beverages: Content and safety. *Mayo Clinic Proceedings* 85:1033, 2010.

Check out the Connect site www.mcgrawhillconnect.com to further explore sports and energy drinks.

heat exhaustion The first stage of heat-related illness that occurs because of depletion of blood volume from fluid loss by the body. This increases body temperature and can lead to headache, dizziness, muscle weakness, and visual disturbances, among other effects.

heat cramps A frequent complication of heat exhaustion. They usually occur in people who have experienced large sweat losses from exercising for several hours in a hot climate and have consumed a large volume of water. The cramps occur in skeletal muscles and consist of contractions for 1 to 3 minutes at a time.

dehydration. Football players wearing equipment for two-a-day practices during the heat of August may need even more than 800 milliliters per hour to prevent dehydration. The best plan is to determine individual rate of fluid losses during training and plan accordingly. In many cases, athletes, especially children and teenagers, need to be reminded to consume fluids during exercise. Colder drinks also enhance body cooling.

• Within 4 to 6 hours after exercise, about 2 to 3 cups of fluid should be consumed for every pound lost. It is important that weight be restored before the next exercise period. Skipping fluids before or during events will almost certainly impair performance.

The popularity of caffeine-containing energy drinks has surged in recent years. Some studies show that caffeine improves athletic performance during endurance events (e.g., cycling) or sports that require a high level of mental alertness (e.g., archery). However, excessive caffeine consumption can lead to shakiness, nervousness, anxiety, nausea, and insomnia. In addition, the diuretic effect of caffeine may not support optimal hydration, particularly for athletes who are not accustomed to caffeine. Compare the caffeine and kilocalorie contents of several top-selling energy drinks (Table 10-6).

As environmental temperature rises above 95°F (35°C), virtually all body heat is lost through the evaporation of sweat from the skin. Sweat rates during prolonged exercise range from 3 to 8 cups (750 to 2000 milliliters) per hour.

Wearing football equipment in hot weather can lead to a loss of 2% of body weight in 30 minutes. Marathon runners have been shown to lose 6% to 10% of body weight during a race. Dehydration reduces endurance, strength, and overall performance. As humidity rises, especially above 75%, evaporation slows and sweating becomes an inefficient way to cool the body. The result is rapid fatigue, increased work for the heart, and difficulty with prolonged exertion. Heat-related injuries—heat exhaustion, heat cramps, and heatstroke—can be as dangerous as extreme cold.

Heat exhaustion occurs when heat stress causes loss of body fluid and then depletion of blood volume. Common symptoms of heat exhaustion include profuse sweating, headache, dizziness, nausea, vomiting, muscle weakness, visual disturbances,

TABLE 10-6 Caffeine, Kilocalorie, and Sugar Content of Popular Energy Drinks

Beverage	Container Size (fl oz)	Caffeine (mg)	Energy (kcal)	Sugars (g)
5-Hour Energy	1.93	80+*	4	0
Amp	16	142	220	58
Full Throttle	16	197	220	58
Monster	16	160	200	54
Red Bull	8.4	80	110	27
Red Bull Sugarfree	8.4	80	10	0
Red Rain Energy Shot	2	80+*	0	0
Rockstar	16	160	280	62
Slap Energy Frost	16	200	220	52
SoBe Energize	20	160	88	23

*Caffeine content is not specified by the manufacturer but rather as part of a total amount of "energy blend." The labels state these products have approximately the same amount of caffeine as a strong cup of coffee (typical range: 80–175 milligrams). An independent lab analysis of 5-Hour Energy determined caffeine content was 207 milligrams.

and flushing of the skin. A person with heat exhaustion should be taken to a cool environment immediately, and excess clothing should be removed. The body should be sponged with tap water. Fluid replacement, as tolerated, then should suffice to correct the condition.

Heat cramps are a frequent complication of heat exhaustion, but they may appear without other symptoms of dehydration. Cramps usually occur in individuals who have exercised for several hours in a hot climate, experienced significant sweating, and have consumed a large volume of water without replacing sodium losses. It is important not to confuse heat cramps with other forms of muscle cramps, such as those caused by GI tract upset. Heat cramps occur in skeletal muscles, including those of the abdomen and extremities. They consist of a contraction lasting 1 to 3 minutes at a time. The cramp moves down the muscle and is associated with excruciating pain. To prevent heat cramps, exercise moderately at first; aim to have adequate salt intake before engaging in long, strenuous activity in the heat; and avoid dehydration.

Heatstroke can occur when the internal body temperature reaches 104°F or more. Related symptoms include nausea, confusion, irritability, poor coordination, seizures, and coma. Exertional heatstroke results from high blood flow to exercising muscles, which overloads the body's cooling capacity. Sweating generally ceases, and the body temperature may become dangerously high. If left untreated, circulatory collapse, nervous system damage, and death are likely. The death rate from heatstroke is high, approximately 10%, making heatstroke the number 3 killer of athletes in the United States. Since 1995, at least 40 football players have died as a result of heatstroke.

Many individuals faint during heatstroke, and their skin becomes hot and dry. Cooling the skin with ice packs or cold water is the usual recommended immediate treatment until medical help can be summoned. To decrease the risk of developing heatstroke, athletes should watch for rapid body-weight changes (2% or more of body weight), replace lost fluids, and avoid exercising under extremely hot, humid conditions.

Sports Drinks

A question that often arises is whether to drink water or a sports-type carbohydrate-electrolyte drink (e.g., All Sport, Exceed Energy Drink, Gatorade, PowerAde, and Amino Force) during competition (Fig. 10-7). For sports that require less than 60 minutes of exertion or when total weight loss is less than 5 to 6 pounds, the primary concern is replacing the water lost in sweat, because losses of carbohydrate stores and electrolytes (sodium, chloride, potassium, and other minerals) are not usually very great. Although electrolytes are lost in sweat, the quantities lost in exercise of brief to moderate duration can be easily replaced later by consuming normal foods, such as orange juice, potatoes, and tomato juice. Keep in mind that sweat is about 99% water and only 1% electrolytes and other substances.

When exercise extends beyond 60 minutes, electrolyte (especially sodium) and carbohydrate replacement becomes increasingly important. Use of sports drinks during long bouts of exercise—especially in hot weather—offers several advantages.

Water by itself, as you have learned, increases blood volume to allow for efficient cooling and transport of fuels and waste products to and from cells. The addition of carbohydrate to a sports drink supplies glucose to muscles as they become depleted of glycogen, and thus can enhance performance when administered during endurance activities (see the later section on carbohydrate replacement). Carbohydrate also adds flavor, which encourages athletes to drink. Finally, the electrolytes in sports drinks help to maintain blood volume, enhance the absorption of water and carbohydrate from the intestine, and stimulate thirst. For these reasons, some experts prefer sports drinks over water for all athletes.

Overall, the decision to use a sports drink hinges primarily on the duration of the activity. As the projected duration of continuous activity approaches 60 minutes or longer, the advantages of the use of a sports drink over plain water clearly emerge. However, athletes should first experiment with sports drinks during practice, instead of trying them for the first time during competition.

heatstroke Heatstroke can occur when internal body temperature reaches 104°F. Sweating generally ceases if left untreated, and blood circulation is greatly reduced. Nervous system damage may ensue, and death is likely. Often the skin of individuals who suffer heatstroke is hot and dry.

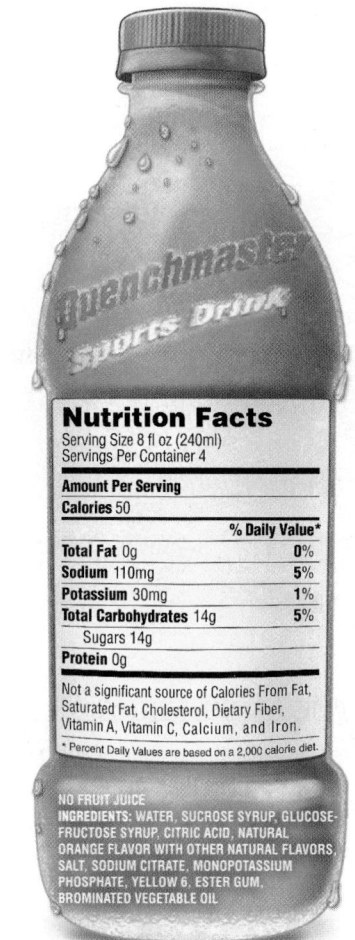

FIGURE 10-7 ▶ Sports drinks for fluid and electrolyte replacement typically contain a form of simple carbohydrate plus sodium and potassium. The various sugars in this product total 14 grams per 1 cup (240 milliliters) serving. In percentage terms based on weight, the sugar content is about 6% ([14 grams sugar per serving ÷ 240 grams per serving] × 100 = 5.8%). Sports drinks typically contain about 6% to 8% sugar. This provides ample glucose and other monosaccharides to fuel working muscles, and it is well tolerated. Drinks with a sugar content above 10%, such as soft drinks or fruit juices, may cause stomach distress and are not recommended.

General Guide for Approximate Pre-event Carbohydrate Intake

Hours Before	Grams per kilogram Body Weight	For a 70-kilogram Person
1	1	70
2	2	140
3	3	210
4	4	280

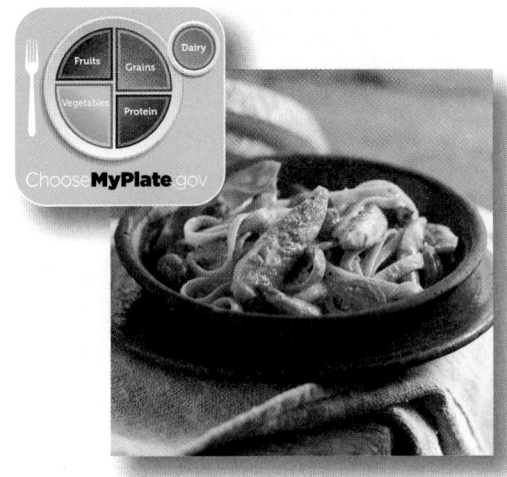

CRITICAL THINKING

Pre-event meals may require a higher proportion of grains than suggested by MyPlate to boost carbohydrate content. Choose starchy vegetables and grain-based snacks to help top off glycogen stores. How does this pasta meal compare to MyPlate?

It is also possible for some athletes to drink too much water and thereby develop water intoxication (hyponatremia). Endurance athletes (especially poorly trained individuals) may compete at relatively low exercise intensities for prolonged periods and therefore may not sweat as much as one might predict. Thus, water losses are not high. Drinking less fluid, choosing a sports drink containing sodium (usually in the form of sodium chloride), and not gaining weight during the activity can help prevent this problem. (A drop in blood sodium can occur in both hot and cold weather.)

10.6 Specialized Dietary Advice for Before, During, and After Endurance Exercise

Pre-event Meals Optimize Performance

A light meal supplying up to 1000 kcal should be eaten about 2 to 4 hours before an endurance event to top off muscle and liver glycogen stores, prevent hunger during the event, and provide extra fluid. The longer the period before an event, the larger the meal can be, because there will be more time available for digestion. A pre-event meal should consist primarily of carbohydrate (about 200 grams), contain little fat or fiber, and include a moderate amount of protein (Table 10-7). A meal eaten 1 hour or so before an event should be blended or liquid to promote rapid stomach emptying. Examples are low-fat smoothies, juices, and sports drinks.

Good food choices for a pre-event meal include spaghetti, muffins, bagels, pancakes with fresh fruit topping, oatmeal with fruit, baked potato topped with a small amount of sour cream, toasted bread with jam, bananas, and low-sugar breakfast cereals with reduced-fat or fat-free milk. Liquid meal-replacement formulas, such as Carnation Instant Breakfast, also can be used. Foods especially rich in fiber should be eaten the previous day to help empty the colon before an event, but they should not be eaten the night before or on the morning of the event. Avoid fatty or fried foods, such as sausage, bacon, sauces, and gravies. Some foods (e.g., dairy products) may cause

TABLE 10-7 Convenient Pre-event Meals

Breakfast	
Cheerios, ¾ cup	450 kcal
Reduced-fat milk, 1 cup	92 grams (82%) carbohydrate
Blueberry muffin, 1	
Orange juice, 4 ounces	
or	
Low-fat fruit yogurt, 1 cup	482 kcal
Plain bagel, ½	84 grams (68%) carbohydrate
Apple juice, 4 ounces	
Peanut butter (for bagel), 1 tbsp	
Lunch or Dinner	
Broiled pork chop, 3 ounces	839 kcal
White rice, 1½ cups	120 grams (57%) carbohydrate
Steamed zucchini, 1 cup	
Chocolate milk, 1 cup	
Jello, ½ cup	
or	
Spaghetti noodles, 2 cups	761 kcal
Spaghetti sauce, 1 cup	129 grams (66%) carbohydrate
Reduced-fat milk, 1½ cups	
Green beans, 1 cup	

With regard to the timing of pre-activity meals, a general guide is to allow 4 hours for a big meal (about 1200 kcal), 3 hours for a moderate meal (about 800 to 900 kcal), 2 hours for a light meal (about 400 to 600 kcal), and an hour or less for a snack (about 300 kcal).

gastrointestinal upset. Athletes should experiment with the size, timing, and composition of pre-event meals during training to determine what will be tolerated.

Replenishing Fuel During Endurance Exercise

We've already established the importance of consuming adequate fluids during endurance exercise. For sporting events longer than 60 minutes, consumption of carbohydrate during activity can also improve athletic performance. This is because prolonged exercise depletes muscle glycogen stores and low levels of blood glucose lead to fatigue, both physical and mental. When the supply of carbohydrate calories runs low, athletes often complain of "hitting the wall," the point at which maintaining a competitive pace seems impossible. One way to overcome this obstacle is to maintain normal blood glucose concentrations by carbohydrate feedings.

A general guideline for endurance events is to consume 30 to 60 grams of carbohydrate per hour. Some experts suggest that consuming protein with carbohydrate during exercise provides added benefit. In particular, branched-chain amino acids, which can be used for fuel, are thought to delay fatigue. This is an area of ongoing research, but there is not enough evidence at this time to support a recommendation for ingesting protein during exercise. Compared to carbohydrates, fat is more slowly digested, absorbed, and metabolized. Thus, although it serves as fuel during prolonged aerobic activity, consumption of fat during activity is not likely to improve athletic performance.

Sports drinks are a good source of carbohydrate calories during endurance events. They supply the necessary fluid, electrolytes, and carbohydrate to keep an athlete performing at his or her best. As an alternative to sports drinks, some athletes use carbohydrate gels (e.g., PowerGel and Clif Shot) and energy bars (e.g., PowerBar). Check the label on these products to gauge the amount of gel or bar that provides 30 to 60 grams of carbohydrate per hour. Whereas sports drinks contain about 14 grams of carbohydrate per 8-oz serving, gels contain about 25 grams of carbohydrate per serving, and depending on the type, popular energy bars range from 2 to 45 grams of carbohydrate per serving (Table 10-8). The wide range of carbohydrate content in energy bars is due to a variety of marketing trends in the sports supplement industry. Overall, choosing a bar with about 40 grams of carbohydrate and no more than 10 grams of protein, 4 grams of fat, and 5 grams of fiber is recommended. The bars may also be fortified with up to 100% of the Daily Values of certain vitamins and minerals. These bars can be seen as a convenient, although somewhat expensive, source of nutrients. Caution should be exercised to avoid toxicities from such fortified products.

If solid sources of carbohydrate are one's preference, Teddy Grahams, Gummy Bears, and jellybeans can also yield a quick source of glucose at a much lower cost. However, any carbohydrate-containing food, including energy bars and gels, must be accompanied by fluid to ensure adequate hydration.

MAKING DECISIONS

Energy Bars

As discussed, food manufacturers have begun to promote meal replacement bars (also called "energy" bars) to all kind of athletes. These bars typically contain about 180 to 250 kcal, with a macronutrient distribution typical of common diets. However, some bars replace much of the carbohydrate with protein. The bars are fortified with vitamins and minerals in amounts ranging from about 25% to 100% of typical human needs. Some people find these bars provide a convenient way to consume a meal (or snack) on the run, while also focusing on certain nutrients they may underconsume, such as the B-vitamin folate or the mineral calcium. These bars generally cost $1 to $2. The energy and nutrient contents of popular energy bars are shown in Table 10-8. Critics suggest these products are essentially the nutritional equivalent of a cup of low-fat yogurt and piece of fruit.

It cannot be emphasized enough that any nutrition strategies should be tested during practice and trial runs before being used in a meet or key event. An athlete should never try a new food or beverage on the day of competition. Some food items and beverages may not be well tolerated, and the day of competition is not the time to find out.

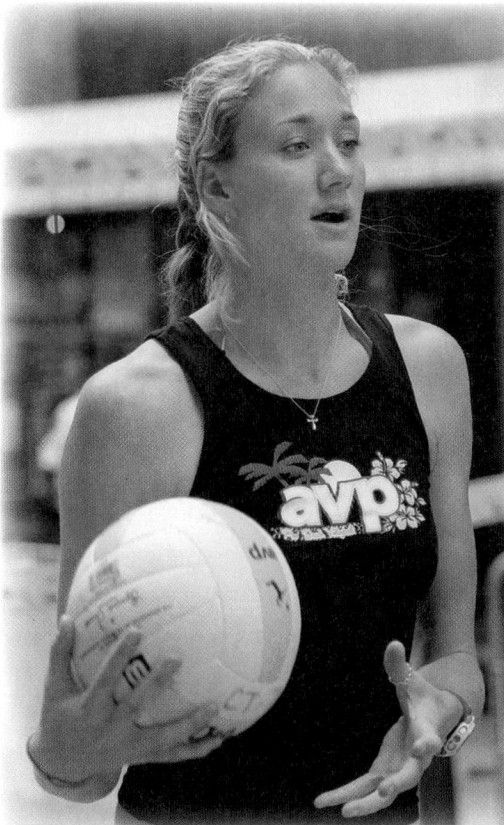

▲ Elite athletes such as Olympic beach volleyball gold medal winner Kerri Walsh are well aware that modifying their diet and training regimen to match the specific needs of their sport is key to optimum performance. Replenishing carbohydrate and fluids is especially important when training.

TABLE 10-8 Energy and Macronutrient Content of Popular Energy Bars, Gels, and Chews

Energy Bars	Serving (oz)	Energy (kcal)	Carbohydrates (g)	Fiber (g)	Protein (g)	Fat (g)
Balance Bar (peanut butter)	1.76	200	21	1	14	7
Clif Bar (chocolate chip)	2.4	240	44	5	10	4.5
Clif Builder's (peanut butter)	2.4	270	30	4	20	8
Clif Kid Z-Bar (honey graham)	1.27	130	26	3	3	2
EAS Myoplex (chocolate peanut butter)	2.65	290	35	1	25	9
Genisoy Bar (cookies & cream)	2.2	230	33	1	14	4.5
Kashi GoLean Bar (malted chocolate chip)	1.94	190	31	5	12	4.5
LARABAR (peanut butter cookie)	1.7	220	23	4	7	12
LUNA Bar (nutz over chocolate)	1.69	180	25	4	9	6
MET-Rx Big 100 Bar (super cookie crunch)	3.52	410	41	3	32	14
Met-Rx Protein Plus (chocolate fudge deluxe)	3.0	310	32	2	32	9
Power Crunch Bar (peanut butter crème)	1.4	200	10	1	13	12
PowerBar Harvest (toffee chocolate chip)	2.29	250	42	5	10	5
PowerBar Performance (peanut butter)	2.3	240	44	1	9	4
PowerBar Pria (French vanilla crisp)	0.98	110	17	1	5	3
PowerBar ProteinPlus (chocolate crisp)	2.75	290	37	2	23	6
PowerBar TripleThreat	1.94	230	31	3	10	9
Premier Nutrition Titan (cookie & cream)	2.8	320	27	<1	26	8
Promax Energy Bar (German chocolate cake)	2.7	280	37	2	20	6
Pure Protein (chocolate deluxe)	1.76	180	17	2	20	4.5
Snickers Marathon Protein Bar (caramel nut rush)	2.82	290	40	10	20	10
Tiger's Milk (peanut butter and honey)	1.23	140	19	<1	5	5
Zone Perfect (chocolate mint)	1.76	210	24	3	14	7
Energy Gels & Chews						
Carb BOOM! Energy Gel (strawberry kiwi)	1.4	110	27	0	0	0
Clif Shot (vanilla)	1.1	100	24	0	0	0
Clif Shot Blocks (cran-razz)	1.0	100	24	0	0	0
GU Energy Gel (lemon sublime)	1.1	100	25	0	0	0
Hammer Gel (raspberry)	1.2	90	21	0	0	0
Honey Stinger Energy Gel (orange blossom)	1.8	160	39	1	1	0
Jelly Belly Sport Beans (berry)	1.0	100	24	0	0	0
PowerBar Energy Bites (chocolate)	3.0	340	58	2	11	7
PowerBar Gel (strawberry banana)	1.44	110	27	0	0	0

Overall, choosing energy bars is preferable to choosing candy bars and packaged cakes. When used in sports situations, energy bars can be handy. Better yet, however, is to eat a variety of wholesome foods; these offer more health-protective compounds. This is also a less expensive choice, especially for day-to-day snacking. An additional concern is that micronutrient toxicity might occur if numerous bars are eaten in a day, as many are highly fortified. Vitamin A and iron are two nutrients of special concern in this regard.

Carbohydrate Intake During Recovery from Prolonged Exercise

An athlete's need for nutrition during recovery from exercise depends on the type of workout completed and the timing of the next workout. For example, multiple events in the same day will require rapid restoration of glycogen stores. However, if an athlete will be able to rest for 1 or 2 days before the next exercise session, immediate consumption of a postworkout meal is not as crucial.

To rapidly restore glycogen stores, carbohydrate-rich foods providing 1 to 1.5 grams of carbohydrate per kilogram body weight should be consumed within 30 minutes after extended (endurance) exercise (Table 10-9). Immediately after exercise is when glycogen synthesis is greatest, because the muscles are insulin-sensitive at this point. This process should then be repeated every 2 hours for the next 4 to 6 hours. Athletes training hard can consume a sugar candy, sugared soft drink, fruit or fruit juice, or a sports-type carbohydrate supplement right after training as they attempt to reload their muscles with glycogen.

Later, enriched bread, mashed potatoes, and short-grain white rice can contribute to additional carbohydrate consumption. These high-glycemic-load carbohydrates especially contribute to glycogen synthesis. Recall that Table 4-4 shows the glycemic load for various foods. Adding an appropriate amount of protein (3 grams of carbohydrate: 1 gram of protein) during recovery can be especially helpful for meeting overall calorie and nutrient needs. For a 154-pound (70-kilogram) athlete, this corresponds to about 70 grams of carbohydrate and 25 grams of protein in each 2-hour interval (Table 10-9 contains sample meals of this composition). In summary, the following are key factors for achieving the most rapid replenishment of muscle glycogen after exercise: (1) availability of adequate carbohydrate, (2) ingestion of carbohydrate as soon as possible after completion of exercise, and (3) selection of high-glycemic-load carbohydrates.

Fluid and electrolyte (i.e., sodium and potassium) intake is also an essential component of an athlete's recovery diet. This helps replenish body fluids as quickly as possible. This is especially important if two workouts a day are performed or if the environment is hot and humid. If food and fluid intake is sufficient to restore weight loss, it generally will also supply enough electrolytes to meet needs during recovery from endurance activities.

TABLE 10-9 Sample Postexercise Meals for Rapid Muscle Glycogen Replacement

Option 1
1 regular bagel
2 tbsp peanut butter, smooth
8 fl oz fat-free milk
1 medium banana
562 kcal, 77 grams carbohydrate, 23 grams protein, 18 grams fat

Option 2 (blend until smooth)
1 packet Carnation Instant Breakfast
8 oz fat-free milk
1 medium banana
1 tbsp peanut butter
438 kcal, 70 grams carbohydrate, 17 grams protein, 10 grams fat

Option 3
1.5 cans GatorPro (11 fl oz per can)
559 kcal, 89 grams carbohydrate, 26 grams protein, 11 grams fat

For more information on sports nutrition, visit the Gatorade Sports Science Institute webpage (www.gssiweb.com). For more information on sports medicine, visit https://physsportsmed.org. This homepage of *The Physician and Sportsmedicine* journal details current issues in sports medicine, including injury prevention, nutrition, and exercise. Also helpful are the webpages of the American College of Sports Medicine (www.acsm.org), Centers for Disease Control and Prevention Division of Nutrition, Physical Activity and Obesity (www.cdc.gov/nccdphp/dnpao), and the American Council on Exercise (www.acefitness.org).

CONCEPT CHECK

All athletes would do well to plan a diet that conforms to MyPlate recommendations. High-carbohydrate foods should be emphasized, and these should dominate in pre-event meals. Protein intake above 1.7 grams per kilogram of body weight is not supported by scientific evidence. Most athletes easily consume enough protein from typical food choices. If nutrient supplements are used, dosages generally should not exceed the Upper Level set for each nutrient. Fluid should be consumed as liberally as possible before, during, and after an event. Carbohydrate and electrolytes in the fluid are especially helpful to help delay fatigue and maintain electrolyte balance when exercise duration exceeds 60 minutes.

Ergogenic Aids and Athletic Performance

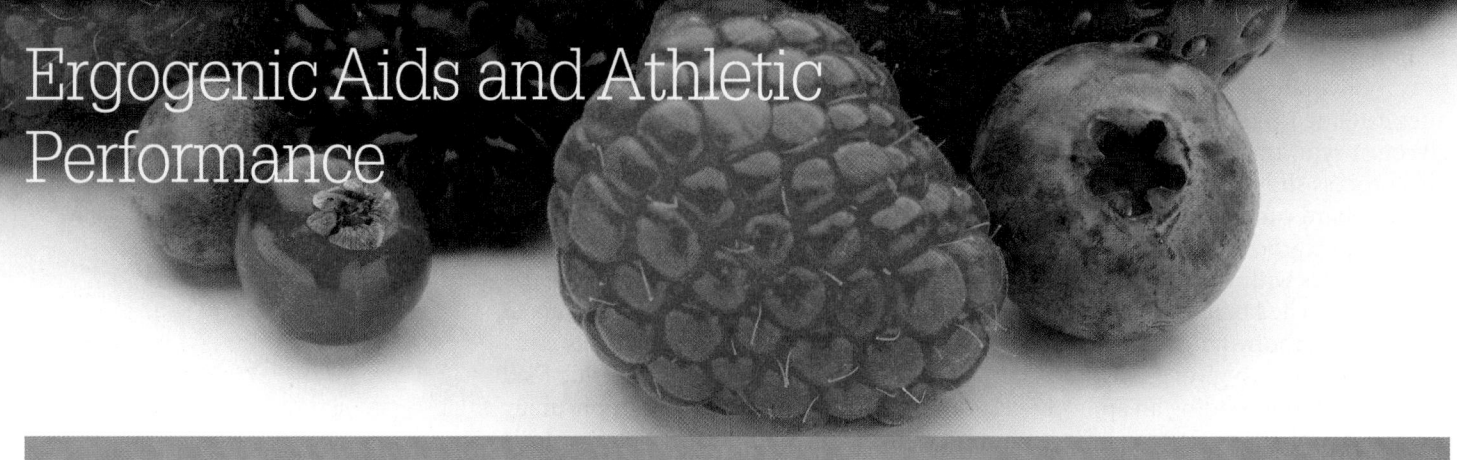

Ergogenic Aids to Enhance Athletic Performance

Extreme diet manipulation to improve athletic performance is not a recent innovation. As long as 30 years ago, American football players were encouraged on hot practice days to "toughen up" for competition by liberally consuming salt tablets before and during practice and by not drinking water. Now it is widely recognized that this practice can be fatal. Today's athletes are as likely as their predecessors to experiment with any substance that promises a competitive advantage. In 2010, consumers spent more than $22.7 billion on sports nutrition and weight loss supplements. Artichoke hearts, bee pollen, dried adrenal glands from cattle, seaweed, freeze-dried liver flakes, gelatin, and ginseng are just some of the ineffective substances used by athletes in hopes of gaining an **ergogenic** (work-producing) edge.

Based on what is known at this time, today's athletes can benefit from scientific evidence documenting the ergogenic properties of a few dietary substances. These ergogenic aids include sufficient water and electrolytes, lots of carbohydrates, and a balanced and varied diet consistent with MyPlate. Protein and amino acid supplements are not among those aids because athletes can easily meet protein needs from foods, as Table 10-3 demonstrated. The use of nutrient supplements should

> **ergogenic** Work-producing. An ergogenic aid is a mechanical, nutritional, psychological, pharmacological, or physiological substance or treatment intended to directly improve exercise performance.

be designed to meet a specific dietary shortcoming, such as an inadequate iron intake. These and other aids, which often have dubious benefits and may pose health risks, must be given close scrutiny before use. The risk-benefit ratio of any ergogenic aid merits careful evaluation (see Further Readings 6 and 13).

As summarized in Table 10-10, no scientific evidence supports the effectiveness of many substances touted as performance-enhancing aids. Many are useless; some are dangerous. Athletes should be skeptical of any substance until its ergogenic effect is scientifically validated. FDA has a limited ability to regulate these dietary supplements (review Chapter 1), and the manufacturing processes for dietary supplements are not as tightly regulated by FDA as they are for prescription drugs. Some supplements may contain substances that will cause athletes to "test positive" for various banned substances. This was demonstrated in the 2002 Winter Olympics. Studies also have called into question the quality control associated with the manufacturing of dietary supplements. Many do not contain the substance and/or the amount listed on the label.

These results add yet another worry for the athlete. Not only must he or she determine whether there is evidence that a dietary supplement is safe and effective, but must also question if the dietary supplement contains what it is supposed to contain.

Even substances whose ergogenic effects have been supported by systematic scientific studies should be used with caution, as the testing conditions may not match those of the intended use. Caution should be exercised when it comes to using the appropriate dose of supplements or using multiple types of supplements concurrently.

Finally, rather than waiting for a magic bullet to enhance performance, athletes are advised to concentrate their efforts on improving their training routines and sport techniques, while consuming well-balanced diets as described in this chapter.

MAKING DECISIONS

NCAA and Supplements

The NCAA's Committee on Competitive Safeguards and Medical Aspects of Sports has developed lists of permissible and nonpermissible supplements for athletic departments to dispense. The NCAA advises students to discuss their use of *any* dietary supplement with their coaches to avoid unknowingly ingesting banned substances. Following are a few key examples:

Permissible	Nonpermissible
Vitamins and minerals	Amino acids
"Energy" bars (if no more than 30% protein)	Creatine
Sports drinks	Glycerol
Meal replacement drinks such as Ensure Plus or Boost	HMB
	L-carnitine
	Protein powders

For a complete explanation of NCAA's rules regarding dietary supplements, see www.ncaa.org.

TABLE 10-10 An Evaluation of Popular Ergogenic Aids

Substance/Practice	Rationale	Reality
Useful in Some Circumstances		
Creatine	Increase phosphocreatine (PCr) in muscles to keep ATP concentration high	Use of 20 grams per day for 5 to 6 days and then a maintenance dose of 2 grams per day may improve performance in those who undertake repeated bursts of activity, such as in sprinting and weight lifting. Vegetarian athletes benefit the most because their diets are low in or devoid of creatine. Some of the muscle weight gain noted with use results from water contained in muscles. Endurance athletes do not benefit from use. Little is known about the safety of long-term creatine use. Continual use of high doses has led to kidney damage in a few cases. Cost: $25 to $65 per month.
Sodium Bicarbonate (baking soda)	Counter lactic acid buildup	Partially effective in some circumstances (when lactic acid is rapidly produced), such as wrestling, but induces nausea and diarrhea. The dose used is 300 milligrams/kilogram, given 1 to 3 hours before exercise. Cost: nil.
Caffeine	Increase use of fatty acids to fuel muscles, promote mental alertness	Drinking two to three 5-ounce cups of coffee (equivalent to 3 to 9 milligrams of caffeine per kilogram of body weight) about 1 hour before events lasting about 5 minutes or longer is useful for some athletes; benefits are less apparent in those who have ample stores of glycogen, are highly trained, or habitually consume caffeine; intake of more than about 600 milligrams (six to eight cups of coffee) elicits a urine concentration illegal under NCAA rules (greater than 15 micrograms per milliliter). Possible side effects include shakiness, nervousness, nausea, anxiety, and insomnia. Cost: $0.08 per 300 milligrams.
Possibly Useful, Still Under Study		
Beta-hydroxy-beta methylbutyric acid (HMB)	Decrease protein catabolism, causing a net growth-promoting effect	Some research suggests that supplementation with this substance may increase muscle mass by 0.5 to 1 kilogram beyond unsupplemented diets when taken during initial phases of weight training. Still, safety and effectiveness of-long term HMB use in humans is unknown. Cost: $100 per month.
Glutamine (an amino acid)	Enhance immune function, preserve lean body mass	Some preliminary studies show decreased occurrence of upper respiratory tract infections in athletes with use. It also may promote muscle growth, but long-term studies are lacking. Protein foods are a rich source of glutamine. Cost: $10 to $20 per month for 1 to 2 grams per day.
Branched-chain amino acids (BCAA) (leucine, isoleucine, valine)	Increase gains in muscle mass during resistance training Important energy source, especially when carbohydrate stores are depleted	Several studies point to positive effects of BCAA on increases in muscle mass when taken before or after resistance training. This effect is most dramatic among untrained athletes who are just beginning a resistance-training program. Protein-rich foods (especially dairy proteins) are also rich in BCAA. Cost: $20 per month. For endurance athletes, supplementation of BCAA (10 to 30 grams per day) during exercise can increase BCAA in the blood when it has been depleted due to exercise, although there is no consistent evidence of improved endurance performance. Carbohydrate feeding, by delaying use of BCAA as fuel, may negate the need for BCAA supplementation in endurance activities.
Dangerous or Illegal Substances/Practices		
Anabolic steroids (and related substances, such as androstenedione and tetrahydrogestrinone)	Increase muscle mass and strength	Although effective for increasing protein synthesis, anabolic steroids are illegal in the United States unless prescribed by a physician. They have numerous potential side effects, such as premature closure of growth plates in bones (thus possibly limiting the adult height of a teenage athlete), bloody cysts in the liver, increased risk of cardiovascular disease, increased blood pressure, and reproductive dysfunction. Possible psychological consequences include increased aggressiveness, drug dependence (addiction), withdrawal symptoms (such as depression), sleep disturbances, and mood swings (known as "roid rage"). Use of needles for injectable forms adds further health risk. Banned by the International Olympic Committee.

TABLE 10-10 *(continued)*

Substance/Practice	Rationale	Reality
Growth hormone	Increase muscle mass	At critical ages, may increase height; may also cause uncontrolled growth of the heart and other internal organs and even death; potentially dangerous; requires careful monitoring by a physician. Use of needles for injections adds further health risk. Banned by the International Olympic Committee.
Blood doping	To enhance aerobic capacity by injecting red blood cells harvested previously from the athlete, or alternately the athlete may use the hormone erythropoietin (Epogen) to increase red blood cell number	May offer aerobic benefit; very serious health consequences are possible, including thickening of the blood, which puts extra strain on the heart; is an illegal practice under Olympic guidelines.
Gamma hydroxybutyric acid (GHB)	Promoted as a steroid alternative for bodybuilding	FDA has never approved it for sale as a medical product; is illegal to produce or sell GHB in the United States. GHB-related symptoms include vomiting, dizziness, tremors, and seizures. Many victims have required hospitalization, and some have died. Clandestine laboratories produced virtually all of the chemical accounting for GHB abuse. FDA is working with the U.S. Attorney's office to arrest, indict, and convict individuals responsible for the illegal operations.

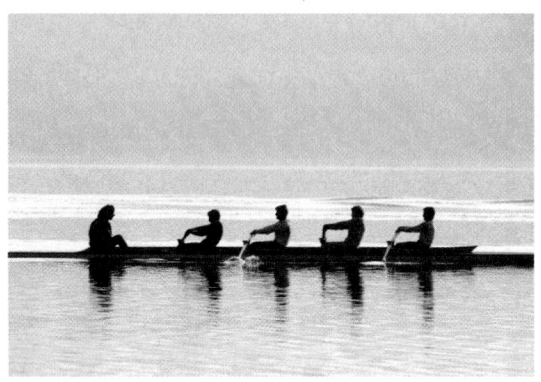

◀ Attention to carbohydrate and fluid needs—along with meeting overall nutrient needs—is the most important ergogenic aid.

Case Study Planning a Training Diet

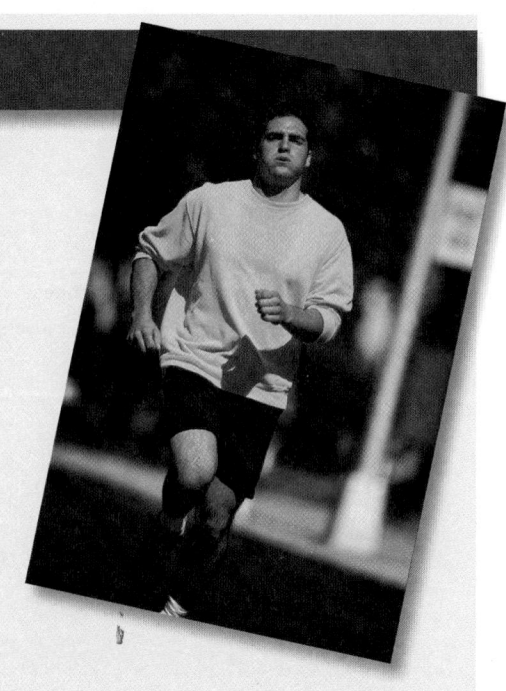

Michael is training for a 10K run coming up in 3 weeks. He has read a lot about sports nutrition and especially about the importance of eating a high-carbohydrate diet while in training. He also has been struggling to keep his weight in a range that he feels contributes to better speed and endurance. Consequently he is also trying to eat as little fat as possible. Unfortunately, over the past week his workouts in the afternoon have not met his expectations. His run times are slower, and he shows signs of fatigue after just 20 minutes into his training program.

His breakfast yesterday was a large bagel, a small amount of cream cheese, and orange juice. For lunch, he had a small salad with fat-free dressing, a large plate of pasta with marinara sauce and broccoli, and a diet soft drink. For dinner, he had a small broiled chicken breast, a cup of rice, some carrots, and iced tea. Later, he snacked on fat-free pretzels.

Answer the following questions, and check your responses in Appendix A.

1. Is the high-carbohydrate diet a good idea during Michael's training?
2. Are there any important components missing in Michael's diet? Are missing components contributing to his fatigue?
3. Describe some changes that should be made in Michael's diet including some specific foods that should be emphasized.
4. How should fluid needs be met during workouts?
5. Should Michael focus on fueling his body before, during, or after workouts?

Summary (Numbers refer to numbered sections in the chapter.)

10.1 A gradual increase in regular physical activity is recommended for all healthy persons. Benefits include improvements in cardiovascular health, gastrointestinal function, blood glucose regulation, and sleep; reduced risk of certain cancers; and enhanced muscle and bone strength.

10.2 The Physical Activity Guidelines for Americans advise adults to do at least 150 minutes of moderate-intensity or 75 minutes of vigorous-intensity aerobic physical activity per week. In addition, adults should perform muscle-strengthening activities at least twice per week. Workouts should allow time for warm-up exercises to increase blood flow and warm the muscles, and then end with cooldown exercises, including stretching.

10.3 Human metabolic pathways extract chemical energy from carbohydrate, fat, and protein to yield ATP, the compound that provides energy for body functions. Phosphocreatine is another high-energy compound that can be used to resupply ATP during short, intense activities. The mix of macronutrients used for fuel depends on the intensity and duration of activity: short-term, intense exercises

primarily use carbohydrate for fuel, whereas low- or moderate-intensity endurance exercises use more fat for fuel. Protein makes a minor contribution as a fuel source.

10.4 To support physical activity, athletes require 5 to 8 kcal per minute of activity above energy needs for a sedentary person. Monitoring weight changes over time is a good way to assess the adequacy of energy intake. Athletes should obtain energy from a varied diet that includes sources of carbohydrates (6 to 10 grams of carbohydrate per kilogram of body weight; usually 60% of total energy), protein (0.8 to 2.0 grams of protein per kilogram, depending on the type of training), and fat (up to 35% of energy, focusing on vegetable oils instead of solid fats). The increased overall food intake of athletes typically furnishes adequate vitamins and minerals. Some micronutrients concern are iron and calcium, especially for women.

10.5 Athletes should consume enough fluid to both minimize loss of body weight and ultimately restore pre-exercise weight. Sports drinks help replace fluid, electrolytes, and carbohydrates lost during workouts that last beyond 60 minutes.

10.6 In the 24 hours before an event, athletes should drink fluids freely and consume plenty of carbohydrates. During endurance events, athletes should consume enough fluid and electrolytes to prevent losses of more than 2% of body weight, as determined by individuals during training. Sports drinks and energy gels are two options for fueling during events. In the recovery period, endurance athletes should consume high-glycemic-load carbohydrates and some protein soon after a workout to begin restoration of muscle glycogen stores. To replace fluid losses, athletes should drink 2 to 3 cups of fluid for every pound lost.

N&YH Athletes can benefit from ergogenic properties of sufficient water and electrolytes, lots of carbohydrates, and a balanced and varied diet consistent with the Dietary Guidelines and MyPlate. Under some circumstances, creatine, sodium bicarbonate, and caffeine are useful for enhancing athletic performance. Protein and amino-acid supplements are not beneficial because athletes meet protein needs from foods.

Check Your Knowledge (Answers to the following questions are below.)

1. An energy-rich compound, phosphocreatine (PCr), is found in _____ tissue.
   a. adipose
   b. muscle
   c. liver
   d. kidney

2. A fitness program should include
   a. aerobic exercises 5 days per week.
   b. strength-training exercises 2 to 3 days per week.
   c. stretching exercises 2 to 3 days per week.
   d. All of the above.

3. During muscle-building regimes, athletes should consume _____ grams of protein per kilogram body weight.
   a. 0.5 to 0.7
   b. 0.8
   c. 1.5 to 1.7
   d. 2 to 2.5

4. Which of these foods is the best choice for carbohydrate loading before endurance events?

   a. potato chips
   b. French fries
   c. All-Bran (high-fiber) cereal
   d. rice

5. As the body adapts to regular exercise, the "training effect" results in
   a. decreased blood flow to muscles.
   b. increased lactic acid production.
   c. decreased muscle triglyceride content.
   d. decreased resting heart rate.

6. A physically active lifestyle leads to
   a. increased bone strength.
   b. decreased risk of colon cancer.
   c. reduced stress.
   d. All of the above.

7. How many cups of fluid are required to replace each pound of weight lost during an athletic event or workout?
   a. 0.5 to 0.75
   b. 1 to 1.5
   c. 2 to 3
   d. 4 to 5

8. The benefit of a "sports" drink is to provide
   a. water to hydrate.
   b. electrolytes to enhance water absorption in the intestine and maintain blood volume.
   c. carbohydrate for energy.
   d. All of the above.

9. Compared to anaerobic glucose metabolism, aerobic glucose metabolism produces more
   a. lactic acid.
   b. ATP.
   c. phosphocreatine.
   d. fatty acids.

10. Caffeine is used as an ergogenic aid by some athletes because it is thought to
    a. increase use of fatty acids.
    b. decrease the buildup of lactic acid.
    c. serve as an energy source.
    d. increase muscle mass and strength.

Answers: 1. b (LO 10.3), 2. d (LO 10.2), 3. c (LO 10.6), 4. d (LO 10.8), 5. d (LO 10.5), 6. d (LO 10.1), 7. c (LO 10.7), 8. d (LO 10.7), 9. b (LO 10.4), 10. a (LO 10.9)

Study Questions (Numbers refer to Learning Outcomes)

1. How does greater physical fitness contribute to better overall health? Explain the process. **(LO 10.1)**

2. You have set a goal to increase muscle mass and decrease body fat. Plan a weekly fitness regime, specifying activity types, frequency, intensity, duration, and progression. **(LO 10.2)**

3. How are carbohydrates, fat, and protein used to supply energy during a 100-meter sprint? During a weight-lifting session? During a 3-mile walk? **(LO 10.3)**

4. What is the difference between anaerobic and aerobic exercise? Explain why aerobic metabolism is increased by a regular exercise routine. **(LO 10.4)**

5. Is fat from adipose tissue used as an energy source during exercise? If so, when? **(LO 10.5)**

6. What are some typical measures used to assess whether an athlete's calorie intake is adequate? **(LO 10.6)**

7. List five specific nutrients that athletes need and the appropriate food sources from which these nutrients can be obtained. **(LO 10.6)**

8. You plan to participate in half-marathon. Plan your menu for the day, being sure to include appropriate levels of macronutrients and fluids before, during, and after the athletic event. **(LO 10.8)**

9. What advice would you give your neighbor, planning to run a 5-kilometer (km) race, concerning fluid intake before and during the event? **(LO 10.7)**

10. One of your friends, a competitive athlete, asks your opinion about an amino-acid supplement sold in a local sporting-goods store. She has read that such supplements can help improve athletic performance. What would you tell her about the general effectiveness of such products? **(LO 10.9)**

What Would You Choose Recommendations

In this chapter, you have learned that it's important to replenish carbohydrates, fluids, and electrolytes for optimal performance during endurance events, like this half-marathon. General guidelines are to consume ½ to 1 ½ cups of fluid every 15 minutes and 30 to 60 grams of carbohydrate per hour. Choosing a sports nutrition product is something you should do during training. With a few weeks to go, you have time to experiment with a product that can help you avoid "hitting the wall" at mile nine.

The PowerBar ProteinPlus energy bar provides 300 kcal, 6 grams of fat, 39 grams of carbohydrate, and 23 grams of protein. This might be a tasty and convenient meal replacement during your busy weeks of training. Alternatively, it could serve as a recovery meal to help replenish your muscle glycogen stores after the race. However, during the race, its high fat and protein content would slow digestion, possibly leading to abdominal cramps. Furthermore, this product would not contribute to fluid replenishment.

The Essential Amino Energy drink provides 2 grams of carbohydrate and 5 grams of essential amino acids in free form, including branched-chain amino acids. The drink may help meet fluid needs, but the carbohydrate content is not sufficient to maintain blood glucose during the race. It is true that BCAAs are utilized for fuel during endurance activities and that they can enhance muscle building during weight

training, but there is no consistent evidence that supplying BCAAs during endurance exercise enhances performance.

A sports drink, such as Powerade, is superior to water for events lasting more than 60 minutes. The added carbohydrates help to supply energy to the brain and muscles. The added flavor encourages consumption. The electrolytes replace those lost in sweating, increase fluid absorption, and stimulate thirst. A 32-ounce bottle of Powerade (4 servings) contains a total of 200 kcal and 56 grams of carbohydrate in 4 cups of fluid. One bottle of Powerade per hour while you compete would meet your fluid and carbohydrate needs, but may be inconvenient to tote while running.

The energy gel is small enough to take along during the race—and the chocolate cherry flavor sounds delicious! The label says it has 110 kcal, 1.5 grams of fat, 22 grams of carbohydrate, 12 grams of sugar, and 100 milligrams of caffeine. A Clif Shot during the race could help replenish blood glucose and electrolytes, but it definitely won't meet your fluid requirements while racing. However, there will be water available at numerous stops along the course.

Some energy gels are caffeine-free, but this one contains as much caffeine as a strong cup of coffee. Research shows that caffeine can increase the ability of muscles to use fatty acids for energy and increase mental alertness among people who are not habitual caffeine consumers. On the other hand, negative effects of excessive

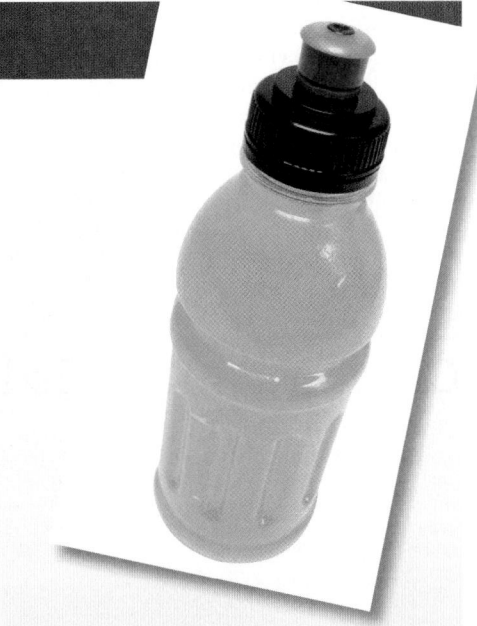

▲ Sports drinks replenish carbohydrates and electrolytes lost during prolonged exercise.

caffeine include dehydration, heart palpitations, and gastrointestinal discomfort, so moderation is necessary.

In summary, both the Powerade and the Clif Shot would replenish carbohydrates and electrolytes. The Powerade would also fulfill your fluid needs, whereas you'd need to grab water along the course if you choose the energy gel. The energy gel has the advantage of being light and portable, plus the caffeine may have an ergogenic effect. Give both the Powerade and the Clif Shot energy gel a trial run during your training sessions and see which one helps you most around mile nine.

Further Readings

1. Adamidou J, Bell-Wilson J: Iron deficiency anemia and exercise. *IDEA Fitness Journal* May:82, 2006.

   This article reviews why athletes may have increased iron requirements. The best food sources to prevent iron depletion and sports anemia are also suggested.

2. DeJonge L, Smith MR: Macronutrients and exercise. *Obesity Management* February:11, 2008.

   Body stores of carbohydrate and fat are used preferentially as fuel for exercising muscles, whereas protein is conserved. Exercise not only leads to increased fat oxidation during exercise, but also in the post-exercise period. Furthermore, the body's ability to burn fat is improved by training.

3. Garber CE and others: American College of Sports Medicine Position Stand: Quantity and quality of exercise for developing and maintaining cardiorespiratory, musculoskeletal, and neuromotor fitness in apparently healthy adults: Guidance for prescribing exercise. *Medicine and Science in Sports and Exercise* 43:1334, 2011.

   These exercise guidelines from the American College of Sports Medicine generally agree with advice conveyed by the 2008 Physical Activity Guidelines for Americans. The benefits of and recommendations for endurance, strength, and flexibility exercises are reviewed. Sedentary behavior is discouraged.

4. Gleeson M: Can nutrition limit exercise-induced immunodepression? *Nutrition Reviews* March:119, 2006.

   Intense or prolonged exercise can lead to immunodepression, resulting in increased incidence of infections among athletes. These effects are due to the activity of stress hormones on immune cells. Optimal nutrition, including adequate habitual dietary intake of protein, essential fatty acids, zinc, iron, and antioxidants supports immune function. Consuming carbohydrate and staying hydrated are important strategies to prevent the stress response that leads to immune dysfunction.

5. Harber VJ: Energy balance and reproductive function in active women. *Canadian Journal of Applied Physiology* 29:48, 2004.

   It is important for female athletes engaged in rigorous training programs to meet their calorie needs. If not, the resulting negative calorie balance will likely lead to a variety of menstrual cycle disturbances that can lead to other health problems.

6. Jenkinson DM, Harbert AJ. Supplements and sports. *American Family Physician* 78:1039, 2008.

   Use of dietary supplements among athletes is widespread and supplement users are often uninformed about the risks and benefits of supplementation. Some supplements, including anabolic steroids and ephedrine, have dangerous effects. Most supplements do not demonstrate consistent benefits for athletic performance. A few substances, including creatine, caffeine, and sodium bicarbonate, are useful under certain circumstances.

7. Kreider RB and others: ISSN exercise and sport nutrition review: Research and recommendations. *Journal of the International Society of Sports Nutrition* 7:7, 2010.

   This detailed and comprehensive review covers fluid and nutrient needs for optimal athletic performance, timing of food intake, and up-to-date research on an array of dietary supplements. Of note, ISSN recommends up to 2.0 grams of protein per kilogram of body weight for some athletes involved in intense training—more than twice the recommendations of the Food and Nutrition Board.

8. Laaksonen DE and others: Physical activity in the prevention of type 2 diabetes: The Finnish Diabetes Prevention Study. *Diabetes* 54:158, 2005.

   Regular physical activity can substantially reduce the risk of developing type 2 diabetes in high risk individuals. People who increased their activity from moderate to vigorous amounts reduced their risk of developing type 2 diabetes by 65% compared to people who remained inactive.

9. Margaritis I, Rousseau AS: Does physical exercise modify antioxidant requirements? *Nutrition Research Reviews* 21:3, 2008.

   Exercise induces oxidative stress, leading to the hypothesis that exercise may increase antioxidant nutrient requirements among athletes. To date, however, research does not support use of antioxidant supplements to enhance athletic performance. In fact, some studies show detrimental effects of supplementation on endpoints such as muscle recovery and even all-cause mortality. Except in cases of pre-existing nutrient deficiencies, consuming a well-balanced diet is the best advice for optimizing athletic performance.

10. Maughan RJ, Shirreffs SM: Development of individual hydration strategies for athletes. *International Journal of Sport and Nutrition and Exercise Metabolism* 18:457, 2008.

    Both dehydration and hyperhydration are detrimental to athletic performance and can be lethal. Despite the popular devaluation of thirst as an indicator of dehydration, recent research demonstrates that adherence to physiologic cues for consumption of fluid and electrolytes supports optimal athletic performance even when 100% body weight is not maintained. For optimal performance, hydration strategies should account for carbohydrate and electrolyte replacements in addition to fluid intake.

11. Nichols DL and others: Bone density and young athletic women. An update. *Sports Medicine* 37:1001, 2007.

    Athletes have 5–30% higher bone density than their non-athletic counterparts. In combination with prolonged negative energy balance, however, high levels of physical activity may lead to the female athlete triad, in which low dietary intake and weight loss lead to amenorrhea and subsequent bone loss. Although current research does not point to augmented requirements for female athletes, meeting DRIs for protein, calcium, and vitamin D intake is an important dietary goal to support optimal bone development.

12. Rodriguez NR and others: Position of the American Dietetic Association, Dietitians of Canada, and the American College of Sports Medicine: Nutrition and athletic performance. *Journal of the American Dietetic Association* 109:509, 2009.

    This position statement summarizes recommendations for nutrient and fluid intake before, during, and after exercise to optimize athletic performance. Guidance for special population groups, such as vegetarian athletes, is provided. Dietary supplements and ergogenic acids are discouraged because food intake usually provides adequate micronutrients and supplements may be contaminated with banned and/or dangerous ingredients.

13. Rosenbloom C, Rosbruck M. Popular dietary supplements used in sports. *Nutrition Today* 43:60, 2008.

    The authors review four dietary supplements that are popular as ergogenic and weight loss aids: creatine, caffeine, epigallocatechin (EGCG), and nitric oxide and its metabolite, L-arginine.

14. Sawka MN and others: American College of Sports Medicine Position Stand: Exercise and fluid replacement. *Medicine and Science in Sports and Exercise* 39:377, 2007.

    This review summarizes the water intake recommendations for healthy humans, emphasizing that hydration is well maintained as long as food and fluid are readily available. The review concludes that exercise and heat can greatly increase water needs, and that the individual variability between athletes can be significant.

15. Williams MH: *Nutrition for health, fitness, & sport.* 9th ed. Boston: McGraw-Hill, 2009.

    Excellent textbook for reviewing nutrient needs of athletes, as well as learning more about ergogenic aids; also provides a detailed look at metabolism in exercise.

To get the most out of your study of nutrition, go to McGraw-Hill's online resources: Connect www.mcgrawhillconnect.com, where you will find NutritionCalc Plus, LearnSmart, and many other dynamic tools.

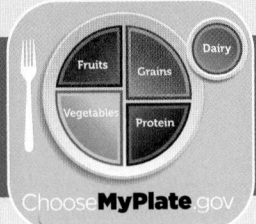

RATE YOUR PLATE

I. Evaluating Protein Intake—A Case Study

Mark is a college student who has been lifting weights at the student recreation center. The trainer at the center recommended a protein drink to help Mark build muscle mass. Answer the following questions about Mark's current food intake and determine whether a protein drink is needed to supplement Mark's diet.

1. The following is a tally of yesterday's intake.

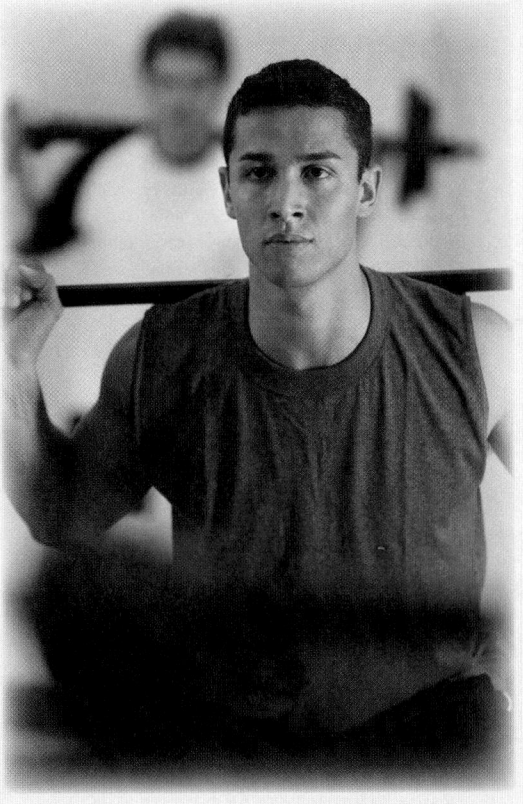

Breakfast	Frosted Mini-Wheats cereal, 2 oz 1% milk, 1½ cups Orange juice, chilled, 6 oz Glazed yeast doughnut, 1 Brewed coffee, 1 cup
Lunch	Double hamburger with condiments, 1 French fries, 30 Cola, 12 oz Medium apple, 1
Dinner	Frozen lasagna w/meat, 2 pieces 1% milk, 1 cup Looseleaf lettuce, chopped, 1 cup Creamy Italian salad dressing, 2 tsp Medium tomato, ½ Whole carrot, raw, 1
Evening snack	Vanilla ice milk, 1 cup Hot fudge chocolate topping, 2 tsp Soft chocolate chip cookies, 2

Evaluate Mark's diet using NutritionCalc Plus—is he meeting the minimum recommendations of MyPlate's Daily Food Plan for his calorie needs?

_____

2. Mark's weight has been stable at 70 kilograms (154 pounds). Determine his protein needs based on the RDA (0.8 grams per kilogram).
   a. Mark's estimated protein RDA: _____
   b. What are the maximum recommendations for protein intake for strength-training athletes (see p. 423)? _____
   c. Calculate the maximum protein recommendation for Mark. _____

   _____

3. An analysis of the total calorie and protein content of Mark's current diet is 3470 kcal, 125 grams of protein (14% of total calories supplied by protein). This diet is representative of the food choices and amounts of food that Mark chooses on a regular basis.
   a. What is the difference between Mark's estimated protein needs as an athlete (from number 2) and the amount of protein that his current diet provides? _____
   b. Is his current protein intake inadequate, adequate, or excessive? _____

4. Mark takes his trainer's advice and goes to the supermarket to purchase a protein drink to add to his diet. Four products are available; they contain the following label information.

	Amino Fuel	Joe Weider's Sugar-Free 90% Plus Protein	Joe Weider's Dynamic Muscle Builder	Victory Super Mega Mass 2000
Serving size	3 tbsp	3 tbsp	3 tbsp	¼ scoop
Kcal	104	110	103	104
Protein (grams)	15	24	10	5

The trainer recommends adding the supplement to Mark's diet two times a day. Mark chooses the Muscle Builder protein drink.
a. How much protein would be added to Mark's diet daily from two servings of the supplement alone (prior to mixing it with a beverage)?

b. Mark mixes the powder with the milk he already consumes at breakfast and dinner. How much protein total would Mark now consume in 1 day? (Add the protein amount from the nutrition analysis to the value from question 4a.)

c. What is the difference between Mark's estimated protein needs as an athlete and this total intake?

5. What is your conclusion—does Mark need the protein supplement?

Answers to Calculations

2a. Mark's estimated protein RDA: 70 kilograms × 0.8 grams per kilogram = 56 grams.
2b. Maximum recommendation for protein intake for athletes = 1.7 grams per kilogram.
2c. Applied to Mark: 1.7 × 70 = 119 grams.
3a. Difference between Mark's estimated maximum protein needs and the amount of protein provided by his current diet: 125−119 = 6 grams protein.
3b. Mark's current protein intake exceeds maximum protein needs.
4a. Two servings of protein supplement alone = 20 grams of protein.
4b. Mark's total protein consumption: 125 grams + 20 grams = 145 grams protein.
4c. Difference between Mark's estimated maximum protein needs for muscle mass gain and total protein consumption with protein supplement (from above): 145 grams −119 grams = 26 grams protein.

II. How Physically Fit Are You?

The fitness assessments presented here are easy to do and require little equipment. Also included are charts to compare your results to those typical of your peers.

Cardiovascular Fitness: One-Mile Walk

Measure a mile on a running track (usually four laps) or on a little-trafficked neighborhood street (use a car's odometer to get the right distance). With a stopwatch or watch with a second hand, walk the mile as fast as you can. Note the time it took.

Strength: Push-ups

Men: Get up on your toes and hands. Keep your back straight, with hands flat on the floor directly below your shoulders. Women: Same position, but you can support your body on your knees if necessary.

Lower your body, bending your elbows, until your chin grazes the floor. Push back up until your arms are straight. Continue until you can't do any more push-ups (you can rest when in the up position).

Strength: Curl-ups

Lie on the floor on your back with your knees bent, feet flat. Your hands should rest on your thighs. Now squeeze your stomach muscles, push your back flat, and raise your upper body high enough for your hands to touch the tops of your knees. Don't pull with your neck or head, and keep your lower back on the floor. Count how many curl-ups you can do in one minute.

Flexibility: Sit-and-Reach

Place a yardstick on the floor and apply a two-foot piece of tape on the floor perpendicular to the yardstick, crossing at the 15-inch mark. Sit on the floor with your legs extended and the soles of your feet touching the tape at the 15-inch mark, the zero-inch facing you. Your feet should be about 12 inches apart. Put one hand on the other, exhale, and very slowly reach forward as far as you can along the yardstick, lowering your head between your arms. Don't bounce! Note the farthest inch mark you reach. Don't hurt yourself by reaching farther than your body wants to. Relax, and then repeat two more times.

Now check your results. Want to improve? You know the answer:

- Do aerobic exercise that makes you breathe hard for at least half an hour on most or all days of the week.
- Lift weights that challenge you two to three times per week.
- Stretch after activity at least a couple of times per week.
- Walk more.

Cardiovascular: One-mile walk (time, in minutes)

	Under 40 Years		Over 40 Years	
	Men	Women	Men	Women
Excellent	13:00 or less	13:30 or less	14:00 or less	14:30 or less
Good	13:01–15:30	13:31–16:00	14:01–16:30	14:31–17:00
Average	15:31–18:00	16:01–18:30	16:31–19:00	17:01–19:30
Below average	18:01–19:30	18:31–20:00	19:01–21:30	19:31–22:00
Poor	19:31 or more	20:01 or more	21:31 or more	22:01 or more

Source: Cooper Institute.

Strength: Push-ups (number completed without rest)

Men						
Age	17–19	20–29	30–39	40–49	50–59	60–65
Excellent	>56	>47	>41	>34	>31	>30
Good	47–56	39–47	34–41	28–34	25–31	24–30
Above average	35–46	30–39	25–33	21–28	18–24	17–23
Average	19–34	17–29	13–24	11–20	9–17	6–16
Below average	11–18	10–16	8–12	6–10	5–8	3–5
Poor	4–10	4–9	2–7	1–5	1–4	1–2
Very poor	<4	<4	<2	0	0	0

Women						
Age	17–19	20–29	30–39	40–49	50–59	60–65
Excellent	>35	>36	>37	>31	>25	>23
Good	27–35	30–36	30–37	25–31	21–25	19–23
Above average	21–27	23–29	22–30	18–24	15–20	13–18
Average	11–20	12–22	10–21	8–17	7–14	5–12
Below average	6–10	7–11	5–9	4–7	3–6	2–4
Poor	2–5	2–6	1–4	1–3	1–2	1
Very poor	0–1	0–1	0	0	0	0

Source: Golding LA, YMCA of the USA: *YMCA Fitness Testing and Assessment Manual*, 4th ed, 2000. www.topendsports.com.

Strength: Curl-ups (number completed in 60 seconds)

	Men					
Age	**18–25**	**26–35**	**36–45**	**46–55**	**56–65**	**65+**
Excellent	>49	>45	>41	>35	>31	>28
Good	44–49	40–45	35–41	29–35	25–31	22–28
Above average	39–43	35–39	30–34	25–28	21–24	19–21
Average	35–38	31–34	27–29	22–24	17–20	15–18
Below average	31–34	29–30	23–26	18–21	13–16	11–14
Poor	25–30	22–28	17–22	13–17	9–12	7–10
Very poor	<25	<22	<17	<13	<9	<7

	Women					
Age	**18–25**	**26–35**	**36–45**	**46–55**	**56–65**	**65+**
Excellent	>43	>39	>33	>27	>24	>23
Good	37–43	33–39	27–33	22–27	18–24	17–23
Above average	33–36	29–32	23–26	18–21	13–17	14–16
Average	29–32	25–28	19–22	14–17	10–12	11–13
Below average	25–28	21–24	15–18	10–13	7–9	5–10
Poor	18–24	13–20	7–14	5–9	3–6	2–4
Very poor	<18	<13	<7	<5	<3	<2

Source: Golding LA, YMCA of the USA: *YMCA Fitness Testing and Assessment Manual*, 4th ed, 2000.

Flexibility: Sit-and-reach (in centimeters)

	Men	Women
Super	>+27	>+30
Excellent	+17 to +27	+21 to +30
Good	+6 to +16	+11 to +20
Average	0 to +5	+1 to +10
Fair	−8 to −1	−7 to 0
Poor	−19 to −9	−14 to −8
Very poor	<−20	<−15

Source: Golding LA, YMCA of the USA: *YMCA Fitness Testing and Assessment Manual*, 4th ed, 2000.

These charts are typical charts used by health and fitness experts. For a more thorough assessment of fitness or for development of an exercise plan appropriate for your fitness level, consult a certified personal trainer or other fitness professional.

Chapter 11 Eating Disorders:
Anorexia Nervosa, Bulimia Nervosa, and Other Conditions

Student Learning Outcomes

Chapter 11 is designed to allow you to:

11.1 Contrast healthy attitudes toward uses of food with behavior patterns that could lead to unhealthy uses of food.

11.2 Outline the causes of, effects of, typical persons affected by, and treatment for anorexia nervosa.

11.3 Outline the causes of, effects of, typical persons affected by, and treatment for bulimia nervosa.

11.4 Describe still other forms of eating disorders: binge-eating disorder, night eating syndrome, and the female athlete triad.

11.5 Relate the presence of eating disorders to current social trends.

11.6 Describe methods to reduce the development of eating disorders, including the use of warning signs to identify early cases.

What Would You Choose?

Your college roommate has been acting strangely lately, and you are starting to suspect she has an eating disorder. Over the first few months at college, she gained the "freshman fifteen." She got kind of depressed about it when her jeans started to fit too snugly and declared she was going on a diet. Her weight has not really changed much since then, but her eating behaviors have. She stopped joining your group of friends for meals in the dining hall, opting instead to eat by herself in your dorm room. She has been spending at least 2 hours a day in the campus recreation center, sometimes going in the morning and evening. A few days ago, you thought you heard her throwing up in the restroom, but when she came out of the stall, she said she was fine. What would you choose to help your roommate?

a Tell her she has bulimia and needs to get some treatment.

b Give her some weight-management advice that you learned in Chapter 7.

c Express your concern and ask her if you can go with her to the student health center to talk to someone about it

d Ignore her behavior; she is just trying to draw attention to herself, and this phase will pass in a few weeks.

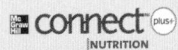 **NUTRITION** **Think about your choice as you read Chapter 11, then see our recommendations at the end of the chapter. To learn more about warning signs of eating disorders, check out the Connect site:** www.mcgrawhillconnect.com

Part Four

Nutrition: Beyond the Nutrients

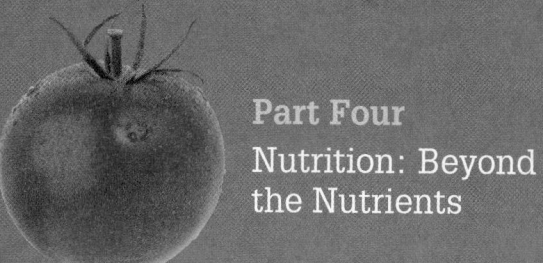

Many of us occasionally eat until we're stuffed and uncomfortable, such as at Thanksgiving dinner. Faced with savory and tempting foods, we find that we can't easily stop eating. Usually we forgive ourselves, vowing not to overeat the next time. Nevertheless, many of us have problems controlling our food intake and body weight. The combination of too many instances of simple overeating, and too little physical activity eventually leads to progressive weight gain.

The obesity epidemic tends to upstage all other nutrition-related problems. However, the eating disorders discussed here are just as serious, if not more, than obesity, and can develop into life-threatening conditions if left untreated. What's most alarming about these disorders—anorexia nervosa, bulimia nervosa, binge-eating disorder, and the female athlete triad—is the increasing number of cases reported each year.

Some people are more susceptible to these eating disorders than other people are—for genetic, psychological, and physical reasons. Successful treatment of eating disorders, therefore, is complex and must go beyond nutritional therapy. Keep in mind that eating disorders are not restricted to any socioeconomic class or ethnicity. They can also strike, as suggested in the comic in this chapter, at any age in both females and males. Let's examine the causes and treatments of these conditions in detail, because eating disorders touch many of our lives.

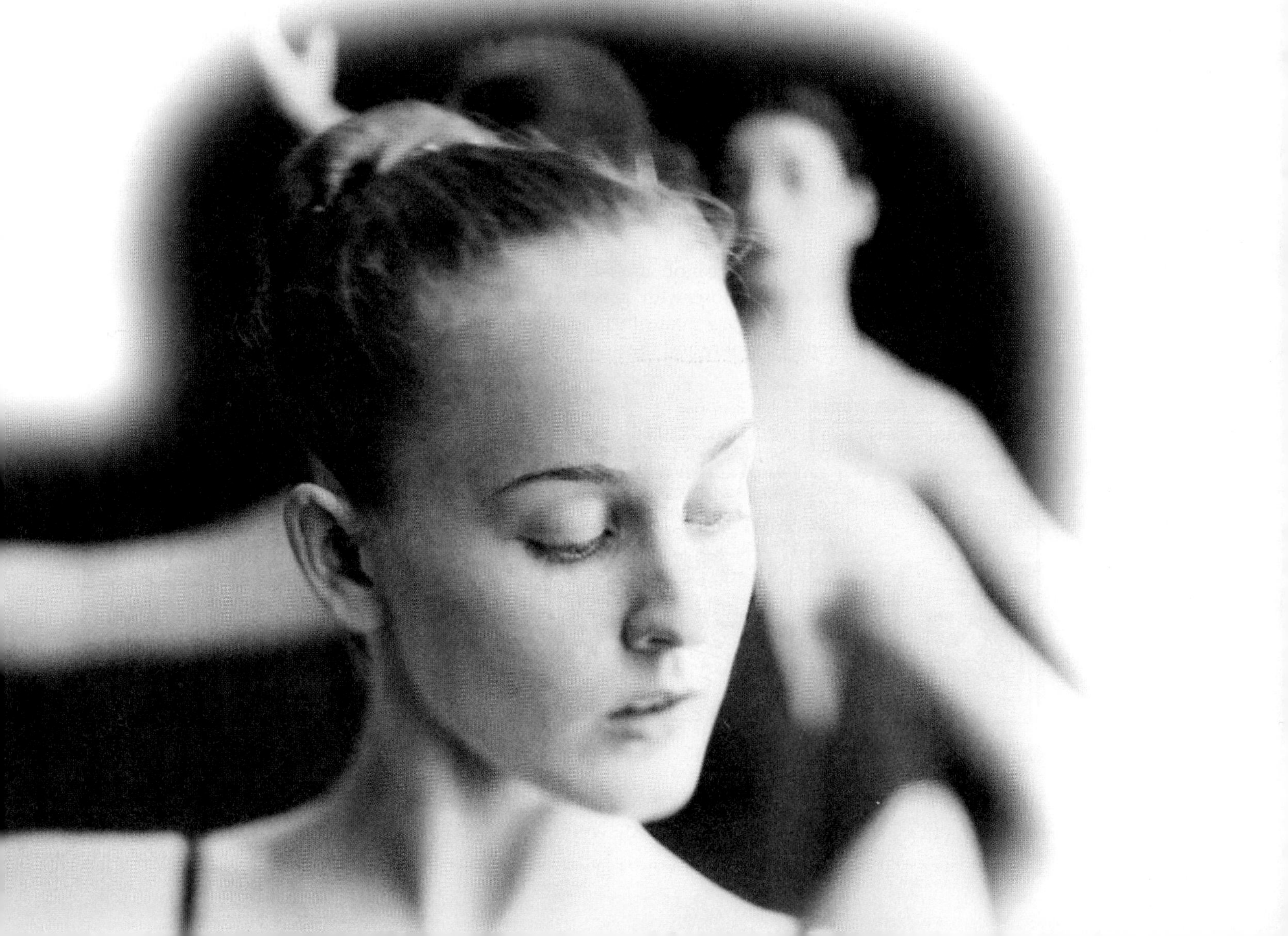

Refresh Your Memory

As you begin your study of eating disorders, such as anorexia nervosa and bulimia nervosa, in Chapter 11, you may want to review:

- The effects of neurotransmitters on food intake in Chapter 1
- The role of genetic risk in disease susceptibility in Chapter 3
- Calculation of BMI in Chapter 7
- The effects and treatment of osteoporosis in Chapter 9
- The effects and treatment of iron-deficiency anemia in Chapter 9

11.1 From Ordered to Disordered Eating Habits

Eating—a completely instinctive behavior for animals—serves an extraordinary number of psychological, social, and cultural purposes for humans. Eating practices may take on religious meanings; signify bonds within families and ethnic groups; and provide a means to express hostility, affection, prestige, or class values. Within the family, supplying, preparing, and distributing food may be a means of expressing love, hatred, or even power.

We are bombarded daily with images of our society's portrayal of the "ideal" body. Dieting is promoted to achieve this ideal body—eternally young and admired. Television programs, billboard and Internet advertisements, magazine pictures, movies, and newspapers suggest that an ultraslim body will bring happiness, love, and ultimately, success. This fantasy notion is contradictory to the fact that much of society is becoming fatter, even obese. In response to this social pressure, some of us take an extreme approach—the pathological pursuit of weight control or weight loss.

Early in life, we develop images of "acceptable" and "unacceptable" body types. Of the attributes that constitute attractiveness, many people view body weight as the most important, partly because we can control our weight somewhat. Fatness is the most dreaded deviation from our cultural ideals of body image, the one most derided and shunned, even among schoolchildren.

It is difficult to resist comparing ourselves to the "ideal" body. Not everyone can look like a fashion model. People who are overly impressed by media messages, especially those with genetic, psychological, and environmental influences, may be more likely than others to develop eating disorders in an effort to close the gap between reality and the perceived ideal.

FOR BETTER OR FOR WORSE

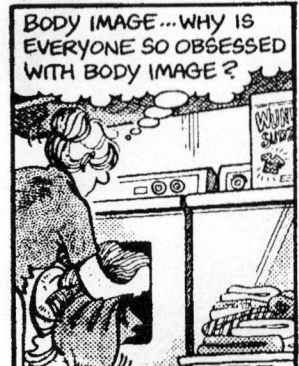
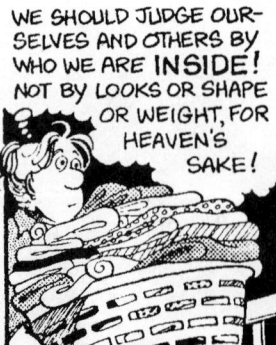
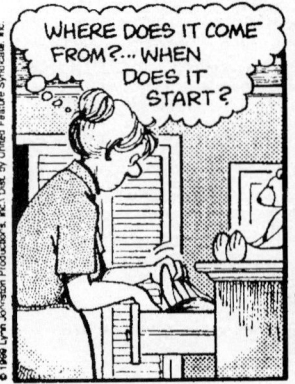
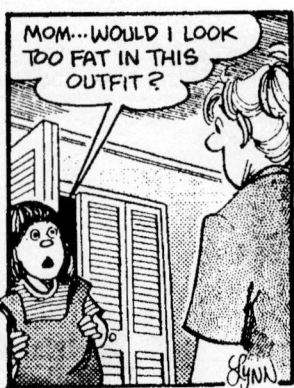

Concern with body image often starts early in life. Why do you think this is so? What societal trends have fostered this concern? Are some people more vulnerable, based on genetics and environment? Chapter 11 provides some answers.

© Lynn Johnston Productions, Inc. Distributed by United Features Syndicate, Inc.

Given the multiple functions associated with normal eating and constant exposure to our culture's ideal body image, it is not surprising that some people progress from typical responses to hunger and satiety cues to obsessive weight-loss behaviors, and then to a full-blown eating disorder.

Food: More than Just a Source of Nutrients

From birth, we link food with personal and emotional experiences. As infants, we associate milk with security and warmth so the breast or bottle becomes a source of comfort as well as food. As noted in Chapter 1, even when older, most people continue to derive comfort and great pleasure from food. This is both a biological and a psychological phenomenon. Food can be a symbol of comfort, but eating can also stimulate the release of certain neurotransmitters (e.g., serotonin) and *natural opioids* (including **endorphins**), which produce a sense of calm and euphoria in the human body. Thus, in times of great stress, some people turn to food for a druglike, calming effect.

Food is also used as a reward or a bribe. Haven't you heard or spoken something similar to the following comments?

You can have your dessert if you eat five more bites of your vegetables.
You can't play until you clean your plate.
I'll eat the broccoli if you let me watch TV.
If you love me, you'll eat your dinner.

On the surface, using food as a reward or bribe seems harmless enough. Eventually, however, this practice encourages both caregivers and children to use food to achieve goals other than satisfying hunger and nutrient needs. Food may then become much more than a source of nutrients. Regularly using food as a bargaining chip can contribute to abnormal eating patterns. Carried to the extreme, these patterns can lead to **disordered eating.**

Disordered eating can be defined as mild and short-term changes in eating patterns that occur in response to a stressful event, an illness, or even a desire to modify the diet for a variety of health and personal appearance reasons (see Further Reading 14). The problem may be no more than a bad habit, a style of eating adapted from friends or family members, or an aspect of preparing for athletic competition. While disordered eating can lead to weight loss or weight gain, as well as certain nutritional problems, it rarely requires in-depth professional attention. If, however, disordered eating becomes sustained, distressing, or starts to interfere with everyday activities and is linked to physiological changes, it may require professional intervention.

Overview of Anorexia Nervosa and Bulimia Nervosa

Given the common practice of dieting in North America, it can sometimes be difficult to tell where disordered eating stops and an **eating disorder** begins. Indeed, many eating disorders start with a simple diet. Eating disorders then go on to involve physiological changes associated with food restriction, binge eating, purging, and fluctuations in weight. They also involve a number of emotional and cognitive changes that affect the way a person perceives and experiences his or her body, such as feelings of distress or extreme concern about body shape or weight. Eating disorders are not due to a failure of will or behavior; rather, they are real, treatable medical illnesses in which certain maladaptive patterns of eating take on a life of their own.

The main types of eating disorders are **anorexia nervosa** and **bulimia nervosa**. Another type, **binge-eating disorder**, is not yet approved as a formal psychiatric diagnoses, but this will likely change with the update of the American Psychiatric Association's *Diagnostic and Statistical Manual of Mental Disorders*, expected in 2013. The various classifications of eating disorders are all rooted in an overvaluation of body shape or body weight as a source of self-identity. Although it is convenient to label patients with a particular diagnosis, the various types of eating disorders have more similarities than distinctions, particularly in the psychological processes that underlie them. Furthermore, people who cope with eating disorders tend to migrate from one type to another.

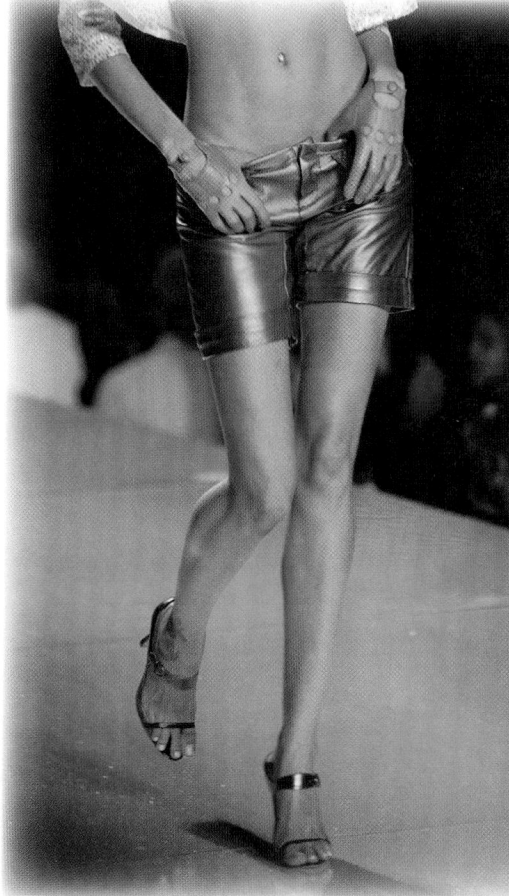

▲ Maintaining an anorexic body type is an all too common goal in today's culture. The media and the fashion world bombard us with body images that are unrealistic for most people.

endorphins Natural body tranquilizers that may be involved in the feeding response and function in pain reduction.

disordered eating Mild and short-term changes in eating patterns that occur in relation to a stressful event, an illness, or a desire to modify one's diet for a variety of health and personal appearance reasons.

eating disorder Severe alterations in eating patterns linked to physiological changes. The alterations are associated with food restriction, binge eating, purging, and fluctuations in weight. They also involve a number of emotional and cognitive changes that affect the way a person perceives and experiences his or her body.

Early detection is important (handwritten annotation)

anorexia nervosa An eating disorder involving a psychological loss or denial of appetite, followed by self-starvation; related in part to a distorted body image and to various social pressures commonly associated with puberty.

bulimia nervosa An eating disorder in which large quantities of food are eaten at one time (binge eating) and then purged from the body by vomiting, or misuse of laxatives, diuretics, or enemas. Alternate means to counteract the binge behavior are fasting and excessive exercise.

binge-eating disorder An eating disorder characterized by recurrent binge eating that is not followed by purging and has lasted at least 6 months. Binge episodes are characterized by loss of control over eating and can be triggered by frustration, anger, depression, anxiety, permission to eat forbidden foods, and excessive hunger.

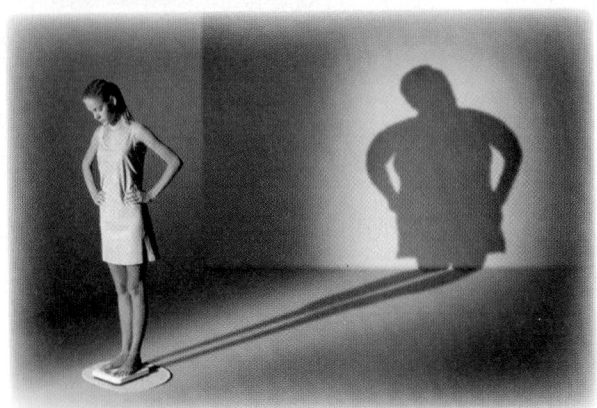

▲ Self-image is an important part of adolescence. For people with eating disorders, the difference between the real and desired body images may be too difficult to accept. See the website www.4women.gov/body-image.

Progression from Ordered to Disordered Eating

Attention to hunger and satiety signals; limitation of calorie intake to restore weight to a healthful level

↓

Some disordered eating habits begin as weight loss is attempted, such as very restricted eating

↓

Clinically evident eating disorder recognized

According to the National Eating Disorders Association, as many as 10 million people in the United States have an eating disorder. Eating disorders typically develop during adolescence or young adulthood, but increasingly, the onset occurs during childhood (an alarming trend; see Further Reading 2). Eating disorders frequently co-occur with other psychological disorders, such as depression, substance abuse, and anxiety disorders. *People who suffer from eating disorders, especially anorexia nervosa and bulimia nervosa, can experience a wide range of health complications, including heart conditions and kidney failure, which may even lead to death.* Recognition of eating disorders as important and treatable diseases, therefore, is critical.

Common to both eating disorders, *nervosa* refers to an attitude of disgust with one's body. The term *anorexia* implies a loss of appetite; however, a denial of one's appetite more accurately describes the behavior of people with anorexia nervosa. Anorexia nervosa is characterized by extreme weight loss; a distorted body image; and an irrational, almost morbid, fear of obesity and weight gain. Anorexic patients irrationally believe they are fat, even though others constantly comment on their thin physique. Some anorexics realize they are thin but continue to be haunted by certain areas of their bodies that they believe to be fat (such as thighs, buttocks, and stomach).

Bulimia nervosa (*bulimia* means "great [ox] hunger") is characterized by episodes of binge eating followed by attempts to purge the calories by vomiting or misusing laxatives, diuretics, or enemas. People with this disorder may be difficult to identify because they keep their binge-purge behaviors secret, and their symptoms are not obvious. Four percent or more of adolescent and college-age women suffer from bulimia nervosa. And, as with anorexia nervosa, about 10% of the cases occur in men.

Specific criteria are used by clinicians to diagnose eating disorders (e.g., *Diagnostic and Statistical Manual of Mental Disorders* of the American Psychiatric Association). Some characteristics are listed in Table 11-1. It is possible that people exhibit some symptoms of eating disorders but not enough to enable a medical worker to diagnose one of the two recognized diseases. Also, as suggested in the diagnostic criteria, some people show characteristics of both anorexia nervosa and bulimia nervosa because the diseases overlap considerably. About half of the women diagnosed as having anorexia nervosa eventually develop bulimic symptoms. As shown in Table 11-1, bulimic characteristics also can be seen in anorexia nervosa, which blurs the distinction. Still, appreciating the differences between the disorders helps us to understand the various approaches to prevention and treatment.

Certainly, women outnumber men when it comes to eating disorders—by at least 5 to 1. Currently, up to 5% of women in North America develop some form of anorexia nervosa or bulimia nervosa during their lifetimes. By rough estimate, approximately 0.5% (1 in 200) of women in North America eventually develop anorexia nervosa. Approximately 2% to 3% of women will develop bulimia nervosa. An estimated 95% of all cases of eating disorders occur among young women (ages 12 to 25). This high number may be due to the tendency of females to blame themselves for weight gain typical of their age group.

Men only account for 10% to 15% of all cases of eating disorders, partly because the image conveyed for men is big and muscular (see Making Decisions on page 463). Among men, exercise status and sexual orientation are factors that particularly influence development of eating disorders. Male athletes are more prone than nonathletes to develop eating disorders, especially those who participate in sports that require weight classes, such as boxers, wrestlers, and jockeys (see Further Readings 3 and 10). The rate of eating disorders among athletes lies between 10% and 20%. Other activities that may foster eating disorders in men include swimming, dancing and modeling. The prevalence of eating disorders in gay men is two to three times that of heterosexual men (see Further Reading 5).

ppl @ risk → (handwritten annotation) Until recently, most researchers have reported that eating disorders primarily affect middle- and upper-class Caucasian women. Now, studies show greater similarities in the rates of body dissatisfaction and disordered eating behaviors across ethnic and cultural groups. Perhaps minorities with eating disorders have been less likely to seek

TABLE 11-1 Typical Characteristics of Anorexic and Bulimic Persons

Anorexia Nervosa	Bulimia Nervosa
• Rigid dieting causing dramatic weight loss, generally to less than 85% of what would be expected for one's age (or BMI of 17.5 or less) • False body perception—thinking "I'm too fat," even when extremely underweight; relentless pursuit of control • Rituals involving food, excessive exercise, and other aspects of life • Maintenance of rigid control in lifestyle; security found in control and order • Feeling of panic after a small weight gain; intense fear of gaining weight • Feelings of purity, power, and superiority through maintenance of strict discipline and self-denial • Preoccupation with food, its preparation, and observing another person eat • Helplessness in the presence of food • Lack of menstrual periods (after what should be the age of puberty) for at least 3 months • Possible presence of bingeing and purging practices	• Secretive binge eating; generally not overeating in front of others • Eating when depressed or under stress • Bingeing on a large amount of food, followed by fasting, laxative or diuretic abuse, self-induced vomiting, or excessive exercise (at least twice a week for 3 months • Feelings of shame, embarrassment, deceit, and depression; low self-esteem and guilt (especially after a binge) • Fluctuating weight (±10 pounds or 5 kilograms) resulting from alternate bingeing and fasting • Loss of control; fear of not being able to stop eating • Perfectionism; "people pleaser"; food as the only comfort/escape in an otherwise carefully controlled and regulated life • Erosion of teeth, swollen glands • Purchase of syrup of ipecac, a compound sold in pharmacies that induces vomiting

Those who exhibit only one or a few of these characteristics may be at risk but probably do not have either disorder. They should, however, reflect on their eating habits and related concerns and take appropriate action, such as seeking a careful evaluation by a physician.

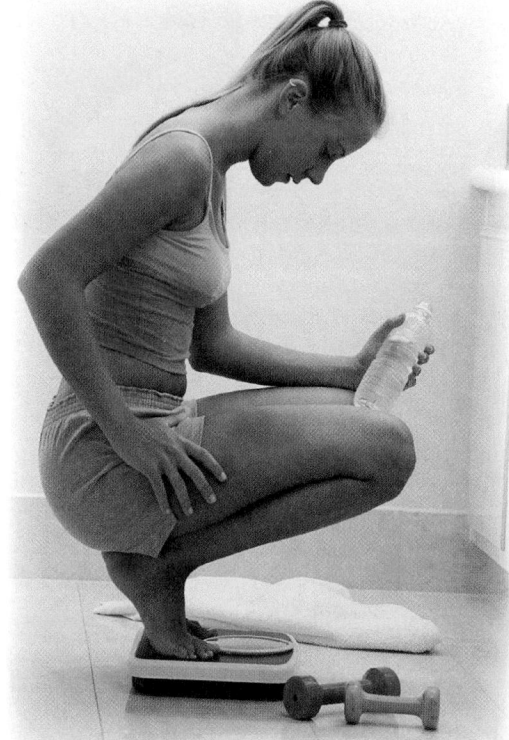

▲ Anorexia nervosa is characterized by a feeling of panic after only a small weight gain; bulimia nervosa is characterized by frequent weight fluctuations from alternate bingeing and fasting.

help in the past due to fear of shame or stigma, lack of resources, or language barriers. It seems more likely, however, that health care workers are less likely to diagnose non-Caucasians as having eating disorders. Previously, it seemed that non-Caucasian cultures were more accepting of larger body shapes, but mainstream pressures for thinness now seem to cut across racial differences. Our overall cultural change may be associated with increased vulnerability to eating disorders.

There are no simple causes of eating disorders, and there are no simple treatments. Stress may have an especially strong role in the development of eating disorders. An underlying commonality seems to be the lack of appropriate coping mechanisms as individuals begin to reach adolescence and young adulthood, coupled with dysfunctional family relationships.

The influence of genetics on the development of eating disorders is an area of active research. In general, twin studies have shown that identical twins have a higher likelihood of sharing eating disorders than do fraternal twins. This indicates that genetics is a strong risk factor in development of such disorders, because identical twins share the same DNA. One study found genetic background to describe 56% of the overall risk of developing anorexia nervosa. A variety of genes could be implicated in the development of eating disorders, including those that code for the expression of hormones and neurotransmitters involved in weight regulation and eating behaviors (review Chapter 1), as well as genes that lead to depression or individual responses to stress. In addition to the genetic code itself, researchers are also studying **epigenetics**, the interaction between genes and environmental influences as it relates to the development of eating disorders see Further Reading 4. Some studies suggest that maternal stress or hormone levels during pregnancy can predict the future development of an eating disorder in the offspring. Identifying genes that cause eating disorders eventually could

Our passion for thinness may have its roots in the Victorian era of the nineteenth century, which specialized in denying "unpleasant" physical realities, such as appetite and sexual desire. Flappers of the 1920s cemented the twentieth century trend for thinness. Since 1922, the BMI values of Miss America winners have steadily decreased; during the last three decades, most winners had a BMI in the "underweight" range (less than 18.5).

epigenetics The study of changes in gene function that are independent of DNA sequence. For example, malnutrition during pregnancy may modify gene expression in the fetus and affect long-term body weight regulation in the offspring.

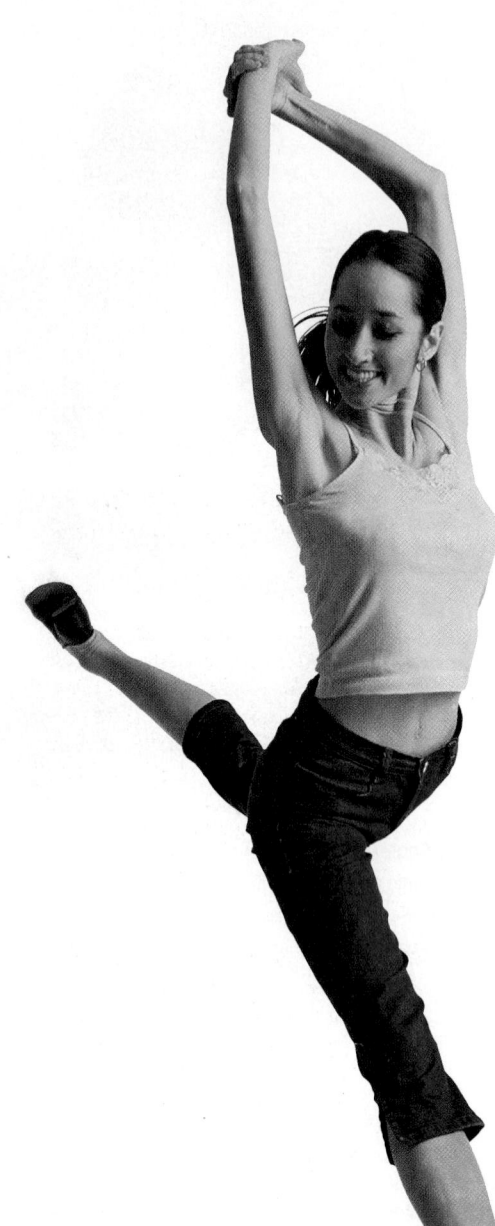

▲ Eating disorders are commonly seen in people who must maintain low body weight, such as ballet dancers (see Further Reading 16).

help in tailoring prevention and treatment efforts for at-risk individuals. However, the psychiatric counseling that is part of current therapy will still be of value.

Do you know someone who is at risk of these eating disorders? If so, suggest that the person seek a professional evaluation because, the sooner treatment begins, the better the chances for recovery. However, do not try to diagnose eating disorders in your friends or family members. Only a professional can exclude other possible diseases and correctly evaluate the diagnostic criteria required to make a diagnosis of anorexia nervosa or bulimia nervosa. Once an eating disorder is diagnosed, immediate treatment is advisable. As a friend, the best you can do is to encourage an affected person to seek professional help. Such help is commonly available at student health centers and student guidance/counseling facilities on college campuses.

11.2 A Closer Look at Anorexia Nervosa

Anorexia nervosa evolves from a dangerous mental state to an often life-threatening physical condition. As first described in the early medical literature in 1689, people suffering from this disorder think they are fat and intensely fear obesity and weight gain. They lose much more weight than is healthful. Although food is entwined in this disease, it stems more from psychological conflict.

About 3% of people with anorexia nervosa eventually die from the disease—from suicide, heart ailments, and infections. About one quarter of those with anorexia nervosa recover within 6 years, whereas the rest simply exist with the disease or go on to develop another form of eating disorder. The longer someone suffers from this eating disorder, the poorer the chances for complete recovery. A young patient with a brief episode and a cooperative family has a better outlook than an older patient with a long history of disordered eating and dysfunctional family relationships. Overall, prompt and vigorous treatment and close long-term follow-up improve the chances for success.

Anorexia nervosa may begin as a simple attempt to lose weight. A comment from a well-meaning friend, relative, or coach suggesting that the person seems to be gaining weight or is too fat may be all that is needed. The stress of having to maintain a certain weight to look attractive or competent on a job can also lead to disordered eating. Physical changes associated with puberty, the stress of leaving childhood, or the loss of a friend are examples of triggers for extreme dieting. Leaving home for college or starting a job can reinforce the desire to appear more "socially acceptable." Still, looking "good" does not necessarily help people deal with anger, depression, low self-esteem, or past experiences with sexual abuse. If these issues are behind the disorder and are not resolved as weight is lost, the individual may intensify efforts to lose weight "to look even better," rather than work through unresolved psychological concerns.

During adolescence, a period of turbulent sexual and social tensions, teenagers seek—and are often expected—to establish separate and independent lives. While declaring independence, they seek acceptance and support from peers and parents and react intensely to how they think others perceive them. At the same time, their bodies are changing, and much of the change is beyond their control. In response to the adolescent's or teenager's lack of control and coping mechanisms, dieting may start and then lead to a failure to gain appropriate weight-for-height. This may not be readily identified as a problem because the child has not actually lost any weight. Stunting (failure to grow in height) may also occur if inadequate calories are ingested during a period of growth. If anorexia develops before puberty, sexual maturation and menstruation also may be delayed.

Teens with chronic illnesses, such as type 1 diabetes or asthma, are at even greater risk for disordered eating. Any evidence of poor weight gain/maintenance or excessive exercise among these individuals needs to be investigated as a possible sign of disordered eating.

Extreme dieting is the most important predictor of an eating disorder. (Adolescents expressing concern about their weight should be advised to focus on exercise, which does not appear to impart a risk for subsequent problems.) Once dieting begins, a person developing anorexia nervosa does not stop. The result is a long period of rigidly self-enforced semistarvation, practiced almost with a vengeance, in a relentless pursuit of control. Anorexia nervosa may eventually lead to bingeing on large amounts of food in a short time, then purging. Purging occurs primarily through vomiting, but laxatives, diuretics, and enemas are also used. Thus, a person with anorexia nervosa may exist in a state of semistarvation or may alternate periods of starvation with periods of bingeing and purging.

Profile of the Typical Person with Anorexia Nervosa

A person with anorexia nervosa refuses to eat enough food to maintain an acceptable weight. This refusal is a hallmark of the disease, whether or not other practices, such as binge-purge cycles, appear. The most typical anorexic person is a Caucasian female from the middle or upper socioeconomic class. Perhaps her mother also has distorted views of desirable body shape and acceptable food habits. The girl is often described by parents and teachers as responsible, meticulous, and obedient.

She is competitive and often obsessive. Her parents set high standards for her. At home, she may not allow clutter in her bedroom. Physicians note that, after a physical examination, she may fold her examination gown very carefully and clean up the examination room before leaving. Even though such behavior may seem odd, only a skilled professional can tell the difference between anorexia nervosa and other adolescent complaints, such as delayed puberty, fatigue, and depression.

A common thread underlying many—but not all—cases of anorexia nervosa is conflict within the family structure, typically with an overbearing mother and an emotionally absent father. When family expectations are always too high—including those regarding body weight—frustration results and leads to fighting. Overinvolvement, rigidity, over-protection, and denial are typical daily transactions of such families.

Issues of control are central to the development of anorexia nervosa. Often, the eating disorder allows an anorexic person to exercise control over an otherwise powerless existence. Losing weight may be the first independent success the person has had. People with anorexia evaluate their self-worth almost entirely in terms of self-control. Some sexually abused children develop anorexia nervosa, believing that if they control their appetite for food, sexual relations, and human contact, they will feel in control and competent and will eliminate shameful feelings. Moreover, food restriction, which arrests development and shuts down sexual impulses, may be a strategy to prevent future victimization and guilt feelings. Often anorexic persons feel hopeless about human relationships and socially isolated because of their dysfunctional families. They focus on food, eating, and weight instead of human relationships.

Early Warning Signs

A person developing anorexia nervosa exhibits important warning signs. At first, dieting becomes the life focus. The person may think, "The only thing I am good at is dieting. I can't do anything else." This innocent beginning often leads to very abnormal self-perceptions and eating habits, such as cutting a pea in half before eating it. Other habits include hiding and storing food or spreading food around a plate to make it look as if much has been eaten. An anorexic person may cook a large meal and watch others eat it while refusing to eat anything. Anorexic persons may also exercise compulsively to the point that it is obsessive. Exercise can interfere with life activities or occur at unusual times or settings—for example, doing squats while brushing teeth.

As the disorder progresses, the range of foods may narrow and be rigidly divided into safe and unsafe ones, with the list of safe foods becoming progressively shorter. For people developing anorexia nervosa, these practices say "I am in control." These people may be hungry, but they deny it, driven by the belief that good things will happen by just becoming thin enough. It becomes a question of willpower.

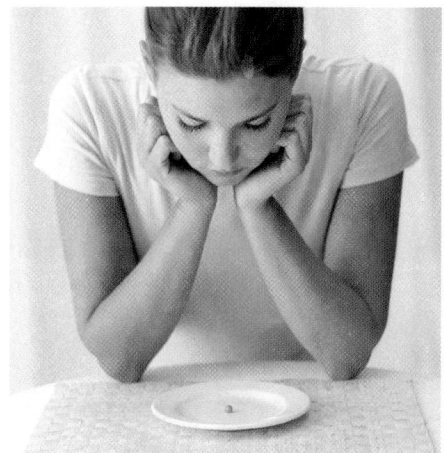

▲ Extreme dietary rules severely limit nutritional intake among people with anorexia nervosa.

Links exist between disordered eating behaviors and substance abuse, particularly alcohol abuse. Some people may use food restriction or purging to offset the calories consumed during drinking binges. Popularly called "drunkorexia," this practice can lead to severe nutrient deficiencies and dehydration.

Anorexia Nervosa

By severely limiting calorie intake for long periods, adolescent girls and young adult women greatly compromise their nutritional status, impair their reproductive systems, and restrict growth. The harm produced by milder, shorter periods of diet restriction is not clear. Evidence, however, suggests that even moderate diet restriction, if continued, contributes to the risks for various forms of anemia, future pregnancy complications and delivery of low-birth-weight infants, and permanently reduced bone mass.

[Handwritten annotations in margins:]
animal products: ready to eat cereal, potato & milk
B6: Spinach, broccoli, banana, sunflower seed

People with anorexia become irritable and hostile and begin to withdraw from family and friends. School performance generally crumbles. They refuse to eat out with family and friends, thinking, "I won't be able to have the foods I want to eat," or "I won't be able to throw up afterward."

Anorexic persons see themselves as rational and others as irrational. They also tend to be excessively critical of themselves and others. Nothing is good enough. Because it cannot be perfect, life appears meaningless and hopeless. A sense of joylessness pervades everything.

As stress increases in the person's life, sleep disturbances and depression are common. Many of the psychological and physical problems associated with anorexia nervosa arise from insufficient calorie intake, as well as deficiencies of nutrients, such as thiamin and vitamin B-6. For a female, the combination of problems—coupled with lower and lower body weight and fat stores—causes menstrual periods to cease. This may be the first sign of the disease that a parent notices and represents an additional hallmark of the disease.

Ultimately, an anorexic person eats very little food; 300 to 600 kcal daily is not unusual. In place of food, the person may consume up to 20 cans of diet soft drinks and chew many pieces of sugarless gum each day.

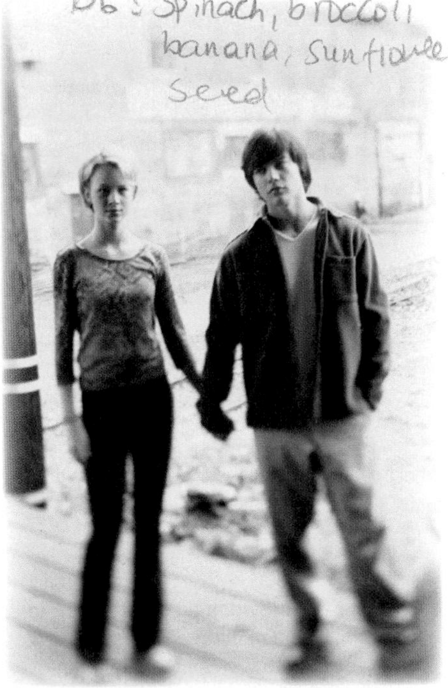

Physical Effects of Anorexia Nervosa

Rooted in the emotional state of the victim, anorexia nervosa produces profound physical effects. The anorexic person often appears to be skin and bones. Body weight less than 85% of that expected is one clinical indicator of anorexia nervosa. This percentage can be calculated using the Metropolitan Life Insurance Company tables (see Appendix G), but body build and weight history should also be used when estimating an appropriate weight. BMI is a more reliable indicator of the degree of malnourishment; generally, a BMI of 17.5 or less indicates a severe case (review Chapter 7 for more on BMI). For children under age 18, growth charts should be used to assess weight status (see Chapter 15).

[Handwritten: Bd weigh in kg/height² in meter or wei hei]

The state of semistarvation disturbs many body systems as it forces the body to conserve energy stores as much as possible (Fig. 11-1). This attempt to conserve energy stores is the cause of most of the physical effects. Thus, many complications can be reversed by returning to a healthy weight, provided the duration of the insult has not been too long. The following are predictable effects caused by hormonal responses to and deficient nutrient intakes from semistarvation:

- Lowered body temperature and cold intolerance from loss of insulating fat layer.
- Slowed metabolic rate from decreased synthesis of thyroid hormones.
- Decreased heart rate as metabolism slows, leading to premature fatigue, fainting, and an overwhelming need for sleep. Other changes in heart function may occur as well, including loss of heart tissue and irregular heart rhythm.
- Iron-deficiency anemia, which leads to further weakness.
- Rough, dry, scaly, and cold skin, which may show multiple bruises because of the loss of the protective fat layer normally present under the skin.
- Low white blood cell count, which increases the risk of infection—one cause of death in people with anorexia nervosa.
- Abnormal feeling of fullness or bloating, which can last for several hours after eating.
- Loss of hair.
- Appearance of **lanugo**—downy hairs on the body that trap air to partially counteract heat loss that occurs with loss of fat tissue.
- Constipation due to deterioration of the gastrointestinal tract and abuse of laxatives.

▲ Anorexia nervosa occurs much more frequently in young women than in young men.

[Handwritten: Thiamin - pork, sunflower, milk, whole & enriched grains, orange juice, organ meat, dried beans, & peanuts, breakfast cereal]

Parents may not consider a teenager mature enough to make decisions. If the teen disagrees and the situation is very tense, she may turn to purging or starving as a way to show her power: "You may try to control my life, but I can do anything I want with my body."

In the words of one young woman, "I couldn't get angry, because it would be like destroying someone else, like my mother. It felt like she would hate me forever. I got angry through anorexia nervosa. It was my last hope. It's my own body and this was my last-ditch effort."

lanugo Downlike hair that appears after a person has lost much body fat through semistarvation. The hair stands erect and traps air, acting as insulation for the body to compensate for the relative lack of body fat, which usually functions as insulation.

- Low blood potassium, worsened by potassium losses during vomiting and use of some types of diuretics. This increases the risk of heart rhythm disturbances, another leading cause of death in anorexic people.
- Loss of menstrual periods because of low body weight, low body fat content, and the stress of the disease. Accompanying hormonal changes contribute to bone loss.
- Changes in neurotransmitter function in the brain, which lead to depression
- Osteopenia (i.e., low bone mass, evident in 90% of adult women with anorexia nervosa) and osteoporosis (evident in at least one site in 40% of adult women with anorexia nervosa). Bone loss is due to decreased body weight and lean mass, several related hormonal changes, and prolonged use of some antidepressant medications.
- Eventual loss of teeth caused by acid erosion of tooth enamel if frequent vomiting occurs. Until vomiting ceases, one way to reduce this effect on teeth is to rinse the mouth with water right away and brush the teeth as soon as possible. Loss of teeth (along with low bone mass) can be lasting signs of the disease, even if the other physical and mental problems are resolved.
- Muscle tears and stress fractures in athletes because of decreased bone and muscle mass.

A person with this disorder is psychologically and physically ill and needs help.

CONCEPT CHECK

Anorexia nervosa is an eating disorder characterized by semistarvation. It is found primarily—but not exclusively—in adolescent girls, starting at or around puberty. People with anorexia dwindle essentially to skin and bones yet still believe they are fat. Semistarvation produces hormonal changes and nutrient deficiencies, which lower body temperature; slow the heart rate; decrease immune response; stop menstrual periods; and contribute to hair, muscle, and bone loss. It is a serious disease, which often produces lifelong consequences and may be fatal.

CRITICAL THINKING

Jennifer is an attractive 13-year-old. However, she's very compulsive. Everything has to be perfect—her hair, her clothes, even her room. Her body is beginning to mature, so she's obsessed with having perfect physical features as well. Her parents are worried about her behavior. Given her behavioral traits, what symptoms of an eating disorder should they watch for? What should Jennifer's parents do if they suspect an eating disorder?

Erika Goodman, former dancer with the Joffrey Ballet, became crippled from osteoporosis resulting from years of restricting food intake to maintain a low body weight. Her food restriction led to irregular or absent menstrual periods for many years. She died in 2004 at the age of 59 after falling in her Manhattan apartment.

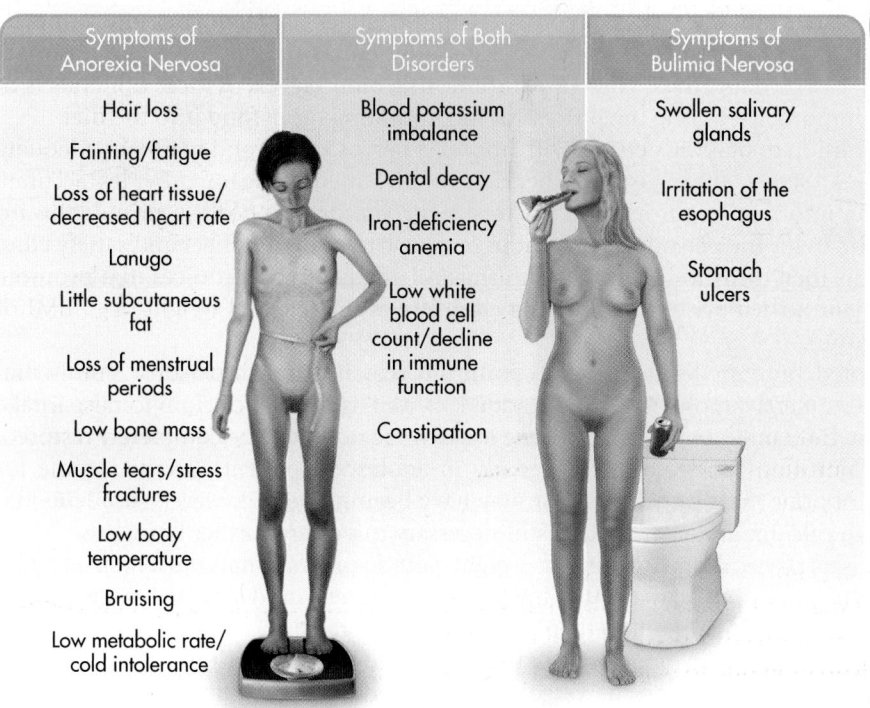

Symptoms of Anorexia Nervosa	Symptoms of Both Disorders	Symptoms of Bulimia Nervosa
Hair loss	Blood potassium imbalance	Swollen salivary glands
Fainting/fatigue	Dental decay	Irritation of the esophagus
Loss of heart tissue/decreased heart rate	Iron-deficiency anemia	Stomach ulcers
Lanugo	Low white blood cell count/decline in immune function	
Little subcutaneous fat		
Loss of menstrual periods	Constipation	
Low bone mass		
Muscle tears/stress fractures		
Low body temperature		
Bruising		
Low metabolic rate/cold intolerance		

FIGURE 11-1 ▶ Signs and symptoms of eating disorders. A vast array of physical effects are associated with anorexia nervosa and bulimia nervosa. This figure contains many but is not an exhaustive list of all potential consequences. These physical effects can also serve as warning signs that a problem exists. Professional evaluation is then indicated.

Singer Karen Carpenter's death from complications of anorexia nervosa in 1983 increased awareness of the serious nature of this disease. Currently, the average time for recovery from anorexia nervosa is 7 years; many insurance companies cover only a fraction of the estimated $150,000 cost of treatment.

A young woman in a self-help group for those with anorexia nervosa explained her feelings to the other group members: "I have lost a specialness that I thought it gave me. I was different from everyone else. Now I know that I'm somebody who's overcome it, which not everybody does."

A disturbing trend is the attempt to promote eating disorders as a way of life. Some anorexic individuals have personified their illness into a role model named "Ana," who tells them what to eat and mocks them when they don't lose weight. Ana websites reject the serious health risks of anorexia behaviors and instead dispense unsafe "thinspiration" to vulnerable individuals (see Further Reading 12).

Treatment of Anorexia Nervosa

People with anorexia often sink into shells of isolation and fear. They deny that a problem exists. Frequently, their friends and family members meet with them to confront the problem in a loving way. This is called an *intervention*. They present evidence of the problem and encourage immediate treatment. Treatment then requires a multidisciplinary team of experienced physicians, registered dietitians, psychologists, and other health professionals working together. An ideal setting is an eating disorders clinic in a medical center. Outpatient therapy generally begins first. This may be extended to 3 to 5 days per week. Day hospitalization (6 to 12 hours) is another option, as is total hospitalization. Hospitalization is necessary once a person falls below 75% of expected weight, experiences acute medical problems, and/or exhibits severe psychological problems or suicidal risk. Still, even in the most skilled hands at the finest facilities, efforts may fail. This tells us that the prevention of anorexia nervosa is of utmost importance.

Once a medical team has gained the cooperation and trust of an anorexic person, the team attempts to work together to restore a sense of balance, purpose, and future possibilities. As previously stated, anorexia nervosa is usually rooted in psychological conflict. However, the anorexic person who has been barely existing in a state of semi-starvation cannot focus on much besides food. Dreams and even morbid thoughts about food will interfere with therapy until sufficient weight is regained.

Nutrition Therapy. The first goal of nutrition therapy is to gain the person's cooperation and trust, with the ultimate objective of increasing oral food intake. Ideally, weight gain must be enough to raise the metabolic rate to normal and reverse as many physical signs of the disease as possible. Food intake is designed first to minimize or stop any further weight loss. Then, the focus shifts to restoring appropriate food habits. After this, the expectation can be switched to slowly gaining weight. A gain of 2 to 3 pounds per week is appropriate. Tube and/or intravenous (IV) feeding is used only if immediate renourishment is required, as this can frighten the person and cause him or her to distrust medical staff.

Persons with anorexia nervosa need considerable reassurance during the refeeding process because of uncomfortable and unfamiliar effects—such as bloating, increase in body heat, and increase in body fat. This is a frightening process because these changes can symbolize a loss of control. Rapid changes in electrolytes and minerals in the blood associated with refeeding, especially potassium, phosphorus, and magnesium, can be dangerous. Therefore, monitoring blood levels of these minerals is of critical importance during the process of incorporating more food into the diet.

In addition to helping persons with anorexia nervosa reach and maintain adequate nutritional status, the registered dietitian on the medical team provides accurate nutrition information throughout the treatment, promotes a healthy attitude toward food, and helps the person learn to eat in response to natural hunger and satiety cues. The focus then turns to identifying healthy and adequate food choices that promote weight gain to achieve and maintain a clinically estimated goal weight (e.g., BMI of 20 or more).

As noted, nutrient deficiencies are commonly seen in anorexic persons. A multivitamin and mineral supplement will be added, as well as enough calcium to raise intake to about 1500 milligrams per day. Bone loss will be not likely be completely restored, even if nutrition is adequate. Particularly in adolescent patients, a critical time for accrual of bone mass or gains height may have been missed. However, supplementation with calcium and vitamin D is still necessary to prevent further bone loss.

Excessive physical activity prevents weight gain, so professionals must help anorexic persons regulate their activity. At many treatment centers, moderate bed rest is used in the early stages of treatment to help promote weight gain.

Experienced professional help is the key (see Further Readings 1 and 11). An anorexic person may be on the verge of suicide and starvation. In addition, anorexic people are often very clever and resistant to therapy. They may try to hide weight loss by wearing many layers of clothes, putting coins in their pockets or underwear, and drinking numerous glasses of water before stepping on the scale.

Psychological and Related Therapy. Once the physical problems of anorexia nervosa are addressed, the treatment focus shifts to the underlying emotional problems that led to excessive dieting and other symptoms of the disorder. To heal, these anorexic persons must reject the sense of accomplishment they have associated with an emaciated body and begin to accept themselves at a healthy body weight. If therapists can discover reasons for the disorder, they can develop strategies for restoring normal weight and eating habits that involve resolving psychological conflicts. Education about the medical consequences of semistarvation is also helpful. A key aspect of psychological treatment is showing affected individuals how to regain control of other facets of their lives and cope with difficult situations. As eating evolves into a normal routine, they can turn to previously neglected activities.

Therapists may use **cognitive behavior therapy,** which involves helping the person confront and change irrational beliefs about body image, eating, relationships, and weight. Underlying issues that may be the cause for the disease, such as sexual abuse, also must be identified and addressed by the therapist.

Family therapy often is important in treating anorexia nervosa, especially for younger persons who still live with their families. It focuses on the role of the illness among family members, the reactions of individual family members and ways in which their subconscious behavior might contribute to the abnormal eating patterns. Frequently, a therapist finds family struggles at the heart of the problem. As the disorder resolves, patients must relate to family members in new ways to gain the attention that was needed and previously tied to the disease. For example, the family may need to help the young person ease into adulthood and accept its responsibilities as well as its advantages. Self-help groups for anorexic (and bulimic) people, as well as their families and friends, represent nonthreatening first steps into treatment.

Food is the drug of choice in the treatment of anorexic patients. Generally, medications are not effective in management of the primary symptoms of anorexia nervosa. Fluoxetine (Prozac®) and related medications may stabilize recovery once 85% of expected body weight has been attained. These medications work by prolonging serotonin activity in the brain, which in turn regulates mood and feelings of satiety. A variety of other pharmacologic agents, such as olanzapine (Zyprexa®), may have some role in treating mood changes, anxiety, or psychotic symptoms associated with anorexia nervosa, but they have limited value unless weight gain is also achieved.

With professional help, many people with anorexia nervosa can lead normal lives. Although they may not be totally cured, anorexic individuals do not have to depend on unusual eating habits to cope with daily problems. They recover a sense of normalcy in their lives. Longer follow-up—sometimes several years—is associated with better outcomes. No universal approach exists, because each case is unique. Establishing a strong relationship with either a therapist or another supportive person is an especially important key to recovery. Once anorexic persons feel understood and accepted by another person, they can begin to build a sense of self and exercise some autonomy. As they learn alternative coping mechanisms, they can relinquish their dysfunctional relationships with food and instead develop healthy personal relationships.

cognitive behavior therapy Psychological therapy in which the person's assumptions about dieting, body weight, and related issues are confronted. New ways of thinking are explored and then practiced by the person. In this way, an individual can learn new ways to control disordered eating behaviors and related life stress.

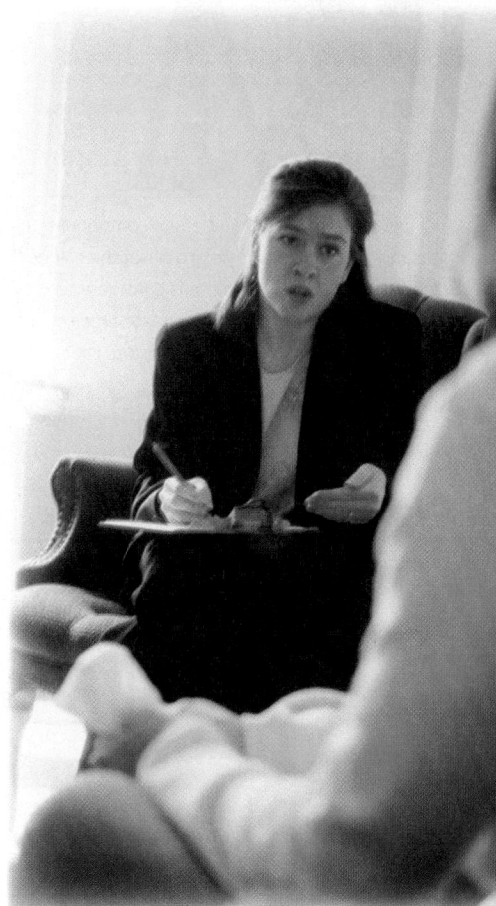

▲ Early treatment for an eating disorder, such as anorexia nervosa, improves chances of success.

CONCEPT CHECK

To relieve the semistarved condition of most anorexic persons, the initial treatment focuses on moderately increased food intake and slow weight gain. Once this is accomplished, psychotherapy can begin to uncover the causes of the disease and help the individual develop the skills needed to return to a healthy life. Family therapy can be an important tool in treatment, whereas medications have a limited role.

Bingeing and purging (via vomiting) was evident in pre-Christian Roman times, but was practiced in a group setting. The eating disorder bulimia nervosa is generally practiced in private. It was first described in the medical literature in 1979.

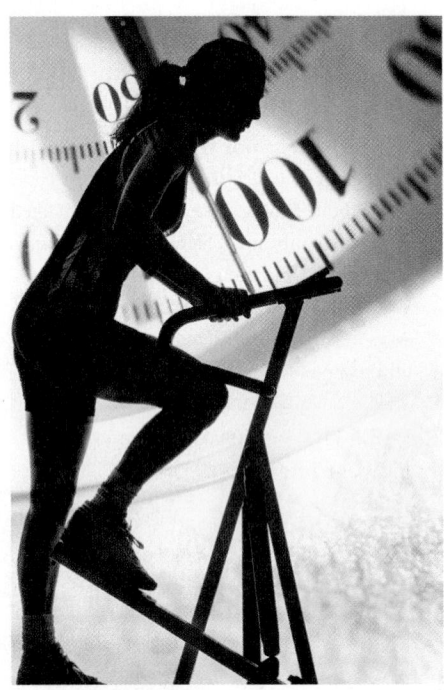

▲ Excessive exercise can be one component of bulimia if it is used as a way to offset the calorie intake from a binge. Exercise is considered excessive when it is done at inappropriate times or settings or when a person does it despite injury or other medical complications.

11.3 A Closer Look at Bulimia Nervosa

Bulimia nervosa involves episodes of binge eating followed by various means to purge the food. It is most common among young adults of college age, although some high school students are also at risk. Susceptible people often have genetic factors and lifestyle patterns that predispose them to becoming overweight, and many try frequent weight-reduction diets as teenagers. Like people with anorexia nervosa, those with bulimia nervosa are usually female and successful. Unlike anorexic individuals, however, they are usually at or slightly above a normal weight. Females with bulimia nervosa are also more likely to be sexually active than those with anorexia nervosa.

The person with bulimia nervosa may think of food constantly. But unlike the anorexic person, who turns away from food when faced with problems, the bulimic person turns toward food in critical situations. Also, unlike those with anorexia nervosa, people with bulimia nervosa recognize their behavior as abnormal. These people often have low self-esteem and are depressed. Approximately half of the people with bulimia nervosa have major depression. Lingering effects of child abuse may be one reason for these feelings. Many bulimic persons report that they have been sexually abused. They appear competent to outsiders, while they actually feel out of control, ashamed, and frustrated.

Bulimic people tend to be impulsive, which may be expressed in behaviors such as stealing, increased sexual activity, drug and alcohol abuse, self-mutilation, or attempted suicide. Some experts have suggested that part of the problem may actually arise from an inability to control responses to impulse and desire. Some studies have demonstrated that bulimic people tend to come from disengaged families—ones that are loosely organized. In these families, roles for family members are not clearly defined, rules are disregarded, and a great deal of conflict exists. (In contrast, anorexic people tend to have families so actively engaged that roles may be too well defined.)

Typical Behavior in Bulimia Nervosa

It is likely that many people with bulimic behavior are never diagnosed; the diagnostic criteria specify that a person must binge and purge at least twice a week for 3 months. People with bulimia nervosa lead secret lives, hiding their abnormal eating habits. Moreover, it is impossible to recognize the disorder simply by appearance. Most diagnoses of bulimia nervosa rely on self-reports, so estimates of the number of cases are probably low. The disorder, especially in its milder forms, may be much more widespread than commonly thought.

For intake to qualify as a binge, an atypically large amount of food must be consumed in a short time and the person must exhibit a lack of control over his or her behavior. Among sufferers of bulimia nervosa, bingeing often alternates with attempts to rigidly restrict food intake. Elaborate food rules are common, such as avoiding all sweets. Thus, eating just one cookie or donut may cause individuals with this disorder to feel as though they have broken a rule. At that point, in the mind of a bulimic person, the objectionable food must be eliminated. Usually this leads to further overeating, partly because it is easier to regurgitate a large amount of food than a small amount.

Binge-purge cycles may be practiced daily, weekly, or across longer intervals. A specific time often is set aside. Most binge eating occurs at night, when other people are less likely to interrupt, and usually lasts from ½ to 2 hours. A binge can be triggered by a combination of stress, boredom, loneliness, and depression. It often follows a period of strict dieting and thus can be linked to intense hunger. The binge is not at all like normal eating; once begun, it seems to propel itself. The person not only loses control, but generally doesn't even taste or enjoy food during a binge. This separates the practice from overeating.

Most commonly, bulimic people consume cakes, cookies, ice cream, and other high-carbohydrate convenience foods during binges because these foods can be purged relatively easily and comfortably by vomiting. In a single binge, foods supplying 3000 kcal or more may be eaten. Purging follows in hopes that no weight will be gained. However, even when vomiting follows the binge, 33% to 75% of the calories taken in are still absorbed, inevitably causing some weight gain. When laxatives or enemas are used, about 90% of the calories are absorbed, as laxatives act in the large intestine, beyond the point of most nutrient absorption. The belief that purging soon after bingeing will prevent excessive calorie absorption and weight gain is a misconception.

At the onset of bulimia nervosa, sufferers often induce vomiting by placing their fingers deep into the mouth. They may bite down on these fingers inadvertently, resulting in bite marks and scars around the knuckles, a characteristic sign of this disorder. Once the disease is established, however, a person may be able to vomit simply by contracting the abdominal muscles. Vomiting may also occur spontaneously.

Another way bulimic persons attempt to compensate for a binge and control their weight is by engaging in excessive exercise to expend a large amount of calories. In this practice, referred to as "debting," bulimic individuals try to estimate the amount of calories eaten during a binge, and then exercise to counteract the excess.

People with bulimia nervosa are not proud of their behavior. After a binge, they usually feel guilty and depressed. Over time, they experience low self-esteem, feel hopeless about their situation, and are caught in a vicious cycle of obsession (Fig. 11-2). Compulsive lying, shoplifting to obtain food, and drug abuse can further intensify these feelings. Bulimic people discovered in the act of bingeing by a friend or family member may order the intruder to "get out" and "go away." Sufferers gradually distance themselves from others, spending more time preoccupied by and engaging in bingeing and purging.

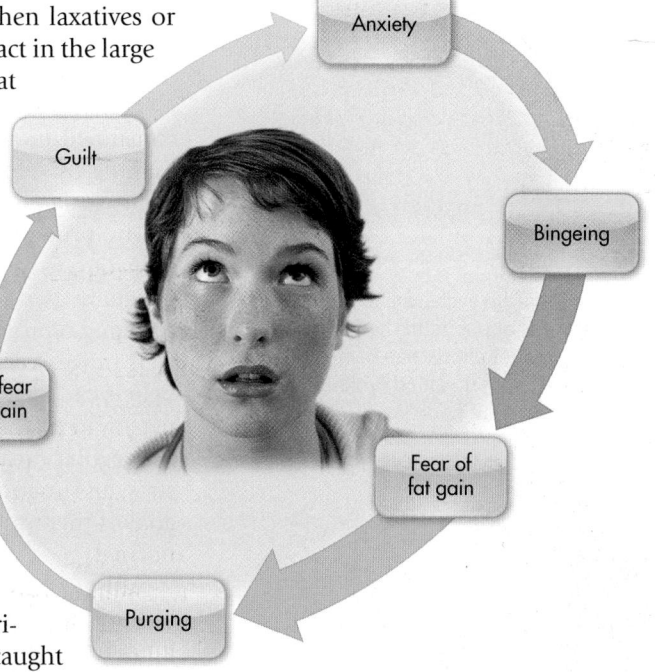

FIGURE 11-2 ▶ Bulimia nervosa's vicious cycle of obsession.

Health Problems Stemming from Bulimia Nervosa

The vomiting that many bulimic sufferers induce is a physically destructive method of purging. Indeed, the majority of health problems associated with bulimia nervosa, as noted here, arise from vomiting:

- Repeated exposure of teeth to stomach acid causes demineralization, making the teeth painful and sensitive to heat, cold, and acids. Eventually, the teeth may decay severely, erode away from fillings, and finally fall out. Dental professionals are sometimes the first health professionals to notice signs of bulimia nervosa. As noted, it is important to rinse the mouth with water after any vomiting episode, especially before brushing the teeth.
- Blood potassium can drop significantly with regular vomiting or the use of certain diuretics. This can disturb the heart's rhythm and even produce sudden death.
- Salivary glands may swell as a result of infection and irritation from persistent vomiting.
- Stomach ulcers and bleeding and tears in the esophagus develop in some cases.
- Constipation may result from frequent laxative use.
- Ipecac syrup, sometimes used to induce vomiting, is toxic to the heart, liver, and kidneys. It has caused accidental poisoning when taken repeatedly.

Overall, bulimia nervosa is a potentially debilitating disorder that can lead to death, usually from suicide, low blood potassium, or overwhelming infections.

Treatment of Bulimia Nervosa

Therapy for bulimia nervosa, as for anorexia nervosa, requires a team of experienced clinicians (see Further Reading 1). Bulimic individuals are less likely than those with anorexia to enter treatment in a state of semistarvation. However, if a bulimic person has lost significant weight, this must be treated before psychological treatment begins.

People with type 1 diabetes may intentionally skip doses of insulin to induce weight loss. This practice, so called "diabulimia," can have dangerous consequences, such as eye damage, kidney damage, diabetic coma, or death (see Further Reading 6).

Although clinicians have yet to agree on the best therapy for bulimia nervosa, they generally agree that treatment should last at least 16 weeks. Hospitalization may be indicated in cases of extreme laxative abuse, regular vomiting, substance abuse, and depression, especially if physical harm is evident.

The first goal of treatment for bulimia nervosa is to decrease the amount of food consumed in a binge session to decrease the risk of esophageal tears from related purging by vomiting. A decrease in the frequency of this type of purging will also decrease damage to the teeth.

The primary aim of psychotherapy is to improve a persons' self-acceptance and help one to be less concerned about body weight. Cognitive behavior therapy is generally used (see Further Reading 11). Psychotherapy helps correct the all-or-none thinking typical of bulimic persons: "If I eat one cookie, I'm a failure and might as well binge." The premise of this psychotherapy is that, if abnormal attitudes and beliefs can be altered, normal eating will follow. In addition, the therapist guides the person in establishing food habits that will minimize bingeing: avoiding fasting, eating regular meals, and using alternative methods—other than eating—to cope with stressful situations. Group therapy is often useful to foster strong social support. One goal of therapy is to help bulimic persons accept some depression and self-doubt as normal.

Although pharmacological agents should not be used as the sole treatment for bulimia nervosa, studies indicate that some medications may be beneficial in conjunction with other therapies. Fluoxetine (Prozac®) is the only antidepressant that has been approved by FDA for use in the treatment of bulimia nervosa, but physicians also may prescribe other similar forms of antidepressants, other classes of psychiatric medications, or certain antiseizure medications, (e.g., topiramate [Topamax®]).

Nutritional counseling has two main goals: correcting misconceptions about food and re-establishing regular eating habits. Bulimic persons are given information about bulimia nervosa and its consequences. Avoiding binge foods and not constantly stepping on a scale may be recommended early in treatment. The primary goal, however, is to develop a normal eating pattern. To achieve this goal, some specialists encourage these individuals to develop daily meal plans and keep a food diary in which they record food intake, internal sensations of hunger, environmental factors that precipitate binges, and thoughts and feelings that accompany binge-purge cycles. Keeping a food diary not only is an accurate way to monitor food intake but also may help identify situations that seem to trigger binge episodes. With the help of a therapist, bulimic persons can develop alternative coping strategies.

In general, the focus is not on stopping bingeing and purging *per se* but on developing regular eating habits. Once this is achieved, the binge-purge cycle should start to break down. Individuals are discouraged from following strict rules about healthy food choices, because this mimics the typical obsessive attitudes associated with bulimia nervosa. Rather, encouraging a mature perspective on nutrient intake—that is, regular consumption of moderate amounts of a variety of foods balanced among the food groups—helps one overcome this disorder.

Setting time limits for the completion of meals and snacks is important for people with eating disorders. Many bulimic persons eat quickly, reflecting their difficulties with satiety. Suggesting that the person put his or her utensil down after each bite is a behavioral technique that a therapist might try during recovery for bulimia. (In comparison, many anorexic persons eat in an excessively slow manner—for example, taking 1 hour to eat a muffin cut into tiny, bite-size pieces.)

People with bulimia nervosa must recognize that they have a serious disorder that can have grave medical complications if not treated. Relapse is likely, so therapy should be long term. Those with bulimia nervosa need professional help because they can be very depressed and are at a high risk for suicide. About 50% of people with bulimia nervosa recover completely from the disorder. Others continue to struggle with it to varying degrees for the rest of their lives. Such a difficult course of treatment underscores the need for prevention.

The binge-purge cycle can create an initial state of euphoria in the person. Giving up this euphoria has been equated to giving up an addiction. Still, it is important to do so.

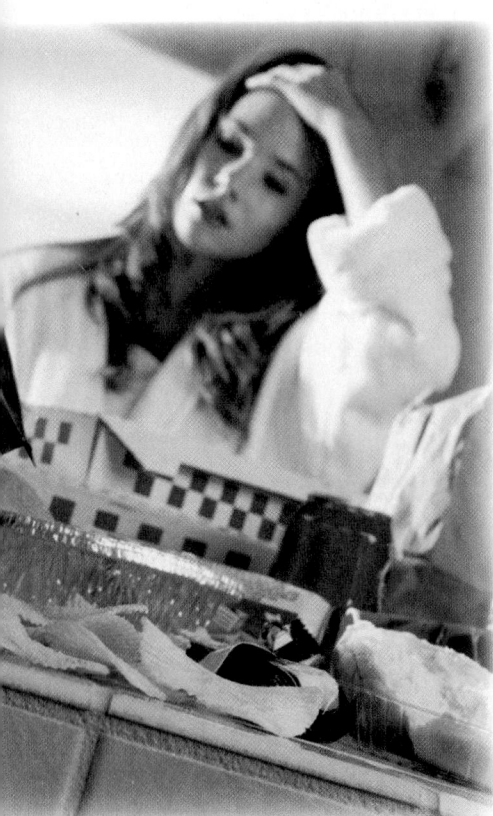

▲ Developing regular eating habits helps a person with bulimia nervosa to stop the binge-purge cycle.

CONCEPT CHECK

Bulimia nervosa is characterized by episodes of binge eating followed by purging, usually by vomiting. Vomiting is very destructive to the body, often causing severe dental decay, stomach ulcers, irritation of the esophagus, and blood potassium imbalances. Treatment using nutrition counseling and psychotherapy attempts to restore normal eating habits, to help the person correct distorted beliefs about diet and lifestyle, and to find tools to cope with the stresses of life. Medications, such as fluoxetine (Prozac®), can aid recovery when added to this regimen.

11.4 Other Disordered Eating Patterns

In recent years, other patterns of disordered eating have been recognized (see Further Readings 6, 8, 9, and 10). Several of these patterns fall under the diagnosic category, *eating disorder not otherwise specified* (EDNOS). EDNOS is described in the American Psychiatric Association diagnostic manual as a "category [of] disorders of eating that do not meet the criteria for any specific eating disorder."

The EDNOS category is frequently used for people who have some, but not all, of the characteristics of anorexia nervosa or bulimia nervosa. Each EDNOS has distinctive qualities. For example, a person may experience episodes of bingeing and purging, but not frequently enough to meet the diagnosis of bulimia nervosa. A person may also engage in bingeing episodes without the use of inappropriate compensatory behaviors; this is referred to as binge-eating disorder. Another disordered eating pattern under study is night eating syndrome. **Night eating syndrome** is characterized by eating a lot of food in the late evening and nocturnal awakening with ingestion of food. Finally, the **female athlete triad** is a condition characterized by disordered eating, lack of menstrual periods, and osteoporosis. These conditions have been recognized as requiring professional treatment and are discussed in the following sections.

Binge-Eating Disorder

The typical characteristics for binge-eating disorder are listed in Table 11-2. Generally, it can be defined as binge-eating episodes not accompanied by purging (as typifies bulimia nervosa) at least two times per week for at least 6 months. First officially described in 1994, today health care professionals recognize binge-eating disorder as a growing, complex, and potentially serious problem. It is likely that binge-eating disorder will move from the EDNOS category and be recognized as a district eating disorder in the *DSM-V*, expected in 2013.

Approximately 30% of subjects in organized weight-control programs have binge-eating disorder, whereas among the general U.S. population, about 4 million have this disorder. However, many more people in the general population are likely to have less severe forms of the disorder that do not meet all the criteria that describe the problem. The number of cases of binge-eating disorder is far greater than that of either anorexia nervosa or bulimia nervosa. This disorder is also more common among the severely obese and those with a long history of frequent restrictive dieting, although obesity is not a criterion for having binge-eating disorder.

Development and Characteristics of Binge-Eating Disorder. Individuals with binge-eating disorder (about 40% of whom are males) often perceive themselves as hungry more often than normal. They usually started dieting at a young age, began bingeing during adolescence or in their early twenties, and did not succeed in commercial weight-control programs. Almost half of those with severe binge-eating disorder exhibit clinical depression. Some people also may have a genetic predisposition for this disorder.

Up to 25% of college-age women exhibit some degree of binge eating. Such behavior may have a negative impact on physical appearance, health, social life, and academics.

night eating syndrome Eating a lot of food in the late evening and nocturnal awakenings with ingestion of food.

female athlete triad A condition characterized by disordered eating, lack of menstrual periods (amenorrhea), and osteoporosis.

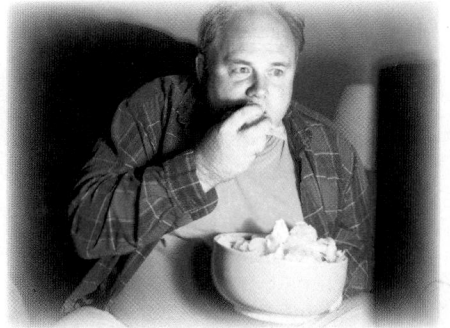

▲ Binge-eating disorder is seen in both men and women.

TABLE 11-2 Some Characteristics of Binge-Eating Disorder

A. Recurrent episodes of binge eating, which is characterized by:
    (1) Eating, in a discrete period (e.g., within any 2-hour period), an amount of food definitely larger than most people would eat during a similar period in similar circumstances
    (2) A sense of lack of control during the episodes (e.g., a feeling that one can't stop eating or control what or how much one is eating)

B. During most binge episodes, at least three of the following occur:
    (1) Eating much more rapidly than usual
    (2) Eating until feeling uncomfortably full
    (3) Eating large amounts of food when not feeling physically hungry
    (4) Eating alone because of being embarrassed by how much one is eating
    (5) Feeling disgusted with oneself, depressed, or guilty after overeating

C. Marked distress regarding binge eating

D. The binge eating occurs, on average, at least 2 days a week for 6 months.

E. The behavior does not occur only during the course of bulimia nervosa or anorexia nervosa.

Based on information from the *Diagnostic and Statistical Manual of Mental Disorders*, Fourth Edition (DSM-IV-TR). Washington DC: American Psychiatric Association, 2000.

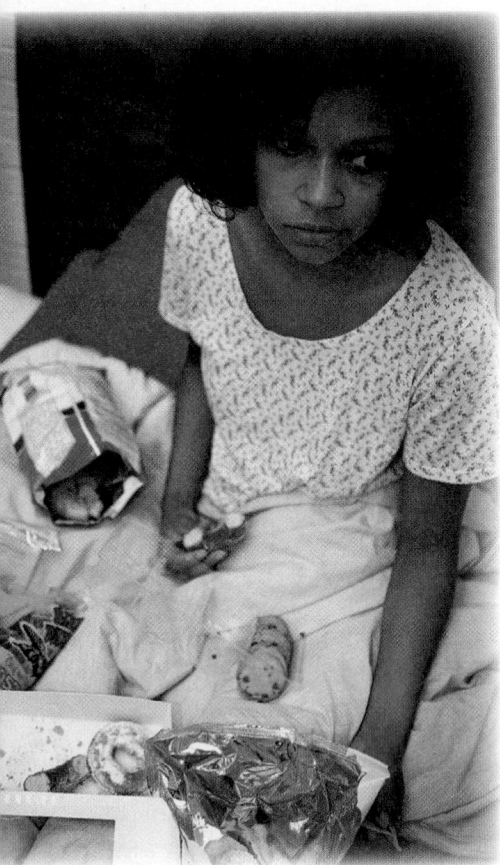

▲ Professional help is advised for people with a binge-eating disorder.

As noted in Chapter 2, spreading one's dietary intake into numerous, small meals (grazing) over a day provides some health advantages if overall calorie intake remains appropriate.

People with binge-eating disorder may come from families with alcoholism or may have suffered sexual abuse. Members of such dysfunctional families often do not know how to deal effectively with emotions. They cope by turning to substances. Family members learn to cover up dysfunctional patterns for the alcoholic person and to nurture him or her at the expense of each other and their own needs.

Typical binge eaters isolate themselves and eat large quantities of a favorite food. Stressful events and feelings of depression or anxiety can trigger this behavior. Giving themselves permission to eat a forbidden food can also precipitate a binge. Other triggers include loneliness, anxiety, self-pity, depression, anger, rage, alienation, and frustration (see Further Reading 15). They sometimes binge on whatever is easy to eat in large amounts—noodles, rice, bread, leftovers. Characteristically, however, binge eaters consume foods that carry the social stigma of "junk" or "bad" foods—ice cream, cookies, sweets, potato chips, and similar snack foods.

In general, people engage in binge eating to induce a sense of well-being and perhaps even numbness, usually in an attempt to avoid feeling and dealing with emotional pain and anxiety. They eat without regard to biological need and often in a recurrent, ritualized fashion. Some people with this disorder eat food continually over an extended period, called *grazing;* others cycle episodes of bingeing with normal eating. For example, someone with a stressful or frustrating job might come home every night and graze until bedtime. Another person might eat normally most of the time but find comfort in consuming large quantities of food when an emotional setback occurs.

Although people with anorexia nervosa and bulimia nervosa exhibit persistent preoccupation with body shape, weight, and thinness, binge eaters do not necessarily share these concerns. Thus, neither purging nor prolonged food restriction is characteristic of binge-eating disorder. Some physicians classify binge-eating disorder as an addiction to food, involving psychological dependence. The person becomes attached to the behavior and has a drive to continue it, senses only limited control over it, and needs to persist at it despite negative consequences. Food is used to reduce stress, produce feelings of power and well-being, avoid feelings of intimacy with others, and avoid life problems. Obesity and binge eating are not necessarily linked. Not all obese people are binge eaters, and, although obesity may result from trying to numb emotional pain with food, it is not necessarily an outcome of binge eating.

Binge-eating disorder is most likely to develop in people who never learned to express and deal appropriately with their feelings. Rather than face their frustration, anger, and pain, they turn to food. The frustration will continue because they never confront the basic problem. Binge eating makes them feel they cannot control the behavior pattern and therefore cannot control their lives. Worse, the binge eating usually increases feelings of guilt, embarrassment, and shame.

Often, people who practice binge eating have been shaped by families who do not address and express feelings in healthful ways. The parents nurture and comfort their children with food rather than engage in healthy exchanges of self-disclosure of feelings and potential solutions. Members of such families learn to eat in response to emotional needs and pain instead of hunger. Those who regularly practice binge eating may grow up nurturing others instead of themselves, avoiding their own feelings and taking little time for themselves. Not knowing how to satisfy their personal and emotional needs in more healthful ways, people in these families turn to food.

For some people, frequent dieting beginning in childhood or adolescence is a precursor to binge-eating disorder. During periods when little food is eaten, they get very hungry and obsessive about food. When allowed to eat more food, they feel driven to eat in a compulsive, uncontrolled way. The pattern of strict dieting alternating with binge eating may continue over time.

Help for the Person with Binge-Eating Disorder. Those with binge-eating disorder must learn to eat in response to hunger—a biological signal—rather than in response to emotional needs or external factors (such as the time of day or the simple presence of food). Counselors often direct binge eaters to record their perceptions of physical hunger throughout the day and at the beginning and end of every meal. These people must learn to respond to a prescribed amount of fullness at each meal. They should initially avoid weight-loss diets because feelings of food deprivation can lead to more disruptive emotions and a greater sense of unmet needs. Diets are likely to encourage more intense problems, such as extreme hunger. Many people with binge-eating disorder may experience difficulty in identifying personal emotional needs and expressing emotions. This problem is a common predisposing factor in binge eating, so communication issues should be addressed during treatment. Binge eaters often must be helped to recognize their buried emotions in anxiety-producing situations, and then encouraged to share them with their therapist or therapy group. Learning simple but appropriate phrases to say to oneself can help stop bingeing when the desire is strong.

Self-help groups, such as Overeaters Anonymous, aim to help recovery from binge-eating disorder. Their treatment philosophy, which parallels that of Alcoholics Anonymous, attempts to create an environment of encouragement and accountability to overcome this eating disorder. Dietary advice typically ranges from avoiding restraint in eating in general to limiting binge foods. Some experts feel that learning to eat all foods—but in moderation—is an effective goal for binge eaters. This practice can prevent the feelings of desperation and deprivation that come from limiting particular foods. Antidepressants, such as fluoxetine (Prozac®), and other types of medications (e.g., topiramate [Topamax®]) also have been found to help reduce binge eating in these individuals by decreasing depression. Overall, people who have this disorder are usually unsuccessful in controlling it on their own. Professional help is advised.

Night Eating Syndrome

Night eating syndrome is characterized by evening hyperphagia (eating more than one-third of total daily calories after the evening meal) and nighttime awakening accompanied by the ingestion of food. Although night eating syndrome was first observed among obese patients, it also occurs among nonobese persons. It has been estimated to occur in 1.5% of the general population and in 8.9% of persons treated in obesity clinics (see Further Reading 8).

Signs and Symptoms of Night Eating Syndrome

- Not feeling hungry in the morning and delaying the first meal until several hours after waking
- Overeating in the evening with more than one-third of daily food intake after dinner

NEWSWORTHY NUTRITION

Strong connection between eating disorders and binge drinking

A survey of 480 college-age women at high risk for eating disorders found a positive correlation between binge drinking (consuming four or more drinks in one sitting) and disordered eating behaviors. At baseline, 67% of the women in the study engaged in binge drinking at least once per month, and 30% did so frequently (three or more times per month). Additional research also supports this interplay between substance abuse and disordered eating behavior—purging, skipping meals, or fasting to compensate for calories consumed during drinking episodes—particularly among women. These studies exemplify how disordered eating behaviors and abuse of substances such as alcohol are used as inappropriate coping mechanisms. The stress of college and the influence of peers in this age group demand university-based intervention programs to educate students on the dangers of both eating disorders and substance abuse and to help students develop effective coping mechanisms.

Sources: Khaylis A and others: Binge drinking in women at risk for developing eating disorders. *International Journal of Eating Disorders* 42:409, 2009.

Kelly-Weeder S: Binge drinking and disordered eating in college students. *Journal of the American Academy of Nurse Practitioners* 23:33, 2011.

connect Check out the Connect site www.mcgrawhillconnect.com to further explore eating disorders and binge drinking.

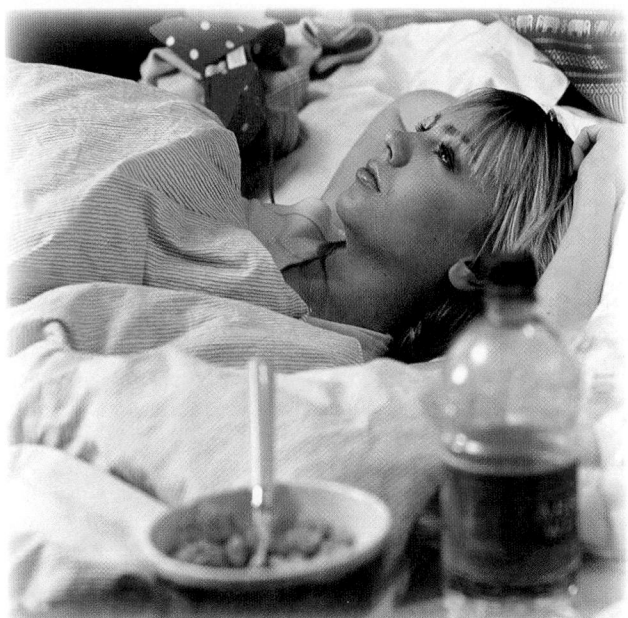

▲ Night eating syndrome is characterized by waking at least once during the night and needing to eat to be able to fall asleep again.

It is often difficult to get female athletes to accept necessary treatment plans. They frequently have a single-minded approach to their sport, while ignoring future health consequences.

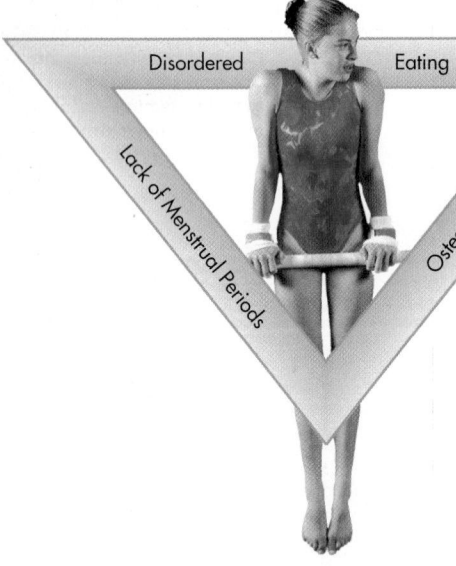

FIGURE 11-3 ▶ The female athlete triad occurs when the athlete has disordered eating, lack of menstrual periods, and osteoporosis. Stress fractures and chronic fatigue also occur. This triad often is seen in appearance-related sports, such as gymnastics. Long-term health is at risk; thus, prevention and early treatment are crucial.

- Difficulty falling asleep and a need to eat something to help fall asleep faster
- Waking at least once during the night with a need to eat to be able to fall asleep again
- Eating produces feelings of guilt and shame
- Feeling depressed, especially at night

Research shows that the cause of night eating syndrome may be an abnormal food cycle in the body, resulting in a delayed intake of food during the day. The circadian rhythm (your body's 24-hour clock) of food intake appears to be disturbed in night eating syndrome. Studies have also shown that night eating syndrome is prevalent among outpatients with psychiatric conditions and that the symptoms, including nocturnal ingestion and evening hyperphagia, are significantly improved with use of the antidepressant setraline (Zoloft®).

Female Athlete Triad

Women participating in appearance-based and endurance sports are at risk of developing an eating disorder. One study of college-age female athletes found that 15% of swimmers, 62% of gymnasts, and 32% of varsity athletes exhibited disordered eating patterns. Estimates of eating disorders for college women not involved in competitive sports are much lower.

In addition to disordered eating, college women athletes tend to experience irregular menstruation more frequently than other college women. Disordered eating, particularly food restriction, and stress can precipitate this, causing women to have less dense and weaker bones than normal because of lower estrogen concentrations in the blood. Some of these young women have bone mass values equivalent to those of 50- to 60-year-olds, increasing their risk for bone and stress fractures during sports as well as general activities. Much of the bone loss is irreversible.

The American College of Sports Medicine (ACSM) has named this syndrome "female athlete triad" because it consists of three parts: disordered eating, lack of menstrual periods, and osteoporosis (Fig. 11-3). The ACSM has issued a plea to teachers, coaches, health professionals, and parents to educate female athletes about the triad and its health consequences.

Many coaches/trainers and even some health professionals wrongly believe that loss of menstrual periods is a normal consequence of a high level of physical activity. However, loss of menstrual periods in female athletes stems from a dramatic decrease in female reproductive hormones, particularly estrogen. Loss of estrogen has other negative consequences on the body, such as fragile bones, as mentioned. Correcting the hormonal imbalance and menstrual irregularities by increasing caloric intake should stabilize bone mass. During therapy, a physician may prescribe a multivitamin and mineral supplement as well as calcium supplements as needed to maintain an intake of 1200 to 1500 milligrams.

Those exhibiting symptoms of the female athlete triad should seek treatment from a multidisciplinary team of health professionals. Involving the coach or trainer in therapy is usually a key factor in the success of the treatment plan. Suggestions for treatment are as follows:

- Reduce preoccupation with food, weight, and body fat.
- Gradually increase meals and snacks to an appropriate amount.
- Achieve an appropriate weight-for-height.
- Establish regular menstrual periods.
- Decrease training time and/or intensity by 10% to 20%.

The tragic case of Christy Henrich illustrates why anyone at risk for the female athlete triad should seek professional help. As a young teenager, Christy weighed 95 pounds and was 4 feet 11 inches tall. She showed promise as a gymnast but was told that she was too fat to excel in gymnastics. Christy continued her training but often starved herself, some days consuming just an apple and frequently purging by vomiting. Her success in gymnastics continued, but at age 22 her weight had fallen to 52 pounds, and she died from the effects of long-term semistarvation.

MAKING DECISIONS

Muscle Dysmorphia: The Pursuit of "Bigness"

Muscle dysmorphia has gained attention as a psychological condition with many similarities to eating disorders. First identified among male bodybuilders in the 1990s, muscle dysmorphia was initially termed "reverse anorexia." Men (and some women) with this disorder perceive themselves as *too thin*, rather than too fat, and are preoccupied with strict weightlifting and diet regimens to achieve a high level of muscularity. Among high school and college-aged men, in particular, body dissatisfaction may lead to disordered eating and exercise practices. In muscle dysmorphia, numerous hours are devoted to working out at the gym; planning and eating low-carbohydrate, high-protein meals; and keeping meticulous records of exercise, body measurements, and food intake. The dietary practices (e.g., high-volume eating, protein intakes of up to 5 grams per kilogram) and use of unproven ergogenic aids or anabolic steroids can result in physical impairment. Such exercise and eating routines also interfere with social, occupational, and recreational activities. People with muscle dysmorphia may avoid social contact, eating in restaurants, and being seen without clothes because of distress over appearing too thin. Considering its many similarities with anorexia nervosa and a tendency for people with muscle dysmorphia to cross over to other forms of eating disorders over time, some experts support recognition of muscle dysmorphia as an eating disorder.

A female high school athlete recently admitted her 3-year struggle with anorexia nervosa and bulimia nervosa. Even after her athletic performance declined and she suffered a sports-related injury, which sidelined her for a year and required surgery, she continued to think that controlling her weight and eating behaviors would make her the best—academically and physically. This example demonstrates several important points about eating disorders: certain groups of people are at greater risk for developing eating disorders; these people are often high achievers and are careful about concealing their eating disorder; and eating disorders such as the female athlete triad, bulimia nervosa, and anorexia nervosa frequently overlap.

11.5 Prevention of Eating Disorders

A key to developing and maintaining healthful eating behavior is to realize that some concern about diet, health, and weight is normal. It is also normal to experience variation in what we eat, how we feel, and even how much we weigh. For example, it is normal to experience some minimal weight change (up to 2 to 3 pounds) throughout the day and even more over the course of a week. A large weight fluctuation or ongoing weight gain or weight loss is more likely to indicate that a problem is present. If you notice a large change in your eating habits, how you feel, or your body weight, it is a good idea to consult your personal physician. Treating physical and emotional problems early helps lead you to peace of mind and good health.

With a view on society as a whole, many people begin to form opinions about food, nutrition, health, weight, and body image prior to or during puberty. Parents, friends, and professionals working with young adults should consider the following advice for preventing eating disorders:

- Discourage restrictive dieting and meal skipping. Fasting is also discouraged (except for religious occasions).
- Provide information about normal changes that occur during puberty.
- Correct misconceptions about nutrition, healthy body weight, and approaches to weight loss.
- Carefully phrase any weight-related recommendations and comments.
- Don't overemphasize numbers on a scale. Instead, primarily promote healthful eating.
- Encourage normal expression of disruptive emotions.
- Encourage children to eat only when they're hungry.
- Teach the basics of proper nutrition and regular physical activity in school and at home.
- Provide adolescents with an appropriate, but not unlimited, degree of independence, choice, responsibility, and self-accountability for their actions.

CRITICAL THINKING

Tom, a high school teacher, is concerned about eating disorders. He wants to try to prevent young adults from falling into the discouraging traps of anorexia nervosa and bulimia nervosa. What are some of the topics and issues he should discuss with students in his health classes?

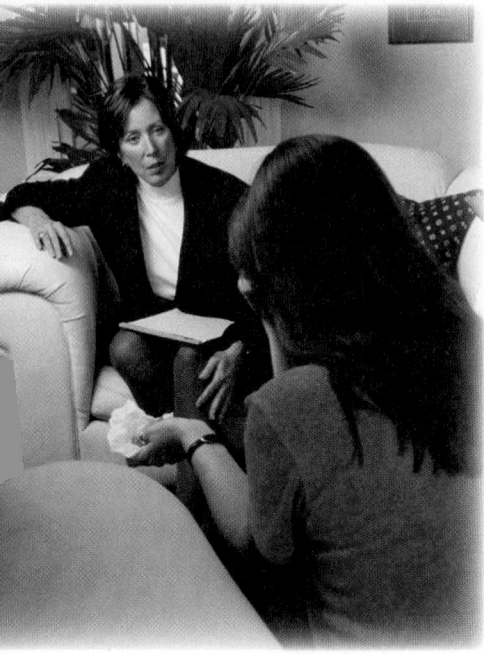

▲ Bulimia nervosa affects many college students. Counselors are aware of this and are available to help.

For further information on eating disorders, contact:

Academy for Eating Disorders, 111 Deer Lake Road, Suite 100, Deerfield, IL 60015 847-498-4274; www.aedweb.org

The National Eating Disorders Association, 603 Stewart St., Suite 803, Seattle, WA 98101; 206-382-3587 or 800-931-EDAP; www.nationaleatingdisorders.org

The National Institute of Mental Health has published a concise review of eating disorders (www.nimh.nih.gov/publicat/eatingdisorders.cfm).

- Increase self-acceptance and appreciation of the power and pleasure emerging from one's body.
- Enhance tolerance for diversity in body weight and shape.
- Build respectful environments and supportive relationships.
- Encourage coaches to be sensitive to weight and body-image issues among athletes.
- Emphasize that thinness is not necessarily associated with better athletic performance.

Our society as a whole can benefit from a fresh focus on nutritious food practices and a healthful outlook toward food and body weight. Not only is treatment of eating disorders far more difficult than prevention, these disorders also have devastating effects on the entire family. For this reason, caregivers and health care professionals must emphasize the importance of an overall healthful diet that focuses on moderation, as opposed to restriction and perfection. Restricted diets are especially detrimental to children because they do not supply enough calories to sustain growth. In response, nutritional counseling can assure caregivers that including some sweets and fast-food in a child's diet is acceptable (see Chapter 15 for more details).

Overall, the challenge facing many North Americans is achieving a healthy body weight without excessive dieting. This means adopting and maintaining sensible eating habits, a physically active lifestyle, and realistic and positive attitudes and emotions while practicing creative ways to handle stress. Eating disorders develop in part from certain cultural values; changing these values might reduce the pressures predisposing some people to various types of disordered eating behavior. Some feminists, for example, assert that true liberation means being free to find one's natural weight. Women who combine careers and motherhood are saying that they have more important things to worry about; some fashion leaders are tolerating more curves; exercise programs are encouraging regular brisk walking, rather than high-intensity activities such as jogging. Finally, writers, therapists, and registered dietitians are working to help women accept their bodies, as noted in the "size acceptance" approach discussed in Chapter 7.

MAKING DECISIONS

Polycystic Ovary Syndrome and Eating Disorders

Polycystic ovary syndrome (PCOS) is a complex hormonal disorder and is the leading cause of infertility. PCOS is characterized by hormonal imbalances in women with high levels of male hormones such as testosterone secreted by the ovaries. The hormonal imbalance causes tiny cysts to surround the ovaries like a strand of pearls. The signs and symptoms of PCOS include difficulty losing weight, intense cravings for carbohydrates, and irregular or absent periods. Most of these have a direct effect on body image and self-esteem, so a relationship between PCOS and eating disorders is suspected. The overlap in symptoms means it is important that persons with these characteristics be screened for both PCOS and eating disorders before recommendations for treatment are made (see Further Reading 7).

CONCEPT CHECK

Food bingeing (without purging) and grazing are two characteristic behaviors of binge-eating disorder. Treatment addresses the deeper emotional issues that undermine healthy eating practices, while shifting the person's focus away from food deprivation and restrictive diets and toward more normal eating behaviors. Night eating syndrome involves overeating in the evening and a need to eat to be able to fall asleep. The female athlete triad consists of disordered eating, amenorrhea, and osteoporosis, and most commonly affects those in appearance-related and endurance sports. Parents, coaches, teachers, and health professionals need to be involved in efforts to prevent and treat this problem.

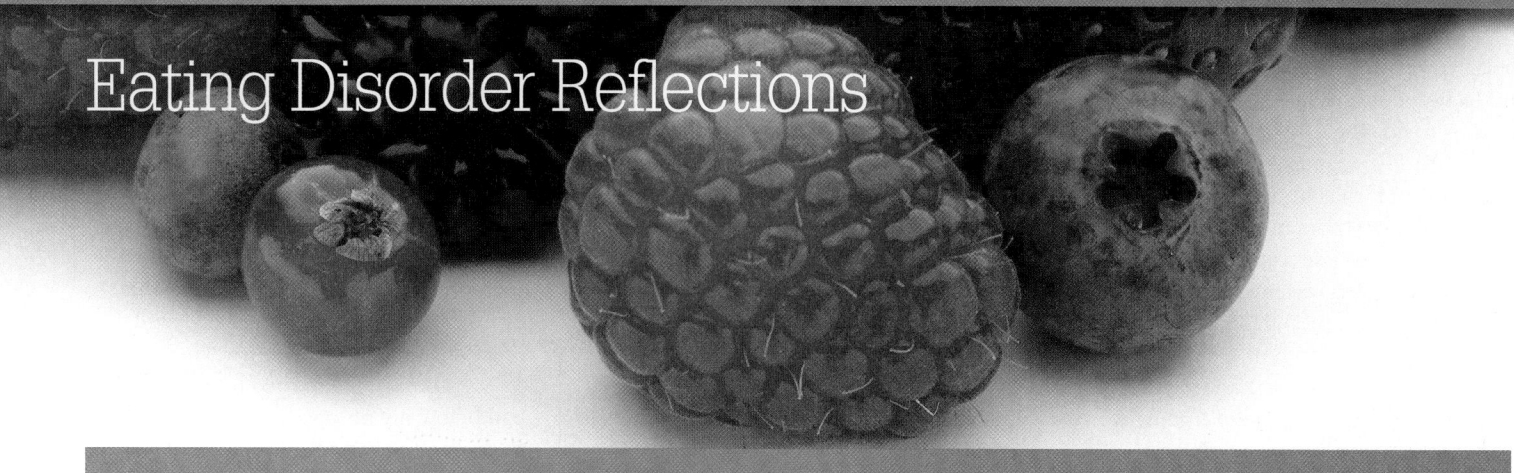

Eating Disorder Reflections

Thoughts of an Anorexic Woman

It was the spring of my freshman year of high school, and I had just turned 15. I wanted to get a leading role in the upcoming high school musical *West Side Story*. I thought I should lose some weight to look more attractive to the student director Shawn, so I decided to give up "junk" food. The next day my friend Sandra looked at my lunch, spread out neatly on a napkin before me, and squawked, "Dill pickles?! Who brings dill pickles for lunch in a zip-lock baggie?" The other girls at the table fell into a fit of hysterics. "Casting for *West Side Story* is coming up,"

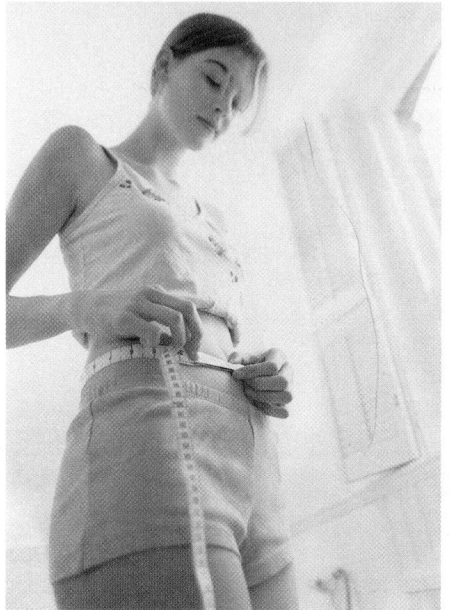

▲ A history of anorexia nervosa can harm physical as well as mental health.

I said, "and I gave up 'junk' food to try to lose a few pounds." One of my friends thought it would be funny to give me an M&M—just to smell. Ha, ha. I put it in a little Tupperware container and kept it for days in my backpack as a reminder. Every once in a while, I did smell it.

For the next few weeks there were times when I would find myself cracking open the refrigerator door and just staring down what I knew to be a deliciously crunchy, crisp, and cold Kit Kat bar in the dairy bin. I didn't eat it though. At the mall with my friends (since at 15, that's about all my parents allowed me to do), Bridgette and Nora wanted to stop and get a cinnamon bun. They chided me, but I didn't budge. The cinnamon bun smelled so good. But as I sat opposite them in the food court and watched them over-dramatize its ooey-gooey goodness, I felt a sense of pride that I could make a decision and stick with it. I could see that they were jealous of my willpower.

When Easter came around, I took a look at the contents of the Easter basket my mom insisted on preparing and turned up my nose at it. I had proven to myself that I could resist temptation . . . why stop now?

I was eventually offered only a minor part in the musical, but I wasn't that disappointed. I was looking so much better as the pounds kept coming off. Every morning, just after going to the bathroom and before getting any breakfast, I would pop onto the scale in my mom's bathroom. One hundred and fifteen pounds and still going. At 5 feet 7 inches, that wasn't too bad.

Also at this time, I started running, and my friend Laura became my running partner. She was getting in shape for the next season of field hockey. After school, we met in the locker room, changed out of our school clothes, and out we went. I had never been much of an athlete—I thought that being part of a team, whether in sports or academics, diluted the excellence I could achieve on my own. Running, however, could just be me and the road—no mediocrity there.

Cheese and butter had made it to the "no" list by the time I was 16 and down to 105 pounds. Fat-free was my mantra. For my 16th birthday, my friends threw a little surprise party for me. Nora, knowing I would put up a fight, made me a cake. "It's your birthday! You can have a piece of cake!" I politely said no, that I would cut it for everyone else, but I really didn't want any. They pestered me and Nora started to feel offended, so finally I took a few bites so she wouldn't burst into tears. It had been so long since I'd had so much sugar. I felt bloated and sick. I ate nothing for the rest of the day, and only 6 saltines, 1 apple, and 2 stalks of celery the next day. Those foods were on the "yes" list. Salads also were okay, but only lettuce with salt and vinegar. I told my parents that the dissections in biology class had given me a distaste for meat, but really, I just didn't want all those calories. For a while, I craved food day and night, but I was getting better and better at holding my ground.

By my senior year, I was skipping lunches altogether, opting instead to hang out in the library and read over my AP Bio text. "Where were you at lunch today?" Bridgette would ask later. "Oh, I had some reading to do. The AP exam is going to be tough." At 100 pounds, I was getting closer to finding out what "tough" really meant.

Even though Laura moved out of state, I didn't give up on exercising. Now, the stair stepper in the gym was my favorite. I'd take my biology notes, prop them up in front of me, and step-step-step until I had burned 400 kcal. I felt so efficient knowing that I could multi-task. Sometimes I'd go twice a day. As senior year wore on, though, it got harder and harder to get up in the morning and put on my tennis shoes. And then one morning, in the shower, I just collapsed under the stream of hot water.

I ended up in this hospital bed with an IV tube in my arm. At 92 pounds, my body was starving. As it turns out, if you don't give your body any fuel, you start to cannibalize yourself, in a sense. My body had been so hungry, my muscles had been wasting away, and the episode in the shower was due to a problem with my heart. It's a problem I have created . . . not my parents or my distant group of friends . . . just me. My mom was there, next to me, caressing the arm with the IV tube, putting her whole life on hold because of me. Isn't this what I'd wanted—to be in control of my own destiny?

Where do I go from here?

Thoughts of a Bulimic Woman

From Hall L, Cohn L: *Bulimia—A Guide to Recovery.* Gurze Books: Carlsbad, CA, 1992.

I am wide awake and immediately out of bed. I think back to the night before, when I made a new list of what I wanted to get done and how I wanted to be. My husband is not far behind me on his way into the bathroom to get ready for work. Maybe I can sneak onto the scale to see what I weigh this morning before he notices me. I am already in my private world. I feel overjoyed when the scale says that I stayed the same weight as I was the night before, and I can feel that slightly hungry feeling. Maybe it will stop today; maybe

today everything will change. What were the projects I was going to get done?

We eat the same breakfast, except that I take no butter on my toast, no cream in my coffee, and never take seconds (until Doug gets out the door). Today I am going to be really good, and that means eating certain predetermined portions of food and not taking one more bite than I think I am allowed. I am very careful to see that I don't take more than Doug. I judge myself by his body. I can feel the tension building. I wish Doug would hurry up and leave so I can get going!

As soon as he shuts the door, I try to get involved with one of the myriad responsibilities on my list. I hate them all! I just want to crawl into a hole. I don't want to do anything. I'd rather eat. I am alone; I am nervous; I am no good; I always do everything wrong anyway; I am not in control; I can't make it through the day, I know it. It has been the same for so long. I remember the starchy cereal I ate for breakfast. I am into the bathroom and onto the scale. It measures the same, but I don't want to stay the same! I want to be thinner! I look into the mirror. I think my thighs are ugly and deformed looking. I see a lumpy, clumsy, pear-shaped wimp. There is always something wrong with what I see. I feel frustrated, trapped in this body, and I don't know what to do about it.

I float to the refrigerator knowing exactly what is there. I begin with last night's brownies. I always begin with the sweets. At first I try to make it look like nothing is missing, but my appetite is huge and I resolve to make another batch of brownies. I know there is half of a bag of cookies in the bathroom, thrown out the night before, and I polish them off immediately. I take some milk so my vomiting will be smoother. I like the full feeling I get after downing a big glass. I get out six pieces of bread and toast one side of each in the broiler, turn them over and load

them with pats of butter, and put them under the broiler again until they are bubbling. I take all six pieces on a plate to the television and go back for a bowl of cereal and a banana to have along with them. Before the last piece of toast is finished, I am already preparing the next batch of six more pieces. Maybe another brownie or five, and a couple of large bowls full of ice cream, yogurt, or cottage cheese.

My stomach is stretched into a huge ball below my rib cage. I know I'll have to go into the bathroom soon, but I want to postpone it. I am in never-never land. I am waiting, feeling the pressure, pacing the floor in and out of the rooms. Time is passing. Time is passing. It is getting to be time. I wander aimlessly through each of the rooms again, tidying, making the whole house neat and put back together. I finally make the turn into the bathroom. I brace my feet, pull my hair back and stick my finger down my throat, stroking twice, and get up a huge pile of food. Three times, four times, and another pile of food. I can see everything come back. I am so glad to see those brownies because they are so fattening. The rhythm of the emptying is broken and my head is beginning to hurt. I stand up feeling dizzy, empty, and weak. The whole episode has taken about an hour.

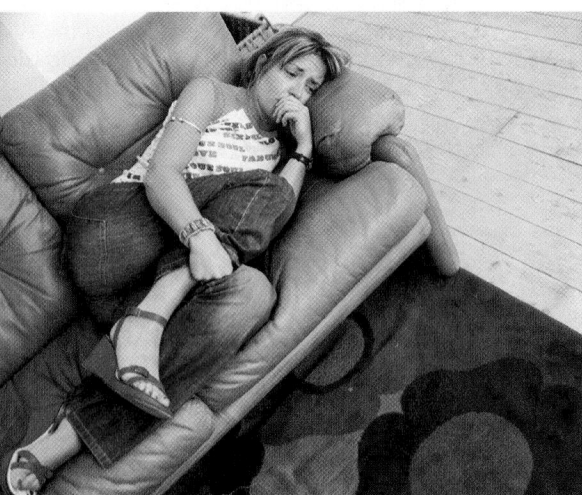

▲ Bulimic episodes add to the despair felt in this disorder.

Case Study Eating Disorders—Steps to Recovery

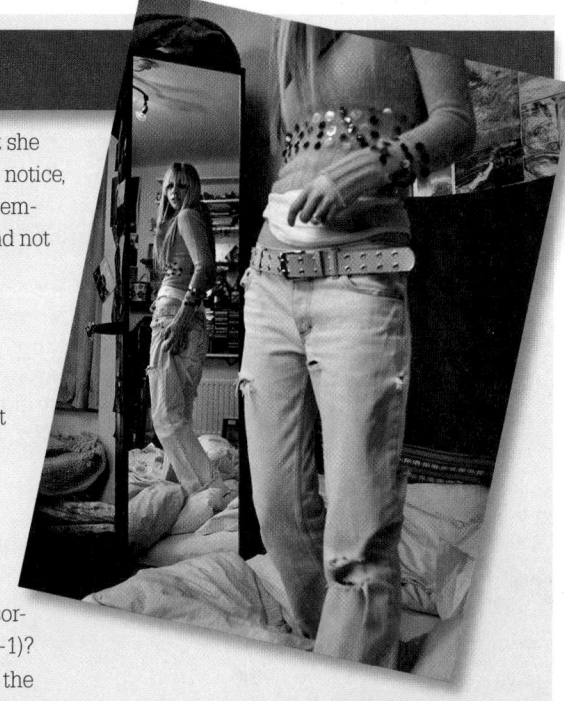

At age 16, Sarah suddenly became self-conscious about her body when her peers teased her about being overweight. She began exercising to an aerobics video for an hour each day and found that she had success in losing weight; this was the beginning of her obsession to be thin. Next, Sarah turned to eating less food to lose even more weight and began eliminating certain foods from her diet, such as candy and meat. She increased her water and vegetable intake and chewed sugarless gum to curb her appetite. Once she began dieting, it was impossible for her to stop. She enjoyed having a high degree of self-control over her body. Still, she was literally obsessed with food, even staring at others while they were eating a meal. She occasionally cooked large meals and then refused to eat all but a few bites. By the time Sarah was 19 years old and 5 feet 6 inches tall, her weight had dropped from 150 pounds to 85 pounds in 20 months. Her family was concerned about her weight status, demanding that she go to a physician for an evaluation. Sarah was not happy about this idea but believed that her family would stop pestering her if she went. Sarah did not think she had a problem; she thought she was still grotesquely overweight. She did notice, however, that she was intolerant of cold temperatures and was concerned that she had not menstruated in a year.

Answer the following questions, and check your responses in Appendix A.

1. Sarah appears to have an eating disorder. Which eating disorder best describes her behavior?

2. List the behaviors that Sarah developed between age 16 and 19 years that are signs of the development of this eating disorder.

3. What physical symptoms of this disorder does Sarah have (review Fig. 11-1)?

4. What types of therapy do you think the physician will suggest for Sarah?

5. Do you think Sarah has developed any vitamin or mineral deficiencies? Which ones would be most likely? How could these deficiencies be best treated?

6. Where could she go for the therapy she needs?

7. What type of professionals would most likely provide therapy for Sarah's condition?

8. What is the likelihood that she will fully recover from her condition?

Summary (Numbers refer to numbered sections in the chapter.)

11.1 Healthy eating, which incorporates the principals of balance, variety, and moderation, provides fuel for the body and a source of pleasure. Disordered eating encompasses mild and short-term changes in eating patterns that occur as a result of life stress, illness, or a desire to change body weight. When carried to the extreme, disordered eating may progress to an eating disorder, in which severe changes in eating patterns have lasting and detrimental effects.

11.2 Anorexia nervosa is most common among high-achieving, perfectionist girls from families marked by conflict, high expectations, rigidity, and denial. The disorder usually starts with dieting in early puberty and proceeds to the near-total refusal to eat. Early warning signs include intense concern about weight gain and dieting, as well as abnormal food habits, such as cooking food that they won't allow themselves to eat.

Anorexia nervosa may be defined as a denial of appetite. Anorexic persons become irritable, hostile, overly critical, and joyless; they tend to withdraw from family and friends. Eventually, anorexia nervosa can lead to numerous physical effects, including a profound decrease in body weight and body fat, a fall in body temperature and heart rate, iron-deficiency anemia, a low white blood cell count, hair loss, constipation, low blood potassium, and the loss of menstrual periods. Those with anorexia nervosa are in a state of physical illness. Treatment of anorexia nervosa includes increasing food intake to support gradual weight gain. Psychological counseling attempts to help establish regular food habits and to find means of coping with the life stresses that led to the disorder. Hospitalization may be necessary, as well as use of certain medications.

11.3 Bulimia nervosa is characterized by secretive bingeing on large amounts of food within a short time span, and then purging by vomiting or misusing laxatives, diuretics, or enemas. Alternately, fasting and excessive exercise may be used. Both men and women are at risk. Vomiting as a means of purging is especially destructive to the body; it can cause severe tooth decay, stomach ulcers, irritation of the esophagus, low blood potassium, and other problems. Bulimia nervosa poses a serious health problem and is associated with significant risk of suicide. Treatment of bulimia nervosa includes psychological as well as nutritional counseling. During treatment, bulimic persons learn to accept themselves and to cope with problems in ways that do not involve food. Regular eating patterns are developed as these bulimic persons begin to plan meals in an informed, healthful manner. Certain medications can be a helpful addition to the regimen.

11.4 Besides anorexia nervosa and bulimia nervosa, there are several categories of eating disorders not otherwise specified (EDNOS). Binge-eating disorder, more widespread than either anorexia nervosa or bulimia nervosa, is most common among people with a history of frequent, unsuccessful dieting. Binge eaters typically either practice bingeing (without purging) or grazing (i.e., eating continually over extended periods). Emotional disturbances are often at the root of this disordered

form of eating. Night eating syndrome is overeating in the evening with more than one-third of daily food intake after dinner, difficulty falling asleep and a need to eat something to help fall asleep faster, and waking at least once during the night and a need to eat to be able to fall asleep again. The female athlete triad consists of disordered eating, loss of menstrual periods, and osteoporosis. It is particularly common in appearance-related and endurance sports. If not corrected, this disorder eventually leads to decreased athletic performance and general health problems.

11.5 Prevention of eating disorders is crucial because treatments are expensive and lengthy and are not 100% effective. Encouraging healthy attitudes about eating and exercise from a young age will aid in preventing the development of eating disorders. Those who work closely with children and young adults should encourage acceptance of diversity in body sizes and carefully phrase comments about body weight. Helping children to develop healthy ways to cope with emotions is also important.

Check Your Knowledge (Answers to the following questions are below.)

1. Anorexia nervosa generally is a disease of
   a. children.
   b. middle-aged women.
   c. young boys.
   d. teenage women.

2. Anorexia nervosa can be defined as
   a. compulsive eating.
   b. hyperactivity.
   c. psychological denial of appetite.
   d. purging.

3. A long-term health consequence of anorexia nervosa could be
   a. fractures resulting from bone loss.
   b. atherosclerotic heart disease.
   c. esophageal ulcers.
   d. cancer.

4. Bulimia is most frequently diagnosed by a
   a. dietitian.
   b. physician.
   c. dentist.
   d. physical therapist.

5. The *major* health risk from frequent vomiting due to bulimia nervosa is
   a. a drop in blood potassium.

   b. constipation.
   c. weight gain.
   d. a swelling of salivary glands.

6. Initial treatment of bulimia nervosa includes all of the following *except*
   a. psychotherapy to improve body image.
   b. emphasis on regular eating habits.
   c. nutritional counseling.
   d. refeeding via tube feedings.
   e. Both a and c.

7. Binge-eating disorder can be characterized as
   a. bingeing accompanied by purging.
   b. secretive eating.
   c. eating to avoid feeling and dealing with emotional pain.
   d. the early phase of bulimia nervosa.

8. Binge-eating disorder is different from anorexia nervosa, and particularly bulimia nervosa, because it doesn't involve
   a. females.
   b. a persistent concern with body shape, weight, and thinness.
   c. purging, such as regular vomiting.

   d. health risks.
   e. Both b and c.

9. Night eating syndrome is characterized by
   a. eating dinner but no breakfast or lunch.
   b. the need to eat to fall asleep.
   c. waking at night to purge by vomiting.
   d. consuming all of the daily calories at night.

10. Female athlete triad consists of
    a. anorexia nervosa, lack of family support, and overtraining.
    b. disordered eating, overtraining, and lack of menstrual periods.
    c. osteoporosis, lack of menstrual periods, and disordered eating.
    d. osteoporosis, lack of sleep, and disordered eating.

Answers: 1. d (LO 11.2), 2. c (LO 11.2), 3. a (LO 11.2), 4. c (LO 11.3), 5. a (LO 11.3), 6. d (LO 11.3), 7. c (LO 11.4), 8. e (LO 11.4), 9. b (LO 11.4), 10. c (LO 11.4)

Study Questions (Numbers refer to Learning Outcomes)

1. What are the typical characteristics of a person with anorexia nervosa? What may influence a person to begin rigid, self-imposed dietary patterns? (LO 11.2)

2. List the detrimental physical and psychological side effects of bulimia nervosa. Describe important goals of the psychological and nutrition therapy used to treat bulimic patients. (LO 11.3)

3. What is the current thinking concerning medication use for anorexia nervosa and bulimia nervosa? (LOs 11.2 and 11.3)

4. Explain the role of excessive exercise in eating disorders. (LO 11.1)

5. How might parents significantly contribute to the development of an eating disorder? Suggest an attitude that a parent or an adult friend of yours

displayed that may not have been conducive to developing a normal relationship to food. (LO 11.5)

6. Based on your knowledge of good nutrition and sound dietary habits, answer the following questions:
   a. How can repeated bingeing and purging lead to significant nutrient deficiencies?

b. How can significant nutrient deficiencies contribute to major health problems in later life?

c. A friend asks you, the nutrition expert, if it is okay to "cleanse" the body by eating only grapefruit for a week. What is your response? **(LO 11.1)**

7. How, in your opinion, has society contributed to the development of various forms of disordered eating? Provide an example. **(LO 11.5)**

8. List the three symptoms that constitute the female athlete triad. What is the major health risk associated with loss of menstrual periods in the female athlete? **(LO 11.4)**

9. How does binge-eating disorder differ from bulimia nervosa? Describe the factors that contribute to the development and treatment of binge-eating disorder. **(LO 11.4)**

10. Provide two recommendations to reduce the problem of eating disorders in our society. **(LO 11.6)**

What Would You Choose Recommendations

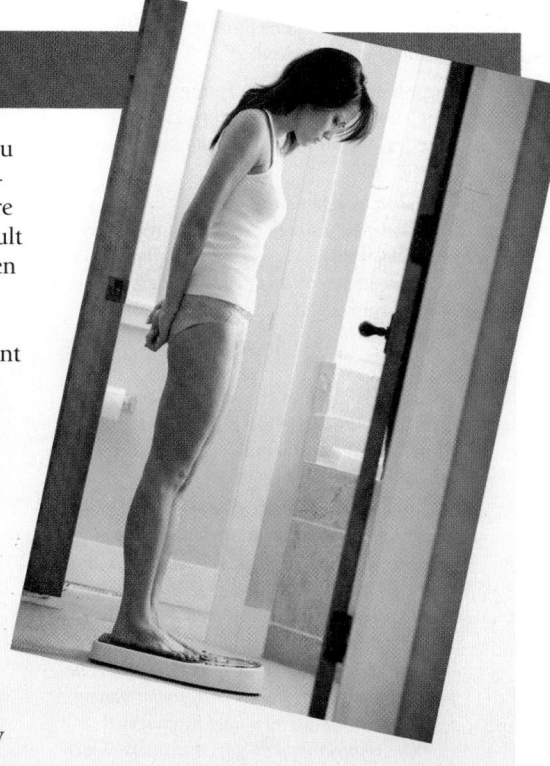

It can be uncomfortable to confront a friend about an unhealthy behavior. You may worry about compromising your friendship. The eating and excessive exercise behaviors you have witnessed may be short-term disordered eating and may pass in a few weeks. On the other hand, they might just be the tip of the iceberg. Ignoring her behavior will not make it go away. As you have learned in this chapter, eating disorders can have very serious consequences, and the earlier they are treated, the better the outcome. If you feel unable to address your concerns one on one with your roommate, you can seek help from a resident assistant in your dorm, a school counselor, or a nurse in the student health center. You will not be betraying your friendship; you will be showing how much you care about her by taking action.

Diagnosing an eating disorder is a complex task. People with eating disorders may deny the problem, hide their behaviors, and be irrational and uncooperative with those who try to help them. Do not try to diagnose your friend, but do try to keep the lines of communication open. Tell her what you have observed and ask her how you can help. She may open up to you and be glad she is not alone in her struggle. Then again, she may get angry and withdraw from you. Try to share what you know about eating disorders without lecturing or admonishing her. Also, be aware that your friend is going through a difficult emotional struggle that has probably been years in the making. Do not assume you know what she is going through.

Discussing healthy weight-management techniques with your roommate is not likely to help her if she has fallen prey to an eating disorder. She is already critical of her appearance and weight; your advice, although well intended and backed by the nutrition knowledge you have picked up in this course, may be construed as judgmental. Eating disorders are not about food. Rather, they involve issues of self-concept and control. It is important to be supportive but not critical. Taking the focus off food and body weight is important. Do not try to force her to eat or slow down on her exercise. If you can help get your roommate to seek professional treatment, psychiatric counseling will help to address her unhealthy relationship with food; eventually, nutrition counseling will help her to establish better eating habits.

Get prepared before you confront your roommate. Find out what information and resources are available on campus so you can share them with her. Recognize that you are not going to cure her disorder—she needs professional help. You can be supportive and patient as she deals with her inner turmoil. Listen and offer to go with her to seek care. Someday, you may be a health professional who is able to diagnose and counsel victims of eating disorders. For now, leave it to a qualified professional.

Further Readings

1. ADA Reports: Position of the American Dietetic Association: Nutrition intervention in the treatment of anorexia nervosa, bulimia nervosa, and other eating disorders. *Journal of the American Dietetic Association* 106:2073, 2006.

   Eating disorders are complex and serious illnesses that span a continuum from extreme dieting to diagnosed conditions. For effective treatment the expert interaction between professionals in many disciplines, including dietetics, is required.

2. American Academy of Pediatrics: Clinical Report—Identification and management of eating disorders in children and adolescents. *Pediatrics* 126:1240, 2010.

   Physicians should screen children and adolescents annually by looking for evidence of disordered eating, delayed development, and especially by monitoring weight and height. In children, eating disorders may appear not as weight loss, but as failure to grow appropriately. Early detection and treatment of eating disorders are especially important for younger patients because problems with growth, brain development, and bone mineralization can be irreversible.

3. Bonci CM: National Athletic Trainers' Association position statement: Preventing, detecting, and managing disordered eating in athletes. *Journal of Athletic Training* 43:80, 2008.

Disordered eating is common among athletes, particularly in sports with weight classifications or those in which appearance is related to success. As training intensity increases nutrient needs, nutrient deficiencies impair athletic performance. Athletic trainers, coaches, and others who regularly interact with athletes should be trained to promote healthful dietary behaviors, recognize signs of eating disorders, and exercise sensitivity to weight issues.

4. Campbell IC and others: Eating disorders, gene-environment interactions and epigenetics. *Neuroscience and Behavioral Reviews* 35:784, 2011.

The role of genetics and epigenetics in the development of eating disorders is a relatively new field of study. Environmental influences, including undernutrition, overnutrition, and stress at various stages of the life cycle, may impact a person's genetic predisposition for eating disorders.

5. Feldman MB, Meyer IH: Eating disorders in diverse lesbian, gay, and bisexual populations. *International Journal of Eating Disorders* 40:218, 2007.

This study assessed prevalence of eating disorders in a diverse community sample. Rates of eating disorders are higher among gay and bisexual men compared to heterosexual men. Whereas many heterosexual men are motivated to attain a large, muscular physique, gay and bisexual men tend to desire a slender build. The prevalence of eating disorders is similar among lesbians, bisexual women, and heterosexual women. Younger lesbian, gay, and bisexual men and women were more susceptible to disordered eating practices than older study participants.

6. Goebel-Fabbri AE: Eating disorders in type 1 diabetes: Clinical significance and treatment recommendations. *Current Diabetes Reports* 9:133, 2009.

Type 1 diabetes increases risk for eating disorders. Dietary restrictions and fear of hypoglycemia may precipitate binge eating. Some individuals may restrict insulin therapy as a means of purging calories without regard to the detrimental outcomes of impaired glucose control. Girls and women with diabetes should be screened for the presence of eating disorders.

7. Grassi A: Are polycystic ovary syndrome & eating disorders related? *Today's Dietitian* p. 32, October 2006.

Polycystic ovary syndrome (PCOS) is a complex hormonal disorder and is the leading cause of infertility. The symptoms of PCOS have a direct effect on body image and self-esteem and may lead to the development of eating disorders.

8. Lundgren JD and others: Prevalence of the night eating syndrome in a psychiatric population. *American Journal of Psychiatry* 163 (1):156, 2006.

Night eating syndrome is characterized by evening hyperphagia and waking during the night to consume food. The results of this study show that night eating syndrome is a common disorder among psychiatric outpatients and is associated with substance use and obesity.

9. Mathieu J: What is orthorexia? *Journal of the American Dietetic Association* 105:1510, 2005.

"Orthorexia," although not currently classified as an eating disorder, describes an emerging condition in which healthful eating becomes an obsession. A need for perfection or purity lies at the heart of orthorexia. Healthful or not, strict dietary practices become a problem when they interfere with a person's ability to take part in society. Such extreme dietary perfectionism may be related to obsessive-compulsive disorder.

10. McFarand MB and Kaminski PL: Men muscles, and mood: The relationship between self-concept, dysphoria, and body image disturbances. *Eating Behaviors* 10:68, 2009.

Just as women are under societal pressure to maintain unnatural thinness. men are unduly influenced by the extremely lean and muscular male body ideal portrayed by the media. This study of college-age men found that body dissatisfaction is predicted by low self-concept and increased levels of interpersonal sensitivity, depression, and anxiety. The study also noted associations between muscle dysmorphia and disordered eating.

11. Murphy R and others: Cognitive behavioral therapy for eating disorders. *Psychiatric Clinics of North America* 33:611, 2010.

The success of cognitive behavioral therapy (CBT) for patients with bulimia nervosa has spawned interest in applying CBT to anorexia nervosa and other eating disorders. This is based on the conclusion that all eating disorders, regardless of classification, stem from placing too much value on body shape and weight. This type of therapy aims to identify and modify the pathological thought patterns, such as strict dieting rules, that support an eating disorder.

12. Norris ML and others: Ana and the Internet: A review of pro-anorexia websites. *International Journal of Eating Disorders* 39:443, 2006.

Searching for "anorexia" using common search engines results in hundreds of links, many of which are "pro-anorexia." These websites provide information that is supportive of anorexia nervosa but is largely controversial and dangerous. Key characteristics of pro-anorexia websites include control, success, and perfection. It is important that health care providers and caregivers be aware of these websites and their content.

13. Ringham R and others: Eating disorder symptomatology among ballet dancers. *International Journal of Eating Disorders* 39:503, 2006.

Ballet dancers are at high risk of developing eating disorders. In this study, 29 female ballet dancers were compared to women with anorexia nervosa, bulimia nervosa, and not eating pathology. The results showed that the eating patterns of dancers were more similar to eating-disordered individuals than to control individuals. The majority of the dancers (83%) met lifetime criteria for eating disorders.

14. Robinson-O'Brien R and others: Adolescent and young adult vegetarianism: Better dietary intake and weight outcomes but increased risk of disordered eating behaviors. *Journal of the American Dietetic Association* 109:648, 2009.

This study of more than 2500 young men and women contributes to the body of evidence demonstrating that appropriately planned vegetarian and vegan lifestyles can be healthfully practiced by people of all ages. However, some young adults may use these socially acceptable eating patterns as a means of unhealthful dietary restriction for extreme weight loss. A history of vegetarian dietary practices is associated with disordered eating practices. If weight loss is the primary motive for choosing a vegetarian lifestyle, parents should be on alert for warning signs of eating disorders.

15. Stuppy P: Eating disorders in women at midlife. *Today's Dietitian* p. 12, January 2006.

Several emotional changes that occur in middle age, such as death of a spouse, divorce, the "empty nest" syndrome, and caring for aging parents, may precipitate eating disorders. Women, who already experience a high level of dissatisfaction with their bodies, may use dietary restriction or bingeing behaviors as coping mechanisms. Registered dietitians can help clients by facilitating recognition of the emotional underpinnings of clients' eating problems and by appropriately referring clients to mental health professionals, when needed.

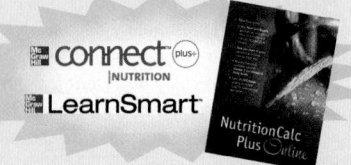

To get the most out of your study of nutrition, go to McGraw-Hill's online resources: Connect www.mcgrawhillconnect.com, where you will find NutritionCalc Plus, LearnSmart, and many other dynamic tools.

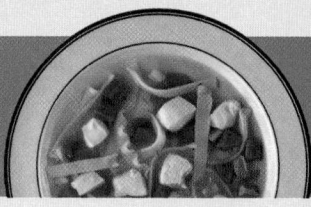
I. Assessing Risk of Developing an Eating Disorder

British investigators have developed a five-question screening tool called the **SCOFF** Questionnaire for recognizing eating disorders:[†]

1. Do you make yourself **S**ick because you feel full?
2. Do you lose **C**ontrol over how much you eat?
3. Have you lost more than **O**ne stone (about 13 pounds) recently?
4. Do you believe yourself to be **F**at when others say you are thin?
5. Does **F**ood dominate your life?

Two or more positive responses suggest an eating disorder.

1. After completing this questionnaire, do you feel that you might have an eating disorder or the potential to develop one?

   _____

   _____

2. Do you think any of your friends might have an eating disorder?

   _____

   _____

3. What counseling and education resources exist in your area or on your campus to help with a potential eating disorder?

   _____

   _____

4. If a friend has an eating disorder, what do you think is the best way to assist him or her in getting help?

   _____

   _____

[†]Morgan JF and others: The SCOFF Questionnaire, *British Medical Journal* 319:1467, 1999.

II. Helping Prevent Eating Disorders

You have been asked to speak to a junior high school class about eating disorders. What are four major points that you would make to help prevent disordered eating in this population?

1. _____
2. _____
3. _____
4. _____

Here are points you may consider:

1. Extreme thinness is oversold in the media. Extremely low weight (i.e., BMI of less than 17.5) is generally not healthy.
2. Self-induced vomiting is dangerous. Damage to the teeth, stomach, and esophagus often results.
3. Loss of menstrual periods is a sign of illness. It is important to see a physician about this. Bone deterioration is a common result.
4. The treatment of eating disorders in early phases aids success. These diseases are difficult to treat once firmly established.

Chapter 12 Undernutrition Throughout the World

Student Learning Outcomes

Chapter 12 is designed to allow you to:

12.1 Define and characterize the terms *hunger, malnutrition,* and *undernutrition.*

12.2 Examine undernutrition in the United States and highlight several programs established to combat this problem.

12.3 Examine undernutrition in the developing world and evaluate the major obstacles that hinder a solution.

12.4 Outline some possible solutions to under-nutrition in the developing world.

12.5 Evaluate the consequences of undernutrition during critical periods in a person's life.

What Would You Choose?

"You'd better clean your plate! There are starving children in Africa who would love to eat that dinner!"

Mom was right—we often overlook the fact that we live in a rich nation with access to plentiful food and clean water, whereas something as simple as clean drinking water is merely a dream in many developing nations. In fact, the problems of hunger and food insecurity exist in your own community. It is probably not feasible (or sanitary) to send your rejected green beans overseas, but there are some simple steps you can take at home to support agencies seeking to provide clean water and nutritious food for people in need. What would you choose to help put an end to world hunger?

a Organize a group of friends to prepare and hand out peanut butter and jelly sandwiches to homeless people downtown.

b Donate $10 per month to an international aid organization that supplies food to starving children in Africa.

c Participate in a 5K run/walk event that raises funds and awareness to combat world hunger.

d Buy locally grown fruits and vegetables at your community's farmers' market.

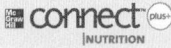 **Think about your choice as you read Chapter 12, then see our recommendations at the end of the chapter. To learn more about combating hunger, check out the Connect site:** www.mcgrawhillconnect.com

Part Four
Nutrition: Beyond the Nutrients

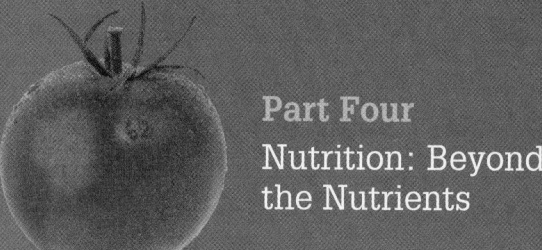

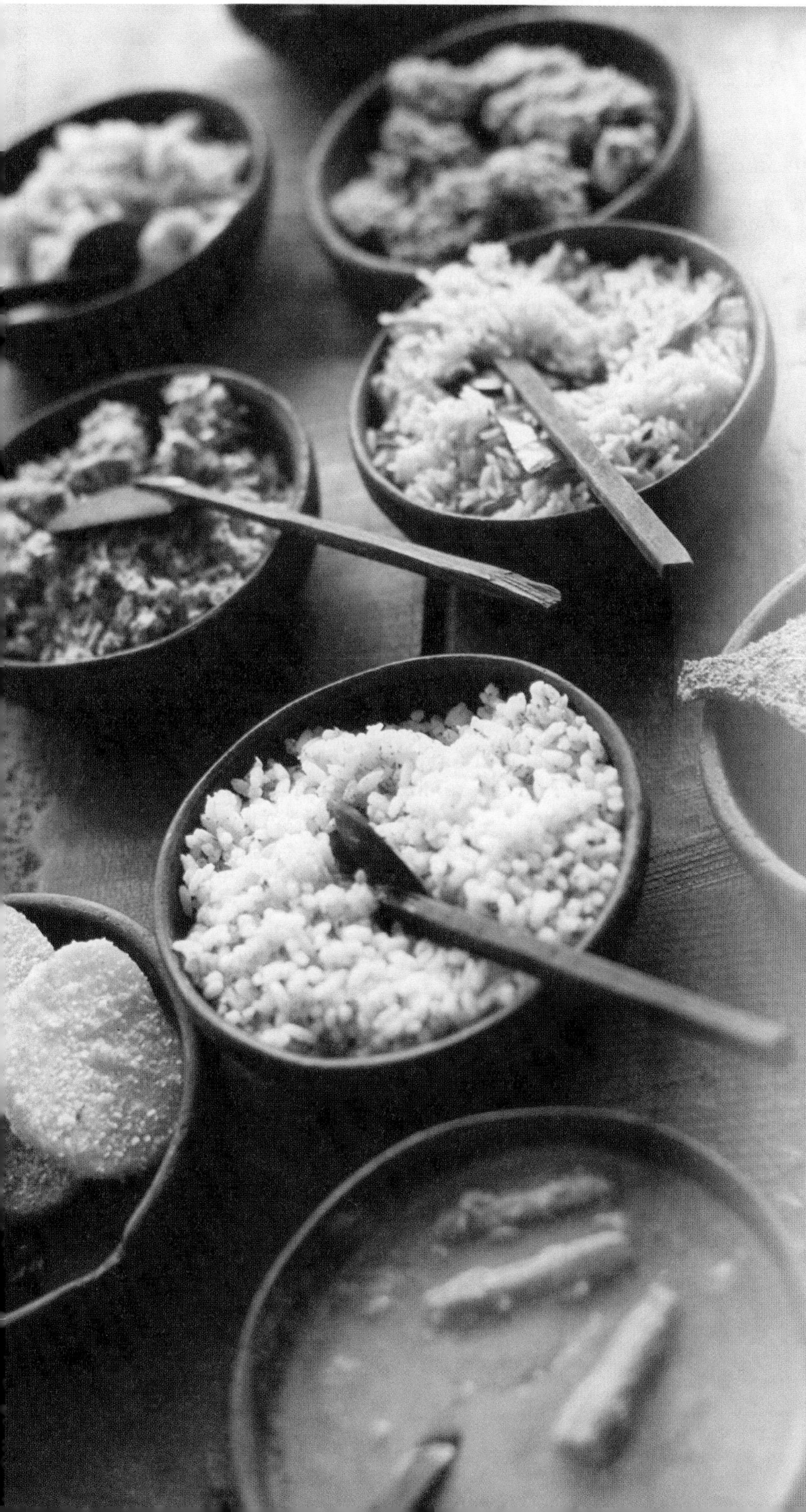

Today, nearly one in six people worldwide is chronically undernourished— too hungry to lead a productive, active life. Over the past 10 years, this problem has worsened. Throughout the world, the problems of poverty and undernutrition are widespread and growing—even though there is enough food available to sufficiently feed all of us.

Within the developing world, approximately 1 billion people are malnourished, with Asia having the largest number. Malnutrition is the main cause of lowered resistance to disease, infection, and death, with children under 5 years being the most susceptible.

Chapter 12 examines the problem of undernutrition, the conditions that create it, and some possible solutions. If we are to eradicate undernutrition, we all have to understand the problem. As the comic in the chapter suggests, we must begin to assume responsibility today, not tomorrow, to work on solutions to hunger close to home and in faraway nations. It is important to recognize that many political, economic, and social factors worldwide contribute directly and indirectly to the hunger problem.

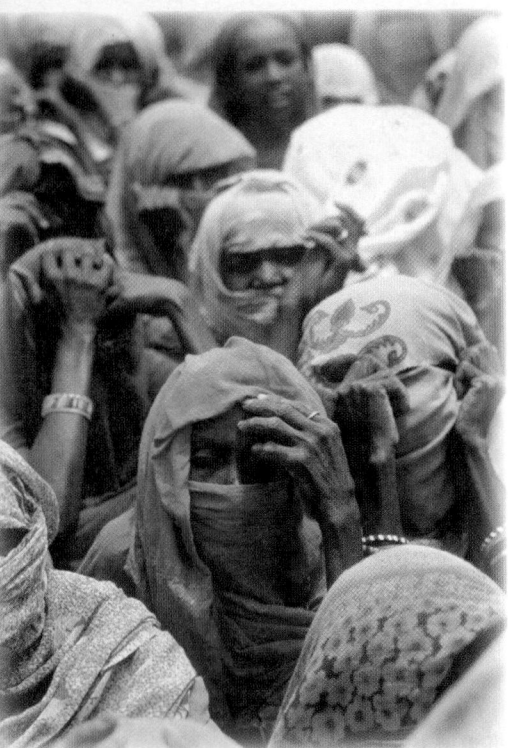

▲ Malnutrition is associated with or exacerbated by overpopulation in some developing countries.

food insecure Condition in which the quality, variety, and/or desirability of the diet is reduced and there is difficulty at times providing enough food for everyone in the household.

hunger The primarily physiological (internal) drive to find and eat food.

 Refresh Your Memory

As you begin your study of world hunger in Chapter 12, you may want to review:

- The health effects of protein-calorie malnutrition in Chapter 6
- The role of vitamin A and rich food sources in Chapter 8
- The roles and rich food sources of iron, zinc, and iodide in Chapter 9

12.1 World Hunger: A Crisis on the Rise

Uncertainty regarding the source of one's next meal remains a daily experience for close to 1 billion people around the world. This situation is troubling considering that worldwide agriculture produces more than enough food to meet the energy requirements of each of the nearly 7 billion persons. Even with this abundance, in 2008, 963 million people were unable to access enough food to lead active, healthy lives—that is, they were **food insecure.** The serious problems of food insecurity and malnutrition exist in virtually every nation. They are most common in the developing world, with Asia having the largest number, along with sub-Saharan Africa, Latin America, and the Caribbean. Nearly all people suffering from food insecurity, hunger, or malnutrition are poor.

Let's begin our look at the problem of world hunger and malnutrition by defining some key terms.

Hunger

The physiological state that results when not enough food is eaten to meet energy needs is **hunger.** It also describes an uneasiness, a discomfort, a weakness, or a pain caused by lack of food. The medical and social costs of the undernutrition that can result from hunger are high—preterm births, mental disabilities, inadequate growth and development in childhood, poor school performance, decreased work output in adulthood, and chronic disease. Although malnutrition does occur in North America, it is not due to extreme poverty over a large section of the population. Instead, there are usually specific causes such as an eating disorder, alcoholism, problems in nursing home settings, or homelessness. There is also some degree of moderate malnutrition in some of the poorer segments of North American society (i.e., those earning less than the current poverty level). Fortunately, there are resources such as food banks and food stamps, though sometimes there are bureaucratic obstacles to getting these

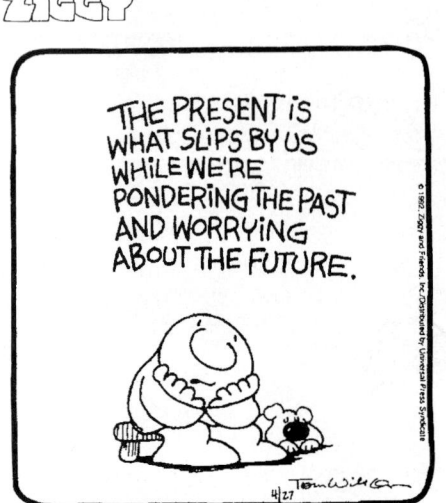

ZIGGY®

THE PRESENT IS WHAT SLIPS BY US WHILE WE'RE PONDERING THE PAST AND WORRYING ABOUT THE FUTURE.

Millions of people worldwide die each year from health problems related to undernutrition. Rising food prices, war, and environmental catastrophe combine with the global threat of AIDS as important causes. Why must we act today to stem this tide of undernutrition? Why is Ziggy's concern an important one? Chapter 12 provides some answers.

ZIGGY © ZIGGY AND FRIENDS, INC. Reprinted with permission of UNIVERSAL PRESS SYNDICATE. All rights reserved.

resources to the people who need them. In addition, there is the problem known as **food insecurity,** which describes a state of anxiety about running out of food or running out of money to buy more food. In 2009, 14.7% of households in the United States reported that they experienced food insecurity. Food insecurity is also a problem in Canada with 8% living in food-insecure households in 2008.

Around the world, poverty is a primary cause of malnutrition. In the United States, at least 13 million children, 18% of all children under the age of 18, are in families living below the federal poverty level, defined as a family of four having an income less than $22,350 a year in 2011 (more information available at http://aspe.hhs.gov/poverty/11poverty.shtml). Research, however, estimates that families need an income of about twice that level to cover basic expenses. Using this income standard, 39% of children live in low-income families. Living in poverty impairs a child's ability to learn and contributes to behavioral problems and poor health. The risks of poverty are greatest for young children. Fortunately, the United States does have food assistance programs for low-income families, and therefore most children in the United States are shielded from hunger.

Malnutrition and Micronutrient Deficiences

A condition of impaired development or function caused by either a long-term deficiency or excess in calorie and/or nutrient intake is **malnutrition.** When food supplies are low and the population is large, **undernutrition** is common, leading to nutritional deficiency diseases, such as goiter (from an iodide deficiency) and xerophthalmia (eye problems caused by poor vitamin A intake). However, when the food supply is ample or overabundant, incorrect food choices coupled with an excessive intake can lead to overnutrition and its related chronic diseases, such as type 2 diabetes.

Undernutrition is the most common form of malnutrition among the poor in both developing and developed countries. Undernutrition is also the primary cause of specific nutrient deficiencies that can result in muscle wasting, blindness, scurvy, pellagra, beriberi, anemia, rickets, goiter, and a host of other problems (Table 12-1).

The most critical micronutrients missing from diets worldwide (see Fig. 12-1) are iron, vitamin A, iodide, zinc, and various B vitamins (e.g., folate), as well as selenium and vitamin C (see Further Readings 7 and 11). About 1 billion people, mostly in the developing world, are affected by iron deficiency. The same is true for zinc deficiencies. With poor iron status, cognitive development will likely be impaired, particularly if prolonged deficiency occurs during early infancy. An estimated 50 million people worldwide also suffer brain damage from preventable maternal iodide deficiency. Although severe vitamin A deficiency, which causes blindness, is on the decline, up to 500,000 preschool-age children are still blinded by it each year. UNICEF reports that the lives of 1 million to 3 million children could be saved annually in the developing world if vitamin A supplements were provided a few times each year. The annual cost per child would be about 6 cents.

Of the 6.4 billion people in the world, about 2 billion may experience episodes of food shortages and be affected by some form of micronutrient malnutrition. Death and disease from infections, particularly those causing acute and prolonged diarrhea or respiratory disease, increase dramatically when the infections occur during a state of chronic undernutrition. Chronic undernutrition leaves many people in the developing world in a continual state of depressed immune function, in turn greatly increasing the risk of death, especially in childhood.

Protein-calorie malnutrition (PCM) is a form of undernutrition caused by an extremely deficient intake of calories or protein generally accompanied by an illness. The dramatic results of PCM—kwashiorkor and marasmus—were described in Chapter 6. This chapter focuses on the more subtle effects of a chronic lack of food.

Famine

The extreme form of chronic hunger is **famine.** Periods of famine are characterized by large-scale loss of life, social disruption, and economic chaos that slows food production. As a result of these extreme events, the affected community experiences

food insecurity A condition of anxiety regarding running out of either food or money to buy more food.

malnutrition Failing health that results from longstanding dietary practices that do not coincide with nutritional needs.

undernutrition Failing health that results from a longstanding dietary intake that is not enough to meet nutritional needs.

famine An extreme shortage of food, which leads to massive starvation in a population; often associated with crop failures, war, and political unrest.

The Irish potato famine of 1840 to 1850 caused an estimated 2 million deaths and resulted in nearly as many people emigrating to other countries, such as the United States and Canada. More than 3 million people may have perished in the great famine of 1943 in Bengal, India. China suffered a famine from 1959 to 1961—estimates of mortality range from 16 million to 64 million. In 1974, another 1.5 million starved in the country of Bangladesh.

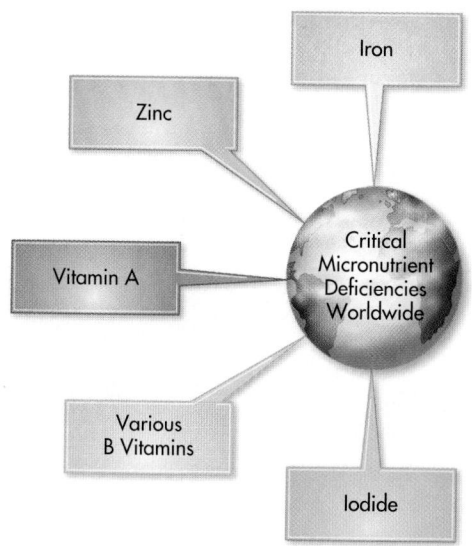

FIGURE 12-1 ▶ Critical micronutrient deficiencies worldwide.

TABLE 12-1 Nutrient-Deficiency Diseases That Commonly Accompany Undernutrition

Disease and Key Nutrient Involved*	Typical Effects	Foods Rich in Deficient Nutrient	Target Populations for Intervention
Xerophthalmia Vitamin A	Blindness from chronic eye infections, restricted growth, dryness and keratinization of epithelial tissues	Fortified milk, sweet potatoes, spinach, greens, carrots, cantaloupe, apricots	Asia, Africa
Rickets Vitamin D	Poorly calcified bones, bowed legs, other bone deformities	Fortified milk, fish oils, sun exposure	Asia, Africa, and parts of the world where religious dress codes prevent women and children from receiving adequate sun exposure; older adults in developed nations
Beriberi Thiamin	Nerve degeneration, altered muscle coordination, cardiovascular problems	Sunflower seeds, pork, whole and enriched grains, dried beans	Victims of famine in Africa
Ariboflavinosis Riboflavin	Inflammation of tongue, mouth, face and oral cavity, nervous system disorders	Milk, mushrooms, spinach, liver, enriched grains	Victims of famine in Africa
Pellagra Niacin	Diarrhea, dermatitis, dementia	Mushrooms, bran, tuna, chicken, beef, peanuts, whole and enriched grains	Victims of famine in Africa, survivors of war-torn Eastern Europe
Megaloblastic anemia Folate	Enlarged red blood cells, fatigue, weakness	Green leafy vegetables, legumes, oranges, liver	Asia, Africa
Scurvy Vitamin C	Delayed wound healing, internal bleeding, abnormal formation of bones and teeth	Citrus fruits, strawberries, broccoli	Victims of famine in Africa
Iron-deficiency anemia Iron	Reduced work output, retarded growth, increased health risk in pregnancy	Meats, seafood, broccoli, peas, bran, whole-grain and enriched breads	Worldwide
Goiter Iodide	Enlarged thyroid gland in teenagers and adults, possible mental retardation, cretinism	Iodized salt, saltwater fish	South America, Eastern Europe, Africa

*Although the nutrients are listed separately to illustrate the important role of each one, often two or more nutrition-deficiency diseases are found in an undernourished person in the developing world.

a downward spiral characterized by human distress; sales of land, livestock, and other farm assets; migration; division and impoverishment of the poorest families; crime; and the weakening of customary moral codes, as seen in Sudan and Rwanda. In the midst of all this, undernutrition rates soar; infectious diseases, such as cholera, spread; and many people die.

Special efforts are needed to eradicate the fundamental causes of famine. Causes vary by region and decade, but the most common is crop failure. The most obvious reasons for crop failure are extreme weather conditions such as floods or drought, war, and civil strife. War deserves a special focus and will be specifically addressed in a separate section on war and political/civil unrest.

General Effects of Semistarvation

In the initial stages, the results of undernutrition from semistarvation are often so mild that physical symptoms are absent and blood tests do not usually detect the slight metabolic changes. Even in the absence of clinical symptoms, however, under-nourishment may affect reproductive capacity, resistance to and recovery from disease, and physical activity and work output, and lead to fatigue and behavior problems. Recall from Chapter 2 that, as tissues continue to be depleted of nutrients, blood tests eventually detect biochemical changes, such as a drop in blood hemoglobin concentration. Physical symptoms, such as body weakness, appear with further depletion. Finally, the full-blown symptoms of the predominating deficiency are recognizable, such as when blindness accompanies a vitamin A deficiency.

When a few people in a population develop a severe deficiency, this may represent only the "tip of the iceberg." Typically, a much greater number have milder degrees of undernutrition. These deficiencies should not, therefore, be dismissed as trivial, especially in the developing world. It is becoming clear that combined deficiencies of specific vitamins and the minerals iron and zinc can seriously reduce work performance, even when they do not cause obvious physical symptoms. This resulting state of ill health, in turn, diminishes the ability of individuals, communities, and even whole countries to perform at peak levels of physical and mental capacity (Fig. 12-2).

Added to their lack of nourishment, the inhabitants of poorer countries must also contend with recurrent infections, poor sanitation, extreme weather conditions, and regular exposure to infectious diseases. They require greater amounts of certain nutrients—especially iron—to combat rampant parasite and other infections. Deficiencies of both iron and zinc can lead to reduced immune function and thereby increase the risk of diseases, such as diarrhea and pneumonia.

The effects of hunger are widespread:
- Reduced energy and strength
- Diminished concentration
- Impaired ability to learn
- Lowered productivity
- Worsening of chronic health conditions
- Increased susceptibility to infectious diseases
- Deterioration of mood
- Slowed recovery from illness and injury

Historical Research on Undernutrition

In the 1940s a group of researchers led by Dr. Ansel Keys examined the general effects of undernutrition on adults. Previously healthy men were fed a diet averaging about 1800 kcal daily for 6 months. During this time, the men lost an average of 24% of their body weight. After about 3 months, the participants complained of fatigue, muscle soreness, irritability, intolerance to cold, and hunger pains. They exhibited a lack of ambition, self-discipline, and concentration, and were often moody, apathetic, and depressed. Their heart rate and muscle tone decreased, and they developed edema. When the men were permitted to eat normally again, feelings of recurrent hunger and fatigue persisted even after 12 weeks of rehabilitation. Full recovery required about 8 months. This study helps us understand the general state of undernourished adults worldwide.

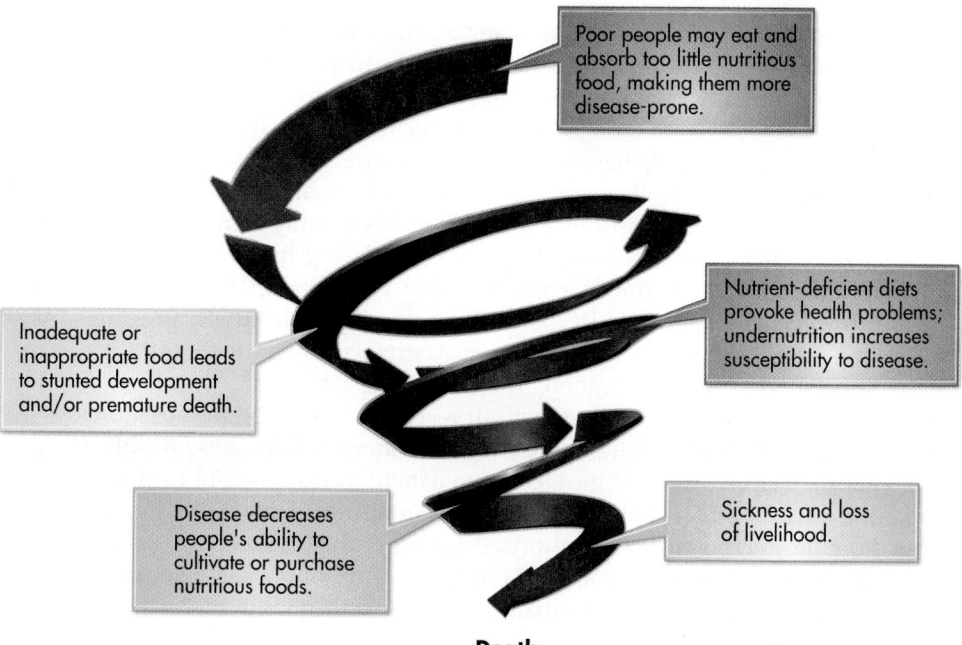

FIGURE 12-2 ▶ The downward spiral of poverty and illness can ultimately end in death (based on World Food Program graphic).

CONCEPT CHECK

Hunger provokes uneasiness and pain when insufficient food is eaten to meet calorie needs. Food insecurity is anxiety about running out of food or money to buy more food. Chronic hunger leads to undernutrition, which can cause growth failure in children and physical weakness in adults. Risk of infection increases, and nutrient-deficiency diseases result. The primary cause of undernutrition is poverty. The critical periods for undernutrition occur during pregnancy, infancy, childhood, and old age. Chronic undernutrition decreases work performance, motivation, and immune function. The adverse effects in pregnancy and infancy are dramatic, as evidenced by mortality rates much higher than those of healthy populations. Irreversible developmental damage in surviving children is also common.

12.2 Undernutrition in the United States

About 50 million (14.7%) people in the United States live at or below the poverty level, estimated at about $22,350 annually for a family of four. Of those 50 million, 17 million (34%) are children. The percentage of the population living in food-insecure households in Canada is lower than in the United States (see Further Reading 14).

Ten percent of Caucasians, 24% of African-Americans, and 20.6% of Hispanics live in poverty. Many Native Americans are also poor, as are 18% of Asian Americans. (Many Native Americans in Canada also live in poverty.)

The poor often face difficult choices: whether to buy groceries for the family or pay this month's rent; whether to have dental work done or pay the current utility bill; whether to replace clothes the children have outgrown or pay for transportation to apply for a job. Food is one of the few flexible items in a poor person's budget. Whereas housing and utility costs, medical care, and transportation fares are non-negotiable, a person can always eat less. The short-term consequences of eating less may be less dramatic than getting evicted, but the long-term cumulative effects are significant.

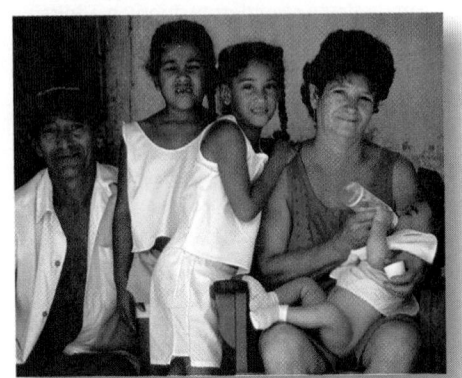

▲ Food insecurity is part of the North American landscape. A "safety net" of programs exists, but it is "porous."

Helping the Hungry in the United States

Until the twentieth century, individuals and a wide variety of charitable, often church-related organizations, provided most of the help to poor, undernourished people in the United States. Early programs rarely distributed direct cash payments to poor people because these were thought to reduce recipients' motivation to improve their circumstances or change behaviors, such as excessive drinking, that contributed to their poverty. Beginning in the early 1900s, the involvement of local, county, and state governments in providing assistance to the poor has steadily increased.

After observing extensive hunger and poverty during his presidential campaign in the 1960s, John F. Kennedy revitalized the Food Stamp Program, which had begun two decades earlier, and expanded commodity distribution programs. As of October 1, 2008, Supplemental Nutrition Assistance Program (SNAP) is the new name for the Food Stamp Program. The new name reflects the program's focus on nutrition and putting healthy food within reach for low-income households. SNAP helps low-income people and families buy food they need for good health. The program allows recipients to use an Electronic Benefit Transfer (EBT) card to purchase food and garden seeds—but not tobacco, cleaning items, alcoholic beverages, and nonedible products—at stores authorized to accept them. In recent years, each participating household received about $190 per month, on average. About 39 million people in the United States participate in this program (Table 12-2). The American Recovery and Reinvestment Act of 2009 increased benefits for SNAP participants. The increase for a participating household of four was $80 in monthly benefits.

The U.S. Congress established the School Breakfast Program in 1965 as politicians became aware of the number of hungry children coming to school. School breakfast and lunch programs still enable low-income students—11.7 million for breakfast

Chapter 12: Undernutrition Throughout the World

TABLE 12-2 Some Current Federally Subsidized Programs That Supply Food for People in the United States

Program	Eligibility	Description
Supplemental Nutrition Assistance Program (formerly Food Stamp Program)*	Low-income families	Electronic Benefit Transfer (debit) cards are given to purchase food at grocery stores; the amount is based on size of household and income.
The Emergency Food Assistance Program (TEFAP)*	Low-income families	Provides nutrition assistance to needy Americans through distribution of USDA food commodities.
Commodity Supplemental Food Program	Certain low-income populations, such as pregnant women, children until the age of 6 years, and seniors	USDA surplus foods are distributed by county agencies; not found in all states; may be based on nutritional risk.
Special Supplemental Nutrition Program for Women, Infants, and Children (WIC)*	Low-income pregnant/lactating women, infants, and children less than 5 years old at nutritional risk	Coupons are given to purchase milk, cheese, fruit juice, cereal, infant formula, and other specific food items at grocery stores; includes nutrition education component. Includes new Farmers' Market Nutrition Program (FMNP).
National School Lunch Program*	Low-income children of school age	Free or reduced-price lunch is distributed by the school; meal follows USDA pattern based on MyPyramid; cost for the child depends on family income. For students who do not participate in the lunch program, special milk program may be available.
School Breakfast Program	Low-income children of school age	Free or reduced-price breakfast is distributed by the school; meal follows USDA pattern; cost for the child depends on family income.
Child and Adult Care Food Program	Child enrolled in organized child-care program and seniors in adult-care programs; income guidelines are the same as those for the School Lunch Program	Reimbursement is given for meals supplied to children at the site; meals must follow USDA guidelines based on MyPlate.
Congregate Meals for the Elderly	Age 60 or over (no income guidelines)	Free noon meal is furnished at a site; meal follows specific pattern based on one-third of nutrient needs.
Home-Delivered Meals	Age 60 or over, homebound	Noon meal is delivered at no cost or for a donation at least 5 days a week. Sometimes additional meals for later consumption are delivered at the same time; often referred to as "Meals on Wheels."
Summer Food Service Program	Residence in a low-income neighborhood or participation in a program	Free, nutritious meals and snacks are given to children in a low-income area at a central site, such as a school or a community center during long school vacations.
Food Distribution Program on Indian Reservations*	Low-income American Indian and non-Indian households on reservations; members of federally recognized tribes	Alternative to Supplemental Nutrition Assistance Program, distribution of monthly food packages; includes nutrition education component.
Fresh Fruit and Vegetable Program	Low-income elementary schools	Provides free fresh fruits and vegetables to increase their consumption and to combat childhood obesity.

* Benefits increased through the American Recovery and Reinvestment Act of 2009.

and 31.7 million for lunch in 2010—to receive meals free or at reduced cost if certain income guidelines are met (under $29,055 to $41,348, respectively, for annual income of a family of four). In the same year, the U.S. Congress funded group noon-time (called *congregate*) meals and home-delivered meals for all citizens over 60 years of age, regardless of income (donations are requested, however). Both remain active programs, serving about 1 million meals each day, but they still do not reach all who need help. In addition, in 1972, the Special Supplemental Nutrition Program for Women, Infants, and Children (WIC) was authorized. This program provides food

CRITICAL THINKING

While studying early childhood development, Nakia was surprised to learn that some children in the United States are undernourished. What evidence might Nakia observe in children that would suggest undernourishment?

vouchers and nutrition education to low-income pregnant and lactating women and their young children. It serves about 9.2 million people. Read more about child and adolescent nutrition assistance programs in Further Reading 4.

Between 1969 and 1971, some already large federal food programs were expanded and others were created. For example, the Food Stamp Program served only 2 million people in 1968, but by 1971 it was serving 11 million. The National School Lunch Program, which served only 2 million poor children before 1970, was serving 8 million children by 1971. Soon after, the School Breakfast Program, a pilot program for children living in impoverished areas, became available nationally.

Sometimes, severe undernutrition due to involuntary hunger does occur in the United States. More often, though, Americans experience periodic episodes of hunger and food insecurity. Unemployment, medical and housing expenses, and even occasional holiday shopping can cause a household to be hungry or food insecure.

Government food assistance programs are like a "safety net"—they are strong, yet porous. The Recovery Act that was signed by President Obama in February 2009 was an unprecedented effort to increase benefits and services offered by the federal food and nutrition programs (Table 12-2). The enhancement of these programs has helped those workers and families hardest hit by the economic crisis. Privately funded programs have stepped in to add to state and federal efforts to combat hunger and related food insecurity in the United States. There are more than 150,000 charitable food providers (such as food banks and food pantries) helping to cope with this problem. They serve about 23 million Americans. Many low-income U.S. households rely on food pantries, and one survey found that slightly more than two of every three people requesting such emergency food assistance are members of families—children and their parents.

MAKING DECISIONS

Food Insecurity and Overweight?

Undernutrition in North America is a much more subtle problem than in developing countries. To the untrained eye, undernourished children may just seem skinny, when, in fact, their growth is being stunted by insufficient nutrients. More likely, though, children from food-insecure households are prone to be overweight. This may be the result of considerable reliance on convenience foods that provide mostly fat and sugar. Also, food-insecure families may buy candies and snack foods as treats when expensive toys and clothing aren't affordable.

The availability of cooking facilities affects nutrient intake among the poor. Without cooking facilities, people may buy expensive convenience foods that require no preparation. These are typically highly processed snack foods, which provide calories but are often lacking in nutrients.

Socioeconomic Factors Related to Undernutrition

In the United States, persistent hunger and food insecurity are largely associated with two interrelated conditions: poverty and homelessness. Thus, the economic, social, and political changes that lead to an increase in the number of poor or homeless people also tend to intensify the problem of undernutrition.

Poverty. Underemployment leads to poverty. This relationship has increased significantly with the economic recession that began late in 2007. The recent economic crisis is the worst in decades and has caused unemployment to soar. Between December 2007 and September 2009, 7.6 million jobs were lost. These job losses occurred across all major private-sector industries, including manufacturing, retail trade, leisure and hospitality, financial, transportation, and warehousing. In June 2011, the number of unemployed persons was 14.1 million, resulting in an unemployment rate of 9.2%. The impact of the increase in unemployment has been enhanced because, during the economic downturn, many states have cut their welfare assistance. This combination of events has resulted in more people living in poverty and in need of food assistance, at risk of homelessness, and without sufficient healthcare.

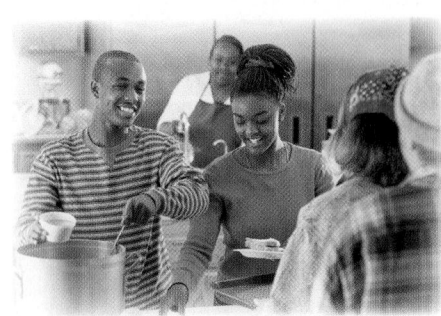

▲ Food pantries and soup kitchens are important sources of nutrients for a growing number of people in the United States. Consider volunteering some of your time to a local program.

Access to Healthy Food. Access to affordable and nutritious foods is also a challenge to many (see Further Reading 6). In 2011, 23.5 million Americans, including 6.5 million children, lived in low-income areas lacking stores likely to sell affordable healthy foods such as fresh fruits and vegetables. These impoverished areas with little access to healthy foods have been named "food deserts." The USDA defines a food desert as an area where 33% or 500 people, whichever is less, live more than a mile from a grocery store in an urban area, or more than 10 miles away in a rural area. In 2011, several national retail stores, including Wal-Mart, Walgreens, and SuperValu, as well as some regional companies, agreed to bring more nutritious and fresh food to underserved communities by opening or expanding more than 1500 stores. These changes were aimed to serve about 9.5 million people and to create tens of thousands of jobs.

food desert An area where 33% or 500 people, whichever is less, live more than a mile from a grocery store in an urban area or more than 10 miles away in a rural area.

Homelessness. The growing shortage of affordable rental housing and a simultaneous increase in poverty are the two trends largely responsible for the rise in homelessness over the past 25 years. The more recent foreclosure and economic crises have added to this situation and created a significant increase in homelessness and the number of families at risk of homelessness across the country. In 2009, data from major cities indicated increases of homelessness by as much as 20% since the foreclosure crisis began in 2007. A study done by the National Law Center on Homelessness and Poverty estimates that 3.5 million people, including 1.35 million children are likely to experience homelessness in a given year. Families with children are one of the fastest growing homeless groups, especially in rural areas, and make up about 23% of the homeless population. Single mothers in their late 20s with approximately two children are the most common heads of homeless families. Poor people must make difficult choices when limited resources cover only some necessities such as housing, food, childcare, health care, and education. Because housing absorbs a high percentage of income, it is often given up. Currently the largest gap on record exists between the number of affordable housing units and the number of people needing them. The homelessness created by this gap impacts the health and well-being of all individuals. Homeless children are most vulnerable and are twice as likely to experience hunger compared to children with a home.

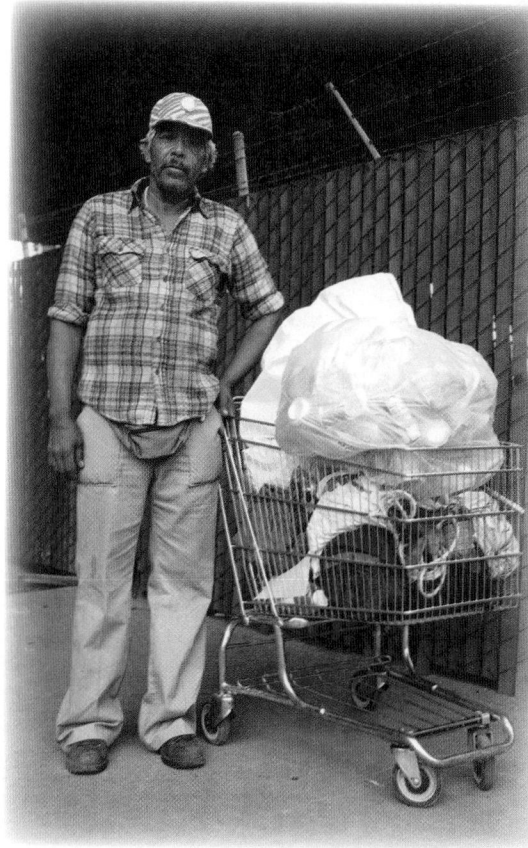

▲ Homelessness can be the result of many problems, including poverty.

Possible Solutions to Poverty and Hunger in the United States

Government-funded food assistance programs have helped to alleviate some problems of undernutrition in the United States. The question is, *Can government programs provide a permanent solution to poverty and undernutrition . . . and should they?* (see Further Reading 2).

It is documented that an increasing number of people who are experiencing poverty are accessing the Supplemental Nutrition Assistance Program (SNAP; formerly called the Food Stamp Program) benefits as well as other federal programs. As a result of the American Recovery and Reinvestment Act of 2009 (www.recovery.gov), more federal funds have been infused into assistance programs. There is no guarantee, however, that benefits from these programs will suitably meet the needs of the poor. In addition, there is a growing sentiment that state and federal support programs and policies are ineffective and inappropriate. These concerns are especially expressed by those who are falling deeper into poverty and those who are at increased risk of poverty and homelessness.

Obtaining food to survive is a tremendous challenge, especially when homeless people are forced to live outside. Surveys on hunger and homelessness in U.S. cities indicate that indoor food programs are not adequate to meet the need in some cities. A national survey by the Interagency Council on Homelessness also revealed that 40% of homeless people did not have anything to eat on one or more days during the month previous to the survey.

Although many people assume that food pantries and soup kitchens are abundant and accessible for every needy person there are many obstacles to these resources. Food pantries are often ineffective because they can give only one box of food to families per month, which does not meet their needs. Furthermore, homeless people lack the cooking facilities necessary to prepare the food. Food availability through soup kitchens is also limited in many cities. An additional challenge is that cities have recently begun to use ordinances and policies to discourage or prohibit the sharing of food with poor or homeless persons by individuals and groups. These laws are troubling, considering that most cities do not have adequate food resources to meet the need of their poor and homeless. Advocacy groups raise questions about individual rights and freedoms and have challenged these practices in court cases. Advocates and food providers appear eager to work with cities and other government agencies to help address the problems of hunger and homelessness by improving access to federal food benefits and other food resources.

Despite even the highest motivation, the outlook is bleak for many people who attempt to gain independence from assistance programs. Teen pregnancy may have cut short the education or vocational training of one or both parents, thwarting efforts to earn adequate income. Often, the expense of reliable and safe child care far exceeds the meager income from a minimum-wage job. Illness of either the parents or children may prevent the adults from holding steady employment. Poor communication skills, inability to relocate, and a lack of economic reserves also complicate financial independence. Regardless of how wasteful government assistance appears to some people, it will probably always be necessary to some extent.

Many consider an increase in individual responsibility as a critical goal. Government programs cannot easily fix poverty and the resulting hunger that stem from irresponsible individual behavior. Government programs can, however, help reduce or prevent the poverty that results largely from lack of education or opportunity.

Long-term undernutrition—especially among children—has both individual and societal consequences, so everyone in the United States is affected by this problem, either directly or indirectly. As government programs are redesigned, it is likely that some will suffer. The hope is that these new approaches will lead to long-term progress and the eventual relief of poverty and hunger.

Two objectives of *Healthy People 2020* are to eliminate very low food security among children from 1.3% of households in 2008 to 0.2% in 2020 and to reduce hunger by reducing household food insecurity from 14.6% of households in 2008 to 6% in 2020.

CONCEPT CHECK

In response to reports of widespread poverty and hunger during the 1960s, the U.S. Congress established several food assistance programs and substantially increased funding for already existing programs. Largely as a result of these federal programs, undernutrition had decreased substantially by the mid-1970s. The presence of poverty, homelessness, and undernutrition is influenced by economic, cultural, and individual factors, as well as government policies. The serious questions about the long-term effectiveness of many government assistance programs are causing major changes in their program design. All citizens can help reduce the problem of undernutrition.

12.3 Undernutrition in the Developing World

Undernutrition in the developing world is also tied to poverty, and any true solution must address this problem. However, these countries have a multitude of problems so complex and interrelated that they cannot be treated separately. Programs that have proved immensely helpful in the United States (and throughout the rest of North America) are only a starting point in this context. The following major obstacles challenge those seeking a solution:

- Extreme imbalances in the food/population ratio in different regions of a country
- War and political/civil unrest, especially in Africa

- The rapid depletion of natural resources, such as farmland, fish, and water
- The disease AIDS, especially in sub-Saharan Africa and Asia
- High external (foreign) debt, much of which is owed to developed nations
- Poor **infrastructure,** especially poor housing, sanitation and storage facilities, education, communications, and transportation systems

Each problem deserves individual consideration (Fig. 12-3).

infrastructure The basic framework of a system of organization. For a society, this includes roads, bridges, telephones, and other basic technologies.

Food/Population Ratio

The world has 6.85 billion inhabitants. Population growth exceeds economic growth in much of the developing world, and as a result, poverty is increasing. This disrupts the balance in the food/population ratio, tipping it toward food shortages. If we want to ensure a decent life for a widening segment of humanity, many experts suggest that the growth in the earth's most vulnerable populations should slow. If not, by 2050 the world may have 1 to 3 billion more people than it does today—most of them in countries where the average person earns less than $2 per day. In developing countries, nearly 29% of people live on less than $1 per day. Unless a catastrophe occurs, more than 9 of 10 infants in the next generation will be born in the poorest parts of the world.

More than three-quarters of people in the world live in developing countries, and more than half live in Asia. A United Nations report on worldwide hunger revealed that almost two-thirds of the world's undernourished live in Asia and the Pacific Rim. The world's food supplies also are not distributed equally among consumers. Gross disparities exist between developed and developing countries, among the rich and the poor within countries, and even within families (males may be fed before females).

Still, economists estimate that world food production will continue to increase more rapidly than the world population in the near future, allowing the food/population ratio to increase through the year 2020. This will come at a high cost, however, in terms of the water, fertilizer, and pesticides needed to allow for this production. Overall, in the short run, the primary problem appears not to be food production *but* distribution and use, especially in poverty-stricken areas of developing nations.

Eventually, though, food production will begin to lag behind population growth. Most good farmland in the world is already in use, and because of poor farming practices or competing land-use demands, the number of farmable acres worldwide decreases annually. For many reasons, sustainable world food output—an amount that doesn't deplete the earth's resources—is now running well behind food consumption. This discrepancy suggests that food production in less-developed countries will barely keep up with population growth and will soon lag behind.

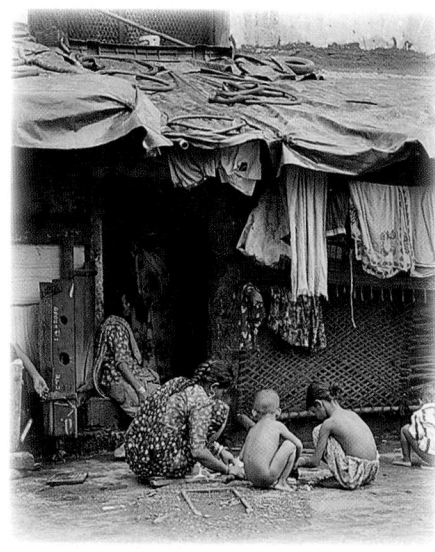

▲ Poverty aggravates the problem of hunger in the developing world

FIGURE 12-3 ▶ Many factors contribute to undernutrition in the developing world. Any solutions to the problem must take these factors into consideration.

AIDS

War and political/civil unrest

Rapid depletion of natural resources, such as farmland, fish, and water

Hunger in the Developing World

Extreme imbalances in the food/population ratio

Poor infrastructure

High external (foreign) debt

Birth control programs, an obvious brake on population expansion, have been effective in developed countries but relatively ineffective in many developing countries that could really benefit from them. Among women, family planning and contraceptive use worldwide has increased to 63% today, up from 10% in 1969. If the United Nations, voluntary organizations, and governments had not started promoting family planning and contraceptive use, the population today might be as high as 7 or 8 billion. However, women (and men) in many developing countries are still lacking adequate access to contraceptives. The United Nations estimates that at least 200 million women want to use safe and effective family planning methods, but they lack access to information and services or the support of their husbands and communities. Organizations such as Population Services International are trying to keep distribution costs low and make the products available to as many people as possible by subsidizing condoms and oral contraceptives to areas such as Bangladesh.

human immunodeficiency virus (HIV) The virus that leads to acquired immune deficiency syndrome (AIDS).

acquired immune deficiency syndrome (AIDS) A disorder in which a virus (human immunodeficiency virus [HIV]) infects specific types of immune system cells. This leaves the person with reduced immune function and, in turn, defenseless against numerous infectious agents; typically contributes to the person's death.

MAKING DECISIONS

Benefits of Breastfeeding

Promoting breastfeeding also contributes to the goal of birth control. Although it is not a completely reliable method of contraception, exclusively breastfeeding an infant lessens ovulation, thereby lowering the likelihood of fertilization, for an average of 6 months. (Women who do not breastfeed generally begin to ovulate within a month or so after giving birth.) When childbirths are more widely spaced, not only do fewer total births occur, but the mother has a longer chance to recover from pregnancy, and the infant receives feeding priority for a longer time. One possible exception to the healthful nature of breastfeeding occurs, however, when mothers are infected with the **human immunodeficiency virus (HIV).** The risk of transferring the virus through human milk is about 10%. Depending on the circumstances, this may outweigh the benefits of breastfeeding.

Experience with family planning programs in developing countries and historical changes in birth rates in many developed countries suggest an important conclusion. Generally, only when people have enough to eat and are financially secure do they feel confident that having fewer children will still result in enough surviving sons and/ or daughters to provide for their care in later years. Increasing per capita income and improving education, especially for women in developing nations, are considered to be the most likely long-term solutions to excessive population growth. In the last few years, this effort has led to a decline in family size in Brazil, Egypt, India, and Mexico. A major concern is whether there are enough resources worldwide to raise per capita income and provide enough education to slow population growth.

CONCEPT CHECK

World food production is sufficient to meet the calorie needs of the world's population. Despite these adequate food resources, undernutrition continues to exist because of poverty, politics, and unequal food distribution. In addition, projected population growth may soon overwhelm food production. Most scientists and world leaders recommend limiting population growth, especially in developing countries where birth rates are high.

▲ Lasting gains have come slowly in the world's battle against undernutrition.

The conflicts in the Darfur region of Sudan have led to high rates of death and undernutrition among people displaced by war.

War and Political/Civil Unrest

The Millennium Summit of the United Nations in September 2000 resulted in the Millennium Declaration that included the resolution to "spare no effort to free our peoples from the scourge of war." Against that background stands the reality that worldwide military spending is reported to be over $2.1 trillion in annual expenditure and has been rising in recent years since 2001. The entire budget of the United Nations is only a fraction of the world's military expenditure at approximately 1.5%. In the twentieth century, deadly weapons of war took an enormous toll on civilians living in poor, politically vulnerable, war-torn nations. Less than one-half of 1% of the world's yearly production of goods and services is devoted to economic development assistance, whereas approximately 6% goes to military expenditures.

Aside from the economic impact of military spending, civil disruptions and wars are setting back the progress of the poor and contributing to massive undernutrition. Many regions of Africa have been involved in numerous civil wars and conflicts in recent years. These include conflicts in the countries directly involved in the Democratic Republic of Congo, the Sierra Leone crisis, and the war in Ethiopia/Eritrea. These conflicts have resulted in millions of deaths as well as over 9 million refugees and internally displaced people. While war has raged, health, education, and public services have declined for African people, and poverty has increased in Sub-Saharan Africa. War-related famine affects at least 20 million people in southern and northeastern Africa. The border war between Ethiopia and neighboring Eritrea has had a tremendous negative impact on food resources. A World Bank official stated that the food shortage in Ethiopia is a problem that will persist until political changes are made. Approximately 12.4 million people in Ethiopia, Eritrea, Djibouti, Kenya, Somalia, and Zimbabwe are at risk for food shortages. Other conflicts continue between Congo (formerly Zaire) and the Republic of Congo, as well as in Angola and Sudan, where millions have been put at risk of starvation (see Further Reading 12). In the capitol of war-torn Iraq, Baghdad, child malnutrition has increased dramatically. Disruptions in infrastructure from bombing and looting limit the safety of water, and as a result, health officials have observed a 250% increase in cases of diarrhea. Furthermore, health facilities needed to cope with undernutrition and dehydration have been damaged and looted throughout Baghdad and the surrounding area. Overall, most people in war-torn areas are without sufficient shelter, clothing, food, or means of obtaining them. Worldwide, this entire problem is projected to worsen over the next 15 years.

Even when food is available, political divisions may impede its distribution to the point that undernutrition will plague many people for years. Especially during emergencies, programs designed to help the poor have been undermined by unstable administration, corruption, and political influence. During such political chaos, relief agencies are often caught between warring factions and those they are trying to help. This has been the case in Sudan where non-governmental relief organizations, such as the Children's Hunger Relief Fund, have been expelled in recent years. This has caused continued deterioration in the Darfur region, and hundreds of thousands of refugees are left without the help they depended on from relief organizations.

During the 1960s and 1970s, the problem of undernutrition in developing countries was perceived as a technical one: how to produce enough food for the growing world population. The problem is now seen as largely political: how to achieve cooperation among and within nations, so that gains in food production and infrastructure are not wiped out by war. The best answer lies in a combination of approaches—finding technical solutions to help with the problems of chronic hunger and poverty and resolving political crises that have pushed developing nations into a state of acute hunger and chaos.

Rapid Depletion of Natural Resources

As we quickly deplete the earth's resources, population control grows increasingly critical. Agriculture production is approaching its limits in many areas worldwide. Environmentally unsustainable farming methods are undermining food production, especially in developing countries.

The **green revolution** was a phenomenon that began in the 1960s when crop yields rose dramatically in some countries, such as the Philippines, India, and Mexico (countries in Africa did not benefit because climates were not compatible with the

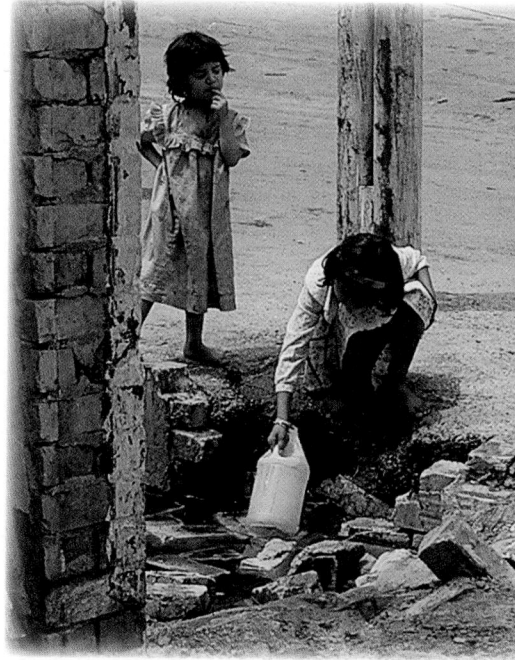

▲ Homes and infrastructure are often damaged during times of war and political unrest.

green revolution This refers to increases in crop yields that accompanied the introduction of new agricultural technologies in less-developed countries, beginning in the 1960s. The key technologies were high-yielding, disease-resistant strains of rice, wheat, and corn; greater use of fertilizer and water; and improved cultivation practices.

crops used). The increased use of fertilizers, irrigation, and the development of superior crops through careful plant breeding made this boost in agricultural production possible. Many of the technologies associated with the green revolution have now achieved their potential. Rice yields, for example, have not increased significantly since the release of superior varieties in 1966. (The green revolution was intended as a stopgap measure until world leaders could control population growth.)

Future gains in productivity may be much harder to accomplish because of the existence of less productive farmland. Until the introduction of another superior strain of rice or other grain, developing countries will not benefit greatly from recent, more modest breakthroughs in biotechnology (see the section on use of biotechnology).

Areas of the world that remain uncultivated or ungrazed are mostly too rocky, steep, infertile, dry, wet, or inaccessible to sustain farming. Nearly all irrigation water available worldwide is being used, and groundwater supplies are becoming depleted at rapid rates in many regions. An eventual water shortage is projected to increase war and civil unrest in arid areas of the world, such as Northern Africa and the Middle East. China, which has more than 20% of the world's irrigated land, is also plagued with a growing scarcity of fresh water. In the future, billions of people will face ongoing water shortages.

The prospects of obtaining substantially more food from the oceans are also poor. In recent years, the amount of fish caught worldwide has leveled off. Fish was once considered the poor person's protein, but this is not likely to continue because farming of fish does not come close to compensating for the degree of reduction in wild fish populations.

Clearly, we can exploit the earth's resources only so far—the world population probably cannot continue to expand as it does today without the potential for serious famine and death. The Food and Agriculture Organization (FAO) of the United Nations works on this principle: "The fight to ensure that all people have enough nutritious food to eat is worthy of our greatest efforts, but it must be fought with the full recognition that it cannot be won unless agricultural, fishery, and forestry production returns to the earth as much as—or more than—it takes." Thus, if food production is to keep up with the expanding population, immediate action is needed to protect the earth's already deteriorated environment from further destruction (see Further Reading 10).

Inadequate Shelter and Sanitation

When people die from undernutrition in developing countries, other factors, such as inadequate shelter and sanitation, almost always contribute. Poor sanitation along with undernutrition particularly raises the risk of infection. Inadequate and deteriorating shelters threaten the lives of more than 500 million people. Many of the 15 million annual deaths of children—half of them under 5 years old—in developing countries could be prevented by improving the standards of environmental hygiene. Urban populations of some developing countries are growing at an annual rate of 5% to 7%. Such a skewed population distribution will result in more poverty. The urban explosion is the result of both high birth rates and continuing migration of people to the cities from rural areas. People go to the cities to find employment and resources the countryside can no longer provide. Worldwide, 38% of people lived in urban areas in 1975. The figure is now about 50% and is expected to reach 70% by 2050. Nine of the world's 10 largest cities will be in poor countries 20 years from now. The World Bank reports that 16 of the 20 most polluted cities in the world are in China.

In developing countries, the poor make up most of the urban population, and their needs for housing and community services often go beyond available governmental resources. Most of these urban poor live in overcrowded, self-made shelters, which lack a safe and adequate water supply and are only partially served by public

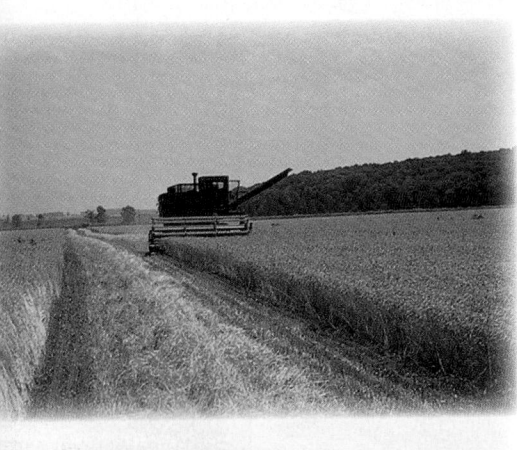

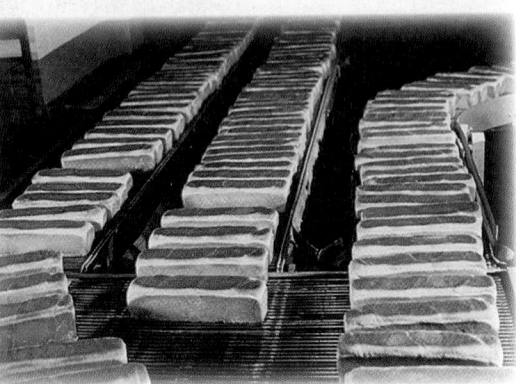

▲ Rich agricultural resources in North America, seen in the wheat fields above, results in a bounty of food to enjoy, such as these loaves of fresh bread.

In Brazil, migrants displaced by multinational land developers have flooded from the north and northeast into Rio de Janeiro and São Paulo, attracted by the prospect of jobs. There they have built shantytowns next to apartment towers and affluent suburbs, but the jobs do not materialize, and urban poverty replaces rural impoverishment.

utilities. The shantytowns and ghettos of the developing world are often worse than the rural areas the people left behind. The urban poor need cash to purchase food, so they often subsist on diets even more meager than the homegrown rural fare. Making matters worse, haphazard shelters often lack facilities to protect food from spoilage or damage by insects and rodents. This inability to protect food supplies in some developing countries leads to the loss of as much as 40% of all perishable foods.

The shift from rural to urban life takes its greatest toll on infants and children. Infants are often weaned early from the breast to infant formula, partly because the mother must find employment and partly because she may be influenced by advertisements depicting images of sophisticated, formula-feeding women. Unfortunately, because infant formulas are relatively expensive, poor parents may try to conserve the formula by either overdiluting the mixture or using too little to meet the infant's needs. The water supply may not be safe, so the prepared formula is also likely to be contaminated with bacteria. Human milk, in contrast, is much more hygienic, readily available, and nutritious. It also provides infants with immunity to some ailments. Promoting breastfeeding is important when it is safe for the infant (review the earlier discussion of AIDS, HIV, and breastfeeding).

Overall, the single most effective health advantage for people, wherever they live, is a safe and convenient water supply. Inadequate sanitation and the consumption of contaminated water cause 75% of all diseases and more than one-third of deaths in developing countries. The World Health Organization (WHO) estimates that 1.1 billion people, about one-sixth of all people, have an unsafe and inadequate water supply. In addition, up to 90% of the diseases seen in developing countries may be attributed to contaminated water.

Poor sanitation, another example of inadequate infrastructure in the developing world, creates a critical public health problem. Human feces, rotting garbage, and associated insect and rodent infestations are potent sources of disease organisms commonly seen in urban areas of the developing world. Two of the most dangerous substances encountered in routine daily living are human urine and feces. The inability to dispose of the massive numbers of dead people (and dead animals) resulting from civil wars causes additional sanitation problems. In some developing countries, diarrheal diseases account for as many as one-third of all deaths in children under 5 years of age. WHO estimates that even with improvements in housing, 2 billion people in the world still lack proper sanitation facilities. Read more about the sanitation crisis in Further Reading 16.

High External Debt

Since the 1970s many developing countries have become trapped in a cycle of borrowing repeatedly from foreign countries and international banks. Servicing these external debts has brought several countries to the verge of economic collapse. About $6 billion is owed to the United States. The external debt of Latin America represents 45% of the region's gross regional output of goods and services.

Many African nations also carry large debt burdens. This problem is made worse by drops in prices for the raw commodities they export, higher prices for imported oil, and embezzlement of funds by high-ranking officials. To make up the difference between export income and import expenses, countries have been forced to borrow millions of dollars from international banks. Although the African debts are much smaller in absolute terms than those of Brazil, Argentina, and Mexico, for example, the burden is greater when national incomes and export earnings are considered. Nearly half the money African nations earn from exports goes to paying off the continent's multibillion-dollar debt. Much of the rest goes to fund imports of machinery, concrete, trucks, and consumer goods from developed countries. This leaves little for domestic programs, necessitating cutbacks that translate into fewer resources to counter already widespread undernutrition.

Blood loss caused by intestinal and blood-borne parasite infections is another common cause of anemia among poor populations, especially when people do not wear shoes. Parasites, such as hookworms, can easily penetrate the soles of the feet and legs and enter the bloodstream. Although hookworm disease has been largely eradicated through improved sanitation in the United States and other industrialized nations, it continues to plague more than one-eighth of the world's population, mostly in tropical regions.

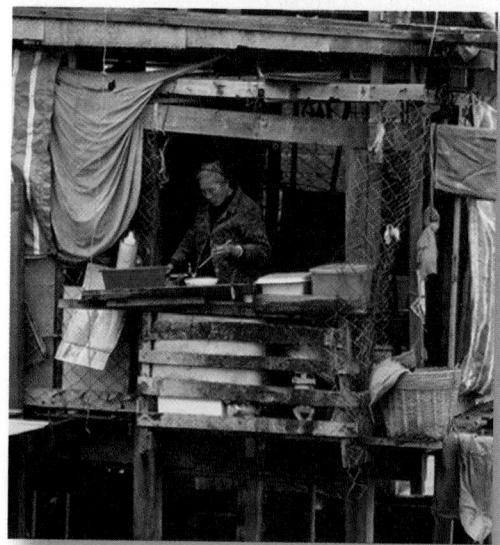

▲ Inadequate sanitation facilities and the consumption of contaminated water cause the majority of all diseases. About 1 billion people in developing countries often lack access to a safe water supply.

CONCEPT CHECK

War and civil strife, along with a decline in the world's natural resources, contribute to the difficulty of ending undernutrition in many developing countries. In addition, substandard housing conditions, impure water, and inadequate sanitation worldwide increase the risk for infection and disease. Infection then combines with undernutrition to compromise further the health of impoverished people. Finally, many developing countries are burdened by extremely high external debts, which severely limit their ability to implement programs to reduce undernutrition.

NEWSWORTHY NUTRITION

Should HIV-positive women choose breastfeeding for their infants?

Exclusive breastfeeding is recommended for infants of HIV-positive women during the first months of life if available replacement feeding methods are not acceptable, feasible, affordable, sustainable, or safe for their circumstances. This study of South African HIV-positive women found that exclusive breastfeeding was successful when the women had a strong belief in the benefits of breastfeeding and a supportive home environment and when they could recall key messages on mother-to-child transmission risks and mixed feeding and could resist pressure from the family to introduce other fluids.

Source: Doherty T and others: A longitudinal qualitative study of infant-feeding decision making and practices among HIV-positive women in South Africa. *Journal of Nutrition* 136:2421, 2006 (see Further Reading 8).

connect NUTRITION **Check out the Connect site** www.mcgrawhillconnect.com **to further explore HIV and breastfeeding.**

The Impact of AIDS Worldwide

About 33 million people around the world are infected with the human immunodeficiency virus (HIV) or have gone on to develop acquired immune deficiency syndrome (AIDS) from the infection. The male to female ratio is about 1:1 but is now increasing faster in women than in men in several countries. Although the annual number of AIDS deaths has declined worldwide since 2005, 1.8 million adults and children died with AIDS in 2009.

An individual can be infected with HIV through contact with bodily fluids including blood, semen, vaginal secretions, and human milk. Thus the virus can be transmitted through sexual contact; through blood-to-blood contact; as well as from a mother to an infant during pregnancy, delivery, or breastfeeding. The virus has a very limited ability to exist outside the body. Read more about HIV and breastfeeding in Newsworthy Nutrition and Further Readings 5 and 8.

Once infected with HIV, the individual is said to be HIV-positive. If untreated, the viral disease progresses over the next few years, and the individual develops symptoms of opportunistic infections such as diarrhea, lung disease, weight loss, and a form of cancer. Once the individual has developed these symptoms, they are said to have AIDS. Without treatment, an individual will likely die from AIDS within 4 to 5 years.

Global efforts are having some effect in that the HIV epidemic worldwide is stabilizing and the rate of new HIV infections has decreased in several countries (see Further Reading 13). From 2001 to 2009 the annual number of new HIV infections decreased from 3.1 to 2.6 million. In Africa, particularly sub-Saharan countries, HIV is rampant throughout the entire population, both in men and women. This region contains over 34% of the world's HIV-positive people (Fig. 12-4). In most areas of sub-Saharan Africa, AIDS is reducing life expectancy by one-half, especially if the person also has tuberculosis. In many countries, AIDS is also creating orphans, with an estimated 12 million in Africa alone.

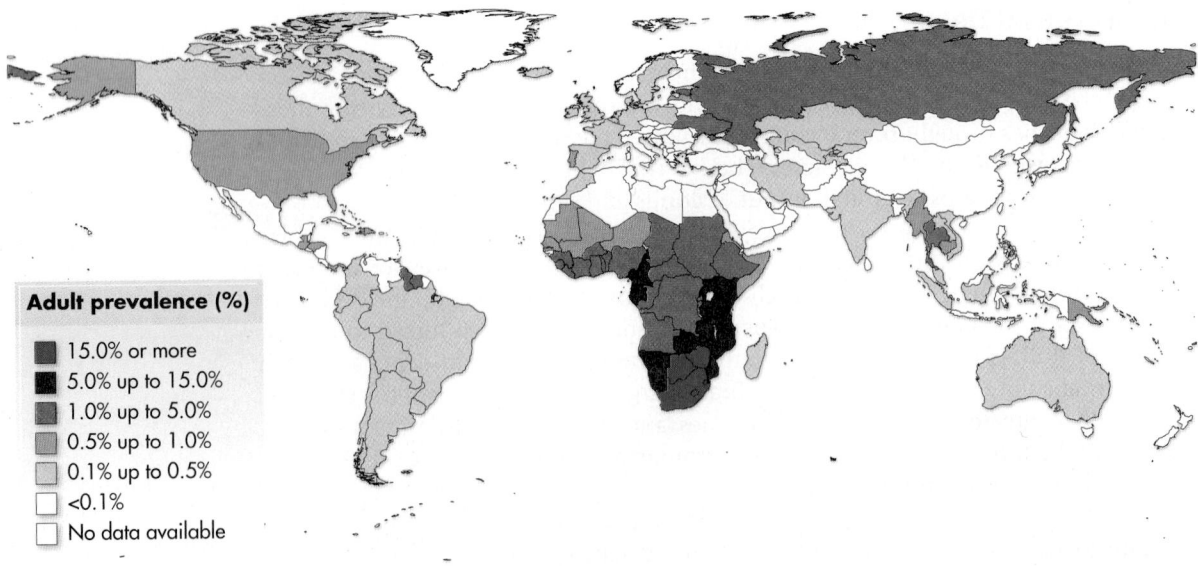

Adult prevalence (%)
- 15.0% or more
- 5.0% up to 15.0%
- 1.0% up to 5.0%
- 0.5% up to 1.0%
- 0.1% up to 0.5%
- <0.1%
- No data available

FIGURE 12-4 ▶ A global view of 33 million people living with HIV infection in 2009.

Source: Report on the Global HIV/AIDS Epidemic 2010: Executive Summary, 2010.

The largest regional increase in HIV prevalence has been in Eastern Europe and Central Asia. The number of people living with HIV in these areas has tripled since 2000.

North America also has an AIDS problem. In the United States, it is estimated that about 1 million people are infected with HIV, with 1 in 5 (21%) unaware of their infections. (Reports show 1 in every 100 persons in New York City is infected with HIV.) About 580,000 people in the United States have died from the disease since it surfaced in the early 1980s, and each year about 56,300 new cases are reported. HIV affects a greater percentage of minority populations in the United States.

The face of AIDS is quickly becoming the face of a child. In 2009, 2.5 million children under 15 years were living with HIV/AIDS globally. Most of those children, almost 9 in 10, live in sub-Saharan Africa. Fortunately there has been an estimated 19% decrease in AIDS-related deaths among children worldwide from 2004 to 2009.

Although no vaccine is available to prevent AIDS, the latest antiviral drugs can significantly slow the progression of the disease. However, there are many barriers to the use of these drugs in the developing world. For example, the newest therapies require a person to take at least three different drugs in the form of about 14 pills each day. A few missed doses can significantly reduce the effectiveness of the drugs and result in faster disease progression. Another barrier is economic: a typical drug regimen can cost approximately $14,000 per year, not including unforeseen hospital stays. Certain drug companies and governments are working to lower the cost of AIDS drugs for developing nations. Still, in most cases, the drugs will remain out of reach to those who need them. It has been suggested that developed nations should step in and cover most or all of the costs. The United Nations is spearheading an effort to raise the $8 to $10 billion needed to fight the disease.

MAKING DECISIONS

Nutrition and AIDS

Can eating a balanced diet prevent AIDS? The answer, unfortunately, is no. Healthy eating does not cure the disease, but it can help to lessen the impact of infections associated with AIDS. Poor nutritional status, such as a low status of vitamin A and vitamin E, contributes to a quicker onset of symptoms such as body wasting and fever, and a more rapid demise. This explains why daily use of a balanced vitamin and mineral supplement was shown to slow health declines in such people in one study. Overall, maintenance of nutritional status should be an integral part of the treatment for AIDS.

The devastating effects of AIDS on our civilization have been rapid when measured by earth's scale of time. One study warns us that 57 countries risk major HIV outbreaks. Reported HIV cases are increasing rapidly in Africa, the Indian subcontinent, Southeast Asia, China, the Caribbean, Russia, and much of Eastern Europe. The main goal for addressing the problem of AIDS in the developing world is prevention of new cases through education regarding safer sex and the importance of clean needles, and other behavior-linked approaches. Providing AIDS drugs to pregnant women is also important. If a woman begins taking AIDS drugs such as zidovudine (AZT) by the fourteenth week of pregnancy, the risk of transferring the virus to her offspring is greatly reduced. Providing the drug immediately before birth also helps (see Further Reading 9).

Behind the mind-boggling statistics on AIDS are less obvious costs to businesses, families, schools and universities, and society in general. For example, worker productivity will plummet because AIDS victims produce less and demand more, especially in the latter stages of the disease. Business productivity drops even further when relatives take time away from work and school to care for family members afflicted with AIDS. Furthermore, AIDS demands a considerable amount of family income. Hard-pressed families, who have to devote much of their income to doctors and medicines, have little left for living expenses. Other family members must struggle to keep up with daily duties because they must care for orphans left behind in the disease's wake. To learn more about AIDS, check out the website www.unaids.org.

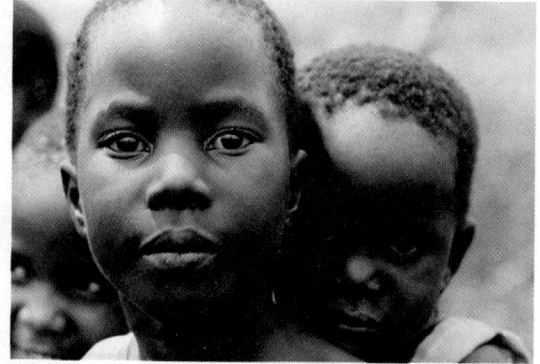

▲ A particularly sad consequence of AIDS in Africa is the number of AIDS orphans, children whose parents have both died of AIDS. The United Nations reports that about 15 million AIDS orphans have become responsible for the care of their siblings and other family members.

CONCEPT CHECK

About 40 million people around the world are infected with the human immunodeficiency virus (HIV) or have gone on to develop acquired immunodeficiency syndrome (AIDS) from the infection. The virus can be transmitted through sexual contact; through blood-to-blood contact; or from a mother to a baby during pregnancy, delivery, and breastfeeding. Without treatment, an individual once infected will likely die from AIDS within 4 to 5 years. The main hope for addressing the problem of AIDS in the developing world is prevention of new cases.

Reducing Undernutrition in the Developing World

As you have probably guessed, greatly reducing undernutrition in the developing world will be complicated and will take considerable time to accomplish (Fig. 12-5). It is a common practice for the more affluent nations to supply famine areas with direct food aid. However, direct food aid is not a long-term solution. Although it reduces the number of deaths from famine, it can also reduce incentives for local production by driving down prices. In addition, the affected countries may have little or no means of transporting the food to those who need it most, and the donated foods may not be culturally acceptable.

In the short run, there is no choice—aid must be given because people are starving (see Further Reading 3). Still, improving the infrastructure for poor people, especially rural people, needs to be the long-term focus. This future-minded approach is

FIGURE 12-5 ▶ Possible solutions to the puzzle of hunger in the developing world. Putting all the pieces together employs the action steps that contribute to meeting the overall goal.

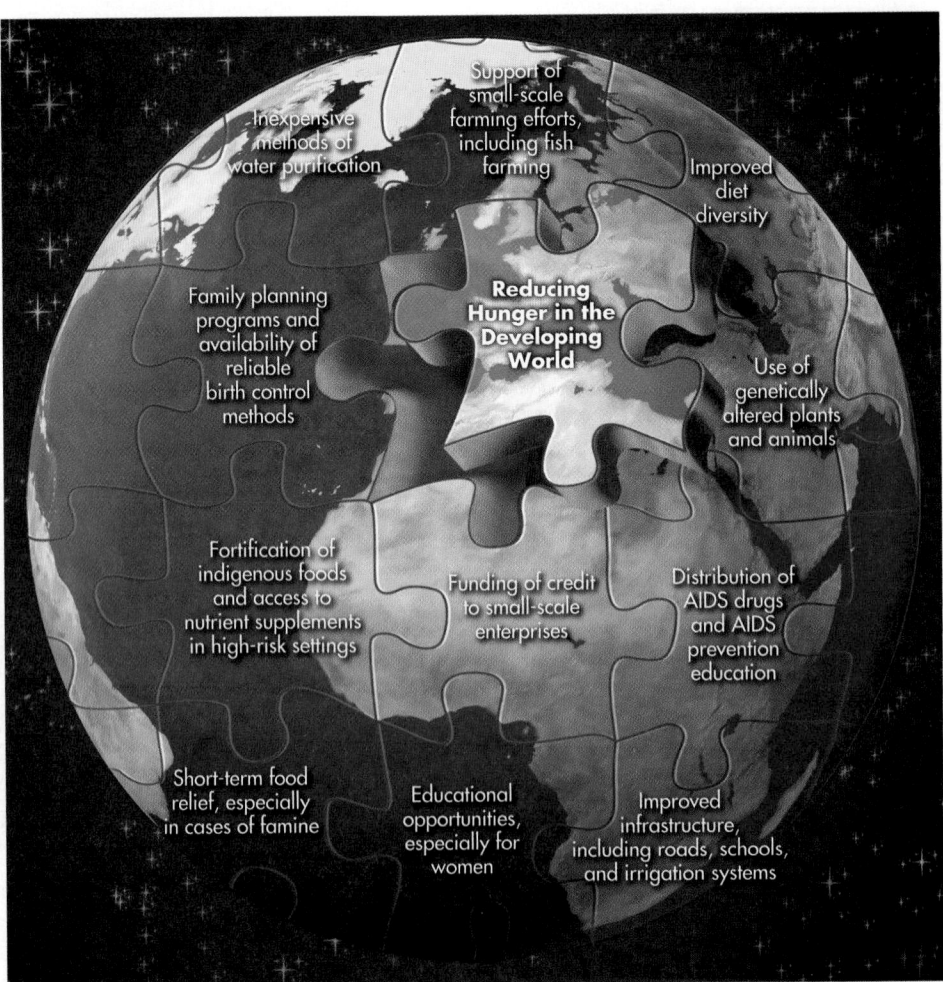

necessary because the most significant factor affecting the undernutrition of people in impoverished areas of the world is their reliance on outside sources for basic needs. Their dependence makes them constantly vulnerable.

Three basic approaches to counteract micronutrient deficiencies are suggested by the World Bank: increase diversity of the food supply; fortify specific foods with nutrients; and provide nutrient supplementation for individuals when necessary.

Development Tailored to Local Conditions Is Important. Recall that, in the past 40 years, world food supplies have grown faster than the population. Thus, the increase in undernutrition during this period has been caused by an increase in the number of people cut off from their share of this supply. Millions of farmers are losing access to resources they need to be self-reliant. There is a growing realization that unless economic opportunities can be created as part of a plan for sustainable development, rural people who own no land will flock to the overcrowded cities. In response, careful, small-scale regional development is one option.

For the most part, the solution lies in helping people meet their own needs and directing them to resources and employment opportunities, rather than giving them resources. Experience has shown that the provision of credit—along with training, food storage facilities, and marketing support—allows rural people to actively participate in their development, which will benefit their families and communities.

One U.S. program, the Peace Corps, has helped improve conditions in developing nations by providing education, distributing food and medical supplies, and building structures for local use. The aim of the Peace Corps is to help create independent, self-sustaining economies around the world.

Impoverished women are a special concern. In addition to working longer hours than men, they grow most of the food for family consumption and make up three-fourths of the labor force in the informal sector of the economy and an increasing proportion in the formal sector. Economic opportunities for women and education regarding family planning must be augmented. Of the 3 billion people in the world living on less than $2 a day, 70% are women. Moreover, among the developing world's 900 million illiterate people, women outnumber men 2 to 1. Thus, an important means of propelling nations out of poverty is to end the cycle of female neglect.

Suitable technologies for processing, preserving, marketing, and distributing nutritious local staples also need to be encouraged, so that small farmers can flourish. Education on how to use these foods to create healthful diets, such as preparing vitamin A-rich vegetables, adds further benefit. Supplementing indigenous foods with nutrients that are in short supply, such as iron, various B vitamins, zinc, and iodide, also deserves consideration. One program involves adding iron to sugar in various parts of the world. The next section examines the role of biotechnology in improving nutrient quality and other plant and animal characteristics, another possible positive step in lessening undernutrition. In addition, advances in water purification need to be employed.

Promoting extensive land ownership may also be one part of the solution. Increasing the availability of food is one of its many advantages. If food resources are concentrated among a minority of people, as often happens with unequal land ownership, food is not likely to be equally distributed unless efficient transportation systems are in place. Inequitable distribution then proves to be a difficult problem to resolve.

Raising the economic status of impoverished people by employing them is as important as expanding the food supply. If an increase in food supply is achieved without an accompanying rise in employment, there may be no long-term change in the number of undernourished people. Although food prices may fall with increased mechanization, use of fertilizers, and other modern technologies, it needs to be realized that these advances can also displace people from jobs, a result that worsens rather than helps the population.

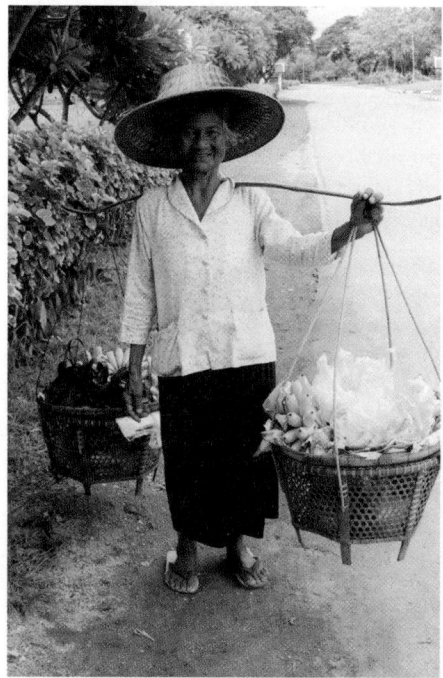

▲ Food security is fostered by communities raising and distributing locally grown food.

CRITICAL THINKING

Stan has read about various relief efforts to help undernourished people in developing countries, especially the emergency food aid programs for famine-ravaged areas. Many of these efforts appear to be only temporary, and he wonders what long-range approaches might help alleviate the problem of undernutrition. What suggestions would you give Stan about possible long-term solutions for undernutrition in developing countries?

sustainable development Economic growth that will simultaneously reduce poverty, protect the environment, and preserve natural capital.

gender and development (GAD) approach Understanding the roles and responsibilities of both men and women in the process of sustainable development.

MAKING DECISIONS

Sustainable Development and the Gender and Development (GAD) Approach

Sustainable development is economic growth that will reduce poverty while at the same time protect the environment and preserve natural capital. In its 2005 World Summit Outcome Document, the United Nations cites economic development, social development, and environmental protection as the "reinforcing pillars" of sustainable development. During the past 20 years, an understanding of the roles and responsibilities of both women and men in the community and the relationship of men and women to each other have been important components of sustainable development. The **gender and development (GAD) approach** works toward improving the status of women through the active participation of both men and women. By increasing women's access to education, information and communication technologies, economic resources, and governance, the GAD approach reduces poverty, promotes development, achieves gender equality, protects women's human rights, and eliminates violence against women.

12.4 The Role of Sustainable Agriculture and Biotechnology in Worldwide Food Availability

Sustainable Agriculture

Over the years, changes in agricultural practices have had many positive results on the availability of food around the world. Along with the positive effects on farming, however, there have been significant negative impacts. Most significant among these are depletion of topsoil, contamination of groundwater, the decline of family farms, neglect of living and working conditions for farm laborers, increasing costs of production, and the lack of integration of economic and social conditions in rural communities.

During the past two decades, the role of the agriculture industry in promoting practices that contribute to environmental and social problems has been debated. As a result, interest in alternative farming practices has grown and a movement toward **sustainable agriculture** has emerged. Sustainable agriculture describes farming systems that can indefinitely maintain their productivity and usefulness to society. Sustainable agriculture depends on the integration of several goals including environmental health, economic profitability, and social and economic equity. It addresses many environmental and social concerns, and offers innovative and economically viable opportunities for many in the food system including growers, laborers, consumers, and policymakers. Today sustainable agriculture is gaining support and acceptance from conventional farmers in many countries.

Sustainable agriculture involves maintaining or enhancing the land and natural resources for use long into the future. In addition, the social responsibilities of human resources, including working and living conditions of laborers, the needs of rural communities, and consumer health and safety, must be considered both in the present and the future. The potential of sustainability is best understood when the consequences of farming practices on both human communities and the environment are considered.

Farmers around the globe can succeed in their transition to sustainable agriculture by taking small realistic steps based on their personal goals and family economics. Reaching the goal of worldwide sustainable agriculture will require participation by all stakeholders including farmers, laborers, retailers, consumers, researchers, and policymakers.

sustainable agriculture Agricultural system that provides a secure living for farm families; maintains the natural environment and resources; supports the rural community; and offers respect and fair treatment to all involved, from farm workers to consumers to the animals raised for food.

The ability of humans to manipulate nature has enabled us to improve the production and yield of many important foods. Traditional **biotechnology** is almost as old as agriculture. The first farmer to improve stock by selectively breeding the best bull with the best cows was implementing biotechnology in a simple sense. The first baker to use yeast to make bread rise took advantage of biotechnology.

By the 1930s, biotechnology made possible the selective breeding of better plant hybrids. As a result, corn production in the United States quickly doubled. Through similar methods, agricultural wheat was crossed with wild grasses to confer more desirable properties, such as greater yield, increased resistance to mildew and bacterial diseases, and tolerance to salt or adverse climatic conditions.

Another type of biotechnology uses hormones rather than breeding. In the last decade, Canadian salmon have been treated with a hormone that allows them to mature three times faster than normal—without changing the fish in any other way. In general terms, biotechnology can be understood as the use of living things—plants, animals, bacteria—to manufacture products.

Biotechnology

The new biotechnology used in agriculture includes several methods that directly modify products. It differs from traditional methods because it more directly changes some of the genetic material (DNA) of organisms to improve characteristics. Crossbreeding plants or animals is no longer the only tool. Development of the new process, called **genetic engineering,** began in the 1970s. The field now features a wide range of cell and subcell techniques for the synthesis and placement of genetic material in organisms (Fig. 12-6).

This process of **recombinant DNA technology** allows access to a wider gene pool, and it permits faster and more accurate production of new and more useful microbial, plant, and animal species. Conventional breeding is inefficient and has inconsistent results; biotechnology uses genetic material more precisely. Scientists select the traits they want and genetically engineer or introduce the gene that produces the desired trait into plants or animals (now called a **genetically modified organism [GMO]** or **transgenic**). Genetic engineering has not replaced conventional breeding practices; both work together.

Biotechnology has been used to enhance crops in three main categories. The primary category is the addition of a unique characteristic called an *input trait* to a crop. These enhanced input traits include herbicide tolerance, insect and virus protection, and tolerance to environmental stressors such as drought. Other categories are

biotechnology A collection of processes that involves the use of biological systems for altering and, ideally, improving the characteristics of plants, animals, and other forms of life.

genetic engineering Manipulation of the genetic makeup of any organism with recombinant DNA technology.

recombinant DNA technology A test tube technology that rearranges DNA sequences in an organism by cutting the DNA, adding or deleting a DNA sequence, and rejoining DNA molecules with a series of enzymes.

genetically modified organism (GMO) Any organism created by genetic engineering.

transgenic Organism that contains genes originally present in another organism.

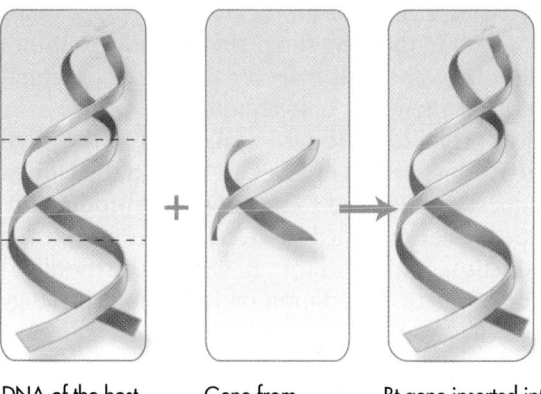

DNA of the host plant, corn.

Gene from bacteria (Bt gene) that produces a protein toxic to the European corn borer.

Bt gene inserted into DNA of corn plant. Now the corn plant is genetically modified. It makes the Bt toxin and, so, is resistant to the European corn borer.

FIGURE 12-6 ▶ Biotechnology involves various techniques for transferring foreign DNA into an organism. In this diagram, a sample of DNA is cleaved out of a larger DNA fragment and inserted into the DNA of a host cell. Thus, the host cell contains new genetic information, with the potential of providing the cell with new capabilities. For corn, this could mean resistance to the European corn borer. The corn plant is now referred to as a genetically modified organism (GMO). In another application, bacteria can be engineered to produce the human form of the hormone insulin.

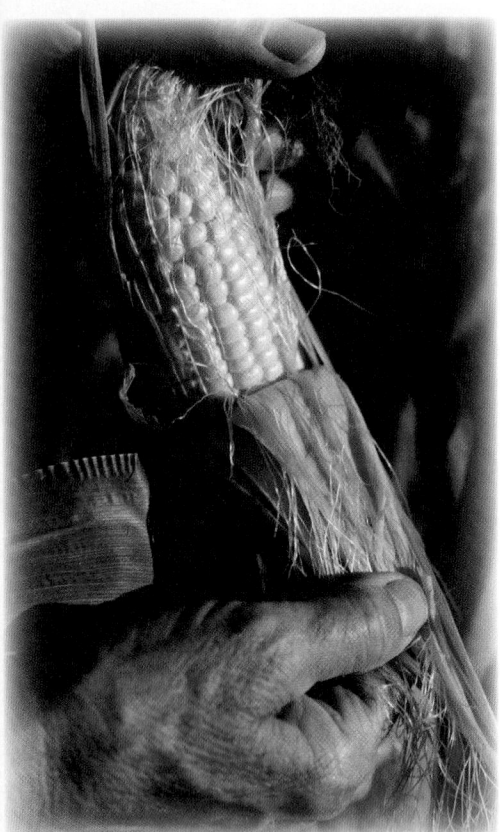

▲ Both traditional plant breeding and biotechnology have produced high-yielding and disease-resistant plant varieties, including new varieties of corn.

value-added output traits, such as plant oils with increased levels of omega-3 fatty acids, and crops that produce pharmaceuticals. Scientists have engineered plants that grow with the use of less pesticides and new forms of potatoes that can be stored longer without preservatives. In addition, biotechnology allows scientists to create fruits and grains with greater amounts of nutrients such as beta-carotene (e.g., "golden rice") and vitamins E and C. Biotechnology is being used cautiously and conservatively, so benefits of the new biotechnology will strike us as only subtly different. The ultimate benefits, however, could be important if foods eaten by people in the developing world can be so enhanced.

Few consumers in the United States realize that at least 72% of corn and 94% of soybeans produced in the United States have been genetically engineered to either resist certain insects, thereby reducing pesticide use, and/or survive when sprayed with herbicides that kill surrounding weeds. Papaya plants have been genetically engineered for viral resistance.

Genetic modification of corn has received a lot of media attention. Corn can be genetically altered by inserting a gene from the bacterium *Bacillus thuringiensis,* usually referred to as the Bt gene, into the corn DNA (Fig. 12-6). The gene allows the corn plant to make a protein lethal to certain caterpillars that destroy the plant. The Bt protein in the corn, however, is present in the plant in low concentrations and has no effect on humans—it is digested along with the other proteins in corn. For many years organic farmers have used the Bt bacteria as a dust on plants to destroy pests. (Dusting crops, however, does not change the DNA of the plant.)

FDA is confident that approved varieties of genetically engineered foods are safe to consume. Food manufacturers, therefore, are not required to disclose the genetically modified ingredient content on food labels. FDA does not believe labeling of GMO products is needed because they pose no health risk.

Public response to use of GMO biotechnology, however, has been mixed. Even the scientific community has conflicting opinions about this technology, with supporters as convinced about the benefits as opponents are of the risks. The biggest debate in the United States surrounds the potential environmental hazards of introducing genes from one species to another. Some challengers even question the reduction in pesticide use that accompanies the cultivation of genetically modified crops. Although the use of genetically modified crops may reduce the need for environmentally harmful activities, such as spraying crops with pesticides, critics point out that seeds produced with additional insecticide potentially will lead to rapid insect resistance because the insecticides are continuously emitted. Use of traditional pesticides involves prudent application, in part to avoid insect resistance. In addition, accidental release of genetically modified animals, such as fish, may go on to harm wild varieties.

Although the risks of biotechnology may appear to be momentarily negligible, they may be cumulative and therefore of concern in the long run. FDA carefully examines all products developed using this technology and will enforce labeling of potential allergens that may be newly present in food altered by biotechnology.

The public has long been opposed to processes perceived as harmful to the environment, such as producing unnatural products. Food reserves are high in the United States, Canada, and Europe, so some question the need to increase food production. Skepticism surrounds unnatural products, as exemplified by Western Europe's ban of hormones used in beef and milk production, and of almost all genetically modified foods. Read the position of the American Dietetic Association on food biotechnology in Further Reading 1.

Role of the New Biotechnology in the Developing World

Twenty-nine countries planted 366 million acres of crops enhanced through biotechnology in 2010. These crops included improved varieties of soybeans, corn, cotton, canola, papaya, and squash. The United States maintained the largest growth of biotech crops with nearly 165 million acres of soybeans, corn, and cotton. Brazil was second with 62 million acres. Developing countries also saw an increase, growing 48% of the biotech crops in 2010. Columbia, Honduras, and Iran were the second leading producers of biotechnology crops with acreage of 13.2 million. These countries aimed to increase crop production in rural areas to improve incomes and supply growing urban populations.

Whether applications of genetic engineering will help to significantly reduce undernutrition in the developing world remains to be seen. Unless price cuts accompany the increased production, only landowners and suppliers of biotechnology will enjoy the benefits. Small farmers may benefit if they can afford to purchase the genetically modified seeds. This point deserves emphasis: The person who cannot afford to buy enough food today will still face that same predicament in the future.

As with most innovations, the more successful farmers—often those with larger farms—will adopt the new biotechnology first. Because of this, the present trend toward fewer and larger farms will continue in the developing world, a movement that undermines the solution to one of the most pressing undernutrition issues there. Furthermore, biotechnology does not promise dramatic increases in the production of most grains and cassava, the primary food resources in developing parts of the world.

With the introduction of drought- and pest-resistant, as well as self-fertilizing crops, agricultural biotechnology may help to lessen world hunger. Perhaps the most promising potential of genetically modified foods today lies within the realm of plant breeding for micronutrients. Developing countries will then have a tool to treat and prevent selected nutrient deficiencies among their populations if they have access to farming resources to augment the micronutrient composition of crops. In addition, greater yields for indigenous plants, such as tomatoes that tolerate high soil salinity, are another hopeful outcome. Biotechnology will likely be a useful tool against the complex scourge of world undernutrition. Improved crops produced by this technology, together with political and other efforts, can contribute to success in the battle against worldwide undernutrition.

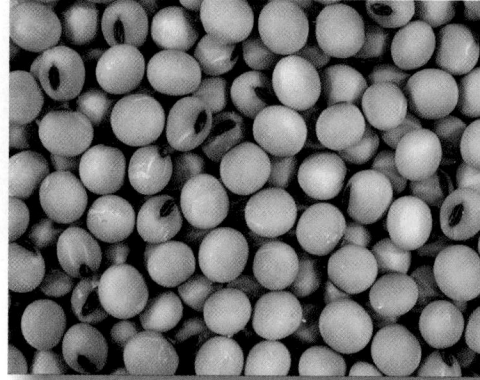

▲ Soybeans are a common GMO food in the marketplace. Over 90% of the soybeans grown in the United States are genetically modified.

Some Concluding Thoughts

The economic loss from undernutrition is staggering, and the amount of human pain and suffering is incalculable. With all the international relief efforts and assistance from governments and private organizations combined, we are still failing in our battle against undernutrition. Read more about the progress toward the goal of halving global hunger by 2015 in Further Reading 15.

Ultimately, the depletion of world resources, the massive debt incurred by poorer countries, the threat of danger to more prosperous countries nearby, and the toll taken in human lives affect the world economy and well-being. The resulting instability can go on to affect the developing world, as has been apparent in recent years. Life is not necessarily fair, but the aim of civilization should be to make it more so. The world has both enough food and the technical expertise to end hunger. What is lacking is the concerted political will to do so.

CONCEPT CHECK

Overall, one important strategy to reducing undernutrition in the developing world lies in providing sufficient employment, so that people can purchase the food their families need. Providing access to land and other food production resources will also counteract undernutrition. Development programs must be sensitive to regional conditions to ensure that the new technologies introduced do not intensify existing problems for the poorest people.

Undernutrition at Critical Life Stages

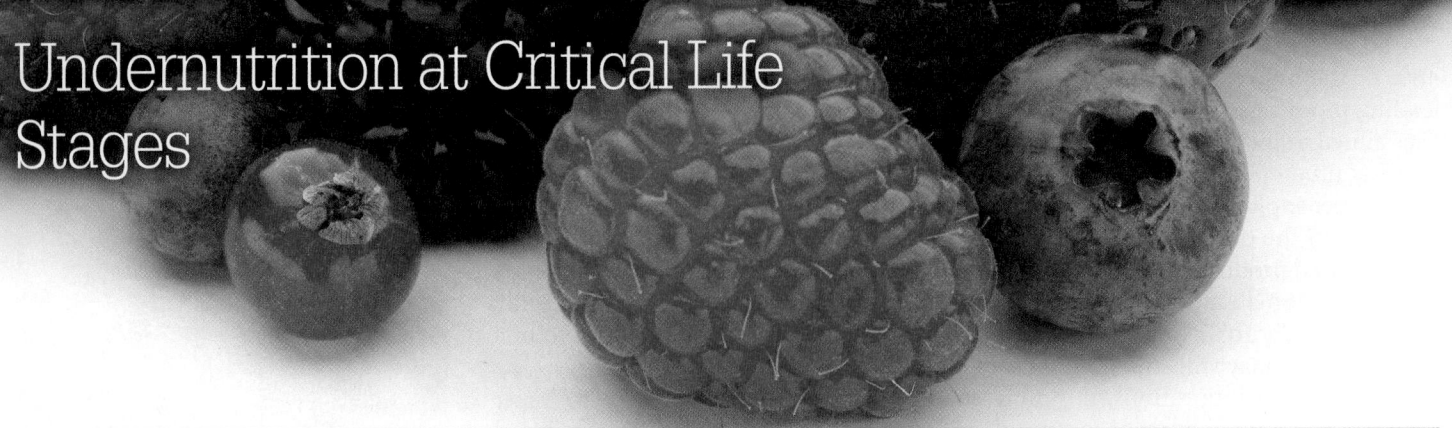

Critical Life Stages When Undernutrition Is Particularly Devastating

Prolonged undernutrition is detrimental to many aspects of human health (Fig. 12-7). It is particularly damaging during some periods of growth and old age. The United Nations Children's Fund developed a conceptual framework of malnutrition in 1990 (Fig. 12-8). According to this framework, the immediate causes of malnutrition (inadequate dietary intake and unsatisfactory health) affect individuals. The underlying causes relate to families and include inadequate access to food, inadequate care for women and children, and insufficient health services. Basic causes relate to human and economic resources and have their effect on communities and nations.

Pregnancy

Undernutrition poses the greatest health risk during pregnancy. About 500,000 women worldwide die each year from complications of pregnancy and childbirth. A pregnant woman needs extra nutrients to meet both her own needs and those of her developing offspring. Nourishing the fetus may deplete maternal stores of nutrients. Maternal iron deficiency anemia is one possible consequence (Chapter 14).

In Africa, women in their lifetimes give birth, on average, to more than six live babies. Coupled with chronic undernutrition, these high birth rates result in a 1 in 20 in chance that a woman will die from pregnancy-related causes. In

contrast, North American women only face a risk of 1 death in about 8000 births from pregnancy-related causes. Pregnancy-related death is the social indicator showing the largest disparity between the developing and industrialized worlds. Smaller differences exist for literacy, life expectancy, and infant mortality.

Fetal and Infant Stages

The fetus faces major health risks from undernutrition during gestation. To support growth and development of the brain and other body tissues, a growing fetus requires a rich supply of protein, vitamins, and minerals. When these needs are not met, the infant is often born before 37 weeks of gestation, well before the ideal 40 weeks of gestation. The consequences of this pre-term birth include reduced lung function and a weakened immune system. These conditions not only compromise health but also increase the likelihood of premature death. Long-term problems in growth and development can result if the infant survives. In extreme cases, low-birth-weight infants (about 5.5 pounds [2.5 kilograms] or less) face 5 to 10 times the normal risk of dying before the age of 1 year, primarily because of reduced lung development. When low birth weight is accompanied by other physical abnormalities, medical intervention can cost $200,000 or more. These costs can be met only in developed countries.

Worldwide, more than 30 million infants are born each year with low birth weight. About 8% of infants born in the

United States and 6% in Canada have low birth weights. In the United States, low birth weight accounts for more than half of all infant deaths and 75% of deaths of infants younger than 1 month old. Whereas undernutrition is a major contributor to low birth weight in developing countries, the primary cause for this problem in industrialized countries is cigarette smoking. Pregnancy during the teenage years, while a girl's body is still growing, contributes to low birth weight in developing and industrialized countries alike.

The percentage of infants born with low birth weight in the United States has been increasing steadily during the past 20 years. One reason is that more twins, triplets, and higher-order multiple births are being born because of improvements in medicine and fertility procedures. Rates of low birth weight also vary by race. About 13% of infants born to African-American women have low birth weights. Among Hispanics in the United States, infants of Mexican origin have the lowest rate of low birth weight (6%), while infants of Puerto Rican heritage have the highest (9%). Among Asian subgroups, low-birth-weight rates range from 5% for infants of Chinese heritage to nearly 9% for Filipino infants.

Childhood

Early childhood, when growth is rapid, is another period when undernutrition is extremely risky. The central nervous system— including the brain—continues to be vulnerable because of rapid growth through early childhood. After the

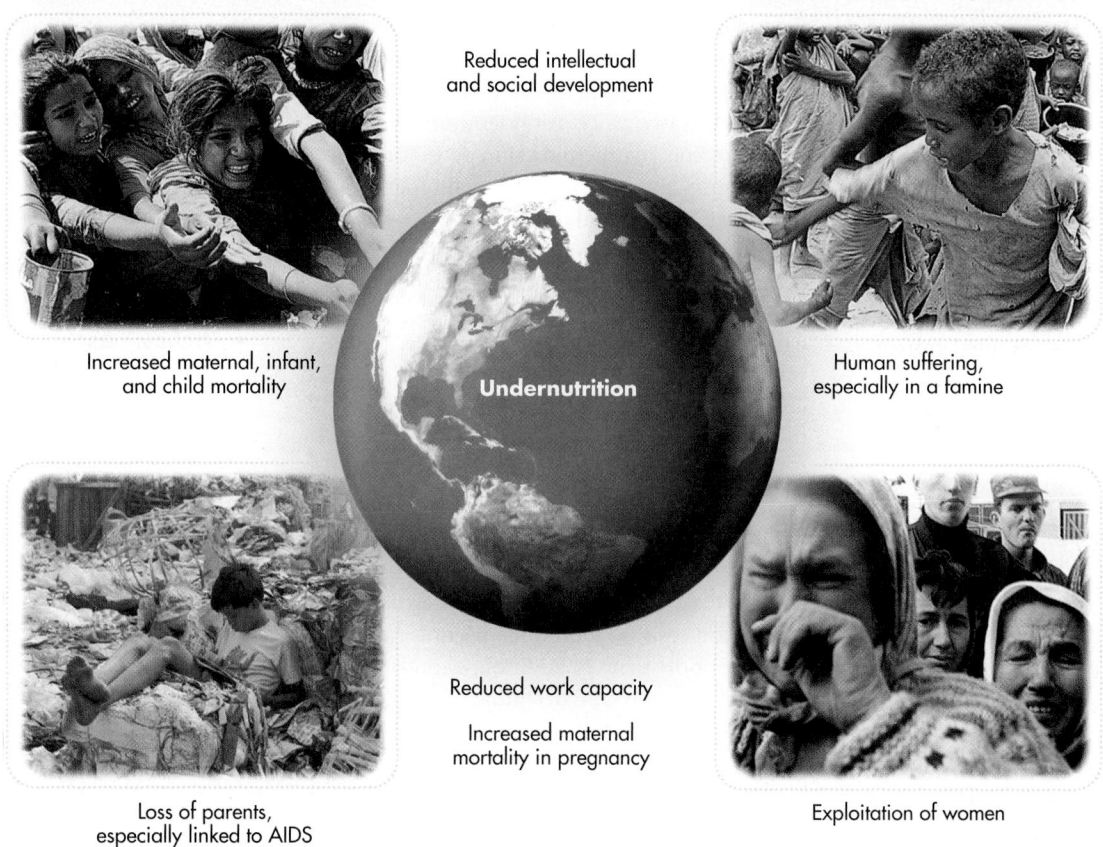

Reduced intellectual
and social development

Undernutrition

Increased maternal, infant,
and child mortality

Human suffering,
especially in a famine

Reduced work capacity

Increased maternal
mortality in pregnancy

Loss of parents,
especially linked to AIDS

Exploitation of women

FIGURE 12-7 ▶ Undernutrition results from and affects many aspects of human health and humanity.

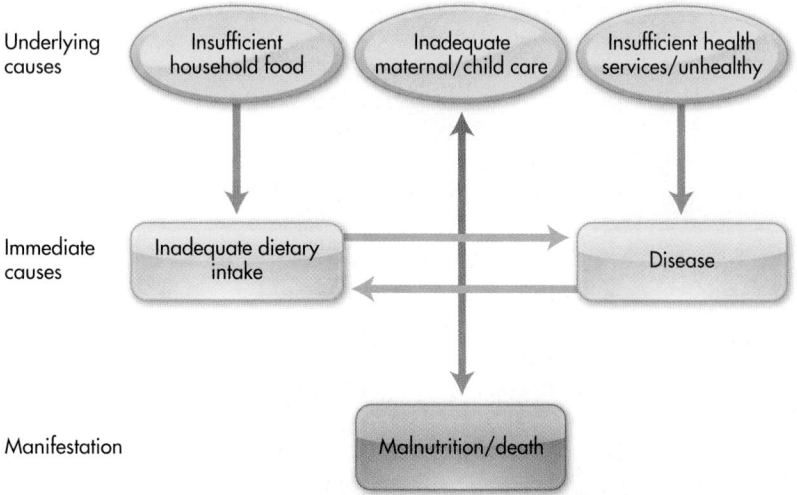

Underlying
causes

Insufficient
household food

Inadequate
maternal/child care

Insufficient health
services/unhealthy

Immediate
causes

Inadequate dietary
intake

Disease

Manifestation

Malnutrition/death

FIGURE 12-8 ▶ The UNICEF conceptual framework of the causes of malnutrition takes into account food, health, and caring practices. The causes are separated into three causes: immediate, underlying, and basic (not shown). Basic causes include human, economic, and organizational resources. The framework is used as a guide in health policy decision making.

preschool years, brain growth and development slow dramatically until maturity. Nutritional deprivation, especially in early infancy, can lead to permanent brain impairment. Without an effective intervention, it is projected that ongoing undernutrition could leave more than 1 billion children with mental impairment by 2020.

In general, poor children are at the greatest risk for nutritional deprivation and subsequent illness. Stunted growth is an obvious effect, seen in about one-third of children under 5 years of age worldwide. In addition, iron-deficiency anemia is much more common among low-income children than children from less deprived families. This deficiency can lead to fatigue upon exertion, reduced stamina, stunted growth, impaired motor development, and learning problems. Undernutrition in childhood can also weaken resistance to infection because immune function decreases when nutrients such as protein, vitamin A, and zinc are low in a diet. Clearly, undernutrition

and illness have a cyclical relationship. Not only does undernutrition lead to illness, but illness, particularly diarrhea and infectious diseases, worsens undernutrition. For this reason, many children in developing countries are dying from the combination of malnutrition and infection. Conversely, when missing nutrients such as vitamin A and zinc are restored to children's diets, improvements in health can be obvious.

Later Years

Older adults, especially older women living alone in poverty, are also at risk for undernutrition. Older adults in general require nutrient-dense foods, in amounts dependent on their state of health and degree of physical activity. Many of them have fixed incomes and incur significant medical costs, so food often becomes a low-priority item. In addition, depression, social isolation, and declining physical and mental health can compound the problem of undernutrition in older adults.

▶ Compared to other children, homeless children suffer higher rates of many medical problems, some of which include:
- Upper respiratory tract infections
- Scabies and lice
- Tooth decay
- Ear and skin infections
- Diaper rash
- Eye infections
- Developmental delays
- Trauma-related injuries

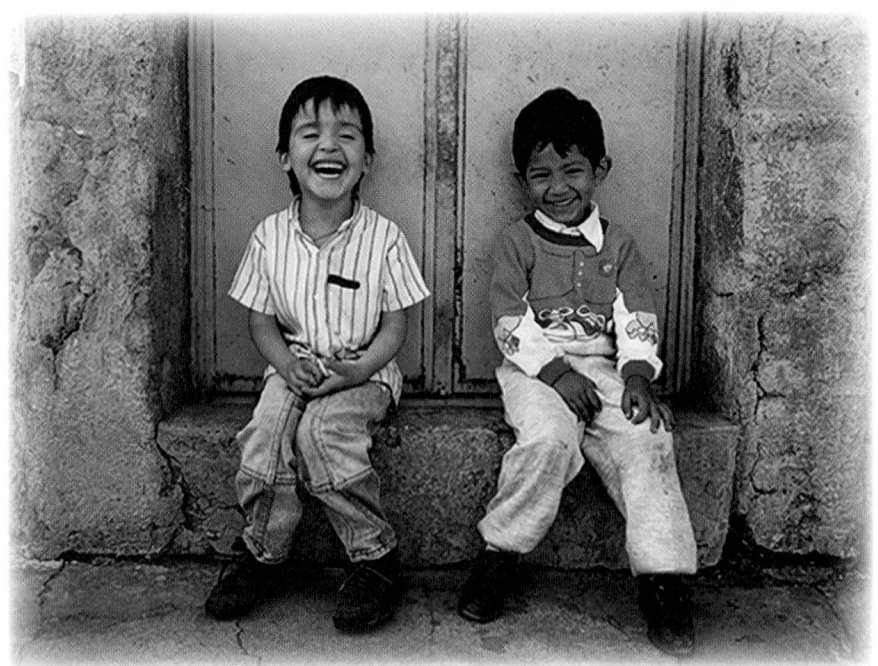

◀ Minimal intakes of protein and zinc limit the growth of children worldwide. About 30% of children in developing countries show evidence of poor growth rates.

Case Study Undernutrition During Childhood

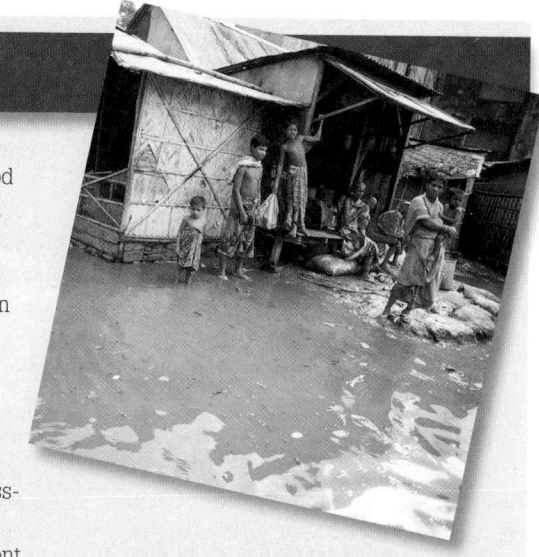

Jamal traveled to the Philippines with his church group last summer. During their stay, they helped build shelters for people in a village where, a few weeks before, a storm had destroyed several houses. Jamal noticed that many of the children were very short, much shorter than the children in his neighborhood in the United States. His group worked in a remote, low-elevation area where the storm and subsequent flooding had caused the most damage. On several occasions he noticed young mothers crouched on curbs or in doorways, holding their children. These children rarely moved—they appeared pale and listless. In contrast to the children Jamal's group had met at a church in the capital city, most of the children in this village were not active and lively. One evening a nurse from the local clinic came to speak to Jamal's group. She said that many children in this area do not get enough to eat and that health problems were rampant. She considered the recent storm a blessing in disguise, hoping

it would spur the Philippine government to send supplies to the village, particularly food and medicines. Jamal is shocked by such a degree of suffering. He wonders why children in the Philippines can be starving to death while many children in his hometown in the United States are overweight.

Answer the following questions, and check your responses in Appendix A.

1. Should Jamal have been surprised by widespread disease and general listlessness in the Philippine children?
2. Which nutrients are likely to be deficient in the diets of these children?
3. Which nutrient deficiencies contribute to poor growth or "stunting" of growth?
4. Which nutrient deficiencies may be causing diarrhea and illness?
5. Are these children likely to be consuming adequate calories? What effect does consumption of inadequate calories have on growth?
6. Why might the recent storm be a blessing for this small village?
7. List some reasons why the children in Jamal's neighborhood at home are more likely to be overweight

Summary (Numbers refer to numbered sections in the chapter.)

12.1 Poverty is commonly linked to chronic or periodic undernutrition. Malnutrition can occur when the food supply is either scarce or abundant. The resulting deficiency conditions and degenerative diseases contribute to poor health.

Undernutrition is the most common form of malnutrition in developing countries. It results from inadequate intake, absorption, or use of nutrients or food energy. Many deficiency conditions consequently appear, and infectious diseases thrive because the immune system cannot function properly.

Undernutrition diminishes both physical and mental capabilities. In poor countries, this is worsened by recurrent infections, unsanitary conditions, extreme weather, inadequate shelter, and exposure to diseases.

12.2 In North America, famine is not seen but food insecurity and undernutrition

remain problems. Soup kitchens, food stamps, the school lunch and breakfast programs, and the Special Supplemental Nutrition Program for Women, Infants, and Children (WIC) have focused on improving the nutritional health of poor and at-risk people. When adequately funded, these programs have proved effective in reducing undernutrition. The need to reduce out-of-wedlock pregnancies remains a national priority because single parents and their children are much more likely to live in poverty.

12.3 Multiple factors contribute to the problem of undernutrition in the developing world. In densely populated countries, food resources, as well as the means for distributing food, may be inadequate. Farming methods often encourage erosion, which deprives the soil of valuable nutrients and thereby hampers future efforts to grow food. Limited water availability

hinders food production. Naturally occurring devastation from droughts, excessive rainfall, fire, crop infestation, and human causes—such as urbanization, war and civil unrest, debt, poor sanitation, and AIDS—all contribute to the major problem of undernutrition.

12.4 Proposed solutions to world undernutrition must consider multiple interacting factors, many thoroughly embedded in cultural traditions. Family planning efforts, for example, may not succeed until life expectancy increases. Through education, efforts should be made to upgrade farming methods, improve crops, limit pregnancies, encourage breastfeeding when it is safe to do so, and improve sanitation and hygiene.

Direct food aid is only a short-term solution. In what may appear to be a step backward, many experts recommend more sustainable subsistence-level farming. Small-scale industrial development is another way to create meaningful employment and purchasing power for vast numbers of the rural poor. Various biotechnology applications may also prove beneficial.

N&YH The greatest risk of undernutrition occurs during critical periods of growth and development: gestation, infancy, and childhood. Low birth weight is a leading cause of infant deaths worldwide. Many

developmental problems are caused by nutritional deprivation during critical periods of brain growth. People in their later years are also at great risk.

Check Your Knowledge (Answers to the following questions are below.)

1. There are an estimated _____ chronically undernourished people in the world.
   a. 14 million
   b. 800 million to 1.1 billion
   c. 3 billion
   d. 6 billion

2. The number one killer of children in developing countries is
   a. xerophthalmia.
   b. iron deficiency anemia.
   c. iodide deficiency.
   d. diarrhea.

3. The human organism is particularly susceptible to the effects of undernutrition during
   a. pregnancy.
   b. infancy.
   c. childhood.
   d. All of the above.

4. A barrier to solving undernutrition in the developing world is NOT
   a. external debt.
   b. poor infrastructure.
   c. a lack of manpower.
   d. expanding population

5. Many of the child deaths each year in developing countries could be prevented if

a. technology was improved.
b. doctors were more specialized.
c. mothers would learn more about nutrition.
d. sanitation and hygiene were improved.

6. The food stamp program, recently renamed the Supplemental Nutrition Assistance Program, allows
   a. low-income families to buy surplus food at government stores with government-issued Electronic Benefit Transfer cards.
   b. low-income people to purchase food, cleaning supplies, alcoholic beverages, and anything else sold in supermarkets with Electronic Benefit Transfer cards.
   c. low-income people to turn in government-issued Electronic Benefit Transfer cards for cash to buy food.
   d. low-income people to purchase food and seeds with government-issued Electronic Benefit Transfer cards.

7. A long-term solution to world hunger is
   a. the green revolution.
   b. cash crops.

c. jobs and self-sufficiency.
d. government/private aid.

8. Bt corn has been genetically modified to make
   a. the bacterium *Bacillus thuringiensis*.
   b. a protein toxic to caterpillars that can destroy the corn plant.
   c. a sugar that makes the corn sweeter.
   d. a fat that makes corn oil healthier.

9. Genetically modified soybeans make up _____% of the soybeans grown in the United States.
   a. 50
   b. 75
   c. 80
   d. 90

10. FDA requires the statement "contains genetically modified ingredients" on the label of all foods containing genetically modified ingredients.
    a. True   b. False

Answer Key: 1. b (LO 12.1), 2. d (LO 12.3), 3. d (LO 12.5), 4. c (LO 12.3), 5. d (LO 12.3), 6. d (LO 12.2), 7. c (LO 12.4), 8. b (LO 12.4), 9. d (LO 12.4), 10. b (LO 12.4)

Study Questions (Numbers refer to Learning Outcomes)

1. Describe the difference between malnutrition and undernutrition. **(LO 12.1)**

2. Describe in a short paragraph any evidence of undernutrition that you saw while you were growing up, such as on television. What are/were the likely roots of these problems? **(LO 12.1)**

3. What do you believe are the major factors contributing to undernutrition in wealthy nations, such as the United States? What are some solutions to this problem? **(LO 12.2)**

4. What three points would you make to a group of seventh grade girls concerning the economic perils of teen pregnancy and parenting? **(LO 12.2)**

5. What federal programs are available to address the problem of under nutrition in the United States? **(LO 12.2)**

6. Outline how war and civil unrest in developing countries have worsened problems of chronic hunger over the past few years. **(LO 12.3)**

7. How important is population control in addressing the problem of world hunger

now and in the future? Support your answer with three main points. **(LO 12.3)**

8. Why is solving the problem of undernutrition a key factor in the ability of developing countries to reach their full potential? **(LO 12.3)**

9. Name three nutrients often lacking in the diets of undernourished people. What effects can be expected with each deficiency? **(LO 12.1)**

10. Describe how sustainable agriculture and biotechnology can improve food availability worldwide. **(LO 12.4)**

What Would You Choose Recommendations

The correct response for the question posed at the beginning of this chapter is *all of the above*! Do what comes naturally to you—whether it is donating your spare change or volunteering your spare time—to move thought into action against world hunger. Indeed, the need is great—both globally and locally—and opportunities to get involved abound.

As you learned in this chapter, there are basically two ways to address the problem of hunger: direct food aid or empowering others to help themselves. Direct aid (e.g., donating money each month) is a short-term solution—one that necessarily fills an immediate gap between resources and requirements. However, in the long run, solving the problem of world hunger will take bottom-up changes that enable struggling communities to provide their own food and clean water.

It may be easier and more comfortable to visualize the hunger problem in a faraway place, such as in a developing country. In reality, however, poverty and hunger lurk in your own community. You can help local efforts by donating nonperishable items to local food pantries, volunteering at Summer Food Service Programs for school-age children, or simply by shopping for locally grown foods direct from farmers in your neighborhood.

In your quest to get involved, look for organizations whose focus is to help set up sustainable solutions in communities—empowering local citizens to grow their own food, maintain their own clean water supplies, or build their own local economies.

Action Against Hunger:
www.actionagainsthunger.org
Alliance to End Hunger:
www.alliancetoendhunger.org
Blood:Water Mission:
www.bloodwatermission.com
Bread for the World: www.bread.org
The Hunger Project: www.thp.org
The International Food Policy Research
Institute: www.ifpri.org

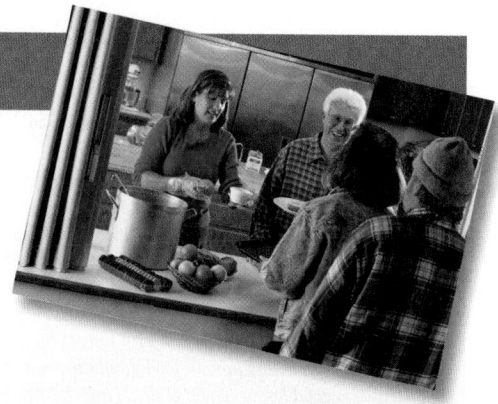

▲ Volunteer your time at a local food pantry or soup kitchen. Check out www.serve.gov/endhunger.asp to find a volunteer opportunity near you.

MAZON: A Jewish Response to Hunger:
http://mazon.org
Stop Hunger Now:
www.stophungernow.org
There are many creative ideas for raising funds and awareness to end world hunger. Check out the Rate Your Plate section at the end of Chapter 12 for more ideas, and put your own talents and passions to work for a good cause!

Further Readings

1. ADA Reports: Position of the American Dietetic Association: Agricultural and food bio-technology. *Journal of the American Dietetic Association* 106:285, 2006.

   It is the position of the American Dietetic Association that agricultural and food biotechnology techniques can enhance the quality, safety, nutritional value, and variety of food available for human consumption and increase the efficiency of food production, food processing, food distribution, and environmental and waste management.

2. ADA Reports: Position of the American Dietetic Association: Food insecurity in the United States. *Journal of the American Dietetic Association* 110:1368, 2010.

   It is the position of the American Dietetic Association that systematic and sustained action is needed to achieve food and nutrition security for all in the United States. Interventions are needed, including adequate funding for and increased use of food and nutrition assistance programs, inclusion of food and nutrition education in such programs, and innovative programs to promote and support individual and household economic self-sufficiency.

3. ADA Reports: Position of the American Dietetic Association: Addressing world hunger, malnutrition and food security. *Journal of the American Dietetic Association* 103:1046, 2003.

   It is the position of the American Dietetic Association that access to adequate amounts of safe, nutritious, and culturally appropriate foods is a fundamental human right. Still, hunger continues to be a worldwide problem of staggering proportions. In response, it is important to encourage programs and practices that combat hunger and malnutrition, increase food security, promote self-sufficiency, and are environmentally and economically sustainable.

4. ADA Reports: Position of the American Dietetic Association: Child and adolescent nutrition assistance programs. *Journal of the American Dietetic Association* 110:791, 2010.

   Children and adolescents should have access to an adequate supply of healthful and safe foods that promote optimal physical, social, and cognitive growth and development. Nutrition assistance programs, such as food assistance and meal service programs and nutrition initiatives, play a vital role in meeting this critical need.

5. Coutsoudis A: Infant feeding dilemmas created by HIV: South African experiences. *Journal of Nutrition* 135:956, 2005.

   This paper discusses the dilemma surrounding the risks and benefits of breastfeeding by an HIV-infected mother. The impact of the South African Safer Breastfeeding Programme, implemented to reduce some of the risk factors associated with HIV transmission, is reported.

6. Dammann KW, Smith C: Race, homelessness, and other environmental factors associated with the food-purchasing behavior of low-income women. *Journal of the American Dietetic Association* 110:1351, 2010.

The hunger-obesity paradox has increased interest in the quality of low-income households' food purchases. This study of low-income, urban women's food purchases showed that rates of "less healthy" food group purchases were higher compared to "healthy" food group purchases. Racial differences were found with respect to purchasing healthy protein food groups but not fruits, vegetables, or whole grains. Homelessness reduced the likelihood of purchasing most food groups, regardless of nutrient density. These findings indicate that we must strategize to help low-income, urban women make best use of food resources within their local food system.

7. Darton-Hill I and others: Micronutrient deficiencies and gender: Social and economic costs. *American Journal of Clinical Nutrition* 81:1198S, 2005.

Micronutrient deficiencies, such as for vitamin A, iodine, iron, and zinc, in developing countries, lead to health problems, especially in females. Addressing these micronutrient deficiencies is important in order to improve economic status at the personal, community, and national level in developing countries.

8. Doherty T and others: A longitudinal qualitative study of infant-feeding decision making and practices among HIV-positive women in South Africa. *Journal of Nutrition* 136:2421, 2006.

HIV-positive women face challenges regarding infant-feeding decisions. This study examined these challenges and found that successful breastfeeding resulted from a supportive home environment, a strong belief in the benefits of breastfeeding, and the ability to resist pressure to introduce other fluids.

9. Dworkin SL, Ehrhardt AA: Going beyond "ABC" to include "GEM": Critical reflections on progress in the HIV/AIDS epidemic. *American Journal of Public Health* 97:13, 2007.

This article discusses the feminization of HIV/AIDS and the limitations of the "ABC" (abstinence, be faithful, condom use) strategy.

Strategies focused on gender relation, economics, and migration (GEM) are suggested as more appropriate prevention measures.

10. Food and Agriculture Organization of the United Nations: *The state of food insecurity in the world 2008: High food prices and food security-threats and opportunities.* FAO, Rome, Italy, 2008

This report of the FAO food security meeting in Rome, Italy in June 2008, emphasizes that in 2008 alone, millions more became food-insecure, demanding urgent action and substantial investments. The worldwide concern about threats to global food security, largely triggered by soaring food prices, is discussed. Representatives of 180 countries plus the European Union met to express their conviction "that the international community needs to take urgent and coordinated action to combat the negative impacts of soaring food prices on the world's most vulnerable countries and populations."

11. Gibson RS: Zinc: The missing link in combating micronutrient malnutrition in developing countries. *Proceedings of the Nutrition Society* 65:51, 2006.

Although zinc deficiency is included as a major risk factor in the global burden of disease, zinc is still not included in the United Nations micronutrient priority list. Certain countries are at risk of zinc deficiency and should be targeted for zinc interventions. Zinc intervention strategies are discussed in this article.

12. Grandesso F and others: Mortality and malnutrition among populations living in South Darfur, Sudan. *Journal of the American Medical Association* 293:1490, 2005.

The conflicts in the Darfur region of Sudan have led to high rates of death and undernutrition among people displaced by war. This article describes what has been seen numerous times in the last 50 years—undernutrition and related death is a typical casualty of war.

13. Joint United Nations Programme on HIV/AIDS (UNAIDS) and World Health Organization. UNAIDS Report on the Global AIDS Epidemic 2010.

This UNAIDS report contains the 2010 global estimates on the scale of the AIDS pandemic. It

is reported that approximately 33 million people were living with HIV in 2009. The world has halted and begun to reverse the spread of HIV. Since 1999, the number of new infections has fallen by 19%.

14. Nord M, Hopwood H: A comparison of household food security in Canada and the United States. *Economic Research Report* 67, December 2008. www.ers.usda.gov/publications/err67/.

Differences in the prevalence of household food insecurity between Canada and the United States are described in this report. The percentage of the population living in food-insecure households was lower in Canada (7.0%) than in the United States (12.6%). The difference between the percentage of children living in food-insecure households in Canada vs. the United States was greater (8.3% vs. 17.9%) than that for adults (6.6% vs. 10.8%).

15. Shetty P: Achieving the goal of halving global hunger by 2015. *Proceedings of the Nutrition Society* 65:7, 2006.

This article reviews the goal of the FAO World Food Summit (WFS) and the United Nations Millennium Development Goals (MDG) to halve the numbers of the global population suffering from hunger by the year 2015. To date, the efforts have fallen short of the pace needed to achieve this goal. Developing countries are facing new challenges of hunger co-existing with new epidemics of diet-related diseases.

16. United Nations: *Tackling a global crisis: International year of sanitation 2008.* UN-Water, 2008. www.unwater.org.

The International Year of Sanitation in 2008 focused global attention on the need for improved health and hygiene. It is estimated that around the world, 2.6 billion people do not have a clean and safe place to perform their bodily functions because they lack access to a basic necessity, a toilet. This report helps to expose the scandal of human indignity, unnecessary child death, and lost economic opportunities associated with the sanitation crisis and provides a call to action for organizations to redouble their efforts and bring this silent crisis to an end.

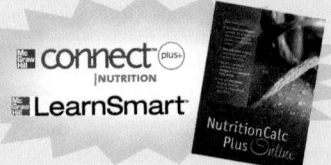

To get the most out of your study of nutrition, go to McGraw-Hill's online resources: Connect www.mcgrawhillconnect.com, **where you will find NutritionCalc Plus, LearnSmart, and many other dynamic tools.**

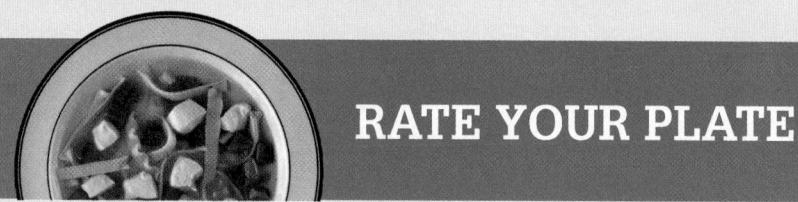

I. Fighting World Undernutrition on a Personal Level

If you want to do something about world and domestic undernutrition, consider the following activities. It is a noble act to try to make a difference, even if you make only one small step. As with any change in behavior, do not try to do too many things at once. Try one or two activities that represent your commitment to solving this problem.

1. Volunteer at a local soup kitchen or homeless shelter for a time (1 month, for example). What insights did you gain?

2. Coordinate the efforts of a campus organization to donate money to an antihunger agency such as the following:

Bread for the World
50 F Street NW, Suite 500
Washington, DC 20001
www.bread.org/

Catholic Relief Services
228 W. Lexington St
Baltimore, MD 21201
www.crs.org

Oxfam America
226 Causeway St., 5th Floor
Boston, MA 02114
www.oxfamamerica.org/

Feeding America
35 E. Wacker Dr., #2000
Chicago, IL 60601
http://feedingamerica.org

CARE USA
151 Ellis Street, NE
Atlanta, GA 30303
www.care.org/

EarthSave International
PO Box 96
New York, NY 10108
www.earthsave.org/

Save the Children Foundation
54 Wilton Rd.
Westport, CT 06880
www.savethechildren.org/

3. Make a contribution of nonperishable foods to the ongoing offering at a place of worship near you. If such an offering does not exist, start one.

4. Get on a food recovery program's mailing list, read its newsletters for information on upcoming fund-raisers and other activities, and become involved.

5. Utilize your love of good food and healthy cooking skills to organize a local meal for the hungry or a benefit dinner to raise money for local food banks. Resources to set up projects may be available from mission organizations. For example, with Blood: Water Mission's Lemon: Aid project, students or families can use something as simple as the sale of a refreshing drink to fund potable drinking water in rural communities in Africa.

6. Participate in food drives organized by local grocery stores by contributing food or services. Food-drive organizers may need volunteers to transport the donations to a food pantry. Pay attention to events around World Food Day, October 16.

7. Point, click, and fight hunger. Internet users can find information on hunger at several sites, including the following:

- Someone somewhere dies of hunger every 3.6 seconds. You can help stop the clock: go to www.thehungersite.com and click on Donate Free Food to send a meal to a needy someone. This site is affiliated with the UN World Food Program, which tracks the number of clicks and then sends a bill to one of its corporate or nonprofit sponsors.

- The Food and Agriculture Organization of the United Nations has worked to alleviate poverty and hunger by promoting agricultural development, improved nutrition, and the pursuit of food security. This website will keep you up-to-date on recent issues and provides an extensive list of publications related to food security. www.fao.org

- America's Second Harvest, the largest domestic hunger-relief organization, shows you how to help online and has information about the latest updates. www.secondharvest.org

- Bread for the World is a nationwide Christian citizens' movement seeking justice for the world's hungry people by lobbying our nation's decision makers. www.bread.org

- CARE is one of the world's largest private international relief and development organizations, with the goal of saving lives, building opportunities, and bringing hope to people in need. www.care.org

- Turn your personal fitness goals into a campaign to raise funds and awareness for projects that provide food and clean water to communities around the world. Water Walks (see www.bloodwatermission.com) or Crop Walks (see www.churchworld service.org) are great ways to walk a mile in someone else's shoes.

II. Joining the Battle Against Undernutrition

Imagine that you recently spent your summer vacation in a developing country and saw evidence of undernutrition and hunger. Then imagine that you are now asking a large corporation to support your efforts to ease hunger and suffering in this area. Develop a two-paragraph statement outlining why addressing hunger issues in this area is important. Include how the corporation could assist you.

Chapter 13 Safety of Our Food Supply

Student Learning Outcomes

Chapter 13 is designed to allow you to:

13.1 List some of the types and common sources of viruses, bacteria, fungi, and parasites that can make their way into food.

13.2 Compare and contrast food-preservation methods.

13.3 Understand the foodborne illnesses caused by bacteria, viruses, and parasites.

13.4 Describe the main reasons for using chemical additives in foods, the general classes of additives, and the functions of each class.

13.5 Identify sources of toxic environmental contaminants in food and the consequences of their ingestion.

13.6 Understand the reasons behind pesticide use, the possible long-term health complications, and the safety limits set for their use.

13.7 Understand the effects of conventional and sustainable agriculture on our food choices.

13.8 Describe the procedures that can be used to limit the risk of foodborne illness.

What Would You Choose?

By now, you have learned the importance of including more fruits and vegetables in your diet. You are choosing fresh or frozen produce more often than canned to cut back on sodium and other preservatives. You are steaming or stir-frying your vegetables to retain nutrients and avoid adding too much fat during preparation. In the grocery store, you have seen the growing selection of organic products including produce. Do they have health benefits that make them worth the extra cost? If cost was not a concern, what type of fruits and vegetables would you choose from the following list to satisfy your desire for increased nutritional value, decreased exposure to preservatives, lower risk for foodborne illness, and decreased exposure to pesticides?

a Canned low-sodium

b Organically grown

c Frozen

d Fresh

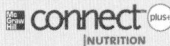 **Think about your choice as you read Chapter 13, then see our recommendations at the end of the chapter. To learn more about organic foods, check out the Connect site:** www.mcgrawhillconnect.com

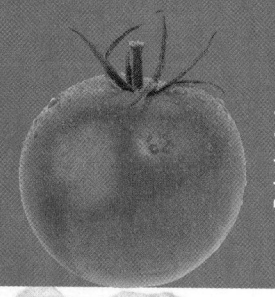

Over 100 years ago, in 1906, increasing public pressure forced the passage of the first Food and Drug Act in the United States and generally improved food preparation standards. Today, warnings about the safety of food and water appear everywhere. Attention has turned to more contemporary concerns, such as microbial and chemical contamination. Whereas we are told to eat more fruits, vegetables, fish, and poultry and to drink more water, we are also warned that these may contain dangerous substances. We still must ask, "How safe is our food and water?"

Scientists and health authorities agree that North Americans enjoy a relatively safe food supply, especially if foods are stored and prepared properly. Over the past 100 or so years, tremendous progress has been made to allow for this. Nonetheless, microorganisms and certain chemicals in foods still can pose a health risk. Thus, the nutritional and health benefits of food must be balanced against any food-related hazards. Chapter 13 focuses on these hazards—how real they are and how you can minimize their effect on your life. As the comic in the chapter suggests, you bear some responsibility for this—government agencies and industry can only do so much. Recall from Chapter 2 that the 2010 Dietary Guidelines for Americans encourage us to prepare and store foods safely.

pasteurizing The process of heating food products to kill pathogenic microorganisms and reduce the total number of bacteria.

virus The smallest known type of infectious agent, many of which cause disease in humans. A virus is essentially a piece of genetic material surrounded by a coat of protein. They do not metabolize, grow, or move by themselves. They reproduce only with the aid of a living cellular host.

bacteria Single-cell microorganisms; some produce poisonous substances, which cause illness in humans. Bacteria can be carried by water, animals, and people. They survive on skin, clothes, and hair and thrive in foods at room temperature. Some can live without oxygen and survive by means of **spore** formation.

spores Dormant reproductive cells capable of turning into adult organisms without the help of another cell. Various bacteria and fungi form spores.

fungi Simple parasitic life forms, including molds, mildews, yeasts, and mushrooms. They live on dead or decaying organic matter. Fungi can grow as single cells, like yeast, or as a multicellular colony, as seen with molds.

parasite An organism that lives in or on another organism and derives nourishment from it.

foodborne illness Sickness caused by the ingestion of food containing harmful substances.

Refresh Your Memory

As you begin your study of food safety in Chapter 13, you may want to review:

- Alternative sweeteners in Chapter 4
- The disease phenylketonuria (PKU) in Chapter 4
- Fat substitutes in Chapter 5
- Food biotechnology in Chapter 12

13.1 Food Safety: Setting the Stage

During the early stages of urbanization in North America, contaminated water and food—notably, milk—were responsible for many large outbreaks of typhoid fever, septic sore throat, scarlet fever, diphtheria, and other devastating human diseases. These experiences led to the development of processes for purifying water, treating sewage, and **pasteurizing** milk. Since that time, safe water and milk have become universally available, with only occasional problems from either.

The greatest health risk from food today is contamination by **viruses** and **bacteria** and, to a lesser extent, by various forms of **fungi** and **parasites.** These microorganisms can all cause **foodborne illness.** In a recent outbreak in the United States, 199 persons in 26 states were infected with *Escherichia coli* (*E. coli*) bacteria O157:H7 from fresh spinach. Of these ill persons, 102 were hospitalized, 31 developed kidney failure, and 22 were children under 5 years. Three deaths were associated with the outbreak. A deadlier outbreak of Escherichia coli O104:H4 occurred in Germany during the summer of 2011, resulting in over 3000 infections, hundreds of cases of kidney failure, and a death toll of at least 36. Read more about this outbreak that was linked to sprouts in Table 13.1.

Although microbial contamination is the cause of most incidents of foodborne illness, North Americans seem more concerned about health risks from chemicals in foods. In the long run, this concern has some merit. On a day-to-day basis, however, food additives cause only about 4% of all cases of foodborne illness in North America. Microbial contamination of food is by far the more important issue for our day-to-day health, so it will be discussed first. Chapter 13 will then cover chemical food safety hazards, including the use and safety of food additives, and discuss the risks of pesticides in foods.

Garfield ® by Jim Davis

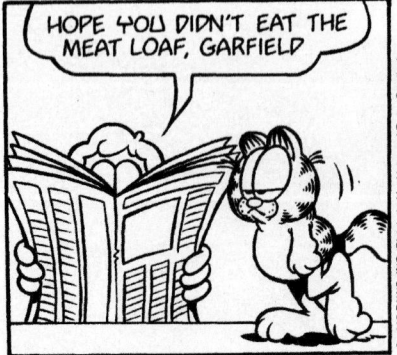
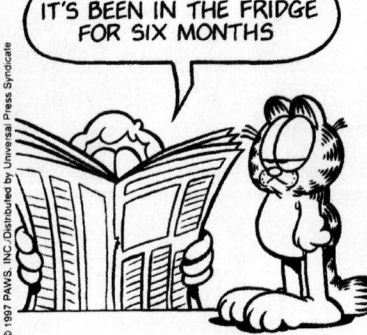
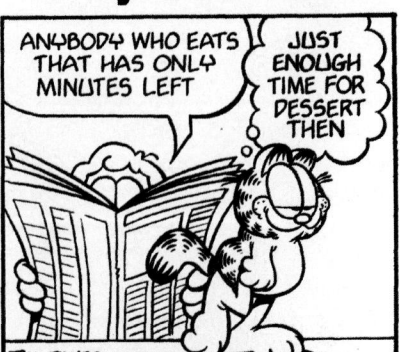

Which foods pose the greatest risk for foodborne illness? Is any food safe after being stored in the refrigerator for 6 months? Are food additives and pesticides an even greater day-to-day concern? Chapter 13 provides some answers.

GARFIELD © Paws, Inc. Reprinted with permission of Universal Press Syndicate. All rights reserved.

Effects of Foodborne Illness

According to the U.S. Centers for Disease Control and Prevention, foodborne illness causes 48 million illnesses, 128,000 hospitalizations, and 3000 deaths in the United States each year. Some people are particularly susceptible to foodborne illness, including the following:

- Infants and children
- Older adults
- Those with liver disease, diabetes, HIV infection (and AIDS), or cancer
- Postsurgical patients
- Pregnant women
- People taking immunosuppressant agents (e.g., transplant patients)

Some bouts of foodborne illness, especially when coupled with ongoing health problems, are lengthy and lead to food allergies, seizures, blood poisoning (from **toxins** or microorganisms in the bloodstream), or other illnesses. Foodborne illnesses often result from the unsafe handling of food at home, so we each bear some responsibility for preventing them (see Further Readings 2 and 10). You can't usually tell so by taste, smell, or sight that a particular food contains harmful microorganisms; therefore, you might not even be aware that food has caused your distress. In fact, your last case of diarrhea may have been caused by foodborne illness (Table 13-1). In response to the significant public health burden of foodborne illness that is largely preventable, the FDA Food Safety Modernization Act was signed into law by President Obama on January 4, 2011. This new law strengthens the food safety system, enabling FDA to better protect public health. It allows FDA to focus on prevention of food safety problems before they occur. The law also provides new tools for inspection and compliance and for holding imported foods to the same standards as domestic foods. The law also directs FDA to build a national food safety system that is integrated and in partnership with state and local authorities. Although government agencies are at work on problems regarding food safety, this does not substitute for individual safety efforts (Table 13-2).

toxins Poisonous compounds produced by an organism that can cause disease.

Read more about the Food Safety Modernization Act at www.fda.gov./Food/FoodSafety/FSMA/default.htm.

Why Is Foodborne Illness So Common?

Foodborne illness is carried or transmitted to people by food. Most foodborne illnesses are transmitted through food in which microorganisms are able to grow rapidly. These foods are generally moist, rich in protein, and have a neutral or slightly acidic pH. Unfortunately, this describes many of the foods we eat every day, such as meats, eggs, and dairy products.

Our food industry tries whenever possible to increase the shelf life of food products; however, a longer shelf life allows more time for bacteria in foods to multiply. Some bacteria even grow at refrigeration temperatures. Partially cooked—and some fully cooked—products pose a particular risk because refrigerated storage may only slow, not prevent, bacterial growth. The risk of contracting foodborne illness also is high because of consumer trends. First, there is greater consumer interest in eating raw or undercooked animal products. In addition, more people receive medication that suppresses their ability to combat foodborne infectious agents. Another factor is the continuing increase in the number of older adults in the population.

The risk of illness from foodborne microorganisms increases as more of our foods are prepared in kitchens outside the home. Supermarkets have become an alternative to cooking at home by offering a variety of prepared foods from specialty meat shops, salad bars, and bakeries. With the increasing number of two-income families, more people are looking for convenient, easy-to-prepare, nutritious foods. Supermarkets offer entrées that can be served immediately or reheated. The foods are usually prepared in central kitchens or processing plants and shipped to individual stores.

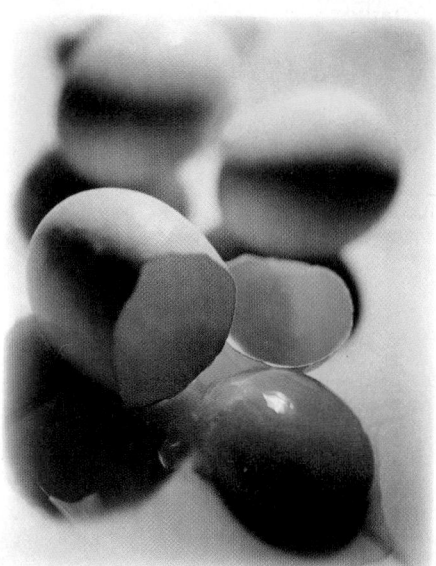

▲ Some restaurants that serve requested undercooked food are now warning patrons (on the menu) of the health risks of ordering such foods, particularly with undercooked eggs and meats.

TABLE 13-1 Some Examples of Cases of Foodborne Illness. We generally have a safe food supply, but there are occasional instances of foodborne illnesses, such as those listed.

Viruses

- *Norovirus:* Over 380 passengers and crew members of the largest cruise ship, Royal Caribbean's Freedom of the Seas, were sickened by *Norovirus*. The ship was sanitized, but one week later a second outbreak of the gastrointestinal illness afflicted 97 passengers and 11 crew members.

- *Hepatitus A:* Over 500 adults in the United States contracted hepatitis A after eating raw green onions in a Mexican restaurant. These were contaminated during growth in Mexico and not properly washed by food service workers.

Bacteria

- *Salmonella:* In 2008–2009, two outbreaks of salmonella cost their industries millions of dollars. The first outbreak was traced to imported jalapeno and serrano peppers from one Mexican farm. Illnesses led to 282 hospitalizations and 2 deaths. The second outbreak, traced to peanut butter from a processing plant in Georgia may have caused at least eight deaths.
- *Shigella:* More than 600 people on a cruise ship developed shigellosis and one person died.
- *Listeria:* Forty-eight deaths were associated with foodborne illness caused by *Listeria* organisms in soft, Mexican-style cheeses. A listeriosis outbreak associated with undercooked hot dogs and cold cuts resulted in more than 82 illnesses and 17 deaths in 19 states.
- *E. coli:* The world's deadliest outbreak of *Escherichia coli* occurred during the summer of 2011 with 3332 persons infected, more than 600 in intensive care, and a death toll of 36. The outbreak occurred mainly in Germany and involved the rare *E. coli* O104:H4 strain. Several hundred also contracted its potentially fatal kidney complication. The *E.coli* infection was caused by tainted vegetable sprouts from a small, rather traditional organic sprout farm. The sprout seeds were mostly imported from overseas and the *E.coli* bacteria were antibiotic

resistant. In the United States, the largest *E. coli* O157:H7 outbreak on record infected more than 1000 people in upstate New York at a county fair. The bacterium was found in infected well water. It killed a 79-year-old man and a 4-year-old girl, and it caused 10 other children to undergo kidney dialysis. Six adults and a 2-year-old child were killed after an *E. coli* outbreak from contaminated drinking water in Canada. The bacteria entered the water supply from animal manure after flooding from a heavy storm. In an outbreak of 199 persons infected with *E. coli* from fresh spinach, *E. coli* O157:H7 was isolated from 13 packages of fresh spinach in 10 states.
- *C. botulinum:* A man in Arkansas developed botulism after eating stew that was cooked and then kept at room temperature for 3 days. He spent—42 days on mechanical ventilation.
- *Vibrio:* Since 1992, 17 people in Florida have died of *Vibrio vulnificus* infections after eating raw oysters.
- *B. cereus:* A teenage boy and his father experienced abdominal pain, vomiting, and diarrhea within 30 minutes of eating 4-day-old homemade pesto that had been reheated and left out a number of times and was apparently contaminated with *Bacillus cereus*. The boy died of liver failure.

Parasites

- *Cryptosporidium:* A group attending a banquet developed diarrhea 3 to 9 days after eating green onions. Stool specimens were positive

for *Cryptosporidium*. Restaurant workers reported they did not consistently wash green onions before using them.

Risks from Seafood

- *Ciguatera:* An outbreak of ciguatera fish poisoning involved 17 crew members of a cargo ship that caught, cooked, and ate a barra-cuda in the Bahamas. All became ill with nausea, vomiting, abdominal

cramps, and diarrhea within hours of eating the fish. Within 2 days, all suffered from muscle pain and weakness; dizziness; and numb or itchy feet, hands, and mouth.

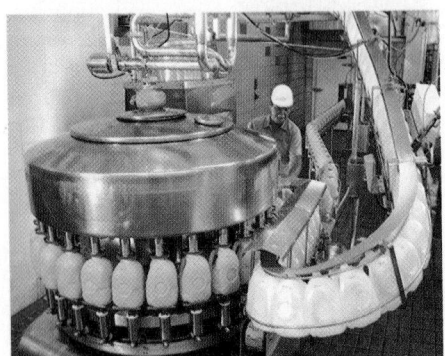

▲ Food contaminated in a central plant can go on to produce illness in people across the nation. In the case of juices, pasteurization is an effective method of reducing the risk of foodborne illness.

This centralization of food production by the food-processing and restaurant industry enhances the risk of foodborne illness. If a food product is contaminated in a central processing plant, consumers over a wide area can suffer foodborne illness. For example, a malfunction in an ice cream plant in Minnesota resulted in 224,000 suspected cases of *Salmonella* bacterial infections, which were linked to use of contaminated ice cream mix. At least 4 people died and 700 became ill in Washington and surrounding western states after eating at a chain of fast-food restaurants. The source of the problem was undercooked hamburger contaminated with the bacterium *E. coli* O157:H7. Restaurants are inspected by health departments only about every 6 months so we must rely on each restaurant to practice good food safety.

Greater consumption of ready-to-eat foods imported from foreign countries is still another cause of increased foodborne illness in North America. In the past, food imports were mostly raw products processed here under strict sanitation standards. Now, however, we import more ready-to-eat processed foods—such as berries from Guatemala and shellfish from Asia—some of which are contaminated. U.S. authorities are re-examining inspection procedures for these imports.

TABLE 13-2 Agencies Responsible for Monitoring the Food Supply in the United States

Agency Name	Responsibilities	Methods	How to Contact
United States Department of Agriculture (USDA)	• Enforces wholesomeness and quality standards for grains and produce (while in the field), meat, poultry, milk, eggs, and egg products	• Inspection • Grading • "Safe Handling Label"	www.fsis.usda.gov
Bureau of Alcohol, Tobacco, Firearms and Explosives (ATF)	• Enforces laws on alcoholic beverages	• Inspection	www.atf.gov
Environmental Protection Agency (EPA)	• Regulates pesticides • Establishes water quality standards	• Approval required for all U.S. pesticides • Sets pesticide residue limits in food	www.epa.gov
Food and Drug Administration (FDA)	• Ensures safety and wholesomeness of all foods in interstate commerce (except meat, poultry, and processed egg products) • Regulates seafood • Controls product labels	• Inspection • Food sample studies • Sets standards for specific foods	www.fda.gov or call 1-800-FDA-4010
Centers for Disease Control and Prevention (CDC)	• Promotes food safety	• Responds to emergencies concerning foodborne illness • Surveys and studies environmental health problems • Directs/enforces quarantines • National programs for prevention and control of foodborne and other diseases	www.cdc.gov
National Marine Fisheries Service or NOAA Fisheries	• Domestic and international conservation and management of living marine resources	• Voluntary seafood inspection program • Can use mark to show federal inspection	www.nmfs.noaa.gov
State and local governments	• Milk safety • Monitors food industry within their borders	• Inspection of food-related establishments	Government pages of telephone book

Government agencies responsible for monitoring food safety in Canada and the specific laws followed are listed in Appendix C.

The use of antibiotics in animal feeds is also increasing the severity of cases of foodborne illness. This antibiotic use encourages bacteria such as *E.coli* O157:H7 and O104:H4 to develop antibiotic-resistant strains, those that can grow even if exposed to typical antibiotic medicines. This issue is receiving considerable attention by scientists in the field.

Finally, more cases of foodborne disease are reported now because scientists are more aware of the roles of various players in the process. Every decade the list of microorganisms suspected of causing foodborne illness lengthens. In addition, physicians are more likely to suspect foodborne contaminants as a cause of illness. Furthermore, we now know that food, besides serving as a good growth medium for some microorganisms, transmits many others as well. Seafood is receiving greater scrutiny and surveillance by FDA as a cause of foodborne illness. For more information about food safety, contact FDA's Center for Food Safety and Applied Nutrition information line at 1-888-SAFEFOOD or log on to www.FoodSafety.gov (see Further Reading 5).

One tool in the battle against foodborne illness is HACCP, or Hazard Analysis Critical Control Point. By applying the principles of HACCP, food handlers critically analyze how they approach food preparation and what conditions may exist that might allow pathogenic microorganisms to enter and thrive in the food system. Once specific hazards and critical control points (potential problems) are identified, preventive measures can be used to reduce specific sources of contamination.

13.2 Food Preservation—Past, Present, and Future

For centuries, salt, sugar, smoke, fermentation, and drying have been used to preserve food. Ancient Romans used sulfites to disinfect wine containers and preserve wine. In the age of exploration, European adventurers traveling to the New World preserved their meat by salting it. Most preserving methods work on the principle of decreasing water content. Bacteria need abundant stores of water to grow; yeasts and molds can grow with less water, but some is still necessary. Adding sugar or salt binds water and so decreases the water available to these microbes. The process of drying evaporates off free water.

Decreasing the water content of some high-moisture foods, however, would cause them to lose essential characteristics. To preserve such foods—cucumber pickles, sauerkraut, milk (yogurt), and wine—fermentation has been a traditional alternative. Selected bacteria or yeast are used to ferment or pickle foods. The fermenting bacteria or yeast make acids and alcohol, which minimize the growth of other bacteria and yeast.

Today we can add pasteurization, sterilization, refrigeration, freezing, food **irradiation,** canning, and chemical preservation to the list of food preservation techniques. An additional method of food preservation—**aseptic processing**—simultaneously sterilizes the food and package separately before the food enters the package. Liquid foods, such as fruit juices, are especially easy to process in this manner. With aseptic packaging, boxes of sterile milk and juices can remain on supermarket shelves, free of microbial growth, for many years.

Food irradiation uses minimal doses of radiation to control pathogens such as *E. coli* O157:H7 and *Salmonella.* The radiation energy used does not make the food radioactive. The energy essentially passes through the food, as in microwave cooking, and no radioactive residues are left behind. However, the energy is strong enough to break chemical bonds, destroy cell walls and cell membranes, break down DNA, and link proteins together. Irradiation thereby controls growth of insects, bacteria, fungi, and parasites in foods.

FDA approved the use of irradiation for raw red meat to reduce risk of *E. coli* and other infectious microorganisms. Other additions to the approved list are shell eggs and seeds. Prior to this, the only animal products so treated were pork and chicken. Irradiation also extends the shelf life of spices, dry vegetable seasonings, meats, and fresh fruits and vegetables.

Irradiated food, except for dried seasonings, must be labeled with the international food irradiation symbol, the Radura, and a statement that the product has been treated by irradiation. Foods treated in this way are safe in the opinion of FDA and many other health authorities, including the American Academy of Pediatrics. Although the demand for irradiated foods is still low in the United States, other countries, including Canada, Japan, Italy, and Mexico, all use food irradiation technology widely. Certain consumer groups continually try to block its use in the United States, claiming that irradiation diminishes the nutritional value of food and that it can lead to the formation of harmful compounds, such as carcinogens. Future research should be able to sort out this controversy, but in any case the risk is very low. Keep in mind that, even when foods, especially meats, have been irradiated, it is still important to follow basic food-safety procedures, as later contamination during food preparation is possible.

13.3 Foodborne Illness Caused by Microorganisms

Most cases of foodborne illness are caused by specific viruses, bacteria, and other fungi. Prions—proteins involved in maintaining nerve cell function—can also turn infectious and lead to diseases such as mad cow disease. Bacteria specifically cause health problems either directly by invading the intestinal wall and producing an *infection* via a toxin contained in the organism, or indirectly by producing a toxin

irradiation A process in which **radiation** energy is applied to foods, creating compounds (free radicals) within the food that destroy cell membranes, break down DNA, link proteins together, limit enzyme activity, and alter a variety of other proteins and cell functions of microorganisms that can lead to food spoilage. This process does not make the food radioactive.

radiation Literally, energy that is emitted from a center in all directions. Various forms of radiation energy include X-rays and ultraviolet rays from the sun.

aseptic processing A method by which food and container are separately and simultaneously sterilized; it allows manufacturers to produce boxes of milk that can be stored at room temperature.

▲ This is the Radura, the international label denoting prior irradiation of the food product.

secreted into the food, which later harms us (called an *intoxication*). The main way to distinguish an infectious route from an intoxication is time: If symptoms appear in 4 hours or less, it is an intoxication.

Bacteria

Bacteria are single-cell organisms found in the food we eat, the water we drink, and the air we breathe. Many types of bacteria cause foodborne illness, including *Bacillus, Campylobacter, Clostridium, Escherichia, Listeria, Vibrio, Salmonella,* and *Staphylococcus* (Table 13-3). Bacteria are everywhere: each teaspoon of soil contains about 2 billion bacteria. Luckily, only a small number of all bacteria pose a threat. Some foodborne bacteria cause infections, whereas others cause intoxications. *Salmonella,* for example, causes an infection because the bacteria cause the illness. *Clostridium botulinum, Staphylococcus aureus,* and *Bacillus cereus* produce toxins and therefore cause illness from intoxication. In addition, while most strains of *E. coli* are harmless, *E. coli* O157:H7 and O104:H4 produce a toxin that can cause severe illness, including severe bloody diarrhea and hemolytic uremic syndrome (HUS). Bacterial foodborne illnesses typically cause gastrointestinal symptoms such as vomiting, diarrhea, and abdominal cramps. *Salmonella, Listeria, E. coli* O157:H7 and O104:H4, and *Campylobacter* are the bacterial foodborne illnesses of particular interest because they are the ones most often associated with death. *E. coli* O157:H7 and O104:H4 has caused deaths when HUS has developed. Of the 1600 cases of Listeriosis in the United States each year, 255 cases are fatal. Listeriosis is of particular concern for pregnant women because they are about 20 times more likely to get this infection than other healthy adults, and Listeriosis can cause spontaneous abortion or stillbirth because the *Listeria* bacteria can cross the placenta and infect the fetus.

To proliferate, bacteria require nutrients, water, and warmth. Most grow best in **danger zone** temperatures of 40° to 140°F (4° to 60°C) (Fig. 13-1). Pathogenic bacteria

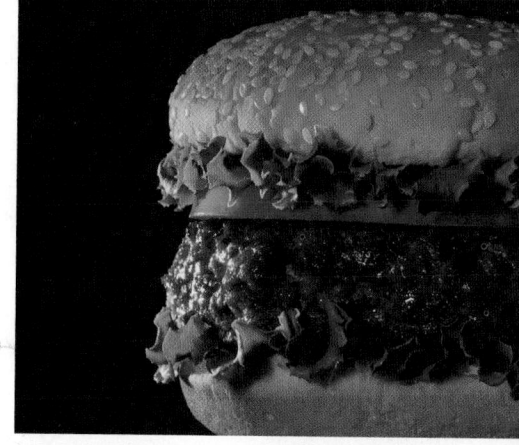

▲ Ground meats are a typical source of foodborne infection because bacteria on the surface of whole meats are distributed throughout the meat during grinding.

FIGURE 13-1 ▶ Effects of temperature on microbes that cause foodborne illness.

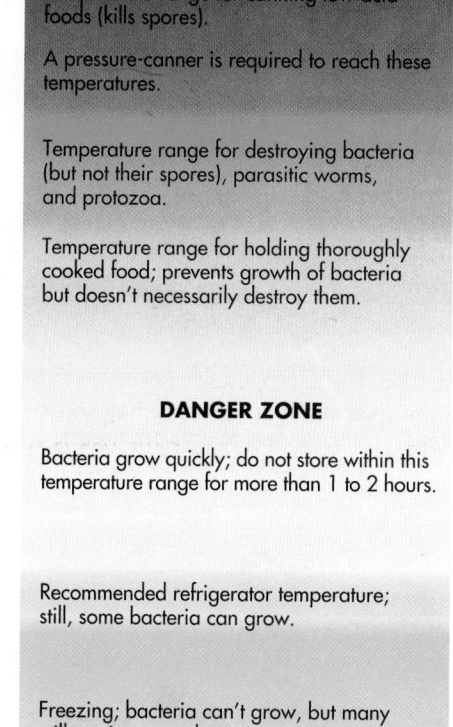

°C	°F	
121	250	Temperature range for canning low-acid foods (kills spores).
116	240	A pressure-canner is required to reach these temperatures.
100	212	
74	165	Temperature range for destroying bacteria (but not their spores), parasitic worms, and protozoa.
		Temperature range for holding thoroughly cooked food; prevents growth of bacteria but doesn't necessarily destroy them.
60	140	
52	125	**DANGER ZONE**
15	60	Bacteria grow quickly; do not store within this temperature range for more than 1 to 2 hours.
4	40	Recommended refrigerator temperature; still, some bacteria can grow.
0	32	
−18	0	Freezing; bacteria can't grow, but many will survive; growth can resume on thawing.

$$C = (F - 32) \times 5/9$$

$$F = \frac{9 \times (C°)}{5} + 32$$

TABLE 13-3 Bacterial Causes of Foodborne Illness

Bacteria	Typical Food Sources	Symptoms	Additional Information
***Salmonella* species** 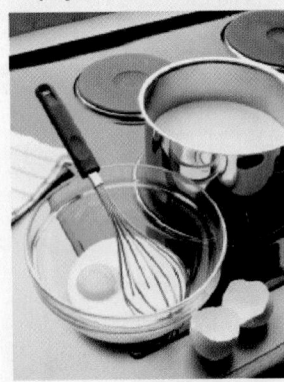	Raw and undercooked meats, poultry, eggs, and fish; produce, especially raw sprouts; peanut butter; unpasteurized milk (see Further Reading 4.)	Onset: 12–72 hours; nausea, fever, headache, abdominal cramps, diarrhea, and vomiting; can be fatal in infants, the elderly, and those with impaired immune systems; lasts 4–7 days	Estimated 1 million infections/year; bacteria live in the intestines of animals and humans; food is contaminated by infected water and feces; about 2000 strains of *Salmonella* bacteria can cause disease, but 3 strains account for almost 50% of cases; *Salmonella enteritidis* infects the ovaries of healthy hens and contaminates eggs; almost 20% of cases are from eating undercooked eggs or egg-containing dishes; reptiles, such as turtles, also spread the disease
Campylobacter jejuni	Raw and undercooked meat and poultry (more than half of raw poultry in the United States is contaminated), unpasteurized milk, contaminated water	Onset: 2–5 days; muscle pain, abdominal cramping, diarrhea (sometimes bloody), fever; lasts 2–7 days	Estimated 845,000 infections/year; produces a toxin that destroys intestinal mucosal surfaces; can cause Guillain-Barré syndrome, a rare neurological disorder that causes paralysis
***Escherichia coli* (O157:H7 O104:H4 and other strains)**	Undercooked ground beef; produce—lettuce, spinach, sprouts; unpasteurized juice and milk	Onset: 1–8 days; bloody diarrhea, abdominal cramps; in children under age 5 and the elderly, hemolytic uremic syndrome (HUS) is a serious complication; red blood cells are destroyed and kidneys fail; can be fatal; lasts 5–10 days	Leading cause of bloody diarrhea in the United States; estimated 73,000 cases/year; lives in the intestine of healthy cattle; cattle and cattle manure are chief sources; illness caused by a powerful toxin made by the bacteria; petting zoos, lakes, and swimming pools can contain pathogenic *E. coli*
***Shigella* species**	Fecal/oral transmission; water supplies, produce, and other foods contaminated by infected food handlers with poor hygiene	Onset: 1–3 days; abdominal cramps, fever, diarrhea (often bloody); lasts 5–7 days	Estimated 448,000 cases/year; humans and primates are the only sources; common in day-care centers and custodial institutions from poor hygiene; traveler's diarrhea often caused by *Shigella dysenteriae*
Staphylococcus aureus	Ham, poultry, egg salads, cream-filled pastries, custards, whipped cream	Onset: 1–6 hours; diarrhea, vomiting, nausea, abdominal cramps; lasts 1–3 days	Bacteria on skin and nasal passages of up to 25% of people; can be passed to foods; multiplies rapidly when contaminated foods are held for extended time at room temperature; illness caused by a heat-resistant toxin that cannot be destroyed by cooking

TABLE 13-3 *(continued)*

Bacteria	Typical Food Sources	Symptoms	Additional Information
Clostridium perfringens	Beef, poultry, gravy, Mexican food	Onset: 8–24 hours; abdominal pain and diarrhea, usually mild; can be more serious in elderly or ill persons; lasts 1 day or less	Estimated 966,000 cases/year; anaerobic bacteria widespread in soil and water; multiplies rapidly in prepared foods, such as meats, casseroles, and gravies, held for extended time at room temperature
Listeria monocytogenes	Unpasteurized milk and soft cheeses, raw meats, uncooked vegetables, ready-to-eat deli meats and hotdogs, refrigerated smoked fish (see Further Reading 6.)	Onset: 9–48 hours for early symptoms, 14–42 days for severe symptoms; fever, muscle aches, headache, vomiting; can spread to nervous system, resulting in stiff neck, confusion, loss of balance, or convulsion; can cause premature birth and stillbirth	Estimated 1600 cases with 260 fatalities/year; widespread in soil and water and can be carried in healthy animals; grows at refrigeration temperatures; about one-third of cases occur during pregnancy; high-risk persons should avoid uncooked deli meats, soft cheeses (e.g., feta, Brie, and Camembert), blue-veined cheeses, Mexican-style cheeses (e.g., queso blanco made from unpasteurized milk), refrigerated meat spreads or pates, uncooked refrigerated smoked fish
Clostridium botulinum	Incorrectly home-canned vegetables, meats, and fish; incorrectly canned commercial foods; herb-infused oils; bottled garlic; potatoes baked in foil and held at room temperature; honey	Onset: 18–36 hours but can be 6 hours to 10 days; neurological symptoms—double and blurred vision, drooping eyelids, slurred speech, difficulty swallowing, muscle weakness, and paralysis of face, arms, respiratory muscles, trunk, and legs; can be fatal; lasts days to weeks	Estimated 100 cases/year; caused by a neurotoxin; *C. botulinum* grows only in the absence of air in non-acidic foods; incorrect home canning causes most botulism, but in 2007 commercially canned chili sauce caused an outbreak; honey can contain botulism spores and should not be given to infants younger than 1 year of age
Vibrio	*V. parahemolyticus:* raw and undercooked shellfish, especially oysters	Onset: 24 hours; watery diarrhea, nausea, vomiting, fever, chills; lasts 3 days	Found in coastal waters; more infections in summer; number of infections hard to determine because it is difficult to isolate in the lab
	V. vulnificus: raw and undercooked shellfish, especially oysters	Onset: 1–2 days; vomiting, diarrhea, abdominal pain; in more severe cases, bloodstream infection with fever, chills, decreased blood pressure, blistering skin lesions; lasts 3 or more days	Estimated 95 cases/year; found in coastal waters; more infections in summer; those with impaired immune systems and liver disease at higher risk of infection; fatality rate of 50% with bloodstream infection
	V. cholerae: contaminated water and food, human carriers	Onset: 2–3 days; severe, dehydrating diarrhea, vomiting; dehydration, cardiovascular collapse, and death can occur	Occurs mainly in countries without adequate water purification and sewage treatment
Yersinia enterocolitica	Raw or undercooked pork, particularly pork intestines (chitterlings); tofu; water; unpasteurized milk	Onset: 4–7 days; fever, abdominal pain, diarrhea (often bloody); lasts 1–3 weeks or longer	Yersinosis most common in children under age 5 years; relatively rare; bacteria live mainly in pigs but can be found in other animals

typically do not multiply when food is held at temperatures above 140°F (60°C) or stored at safe refrigeration temperatures, 32° to 40°F (0° to 4.4°C). One important exception is *Listeria* bacteria, which can multiply at refrigeration temperatures. Also note that high temperatures can kill toxin-producing bacteria, but any toxin produced in the food will not be inactivated by high temperatures. Most pathogenic bacteria also require oxygen for growth, but *Clostridium botulinum* and *Clostridium perfringens* grow only in anaerobic (oxygen-free) environments, such as those found in tightly sealed cans and jars. Food acidity can affect bacterial growth, too. Although most bacteria do not grow well in acidic environments, some, such as disease-causing *E. coli*, can grow in acidic foods, such as fruit juice.

Viruses

Viruses, like bacteria, are widely dispersed in nature. Unlike bacteria, however, viruses can reproduce only after invading body cells, such as those that line the intestines. Experts speculate that about 70% of foodborne illness cases go un-diagnosed because they result from viral causes, and there is no easy way to test for these pathogens. Table 13-4 describes the two most common viral causes of foodborne illness and describes typical food sources and symptoms of the illnesses they cause. Norovirus is the number one pathogen contributing to domestically acquired foodborne illnessses. It causes an illness commonly misdiagnosed as the "stomach flu." Norovirus infection has a sudden onset and usually a short duration of only one to two days. Noroviruses have become a problem on cruise ships. They are hardy and survive freezing, relatively high temperatures, and chlorination up to 10 ppm. A website coordinating the U.S. efforts on food safety is the www.FoodSafety.gov site mentioned earlier. Another useful website is www.homefoodsafety.org.

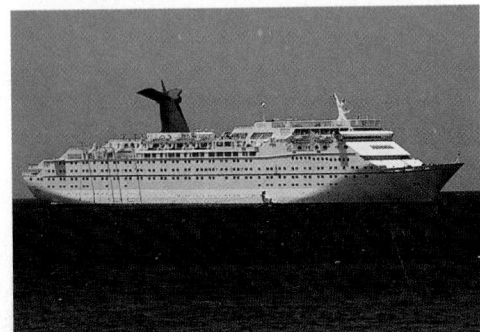

▲ Norovirus epidemics commonly occur on cruise ships. Noroviruses were originally called "Norwalk viruses" from Norwalk, Ohio, where they were first known to cause an epidemic of gastroenteritis.

TABLE 13-4 Viral Causes of Foodborne Illness

Viruses	Typical Food Sources	Symptoms	Additional Information
Norovirus (Norwalk and Norwalk-like viruses), human rotavirus	Foods prepared by infected food handlers; shellfish from contaminated waters; vegetables and fruits contaminated during growing, harvesting, and processing (see Further Reading 13.)	Onset: 1–2 days; "stomach flu"— severe diarrhea, nausea, vomiting, stomach cramping, low-grade fever, chills, muscle aches; lasts 1–2 days or longer	Estimated over 5 million cases per year and 150 deaths. Viruses found in stool and vomit of infected persons; food handlers can contaminate foods or work surfaces; noroviruses are very infectious—as few as 10–100 particles can lead to infection; workers with norovirus symptoms should not work until 2 or 3 days after they feel better.
Hepatitis A virus	Foods prepared by infected food handlers, especially uncooked foods or those handled after cooking, such as sandwiches, pastries, and salads; shellfish from contaminated waters; vegetables and fruits contaminated during growing, harvesting, and processing	Onset: 15–50 days; anorexia, diarrhea, fever, jaundice, dark urine, fatigue; may cause liver damage and death; lasts several weeks up to 6 months	Infected food handlers contaminate food and transmit the disease to dozens of persons; children and young adults are more susceptible; a vaccine is available, decreasing the number of infections dramatically; immunoglobulin given within 1 week to those exposed to hepatitis A virus can also decrease infection.

[handwritten: eating disorder]

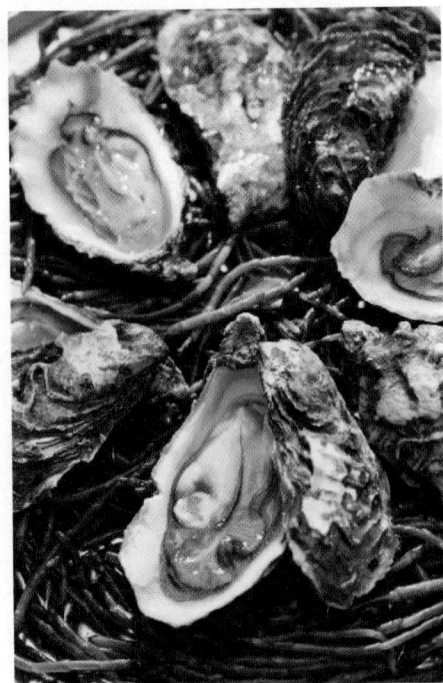

▲ Raw shellfish, especially bivalves (e.g., oysters and clams), present a particular risk related to foodborne viral disease. These animals filter feed, a process that concentrates viruses, bacteria, and toxins present in the water as it is filtered for food. Adequate cooking of shellfish will kill viruses and bacteria, but toxins may not be affected. It's important to buy shellfish from reliable sources who have harvested these foods from safe areas.

CONCEPT CHECK

Viruses and bacteria pose the greatest risk for foodborne illness. In the past, the addition of sugar and salt to foods, as well as smoking and drying, were used to prevent the growth of microorganisms. Commercial processes, such as pasteurization and irradiation, offer protection from foodborne illness. Treat all raw animal products, cooked food, and raw fruits and vegetables as potential sources of foodborne illness.

Parasites

Parasites live in or on another organism, known as the host, from which they absorb nutrients. Humans may serve as a host to parasites. These tiny ravagers rob millions of people around the globe of their health and, in some cases, their lives. Those hardest hit live in tropical countries where poor sanitation fosters the growth of parasites.

The more than 80 foodborne parasites known to affect humans include mainly **protozoa** (one-celled animals), such as *Cryptosporidium* and *Cyclospora*, and **helminths,** such as tapeworms and the roundworm *Trichinella spiralis*. Table 13-5 describes common parasites and typical food sources and symptoms of the illnesses they cause. Parasitic infections spread via person-to-person contact and contaminated food, water, and soil.

13.4 Food Additives

By the time you see a food on the market shelf, it usually contains substances added to make it more palatable or increase its nutrient content or shelf life. Manufacturers also add some substances to foods to make them easier to process. Other substances may have accidentally found their way into the foods you buy. All of these extraneous substances are known as **additives,** and, although some may be beneficial, others, such as sulfites, may be harmful for some people. All purposefully added substances must be evaluated by FDA.

Why Are Food Additives Used?

Most additives are used to limit food spoilage. Common food additives serve the general function of **preservatives,** including acidic or alkaline agents, antioxidants, antimicrobial agents, curing and pickling agents, and **sequestrants.** Table 13-6 helps you to understand exactly why these are used and to learn more about the specific substances used. Food additives, such as potassium sorbate, are used to maintain the safety and acceptability of foods by retarding the growth of microbes implicated in foodborne illness.

Additives are also used to combat some enzymes that lead to undesirable changes in color and flavor in foods but don't cause anything as serious as foodborne illness. This second type of food spoilage occurs when enzymes in a food react to oxygen—for example, when apple and peach slices darken or turn rust color as they are exposed to air. Antioxidants are a type of preservative that slow the action of oxygen-requiring enzymes on food surfaces. These preservatives are not necessarily novel chemicals. They include vitamins E and C and a variety of sulfites.

Without the use of some food additives, it would be impossible to produce massive quantities of foods and safely distribute them nationwide or worldwide, as is now done. Despite consumer concerns about the safety of food additives, many have been extensively studied and proven safe when FDA guidelines for their use are followed.

---

protozoa One-celled animals that are more complex than bacteria. Disease-causing protozoa can be spread through food and water.

helminth Parasitic worm that can contaminate food, water, feces, animals, and other substances.

additives Substances added to foods, such as preservatives.

preservatives Compounds that extend the shelf life of foods by inhibiting microbial growth or minimizing the destructive effect of oxygen and metals.

sequestrants Compounds that bind free metal ions. By so doing, they reduce the ability of ions to cause rancidity in foods containing fat.

TABLE 13-5 Parasitic Causes of Foodborne Illness

Parasite	Typical Food Sources	Symptoms	Additional Information
Trichinella spiralis	Pork, wild game	Onset: weeks to months; GI symptoms followed by muscle weakness, fluid retention in the face, fever, flulike symptoms	The number of trichinosis infections has decreased greatly because pigs are now less likely to harbor this parasite; cooking pork to 160°F (72°C) will kill *trichinella*, as will freezing it for 3 days at −4°F (−20°C).
Anisakis	Raw or undercooked fish	Onset: 12 hours or less; violent stomach pain, nausea, vomiting	Caused by eating the larvae of roundworms; the infection is more common where raw fish is routinely consumed.
Tapeworms	Raw beef, pork, and fish	Abdominal discomfort, diarrhea	
Toxoplasma gondii	Raw or undercooked meat, unwashed fruits and vegetables	Onset: 5–20 days; most people are asymptomatic; those with symptoms have fever, headache, sore muscles, diarrhea; can be fatal to the fetus of pregnant women	Parasite is spread to humans from animals, including cats, the main reservoir of the disease; humans acquire the disease from ingesting contaminated meat or from fecal contamination from handling cat litter.
Cyclospora cayetanensis	Water, contaminated food	Onset: 1 week; watery diarrhea, vomiting, muscle aches, fatigue, anorexia, weight loss; lasts 10–12 weeks	Most common in tropical and subtropical areas, but since 1990 about a dozen outbreaks, affecting 3600 people, have occurred in the United States and Canada.
Cryptosporidium	Water, contaminated food	Onset: 2–10 days; watery diarrhea, abdominal pain, fever, nausea, vomiting, weight loss; those with impaired immune systems become more ill; lasts 1–2 weeks in otherwise healthy persons	Outbreaks occur worldwide; the largest U.S. outbreak was in 1993 in Milwaukee, with more than 443,000 persons affected; also can be spread in water parks and community swimming pools.

TABLE 13-6 Types of Food Additives—Sources and Related Health Concerns

Food Additive Class	Attributes	Health Risks
Acidic or alkaline agents, such as citric acid, calcium lactate, and sodium hydroxide	Acids impart a tart taste to soft drinks, sherbets, and cheese spreads; inhibit mold growth; lessen discoloration and rancidity. They also reduce the risk of botulism in naturally low-acid vegetables, such as canned green beans. Alkaline agents neutralize acids produced during fermentation, and so improve flavor.	No known health risks when used properly.
Alternative low-calorie sweeteners, such as saccharin, sucralose, ascesulfame potassium, aspartame, neotame, and tagatose	Sweeten foods without adding more than a few calories	Moderate use of these alternative sweeteners is considered safe (except for use of aspartame by people with the disease PKU).
Anticaking agents, such as calcium silicate, magnesium stearate, and silicon dioxide	Absorb moisture to keep table salt, baking powder, or powdered sugar and powdered food products free-flowing and prevent caking and lumping	No known health risks when used properly.
Antimicrobial agents, such as salt, sodium benzoate, sorbic acid, and calcium propionate	Inhibit mold and fungal growth	Salt increases the risk of developing hypertension, especially in some individuals. No known health risks from other agents when used properly.
Antioxidants, such as BHA (butylated hydroxyanisole), BHT (butylated hydroxytoluene), alpha-tocopherol (vitamin E), ascorbic acid (vitamin C), and sulfites	Delay food discolorations from oxygen exposure; Reduce rancidity from the breakdown of fats; Maintain the color of luncheon meats; Prevent the formation of cancer-causing nitrosamines	Sulfites can cause an allergic reaction in about 1 in every 100 people. Symptoms include difficulty breathing, wheezing, hives, diarrhea, abdominal pain, cramps, and dizziness. Salad bars, dried fruit, and wine are typical sources of sulfites.
Color additives, such as tartrazine	Make foods more appealing	Tartrazine (FD&C yellow number 5) can cause allergic symptoms such as hives and nasal discharge in some people, especially those allergic to aspirin. FDA requires manufacturers to list all forms of synthetic colors on the labels of foods that contain them.
Curing and pickling agents, such as salt, nitrates, and nitrites	Nitrates and nitrites act as preservatives, especially to prevent the growth of *Clostridium botulinium;* often used in conjunction with salt	Salt increases the risk of developing hypertension, especially in some individuals. Nitrate and nitrite consumption from both cured foods and that found naturally in some vegetables has been associated with synthesis of nitrosamines. (An adequate

Sugar, salt, corn syrup, and citric acid constitute 98% of all additives (by weight) used in food processing.

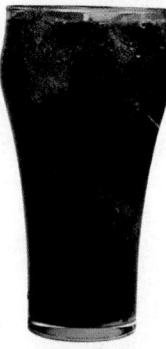

▲ Soft drinks are typical sources of alternative sweeteners for many of us. Moderate use of these products generally poses no health risk in most people.

You might wonder why, if nitrates and nitrites form chemical substances that can cause cancer, they aren't banned by the Delaney Clause. In the United States, USDA regulates the use of chemicals in meats. The laws that govern USDA regulation of foods are separate from those that govern FDA regulation. Because of this, the Delaney Clause does not apply to USDA actions. USDA sees no clear threat to public safety from the regulated use of nitrates and nitrites in meats, so no action has been taken.

TABLE 13-6 *(continued)*

Food Additive Class	Attributes	Health Risks
		vitamin C intake may reduce this synthesis.) Some nitrosamines are cancer-causing agents, particularly for the stomach, esophagus, and colon, but the risk is low. The National Cancer Institute advises consuming these foods in moderation.
Emulsifiers, such as monoglycerides and lecithins	Suspend fat in water to improve uniformity, smoothness, and body of foods, such as baked goods, ice cream, and mayonnaise	No known health risks when used properly.
Fat replacements, such as Paselli SA2, Dur-Low, Oatrim, Sta-Slim 143, Stellar, and Olean	Limit calorie content of foods by reducing some of the fat content	Generally no known health risks when used properly.
Flavor and flavoring agents (such as natural and artificial flavors), sugar, and corn syrup	Impart more or improve flavor of foods	Sugar and corn syrup can increase risk for dental caries. Generally no known health risks for flavoring agents when used properly.
Flavor enhancers, such as monosodium glutamate (MSG) and salt	Help bring out the natural flavor of foods, such as meats	Some people (especially infants) are sensitive to the glutamate portion of MSG and after exposure experience flushing, chest pain, facial pressure, dizziness, sweating, rapid heart rate, nausea, vomiting, increase in blood pressure, and headache. Those so affected should look for the word glutamate on food labels, as well as isolated protein, yeast extract, bullion, and soup stock. Salt increases the risk of developing hypertension, especially in some people.
Humectants, such as glycerol, propylene glycol, and sorbitol	Retain more moisture, texture, and fresh flavor in foods such as candies, shredded coconut, and marshmallows	No known health risk when used properly.
Leavening agents, such as yeast, baking powder, and baking soda	Introduce carbon dioxide into food products	No known health risk when used properly.
Maturing and bleaching agents, such as bromates, peroxides, and ammonium chloride	Shorten the time needed for maturation of flour to become usable for baking products	No known health risk when used properly.
Nutrient supplements, such as vitamin A, vitamin D, and potassium iodide	Enhance the nutrient content of foods such as margarine, milk, and ready-to-eat breakfast cereals	No known health risk if intake from such supplemental sources combined with other natural food sources of a nutrient does not exceed the Upper Level set for a particular nutrient (iron may be one exception; review Chapter 9).

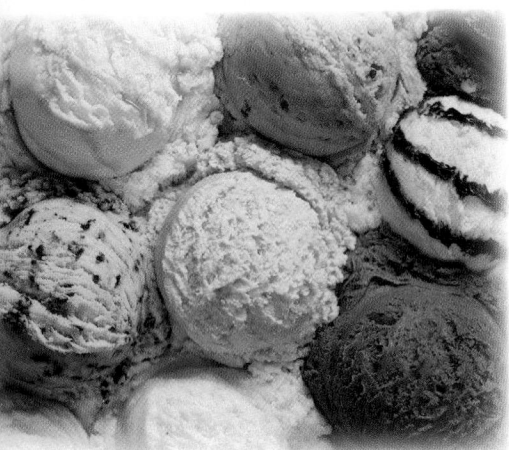

▲ Emulsifiers improve the texture of foods such as ice cream, baked goods, and cookies.

CRITICAL THINKING

Recognizing that Joseph is taking a nutrition class, his roommate asks him, "What is more risky: the bacteria that can be present in food or the additives listed on the label of my favorite snack cake?" How should Joseph respond? On what information should he base his conclusions?

TABLE 13-6 *(continued)*

Food Additive Class	Attributes	Health Risks
Stabilizers and thickeners, such as pectins, gums, gelatins, and agars	Impart a smooth texture and uniform color and flavor to candies, ice cream and other frozen desserts, chocolate milk, and beverages containing alternative sweeteners. Prevent evaporation and deterioration of flavorings used in cakes, puddings, and gelatin mixes	No known health risk when used properly.
Sequestrants, such as EDTA and citric acid	Bind free ions, helping preserve food quality by reducing ability of ions to cause rancidity in products containing fat	No known health risk when used properly.

[handwritten:] marbling - is fat

[handwritten:] product of decomposed fatty acid that have unpleasant flavor/ odor

Intentional Versus Incidental Food Additives

Food additives are classified into two types: **intentional food additives** (directly added to foods) and **incidental food additives** (indirectly added as contaminants). Both types of agents are regulated by FDA in the United States. Currently, more than 2800 different substances are intentionally added to foods. As many as 10,000 other substances enter foods as contaminants. This includes substances that may reasonably be expected to enter food through surface contact with processing equipment or packaging materials.

The GRAS List

In 1958, all food additives used in the United States and considered safe at that time were put on a **generally recognized as safe (GRAS)** list. The U.S. Congress established the GRAS list because it believed manufacturers did not need to prove the safety of substances that had been used for a long time and were already generally recognized as safe. Since that time, FDA has been responsible for proving that a substance does not belong on the GRAS list. Substances may be added to the GRAS list if data and information about the use of the substance are known and accepted widely by qualified experts, and establish that the substance is safe under the conditions of its intended use.

Since 1958, some substances on the list have been reviewed. A few, such as cyclamates, failed the review process and were removed from the list. The additive red dye #3 was removed because it is linked to cancer. Many chemicals on the GRAS list have not yet been rigorously tested, primarily because of expense. These chemicals have received a low priority for testing, mostly because they have long histories of use without evidence of toxicity or because their chemical characteristics do not suggest they are potential health hazards.

Are Synthetic Chemicals Always Harmful?

Nothing about a natural product makes it inherently safer than a synthetic product. Many synthetic products are laboratory copies of chemicals that also occur in nature (see the discussion in Chapter 12 on biotechnology for some examples). Moreover, although human endeavors contribute some toxins to foods, such as synthetic pesticides and industrial chemicals, nature's poisons are often even more potent and

intentional food additives Additives knowingly (directly) incorporated into food products by manufacturers.

incidental food additives Additives that appear in food products indirectly, from environmental contamination of food ingredients or during the manufacturing process.

generally recognized as safe (GRAS) A list of food additives that in 1958 were considered safe for consumption. Manufacturers were allowed to continue to use these additives, without special clearance, when needed for food products. FDA bears responsibility for proving they are not safe, but can remove unsafe products from the list.

Some important definitions:

toxicology	Scientific study of harmful substances
safety	Relative certainty that a substance won't cause injury
hazard	Chance that injury will result from use of a substance
toxicity	Capacity of a substance to produce injury or illness at some dosage

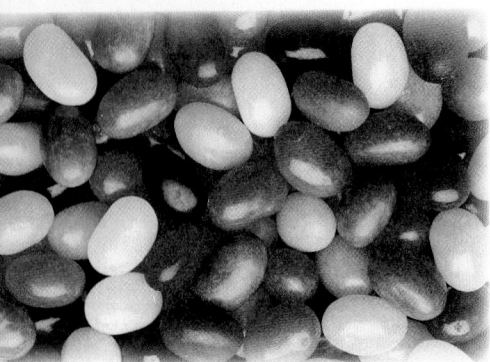

▲ Color additives make some foods more desirable.

The 100-fold margin of safety is 25 times less than that for vitamin A, when you compare the RDA for healthy women (700 micrograms) to a potentially harmful dose of vitamin A for pregnant women (3000 micrograms).

Delaney Clause A clause to the 1958 Food Additives Amendment of the Pure Food and Drug Act in the United States that prevents the intentional (direct) addition to foods of a compound shown to cause cancer in laboratory animals or humans.

widespread. Some cancer researchers suggest that we ingest at least 10,000 times more (by weight) natural toxins produced by plants than we do synthetic pesticide residues. (Plants produce these toxins to protect themselves from predators and disease-causing organisms.) This comparison does not make synthetic chemicals any less toxic, but it does put them in a more accurate perspective.

Consider vitamin E, often added to food to prevent rancidity of fats. This chemical is safe when used within certain limits. However, high doses have been associated with health problems, such as interfering with vitamin K activity in the body (review Chapter 8). Thus, even well-known chemicals we are comfortable using can be toxic in some circumstances and at some concentrations.

Tests of Food Additives for Safety

Food additives are tested by FDA for safety on at least two animal species, usually rats and mice. Scientists determine the highest dose of the additive that produces *no observable effects* in the animals. These doses are proportionately much higher than humans are ever exposed to. The maximum dosage that produced no observable effects is then divided by at least 100 to establish a margin of safety for human use. This 100-fold margin is used because it is assumed that we are at least 10 times more sensitive to food additives than are laboratory animals and that any one person might be 10 times more sensitive than another. This broad margin essentially ensures that the food additive in question will cause no harmful health effects in humans. In fact, many synthetic chemicals are probably less dangerous at these low doses than some of the natural compounds in common foods such as apples or celery.

One important exception applies to the schema for testing intentional food additives: If an additive is shown to cause cancer, even though only in high doses, no margin of safety is allowed. The food additive cannot be used, because it would violate the **Delaney Clause** in the 1958 Food Additives Amendment. This clause prohibits intentionally adding to foods a compound introduced after 1958 and that causes cancer at any level of exposure. Evidence for cancer could come from either laboratory animal or human studies. Few exceptions to this clause are allowed; exceptions are discussed regarding curing and pickling agents in Table 13-6.

Incidental food additives are another matter. FDA cannot ban various industrial chemicals, pesticide residues, and mold toxins from foods, even though some of these contaminants can cause cancer. These products are not purposely added to foods. FDA sets an acceptable level for these substances. An incidental substance found in a food cannot contribute to more than one cancer case during the lifetimes of 1 million people. If a higher risk exists, the amount of the compound in a food must be reduced until the guideline is met.

In general, if you consume a variety of foods in moderation, the chances of food additives jeopardizing your health are minimal. Pay attention to your body. If you suspect an intolerance or a sensitivity, consult your physician for further evaluation. Remember that in the short run, you are more likely to suffer either from foodborne illness due to poor food-handling practices that allow viral and bacterial contamination in food, or from the consumption of raw animal foods, than from consuming additives. Excess calories, saturated fat, cholesterol, *trans* fat, salt, and other potential "problem" nutrients in our diets pose the greatest long-term health risk.

Approval for a New Food Additive

Before a new food additive can be added to foods, FDA must approve its use. Besides rigorously testing an additive to establish its safety margins, manufacturers must give FDA information that (1) identifies the new additive, (2) gives its chemical composition, (3) states how it is manufactured, and (4) specifies laboratory methods used to measure its presence in the food supply at the amount of intended use.

Manufacturers must also offer proof that the additive will accomplish its intended purpose in a food, that it is safe, and that it is to be used in no higher amount than needed. Additives cannot be used to hide defective food ingredients, such as rancid oils; to deceive customers; or replace good manufacturing practices. A manufacturer must establish that the ingredient is necessary for producing a specific food product.

MAKING DECISIONS

Processed or Whole Foods?

If you are bewildered or concerned about all the additives in your diet, you can easily avoid most of them by consuming unprocessed whole foods. However, no evidence shows that this will necessarily make you healthier, nor can you avoid all additives, because some are used even on whole foods, such as with pesticides. It amounts to a personal decision. Do you have confidence that FDA and food manufacturers are adequately protecting your health and welfare, or do you want to take more personal control by minimizing your intake of compounds not naturally found in foods?

CONCEPT CHECK

Food additives are used to reduce spoilage from microbial growth, oxygen, metals, and other compounds. Additives are also used to adjust acidity, improve flavor and color, leaven, provide nutritional fortification, thicken, and emulsify food components. Additives are classified as intentional (direct; purposely added to foods), and incidental (indirect; present in foods from environmental contamination or various manufacturing practices). The amount of an additive allowed in a food is limited to one-one-hundredth of the highest amount that has no observable effect when fed to animals. The Delaney Clause allows FDA to limit intentional addition of cancer-causing compounds to food in the United States under its jurisdiction. Also set by law in the United States are the permissible amounts of carcinogens that incidentally enter foods.

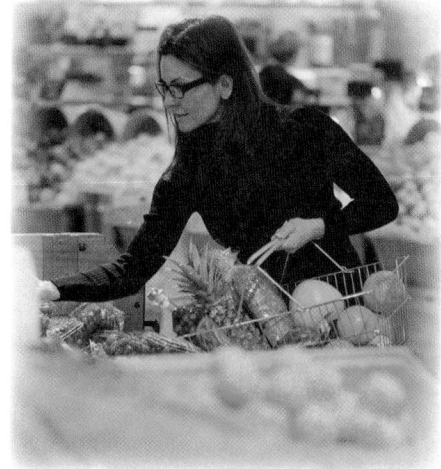

▲ Depending on whether you choose fresh versus processed foods, a diet can be either essentially free of or contain food additives. For most of us, this specific concern regarding food choice is not worth worrying about.

13.5 Substances That Occur Naturally in Foods and Can Cause Illness

Foods contain a variety of naturally occurring substances that can cause illness. Here are some of the more important examples:

- *Safrole*—found in sassafras, mace, and nutmeg; causes cancer when consumed in high doses
- *Solanine*—found in potato shoots and green spots on potato skins; inhibits the action of neurotransmitters
- *Mushroom toxins*—found in some species of mushrooms such as aminita; can cause stomach upset, dizziness, hallucinations, and other neurological symptoms. The more lethal varieties can cause liver and kidney failure, coma, and even death. FDA regulates commercially grown and harvested mushrooms. These are cultivated in concrete buildings or caves. However, there are no systematic controls on individual gatherers harvesting wild species, except in Illinois and Michigan.
- *Avidin*—found in raw egg whites (cooking destroys avidin); binds the vitamin biotin in a way that prevents its absorption, so a biotin deficiency may ultimately develop over the long term
- *Thiaminase*—found in raw fish, clams, and mussels; destroys the vitamin thiamin
- *Tetrodotoxin*—found in puffer fish; causes respiratory paralysis
- *Oxalic acid*—found in spinach, strawberries, sesame seeds, and other foods; binds calcium and iron in the foods, and so limits absorption of these nutrients
- *Herbal teas* containing senna or comfrey—can cause diarrhea and liver damage

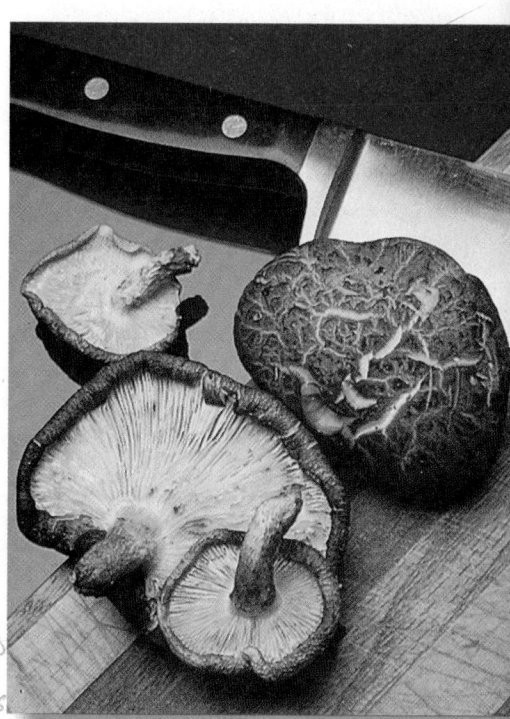

▲ When hunting wild mushrooms, know what you are looking for. Many varieties contain deadly toxins.

People have coexisted for centuries with these naturally occurring substances and have learned to avoid some of them and limit intake of others. They pose little health risk. Farmers know potatoes must be stored in the dark, so that solanine won't be synthesized. Furthermore, we've developed cooking and food-preparation methods to limit the potency of other substances, such as thiaminase. Spices are used in such small amounts that health risks don't result. Nevertheless, it's important to understand that some potentially harmful chemicals in foods occur naturally.

Is Caffeine a Cause for Concern?

Why all the controversy over a cup of coffee? Researchers have spent a great deal of time on the study of caffeine, the substance of greatest concern in the favorite beverage of many of us. So why do caffeine recommendations change from year to year?

Caffeine is a stimulant found as a natural or added ingredient in many beverages and chocolate. On average, we consume 75% of our caffeine intake as coffee, 15% as tea, 10% as soft drinks, and 2% as chocolate (Table 13-7). (For teenagers and young adults this ratio is often relatively higher for soft drinks and lower for coffee.)

Caffeine is not often consumed by itself. With the popularity of trendy coffee shops that serve everything from mocha java to flavored lattes, it is difficult to separate caffeine intake from cream, sugar, alternative sweeteners, and flavorings. So what is the conscientious coffee drinker to think? Let's explore the myths and facts of caffeine intake.

Caffeine does not accumulate in the body and is normally excreted within several hours following consumption. Caffeine can cause anxiety, increased heart rate, insomnia, increased urination (possibly resulting in dehydration), diarrhea, and gastrointestinal upset in high doses. In addition, those already suffering from ulcers may experience irritation due to increased acid production; those who have anxiety

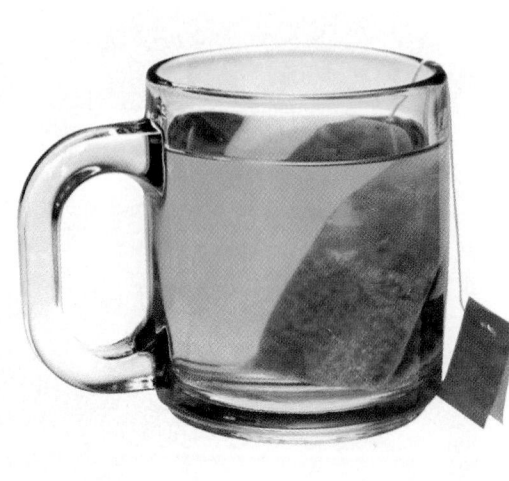

TABLE 13-7 Caffeine Content of Common Sources

Item	Milligrams of Caffeine	
	Typical	Range*
Coffee (8 fl oz)		
Brewed, drip method	85	65–120
Brewed, percolator	75	60–85
Decaffeinated, brewed	3	2–4
Espresso (1 fl oz serving)	40	30–50
Teas (8 fl oz)		
Brewed, Black tea	40	20–90
Brewed, Green tea	20	8–30
Iced	25	9–50
Instant	28	24–31
Some soft drinks (8 fl oz)	24	20–40
"Energy drinks" such as Red Bull (8.3 fl oz)	80	0–80
Cocoa beverage (8 fl oz)	6	3–32
Chocolate milk beverage (8 fl oz)	5	2–7
Milk chocolate (1 oz)	6	1–15
Dark chocolate, semi-sweet (1 oz)	20	5–35
Baker's chocolate (1 oz)	26	26
Chocolate-flavored syrup (1 fl oz)	4	4

*For the coffee and tea products, the range varies due to brewing method, plant variety, brand of product, and so on.

Source: International Food Information Council. *Caffeine and women's health,* August 2002.

or panic attacks may find that caffeine worsens their symptoms; and those prone to heartburn may find that caffeine worsens this symptom because it relaxes sphincter muscles in the esophagus. Some people need little caffeine to feel such effects, and the dosage for children is likely even lower than that for adults.

Withdrawal symptoms are also real. Former coffee drinkers may experience headache, nausea, and depression for a short time after discontinuing use. These symptoms can be expected to peak at 20 to 48 hours following the last intake of caffeine. Symptoms hold true even for those trying to quit as little as one cup of coffee per day. Slow tapering of use over a few days is recommended to avoid these problems.

Are there more serious consequences of consuming caffeine regularly? It has been hypothesized that caffeine consumption can lead to certain types of cancer, such as pancreatic and bladder cancers. The association of caffeine with cancer has not been supported in recent literature. In fact, regular coffee consumption has been linked to a decreased risk of colon cancer.

Negative press has dwindled with regard to a link between cardiovascular disease and moderate coffee consumption. Heavy use does increase blood pressure for a short period of time. Coffee consumption also has been linked to increased LDL-cholesterol and triglycerides in the blood. This association was found to be caused by cafestol and kahweol, two oils in ground coffee. However, filtered and instant coffees do not contain the harmful oils. It is prudent, though, to limit the amount of coffee in general, especially from French coffee presses and from espresso as these beverages are not filtered.

Women are thought to be at higher risk for a variety of deleterious effects with caffeine consumption, including miscarriages, osteoporosis, and birth defects in their offspring. It is true that heavy caffeine use mildly increases the amount of calcium excreted in urine. For this reason, it is important that heavy coffee drinkers check their diets for adequate calcium sources. Some studies do show a higher likelihood for miscarriages in women consuming more than 500 milligrams of caffeine per day (about five 8-ounce cups of coffee). FDA warns women to consume caffeine in moderation (no more than the equivalent of one to two 8-ounce cups of coffee per day).

In contrast to these possibly harmful effects of caffeine consumption, many people are convinced of the benefits of a "cup of joe." Though some women testify to the idea that caffeine improves premenstrual symptoms, no study proves this theory. Some weight-loss drugs previously contained caffeine, under the assumption that it made the drugs more effective. FDA has since banned this use as it was found to be ineffective. Some newer research findings suggest caffeine may reduce the risk of developing headaches, cirrhosis of the liver, some forms of kidney stones, gallbladder stones, some nerve-related diseases, and furthermore, that it aids in blood glucose regulation. You may have heard that caffeine can improve physical performance. This has been shown in highly trained athletes; recall that use of large amounts of caffeine is banned by the NCAA (review Chapter 10). For those below professional status, though, no benefit has been shown. Also keep in mind that coffee will not "sober up" a person who is drunk.

Though the debate over caffeine will likely continue as long as North Americans drink coffee, research does not support many of the concepts previously thought of as fact. These studies are reinforcing the idea of moderation—the equivalent of about two to three 8-ounce cups of coffee per day. A prudent dose of caffeine is 200 to 300 milligrams per day. Review Table 13-7 concerning the caffeine content of typical sources.

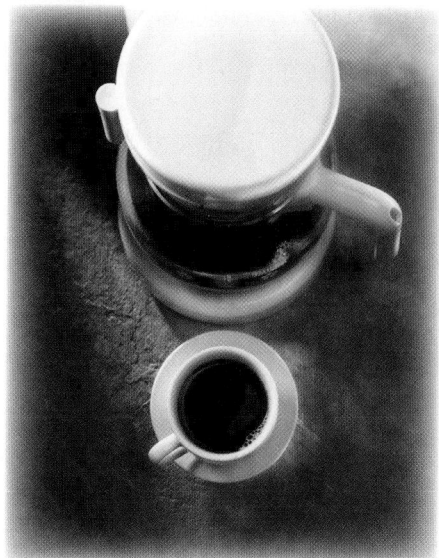

▲ Coffee is a common source of caffeine for many adults.

13.6 Environmental Contaminants in Food

A variety of environmental contaminants can be found in foods. Aside from pesticide residues, other potential contaminants that deserve attention are listed in Table 13-8. To reduce exposure to environmental toxins present in our foods that cause disease, find out which foods pose a risk. In addition, emphasize variety and moderation in food selection. Tips provided in Tables 13-8 and 13-9 also apply to reducing exposure to environmental contaminants.

Genetic alteration of foods such as corn and soybeans has created concern, especially in Europe. FDA considers genetically altered products safe if approval for human use has been granted (see Chapter 12 for details).

TABLE 13-8 Potential Environmental and Other Contaminants in Our Food Supply

Chemical Substance	Sources	Toxic Effects	Preventive Measures
Acrylamide	Fried foods rich in carbohydrate cooked at high temperatures for extended periods, such as French fries and potato chips	Potential neurotoxin and carcinogen. Known carcinogen for laboratory animals; however, studies have not clearly proven the relationship between acrylamide ingestion and the development of cancer in humans.	Limit intake of deep-fat fried foods rich in carbohydrate.
Cadmium	Plants in general if much cadmium is in the soil Clams, shellfish, tobacco smoke Occupational exposure in some cases	Kidney disease Liver disease Prostate cancer (debatable) Bone deformities Lung disease (when inhaled)	Consume a wide variety of foods, including seafood sources.
Dioxin	Trash-burning incinerators Bottom-feeding fish from the Great Lakes Animal fats from animals exposed to such contamination via water or soil	Abnormal reproduction and fetal/infant development Immune suppression Cancer (to date only clearly shown in laboratory animals)	Pay attention to warnings of dioxin risks from local fish; if risk exists, limit intake as suggested on the fishing license. Consume a variety of fish from local waters rather than mostly one specific species.
Lead	Lead-based paint chips and related dust in older homes Occupational exposure (e.g., radiator repair) Lead caps on wine bottles Fruit juices and pickled vegetables stored in galvanized or tin containers or leaded glass Some types of solder used in joining copper pipes (mostly in older homes) Mexican pottery dishes Koo Soo herbal remedies Leaded glass containers (see Further Reading 8.)	Anemia Kidney disease Nervous system damage (tiredness and changes in behavior are symptoms) Reduced learning capacity in childhood (even from mild lead exposure)	Avoid paint chips and related dust in older homes; regular cleaning of these homes is also important (see **www.hud.gov/offices/lead**). Meet iron and calcium needs to reduce lead absorption. Wipe the inside and outside neck of wine bottles before use if the bottle has a lead cap. Store fruit juices and pickled vegetables in glass or plastic or waxed paper containers. Let water run 1 minute or so if off for more than 2 hours, and use only cold water for cooking; do not soften drinking water. Do not store alcoholic beverages in leaded glass containers.
Mercury	Swordfish, shark, king mackerel, and tilefish. Fresh and canned albacore tuna also is a possible source. (In contrast, the more typical light chunk tuna is very low in mercury.)	Reduced fetal/child development and birth defects; toxic to nervous system	Consume these sources no more than once per week, no more than two times per week for albacore tuna. Pregnant women should avoid these species of fish, but some albacore tuna consumption is fine. Two to three fish meals per week is appropriate for pregnant (and nursing) women if different types of fish are eaten.
Polychlorinated biphenyls (PCBs)	Fish from the Great Lakes and Hudson River Valley (e.g., coho salmon) Farmed salmon are a possible source, but less so	Cancer (to date only clearly shown in laboratory animals), as well as a potential for liver, immune, and reproductive disorders	Pay attention to warnings of PCB contamination from local fish; if risk exists, limit intake as suggested on the fishing license or on state advisories. Vary the type of fish eaten during a specific week.
Urethane	Alcoholic beverages such as sherry, bourbon, sake, and fruit brandies	Cancer (to date only clearly shown in laboratory animals)	Avoid generous amounts of typical sources.

CONCEPT CHECK

A general program to minimize exposure to environmental contaminants includes knowing which foods pose greater risks and consuming a wide variety of foods in moderation.

Pesticides in Food

Pesticides used in food production produce both beneficial and unwanted effects (see Further Reading 3). Most health authorities believe that the benefits outweigh the risks. Pesticides help ensure a safe and adequate food supply and help make foods available at reasonable cost. However, there is sentiment nationwide that pesticides pose avoidable health risks. Consumers have come to assume that synthetic is dangerous and organic is safe. Some researchers believe this sentiment is grounded in fear and fueled by unbalanced reports. Other researchers say concern about pesticides is valid and overdue.

Most concern about pesticide residues in food appropriately focuses on chronic rather than acute toxicity because the amounts of residue present, if any, are extremely small. These low concentrations found in foods are not known to produce adverse effects in the short term, although harm has been caused by the high amounts that occasionally result from accidents or misuse. For humans, pesticides pose a danger mainly in their cumulative effects, so their threats to health are difficult to determine. However, growing evidence, including the problems of the contamination of underground water supplies and destruction of wildlife habitats, indicates that North Americans would probably be better off if we could reduce our use of pesticides. Both the U.S. federal government and many farmers are working toward that end. Chapter 12 discussed the lastest use of biotechnology to reduce pesticide use.

What Is a Pesticide?

Federal law defines a pesticide as any substance or mixture of substances intended to prevent, destroy, repel, or mitigate any pest. The built-in toxic properties of pesticides lead to the possibility that other, nontarget organisms, including humans, might also be harmed. The term *pesticide* tends to be used as a generic reference to many types of products, including insecticides, herbicides, fungicides, and rodenticides. A pesticide product may be chemical or bacterial, natural or synthetic. For agriculture, EPA allows about 10,000 pesticides to be used, containing some 300 active ingredients. About 1.2 billion pounds of pesticides are used each year in the United States, much of which is applied to agricultural crops.

Once a pesticide is applied, it can turn up in a number of unintended and unwanted places. It may be carried in the air and dust by wind currents, remain in soil attached to soil particles, be taken up by organisms in the soil, decompose to other compounds, be taken up by plant roots, enter groundwater, or invade aquatic habitats. Each is a route to the food chain; some are more direct than others.

Why Use Pesticides?

In the United States, pests destroy nearly $20 billion of food crops yearly, despite extensive pesticide use. The primary reason for using pesticides is economic—the use of agricultural chemicals increases production and lowers the cost of food, at least in the short run. Many farmers believe that it would be impossible to stay in business without pesticides, which help protect farmers from ruinous losses.

Consumer demands also have changed over the years. At one time, we wouldn't have thought twice about buying an apple with a worm hole; we took it home, cut out

One of the problems with pesticides is that they create new pests because they destroy the predators (spiders, wasps, and beetles) that naturally keep most plantfeeding insect populations in check. The brown plant hopper, which has plagued Indonesian rice fields, was not a serious problem before heavy pesticide use began to kill its predators in the early 1970s. In the United States, such major pests as spider mites and the cotton bollworm were merely nuisances until pesticides decimated their predators.

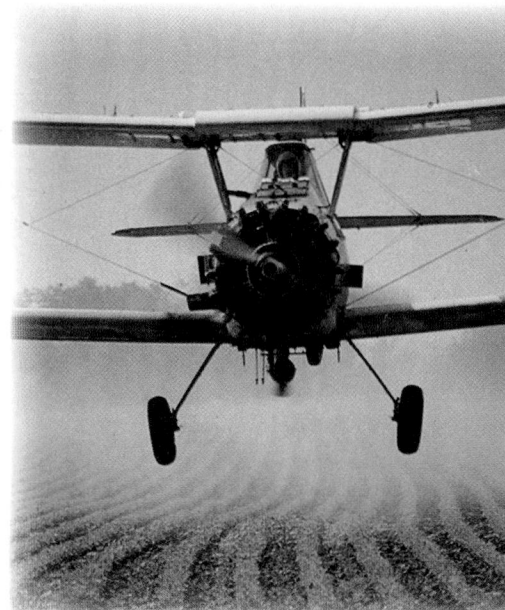

▲ Pesticide use poses a risk-versus-benefit question. Each side has points that deserve to be considered. Rural communities, where exposure is more direct, experience the greatest short-term risk.

the wormy part, and ate the apple. Today, consumers find worm holes less acceptable, so farmers rely more on pesticides to produce cosmetically attractive fruits and vegetables. On the practical side, pesticides can protect against the rotting and decay of fresh fruits and vegetables. This is helpful because our food distribution system doesn't usually permit consumer purchase within hours of harvest. Also, food grown without pesticides can contain naturally occurring organisms that produce carcinogens at concentrations far above current standards for pesticide residues. For example, fungicides help prevent the carcinogen aflatoxin (caused by growth of a fungus) from forming on some crops. Thus, although some pesticides may do little more than improve the appearance of food products, others help keep foods fresher and safer to eat.

Regulation of Pesticides EPA

The responsibility for ensuring that residues of pesticides in foods are below amounts that pose a danger to health is shared by FDA, EPA, and the Food Safety and Inspection Service of USDA in the United States. Table 13-2 listed the roles of various food protection agencies. FDA is responsible for enforcing pesticide tolerances in all foods except meat, poultry, and certain egg products, which are monitored by USDA. A newly proposed pesticide is exhaustively tested, perhaps over 10 years or more, before it is approved for use. EPA must decide that the pesticide causes no unreasonable adverse effects on people and the environment and that benefits of use outweigh the risks of using it. However, there is concern about older chemicals registered before 1970, when less stringent testing conditions were permitted. EPA is now asking chemical companies to retest the old compounds using more rigorous tests. Unfortunately, inadequate funding at EPA has hampered the review of older pesticides. The slow pace of this retesting has angered the critics of pesticide use. When weighing whether to approve or cancel a pesticide, EPA considers how much more it would cost the farmer to use an alternative pesticide or process and whether cancellation would decrease productivity. After determining the dollar cost to the farmer, EPA then looks at costs to processors and consumers. Once a pesticide is approved for use, it must follow the margin of safety provisions required of food additives (see previous section, "Tests of Food Additives for Safety").

How Safe Are Pesticides?

Dangers from exposure to pesticides through food depend on how potent the chemical toxin is, how concentrated it is in the food, how much and how frequently it's eaten, and the consumer's resistance or susceptibility to the substance. Accumulating information links pesticide use to increased cancer rates in farm communities. For rural counties in the United States, the incidence of lymph, genital, brain, and digestive tract cancers increases with higher-than-average pesticide use. Respiratory cancer cases increase with greater insecticide use. In tests using laboratory animals, scientists have found that some of the chemicals present in pesticide residues cause birth defects, sterility, tumors, organ damage, and injury to the central nervous system. Some pesticides persist in the environment for years.

Still, some researchers argue that the cancer risk from pesticide residues is hundreds of times less than the risk from eating such common foods as peanut butter, brown mustard, and basil. Plants manufacture toxic substances to defend themselves against insects, birds, and grazing animals (including humans). When plants are stressed or damaged, they produce even more of these toxins. Because of this, many foods contain naturally occurring chemicals considered toxic, and some are even carcinogenic. Other scientists argue that if natural carcinogens are already in the food supply, then we should reduce the number of added carcinogens whenever possible. In other words, we should do what we can to decrease our overall exposure.

Tests of the Amounts of Pesticides in Foods

FDA tests thousands of raw products each year for pesticide residues. (A pesticide is considered illegal in this case if it is not approved for use on the crop in question or

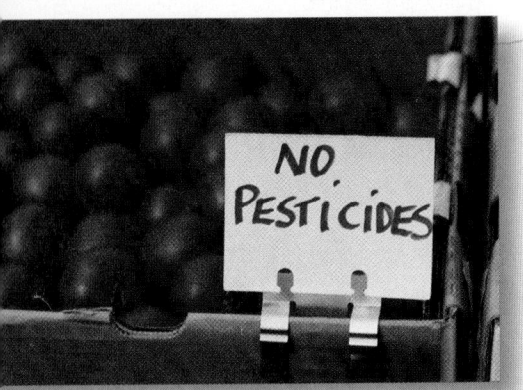

▲ Fruits and vegetables grown without use of pesticides are available and may bear an "organic" label (see Table 2-10 for rules regarding the use of the term "organic" on food labels). These products generally are more expensive than those grown using pesticides. Consumers need to decide if the potential benefits of the products are worth the extra cost.

if the amount used exceeds the allowed tolerance.) The latest FDA studies show no residues in about 60% of samples. Less than 1% of domestic and about 3% of import samples have residues continually over tolerance. These findings continue to support previous FDA studies over the past 10 years that pesticide residues in food are generally well below EPA tolerances, and they confirm the safety of the food supply relative to pesticide residues.

Personal Action

We often take risks in our lives, but we prefer to have a choice in the matter after weighing the pros and cons. With regard to pesticides in food, however, someone else is deciding what is acceptable and what is not. Our only choice is whether to buy or avoid pesticide-containing foods. In reality, it's almost impossible to avoid pesticides entirely, because even organic produce often contains traces of pesticides, probably as the result of cross-contamination from nearby farms.

Short-term studies of the effects of pesticides on laboratory animals cannot precisely pinpoint long-term cancer risks in humans. It should be clearly understood, however, that the presence of minute traces of an environmental chemical in a food does not mean that any adverse effect will result from eating that food.

FDA and other scientific organizations believe that the hazards are comparatively low and in the short run are less dangerous than the hazards of foodborne illness created in our kitchens. We cannot avoid pesticide risks entirely, but we can limit exposure by following some simple advice (Table 13-9).

We can also encourage farmers to use fewer pesticides to reduce exposure to our foods and water supplies, but we'll have to settle for produce that isn't perfect in appearance or that has been grown with the aid of biotechnology (again, see Chapter 12 for details). Are you concerned enough about pesticides on food to change your shopping habits or take more political action?

13.7 Food Production Choices

Agriculture, the production of food and livestock, has supplied humans with food for millennia. At one time, nearly everyone was involved in food production. Only about 1 in 3 people around the globe and far fewer in the United States (less than 1%), is now involved in farming. Today, numerous advances in agricultural sciences are affecting our food supply; of particular note are organic food production and sustainable agriculture.

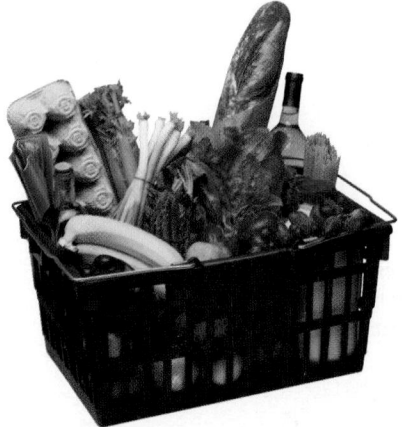

▲ FDA's yearly evaluation of a "market basket" of typical foods shows that pesticide content is minimal in most foods.

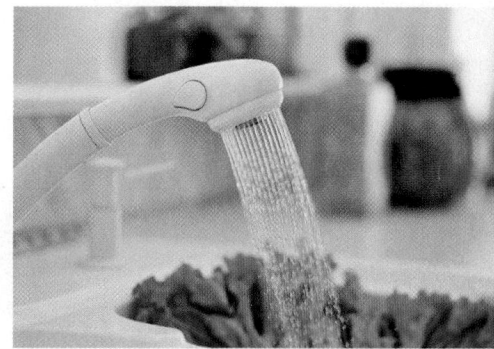

▲ Wash fresh fruits and vegetables under running water to remove bacteria and soil. Special antibacterial washing products are not necessary.

TABLE 13-9 What You Can Do to Reduce Exposure to Pesticides

FDA's sampling and testing show that pesticide residues in foods do not pose a health hazard. Nevertheless, if you want to reduce dietary exposure to pesticides, follow this advice from the Environmental Protection Agency:

- Consume a wide variety of foods, especially regarding fruits, vegetables, and fish.
- Thoroughly rinse and scrub (with a brush if possible) fruits and vegetables. Peel them, if appropriate—although some nutrients will be peeled away.
- Remove the outer leaves of leafy vegetables, such as lettuce and cabbage.
- Residues of some pesticides in animal feed concentrate in the animals' fat, so trim fat from meat, poultry, and fish; remove skin (which contains most of the fat) from poultry and fish; and discard fats and oils in broths and pan drippings.
- When fishing, throw back the big fish—the little ones have had less time to take up and concentrate pesticides and other harmful residues. In addition, pay attention to any warnings by local authorities (and on the fishing license) about the high risk for contamination in specific waters or species of fish.
- Avoid lawns, gardens, and flower beds that have recently been treated with pesticides and herbicides.

Adapted from Food and Drug Administration: Safety first: Protecting America's food supply, *FDA Consumer,* p. 26, November 1988.

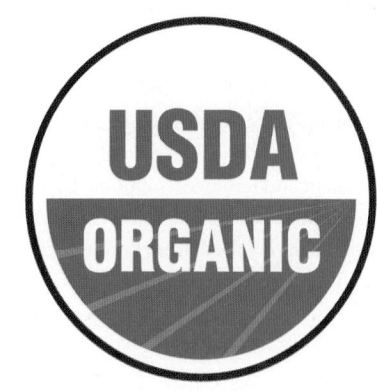

▲ The USDA organic seal identifies organic foods grown on USDA-certified organic farms.

Organic Foods

Organic foods are increasingly available in supermarkets, specialty stores, farmers' markets, and restaurants (see Further Readings 11 and 14). Consumers can select organic fruits, vegetables, grains, dairy products, meats, eggs, and many processed foods, including sauces and condiments, breakfast cereals, cookies, and snack chips. Interest in personal and environmental health has contributed to the increasing availability and sales of organic foods. According to the Organic Trade Association, U.S. sales of organic foods reached $26.7 billion by the end of 2010. This was a 7.7% increase over 2009 sales, despite tough economic times. Despite this rapid growth, only 4% of foods sold are organic. Organic foods, because they often cost more to grow and produce, are typically more expensive than comparable conventional foods.

The term **organic** refers to the way agricultural products are produced. Organic production relies on farming practices such as **biological pest management**, composting, manure applications, and crop rotation to maintain healthy soil, water, crops, and animals. Synthetic pesticides, fertilizers, and hormones; antibiotics; sewage sludge (used as fertilizer); genetic engineering; and irradiation are not permitted in the production of organic foods. Additionally, organic meat, poultry, eggs, and dairy products must come from animals allowed to graze outdoors and are fed only organic feed.

The Organic Foods Production Act of 1990 established standards for the production of foods that bear the USDA organic seal. Foods labeled and marketed as organic must be grown on farms that are certified by the USDA as following all of the rules established in the 1990 act. Foods made from multiple ingredients (e.g., breakfast cereal) labeled as organic must have at least 95% of their ingredients (by weight) meet organic standards. The term "made with organic" can be used if at least 70% of the ingredients are organic. Small organic producers and farmers with sales less than $5000 per year are exempt from the certification regulation. Some farmers use organic production methods but choose not to be USDA certified. Their foods cannot be labeled as organic, but many of these farmers market and sell to those seeking organic foods.

The organic food market received a boost in 2009 when USDA offered $50 million in new funding to encourage greater production of organic food in the United States. The Organic Trade Association (www.ota.com/index.html) believes that this funding will further encourage farmers to use organic practices and help increase the U.S. production of organic food to meet growing consumer demand. With tough economic times, consumers have used various strategies in continuing to buy organic products. Because most stores now offer organic products, consumers have the opportunity to shop around. Increased availability and use of coupons, the proliferation of private label and store brands, and better value products offered by major organic brands all have contributed to increased sales.

Organic Foods and Health Consumers may choose to eat organic foods to reduce their pesticide intake, to protect the environment, and to improve the nutritional quality of their diets. Those who consume organic produce do ingest lesser amounts of pesticides (only 1 in 4 organically grown fruits and vegetables contains pesticides and in lower amounts than conventional produce), but it's still not known whether or how this affects the health of most consumers. However, organic foods may be a wise choice for young children because pesticide residues may pose a greater risk to them. Consumers also may opt for organic foods to encourage environmentally friendly **sustainable agriculture** practices.

Most studies do not show that organic foods have higher amounts of vitamins and minerals (see Further Reading 5). However, researchers have found that, in some cases, organic fruits and vegetables contain more vitamin C and antioxidants that help protect cells against damage. At this point, it's not possible to recommend organic foods over conventional foods based on nutrient content—both can meet nutritional needs. A healthy dose of common sense also is important—an "organic" label does not change a less healthy food into a more healthy food. Organic potato chips have the same calorie and fat content as conventional potato chips.

▲ Organic fruits and vegetables experienced the highest growth in food sales at 11.8% over 2009 sales and representing over 11% of all fruit and vegetable sales.

biological pest management Control of agricultural pests by using natural predators, parasites, or pathogens. For example, ladybugs can be used to control an aphid infestation.

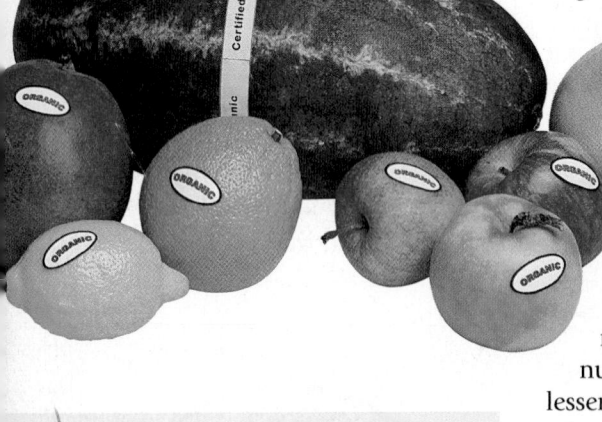

sustainable agriculture Agricultural system that provides a secure living for farm families; maintains the natural environment and resources; supports the rural community; and offers respect and fair treatment to all involved, from farm workers to consumers to the animals raised for food.

One concern raised about organic foods is that food safety may be jeopardized because animal manures used for fertilizers might cause more pathogen contamination of food. The recent outbreaks of foodborne illness linked to organically grown sprouts in Europe confirm that an organic label does not guarantee good health. However, research does not show that certified organic food has higher contamination with bacterial pathogens. Consumers should wash or scrub all produce—organic as well as conventional—under running water.

The term "natural" is not regulated. Products labeled as "natural" are generally those derived from natural ingredients, such as a plant source, which retain their natural properties in the finished product. Meat or poultry labeled "natural" must be minimally processed, and contain no artificial flavoring, coloring, chemical preservative, or other artificial or synthetic ingredient. No one is really checking these products, and there is some debate over what constitutes "minimally processed." Although all organic products fit this definition of natural, not all natural products are necessarily organic.

Sustainable Agriculture

Conventional agriculture focuses on maximizing production through the use of large acreages, powerful machines, chemicals to control pests, and petroleum-based fertilizers to boost growth. In contrast, sustainable agriculture is an integrated system of plant and animal production that will, over the long-term, satisfy human food needs, enhance environmental quality, efficiently use nonrenewable resources, sustain the economic viability of farm operations, and enhance the quality of life for farmers and society as a whole. A culture of sustainability has emerged, including a clear trend for sustainable food choices manufactured in an environmentally responsible way. The food industry has responded with a move toward "green" initiatives that should be sustainable for the long-term. A new demographic term, LOHAS (Lifestyle of Health and Sustainability), describes a growing demographic group focused on sustainable living. An increasing number of today's college students are joining this market segment and developing behaviors associated with social responsibility. These consumers are driving changes in many areas, including the food industry. Slow Food Nation is an example of a non-profit group dedicated to creating a framework for a deeper environmental connection to our food and aiming to inspire and empower Americans to build a food system that is sustainable, healthy, and delicious.

Locally Grown Foods

With people everywhere more interested in the origins of their food, more grocery store shelves are devoted to "locally grown" products. Consumers are demanding increased transparency with the food supply, and local food helps answer questions about where food comes from and how it was grown. Retailers are using the "locally grown" label to respond to consumer desires for fresh, safe products that also support small, local farmers and help the environment. Local products provide fresher options, do not have the added costs of long transportation, and thus, use less fossil fuel. Foodservice establishments are giving greater emphasis to local producers, focusing on where food was grown and how it was handled.

Farmers' markets are the most obvious way that consumers have access to locally grown, farm-fresh produce. Farmers' markets are also an integral part of the urban/farm linkage and continue to gain popularity. In 2010 there were 6132 farmers' markets operating throughout the United States, which was a 16% increase from 2009.

The interest in "local" foods has become such a phenomenon that the term "locavore" was the 2007 Word of the Year in the New Oxford American Dictionary. **Locavore** is defined as someone who eats food grown or produced locally or within a certain radius such as 50, 100, or 150 miles. The locavore movement has gained prominence due to food-safety concerns by consumers and the search for local, sustainable foods. It encourages consumers to buy from farmers' markets or even to produce their own food, with the argument that fresh, local products are more nutritious and taste better.

CRITICAL THINKING

Stephanie, a college sophomore, is adamant about eating only organic foods. She frequently states that conventionally grown and processed foods are unhealthy, full of harmful chemicals, and almost nutrient-free. Knowing that you are studying nutrition, Stephanie discusses her beliefs with you and asks for your opinion. What are some ways you might respond to her?

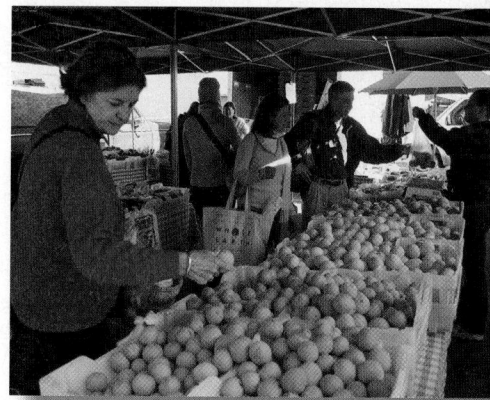

▲ The locavore movement is based on the assumption that local products are more nutritious and taste better and encourages consumers to buy from farmers' markets or even to produce their own food.

locavore Someone who eats food grown or produced locally or within a certain radius such as 50, 100, or 500 miles.

NEWSWORTHY
NUTRITION

German organic sprouts cause deadly *E. coli* outbreak

The world's deadliest outbreak of *Escherichia coli* occurred during the summer of 2011. The outbreak occurred mainly in Germany and involved a rare enterohemorrhagic strain of *E. coli* known as O104:H4. In June 2011, 3332 persons had been infected, more than 600 were in intensive care, and the death toll from the outbreak had reached 36. Several hundred also contracted its potentially fatal kidney complication, known as hemolytic uremic syndrome. The European Centre for Disease Prevention and Control concluded that the *E. coli* infection was caused by tainted vegetable sprouts from a small, rather traditional organic sprout farm. The sprout seeds were mostly imported from overseas and the *E. coli* bacteria were antibiotic resistant. Experts say these types of outbreaks are becoming more common due to large-scale industrial farming and the widespread use of antibiotics.

Source: Dempsey J, Neuman W: Deadly *E. coli* outbreak linked to German sprouts. *New York Times*, June 5, 2011.

connect NUTRITION   **Check out the Connect site**
www.mcgrawhillconnect.com
to further explore *E. coli*.

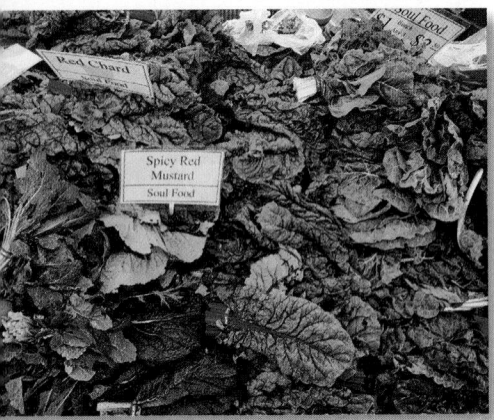

▲ Farmers participating in community supported agriculture (CSA) offer a share of foods from each growing season, to individuals, families or companies who support the CSA financially and/or by working for the CSA.

There is no evidence, however, that locally grown products are safer. Although many small producers have good food-safety practices, they often lack the expensive food-safety audits more common among big producers. Food-safety auditors determine such things as whether or not there is evidence of insects on produce and whether or not producers have enough bathrooms for workers. In addition, undetected foodborne illness outbreaks are more likely with "local" products delivered in small quantities and sold in a small area. Local products are not necessarily pesticide-free and may not be cheaper, given that smaller growers lack the economic advantages of bigger growers. Read about the outbreak of foodborne illness linked to a local organic farm in Newsworthy Nutrition.

Unlike organic products, there are no regulations specifying the meaning of "locally grown." Whole Foods Market, Inc. is the biggest retailer of natural and organic food and probably the best-known for buying and selling locally grown produce. Whole Foods considers local to be anything produced within seven hours of one of its stores, with most local producers within 200 miles of a store. Wal-Mart, the world's largest retailer, has also become a large buyer of locally grown fruits and vegetables and considers anything local if it is grown in the same state as it is sold. Searchable databases and mapping resources such as MarketMaker (http://national.marketmaker.uiuc.edu/) are now available to connect growers with buyers, restaurants with distributors, and consumers with local farmers' markets. These tools make it easier for people to find and sell locally grown foods.

Community Supported Agriculture

Consumers are not only taking comfort in knowing where their food comes from, but are also starting to have interest in community connections with local/regional farmers. Stemming from the interest in locally grown food, there is growing national support for local food collaboratives and community supported agriculture. Community Supported Agriculture programs (CSA) involve a partnership between local food producers and local consumers. During each growing season, CSA farmers offer a share of foods to individuals, families, or companies who have pledged support to the CSA either financially and/or by working for the CSA.

Another example of a farm-community partnership is the National Farm to School Program (www.farmtoschool.org/), a nonprofit effort to connect farmers with nearby school cafeterias. Between 1997 and 2011, this program grew from only six local programs to 2352 programs in 48 states resulting in 9756 schools incorporating the local bounty into their menus. Administrators of the program have found that if kids can meet the farmer who actually grew the food, they are much more likely to eat it.

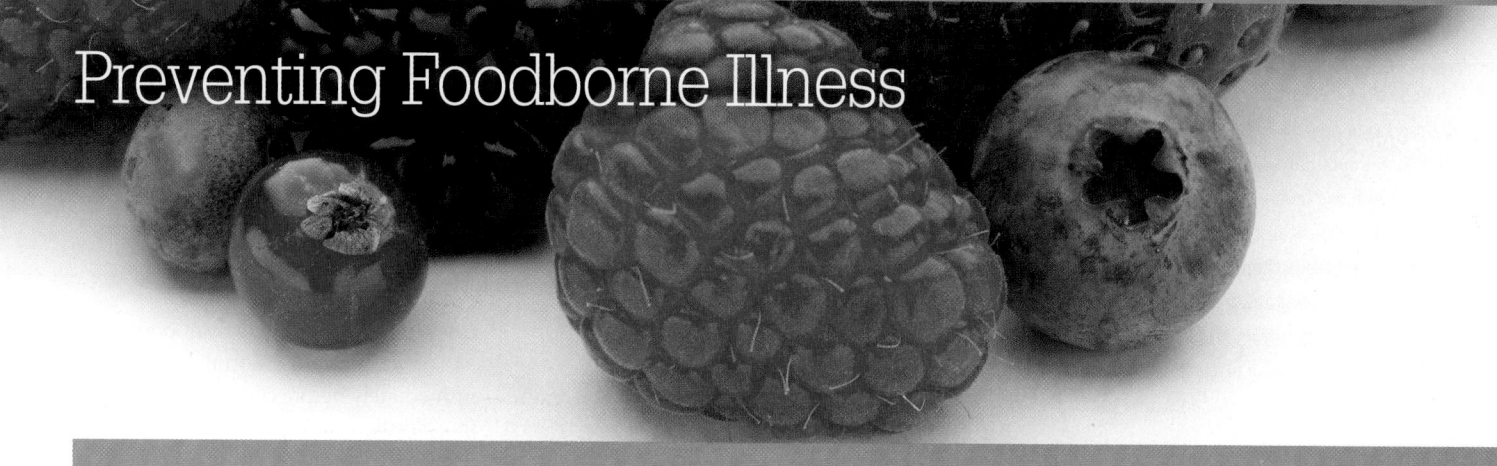

Preventing Foodborne Illness

General Rules for Preventing Foodborne Illness

You can greatly reduce the risk of foodborne illness by following some important rules (see Further Reading 7). It's a long list, because many risky habits need to be addressed.

Purchasing Food

- When shopping, select frozen foods and perishable foods, such as meat, poultry, or fish, last. Always have these products put in separate plastic bags, so that drippings don't contaminate other foods in the shopping cart. Don't let groceries sit in a warm car; this allows bacteria to grow. Get the perishable foods such as meat and egg and dairy products home and promptly refrigerate or freeze them.
- Don't buy or use food from damaged containers that leak, bulge, or are severely dented or from jars that are cracked or have loose or bulging lids. Don't taste or use food that has a foul odor or spurts liquid when the can is opened; the deadly *Clostridium botulinum* toxin may be present.
- Purchase only pasteurized milk and cheese (check the label). This is especially important for pregnant women because highly toxic bacteria and viruses that can harm the fetus thrive in unpasteurized milk.
- Purchase only the amount of produce needed for a week's time. The longer you keep fruits and vegetables, the more time is available for bacteria to grow.
- When purchasing precut produce or salads, avoid those that look slimy,

brownish, or dry; these are signs of improper holding temperatures.
- Observe sell-by and expiration dates on food labels.

Preparing Food

- Thoroughly wash your hands for 20 seconds with hot, soapy water before and after handling food. This practice is especially important when handling raw meat, fish, poultry, and eggs, after using the bathroom, after playing with pets, or after changing diapers (see Further Reading 2).
- Make sure counters, cutting boards, dishes, and other equipment are thoroughly sanitized and rinsed before use. Be especially careful to use hot, soapy water to wash surfaces and equipment that have come in contact with raw meat, fish, poultry, and eggs as soon as possible to remove *Salmonella* bacteria that may be present. Otherwise, bacteria on the surfaces will infect the next foods that come in contact with the surface, a process called cross-contamination. In addition, replace sponges and wash kitchen towels frequently. (Microwaving sponges for 30 to 60 seconds also helps rid them of live bacteria.)
- If possible, cut foods to be eaten raw on a clean cutting board reserved for that purpose. Then clean this cutting board using hot, soapy water. If the same board must be used for both meat and other foods, cut any potentially contaminated items, such as meat, last. After cutting the meat, wash the cutting board thoroughly.

FDA recommends cutting boards with unmarred surfaces made of easy-

to-clean, non-porous materials, such as plastic, marble, or glass. If you prefer a wooden board, make sure it is made of a nonabsorbent hardwood, such as oak or maple, and has no obvious seams or cracks. Then reserve it for a specific purpose; for example, set it aside for cutting raw meat and poultry. Keep a separate wooden cutting board for chopping produce and slicing bread to prevent these products from picking up bacteria from raw meat. Many foods are served raw, so any bacteria clinging to them are not destroyed.

Furthermore, FDA recommends that all cutting boards be replaced when they become streaked with hard-to-clean grooves or cuts, which may harbor bacteria. In addition, cutting boards should be sanitized once a week in a dilute bleach solution. Flood the board with the solution, let it sit a few minutes, then rinse thoroughly.

- When thawing foods, do so in the refrigerator, under cold potable running water, or in a microwave oven. Also, cook foods immediately after thawing under cold water or in the microwave. Never let frozen foods thaw unrefrigerated all day or night. Also, marinate food in the refrigerator.
- Avoid coughing or sneezing over foods, even when you're healthy. Cover cuts on hands with a sterile bandage. This helps stop *Staphylococcus* from entering food.
- Carefully wash fresh fruit and vegetables under running water to remove dirt and bacteria clinging to the surface, using a vegetable brush if the skin is to

▶ The World Health Organization's Golden Rules for Safe Food Preparation

1. Choose foods processed for safety.
2. Cook food thoroughly.
3. Eat cooked foods immediately.
4. Store cooked foods carefully.
5. Reheat cooked foods thoroughly.
6. Avoid contact between raw and cooked foods.
7. Wash hands repeatedly.
8. Keep all kitchen surfaces meticulously clean.
9. Protect foods from insects, rodents, and other animals.
10. Use pure water.

The USDA simplified these rules into four actions as a part of their Fight BAC! Program (check out www.fightbac.org):

1. Clean. Wash hands and surfaces often.
2. Separate. Don't cross-contaminate.
3. Cook. Cook to proper temperatures.
4. Chill. Refrigerate promptly.

The 2010 Dietary Guidelines for Americans also stress the importance of these four actions.

be eaten. People have become ill from *Salmonella* introduced from melons used in making a fruit salad and from oranges used for fresh-squeezed orange juice. The bacteria were on the outside of the melons and oranges (see Further Reading 10).

• Completely remove moldy portions of food or don't eat the food. *When in doubt, throw the food out.* Mold growth is prevented by properly storing food at cold temperatures and using the food promptly.

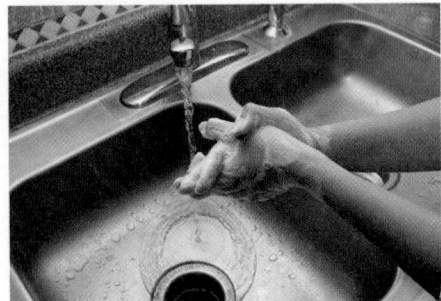

▲ Washing hands thoroughly (for at least 20 to 30 seconds) with hot water and soap should be the first step in food preparation. The 4 "F's" of food contamination are fingers, foods, feces, and flies. Handwashing especially combats the finger and fecal routes.

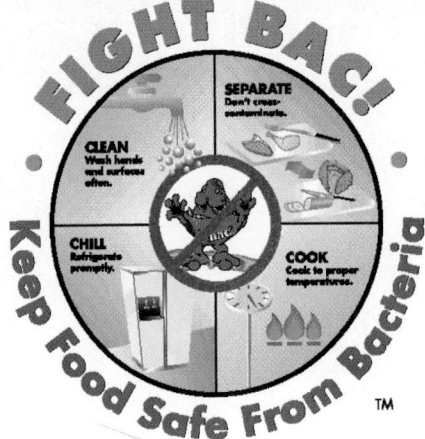

▲ Food safety logo of USDA.

• Use refrigerated ground meat and patties in 1 to 2 days and frozen meat and patties within 3 to 4 months. The 6-month interval mentioned in the comic at the beginning of this chapter is too long a time to be safe.

Cooking Food

• Cook food thoroughly using a bimetallic thermometer to check for doneness, especially for fresh beef and fish (145°F [63°C]), pork (160°F [71°C]), and poultry (165°F [74°C]) (Fig. 13-2). Eggs should be cooked until the yolk and white are hard. Alfalfa sprouts and other types of sprouts should be cooked until they are steaming. Cooking is by far the most reliable way to destroy foodborne viruses and bacteria, such as Norovirus and toxic strains of *E. coli*. Freezing only halts viral and bacterial growth. FDA does not recommend that eggs be prepared sunny-side-up.

As noted, many restaurants now include an advisory on menus stating that an increased risk of foodborne illness is associated with eating undercooked eggs. As long as restaurants provide this warning on their menus, however, they are allowed to cook eggs to any temperature requested by the consumer. FDA warns us not to consume homemade ice cream, eggnog, and mayonnaise if made with unpasteurized, raw eggs because of the risk of *Salmonella* foodborne illness. It is safer to use eggs or egg products that have been pasteurized, which kills *Salmonella* bacteria. Overall, a good general precaution is to eat no raw animal products.

USDA answers questions about the safe use of animal products (800-535-4555, 10 A.M. to 4 P.M. weekdays, Eastern time).

Seafood also poses a risk of foodborne illness, especially oysters. Properly cooked seafood should flake easily and/or be opaque or dull and firm. If it's translucent or shiny, it's not done.

• Cook stuffing separately from poultry (or wash poultry thoroughly, stuff immediately before cooking, and then transfer the stuffing to a clean bowl immediately after cooking). Make sure the stuffing reaches 165°F (74°C). *Salmonella* is the major concern with poultry.

• Once a food is cooked, consume it right away, or cool it to 40°F (4°C) within 2 hours. If it is not to be eaten immediately, in hot weather (80°F and above) make sure this cooling is done within 1 hour. Do this by separating the food into as many shallow pans as needed to provide a large surface area for cooling. Be careful not to recontaminate cooked food by contact with raw meat or juices from hands, cutting boards, dirty utensils, or in other ways.

• Serve meat, poultry, and fish on a clean plate—never the same plate used to hold the raw product. For example, when grilling hamburgers, don't put cooked items on the same plate used to carry the raw product out to the grill.

• For outdoor cooking, cook food completely at the picnic site, with no partial cooking in advance.

Storing and Reheating Cooked Food

• Keep foods out of the "danger zone" (Fig.13-1) by keeping hot foods hot and cold foods cold. Hold food below 40°F (4°C) or above 140°F (60°C). Foodborne microorganisms thrive in more moderate temperatures (60°F to 110°F [16°C to 43°C]). Some microorganisms can even grow in the refrigerator. Again, don't leave cooked or refrigerated foods, such as meats and salads, at room temperature for more than 2 hours (or 1 hour in hot weather) because that gives microorganisms an opportunity to grow. Store dry food at 60°F to 70°F (16°C to 21°C).

• Reheat leftovers to 165°F (74°C); reheat gravy to a rolling boil to kill *Clostridium*

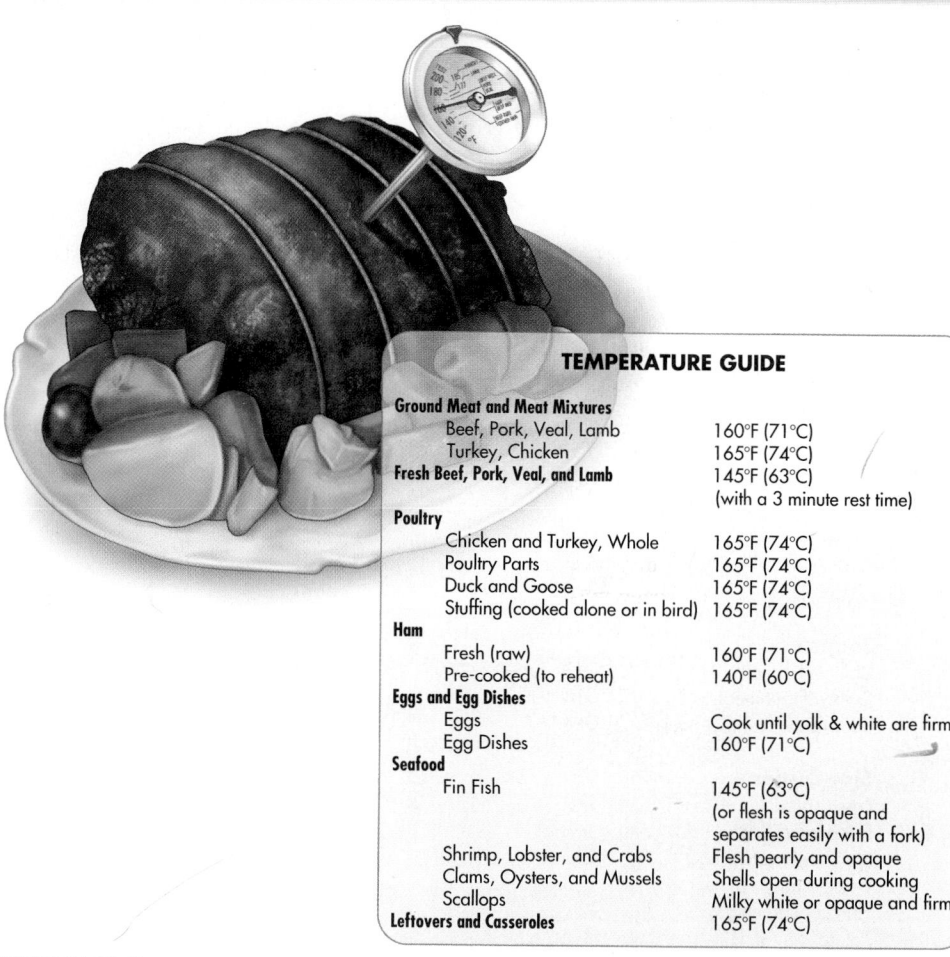

TEMPERATURE GUIDE

Ground Meat and Meat Mixtures	
Beef, Pork, Veal, Lamb	160°F (71°C)
Turkey, Chicken	165°F (74°C)
Fresh Beef, Pork, Veal, and Lamb	145°F (63°C)
	(with a 3 minute rest time)
Poultry	
Chicken and Turkey, Whole	165°F (74°C)
Poultry Parts	165°F (74°C)
Duck and Goose	165°F (74°C)
Stuffing (cooked alone or in bird)	165°F (74°C)
Ham	
Fresh (raw)	160°F (71°C)
Pre-cooked (to reheat)	140°F (60°C)
Eggs and Egg Dishes	
Eggs	Cook until yolk & white are firm
Egg Dishes	160°F (71°C)
Seafood	
Fin Fish	145°F (63°C)
	(or flesh is opaque and separates easily with a fork)
Shrimp, Lobster, and Crabs	Flesh pearly and opaque
Clams, Oysters, and Mussels	Shells open during cooking
Scallops	Milky white or opaque and firm
Leftovers and Casseroles	165°F (74°C)

▲ Sushi, like all raw fish or meat dishes, is a high-risk food. For maximum protection from food-borne illness, animal foods should be cooked thoroughly before eating.

FIGURE 13-2 ▶ Minimum internal temperatures when cooking or reheating foods.

Source: "Safe Cooking Temperatures as Measured with a Food Thermometer." (FDA, 2011)

perfringens bacteria, which may be present. Merely reheating to a good eating temperature isn't sufficient to kill harmful bacteria.

- Store peeled or cut-up produce, such as melon balls, in the refrigerator.
- Make sure the refrigerator stays below 40°F (4°C). Either use a refrigerator thermometer or keep it as cold as possible without freezing milk and lettuce.
- Keep leftovers in the refrigerator only for the recommended length of time (Fig. 13-3).

Cross-contamination is not only a threat during food preparation; it can also become a problem during food storage. Make sure all foods, including leftovers, are contained and covered in the refrigerator to prevent drippings from uncooked and potentially hazardous foods from tainting other foods. It is a good idea to store foods likely to pose risk of foodborne illness on lower shelves of the refrigerator, beneath other foods to be eaten raw.

MAKING DECISIONS

Raw Fish

Raw fish dishes, such as sushi, can be safe for most people to eat if they are made with very fresh fish that has been commercially frozen and then thawed. The freezing is important to eliminate potential health risks from parasites. FDA recommends that the fish be frozen to an internal temperature of −10°F for 7 days. If you choose to eat uncooked fish, purchase the fish from reputable establishments that have high standards for quality and sanitation. If you are at high risk for foodborne illness, it is wise to avoid raw fish products.

FIGURE 13-3 ▶ Length of time to keep leftovers in the refrigerator.

▶ **Current Safe Handling Instructions Issued by USDA for Labeling Meat and Poultry Products**

This product was prepared from inspected and passed meat and/or poultry. Some food products may contain bacteria that could cause illness if the product is mishandled or cooked improperly. For your protection, follow these handling instructions.

Keep refrigerated or frozen.

Thaw in refrigerator or microwave.

Keep raw meat and poultry separate from other foods.

Wash working surfaces (including cutting boards), utensils, and hands after touching raw meat or poultry.

Cook thoroughly.

Keep hot foods hot. Refrigerate leftovers immediately or discard.

▶ **Safe Handling Instructions for Eggs**

To prevent illness from bacteria: keep eggs refrigerated, cook eggs until yolks are firm, and cook foods containing eggs thoroughly.

▶ To reduce the risk of bacteria surviving during microwave cooking,

- Cover food with glass or ceramic when possible to decrease evaporation and heat the surface.

- Stir and rotate food at least once or twice for even cooking. Then, allow microwaved food to stand, covered, after heating is completed to help cook the exterior and equalize the temperature throughout.

- Use the oven temperature probe or a meat thermometer to check that food is done. Insert it at several spots.

- If thawing meat in the microwave, use the oven's defrost setting. Ice crystals in frozen foods are not heated well by the microwave oven and can create cold spots, which later cook more slowly.

▶ Regularly cleaning surfaces and equipment with a dilute bleach solution (1:10) is helpful in reducing the risk of cross-contamination of foods.

When in doubt, throw it out!

Food	Refrigerator Storage Time (days)
Meats	
Cooked ground beef/turkey	3–4
Deli meat	2–3
Cooked pork	3–4
Cooked poultry	3–4
Cooked beef, bison, lamb	3–4
Seafood	
Raw (e.g. sushi/sashimi)	Must consume on day of purchase
Cooked	2
Other Entrees	
Pizza	1–2
Pasta/rice	1–2
Casserole	3–4
Soups and Chili	
Chili with meat	2–3
Chili without meat	3–4
Soup/stew	3–4
Side Dishes	
Fresh salad	1–2
Fresh vegetables	1–2
Pasta or potato salad	2–3
Deviled egg	2–3
Hard boiled egg	7
Potato (any style)	3–4
Cooked vegetables	3–4
Dessert	
Cream pie	2–3
Fruit pie	2–3
Pastries	7
Cake	7
Cheesecake	7

CONCEPT CHECK

Thoroughly cook all meat and poultry to reduce the risk of foodborne illness from *E. coli*, and *Salmonella*. In addition, always separate raw meats and poultry products from cooked foods. To prevent foodborne intoxication from *Staphylococcus* organisms, cover cuts on hands and avoid sneezing on foods. To avoid intoxication from *Clostridium perfringens*, rapidly cool leftover foods and thoroughly reheat them. To avoid intoxication from *Clostridium botulinum*, carefully examine canned foods. Overall, don't allow cooked food to stand for more than 1 to 2 hours at room temperature. For other causes of foodborne illness, precautions already mentioned generally apply as well. In addition, thoroughly cook fish and other seafood; consume only pasteurized dairy products; wash all fruits and vegetables; and thoroughly wash your hands with soap and water before and after preparing food and after using the bathroom.

Case Study Preventing Foodborne Illness at Gatherings

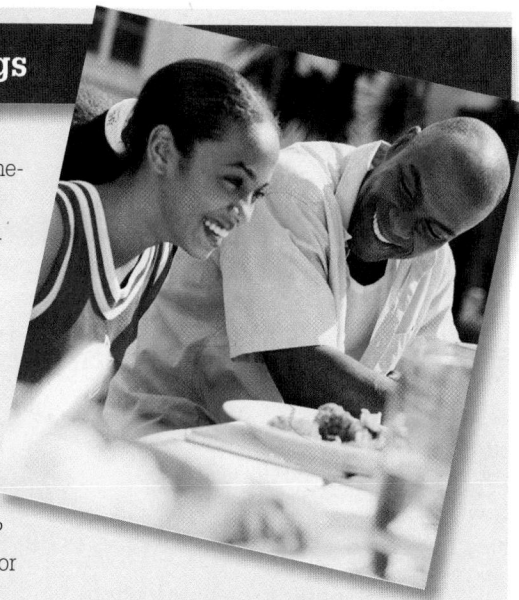

Nicole attended a gathering of her co-workers on a warm Saturday in July. The theme of the party was international dining. Nicole and her husband were asked to bring an Argentinian dish, potato and beef empanadas. They followed the recipe and cooking time carefully, removing the dish from the oven at 1 P.M. and keeping it warm by wrapping the pan in a towel. They traveled in their car to the party and set the dish out on the buffet table at 3 P.M. Dinner was to be served at 4 P.M. However, the guests were enjoying themselves so much lounging around the host's pool and drinking ginger beer (also on the menu) that no one began to eat until 6 P.M. Nicole made sure she sampled the empanadas that she and her husband made, while her husband did not. She also had some salad, garlic bread, and a sweet dessert made with coconut.

The couple returned home at 11 P.M. and went to bed. At about 2 A.M., Nicole knew something was wrong. She had severe abdominal pain and had to make a dash to the bathroom. She spent most of the next 3 hours in the bathroom with severe diarrhea. By dawn, the diarrhea subsided and she started to feel better. After a few cups of tea and a light breakfast, she was feeling like herself by noon.

Answer the following questions, and check your responses in Appendix A.

1. Based on her symptoms, what type of foodborne illness did Nicole contract?
2. Why is the beef the most likely vehicle for this type of foodborne illness?
3. Why is consuming food at large gatherings risky?
4. What precautions for avoiding foodborne illness were ignored by Nicole and the rest of the people at the party?
5. How could this scenario be rewritten to substantially reduce the risk of foodborne illness?

Summary (Numbers refer to numbered sections in the chapter.)

13.1, 13.3 Viruses, bacteria, and other microorganisms in food pose the greatest risk for foodborne illness. Major causes of foodborne illness are Norovirus and the bacteria *Campylobacter jejuni*, *Salmonella*, *Staphylococcus aureus*, and *Clostridium perfringens*. In addition, such bacteria as *Clostridium botulinum*, *Listeria monocytogenes*, and *Escherichia coli* have been found to cause illness.

13.2 In the past, salt, sugar, smoke, fermentation, and drying were used to protect against foodborne illness. Today, careful cooking, pasteurization, keeping hot foods hot and cold foods cold, and thorough handwashing provide additional insurance.

13.4 Food additives are used primarily to extend shelf life by preventing microbial growth and the destruction of food components by oxygen, metals, and other substances. Food additives are classified as those intentionally added to foods and those that incidentally appear in foods. An intentional additive is limited to no more

than one-one-hundredth of the greatest amount that causes no observed symptoms in animals. Under its jurisdiction in the United States, the Delaney Clause allows FDA to ban the use of any intentional food additive that causes cancer.

Antioxidants, such as BHA, BHT, vitamins E and C, and sulfites, prevent oxygen and enzyme destruction of food products. Emulsifiers suspend fat in water, improving the uniformity, smoothness, and body of foods such as ice cream. Common preservatives include salt, sodium benzoate, and sorbic acid, which prevent bacterial growth. Sequestrants bind metals and thus prevent spoilage of food from metal contamination. Various natural products such as natural flavors, sugar, and corn syrup, as well as artificial flavors and sweeteners, such as aspartame, improve the flavor of food.

13.5 Toxic substances occur naturally in a variety of foods, such as green potatoes, raw fish, mushrooms, and raw egg whites. Cooking foods limits their toxic effects in

some cases; others are best to avoid altogether, such as toxic mushroom species and the green parts of potatoes.

13.6 A variety of environmental contaminants and pesticide residues can be found in foods. It is helpful to know which foods pose the greatest risks and act accordingly to reduce exposure, such as washing fruits and vegetables before use.

13.7 Conventional agriculture focuses on maximizing production through the use of large farms, machines, and chemicals. A more recent culture of sustainability demands food choices produced in an environmentally responsible way. U.S. sales of organic foods have grown dramatically in recent years, despite tough economic times. Consumers are more interested in the origins of their food, resulting in grocery stores providing more "locally grown" products. Although there is no evidence that locally grown products are safer, local products provide fresher options and do not have the added transportation costs. Consumers also have an interest in connecting with local/regional farmers, resulting in growing national support for community-supported agriculture.

N&YH To protect against viruses and bacteria, cook susceptible foods thoroughly. In addition, cover cuts on the hands, do not sneeze or cough on foods, avoid contact between raw meat or poultry products and other food products, rapidly cool and thoroughly reheat leftovers, and use pasteurized dairy products. Overall, be careful when foods are in the "danger zone" (40°F to 140°F).

Cross-contamination commonly causes foodborne illness. It occurs particularly when bacteria on raw animal products contact foods that can support bacterial growth. Because of the risk of cross-contamination, no perishable food should be kept in the "danger zone" for more than 1 to 2 hours (depending on the environmental temperature), especially if it may have come in contact with raw animal products.

Check Your Knowledge (Answers to the following questions are below.)

1. Nitrite prevents the growth of *Canned Food*
   a. *Clostridium botulinum.*
   b. *Escherichia coli.*
   c. *Staphylococcus aureus.*
   d. yeasts.

2. Substances used to preserve foods by lowering the pH are
   a. smoke and irradiation.
   b. baking powder and soda.
   c. salt and sugar.
   d. vinegar and citric acid.

3. Food additives widely used for many years without apparent ill effects are on the _____ list.
   a. FDA
   b. GRAS
   c. USDA
   d. Delaney

4. The foodborne illness organism often associated with small cuts and boils is
   a. *Listeria.*
   b. *Staphylococcus.*
   c. *C. botulinum.*
   d. *Salmonella.*

5. Salmonella bacteria are usually spread via
   a. raw meats, poultry, and eggs.
   b. pickled vegetables.
   c. home-canned vegetables.
   d. raw vegetables.

6. It is unwise to thaw meats or poultry *- warm*
   a. in a microwave oven.
   b. in the refrigerator.
   c. under cool running water.
   d. at room temperature.

7. Milk that can remain on supermarket shelves, free of microbial growth, for many years has been processed by which of the following methods?
   a. use of humectants
   b. using antibiotics in animal feed
   c. use of sequestrants
   d. aseptic processing

8. Those at greatest risk for food-borne illness include
   a. pregnant women.
   b. infants and children.
   c. immunosuppressed individuals.
   d. All of the above.

9. Pasteurization involves the
   a. exposure of food to high temperatures for short periods to destroy harmful microorganisms.
   b. exposure of food to heat to inactivate enzymes that cause undesirable effects in foods during storage.
   c. fortification of foods with vitamins A and D.
   d. use of irradiation to destroy certain pathogens in foods.

10. Food can be kept for long periods by adding salt or sugar because these substances
    a. make the food too acidic for spoilage to occur.
    b. bind to water, thereby making it unavailable to the microorganisms.
    c. effectively kill microorganisms.
    d. dissolve the cell walls in plant foods.

Answers: 1. a (LO 13.4), 2. d (LO 13.2), 3. b (LO 13.4), 4. b (LO 13.1), 5. a (LO 13.1), 6. d (LO 13.8), 7. d (LO 13.2), 8. d (LO 13.3), 9. a (LO 13.2), 10. b (LO 13.4)

Study Questions (Numbers refer to Learning Outcomes)

1. What three trends in food purchasing and production have led to a greater number of cases of foodborne illness? (**LO 13.1**)

2. Which types of foods are most likely to be involved in foodborne illness? Why are they targets for contamination? (**LO 13.2**)

3. Identify three major classes of microorganisms responsible for foodborne illness. (**LO 13.3**)

4. Define the term *food additive,* and give examples of four intentional food additives. What are their specific functions in foods? What is their relationship to the GRAS list? (**LO 13.4**)

5. Describe the federal process that governs the use of food additives, including the Delaney Clause. (**LO 13.4**)

6. Put into perspective the benefits and risks of using additives in food. Point out an easy way to reduce the consumption of food additives. Do you think this is worth the effort in terms of maintaining health? Why or why not? (**LO 13.4**)

7. Name some substances that occur naturally in foods but may cause illness (**LO 13.5**).

8. Describe four recommendations for reducing the risk of toxicity from environmental contaminants. (**LO 13.6**)

9. Why is thoroughly cooking food an important practice for reducing the risk of foodborne illness? (**LO 13.8**)

10. List four techniques other than thorough cooking that are important in preventing foodborne illness. (**LO 13.8**)

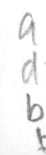
a
d
b
b
a
d

What Would You Choose Recommendations

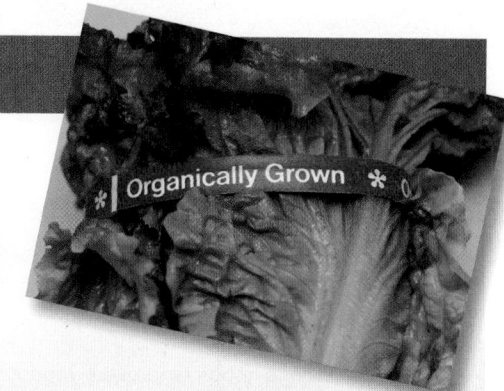

Some organic fruits and vegetables do have higher levels of vitamin C, iron, phosphorus, magnesium, and phytochemicals. Exposure to environmental stressors may cause plants to produce more phytochemicals that have a positive impact on human health. However, current research is insufficient to recommend organic over conventional produce on the basis of nutrient content. Canned and frozen fruits and vegetables have greater nutrient content compared to fresh or organic products that are purchased several days or weeks after harvest.

Products labeled organic must comply with standards regarding use of fertilizers, pesticides, hormones, antibiotics, genetic engineering, and irradiation. Organic food

producers may use natural preservatives. Most preservatives are used to prevent food spoilage and are not linked to negative health effects. Buying fresh or frozen produce and preparing meals at home are the best ways to avoid excessive preservative intake.

Organic produce is no less likely to be contaminated with microorganisms than conventionally grown foods. Although manure is used as organic fertilizer, statistics show similar levels of foodborne pathogens from either type of food. It is still important to follow food-safety advice, such as washing all fresh produce before eating it.

Exposure to pesticides makes organically grown produce stand apart. Because of

▲ Exposure to pesticides is lower from organic foods.

strict production standards we can expect a dramatically lower intake of pesticides from organic produce compared to conventionally grown produce. The health benefits of lower pesticide intake is greatest for children.

Further Readings

1. ADA Reports: Position of the American Dietetic Association: Food and water safety. *Journal of the American Dietetic Association* 109:1449, 2009.

   The public has a right to a safe food and water supply. The ADA supports collaboration among food and nutrition professionals, academics, representatives of the agriculture and food industries, and appropriate government agencies to ensure the safety of the food and water supply.

2. Anderson JB and others: A camera's view of consumer food-handling behaviors. *Journal of the American Dietetic Association* 104:186, 2004.

   Improper food handling was common in households studied. Implementing Fight BAC! recommendations would improve food handling practices.

3. Calvert GM: Health effects of pesticides. *American Family Physician* 69:1613, 2004.

   Clear cases of disease from high pesticide exposure are seen. Effects of low dose, chronic exposure have been hard to quantify, but most adults have detectable pesticide levels in their blood.

4. Consumers Union: Dirty birds: Even "premium" chickens harbor dangerous bacteria. *Consumer Reports* p. 20, January 2007.

   An analysis of fresh, whole chickens bought in the United States revealed that 83% contained two leading causes of foodborne disease.

5. Dangour AD and others: Nutritional quality of organic foods: A systematic review. *American Journal of Clinical Nutrition* 90:680, 2009.

   This systematic review found there is inadequate evidence of a nutritional benefit to consuming organic foods over conventionally produced foods. Organic and conventional food production methods had minimal impact on the nutrient content and therefore minimal health benefit.

6. Food Safety and Inspection Service: A century of progress in food safety. *Be Food Safe* Fall:12, 2006.

   This article summarizes the 100-year history of federal inspection of meat and poultry.

7. Gerner-Smidt P and others: Invasive listeriosis in Denmark 1994–2003: A review of 299 cases with special emphasis on risk factors for mortality. *Clinical Microbiological Infections* 11:618, 2005.

   Listeria infections lead to death primarily in older people and those with underlying cases of cancer.

8. McCabe-Sellers BJ, Beattie SF: Food safety: emerging trends in foodborne illness surveillance and prevention. *Journal of the American Dietetic Association* 104:1708, 2004.

   Recommendations are given to reduce risk of foodborne illness, with proper personal hygiene being a major focus.

9. Schardt D: Get the lead out—What you don't know can hurt you. *Nutrition Action Healthletter* p. 1, March 2005.

   Hypertension, renal disease, impaired brain function, and cataracts have been linked to lead exposure.

10. Sivapalasingam S and others: Fresh produce: A growing cause of outbreaks of foodborne illness in the United States. *Journal of Food Protection* 67:2342, 2004.

    Caution should be used with fresh produce, just as one would with raw meat and dairy products.

11. Spano M: Organics in overdrive—the explosion of natural food products. *Today's Dietitian* 9:66, October 2007.

    Increased availability of organic products and fear of hormones and antibiotics, has led to a dramatic growth in organic food sales.

12. U.S. Food and Drug Administration: *Food Code*. U.S. Department of Health and Human Services, Public Health Service, Food and Drug Administration: College Park, MD, 2009.

    The FDA Food Code is the model for local, state, tribal, and federal regulators to develop or update their food safety rules consistent with national policy.

13. Widdowson MA and others: Norovirus and foodborne disease, United States, 1991–2000. *Emerging Infectious Diseases* 11:95, 2005.

    The Norovirus leads to more causes of foodborne illness than any other agent.

14. Yeager D: Got organic? *Today's Dietitian* 10:60, October 2008.

    The USDA regulates the organic industry and the National Organic Program certifies that food is produced using organic practices.

connect plus+
NUTRITION
LearnSmart
NutritionCalc Plus Online

To get the most out of your study of nutrition, go to McGraw-Hill's online resources: Connect www.mcgrawhillconnect.com, where you will find NutritionCalc Plus, LearnSmart, and many other dynamic tools.

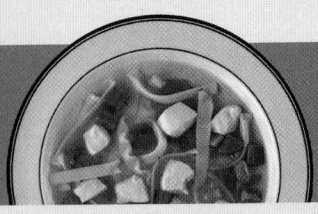

RATE YOUR PLATE

I. Can You Spot the Improper Food-Safety Practices?

In this chapter you learned that (1) foodborne illness strikes up to 76 million U.S. citizens each year and (2) about 5000 deaths each year in the United States are caused by foodborne organisms.

Carefully preparing foods to prevent foodborne illness can minimize its occurrence for most of us. Read the following excerpt and find the food-safety violations that could lead to illness.

A Local Health Department Inspector Gives the Following Account of His Visit to a Local Diner

As I walked through the kitchen of the Morningside Diner, I noticed that all food handlers washed their hands thoroughly with hot, soapy water before handling the food, especially after handling raw meat, fish, poultry, or eggs. Before preparing raw foods, they also thoroughly washed the cutting boards, dishes, and other equipment. As they used their cutting boards after cutting foods, they wiped them with a damp rag and used them again to cut more food.

When preparing fresh fruits and vegetables, they washed them but were careful to leave a little dirt on for fear of washing important nutrients from the outside. The cooks generally cooked meats to an internal temperature of 180°F (82°C). However, to preserve the flavor, pork was cooked to an internal temperature of 140°F (60°C). Some cooked foods to be served later were cooled to below 41°F (5°C) within 2 hours, and foods like beef stew were cooled in shallow pans.

The diner served canned foods, even when the cans were dented. When leftovers were reheated, they were raised to an internal temperature of 130°F (55°C) and served immediately. Food handlers took great care to remove moldy portions of food. The cooks prepared stuffing separately from the poultry. The temperature of refrigerators was approximately 45°F (7°C).

1. List the violations of food-safety practices that could contribute to foodborne illness.

_____
_____
_____
_____

2. If you were writing a report describing ways to correct these practices, what would you say?

_____
_____
_____
_____

3. List the food-safety practices that follow the general rules for preventing foodborne illness.

_____
_____
_____
_____

II. Take a Closer Look at Food Additives

Evaluate a food label of a convenience food item (e.g., frozen entree, ready-to-eat baked good) either in the supermarket or one you have available.

1. Write out the list of ingredients.

_____

_____

_____

_____

2. Identify the ingredients that you think may be food additives.

_____

_____

_____

_____

_____

3. Based on the information available in this chapter, what are the functions of these food additives?

_____

_____

_____

_____

4. How might this food product differ without these ingredients?

_____

_____

_____

_____

III. Take a Closer Look at Organic Foods

Visit one or more supermarkets to see what organic foods are available. Note your findings below.

	Available	Not Available
Meat		
Poultry		
Milk		
Eggs		
Cheese		
Lettuce		
Apples		
Bananas		
Broccoli		
Other produce		
Breakfast cereal		
Snack chips		
Crackers		
Bread		
Pasta		
Beer		

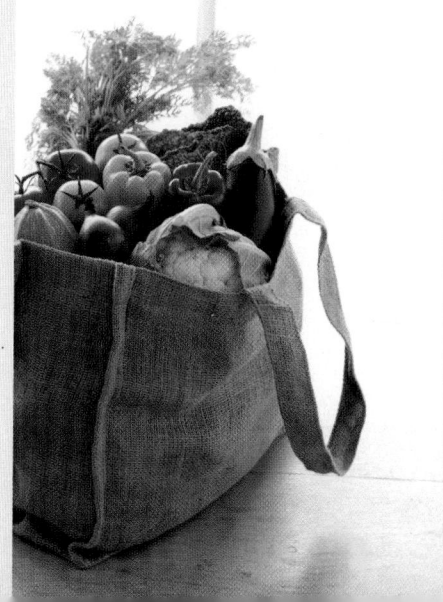

Do you currently purchase organic foods? Why or why not?

Chapter 14 Pregnancy and Breastfeeding

Student Learning Outcomes

Chapter 14 is designed to allow you to:

14.1 List major physiological changes that occur in the body during pregnancy and how nutrient needs are altered.

14.2 List factors that predict a successful pregnancy outcome and some that do not.

14.3 Specify the optimal weight gain during pregnancy for a healthy adult woman.

14.4 Design an adequate, balanced meal plan for a pregnant or breastfeeding woman based on the Dietary Guidelines and MyPlate.

14.5 Identify the nutrients that may need to be supplemented during pregnancy and explain the reason for each.

14.6 Explain the typical discomforts of pregnancy that can be minimized by dietary changes.

14.7 Describe the physiological processes involved in breastfeeding, as well as some advantages of breastfeeding for both the infant and mother.

What Would You Choose?

As a pregnant vegetarian, which of the following meals would you choose as the best source of iron?

a Spinach salad with hard boiled eggs and a whole-wheat roll

b Lean hamburger with cheese, lettuce, and tomato and roasted red potatoes

c Bean and cheese soft taco and stewed tomatoes

d Kellogg's Smart Start cereal, fat-free milk, and orange juice

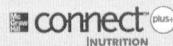 **Think about your choice as you read Chapter 14, then see our recommendations at the end of the chapter. To learn more about pregnancy and vegetarian diets, check out the Connect site:** www.mcgrawhillconnect.com

Part Five

Nutrition: A Focus on Life Stages

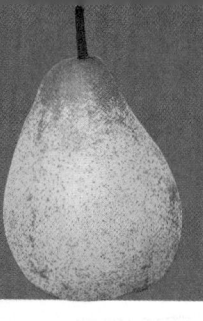

Pregnancy can be a special time. Exhilaration and amazement accompany parents' tremendous responsibility of helping a child develop and grow. Parents-to-be often feel an overriding desire to produce a healthy baby, which can arouse new interest in nutrition and health information. They usually want to do everything possible to maximize their chances of having a robust, lively newborn.

Despite these intentions, the infant mortality rate in North America is higher than that seen in many other industrialized nations. In Canada, about 6.1 of every 1000 infants per year die before their first birthday, while in the United States, it is 6.9. These are alarming statistics for two countries that have such a high per capita expenditure for health care compared to many other countries in the world. Comparatively, the rate of infant mortality in Sweden is roughly 3 of every 1000 infants. In addition, in the United States, about 20% of pregnant women receive inadequate prenatal care in the early months of pregnancy. Expectant teenagers are at the highest risk for this.

Producing a healthy baby is not just a matter of luck. True, some aspects of fetal and newborn health are beyond our control. Still, as the comic in this chapter suggests, conscious decisions about social, health, environmental, and nutritional factors during pregnancy significantly affect the baby's future. Choosing to breastfeed the infant adds further benefits. Let's examine how eating well during pregnancy and breastfeeding can help a baby to have a healthy start in life.

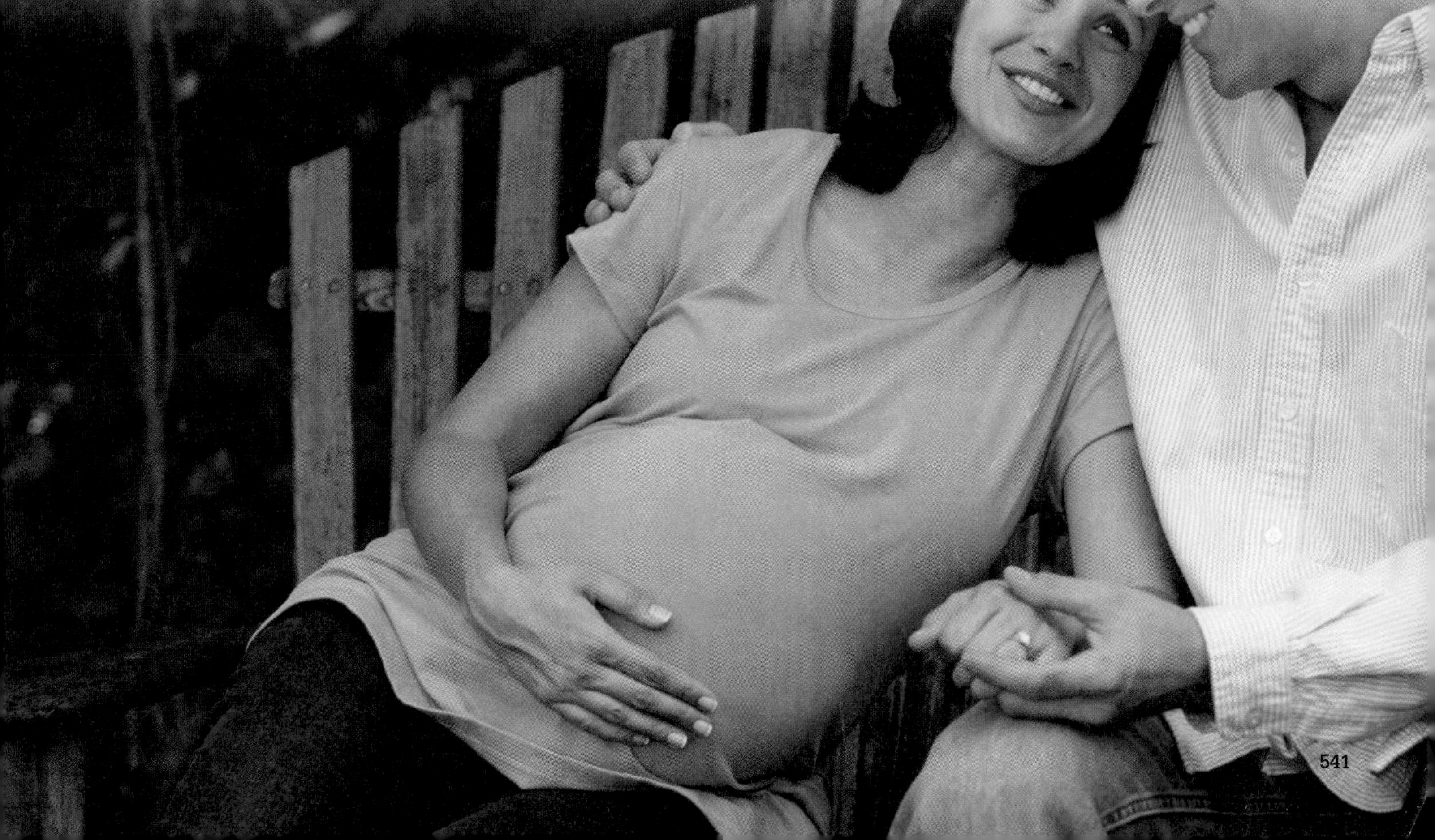

Refresh Your Memory

As you begin your study of nutrition in pregnancy and breastfeeding in Chapter 14, you may want to review:

- Typical fortification in meal replacement bars in Chapter 1 and ready-to-eat breakfast cereals in Chapter 2
- Causes and effects of ketosis in Chapter 4
- Components of the macronutrient classes—carbohydrates, proteins, and lipids—in Chapters 4 to 6, especially omega-3 fatty acids
- Calculation of body mass index in Chapter 7
- Food sources of folate in Chapter 8 and calcium, iron, and zinc in Chapter 9

14.1 Planning for Pregnancy

In an effort to reduce the occurrence of neural tube defects, *Healthy People 2020* includes a goal of increasing by 10% the proportion of women of child-bearing potential who consume at least 400 micrograms of folic acid per day. Currently, about 24% of women of child-bearing potential consume adequate folic acid from fortified foods or dietary supplements.

Controlling or correcting existing health conditions and modifying potentially harmful habits before conception can improve the chances for a successful pregnancy. About 50% of all pregnancies are unplanned. Even when planned, women often do not suspect they are pregnant during the first few weeks after conception. They may not seek medical attention until after the first 2 to 3 months of pregnancy. Still, even without fanfare, the child-to-be grows and develops daily. For that reason, the health and nutrition habits of a woman who is trying to become pregnant—or who has the ability to become pregnant—are particularly important. Although some aspects of fetal and newborn health are beyond the parents' control, a woman's conscious decisions about social, health, environmental, and nutritional factors affect her infant's health and future.

The time to address ongoing health concerns is before conception. Poor control of existing diabetes, hypertension, phenylketonuria, and HIV-positive status or AIDS may lead to serious complications in pregnancy, including birth defects and fetal death. In addition, women should aim to achieve a healthy weight prior to becoming pregnant. Prepregnancy weight and nutrient stores affect the woman's ability to become pregnant. Many underweight women experience amenorrhea, which may reduce their ability to ovulate. The chances of ovulating and becoming pregnant improve when body fat increases to a healthy level.

Infants born to women who began pregnancy substantially above or below a healthy weight are more likely to experience problems than women who began

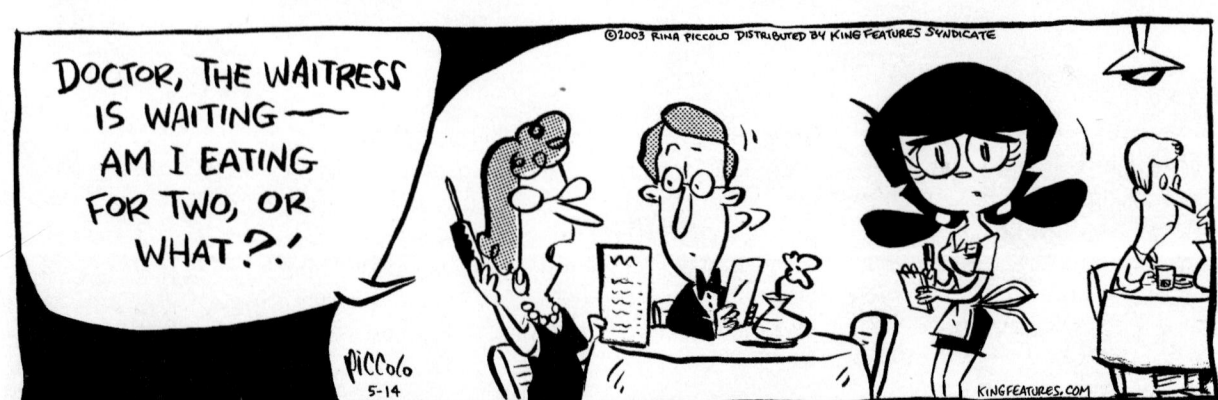

Which diet and lifestyle habits contribute to a successful pregnancy? Which are likely to be harmful?

Why should a woman begin to prepare for pregnancy months before conception of her new baby?

When pregnant, does the mother need to "eat for two?" Chapter 14 provides some answers.

© Rina Piccolo. Reprinted with special permission of King Features Syndicate.

pregnancy at a normal weight. For instance, babies born to obese women are at increased risk of having birth defects, death in the first few weeks after birth, and obesity in childhood. Many obese pregnant women experience high blood pressure, gestational diabetes, and difficult deliveries. At the other extreme, women who begin pregnancy underweight (BMI < 18.5) are more likely to have infants who are low birth weight and preterm than women at a normal weight. These differences may be because underweight women tend to have lighter placentas and lower nutrient stores, especially iron, than heavier women, which can affect fetal growth negatively. An underweight woman can improve her nutrient stores and pregnancy outcome by gaining weight before pregnancy or gaining extra weight during pregnancy.

Figure 14-1 depicts how and when toxic agents can harm the developing fetus. To prepare for a healthy pregnancy, the mother should undoubtedly eliminate tobacco, alcohol, and illicit drugs (e.g., marijuana and cocaine). Certain medicines, such as aspirin and related NSAIDs (e.g., ibuprofen [Advil]), as well as typical medicines to treat the common cold and many herbal therapies, have the potential to damage the fetus. Lower doses and/or safer alternatives should be used when planning for pregnancy. Health hazards in the mother's environment, including job-related hazards and exposure to x-rays, should be minimized. Caffeine intake also should be limited.

Much research suggests that an adequate vitamin and mineral intake at least 8 weeks before conception and then during pregnancy can improve outcomes of pregnancy. In particular, meeting folate needs (400 micrograms of synthetic folic acid per day) helps to prevent birth defects such as neural tube defects (review Fig. 8-27 in Chapter 8) and decrease the risk of preterm delivery. Recall from Chapter 8 that adequate folate status before and during pregnancy reduces the risk of neural tube defects by about 70%. Low intakes of calcium and iron or excessive intakes of vitamin A also are cause for concern during pregnancy. Careful dietary choices, often with the help of a balanced multivitamin and mineral supplement, will contribute to a healthy pregnancy for both mother and infant.

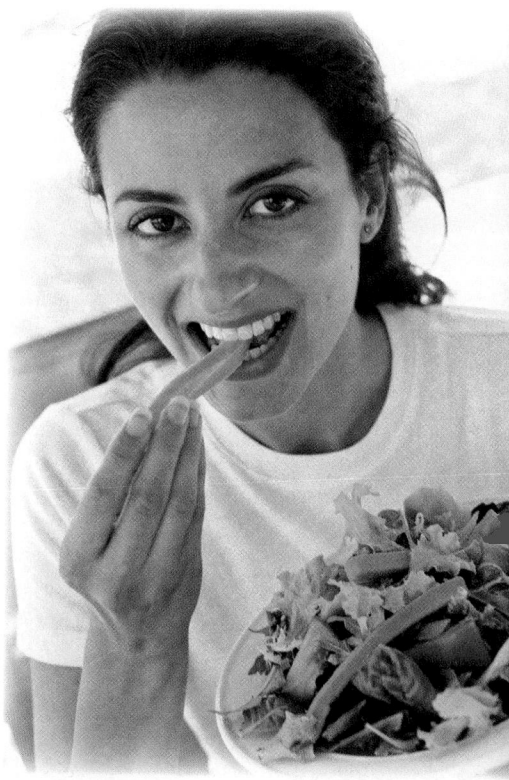

▲ The time to begin thinking about prenatal nutrition is before becoming pregnant. This includes making sure folic acid intake is adequate (400 micrograms of synthetic folic acid per day) and that any supplemental intake of preformed vitamin A does not exceed 100% of the Daily Value (1000 micrograms RAE or 5000 IU).

MAKING DECISIONS

Folate Supplements

Women who have previously given birth to an infant with a neural tube defect such as spina bifida should consult their physician about the need for folate supplementation; an intake of 4 milligrams of synthetic folic acid per day at least one month prior to conception is recommended for these women, but must be taken under a physician's supervision.

14.2 Prenatal Growth and Development

For 8 weeks after conception, a human **embryo** develops from a fertilized **ovum** into a **fetus.** For about another 32 weeks, the fetus continues to develop. When its body finally matures, the infant is born. Until birth, the mother nourishes it via a **placenta,** an organ that forms in her uterus to accommodate the growth and development of the fetus (Fig. 14-2). The role of the placenta is to exchange nutrients, oxygen and other gases, and waste products between the mother and the fetus. This occurs through a network of capillaries that bring the fetal blood close to the maternal blood supply, but the two blood supplies do not mix.

Early Growth—The First Trimester Is a Very Critical Time

In the formation of the human organism, egg and sperm unite to produce the **zygote** (Fig. 14-1). From this point, the reproductive process occurs very rapidly:

• Within 30 hours—zygote divides in half to form 2 cells.
• Within 4 days—cell number climbs to 128 cells.

embryo In humans, the developing offspring in utero from about the beginning of the third week to the end of the eighth week after conception.

ovum The egg cell from which a fetus eventually develops if the egg is fertilized by a sperm cell.

fetus The developing life form from about the beginning of the ninth week after conception until birth.

placenta An organ that forms in the uterus in pregnant women. Through this organ, oxygen and nutrients from the mother's blood are transferred to the fetus, and fetal wastes are removed. The placenta also releases hormones that maintain the state of pregnancy.

zygote The fertilized ovum; the cell resulting from the union of an egg cell (ovum) and sperm until it divides.

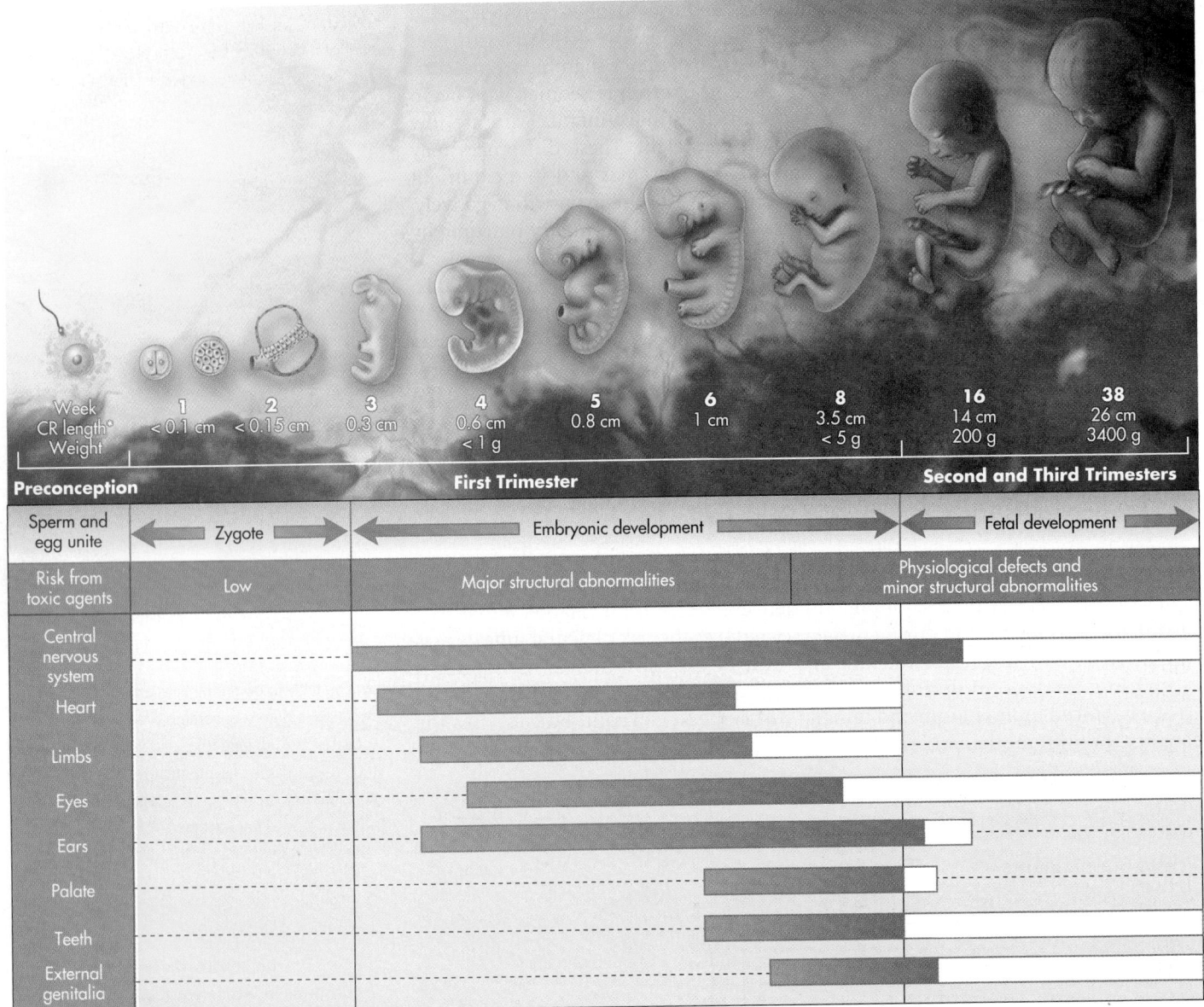

	Week	1	2	3	4	5	6	8	16	38
	CR length*		<0.1 cm	<0.15 cm	0.3 cm	0.6 cm	0.8 cm	1 cm	3.5 cm	14 cm	26 cm
	Weight					<1 g			<5 g	200 g	3400 g

| | **Preconception** | | **First Trimester** | | | **Second and Third Trimesters** |

FIGURE 14-1 ▶ Harmful effects of toxic agents during pregnancy. Vulnerable periods of fetal development are indicated with purple bars. The purple shading indicates the time of greatest risk to the organ. The most serious damage to the fetus from exposure to toxins is likely to occur during the first 8 weeks after conception, two-thirds of the way through the first trimester. As the white bars in the chart show, however, damage to vital parts of the body—including the eyes, brain, and genitals—can also occur during the later months of pregnancy.

trimesters Three 13- to 14-week periods into which the normal pregnancy (the length of a normal pregnancy is about 40 weeks, measured from the first day of the woman's last menstrual period) is divided somewhat arbitrarily for purposes of discussion and analysis. Development of the offspring, however, is continuous throughout pregnancy, with no specific physiological markers demarcating the transition from one trimester to the next.

- At 14 days—the group of cells is called an embryo.
- Within 35 days—heart is beating, embryo is 1/30 of an inch (8 millimeters) long, eyes and limb buds are clearly visible.
- At 8 weeks—the embryo is known as a fetus.
- At 13 weeks (end of first trimester)—most organs are formed, and the fetus can move.

For purposes of discussion, the duration of pregnancy—normally, 38 to 42 weeks—is commonly divided into three periods, called **trimesters.** Growth begins in the first trimester with a rapid increase in cell number. This type of growth dominates embryonic and early fetal development. The newly formed cells then begin to grow larger. Further growth is a mix of increases in cell number and cell size. By the end of 13 weeks—the first trimester—most organs are formed and the fetus can move (see Fig. 14-1).

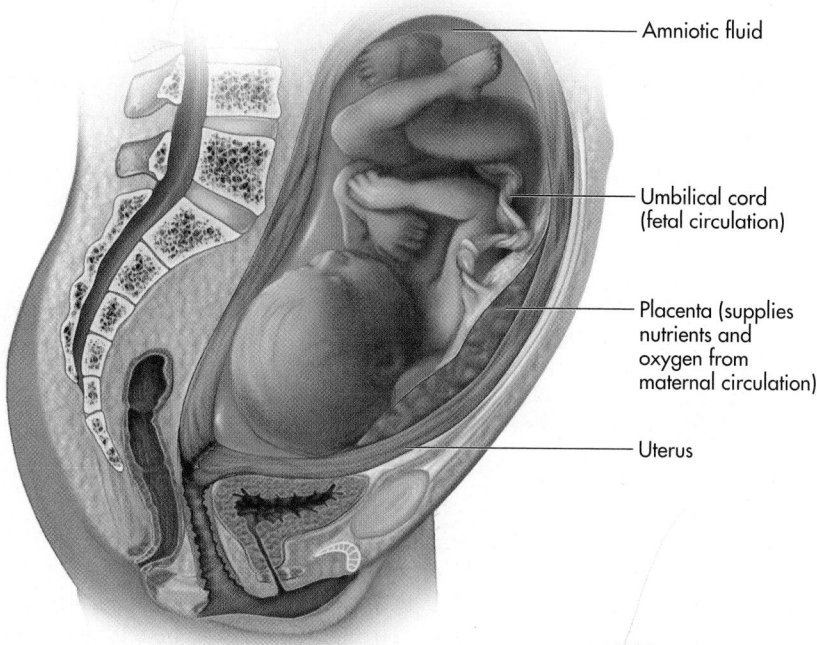

Amniotic fluid

Umbilical cord
(fetal circulation)

Placenta (supplies
nutrients and
oxygen from
maternal circulation)

Uterus

FIGURE 14-2 ▶ The fetus in relationship to the placenta. The placenta is the organ through which nourishment flows to the fetus.

As the embryo or fetus develops, nutritional deficiencies and other insults have the potential to impose damage or risk to organ systems. For example, adverse reactions to medications, high intakes of vitamin A, exposure to radiation, or trauma can alter or arrest the current phase of fetal development, and the effects may last a lifetime (review Fig. 14-1). The most critical time for these potential problems is during the first trimester. Most **spontaneous abortions**—premature terminations of pregnancy that occur naturally—happen at this time. About one-half or more pregnancies end in this way, often so early that a woman does not even realize she was pregnant. (An additional 15% to 20% are lost before normal delivery.) Early spontaneous abortions usually result from a genetic defect or fatal error in fetal development. Smoking, alcohol abuse, use of aspirin and NSAIDs, and illicit drug use raise the risk for spontaneous abortion.

A woman should avoid substances that may harm the developing fetus, especially during the first trimester. This holds true, as well, for the time when a woman is trying to become pregnant. As previously mentioned, she is unlikely to be aware of her pregnancy for at least a few weeks. In addition, the fetus develops so rapidly during the first trimester that, if an essential nutrient is not available, the fetus may be affected even before evidence of the nutrient deficiency appears in the mother.

For this reason, the *quality*—rather than the *quantity*—of the woman's nutritional intake is most important during the first trimester. In other words, women should consume the same amount of calories, but the foods chosen should be more nutrient dense. Although some women lose their appetite and feel nauseated during the first trimester, they should be careful to meet nutrient needs as much as possible.

Although a mother's decisions, practices, and precautions during pregnancy contribute to the health of her fetus, she cannot guarantee her fetus good health because some genetic and environmental factors are beyond her control. She and others involved in the pregnancy should not hold an unrealistic illusion of total control.

Second Trimester

By the beginning of the second trimester, a fetus weighs about 1 ounce. Arms, hands, fingers, legs, feet, and toes are fully formed. The fetus has ears and begins to form tooth sockets in its jawbone. Organs continue to grow and mature, and, with a stethoscope or Doppler instrument, physicians can detect the fetal heartbeat. Most bones

spontaneous abortion Cessation of pregnancy and expulsion of the embryo or nonviable fetus prior to 20 weeks gestation. This is the result of natural causes, such as a genetic defect or developmental problem; also called *miscarriage*.

▶ A healthy 1-week-old baby. At birth, a baby usually weighs about 7.5 pounds and is 20 inches long.

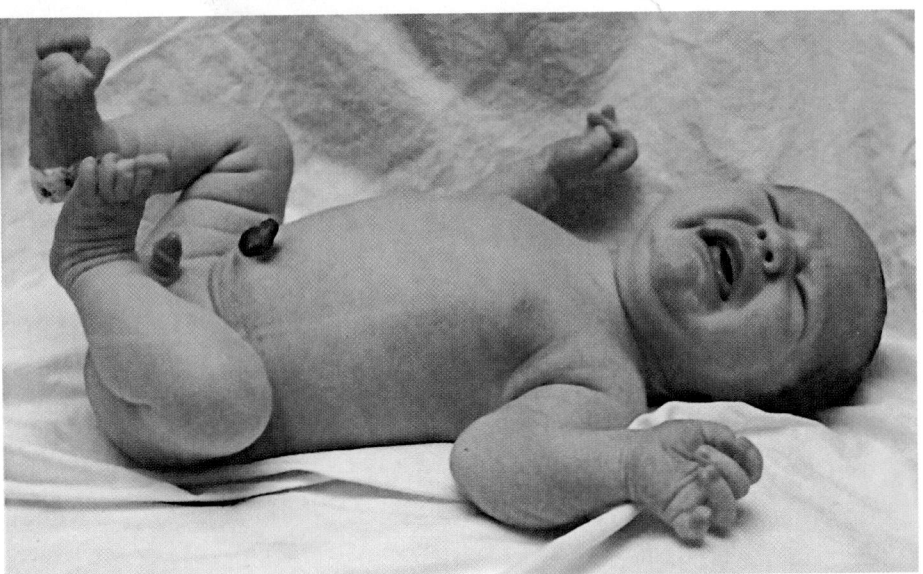

lactation The period of milk secretion following pregnancy; typically called *breastfeeding.*

gestation The period of intrauterine development of offspring, from conception to birth; in humans, gestation lasts for about 40 weeks after the woman's previous menstrual period.

A goal of *Healthy People 2020* is to reduce low birth weight by 5% and preterm births by 10%. Currently about 8% of live births are of low birth weight and about 13% are preterm.

are distinctly evident through the body. Eventually, the fetus begins to look more like an infant. It may suck its thumb and kick strongly enough to be felt by the mother. As was shown in Figure 14-1, the fetus can still be affected by exposure to toxins, but not to the degree seen in the first trimester.

During the second trimester, the mother's breast weight increases by approximately 30% due to the development of milk-producing cells and the deposition of 2 to 4 pounds of fat for **lactation.** This stored fat serves as a reservoir for the extra calories needed to produce breast milk.

Third Trimester

By the beginning of the third trimester, a fetus weighs about 2 to 3 pounds. The third trimester is a crucial time for fetal growth. The fetus will double in length and will increase its weight by three to four times. The fetus takes higher priority than the mother with regard to iron and will deplete the stores of the mother. If the mother is not meeting her iron needs, she can be severely depleted after delivery. An infant born after about 26 weeks of **gestation** has a good chance of survival if cared for in a nursery for high-risk newborns. However, the infant will not contain the stores of minerals (mainly iron and calcium) and fat normally accumulated during the last month of gestation. This and other medical problems, such as a poor ability to suck and swallow, complicate nutritional care for preterm infants.

By full term, the fetus usually weighs about 7 to 9 pounds (3 to 4 kilograms) and is about 20 inches (50 centimeters) long. A soft spot on the top of the head indicates where the skull bones (fontanels) are growing together. The bones finally close by the time the baby is about 12 to 18 months of age.

14.3 Success in Pregnancy

The goal of pregnancy is to achieve optimal health for both the baby and the mother. For the mother, a successful pregnancy is one in which her physical and emotional health is protected so that she can return to her prepregnancy health status. For the infant, two widely accepted criteria are (1) a gestation period longer than 37 weeks and (2) a birth weight greater than 5.5 pounds (2.5 kilograms). Sufficient lung development, likely to have occurred by 37 weeks of gestation, is critical to the survival of a newborn. The longer the gestation, the greater the ultimate birth weight and maturation state, leading to fewer medical problems and better quality of life for the infant. Overall, a successful pregnancy is the outcome of a complex interplay between genes, various lifestyle practices, and the environment.

Infant Birthweight

Low-birth-weight (LBW) infants are those weighing less than 5.5 pounds (2.5 kilograms) at birth. Most commonly, LBW is associated with **preterm** birth. Medical costs during the first year of life for LBW infants are higher than those for normal-weight infants. In fact, hospital-related costs of caring for LBW newborns total more than $4 billion per year in the United States. Full-term and preterm infants who weigh less than the expected weight for their duration of gestation, the result of insufficient growth, are described as **small for gestational age (SGA).** Thus, a full-term infant weighing less than 5.5 pounds at birth is SGA but not preterm, whereas a preterm infant born at 30 weeks' gestation is probably LBW without being SGA. Infants who are SGA are more likely than normal-weight infants to have medical complications, including problems with blood glucose control, temperature regulation, growth, and development in the early weeks after birth.

Prenatal Care and Counseling

Adequate prenatal care is a primary determinant of success in pregnancy. Ideally, women should receive examinations and counseling before becoming pregnant and continue regular prenatal care throughout pregnancy. If prenatal care is inadequate, delayed, or absent, untreated maternal nutritional deficiencies can deprive a developing fetus of needed nutrients. In addition, untreated health conditions, such as anemia, AIDS, hypertension, or diabetes, must be carefully addressed to minimize complications of pregnancy. Treating ongoing infections will also decrease risks of fetal damage. Without prenatal care, a woman is three times more likely to deliver an LBW baby—one who will be 40 times more likely to die during the first 4 weeks of life than a normal-birth-weight infant. According to the Physicians Committee for Responsible Medicine, early and consistent prenatal care could reduce the number of LBW births by 12,600 per year in the United States. Although the ideal time to start prenatal care is before conception, about 20% of women in the United States receive *no* prenatal care throughout the first trimester—a critical time to positively influence the outcome of pregnancy.

Food habits cannot be predicted from income, education, or lifestyle. Although some women already have good dietary habits, most can benefit from nutritional advice. All should be reminded of habits that may harm the growing fetus, such as severe dieting or fasting. By focusing on appropriate prenatal care, nutrient intake, and health habits, parents give their fetus—and later, their infant—the best chance of thriving. Overall, the chances of producing a healthy baby are maximized with education, an adequate diet, and early and consistent prenatal medical care.

Effects of Maternal Age

The age of the mother is another factor that determines pregnancy outcome. The ideal age for pregnancy is between 20 and 35 years of age. Outside that age range—at either extreme—complications are more likely to arise. The rates of teen pregnancy have declined since 1990; still, approximately 400,000 babies are born to teen mothers each year—the highest of any industrialized country. Teen pregnancy increases risk for negative outcomes for both mother and child (Table 14-1) and costs taxpayers an estimated $9.1 billion each year. A portion of these burdens stems from a disadvantaged background, but teenage pregnancy cuts across socioeconomic classes and the effects are evident even after controlling for background factors. Pregnant teens frequently exhibit a variety of risk factors that can complicate pregnancy and pose risk to the fetus. For instance, teenagers are more likely than adult women to be underweight at the start of pregnancy and to gain too little weight during pregnancy. In addition, their bodies lack the physical maturity needed to carry a fetus safely. Even with prenatal care—and 7% of teenage mothers receive none at all—10% of children born to teenage mothers are of low birth weight and 15% are preterm.

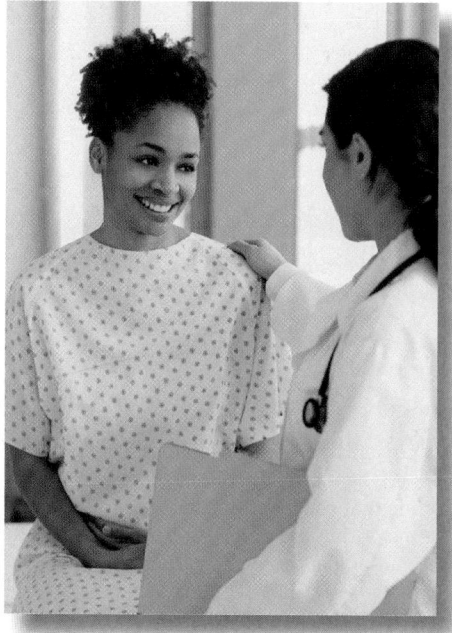

▲ To ensure optimal health and rapid treatment of medical conditions that develop during pregnancy, a pregnant woman should consult with her health-care provider on a regular basis. Ideally, this consultation should begin before she becomes pregnant.

low birth weight (LBW) Referring to any infant weighing less than 2.5 kilograms (5.5 pounds) at birth; most commonly results from preterm birth.

preterm An infant born before 37 weeks of gestation; also referred to as *premature*.

small for gestational age (SGA) Referring to infants who weigh less than the expected weight for their length of gestation. This corresponds to less than 2.5 kilograms (5.5 pounds) in a full-term newborn. A preterm infant who is also SGA will most likely develop some medical complications.

TABLE 14-1 The Burdens of Teenage Pregnancy

For Mother	For Child
↑ Depression and other mental health problems	↓ Birth weight
↑ Use of illicit drugs and alcohol	↑ Preterm birth
↑ Poverty and reliance on public assistance	↑ Infant mortality
↓ Graduation rates from high school and college	↑ Hospital admissions during childhood
↑ Single parenthood	↓ Academic performance
	↓ Nutritional status
	↑ Rates of imprisonment during adulthood

Women with acquired immune deficiency syndrome (AIDS) may pass the virus that causes this disease to the fetus during pregnancy or delivery. About one in three infected newborns will develop AIDS symptoms and die within just a few years. Studies show that these odds of mother-infant transmission can be cut significantly if the woman begins taking highly active antiretroviral therapy (HAART) and receiving routine obstetrical care. Before HAART was available, up to 45% of babies born to mothers with the AIDS virus were infected. Now, transmission is less than 2%. Thus, screening pregnant women for AIDS and providing HAART to those with AIDS are advocated by many experts.

At the other end of the spectrum, advanced maternal age poses special risks for pregnancy. The risks of LBW and preterm delivery increase modestly, but progressively, with maternal age beyond 35 years. Given close monitoring, however, a woman older than 35 years has an excellent chance of producing a healthy infant.

Closely Spaced and Multiple Births

Siblings born in succession to a mother with less than a year between birth and subsequent conception are more likely to be born with low birth weights than are those farther apart in age. The risks of low birth weight, preterm birth, or small size for gestational age are 30% to 40% higher for infants conceived less than 6 months following a birth compared to those conceived 18 to 23 months following a birth. These poor outcomes are probably linked to a lack of enough time to rebuild nutrient stores depleted by the pregnancy. Similarly, multiple births (i.e., twins) increase the risk for preterm birth.

Smoking, Medication Use, and Drug Abuse

Smoking, use of some medications, and illicit drug use during pregnancy all lead to harmful effects. Smoking is linked to preterm birth and appears to increase the risk of birth defects, sudden infant death, and childhood cancer. Problem drugs include aspirin (especially when used heavily), hormone ointments, nose drops and related "cold" medications, rectal suppositories, weight-control pills, antidepressants, and medications prescribed for previous illnesses. Illicit drug use is particularly harmful during pregnancy. Many chemicals in recreational drugs cross the placenta and affect the fetus, whose detoxification systems are immature. During organ development, such insults can cause malformations. Marijuana, the most common illegal drug used during the reproductive years, can result in reduced blood flow to the uterus and placenta, leading to poor fetal growth. Low birth weight and higher risk of preterm delivery often are seen in infants whose mothers used marijuana during pregnancy. Use of psychoactive drugs, such as cocaine and methamphetamines, restricts fetal growth and brain development, the effects of which may plague the child for a lifetime.

Food Safety

The USDA warns pregnant women to thoroughly cook (e.g., microwave) all ready-to-eat meats, including hot dogs and cold cuts, until they are steaming to reduce risk of *Listeria* infections.

Any foodborne illness during any stage of life is a concern. One type of foodborne illness that poses particular danger for pregnant women is caused by the bacterium *Listeria monocytogenes* (review Chapter 13). Infection with this microorganism typically causes mild flulike symptoms, such as fever, headache, and vomiting, about 7 to 30 days after exposure. However, pregnant women, newborn infants, and people with depressed immune function may suffer more severe symptoms, including spontaneous abortion and serious blood infections. In these high-risk people, 25% of infections may be fatal. Unpasteurized milk, soft cheeses made from raw milk (e.g., brie, Camembert, feta, and blue cheeses), and raw cabbage can be sources of *Listeria* organisms, so it is especially important that pregnant women (and other people at high risk for infection) avoid these products. Experts advise consuming only pasteurized milk products and cooking meat, poultry, and seafood thoroughly to kill this and other foodborne organisms. It is unsafe in pregnancy to eat any raw meats or other raw animal products, uncooked hot dogs, or undercooked poultry. These food safety recommendations are included in the Dietary Guidelines for Americans discussed later in the chapter (Table 14-3 on page 554).

Nutritional Status

Is attention to good nutrition worth the effort? Yes; evidence shows that the effort is justified (see Further Readings 3, 5, and 19). Extra nutrients and calories are used for fetal growth, as well as for the changes the mother's body undergoes to accommodate the fetus. Her uterus and breasts grow, the placenta develops, her total blood volume increases, the heart and kidneys work harder, and stores of body fat increase.

Although it is difficult to predict to what degree poor nutrition will affect each pregnancy, a daily diet containing only 1000 kcal has been shown to greatly restrict fetal growth and development. Increased maternal and infant death rates seen in famine-stricken areas of Africa provide further evidence.

Genetic background can explain little of the observed differences in birth weight between developed and developing countries. Both environmental factors and nutritional factors are important. The worse the nutritional condition of the mother at the beginning of pregnancy, the more valuable a healthy prenatal diet and/or use of prenatal supplements are in improving the course and outcome of her pregnancy.

Nutrition Assistance for Low-Income Families

A low socioeconomic status is also associated with problems in pregnancy. Typical characteristics of low socioeconomic status include poverty, inadequate health care, poor health practices, lack of education, and unmarried status. In the United States, about 4 of every 10 births are to unwed mothers, and about 25% of unwed mothers and children live in poverty.

Several U.S. government programs provide high-quality health care and foods to reduce infant mortality. These are designed to alleviate the negative impact of poverty, insufficient education, and inadequate nutrient intake on pregnancy outcome. An example of such a program is the Special Supplemental Nutrition Program for Women, Infants, and Children (WIC). This program offers health assessments and vouchers for foods that supply high-quality protein, calcium, iron, and vitamins A and C to pregnant women, infants, and children (up to age 5 years) from low-income populations. The WIC program is available in all areas of the United States and has a staff trained to help women have healthy babies. More than 9 million women, infants, and young children are benefiting from this program, but many eligible pregnant women are not participating.

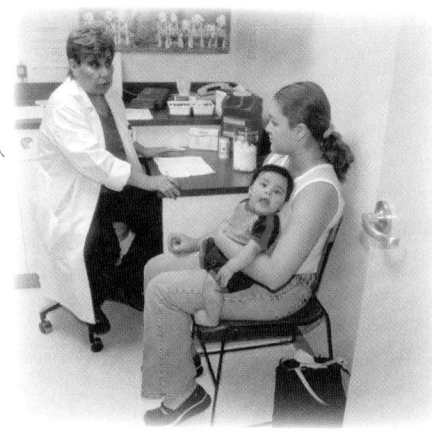

▲ In the United States, low-income pregnant women and their infants (and children) benefit from the nutritional and medical attention provided by the WIC program.

CONCEPT CHECK

To help ensure the optimal health of both the mother and her offspring, adequate nutrition is vital both before and during pregnancy. In particular, meeting folate needs from a synthetic source starting at least 3 months before pregnancy begins, is effective at preventing a variety of fetal malformations. The first trimester is a critical period when inadequate nutrient intake or alcohol and drug use can result in birth defects.

Infants born after 37 weeks of gestation who weigh more than 5.5 pounds (2.5 kilograms) have the fewest medical problems at birth. To reduce infant and maternal medical problems or death, the expectant mother, family, and medical care providers should take the steps necessary to allow the mother to carry the baby in her uterus for the entire 40 weeks. Good nutrition and health practices aid in this goal.

14.4 Increased Nutrient Needs to Support Pregnancy

Pregnancy is a time of increased nutrient needs. It is important to recognize the need for individual assessment and counseling of mothers-to-be, as the nutritional and health status of each woman is different. Still, there are some general principles true for most women with regard to increased nutrient needs.

CRITICAL THINKING

Alexandra wants to have a baby. She has read that it is very important for the woman to be healthy during the pregnancy. However, Jane, her sister, tells her that the time to begin to assess her nutritional and health status is before she becomes pregnant. What additional information should Jane have given Alexandra?

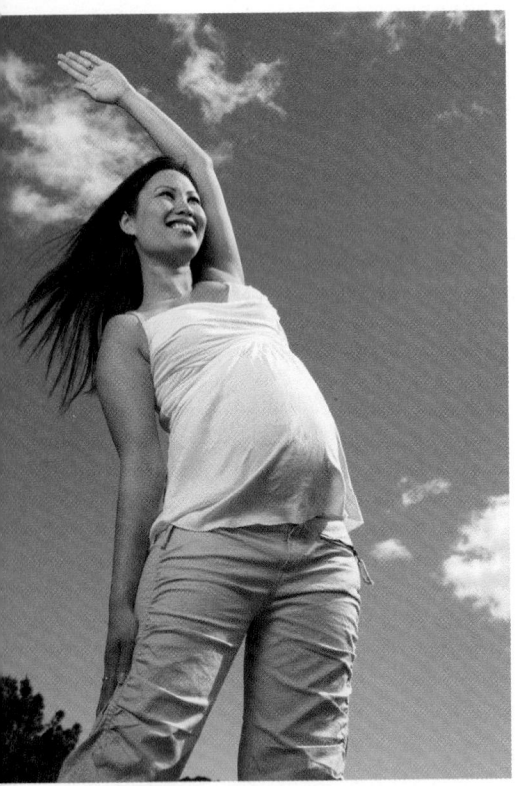

▲ The 2008 Physical Activity Guidelines for Americans recommend that healthy women should get at least 150 minutes of moderate-intensity aerobic activity each week during pregnancy.

Increased Calorie Needs

To support the growth and development of the fetus, pregnant women need to increase their calorie intake. Calorie needs during the first trimester are essentially the same as for nonpregnant women. However, during the second and third trimesters, it is necessary for a pregnant woman to consume approximately 350 to 450 kcal more per day than her prepregnancy needs (the upper end of the range is needed in the third trimester).

Rather than seeing this as an opportunity to fill up on sugary desserts or fat-filled snacks, these extra calories should be in the form of nutrient-dense foods. For example, throughout the day, about six whole-wheat crackers, 1 ounce of cheese, and ½ cup of fat-free milk would supply the extra calories (and also some calcium). Although she "eats for two," the pregnant woman must not double her normal calorie intake. The "eating for two" concept refers more appropriately to increased needs for several vitamins and minerals. Micronutrient needs are increased by up to 50% during pregnancy, whereas calorie needs during the second and third trimesters represent only about a 20% increase.

If a woman is active during her pregnancy, she may need to increase her calorie intake by even more than the estimated 350 to 450 kcal per day. Her greater body weight requires more calories for activity. Many women find that they are inactive during the later months, partly because of their increased size, so an extra 350 to 450 kcal in their daily diets is usually enough.

MAKING DECISIONS

Staying Active During Pregnancy

While pregnancy is not the time to begin an intense fitness regimen, women can generally take part in most low- or moderate-intensity activities during pregnancy. Walking, cycling, swimming, or light aerobics for at least 150 minutes per week is generally advised. Such exercise may prevent pregnancy complications and promote an easier delivery. Some research indicates that regular physical activity during pregnancy lowers a woman's risk of developing gestational diabetes by 50% and preeclampsia by 40%. Women who were highly active prior to pregnancy can maintain their activities as long as they remain healthy and discuss with their health care providers. A few types of activities can potentially harm the fetus and should be avoided, especially those with inherent risk of falls and abdominal trauma. Examples of exercises to avoid, especially during the second and third trimesters, include downhill skiing, weightlifting, soccer, basketball, horseback riding, certain calisthenics (e.g., deep knee bends), any contact sports (e.g., hockey), and SCUBA diving.

Women with high-risk pregnancies, such as those experiencing preterm labor contractions, may need to restrict their physical activity. To ensure optimal health for both herself and her infant, a pregnant woman should first consult her physician about physical activity and possible limitations (see Further Reading 13).

Adequate Weight Gain

Key recommendations for weight management during pregnancy and lactation are included in the Dietary Guidelines for Americans (see Table 14-3 on page 554). Healthy prepregnancy weight and appropriate weight gain during pregnancy are excellent predictors of pregnancy outcome (see Further Readings 8, 10, and 11). Her diet should allow for approximately 2 to 4 pounds (0.9 to 1.8 kilograms) of weight gain during the first trimester and then a subsequent weight gain of 0.8 to 1 pound (0.4 to 0.5 kilogram) weekly during the second and third trimesters (Fig. 14-3). A healthy goal for total weight gain for a woman of normal weight (based on BMI; Table 14-2) averages about 25 to 35 pounds (11.5 to 16 kilograms). Pregnant adolescents and women of various racial and ethnic groups are advised to meet these weight gain goals until further research determines any special recommendations. Women of normal prepregnancy BMI carrying twins should aim to gain within the range of 37 to

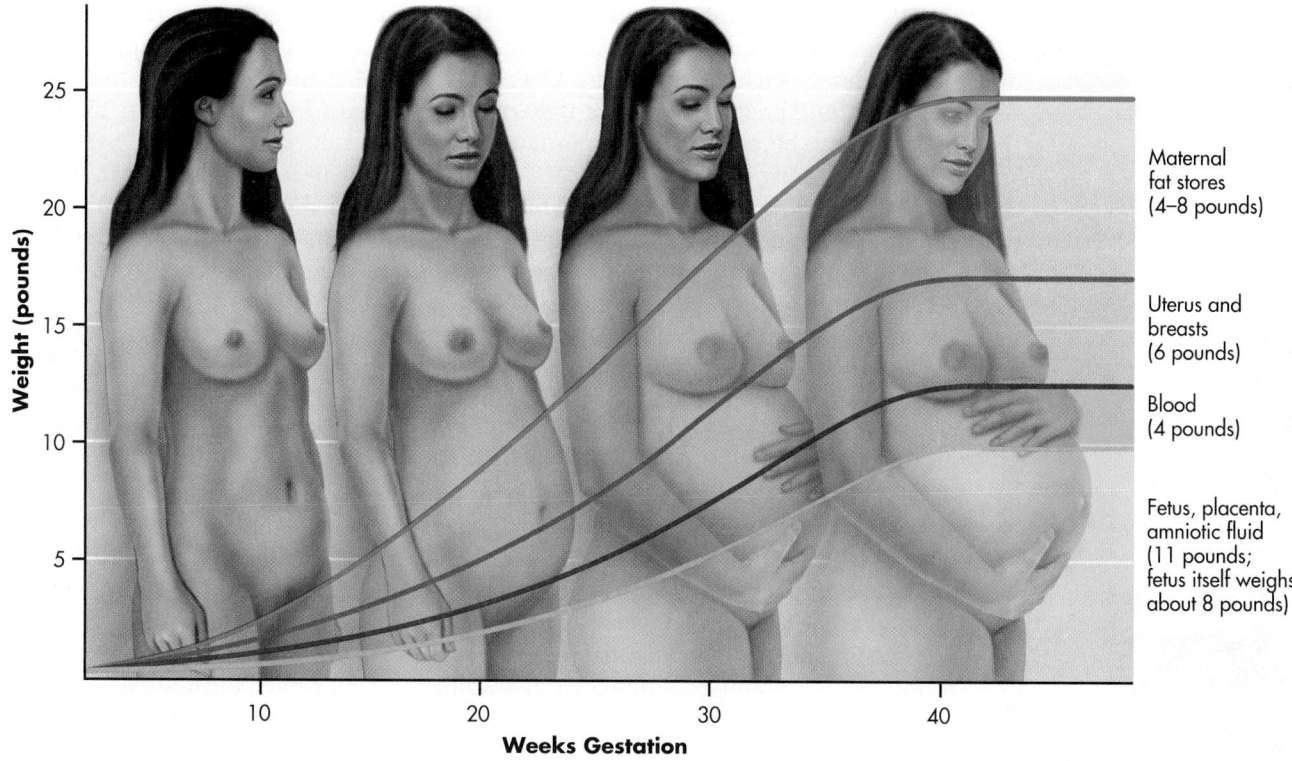

FIGURE 14-3 ▶ The components of weight gain in pregnancy. A weight gain of 25 to 35 pounds is recommended for most women. The various components total about 25 pounds.

54 pounds, whereas overweight or obese women should gain less (31 to 50 pounds or 25 to 42 pounds, respectively).

For women who begin pregnancy with a low BMI, the goal increases to 28 to 40 pounds (12.5 to 18 kilograms). The goal decreases to 15 to 25 pounds (7 to 11.5 kilograms) for overweight women. Target weight gain for obese women is 11 to 20 pounds (5 to 9 kilograms). Figure 14-3 shows why the typical recommendation begins at 25 pounds.

A weight gain of between 25 and 35 pounds for a woman starting pregnancy at normal weight has repeatedly been shown to yield optimal health for both mother and fetus if gestation lasts at least 38 weeks. The weight gain should yield a birth weight of 7.5 pounds (3.5 kilograms). Although some extra weight gain during pregnancy is

TABLE 14-2 Recommended Weight Gain in Pregnancy Based on Prepregnancy Body Mass Index (BMI)

Prepregnancy BMI Category	Total Weight Gain*	
	(pounds)	(kilograms)
Low (BMI less than 18.5)	28 to 40	12.5 to 18
Normal (BMI 18.5 to 24.9)	25 to 35	11.5 to 16
High (BMI 25.0 to 29.9)	15 to 25	7 to 11.5
Obese (BMI greater than 30.0)	11 to 20	5 to 9

*The listed values are for pregnancies with one fetus. For women of normal BMI carrying twins, the range is 37 to 54 pounds (17 to 24.5 kilograms), or less for heavier women.

Reprinted in part with permission from *Weight Gain During Pregnancy: Reexamining the Guidelines*, Copyright 2009 by the Institute of Medicine and National Research Council of the National Academies. Courtesy of the National Academies Press, Washington, DC.

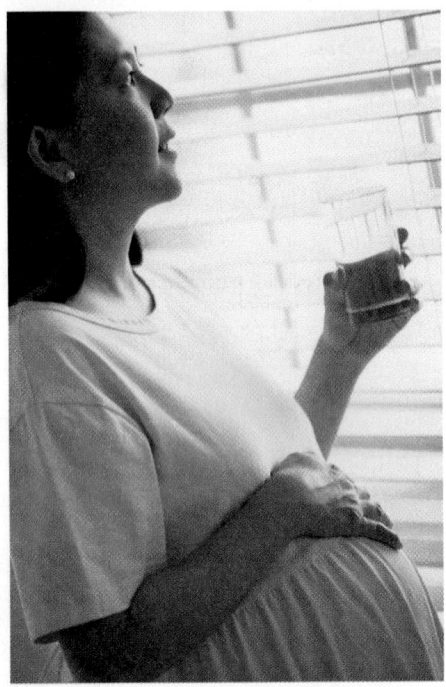

During pregnancy, women in North America are more likely to gain excess weight and make poor food choices than to eat too little.

▲ During pregnancy, the Adequate Intake for total water increases 0.3 liters (1¼ cups) above prepregnancy needs to 3.0 liters (about 12½ cups) per day. For breastfeeding, consume 3.8 liters (16 cups) daily.

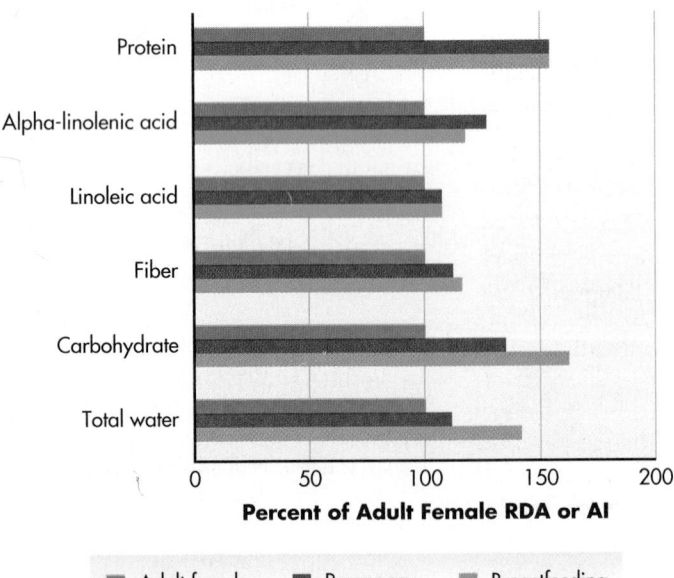

FIGURE 14-4 ▶ Relative macronutrient and water requirements for pregnancy and breastfeeding. Note that there is no RDA or AI for total fat.

usually not harmful (about 5 to 10 pounds), it can set the stage for a pattern of weight gain during the child-bearing years if the mother does not return to her approximate prepregnancy weight after delivery. Overweight and obesity do contribute to complications during pregnancy. Excess maternal body weight increases risk for diabetes, hypertension, blood clots, and spontaneous abortions during pregnancy. Even after childbirth, lasting effects of excess gestational weight gain include high BMI, central body fat distribution, and elevated blood pressure. For the baby, there is a greater chance of birth defects and macrosomia, in which the fetus grows larger than average in utero. Larger infants contribute to a greater need for surgical delivery (i.e., Cesarean sections) among overweight and obese mothers.

Weight gain during pregnancy should generally follow the pattern in Figure 14-3. Monitoring weekly records of a pregnant woman's weight gain helps assess how much to adjust her food intake. Weight gain is a key issue in prenatal care and a concern of many mothers-to-be. Remember that inadequate weight gain can cause many problems.

If a woman deviates from the desirable pattern, she should make the appropriate adjustment. For example, if a woman begins to gain too much weight during her pregnancy, she should not lose weight to get back on track. Even if a woman gains 35 pounds in the first 7 months of pregnancy, she must still gain more during the last 2 months. She should, however, slow the increase in weight to parallel the rise on the prenatal weight gain chart. In other words, the sources of the unnecessary calories should be found and minimized. Alternately, if a woman has not gained the desired weight by a given point in pregnancy, she shouldn't gain the needed weight rapidly. Instead, she should slowly gain a little more weight than the typical pattern to meet the goal by the end of the pregnancy. A registered dietitian can help make any needed adjustments.

Increased Protein and Carbohydrate Needs

The RDA for protein increases by an additional 25 grams per day during pregnancy. A cup of milk alone contains 8 grams. Many nonpregnant women already consume protein in excess of their needs and therefore do not need to increase protein intake any further. However, all women should check to make sure they are eating enough protein as well as enough calories, so this protein is not used to meet energy needs.

The RDA for carbohydrate increases to 175 grams daily, primarily to prevent ketosis. Ketone bodies, a by-product of metabolism of fat for energy, are thought to be poorly used by the fetal brain, implying possible slowing of fetal brain development. Carbohydrate intakes of most women, pregnant or not, already exceed the RDA (Fig. 14-4).

A Word About Lipids

Fat intake should increase proportionally with calorie intake during pregnancy to maintain around 20% to 30% of total calories from fat. Pregnancy is not a time for a low-fat diet, as lipids are a source of extra calories and essential fatty acids needed during pregnancy. Recommendations for the types of lipids during pregnancy are generally the same as for nonpregnant adults. To reduce risk for cardiovascular disease, the American Heart Association recommends no more than 7% of total calories from saturated fat and no more than 1% from *trans* fat. Consumption of dietary cholesterol is not required, but keeping cholesterol intake at a maximum of 300 milligrams per day is also a good goal for maintenance of maternal cardiovascular health.

During pregnancy, it is particularly important to make sure to consume adequate essential fatty acids—linoleic acid (omega-6) and alpha-linolenic acid (omega-3). As you learned in Chapter 5, essential fatty acids cannot be synthesized in the body and must be consumed in the diet. For the developing fetus, essential fatty acids are required for growth, brain development, and eye development. Recommendations are slightly increased by pregnancy: 13 grams per day of omega-6 fatty acids and 1.4 grams per day of omega-3 fatty acids. These needs can be met by consuming 2 to 4 tablespoons per day of plant oils. Consumption of fish at least two times per week is also helpful in meeting needs for essential fatty acids in the diet (see Further Reading 15). (See the "Nutrition and Your Health" section at the end of this chapter for a discussion of mercury in fish.)

Increased Vitamin Needs

Vitamin needs generally increase from prepregnancy RDAs/Adequate Intakes by up to 30% for most of the B vitamins and even greater for vitamin B-6 (45%) and folate (50%) (Fig 14-5). Vitamin A needs only increase by 10%, so a specific focus on this vitamin is not needed. And remember, excess amounts of vitamin A are harmful to the developing fetus.

The extra amount of vitamin B-6 and other B vitamins (except folate) needed in the diet is easily met via wise food choices, such as a serving of a typical ready-to-eat breakfast cereal and some animal protein sources. Folate needs, however, often merit specific diet planning and possible vitamin supplementation. The synthesis of DNA, and therefore cell division, requires folate, so this nutrient is especially crucial during pregnancy. Ultimately, both fetal and maternal growth depend on an ample supply of folate. Red blood cell formation, which requires folate, increases during pregnancy. Serious folate-related anemia therefore can result if folate intake is inadequate. The RDA for folate increases during pregnancy to 600 micrograms DFE per day (review Chapter 8 for calculation of DFE). This is a critical goal in the nutritional care of a pregnant woman. Increasing folate intakes to meet 600 micrograms DFE per day for a pregnant woman can be achieved through dietary sources, a supplemental source of folic acid, or a combination of both. Choosing a diet rich in synthetic folic acid, such as from ready-to-eat breakfast cereals or meal replacement bars (look for approximately 50% to 100% of the Daily Value), is especially helpful in meeting folate needs. Recall from Chapter 8 that synthetic folic acid is much more easily absorbed than the various forms of folate found naturally in foods (see Further Readings 14 and 17).

Increased Mineral Needs

Mineral needs generally increase during pregnancy, especially the requirements for iodide and iron (Fig. 14-6). Zinc needs also increase. (Calcium needs do not increase but still may deserve special attention because many women have deficient intakes.)

Pregnant women need the extra iodide (total of 220 micrograms per day) for prevention of goiter. Typical iodide intakes are enough if the woman uses iodized salt. Animal proteins or a fortified ready-to-eat breakfast cereal in the diet can easily provide enough extra zinc. The extra iron (total of 27 milligrams per day) is needed to synthesize the greater amount of hemoglobin needed during pregnancy and to provide iron stores for the fetus. Women often need a supplemental source of iron, especially if they do not consume iron-fortified foods, such as highly fortified breakfast cereals containing close to 100% of the Daily Value for iron (18 milligrams). Iron supplements decrease appetite and can cause nausea and constipation, so if used, these should be taken between meals or just before going to bed. Milk, coffee, or tea should not be consumed with an iron supplement because these beverages have substances that interfere with iron absorption. Eating foods rich in vitamin C along with nonheme iron-containing foods and iron supplements helps increase iron absorption from those sources. Pregnant women who are not anemic may wait until the second trimester, when pregnancy-related nausea generally lessens, to start iron supplementation if needed.

The consequences of iron-deficiency anemia—especially during the first trimester—can be severe. Negative outcomes include preterm delivery, LBW infants, and increased risk for fetal death in the first weeks after birth.

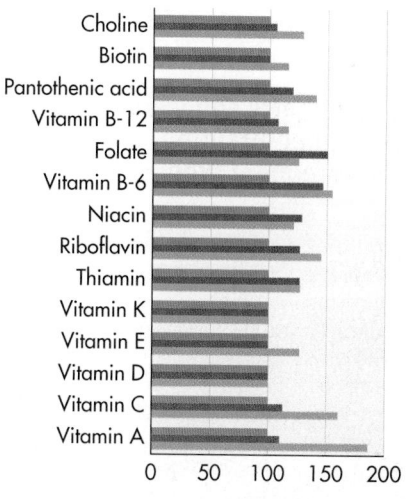

Percent of Adult Female RDA or AI

- Adult female
- Pregnancy
- Breastfeeding

FIGURE 14-5 ▶ Relative vitamin requirements for pregnancy and breastfeeding.

The Dietary Guidelines for Americans recommend that women who may become pregnant eat foods high in iron and consume adequate amounts of the synthetic form of folate (see Table 14-3).

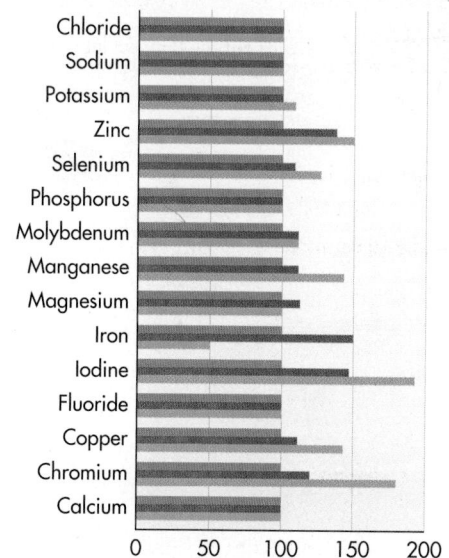

Percent of Adult Female RDA or AI

- Adult female
- Pregnancy
- Breastfeeding

FIGURE 14-6 ▶ Relative mineral requirements for pregnancy and breastfeeding.

NEWSWORTHY
NUTRITION

Experts advocate higher vitamin D for pregnant women

Emerging evidence indicates that low maternal levels of vitamin D during pregnancy affect multiple health parameters in their children. Aside from its well-known role in bone health and prevention of rickets, poor vitamin D status is implicated in serious complications of pregnancy, including higher rates of gestational diabetes, pregnancy-induced hypertension, and a fourfold increased rate of Cesarean section. Vitamin D's role in immune regulation is underscored by higher rates of respiratory infections and mother-to-child transmission of HIV. Because of the ability of vitamin D to modulate gene expression, vitamin D status is critically important during early fetal development through infancy. Diseases that develop later in childhood or adulthood, such as type 1 diabetes, multiple sclerosis, asthma, schizophrenia, and certain types of cancer, are associated with low vitamin D status during gestation. The RDA for pregnant women is 15 micrograms (600 IU) of vitamin D daily, but many experts advocate increasing this recommendation to 25 micrograms (1000 IU) or more.

Source: Dror DK, Allen LH. Vitamin D inadequacy in pregnancy: Biology, outcomes, and interventions. *Nutrition Reviews* 68: 464, 2010.

connect NUTRITION **Check out the Connect site** www.mcgrawhillconnect.com **to further explore vitamin D and pregnancy.**

TABLE 14-3 Targeted Recommendations for Women from the Latest Dietary Guidelines for Americans

Balancing Calories to Manage Weight

Women capable of becoming pregnant
- Achieve and maintain a healthy weight before becoming pregnant.

Women who are pregnant
- Gain weight within the 2009 Institute of Medicine gestational weight-gain guidelines (review Table 14-2).

Foods and Food Components to Reduce

Women capable of becoming pregnant and women who are pregnant
- During pregnancy or when conception is possible, avoid alcohol. No safe level of alcohol consumption during pregnancy has been established.

Women who are pregnant
- Only eat foods with seafood, meat, poultry, or eggs that have been cooked to recommended safe minimum internal temperatures.
- Do not consume unpasteurized (raw) juice or milk or foods made from unpasteurized milk, like some soft cheeses (e.g., feta, queso blanco, queso fresco, Brie, Camembert, blue-veined cheeses, and Panela).
- Reheat deli and luncheon meats and hot dogs to steaming hot to kill *Listeria* and do not eat raw sprouts).

Women who are breastfeeding
- Wait at least 4 hours after drinking alcohol before breastfeeding.
- Alcohol should not be consumed at all until consistent latch on and breastfeeding patterns are established.

Foods and Nutrients to Increase

Women capable of becoming pregnant
- Choose foods that supply heme iron, which is more readily absorbed by the body, additional iron sources, and enhancers of iron absorption such as vitamin C–rich foods.
- Consume 400 micrograms per day of synthetic folic acid (from fortified foods and/or supplements) in addition to food forms of folate from a varied diet.

Women who are pregnant
- Take an iron supplement, as recommended by an obstetrician or other health care provider.
- Consume 600 micrograms of dietary folate equivalents daily from all food sources.

Women who are pregnant or breastfeeding
- Consume 8 to 12 ounces of seafood per week from a variety of seafood types.
- Due to their methyl mercury content, limit white (albacore) tuna to 6 ounces per week and do not eat the following four types of fish: tilefish, shark, swordfish, and king mackerel.

Use of Prenatal Vitamin and Mineral Supplements

Special supplements formulated for pregnancy are prescribed routinely for pregnant women by most physicians. Some are sold over the counter, while others are dispensed by prescription because of the high synthetic folic acid content (1000 micrograms), which could pose problems for others, such as older people (see Chapter 16). These supplements are high in iron (27 milligrams per pill). There is no evidence that use of such supplements causes significant health problems in pregnancy, aside perhaps from the combined amounts of supplementary and dietary vitamin A (see Nutrition and Your Health at the end of this chapter).

Instances when prenatal supplements may especially contribute to a successful pregnancy are with poor women, teenagers, those with a generally deficient diet, women carrying multiple fetuses, those that smoke or use alcohol or illegal drugs, and vegans. In other cases, healthy diets can provide the needed nutrients. When choosing a multivitamin, rely on brands that display the USP symbol on their label, signifying that the supplement meets the content, quality, purity, and safety standards of the

U.S. Pharmacopoeia. Also, avoid megadoses of any nutrient. In particular, toxicity of vitamin A is linked with birth defects. Skip supplements containing herbs, enzymes, and amino acids. Many of these ingredients have not been evaluated for safety during pregnancy or breastfeeding and may be toxic to the fetus. Furthermore, discard supplements that are past the expiration date, as some ingredients lose potency over time.

14.5 Food Plan for Pregnant Women

One dietary approach to support a successful pregnancy is based on MyPlate. For an active 24-year-old woman, about 2200 kcal is recommended during the first trimester (the same as recommended for such a woman when not pregnant). The plan should include:

- 3 cups of calcium-rich foods from the dairy group or use of calcium-fortified foods to make up for any gap between calcium intake and need
- 6 ounce-equivalents from the protein group
- 3 cups from the vegetables group
- 2 cups from the fruits group
- 7 ounce-equivalents from the grains group
- 6 teaspoons of vegetable oil

MAKING DECISIONS

Cravings During Pregnancy

It is a common myth that women instinctively know what to eat during pregnancy. Cravings of the last two trimesters are often related to hormonal changes in the mother, or family traditions. Such "instinct" cannot be trusted, however, based on observations that some women crave nonfood items (called **pica**) such as laundry starch, chalk, cigarette ashes, and soil (clay). This practice can be extremely harmful to the mother and the fetus. Overall, though women may have a natural instinct to consume the right foods in pregnancy, humans are so far removed from living by instinct that relying on our cravings to meet nutrient needs is risky. Nutrition advice by experts is more reliable.

Specifically, choices from the dairy group should include low-fat or fat-free versions of milk, yogurt, and cheese. These foods supply extra protein, calcium, and carbohydrate, as well as other nutrients. Choices from the protein group should include both animal and vegetable sources. Besides protein, these foods help provide the extra iron and zinc needed. The vegetables and fruits group choices provide a variety of vitamins and minerals. One cup from this combination should be a good vitamin C source, and 1 cup should be a green vegetable or other rich source of folate. Choices from the grains group should focus on whole-grain and enriched foods. One ounce of a whole-grain, ready-to-eat breakfast cereal significantly contributes to meeting many vitamin and mineral needs. Finally, inclusion of plant oils in the diet contributes essential fatty acids. Calories from solid fats and added sugars should be limited to 270 kcal per day.

In the second and third trimesters, about 2600 kcal is recommended for this woman. The plan should now include:

- 3 cups of calcium-rich foods from the dairy group or use of calcium-fortified foods
- 6 ½ ounce-equivalents from the protein group
- 3 ½ cups from the vegetables group
- 2 cups from the fruits group
- 9-ounce equivalents from the grains group
- 8 teaspoons of vegetable oil

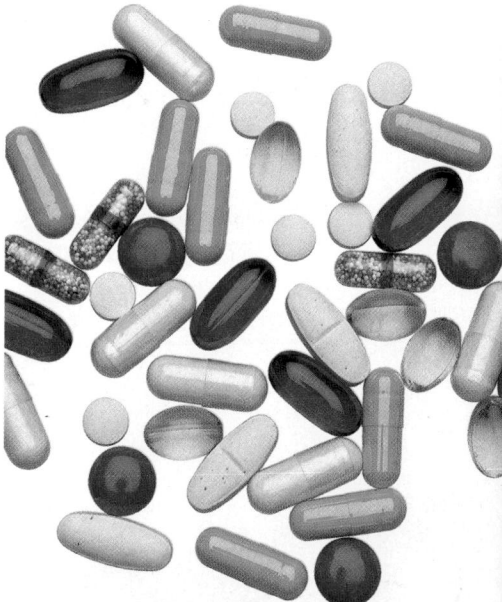

▲ Pregnancy, in particular, is not a time to self-prescribe vitamin and mineral supplements. For example, although vitamin A is a routine component of prenatal vitamins, intakes over three times the RDA for vitamin A have been shown to have toxic effects on the fetus.

pica The practice of eating nonfood items, such as dirt, laundry starch, or clay.

At www.ChooseMyPlate.gov, moms-to-be can find individualized dietary information by clicking on the link for Daily Food Plans for Moms. Based on age, height, physical activity, and prepregnancy weight, calorie and food group recommendations are generated for each trimester.

Solid fats and added sugars should contribute no more than 360 kcal per day. Table 14-4 illustrates one daily menu based on the 2600 kcal plan for pregnancy for women in the second or third trimesters. This menu meets the extra nutrient needs associated with pregnancy. Women who need to consume more than this—and some do for various reasons—should incorporate additional fruits, vegetables, and whole-grain breads and cereals, not poor nutrient sources such as desserts and sugared soft drinks.

Pregnant Vegetarians

pl dairy egg   *pl & dairy*

Women who are either lactoovovegetarians or lactovegetarians generally do not face special difficulties in meeting their nutritional needs during pregnancy. Like

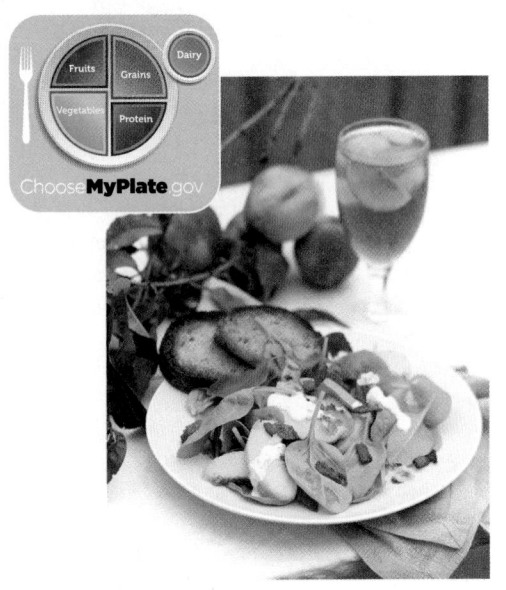

CRITICAL THINKING

How does this lunch of spinach and fruit salad and whole-wheat toast compare to MyPlate? Is iced tea a good beverage choice? Why or why not?

TABLE 14-4 Sample 2600 kcal Daily Menu That Meets the Nutritional Needs of Most Pregnant and Breastfeeding Women

	Vitamin B-6	Folate	Iron	Zinc	Calcium
Breakfast					
1 cup Kellogg's Smart Start cereal	✓	✓	✓	✓	✓
1 cup orange juice		✓			
1 cup fat-free milk	✓				✓
Snack					
2 tbsp peanut butter	✓	✓	✓	✓	
2 stalks of celery		✓			
1 slice whole-wheat toast		✓	✓	✓	
1 cup plain low-fat yogurt	✓				✓
½ cup strawberries		✓			
Lunch					
2 cups spinach and fruit salad with 2 tbsp oil and vinegar dressing		✓			✓
2 slices whole-wheat toast		✓	✓	✓	
1 ½ ounces provolone cheese	✓				✓
Snack					
5 whole-wheat crackers		✓	✓	✓	
1 cup grape juice					
Dinner					
3 ounces lean hamburger, broiled (with condiments)	✓		✓	✓	
½ cup baked beans	✓	✓	✓	✓	
1 hamburger bun		✓	✓		
½ sliced tomato					
1 cup cooked broccoli		✓			✓
1 tsp soft margarine					
Iced tea					
Snack					
Granola bar (2 ounces)		✓	✓	✓	
½ banana	✓				
Foods or beverages containing solid fats or added sugars can be included (up to 360 kcal per day) to support adequate weight gain.					

*Amount of solid fats and added sugars will vary based on the actual food choices made within each MyPlate group.

This diet meets nutrient needs for pregnancy and breastfeeding. Lack of a check (✓) indicates a poor source of the nutrient. The vitamin- and mineral-fortified breakfast cereal used in this example makes an important contribution to meeting nutrient needs. Fluids can be added as desired. Total intake of fluids, such as water, should be 10 cups per day for pregnant women or about 13 cups per day for breastfeeding women.

nonvegetarian women, they should be concerned primarily with meeting vitamin B-6, iron, folate, and zinc needs.

On the other hand, for a vegan, careful diet planning during preconception and pregnancy is crucial to ensure sufficient protein, vitamin D (particularly in the absence of sufficient sun exposure), vitamin B-6, iron, calcium, zinc, and especially a supplemental source of vitamin B-12. The basic vegan diet listed in Chapter 6 should be modified to include more grains, beans, nuts, and seeds to supply the necessary extra amounts of some of these nutrients. As mentioned, use of a prenatal multivitamin and mineral supplement also is generally advocated to help fill micronutrient gaps. However, although these are high in iron, this is not true for calcium (200 milligrams per pill). If iron and calcium supplements are used, they should not be taken together, to avoid possible competition for absorption.

CONCEPT CHECK

Calorie needs increase by an average of about 350 to 450 kcal per day during the second and third trimesters of pregnancy, respectively. Weight gain should be slow and steady up to a total of 25 to 35 pounds for a woman of normal weight (i.e., prepregnancy BMI of 18.5 to 24.9). Protein and certain vitamin and mineral needs increase during pregnancy. Most important to consider are vitamin B-6, folate, iron, iodide, and zinc. A pregnant woman's diet should be varied and generally comply with MyPlate standards. A prenatal multivitamin and mineral supplement is commonly prescribed but may not be necessary, depending on one's diet and health status. Taking too many supplements—especially vitamin A—can be hazardous to the fetus.

14.6 Physiological Changes of Concern During Pregnancy

During pregnancy, the fetus's needs for oxygen and nutrients, as well as excretion of waste products increase the burden on the mother's lungs, heart, and kidneys. Although a mother's digestive and metabolic systems work efficiently, some discomfort accompanies the changes her body undergoes to accommodate the fetus.

Heartburn, Constipation, and Hemorrhoids

Hormones (such as progesterone) produced by the placenta relax muscles in the uterus and the gastrointestinal tract. This often causes heartburn as stomach acid refluxes into the esophagus (review Chapter 3). When this occurs, the woman should avoid lying down after eating, eat less fat so that foods pass more quickly from the stomach into the small intestine, and avoid spicy foods she cannot tolerate. She should also consume most liquids between meals to decrease the volume of food in the stomach after meals, and thus relieve some of the pressure that encourages reflux. Women with more severe cases may need antacids or related medications.

Constipation often results as the intestinal muscles relax during pregnancy. It is especially likely to develop late in pregnancy, as the fetus competes with the GI tract for space in the abdominal cavity. To offset these discomforts, a woman should perform regular exercise and consume more fluid, fiber, and dried fruits, such as prunes (dried plums). The Adequate Intake for fiber in pregnancy is 28 grams, slightly more than for the nonpregnant woman. Fluid needs are 10 cups per day. These practices can help prevent constipation and a problem that frequently accompanies it, hemorrhoids. Straining during elimination can lead to hemorrhoids, which are more likely to occur during pregnancy because of other body changes. A re-evaluation of the need for and dose of iron supplementation also should be considered, as high iron intakes are linked to constipation.

Edema

Placental hormones cause various body tissues to retain fluid during pregnancy. Blood volume also greatly expands during pregnancy. The extra fluid normally causes some swelling (edema). There is no reason to restrict salt severely or use diuretics to limit mild edema. However, the edema may limit physical activity late in pregnancy and occasionally requires a woman to elevate her feet or wear compression stockings to control the symptoms. Overall, edema generally spells trouble only if hypertension and the appearance of extra protein in the urine accompany it (see a following section, "Pregnancy-Induced Hypertension").

Morning Sickness

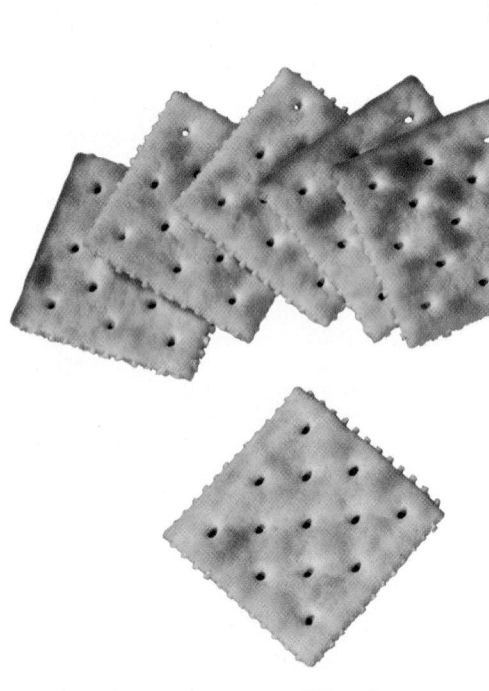

About 70% to 85% of pregnant women experience nausea during the early stages of pregnancy. This nausea may be related to the increased sense of smell induced by pregnancy-related hormones circulating in the bloodstream. Although commonly called "morning sickness," pregnancy-related nausea may occur at any time and persist all day. It is often the first signal to a woman that she is pregnant. To help control mild nausea, pregnant women can try the following: avoiding nauseating foods, such as fried or greasy foods; cooking with good ventilation to dissipate nauseating smells; eating saltine crackers or dry cereal before getting out of bed; avoiding large fluid intakes early in the morning; and eating smaller, more frequent meals. The iron in prenatal supplements triggers nausea in some women, so changing the type of supplement used or postponing use until the second trimester may provide relief in some cases. If a woman thinks her prenatal supplement is related to morning sickness, she should discuss switching to another supplement with her physician.

Overall, if a food sounds good to a pregnant woman with morning sickness, whether it is broccoli, soda crackers, or lemonade, she should eat it and eat when she can, while also striving to follow her prenatal diet. The American College of Obstetricians and Gynecologists recommends the following for the prevention and treatment of nausea and vomiting of pregnancy:

▲ A few saltine crackers upon waking or between meals can help lessen pregnancy-related nausea.

- History of use of a balanced multivitamin and mineral supplement at the time of conception
- Use of megadoses of vitamin B-6 (10–25 milligrams taken three to four times a day), especially coupled with the antihistamine doxylamine (10 milligrams) with each dose
- Ginger may also be helpful (350 milligrams taken three times per day)

Usually, nausea stops after the first trimester; however, in about 10% to 20% of cases, it can continue throughout the entire pregnancy. In cases of serious nausea, the preceding practices offer little relief. Excessive vomiting can cause dangerous dehydration and must be avoided. When vomiting persists (about 0.5% to 2% of pregnancies), medical attention is needed.

Anemia

physiological anemia The normal increase in blood volume in pregnancy that dilutes the concentration of red blood cells, resulting in anemia; also called *hemodilution*.

To supply fetal needs, the mother's blood volume expands to approximately 150% of normal. The number of red blood cells, however, increases by only 20% to 30%, and this occurs more gradually. As a result, a pregnant woman has a lower ratio of red blood cells to total blood volume in her system. This hemodilution is known as **physiological anemia**. It is a normal response to pregnancy, rather than the result of inadequate nutrient intake. If during pregnancy, however, iron stores and/or dietary iron intake are not sufficient to meet needs, any resulting iron-deficiency anemia requires medical attention. The Dietary Guidelines for Americans recommend that women who may become pregnant eat foods high in iron (Table 14-3).

Gestational Diabetes

Hormones synthesized by the placenta decrease the efficiency of insulin. This leads to a mild increase in blood glucose, which helps supply calories to the fetus. If the rise in blood glucose becomes excessive, this leads to **gestational diabetes,** often beginning in weeks 20 to 28, particularly in women who have a family history of diabetes or who are obese. Other risk factors include maternal age over 35 and gestational diabetes in a prior pregnancy. In North America, gestational diabetes develops in about 4% of pregnancies; however, it increases to 7% in the Caucasian population. Today, pregnant women with risk factors for type 2 diabetes (e.g., obesity, family history) should be screened for undiagnosed type 2 diabetes at the first prenatal visit. Pregnant women without type 2 diabetes should be screened for diabetes at 24 to 28 weeks by checking for elevated blood glucose concentration 1 to 2 hours after consuming 75 grams of glucose (see Further Reading 16). If gestational diabetes is detected, a special diet that distributes low glycemic load carbohydrates throughout the day needs to be implemented. Sometimes insulin injections or oral medications are also needed. Regular physical activity also helps control blood glucose.

The primary risk of uncontrolled diabetes during pregnancy is that the fetus can grow quite large. This is a result of the oversupply of glucose from maternal circulation coupled with an increased production of insulin by the fetus, which allows fetal tissues to take up an increased amount of building materials for growth. The mother may require a Cesarean section if the size of the fetus is not compatible with a vaginal delivery. Another threat is that the infant may have low blood glucose at birth, because of the tendency to produce extra insulin that began during gestation. Other concerns are the potential for early delivery and increased risk of birth trauma and malformations. Although gestational diabetes often disappears after the infant's birth, it increases the mother's risk of developing diabetes later in life, especially if she fails to maintain a healthy body weight. Studies show that infants of mothers with gestational diabetes may also have higher risks of developing obesity and type 2 diabetes as they grow to adulthood. For all these reasons, proper control of gestational diabetes (and any diabetes present in the mother before pregnancy) is extremely important.

Pregnancy-Induced Hypertension

Pregnancy-induced hypertension is a high-risk disorder that occurs in about 3% to 5% of pregnancies. In its mild forms, it is also known as *preeclampsia* and, in severe forms, as *eclampsia*. Early symptoms include a rise in blood pressure, excess protein in the urine, edema, changes in blood clotting, and nervous system disorders. Very severe effects, including convulsions, can occur in the second and third trimesters. If not controlled, eclampsia eventually damages the liver and kidneys, and mother and fetus may die. The populations most at risk for this disorder are women under age 17 or over age 35, overweight or obese women, and those who have had multiple-birth pregnancies. A family history of pregnancy-induced hypertension in the mother's or father's side of the family, diabetes, African-American race, and a woman's first pregnancy also raise risk.

Pregnancy-induced hypertension resolves once the pregnancy ends, making delivery the most reliable treatment for the mother. However, because the problem often begins before the fetus is ready to be born, physicians in many cases must use treatments to prevent the worsening of the disorder. Bed rest and magnesium sulfate are the most effective treatment methods, although their effectiveness varies. Magnesium likely acts to relax blood vessels, and so leads to a fall in blood pressure. There is good evidence of the role of adequate calcium intake in reducing incidence of pregnancy-induced hypertension. However, results of a recent trial showed that vitamin C and E supplementation during pregnancy is not effective in preventing the disorder. Several other treatments, such as various antiseizure and antihypertensive medications, fish oils, selenium, and vitamin D are under study (see Further Reading 6).

gestational diabetes A high blood glucose concentration that develops during pregnancy and returns to normal after birth; one cause is the placental production of hormones that antagonize the regulation of blood glucose by insulin.

pregnancy-induced hypertension A serious disorder that can include high blood pressure, kidney failure, convulsions, and even death of the mother and fetus. Although its exact cause is not known, an adequate diet (especially adequate calcium intake) and prenatal care may prevent this disorder or limit its severity. Mild cases are known as *preeclampsia;* more severe cases are called *eclampsia* (formerly called *toxemia*).

CRITICAL THINKING

Sandy, 4 months pregnant, has been having heartburn after meals, constipation, and difficult bowel movements. As a student of nutrition, you understand the digestive system and the role of nutrition in health. What remedies might you suggest to Sandy to relieve her problems?

CONCEPT CHECK

Heartburn, constipation, hemorrhoids, nausea and vomiting, edema, anemia, and gestational diabetes are possible discomforts and complications of pregnancy. Changes in food habits can often ease these problems. Pregnancy-induced hypertension, with high blood pressure and kidney failure, can lead to severe complications or even death of the mother and fetus if not treated.

14.7 Breastfeeding

Breastfeeding the new infant further fosters his or her health, and so complements the attention given to diet during pregnancy. The American Dietetic Association and the American Academy of Pediatrics (AAP) recommend breastfeeding exclusively for the first 6 months, with the continued combination of breastfeeding and infant foods until 1 year (see Further Readings 2 and 4). The World Health Organization goes beyond that to recommend breastfeeding (with appropriate solid food introduction; see Chapter 15) for at least 2 years. Still, surveys show that only about 70% of North American mothers now begin to breastfeed their infants in the hospital, and at 4 and 6 months only 33% and 20%, respectively, are still breastfeeding their infants. The number falls to 18% at 1 year of age. These statistics refer to Caucasian women; minority women are even less likely to be breastfeeding at these time intervals.

Women who choose to breastfeed usually find it an enjoyable, special time in their lives that strengthens the bond with their new infant. Although bottle feeding with an infant formula is also safe for infants, as discussed in Chapter 15, it does not equal the benefits derived from human milk in all aspects. If a woman doesn't breastfeed her child, breast weight returns to normal soon after birth.

Planning to Breastfeed

Almost all women are physically capable of breastfeeding their children (see later section "Medical Conditions Precluding Breastfeeding" for exceptions). In most cases, problems encountered in breastfeeding are due to a lack of appropriate information. Anatomical problems in breasts, such as inverted nipples, can be corrected during pregnancy. Breast size generally increases during pregnancy and is no indication of success in breastfeeding. Most women notice a dramatic increase in the size and weight of their breasts by the third or fourth day of breastfeeding. If these changes do not occur, a woman needs to speak with her physician or a lactation consultant.

Breastfed infants must be followed closely over the first days of life to ensure that feeding and weight gain are proceeding normally. Monitoring is especially important with a mother's first child, because the mother will be inexperienced with the technique of breastfeeding. Mothers and healthy infants are commonly discharged from the hospital 1 to 2 days after delivery, whereas 20 years ago they stayed in the hospital for 3 or 4 days or longer. One result of such rapid discharge is a decreased period of infant monitoring by health care professionals. Incidents have been reported of infants developing dehydration and, in turn, blood clots soon after hospital discharge when breastfeeding did not proceed smoothly. Careful monitoring in this first week by a physician or lactation consultant is advised.

First-time mothers who plan to breastfeed should learn as much as they can about the process early in their pregnancy. Interested women should learn the proper technique, what obstacles to anticipate, and how to respond to them. Overall, breastfeeding is a learned skill, and mothers need knowledge to breastfeed, especially with the first child.

Many of the benefits of breastfeeding can be found in Table 14-5 and at www.womenshealth.gov/Breastfeeding/index.cfm, sponsored by the U.S. Surgeon General.

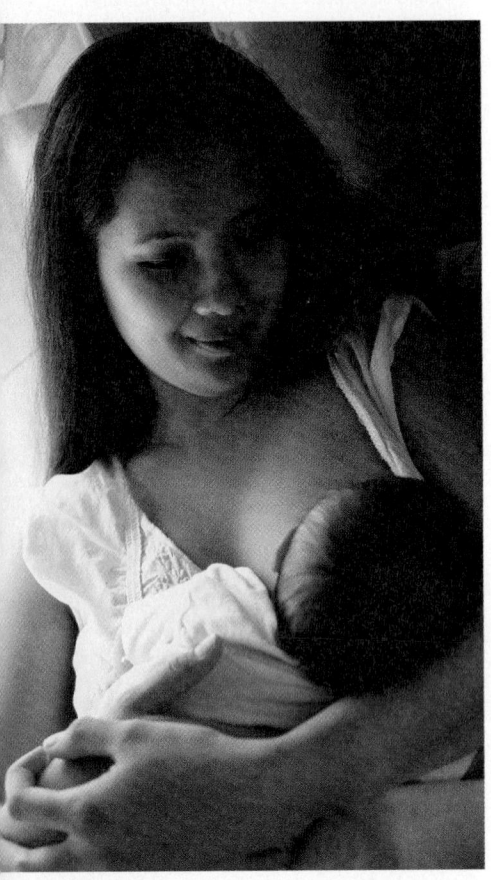

▲ Breastfeeding is the preferred way to feed a young infant.

Healthy People 2020 has set a goal of 82% of women breastfeeding their infants at time of hospital discharge, 60% breastfeeding for 6 months, and 34% still breastfeeding at 1 year.

Production of Human Milk

During pregnancy, cells in the breast form milk-producing cells called **lobules** (Fig. 14-7). Hormones from the placenta stimulate these changes in the breast. After birth, the mother produces more **prolactin** hormone to maintain the changes in the breast and therefore the ability to produce milk. During pregnancy, breast weight increases by about 1 to 2 pounds.

The hormone prolactin also stimulates the synthesis of milk. Infant suckling stimulates prolactin release from the pituitary gland. Milk synthesis then occurs as an infant nurses. The more the infant suckles, the more milk is produced. Because of this, even twins (and triplets) can be breastfed adequately.

Most protein found in human milk is synthesized by breast tissue. Some proteins also enter the milk directly from the mother's bloodstream. These proteins include immune factors (e.g., antibodies) and enzymes. Fats in human milk come from both the mother's diet and those synthesized by breast tissue. The sugar galactose is synthesized in the breast, whereas glucose enters from the mother's bloodstream. Together, these sugars form lactose, the main carbohydrate in human milk.

Let-Down Reflex

An important brain-breast connection—commonly called the **let-down reflex**—is necessary for breastfeeding. The brain releases the hormone **oxytocin** to allow the breast tissues to let down (release) the milk from storage sites (Fig. 14-8). It then travels to the nipple area. A tingling sensation signals the let-down reflex shortly before milk flow begins. If the let-down reflex doesn't operate, little milk is available to the infant. The infant then gets frustrated, and this can frustrate the mother.

The let-down reflex is easily inhibited by nervous tension, a lack of confidence, and fatigue. Mothers should be especially aware of the link between tension and a weak let-down reflex. They need to find a relaxed environment where they can breastfeed.

lobules Saclike structures in the breast that store milk.

prolactin A hormone secreted by the pituitary gland that stimulates the synthesis of milk in the breast.

let-down reflex A reflex stimulated by infant suckling that causes the release (ejection) of milk from milk ducts in the mother's breasts; also called *milk ejection reflex*.

oxytocin A hormone secreted by the pituitary gland. It causes contraction of the muscle-like cells surrounding the ducts of the breasts and the smooth muscle of the uterus.

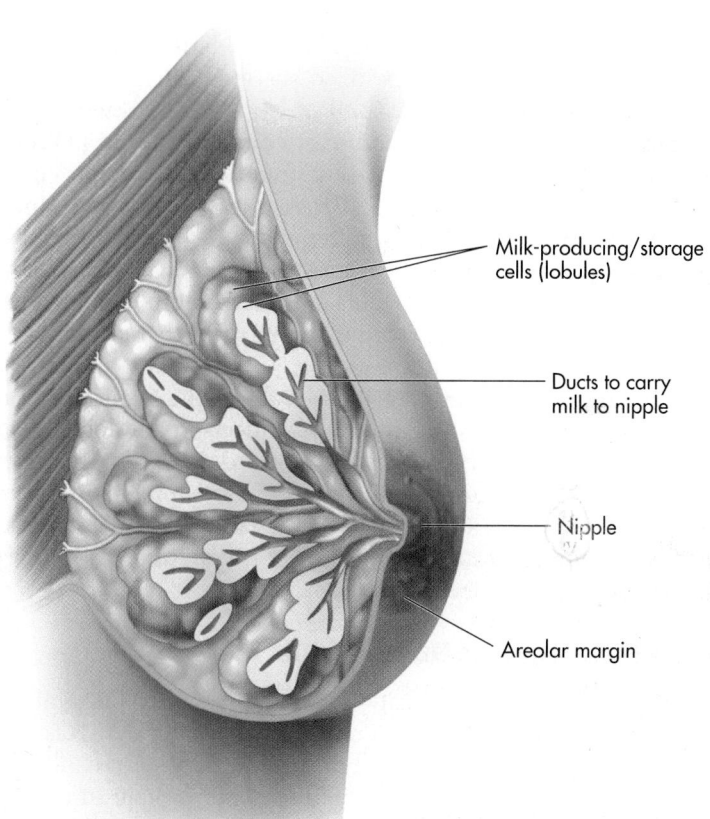

FIGURE 14-7 ▶ The anatomy of the breast. Many types of cells form a coordinated network to produce and secrete human milk.

Milk-producing/storage cells (lobules)

Ducts to carry milk to nipple

Nipple

Areolar margin

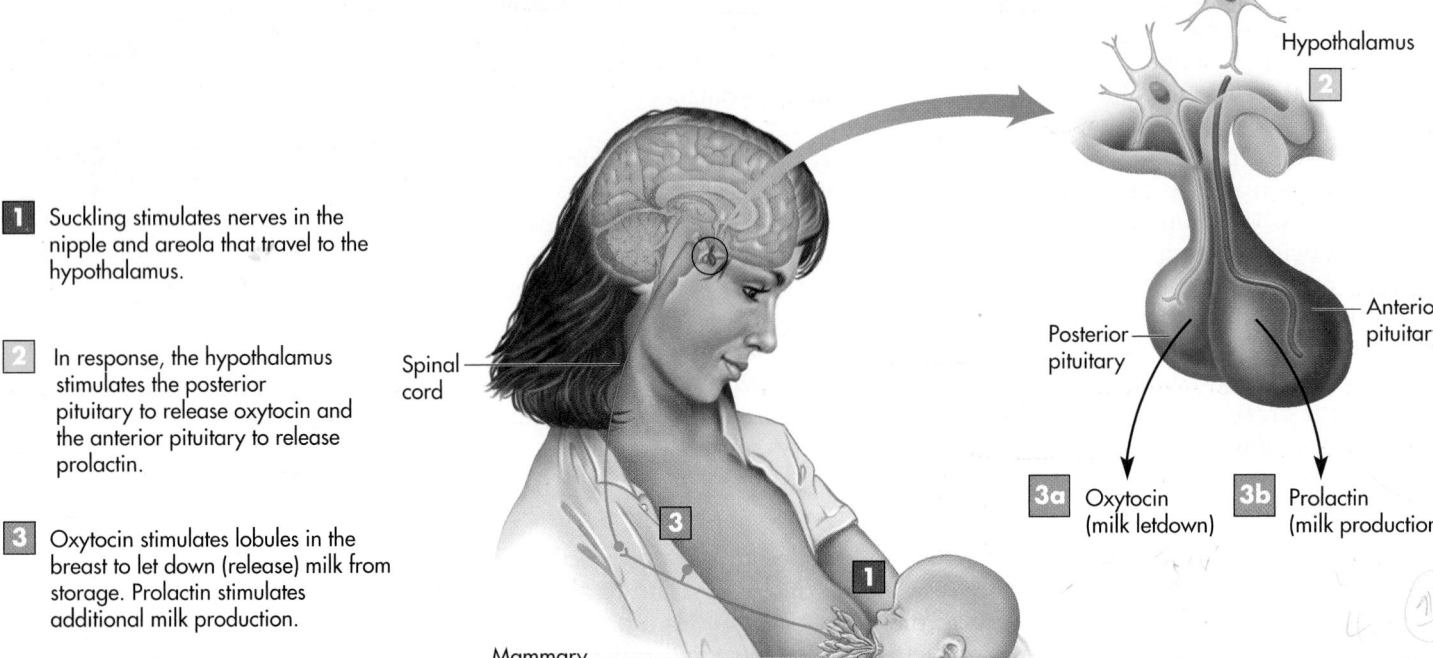

1 Suckling stimulates nerves in the nipple and areola that travel to the hypothalamus.

2 In response, the hypothalamus stimulates the posterior pituitary to release oxytocin and the anterior pituitary to release prolactin.

3 Oxytocin stimulates lobules in the breast to let down (release) milk from storage. Prolactin stimulates additional milk production.

FIGURE 14-8 ▶ Let-down reflex. Suckling sets into motion the sequence of events that lead to milk let-down, the flow of milk into ducts of the breast.

Disposable diapers can absorb so much urine that it is difficult to judge when they are wet. A strip of paper towel laid inside a disposable diaper makes a good wetness indicator. Alternatively, cloth diapers may be used for a day or two to assess whether nursing is supplying sufficient milk.

After a few weeks, the let-down reflex becomes automatic. The mother's response can be triggered just by thinking about her infant or seeing or hearing another one cry. At first, however, the process can be a bit bewildering. A mother cannot measure the amount of milk the infant takes in, so she may fear that she is not adequately nourishing the infant.

As a general rule, a well-nourished breastfed infant should (1) have three to five wet diapers per day by 3 to 5 days of age and four to six wet diapers per day thereafter, (2) show a normal weight gain, and (3) pass at least one or two stools per day that look like lumpy mustard. In addition, softening of the breast during the feeding helps indicate that enough milk is being consumed. Parents who sense their infant is not consuming enough milk should consult a physician immediately because dehydration can develop rapidly. Losing more than 7% of birth weight is an indicator of a feeding problem that requires intervention.

It generally takes 2 to 3 weeks to fully establish the feeding routine: Infant and mother both feel comfortable, the milk supply meets infant demand, and initial nipple soreness disappears. Establishing the breastfeeding routine requires patience, but the rewards are great. The adjustments are easier if supplemental formula feedings are not introduced until breastfeeding is well established, after at least 3 to 4 weeks. Then it is fine if a supplemental bottle or two of infant formula per day is needed, but supplemental feedings will decrease milk production.

Nutritional Qualities of Human Milk

Human milk is different in composition from cow's milk. Unless altered, cow's milk should never be used in infant feeding until the infant is at least 12 months old. Cow's milk is too high in minerals and protein and does not contain enough carbohydrate to meet infant needs. In addition, the major protein in cow's milk is harder for an infant to digest than the major proteins in human milk. The proteins in cow's milk also may spur allergies in the infant. Finally, certain compounds in human milk presently under study show other possible benefits for the infant.

Colostrum. At the end of pregnancy, the first fluid made by the human breast is **colostrum.** This thick, yellowish fluid may leak from the breast during late pregnancy and is produced in earnest for a few days to a week after birth. Colostrum contains antibodies and immune system cells, some of which pass unaltered through the infant's immature GI tract into the bloodstream. The first few months of life are the only time when we can readily absorb whole proteins across the GI tract. These immune factors and cells protect the infant from some GI tract diseases and other infectious disorders, compensating for the infant's immature immune system during the first few months of life.

One component of colostrum, the *Lactobacillus bifidus* **factor,** encourages the growth of *Lactobacillus bifidus* bacteria. These bacteria limit the growth of potentially toxic bacteria in the intestine. Overall, breastfeeding promotes the intestinal health of the breastfed infant in this way.

Mature Milk. Human milk composition gradually changes until it achieves the normal composition of mature milk several days after delivery. Human milk looks very different from cow's milk. (Table 15-1 in Chapter 15 provides a direct comparison.) Human milk is thin and almost watery in appearance and often has a slightly bluish tinge. Its nutritional qualities, however, are impressive.

Human milk's proteins form a soft, light curd in the infant's stomach and are easy to digest. Some human milk proteins bind iron, reducing the growth of iron-requiring bacteria, some of which can cause diarrhea. Still other proteins offer the important immune protection already noted.

The lipids in human breast milk are high in linoleic acid and cholesterol, needed for brain development. Breast milk also contains long-chain omega-3 fatty acids, such as docosahexaenoic acid (DHA). This polyunsaturated fatty acid is used for the synthesis of tissues in the brain and the rest of the central nervous system and in the retina of the eye.

The fat composition of human milk changes during each feeding. The consistency of milk released initially (fore milk) resembles that of skim milk. It later has a greater fat proportion, similar to whole milk. Finally, the milk released after 10 to 20 minutes (hind milk) is essentially like cream. Babies need to nurse long enough (e.g., a total of 20 or more minutes) to get the calories in the rich hind milk to be satisfied between feedings and to grow well. The overall calorie content of human milk is about the same as that of infant formulas (67 kcal per 100 milliliters).

Human milk composition also allows for adequate fluid status of the infant, provided the baby is exclusively breastfed. A question commonly asked is whether the infant needs additional water if stressed by hot weather, diarrhea, vomiting, or fever. The AAP recommends against supplemental water or juice during the first 6 months of life. The practice may unnecessarily introduce pathogens or allergens. Excessive water can lead to brain disorders, low blood sodium, and other problems. Thus, supplemental water and juice should be given only with a physician's guidance before 6 months of age.

Food Plan for Women Who Breastfeed

Nutrient needs for a breastfeeding mother change to some extent from those of the pregnant woman in the second and third trimester (see the inside cover of this book). There is a decrease in folate and iron needs and an increase in the needs for calories, vitamins A, E, and C, riboflavin, copper, chromium, iodide, manganese, selenium, and zinc. Still, these increased needs of the breastfeeding mother will be met by the general diet plan proposed for a woman in the latter stages of pregnancy. Recall that each day of this diet plan includes at least:

- 3 cups of calcium-rich foods such as from the dairy group or use of calcium-fortified foods to make up for any gap between calcium intake and need
- 6 ½ ounce-equivalents from the protein group
- 3 ½ cups from the vegetables group

colostrum The first fluid secreted by the breast during late pregnancy and the first few days after birth. This thick fluid is rich in immune factors and protein.

Lactobacillus bifidus **factor** A protective factor secreted in the colostrum that encourages growth of beneficial bacteria in the newborn's intestines.

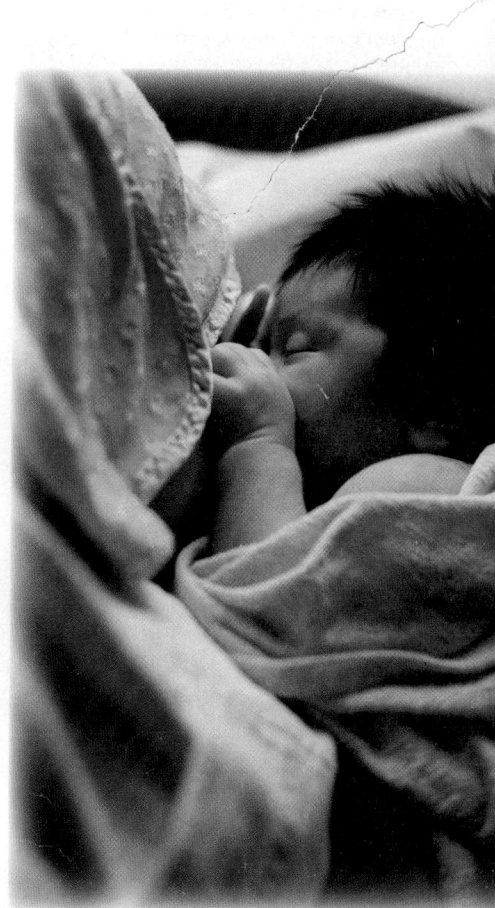

▲ Breastfeeding promotes the intestinal health of the breastfed infant.

Most substances that the mother ingests are secreted into her milk. For this reason, she should limit intake of or avoid all alcohol and caffeine and check all medications with a pediatrician. Some mothers believe that certain foods, such as garlic and chocolate, flavor the breast milk and upset the infant. If a woman notices a connection between a food she eats and the infant's later fussiness, she could consider avoiding that food. However, she might experiment again with it later, as infants become fussy for other reasons. Some researchers, on the other hand, feel that the passage of flavors from the mother's diet into her milk affords an opportunity for the infant to learn about the flavor of the foods of its family long before solids are introduced. These researchers suspect that bottle-fed infants are missing significant sensory experiences that, until recent times in human history, were common to all infants.

- 2 cups from the fruits group
- 9 ounce-equivalents from the grains group
- 8 teaspoons of vegetable oil

Foods containing solid fats and added sugars (up to about 360 kcal) can then be added to allow for weight maintenance or gradual weight loss, whichever is needed.

Table 14-4 provided a menu for such a plan. Substituting a soyburger (veggie burger) for the hamburger in that menu would make this a practical guide for a lacto-vegetarian woman as well.

As in pregnancy, a serving of a highly fortified ready-to-eat breakfast cereal (or use of a balanced multivitamin and mineral supplement) is advised to help meet extra nutrient needs. And, as mentioned for pregnant women, breastfeeding mothers should consume fish at least twice a week (or 1 gram per day of omega-3 fatty acids from a fish oil supplement) because the omega-3 fatty acids present in fish are secreted into breast milk and are likely to be important for development of the infant's nervous system.

Milk production requires approximately 800 kcal every day. The Estimated Energy Requirement during lactation is an extra 400 to 500 kcal daily above prepregnancy recommendations. The difference between that needed for milk production and the recommended intake—about 300 kcal—should allow a gradual loss of the extra body fat accumulated during pregnancy, especially if breastfeeding is continued for 6 months or more and the woman performs some physical activity. This shows just one of the natural benefits of following pregnancy with at least several months of breastfeeding.

After giving birth, women are often eager to shed the excess "baby fat." Breastfeeding, however, is no time for crash diets. A gradual weight loss of 1 to 4 pounds per month by the nursing mother is appropriate. At significantly greater rates of weight loss—when calories are restricted to less than about 1500 kcal per day—milk output decreases. A reasonable approach for a breastfeeding mother is to eat a balanced diet that supplies at least 1800 kcal per day; has moderate fat content; and includes a variety of dairy products, fruits, vegetables, and whole grains.

To promote the best possible feeding experience for the infant, there are several other dietary factors to consider. Hydration is especially important during breastfeeding; the woman should drink fluids every time her infant nurses. Drinking about 13 cups of fluids per day encourages ample milk production. Poor health habits, such as smoking cigarettes or drinking more than two alcoholic drinks a day, can decrease milk output. (Even less alcohol can have a deleterious effect on milk output in some women.) To avoid exposure to harmful levels of mercury, precautions concerning fish likely to contain mercury should extend past pregnancy for the breastfeeding mother. There is no evidence that maternal diet restrictions (e.g., peanuts, eggs, fish) during pregnancy or breastfeeding prevent food allergies in their infants. The AAP recommends exclusive breastfeeding and delaying introduction of solid foods until 4 to 6 months of age as the best approaches for preventing **atopic diseases** (see Further Reading 9).

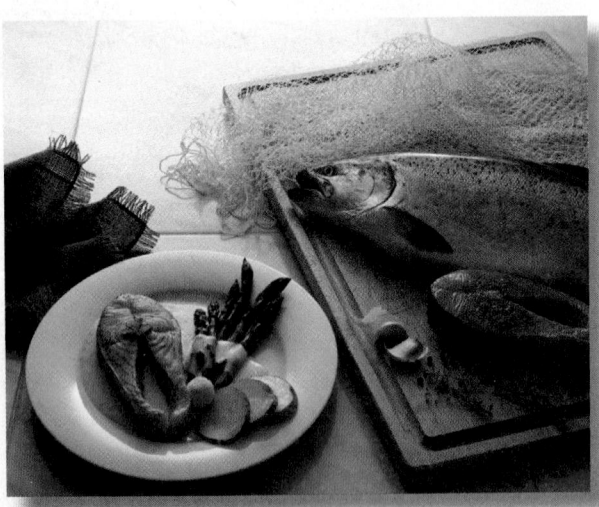

▲ Eating fish at least twice a week will help breastfeeding women ensure that their infants receive important omega-3 fatty acids. It is important, however, to avoid those fish likely to be contaminated with mercury (swordfish, shark, king mackerel, and tile fish).

atopic disease Condition resulting from an inappropriate immune response, such as asthma, allergic rhinitis, food allergies, or eczema.

CONCEPT CHECK

Recognition of the importance of breastfeeding has contributed to its greater popularity. Almost all women have the ability to breastfeed. The hormone prolactin stimulates breast tissue to synthesize milk. Infant suckling triggers a let-down reflex, which releases the milk. The more an infant nurses, the more milk is synthesized. Some components of human milk come directly from the mother's bloodstream. The nutrient composition of human milk is different from that of cow's milk and changes as the infant matures. The first fluid produced, colostrum, is rich in immune factors. The mother's diet during breastfeeding is generally similar to that for pregnancy, except for necessary additional fluids.

Breastfeeding Today

As noted, the vast majority of women are capable of breastfeeding and their infants benefit from it (see Table 14-5 and Further Reading 18). Nonetheless, some circumstances may make breastfeeding impractical or undesirable for a woman. Mothers who don't want to breastfeed their infants should not feel pressured to do so. Breastfeeding provides advantages, but none so great that a woman who decides to bottle feed should feel she is compromising her infant's well being.

Advantages of Breastfeeding. Human milk is tailored to meet infant nutrient needs for the first 4 to 6 months of life. However, there are some cases when infant dietary supplements, used under a pediatrician's guidance, are recommended:

- The AAP recommends all infants, including exclusively breastfed infants, be given 400 IU of vitamin D per day, beginning shortly after birth and continuing until the infant consumes that much from food (e.g., at least 2 cups (0.5 liters) of infant formula per day). Some sun exposure also helps in meeting vitamin D needs.
- Iron supplements are generally necessary for infants who were preterm, LBW, have blood disorders, or who were born with low iron stores.
- The AAP does not advise fluoride supplements before 6 months of age. After 6 months, the pediatrician or dentist may recommend supplemental fluoride if the infant's intake of fluoridated water, food sources, and use of toothpaste is insufficient.
- Vitamin B-12 supplements are recommended for the breastfed infant whose mother is a complete vegetarian (vegan).

Fewer Infections. Due in part to the antibodies in human milk, breastfeeding reduces the infant's overall risk of developing infections (see Further Reading 7). Breastfed

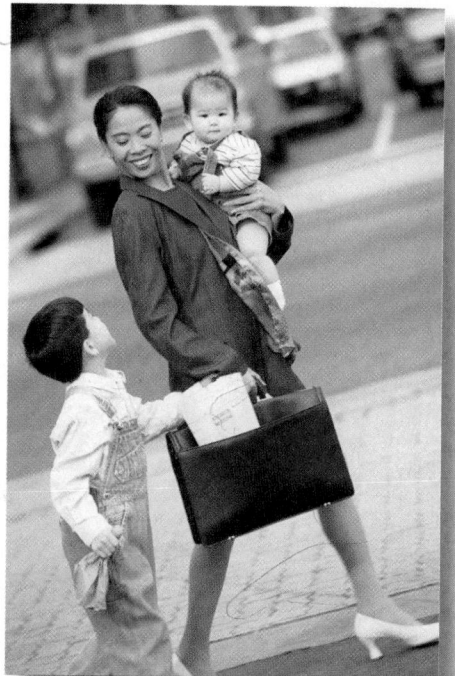

▲ Mothers who return to work outside the home can continue to breastfeed with the aid of a breastpump. In 2010, President Obama signed an amendment to the Fair Labor Standards Act that requires most U.S. employers to allow break time and a private setting for breastfeeding mothers to express milk.

TABLE 14-5 Advantages of Breastfeeding

For Infant
• Bacteriologically safe
• Always fresh and ready to go
• Provides antibodies and substances that contribute to maturation of the immune system
• Contributes to maturation of gastrointestinal tract via *Lactobacillus bifidus* factor; decreases incidence of diarrhea and respiratory disease
• Reduces risk of food allergies and intolerances, as well as some other allergies
• Establishes habit of eating in moderation, linked to 20% lower risk of obesity later in life
• Contributes to proper development of jaws and teeth for better speech development
• Decreases ear infections
• May enhance nervous system development (by providing DHA) and eventual learning ability
• May reduce the risk of chronic diseases (e.g., hypertension and diabetes)

For Mother
• Contributes to earlier recovery from pregnancy due to the action of hormones that promote a quicker return of the uterus to its prepregnancy state
• Decreases the risk of ovarian and premenopausal breast cancer
• Potential for quicker return to prepregnancy weight
• Potential for delayed ovulation, thus reducing chances of pregnancy in the short term

infants also have fewer ear infections (otitis media) because they do not sleep with a bottle in their mouths. Experts strongly discourage allowing any infants to sleep with a bottle in their mouths; milk can pool in the mouth, throat, and inner ear, creating a growth medium for bacteria. By reducing these common infections parents can decrease discomfort for the infant, avoid related trips to the doctor, and prevent possible hearing loss. Tooth decay from nighttime bottles is another likely consequence of sleeping with a bottle in the mouth (see Chapter 15).

Fewer Allergies and Intolerances. Breastfeeding also reduces the chances of some allergies, especially in allergy-prone infants (see Chapter 15). The key time to attain this benefit from breastfeeding is during the first 4 to 6 months of an infant's life. A longer commitment is best, but breastfeeding for even a few weeks is beneficial. Infants are also better able to tolerate human milk than formulas. Formulas sometimes must be switched several times until caregivers find the best one for the infant.

Convenience and Cost. Breastfeeding frees the mother from the time and expense involved in buying and preparing formula and washing bottles. Human milk is ready to go and sterile. This allows the mother to spend more time with her baby.

Possible Barriers to Breastfeeding. Widespread misinformation, the mother's need to return to a job, and social reticence serve as barriers to breastfeeding.

Misinformation. The major barriers to breastfeeding are misinformation, such as the idea that one's breasts are too small, and the lack of role models. One positive note has been the widespread increase in the availability of lactation consultants over the past several years. First-time mothers who are interested in breastfeeding can find invaluable support from lactation consultants or by talking to women who have experienced it successfully. In almost every community, a group called La Leche League offers classes in breastfeeding and advises women who have problems with it (800-LALECHE or www.lalecheleague.org). Online resources are listed in the margin.

Return to an Outside Job. Working outside the home can complicate plans to breastfeed. One possibility after a month or two of breastfeeding is for the mother to express and save her own milk. She can use a breast pump or manually express milk into a sterile plastic bottle or nursing bag (used in a disposable bottle system). Saving human milk requires careful sanitation and rapid chilling. It can be stored in the refrigerator for 3 to 5 days or be frozen for 3 to 6 months. Thawed milk should be used within 24 hours. There is a knack to learning how to express milk, but the freedom can be worth it, because it allows others to feed the infant the mother's milk. A schedule of expressing milk and using supplemental formula feedings is most successful if begun after 1 to 2 months of exclusive breastfeeding. After 1 month or so, the baby is well adapted to breastfeeding and probably feels enough emotional security and other benefits from nursing to drink both ways.

Some women can juggle both a job and breastfeeding, but others find it too cumbersome and decide to formula-feed. A compromise—balancing some breastfeedings, perhaps early morning and night, with infant formula feedings during the day—is possible. However, too many supplemental infant formula feedings decrease milk production.

Social Concerns. Another barrier for some women is embarrassment about nursing a child in public. Historically, our society has stressed modesty and has discouraged public displays of breasts—even for as good a cause as nourishing babies. In the United States, no state or territory has a law prohibiting breastfeeding. However, indecent exposure (including the exposure of women's breasts) has long been a common law or statutory offense. Now, 45 states, the District of Columbia, and the Virgin Islands have specific laws that protect a woman's right to breastfeed in any location. Women who feel reluctant should be reassured that they do have social support and that breastfeeding can be done discreetly with little breast exposure.

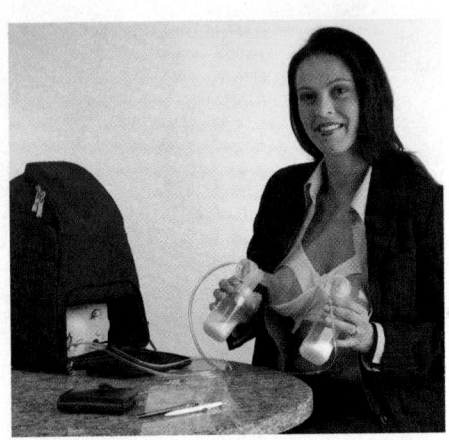

▲ Breast milk can be expressed by the mother using a manual, battery-operated, or electric (shown) breast pump. The expressed milk can be stored for times when the mother is not available to breastfeed the infant.

Useful breastfeeding resources on the Web:

www.lalecheleague.org

www.breastfeeding.com

www.breastfeeding.org

nal.usda.gov/wicworks

www.cdc.gov/breastfeeding

www.usbreastfeeding.org

www.breastfeedinginc.ca

Nipple piercings should have no impact on a woman's ability to breastfeed, but the jewelry should be removed before each feeding. Repeated removal and reinsertion of the jewelry may be inconvenient and irritating, so it may be best to leave the jewelry out for the entire period of breastfeeding. Breast tattoos will not impair breastfeeding, either. However, getting a new nipple piercing or breast tattoo while breastfeeding is not advised due to the pain of healing and possibility of infection. Past breast augmentation or reduction surgeries may impair a woman's ability to breastfeed if milk-producing tissue was damaged during the surgery.

Medical Conditions Precluding Breastfeeding. Breastfeeding may be ruled out by certain medical conditions in either the infant or mother. For example, breastfeeding is contraindicated for infants with galactosemia, an inherited disorder in which the body cannot break down galactose. Recall from Chapter 4 that lactose, the main carbohydrate in human breast milk, is made of glucose and galactose. When galactose is not properly broken down, its by-products can damage body organs.

Certain medications, which pass into the milk and adversely affect the nursing infant, are best avoided while breastfeeding. In addition, a woman in North America or other developed region of the world who has a serious chronic disease (such as tuberculosis, AIDS, or HIV-positive status) or who is being treated with chemotherapy medications should not breastfeed.

Environmental Contaminants in Human Milk. There is some legitimate concern over the levels of various environmental contaminants in human milk. However, the benefits of human milk are well established and the risks from environmental contaminants are still largely theoretical. Thus, it is probably best to continue with what has been shown to work until sufficiently strong research data contradict it. A few measures a woman could take to counteract some known contaminants are to (1) consume a variety of foods within each food group; (2) avoid freshwater fish from polluted waters; (3) carefully wash and peel fruits and vegetables; and (4) remove the fatty edges of meat, as pesticides concentrate in fat. In addition, a woman should not try to lose weight rapidly while nursing (more than ¾ to 1 pound per week) because contaminants stored in her fat tissue might then enter her bloodstream and affect her milk. If a woman questions whether her milk is safe, especially if she has lived in an area known to have a high concentration of toxic wastes or environmental pollutants, she should consult her local health department.

Phenylketonuria (PKU), a disorder of phenylalanine metabolism described in Chapter 6, was once thought to be a contraindication for breastfeeding. However, with complementary use of specialized phenylalanine-free formulas, infants with PKU can now enjoy the health and emotional benefits of breastfeeding.

MAKING DECISIONS

Breast Milk for Preterm Infants

There is no universal answer to whether a woman can breastfeed a preterm infant. In some cases, human milk is the most desirable form of nourishment, depending on infant weight and length of gestation. If so, it must usually be expressed from the breast and fed through a tube until the infant's sucking and swallowing reflex develops. This type of feeding demands great maternal dedication. Fortification of the milk with such nutrients as calcium, phosphorus, sodium, and protein is often necessary to meet the needs of a rapidly growing preterm infant. In other cases, special feeding problems may prevent the use of human milk or necessitate supplementing it with specialized formula. Sometimes total parenteral nutrition (intravenous feeding) is the only option. Working as a team, the pediatrician, neonatal nurses, and registered dietitian must guide the parents in this decision.

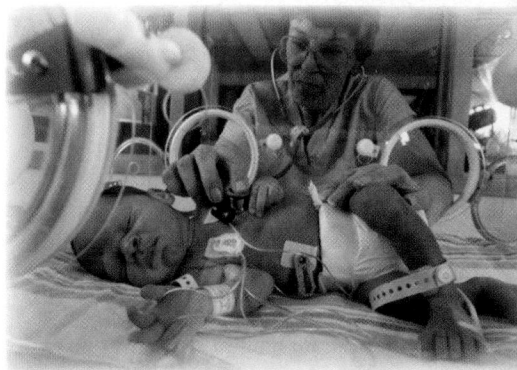

▲ If human milk is used to feed the preterm infant, fortification of the milk with certain nutrients is often needed.

CONCEPT CHECK

Human milk supplies most of an infant's nutritional needs for the first 6 months, although supplementation with vitamin D, iron, and fluoride may be needed. Breastfeeding is often more convenient than formula feeding. Compared with formula-fed infants, breastfed infants have fewer intestinal, respiratory, and ear infections and are less susceptible to some allergies and food intolerances. Despite the advantages of breastfeeding, misinformation, job responsibilities, and social reticence may dissuade a mother from breastfeeding. A combination of breastfeeding and formula feeding is possible when a mother is regularly away from the infant and is not able to express and store her milk for later use. Breastfeeding is not desirable if a mother has certain diseases or must take medication potentially harmful to the infant. The preterm infant, depending on its condition, may benefit from consuming human milk.

Preventing Birth Defects

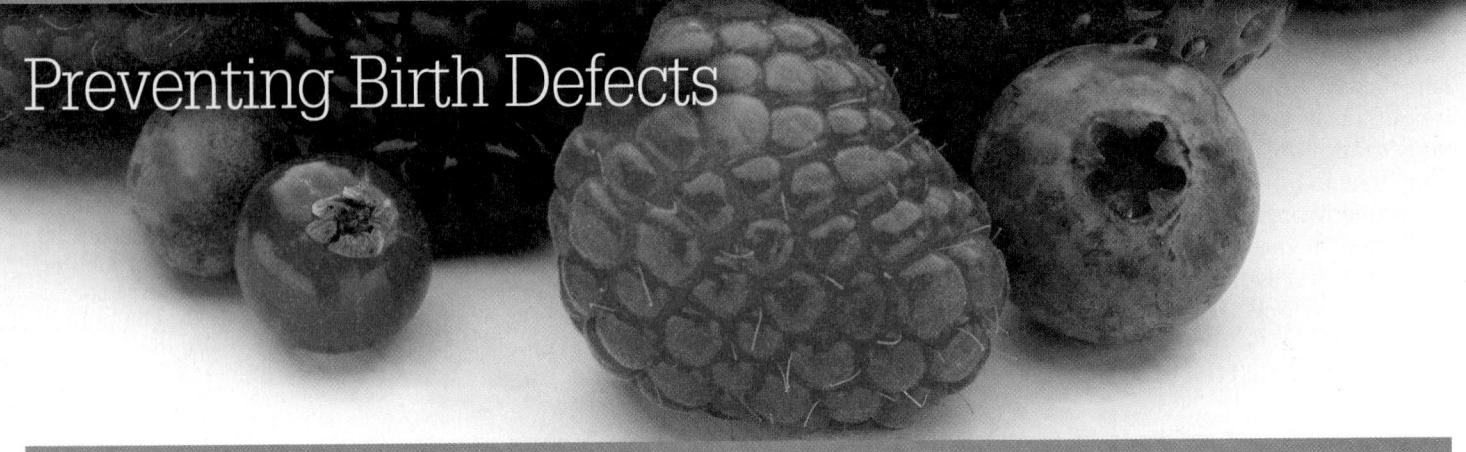

Eating well for a healthy pregnancy not only supplies materials for fetal growth and development, but also helps to direct the amazing process of building a new life. Considering the complexity of the human body and its more than 20,000 genes, it's not surprising that abnormalities of structure, function, or metabolism are sometimes present at birth. Birth defects impact one of every 33 babies born in the United States. In some cases, they are so severe that a baby cannot survive or thrive. Birth defects are the presumed cause of many spontaneous abortions and are at the root of about 20% of infant deaths before one year of age. However, with medical intervention, many babies with birth defects can go on to live healthy and productive lives.

A wide range of physical or mental disabilities result from birth defects. Heart defects are present in approximately 1 of every 100 to 200 newborn babies, accounting for a large proportion of infant deaths. Cleft lip and/or cleft palate are malformations of the lip or roof of the mouth and occur in approximately 1 in 700 to 1000 births. Neural tube defects are malformations of the brain or spinal cord that occur in early stages of pregnancy, during embryonic development. Examples include spina bifida, in which all or part of the spinal cord is exposed, and anencephaly, in which some or all of the brain is missing. Babies born with spina bifida can survive to adulthood, but in many cases, have extreme disabilities. Babies born with anencephaly die soon after birth. Neural tube defects occur in 1 in 1000 births. Down syndrome, a condition in which an extra chromosome

leads to mental retardation and other physical alterations, occurs in about 1 in 800 births. Other common birth defects include musculoskeletal defects, gastrointestinal defects, and metabolic disorders.

What causes a birth defect? About 15%–25% of birth defects are known to be genetic (i.e., inherited or spontaneous mutations of the genetic code). Another 10% are due to environmental influences (e.g., exposure to **teratogens**). The specific cause of the remaining 65%–75% of birth defects is unknown. Although the etiology of birth defects is multifactorial and many elements are beyond human control, good nutrition practices are an important way a mother-to-be can have a positive influence on the outcome of her pregnancy.

Folic Acid

During the 1980s, researchers in the United Kingdom noticed a relationship between poor dietary habits and a high rate of neural tube defects among children of impoverished women. Subsequent intervention studies demonstrated that administration of a multivitamin supplement during the periconceptional period—the months before conception and during early pregnancy—reduced the recurrence of these birth defects. The specific link between dietary folic acid and neural tube defects was tested and confirmed in several follow-up studies. As you learned in Chapter 8, folate plays a leading role in the synthesis of DNA and the metabolism of amino acids. The rapid cell growth of pregnancy increases needs for folate during pregnancy to 600 micrograms DFE per day. Some women, for genetic reasons,

may have an even higher requirement. Adequate folic acid in the periconceptional period decreases the risk of neural tube defects by about 70% and has also been associated with decreased risk of cleft lip/palate, heart defects, and Down syndrome.

In 1998, the FDA mandated fortification of grain products to provide 140 micrograms of folic acid per 100 grams of grain consumed. In Canada, the level of fortification is 150 micrograms of folate per 100 grams of grain consumed. In general, this increases the average consumption of dietary folic acid by 100 micrograms per day.

A well-planned diet can meet the RDA for folic acid, but the U.S. Public Health Service and the March of Dimes recommend that all women of childbearing age take a daily multivitamin and mineral supplement that contains 400 micrograms of folic acid. A physician may recommend prenatal vitamins or a higher dose of folic acid for some women, particularly those who have had a prior pregnancy complicated by a neural tube defect. The Dietary Guidelines for Americans recommend that women who may become pregnant and those in the first few months of pregnancy consume an adequate amount of the synthetic form of folate, folic acid (Table 14-3).

teratogen A substance that may cause or increase the risk of a birth defect. Exposure to a teratogen does not always lead to a birth defect; its effects on the fetus depend on the dose, timing, and duration of exposure.

Iodide

The relationship between folic acid and neural tube defects is a dramatic example of how a nutrient deficiency can negatively impact pregnancy outcome, but it is not the only nutrient of concern. Low iodide status during the first trimester of pregnancy—a critical period of brain development—may lead to cretinism (see Further Reading 20). This is a congenital form of hypothyroidism that leads to diminished physical and mental development if left untreated. When the defect is identified early (by newborn screening tests), cretinism can be prevented by treatment with thyroid hormones. With use of iodized salt, however, iodide deficiencies are rare.

Antioxidants

A case can be made for antioxidants in the prevention of birth defects as well. Free radicals are constantly generated within the body as a result of normal metabolic processes. An abundance of free radicals results in damage of cells and their DNA, which can lead to gene mutations or tissue malformations. Some research points to free radicals as a source of damage during embryo development and organogenesis. Antioxidant systems within the body act to minimize the damage caused by free radicals, and researchers hypothesize that dietary sources of antioxidants may aid in the prevention of birth defects. At this time, there is insufficient evidence to support supplementation of individual nutrients that participate in antioxidant systems—vitamin E, vitamin C, selenium, zinc, and copper—for the prevention of birth defects. However, use of a balanced multivitamin and mineral supplement while consuming a diet rich in whole grains, legumes, and a variety of fruits and vegetables will provide enough of these nutrients to meet current recommendations.

Vitamin A

Whereas the needs for most vitamins and minerals increase by about 30% during pregnancy, the requirement for vitamin A increases by only 10%. Studies have shown the teratogenic potential of vitamin A in doses as low as approximately 3000 micrograms RAE per day. This is just over three times the RDA of 770 micrograms RAE/per day for pregnant adult women.

Fetal abnormalities resulting from vitamin A toxicity primarily include facial and cardiac defects, but a wide range of defects have been reported. It is rare that food sources of vitamin A would lead to toxicity. Recall from Chapter 8 that preformed vitamin A is found in liver, fish, fish oils, fortified milk and yogurt, and eggs. Carotenoids, found in fruits and vegetables, are precursors of vitamin A that are converted to vitamin A in the small intestine. However, the efficiency of absorption of carotenoids decreases as intake increases. Vitamin A excesses typically arise from high-dose dietary supplements rather than food sources. Typical North American diets supply adequate vitamin A from foods, so supplemental use is not generally necessary. During pregnancy, supplemental preformed vitamin A should not exceed 3000 micrograms RAE per day (15,000 IU per day). Most multivitamins and prenatal vitamins supply less than 1500 micrograms RAE per day. A balanced diet and prudent use of dietary supplements are actions that can sidestep potential problems with vitamin A toxicity.

Caffeine

Caffeine has been scrutinized for its safety during pregnancy, especially for any link with rate of birth defects. Caffeine decreases the mother's absorption of iron and may reduce blood flow through the placenta. In addition, the fetus is unable to detoxify caffeine. Research shows that as caffeine intake increases, so does the risk of miscarriage or delivering an LBW infant. Heavy caffeine use during pregnancy may also lead to caffeine withdrawal symptoms in the newborn. These risks are reported with caffeine intakes in excess of 500 milligrams, or the equivalent of about 5 cups of coffee per day. Moderate use of caffeine (up to the equivalent of 3 cups of coffee per day), however, is not associated with risk for birth defects. Based on current evidence, drinking no more than three cups of coffee and no more than four cups of caffeinated soft

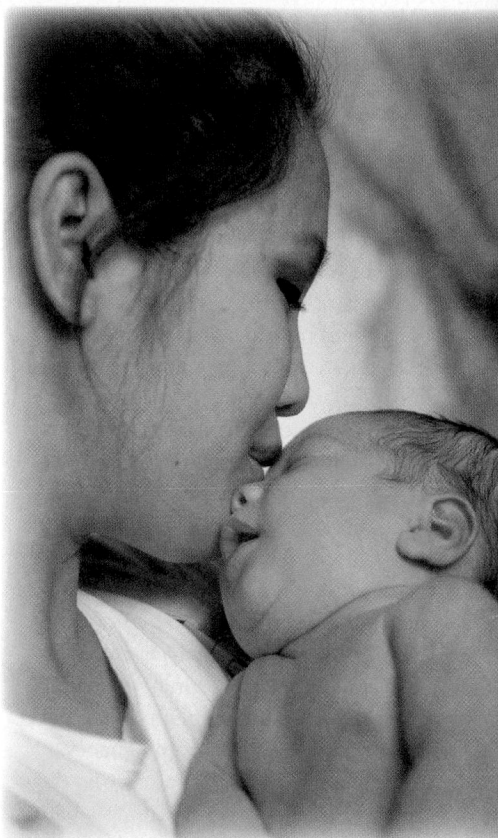

▲ Delivering a healthy baby is more than just luck. Many nutrition- and health-related practices need to be considered.

drinks per day during pregnancy (or when pregnancy is possible) is advocated. Paying attention to caffeine intake from tea, over-the-counter medicines containing caffeine, and chocolate is also important.

Aspartame

Phenylalanine, a component of the artificial sweetener aspartame (NutraSweet® and Equal®), causes concern for some pregnant women. High amounts of phenylalanine in maternal blood disrupt fetal brain development if the mother has a disease known as *phenylketonuria* (see next section). If the mother does not have this condition, however, it is unlikely that the baby will be affected by moderate aspartame use.

For most adults, diet soft drinks are the primary source of artificial sweeteners. Of greater concern than the safety of sweeteners during pregnancy is the quality of foods and beverages consumed. A high intake of diet soft drinks may crowd out healthier beverages, such as water and low-fat milk.

Obesity and Chronic Health Conditions

Even before becoming pregnant, women of childbearing age should have regular medical checkups to keep an eye on any health conditions that already exist or to identify any developing health problems. In some cases, the condition itself increases risk for birth defects. Obesity, high blood pressure, and uncontrolled diabetes are common health problems known to increase the risk for birth defects, including neural tube defects. In other cases, medications used to control illnesses may pose a risk to the developing fetus. Other health issues, such as seizure disorders and metabolic disorders, could also affect fetal development. A preconception visit with a health professional can help to sort out and make plans to minimize such risks. Once a woman has become pregnant, early and regular prenatal care can aid in the success of a pregnancy.

Women with diabetes are two to three times more likely to give birth to a baby with birth defects compared to women with normal glucose metabolism. Examples of birth defects common in this group include malformations of the spine, legs, and blood vessels of the heart. Some experts speculate that the mechanism by which diabetes increases birth defects is via excessive free radicals, which lead to oxidative damage of DNA during early gestation. Careful control of blood glucose drastically lowers risk for women with diabetes. Optimal blood glucose control can be achieved through a combination of dietary modifications and medications. Given that diabetes is on the rise among women of childbearing age, this elevated rate of birth defects has become an area of heightened awareness.

Another health condition for which maternal nutritional control is of utmost importance is PKU. Recall from Chapter 6 that PKU is an error of metabolism in which the liver lacks the ability to process phenylalanine, leading to an accumulation of this amino acid and its metabolites in body tissues. Babies born to women who have phenylketonuria that is not controlled by diet are at heightened risk for brain defects, such as microcephaly and mental retardation (see Further Reading 1).

Alcohol

Conclusive evidence shows that repeated consumption of four or more alcoholic drinks at one sitting harms the fetus (see Further Reading 12). Such binge drinking is especially perilous during the first 12 weeks of pregnancy, as this is when critical early developmental events take place in utero. Although scientists don't know whether pregnant women must totally eliminate alcohol use to avoid risk of damage to the fetus, women are advised not to drink any alcohol during pregnancy or when there is a chance pregnancy might occur—until a safe level can be established. The embryo (and, at later stages, the fetus), has no means of detoxifying alcohol.

Women with chronic alcoholism produce children with a variety of physical and intellectual problems collectively called **fetal alcohol spectrum disorders (FASDs)**. The most severe of these disorders is **fetal alcohol syndrome (FAS)**. A diagnosis of FAS is based mainly on poor fetal and infant growth, physical deformities (especially of facial features), and mental retardation (Fig. 14-9). Irritability, hyperactivity, short attention span, and limited hand-eye coordination are other symptoms of FAS. Defects in vision, hearing, and mental processing may also develop over time. Other FASDs consist of some but not all of the defects of FAS. **Alcohol-related neurodevelopmental disorders (ARNDs)** include behavior and learning problems resulting from exposure to alcohol in utero. **Alcohol-related birth defects (ARBDs)** typically include malformations of the heart, kidneys, bones, and/or ears.

Exactly how alcohol causes these defects is not known. One line of research suggests that alcohol, or products produced by the metabolism of alcohol (e.g., acetaldehyde), cause faulty movement of cells in the brain during early stages of nerve cell development or block the action of certain brain neurotransmitters. In addition, inadequate nutrient intake, reduced nutrient and oxygen transfer across the placenta, cigarette smoking commonly associated with alcohol intake, drug use, and possibly other factors contribute to the overall result.

The Dietary Guidelines for Americans recommend that alcoholic beverages not be consumed by pregnant women (Table 14-3). For more information about fetal alcohol syndrome, visit the website www.cdc.gov/ncbddd/fasd/.

Environmental Contaminants

There is little evidence to link birth defects with the amounts of pesticides, herbicides, or other contaminants in foods or public water supplies in North America. However, evaluating such a link can be methodologically difficult and many would argue that regulations concerning contaminants in the food and water supply are too permissive. Thus, it seems prudent to take measures to decrease intake of pesticides and herbicides wherever possible. For fruits and vegetables, peeling, removing outer leaves, and/or thoroughly rinsing and scrubbing with a brush under running water will remove the majority of contaminants. In animal products, pesticides and other contaminants are most likely to accumulate in fatty tissues. Therefore, removing skin, discarding drippings, and trimming visible fat will decrease exposure from meat, poultry, and fish.

For fish, mercury is of particular concern because it can harm the nervous system of the fetus. Thus, FDA warns pregnant women to avoid swordfish, shark, king mackerel, and tile fish because of possible high mercury contamination. Largemouth bass are also implicated. In general, intake of other fish and shellfish

▶ A goal of *Healthy People 2020* is 98.3% abstinence from alcohol, cigarettes, and illicit drugs by pregnant women, a 10% improvement over current statistics.

fetal alcohol spectrum disorders (FASDs) A group of irreversible physical and mental abnormalities in the infant that result from the mother's consuming alcohol during pregnancy.

fetal alcohol syndrome (FAS) Severe form of FASD that involves abnormal facial features and problems with development of the nervous system and overall growth as a result of maternal alcohol consumption during pregnancy.

should not exceed 12 ounces per week. Canned albacore tuna is a potential mercury source, so it should not be consumed in amounts exceeding 6 ounces per week. As a rule of thumb, consuming a variety of foods minimizes risk of exposure to contaminants from the food supply.

Summing Up

Although many risk factors for birth defects are beyond our control, a woman of childbearing potential can make some wise nutrition choices to improve her chances of having a healthy baby without birth defects. A varied and balanced diet, such as the food plan for pregnant women described in this chapter, along with a daily multivitamin and mineral supplement with 400 micrograms of folic acid will ensure adequate nutrient status. It is estimated that daily use of a multivitamin and mineral supplement containing folic acid will decrease the rate of all birth defects by 50%. Discuss use of any other

dietary supplements with a physician to be sure that the fetus will not be exposed to toxic levels of vitamin A or other dangerous ingredients. Early and consistent prenatal care can help control obesity and any chronic health conditions that may complicate a pregnancy. Also, avoiding alcohol during pregnancy will eliminate any risk for fetal alcohol spectrum disorders.

Although it seems that advice for a healthy pregnancy is always directed at the mother, fathers-to-be are not off the hook. Health is a family affair, so encouraging healthy eating habits and avoiding smoking and alcohol are important for fathers, too. Less research has been done in the area, but the genetics of the baby are certainly an outcome of both parents. Indeed, inadequate supplies of zinc, folate, and vitamin C affect the quality of sperm, which may impair fertility. Considering that spermatogenesis takes approximately 70 days, the periconceptional period is a time for good nutrition and careful lifestyle practices for the father as well.

▶ In North America, maternal death as a result of childbirth is uncommon—only about 11 deaths in every 100,000 live births. The infant mortality rate, however, is much higher: for each 100,000 live births, about 600 to 700 infants die within the first year. The infant death rate among African-Americans is more than double the rates among Whites and Hispanics in the United States.

▶ Pregnant women should recognize that many cough syrups contain alcohol. Cases have been reported of infants with FASDs born to mothers who consumed generous amounts of such cough syrups but no other alcoholic beverages.

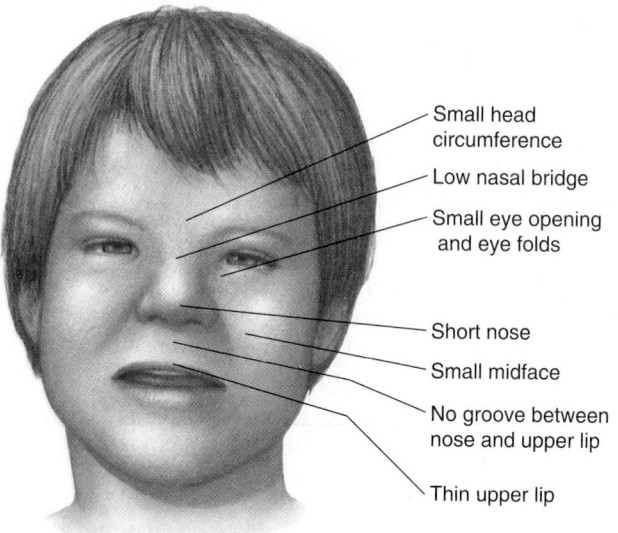

Small head circumference

Low nasal bridge

Small eye opening and eye folds

Short nose

Small midface

No groove between nose and upper lip

Thin upper lip

FIGURE 14-9 ▶ Fetal alcohol syndrome. The facial features shown are typical of affected children. Additional abnormalities in the brain and other internal organs accompany fetal alcohol syndrome but are not immediately apparent from simply looking at the child. Milder forms of alcohol-induced changes from a lower alcohol exposure to the fetus are known as alcohol-related neurodevelopmental disorders (ARNDs) and alcohol-related birth defects (ARBDs).

Case Study Preparing for Pregnancy

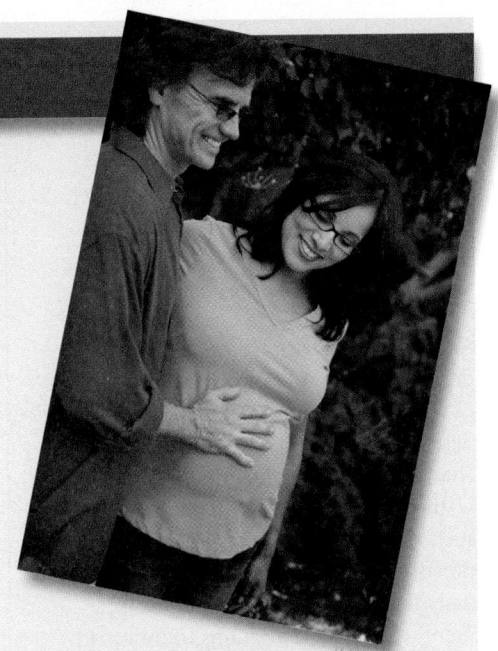

Lily and her husband have decided that they are ready to prepare for Lily's first pregnancy. She is 25 years old, weighs 135 pounds, and is 67 inches tall. Lily has been reading everything she can find on pregnancy because she knows that her prepregnancy health is important to the success of her pregnancy.

She knows she should avoid alcohol, especially because alcohol is potentially toxic to the growing fetus in the first weeks of pregnancy, and she could become pregnant and not know about it right away. Lily is not a smoker, does not take any medications, and limits her coffee intake to 4 cups a day and soft drink intake to 3 colas per day. Based on her reading, she has decided to breastfeed her infant and has already inquired about childbirth classes. She has modified her diet to include some extra protein, along with more fruits and vegetables. She has also started taking an over-the-counter vitamin and mineral supplement. Lily has always kept in good shape, and

she is admittedly worried about gaining too much weight during pregnancy. Recently, she started a running program 5 days a week, and she plans to continue running throughout her pregnancy.

Answer the following questions, and check your responses in Appendix A.

1. What recommendations do you have regarding Lily's use of dietary supplements?
2. What is Lily doing to prevent neural tube defects? What else could she do?
3. What recommendations would you make regarding Lily's caffeine consumption?
4. Lily is wise to pay attention to her protein intake to prepare for pregnancy and breastfeeding. Should she include fish as a source of protein in her diet? Why or why not?
5. Constipation is a common complaint during pregnancy. What suggestions do

you have to help Lily avoid this health concern?
6. What information would you share with Lily about appropriate weight gain during pregnancy?

Summary (Numbers refer to numbered sections in the chapter.)

14.1 The best time to prepare for pregnancy is before conception even occurs. Achieving a healthy body weight, avoiding toxic agents, correcting nutritional deficiencies, and controlling existing medical conditions will set the stage for a successful pregnancy.

14.2 Pregnancy is arbitrarily divided into three trimesters of 13 to 14 weeks each. The first trimester is characterized by a rapid increase in cell number as the zygote grows to be an embryo, then a fetus. During the first trimester, the growing organism is most susceptible to damage from exposure to toxic agents or nutrient deficiencies. By the start of the second trimester, the organs and limbs have formed and will continue to grow and develop. The third trimester is marked by rapid fetal growth and storage of nutrients in preparation for life outside the womb.

14.3 A successful pregnancy results in optimal health for both the infant and

the mother. Pregnancy success is defined as (1) gestation longer than 37 weeks and (2) birth weight greater than 5.5 pounds (2.5 kilograms). Factors that predict pregnancy success include early and regular prenatal care, maternal age within the range of 20 to 35 years, and adequate nutrition. Factors that contribute to poor pregnancy outcome include inadequate prenatal care, obesity, underweight, teenage pregnancy, smoking, alcohol consumption, use of certain prescription medications and all illicit drugs, inadequate nutrition, heavy caffeine use, and various infections, such as listeriosis.

14.4 For women with a healthy prepregnancy BMI (18.5 to 24.9), total weight gain should be within the range of 25 to 35 pounds. Underweight women and those carrying multiple fetuses should gain more; overweight and obese women should gain less. During the first trimester, although she need not increase diet

quantity, the woman should focus on diet quality to meet increased requirements for protein, carbohydrate, essential fatty acids, fiber, water, and many vitamins and minerals. A woman typically needs an additional 350 to 450 kcal per day during the second and third trimesters.

14.5 Following a plan based on the Dietary Guidelines for Americans as exemplified by MyPlate is recommended for pregnant and breastfeeding women. The mother-to-be should especially emphasize good sources of vitamin B-6, folate, iron, zinc, and calcium. Vegetarian diets are safe during pregnancy, but vegan mothers should specifically seek out good sources of vitamin B-12 and vitamin D. Prenatal multivitamin and mineral supplements are useful for meeting increased nutrient requirements during pregnancy.

14.6 Pregnancy-induced hypertension, gestational diabetes, heartburn, constipation, nausea, vomiting, edema, and anemia are all possible discomforts and complications of pregnancy. Nutrition therapy can help minimize some of these problems.

14.7 Almost all women are able to breastfeed their infants. The nutritional composition of human milk is different from that of unaltered cow's milk and is much more desirable for the infant.

For the infant, the advantages of breastfeeding over formula feeding are numerous, including fewer intestinal, respiratory,

and ear infections and fewer allergies and food intolerances. Benefits for the mother include reduced risk of certain cancers, earlier recovery from pregnancy, and faster return to prepregnancy weight. For mothers who choose not to breastfeed or in medical situations that contraindicate breastfeeding (e.g., galactosemia), infants can be adequately nourished with formula.

N&YH There are several steps pregnant women can take to help prevent birth

defects. Achieve a healthy body weight before pregnancy and strive to gain weight within the ranges recommended by the Institute of Medicine. Adequate intakes of folic acid, iodide, and antioxidant nutrients are essential for prevention of many types of birth defects. Excesses of vitamin A and caffeine should be avoided. There is no safe level of alcohol intake known during pregnancy. Dietary control of diseases (e.g., diabetes and PKU) will also protect the fetus.

Check Your Knowledge (Answers to the following multiple choice questions are below.)

1. The fetus is most susceptible to damage from nutrient deficiencies; teratogens; and use of certain medications, alcohol, and illicit drugs during
   a. the first trimester.
   b. the second trimester.
   c. the third trimester.
   d. labor and delivery.

2. An infant born at 38 weeks' gestation weighing 5.0 pounds can be described as
   a. preterm.   c. SGA.
   b. LBW.   d. LBW and SGA.

3. If a woman is 5'2" and weighs 150 pounds before becoming pregnant, how much weight should she gain during pregnancy?
   a. 28 to 40 pounds (12.5 to 18 kilograms)
   b. 25 to 35 pounds (11.5 to 16 kilograms)
   c. 15 to 25 pounds (7 to 11.5 kilograms)
   d. As little as possible

4. Increased carbohydrate needs during pregnancy are set to
   a. prevent ketosis.
   b. alleviate nausea.

   c. prevent pregnancy-induced hypertension.
   d. supply adequate folate.

5. Which of the following is best paired with an iron supplement during pregnancy?
   a. skim milk
   b. orange juice
   c. coffee
   d. tea

6. A food plan for a woman in the third trimester of pregnancy differs from her prepregnancy diet in that
   a. fluid needs are higher.
   b. additional solid fats and added sugars are allowed.
   c. there are more servings from the grains group.
   d. All of the above.

7. Consuming one cup of coffee per day is associated with
   a. spontaneous abortions.
   b. LBW.
   c. birth defects.
   d. None of the above.

8. Which of the following may help to alleviate nausea during pregnancy?

   a. postponing meals until the afternoon
   b. drinking large amounts of water
   c. postponing use of iron supplements until the second trimester
   d. All of the above.

9. Which of the following conditions medically prevents a woman from breastfeeding her infant?
   a. breasts are too small
   b. infant has galactosemia
   c. inverted nipples
   d. None of the above.

10. Physiologically, milk production requires _____ kcals per day.
    a. 300
    b. 500
    c. 800
    d. 1000

Answer Key: 1. a (LO 14.2), 2. d (LO 14.2), 3. c (LO 14.3), 4. a (LO 14.1), 5. b (LO 14.5), 6. d (LO 14.4), 7. d (LO 14.2), 8. c (LO 14.6), 9. b (LO 14.7), 10. c (LO 14.4)

Study Questions (Numbers refer to Learning Outcomes)

1. Provide three key pieces of advice for parents seeking to maximize their chances of having a healthy infant. Why did you identify those specific factors? (LO 14.2)

2. Outline current weight-gain recommendations for pregnancy. What is the basis for these recommendations? (LO 14.3)

3. Identify four key nutrients for which intake should be significantly increased during pregnancy. (LO 14.1)

4. Describe a diet based on the Dietary Guidelines as exemplified by MyPlate that meets the increased nutrient needs of pregnancy. (LO 14.4)

5. Why does teenage pregnancy receive so much attention these days? At what age do you think pregnancy is ideal? Why? (LO 14.2)

6. Give three reasons a woman should give serious consideration to breastfeeding her infant. (LO 14.7)

7. Describe the physiological mechanisms that stimulate milk production and release. How can knowing about these help mothers breastfeed successfully? **(LO 14.7)**

8. Describe two nutrients that may require supplementation during pregnancy and give reasons for each. **(LO 14.5)**

9. How should the basic food plan suitable for pregnancy be modified during breastfeeding? **(LO 14.4)**

10. What nutrition advice would you give to a friend who suffers from morning sickness? **(LO 14.6)**

What Would You Choose Recommendations

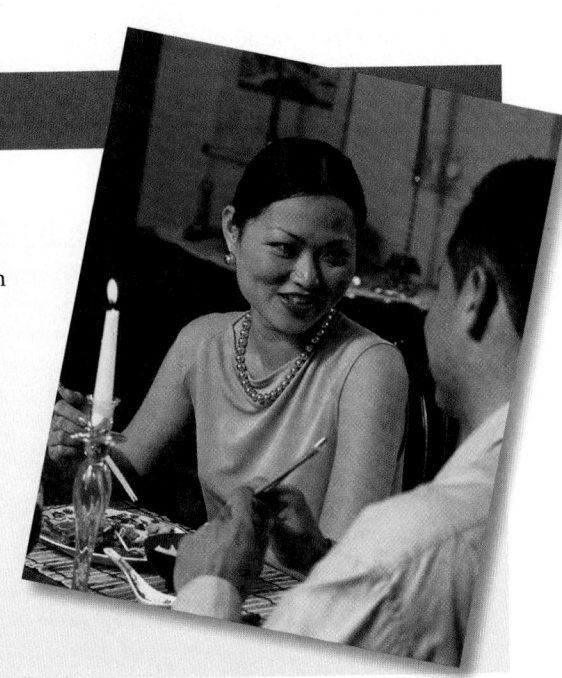

The spinach salad meal with hard-boiled egg and whole-wheat roll provides only about 2 grams of iron. It is a healthy, nutrient-dense choice that provides some protein, but does not make a significant contribution to meeting iron needs.

A hamburger is a source of iron—this meal would provide about 4.5 milligrams of iron—but it would not be a choice for a person who follows a vegetarian diet.

The bean and cheese taco option provides just as much iron (4.5 milligrams) as the hamburger meal and would be appropriate for a vegetarian.

Even though the nonheme iron in beans is not as well absorbed as the heme iron in beef, the 20 milligrams of vitamin C in the stewed tomatoes will enhance iron absorption.

All of these meals, however, pale in comparison to the iron contribution of the fortified, ready-to-eat breakfast cereal. One cup of Kellogg's Smart Start cereal provides 18 milligrams of iron, and the 72 milligrams of vitamin C in 1 cup of orange juice will enhance iron absorption. In one easy meal, any pregnant woman could obtain more than half of the 27-milligram RDA for iron during pregnancy.

Further Readings

1. AAP Committee on Genetics: Policy Statement: Maternal phenylketonuria. *Pediatrics* 122:445, 2008.

   Uncontrolled maternal phenylketonuria (PKU) leads to exposure of the fetus to elevated phenylalanine levels in the blood, which can lead to birth defects, poor physical growth, and altered brain development. All girls and women with PKU should be educated and counseled throughout life about controlling phenylalanine levels to minimize risks during pregnancy.

2. AAP Section on Breastfeeding: American Academy of Pediatrics Policy Statement: Breastfeeding and the use of human milk. *Pediatrics* 115:496, 2005.

   AAP firmly supports breastfeeding as the ideal nutrition for infants. A few contraindications to breastfeeding are discussed, such as HIV infection and galactosemia. Exclusive breastfeeding is recommended for the first 6 months of life. Breastfeeding should continue with age-appropriate introduction of complementary solid foods until 1 year of age or longer. Guidelines are provided for infant nutrient supplementation.

3. ADA Reports: Position of the American Dietetic Association: Nutrition and lifestyle for a healthy pregnancy outcome. *Journal of the American Dietetic Association* 108:553, 2008.

   The key components of a healthy lifestyle during pregnancy include appropriate weight gain; consumption of a variety of foods; appropriate and timely vitamin and mineral intake; avoidance of alcohol, tobacco, and other harmful substances; and safe food handling. Supplementation is appropriate for some nutrients.

4. James DC and others: Position of the American Dietetic Association: Promoting and supporting breastfeeding. *Journal of the American Dietetic Association* 109:1926, 2009.

   The American Dietetic Association strongly supports the breastfeeding of infants. This article discusses the benefits of breastfeeding for the mother and infant, as well as dietary considerations that need to be addressed, such as avoiding consumption of species of fish known to contain high amounts of mercury.

5. Barger MK. Maternal nutrition and perinatal outcomes. *Journal of Midwifery and Women's Health* 55:502, 2010.

   This review details the roles and requirements of various nutrients during pregnancy with an emphasis on the developmental origins of disease hypothesis. Nutritional status influences infant growth, length of gestation, and several pregnancy complications, such as gestational diabetes and preeclampsia.

6. Bodnar LM and others: Periconceptional multivitamin use reduces the risk of preeclampsia. *American Journal of Epidemiology* 164:470, 2006.

   In the Pregnancy Exposures and Preeclampsia Prevention Study, women who regularly consumed a multivitamin during the periconceptional period had a 45% lower risk of developing preeclampsia during their first pregnancy than those who did not consume multivitamins. Women with BMI less than 25 benefited most from multivitamin use.

7. Field CJ: The immunological components of human milk and their effect on immune development in infants. *Journal of Nutrition* 135:1, 2005.

   Human milk contains many factors that improve immune function in the infant. This article reviews a number of these complex factors.

8. Fraser A and others: Associations of gestational weight gain with maternal body mass index, waist circumference, and blood pressure measured 16 years after pregnancy: The Avon Longitudinal Study of Parents and Children (ALSPAC). *American Journal of Clinical Nutrition* 93:1285, 2011.

Researchers examined long-term health effects of prepregnancy weight and gestational weight gain. Mothers with high prepregnancy BMI and gestational weight gain above recommended ranges had higher BMI, waist circumference, and blood pressure measurements 16 years after pregnancy. Of interest, even among women with normal prepregnancy weight, high rates of weight gain during midpregnancy were associated with higher blood pressure later in life. The results confirm that adherence to the 2009 IOM guidelines for prepregnancy weight and weight gain during pregnancy optimizes long-term maternal health.

9. Greer FR and others: Effects of early nutritional interventions on the development of atopic disease in infants and children: The role of maternal dietary restriction, breastfeeding, timing of introduction of complementary foods, and hydrolyzed formulas. *Pediatrics* 121:183, 2008.

The American Academy of Pediatrics revised previous recommendations for prevention of atopic disease. Current evidence does not support a role of maternal dietary restrictions in prevention of atopic disease in children. The best course of action for at-risk infants is to breastfeed exclusively and delay introduction of solid foods until 4 to 6 months of age. Delaying introduction of complementary feedings beyond 6 months is not advantageous.

10. Han Z and others: Maternal underweight and the risk of preterm birth and low birth weight: A systematic review and meta-analysis. *International Journal of Epidemiology* 40:65, 2011.

Despite the increasing prevalence of overweight and obesity among women of childbearing age, maternal underweight is related to higher risk of preterm birth and low birth weight.

11. Institute of Medicine and National Research Council: *Weight gain during pregnancy: Reexamining the guidelines.* Washington, DC: The National Academies Press, 2009.

Excess maternal weight affects the health of both the fetus (size at birth, gestational age, and impact on childhood obesity) and the mother (postpartum weight retention and requirement for surgical delivery). The revised guidelines for weight gain during pregnancy recommended relatively narrow ranges based on mother's prepregnancy BMI, which was found to be an important predictor of pregnancy outcome. New guidelines for obese mothers now advise a weight gain of only 11 to 20 pounds (5 to 9 kilograms). Provisional recommendations are given for women carrying multiple fetuses.

12. Jones KL: The effects of alcohol on fetal development. *Birth Defects Research (Part C)* 93:3, 2011.

This comprehensive review traces research on fetal alcohol spectrum disorders and describes its many physiological and neurological defects with color photos. Several maternal risk factors can increase risk for FASD, including maternal age >30 years, low socioeconomic status, previous children with FASD, genetics, and malnutrition.

13. Kelly, AKW: Practical exercise advice during pregnancy. *The Physician and Sports Medicine* 33(6):24, 2005.

It is safe for pregnant women to exercise if they are experiencing uncomplicated pregnancies. Most non-weight-bearing exercises (e.g., swimming) and walking are safe for pregnant women. Women should begin with 15 minutes of exercise three times a week and progress as tolerated.

14. Lucas RM and others: Future health implications of prenatal and early-life vitamin D status. *Nutrition Reviews* 66:710, 2008.

In addition to its role in bone health, preventive effects of vitamin D on autoimmune disorders, diabetes, cancer, cardiovascular disease, osteoporosis, and psychiatric illness are mediated by the vitamin's involvement in gene expression. Maternal vitamin D supplementation could lead to widespread improvements in public health.

15. Makrides M: Outcomes for mothers and their babies: Do n-3 long-chain polyunsaturated fatty acids and seafoods make a difference? *Journal of the American Dietetic Association* 108: 1622, 2008

Omega-3 fatty acids are important for brain and eye development of the fetus and infant. These fats have been implicated in prevention of preeclampsia, preterm birth, LBW, and SGA, but current evidence does not support supplementation for these purposes. Despite the importance of n-3 fatty acids for fetal development, many women have inadequate intakes of these fats. Available data indicate that pregnant and lactating women should aim to consume at least 200 milligrams per day of omega-3 fatty acids from dietary sources, including oily fish, eggs, and lean red meats.

16. Rubin RC: Change is good—evidence to support lowering the diagnostic threshold for GDM. *Today's Dietitian* 13:10, 2011.

Gestational diabetes may lead to macrosomia, birth injuries, and postnatal hypoglycemia for infants. For mothers, GDM increases risk of type 2 diabetes later in life. The American Diabetes Association updated its guidelines on diagnosis and treatment of GDM: high-risk women should be screened for undiagnosed type 2 diabetes at their first prenatal visit; all women should undergo a standardized 75-gram oral glucose tolerance test to screen for GDM between 24 and 28 weeks of gestation; after birth, mothers with GDM should be monitored for development of type 2 diabetes.

17. Tamura T, Picciano MF: Folate and human reproduction. *American Journal of Clinical Nutrition* 83:993, 2006.

Folic acid supplementation for the prevention of megaloblastic anemia and neural tube defects represents a major public health advancement. Folate status may also be linked to placental abruption, preeclampsia, spontaneous abortion, stillbirth, low birth weight, and risk for birth defects other than neural tube defects.

18. Taylor JS and others: A systematic review of the literature associating breastfeeding with type 2 diabetes and gestational diabetes. *Journal of the American College of Nutrition* 24:320, 2005.

Breastfed infants have lower rates of obesity, type 1 diabetes, and type 2 diabetes in adulthood compared to formula-fed infants. In addition, mothers who breastfeed have improved glucose tolerance and lower risk for postpartum diabetes compared to nonlactating mothers.

19. Ward EM: Prime the body for pregnancy—preconception care and nutrition for moms-to-be. *Today's Dietitian* 10:26, 2008.

Women of childbearing potential should take steps to ensure a healthy pregnancy before becoming pregnant. The article provides practical guidelines for intakes of key nutrients (e.g., folic acid and iron), supplement use, weight management, physical activity, and caffeine and alcohol consumption.

20. Zimmerman MB: Iodine deficiency in pregnancy and the effects of maternal iodine supplementation on the offspring: A review. *American Journal of Clinical Nutrition* 89(suppl):668S, 2009.

Iodine deficiency leads to cretinism or more subtle deficits in brain function. Recently, the World Health Organization augmented recommendations for iodine deficiency during pregnancy from 200 to 250 micrograms per day. Annual supplementation with 400 milligrams of iodine in the form of iodized oil or daily supplementation with potassium iodide are effective strategies for reducing maternal iodine deficiency and associated birth defects.

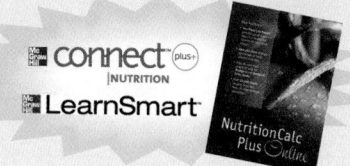

To get the most out of your study of nutrition, go to McGraw-Hill's online resources: Connect www.mcgrawhillconnect.com, where you will find NutritionCalc Plus, LearnSmart, and many other dynamic tools.

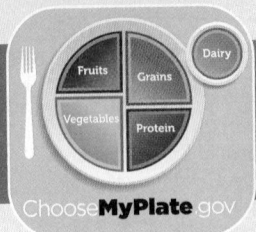
RATE YOUR PLATE

I. Targeting Nutrients Necessary for Pregnant Women

This chapter mentioned that pregnant women may have difficulty meeting their increased needs for folate, vitamin B-6, iron, and zinc. List six foods rich in each of these nutrients next to the appropriate heading. Refer to Chapters 8 and 9 if necessary.

Nutrient	Foods	Nutrient	Foods
Folate	_____	Iron	_____
	_____		_____
	_____		_____
	_____		_____
	_____		_____
	_____		_____
Vitamin B-6	_____	Zinc	_____
	_____		_____
	_____		_____
	_____		_____
	_____		_____
	_____		_____

1. Foods rich in more than one of these nutrients would be especially valuable for pregnant women. Write on the line any foods you listed that are good sources of more than one of these critical nutrients.

   _____

2. The needs for folate, vitamin B-6, iron, and zinc increase during pregnancy. For which of these nutrients can pregnant women usually obtain adequate intakes from dietary sources?

   _____

3. Which of these nutrients are commonly taken in supplement form during pregnancy?

   _____
   _____

4. Why might it be hard for pregnant women to meet their increased needs for these nutrients from food alone?

   _____
   _____
   _____

II. Putting Your Knowledge About Nutrition and Pregnancy to Work

A college friend, Angie, tells you that she is newly pregnant. You are aware that she usually likes to eat the following foods for her meals:

Breakfast

Skips this meal, or eats a granola bar
Coffee

Lunch

Sweetened yogurt, 1 cup
Small bagel with cream cheese
Occasional piece of fruit
Regular caffeinated soda, 12 ounces

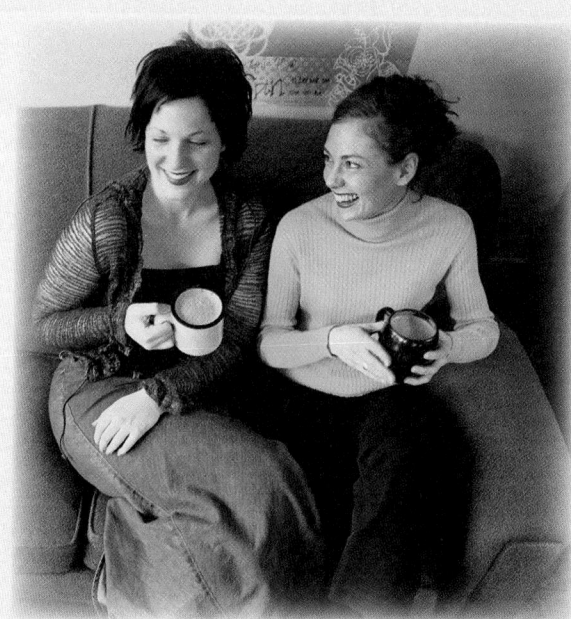

Snack

Chocolate candy bar

Dinner

2 slices of pizza, macaroni and cheese, or 2 eggs with 2 slices of toast
Seldom eats a salad or vegetable
Regular caffeinated soda, 12 ounces

Snacks

Pretzels or chips, 1 ounce
Regular caffeinated soda, 12 ounces

1. Using NutritionCalc Plus software, evaluate Angie's diet for protein, carbohydrate, folate, vitamin B-6, iron, and zinc. How does her intake compare with the recommended amounts for pregnancy?

   _____

   _____

   _____

2. Now redesign her diet and make sure that her intake meets pregnancy needs for protein, carbohydrate, folate, vitamin B-6, and zinc. (Hint: Fortified foods, such as breakfast cereal, are generally nutrient-rich foods, which can more easily help meet one's needs.) Increase the iron content as well, but it still may be below the RDA for pregnancy.

   _____

   _____

   _____

Chapter 15 Nutrition from Infancy Through Adolescence

Student Learning Outcomes

Chapter 15 is designed to allow you to:

15.1 Describe the extent to which nutrition affects infant and child growth and physiological development.

15.2 Identify diet guidelines to meet the basic nutritional needs for normal growth and development for an infant and discuss some do's and don'ts associated with infant feeding.

15.3 List several challenges parents might face in dealing with childhood eating habits.

15.4 List the nutrients often found to be lacking in the diets of infants, toddlers, preschoolers, and teenagers and make recommendations to remedy the problems.

15.5 Describe the long-term effects of childhood obesity and suggest ways to prevent or treat the problem.

15.6 Identify common food allergens and suggest several practices that may reduce the risk of developing a food allergy.

What Would You Choose?

Your brother and his wife have asked you to watch your 18-month-old niece, Lila, while they enjoy a weekend getaway at the lake to celebrate their anniversary. Before they drop her off, you make a trip to the grocery store to pick up some kid-friendly foods. Lila does not have any food allergies, but your brother warned you that she has gotten into some picky eating behaviors. Which of the following snack foods would you choose for your little houseguest?

a Reduced-fat popcorn

b Raw baby carrots with ranch dressing

c Fat-free light yogurt

d Whole-grain crackers with sliced cheddar cheese

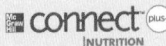 **connect** PLUS+ | NUTRITION

Think about your choice as you read Chapter 15, then see our recommendations at the end of the chapter. To learn more about appropriate feeding practices for infants and preschoolers, check out the Connect site: www. mcgrawhillconnect.com

Part Five
Nutrition: A Focus on Life Stages

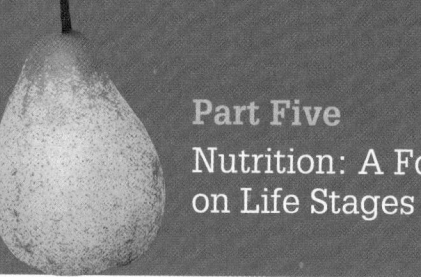

From infancy through adolescence, rapid growth dictates calorie, protein, vitamin, and mineral requirements. The growth rate of infants is the highest of any life stage, so nutrient needs per pound of body weight are highest. As a child gets older, the rate of growth slows and nutrient needs per pound of body weight decrease proportionately. As the chapter comic suggests, this can lead to picky eating behaviors, which can be a source of frustration for parents and other caregivers. Nonetheless, these early years of life are an important time to establish healthful eating and exercise habits.

Influences on eating behaviors shift over time. During infancy and early childhood, the family mostly controls food intake, informs food preferences, and models eating behaviors. For school-age children and adolescents, peer and media influences take on more importance. Education designed to change the nutrition habits of children should start early and involve the family. Whenever possible, families should share meals together. Family mealtimes help children establish healthy eating habits; aid in prevention of childhood obesity; and, as children grow older, teach communication skills and improve self-esteem. Chapter 15 examines the specific nutrition issues facing each of these life stages and demonstrates how food choices should be tailored to adapt to changing needs of growing children.

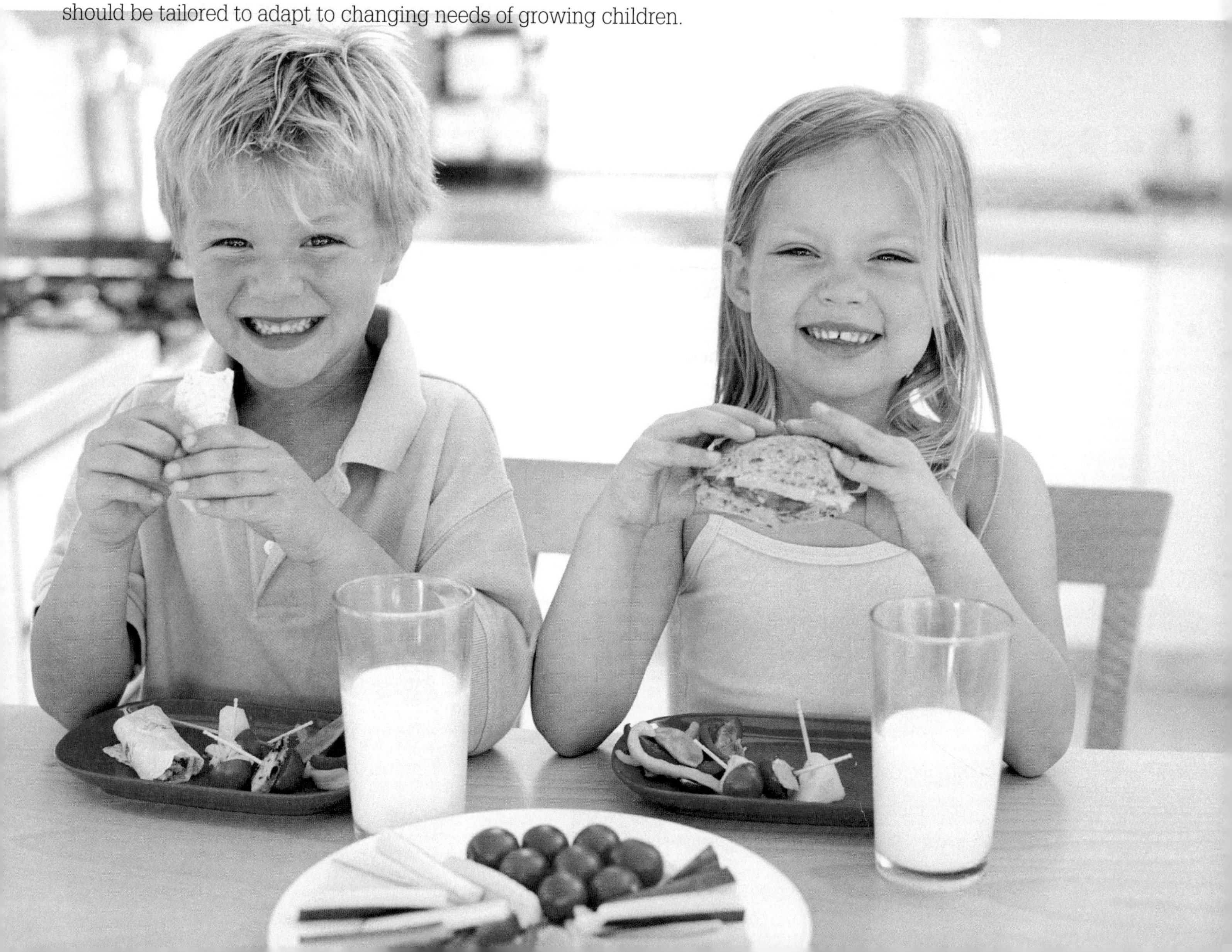

Refresh Your Memory

As you begin your study of nutrition from infancy through adolescence in Chapter 15, you may want to review:

- MyPlate and the 2010 Dietary Guidelines in Chapter 2
- The immune system in Chapter 3
- Diagnosis and treatment of type 2 diabetes in Chapter 4
- Common sources of saturated fat, cholesterol, and *trans* fat in Chapter 5
- Vegetarianism in Chapter 6

15.1 Nutrition and Child Health— an Introduction

Current statistics describing nutrition and overall health among children and adolescents in North America have shown both positive and negative trends. On a positive note, more children are receiving vaccinations than ever before and fewer teenagers are giving birth. In contrast to this good news, the number of children and teenagers with obesity and type 2 diabetes is rising, and physical activity in general is on the decline as more time is spent sitting in front of computer screens and television sets. Low calcium intakes are also receiving much attention, as soft drinks and energy drinks have replaced much of the milk that children and teenagers previously consumed on a daily basis. Fruits, vegetables, and whole grains are also often in short supply in their diets. In this chapter, we will look at these trends and their effects on nutrition and overall health of this age group.

15.2 Infant Growth and Nutrition Needs

During infancy, attitudes toward foods and the eating process begin to take shape. If parents and other caregivers practice good nutrition and are flexible, they can lead an infant into lifelong healthful food habits. A family environment that encourages healthy eating will provide the nutrients needed to optimize physical growth and development. However, these advantages don't guarantee that a child will thrive.

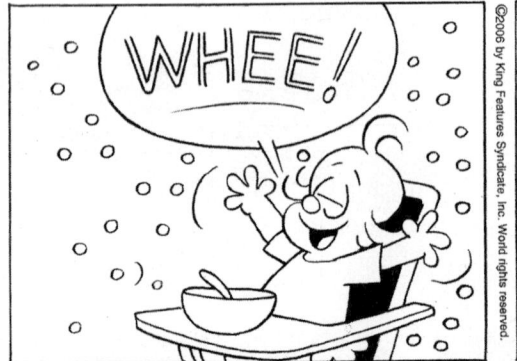
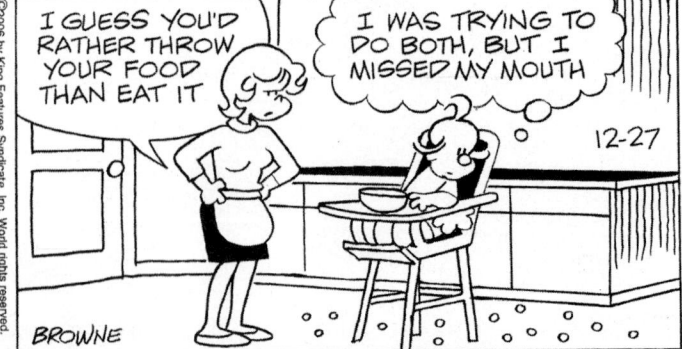

At what age should an infant be fed solid foods? Which foods are most appropriate for those early stages of solid food introduction? Which foods should not be fed to infants? Why? Chapter 15 provides some answers.

MARVIN © Reprinted with special permission of King Features Syndicate, Inc.

Children also need specific attention focused on them; they need to grow in a stimulating environment, and they need a sense of security. For example, children hospitalized for growth failure gain weight more quickly when more caring stimulation, such as holding and rocking the infant, accompanies needed nutrients.

The Growing Infant

All babies seem to do is eat and sleep. There's a good reason for this. An infant's birth weight doubles in the first 4 to 6 months and triples within the first year. Never again is growth so rapid. Such rapid growth requires a lot of nourishment and sleep. After the first year, growth is slower; it takes 5 more years to double the weight seen at 1 year. An infant also increases in length in the first year by 50% and then continues to gain height through the teen years. These gains are not necessarily continuous—spurts of growth alternate with plateaus. Height is essentially maximized by age 19, although increases of several inches may occur in the early twenties, especially for boys (Fig. 15-1). Head size in proportion to total height shrinks from one-fourth to one-eighth during the climb from infancy to adulthood.

The human body needs a lot more food to support growth and development than it does to merely maintain its size once growth ceases. When nutrients are missing at critical phases of this process, growth and development may slow or even stop.

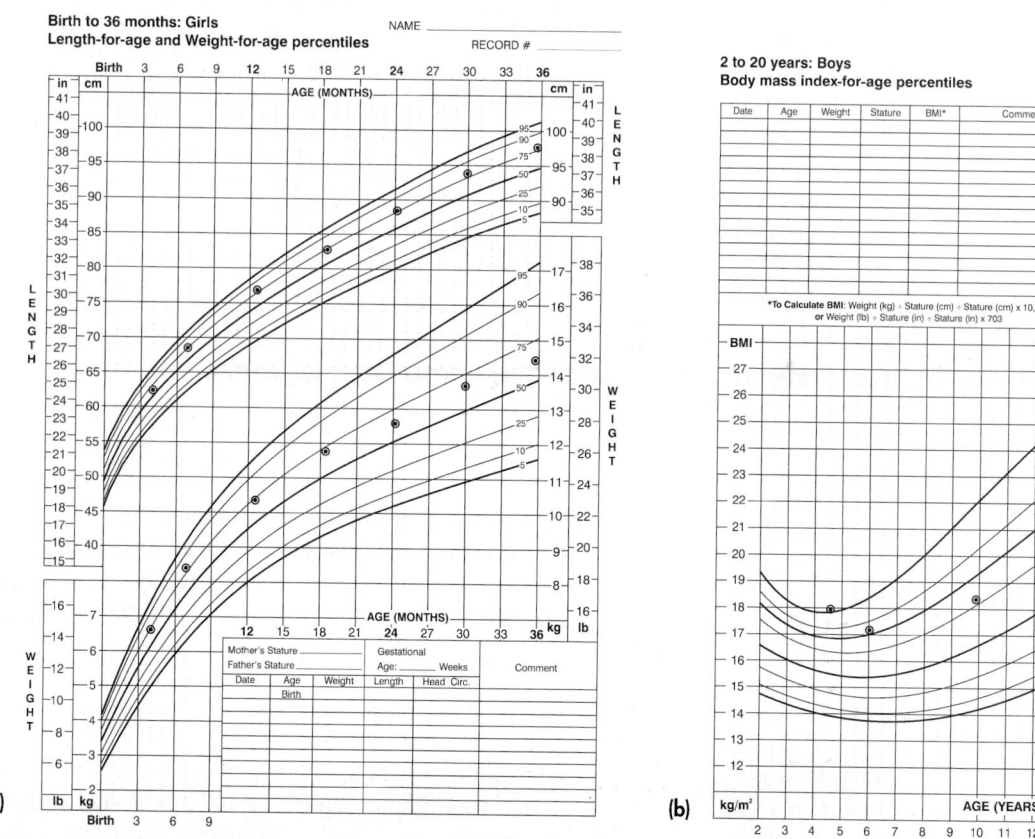

FIGURE 15-1 ► Growth charts for assessment of children in the growing years. The growth of a youngster is plotted to show how the charts are used in health care settings. (a) Growth charts used to assess length (height) and weight in young girls. A certain length (height) and weight correspond to a percentile value (i.e., a ranking of the person among 100 peers). This chart shows that at 36 months of age, the girl was at the 75th percentile for length and the 62nd percentile for weight. (b) Growth charts used to assess weight-for-height relationships in boys ages 2 to 20 years. Today, growth charts for older children and adolescents typically use BMI for evaluation purposes. At 6 years of age, the boy was at the 85th percentile for BMI.

Source: Developed by the National Center for Health Statistics in collaboration with the National Center for Chronic Disease Prevention and Health Promotion (2000). www.cdc.gov/growthcharts. *Revised November 21, 2000.*

undernutrition Failing health that results from a long-standing dietary intake that is not enough to meet nutritional needs.

percentile Classification of a measurement of a unit into divisions of 100 units.

In countries of the developing world, about one-third of the children under 5 years of age are short and underweight for their ages. Poor nutrition—called **undernutrition**—is at the heart of the problem. This occurs to a lesser extent in North America. The undernourished children are smaller versions of nutritionally fit children. In poorer countries, when breastfeeding ceases, children are often fed a high-carbohydrate, low-protein diet. This diet supports some growth but does not allow children to attain their full genetic potential. To grow, children must consume adequate amounts of calories, protein, calcium, iron, zinc, and other nutrients.

Effect of Undernutrition on Growth

As with the fetus in utero, the long-term effects of nutritional problems in infancy and childhood depend on the severity, timing, and duration of the nutritional insult to cell processes.

The single best indicator of a child's nutritional status is growth, particularly weight gain in the short run and length (height) in the long run. Mild zinc deficiencies in North American children have been linked to poor growth. Improving the diets of these children then leads to improved growth. Overall, eating a poor diet during a critical stage of infancy or childhood hampers the cell division that occurs at that stage. Consuming an adequate diet later usually won't compensate for lost growth, however, as the hormonal and other conditions needed for growth will not likely be present. In addition, growth ceases in girls and boys when the skeleton reaches its final size. This happens as growth plates at the ends of the bones fuse, which begins around 14 years of age in girls and 15 years of age in boys. The final stages of this process end at about 19 years of age in girls and 20 years of age in boys. Furthermore, muscles can increase in diameter later in life but their linear growth is limited by the length of the bone.

For these reasons, a 15-year-old Central American girl who is 4 feet 8 inches tall cannot attain the adult height of a typical North American girl simply by eating better. Girls experience their peak rate of growth right before the onset of menses. Once the time for growth ceases (in women, this is about 5 years after they start menstruating), a sufficient nutrient intake helps maintain health and weight but cannot make up for lost growth.

Assessment of Infant Growth and Development

Health professionals assess a child's increases in height and weight by comparing them with typical growth patterns recorded on charts (review Fig. 15-1). The charts contain **percentile** divisions, which represent the typical measurements for 90% to 96% of children. A percentile represents the rank of the person among 100 peers matched for age and gender. If a young boy, for example, is at the 90th percentile of height-for-age, he is shorter than 10% and taller than 89% of children his age. A child at the 50th percentile is considered average. Fifty of 100 children will be taller than this child; 49 will be shorter.

Individual growth charts are available for both males and females from the National Center for Health Statistics (as shown in Fig. 15-1). For ages ranging from birth to 36 months, options for growth charts include weight-for-age, length-for-age, weight-for-length, and head circumference-for-age. For males and females who are 2 to 20 years old, growth charts are available to determine weight-for-age and height-for-age; however, the preferred growth chart for children and adolescents is body mass index (BMI)-for-age. For adults, BMI has fixed cutoff points (for example, a BMI of 25 for an adult is considered overweight). As Figure 15-1 shows, this is not true for children, as BMI reference ranges are both gender- and age-specific.

In 2006, the World Health Organization released a new set of growth standards for children from birth through five years of age to replace the NCHS charts currently in use. The WHO growth charts provide a way to assess the same parameters listed (e.g., height or length, weight, BMI, and head circumference) but they are based on data collected from children from various regions of the world raised under conditions for optimal growth and development: breastfed as infants, followed recommended infant and child feeding practices set forth by WHO, had adequate health care, and mothers did not use tobacco during or after pregnancy. In contrast, the NCHS growth charts are based on data from primarily Caucasian children who were mostly formula-fed during infancy. The new WHO growth standards stress that breastfeeding is the biological norm for infant nutrition. The CDC advises clinicians to use WHO growth charts to monitor growth in infants and children from birth to 2 years, then use NCHS growth charts for children from 2 to 19 years.

Infants and children should have their growth assessed during regular health checkups. It takes 1 to 3 years for the genetic potential (in terms of percentile ranking on growth charts) of infant growth to be established. By 3 years of age, a child's measurements, such as length (height) for age, should generally track along the established percentile. If the child's growth does not keep up with his or her length for age percentile, the physician needs to investigate whether a medical or nutritional problem is impeding the predicted growth. Inappropriate weight gain—too little or too much—should also be investigated.

Infants born preterm may catch up in growth in 2 to 3 years. This requires that the child move up in the percentiles. If this occurs—especially in length for age—it is usually no cause for alarm. On the other hand, moving up in the percentiles for weight for height can be disturbing if the child approaches the 80th to 90th percentiles. A child between the 85th and 95th percentile for BMI is considered overweight. At or above the 95th percentile, the child is considered obese. At the 95th percentile, the diagnosis of obesity can also be established if the physical exam of the child indicates he or she is truly overfat. This is generally the case at this percentile.

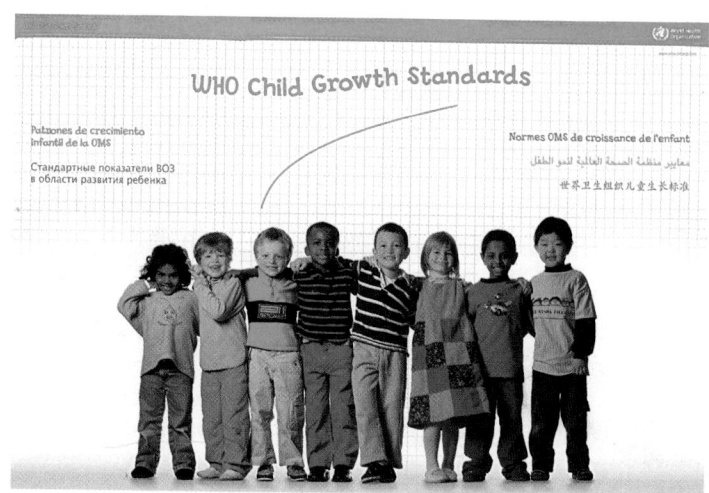

▲ The new WHO Growth Standards for Children differ from previous standards in part because they reflect data gathered from children from around the world who were raised in conditions for optimal growth and development. Go to www.who.int/childgrowth/en/ for more information on the WHO Child Growth Standards.

Children under 2 to 3 years of age are measured lying on their backs with knees unflexed, so the term *length* is used rather than *height*.

MAKING DECISIONS

Head Circumference and Brain Development

The brain grows faster in infancy than at any other time of life. To accommodate this growth, an infant's head circumference must be very large in proportion to the rest of the body. The rapid growth stops at about 18 months of age. In early physical checkups, a health professional usually measures the head circumference as one means of assessing growth, especially brain growth. How nutritional status affects brain development and intelligence quotient (IQ) is difficult to measure because scientists have not determined how to separate the effects of nature from those of nurture. However, several studies have determined that breastfed babies have higher IQs than do babies who were fed with infant formula. At the same time, studies from Central America suggest that IQ after age 5 years relates more closely to the amount of schooling a child receives than to nutritional intake during early childhood.

Adipose Tissue Growth

Since 1970, researchers have speculated that overfeeding during infancy may increase the number of adipose tissue cells. Today, we know that the number of adipose cells can also increase as adulthood obesity develops. Still, if calorie intake is limited during infancy to keep down the number of adipose cells, the growth of other organ systems may also be severely restricted. Special concern revolves around body growth and development, especially brain and nervous system development. In addition, most overweight infants become normal-weight preschoolers without excessive diet restrictions. For these reasons, it is unwise to greatly restrict diet, and especially fat intake in infants. After the first 12 months, fat intake can range from 30% to 40% of total kcal for ages 1 to 3 years, and 25% to 35% of calorie intake for older children (and teenagers).

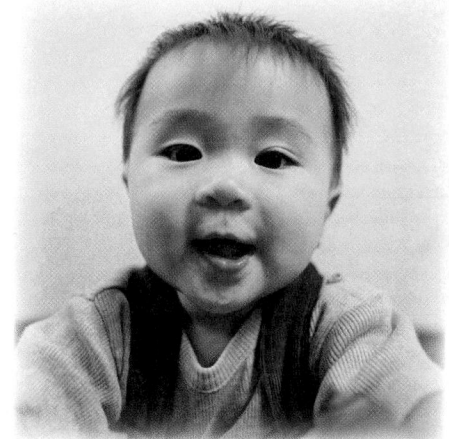

▲ Brain growth is faster in infancy than in any other stage of life. Therefore an infant's head needs to be larger in comparison to the body to allow for such growth.

Failure to Thrive

Occasionally, an infant doesn't grow much in the first few months. Physical problems that may contribute to restricted growth range from poor oral cavity development, infections, and heart irregularities to constant diarrhea associated with intestinal problems. However, more than half the infants who fail to thrive have no apparent disease. Sometimes the cause is poor infant-parent interaction. This stems from misinformation, lack of a parent role model, too little concern about the child's welfare, or even from exerting too much control over feedings (e.g., maternal anxiety, force feeding). Poverty or food insecurity may also be at the root of infant or child undernutrition. In general, the problems arise from the parents' inexperience, rather than intentional negligence. Consequences of failure to thrive include poor physical growth, impaired mental development, and behavioral problems. When health professionals encounter an infant failing to thrive, the true causes need to be identified and then treated.

CONCEPT CHECK

Growth occurs rapidly during infancy: Birth weight doubles in about 4 to 6 months and triples within the first year. Undernutrition in childhood can irreversibly inhibit growth and maturation, so that an individual never attains his or her full genetic potential for height. Infant and child growth is assessed by tracking body weight, length (height), and head circumference over time. Body mass index (BMI) is generally used to assess weight-for-height after 2 years of age. It is not desirable for infants to become overweight, although no evidence strongly indicates that overweight infants become overweight adults. Severe calorie restriction is not recommended for infants because it may slow the growth of organ systems. When infants do not grow properly, their failure to thrive may stem from physical disorders or inadequate care, including inappropriate feeding practices.

Infant Nutritional Needs

Infants' nutritional needs vary as they grow. Initially, human milk or infant formula (usually made from heat-treated cow's milk) supplies needed nutrients. Solid foods are not needed until around 6 months. Even after solid foods are added, the basis of an infant's diet for the first year is still human milk or infant formula. Because of the critical importance of adequate nutrition in infancy and the difficulties encountered in feeding some infants, there is more discussion in this chapter on this developmental period than on the later periods of childhood.

Calories. During infancy, energy needs per pound of body weight are the highest of any life stage. For example, a 6-month-old infant requires two to four times more kcal per pound of body weight than an adult:

Healthy 6-month-old infant
700 kcal/15 pounds = 47 kcal/pound

Healthy 20-year-old woman
2200 kcal / 135 pounds = 16 kcal/pound

Infants need a concentrated source of calories to meet these high demands. Exclusive feeding of either human milk or infant formula is ideal for the first 6 months of life; both are high in fat and supply about 640 kcal/quart (670 kcal/liter; Table 15-1). After 6 months of age, human milk or infant formula, supplemented by developmentally appropriate solid foods, can provide more calories, nutrients, and variety for the developing infant.

The infant's high calorie needs are primarily driven by rapid growth and high metabolic rate. The high metabolic rate is caused in part by the ratio of the infant's body surface area to its weight. More body surface area allows more heat loss from the skin; the body must use extra calories to replace that heat.

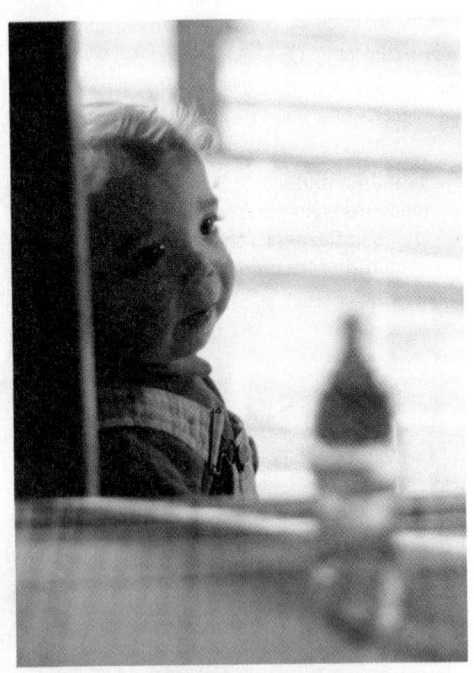

▲ Children older than 2 years are less likely to experience failure to thrive because they can often get food for themselves. Younger children, for the most part, are limited to what caregivers provide.

Age	EER* Equation
0 to 3 months	(89 kcal × weight**) + 75
4 to 6 months	(89 kcal × weight) - 44
7 to 12 months	(89 kcal × weight) – 78
13 to 35 months	(89 kcal × weight) – 80

*EER = Estimated Energy Requirements
**Weight is in kilograms.

TABLE 15-1 Composition of Human and Cow's Milk and Infant Formulas per liter. At 3 Months of Age, Infants Typically Consume 0.75 to 1 liter of Human Milk or Formula per Day.

	Energy (kcal)	Protein (grams)	Fat (grams)	Carbohydrate (grams)	Minerals* (grams)
Milk					
Human milk	670**	11	45	70	2
Cow's milk, whole†	670	36	36	49	7
Cow's milk, fat-free†	360	36	1	51	7
Casein/Whey-Based Formulas					
Similac	680	14	36	71	3
Enfamil	670	15	37	69	3
Good Start	670	16	34	73	3
Soybean Protein-Based Formulas					
ProSobee	670	20	35	67	4
Isomil	680	16	36	68	4
Transition Formulas/Beverages‡					
Similac Toddler's Best	670	25	33	75	3
Enfamil Next Step	670	17	33	74	3
Carnation Follow-Up	670	17	27	88	3

*Calcium, phosphorus, and other minerals.

**Rough estimate; ranges from 650–700 kcal per liter.

†Not appropriate for infant feeding, based primarily on high protein and mineral content.

‡For use after 6 months of age or later (see label).

Carbohydrate. Carbohydrate needs in infancy are 60 grams per day at 0 to 6 months and 95 grams per day at 7 to 12 months. These needs are based on the typical intakes of human milk by breastfed infants and their eventual use of solid foods. Both carbohydrate goals are satisfied by usual intakes of infants on a proper diet.

Protein. Daily protein needs in infancy are about 9 grams per day for younger infants and about 14 grams per day for older infants. These needs also are based on the typical intakes of human milk by breastfed infants for 0 to 6 months, and then on the needs for growth for older infants. About half of total protein intake should come from essential (indispensable) amino acids. As with carbohydrate, protein needs are easily satisfied by either human milk or infant formula. Protein intake should not greatly exceed this standard. Excess nitrogen and minerals supplied by high-protein diets would exceed the ability of an infant's kidneys to excrete the waste products of protein metabolism, thus putting much stress on overall kidney function.

In North America, infant protein deficiency is unlikely, except in cases of mistakes in formula preparation, such as when an infant's formula is excessively diluted with water. Protein deficiency may also be induced by elimination diets used to detect food **allergies** (hypersensitivities). As foods are eliminated from the diet, infants may not be offered enough protein to compensate for the high-protein sources no longer present (see the "Nutrition and Your Health" section later in this chapter).

Fat. Infants need about 30 grams of fat per day. Essential fatty acids should make up about 15% of total fat intake (about 5 grams per day). Both recommendations are again based on the typical intakes of human milk by breastfed infants and the eventual intake of solid foods. Fats are an important part of the infant's diet because they are vital to the development of the nervous system. As a concentrated source of calories, fat also helps resolve the potential problem of the infant's high calorie needs and small stomach capacity. Again, restriction of fat intake is not advised for infants or children under age 2 (Fig. 15-2).

Looking at Table 15-1, it is easy to see why fat-free milk products are not recommended for infants—these do not supply adequate fat and calories to meet needs. Fat-free milk (and reduced fat and whole milk as well) also would provide too much protein and minerals if it were used to meet calorie needs.

See Nutrition and Your Health:
Food Allergies and Intolerances at the end of this chapter.

allergy A hypersensitive immune response that occurs when immune bodies produced by us react with a protein we sense as foreign (an antigen).

FIGURE 15-2 ► The labels on infant foods, like those on adult foods, contain a Nutrition Facts panel. However, the information provided on infant food labels differs from that on adult food labels, especially with respect to total fat, saturated fat, and cholesterol content (see Fig. 2-16 for a comparison). Some cereal brands are fortified with various other micronutrients.

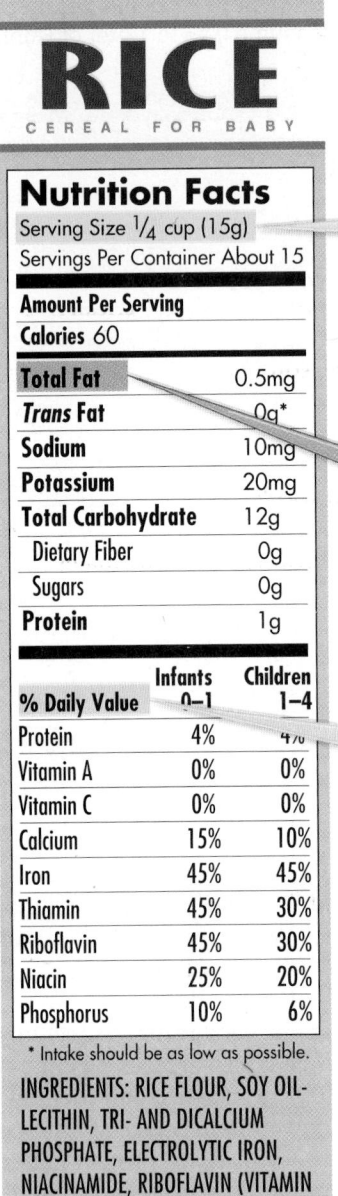

Serving Size

Serving sizes for infant foods are based on the average amount eaten at one time by a child under 2 years.

Total Fat

Shows the amount of total fat in a serving of the food. Unlike adult food labels, labels on infant foods do not list calories from fat, saturated fat, or cholesterol, since infants and toddlers under 2 years need fat. Parents should not attempt to limit their infant's fat intake.

Daily Values

Food labels for infants and children under 4 years list the Daily Value percentages for protein, vitamins, and minerals. Unlike adult food labels, Daily Values for fat, cholesterol, sodium, potassium, carbohydrate, and fiber are not listed.

Arachidonic acid (AA) and docosahexaenoic acid (DHA) are two long-chain fatty acids that have important roles in infant development. The nervous system, especially the brain and eyes, depend on these fatty acids for proper development. During the last trimester, DHA and AA provided by the mother accumulate in the brain and retinas of the eyes in the fetus. Breastfed infants are able to continue to acquire these fatty acids from human milk, especially if their mothers are regularly eating fish. Until recently, no infant formulas sold in the United States included AA or DHA, but many brands are now available with both AA and DHA. These are particularly useful for feeding preterm infants.

Vitamins of Special Interest. As noted in Chapter 8, vitamin K is routinely given by injection to all infants at birth. Formula-fed infants receive the rest of the vitamins they need from the formula. For bone health, immune function, and chronic disease prevention, the American Academy of pediatrics recommends that all infants and children consume 400 IU vitamin D per day starting soon after birth. For all breastfed infants and formula-fed infants who consume less than 1 quart of formula per day, supplemental vitamin D is necessary until they are weaned to infant formula and are consuming at least

500 milliliters of it per day (see Further Reading 14). Breastfed infants whose mothers are total vegetarians (vegans) should also receive vitamin B-12 in supplement form.

Minerals of Special Interest. Infants are born with some internal stores of iron. However, by the time birth weight doubles (4 to 6 months of age), iron stores are generally depleted if not otherwise part of the diet. If the mother was iron deficient during the pregnancy, these iron stores will be exhausted even sooner. As you will recall from Chapter 9, iron-deficiency anemia can lead to poor mental development in infants. Several studies indicate that iron deficiency anemia during infancy, even if corrected, has a lasting impact in terms of impaired cognition, motor development, and behavioral problems later in life. To maintain a desirable iron status, the American Academy of Pediatrics recommends that formula-fed infants should be given an iron-fortified formula from birth. Low-iron infant formulas are sometimes prescribed to treat infants with various GI tract problems, but otherwise their use is discouraged. In contrast, breastfed infants at about 4 to 6 months of age need solid foods to supply extra iron. This need for iron is a major consideration in the decision to introduce solid foods. Liquid iron supplements may be needed until food intake provides sufficient iron. Supplements are also indicated for preterm or LBW infants, those with blood disorders, or those born with inadequate stores of iron (i.e., due to maternal iron deficiency during pregnancy) (see Further Reading 2).

Breast milk is a poor source of fluoride—and formula manufacturers use fluoride-free water in formula preparation, so intake of this mineral during the first 6 months of life is low. However, fluoride supplementation is not advised before 6 months of age. After 6 months, the pediatrician or dentist may recommend fluoride supplements to aid in tooth development if fluoride supplied by tap water, foods, and toothpaste is inadequate.

Infants also need adequate amounts of zinc and iodide to support growth. However, when human milk and infant formula are provided in quantities to meet calorie needs, sufficient zinc and iodide are generally supplied.

Water. An infant needs about 3 cups (700 to 800 milliliters) of water per day. Infants typically consume enough human milk or formula to supply this amount. Even in hot weather, the American Academy of Pediatrics does not recommend supplemental water or juice during the first 6 months. Excess water can cause hyponatremia in infants.

Infants are easily dehydrated, a condition that has serious effects if not remedied. Early signs of dehydration in infants include:

- More than 6 hours without a wet diaper
- Dark yellow or strong-smelling urine
- Unusual lethargy
- Dry mouth and lips
- Absence of tears when crying

Special fluid-replacement formulas containing electrolytes such as sodium and potassium are available in supermarkets and pharmacies to treat mild to moderate dehydration. A physician should guide any use of these products. As dehydration becomes more severe, the infant's eyes and/or the soft spot on the head may appear sunken, hands and feet may be cold and splotchy, and he or she may be excessively tired and

The American Dental Association does not recommend fluoridated bottled water for use by infants because it creates risk for enamel fluorosis during early tooth development.

MAKING DECISIONS

Extra Fluid for Infants

In some stores, bottled water products marketed specifically for infants may be placed alongside infant formulas and electrolyte-replacement solutions. This placement may give parents and caregivers the mistaken impression that bottled water products are an appropriate feeding supplement or substitute for fluid replacement for infants; they are not and should not be used for such purposes. It is important to remember that excessive fluid can also be harmful, especially to the brain.

fussy. Such severe dehydration can result in rapid loss of kidney function and warrants medical intervention. Hospitalization and intravenous fluid treatment may be necessary for extreme cases or when the infant is unable to keep anything in the stomach.

Overall, it is best to rely exclusively on breast milk or infant formula to meet infant fluid needs up to 6 months of age unless a physician suggests otherwise. In sum, extremes in fluid intake—either too little or too much—can lead to health problems.

CONCEPT CHECK

Most nutrient needs in the first 6 months are met by human milk or infant formula. All infants and children should receive 400 IU of vitamin D, which necessitates supplementation for breastfed and some formula-fed infants. Some infants, especially after 4 months of age, with low iron stores may require iron supplements. Formula-fed infants and breastfed infants may need fluoride supplements after 6 months of age. Infants usually receive enough water from the human milk or infant formula they drink.

Formula Feeding for Infants

Breastfeeding was covered in detail in Chapter 14. Let's now focus on formula feeding. You'll recall that a major advantage of breastfeeding is the provision of immune protection to the infant. Although it lacks the full spectrum of benefits of breastfeeding, formula feeding is a safe alternative for infants in areas of the world with clean water supplies.

Formula Composition. Infants cannot tolerate cow's milk as such because of its high protein and mineral content. Cow's milk is perfect for the greater growth needs of calves, but not for human infants. Thus, cow's milk must be altered by formula manufacturers to be safe for infant feeding. Altered forms of cow's milk, known as infant formulas, must conform to strict federal guidelines for nutrient composition and quality. Formulas generally contain lactose and/or sucrose for carbohydrate, heat-treated proteins from cow's milk, and vegetable oils for fat (review Table 15-1). Soy protein–based formulas are available for infants who can't tolerate lactose or the types of proteins found in cow's milk. If the soybean-based formula is not tolerated, the next step is to try a predigested formula in which the proteins have been broken down into small polypeptides and amino acids. A variety of other specialized formulas also are available for specific medical conditions. In any case, it is important to use an iron-fortified formula unless a physician recommends otherwise.

Some transition formulas/beverages have been introduced for older infants and toddlers (review Table 15-1). Some of these products are intended for use after 6 months of age if the infant is consuming solid foods, whereas others are intended for use only by toddlers. These transition products are lower in fat than human milk or standard infant formulas; their iron content is higher than that of cow's milk; and their overall mineral content is generally more like that of human milk than cow's milk. According to the manufacturers, the advantages of these transition formulas/beverages over standard formulas for older infants and toddlers include reduced cost and better flavor. Parents should consult their physician with regard to the use of these products.

Formula Preparation. Some infant formulas come in ready-to-feed form. These are poured into a clean bottle and fed immediately. Room-temperature formula is acceptable for many infants. Otherwise, to warm a bottle of formula, a caregiver can run hot water over it or place it briefly in a pan of simmering water. Infant formulas should not be heated in a microwave oven because hot spots may develop, which can burn the infant's mouth and esophagus.

Powdered and concentrated fluid formula preparations are also commonly used. All utensils used to prepare formula should be washed and thoroughly rinsed.

Parents should consult a physician when choosing an appropriate infant formula. Not all formula-like products are designed for infant use. A 5-month-old girl was admitted to a hospital in Arkansas with symptoms of heart failure, rickets, inflamed blood vessels, and possible nerve damage after being fed Soy Moo (a soy beverage sold in health stores) since 3 days of age. The symptoms suggest severe vitamin deficiencies.

Bisphenol A (BPA) is a chemical used in the manufacture of many plastics, including some baby bottles. Human exposure to BPA, mainly through leaching of the chemical from packaging into foods and beverages, is widespread. Concern about exposure stems from animal studies that link BPA with reproductive and developmental defects. However, the consensus among regulatory agencies in the United States and Canada is that current levels of BPA exposure are not harmful, even for infants. For parents who wish to limit exposure, BPA-free baby bottles are available.

Powdered or concentrated formulas should be combined with clean, cold water, exactly following the directions on the formula label. The formula is then warmed, if desired, and fed immediately to the infant. Hot water from the faucet should not be used to make formula, since it poses a risk for high lead content (see Chapter 13). Cold water poses much less risk. For infants up to 6 months of age, pediatricians commonly recommend boiling (and then cooling) the water to be used in formula preparation and sterilizing bottles and utensils by immersion in boiling water.

Refrigerating prepared formula for 1 day is safe. However, formula left over from a feeding should be discarded because it will be contaminated by bacteria and enzymes from the infant's saliva. If well water is used, it should be boiled before making formula for at least the infant's first 3 months of life, and it should be analyzed for excessive concentration of naturally occurring nitrates, which can lead to a severe form of anemia. If nitrates are high in municipal water systems, consumers will be warned (such as in a local newspaper) not to use the water for making infant formula until the concentration falls to a safe amount. The American Dental Association does not recommend that formula be mixed with bottled nursery water, available alongside infant formula in most supermarkets, to limit risk of tooth discoloration from high fluoride levels.

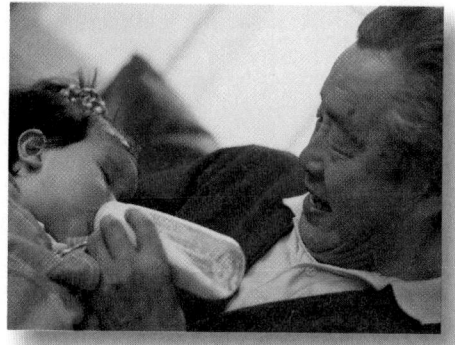

▲ Careful attention during feeding allows the caregiver to notice the infant's signal as to when the feeding should cease.

Feeding Technique

Infants swallow a lot of air as they ingest either formula or human milk, so it's important to burp an infant after either 10 minutes of feeding or 1 to 2 ounces (30 to 60 milliliters) has been consumed from a bottle and again at the end of feeding. Spitting up a bit of milk is normal at this time.

When the infant begins acting full, bottle feeding should be stopped, even if some milk is left in the bottle. Common cues that signal that an infant has had enough include turning the head away, being inattentive, falling asleep, and becoming playful. Generally, the infant's appetite is a better guide than standardized recommendations concerning feeding amounts. Breastfeeding infants usually have had enough to eat after about 20 minutes. Although it's difficult to tell how much milk breastfed infants are getting, they also give signs when full. By carefully observing bottle-feeding or breastfeeding infants and responding to their cues appropriately, caregivers not only can be assured that the infants' calorie needs are being met but also can foster a climate of trust and responsiveness.

Once fed, an infant should not be placed on its stomach. Placing the infant on its back is recommended by the American Academy of Pediatrics. The reason that an infant should not be placed on its stomach is because this sleeping position has been linked to sudden infant death syndrome (SIDS). The Back to Sleep campaign, started in 1994 in the United States, has reduced SIDS by 40%.

The Back to Sleep campaign, however, has led to a problem known as flattened head syndrome (clinically known as positional plagiocephaly). Infant skulls are soft and therefore can change in shape. Flattened head syndrome can occur if an excessive amount of an infant's day is spent on his or her back or against a highchair/car seat. In response to this concern, the American Academy of Pediatrics has recommended periodic repositioning of an infant's head while asleep and allowing for supervised time on his or her stomach while awake. In addition, some infants may need to wear specially fitted helmets to correct the shape of their heads.

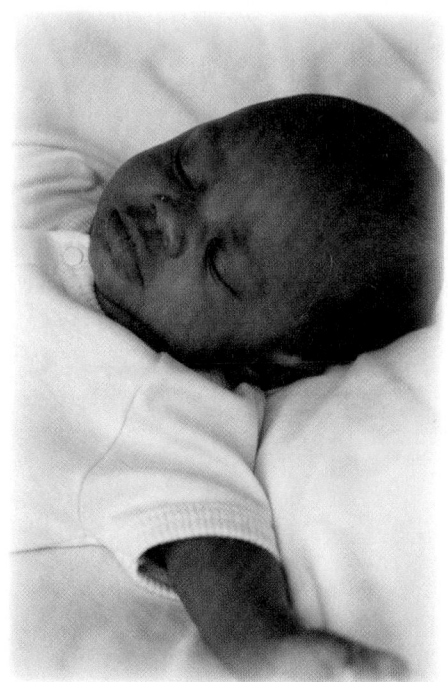

▲ The Back to Sleep campaign aims to reduce risk of sudden infant death syndrome.

Expanding the Infant's Mealtime Choices

By about 6 months of age, the infant is ready to start eating "table food." Initially, table foods add to—rather than replace—formula or human milk. In the first attempts to introduce solid foods, just getting the food into the infant's mouth may prove to be a challenge. By the end of the first year, though, the infant should be eating a variety of protein sources, vegetables, fruits, and grains so that the diet begins to resemble a balanced pattern, setting the stage for lifelong preferences and dietary habits (Table 15-2).

TABLE 15-2 Sample Daily Menu for a 1-Year-Old Child*

Breakfast	**Snack**
1 to 2 tbsp applesauce	½ ounce cheddar cheese
¼ cup Cheerios	4 wheat crackers
½ cup whole milk	½ cup whole milk

Snack	**Dinner**
½ hard-cooked egg	1 ounce hamburger (crumbled)
½ slice wheat toast with ½ tsp margarine	1 to 2 tbsp mashed potatoes with ½ tsp margarine
½ cup orange juice	1 to 2 tbsp cooked carrots (cut in strips, not coins)
	½ cup whole milk

Lunch	**Snack**
1 ounce roasted chicken, minced	½ banana
1 to 2 tbsp rice with ½ tsp margarine	2 oatmeal cookies (no raisins)
1 to 2 tbsp cooked peas	½ cup whole milk
½ cup whole milk	

Nutritional Analysis	
Total energy (kcal)	1100
% energy from	
Carbohydrate	40%
Protein	19%
Fat	41%

*This diet is just a start. A 1-year-old may need more or less food. In those cases, serving sizes should be adjusted. The milk can be fed by cup; some can be put into a bottle if the child has not been fully weaned from the bottle. The juice should be fed in a cup.

Throughout the process of expanding the infant's mealtime choices, it is essential to allow the infant to control the situation—the caregiver must proceed slowly and respond to the infant's cues that he or she is hungry or has had enough to eat.

Recognizing the Infant's Readiness for Solid Foods. How does the caregiver know it is time to introduce solid foods? Infant size can serve as a rough indicator of readiness—reaching a weight of at least 13 pounds (6 kilograms) is a preliminary sign of readiness for solid foods. Another physiological cue is frequency of feeding, such as consuming more than 32 ounces (1 liter) of formula daily or breastfeeding more than 8 to 10 times within 24 hours. Underlying these noticeable signals are several important developmental factors:

1. *Nutritional need.* Before the infant is 6 months old, nutritional needs can generally be met with human milk and/or formula. After 6 months of age, however, many infants need the additional calories supplied by solid foods. In terms of individual nutrients, iron stores are exhausted by about 6 months of age. Either solid foods or iron supplements are then needed to supply iron if the child is breastfed or fed a low-iron or iron-free formula. (As previously mentioned, a vitamin D supplement should also be provided.)

2. *Physiological capabilities.* As the infant ages, the ability to digest and metabolize a wider range of food components improves. Before about 3 months of age, an infant's digestive tract cannot readily digest starch. Also, kidney function is limited until about 4 to 6 weeks of age. Until then, waste products from excessive amounts of dietary protein or minerals are difficult to excrete.

3. *Physical ability.* Three physical markers indicate that a child is ready for solid foods: (1) the disappearance of the extrusion reflex (thrusting the tongue forward and pushing food out of the mouth), (2) head and neck control, and (3) the ability to sit up with support. These usually occur around 4 to 6 months of age, but they vary with each infant.

4. *Allergy prevention.* An infant's intestinal tract is "leaky"—whole proteins can readily be absorbed from birth until 4 to 5 months of age. If the infant is exposed too early to some types of proteins—particularly those in cow's milk

and egg whites—the infant may be predisposed to future allergies and other health problems, such as diabetes. For this reason, it is best to minimize the number of different types of proteins in an infant's diet, especially during the first 3 months (see the "Nutrition and Your Health" section on food allergies at the end of this chapter for details).

With these considerations in mind—nutritional need, physiological and physical readiness, and allergy prevention—the American Academy of Pediatrics recommends that solid foods not be introduced until about 6 months of age and that infants receive no unaltered cow's milk before 1 year.

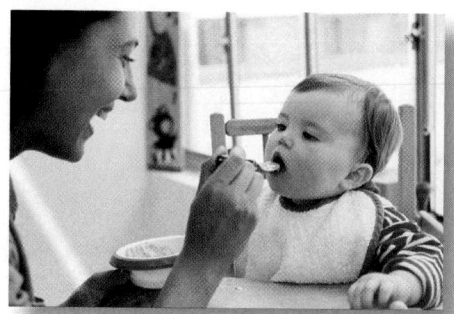

▲ Iron-fortified rice cereal is recommended as the first solid food to be fed to infants.

MAKING DECISIONS

Introducing Solid Foods

Parents may believe that the early addition of solid foods will help an infant sleep through the night. Actually, this achievement is a developmental milestone, and the amount of food consumed by the infant is of little relevance to the achievement of a good night's sleep. Before 4 to 6 months of age, infants are not physically mature enough to consume much solid food. Only occasionally does a rapidly growing infant need solid foods to meet calorie and nutrient needs before 6 months of age.

Foods to Match Needs and Developmental Abilities During the First Year. If solid foods are introduced before 6 months of age, the primary goal of the food should be to meet iron needs. Therefore, the first solid foods should be iron-fortified cereals. Some pediatricians may recommend lean ground (strained) meats for more absorbable forms of iron. Rice is the best cereal to begin with because it is least likely to cause allergies.

When starting solid foods, it is important to start with a teaspoon serving size of a single-ingredient food item, such as rice cereal, and increase the serving size gradually. Once the new food has been fed for about a week without ill effects, another food can be added to the infant's diet. At first, this can be another type of cereal or perhaps a cooked and strained (or mashed) vegetable, meat, fruit, or egg yolk.

Waiting about 7 days between the introduction of each new food is important because it can take that long for evidence of an allergy or intolerance to develop. Also, it is important to avoid introducing mixed foods until each component of the combination dish has been given separately without an adverse reaction. Signs of food allergies include diarrhea, vomiting, a rash, or wheezing. If one or more of these signs appears, the suspected problem food should be avoided for several weeks and then reintroduced in a small quantity. If the problem continues, a physician should be consulted. Fortunately, many babies outgrow food allergies later in childhood.

Until recently, parents and caregivers were advised to avoid feeding children a wide range of highly allergenic foods, including egg whites, chocolate, peanuts, tree nuts, fish, and other seafood. Now, the American Academy of Pediatrics acknowledges that there is no evidence that delaying introduction of solid foods—including these highly allergenic foods—beyond 6 months of age is of any benefit for prevention of food allergies and other atopic diseases. (See Nutrition and Your Health at the end of this chapter.)

Many strained foods for infant feeding are available at the supermarket. Single-food items are more desirable than mixed dinners and desserts, which are less nutrient-dense. Most brands have no added salt, but some fruit desserts contain a lot of added sugar.

As an alternative, plain, unseasoned cooked foods—vegetables, fruits, and meats— can be ground up in an inexpensive plastic baby food grinder/mill. Another option is to puree a larger amount of food in a blender, freeze it in ice-cube portions, store in plastic bags, and defrost and warm as needed. Careful attention to cleanliness is necessary. Seasonings that may please the rest of the family should not be added to infant foods made at home. The infant doesn't notice the difference if salt, sugar, or

▶ **Typical Solid Food Progression, Starting at 6 Months***

Week 1	Rice cereal
Week 2	Add strained carrots
Week 3	Add applesauce
Week 4	Add oat cereal
Week 5	Add cooked egg yolk
Week 6	Add strained chicken
Week 7	Add strained peas
Week 8	Add plums

*Extending the rice cereal step for a month or so is advised if solid food introduction begins at 4 months of age. Also, if at any point signs of allergy or intolerance develop, substitute another similar food item.

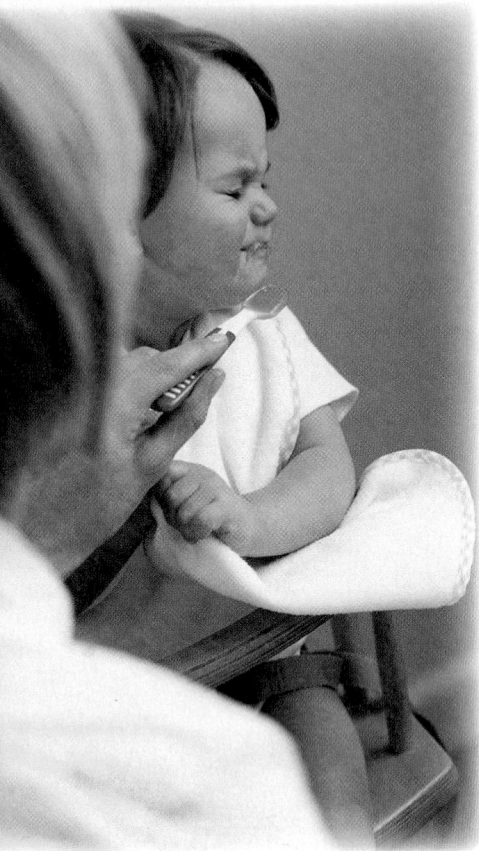

▲ Repeated exposure fosters acceptance of new tastes and textures.

early childhood caries Tooth decay that results from formula or juice (and even human milk) bathing the teeth as the child sleeps with a bottle in his or her mouth. The upper teeth are mostly affected as the lower teeth are protected by the tongue; formerly called *nursing bottle syndrome* and *baby bottle tooth decay*.

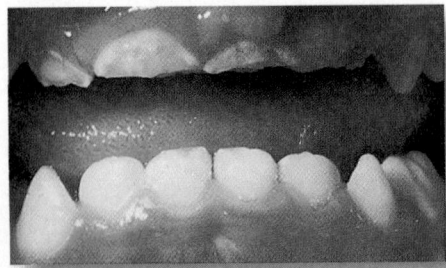

▲ Early childhood caries. An extreme example of tooth decay probably resulting from frequently putting the child to bed with a bottle. The upper teeth have decayed almost all the way to the gum line.

spices are omitted. It is best to introduce infants to a variety of foods, so that by the end of the first year, the infant is consuming many foods—human milk or formula, meats, fruits, vegetables, and grains.

Self-feeding skills require coordination and can develop only if the infant is allowed to practice and experiment. By 6 to 7 months of age, the infant has learned to handle finger foods and transfer objects from one hand to the other with some dexterity. At about this time, teeth also begin to appear. Dry toast, sliced in strips, offers hours of enjoyment. By age 7 to 8 months, infants can push food around on a plate, play with a drinking cup, hold a bottle, and self-feed a cracker or a piece of toast. Through mastery of these manipulations, infants develop confidence and self-esteem. It is important that parents be patient and support these early feeding attempts, even though they appear inefficient.

At 9 to 10 months of age, the infant's desire to explore, experience, and play with foods may hinder feeding. Food is used as a means to explore the environment, and therefore feeding time is often very messy—a bowl of macaroni may end up in the child's hair. Presenting a new food on several consecutive days can aid in an infant's acceptance of that food. Caregivers need to relax and take this phase of infant development in stride. Sloppy, friendly mealtimes make for good memories. By the end of the first year, finger-feeding becomes more efficient and chewing is easier as more teeth erupt. Still, experimentation and unpredictability are to be expected.

To ease the efforts in feeding solid foods, consider the following tips:

- Use a baby-sized spoon; a small spoon with a long handle is best.
- Hold the infant comfortably on the lap, as for breastfeeding or bottle feeding, but a little more upright to ease swallowing. When in this position, the infant expects food.
- Put a small dab of food on the spoon tip and gently place it on the infant's tongue.
- Convey a calm and casual approach to the infant, who needs time to get used to food.
- Expect the infant to take only two or three bites of the first meals.

Weaning from the Breast or Bottle

Around the age of 6 months, juices can be offered in a sippy cup with a wide, flat bottom. Drinking from a cup rather than from a bottle helps prevent **early childhood caries.** If an infant drinks continuously from a bottle, the carbohydrate-rich fluid bathes the teeth, providing an ideal growth medium for bacteria adhering to the teeth. These bacteria then make acids, which dissolve tooth enamel. To avoid dental caries, infants should not be put to bed with a bottle or placed in an infant seat with a bottle propped up.

By about 10 months of age, infants are learning to self-feed and likewise to drink independently from a cup. As children drink from a cup more frequently, fewer bottle feedings and/or breastfeedings are necessary. The added mobility of crawling and walking should naturally lead to gradual weaning from the bottle or breast. Even so, getting a baby out of the bedtime-bottle habit can be difficult. Determined caregivers can either wince through a few nights of their baby's crying or slowly wean the baby away from the bottle with either a pacifier or water (for a week or so).

Dietary Guidelines for Infant Feeding

It can be difficult for new parents to make sense of nutrition goals for infants in the face of changing dietary recommendations from health authorities, cultural preferences, and outdated advice from friends and family. In response to various controversies surrounding infant feeding, the American Academy of Pediatrics has issued a number of statements concerning infant diets. The following guidelines are based on these statements:

- *Build to a variety of foods.* For the first months of life, human milk (or infant formula) is all an infant needs. (Vitamin D supplementation is an exception.)

When the infant is ready, start adding new foods, one at a time. During the first year, the goal is to teach an infant to enjoy a variety of nutritious foods. A lifetime of healthy eating habits begins with this important first step.

- *Pay attention to your infant's appetite to avoid overfeeding or underfeeding.* Feed infants when they are hungry. Never force an infant to finish an unwanted serving of food. Watch for signs that indicate hunger or fullness. This will reinforce the infant's natural capability to self-regulate food intake.
- *Infants need fat.* Although fat contributes to many adult health problems, it's an essential source of calories for growing infants. Fat also helps the nervous system develop.
- *Choose fruits, vegetables, and grains, but don't overdo high-fiber foods.* During the second half of the first year, infants are fed a variety of fruits and vegetables. However, studies show that by 1 year of age, vegetable choices are dominated by white potatoes. Continuing to offer choices of green and yellow vegetables during infancy and the toddler years will enhance intake of important vitamins, minerals, and phytochemicals. In terms of fiber, although many adults benefit from high-fiber diets, they are not good for infants. They are bulky, filling, and often low in calories. The natural amounts of fiber and nutrients in fruits, vegetables, and grains are appropriate as part of a healthy infant diet.
- *Infants need sugars in moderation.* Sugars are an additional source of calories for active, rapidly growing infants. Foods such as human milk, fruits, and 100% juices are natural sources of sugars and other nutrients as well. Foods that contain artificial sweeteners should be avoided; they don't provide the calories growing infants need. On the other hand, excessive intake of sugars, particularly from fruit-flavored drinks and soft drinks, contribute to the epidemic of childhood obesity.
- *Infants need sodium in moderation.* Sodium is a necessary mineral found naturally in almost all foods. As part of a healthy diet, infants need sodium for their bodies to work properly. However, average intakes of sodium among infants and toddlers are above the AI. Caregivers should delay introduction of cow's milk (a source of sodium for infants) until 1 year of age and refrain from offering heavily-seasoned and processed foods.
- *Choose foods containing iron, zinc, and calcium.* Infants need good sources of iron, zinc, and calcium for optimum growth in the first 2 years. These minerals are important for healthy blood, optimal growth, and strong bones. Many infant and toddler foods (e.g., cereal, crackers, and biter biscuits) are fortified with these minerals.

In essence, there is no evidence that restrictive diets during infancy have positive effects, whereas their hazards are well documented.

What Not to Feed an Infant

Following are several foods and practices to avoid when feeding an infant:

- *Honey.* This product may contain spores of *Clostridium botulinum*. The spores can eventually develop into bacteria in the stomach and lead to a foodborne illness known as *botulism*. This can be fatal, especially in children under 1 year old (see Chapter 13).
- *Excessive infant formula or human milk.* After 6 to 8 months, solid foods should play a greater role in satisfying an infant's increasing appetite. The main reason to switch is that solid foods contain considerably more bioavailable iron than do human milk and low-iron formulas. About 24 to 32 ounces (¾ to 1 liters) of human milk or formula daily is ideal after 6 months, with food supplying the rest of the infant's calorie needs.
- *Foods that tend to cause choking.* These foods include hot dogs (unless finely cut into sticks, not coin shapes), candy, whole nuts, grapes, coarsely cut meats, raw carrots, popcorn, and peanut butter. Caregivers should not allow younger children to gobble snack foods during playtime and should supervise all meals.

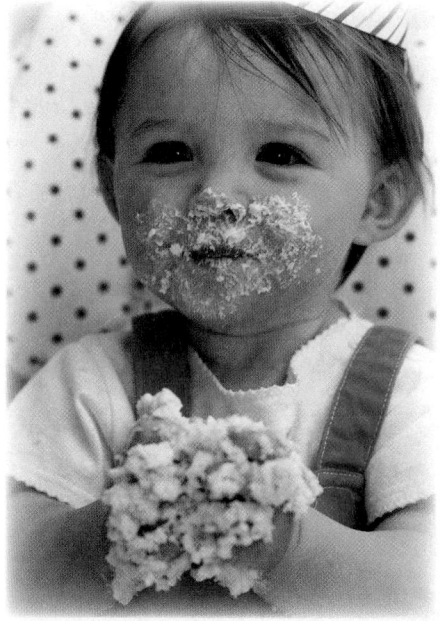

▲ Early feeding attempts should be encouraged, even though they're messy.

▶ A Summary of Infant Feeding Recommendations

Breastfed Infants

- Breastfeed for 6 months or longer, if possible. Then introduce infant formula if and when breastfeeding declines or ceases. (Breast milk can also be pumped and placed in a bottle for later use.)
- Provide a vitamin D supplement (400 IU per day).
- Investigate the need for vitamin B-12, fluoride, and iron supplementation to prevent deficiencies.

Formula-Fed Infants

- Use infant formula for the first year of life, preferably an iron-fortified type.
- Provide a vitamin D supplement if formula intake provides less than 400 IU per day.
- Investigate the need for a fluoride supplement if the water supply is not fluoridated.

All Infants

- Add iron-fortified cereal at about 6 months of age.
- Provide a variety of basic, soft foods after 6 months of age, advancing to a varied diet.

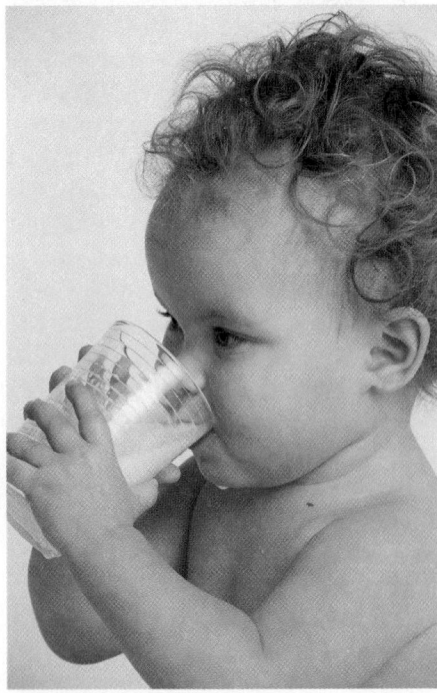

▲ Infants should begin drinking from a cup by 1 year of age. Cups with lids help to prevent spills, but allow a toddler to practice without a lid as his dexterity and coordination improve.

- *Cow's milk, especially low-fat or fat-free cow's milk.* The American Academy of Pediatrics strongly urges parents not to give children under age 2 fat-reduced, 1%, or fat-free milk. Before age 2, the amount of this milk needed to meet calorie needs would supply too many minerals and in turn could overwhelm the kidneys' ability to excrete the excess. The lower fat intake might also harm nervous system development. Beyond 2 years, children can drink fat-reduced, 1%, or fat-free milk, because by this age they are consuming enough solid foods to supply calorie and fat needs.
- *Feeding excessive fruit juice.* The fructose and sorbitol contained in some fruit juices, especially apple and pear juices, can lead to diarrhea because they are slowly absorbed. Also, if fruit juice or related drink products are replacing formula or milk in the diet, the infant may not be receiving adequate calories, calcium, or other nutrients essential for proper growth. Studies have shown a link between excessive amounts of fruit juice and failure to thrive, GI tract complications, obesity, short stature, and poor dental health. Thus, these substances should be used sparingly. Limit fruit juice to 4 to 6 ounces per day for infants from 6 months to 6 years of age.

Inappropriate Infant Feeding Practices

Parents and other caregivers should be aware of a variety of potential health problems related to infant nutrition, so that corrective action can be taken quickly. In some cases, such problems stem from inappropriate feeding practices and inadequate nutrient intakes, including the following:

- Diet providing insufficient iron
- Absence from the diet of an entire MyPlate food group as solid foods are introduced and become the main source of nutrients
- Use of cow's milk before 1 year of age
- Introduction of potential allergy-causing foods, such as egg whites and nuts, prior to 6 months of age
- Drinking raw (unpasteurized) milk, which may be contaminated with bacteria or viruses
- Drinking goat's milk, which is low in folate, iron, vitamin C, and vitamin D
- Failure to begin drinking from a cup by 1 year of age
- Continuing to feed from a bottle past 18 months of age
- Intake of supplemental vitamins or minerals above 100% of the appropriate RDA or other nutrient standard
- Drinking more than 6 ounces of fruit juice per day after 6 months of age, especially as a substitute for infant formula or human milk. (Recall that fruit juice is not to be fed at all before 6 months of age.)

The website of the American Academy of Pediatrics (www.aap.org) can also provide useful information on these and other nutrition-related problems in infancy.

CONCEPT CHECK

Infant formulas generally contain lactose or sucrose, heat-treated proteins from cow's milk, and vegetable oil. Formulas may or may not be fortified with iron. Sanitation is important in preparing and storing formula. Solid foods should not be added to an infant's diet until the child is both ready for and needs solid food, usually at about 6 months of age. The first solid foods can be iron-fortified infant cereals, with gradual additions of other foods—one at a time. Some foods to avoid giving to infants in the first year are honey, cow's milk (particularly fat-reduced, 1%, or fat-free milk), foods that may cause the child to choke, and excessive amounts of fruit juice or related products (e.g., fruit drinks).

15.3 Preschool Children: Nutrition Concerns

The rapid growth rate that characterizes infancy tapers off quickly during the subsequent few years. The average annual weight gain is only 4.5 to 6.6 pounds (2 to 3 kilograms), and the average annual height gain is only 3 to 4 inches (7.5 to 10 centimeters) between the ages of 2 and 5. As a toddler's growth rate tapers off, eating behavior changes. For example, the decreased growth rate leads to a decreased appetite, often called "picky eating," compared with infants.

Because of a reduced appetite, planning a diet that meets the nutrient needs of a preschool child poses a special challenge to caregivers. The USDA's MyPlate, in combination with Team Nutrition, available at www.teamnutrition.usda.gov, offers resources for planning nutritious, age-appropriate meals and snacks. Additional nutrition guidance, starting with pregnancy and extending through the preschool years, is available from the *Start Healthy, Stay Healthy* Resource Center at www.gerber.com. Choosing nutrient-dense foods is particularly important with children who eat relatively little. This is a good time to emphasize some whole grains, fruits, and vegetables without increasing fat and simple sugar intake. A whole-grain ready-to-eat breakfast cereal with limited fat and sugar is an excellent choice. There is no need to decrease fat or simple sugar intake severely, but fatty and sweet food choices should not overwhelm more nutritious ones.

Excessive sodium intake is a concern for preschool children as well (see Further Reading 11). Caregivers can lower sodium intake by limiting salt added during cooking and at the table; cutting back on use of processed foods (e.g., luncheon meats, hot dogs); rinsing canned beans and vegetables before cooking; and encouraging consumption of fruits, vegetables, and whole grains in place of prepackaged snacks. The preschool years are the best time for a child to start a healthful pattern of living and eating, focusing on regular physical activity and nutritious foods. Parents and other caregivers are role models: If they eat a variety of foods, the children will eat a variety of foods. One possible policy is the one-bite rule: Within reason, children should take at least one bite or taste of the foods presented to them. For snacks, parents should select several possibilities of acceptable choices and allow children to choose one; responsibility for food choice by the child ideally should start early.

How to Help a Child Choose Nutritious Foods

One way adults can encourage young children to eat nutritious, well-balanced meals is to serve new foods and repeat exposure to them. The dinner hour is a good time for children to experience new foods and to develop food preferences. Preschool children especially tend to be wary of new foods. One reason is that they have more taste buds, and their taste buds are more sensitive than those of adults. In addition, they have a general distrust of unfamiliar foods. If adults can be patient and persevere, children will build good food habits. It may take 8 to 10 exposures to a new food before a child finds it acceptable. Above all, the dinner table should not become a battleground, and using one food as a bribe to eat another—for example, a piece of pie for peas—is strongly discouraged.

Certain food characteristics, such as crisp textures and mild flavors, are appealing to children. Familiarity also plays an important role in food acceptance. In contrast, young children are especially wary of hot-temperature foods and tend to reject them.

Preschoolers eventually develop skill with spoons and forks and can even use dull knives. However, it's still a good idea to serve some finger foods. A goal should be to make mealtime a happy, social time to share and enjoy healthful foods (see Further Readings 1 and 9).

Childhood Feeding Problems

Tensions between parents, or between parents and children, especially during mealtime, often contribute to eating problems. Getting to the root of family problems and

▶ **Quick Guide to Child Nutrition Needs**

Carbohydrates

- 130 grams per day to supply energy for the central nervous system and prevent ketosis

Protein

- 13–19 grams per day (ages 1–3)
- 34–52 grams per day (older children)

Fat

- at least 5 grams per day of essential fatty acids
- eventually aim for 20% to 35% of total calorie intake by age 19

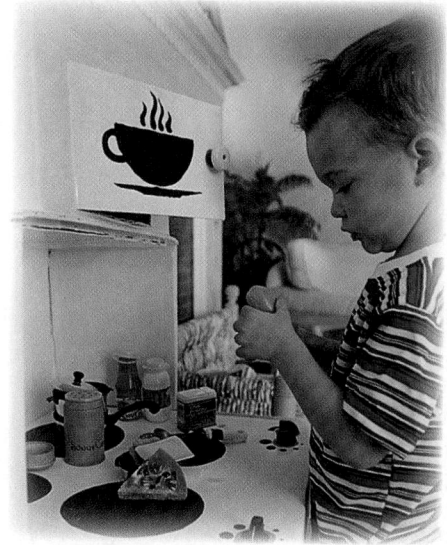

▲ Interest in food starts early in life.

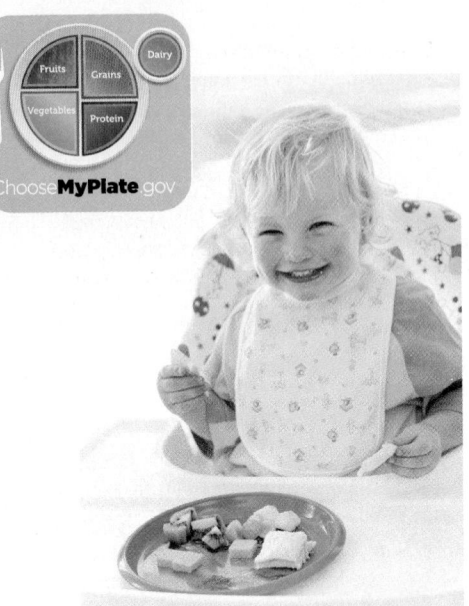

▲ How does this toddler's lunch of a peanut butter sandwich, cubed cheese, kiwi, and grapes compare to MyPlate?

creating a more harmonious family atmosphere are important steps toward resolving many childhood feeding problems. In addition, many parents must be educated as to what to expect of a preschool child and what food-related goals to set. Let's consider some typical complaints and concerns of parents, the causes of the problems, and suggestions for correcting them.

"My Child Won't Eat as Much or as Regularly as He Did as an Infant." This behavior is typical of preschoolers, because their growth rate slows after infancy; thus, they don't need as much food. Parents often need reminding that a 3-year-old can't be expected to eat as voraciously as an infant or to eat adult-size portions. MyPlate is a useful easy-to-understand tool for children, too. The proportions apply to all ages even though the portions will be smaller. Table 15-3 shows a general food plan that conforms to MyPlate proportions and is appropriate for preschool and school-age children. Until about 5 years of age, portion sizes in the vegetables group, fruits group, and protein group should be about 1 tablespoon per year of life, and can be increased as needed. The same advice does not apply to the grains or dairy groups, but consuming too much milk can leave the diet short on iron. Luckily, normal-weight children have a built-in feeding mechanism, which adjusts hunger to regulate food intake at each stage of growth. If a child is developing and growing normally and the caregiver is providing a variety of healthful foods, all can be confident of the child's well-being.

A pattern of picky eating is usually just another expression of independence for children, who have a strong desire to establish a self-determined routine. Caregivers should avoid nagging, forcing, and bribing children to encourage eating. Indirectly, these tactics reinforce picky-eating behaviors due to the added attention given to them. Overall, parents should focus on offering a variety of healthy choices, allowing the child to exert some autonomy over the specific type of food and the amount eaten. A child's sudden loss of appetite, however, may be reason for concern, as a poor appetite may be a sign of underlying illness.

Parents should also be reminded that food likes and dislikes change rapidly in childhood and are influenced by food temperature, appearance, texture, and taste. Sometimes children object to having foods mixed, as in stews and casseroles, even if they normally like the ingredients separately.

In addition, parents should recognize that this is an important age for children to explore the world around them. Even good eaters are sometimes more interested in

TABLE 15-3 Food Plans for Children Based on MyPlate Daily Food Plans

Food Group	Serving Size	Approximate Number of Servings [1]				
		Age 2 [2]	Age 5 [3]	Age 8 [3]	Age 12 [3,4]	Age 16 [3,4]
Grains	ounce	3	5	5	6–7	6–10
Vegetables	cup	1	1.5	2	2.5–3	2.5–3.5
Fruits	cup	1	1.5	1.5	2	2–2.5
Dairy	cup	2	2.5	3	3	3
Protein	ounce	2	4	5	5.5–6	5.5–7
Oils	teaspoon	3	4	5	6	6–8
Solid fats and added sugars	kcal	up to 140	up to 120	up to 120	up to 260–270	up to 260–400

[1]Log on to www.chooseMyPlate.gov for other ages and other physical activity levels.

[2]Based on less than 30 minutes of physical activity.

[3]Based on 30–60 minutes of physical activity.

[4]The lower amounts refer to girls.

exploring than eating. There's room for occasional indulgences, a skipped meal or two, or once in a while "less than ideal" choices. It's eating and lifestyle habits over the course of a month (and lifetime) that matter. Children master their eating when adults set a good example, provide opportunities to learn, give support for exploration, and limit inappropriate behavior.

"My Child Is Always Snacking, Yet She Never Finishes Her Meal." Children have small stomachs. Offering them six or so small meals succeeds better than limiting them to three meals each day. Sticking to three meals a day offers no special nutritional advantages; it's just a social custom. Snacking is fine, as long as good dental habits are practiced. When we eat isn't nearly as important as what we eat. If nutritious snacks are readily available, these are good to offer at midmorning or midafternoon when the child becomes hungry. Fruits and vegetables (fresh, frozen, or canned) and whole-grain breads and crackers are good snack choices. It is important that these snack choices be planned ahead in order to have healthy choices available. Working parents should make sure their children are provided with nutritious snacks to tide them over until dinnertime.

When a child refuses to eat, it's best not to overreact. Doing so may give the child the idea that not eating is a means of getting attention or manipulating a scene. Most children don't starve themselves to any point approaching physical harm. When children refuse to eat, have them sit at the table for a while; if they still aren't interested in eating, remove the food and wait until the next scheduled meal or snack.

"My Child Never Eats Vegetables." Children generally eat enough fruit but not an adequate amount of vegetables. Again, the one-bite policy can be used, including vegetable servings. It takes time for a child to become enthusiastic about a new food; however, with continual exposure and a positive role model, chances are the child may even grow to like it.

Children cannot and should not be forced to eat. They need to develop independence and identities separate from their parents. As stated earlier, children have to choose for themselves—a practice that should be encouraged. No one food is an essential part of a diet. Hunger is still the best means for getting a child to eat. It may be effective to feed children vegetables at the start of a meal, when they are hungriest. Offer new foods with familiar ones. A platter of raw or lightly cooked carrots, broccoli, green and red peppers, cabbage, and mushrooms eaten as a snack with friends may be accepted. A 4- or 5-year-old child can safely eat raw vegetables without fear of choking. Recall that children often are more sensitive than adults to strong flavors and odors. Nutritious dips, such as Ranch dressing, "sell" vegetables to many children. Vegetables may acquire more appeal when children help prepare them. And, as with any food, it is important to remember that children are entitled to their own likes and dislikes, too.

Do Children Need a Multivitamin and Mineral Supplement?

Major scientific groups, such as the American Dietetic Association and the American Society for Clinical Nutrition, believe that multivitamin and mineral supplements are generally unnecessary for healthy children; it's better to emphasize good foods. In fact, consuming fortified foods as well as supplements may lead to intakes above the UL for some nutrients, such as vitamin A and zinc. Children's supplements that are made to look like candy may result in accidental overdose, such as for iron. Fortified ready-to-eat breakfast cereals with milk are especially helpful in closing any gap between current micronutrient intake and needs, such as for vitamin E, folate, and vitamin D. Two micronutrients of particular concern are iron and zinc. These may be lacking in children's diets because they consume such small portions of rich sources, such as animal protein foods. In addition, since the 2010 Dietary Guidelines for Americans suggest that all Americans ages 2 years and older follow a diet low in saturated fat and cholesterol, rich sources of iron and zinc may be lacking in their diets. To compensate,

Food jags, common among preschoolers, are no cause for alarm. A child may switch from one specific food focus to another with equal intensity (older infants may also act this way). If the caregiver continues to offer choices, the child will soon begin to eat a wider variety of foods again, and the specific food focus will disappear as suddenly as it appeared.

Choking is a very preventable hazard for young children. Some suggestions for caregivers include:

- Set a good example at the table by taking small bites and chewing foods thoroughly.
- Have children sit at the table, take their time, and focus on their food during meals and snacks.
- Avoid giving children any foods that are round, firm, sticky, or cut into large chunks. Some examples of foods to avoid are nuts, grapes, raisins, popcorn, peanut butter, and hard pieces of raw fruits or vegetables.

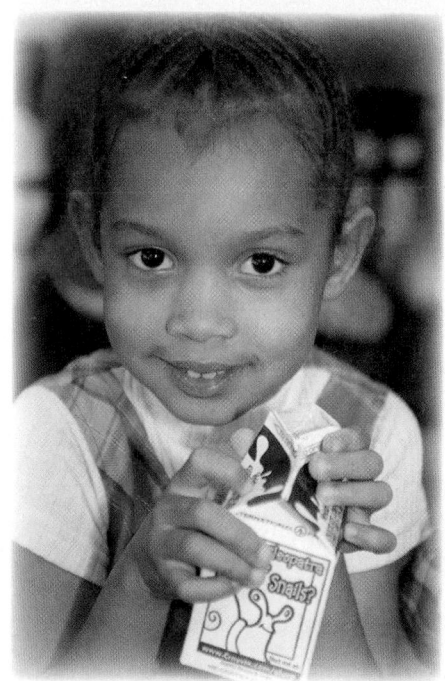

▲ Milk is a nutrient-dense source of protein, calcium, zinc, and other nutrients to support growth. It is especially challenging to meet calcium needs in childhood without regular dairy product consumption (see Chapter 9 for alternative sources of calcium).

parents can search for a whole-grain breakfast cereal that the child likes that also has about 50% of the Daily Value for iron and 25% of the Daily Value for zinc. (This will supply sufficient amounts of both nutrients because the Daily Values are based on the higher needs of adults.) If that's not possible, especially for a child who is ill, has a very erratic food preference pattern or appetite, or is on a weight-loss diet, the American Academy of Pediatrics states that the child may benefit from a children's multivitamin and mineral supplement not exceeding 100% of Daily Values on the label, especially if these conditions persist. Still, as mentioned many times in this textbook, such a practice does not substitute for an otherwise healthy diet—children included.

If current childhood feeding practices are to become more healthful, the focus should be on whole-grain breads and cereals, fruits, vegetables, and low-fat milk and milk products. Children do not need to be severely restricted but, rather, should modify food habits with small changes. Some easy diet changes to begin with are bagels instead of doughnuts, fat-free frozen yogurt instead of ice cream, fat-reduced or 1% milk instead of whole milk, dried fruit instead of candy for snacks, and air-popped popcorn instead of chips.

Nutritional Problems in Preschool Children

Three nutrition-related problems found in preschool children are iron-deficiency anemia, constipation, and dental caries. Proper diet can help correct or relieve these conditions. Vegetarian diets can also pose problems. Autism and lead poisoning are additional conditions that can be affected by nutritional status.

Iron-Deficiency Anemia. The best way to prevent iron-deficiency anemia in children is to provide foods that are adequate sources of iron. Iron-fortified breakfast cereals and a few ounces of lean meat are convenient means of increasing iron in a child's diet. The high proportion of heme iron in many animal foods allows the iron to be more readily absorbed than is iron from plant foods. Consuming a vitamin C source along with the less readily absorbed iron in plants and supplements aids absorption.

Childhood iron-deficiency anemia is most likely to appear in children between the ages of 6 and 24 months. It can lead to decreases in both stamina and learning ability because the oxygen supply to cells decreases. Another effect is lowered resistance to disease. Fortunately, childhood anemia is not common today in North America, probably because of children's use of iron-fortified breakfast cereals. Also deserving of credit in the United States is the Special Supplemental Nutrition Program for Women, Infants, and Children (WIC), sponsored by the U.S. federal government. This program emphasizes the importance of iron-fortified formulas and cereals and distributes these foods—along with nutrition education—to low-income parents of infants and preschool children considered to be at nutritional risk.

Constipation. Constipation may be associated with a more serious disease, yet some young children experience constipation unrelated to any medical condition. When presented with a constipated child, a physician first has to rule out a medical cause, such as intestinal blockage. And, although the most common GI tract symptom that reflects intolerance to cow's milk is diarrhea, chronic constipation may also result. Treatment for constipation generally consists of first evacuating the bowels, generally with an enema. The promotion of regular bowel habits then follows, with laxative use as directed by the physician. Several months to years of supportive intervention may be required for effective treatment.

The primary dietary interventions to alleviate constipation include eating more fiber and drinking more fluids. In the initial stages of treatment, providing certain fruit juices (e.g., prune, grape, and apple) and substituting soy milk for cow's milk may relieve constipation. In the long run, however, whole fruits (e.g., plums, peaches, and apricots) are better choices than juices because whole fruits are less concentrated sources of calories. Other foods to emphasize for fiber include vegetables,

For children who follow a totally vegetarian diet, attention should also focus on protein and vitamin B-12 intake.

Chapter 4 noted that it's unlikely that the use of sugar is the cause of hyperactivity or antisocial behavior in most children.

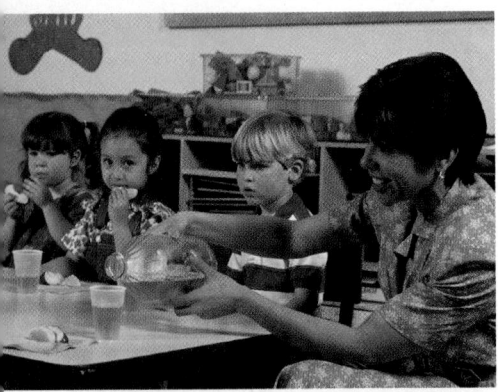

▲ Excessive fruit drink and fruit juice use is another potential problem in preschool (and later adolescent) years. The American Academy of Pediatrics recommends no more than 4 to 6 ounces per day for children 1 to 6 years (and 8 to 12 ounces per day for ages 7 to 18 years). Sweetened soft drinks should also be limited.

whole-grain breads and cereals, and beans. The daily fiber goals for children set by the Food and Nutrition Board vary by age (see margin). Few children meet these goals. Accompanying fluid recommendations are 4 cups (900 milliliters) per day for toddlers and about 5 cups (1200 milliliters) per day for older children.

Dental Caries. A proper diet goes a long way in reducing the risk for dental caries in young children. The following tips can help reduce dental problems in children:

- Begin oral hygiene when teeth start to appear.
- Seek early pediatric dental care.
- Drink fluoridated water.
- Use small amounts of fluoridated toothpaste twice daily.
- Snack in moderation.
- Have a dentist apply tooth sealants if needed.
- Avoid sticky, high-sugar snacks, especially between meals.
- If toddlers or preschoolers are chewing gum, sugarless gum is the best choice, as this has been shown to reduce the incidence of dental caries.

Vegetarianism in Childhood. Vegetarian diets can pose several risks for young children. These include the possibility of developing iron-deficiency anemia, a deficiency of vitamin B-12, and rickets from a vitamin D deficiency. During the first few years of life, children also may not consume enough calories when following a bulky vegetarian diet. These known pitfalls are easily avoided by informed diet planning (see Nutrition and Your Health: Vegetarian and Plant-Based Diets in Chapter 6). Diets for children who eat totally vegetarian fare should focus on protein, vitamin B-12, iron, and zinc content, with additional emphasis on vitamin D (or regular sun exposure) and calcium. Some of these dietary inadequacies can be compensated for by increasing oils, nuts, seeds, ready-to-eat breakfast cereals, and fortified soy milk in the diet.

Autism. Autism spectrum disorder (ASD) is characterized by a range of problems with social interaction, verbal and nonverbal communication, and/or unusual, repetitive, or limited activities and interests. These disorders usually are diagnosed in early childhood and affect an estimated 1 in every 150 children, with higher prevalence in boys than girls. The causes for ASD are not well understood, but there is a definite genetic component.

ASD can both affect and be affected by nutritional status (see Further Reading 6). In addition to developmental and behavioral abnormalities, many children with ASD also experience GI disorders, such as constipation, diarrhea, or reflux disease. Such disorders may impair nutrient intake or absorption. Some autistic children may have feeding problems related to developmental impairments. Also, picky eating behaviors may affect nutrient intake. Thus, careful attention to nutrient-dense food choices is warranted.

There are many nutrient-based theories concerning the causes and treatment of ASD. Nutritional interventions, such as dietary restrictions or nutrient supplements, are commonly employed by families affected by ASD. A widely used nutritional intervention is the gluten-free, casein-free (GFCF) diet, which eliminates all wheat, barley, rye, and milk products (see Further Reading 8). Proponents of this treatment propose that sensitivities to certain food proteins may have effects on neurotransmitter synthesis, thereby altering nervous system function. Clinical evidence supporting the effectiveness of the GFCF diet is limited, but promising. If the GFCF diet is used, families should enlist the aid of a registered dietitian to ensure dietary adequacy, particularly for protein, calcium, vitamin D, folic acid, and some B vitamins.

Other popular therapies for ASD include supplementation with probiotics, vitamin B-6 (0.6 mg/kg/d), magnesium (6.0 mg/kg/d), and omega-3 fatty acids (not exceeding 800 mg/d). Although sparse, research on these therapies is encouraging. There is evidence of altered absorption or metabolism of nutrients among children

▶ **Food and Nutrition Board Fiber Recommendations for Children**

Young Children

1–3 years	19 grams/day
4–8 years	25 grams/day

Boys

9–13 years	31 grams/day
14–18 years	38 grams/day

Girls

9–13 years	26 grams/day
14–18 years	26 grams/day

Despite a popularly held belief, scientific evidence does not support a causal relationship between mercury in vaccines and autism. Although small risks are inherent with routine vaccinations, the risks of infectious diseases are far worse.

with autism, so even with adequate nutrient intake, availability of some nutrients for metabolic processes may be low. Even though these supplements carry a low risk of adverse effects, caution is warranted to avoid overdoses. Because of the rising incidence of ASD and the lack of curative treatments, nutritional interventions for ASD will continue to be an active area of research.

Lead Poisoning. Humans may be exposed to lead from drinking contaminated water, consuming or inhaling lead dust (e.g., from cracked and peeling lead paint), contaminated dietary supplements (e.g., calcium supplements derived from bone meal), or foods stored or prepared in lead-containing vessels. In 2008, nearly 30,000 children were diagnosed with lead poisoning in the United States. Young children are particularly susceptible to the damaging effects of lead poisoning, which include long-term intellectual and behavioral impairments as well as increased risk for several chronic diseases in adulthood. Although it does not address the source of exposure, proper nutrition can reduce the risks of lead poisoning for children. Consuming regular meals, moderating fat intake, and ensuring adequate iron and calcium status are dietary practices known to reduce lead absorption. Adequate zinc, thiamin, and vitamin E intakes also reduce the harmful effects of absorbed lead. For lowest lead levels, only cold water should be used for drinking and preparation of formula or food. Letting cold water run from the tap for 2 to 3 minutes after a long period of inactivity (e.g., overnight) will limit the amount of lead that has accumulated in tap water. If the public water supply contains a high concentration of lead, bottled water is a safer alternative, particularly for formula preparation. Overall, a balanced meal plan that offers a variety of whole grains, lean meats, and low-fat dairy products is especially useful for protecting children from lead poisoning.

Objectives of *Healthy People 2020* include reducing mean blood lead level by 10% and eliminating elevated blood lead levels in children.

CONCEPT CHECK

The rapid growth rate of an infant's first year slows during the toddler and preschool years (ages 1 to 5). As a child's appetite decreases, adults need to serve nutrient-dense foods and allow the child to decide how much to eat. Sudden shifts in food preferences are to be expected. Snacking is fine if attention is given to the selection of healthful foods and good dental hygiene. Although a children's multivitamin and mineral supplement is usually not needed—a plan following MyPlate's Daily Food Plan that includes a serving of fortified ready-to-eat breakfast cereal should meet nutrient needs—use of such a supplement is a reasonable practice. Children need plenty of iron-rich food to prevent iron-deficiency anemia, as well as zinc for growth. Adequate mineral status also reduces risk of lead poisoning. Adequate fiber and fluid help prevent constipation. Diets for children who eat totally vegetarian fare should focus on meeting needs for protein, vitamin D, vitamin B-12, calcium, iron, and zinc. Potentially useful nutritional treatments for autism include the gluten-free, casein-free diet and supplementation with vitamin B-6, magnesium, probiotics, and essential fatty acids; research in this area is ongoing.

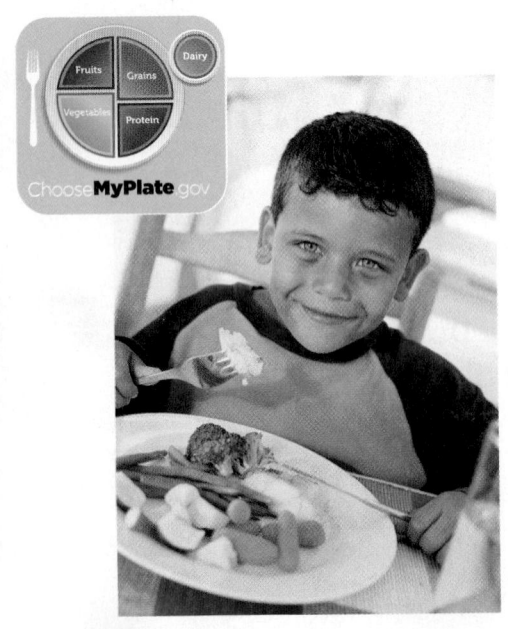

▲ How does this boy's dinner of broiled fish, broccoli, green beans, carrots, and zucchini compare to MyPlate?

15.4 School-Age Children: Nutrition Concerns

The diets of many school-age students can stand general improvement, particularly with regard to fruit, vegetable, whole-grain, and dairy choices. Drinking minimal amounts of sugared soft drinks is also advised. One survey of U.S. schoolchildren revealed that on the day of the survey, 40% of the children ate no vegetables, except for potatoes or tomato sauce, and 20% ate no fruits. Less than 20% of school-age girls consume adequate calcium. In general, the nutritional concerns and goals applicable to school-age children are the same as those discussed in relation to preschoolers. However, with the added pressures of peers, health messages from the media, and an increasing desire for independence, these goals may be harder to achieve as children grow older. MyPlate's daily food plans, which are tailored to age, gender, height, weight, and activity level, continue to be a good basis for diet planning, with an emphasis on moderating fat and sugar intake and ensuring adequate iron, zinc, and calcium intake (Fig. 15-3). Now let's look at several nutritional issues of particular concern during the school-age years.

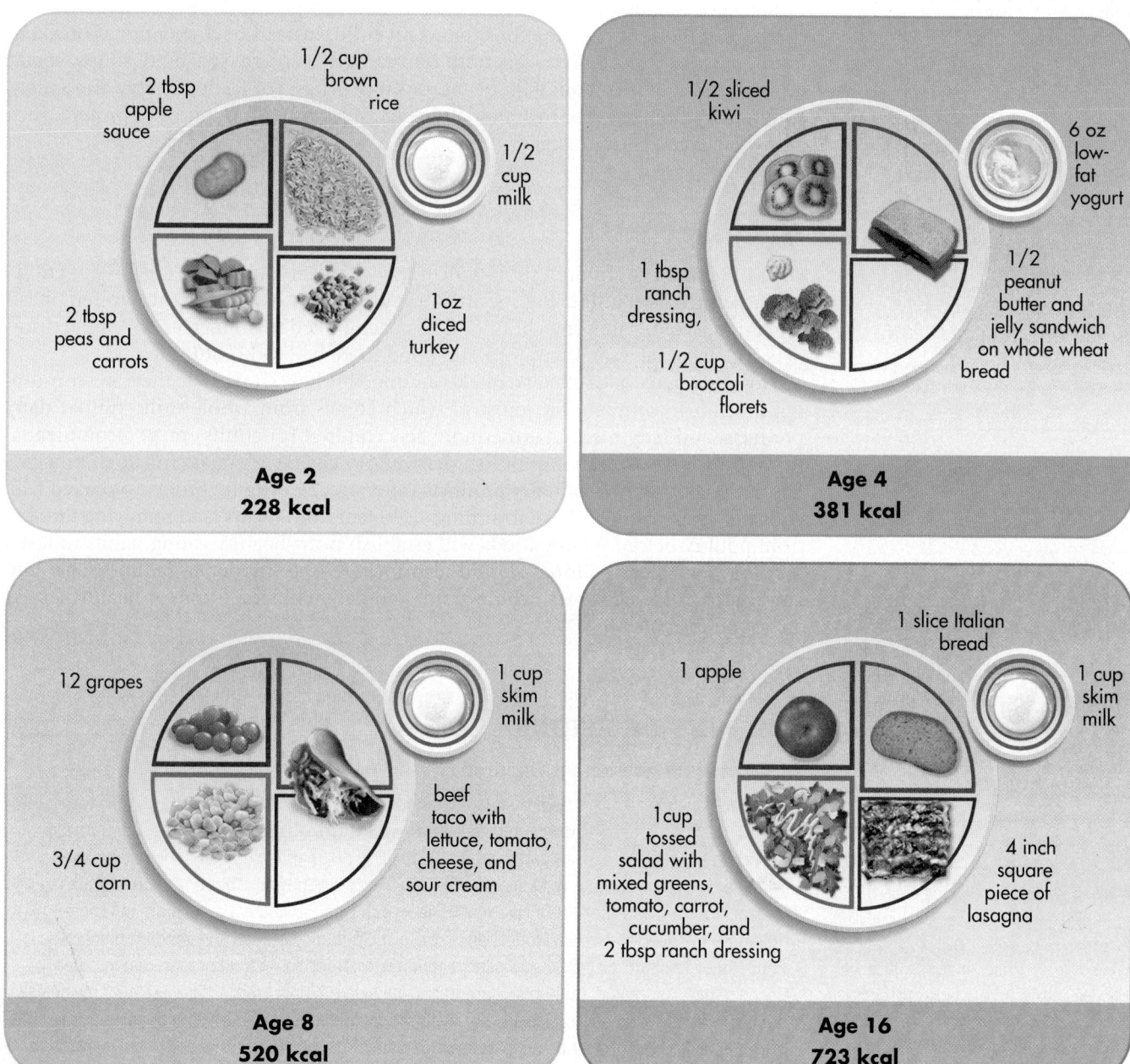

FIGURE 15-3 ▶ Using MyPlate to build a healthy meal for children. MyPlate is useful tool for all Americans, ages 2 and older. MyPlate proportions apply to children as well as adults, but portion sizes and food choices may vary by age.

NEWSWORTHY
NUTRITION

Healthy eating behaviors start at home

Parenting style and frequency of family meals are two important predictors of healthy eating behaviors among children, according to a recent review of family correlates of pediatric obesity. Of four basic parenting styles, authoritative parenting, which is demanding yet responsive to children, promotes healthy eating and physical activity and is associated with low rates of pediatric obesity. Eating family meals is also associated with healthy eating and lower BMI in children. When parents and children enjoy meals together, children are supervised and engaged while parents have the opportunity to communicate and model healthy behaviors. Thus, children eat more fruits and vegetables, leading to better nutrient intake, and are less likely to have disordered eating behaviors. Family meals and an authoritative parenting style promote health at the table and beyond.

Source: Berge JM: A review of family correlates of child and adolescent obesity: What has the 21st century taught us so far? *International Journal of Adolescent Medicine and Health* 21:457, 2009.

connect Check out the Connect site
www.mcgrawhillconnect.com
to further explore healthy eating behaviors.

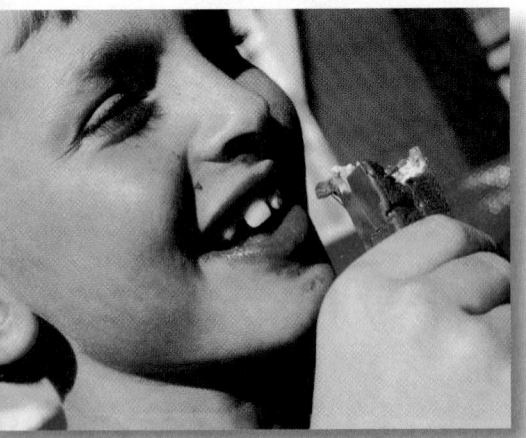

▲ Sweets should be consumed in moderation in childhood, but do not have to be avoided altogether.

CRITICAL THINKING

Tim refuses to eat breakfast before school. He doesn't like cereal, toast, or any of the other usual breakfast foods. What can Tim's parents do to ensure that he eats nutritious foods before leaving for school?

Breakfast

Once children enter school, their eating patterns become more scheduled, and the consumption of regular meals—especially breakfast—becomes an important focus. A fortified ready-to-eat breakfast cereal is typically the greatest source of iron, vitamin A, and folic acid for children ages 2 to 18. Although there is controversy over the true benefit of breakfast for cognitive ability, children who eat breakfast are more likely to meet their daily needs for vitamins and minerals compared to children not eating breakfast. To influence morning test performance, it appears that breakfast must be eaten within a few hours of a test; the subsequent rise in blood glucose is thought to enhance performance.

Breakfast menus need not be limited to traditional fare. A little imagination can spark the interest of even the most reluctant child. Instead of conventional breakfast foods, parents can offer leftovers from dinner, such as pizza, spaghetti, soups, yogurt topped with trail mix, chili with beans, or sandwiches. For lasting energy and satiety, combine traditional carbohydrate-rich breakfast foods with a source of protein, such as low-fat cheese, nuts, or eggs.

Fat Intake

Diets of school-age children should include a variety of foods from each major group, not necessarily excluding any specific food because of its fat content. Overemphasis on fat-reduced diets during childhood has been linked to an increase in eating disorders and encourages an inappropriate "good food, bad food" attitude.

However, surveys of dietary intake among children show that they are consuming too much saturated fat, most of which comes from whole milk, full-fat dairy products, and fatty meats. Furthermore, few children (or adults) meet recommendations to include two servings of fish per week to ensure adequate intake of omega-3 fats. Emphasizing low-fat dairy products (after age 2), offering broiled or baked fish, choosing leaner cuts of meat, trimming visible fat from meats, and removing the skin from poultry before serving foods will establish heart-healthy eating habits to last a lifetime. Snacks for children should also include only moderate fat and sugar and emphasize fruit, vegetables, whole grain, and dairy choices. Ideas for healthy snacks are found in Table 15-4.

MAKING DECISIONS

Nutrition Education for Children

Children spend the majority of their waking hours in school, so it is a great place to learn about positive, healthy eating habits (see Further Reading 3). A strong emphasis on nutrition in schools can help children understand why healthy diet habits will make them feel more energetic, look better, and work more efficiently. Federally-funded programs such as USDA's Team Nutrition and the CDC's National Bone Health Campaign are a good start, but more changes are needed. School foodservice outlets, including cafeterias and vending machines, must present healthier options for school children. Instruction on food preparation in home economics classes and after-school programs will help children learn to prepare healthy meals and snacks. Increased participation in physical education classes and recreational sports is more likely to improve academic performance than detract from it. However, positive nutrition influences must extend beyond the classroom to change persistent trends toward obesity and chronic diseases. Caregivers and other adult role models need to create safe opportunities for children to be active and must practice what they preach when it comes to healthy habits.

TABLE 15-4 Twenty Healthy Snack Ideas for School-Age Children

	Iron	Zinc	Calcium	Vitamin C	Fiber
Almonds (1 oz)			✓		✓
Applesauce (1/2 cup)				✓	✓
Bean and cheese burrito (1)	✓	✓	✓		✓
Cheese (1 oz) and whole-wheat crackers (6)	✓	✓	✓		✓
Dried cranberries (1/4 cup)				✓	✓
Frozen fruit pieces (1 cup)				✓	✓
Fruit salad (1 cup)				✓	✓
Fruit smoothie (1 cup)				✓	✓
Hard-boiled egg	✓	✓			
Hummus (2 tbsp) with bell pepper rings (1 cup)				✓	✓
Low-fat microwave popcorn (3 tbsp unpopped)					✓
Mini-pizzas on whole-grain English muffins (2)	✓	✓	✓	✓	✓
Peanut butter (2 tbsp) and apple slices (1 cup)		✓		✓	✓
Quick breads, such as banana bread, 1 slice	✓				✓
String cheese (1 stick)			✓		
Trail mix (1/4 cup)	✓	✓		✓	✓
Tuna salad (1/2 cup) in whole-wheat pita pocket	✓	✓			✓
Whole-grain cereal (1 cup)	✓	✓			✓
Whole-wheat pasta salad with veggies (1 cup)	✓	✓		✓	✓
Yogurt (8 oz) with granola (2 tbsp)		✓	✓		✓

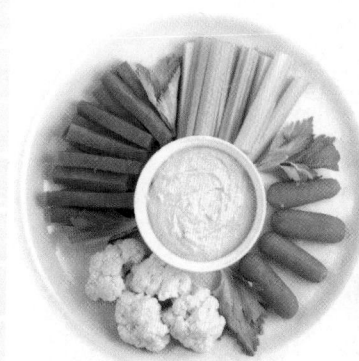

Type 2 Diabetes

Type 2 diabetes is generally thought to be an adult condition. As reviewed in the Nutrition and Your Health section, Diabetes—When Blood Glucose Regulation Fails in Chapter 4, it frequently occurs in overweight people older than 40. However, physicians have noted an alarming increase in the frequency of the disease among children (and teenagers). This is primarily due to the rise in obesity in this age group, coupled with minimal physical activity. Up to 85% of children with the disease are overweight at diagnosis. Experts are calling for screening for diabetes in at-risk children every 2 years, starting at age 10 or at the onset of puberty. Besides obesity and a sedentary lifestyle, other risk factors include having a first- or second-degree relative with the disease or belonging to a nonwhite population. Appropriate diet and lifestyle intervention should be implemented, along with the use of diabetes medications when necessary. A regular intake of low-glycemic-load fruits, vegetables, and whole-grain breads and cereals is especially recommended.

Early Signs of Cardiovascular Disease

Also paralleling the increase in childhood obesity, early signs of cardiovascular disease have become increasingly prevalent among children and adolescents. One out of five youths between the ages of 12 and 19 years has abnormal blood lipids. Therefore, lifestyle modifications to delay the progression of the disease are important throughout the lifespan. The American Academy of Pediatrics now recommends that at-risk children first undergo cholesterol screening sometime between the ages of 2 and 10, followed by repeated cholesterol screening every 3 to 5 years (see Further Reading 7). Children are considered "at risk" if they are overweight, have high blood pressure, smoke, or have diabetes; if they have a family history of cardiovascular disease; or if family history is unknown. For children whose cholesterol is elevated, lifestyle approaches, such as weight management through dietary modification and increased physical activity, are the first line of therapy. Following a meal plan that is based on the Dietary Guidelines and conforms to MyPlate's Daily Food Plan would be appropriate for prevention of cardiovascular disease. Some high-risk children may be candidates for cholesterol-lowering medications.

Overweight and Obesity

In the United States, more than 30% of school-age children are overweight or obese. The number of cases is increasing, especially in minority populations. In the short run, ridicule, embarrassment, possibly depression, and short stature linked to early puberty are the main consequences of such obesity. In the long run, significant health problems associated with obesity, such as cardiovascular disease, type 2 diabetes, and hypertension, usually will appear in adulthood or earlier. Childhood obesity is a serious health threat because about 40% of obese children (and about 80% of obese adolescents) become obese adults. Significant weight gain generally begins between ages 5 and 7, during puberty, or during the teenage years.

Research points to many potential causes of childhood obesity. Recall the nature versus nurture discussion in Chapter 7. Some infants are born with lower metabolic rates; they use calories more efficiently and in turn can more easily produce fat stores. Studies also suggest, though, that this genetic link accounts for only one-third of individual differences in body weight.

Researchers believe that, although diet is an important factor, inactivity is also a contributor to the increase in childhood obesity (see Further Readings 4 and 5). Studies show that as children age, physical activity steadily declines. By age 15, only one-third of children are getting the recommended 60 minutes of exercise per day. It doesn't help that physical education classes are now elective in many high schools. Today's generation of children now glues itself to the TV for an average of 24 hours per week; many children spend another 10 hours or so playing computer and video games. The American Academy of Pediatrics recommends a limit of 14 hours of TV and video time per week for children over age 2 (no television is recommended for children younger than 2 years). In addition, excessive snacking, overreliance on fast-food restaurants, parental neglect, the media in general, lack of safe areas to play, and the abundant availability of high-calorie food choices contribute to childhood obesity. Soft drinks and other sugared beverages are especially implicated.

The initial approach in treating an obese child is to assess how much physical activity he or she engages in. If a child spends much free time in sedentary activities (such as watching television or playing video games), more physical activities should be encouraged. The Physical Activity Guidelines for Americans recommend 60 minutes or more of moderate to intense physical activity per day for children and adolescents. Learning to engage in and enjoy regular physical activity will help children not only to attain a healthy body weight but also to keep a similar body weight later in life. An increase in physical activity won't just happen; parents and other caregivers need to plan for it. Getting the family together for a brisk walk after dinner

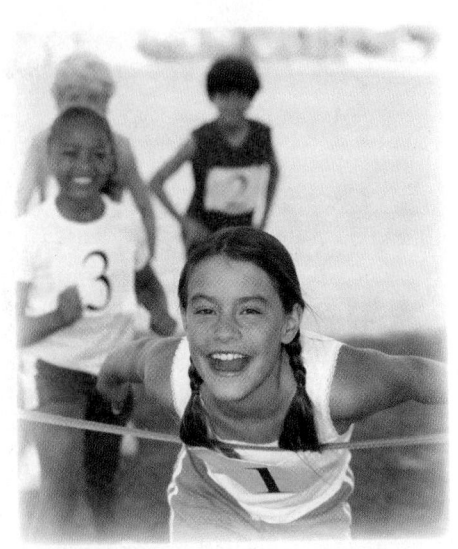

▲ Regular physical activity is an important part of prevention and treatment of weight problems in childhood. The goal is about 60 minutes of such activity each day. Many children do not meet this goal.

encourages healthy habits for all involved. Age-appropriate activities for elementary school-age children include walking, dancing, jumping rope, and participation in organized sports that focus on fun rather than intense competition. For middle school-age children, more complex organized sports (e.g., football and basketball) are of interest and some weight training with small weights can also be beneficial.

Moderation in calorie intake is important, especially the limitation of high-calorie foods, such as sugared soft drinks and whole milk. The focus should be on more vitamin- and mineral-dense foods and healthy snacks. An emphasis on appropriate portion sizes may help youth learn to curb excessive food intake. Making small changes such as substituting low-fat for whole milk, or canned fruit in its own juice instead of heavy syrup, can moderately cut calories without sacrificing taste or disrupting normal eating patterns. To specifically address the increased burden of overweight and obesity among minority populations, health professionals must become versed in varied cultural food preferences.

Resorting to a weight-loss diet is usually not necessary—it is best to emphasize changing habits that allow for weight maintenance. Children have an advantage over adults in dealing with obesity; their bodies can use stored energy for growth. Thus, if weight gain can be moderated, increases in height and resulting lean body tissue may reduce the percentage of body weight accounted for as stored fat, yielding a more healthful weight-to-height ratio. This is one reason it is desirable to treat obesity in childhood. Further growth can contribute to success. If weight loss is necessary in younger children, it should be gradual, about ½ to 1 pound per week. In some cases, the child should be watched closely to ensure that the rate of growth continues to be normal. The child's calorie intake should not be so low that gains in height diminish. In some cases, medications may be prescribed under a physician's care (e.g., orlistat [Xenical]). For the 3% of American children who are morbidly obese, bariatric surgery may be an option for weight management (see Further Readings 12 and 13).

To get kids involved in exercise, new physical education classes have been introduced into schools. These classes provide lifelong fitness lessons in such activities as rock climbing, in-line skating, and recreational jogging. These classes help promote activity because they take the focus away from teams and competition, which often discourage and embarrass kids who lack athletic talent.

CONCEPT CHECK

The school-age child is advised to use MyPlate as a guide for eating and especially moderate choices high in fat and simple sugars. Breakfast is an important meal to refuel the body for a new school day and to help ensure fulfilling nutrient needs for the day. Attention to regular physical activity and healthy diet should help prevent/treat childhood obesity and build a desirable lifestyle pattern for later life.

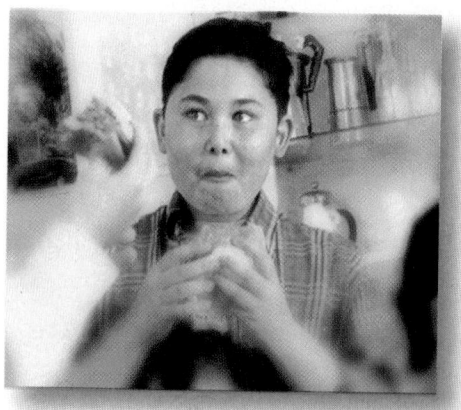

▲ Supersized portions of foods such as hamburgers and sugared soft drinks served to children are contributing to the obesity and type 2 diabetes epidemics they are experiencing.

15.5 Teenage Years: Nutrition Concerns

Most girls begin a rapid growth spurt between the ages of 10 and 13, and most boys experience rapid growth between the ages of 12 and 15. Nearly every organ in the body grows during these periods. Most noticeable are increases in height and weight and the development of secondary sexual characteristics. Girls usually begin menstruating (reach **menarche**) during this growth spurt, and they grow very little beyond 2 years after menarche. Early-maturing girls may begin their growth spurt as early as age 7 to 8, whereas early-maturing boys may begin growing by age 9 to 10.

During this adolescent growth spurt, girls gain about 10 inches (25 centimeters) in height, and boys gain about 12 inches (30 centimeters). Girls also tend to accumulate both lean and fat tissue, whereas boys tend to gain mostly lean tissue. This growth spurt provides about 50% of ultimate adult weight and about 15% of ultimate adult height (review Fig. 15-1).

As the growth spurt begins, teenagers begin to eat more. If teens choose nutritious food, they can take advantage of their increased hunger and easily satisfy their nutrient

menarche The onset of menstruation. Menarche usually occurs around age 13, 2 or 3 years after the first signs of puberty start to appear.

Drinking soft drinks in place of milk causes many teenagers to have inadequate calcium intake. Over the last 20 years, soft drinks have been replacing milk as the preferred beverage of adolescents. Only half of school-age boys and 20% of girls meet recommendations for calcium intake. This trend has been linked to decreased bone mass and increased bone fractures in this age group.

A strictly vegetarian diet must be monitored for adequate energy, protein, iron, vitamin B-12, calcium, and vitamin D (the latter if sun exposure is not sufficient). These nutrients become particularly important in teenagers, as their diets are often already compromised.

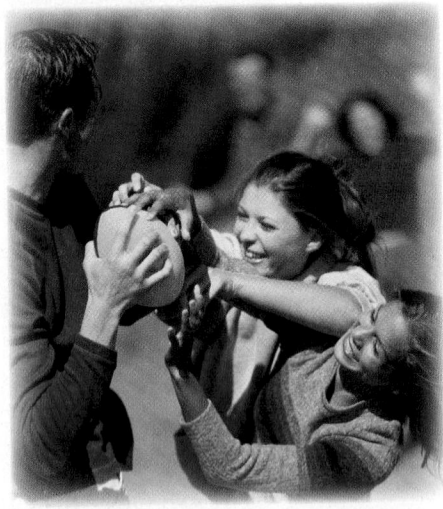

▲ An active lifestyle coupled with a healthy diet should be part of the teen years. Both habits contribute to bone development and bone strength.

Alcoholism is a significant health problem that may have its roots in the teen years. Smoking—another habit that compromises health—also often begins in teen years. Some of the impetus for smoking is the desire to control body weight—but this is not an advisable method.

needs. As discussed for younger age groups, MyPlate can serve as a guide for meeting these nutrient needs (Table 15-3). Following such a plan will meet carbohydrate needs (130 grams per day) and protein needs (52 grams per day for males and 46 grams per day for females).

Nutritional Problems and Concerns of Teens

Anorexia nervosa and bulimia nervosa are nutritional concerns of the teen years, as covered in detail in Chapter 11. Other nutritional problems are more common during the teen years. A survey of high school students showed that only a little over 25% had eaten five servings of fruits and vegetables on the previous day, and they are consuming approximately 25% more sodium than recommended. Another concern is that many teenage girls stop drinking milk, so they may not consume enough calcium to allow for maximal mineralization of bones through their early twenties. Inadequate calcium intake during the teenage years sets the stage for development of osteoporosis later in life.

Inadequate Calcium Intake. Many teenagers are not meeting their needs for calcium. The RDA for calcium for both males and females between ages 9 and 18 years is 1300 milligrams per day, compared with only 1000 milligrams per day for younger children. Three servings per day from the dairy group are recommended for all teenagers and young adults to meet calcium needs. Figure 2-1 in Chapter 2 shows the stark contrast between milk and typical soft drinks with respect to calcium and other nutrients. If dairy products are not consumed, alternative calcium sources need to be included.

Iron Deficiency. A further concern is iron deficiency. Iron-deficiency anemia sometimes appears in girls after they start menstruating (menarche) and in boys during their growth spurt. About 10% of teenagers have low iron stores or related anemia. Teens who strive to forge an identity by adopting dietary patterns unfamiliar to their families—vegetarianism, for example—may not know enough about the alternative diet pattern to keep from developing health problems, such as iron-deficiency anemia. It's important that teenagers choose good food sources of iron, such as lean meats, whole grains, and enriched cereals. Teenage girls, particularly those with heavy menstrual flows, need to eat good sources of iron (or regularly consume an iron supplement). Iron-deficiency anemia is a highly undesirable condition for a teen. It can produce increased fatigue and decreased ability to concentrate and learn. School and physical performance may suffer.

MAKING DECISIONS

Nutrition and Acne

Acne is a common teen concern—about 80% of teens experience it. Although it's popularly believed that eating nuts, chocolate, and pizza can make acne worse, scientific studies have failed to show a strong link between these dietary factors and acne. Based on the results of observational research, two dietary practices currently under study for possible roles in the development of acne include high glycemic load and consumption of cow's milk or whey protein-based product (e.g., body building supplements). However, sufficient evidence is not currently available to support any drastic dietary changes to control acne. A balanced diet and adequate fluid intake combined with sensible hygiene practices remain the best practices to promote skin health.

Acne medications, such as Accutane, contain analogs of vitamin A (e.g., 13-*cis* retinoic acid). Although these treatments can be effective, close supervision by a physician is crucial, as vitamin A analogs can be toxic. Vitamin A itself is no help in treating acne, and excess amounts of vitamin A or related analogs taken during pregnancy can cause birth defects. Thus, girls taking these vitamin A medications should not become pregnant.

Helping Teens Eat More Nutritious Foods

Teenagers face a variety of challenges. They pursue their independence, experience identity crises, seek peer acceptance, and worry about physical appearance. These factors affect food choice. Advertisers take advantage of this by pushing a vast array of products—candy, gum, soft drinks, and snacks—at the teenage market. Potato chips and French fries make up more than one-third of the vegetable servings consumed by teens. Additionally, many schools offer French fries on a regular basis, and soft drink machines can be found in school hallways and cafeterias, in turn competing with the school lunch. The increased consumption of fast-foods, sugary beverages, and snack foods crowds out nutrient-dense foods, thus limiting intake of calcium, iron, zinc, fat-soluble vitamins, and folate.

Teens often do not think about the long-term benefits of good health. They have a hard time relating today's actions to tomorrow's health outcomes. Many teenagers tend to think they can change habits later; there's no hurry.

Still, healthful teen food habits do not require giving up favorite foods. Small portions of fatty foods can complement larger portions of fat-free and reduced-fat dairy products, lean meats, vegetable proteins, fruits, vegetables, and whole-grain products. An example of this type of meal is a plain hamburger with a garden salad (minimize the amount of regular dressing or use a low-fat variety), small order of French fries or chili, and a medium diet soft drink or reduced-fat or fat-free milk.

Obesity is a growing problem among teenagers, and about 30% of obese teenagers have the metabolic syndrome (Syndrome X) discussed in Chapters 4 and 5. If a teen attains ultimate adult height and is still obese, a weight-loss regimen may be necessary. This is especially appropriate after the adolescent growth spurt. Weight loss should be gradual, perhaps 1 pound per week, and generally follow the advice in Chapter 7. Weight loss medications may also be prescribed.

Are Teenage Snacking Practices Harmful?

Teens often obtain one-fourth to one-third of all their calories and major nutrients from snacks. Unfortunately, studies have found just what you might expect—that teens snack mostly on potato and corn chips, cookies, candies, and ice cream. Key reasons for snacking include an opportunity to get out and socialize with friends, accessibility, hunger, and celebration of a special event. Teenagers can obtain many nutrients from snacking. Even fast-food restaurants offer some good food choices. By choosing wisely and eating in moderation, teens can eat at fast-food restaurants occasionally and still consume a very healthful diet. Snacks and fast-food restaurants themselves are not the problem; poor food choices in terms of type and quantity are.

Lack of exercise and poor dietary habits formed during teenage years often continue into adulthood and may increase risk of chronic diseases, such as cardiovascular disease, osteoporosis, and some types of cancer. Getting this message across to teenagers is an important and challenging task for parents and educators.

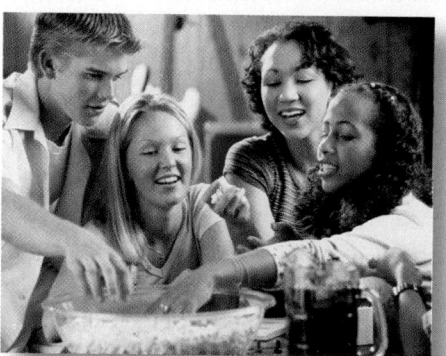
▲ The teenage years are noted for snacking. With reasonable food choices, teenagers can have healthful diets.

CONCEPT CHECK

A second period of rapid growth occurs during the teen years. Girls generally start this growth spurt earlier than boys. MyPlate's Daily Food Plan can direct meal planning. Common nutritional problems in these years arise from poor food choices and include inadequate calcium intake in girls and iron-deficiency anemia. Changes occur so rapidly during these years, and in so many areas—psychological, social, and physical—it may be difficult to stress the relevance of nutrition to teenagers. Moderation in fat and sugar intake are important goals to consider when choosing snacks.

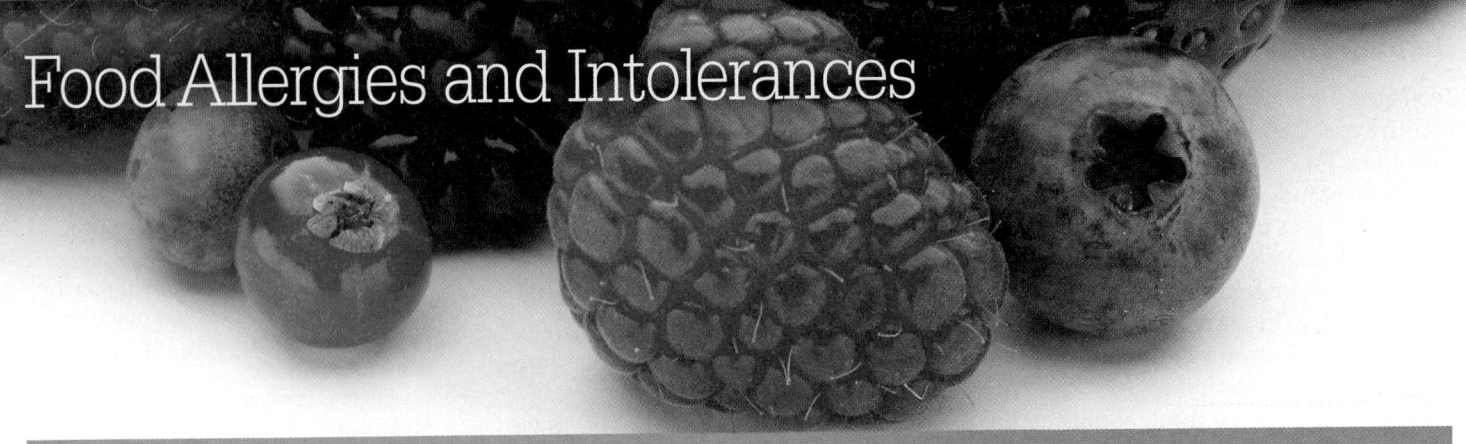

Food Allergies and Intolerances

Food allergies are on the rise. Between 1997 and 2007, food allergies among children increased by 18%. What used to be a rare medical incident is now the cause for 30,000 emergency room visits and 150 to 200 deaths per year. Food allergies cost Americans more than $500 million per year. Today, food allergies affect about 8% (5.9 million) of children in the United States, one-third of whom suffer from multiple food allergies (see Further Reading 10).

Adverse reactions to foods—indicated by sneezing, coughing, nausea, vomiting, diarrhea, hives, and other rashes—are broadly classed as food allergies (also called hypersensitivities) or **food intolerances.** Whereas allergies involve an immune response to a foreign protein (**allergen**), intolerances are caused by an individual's inability to digest a certain food component or by the direct effect of a food component or contaminant on the body. Let's examine each process, first allergies and then intolerances.

FOOD ALLERGIES: SYMPTOMS AND MECHANISM

Allergic reactions to foods are common (Fig. 15-4) and occur more frequently in females than males. Food allergies occur most often during infancy and young adulthood. Three types of reactions may occur after the ingestion of problem foods by susceptible people:

- *Classic*–itching, reddening skin, asthma, swelling, choking, and a runny nose
- *GI tract*–nausea, vomiting, diarrhea, intestinal gas, bloating, pain, constipation, and indigestion

- *General*–headache, skin reactions, tension and fatigue, tremors, and psychological problems

Any reaction milder than these is a **food sensitivity.**

Allergic reactions vary not only in the body system affected, but also in their duration, ranging from seconds to a few days. A generalized, all-systems reaction is called **anaphylactic shock.** This severe allergic response results in low blood pres-

food intolerance An adverse reaction to food that does not involve an allergic reaction.

allergen A foreign protein, or antigen, that induces excess production of certain immune system antibodies; subsequent exposure to the same protein leads to allergic symptoms. Whereas all allergens are antigens, not all antigens are allergens.

food sensitivity A mild reaction to a substance in a food that might be expressed as slight itching or redness of the skin.

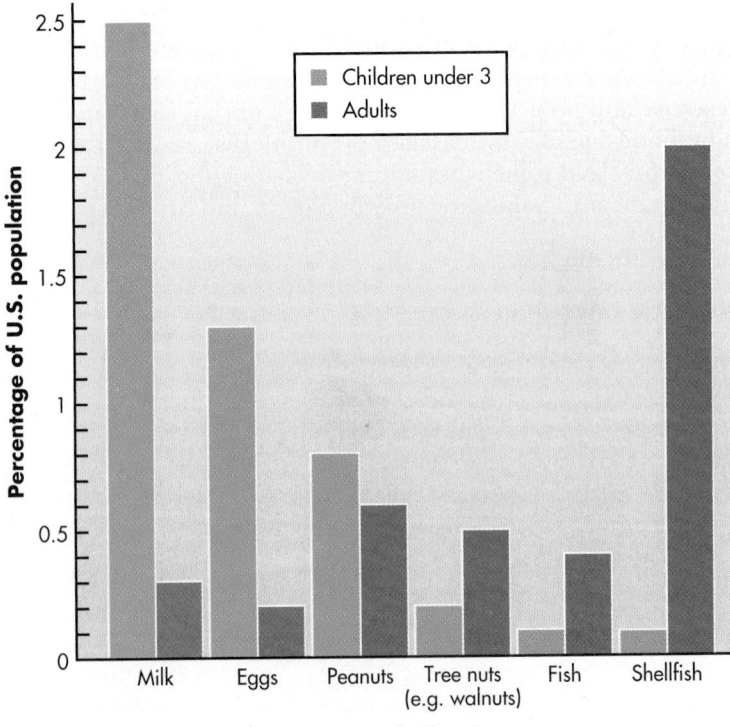

FIGURE 15-4 ▶ Types of allergies and percentage of U.S. population with those allergies.

Source: Journal of Allergy and Clinical Immunology (study done by Mount Sinai School of Medicine).

sure and distress of the respiratory system and GI tract. It can be fatal. A person who is extremely sensitive to a food may not be able to touch the food or even be in the same room where it is being cooked without reacting to it. Although any food can trigger anaphylactic shock, the most common culprits are peanuts (a legume, not a nut), tree nuts (e.g., walnuts, pecans, etc.), shellfish, milk (look for an ingredient called casein on the label), eggs (look for the ingredient albumin on the label), soybeans, wheat, and fish. Other foods frequently identified with adverse reactions include meat and meat products, fruits, and cheese. For a small number of people, avoiding foods such as peanuts or shellfish is a matter of life and death.

Basically, allergies are an inappropriate response of the immune system. When immune cells identify a harmful foreign protein (**antigen**), they destroy it and produce antibodies to it, so that the next response to the harmful substance will be swift and effective. Almost all food allergies are caused by proteins in foods that act as antigens (also called **allergens**). In these cases, the immune system mistakes the food protein for a harmful substance and mounts an immune response, leading to symptoms such as hives, runny nose, and GI disturbances.

No one is sure why the immune system sometimes overreacts to harmless proteins. The early introduction (e.g., before 4 to 6 months of age) of solid foods to infants may trigger food allergies. The reasoning is that the infant's GI tract is immature and "leaky," allowing some undigested proteins to be absorbed into the bloodstream. This is beneficial for breastfed infants, who can absorb immune proteins from breast milk. However, if some food proteins are introduced before the GI tract has matured, these antigens may enter the bloodstream and stimulate an immune response.

The hygiene hypothesis offers another interesting explanation: in our "germophobic" society, with the protection of antibiotics, hand sanitizers, and antimicrobial soaps and cleaners, our immune systems aren't vigorously challenged by antigens. As a result, the immune system may become sensitized to innocuous substances, such as food proteins. Recent research supports the hygiene hypothesis. Children who

grow up on farms or who have pets, and are thereby exposed to many antigens, have fewer allergies and asthma than children who grow up in more sterile environments.

Recently, researchers have proposed a link between low levels of vitamin D and food allergies. The rise in incidence of food allergies has paralleled an increase in vitamin D deficiency. The relationship between vitamin D and food allergies may be mediated by the vitamin's role in immune function.

Whatever the explanation, one thing is clear: food allergies are an important concern for many parents and others who work with children.

Testing for a Food Allergy

The diagnosis of a food allergy can often be a difficult task (Table 15-5). It requires the participation of a skilled physician. The first step in determining whether a food allergy is present is to record a detailed history of symptoms, including the time from ingestion to onset of symptoms, duration of symptoms, most recent reaction, food suspected of causing a reaction, and quantity and nature of food needed to produce a reaction. A family history of allergic diseases can also help, as allergic reactions tend to run in families. A physical examination may reveal evidence of an allergy, such as skin diseases and asthma. Various diagnostic tests can rule out other conditions. The diagnostic first step is to eliminate from the diet—for 1 to 2 weeks—all tested compounds that appear to cause allergic symptoms, plus all other foods suspected of causing an allergy based on the person's food history. The person generally starts out eating foods to which almost no one reacts, such as rice, vegetables, noncitrus fruits, and fresh meats and poultry. If symptoms are still present, the person can more severely restrict the diet or even use special formula diets that are hypoallergenic.

Once a diet is found that causes no symptoms, called an **elimination diet,** foods can be added back one at a time. This type of food challenge is an option only when the culprit foods are known to pose no risk of anaphylactic shock in the person. Doses of ½ to 1 teaspoon (2.5 to 5 milliliters) are given at first. The amount is increased until the dose approximates usual intake. Any reintroduced food that

anaphylactic shock A severe allergic response that results in lowered blood pressure and respiratory and gastrointestinal distress. This can be fatal.

antigen Any substance that induces a state of sensitivity and/or resistance to microorganisms or toxic substances after a lag period; substance that stimulates a specific aspect of the immune system.

▶ People with a history of serious allergic reactions and those who have asthma should carry a self-administered form of epinephrine, such as EpiPen, to subside an episode of anaphylactic shock, should it occur.

▶ The American Academy of Allergy, Asthma, and Immunology has a 24-hour toll-free hot line (800-822-2762) to answer questions about food allergies and to help direct people to specialists. Free information on food allergies is available by contacting The Food Allergy & Anaphylaxis Network. The telephone number is (800-929-4040); the website is www.foodallergy.org.

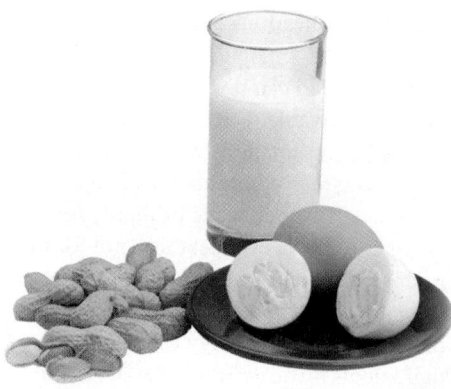

▲ Eggs, milk, and peanuts are three of the foods that pose the greatest risk for food allergies in childhood.

TABLE 15-5 Assessment Strategies for Food Allergies

History	Include description of symptoms, time between food ingestion and onset of symptoms, duration of symptoms, most recent allergic episode, quantity of food required to produce reaction, suspected foods, and allergic diseases in other family members.
Physical examination	Look for signs of an allergic reaction (rash, itching, intestinal bloating, etc.).
Elimination diet	Establish a diet lacking the suspected offending foods and stay on it for 1 to 2 weeks or until symptoms clear.
Food challenge	Add back small amounts of excluded foods, one at a time, as long as anaphylactic shock is not a possible consequence.
Blood test	Determine presence of antibodies in blood that bind to food antigens tested.
Skin test	Place a sample of the suspected allergen under the skin and watch for an inflammatory reaction.

causes significant symptoms to appear is identified as an allergen for the person.

Laboratory tests can also aid in diagnosis of food allergies. Skin testing involves pricking the skin with a small amount of purified food extract and observing any allergic response (e.g., a red eruption at the prick site). These types of tests are easy and safe, even for infants, but they may not clearly diagnose a food allergy. A positive skin-prick test merely indicates that a person has been sensitized to a food; it can't definitively identify if that food is the cause for the symptoms in question. Newer types of blood testing, however, have more diagnostic value. Blood tests estimate the blood concentration of antibodies that bind certain foodborne antigens.

Living with Food Allergies

Once potential allergens are identified, dietary modifications must be made. In some cases, small amounts of the offending food can be consumed without an observable reaction. Also, some food allergens are destroyed by heating, so cooking may eliminate the allergic response. This is effective primarily for allergies to fruits or vegetables, not for the more common allergies to milk, peanuts, or seafood. For most cases, though, complete avoidance of allergy-causing food ingredients is the safest course of action. This makes careful reading of food labels essential. As of 2006, the Food Allergen Labeling and Consumer Protection Act now requires manufacturers to clearly identify the presence of major food allergens (milk, eggs, fish, shellfish, peanuts, tree nuts, wheat, and soy) on food product labels.

A major challenge when treating a person with a food allergy is to make sure that what remains in the diet can still provide essential nutrients. The small food intake of children permits less leeway in removing offending foods that may contain numerous nutrients. A registered dietitian can help guide the diet-planning process to ensure that the remaining food choices still meet nutrient needs or to guide supplement use, if that is necessary.

About 80% of young children with food allergies outgrow them before 3 years. Parents should be made aware of this and not assume the allergy will be long-lived. Food allergies diagnosed after 3 years of age are often more long-lived, but not always. In these cases, about 33% of people outgrow their food allergies within 3 years. For others, the condition may be prolonged; some food allergies can last a lifetime, such as those for peanuts, tree nuts, and shellfish. Periodic reintroduction of offending foods can be tried every 6 to 12 months or so to see whether the allergic reaction has decreased. If no symptoms appear, tolerance to the food has developed.

Several strategies are under study to ease the dietary restrictions imposed by food allergies. One possibility includes treatment with antibodies that will increase the threshold at which an allergic response occurs. For a person with an allergy to peanuts, for example, this would alleviate some anxiety about severe reactions to trace amounts of peanuts found in foods. Similarly, immunotherapy, which exposes allergic individuals to very small, but progressively larger amounts of food allergens, may help some people build up a tolerance to certain food components. Vaccines are another area of research. Also, scientists are working on genetically engineered foods that do not contain common allergens.

Preventing Food Allergies

With the rising number of cases of food allergies, many new parents wonder when and how to introduce new foods during infancy and early childhood. It is evident that introducing foods other than human milk or infant formula before 4 months of age is associated with higher risk of allergic diseases. Most experts, including the American Academy of Pediatrics and the American College of Allergy, Asthma, and Immunology, advise waiting to introduce solid foods until 4 to 6 months of age for lowest risk of food allergies. Delaying introduction of solid foods beyond 6 months of age is not advised.

Any food can contain a potential allergen, but certain foods have been found to have high allergenic potential: peanuts, tree nuts, eggs, cow's milk, fish, and seafood. The American Academy of Pediatrics and the National Institute of Allergy and Infectious Disease no longer advise delaying introduction of highly allergenic foods beyond 6 months of age, even for infants with a family history of food allergies.

Until recently, allergy-prone women were advised to avoid highly allergenic foods during pregnancy and breastfeeding. Allergens can cross the placenta during

elimination diet A restrictive diet that systematically tests foods that may cause an allergic response by first eliminating them for 1 to 2 weeks and then adding them back, one at a time.

pregnancy and are secreted in breast milk. However, research does not demonstrate a benefit of maternal dietary restrictions in preventing food allergies in infants.

The best course of action is to breastfeed the infant exclusively for 6 months and continue to breastfeed through 12 months with appropriate introduction of solid foods to meet the infant's nutritional needs. Human milk contains factors that play a role in the maturation of the small intestine. Formula-fed infants, especially those on cow's milk–based formulas, have a greater risk for developing food allergies. There is evidence that hydrolyzed infant formulas (in which the large proteins have been broken down into smaller peptides) may be useful in allergy prevention for infants at risk of developing food allergies. However, hydrolyzed formulas are about three times as costly as iron-fortified cow's milk–based formulas.

Food Intolerances

Food intolerances are adverse reactions to foods that do not involve allergic mechanisms. Generally, larger amounts of an offending food are required to produce the symptoms of an intolerance than to trigger allergic symptoms. Common causes of food intolerances include:

- Constituents of certain foods (e.g., red wine, tomatoes, pineapples) that have a druglike activity, causing physiological effects such as changes in blood pressure
- Certain synthetic compounds added to foods, such as sulfites, food-coloring agents, and monosodium glutamate (MSG)
- Food contaminants, including antibiotics and other chemicals used in the production of livestock and crops, as well as insect parts not removed during processing
- Toxic contaminants, which may be ingested with improperly handled and prepared foods containing *Clostridium botulinum*, *Salmonella* bacteria, or other foodborne microorganisms (see Chapter 13)
- Deficiencies in digestive enzymes, such as lactase (review Chapter 4)

Almost everyone is sensitive to one or more of these causes of food intolerance, many of which produce GI tract symptoms.

Sulfites, added to foods and beverages as antioxidants, cause flushing, spasms of the airway, and a loss of blood pressure in susceptible people. Wine, dehydrated potatoes, dried fruits, gravy, soup mixes, and restaurant salad greens commonly contain sulfites. A reaction to MSG may include an increase in blood pressure, numbness, sweating, vomiting, headache, and facial pressure. MSG is commonly found in restaurant food and many processed foods (e.g., soups). A reaction to tartrazine, a food-coloring additive, includes spasm of the airway, itching, and reddening skin. Tyramine, a derivative of the amino acid tyrosine, is commonly found in "aged" foods, such as cheeses and red wines. This natural food constituent can cause high blood pressure in people taking monoamine oxidase (MAO) inhibitor medications, which may be prescribed for clinical depression.

The basic treatment for food intolerances is to avoid specific offending components. However, total elimination often is not required because people generally are not as sensitive to compounds causing food intolerances as they are to allergens.

Case Study Undernutrition During Infancy

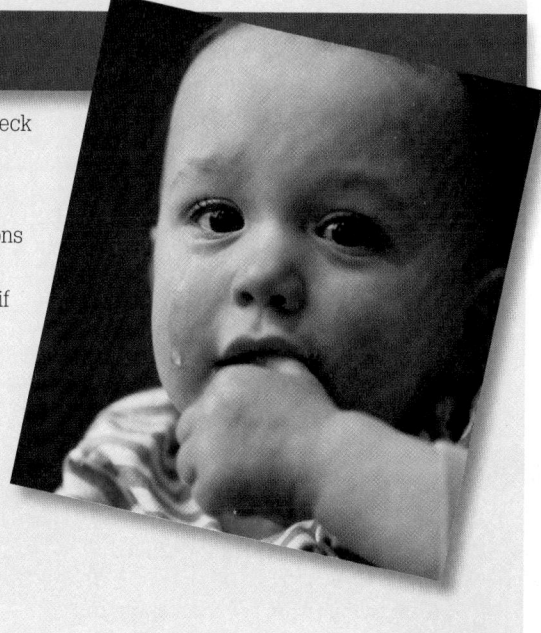

Damon is a 7-month-old boy who has been taken into a clinic for a routine checkup. On examination, he was found to be moderately underweight relative to his age and body length. His physician scheduled a follow-up appointment in 3 months. At the 10-month visit, Damon appeared sluggish and was now even more underweight for his age and length.

A registered dietitian interviewed Damon's 16-year-old mother to collect information on Damon's dietary intake. His intake over the previous 24 hours consisted of two bottles of infant formula, three 8-ounce bottles of Kool-Aid, and a hot dog. However, the mother was still in school, and at night she often left Damon with the neighbor, so that she could go out with friends for a few hours. Thus, she was not aware of all that he ate.

Answer the following questions, and check your responses in Appendix A.

1. Damon's mother did not specify what type of formula he takes. What questions would you ask about his formula?
2. What potential dangers await Damon if his growth continues to lag behind?
3. What foods should Damon's caregivers offer that are appropriate for his age and nutritional needs?
4. What problems might arise from consumption of sugary drinks from a bottle?
5. Does Damon need any vitamin or mineral supplements?

Summary (Numbers refer to numbered sections in the chapter.)

15.1 Alarming trends in child nutrition include an increase in childhood overweight and obesity, cardiovascular disease, and type 2 diabetes. A general lack of physical activity and failure to follow a healthy dietary pattern, such as that suggested by MyPlate's Daily Food Plan, are to blame.

15.2 Growth is rapid during infancy; birth weight doubles in 4 to 6 months, and length increases by 50% in the first year. An adequate diet, especially in terms of calories, protein, and zinc, is essential to support normal growth. Growth charts aid nutritional assessment of infants and children by tracking changes in body weight, height (or length), head circumference, and body mass index over time.

Nutrient needs in the first 6 months can be met by human milk or iron-fortified infant formula. Supplementation with vitamin D, iron, and fluoride may be appropriate for some infants.

Most infants do not need solid foods before 6 months of age. Introduction of solid foods should be based on an infant's nutritional needs, physical and physiological abilities, and developmental readiness. Solid foods should be introduced one at a time, starting with iron-fortified infant cereals or ground meats (sources of iron). Some foods to avoid giving infants in the first year include honey, cow's milk (especially fat-reduced varieties), foods with added salt or sugar, and foods that may cause choking.

15.3 A slower growth rate results in decreased appetite among preschool children. Other common nutrition-related concerns include iron-deficiency, constipation, and dental caries. With smaller portion sizes and picky eating behaviors, it is crucial to offer several small meals and snacks with a variety of nutrient-dense foods. Follow the example set forth by MyPlate, but use smaller portions (e.g., 1 tablespoon of food per year of life). For autism spectrum disorders, several nutritional interventions, including the gluten-free, casein-free diet and some dietary supplements, are under study.

15.4 Among school-age children, excessive energy and fat intakes have led to an alarming increase in overweight, obesity, type 2 diabetes, and cardiovascular disease. Parents can provide healthful food choices and encourage at least 60 minutes of physical activity per day. When controlled early through diet and exercise interventions, the problem of obesity may correct itself as the child continues to grow in height.

15.5 During the adolescent growth spurt, both boys and girls have increased needs for iron and calcium. Inadequate calcium intake by teenage girls is a major concern because it can set the stage for the development of osteoporosis later in life. Teenagers generally should moderate their intake of high-fat and sugar-rich foods—especially snacks and fast-food, which they often consume in abundance—and perform regular physical activity.

N&YH The most common food allergies are associated with peanuts, tree nuts, shellfish, milk, eggs, soybeans, wheat, and fish. Food allergies occur most often during infancy and young adulthood.

Check Your Knowledge (Answers to the following questions are below.)

1. Inadequate intake of which of the following results in poor growth?
   a. calories
   b. iron
   c. zinc
   d. All of the above.

2. An 11-month-old girl who weighs 19 pounds needs approximately _____ kcal per day.
   a. 690
   b. 810
   c. 845
   d. 930

3. Introduction of cow's milk should be delayed until 12 months of age because it
   a. contains too much fat.
   b. supplies too much lactose.
   c. contains too much protein.
   d. All of the above.

4. You are trying to introduce an apple and blueberry puree to a seven-month-old infant, but she rejects it. You should
   a. assume she doesn't like apples and blueberries.
   b. offer the food again on another day.
   c. force a spoonful into her mouth.
   d. None of the above.

5. Milk is a nutrient-dense source of all of the following except
   a. protein.
   b. iron.
   c. calcium.
   d. zinc.

6. A gluten-free, casein-free diet may be used to treat
   a. rickets.
   b. anemia.
   c. lead poisoning.
   d. autism.

7. To ensure adequate vitamin and mineral intake for a picky eater,
   a. provide a fortified breakfast cereal.
   b. promise dessert as a reward for eating meats and vegetables.
   c. use a multivitamin and mineral supplement.
   d. None of the above.

8. For treatment of overweight, school-age children should
   a. eat fewer meals.
   b. follow a low-carbohydrate eating plan.
   c. exercise for 60 minutes per day or more.
   d. avoid dairy products.

9. The prevailing dietary habits of North American teenagers contribute to all of the following except
   a. acne.
   b. high blood pressure.
   c. low bone mass.
   d. type 2 diabetes.

10. Your niece breaks out in hives and feels nauseous after eating a salad containing mango. She probably has a food
    a. sensitivity.
    b. allergy.
    c. intolerance.
    d. All of the above.

Answer key: 1. d (LO 15.1), 2. a (LO 15.2), 3. c (LO 15.2), 4. b (LO 15.2), 5. b (LO 15.4), 6. d (LO 15.3), 7. a (LO 15.3), 8. c (LO 15.5), 9. a (LO 15.4), 10. b (LO 15.6)

Study Questions (Numbers refer to Learning Outcomes)

1. List two factors that limit "catch-up" growth when a nutrient-deficient diet has been consumed throughout childhood. (LO 15.1)

2. Outline three key factors that help determine when to introduce solid foods into an infant's diet. (LO 15.2)

3. A 3-month-old infant is taken to a clinic with failure to thrive. What are two possible explanations? (LO 15.2)

4. List three reasons why preschoolers are noted for "picky" eating. For each, describe an appropriate parent response. (LO 15.3)

5. What three factors are likely to contribute to obesity in a typical 10-year-old child? (LO 15.5)

6. Compare the guidelines for infant feeding summarized in Chapter 15 with the 2010 Dietary Guidelines for Americans for children over age 2 and adults discussed in Chapter 2. Which guidelines are similar? Do any contradict each other? If so, why? (LO 15.2)

7. Describe three pros and cons of snacking. What is the basic advice for healthful snacking from childhood through the teenage years? (LO 15.3)

8. Which two nutrients are of particular concern in planning diets for teenagers? Why does each deserve to be singled out? (LO 15.4)

9. List three nutrients of concern for a teenage vegetarian. (LO 15.4)

10. Recommend two steps that a woman with a family history of food allergies can take to reduce risk of food allergies in her infant. (LO 15.6)

What Would You Choose Recommendations

At 18 months of age, Lila's diet should include small portions of a variety of foods from each MyPlate food group. She should have several teeth by now, but her chewing ability is still limited. As a young child, Lila has high nutrient needs and yet has a small stomach capacity, so snacking makes an important contribution to meeting overall nutrient needs.

Reduced-fat popcorn is a healthy, low-fat snack for older children and adults. Feeding children bulky foods with low energy density, however, can lead to fullness without meeting nutritional needs. Furthermore, popcorn is a choking hazard.

Although baby carrots with ranch dressing would be a good source of beta-carotene and healthy vegetable oils, toddlers are not expert chewers just yet, and large pieces of hard, crunchy foods present a choking hazard. Slicing the carrots into long, thin strips would be a better idea.

Fat-free, light yogurt is a good source of calcium and vitamin D for building healthy bones and certainly does not present choking risk. However, infants and toddlers need the fat and sugar in dairy products to supply calories for their growing bodies. Whole-milk yogurt, such as YoBaby, would be a better choice.

Whole-grain crackers with sliced cheddar cheese would be an excellent snacking option for Lila. This snack provides a healthy balance of carbohydrates, protein, and fat. Using whole-grain crackers, rather than those made with refined flour, will boost the vitamin and mineral content (review Chapter 4).

Toddlers are known for picky eating behaviors. Lila's slower pace of growth may reduce her appetite and she may be more

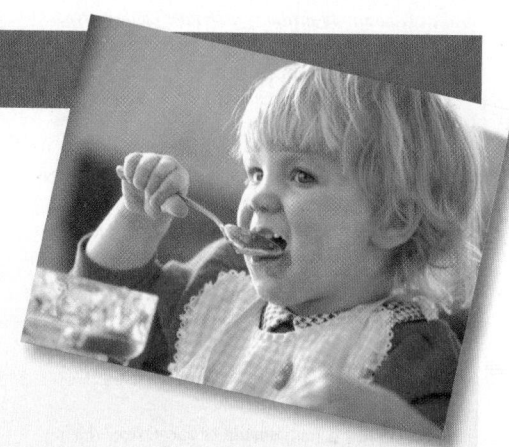

interested in exploring the world around her than sitting down for a meal. Make sure Lila sits down to eat and supervise her while she is eating. Finally, be a good role model. If she sees you eat the healthy snacks you have offered, she will be more likely to accept them.

Further Readings

1. ADA Reports: Position of the American Dietetic Association: Nutrition guidance for healthy children ages 2 to 11 years. *Journal of the American Dietetic Association* 108:1716, 2008.

   MyPyramid combined with the Dietary Guidelines for Americans provide an appropriate blueprint for feeding children. Diets of many children are not following this advice and in turn are contributing to the nutritional problems common in childhood and later adulthood.

2. Baker RD and others: Clinical report—Diagnosis and prevention of iron deficiency and iron-deficiency anemia in infants and young children (0–3 years of age). *Pediatrics* 126:1040, 2010.

   Healthy, full-term infants are born with sufficient iron stores to last through 4 months of age. After 4 months, exclusively and partially breastfed infants need additional iron from liquid iron supplements until consumption of solid foods provides a daily iron intake of 1 milligram per kilogram of body weight. For formula-fed infants, use of iron-fortified infant formula through 12 months of age will meet iron needs. Between 6 and 12 months of age, iron intake should be 11 milligrams per day from iron-rich foods or liquid iron supplements. Preterm infants require 2 milligrams of iron per kilogram for the first 12 months, provided as liquid supplements by 1 month of age until food and/or formula intake provides sufficient iron. Between 1 and 3 years of age, iron intake should be 7 milligrams per day from iron-rich foods, augmented by vitamin C-rich foods, and/or use of a liquid iron supplement.

3. Briggs M and others: Position of the American Dietetic Association, School Nutrition Association, and Society for Nutrition Education: Comprehensive school nutrition services. Journal of the American Dietetic Association 110:1738, 2010.

   More than 31 million children participate in the National School Lunch Program. In addition, school-based nutrition education programs (e.g., garden-based education and farm-to-school programs), increased availability of healthy food choices on school campuses, school-home-community partnerships, and school-based health services for children in need can foster healthy behaviors.

4. Council on Communications and Media: Children, adolescents, obesity, and the media. Pediatrics 128:201, 2011.

   Exposure to media is associated with increases in obesity among children and adolescents. This relationship may be mediated by a sedentary lifestyle, the influence of food advertising, unhealthful snacking practices, or poor sleep habits. The American Academy of Pediatrics urges health care providers to curb media exposure by counseling children and their parents, lobbying government, and initiating public health campaigns.

5. Council on Sports Medicine and Fitness and Council on School Health. Active healthy living: Prevention of childhood obesity through increased physical activity. Pediatrics 117:1834, 2006.

   Physical activity should be encouraged during and after school and as part of home life. Benefits of regular physical activity among children and adolescents include physical changes (e.g., improved insulin sensitivity, lowered blood pressure) and psychological improvements (e.g., increased self-esteem, less depression).

6. Curtis LT and others: Nutritional and environmental approaches to preventing and treating autism and attention-deficit hyperactivity disorder (ADHD): A review. Journal of Alternative and Complementary Medicine 14:79, 2008.

   This article reviews hypothesized environmental and nutritional links to autism and attention-deficit hyperactivity disorder. Evidence does not support a relationship between autism and environmental exposure to mercury. Nutritional interventions of scientific merit in the treatment of autism include avoidance of food allergens and correcting deficiencies of some B vitamins, magnesium, iron, zinc, and omega-3 fatty acids. For treatment of ADHD, some studies show a benefit of eliminating refined sugars and food additives such as coloring agents and preservatives.

7. Daniels SR and others: Lipid screening and cardiovascular health in childhood. Pediatrics 122:198, 2008.

   In light of evidence of cardiovascular disease among youth, the American Academy of Pediatrics urges children with risk factors for cardiovascular disease to undergo regular lipid screening starting by age 10. Treatments for dyslipidemia in children include dietary modifications, physical activity, and lipid-lowering medications.

8. Elder JH: The gluten-free, casein-free diet in autism: An overview with clinical implications. Nutrition in Clinical Practice 23:583, 2008.

   The gluten-free, casein-free (GFCF) diet is a popular but intense treatment for children with autism spectrum disorders. Some researchers hypothesize that intestinal absorption in autistic children is altered (i.e., "leaky gut syndrome"), such that food sensitivities to wheat and dairy proteins develop, leading to inflammation and other effects on the central nervous system. The GFCF diet may be useful for alleviating symptoms in some children with autism, but proper dietary planning is essential to prevent nutrient deficiencies.

9. Gidding SS and others: Dietary recommendations for children and adolescents: A guide for practitioners. Pediatrics 117:544, 2006.

   The American Heart Association recognizes that the dietary patterns of children and adolescents put them at risk for cardiovascular diseases in adulthood and even during childhood. Age-appropriate recommendations are provided for total energy intake, dietary fats, added sugars, sodium, and physical activity.

10. Gupta RS and others: The prevalence, severity, and distribution of childhood food allergy in the United States. Pediatrics 128:e9, 2011.

    Based on data collected from more than 38,000 children, the prevalence of food allergies is now estimated at 8% of children in the United States. About 40% of these children experience severe food allergies, and about one-third have multiple food allergies. Racial and income disparities are discussed.

11. Monsen ER: New findings from the Feeding Infants and Toddlers Study. Journal of the American Dietetic Association 106:S5, 2006.

    The Gerber-sponsored Feeding Infants and Toddlers Study (FITS) examined usual intakes of nutrients from foods and supplements, as well as other dietary practices, with an emphasis on dietary habits of Hispanic infants and children. Infants and toddlers do not consume enough fruits, vegetables, or fiber, and that intakes of total kilocalories, dietary fats, and sodium are on the rise.

12. Rao G: Childhood obesity: Highlights of AMA expert committee recommendations. American Family Physician 78:56, 2008.

    Weight management should be addressed yearly at medical checkups with all children. For those children who are overweight or obese (based on BMI for age), additional screening of blood lipids, glucose, and liver and kidney function is warranted. The four-stage approach for treatment of childhood obesity includes reducing consumption of sweetened beverages and fast foods; limiting time spent watching TV, playing video games, and sitting at the computer; participating in 60 minutes or more of physical activity each day; and encouraging family meals.

13. Spruijt-Metz D: Etiology, treatment, and prevention of obesity in childhood and adolescence: A decade in review. Journal of Research on Adolescence 21:129, 2011.

    This comprehensive review of pediatric obesity provides demographic data on obesity and associated health problems in children and adolescents, and discusses etiological factors contributing to the condition (e.g., genetics and environment), physical and mental health consequences, and strategies for prevention and treatment.

14. Wagner CL and others: Prevention of rickets and vitamin D deficiency in infants, children, and adolescents. Pediatrics 122(5):1142, 2008.

    Rickets and vitamin D deficiency are of concern for infants as well as older children and adolescents in the United States and are attributable to inadequate vitamin D intake and decreased exposure to sunlight. The American Academy of Pediatrics recommends that all infants and children, including adolescents, have a minimum daily intake of 400 IU of vitamin D beginning soon after birth.

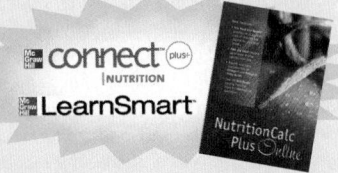

To get the most out of your study of nutrition, go to McGraw-Hill's online resources: Connect www.mcgrawhillconnect.com, where you will find NutritionCalc Plus, LearnSmart, and many other dynamic tools.

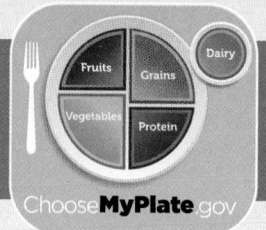

RATE YOUR PLATE

I. Getting Young Bill to Eat

Bill is 3 years old, and his mother is worried about his eating habits. He refuses to eat vegetables, meat, and dinner in general. Some days he eats very little food. He wants to eat snacks most of the time. Mealtime is a battle because Bill says he isn't hungry, and his mother wants him to eat a sit-down lunch and dinner to make sure he gets all the nutrients he needs and to eat everything served on his plate. He drinks five or six glasses of whole milk per day because that is the one food he likes.

When his mother prepares dinner, she makes plenty of vegetables, boiling them until they are soft, hoping this will appeal to Bill. Bill's dad waits to eat his vegetables last, regularly telling the family that he eats them only because he has to. He also regularly complains about how dinner has been prepared. Bill saves his vegetables until last and usually gags when his mother orders him to eat them. Bill has been known to sit at the dinner table for an hour until the war of wills ends. Bill's mother serves casseroles and stews regularly because they are convenient. Bill likes to eat breakfast cereal, fruit, and cheese and regularly requests these foods for snacks. However, his mother tries to deny his requests, so that he will have an appetite for dinner. Bill's mother comes to you and asks you what she should do to get Bill to eat.

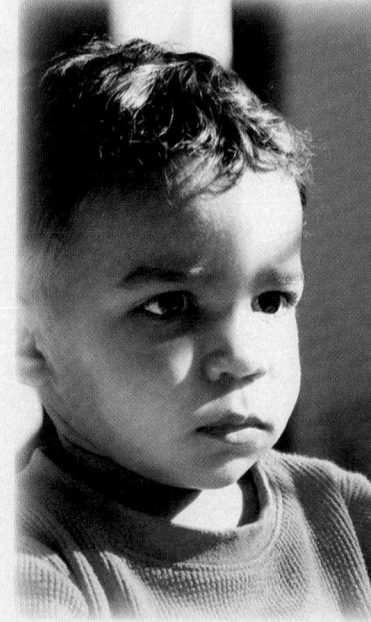

Analysis

1. List four mistakes Bill's parents are making that contribute to Bill's poor eating habits.

_____

_____

_____

_____

2. List four strategies they might try to promote good eating habits in Bill.

_____

_____

_____

_____

II. Evaluating a Teen Lunch

The following are two typical teen lunches and nutritional information for each:

Meal 1	Meal 2
2 pieces cheese pizza	1 large hamburger sandwich with condiments
1 milk chocolate candy bar	30 French fries
20 fluid ounces cola	20 fluid ounces cola

	Meal 1	Meal 2	Nutrient Needs for Teens
Energy (kcal)	990	1000	Males: 3000 Females: 2200
Protein	32	20	Males: 59 Females: 44
Vitamin C (milligrams)	5	18	Both genders: 45 to 75
Vitamin A (micrograms RAE)	300	10	Males: 900 Females: 700
Iron (milligrams)	3	4	Males: 11 Females: 15
Calcium (milligrams)	545	100	Both genders: 1300

1. Keeping in mind that meals should meet about one-third of nutrient needs, what are the shortcomings and excesses of these meals (i.e., given the nutritional information, compare these meals with one-third the RDA for protein, vitamin C, vitamin A, iron, and calcium)?

   _____

   _____

   _____

2. How would you change these meals to improve balance and to meet the nutrient needs above? (Hint: Use NutritionCalc Plus.)

   _____

   _____

   _____

3. Reflect on your food choices as a teenager. Do you think your meal choices were balanced and varied? Why or why not? What could you have done to improve your nutritional habits at that time?

   _____

   _____

   _____

III. Public Health Efforts to Combat Childhood Obesity

Major public health initiatives aim to counter the rapid rise in childhood obesity and related health conditions. Whether school-based, community-driven, or targeted at families, the overarching goals are to promote healthy eating habits and increased physical activity.

1. Find out what is going on in your area to combat childhood obesity. As a starting point, here are a few examples:

    - *We Can!*™ (Ways to Enhance Children's Activity and Nutrition): http://wecan.nhlbi.nih.gov

    - **HealthCorps:** www.healthcorps.net

    - **Action for Healthy Kids:** www.actionforhealthykids.org

    - **The President's Council on Fitness, Sports, and Nutrition:** www.fitness.gov

    _____

    _____

    _____

    _____

Imagine that you have been appointed to develop a public health campaign to decrease childhood obesity in your community.

2. What are the specific needs in your community (e.g., lack of safe space for physical activity, overabundance of fast-food outlets)?

    _____

    _____

    _____

    _____

3. Who will be your target audience? Why?

    _____

    _____

    _____

    _____

4. What activities will you undertake to reach your target audience? What will set your program apart from other efforts in your community?

    _____

    _____

    _____

    _____

5. How will you define the success of your program? List two or more measurable objectives for your campaign.

    _____

    _____

    _____

    _____

Chapter 16 Nutrition During Adulthood

Student Learning Outcomes

Chapter 16 is designed to allow you to:

16.1 Discuss demographic trends among adults in North America and how they impact health care.

16.2 List several hypotheses about the causes of aging.

16.3 Describe how physiological changes that occur during adulthood affect nutritional needs.

16.4 Compare the dietary intake of adults with current recommendations.

16.5 Make recommendations for lifestyle changes in the prevention and treatment of nutritional problems in older adults.

16.6 Identify nutrition-related health issues of the adult years and describe the prevention and treatment options.

16.7 Compare benefits of moderate alcohol use to risks of alcohol abuse.

16.8 List several nutritional programs available to help meet nutritional needs of older adults.

What Would You Choose?

In your family, there is a history of colon cancer. Your grandmother died from complications of colon cancer, and your father has already had some polyps removed from his colon. Even though you have not experienced any digestive abnormalities that would indicate a problem, your desire to learn about the role of lifestyle choices in disease prevention is part of what prompted you to take this nutrition course. What would you choose as the best nutrition strategy for cancer prevention?

a Take a variety of phytochemical supplements.

b Buy a juicer to make antioxidant-rich fruit and vegetable concoctions.

c Focus on filling half your plate at mealtimes with fruits and vegetables.

d Don't worry about making changes now, because colon cancer occurs in older adults.

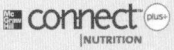 **connect** plus+ |NUTRITION

Think about your choice as you read Chapter 16, then see our recommendations at the end of the chapter. To learn more about links between nutrition and cancer, check out the Connect site: www.mcgrawhillconnect.com

Part Five
Nutrition: A Focus on Life Stages

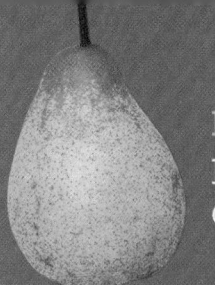

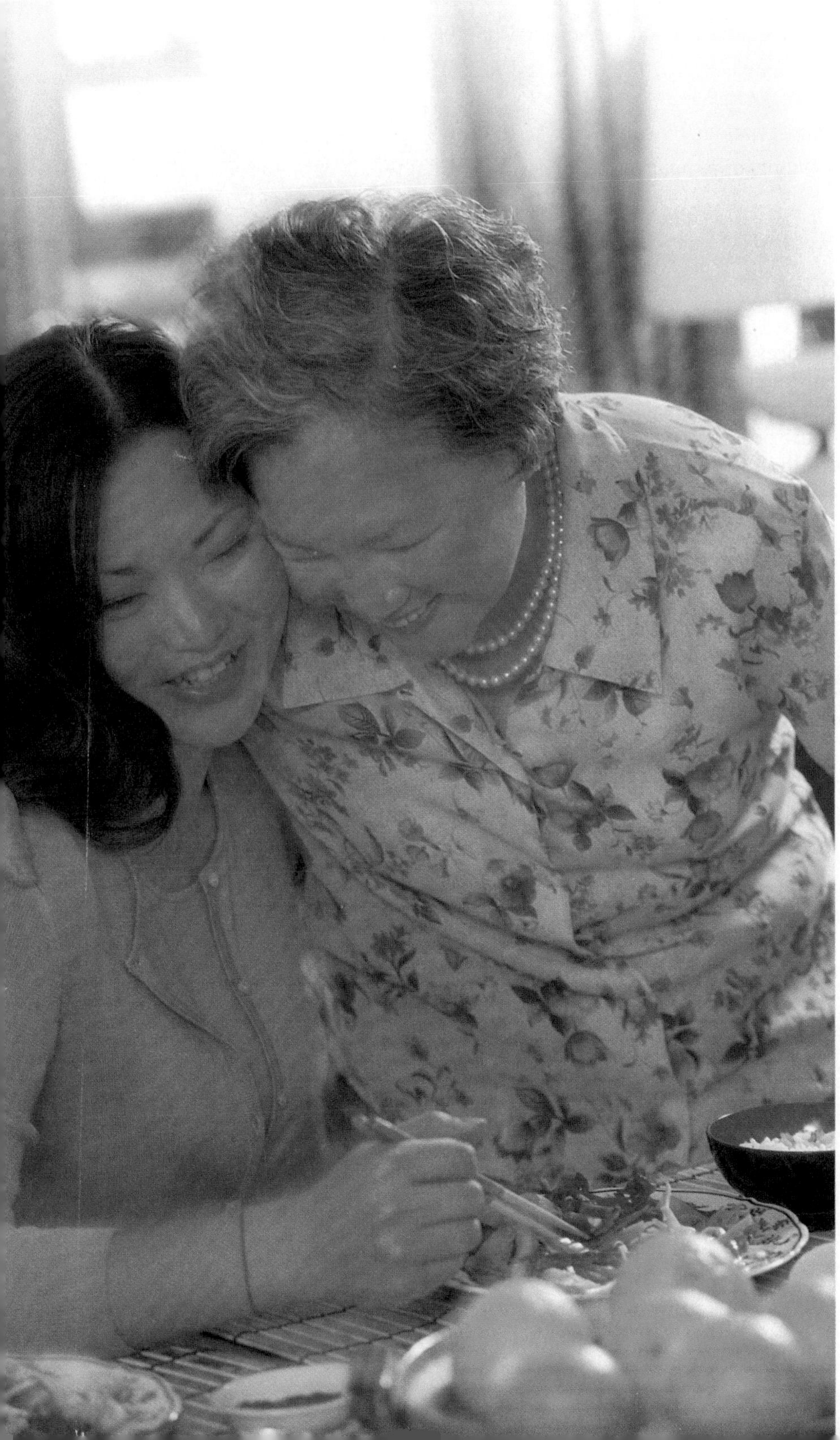

Eating is one of our great pleasures. Guided by common sense and moderation, eating well is also a means to good health. Most of us want a long, productive life, free of illness. Yet, as the comic in this chapter suggests, aging is inevitable. Unfortunately, many people from early middle age onward suffer from obesity, cardiovascular disease, hypertension and strokes, type 2 diabetes, osteoporosis, and other chronic diseases. We can slow the development of—and in some cases even prevent—these diseases by following a dietary pattern such as that exemplified by MyPlate. The effect of such a diet is most profitable if we begin early and continue throughout adulthood. We serve ourselves best—as individuals and as a nation—by striving to maintain vitality even in the later decades of life. This concept was first explored in Chapter 1 and is discussed again in this chapter, in light of the nutrition needs of adults.

Keep in mind that present day-to-day health practices can significantly influence health during later life. Although genetics does play a role, as discussed in Chapter 3, many of the health problems that occur with age are not inevitable; they result from diet-related disease processes that influence physical health. Much can be learned from healthy older people whose attention to a healthy diet and physical activity—along with a little luck—keeps them active and vibrant well beyond typical retirement years. Successful aging is the goal. Age quickly or slowly—it is partly your choice.

Refresh Your Memory

As you begin your study of adult nutrition issues in Chapter 16, you may want to review:

- Implications of the 1994 Dietary Supplement Health and Education Act in Chapter 1
- The effect of genetics on health in Chapter 3
- The various body systems covered in Chapter 3
- The sources of fiber and sugar in Chapter 4
- Definition of healthy body weight in Chapter 7
- The dietary sources of vitamin D, the various B vitamins, and calcium in Chapters 8 and 9
- Recommendations for salt intake in Chapter 9
- The benefits of regular physical activity in Chapter 10

16.1 The Graying of North America

Due to advances in health care and sanitation, the demographics of developed countries are shifting so that as a population, we are getting older. In North America, the group constituting those aged 85+ years is the fastest growing segment. Between 1997 and 2050, the population aged 85+ years in the United States is expected to increase from 3.4 million to 19 million. Even more amazing, 1 million or more people in the United States could be over 100 years old in 2050.

This "graying" of North America poses some problems. Although people older than age 65 account for just 13% of the U.S. population, they account for more than 25% of all prescription medications used, 40% of acute hospital stays, and 50% of the federal health budget. Hip fractures alone cost the nation about $12 billion per year. Of older persons, 65% or more have nutrition-related problems, such as cardiovascular disease, type 2 diabetes, hypertension, and osteoporosis.

Postponing these chronic diseases for as long as possible will help control health care costs. Health and independence contribute quality—not just quantity—to life as

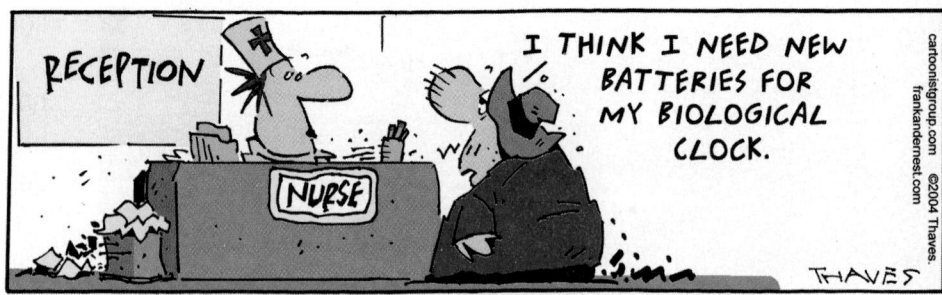

Is a decline in health inevitable as we age? Which diet and lifestyle interventions have been shown to slow (or reverse) the aging process? Which nutrition problems are typically seen in older adults? How should one compensate for these? Chapter 16 provides some answers.

"Frank and Ernest" used with the permission of the Thaves and the Cartoonist Group. All rights reserved. 2/28/1997

age advances and lessen the load on an already overburdened healthcare system. Keep in mind that aging is not a disease. Furthermore, diseases that commonly accompany old age—osteoporosis and atherosclerosis, for example—are not an inevitable part of aging. Many can be prevented or managed. Some people do die of old age, not as a direct result of disease.

16.2 Physiological Changes During Adulthood

Adulthood, the longest stage of the life cycle, begins when an adolescent completes his or her physical growth. Unlike earlier stages of the life cycle, nutrients are used primarily to maintain the body rather than support physical growth. (Pregnancy is the only time during adulthood when substantial amounts of nutrients are used for growth.) As adults get older, nutrient needs change. For example, vitamin D needs increase for older adults. Based on the needs for various nutrients, the Food and Nutrition Board divided the adult years into four stages: ages 19 to 30, 31 to 50, 51 to 70, and beyond 70 years of age. The intervals encompassing ages 19 through 50 are often referred to as young adulthood, 51 to 70 as middle adulthood, and beyond 70 years of age as older adulthood.

Adulthood is characterized by body maintenance and gradual physical and physiological transitions, often referred to as aging. **Aging** can be defined as the time-dependent physical and physiological changes in body structure and function that occur normally and progressively throughout adulthood as humans mature and become older. One view of aging describes it as a process of slow cell death, beginning soon after fertilization. When we are young, aging is not apparent because the major metabolic activities are geared toward growth and maturation. We produce plenty of active cells to meet physiological needs. During late adolescence and adulthood, the body's major task is to maintain cells. From the beginning of adulthood until age 30 or so, body systems are at their peak efficiency rate. Stature, stamina, strength, endurance, efficiency, and health are at their lifetime highs. Rates of cell synthesis and breakdown are balanced in most tissues. Inevitably, though, cells age and die. After about age 30, the rate of cell breakdown slowly begins to exceed the rate of cell renewal, leading to a gradual decline in organ size and efficiency. Eventually, the body can't adjust to meet all physiological demands, and body functioning begins to decrease (Fig. 16-1). Still, body systems and organs usually retain enough **reserve capacity** to handle normal, everyday demands throughout one's entire lifetime.

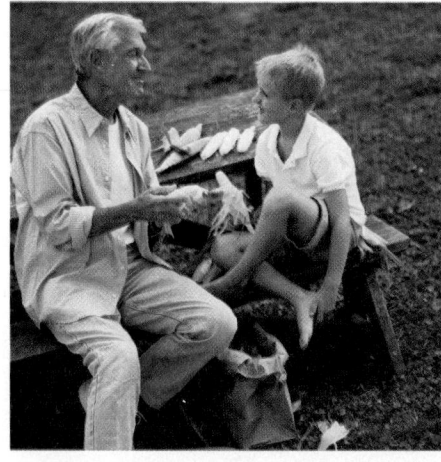

▲ The "baby boom" turned 65 in 2011, and now the health concerns of an aging population will demand increasing attention.

aging Time-dependent physical and physiological changes in body structure and function that occur normally and progressively throughout adulthood as humans mature and become older.

reserve capacity The extent to which an organ can preserve essentially normal function despite decreasing cell number or cell activity.

FIGURE 16-1 ▶ Declines in physiological function seen with aging. The decline in many body functions is especially evident in sedentary people.

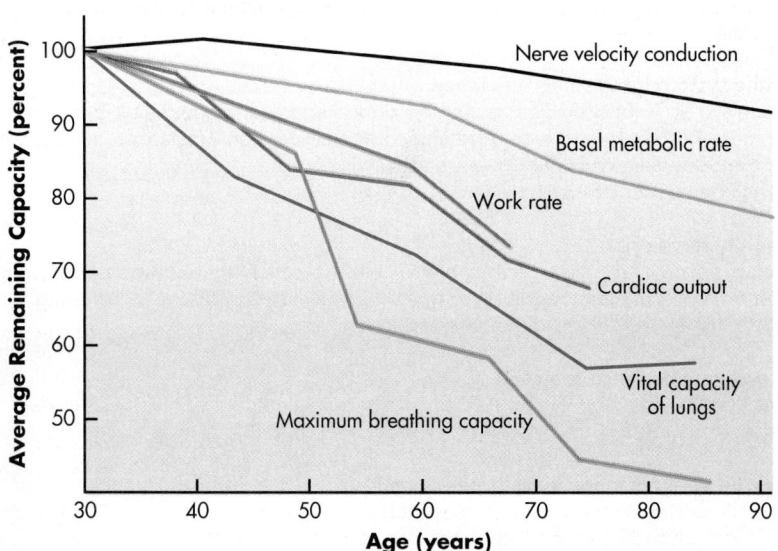

Problems caused by diminished capacity typically don't arise unless severe demands are placed on the aging body. For example, alcohol intake can overtax an aging liver. The stress of shoveling a snow-covered sidewalk can exceed the capacity of the heart and lungs. Coping with an illness also can push an older body beyond its capacity.

The causes of aging remain a mystery. Most likely, the physiological changes of aging are the sum of automatic cellular changes, lifestyle practices, and environmental influences, as listed in Table 16-1. Even with the most supportive environment and healthy lifestyle, cell structure and function still decline over time. The eventual death of deteriorating cells is actually beneficial because it likely prevents diseases such as cancer. Unfortunately, there are negative consequences to this natural cell progression because, as more and more cells in an organ die, organ function decreases. For example, **kidney nephrons** are continually lost as we age. In some people, this loss exhausts the kidneys' reserve capacity and ultimately leads to kidney failure. Most people, however, maintain sufficient kidney function throughout life.

The diseases and degenerative processes commonly observed in older people have long been assumed to be unavoidable consequences of aging. Certainly, some of the declines we blame on aging may be inevitable, such as gradual reductions in tissue

kidney nephrons The units of kidney cells that filter wastes from the bloodstream and deposit them into the urine.

glycosylation The process by which glucose attaches to (glycates) other compounds, such as proteins.

TABLE 16-1 Current Hypotheses About the Causes of Aging

Errors occur in copying the genetic blueprint (DNA).
Once sufficient errors in DNA copying accumulate, a cell can no longer synthesize the major proteins needed to function, and it therefore dies.

Connective tissue stiffens.
Parallel protein strands, found mostly in connective tissue, cross-link to each other. This decreases flexibility in key body components.

Electron-seeking compounds damage cell parts.
Electron-seeking free radicals can break down cell membranes and proteins. One way to prevent some damage from these compounds is to consume adequate amounts of vitamins E and C, selenium, and carotenoids.

Hormone function changes.
The blood concentration of many hormones, such as testosterone in men, falls during the aging process. Replacement of these and other hormones is possible, but the resulting risks and benefits are largely unknown.

Glycosylation of proteins.
Blood glucose, when chronically elevated, attaches to (glycates) various blood and body proteins. This decreases protein function and can encourage immune system attack on such altered proteins.

The immune system loses some efficiency.
The immune system is most efficient during childhood and young adulthood, but with advancing age, it is less able to recognize and counteract foreign substances, such as viruses, that enter the body. Nutrient deficiencies, particularly of protein, vitamin E, vitamin B-6, and zinc, also hamper immune function.

Autoimmunity develops.
Autoimmune reactions occur when white blood cells and other immune system components begin to attack body tissues in addition to foreign proteins. Many diseases, including some forms of arthritis, involve this autoimmune response.

Death is programmed into the cell.
Each human cell can divide only about 50 times. Once this number of divisions occurs, the cell automatically succumbs.

Excess calorie intake speeds body breakdown.
Experimentally, underfed animals, such as spiders, mice, and rats, live longer. Usual calorie intake must be reduced by about 30% to see this effect. This approach is the only proven way to substantially slow the aging process (see Further Readings 8 and 11).

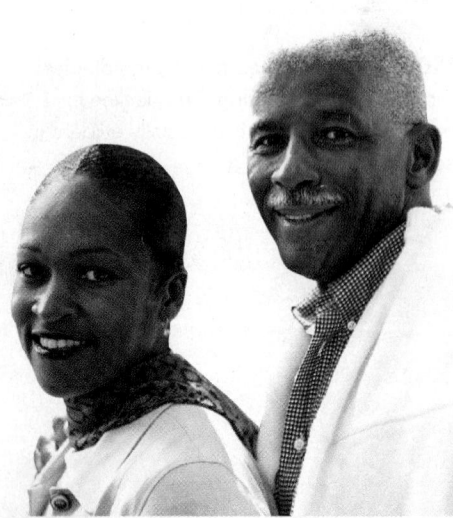

▲ Adopting diet and lifestyle practices that minimize a decline in body function is an investment in your future health. Visit www.nia.nih.gov for a free fact sheet on healthy aging.

and organ cell numbers, graying hair, and reduced lung capacity. However, many of the so-called usual or degenerative age-related changes can, in fact, be minimized, prevented, and/or reversed by healthy lifestyles (e.g., eating nutritious diets, exercising regularly, getting enough sleep) and avoiding adverse environmental factors (e.g., excessive exposure to sunlight and cigarette smoke). These discoveries have led researchers to introduce the concepts of "usual aging" and "successful aging."

Usual and Successful Aging

Body cells age, no matter what health practices we follow. However, to a considerable extent, you can choose how quickly you age throughout your adult years. *Usual aging* refers to those changes commonly thought to be a typical or expected part of aging, such as increasing body fatness, decreasing lean body mass, rising blood pressure, declining bone mass, and increasingly poor health. Researchers point out that many of these changes really represent an acceleration of the aging process induced by unhealthy lifestyle choices, adverse environmental exposures, and/or chronic disease. For instance, blood pressure does not tend to rise with age among people whose diets are traditionally low in sodium. Also, lean body mass is maintained much better in older people who exercise than in those who don't.

Successful aging, on the other hand, describes physical and physiological function declines that occur only because one grows older, not because lifestyle choices, environmental exposures, and chronic disease have aggravated or sped up the rate of aging. Those who are successful agers experience age-related declines at a slower rate and the onset of chronic disease symptoms at a later age than usual agers. Striving to have the greatest number of healthy years and the fewest years of illness is often referred to as **compression of morbidity**. In other words, a person tries to delay the onset of disabilities caused by chronic disease and to compress significant sickness related to aging into the last few years–or months–of life.

Factors Affecting the Rate of Aging

Life span refers to the maximum number of years a human can live. As far as we know, this hasn't changed in recorded time. The longest human life documented to date is 122 years for a woman and 114 years for a man. **Life expectancy**, alternatively, is the time an average person born in a specific year, such as 2009, can expect to live. Life expectancy in North America is about 75 years for men and about 80 years for women, with a span of "healthy years" of about 64. Furthermore, a person who survives to age 80 can expect to live an additional 7 to 10 years.

The rate at which one ages is individual; it is determined by heredity, lifestyle, and environment. With the exception of heredity, most of the factors that influence the rate of aging are directly linked to choices that are under our control.

Heredity

Heredity defines who you are biochemically and, to some extent, it defines how long you will live (longevity). Living to an old age tends to run in some families. If your parents and grandparents lived a long time, you are likely to have the potential to live to an old age, too. One of the most obvious genetic characteristics influencing longevity is gender. In the case of humans, as well as most other species, females tend to live longer than males.

Another genetic characteristic that can influence longevity is metabolic efficiency. Individuals with a "thrifty metabolism" require fewer calories for metabolic processes and are able to store body fat more easily than those with faster metabolic rates. Throughout history, it was the individuals with thrifty metabolism who tended to live the longest because they efficiently stored fat during times of plenty and thus had the energy stores needed to survive frequent periods of food scarcity. In today's

Keep in mind that extending life without delaying onset of chronic disease prolongs suffering in many cases. In addition, the greater number of disabled years is costly to all North Americans. For these reasons, prolonging life without compressing the number of disabled years is called the "failure of success."

compression of morbidity Delay of the onset of disabilities caused by chronic disease.

life span The potential oldest age a person can reach.

life expectancy The average length of life for a given group of people born in a specific year (such as this year).

Besides having other long-lived family members, people who live to 100 years generally:

- Do not smoke and do not drink heavily
- Gain little weight in adulthood
- Eat many fruits and vegetables
- Perform daily physical activity
- Challenge their minds
- Have a positive outlook
- Maintain close friendships
- Are (or were) married (especially true for men)
- Have a healthy rate of HDL cholesterol production

environment of labor-saving devices and abundant, energy-dense foods, however, a thrifty metabolism may actually reduce longevity. Accumulation of excessive body fat increases the risk of developing health problems that reduce life expectancy (e.g., heart disease, hypertension, and certain cancers).

As you know, heredity is largely unchangeable. However, heredity is not necessarily destiny—individuals can exert some control over the expression of their genetic potential. Lifestyle and environment both can modify the expression of genetic potential.

Lifestyle

Lifestyle is one's pattern of living—it includes food choices, exercise patterns, and substance use (e.g., alcohol, drugs, and tobacco). Lifestyle choices can have a major impact on health and longevity, as well as on the expression of genetic potential. If individuals have a family history of premature heart disease, they can adjust their diet, exercise, and tobacco use patterns to slow the progression of the disease, get needed medical care, and possibly extend their lifetime. The converse is true, too. That is, lifestyle choices (e.g., high-fat diet and couch potato mentality) can increase susceptibility to diseases that hasten the rate of aging, ultimately shortening life expectancy, even if a person's genetic potential is for a very long life.

Worldwide, the highest average life expectancy is in Okinawa, a stretch of islands off the coast of Japan: 86 years for women and 78 years for men. Researchers suggest that these statistics are rooted in the traditional diet and lifestyle of inhabitants of Okinawa. The Okinawan diet is based on rice, fish, vegetable protein sources, fruits, vegetables, tea, herbs for seasonings, and small amounts of meat. Alcohol and salt intake is minimal. The low energy density translates into a generally low calorie intake, and BMI averages 21 kg/m². A desire to mimic their weight management success, compression of morbidity, and longevity has given rise to several popular books and websites that promote Okinawan dietary practices.

Followers of the traditional Mediterranean Diet also enjoy some of the lowest recorded rates of chronic disease in the world (See Chapter 2, p. 63). As introduced in Chapter 5, the Mediterranean Diet features the following:

- Olive oil, a source of heart-healthy monounsaturated fat, as the main dietary fat
- Abundant daily intake of fruits, vegetables (especially leafy greens), whole grains, beans, nuts, and seeds
- An emphasis on minimally processed and, wherever possible, seasonally fresh and locally grown foods
- Daily intake of small amounts of cheese and yogurt
- Weekly intake of low to moderate amounts of fish
- Limited use of eggs and red meat
- Regular exercise
- Moderate drinking of wine at mealtime

Common themes among these life-prolonging dietary practices are their focus on unprocessed, fiber-rich foods, healthy sources of fat (e.g., vegetable oils and fish), and lean sources of protein. Besides diet, populations who enjoy extended quality and quantity of life include physical activity as a major part of their daily routines. Compare these lifestyle choices with those of typical North Americans.

Environment

Some aspects of the environment that exert a powerful influence on the rate of aging are income, education level, health care, shelter, and psychosocial factors. For instance, being able to purchase nutritious foods, quality health care, and safe housing helps decrease the rate of aging. Having the education needed to earn a sufficient income, as well as the knowledge required to select a nutritious diet and make

CRITICAL THINKING

The "fountain of youth" remains a mystery. Many people believe a source exists that can stop the aging process, allowing youth to remain. However, Neil, a history student, asserts that the fountain of youth is not a place or a particular thing but, rather, a combination of diet and lifestyle. How can he justify this claim?

wise lifestyle choices, also can slow the aging process. In addition, the willingness to seek health care promptly when it is needed, the capacity to follow the instructions of a health-care provider, and the desire to accept the responsibility for one's own health can slow the rate of aging. Likewise, shelter that protects individuals from physical danger, climatic extremes, and solar radiation helps slow the aging process. Allowing people to make at least some decisions for themselves and control their own activities (autonomy) and providing psychosocial support (informational and emotional resources) promote successful aging and psychological well-being. In contrast, aging is likely to accelerate if any or all of the converse (i.e., insufficient income, low education level, lack of health care, inadequate shelter, and/or lack of autonomy and psychosocial support) are true.

CONCEPT CHECK

Although lifespan has not changed, life expectancy has increased dramatically over the past century. This means an increasing proportion of the North American population is over 65 years of age and will live for decades longer. Avoiding continually rising health care costs and maximizing satisfaction with life require postponing and minimizing chronic illness. Aging begins early in life and is influenced by heredity, lifestyle, and environment. A healthy diet and regular physical activity can play a pivotal role in slowing the aging process.

16.3 Nutrient Needs During Adulthood

The challenge of the adult years is to maintain the body, preserve its function, and avoid chronic disease—that is, to age successfully. A healthy diet can help achieve this goal. One blueprint for a healthy diet comes from the 2010 Dietary Guidelines for Americans, discussed in Chapter 2. The advice from those guidelines can be summarized into three main goals:

1. Balance calories with physical activity to manage weight.
2. Consume more of certain foods and nutrients, such as fruits, vegetables, whole grains, fat-free and low-fat dairy products, and seafood.
3. Consume fewer foods with sodium, saturated fats, *trans* fats, cholesterol, added sugars, and refined grains.

Overall, good nutrition benefits adults in many ways. Meeting nutrient needs delays the onset of certain diseases; improves the management of some existing diseases; speeds recovery from many illnesses; increases mental, physical, and social well-being; and often decreases the need for and length of hospitalization (see Further Readings 1 and 9). As you know, American adults are fairly well nourished, although some dietary excesses and inadequacies do exist. For instance, common dietary excesses are calories, fat, sodium, and, for some, alcohol. The diets of adult women tend to fall short of the recommended amounts of vitamins D and E, folate, magnesium, calcium, zinc, and fiber. The diets of adult men tend to be low in the same nutrients, except vitamin D, which does not become problematic until age 50. The iron intake of most women during their childbearing years (19 to 50) is insufficient to meet their needs; however, due to a reduced iron need after **menopause,** older women do get enough iron (see Further Reading 3).

People age 65 and up, particularly those in long-term care facilities and hospitals, are the single largest group at risk of malnutrition. They may become underweight and show signs of numerous micronutrient deficiencies (e.g., vitamins B-6 and B-12 and folate). Friends, relatives, and health care professionals should monitor nutrient intake in all older people, including those who live in long-term care facilities. Family

menopause Cessation of menses in women, usually beginning at about age 50.

FIGURE 16-2 ▶ A nutrition checklist for older adults.

Reprinted with permission by the Nutrition Screening Initiative, a project of the American Academy of Family Physicians, the American Dietetic Association, and the National Council on Aging, Inc., and funded in part by a grant from Ross Products Division, Abbott Laboratories.

A Nutrition Test for Older Adults

Here's a nutrition check for anyone over age 65. Circle the number of points for each statement that applies. Then compute the total and check it against the nutritional score.

	Points	
	2	1. The person has a chronic illness or current condition that has changed the kind or amount of food eaten.
	3	2. The person eats fewer than two full meals per day.
	2	3. The person eats few fruits, vegetables, or milk products.
	2	4. The person drinks three or more servings of beer, liquor, or wine almost every day.
	2	5. The person has tooth or mouth problems that make eating difficult.
	4	6. The person does not have enough money for food.
	1	7. The person eats alone most of the time.
	1	8. The person takes three or more different prescription or over-the-counter drugs each day.
	2	9. The person has unintentionally lost or gained 10 pounds within the last 6 months.
	2	10. The person cannot always shop, cook, or feed himself or herself.
Total		

Nutritional score:

0–2: Good. Recheck in 6 months.

3–5: Marginal. A local agency on aging has information about nutrition programs for the elderly. The National Association of Area Agencies on Aging can assist in finding help; call (800) 677-1116. Recheck in 6 months.

6 or more: High risk. A doctor should review this test and suggest how to improve nutritional health.

members can play a valuable role in making sure nutrient needs are met by looking for weight maintenance and regular, healthful meal patterns. To pinpoint those over age 65 at risk of nutrient deficiencies, the American Academy of Family Physicians, the American Dietetic Association, and the National Council on Aging developed the Nutrition Screening Initiative checklist (Fig. 16-2). Older Americans, family members, and health care providers can use the checklist to identify those at nutritional risk *before* health deteriorates significantly. If problems arise in consuming a healthful diet, registered dietitians can offer professional and personalized advice.

Defining Nutrient Needs

The DRIs for adults are divided by gender into four age groups to reflect how nutrient needs change as adults grow older. These changes in nutrient needs take into consideration aging-related physiological alterations in body composition, metabolism, and organ function.

Calories. After age 30 or so, total calorie needs of physically inactive adults fall steadily throughout adulthood. This is caused by a gradual decline in basal metabolism. To a considerable extent, adults can exert control over this reduction in calorie need by

ostomy Surgically created short circuit in intestinal flow where the end point usually opens from the abdominal cavity rather than the anus—for example, a colostomy. Short circuiting the intestinal flow means more water is lost in fecal matter than would be if the intestinal tract were intact.

exercising. Exercise can halt, slow, and even reverse reductions in lean body mass and subsequent declines in calorie need. Also, keeping calorie needs high makes it easier to meet one's nutrient needs and avoid becoming overweight.

Protein. The protein intake of adults of all ages in North America tends to exceed current recommended levels. However, some recent studies indicate that consuming protein in amounts slightly higher than the RDA may help preserve muscle and bone mass (see Further Reading 5). Adults who have limited food budgets, have difficulty chewing meat, or are lactose intolerant may not get enough protein. Recall from Chapter 6 that any protein consumed in excess of that needed for the maintenance of body tissue will be broken down and used as energy or stored as fat. The waste products of metabolism of protein must be removed by the kidneys; excessive protein intake may accelerate kidney function decline.

Fat. The fat intake of adults of all ages is often at or above the recommendations. It's a good idea for almost all adults to reduce their fat intake because of the strong link between high-fat diets and obesity, heart disease, and certain cancers. In addition, reducing fat intake "frees up" some calories that can be better "spent" on complex carbohydrates (see Further Reading 12).

Carbohydrates. The total carbohydrate intake of adults of all ages in North America is often lower than recommended. In addition, many adults need to shift the carbohydrate composition of their diets to emphasize complex carbohydrates while minimizing intake of sugary, simple carbohydrates. A diet rich in complex carbohydrates helps us achieve nutrient needs and stay within calorie bounds because many highly sweetened foods are low in nutrients and high in calories. Substituting foods rich in complex carbohydrates for sweets also makes it easier for the body to control blood glucose levels—a function that becomes less efficient as the increases in body fatness and inactivity associated with usual aging occur. Declines in carbohydrate metabolism are so common that more than 25% of those age 65 years or older have diabetes. A diet rich in fiber helps adults reduce their risk of colon cancer and heart disease, lower their blood cholesterol levels, and avoid constipation. The typical American adult gets slightly more than half the recommended amount of dietary fiber.

Water. Many adults, especially those in the later years, fail to consume adequate quantities of water. In fact, many are in a constant state of mild dehydration and at risk of electrolyte imbalances. Low fluid intakes in older adults may be caused by a fading sensitivity to thirst sensations, chronic diseases, and/or conscious reductions in fluid intake in order to reduce the frequency of urination. Some also may have increased fluid output because they are taking certain medications (i.e., diuretics and laxatives), have an **ostomy,** and/or experience an age-related decline in the kidneys' ability to concentrate urine. Dehydration is very dangerous and, among other symptoms, can cause disorientation and mental confusion, constipation, impacted fecal matter, and death.

Minerals and Vitamins. Adequate intake of all vitamins and minerals is important throughout the adult years (Figs. 16-3 and 16-4). The micronutrients that need special attention because they tend to be present in less than optimal amounts in the diets of many adults are calcium, vitamin D, iron, zinc, magnesium, folate, and vitamins B-6, B-12, and E. Adults with impaired absorption or who are unable to consume a nutritious diet may benefit from mineral or vitamin supplements matched with their needs. In fact, many nutrition experts recommend a daily balanced multivitamin and mineral supplement for older adults, especially for those 70 years of age and older. Supplements or fortified foods can be especially helpful when it comes to meeting vitamin D and vitamin B-12 needs.

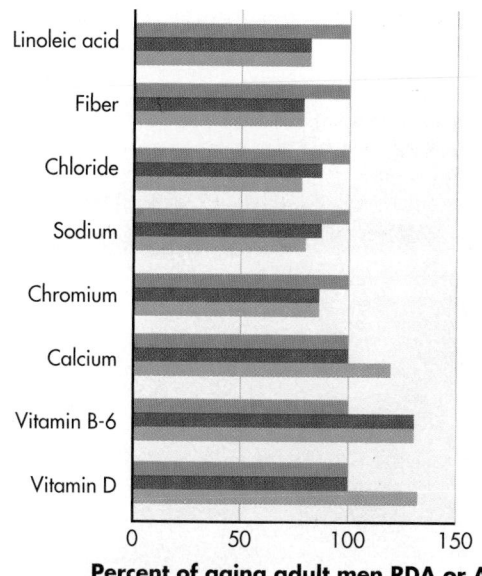

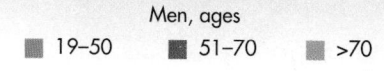

FIGURE 16-3 ▶ Relative nutrient requirements for aging adult men. Only nutrients that vary by age are shown.

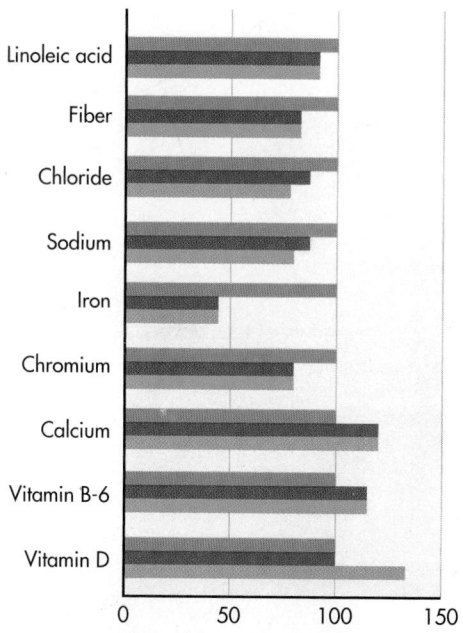

FIGURE 16-4 ▶ Relative nutrient requirements for aging adult women. Only nutrients that vary by age are shown.

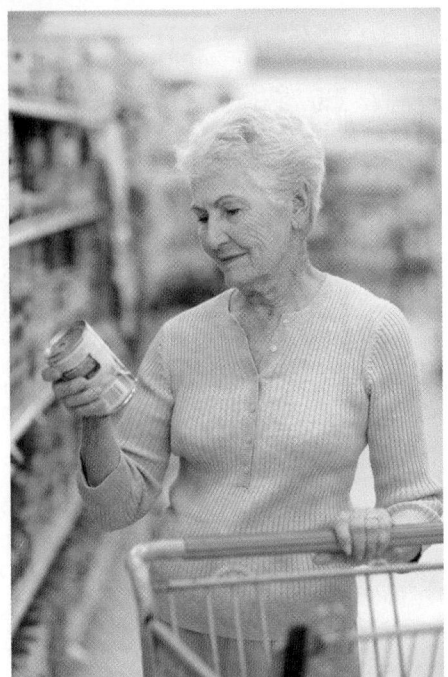

▲ Sodium needs for older adults are 1200 to 1300 milligrams per day. Older adults routinely consume at least this much sodium. Potassium needs are 4700 milligrams per day. Many older adults do not meet this goal.

Calcium and Vitamin D These bone-building nutrients tend to be low in the diets of all adults. They become particularly problematic after age 50. Inadequate intake of these nutrients, coupled with their reduced absorption, the reduced synthesis of vitamin D in the skin, and the kidneys' decreased ability to put vitamin D in its active form, greatly contributes to the development of osteoporosis. Getting enough of these nutrients is a challenge for many older adults because food sources of vitamin D are limited in the North American diet, and the major sources—fatty fish and fortified milk—are not widely consumed by older adults. Plus, with increasing age, lactase production frequently decreases. As you know, one of the richest and most absorbable sources of these nutrients, milk, contains lactose. To get the vitamin D and calcium needed, many with lactose intolerance can consume small amounts of milk at mealtime with no ill effects. Calcium-fortified foods, cheese, yogurt, fish eaten with bones (e.g., canned sardines or salmon), and dark green leafy vegetables can help those with lactose intolerance meet calcium needs—but these foods often do not provide vitamin D. Just 10 to 15 minutes per day of sunlight can make a large difference in vitamin D status.

Iron Iron deficiency anemia, the most common type of malnutrition during the adult years, is found most frequently in women in their reproductive years because their diets do not provide enough iron to compensate for the iron lost monthly during menstruation. Other common causes of iron deficiency in adults of all ages include digestive tract injuries that cause bleeding (i.e., bleeding ulcers or hemorrhoids) and the use of medicines, such as aspirin, that cause blood loss. Impaired iron absorption due to age-related declines in stomach acid production may contribute to iron deficiency in older adults.

Zinc In addition to less than optimal dietary zinc intake during adulthood, zinc absorption declines as stomach acid production diminishes with age. Poor zinc status may contribute to the taste sensation losses, mental lethargy, and delayed wound healing many elderly adults experience.

Magnesium This mineral tends to be low in adults' diets. Inadequate magnesium intakes may contribute to the bone loss muscular weakness, and mental confusion seen in some elderly adults. It also can lead to sudden death from poor heart rhythm and is linked to cardiovascular disease, osteoporosis, and diabetes. The best source of magnesium is the diet; supplements can cause loose stools and diarrhea.

Folate and Vitamins B-6 and B-12 Sufficient folate, because of its role in prevention of neural tube defects, is very important to women during the childbearing years. In later years, folate and vitamins B-6 and B-12 are especially important because they are required to clear homocysteine from the bloodstream. Introduced in Chapter 5, elevated blood concentrations of homocysteine are associated with the increased risk of cardiovascular disease, stroke, bone fracture, and neurological decline seen in some elderly people. Vitamin B-12 is a particular problem for the older population because a deficiency may exist even when intake appears to be adequate. As people age, the stomach slows its production of acid and intrinsic factor, which leads to poor absorption of vitamin B-12 and eventually pernicious anemia. Adults age 51 years and older need to meet vitamin B-12 needs with supplements or foods fortified with synthetic vitamin B-12.

Vitamin E The dietary intake of most of the population falls short of recommendations for vitamin E. Low vitamin E intake means the body has a reduced supply of antioxidants, which may increase the degree of cell damage caused by free radicals, promote the progression of chronic diseases and cataracts, and speed aging. In addition, low vitamin E levels can lead to declines in physical abilities.

Carotenoids. Dietary intakes of certain carotenoids have been shown to have a variety of important anti-aging and health protective effects. Specifically, lutein and zeaxanthin have been linked with the prevention of cataracts and age-related macular degeneration. Diets high in fruit and vegetables, the major sources of carotenoids and other beneficial phytochemicals, are consistently shown to be protective of a wide variety of age-related conditions.

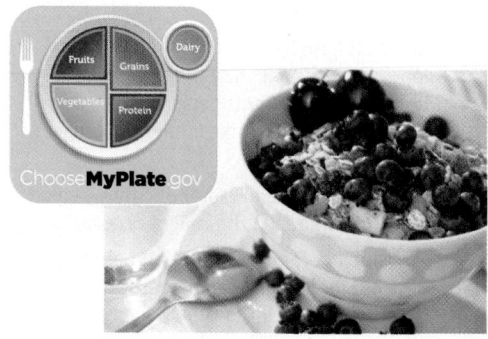

▲ How does this breakfast of whole-grain cereal, fruit, and milk compare to MyPlate?

Are Adults Following Current Dietary Recommendations?

In general, adults in North America are trying to follow many of the diet recommendations described in this chapter. Since the mid-1950s, they have consumed less saturated fat as more people substitute fat-free and low-fat milk for cream and whole milk. However, they eat more cheese, usually a concentrated form of saturated fat. Since 1963, they have eaten less butter, fewer eggs, less animal fat, and more vegetable oils and fish. These changes generally follow recommendations to reduce the intake of saturated fat and cholesterol in favor of unsaturated fat choices. Animal breeders are raising much leaner cattle and hogs than those produced in 1950, which also helps reduce saturated fat intake.

Other aspects of the average adult diet are less promising. The latest nutrition survey of eating habits in the United States shows that the major contributors of calories to the adult diet are white bread, beef, doughnuts, cakes and cookies, soft drinks, milk, chicken, cheese, alcoholic beverages, salad dressing, mayonnaise, potatoes, and sugars/syrups/jams. If the trend in diets were truly toward decreasing sugar and saturated fat intake, and increasing fiber intake, many of these foods would not appear at the top of the list.

CONCEPT CHECK

The 2010 Dietary Guidelines for Americans direct people to maintain healthy weight; choose more vegetables, fruits, legumes (beans), whole-grain products, fat-free and low-fat dairy products, and seafood; and choose fewer foods with sodium, saturated fats, *trans* fats, added sugars, and refined grains. Micronutrients of concern for an aging population include calcium, iron, zinc, magnesium, folate, carotenoids, and vitamins D, B-6, B-12, and E.

16.4 Factors Related to Food Intake and Nutrient Needs

Diet is one of the main factors directly involved in the development of several health conditions during adulthood. The effects of diet and nutrients on many of these conditions, including atherosclerosis, cancer, constipation, diabetes, diverticular disease, heartburn, hypertension, obesity, and osteoporosis, were discussed in earlier chapters. Still other health problems, including arthritis, Alzheimer's disease, and depression, are not directly diet-related, but nutrition is implicated in their prevention and/or treatment.

An important concept to remember is that an aging body loses resilience—it becomes less able to handle stressors and restore balance (homeostasis). For example, compared to a healthy 30-year-old adult, it takes twice as long for the kidneys of an 80-year-old to remove wastes and restore blood levels to normal after eating excess protein. Similarly, the breakdown of alcohol, drugs, and even nutrient supplements is

Researchers believe that maintaining lean muscle mass may be the most important strategy for successful aging. This is because maintaining lean muscle mass:

- Maintains basal metabolic rate, which helps decrease the risk of obesity
- Keeps body fat low, which helps control blood cholesterol levels and helps avoid the onset of type 2 diabetes
- Maintains body water, which decreases the risk of dehydration and improves body temperature regulation

sarcopenia In general, loss of muscle tissue. Among older adults this loss of lean mass greatly increases their risk of illness and death.

sarcopenic obesity Loss of muscle mass accompanied by gains in fat mass.

slowed. Consequently, blood levels of these substances rise higher and have a stronger and longer effect in older adults than in younger people. Taking steps to avoid stressing the body's capabilities (e.g., avoiding excessive protein intake or megadose dietary supplements) can help preserve optimal physiological function in older adults.

Like those of other age groups, the food choices and nutritional adequacy of adults' diets depend on the interplay of physiological, psychosocial, and economic factors. Alterations in any one of these factors can result in deteriorations in the quality of dietary intake, nutritional status, and health.

Physiological Factors

The implications of many of the physiological changes that occur during adulthood on dietary intake and nutrient needs are summarized in Table 16-2. Some of the changes listed (e.g., tooth loss, loss in taste and smell perceptions) can influence dietary intake. Other changes (e.g., loss of lean body tissue) can alter nutrient and/or calorie needs. Still other changes (e.g., reduced stomach acidity, diminished kidney function) can cause changes in nutrient utilization. Chronic diseases and the need for medications are additional physiological changes many adults experience that can influence food intake and nutrient needs. The following section details the interactions of several of these factors on nutritional status during adulthood.

Body Composition. The primary changes in body composition that occur as the adult years progress are diminished lean body mass, increased fat stores, and decreased body water. The loss of lean body mass is termed **sarcopenia.** Some muscle cells shrink and others are lost as muscles age; some muscles lose their elasticity as they accumulate fat and collagen. Loss of muscle mass leads to a decrease in basal metabolism, muscle strength, and energy needs. Less muscle mass also leads to lower physical activity, which makes the prognosis for maintaining muscle even worse. Clearly, it is best to avoid this downward spiral.

Lifestyle greatly determines the rate of muscle mass deterioration. As you might predict, an active lifestyle helps maintain muscle mass, whereas an inactive one encourages its loss. In fact, much of what we associate with old age is due to a lifetime of physical inactivity. Ideally, an active lifestyle should be maintained throughout life and include both aerobic and strength training (see Making Decisions). Physical activity increases muscle strength and mobility, improves balance and decreases the risk of falling, eases daily tasks that require some strength, improves sleep, slows bone loss, and increases joint movement, thus reducing injuries. It also has a positive impact on a person's mental outlook. Strength training (resistance) helps reverse some of the decline in daily function associated with the muscle loss typically seen in older adulthood.

As lean tissue declines with age, body fat often increases, a condition called **sarcopenic obesity** (see Further Reading 13). Much of this increase in body fat results from overeating and limited physical activity, although even athletic men and lean women typically gain some degree of midsection fat after age 50. A small fat gain in adulthood may not compromise health, but large gains are problematic. Recall that obesity can raise blood pressure and blood glucose and make walking and performing daily tasks more difficult.

Decreases in body weight are common in adults age 70 and older. Weight loss is a problem for older people in particular because it increases the risk of nutrition-related illness and death. It may indicate illness, reduced tolerance to medication, or withdrawal from life. The effects of current medication, as well as changes in taste and smell, may inhibit appetite, too. In addition, many older people live alone, a circumstance associated with depressed appetite.

Skeletal System. Recall from Chapter 9 that bone loss in women occurs primarily after menopause. Bone loss in men is slow and steady from middle age throughout later life. Many older people may suffer from undiagnosed osteomalacia, a condition

TABLE 16-2 Typical Physiological Changes of Aging and Recommended Diet and Lifestyle Responses

Physiological Changes	Recommended Responses
Appetite (↓)	• Monitor weight and strive to eat enough to maintain healthy weight. • Use meal replacement products, such as Boost® and Ensure Plus®.
Sense of taste and smell (↓)	• Vary the diet. • Experiment with herbs and spices.
Chewing ability (↓)	• Work with a dentist to maximize chewing ability. • Modify food consistency as necessary. • Eat calorie-rich snacks.
Sense of thirst (↓)	• Consume plenty of fluid each day. • Stay alert for evidence of dehydration (e.g., minimal output or dark-colored urine).
Stomach acidity (↓)	• Consume iron-rich foods with a source of vitamin C. • Choose foods fortified with vitamin B-12 or use a supplemental source of vitamin B-12.
Bowel function (↓)	• Consume enough fiber daily, choosing primarily fruits, vegetables, and whole-grain breads and cereals. • Meet fluid needs.
Lactase production (↓)	• Limit milk serving size at each use. • Substitute yogurt or cheese for milk. • Use reduced-lactose or lactose-free products. • Seek nondairy calcium sources.
Iron status (↓)	• Include some lean meat and iron-fortified foods in the diet. • Ask physician to monitor blood iron status.
Liver function (↓)	• Consume alcohol in moderation, if at all. • Avoid consuming excess vitamin A.
Insulin function (↓)	• Maintain healthy body weight. • Perform regular physical activity.
Kidney function (↓)	• If necessary, work with physician and registered dietitian to modify protein and other nutrients in diet.
Immune function (↓)	• Meet nutrient needs, especially protein, vitamin E, vitamin B-6, and zinc. • Perform regular physical activity.
Lung function (↓)	• Avoid tobacco products. • Perform regular physical activity.
Vision (↓)	• Regularly consume sources of carotenoids, vitamin C, vitamin E, and zinc (e.g., fruits, vegetables and whole-grain breads and cereals). • Moderate total fat intake. • Wear sunglasses in sunny conditions. • Avoid tobacco products. • Perform regular physical activity (to lessen insulin resistance). • In the case of diagnosed moderate macular degeneration, talk with a physician about following a protocol of zinc, copper, vitamin E, vitamin C, and beta-carotene supplementation.
Lean tissue (↓)	• Meet nutrient needs, especially protein and vitamin D. • Perform regular physical activity, including strength training.
Cardiovascular function (↓)	• Use diet modifications or physician-prescribed medications to keep blood lipids and blood pressure within desirable ranges. • Stay physically active. • Achieve and maintain a healthy body weight.
Bone mass (↓)	• Meet nutrient needs, especially calcium and vitamin D (regular sun exposure helps meet needs for vitamin D). • Perform regular physical activity, especially weight-bearing exercise. • Women should consider use of approved osteoporosis medications at menopause. • Remain at a healthy weight (especially avoid unneeded weight loss).
Mental function (↓)	• Meet nutrient needs (e.g., vitamin E, vitamin C, vitamin B-6, folate, and vitamin B-12) and consume seafood twice a week. • Strive for lifelong learning. • Perform regular physical activity. • Obtain adequate sleep.
Fat stores (↓)	• Avoid overeating. • Perform regular physical activity.

Registered dietitians, physicians, and pharmacists can help with any needed adjustments arising from these and other drug-related problems.

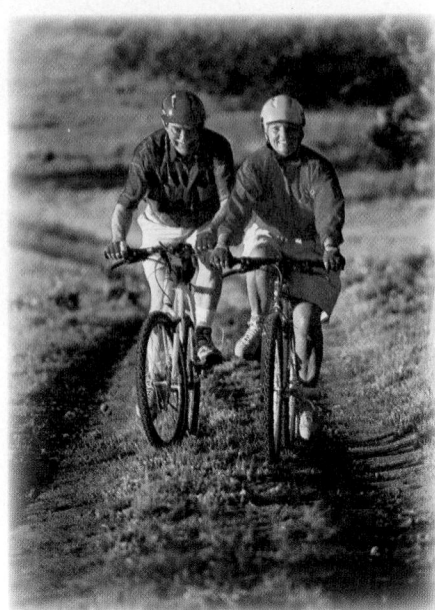

▲ Older people benefit from aerobic and strength-training (resistance) exercises. Download a free copy of *Exercise & Physical Activity: Your Everyday Guide* from the National Institute on Aging at www.nia.nih.gov.

The 2008 Physical Activity Guidelines for Americans provide the following guidelines specifically for older adults:

- When older adults cannot do 150 minutes of moderate-intensity aerobic activity a week because of chronic conditions, they should be as physically active as their abilities and conditions allow.

- Older adults should do exercises that maintain or improve balance if they are at risk of falling.

- Older adults should determine their level of effort for physical activity relative to their level of fitness.

- Older adults with chronic diseases should understand whether and how their conditions affect their ability to do regular physical activity safely.

mainly caused by insufficient vitamin D. Osteoporosis can limit the ability of older people to move about, shop, prepare food, and live normally. Consuming adequate vitamin D, calcium, and protein; not smoking; drinking alcohol moderately or not at all; and engaging in weight-bearing exercises can help preserve bone mass. Medications also can help lessen bone loss.

MAKING DECISIONS

Exercise Guidelines for Older Adults

Aerobic Exercise: All adults should engage in moderate-intensity aerobic exercise for at least 150 minutes per week, or vigorous intensity aerobic exercise for 75 minutes per week, or an equivalent combination of the two. This amount of aerobic activity aids in prevention of chronic diseases. Longer duration of daily exercise may be required for weight loss or weight maintenance. Weight bearing exercises are particularly helpful for preservation of bone mass.

Strength Training: To maintain lean tissue and basal metabolic rate, strength training should include eight to ten different exercises (each with two sets of eight to fifteen repetitions), performed two to three times per week. Exercises that involve the large muscle groups (e.g., arms, back, and legs) and exercises that enhance grip strength should be emphasized. Start slowly, concentrate on breathing, rest between sets, avoid locking joints in the arms and legs, and stop an exercise if it becomes painful.

Flexibility Exercises: To prevent injuries, stretching exercises for each major muscle group should accompany aerobic or strength exercises at least 2 days per week.

Balance Exercises: For those over age 65 who are at risk for falling, exercises that improve balance (e.g., yoga, tai chi) are recommended in addition to aerobic, strength, and flexibility exercises.

All older adults should avoid inactivity. Having an exercise plan, developed with a health professional to accommodate individual health risks and needs, will enhance success for older adults. Men older than age 40; women older than age 50; those with heart conditions, diabetes, or joint problems; and anyone who has been sedentary should consult a physician before beginning an exercise program.

Learn more at www.acsm.org and see Further Reading 4.

Digestive System. The production of HCl, intrinsic factor, and lactase declines with advancing age and, as a result, impairs the absorption of several nutrients. Constipation is the main intestinal problem for older people. To prevent constipation, older people should meet fiber needs, drink enough fluids, and exercise. Fiber medications are generally unnecessary but may be useful when total energy consumption does not allow for enough fiber intake. Because some medications can cause constipation, a physician should be consulted to determine if a laxative or stool softener is needed.

In addition to changes in the GI tract, the functions of the accessory organs decline as we age. For instance, the liver functions less efficiently. A history of significant alcohol consumption or liver disease will cause the liver to function even less efficiently. As liver efficiency declines, its ability to detoxify many substances, including medications, alcohol, and vitamin and mineral supplements, drops. The possibility for vitamin toxicity increases.

The gallbladder also functions less efficiently in later years. Gallstones can block the flow of bile out of the gallbladder into the small intestine, thereby interfering with fat digestion. Obesity is a major risk factor for gallbladder disease, especially in older women. A low-fat diet or surgery to remove the gallbladder may be necessary.

Although pancreatic function may decline with age, this organ has a large reserve capacity. One sign of a failing pancreas is high blood glucose, although this can occur as the result of several conditions. The pancreas may be secreting less insulin, or cells may be resisting insulin action (as is commonly seen in obese people with upper-body fat storage). Where appropriate, improved nutrient intake, regular physical activity, and loss of excess body weight can improve insulin action and blood glucose regulation.

Nervous System. A gradual loss of nerve cells that transmit signals may decrease taste and smell perceptions and impair neuromuscular coordination, reasoning, and memory. Both hearing and vision decline with age. Hearing impairment is greatest in those who have been exposed constantly to loud noises, such as urban traffic, aircraft noise, and music. Because they cannot hear well, older people may avoid social contacts, which increases their risk of poor dietary intake.

Declining eyesight, frequently caused by retina degeneration and cataracts, can affect a person's abilities to grocery shop, locate desired foods, read labels for nutritional content, and prepare foods at home. Vision losses also may cause people to curtail social contacts, reduce physical activity, and not practice daily personal health and grooming routines. Macular degeneration, one form of failing eyesight in old age, is quite common, affecting about 9.1 million adults in the United States. A major risk factor is cigarette smoking. Diets rich in carotenoids help reduce the risk of macular degeneration. The risk of developing cataracts is decreased by consuming a diet rich in fruits and vegetables.

Neuromuscular coordination losses may make it difficult to shop for and prepare food. Physical tasks as simple as opening food packages can become so difficult that individuals restrict dietary intake to foods that require little preparation and depend on others to provide food that is ready to eat. Eating may become difficult, too. Loss of coordination makes it a challenge to grasp cup handles and manipulate eating utensils. As a result, older adults may avoid foods that can be easily spilled (e.g., soups and juices) or that need to be cut (e.g., meats, large vegetable pieces) and restrict food intake to easy-to-eat finger foods. Some may even withdraw from social interaction and eat alone, which can lead to inadequate nutrient intake.

Immune System. With age, the immune system often operates less efficiently. Consuming adequate protein, vitamins (especially folate and vitamins A, D, and E), iron, and zinc helps maximize immune system function. Recurrent sicknesses and poor wound healing are warning signs that a deficient diet (especially of protein and zinc) may be hindering the function of the immune system. On the other hand, overnutrition appears to be equally harmful to the immune system. For example, obesity and excessive fat, iron, and zinc intakes can suppress immune function.

Endocrine System. As adulthood progresses, the rate of hormone synthesis and release can slow. A decrease in insulin release or sensitivity to insulin, for instance, means that it takes longer for blood glucose levels to return to normal after a meal. Maintaining a healthy weight, exercising regularly, eating a diet low in fat and high in fiber, and avoiding foods with a high glycemic index can enhance the body's ability to use insulin and restore elevated blood glucose levels to normal after a meal.

Chronic Disease. The prevalence of obesity, heart disease, osteoporosis, cancer, hypertension, and diabetes rises with age. More than eight out of every ten elderly people have one of these chronic and potentially debilitating diseases. Half of all elderly people have at least two chronic conditions. Chronic diseases may have a strong impact on dietary intake. For instance, excessive fatness, heart disease, and osteoporosis may impair physical mobility to the extent that victims are unable to shop for and prepare food. Chronic disease also can influence nutrient and calorie needs. Cancer, for example, boosts both nutrient and calorie needs. Hypertension may indicate a need to lower sodium intake. Nutrient utilization can be affected by chronic disease, too. For instance, diabetes alters the body's ability to utilize glucose. In addition, the effects of heart disease on the kidneys may impair their ability to reabsorb glucose, amino acids, and vitamin C.

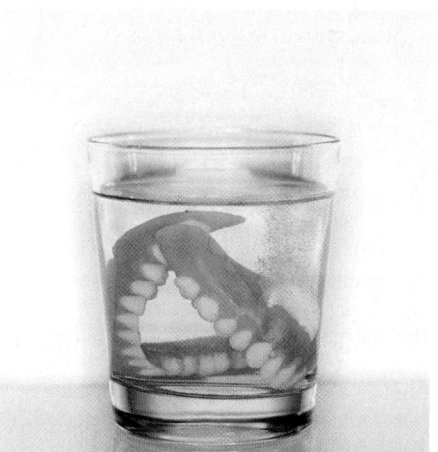

▲ Poor dental health contributes to decreased food intake and digestive problems. Serving softer, easier to chew foods and allowing extra time for chewing and swallowing improves food intake.

MAKING DECISIONS

Nutrition Interventions for Arthritis

There are over 100 forms of arthritis, a disease that causes the degeneration and roughening of the cartilage that covers and cushions the joints. Such changes in the joints cause them to ache and become inflamed and painful to move. Osteoarthritis, which increases in prevalence with advancing age, is the leading cause of disability among older persons. Rheumatoid arthritis, which is not as common, is more prevalent in younger adults.

Although precise causes or cures are unknown, many unproven "remedies" have been publicized. Unusual diets, food restrictions, and nutrient supplements are some of the more popular treatments. However, no special diet, food, or nutrient has been proven to reliably prevent, relieve, or cure arthritis in humans. As far as supplements go, glucosamine and/or chondroitin have been most extensively studied in relation to arthritis. Many but not all studies demonstrate these supplements can relieve pain, slow the progression of joint degeneration, or rebuild cartilage. Maintaining a healthy weight, which reduces stress on painful arthritic joints, is the only diet-related treatment known to offer some relief. MyPlate can be used as a guide in making healthy food choices for weight management.

CRITICAL THINKING

Jamila went to her local pharmacy yesterday to look for a product to help her stay awake while studying. On the shelves she found a dietary supplement claiming to be a Chinese herbal remedy for sleepiness and fatigue. She thought that because a pharmacy carried the product, it should be safe and work as indicated on the label.

Is she correct in these assumptions? Are there specific risks associated with taking such herbal remedies?

N umerous reports have documented significant health risks associated with the use of some herbal and alternative remedies, sometimes resulting in death. Studies especially implicate germander, pokeroot, sassafras, mandrake, pennyroyal, comfrey, chaparral, yohimbe, lobelia, jin bu huan, kava kava, products containing stephanie and magnolia, senna, hai gen fen, paraguay tea, kombucha tea, tung shueh (Chinese black balls), and willow bark.

Medications. Older adults are major consumers of medications (prescription and over-the-counter) and nutrient supplements. Half of all people over age 65 take several medicines each day. The rate of supplement use increases throughout adulthood, such that by age 50, approximately half of all adults are using supplements daily. Physiological declines that occur during aging (e.g., reduced body water, reduced liver and kidney function) cause the effects of medications and nutrient supplements to be exaggerated and persist longer in older adults.

Medications can improve health and quality of life, but some also adversely affect nutritional status, particularly of those who are older and/or take many different medications. For instance, some medications depress taste and smell acuity or cause anorexia or nausea that can blunt interest in eating and lead to reduced dietary intake. Some medications alter nutrient needs. Aspirin, for example, increases the likelihood of stomach bleeding, so long-term use may elevate the need for iron, as well as other nutrients. Antibiotics may deplete the body of vitamin K. Some medications may impair nutrient utilization—diuretics and laxatives may cause excessive excretion of water and minerals. Even vitamin and mineral supplements may have unanticipated effects on nutritional status. Iron supplements taken in large doses can interfere with the functioning of zinc and copper. Folate supplements can mask vitamin B-12 deficiencies.

People who must take medications should eat nutrient-dense foods and avoid any specific food or supplement that interferes with the function of their medications. For example, vitamin K can reduce the action of oral anticoagulants, aged cheese can interfere with certain drugs used to treat hypertension and depression, and grapefruit can interfere with medications such as tranquilizers and those that lower cholesterol levels. A physician or pharmacist should be consulted about any restrictions on food and/or supplements.

Alternative Medicine and Aging

At least half of adults report using some kind of dietary or herbal supplement. Recall from Chapter 2 that these products are not evaluated by FDA for effectiveness or safety since they are governed by the 1994 Dietary Supplement Health and Education Act (DSHEA). Purity and quantity of the product in the bottle are also suspect. Table 16-3 reviews some popular herbal remedies used by older adults. Note from the table that these products can pose health risks in certain people. In addition, they may be expensive ($100 per month or more in some cases) and are not covered by health insurance plans. Use of many herbal products has declined because of expense and questionable benefits. Instead, consumers are opting to spend their money on tried-and-true products, such as multivitamins, vitamin D, omega-3 fatty acids, fiber, and probiotics.

A rational approach to the use of herbal products is to use only one product at a time, keep a diary of symptoms, and check with one's physician first before discontinuing a prescribed medication. In addition, FDA advises anyone who experiences adverse side effects from an herbal remedy to contact a physician. Physicians are then encouraged to report such adverse events to FDA, state and local health departments, and consumer protection agencies.

For additional information about herbal remedies, access the following websites. These are regularly updated and cover the herbals listed in Table 16-3, as well as many others.

National Institutes of Health National Center for Complementary and Alternative Medicine (NCCAM)
www.nccam.nih.gov/
American Botanical Council
http://abc.herbalgram.org/
Complementary and Alternative Medicine Program at Stanford (CAMPS)
http://camps.stanford.edu/
National Institutes of Health Office of Dietary Supplements
http://ods.od.nih.gov/
Natural Medicines Comprehensive Database
www.naturaldatabase.com

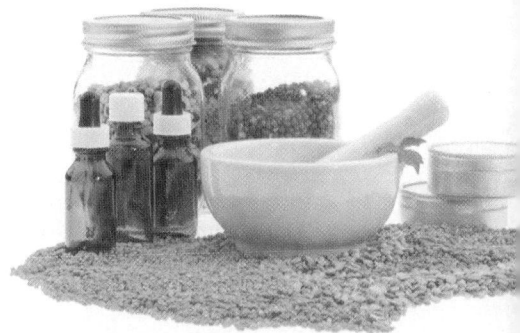

▲ Some herbal products are effective for treating specific medical problems. Follow label instructions carefully. Note potential side effects listed, as well as who should not use the product. The best advice is to only use these substances under strict supervision of a physician.

TABLE 16-3 A Close Look at Some Popular Herbal Remedies

Product	Purported Effects	Side Effects	Who Should Especially Seek Physician Guidance Before Use
Black cohosh	• Mild reduction of postmenopausal symptoms (shown to be effective in some but not all women; use should not go beyond 6 months in general)	• Nausea • Liver damage	• Women who have had breast cancer • Pregnant women • Anyone taking estrogen, hypertension medications, or blood-thinning medications*
Cranberry	• Prevention or treatment of urinary tract infections (some evidence of efficacy)	• Use of concentrated tablets may increase risk of kidney stones	• People susceptible to kidney stones • Anyone taking antidepressants or prescription painkillers
Echinacea	• Stimulation of the immune system • Prevention or treatment of colds or other infections (mild effect at best)	• Nausea • Skin irritation • Allergic reactions • Minor GI tract upset • Increased urination	• Anyone with an autoimmune disease • Pre- or postsurgical patients • Anyone with allergies to daisies
Garlic	• Antibiotic properties • Slight reduction of blood cholesterol or blood pressure in some, but not all, studies	• GI tract upset (e.g., heartburn, flatulence) • Unpleasant odor	• Pre- or postsurgical patients • Perinatal women • People with a history of gallstones • Anyone taking blood-thinning medications or AIDS medications
Ginkgo biloba	• Increased circulation • Improvement of memory (especially for people with Alzheimer's disease; low evidence of efficacy)	• Mild headache • GI tract upset • Allergic reactions • Irritability • Reduced blood clotting • Seizures (if contaminated with toxic ginkgo seeds)	• People with bleeding disorders • Pre- or postsurgical patients • Anyone with allergies to the plant • Concurrent use of feverfew, garlic, ginseng, dong quai, or red clover • Anyone taking diabetes medications, blood-thinning medications, vitamin E supplements, antidepressants, or diuretics

TABLE 16-3 *(continued)*

Product	Purported Effects	Side Effects	Who Should Especially Seek Physician Guidance Before Use
Ginseng	• Increased energy • Stress relief • Decreased weakness and fatigue (efficacy largely unknown)	• Hypertension • Asthma attacks • Irregular heartbeat • Insomnia • Headache • Nervousness • GI tract upset • Reduced blood clotting • Menstrual irregularities and breast tenderness	• Anyone who takes a prescription drug should consult a physician before using • Women on hormone replacement therapy • Women who have had breast cancer • Anyone with chronic GI tract disease • Anyone with uncontrolled hypertension • Anyone taking blood-thinning medications, diabetes medications, antidepressants, or heart failure medications
St. John's wort	• Alleviation of depression (mild effect at best)	• Mild GI tract upset • Rash • Tiredness • Restlessness • Increased sensitivity to sunlight	• Anyone who takes a prescription drug • People with UV sensitivity, including that induced by medications or other treatments** • People with bipolar disorder • Anyone recovering from a graft or organ transplant • Anyone taking ritalin, caffeine, HIV medications, heart failure medications, cholesterol-lowering medications, blood-thinning medications, chemotherapy, oral contraceptives, antidepressants, antipsychotic medications, or asthma medications
Valerian	• Alleviation of restlessness and other sleeping disorders that stem from nervous conditions • Reduction of anxiety (some evidence of efficacy)	• Impaired attention • Headache • Morning grogginess • Irregular heartbeat • GI tract upset • Disagreeable odor • Withdrawal delerium	• Anyone taking central nervous system depressants*** • Anyone who drinks alcohol • People about to operate heavy machinery or drive

Pregnant or breastfeeding women, children under 2 years of age, anyone over the age of 65 years, and anyone with a chronic disease should never take supplements unless under the guidance of a physician. A concern has been raised with regard to patients who abruptly end alternative medicines at the start of hospital treatments or deny that they are involved in alternative therapy. Interactions between alternative therapies and pharmaceutical drugs can be drastic and include complications such as delirium, clotting abnormalities, and rapid heartbeat, resulting in the need for intensive care. Full disclosure of all prescription and nonprescription treatments aids in prevention of such complications. Experts recommend that, if time permits, patients stop taking herbal products for about a week before a scheduled surgery or otherwise take all original supplement containers to the hospital, so that the anesthesiologist can evaluate what was taken.

*Coumadin, aspirin, Heparin, Lovenox, or Fragmin

**Sulfa medications, anti-inflammatory medications, or acid-reflux medications

***Valium, halcion, seconal

Psychosocial Factors

Worries about possible embarrassment caused by deteriorating physical capabilities may cause older adults to withdraw from social interaction and eat alone rather than with others. Those who eat alone, regardless of the reason, seldom eat as much or as nutritiously as they should. Both young and old people who eat without companionship tend to feel unmotivated to shop for or prepare foods. Many become apathetic toward life, which over time causes health and nutritional status to decline. As you'll see later in the chapter, several nutrition assistance programs can help older people obtain the food and social support needed for good health.

Depression A positive outlook on life and intact support networks help make food and eating interesting and satisfying. In contrast, social isolation, grief, chronic pain and infirmity, or a change in lifestyle can lead to depression, loss of appetite, lack of interest in food, and disability. Major depression affects 5% to 8% of adults in the United States. This statistic increases to about 18% among Americans ages 65 or older. Left untreated, depression can lead to a continual decline in appetite, which results in weakness, poor nutrition, mental confusion, and increased feelings of isolation and loneliness (Fig. 16-5). In contrast, some people cope by overeating, which can lead

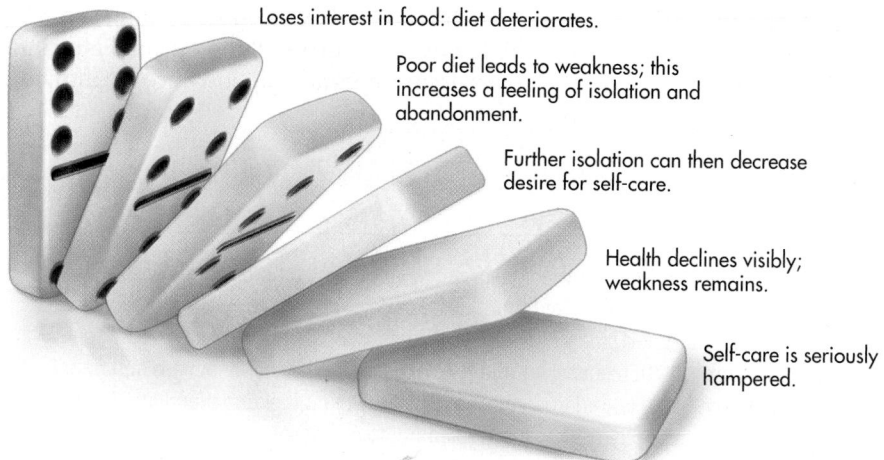

Social isolation; perhaps spouse has died.

Loses interest in food: diet deteriorates.

Poor diet leads to weakness; this increases a feeling of isolation and abandonment.

Further isolation can then decrease desire for self-care.

Health declines visibly; weakness remains.

Self-care is seriously hampered.

FIGURE 16-5 ▶ The decline of health often seen in older adults. A small change leads to a chain of events or "domino effect" that results in poor health. Early intervention can prevent declines in physical health related to psychosocial factors.

to obesity and its associated problems. Depression may signal an underlying illness and can also impair recovery from other illnesses or injuries. As many as 15% of cases end in suicide. For these reasons, early detection of depression is important in older adults. Depression is often treatable, but medication alone will not help those experiencing major life changes, such as the death of a spouse. Adequate social support and/or psychological intervention are also essential.

Alzheimer's Disease. Alzheimer's disease is an irreversible, abnormal, progressive deterioration of the brain that causes victims to steadily lose the ability to remember, reason, and comprehend. Alzheimer's disease often takes a terrible toll on the mental and eventual physical health of older people. About 5.4 million adults in the U.S. have the disease.

The 10 warning signs of Alzheimer's disease are listed in the margin. No one is sure exactly what causes this disease, but scientists have proposed various causes, including alterations in cell development or protein production in the brain, strokes, altered blood lipoprotein composition, obesity, poor blood glucose regulation (e.g., diabetes), high blood pressure, high blood cholesterol, and high free radical levels.

Early efforts at prevention are key, because the process of cognitive decline begins 10 to 20 years before warning signs appear. Preventive measures for Alzheimer's disease focus on maintaining brain activity through lifelong learning, eating a diet rich in fruits and vegetables, and taking ibuprofen. The role of nutrition in preventing or minimizing the risk of this disease is being investigated. Getting enough antioxidant nutrients, such as vitamin C, vitamin E, and selenium, helps protect the body from the damaging effects of free radicals. Adequate intakes of folate and vitamins B-6 and B-12 are especially important because elevated blood homocysteine is also a risk factor. Dietary fats, too, may play a role in keeping this disease at bay. Individuals with diets rich in omega-3 and omega-6 foods and low in saturated and *trans* fatty acids have a reduced risk of Alzheimer's disease.

The dietary intakes of those with Alzheimer's disease are poor, compared with those of a similar age without this disease. Caregivers of those who have Alzheimer's disease need to monitor the patient's weight to ensure maintenance of a healthy weight and nutritional state. Other tips are serving omega-3 rich fish in meals twice per week and making sure eating habits do not pose a health risk (e.g., holding food in one's mouth or forgetting to swallow). Regular physical activity has also been shown to improve mental status in people afflicted with this disease (see Further Reading 6).

Economic Factors. The amount of money available for purchasing food can have a great impact on the types and amounts of food one eats. Unemployment, underemployment, retirement, death of a wage earner, or anything else that limits

Ten Warning Signs of Alzheimer's Disease

1. Recent memory loss that affects job performance
2. Difficulty performing familiar tasks
3. Problems with language
4. Disorientation to time and place
5. Faulty or decreased judgment
6. Problems with abstract thinking
7. Tendency to misplace things
8. Changes in mood or behavior
9. Changes in personality
10. Loss of initiative

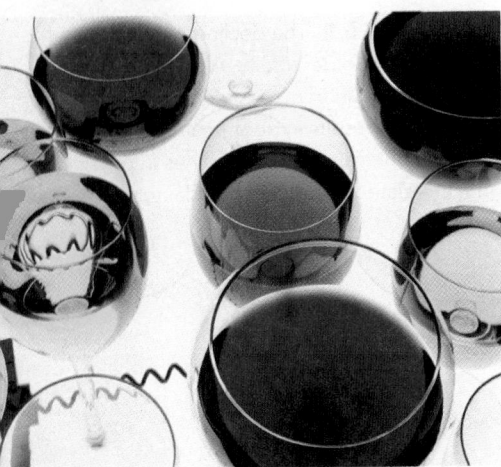

▲ Of all the alcohol sources, red wine in moderation is often singled out as the best choice because of the added bonus of the many phytochemicals present (e.g., resveratrol). These are leached out from the grape skins as the red wine is fermented. Dark beer is also a source of phytochemicals.

ethanol Chemical term for the form of alcohol found in alcoholic beverages.

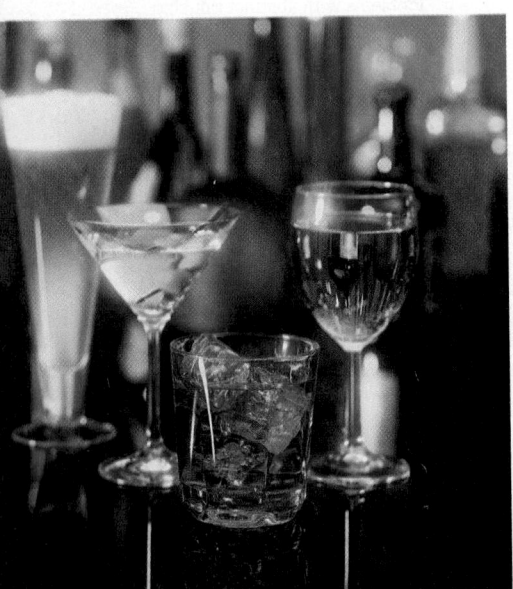

▲ One standard drink is universally defined as one 12-ounce bottle of beer or wine cooler, one 5-ounce glass of wine, 3 ounces of sherry or liqueur, or 1.5 ounces of 80-proof distilled spirits.

income makes it difficult to get the best, most healthful foods and can diminish nutritional status and health. Insufficient income is a particular problem among those ages 65 and up and, as a result, they frequently have trouble making sure they remain well nourished. The Commodity Foods Program and Supplemental Nutrition Assistance Program are two federal U.S. programs that can help low-income individuals of all ages procure the foods they need.

CONCEPT CHECK

Physiological, psychosocial, and economic factors impact the nutritional status of older adults. The following organ systems and functions can decrease as we age: appetite; sense of taste, smell, thirst, hearing, and sight; digestion and absorption; liver, gallbladder, pancreatic, kidney, lung, and heart function; and the immune system. In addition, bone mass and muscle mass gradually decrease, the latter largely because of a deficient diet and inactivity. Appropriate dietary changes, regular physical activity, maintaining social contacts, and participating in nutrition assistance programs can often help reduce the impact of these factors.

16.5 Nutrition Implications of Alcohol Consumption

Given the wide spectrum of alcohol use and abuse, knowledge of alcohol consumption and its relationship to overall health is essential to the study of nutrition. Alcoholic beverages contain the chemical form of alcohol known as **ethanol.** Although not a nutrient *per se*, alcohol is a source of calories (about 7 kcal per gram) for approximately half of adults, constituting about 3% of total calories in the average North American diet (Table 16-4). Bear in mind that alcoholic beverages served in bars and restaurants can be 20% to 45% larger than the "standard drinks" described below.

Moderate consumption of alcohol by a person of legal age is an acceptable practice and even has some health benefits (see Further Reading 2). However, only about half

TABLE 16-4 Alcohol, Carbohydrate, and Calorie Content of Alcoholic Beverages*

Beverage	Amount (fluid ounces)	Alcohol (grams)	Carbohydrates (grams)	Calories (kcal)
Beer				
Regular	12.0	13	13	146
Light	12.0	11	5	99
Distilled Spirits				
Gin, rum, vodka, bourbon, whiskey (80 proof), brandy, cognac	1.5	14	—	96
Wine				
Red	5	14	2	102
White	5	14	1	100
Dessert, sweet	5	23	17	225
Rosé	5	14	2	100
Mixed Drinks				
Manhattan	3.0	26	3	191
Martini	3.0	27	—	189
Bourbon and soda	3.0	11	—	78
Whiskey sour	3.0	13	14	147

*There is little to no fat or protein contribution to calorie content.
Source: USDA.

of alcohol consumed is done so in moderation. About 17.6 million people in the United States suffer from alcohol abuse or alcohol dependence. About one in five people over the age of 12 report binge drinking in the last 30 days. Alcohol by far is the most commonly abused drug.

How Alcoholic Beverages Are Produced

The basis of alcohol production is fermentation, a process by which microorganisms break down simple sugars (e.g., glucose or maltose) to alcohol, carbon dioxide, and water in the absence of oxygen. High-carbohydrate foods especially encourage the growth of yeast, the microorganism responsible for alcohol production. Wine is formed by the fermentation of grape or other fruit juices. Beer is made from malted cereal grain. Distilled spirits (e.g., vodka, gin, whiskey) are made from any number of fruits, vegetables, and grains. Production temperatures, the composition of the food used for fermentation, and aging techniques determine the characteristics of the product.

Absorption and Metabolism of Alcohol

Alcohol requires no digestion. It is absorbed rapidly from the GI tract by diffusion, making it the most efficiently absorbed of all calorie sources. Once absorbed, alcohol is freely distributed into all the fluid compartments within the body. About 1% to 3% of alcohol is excreted via urine and about 1% to 5% evaporates via the breath, the basis for the breathalyzer test. Most alcohol (90% to 98%), however, is metabolized. The liver is the primary site for alcohol metabolism, and some may also be metabolized by the cells lining the stomach. The main pathway of alcohol metabolism involves the enzymes **alcohol dehydrogenase** and **acetaldehyde dehydrogenase**. Alcohol cannot be stored in the body, so it takes absolute priority over other energy sources for metabolism.

As a person's alcohol consumption exceeds the body's capacity to metabolize it, blood alcohol concentration rises, the brain is exposed to alcohol, and symptoms of intoxication appear (see Table 16-5). Absorption and metabolism of alcohol depend on numerous factors: gender, race, body size, physical condition, meal composition, rate of gastric emptying, the alcohol content of the beverage, use of certain drugs,

Alcohol proof represents twice the volume of alcohol in percentage terms. Thus, 80 proof vodka is 40% alcohol.

alcohol dehydrogenase An enzyme used in alcohol (ethanol) metabolism that converts alcohol into acetaldehyde.

acetaldehyde dehydrogenase An enzyme used in ethanol metabolism that eventually converts acetaldehyde into carbon dioxide and water.

alcohol abuse Excessive alcohol consumption that leads to severe alcohol-related health and other problems, such as recurrent sickness, inability to fulfill major obligations, use in hazardous situations (e.g., driving), related legal problems, or use despite social and interpersonal difficulties.

cirrhosis A loss of functioning liver cells, which are replaced by nonfunctioning connective tissue. Any substance that poisons liver cells can lead to cirrhosis. The most common cause is a chronic, excessive alcohol intake. Exposure to certain industrial chemicals also can lead to cirrhosis.

TABLE 16-5 Blood Alcohol Concentration and Symptoms

Concentration*	Sporadic Drinker	Chronic Drinker	Hours for Alcohol to Be Metabolized**
50 (party high) (0.05%)	Congenial euphoria; decreased tension; noticeable impairment in driving and coordination	No observable effect	2–3
75 (0.075%)	Gregarious	Often no effect	3–4
80 to 100 (0.08%–0.1%)	Uncoordinated; 0.08% is legally drunk (as in drunk driving) in the United States and Canada.	Minimal signs	4–6
125–150 (0.125%–0.15%)	Unrestrained behavior; episodic uncontrolled behavior	Pleasurable euphoria or beginning of uncoordination	6–10
200–250 (0.2%–0.25%)	Alertness lost; lethargic	Effort is required to maintain emotional and motor control	10–24
300–350 (0.3%–0.35%)	Stupor to coma	Drowsy and slow	10–24
>500 (>0.5%)	Some will die	Coma	>24

*Milligrams of alcohol per 100 milliliters of blood.

**For a social drinker; alcohol metabolism is somewhat faster in chronic alcohol abusers.

Modified from Wyngaarder JB, Smith LH: *Cecil Textbook of Medicine*, fourth edition, Philadelphia, 1988, WB Saunders. Used with permission.

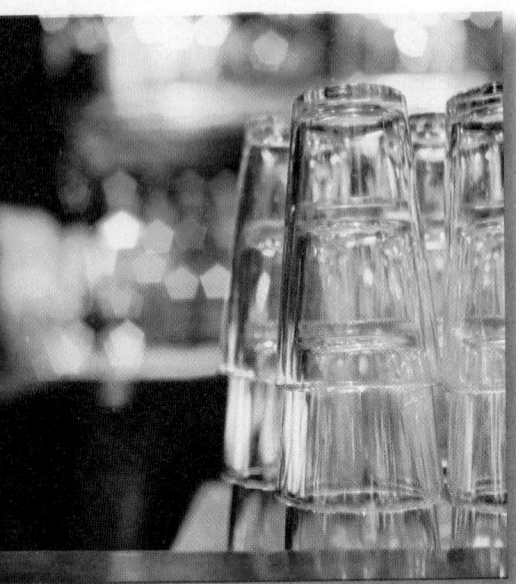

▲ There is no such thing as controlled drinking once a person has alcoholism. Total abstinence is mandatory for recovery.

alcohol dependence The person experiences repeated alcohol-related difficulties, such as an inability to control use, spending a great deal of time associated with alcohol use, continued use of alcohol despite physical or psychological consequences, persistent desire or unsuccessful efforts to cut down or control alcohol use, and withdrawal symptoms. Tolerance is also seen.

alcoholism As defined by the American Medical Association, an illness characterized by significant impairment directly related to persistent and excessive use of alcohol.

CRITICAL THINKING

For many people, drinking and smoking go hand-in-hand. What risks and diseases could correlate with the combination of these behaviors?

chronic alcohol abuse, and even how much sleep one has had. Women absorb and metabolize alcohol differently than men. The amount of alcohol metabolized by the cells lining the stomach is greater in men than in women. Women also have less body water in which to dilute the alcohol than do men. Overall, women develop alcohol-related ailments, such as cirrhosis of the liver, more rapidly than men do with the same alcohol-consumption habits.

Benefits of Moderate Alcohol Use

When used in moderation, alcohol is linked to several health benefits. Benefits of alcohol use are associated with specific intakes of about one drink per day for men and slightly less than one for women. Socialization and relaxation are among the intangible benefits of moderate alcohol use by people of legal drinking age. In terms of physiological benefits, moderate drinkers experience lower risk of developing cardiovascular diseases and type 2 diabetes. Previous consumers of alcohol no longer experience the benefits of alcohol when consumption ceases. See Table 16-6 for additional benefits of alcohol consumption.

Risks of Alcohol Abuse

Despite the few benefits of regular, moderate use, the risks of **alcohol abuse** are more numerous and harmful. Although it is one of the most preventable health problems, excessive consumption of alcohol contributes significantly to 5 of the 10 leading causes of death in North America: heart failure, certain forms of cancer, **cirrhosis of the liver**, motor vehicle and other accidents, and suicides (review Table 16-6 for additional health risks). In the United States, about $185 billion is spent annually in terms of lost productivity, premature deaths, direct treatment expenses, and legal fees associated with alcoholism. Overall, alcohol abuse typically reduces a person's life expectancy by 15 years.

Alcoholic beverages have little nutritional value and, thus, nutrient deficiencies are a common result of alcoholism. The protein and vitamin content is extremely low, except in beer, where it is marginal. Iron content varies from drink to drink, with red wine ranking especially high in iron. Typical deficiencies seen in alcoholism arise mostly from poor nutrient intakes, but increased urinary losses and fat malabsorption (linked to poor pancreatic function) are also to blame. Vitamins most susceptible to depletion in alcoholism include vitamins A, D, E, and K; thiamin; niacin; folate; vitamin B-6 and B-12, and vitamin C. Mineral deficiencies of calcium, phosphorus, potassium, magnesium, zinc, and iron are possible. On the other hand, vitamin and mineral toxicity is also of concern. Damage to the GI tract and liver, as well as high levels of some minerals in alcoholic beverages, may lead to toxicity of vitamin A, iron, lead, or cobalt. In nutritional treatment of alcoholism, the immediate aim is eliminating alcohol intake, followed by replenishment of nutrient stores.

Alcohol dependence is the most common psychiatric disorder, affecting 13% of the North American population. Studies suggest that about 40% of a person's risk for developing alcoholism comes from genetic factors. Certainly, genetic variations coding for the enzymes of alcohol metabolism are involved, but many other genes are also under study. Therefore, people with a family history of alcoholism, particularly children of alcoholics, should be especially aware of their alcohol consumption.

Early diagnosis of **alcoholism** can prevent multiple health problems and save millions in health care costs. Asking a person about the quantity and frequency of alcohol consumption is an important means of detecting abuse and dependence (see the margin note on the CAGE questionnaire on page 642). Alcoholics may exhibit some or all of the following criteria:

- Physiological dependence on alcohol with evidence of withdrawal symptoms when intake is interrupted
- Tolerance to the effects of alcohol, prompting greater alcohol intake to achieve the desired effect

TABLE 16-6 A Summary of Benefits and Risks of Alcohol Use

	Moderate Use*	Alcohol Abuse**
Coronary heart disease	Decreased risk of death in those at high risk for coronary heart disease-related death, primarily by increasing HDL-cholesterol in some people, decreasing blood clotting, and relaxing blood vessels	Heart rhythm disturbances, heart muscle damage, increased blood triglycerides, and increased blood clotting
Hypertension and stroke	Mild decrease in blood pressure; less ischemic stroke in people with normal blood pressure	Increased blood pressure (hypertension); more ischemic and hemorrhagic stroke
Peripheral vascular disease	Decreased risk due to reduced blood clotting	No benefit
Blood glucose regulation and type 2 diabetes	Decreased risk of developing type 2 diabetes; decreased risk of death from cardiovascular disease	Hypoglycemia; reduced insulin sensitivity; damage to pancreas (site of insulin production)
Bone and joint health	Some increase in bone mineral content in women, linked to estrogen output	Loss of active bone-forming cells and eventual osteoporosis (many nutrient deficiencies also contribute to this problem); increased risk of gout
Brain function	Enhanced brain function and decreased risk of dementia by increasing blood circulation in the brain	Brain tissue damage and decreased memory
Skeletal muscle health	No benefit	Skeletal muscle damage
Cancer	No benefit	Increased risk of oral, esophageal, stomach, liver, lung, colorectal, and breast cancer, to name a few (especially if the diet is deficient in the vitamin folate)
Liver function	No benefit	Fatty infiltration and eventual liver cirrhosis, especially if a person is also infected with hepatitis C; iron toxicity
GI tract disease	Decreased risk of certain bacterial infections in the stomach	Inflammation of the stomach (and pancreas); absorptive cell damage leading to malabsorption of nutrients
Immune system function	No benefit	Reduced function and increased infections
Nervous system function	No benefit	Loss of nerve sensation and nervous system control of muscles
Sleep disturbances	Some relaxation	Fragmented sleep patterns; worsens sleep apnea
Impotence and decreased libido	No benefit	Contributes to the problem in both men and women
Drug overdose	No benefit	Contributes to the problem, especially in combination with sedatives
Obesity	No benefit	Increased abdominal fat deposition, contributes to weight gain as calories from alcoholic beverages quickly add up
Nutrient intake	May supply some B vitamins and iron	Leads to numerous nutrient deficiencies: protein, vitamins, and minerals
Alcoholism	No benefit.	Increased risk of developing alcoholism, including the teenage and young adult years
Fetal health	No benefit	Variety of toxic effects on the fetus when alcohol is consumed by pregnant women (see Chapter 14)
Socialization and relaxation	Provides some benefit to socialization and leads to relaxation by increasing brain neurotransmitter activity	Contributes to violent behavior and agitation
Traffic deaths and other violent deaths	No benefit	Contributes to both traffic death and violent death

*About one drink per day for men and slightly less than one for women.

**The risks from alcohol abuse begin at an intake of more than two to three drinks per day for men or one to two drinks per day for women and all adults age 65 and older. Binge drinking (more than four drinks in a row for women or more than five drinks for men) can be especially harmful.

The CAGE questionnaire is used to identify alcohol abuse. More than one positive response suggests an alcohol problem.

C: Have you ever felt you ought to *cut* down on drinking?

A: Have people *annoyed* you by criticizing your drinking?

G: Have you ever felt bad or *guilty* about your drinking?

E: Have you ever had a drink first thing in the morning to steady your nerves or get rid of a hangover (*eye-opener*)?

Ethnicity plays an important role in both the probability of and health risks associated with alcohol dependency and abuse. Native Americans suffer the highest rates of unintentional injuries, suicide, homicide, and domestic abuse related to alcohol use. African-American alcoholics are at greater risk than other racial groups for tuberculosis, hepatitis C, HIV/AIDS, and other infectious diseases. Hispanic Americans are at particular risk for cirrhosis-related death.

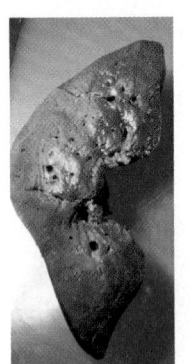 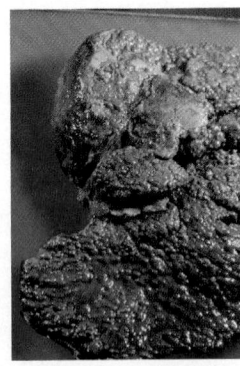

▲ Alcohol is particularly damaging to the liver. Pictured are (a) healthy liver, (b) liver with cirrhosis. There is no cure for this disease except a liver transplant.

- Evidence of alcohol-associated illnesses such as alcoholic liver disease or irreversible brain damage exhibited by memory loss, inability to concentrate, and decline in intellectual functions
- Continued drinking in defiance of strong medical and social contraindications and disruptions in normal life
- Depression, blackouts, and impairment in social and occupational functioning

Other signs of alcoholism include: alcohol odor on the breath; flushed face and reddened skin; and nervous system disorders, such as tremors. Unexplained work absences, frequent accidents, and falls or injuries of vague origin are possible signs of alcoholism. Laboratory evidence (e.g., impaired liver function, enlarged red blood cells, and elevated triglycerides) are also helpful for diagnosis of alcoholism.

Older adults are uniquely vulnerable to alcoholism, perhaps due to an abundance of free time, social events involving drinking, loneliness, or depression. Common symptoms of alcoholism—trembling hands, slurred speech, sleep problems, memory loss, and unsteady gait—can be easily overlooked as signs of old age. Slower alcohol metabolism and decreased body water allow older adults to become intoxicated from a smaller amount of alcohol than their younger counterparts. Even moderate alcohol consumption can exacerbate some chronic health conditions, such as diabetes and osteoporosis. As well, even small amounts of alcohol can react negatively with various medications used by older persons. The adverse health effects of drinking may be amplified in older adults, so people over the age of 65 should limit alcohol consumption to no more than one drink per day.

Once a diagnosis of alcohol abuse or dependence is established, a physician can arrange appropriate treatment and counseling for the person and family. Treatment of alcoholism often includes the use of certain medications, counseling, and social support. Total abstinence must be the ultimate objective. Alcoholics Anonymous (AA) or other reputable therapy programs can support alcoholics and their families as they recover from this devastating disease.

MAKING DECISIONS

Liver Cirrhosis

Alcohol is most damaging to the liver. Cirrhosis develops in up to 20% of cases of alcoholism and is the second leading reason for liver transplants, affecting about 2 million people in the United States. This chronic and usually relentlessly progressive disease is characterized by fatty infiltration of the liver. Fatty liver occurs in response to increased synthesis of fat and decreased use of it for energy by the liver. Eventually, the enlarged fat deposits choke off the blood supply, depriving the liver cells of oxygen and nutrients. Liver cells can accumulate so much fat that they burst and die and are replaced by connective (scar) tissue. At this stage, the liver is deemed cirrhotic. Early stages of alcoholic liver injury are reversible, but advanced stages are not. Once a person has cirrhosis, there is a 50% chance of death within 4 years, a far worse prognosis than many forms of cancer. While no specific level of alcohol consumption guarantees cirrhosis, some evidence suggests that damage is caused by a dose as low as 40 grams per day for men (3 beers) and 20 grams per day for women (1½ beers).

Guidance Regarding Alcohol Use

No government agencies recommend drinking alcohol. The 2010 Dietary Guidelines for Americans provide the following advice regarding use of alcoholic beverages:

- Those who choose to drink alcoholic beverages should do so sensibly and in moderation—defined as the consumption of up to one drink per day for women and up to two drinks per day for men.
- Alcoholic beverages should not be consumed by some individuals, including those who cannot restrict their alcohol intake, women who are pregnant or may

become pregnant, children and adolescents, individuals taking medications that can interact with alcohol, and those with specific medical conditions.

- Alcoholic beverages should be avoided by individuals engaging in activities that require attention, skill, or coordination, such as driving or operating machinery.
- For weight management, monitor calorie intake from alcoholic beverages.

As the understanding of the relationship between drinking alcohol and health grows, registered dietitians and other health professionals can promote healthy lifestyles—not by encouraging indiscriminate drinking, but rather by reassuring adults that moderate alcohol consumption may have beneficial health outcomes.

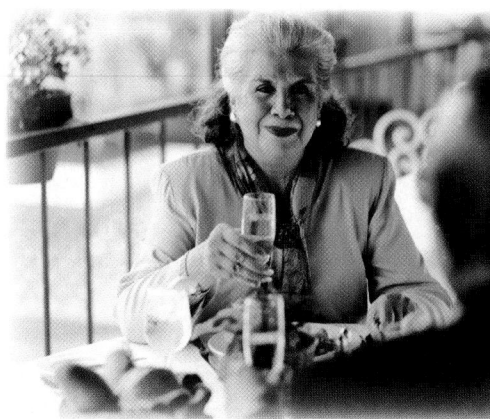

▲ The limit for alcohol intake for older adults is one drink per day.

CONCEPT CHECK

Alcohol is not an essential nutrient but does supply calories for the body. It requires no digestion, and alcohol metabolism takes precedence over metabolism of the other energy-yielding nutrients. Alcohol is primarily metabolized in the liver by alcohol dehydrogenase and acetaldehyde dehydrogenase. A number of individual factors, such as gender, race, and body composition, determine how a person reacts to alcohol. Despite modest benefits of moderate alcohol use, alcoholism interferes with all aspects of family, professional, and social life. Excessive alcohol use increases the risk of hypertension, strokes, heart damage, birth defects, inflammation of the pancreas, brain damage, and malnutrition, to name a few. Treatment of alcoholism often includes the use of certain medications, counseling, and social support.

Healthy People 2020 set an important goal regarding alcohol use: Reduce annual alcohol consumption by 10% (currently, 2.3 gallons per person ages 14 and older).

16.6 Ensuring a Healthful Diet for the Adult Years

Recommended dietary practices for later years would be to increase the diet's nutrient density and to make sure fiber and fluid intakes are adequate. In addition, some protein should come from lean meats to help meet protein, vitamin B-6, vitamin B-12, iron, and zinc needs.

Singles of all ages face logistical problems with food: Purchasing, preparing, storing, and using food with minimal waste are challenging. Economy packages of meats and vegetables are normally too large to be useful for a single person. Many singles live in small dwellings, some without kitchens and freezers. Creating a diet to accommodate a limited budget and facilities and a single appetite requires special considerations. The following are some practical suggestions for diet planning for singles:

- If one owns a freezer, cook large amounts, divide into portions, and freeze.
- Buy only what one uses; small containers may be expensive, but letting food spoil is also costly.
- Ask the grocer to break open a family-sized package of wrapped meat or fresh vegetables and separate it into smaller units.
- Buy only several pieces of fruit—perhaps a ripe one, a medium-ripe one, and an unripe one—so that the fruit can be eaten over a period of several days.
- Keep a box of dry milk handy to add nutrients to recipes for baked foods and other foods for which this addition is acceptable.

Table 16-7 provides more ideas for healthful eating in later years.

Nutritional deficiencies and protein-calorie undernutrition have been identified among some aging populations, particularly those in hospitals, nursing homes, or long-term care facilities. These nutritional problems increase the risk for many diseases, including bed sores (pressure ulcers), and compromise recovery from illness and surgery. Friends, relatives, and health care professionals should monitor nutrient intake in all older people, including those who live in long-term care facilities. Family members can play a valuable role in making sure nutrient needs are met by looking for weight maintenance based on regular, healthful meal patterns. If problems arise in consuming a healthful diet, registered dietitians can offer professional and personalized advice.

To learn more about alcoholism, visit these websites:

National Institute on Alcohol Abuse and Alcoholism; www.niaaa.nih.gov

American Society of Addiction Medicine; www.asam.org

American Self-Help Clearinghouse; www.mentalhelp.net/selfhelp.

Appendix C reviews diet planning guidelines issued by the Canadian government for Canadians. In addition, Chapter 1 discussed *Healthy People 2020*, a U.S. federal agenda aimed at disease prevention and health promotion.

Determine:

- Disease
- Eating poorly
- Tooth loss or mouth pain
- Economic hardship
- Reduced social contact and interaction
- Multiple medications
- Involuntary weight loss or gain
- Need for assistance with self-care
- Elder at an advanced age

To learn about meal programs for senior citizens in your area, call the *Administration on Aging's Elder Care Locator*, (800) 677-1116 or see www.eldercare.gov. For general information on programs for older persons, visit the following websites: *National Institute on Aging*, www.nia.nih.gov; *American Geriatrics Society*, www.americangeriatrics.org; and *Administration on Aging*, www.aoa.gov.

TABLE 16-7 Guidelines for Healthful Eating in Later Years

- Eat regularly; small, frequent meals may be best. Use nutrient-dense foods as a basis for menus.
- Use labor-saving devices and some convenience foods, but try to incorporate some fresh foods into daily menus.
- Try new foods, new seasonings, and new ways of preparing foods. Use canned goods in moderation or choose those low in sodium.
- Keep easy-to-prepare foods on hand for times when you feel tired.
- Have a treat occasionally, perhaps an expensive cut of meat or a favorite fresh fruit.
- Eat in a well-lit or sunny area; serve meals attractively; use foods with different flavors, colors, shapes, textures, and smells.
- Arrange kitchen and eating area so that food preparation and cleanup are easier.
- Eat with friends, relatives, or at a senior center when possible.
- Share cooking responsibilities with a neighbor.
- Use community resources for help in shopping and other daily care needs.
- Stay physically active.
- If possible, take a walk before eating to stimulate appetite.
- When necessary, chop, grind, or blend hard-to-chew foods. Softer, protein-rich foods (e.g., shredded meats, eggs) can be substituted for meat when poor dental function limits normal food intake. Prepare soups, stews, cooked whole-grain cereals, and casseroles.
- If your dexterity is limited, cut the food ahead of time, use utensils with deep sides or handles, and obtain more specialized utensils if needed.

NEWSWORTHY NUTRITION | Calorie restriction: Is your diet a fountain of youth?

Animal studies show that long-term calorie restriction increases longevity. Researchers for the Comprehensive Assessment of the Long-Term Effects of Reducing Intake of Energy (CALERIE) study explored the possibility that 25% calorie restriction for 6 months would alter biomarkers of longevity in humans. Forty-six overweight adults completed the study. Subjects were randomized to one of four groups: control (no caloric restriction), CR (25% calorie restriction), CREX (12.5% calorie restriction + 12.5% increased energy expenditure by structured exercise), and LCD (low-calorie diet followed by weight-maintenance diet after 15% weight loss was achieved). Subjects followed controlled diets that were deficient in calories but otherwise nutritionally adequate and underwent numerous measurements, including body composition, calorimetry (review Chapter 7), body temperature, and various blood tests. Fasting levels of insulin, energy expenditure (i.e., metabolic rate), and a marker of DNA damage decreased in all three intervention groups. Among the CR and CREX groups, core body temperature also decreased. These results indicate that prolonged calorie restriction in humans reduces metabolic rate and decreases fasting insulin and body temperature, two biomarkers of longevity. Further research is needed to distinguish effects of calorie restriction on other biomarkers and to measure life span. For this study, diet was carefully controlled and monitored frequently and all foods were provided. If calorie restriction does prove to increase longevity, could you stick with it?

Source: Heilbronn LK and others: Effect of 6-month calorie restriction on biomarkers of longevity, metabolic adaptation, and oxidative stress in overweight subjects. *Journal of the American Medical Association* 295:1539, 2006.

connect NUTRITION **Check out the Connect site** www.mcgrawhillconnect.com **to learn more about theories of aging.**

Overall, older adults benefit from good nutrition in many ways. As we discussed for younger adults, meeting nutrient needs delays the onset of some diseases; improves the management of some existing diseases; hastens recovery from many illnesses; increases mental, physical, and social well-being; and often decreases the need for and length of hospitalization. Older adults should use MyPlate as a guide to healthy meals, but emphasize nutrients of special concern (e.g., calcium, vitamin D, vitamin B-12). Daily Food Plans are available from www.ChooseMyPlate.gov for older adults, based on age, weight, height, gender, and activity level. A focus on nutrient-dense food choices, plenty of fluids, modified physical activity goals, and use of certain dietary supplements address the unique needs of older adults.

Obtaining enough food may be difficult for some older persons, especially if they are unable to drive and relatives do not live close enough to help with cooking or shopping. For an older person, a request for help may be equated to a loss of independence. Pride, or fear of being victimized by those they hire, may stand in the way of much-needed help. In these cases, friends can be a big help. Special transportation arrangements may also be available through a local transit company or taxi service.

Many eligible older people are missing meals and are poorly nourished because they don't know of available programs to help them. Irregular meal patterns and weight loss, often caused by difficulties in preparing food, are warning signs that undernutrition may be developing. An effort should be made to identify poorly nourished people and inform them of community services.

Community Nutrition Services for Older People

Health care advice and services for older people can come from clinics, private practitioners, hospitals, and health maintenance organizations. Home health care agencies, adult day-care programs, adult overnight-care programs, and **hospice care** (for the terminally ill) can provide daily care.

The Nutrition Screening Initiative, a nutrition checklist for health care workers, family members, and older persons, can be used as a tool to increase health and nutrition awareness and to plan related education of older persons (See Fig. 16-2). The Nutrition Screening Initiative uses the acronym "DETERMINE" (see margin on previous page) to help identify older people whose health needs require extra attention.

Nutrition programs for those age 60 and over in the United States include congregate meal programs, which provide lunch at a central location, and home-delivered meals (often known as Meals on Wheels if sponsored by the local private or public agencies). About 2.6 million older adults are served each year. About half of the meals use the home-delivered method.

The U.S. federal government sets specific standards for home-delivered meals and for those served in congregate feeding centers. The meals are designed to provide one-third of RDA/AI. The social aspect often improves appetite and general outlook on life.

Still, congregate meal programs generally provide one meal a day (some provide more) and usually just 5 days per week. Another problem with home-delivered meals is that the one or two meals delivered may never be eaten, and, if not eaten on delivery and left at room temperature, they may become unsafe to eat later. Thus, these programs can help older adults but probably don't meet all their nutritional needs.

In addition to congregate and home-delivered meals, federal commodity distribution is available in some areas of the United States to low-income older people. Older people whose incomes are below the poverty level can benefit from the SNAP program (food stamps) (see Chapter 12 for details on these programs). Food cooperatives and a variety of clubs and religious and social organizations provide additional aid.

▲ Immune function declines with age, so food safety become increasingly important for older adults. Chapter 13 provides advice on this topic, such as washing one's hands and work surfaces before preparing food.

hospice care A program offering care that emphasizes comfort and dignity in death.

CONCEPT CHECK

A nutrient-dense diet helps meet the unique needs of aging adults. Carefully planned use of multivitamin and mineral supplements can also help, especially for adults 70 years of age and older. Diet planning should be tailored to the individual's physiological, psychosocial, and economic status. In the United States, many nutrition services—such as congregate and home-delivered meals—are available to help the aging population obtain a healthful diet.

Nutrition and Cancer

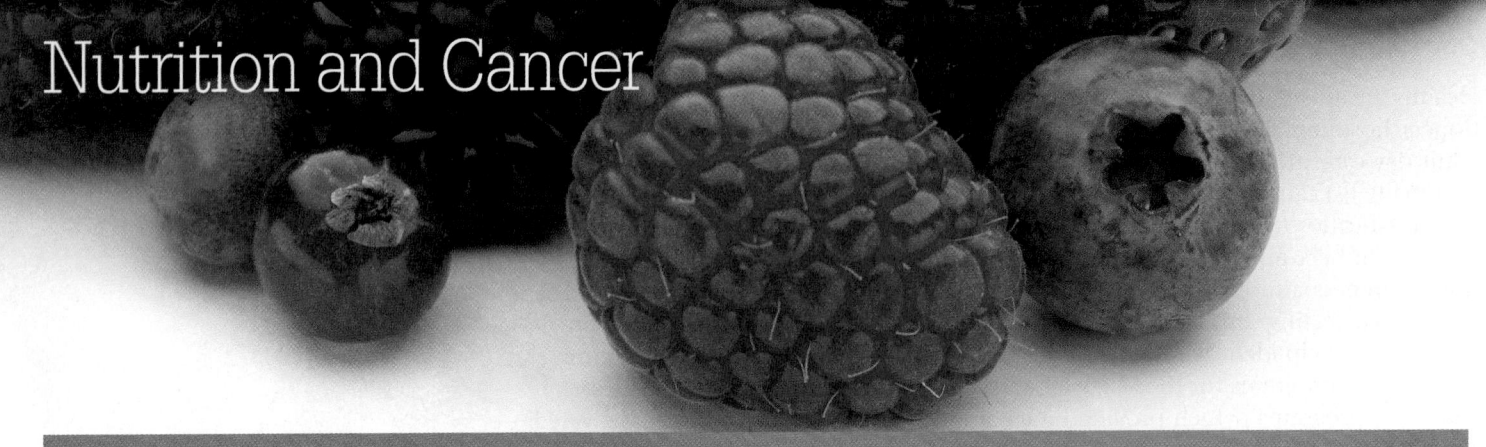

Cancer is the second leading cause of death for North American adults. It is further estimated that more than 1500 people die each day of cancer in the United States. Cancer-related expenses exceed $100 billion each year. The top four cancers, causing more than 50% of cancer deaths, are lung, colorectal, breast, and prostate cancers. Of those, lung cancer in female smokers is the only form increasing on a yearly basis.

Cancer is many diseases; these differ in the types of cells affected and, in some cases, in the factors contributing to cancer development (Fig. 16-6). For example, the factors leading to skin cancer differ from those leading to breast cancer. Similarly, the treatments for the different types of cancer often vary.

Cancer essentially represents abnormal and uncontrollable division of cells that results from mutations in DNA. This initiates the cancer process. The cells then go through a variety of steps (called promotion and progression). A cancer cell is the result. Without effective treatment, cancer then typically leads to death. Most cancers take the form of tumors, although not all tumors are cancers. A **tumor** is spontaneous new tissue growth that serves no physiological purpose. It can be **benign**, like a wart, or **malignant**, like most lung cancers. The terms *malignant tumor* and *malignant neoplasm* are synonymous with cancer.

Whereas benign tumors are only dangerous if their presence interferes with normal body functions, malignant (cancerous) tumors are capable of invading surrounding structures, including blood vessels, the lymph system, and nervous tissue. Cancer can also spread, or **metastasize,** to distant sites via the blood and lymphatic circulation, thereby producing invasive tumors in almost any part of the body. Metastasis then makes the cancer much more difficult to treat. That cancer can spread explains why early detection of cancer is so important. Cancers that can be diagnosed in the early stages are those in the colon, breast, and cervix.

Genetics, environment, and lifestyle are potent forces that influence the risk for developing cancer. A genetic predisposition is especially important in development of colon cancer, some types of breast cancer (e.g., mutated BRCA1 or BRCA2 gene) and prostate cancer (35%, 27%, and 42%, respectively). About 30 cancer-susceptibility genes have been identified. However, experts estimate that only 1% to 5% of most cancers can be explained by the inheritance of a cancer gene. Overall, lifestyle and environmental exposures are also critical factors in most forms of cancer, as evidenced by the variation in cancer rates from country to country. In fact, diet likely accounts for 30% to 40% or more of all cancers.

Although we have little control over our genetic risks for cancer, we can exert a great deal of authority when making decisions about lifestyle risks, especially with regard to smoking, alcohol abuse, physical activity, and nutrient intake (food choice). It is well established that one-third of all cancers in North America are due directly to tobacco use. About half of the cancers of the mouth, pharynx, and larynx are associated with heavy use of alcohol. A combination of alcohol use and smoking increases cancer risks even higher.

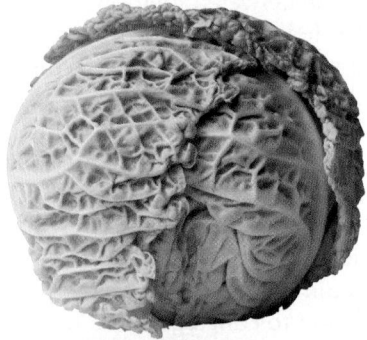

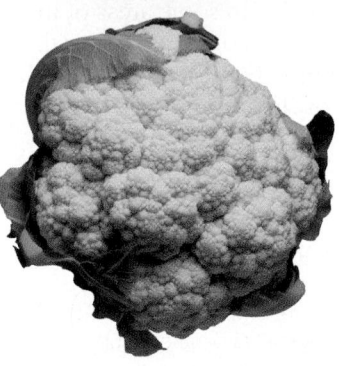

▲ Cruciferous vegetables such as cabbage and cauliflower are rich in cancer-preventing phytochemicals.

tumor Mass of cells; may be cancerous (malignant) or noncancerous (benign).

benign Noncancerous; tumors that do not spread.

malignant Malicious; in reference to a tumor, the property of spreading locally and to distant sites.

metastasize The spreading of disease from one part of the body to another, even to parts of the body that are remote from the site of the original tumor. Cancer cells can spread via blood vessels, the lymphatic system, or direct growth of the tumor.

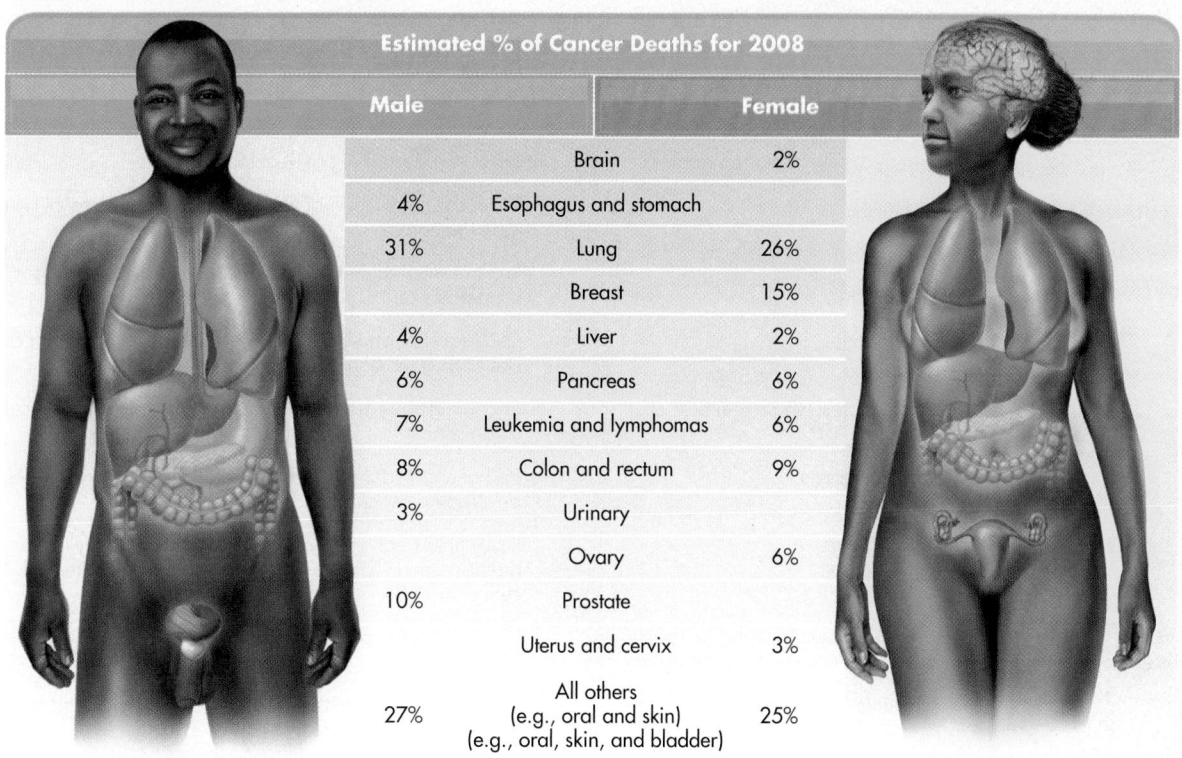

Estimated % of Cancer Deaths for 2008		
Male		**Female**
	Brain	2%
4%	Esophagus and stomach	
31%	Lung	26%
	Breast	15%
4%	Liver	2%
6%	Pancreas	6%
7%	Leukemia and lymphomas	6%
8%	Colon and rectum	9%
3%	Urinary	
	Ovary	6%
10%	Prostate	
	Uterus and cervix	3%
27%	All others (e.g., oral and skin) (e.g., oral, skin, and bladder)	25%

FIGURE 16-6 ▶ Cancer is many diseases. Numerous types of cells and organs are its target. About one-third of all cancers arise from smoking (primarily lung cancer).

A Closer Look at Diet and Cancer

Some food constituents may contribute to cancer development, whereas others have a protective effect (Table 16-8). First the association between fat/calorie intake and cancer risk is discussed, and then some of the food constituents that may reduce the risk for cancer are presented (see Further Reading 10).

Contribution of Calorie and Fat Intakes to Cancer Risk

An excess calorie intake, leading eventually to obesity, is responsible for an estimated 14% of cancer deaths among men and as many as 20% among women. This is the main diet-cancer risk factor. This includes cancer of the breast (especially in post-menopausal women), pancreas, kidney, gallbladder, colon, **endometrium,** and prostate gland. The link probably occurs between adipose tissue and the synthesis of estrogen. High concentrations of circulating estrogen in the blood over time promote cancer. Excess insulin output resulting from an obese, insulin-resistant state is also implicated.

The National Cancer Institute (NCI) also believes there is sufficient evidence for a link between dietary fat and cancer to encourage North Americans to reduce fat intake. It recommends initially decreasing dietary fat to about 30% of total calorie intake and eventually to 20% or less of total calories if the person is at high risk and can follow such a dietary pattern.

Some scientists, however, believe that the NCI has overreacted to the fat and cancer issue. Although epidemiological evidence does link fat and certain forms of cancer, the evidence is not strong. A stronger link exists between cancer and excess calories in the diet. In animal experiments, restricting total calorie intake to about 70% of usual intake results in about a 40% reduction in tumor development, regardless of the amount of fat in the diet. Calorie restriction is the most effective technique for preventing cancer in laboratory animals.

Unfortunately, it is difficult for humans to reduce dietary calories to 70% of usual intake. So while the data obtained from laboratory animal studies are interesting, nutritionists do not see any practical way to make recommendations

on the basis of these studies. In addition, once cancer is present, calorie restriction is no longer helpful.

Cancer-Inhibiting Food Constituents

Many single nutrients may have cancer-inhibiting properties. These anticarcinogens include antioxidants and certain phytochemicals (review Table 16-8).

The antioxidant activity of vitamin C and vitamin E helps to prevent formation of **nitrosamines** in the GI tract, thus preventing formation of a potent carcinogen. Vitamin E also helps protect unsaturated fatty acids from damage by free radicals. Overall, carotenoids, vitamin E, vitamin C, and selenium function as

endometrium The membrane that lines the inside of the uterus. It increases in thickness during the menstrual cycle until ovulation occurs. The surface layers are shed during menstruation if conception does not take place.

nitrosamine A carcinogen formed from nitrates and breakdown products of amino acids; can lead to stomach cancer.

TABLE 16-8 Some Food Constituents Suspected of Having a Role in Cancer

Constituent	Dietary Sources	Action
Possibly Protective*		
Vitamin A	Liver, fortified milk, fruits, vegetables	Encourages normal cell development.
Vitamin D	Fortified milk	Increases production of a protein that suppresses cell growth, such as in the colon.
Vitamin E	Whole grains, vegetable oils, green leafy vegetables	Prevents formation of nitrosamines; general antioxidant properties.
Vitamin C	Fruits, vegetables	Can block conversion of nitrites and nitrates to potent carcinogens; likely has general antioxidant properties.
Folate	Fruits, vegetables, whole grains	Encourages normal cell development; especially reduces the risk of colon cancer.
Selenium	Meats, whole grains	Part of antioxidant system that inhibits tumor growth and kills developing cancer cells.
Carotenoids, such as lycopene	Fruits, vegetables	Likely act as antioxidants; some of these possibly influence cell metabolism. Lycopene in particular may reduce the risk of prostate cancer.
Flavonoids, indoles, phenols, and other phytochemicals	Vegetables, especially cabbage, cauliflower, broccoli, brussels sprouts, garlic, onions, tea	May reduce cancer in the stomach and other organs.
Calcium	Milk products, green vegetables	Slows cell division in the colon, binds bile acids and free fatty acids, thus reducing colon cancer risk.
Omega-3 fatty acids	Cold-water fish, such as salmon and tuna	May inhibit tumor growth.
Soy products	Tofu, soy milk, tempeh, soy nuts	Phytic acid present possibly binds carcinogens in the intestinal tract; the genistein component possibly reduces growth and metastasis of malignant cells.
Conjugated linoleic acid	Milk products, meats	May inhibit tumor development and act as an antioxidant.
Fiber-rich foods	Fruits, vegetables, whole-grain breads and cereals, beans, nuts	Colon and rectal cancer risk may be decreased by accelerating intestinal transit or binding carcinogens such that they are excreted.
Possibly Carcinogenic		
Excessive calorie intake	All macronutrients can contribute	Excess fat mass leading to obesity; linked to increased synthesis of estrogen and other sex hormones, which in excess may themselves increase the risk for cancer. Resulting excess insulin output from creation of an insulin-resistant state is also implicated.
Total fat	Meats, high-fat milk and milk products, animal fats and vegetable oils	The strongest evidence is for excessive saturated and polyunsaturated fat intake. Saturated fat is linked to an increased risk of prostate cancer.
High glycemic load carbohydrates	Cookies, cakes, sugared soft drinks, candy	Insulin surges associated with these foods may increase tumor growth, such as in the colon.
Alcohol	Beer, wine, liquor	Contributes to cancers of the throat, liver, bladder, breast, and colon (especially if the person does not consume enough folate).
Nitrites, nitrates	Cured meats, especially ham, bacon, and sausages	Under very high temperatures will bind to amino acid derivatives to form nitrosamines, potent carcinogens.
Multi-ring compounds: Aflatoxin	Formed when mold is present on peanuts or grains	May alter DNA structure and inhibit its ability to properly respond to physiologic controls; aflatoxin in particular is linked to liver cancer.
Benzo(a)pyrene and other heterocyclic amines	Charcoal-broiled foods, especially meats	Linked to stomach and colon cancer. To limit this risk, trim fat from meat before cooking, cut barbecuing time by partially cooking meat (such as in a microwave oven), and don't consume blackened parts.

*Many of the actions listed for these possibly protective agents are speculative and have been verified only by experimental animal studies. The best evidence supports obtaining these nutrients and other food constituents from foods. The U.S. Preventive Services Task Force (USPSTF) supports this statement, noting there is no clear evidence that nutrient supplements provide the same benefits.

or contribute to antioxidant protection for the body. Some of these antioxidant systems help prevent DNA mutations by electron-seeking compounds, the main way that cancer develops in the first place.

In addition, phytochemicals from fruits and vegetables, and even tea, block cancer development in some types of cells. Numerous studies suggest that fruit and vegetable intake reduces the risk of nearly all types of cancer. These foods are normally rich in carotenoids, vitamin C, and vitamin E. Adequate vitamin D intake is suspected of reducing breast, colon, prostate, and other forms of cancer. Calcium is also linked to a decreased risk for developing colon cancer. In sum, a diet that conforms to MyPlate, so that fruits, vegetables, whole grains, low-fat and fat-free dairy products, and some plant oils are eaten daily, is aimed at cancer prevention. It is likely that all of these foods have a "cocktail" effect, and that no one particular food can make as strong a claim (see Further Reading 7).

Nutrition Concerns During Cancer Treatment

Nutrition concerns during cancer treatment may vary depending on the site of the cancer, but the overall goals of medical nutrition therapy are to minimize weight loss and prevent nutrient deficiencies. Weight loss, particularly loss of muscle mass, is a major concern during cancer treatment because poor nutrition status can limit recovery from illness. Common effects of cancer and/or cancer treatments include fatigue, mouth sores, dry mouth, taste abnormalities, nausea, and diarrhea– all of which can lead to poor food intake.

During cancer treatment, the best food to eat is any food the patient can tolerate. Food choices vary based on each patient's individual symptoms, but cool, non-acidic liquids and soft, mildly-flavored foods are generally well-accepted. Small, frequent meals and foods with high nutrient density and calorie density should be emphasized to meet calorie and protein needs. Often, liquid nutritional supplements are needed. Because immunity may be suppressed during cancer treatment, safe food handling practices also are extremely important (review Chapter 13).

The Bottom Line

Given the toll of cancer treatment and lack of a definitive cure, efforts at prevention are key. A variety of dietary changes will reduce your risk for cancer. Start by making sure that your diet is moderate in calorie and fat content and that you consume many fruits and vegetables, whole-grain breads and cereals, beans, some fish, and low-fat or fat-free milk products. In addition, remain physically active; avoid obesity; consume alcohol in moderation (if at all); and limit intake of animal fat and salt-cured, smoked, and nitrate-cured foods.

Remember also that if a cancer is left untreated, it can spread quickly throughout the body. When this happens, it is much more likely to lead to death. Thus early detection is critical. Aids to early detection include the following warning signs (acronym is CAUTION):

- A **C**hange in bowel or bladder habits
- **A** sore that does not heal
- **U**nusual bleeding or discharge
- A **T**hickening or lump in the breast or elsewhere
- **I**ndigestion or difficulty in swallowing
- An **O**bvious change in a wart or mole
- A **N**agging cough or hoarseness

Unexplained weight loss is an additional warning sign.

There are still other ways to detect cancer early. Colonoscopy examinations for middle-aged and older adults, PSA (prostate-specific antigen) tests for middle-aged and older men, and Papanicolaou tests (Pap smears) and regular breast examinations (and mammograms starting about age 40) for women are recommended by the American Cancer Society. Finally, to learn still more about cancer, review these sources of credible cancer information on the Internet:

American Cancer Society
www.cancer.org
National Cancer Institute
www.cancer.gov
Oncolink
www.oncolink.org
Harvard University Center for Cancer Prevention
www.diseaseriskindex.harvard.edu

▶ **American Institute for Cancer Research Diet and Health Guidelines for Cancer Prevention**

1. Choose a diet rich in a variety of plant-based foods.
2. Eat plenty of vegetables and fruits.
3. Maintain a healthy weight and be physically active.
4. Drink alcohol only in moderation, if at all.
5. Select foods low in fat and salt.
6. Prepare and store food safely.

And always remember …

Do not use tobacco in any form.

Case Study Dietary Assistance for an Older Adult

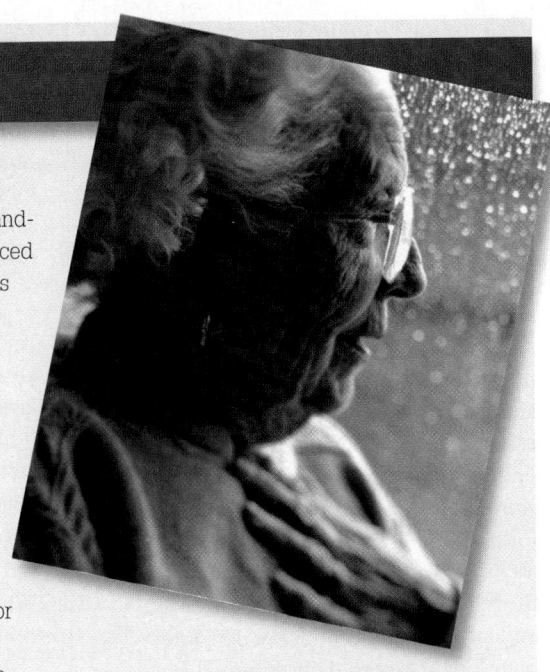

Frances is a 78-year-old woman who suffers from macular degeneration, osteoporosis, and arthritis. Since her husband died a year ago, she has moved from their family house to a small one-bedroom apartment. Her eyesight is progressively getting worse, making it hard to go to the grocery store or even to cook (for fear of burning herself). She is often lonely; her only son lives 1 hour away and works two jobs, but he visits her as often as he can. Frances has lost her appetite and, as a result, often skips meals during the week. She has resorted to eating mostly cold foods, simple to prepare but seriously limiting variety and palatability in her diet. She is slowly losing weight as a result of her dietary changes and loss of appetite.

Her typical diet usually consists of a breakfast that may include 1 slice of wheat toast with margarine, honey, and cinnamon, and 1 cup of hot tea. If she has lunch, she normally has ½ can of peaches, half of a turkey and cheese sandwich, and ½ glass of water. For dinner, she might have half of a tuna fish sandwich made with mayonnaise and 1 cup of iced tea. She usually includes one or two cookies at bedtime.

Answer the following questions, and check your responses in Appendix A.

1. What nutrients are likely to be inadequate in her current diet?
2. What potential effects will Frances' poor dietary pattern have on her health status?
3. Which physiological changes of aging will add to the effects of her poor diet (review Table 16-2)?
4. What services are available in the community that could help Frances improve her diet and possibly increase her appetite?
5. What other convenience foods could be included in her diet to make it more healthful and more varied?

Summary (Numbers refer to numbered sections in the chapter.)

16.1 Although maximum life span hasn't changed, life expectancy has increased dramatically over the past century. For many societies, this means that an increasing proportion of the population is over 65 years of age. As health care costs rise, the goal of delaying disease becomes ever important.

16.2 During adulthood, nutrients are used primarily to maintain the body rather than support physical growth. As adults get older, nutrient needs change. Adulthood is characterized by body maintenance and gradual physiological transitions, often referred to as "aging." The physiologic changes of aging are the sum of cellular changes, lifestyle practices, and environmental influences. Many of these changes can be minimized, prevented, and/or reversed by healthy lifestyles. Usual aging refers to the age-related physical and physiological changes that are commonly thought to be typical of aging. Successful aging describes the declines in physical

and physiological function that occur because one grows older. Striving to have the greatest number of healthy years and the fewest of illness is referred to as compression of morbidity. The rate at which one ages is individual; it is determined by heredity, lifestyle, and environment.

16.3 A healthy diet based on MyPlate and the 2010 Dietary Guidelines for Americans can help one to preserve body function, avoid chronic disease, and age successfully. These guidelines recommend that individuals eat a variety of foods; balance the food eaten with physical activity to maintain or improve weight; choose a diet with plenty of whole grains, vegetables, and fruits; choose a diet low in saturated fat, *trans* fat, and cholesterol; limit sugars and salt; and moderate alcoholic beverage intake. Regular physical activity is also important, as is safe food preparation. American adults are fairly well nourished, although common dietary excesses are calories, fat, sodium, and for some, alcohol. Common

dietary inadequacies include vitamins D and E, folate, magnesium, calcium, zinc, and fiber. People ages 65 and older, particularly those in long-term care facilities and hospitals, are at risk for malnutrition. The Nutrition Screening Initiative checklist can help identify older adults at risk of nutrient deficiencies. The DRIs for adults are divided by gender and age to reflect how nutrient needs change as adults grow older. These changes in nutrient needs take into consideration the aging-related physiological alterations in body composition, metabolism, and organ function.

16.4 The food choices and nutritional adequacy of adults' diets depend on physiological, psychosocial, and economic factors. Alterations in any of these factors can result in deteriorations in the quality of dietary intake, nutritional status, and health. Physiological factors include changes in body composition, body systems, and chronic diseases that influence dietary intake and alter nutrient needs and/or nutrient utilization. Of particular concern is sarcopenia, or loss of muscle mass that frequently accompanies aging. The use of medications and supplements can improve health and quality of life, but some also adversely affect nutritional status. Herbal products should be used with caution. Psychosocial influences on nutritional status include changes in lifestyle and social interaction and the presence of mental health issues, such as depression and Alzheimer's disease. Economic factors may also have a great impact on the types and amounts of food one eats.

16.5 Alcohol use is a complex issue because it involves psychological, social, economic, health, legal, and family issues. Alcohol is metabolized in the liver and other tissues. The benefits of alcohol use are associated with low to moderate alcohol consumption. These benefits include the pleasurable and social aspects of alcohol use, a reduction in various forms of cardiovascular disease, increase in insulin sensitivity, and protection against some harmful stomach bacteria. Alcohol has the potential to worsen health as well. Excessive consumption of alcohol contributes significantly to five of the ten leading causes of death in North America. Alcohol increases the risk of developing certain forms of heart damage, inflammation of the pancreas, GI tract damage, vitamin and mineral deficiencies, cirrhosis of the liver, certain forms of cancer, hypertension, and hemorrhagic stroke—to name a few.

If alcohol is consumed, it should be consumed in moderation with meals. Women are advised to drink no more than one drink per day, as are adults 65 years and older; men are advised to limit intake to two drinks per day.

16.6 Diet plans for adults should be based on nutrient-dense foods and need to be individualized for existing health problems, physical abilities, presence of drug-nutrient interactions, possible depression, and economic constraints. A balanced multivitamin and mineral supplement can be used to help meet needs, especially for adults age 70 years and older. Most communities have congregate or home-delivered meal systems, food stamps, and other provisions to provide nutrition aid for those who qualify.

Check Your Knowledge (Answers to the following questions are below.)

1. Among the older population of the United States, the age of the fastest growing segment is _____ years.
   a. 65
   b. 74
   c. 79
   d. 85+

2. The diets of adults tend to be low in _____.
   a. vitamin E
   b. calcium
   c. fiber
   d. All of the above.

3. The reason the incidence of obesity increases with age is that
   a. the basal metabolic rate decreases with age.
   b. physical activity often decreases with age.
   c. energy intake exceeds energy expenditure.
   d. All of the above.

4. The immune system becomes less efficient with age, so it is especially important to consume adequate _____ and _____, nutrients that contribute to immune function.
   a. vitamin A, vitamin B-6
   b. protein, zinc

   c. zinc, iodide
   d. vitamin A, vitamin K

5. Which of the following accurately portrays a theory about the causes of aging?
   a. Increases in testosterone and estrogen affect cell processes.
   b. Blood sugar decreases, failing to supply adequate energy to brain cells.
   c. Inadequate calorie intake speeds body breakdown.
   d. Excess free radicals damage cell components.

6. To maintain optimal nutritional status and healthy weight, the diet of an older person should have a _____ nutrient density and be _____ in energy content.
   a. low, high
   b. low, low
   c. high, moderate
   d. high, high

7. Nutrition programs such as congregate meals or home-delivered meals provide which of the following?
   a. an improved nutritional status
   b. a social atmosphere

   c. an economical meal for low-income elderly
   d. All of the above.

8. During aging, the needs for vitamins and minerals
   a. continually fluctuate.
   b. greatly decrease.
   c. somewhat increase in some cases.
   d. greatly increase.

9. Alcohol is digested in the
   a. stomach.
   b. small intestine.
   c. liver.
   d. None of the above; alcohol requires no digestion.

10. Alcohol is most damaging to the
    a. brain cells because alcohol can be used as an energy source even before glucose.
    b. kidney cells because this is where alcohol is excreted.
    c. cells of the gastrointestinal tract because they are in direct contact with ingested alcohol.
    d. liver cells where alcohol is metabolized.

Answers: 1. d (LO 16.1), 2. d (LO 16.4), 3. d (LO 16.3), 4. b (LO 16.6), 5. d (LO 16.21), 6. c (LO 16.5), 7. d (LO 16.8), 8. c (LO 16.3), 9. d (LO 16.7), 10. d (LO 16.7)

Study Questions (Numbers refer to Learning Outcomes)

1. List three important points made by the Dietary Guidelines for Americans for the general population and give an example of why each one may be difficult for older adults to implement. What are some suggestions for overcoming these barriers? (LO 16.4)

2. What is the difference between life span and life expectancy? (LO 16.1)

3. List five general guidelines for cancer prevention. (LO 16.6)

4. Describe two hypotheses proposed to explain the causes of aging, and note

evidence for each in your daily life experiences. (LO 16.2)

5. List four organ systems that can decline in function in later years, along with a diet/lifestyle response to help cope with the decline. (LO 16.3)

6. Defend the recommendation for regular physical activity during older adulthood, including some resistance activity (weight training). (LO 16.5)

7. How might the nutritional needs of older people differ from those of

younger people? How are their needs similar? Be specific. (LO 16.3)

8. What three resources in a community are widely available to aid older adults in maintaining nutritional health? (LO 16.8)

9. List two benefits of moderate alcohol intake. List two risks of alcohol abuse. Should a non-drinker take up drinking for the health benefits? (LO 16.7)

10. List four warning signs of undernutrition in older people that are part of the acronym DETERMINE. Briefly justify the inclusion of each. (LO 16.6)

What Would You Choose Recommendations

Lifestyle factors, including diet, are among the most important determinants of cancer risk, so your interest in dietary changes to prevent cancer is wise. Cancer seems like a health problem that strikes mostly in older adults, but you have learned that your lifestyle choices right now will impact your health in the future. Having a genetic predisposition for a certain condition does not predetermine an adverse outcome. You can take charge of modifiable risk factors by eating well and exercising now.

Many phytochemicals are implicated in cancer prevention. For example, lycopene in tomatoes has been associated with lower risk of prostate cancer in men. Compounds in garlic and onions have been linked to reduced risk of several types of cancer. Phytochemical supplements contain isolated plant compounds with purported health benefits. As you learned in Chapter 2, dietary supplements are not tightly regulated in the United States, so the quality and composition of any dietary supplement

are questionable. In addition, there are components of whole foods that likely contribute to cancer prevention beyond the effects of an isolated phytochemical. Fruits, vegetables, and whole grains contain a variety of phytochemicals that likely work synergistically. In addition, the fiber and antioxidants (e.g., vitamins C and E) in fruits and vegetables are also beneficial for cancer prevention. In research studies, supplemental sources of certain nutrients or phytochemicals often come up short in comparison to the positive health effects of whole-food sources.

Fruit juicers are household appliances that can be used to extract juice fresh from fruits or vegetables rather than buying it in bottled or concentrated form. Freshly made juice likely does have more of some vitamins than juice that has been sitting on a shelf because, as you learned in Chapter 8, many vitamins break down over time with exposure to heat, light, or air. You can also control the amount of added sugars in the

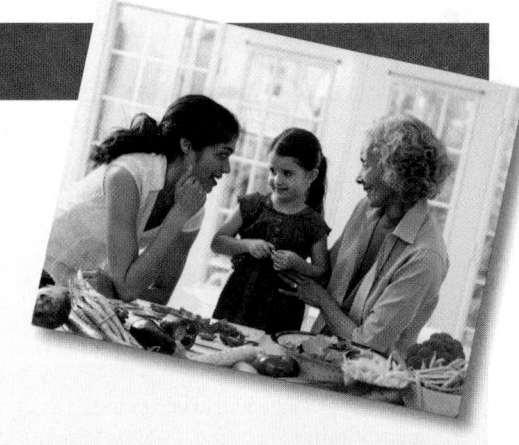

final product. Juicer manufacturers suggest using the leftover pulp as an ingredient in other foods, such as baked goods, but most of it usually ends up being discarded. Thus, much of the fiber and some healthful compounds may be lost.

When it comes to getting the most nutrients from your calories, whole fruits and vegetables offer phytochemicals, antioxidants, and fiber in a low-calorie package. Follow the suggestion of MyPlate to fill half your plate with fruits and vegetables.

Further Readings

1. ADA Reports: Position of the American Dietetic Association: Nutrition across the spectrum of aging. *Journal of the American Dietetic Association* 105:616, 2005.

Behaviors such as a healthful diet, being physically active, and not using tobacco in any form are three keys to healthful aging. The American Dietetic Association supports these

practices, as well as encourages older adults to seek medical and nutritional care to treat ongoing health problems, such as diabetes and hypertension.

2. Brannon CA: Alcohol: Functional food or addictive drug? *Today's Dietitian* 10(12):8, 2008.

   Alcohol has a long history as a functional and medicinal agent, but potential for abuse is high. This article describes the process of ethanol production, health benefits, and risks of alcohol use. A moderate intake of one to two drinks per day, particularly red wine at mealtimes, appears to be beneficial.

3. Brannon CA: Perimenopause: Nutritional management. *Today's Dietitian* 8(10):10, 2006.

   For most women, perimenopause begins in the mid-40s to early 50s. The most significant change during perimenopause is fluctuating levels of estrogen and progesterone. This article reviews several nutrition-related symptoms of this stage of the female life cycle and offers suggestions of several functional foods that contain components that may decrease these unpleasant symptoms.

4. Chodzko-Zajko WJ and others: American College of Sports Medicine Position Stand: Exercise and physical activity for older adults. *Medicine & Science in Sports & Exercise* 41:1510, 2009.

   The American College of Sports Medicine supports the advice of the 2008 Physical Activity Guidelines for Americans. Older adults should avoid inactivity and, instead, participate in physical activity for at least 150 minutes per week. A balanced routine should incorporate aerobic, strength, and flexibility exercises. Physical activity maintains physiological and cognitive functioning among aging adults.

5. De Souza Genaro P, Martini LA: Effect of protein intake on bone and muscle mass in the elderly. *Nutrition Reviews* 68:616, 2010.

   The RDA for protein for older adults is 0.8 grams per kilogram, but a growing body of research demonstrates that a slightly higher protein intake may be beneficial for preventing muscle loss (sarcopenia) and bone loss (osteopenia) during aging.

6. Eat like a Mediterranean to protect your aging brain. *Tufts University Health & Nutrition Letter* 10G:1, 2010.

   Adherence to a Mediterranean Diet is linked to lower risk of Alzheimer's disease and improved mental performance among older adults.

7. Eating to Beat Cancer. *Tufts University Health & Nutrition Letter* May Supplement:S1, 2007.

   Fruits and vegetables, especially tomatoes, cruciferous vegetables, berries, grapes, onions, and garlic, contain many phytochemicals that reduce cancer risk. Consuming fish or fish oils and adequate calcium is associated with reduced risk of colorectal cancer. The monounsaturated fats in olive oil are implicated in lowering cellular DNA damage. Green and black tea are also under study for anticancer activity.

8. Esposito K and others: Long-term effect of Mediterranean-style diet and calorie restriction on biomarkers of longevity and oxidant stress in overweight men. *Cardiology Research and Practice* 2011:1, 2010.

   After 2 years of intervention, overweight men who followed a Mediterranean-style diet with or without caloric restriction improved markers of cardiovascular health, oxidative stress, and insulin sensitivity. While long-term adherence to a calorie-restricted diet may be difficult, following a Mediterranean-style diet offers a beneficial alternative to achieving many of the same benefits as caloric restriction.

9. Grieger L: Dietary tips for baby boomers: Ageless advice for an aging generation. *Today's Dietitian* 10(3):38, 2008.

   Maintaining a healthy weight is considered to be the most important strategy for reducing chronic disease risk. Dietary practices that support and complement this advice include replacing calorie-rich, processed foods with nutrient-dense, unprocessed foods. Plant foods are emphasized because they are low in calories, yet high in vitamins, minerals, fiber, and phytochemicals. Fish is advocated as a source of omega-3 fatty acids.

10. Kushi LH and others: American Cancer Society guidelines on nutrition and physical activity for cancer prevention: Reducing the risk of cancer with healthy food choices and physical activity. *CA: A Cancer Journal for Clinicians* 56:254, 2006.

    Four general guidelines are presented as lifestyle modifications to reduce cancer risk: Maintain a healthy body weight; consume a diet low in red and processed meats and rich in fruits, vegetables, and whole grains; perform regular physical activity; and consume alcohol in moderation, if at all. ACS emphasizes the importance of a supportive social environment for incorporating such changes into a healthy lifestyle.

11. Redman LM and others: Effect of calorie restriction in non-obese humans on physiological, psychological, and behavioral outcomes. *Physiology & Behavior* 94:643, 2008.

    Although prospective, long-term studies of calorie restriction in humans are not feasible, evidence from epidemiological studies and short-term clinical trials indicate that calorie restriction decreases risk for diabetes and cardiovascular disease and improves biomarkers of aging without inducing disordered eating behaviors, constant feelings of hunger, depression, or cognitive decline. The authors point out, however, that the ability to adhere to a calorie-restricted diet will be low in an obesogenic environment. Research continues for an "anti-aging" pill that mimics the effects of calorie restriction in humans.

12. Riediger ND and others: A systemic review of the roles of n-3 fatty acids in health and disease. *Journal of the American Dietetic Association* 109: 668, 2009.

    Omega-3 fatty acids, abundant in fish, fish oils, some plant oils, and now fortified foods (e.g., eggs, spreads), have been shown to improve cardiovascular risk, cancer risk, and several mental health disorders (including depression and Alzheimer's disease). Complaints regarding consumption of fish oils include nausea and fishy burps. Megadose supplements may lead to excessive bleeding. Avoiding shark, swordfish, king mackerel, tilefish, and any fish harvested from contaminated waters can reduce the risk of consuming environmental toxins, including mercury. Typical North American diets are deficient in these healthy fats, but increased availability of fortified foods will support adequate consumption of omega-3 fatty acids.

13. Stenholm S and others: Sarcopenic obesity—definition, etiology, and consequences. *Current Opinions in Clinical Nutrition and Metabolic Care* 11:693, 2008.

    Older adults suffer from loss of muscle mass accompanied by gains in fat mass. Such body composition changes dramatically increase risks for disease and disability. The authors review potential causes for sarcopenic obesity, including changes in diet, physical activity, hormone levels, and inflammation.

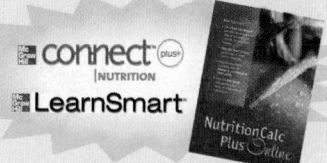

To get the most out of your study of nutrition, go to McGraw-Hill's online resources: Connect www.mcgrawhillconnect.com, **where you will find NutritionCalc Plus, LearnSmart, and many other dynamic tools.**

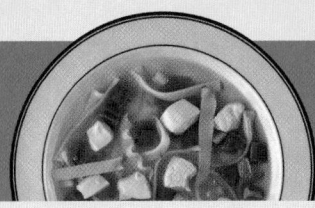

RATE YOUR PLATE

I. Am I Aging Healthfully?

Take Control of Your Aging by Dr. William B. Malarkey (Wooster Book Co., Wooster OH, 1999) includes a plan that incorporates various diet and lifestyle factors associated with successful aging. Indicate the degree to which you are following such a plan (or alternatively fill this out with a parent or another older relative in mind).

Physical: Do you eat a well-balanced diet, exercise on a regular basis, remain free of illness, abstain from smoking, refrain from drinking alcohol excessively, and experience refreshing sleep?

_____

_____

Intellectual: Are you analytical, do you read regularly, do you learn new things each day, do you engage your mental ability at work (or at school), and do you often reflect on your life?

_____

_____

_____

Emotional: Are you at peace, do you like who you are, are you optimistic, and do you laugh and relax regularly?

_____

_____

_____

Relational: Are you a good listener, do you feel supported by friends, do you attend social functions, do you talk with family members often, and do you feel close to coworkers (or fellow students)?

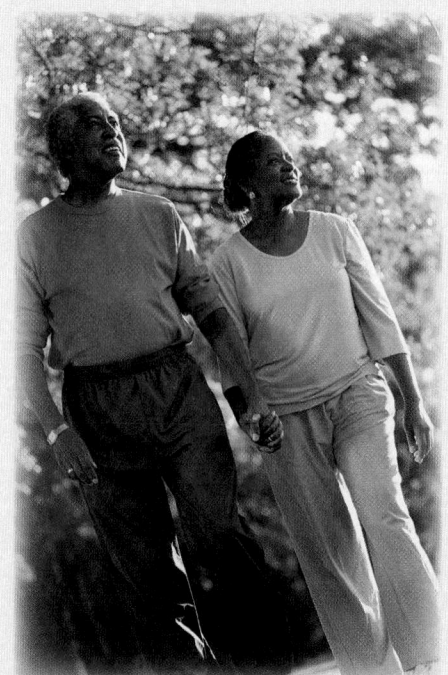

_____

_____

_____

Spiritual: Do you appreciate nature, give to or serve others, meditate or seek religious worship, and feel life has meaning?

_____

_____

_____

The more of these factors that you include in your life, the more well-rounded your plan is for maintaining overall health. Any one of the five areas in which you are not achieving success should show you characteristics to work on in the future.

II. Helping Older Adults Eat Better

During their lifetimes, most people usually eat meals with families or loved ones. As people reach their older ages, many of them are faced with living and eating alone. In a study of the diets of 4400 older adults in the United States, one man in every five living alone and over age 55 ate poorly. One of four women between the ages of 55 and 64 years followed a low-quality diet. These poor diets can contribute to deteriorating mental and physical health. Consider the following example of the living situation of an older adult.

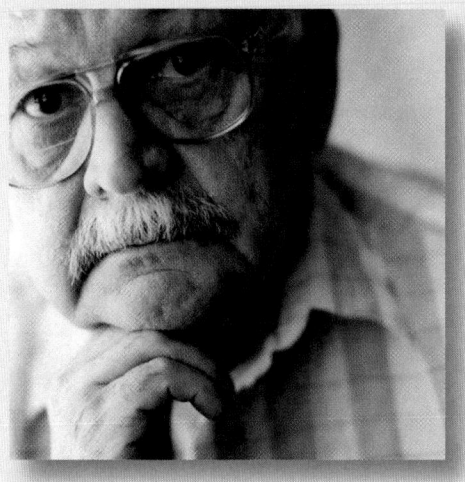

Neal, a 70-year-old man, lives alone in a home in a local suburban area. His wife died 1 year ago. He doesn't have many friends; his wife was his primary confidante. His neighbors across the street and next door are friendly, and Neal used to help them with yard projects in his spare time. Neal's health has been good, but he has had trouble with his teeth recently. His diet has been poor, and in the past 3 months his physical and mental vigor have deteriorated. He has been slowly lapsing into a depression and, so, keeps the shades drawn and rarely leaves his house. Neal keeps very little food in the house because his wife did most of the cooking and shopping, and he just isn't that interested in food.

If you were one of Neal's relatives and learned of Neal's situation, what six things could you do or suggest to help improve his nutritional status and mental outlook? Look back into this chapter to get some ideas.

1. _____

2. _____

3. _____

4. _____

5. _____

6. _____

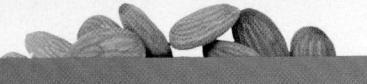

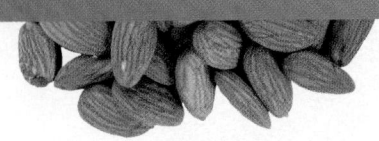

CASE STUDY SOLUTIONS

Chapter 1: Eating Habits in College

1. The most positive aspect of Andy's diet is that it contains good sources of protein from animal products also rich in zinc and iron. Alternating his hamburger and fries for lunch with pizza or tacos is a move in the right direction.

2.a. On the downside, Andy's diet is low in dairy products, fruits, and vegetables. This will result in a low intake of calcium, several of the vitamins and the phytochemical (plant-based) substances discussed in Chapter 1. His diet is also low in fiber because fast-food restaurants primarily use refined grain products, rather than whole-grain products and have few fruit and vegetable choices on the menu. Most of the beverages are soft drinks loaded with sugar. Many menu items, especially fries and chicken nuggets, are high in fat.

2.b. Most value menu options apply to foods rich in fat (French fries) and sugar (soft drinks) resulting in excessive amounts of these two components.

2.c. He could choose a low-fat granola bar instead of the candy bar for breakfast, or he could take the time to eat a bowl of whole-grain breakfast cereal with low-fat or fat-free milk to increase fiber and calcium (in the latter case) intake. Overall, Andy could improve his intake of fruits, vegetables, and dairy products by focusing on variety in food choice and balance among the food groups.

2.d. Andy could alternate between tacos and bean burritos to gain the benefits of plant proteins in a diet. When choosing pizza, he can replace high-fat toppings (e.g., pepperoni), and extra cheese with veggies (e.g., green peppers and onions). Many sub shops and delis offer several low-fat sandwiches, emphasizing lean meats such as turkey and vegetable toppings. For his beverages, Andy could order milk at least half of the time at his restaurant visits and substitute diet soft drinks for the regular variety. This would help moderate his sugar intake.

Chapter 2: Dietary Supplements

1. Whitney should be cautious about taking any supplement, especially one advertised as a "recent breakthrough." As you have read, dietary supplements are not closely regulated by FDA.

2. A general statement such as "increases energy" would be considered a structure/function claim and therefore does not require prior approval by FDA with regard to product labeling.

3. FDA will not have evaluated either the safety or effectiveness of such a product, and even harmful dietary supplements are difficult for FDA to recall.

4. There is a chance that the supplement, if effective, would contain little or none of the purported active ingredients.

5. Unfortunately, Whitney will find out all of this the hard way and will be out $60.

6. Whitney's hard-earned money would be better spent on a medical checkup at the Student Health Center. Consumers need to be cautious about nutrition information, especially regarding dietary supplements marketed as cure-alls and breakthroughs. Let the buyer beware!

Chapter 3: Gastroesophageal Reflux Disease

1. Overeating at mealtimes appears to bring on Caitlin's regular bouts of heart-burn.
2. Typical dietary advice includes consuming smaller, more frequent meals low in fat, not overeating at mealtimes, waiting about 2 hours after meals before lying down, and elevating the head of the bed about 6 inches (review Table 3-5). These recommendations reduce the risk of stomach contents forcing their way back up the esophagus. In addition, losing excess weight (if overweight) can alleviate GERD.
3. If dietary advice does not control symptoms, the primary medication used to control GERD inhibits acid production in the stomach (see earlier discussion on the proton pump inhibitors such as omeprazole [Prilosec] also used to treat peptic ulcers). If this and other medical therapy fails to control the problem, surgery to strengthen the lower esophageal sphincter is possible.
4. Caitlin's GERD can be treated, but most likely will be a lifelong condition. Even surgery will generally not cure the problem. Lifetime diet and lifestyle management, and most likely medications, will still be needed to manage the problem.
5. Lifelong management of GERD is important because long-standing GERD increases the risk of esophageal cancer.

Chapter 4: Problems with Milk Intake

1. Myeshia suspected that she was sensitive to milk because she developed bloating and gas when she consumed milk during one meal.
2. The disaccharide, lactose, is the most likely cause of Myeshia's symptoms.
3. When the enzyme lactase is missing or in short supply in the small intestine, undigested lactose travels to the large intestine and is fermented by bacteria there. The fermentation of lactose by bacteria produces abdominal gas, bloating, and pain. Diarrhea can also occur because the presence of lactose in the colon draws water from the blood vessels into the large intestine.
4. Lactose maldigestion is a normal pattern of physiology that often begins to develop at about ages 3 to 5 years in populations that do not rely on milk and other dairy foods as a main food source. When significant symptoms develop after lactose intake, it is then called lactose intolerance.
5. The primary form of lactose maldigestion is estimated to occur in about 75% of the world's population. Most lactose maldigesters are African-Americans (like Myeshia), Asian-Americans, and Latino/Hispanic Americans. The occurrence of lactose maldigestion also increases as people age.
6. The active bacteria cultures in yogurt digest the lactose when these bacteria are broken apart in the small intestine and release their lactase.
7. Many products, such as low-lactose milk and lactase pills, are available to enable lactose maldigesters to tolerate milk.
8. Many lactose maldigesters can consume moderate amounts of lactose with minimal or no intestinal discomfort because of the eventual lactose breakdown by bacteria in the large intestine.
9. In North America and Western Europe, milk and other dairy products are important sources of calcium and vitamin D. These are important for maintaining bone health.

10. Secondary lactose maldigestion occurs when a condition (e.g., long-standing diarrhea from a viral infection), results in a significant decline in lactase production.

Chapter 5: Planning a Heart-Healthy Diet

1. Jackie's approach to lowering blood cholesterol does not incorporate the best choices. She has excluded a great deal of fat in her diet, perhaps more than necessary, and has failed to include some key food groups that have cholesterol-lowering components.
2. Lowering fat as drastically as she has is not really necessary, especially for a physically active 21-year-old female.
3. Jackie could allow a more liberal amount of fat in her diet by including more monounsaturated fats. Canola oil and olive oil, as well as fats found in nuts and avocados, are rich sources of monounsaturated fats. These fats do not increase blood cholesterol. In addition she should include good sources of omega-3 fatty acids such as fatty fish, walnuts, flaxseeds, or soybean oil. One option is to use a canola oil-and-vinegar dressing on her salad, rather than lemon juice.
4. She has excluded a great deal of fat in her diet by merely replacing it with refined carbohydrates.
5. To make a shift to a more heart-healthy diet, Jackie would need to include at least 2 cups of fruit and 3 cups of vegetables a day, along with more whole-grain products. She should use whole-wheat bread instead of white bread for her sandwiches and eat a breakfast cereal that has at least 3 grams of fiber per serving.
6. Taking a brisk walk each morning is an excellent way to guarantee at least 30 minutes of activity on most days of the week. Exercise has been shown to increase concentration of HDL-cholesterol in the blood and decrease risk of cardiovascular disease.

Chapter 6: Planning a Vegetarian Diet

1. Studies show that the incidence of and the death rates from some chronic diseases, such as certain cardiovascular diseases, hypertension, many forms of cancer, type 2 diabetes, and obesity, are lower for vegetarians than for nonvegetarians.
2. Many components of a healthy vegetarian diet—whole grains, nuts, soy products, beans, 2 to 4 servings of fruits, and 3 to 5 servings of vegetables per day—are missing. With so few fruits and vegetables, his diet is also low in the many phytochemicals under study for numerous health benefits.
3. Protein appears to be low in the diet because Jordan has not replaced meat with a good plant source of protein. Vitamin B-12, iron, and zinc are also missing from the foods he is choosing. His diet seems to be adequate in calcium and riboflavin because he is including dairy products (milkshake and cheese).
4. Some of Jordan's food choices are high in fat (Danish pastry, milkshake, cookies) and sugar (fruit punch).
5. A healthy vegetarian diet includes whole grains, nuts, soy products, beans, 2 to 4 servings of fruits, and 3 to 5 servings of vegetables per day. It is apparent that he has not yet learned to implement the concept of complementary proteins, so the quality of protein in his diet is low. Meals that combine legumes or vegetables with grains or nuts (see Fig. 6-13) will provide the needed amounts of all amino acids.

Chapter 7: Choosing a Weight-Loss Program

1. Joe's weight has been climbing, so he has been experiencing positive energy balance.
2. When Joe is not working, his activity level is low. His time watching TV and studying does not use much energy. Joe should try to find time for physical activity after work and on weekends.

3. Balancing calorie intake with energy expenditure is the main key to weight loss and weight maintenance. Changes that Joe could make to his diet include a decrease in high-fat and -calorie items in his take-out meals. He should include more fruits, vegetables, and whole grains in his meals. A whole-grain cereal with fruit would be a healthy and convenient substitute for his pastry for breakfast. A grilled chicken sandwich or a taco salad would be a nutritious change for lunch. Grilled chicken or chili with a baked potato or salad would be healthier choices for dinner. Table 7-3 includes many ideas for food substitutions that will lower calories.

4. Joe will be wasting his money if he buys the product seen in the infomercial. Unfortunately, regulation of the supplement industry is woefully lacking. In the future, if there is a meaningful breakthrough in weight loss and weight control, health authorities such as the Surgeon General's Office or the National Institutes of Health will make North Americans aware of that fact.

5. The characteristics of a sound weight-loss diet are shown in Figure 7-15. These characteristics include a slow and steady rate of loss, flexibility relative to your habits and tastes, nutritional adequacy, behavior modification, physical activity, and maintenance of overall health.

Chapter 8: Choosing a Dietary Supplement

1. The maintenance dose of two to three tablets per day poses no risk *per se* because this dose of Nutramega does not exceed the Tolerable Upper Intake levels for vitamin A, vitamin C, niacin, or vitamin B-6.

2. a. **Vitamin A**
   33% (0.33) times the Daily Value of 1000 micrograms RAE equals 330 micrograms RAE per tablet. Sixteen tablets would yield 5280 micrograms RAE. The Upper Level is 3000 micrograms RAE for preformed vitamin A. Seventy-five percent of the vitamin A is preformed vitamin A, so this yields 3960 micrograms RAE of preformed vitamin A ($5280 \times 0.75 = 3960$), or 1.3 times the Upper Level ($3960/3000 = 1.3$).

   b. **Vitamin C**
   700% (7) times the Daily Value of 60 milligrams equals 420 milligrams per tablet. 16 tablets would yield 6720 milligrams. The Upper Level is 2000 milligrams. This would then yield 3.4 times the Upper Level ($6720/2000 = 3.4$).

   c. **Niacin**
   200% (2) times the Daily Value of 20 milligrams equals 40 milligrams per tablet. 16 tablets would yield 640 milligrams. The Upper Level is 35 milligrams. This would then yield 18.3 times the Upper Level ($640/35 = 18.3$).

   d. **Vitamin B-6**
   100% (1) times the Daily Value of 2 milligrams equals 2 milligrams per tablet. 16 tablets would yield 32 milligrams. This is less than the Upper Level of 100 milligrams.

   e. The suggested use of Nutramega "at the first sign of feeling ill" poses some health risks for Amy. Taking two to three tablets every 3 hours would mean taking at least 16 tablets per day. This dosage would provide an intake of vitamin A, vitamin C, and niacin well in excess of the Upper Levels for these nutrients.

3. Nutramega is expensive compared to the cost of the typical multivitamin and mineral supplement (a 1-month supply would cost about $2 compared to about $50 for Nutramega).

4. Overall, Amy is smart to be concerned about meeting her nutrient needs, but the stress she is under does not increase nutrient needs.

5. A healthy diet as suggested by MyPlate should be Amy's primary focus. Taking a balanced multivitamin and mineral supplement is also a reasonable practice.

Chapter 9: Giving Up Milk

1. Factors contributing to her potential risk of osteoporosis include a poor dietary intake of calcium and vitamin D. Her diet also is low in protein, an important nutrient for the synthesis of connective tissue important in the skeletal system.
2. Ashley is increasing her chances of developing osteoporosis later in life because of her current high-risk lifestyle. Her new smoking habit and her low level of daily physical activity increase her risk of developing osteoporosis.
3. Ashley should rethink her rationale for avoiding milk. Fat-free milk is low in calories and provides much calcium. Dairy products such as milk do not lead to weight gain *per se*. There are even some studies suggesting that a regular intake of dairy products rich in calcium may aid in weight loss when on an otherwise calorie-restricted diet.
4. Ashley needs to find some reliable sources of calcium and vitamin D. These could include calcium-fortified juices, calcium-fortified bread and snack bars, and calcium-fortified chewable chocolate candies. Tofu (made with calcium) is another potential source, as well as calcium-fortified soy milk. Tofu and soy milk are also good sources of high-quality plant protein. Meeting the Adequate Intake of 1000 milligrams of calcium per day for her age would not be that hard if she were to make an effort to use these calcium-rich foods and/or incorporate other rich sources.
5. To decrease her risk of osteoporosis and several other chronic diseases, Ashley should stop smoking. In addition, including at least 30 minutes of physical activity on most days of the week will decrease her risk of osteoporosis and help her maintain a healthy weight.

Chapter 10: Planning a Training Diet

1. Michael is correct in following a high-carbohydrate diet.
2. In his effort to minimize his fat intake, he is probably not consuming enough calories, protein, iron, and calcium to support his training routine. He has fallen into the bagel, pasta, and pretzel routine that sports nutritionists warn is not conducive to peak performance. Low protein, iron, and overall calories may contribute to fatigue.
3. Michael's performance would improve if he also had a high-protein source at each meal. He could include milk with breakfast and possibly some low-fat yogurt or low-fat cheese at lunch. He should have a carbohydrate/protein snack before his workout, such as half a sandwich with fruit and some water. The sandwich and fruit will help provide him with fuel to support his vigorous training. In the evenings, he could substitute oil and vinegar dressing for the fat-free dressing on his salad and cheese and crackers for the pretzels to improve protein intake.
4. During his workouts, he could consume a sports drink to meet fluid needs and supply some carbohydrate, or he could consume water, along with a few graham crackers or other high-carbohydrate food.
5. Overall, it is important for Michael to fuel his body before, during, and after workouts. Before and during exercise, carbohydrates and fluid will improve athletic performance. After exercise, carbohydrates coupled with protein will enhance muscle recovery. Before and during exercise, carbohydrates and fluid will improve athletic performance. After exercise, carbohydrates coupled with protein will enhance muscle recovery.

Chapter 11: Eating Disorders—Steps to Recovery

1. Sarah has the characteristics to be diagnosed with anorexia nervosa.
2. Sarah's disordered eating habits began when she became self-conscious about her body when her peers teased her about being overweight. She began exercising each day and was successful at losing weight. Her disordered eating then

began with restricting her food intake more. She enjoyed the self-control she had over her body.

3. Sarah has the following physical symptoms of anorexia nervosa: she refuses to maintain a healthy weight-for-height, is at a weight below 85% of that expected, has a distorted view of her appearance, and has had no menstrual periods for over 3 consecutive months.
4. Her treatment would most likely consist of moderate bed rest to promote weight gain and an intake of 1000 to 1600 kcal initially, then increased by increments of about 100 to 200 kcal every few days until an acceptable rate of weight gain is achieved. The goal is to achieve a body weight that is at least 90% of an expected weight for her height, such as a BMI of at least 19.
5. Several nutrient deficiencies are likely in this case. Deficiencies of calcium and iron are probably most likely. The physician would likely prescribe a multivitamin and mineral supplement, along with an additional supplement of calcium as needed to make sure intake is in the range of 1200 to 1500 milligrams per day. Additional iron may be needed if Sarah is anemic. This overall practice will correct vitamin and mineral deficiencies that exist. The calcium in particular will contribute to bone maintenance.
6. Sarah would need to be hospitalized initially, due to her low BMI of 13.8 kg/m².
7. A team of health professionals, most likely consisting of a physician, registered dietitian, and psychologist, would provide therapy. Sarah's cooperation would be the most important element for therapy to be successful. She needs to realize that she has a problem and that she needs help. She must be willing to accept the assistance these professionals are willing to offer. The team, especially the psychologist, may use cognitive behavior therapy to help Sarah improve her self-image.
8. Sarah's outlook for recovery is not good unless she realizes she has a problem. Even if she is willing to accept the therapy and counseling, a relapse is likely to occur. Only 50% of anorexia nervosa patients have been found to recover fully from the disease. Sarah's disordered eating habits have been in place for about 6 years, so her problem is deep-rooted. The chances of recovery are greater if a vigorous treatment program is reinforced with close follow-up.

Chapter 12: Undernutrition During Childhood

1. Jamal should not be surprised that the children in the village were often sick and listless. The living conditions and recent natural disaster have added to the already poor conditions in this village. We know that children are especially susceptible to the effects of poverty and undernutrition.
2. Based on the reports that the children do not get enough to eat and on the outward signs of the children's health, protein, vitamin A, iron, iodide, and zinc are likely to be deficient in the diets of these children.
3. Protein, vitamin A, iron, iodide, and zinc deficiencies contribute to poor growth and stunting because of their essential functions in the body. One or more of these deficiencies is likely present in many children in the village.
4. Protein, vitamin A, iron, iodide, and zinc deficiencies may also contribute to depressed immune function, which can cause diarrhea and illness. These deficiencies are particularly risky in children.
5. The diets of these children are most likely also marginal in caloric content. A low-calorie intake during childhood will further depress the growth and overall health compromised by the protein and micronutrient deficiencies. Recall from Chapter 6 that protein-calorie malnutrition (PCM) is a form of undernutrition caused by an extremely deficient intake of calories or protein and generally is accompanied by an illness.
6. The recent storm will hopefully cause the Philippine government to send food and medicines to the village, which will be a short-term solution to some of their nutrition and health needs.

7. Poverty and undernutrition occur at much lower rates in the United States and other developed countries. Childhood nutrition concerns in developed countries are more likely to be the increasing incidence of overweight and obesity. As we discussed in Chapter 7, maintaining a healthy weight requires the proper balance of calories in and calories out. In Chapter 15 we will learn that overweight children are becoming more common because the typical number of calories they consume per day has increased at the same time that calorie expenditure in physical activity has decreased.

Chapter 13: Preventing Foodborne Illnesses at Gatherings

1. Nicole likely contracted *Clostridium perfringens,* based on the fact that she had diarrhea but did not vomit and the symptoms occurred about 8 hours after consuming the contaminated food (review Table 13-3).

2. Spores of *Clostridium perfringens* are typically present in meat. Thorough cooking will kill any of the live bacteria present, but the product may still contain spores. These can later develop into bacteria if the food is kept in a warm setting for a few hours. The beef in the empanadas was likely the bearer of the spores, and they likely germinated and produced a toxin as the beef sat in the car and on the buffet table.

3. Consuming food at large gatherings is risky for several reasons. First, foods for these events are typically cooked ahead of time and not consumed right away. Unfortunately, the foods end up remaining in the "danger zone" between 40°F and 140°F. Hot foods should be kept hot and cold foods cold. Unfortunately, proper refrigeration or heating equipment is not always available at these events. In addition, many people handle foods and serving utensils at large gatherings. It is important for anyone handling food or serving utensils to thoroughly wash their hands before and after handling food and to avoid coughing or sneezing over foods. Also, when returning to the "buffet" table, always use a clean plate to avoid cross-contamination. Finally, the focus at these events is usually on having fun and socializing and not on food safety.

4. The main precaution that was ignored was keeping the food out of the "danger zone." Overall, it is risky to leave perishable items such as meat, fish, poultry, eggs, and dairy products at room temperature for more than 1 to 2 hours.

5. Ideally, the cooked food should have remained at room temperature for no longer than 1 hour. Thus, soon after Nicole and her husband took it out of the oven, it should have been separated into a few smaller pans to speed cooling and then refrigerated because they knew it was not going to be served within 1 to 2 hours. Before leaving, they could have recombined the dish into one clean pan. Once they arrived at the party, the dish should have been refrigerated again, and then thoroughly reheated when it was time to eat.

Chapter 14: Preparing for Pregnancy

1. Lily's use of an over-the-counter vitamin and mineral supplement provides ample synthetic folic acid and can help fill some gaps between dietary intakes and requirements for various nutrients. Still, she should discuss this supplement use with her physician and would eventually benefit more from a prenatal supplement, as this will have more iron than the over-the-counter supplement. She should be sure not to exceed 100% of the Daily Value for preformed vitamin A because toxicities of this vitamin could cause birth defects. Lily is wise to avoid use of herbal supplements during pregnancy unless her physician approves of them.

2. Folate deficiency is known to be linked to neural tube defects. The synthetic folic acid in vitamin and mineral supplements is well absorbed and will certainly help to meet her needs for this nutrient. Consuming more fruits and vegetables—especially green leafy vegetables—is also a wise choice. A fortified, ready-to-eat

breakfast cereal also contributes to vitamin and mineral intake. Her physician may recommend a prenatal supplement instead of the over-the-counter supplement.

3. Many experts would say that she is consuming too much caffeine and would be wise to cut down coffee and caffeine-containing soft drinks to a total of three servings or fewer per day.

4. If Lily likes fish, she could include two servings of fish per week in her diet plan for pregnancy and breastfeeding. Fish are a good source of protein and also supply healthy fats, including omega-3 fatty acids, linked to brain and eye development in the fetus. However, Lily should avoid some types of fish that may have high mercury content, which can harm the nervous system of the developing fetus. Fish that typically have high levels of mercury include swordfish, shark, king mackerel, tile fish, largemouth bass, and canned albacore tuna.

5. The additional fruits and vegetables Lily is consuming will provide some fiber to help prevent constipation. Other ideas to increase her fiber intake include consuming a variety of whole grains and incorporating beans and legumes into her diet plan. Lily should also increase her fluid intake and be sure to maintain regular exercise, such as walking.

6. Lily expressed concern about her weight gain during pregnancy. Research clearly shows that adequate weight gain during pregnancy is critical for growth and development of the fetus. Inadequate weight gain contributes to risk for delivering a low-birth-weight or small-for-gestational-age baby. On the other hand, excessive weight gain during pregnancy can present problems as well. Excessive weight gain may promote long-term health problems and complicate the pregnancy with gestational diabetes or large-for-gestational age babies. At her pre-pregnancy weight and height, Lily's BMI (21 kg/m²) is within the normal range, so she should aim to gain 25–35 pounds during the entire pregnancy. During the second and third trimesters, consuming an extra 350–450 kilocalories per day of nutrient-dense foods will help her to meet this goal. Regular, moderate exercise is also recommended throughout pregnancy. However, pregnancy is not a time to begin a vigorous exercise routine. Walking or riding a stationary bike are good activities to regulate weight gain. Lily should be reassured that her choice to breastfeed her baby will help her to lose those extra pounds after the baby is born.

Chapter 15: Undernutrition During Infancy

1. Ask if the formula is iron-fortified. Also, verify that Damon's caregivers are appropriately preparing his formula—adding the correct amount of powder or concentrated liquid to water. Be sure that Damon's caregivers plan to continue giving him formula until 1 year of age.

2. The scenario described puts Damon at risk for failure to thrive, likely due to his caregiver's lack of knowledge about appropriate infant feeding practices. His diet is probably lacking in total calories as well as calcium, iron, and zinc. Inadequacies may lead to stunted growth, cognitive problems, behavioral problems, and weak bones.

3. In addition to an iron-fortified infant formula, Damon should be eating fortified infant cereals, pureed fruits, vegetables, and meats, and even some table foods that are soft and cut into small pieces. After six months of age, solid foods help to meet increased nutrient demands. Processed foods, such as the hot dog described in the scenario, are usually high in sodium, fat, or sugars. These are not ideal for meeting Damon's nutritional needs. Allowing Damon to self-feed to some extent will help him to develop motor skills and build confidence.

4. Infants should not be drinking sugary beverages such as colas or fruit-flavored drinks, as these items lack the nutrient density essential to meeting Damon's needs. His caregivers should provide him no more than 4 to 6 ounces of 100% fruit juice. To prevent early childhood caries and develop self-feeding skills, Damon should be learning to drink from a cup rather than a bottle.

5. The combination of an appropriately-prepared, iron-fortified infant formula and a variety of solid foods should provide Damon all the nutrients he needs. However, if he is anemic, he may need an iron supplement.

Chapter 16: Dietary Assistance for an Older Adult

1. Frances' typical diet is low in many nutrients, including protein, calcium, iron, zinc, and vitamins B-12 and D.
2. Her poor diet will cause a more rapid decline in her lean tissue and bone mass, as well as decrease her iron status, vision, and mental function.
3. Physiological changes that will exacerbate the effects of her poor diet include increases in fat stores and decreases in her appetite; sense of taste, smell and thirst; chewing ability; bowel function; lactase production; iron status; liver, kidney, lung, cardiovascular, and immune function; vision; lean tissue; bone mass; and mental function. Review Table 16-2 for the recommended responses to these changes.
4. Frances could contact a local government office that offers congregate meal programs at a central location. She could inquire about location and availability of transportation to the site. This would give her social contact with other older persons, probably an important element missing in her life. This could help alleviate her loneliness. She could also request Meals on Wheels (if available) to provide one hot meal per day. One hot meal per day prepared for her may be what she needs to help stimulate her appetite. She could also have groceries delivered to her home if her budget could withstand the extra cost.
5. Other convenience foods that could be added to her diet include milk; assorted nuts; peanut butter; breakfast cereals; canned chicken or deli meats; yogurt; sliced cheese; cottage cheese; calcium-fortified orange juice; canned or frozen fruits and vegetables; and some fresh fruits and vegetables that do not require preparation, such as prewashed lettuce and bananas. A further possibility is a nutrition bar or a liquid nutritional supplement, such as a can of Ensure® Plus. The resulting increase in her nutrient intake would help prevent disease in the future and increase her sense of well-being.

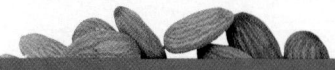

APPENDIX B Daily Values Used on Food Labels

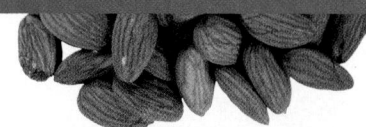

The Daily Values Used on Food Labels in the United States, with a Comparison to the Latest RDAs and Other Nutrient Standards*

Dietary Constituent	Unit of Measure	Current Daily Values for People Over 4 Years of Age	RDA or Other Current Dietary Standard	
			Males 19–30 Years Old	Females 19–30 Years Old
Total Fat[†]	g	<65	—	—
Saturated fatty acids[†]	g	<20	—	—
Protein[†]	g	50	56	46
Cholesterol[§]	mg	<300	—	—
Carbohydrate[†]	g	300	130	130
Dietary Fiber	g	25	38	25
Vitamin A	µg Retinol activity equivalents	1000	900	700
Vitamin D	International units	400	600	600
Vitamin E	International units	30	22–33	22–33
Vitamin K	µg	80	120	90
Vitamin C	mg	60	90	75
Folate	µg	400	400	400
Thiamin	mg	1.5	1.2	1.1
Riboflavin	mg	1.7	1.3	1.1
Niacin	mg	20	16	14
Vitamin B-6	mg	2	1.3	1.3
Vitamin B-12	µg	6	2.4	2.4
Biotin	µg	300	30	30
Pantothenic acid	mg	10	5	5
Calcium	mg	1000	1000	1000
Phosphorus	mg	1000	700	700
Iodide	µg	150	150	150
Iron	mg	18	8	18
Magnesium	mg	400	400	310
Copper	mg	2	0.9	0.9
Zinc	mg	15	11	8
Sodium[‡]	mg	<2400	1500	1500
Potassium[‡]	mg	3500	4700	4700
Chloride[‡]	mg	3400	2300	2300
Manganese	mg	2	2.3	1.8
Selenium	µg	70	55	55
Chromium	µg	120	35	25
Molybdenum	µg	75	45	45

Abbreviations: g = gram, mg = milligram, µg = microgram

*Daily Values are generally set at the highest nutrient recommendation in a specific age and gender category. Many Daily Values exceed current nutrient standards. This is in part because aspects of the Daily Values were originally developed in the early 1970s using estimates of nutrient needs published in 1968. The Daily Values have yet to be updated to reflect the current state of knowledge.

[†]These Daily Values are based on a 2000 kcal diet, instead of RDAs, with a caloric distribution of 30% from fat (and one-third of this total from saturated fat), 60% from carbohydrate, and 10% from protein.

[‡]The considerably higher Daily Values for sodium and chloride are there to allow for more diet flexibility, but the extra amounts are not needed to maintain health.

[§]Based on recommendations of U.S. federal agencies.

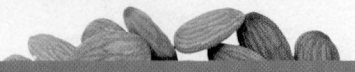

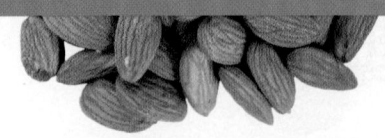

The information in this appendix includes advice on dietary patterns, as well as regulations that apply to food labeling. Previous **Recommended Nutrient Intakes (RNIs)** for nutrients have been replaced by the Dietary Reference Intakes (DRIs) that apply to Canadian and U.S. citizens. These are listed in the back of the text. Both Canadian and American scientists worked on the various DRI committees, coming up with a set of harmonized Dietary Reference Intakes for both countries.

Recommended Nutrient Intake (RNI)
The Canadian version of RDA published in 1990.

SUMMARY OF THE NUTRITION RECOMMENDATIONS FOR CANADIANS

▶ Excellent World Wide Web resources for Canadians are Health Canada (www.hc-sc.gc.ca), Dietitians of Canada (www.dietitians.ca), and the Institute of Nutrition, Metabolism, and Diabetes (www.cihr-irsc.gc.ca).

The Canadian federal department responsible for helping Canadians maintain and improve their health is Health Canada. The Office of Nutrition Policy and Promotion is within the Health Products and Food Branch of Health Canada and focuses on nutrition. Health Canada's National Dietary Guidance programs have been in existence since the 1930s and have always relied on scientific and other related evidence. Since 1977, a pattern of eating that meets nutrient needs and reduces the risk of chronic diseases has been promoted. In the 1990s, dietary guidance included *Canada's Guidelines for Healthy Eating* and *Food Guide to Healthy Eating* as well as *Nutrition for a Healthy Pregnancy* and *Nutrition for Healthy Term Infants*. The *Recommended Nutrient Intake* (RNI), a Canadian version of the RDA, was published in 1990.

In 1995, the U.S. Institutes of Medicine (IOM) brought together Canadian and American scientists to work on various committees, which came up with a set of harmonized Dietary Reference Intakes for both countries. The DRIs replaced the previous RNIs, and a new set of recommendations (EAR, AI, RDA, UL) similar to those in the United States were adopted in Canada. This led to a review and subsequent revision of *Canada's Food Guide to Healthy Eating* and *Guidelines for Healthy Eating*.

The revised *Canada's Food Guide* (Fig. C-1) was released in early 2007. The basic message to Canadians is to "Eat Well" with *Canada's Food Guide.* Learning more about *Canada's Food Guide* will help Canadians know how much food they need, what types of foods are better for them, and the importance of physical activity in their day.

In addition, if Canadians have the amount and type of food recommended and follow the tips included in *Canada's Food Guide,* this will help them:

- Meet their needs for vitamins, minerals, and other nutrients.
- Reduce their risk of obesity, type 2 diabetes, heart disease, certain types of cancer, and osteoporosis.
- Contribute to their overall health and vitality.

▶ A downloadable copy of *Canada's Food Guide* is available at www.hc-sc.gc.ca

Canada's Food Guide places foods into four groups: vegetables and fruits; grain products; milk and alternatives; and meat and alternatives. *Canada's Food Guide* also includes information on the recommended number of Food Guide Servings per day, examples of what is one Food Guide Serving and how to make each Food Guide Serving count within each food group (Fig. C-2) and at each meal (Fig. C-3). Recommendations are also included about the types and amounts of oils and fats to consume, along with guidance to enjoy a variety of foods and to satisfy your thirst with water. Similar to the Dietary Guidelines for Americans recommendations, *Canada's Food Guide* emphasizes the combination of eating well and being active every day (Fig. C-4). The new Canadian Nutrition Facts label is also highlighted in *Canada's Food Guide* with the message to "Read the label." Finally, specific nutrition advice for different ages and stages is included (Fig. C-5). Similar to MyPlate, "My Food Guide" is a web-based interactive tool that will help you personalize the information found in *Canada's Food Guide.* Check out "My Food Guide" at http://www.hc-sc.gc.ca/fn-an/food-guide-aliment/myguide-monguide/index-eng.php.

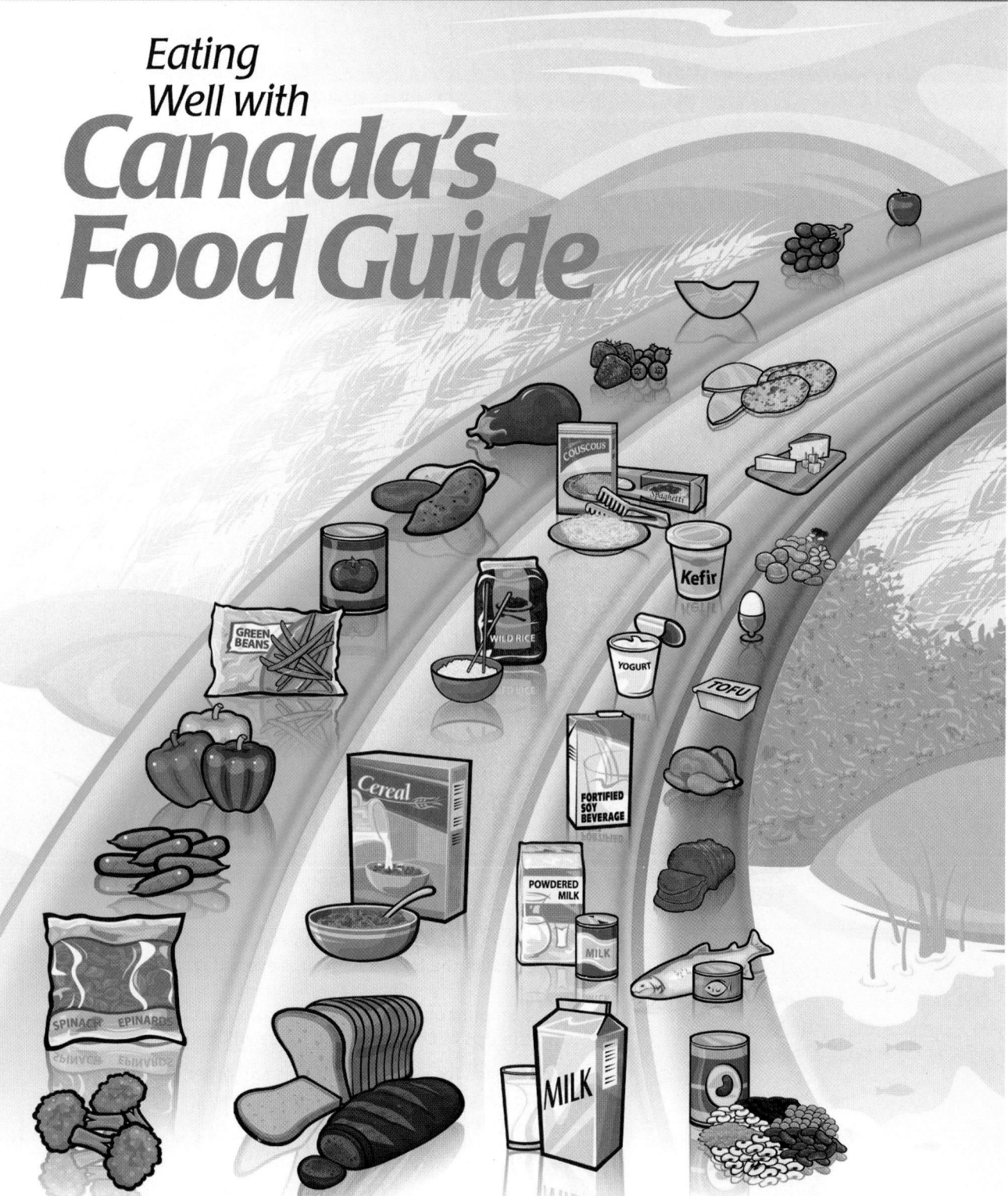

Health Canada Santé Canada

Your health and safety... our priority. *Votre santé et votre sécurité... notre priorité.*

Eating Well with **Canada's Food Guide**

Canada

FIGURE C-1 ▶ Eating Well with Canada's Food Guide.

Recommended Number of *Food Guide Servings* per Day

	Children			Teens		Adults			
Age in Years	2-3	4-8	9-13	14-18		19-50		51+	
Sex	Girls and Boys			Females	Males	Females	Males	Females	Males
Vegetables and Fruit	4	5	6	7	8	7-8	8-10	7	7
Grain Products	3	4	6	6	7	6-7	8	6	7
Milk and Alternatives	2	2	3-4	3-4	3-4	2	2	3	3
Meat and Alternatives	1	1	1-2	2	3	2	3	2	3

The chart above shows how many Food Guide Servings you need from each of the four food groups every day.

Having the amount and type of food recommended and following the tips in *Canada's Food Guide* will help:

• Meet your needs for vitamins, minerals and other nutrients.
• Reduce your risk of obesity, type 2 diabetes, heart disease, certain types of cancer and osteoporosis.
• Contribute to your overall health and vitality.

FIGURE C-2 ▶ Information about Food Guide Servings from *Canada's Food Guide.*

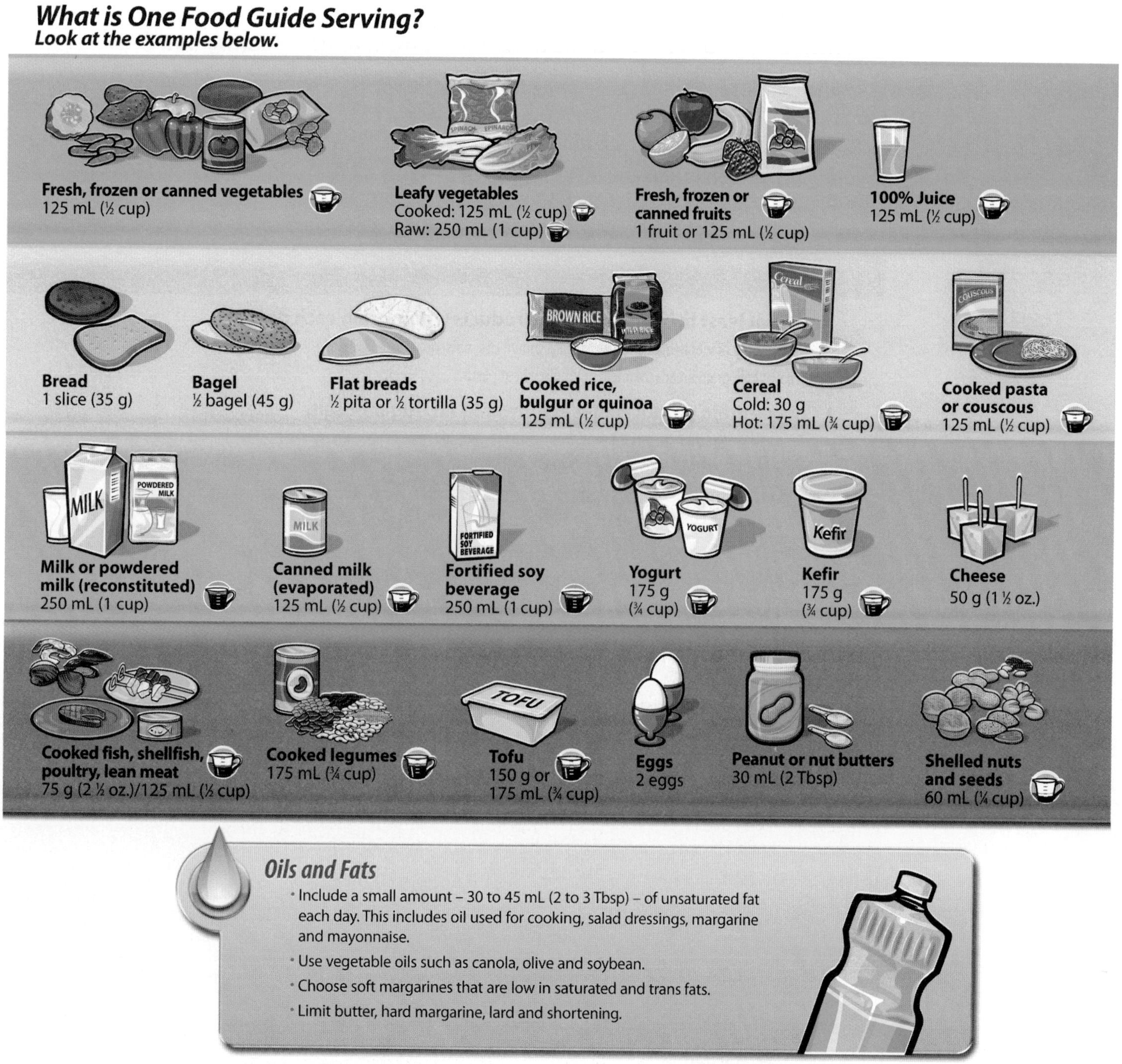

What is One Food Guide Serving?
Look at the examples below.

Fresh, frozen or canned vegetables
125 mL (½ cup)

Leafy vegetables
Cooked: 125 mL (½ cup)
Raw: 250 mL (1 cup)

Fresh, frozen or canned fruits
1 fruit or 125 mL (½ cup)

100% Juice
125 mL (½ cup)

Bread
1 slice (35 g)

Bagel
½ bagel (45 g)

Flat breads
½ pita or ½ tortilla (35 g)

Cooked rice, bulgur or quinoa
125 mL (½ cup)

Cereal
Cold: 30 g
Hot: 175 mL (¾ cup)

Cooked pasta or couscous
125 mL (½ cup)

Milk or powdered milk (reconstituted)
250 mL (1 cup)

Canned milk (evaporated)
125 mL (½ cup)

Fortified soy beverage
250 mL (1 cup)

Yogurt
175 g
(¾ cup)

Kefir
175 g
(¾ cup)

Cheese
50 g (1 ½ oz.)

Cooked fish, shellfish, poultry, lean meat
75 g (2 ½ oz.)/125 mL (½ cup)

Cooked legumes
175 mL (¾ cup)

Tofu
150 g or
175 mL (¾ cup)

Eggs
2 eggs

Peanut or nut butters
30 mL (2 Tbsp)

Shelled nuts and seeds
60 mL (¼ cup)

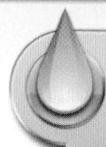

Oils and Fats

- Include a small amount – 30 to 45 mL (2 to 3 Tbsp) – of unsaturated fat each day. This includes oil used for cooking, salad dressings, margarine and mayonnaise.
- Use vegetable oils such as canola, olive and soybean.
- Choose soft margarines that are low in saturated and trans fats.
- Limit butter, hard margarine, lard and shortening.

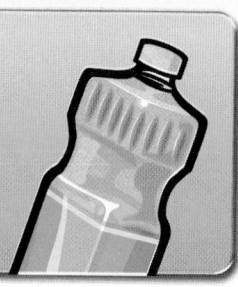

FIGURE C-2 ▶ *(continued)*

Make each Food Guide Serving count...
wherever you are – at home, at school, at work or when eating out!

▶ **Eat at least one dark green and one orange vegetable each day.**
- Go for dark green vegetables such as broccoli, romaine lettuce and spinach.
- Go for orange vegetables such as carrots, sweet potatoes and winter squash.

▶ **Choose vegetables and fruit prepared with little or no added fat, sugar or salt.**
- Enjoy vegetables steamed, baked or stir-fried instead of deep-fried.

▶ **Have vegetables and fruit more often than juice.**

▶ **Make at least half of your grain products whole grain each day.**
- Eat a variety of whole grains such as barley, brown rice, oats, quinoa and wild rice.
- Enjoy whole grain breads, oatmeal or whole wheat pasta.

▶ **Choose grain products that are lower in fat, sugar or salt.**
- Compare the Nutrition Facts table on labels to make wise choices.
- Enjoy the true taste of grain products. When adding sauces or spreads, use small amounts.

▶ **Drink skim, 1%, or 2% milk each day.**
- Have 500 mL (2 cups) of milk every day for adequate vitamin D.
- Drink fortified soy beverages if you do not drink milk.

▶ **Select lower fat milk alternatives.**
- Compare the Nutrition Facts table on yogurts or cheeses to make wise choices.

▶ **Have meat alternatives such as beans, lentils and tofu often.**

▶ **Eat at least two Food Guide Servings of fish each week.***
- Choose fish such as char, herring, mackerel, salmon, sardines and trout.

▶ **Select lean meat and alternatives prepared with little or no added fat or salt.**
- Trim the visible fat from meats. Remove the skin on poultry.
- Use cooking methods such as roasting, baking or poaching that require little or no added fat.
- If you eat luncheon meats, sausages or prepackaged meats, choose those lower in salt (sodium) and fat.

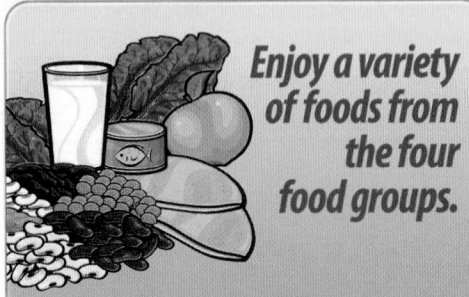

Enjoy a variety of foods from the four food groups.

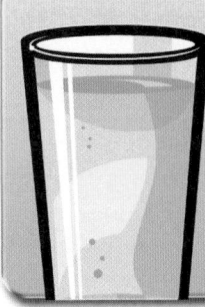

Satisfy your thirst with water!

Drink water regularly. It's a calorie-free way to quench your thirst. Drink more water in hot weather or when you are very active.

* Health Canada provides advice for limiting exposure to mercury from certain types of fish. Refer to www.healthcanada.gc.ca for the latest information.

FIGURE C-2 ▶ *(continued)*

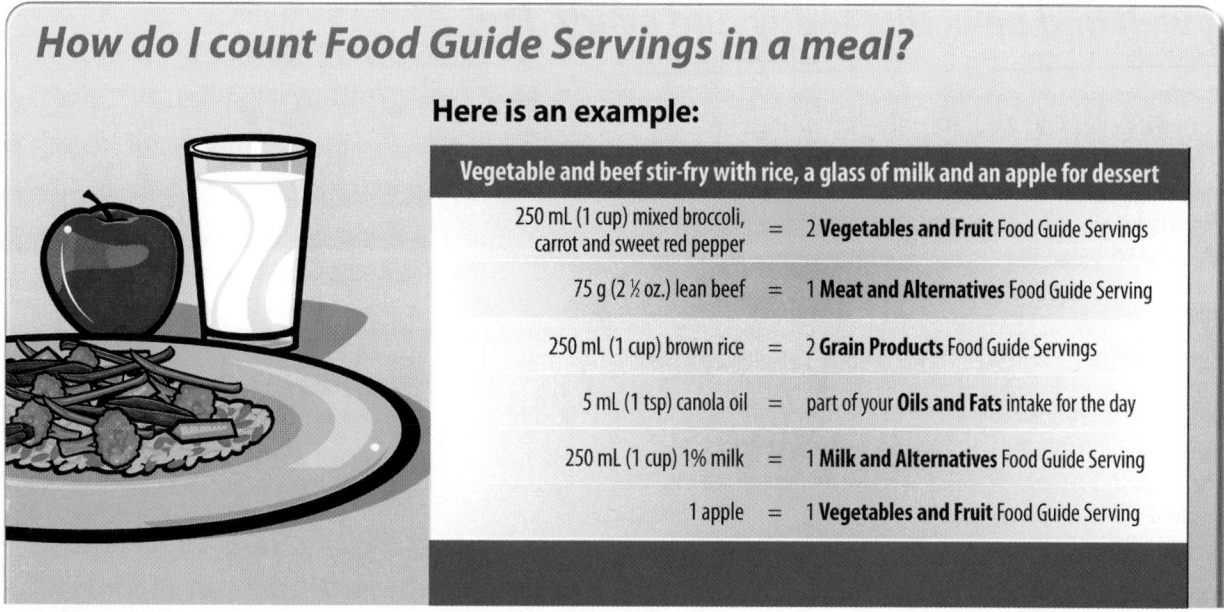

How do I count Food Guide Servings in a meal?

Here is an example:

Vegetable and beef stir-fry with rice, a glass of milk and an apple for dessert		
250 mL (1 cup) mixed broccoli, carrot and sweet red pepper	=	2 **Vegetables and Fruit** Food Guide Servings
75 g (2 ½ oz.) lean beef	=	1 **Meat and Alternatives** Food Guide Serving
250 mL (1 cup) brown rice	=	2 **Grain Products** Food Guide Servings
5 mL (1 tsp) canola oil	=	part of your **Oils and Fats** intake for the day
250 mL (1 cup) 1% milk	=	1 **Milk and Alternatives** Food Guide Serving
1 apple	=	1 **Vegetables and Fruit** Food Guide Serving

FIGURE C-3 ▶ How to count Food Guide Servings in a meal.

Nutrition Labels

New labeling requirements were published on January 1, 2003. The new regulations require most food labels to carry a mandatory Nutrition Facts table listing Calories and 13 key nutrients.

How to Read the Canadian Nutrition Label

The Regulations provide for the optional declaration of the number of Calories both from fat and from saturates plus *trans*. Recommendations on the % of Calories from fat apply to the total diet rather than to an individual food. Therefore, inclusion of the % of Calories from fat in the Nutrition Facts table may be confusing and is not permitted.

The Nutrition Facts table provides information on saturated and *trans* fatty acids, shown to raise serum cholesterol levels. The declaration of the other groups of fatty acids, monounsaturates, omega-3, and omega-6 polyunsaturates, is optional unless claims are made, in which case all three must be declared.

Potassium is not included as a mandatory nutrient of the Nutrition Facts table because it is not considered to be a nutrient of general public health importance. The declaration of potassium, however, is mandatory when a claim is made for the sodium or salt content of a food that contains an added potassium salt.

Daily Value is a comparison standard comprised of
(*a*) vitamin or mineral amounts referred to in the definition of a recommended daily intake for that vitamin or mineral
(*b*) nutrient amounts referred to in the definition of reference standard for that nutrient

Serving size is stipulated for various foods.

The amount of vitamins and minerals is expressed as a percentage of the Daily Value per serving of stated size.

Nutrition Facts
Per 1 cup (264g)

Amount	% Daily Value
Calories 260	
Fat 13g	20%
Saturated Fat 3g + *Trans* Fat 2g	25%
Cholesterol 30mg	
Sodium 660mg	28%
Carbohydrate 31g	10%
Fibre 0g	0%
Sugars 5g	
Protein 5g	
Vitamin A 4% Vitamin C 2%	
Calcium 15% Iron 4%	

g = gram
mg = milligram

Eat well and be active today and every day!

The benefits of eating well and being active include:

- Better overall health.
- Lower risk of disease.
- A healthy body weight.
- Feeling and looking better.
- More energy.
- Stronger muscles and bones.

Be active

To be active every day is a step towards better health and a healthy body weight.

Canada's Physical Activity Guide recommends building 30 to 60 minutes of moderate physical activity into daily life for adults and at least 90 minutes a day for children and youth. You don't have to do it all at once. Add it up in periods of at least 10 minutes at a time for adults and five minutes at a time for children and youth.

Start slowly and build up.

Eat well

Another important step towards better health and a healthy body weight is to follow *Canada's Food Guide* by:

- Eating the recommended amount and type of food each day.
- Limiting foods and beverages high in calories, fat, sugar or salt (sodium) such as cakes and pastries, chocolate and candies, cookies and granola bars, doughnuts and muffins, ice cream and frozen desserts, French fries, potato chips, nachos and other salty snacks, alcohol, fruit flavoured drinks, soft drinks, sports and energy drinks, and sweetened hot or cold drinks.

Read the label

- Compare the Nutrition Facts table on food labels to choose products that contain less fat, saturated fat, trans fat, sugar and sodium.
- Keep in mind that the calories and nutrients listed are for the amount of food found at the top of the Nutrition Facts table.

Limit trans fat

When a Nutrition Facts table is not available, ask for nutrition information to choose foods lower in trans and saturated fats.

Nutrition Facts

Per 0 mL (0 g)

Amount	% Daily Value
Calories 0	
Fat 0 g	0 %
Saturates 0 g	0 %
+ Trans 0 g	
Cholesterol 0 mg	
Sodium 0 mg	0 %
Carbohydrate 0 g	0 %
Fibre 0 g	0 %
Sugars 0 g	
Protein 0 g	

Vitamin A	0 %	Vitamin C	0 %
Calcium	0 %	Iron	0 %

Take a step today...

- ✓ Have breakfast every day. It may help control your hunger later in the day.
- ✓ Walk wherever you can – get off the bus early, use the stairs.
- ✓ Benefit from eating vegetables and fruit at all meals and as snacks.
- ✓ Spend less time being inactive such as watching TV or playing computer games.
- ✓ Request nutrition information about menu items when eating out to help you make healthier choices.
- ✓ Enjoy eating with family and friends!
- ✓ Take time to eat and savour every bite!

For more information, interactive tools, or additional copies visit Canada's Food Guide on-line at:
www.healthcanada.gc.ca/foodguide

or contact:

Publications
Health Canada
Ottawa, Ontario K1A 0K9
E-Mail: publications@hc-sc.gc.ca
Tel.: 1-866-225-0709
Fax: (613) 941-5366
TTY: 1-800-267-1245

Également disponible en français sous le titre :
Bien manger avec le Guide alimentaire canadien

This publication can be made available on request on diskette, large print, audio-cassette and braille.

© Her Majesty the Queen in Right of Canada, represented by the Minister of Health Canada, 2007. This publication may be reproduced without permission. No changes permitted.   HC Pub.: 4651   Cat.: H164-38/1-2007E   ISBN: 0-662-44467-1

FIGURE C-4 ▶ Recommendations to eat well and be active from *Canada's Food Guide*.

Advice for different ages and stages...

Children

Following *Canada's Food Guide* helps children grow and thrive.

Young children have small appetites and need calories for growth and development.

- Serve small nutritious meals and snacks each day.
- Do not restrict nutritious foods because of their fat content. Offer a variety of foods from the four food groups.
- Most of all... be a good role model.

Women of childbearing age

All women who could become pregnant and those who are pregnant or breastfeeding need a multivitamin containing **folic acid** every day. Pregnant women need to ensure that their multivitamin also contains **iron**. A health care professional can help you find the multivitamin that's right for you.

Pregnant and breastfeeding women need more calories. Include an extra 2 to 3 Food Guide Servings each day.

Here are two examples:
- Have fruit and yogurt for a snack, or
- Have an extra slice of toast at breakfast and an extra glass of milk at supper.

Men and women over 50

The need for **vitamin D** increases after the age of 50.

In addition to following *Canada's Food Guide*, everyone over the age of 50 should take a daily vitamin D supplement of 10 µg (400 IU).

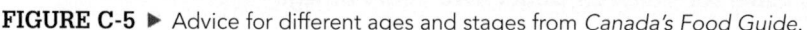

FIGURE C-5 ▶ Advice for different ages and stages from *Canada's Food Guide.*

The new regulations make nutrition labeling mandatory on most food labels using a new format. The regulations also update requirements for nutrient content claims and permit, for the first time in Canada, diet-related health claims for foods.

Templates for Canadian "Nutrition Facts" Tables

Bilingual Label

Nutrition Facts
Valeur nutritive
Per 125 mL (87 g) / 0par 125 mL (87 g)

Amount / Teneur	% Daily Value / % valeur quotidienne
Calories / Calories 80	
Fat / Lipids 0.5 g	**1** %
Saturated / saturés 0 g + *Trans* / trans 0 g	**0** %
Cholesterol / Cholestérol 0 mg	
Sodium / Sodium 0 mg	**0** %
Carbohydrate / Glucides 18 g	**6** %
Fibre / Fibres 2 g	**8** %
Sugars / Sucres 2 g	
Protein / Protéines 3 g	
Vitamin A / Vitamine A	2 %
Vitamin C / Vitamine C	10 %
Calcium / Calcium	0 %
Iron / Fer	2 %

English Label

Nutrition Facts
Per 125 mL (87 g)

Amount	% Daily Value
Calories 80	
Fat 0.5 g	**1** %
Saturated 0 g + *Trans* 0 g	**0** %
Cholesterol 0 mg	
Sodium 0 mg	**0** %
Carbohydrate 18 g	**6** %
Fibre 2 g	**8** %
Sugars 2 g	
Protein 3 g	
Vitamin A 2 %	Vitamin C 10 %
Calcium 0 %	Iron 2 %

French Label

Valeur nutritive
par 125 mL (87 g)

Teneur	% valeur quotidienne
Calories 80	
Lipids 0,5 g	**1** %
saturés 0 g + trans 0 g	**0** %
Cholestérol 0 mg	
Sodium 0 mg	**0** %
Glucides 18 g	**6** %
Fibres 2 g	**8** %
Sucres 2 g	
Protéines 3 g	
Vitamine A 2 %	Vitamine C 10 %
Calcium 0 %	Fer 2 %

g = gram
mg = milligram

New Canadian Nutrition Facts Label for Children Under Two Years of Age

Nutrition Facts
Per 1 jar (126 mL)

	Amount
Calories	110
Fat	0g
Sodium	10 mg
Carbohydrate	27g
Fibre	4g
Sugars	18g
Protein	0g
% Daily Value	
Vitamin A 6%	Vitamin C 45%
Calcium 2%	Iron 2%

g = gram
mg = milligram

Recommended Daily Intakes and Reference Standards

The following are the Recommended Daily Intakes and Reference Standards used on Nutrition Labels for persons 2 years of age and older.* † ‡

Dietary Constituent	Amount	Dietary Constituent	Amount
Fat	**65 g**	Folacin	220 µg
The sum of saturated fatty acids and *trans* fatty acids	**20 g**	Vitamin B$_{12}$	2 µg
Cholesterol	**300 mg**	Pantothenic acid or pantothenate	7 mg
Carbohydrate	**300 g**	Vitamin K	**80 mg**
Fibre	**25 g**	Biotin	**30 µg**
Sodium	**2400 mg**	Calcium	1100 mg
Chloride	**3400 µg**	Phosphorus	1100 mg
Potassium	**3500 mg**	Magnesium	250 mg
Vitamin A	1000 RE	Iron	14 mg
Vitamin D	5 µg	Zinc	9 mg
Vitamin E	10 mg	Iodide	160 µg
Vitamin C	60 mg	Selenium	**50 µg**
Thiamin, thiamine or vitamin B$_1$	1.3 mg	Copper	**2 mg**
Riboflavin or vitamin B$_2$	1.6 mg	Manganese	**2 mg**
Niacin	23 NE	Chromium	**120 µg**
Vitamin B$_6$	1.8 mg	Molybdenum	**75 µg**

*RE = retinol equivalents
†NE = niacin equivalents
‡Together these constitute the Daily Values used on the Canadian Nutrition Facts Label. Reference Standards are bolded.

Approved Nutrient Content Claims for Canada

The following is a sample of approved nutrient content claims for food labels (for the complete list of regulations see the website http://gazette.gc.ca/archives/p1/2005/2005-05-07/html/reg4-eng.html).

Energy

- *Free of energy:* The food provides less than 5 Calories or 21 kilojoules per reference amount and serving of stated size.
- *Low in energy:* The food provides 40 Calories or 167 kilojoules or less per reference amount and serving of stated size.
- *Reduced in energy:* The food is processed, formulated, reformulated, or otherwise modified so that it provides at least 25% less energy per reference amount of a similar food.
- *Lower in energy:* The food provides at least 25% less energy per reference amount of a similar food.

- *Source of energy:* The food provides at least 100 Calories or 420 kilojoules per reference amount and serving of stated size.
- *More energy:* The food provides at least 25% more energy, totalling at least 100 more Calories or 420 more kilojoules per reference amount of a similar food.

Protein

- *Low in protein:* The food contains no more than 1 gram of protein per 100 grams of the food.
- *Source of protein:* The food has a protein rating of 20 or more, as determined by official method

FO-1, *Determination of Protein Rating,* October 15, 1981, (*a*) per reasonable daily intake; or (*b*) per 30 grams combined with 125 milliliters of milk, if the food is a breakfast cereal.

- *Excellent source of protein:* The food has a protein rating of 40 or more, as determined by official method FO-1, *Determination of Protein Rating,* October 15, 1981, (*a*) per reasonable daily intake; or (*b*) per 30 grams combined with 125 milliliters of milk, if the food is a breakfast cereal.
- *More protein:* The food (*a*) has a protein rating of 20 or more, as determined by official method

FO-1, *Determination of Protein Rating*, October 15, 1981, (i) per reasonable daily intake, or (ii) per 30 grams combined with 125 milliliters of milk, if the food is a breakfast cereal; and (*b*) contains at least 25% more protein, totalling at least 7 grams more, per reasonable daily intake compared to the reference food of the same food group or the similar reference food.

Fat

- *Free of fat:* The food contains less than 0.5 grams of fat per reference amount and serving of stated size.
- *Low in fat:* The food contains 3 grams or less of fat per reference amount and serving of stated size and, if the reference amount is 30 grams or 30 milliliters or less, per 50 grams.
- *Reduced in fat:* The food is processed, formulated, reformulated, or otherwise modified so that it contains at least 25% less fat than the reference amount of a similar food.
- *Lower in fat:* The food contains at least 25% less fat per reference amount of the food, than the reference amount of the reference food of the same food group.
- *100% fat-free:* The food (*a*) contains less than 0.5 grams of fat per 100 grams; (*b*) contains no added fat.
- *No added fat:* The food contains no added fats or oils set out in Division 9, or added butter or ghee, or ingredients that contain added fats or oils, or butter or ghee.
- *Free of saturated fatty acids:* The food contains less than 0.2 grams saturated fatty acids and less than 0.2 grams *trans* fatty acids per reference amount and serving of stated size.
- *Low in saturated fatty acids:* (1) The food contains 2 grams or less of saturated fatty acids and *trans* fatty acids combined per reference amount and serving of stated size. (2) The food provides 15% or less energy from the sum of saturated fatty acids and *trans* fatty acids.

- *Reduced in saturated fatty acids:* The food is processed, formulated, reformulated, or otherwise modified without increasing the content of *trans* fatty acids, so that it contains at least 25% less saturated fatty acids per reference amount of the food than the reference amount of the similar reference food.
- *Lower in saturated fatty acids:* The food contains at least 25% less saturated fatty acids and the content of *trans* fatty acids is not higher per reference amount of the food, than the reference amount of the reference food of the same food group.
- *Free of* trans *fatty acids:* The food contains less than 0.2 grams of *trans* fatty acids per reference amount and serving of stated size.
- *Reduced in* trans *fatty acids:* The food is processed, formulated, reformulated, or otherwise modified without increasing the content of saturated fatty acids, so that it contains at least 25% less *trans* fatty acids per reference amount of the food than the reference amount of the similar reference food.
- *Lower in* trans *fatty acids:* The food contains at least 25% less *trans* fatty acids and the content of saturated fatty acids is not higher per reference amount of the food compared to the reference amount of a similar food.
- *Source of omega-3 polyunsaturated fatty acids:* The food contains 0.3 grams or more of omega-3 polyunsaturated fatty acids per reference amount and serving of stated size.
- *Source of omega-6 polyunsaturated fatty acids:* The food contains 2 grams or more of omega-6 polyunsaturated fatty acids per reference amount and serving of stated size.

Cholesterol

- *Free of cholesterol:* The food contains less than 2 milligrams of cholesterol per reference amount and serving of stated size.
- *Low in cholesterol:* The food contains 20 milligrams or less of cholesterol per reference amount and serving of

stated size (if the reference amount is 30 grams or 30 milliliters or less, per 50 grams).
- *Reduced in cholesterol:* The food is processed, formulated, reformulated, or otherwise modified so that it contains at least 25% less cholesterol per reference amount of a similar food.
- *Lower in cholesterol:* The food contains at least 25% less cholesterol per reference amount of a similar food.

Sodium or Salt

- *Free of sodium or salt:* The food contains less than 5 milligrams of sodium per reference amount and serving of stated size.
- *Low in sodium or salt:* The food contains 140 milligrams or less of sodium per reference amount and serving of stated size.
- *Reduced in sodium or salt:* The food is processed, formulated, reformulated, or otherwise modified so that it contains at least 25% less sodium per reference amount of a similar food.
- *Lower in sodium or salt:* The food contains at least 25% less sodium per reference amount of the food.
- *No added sodium or salt:* The food contains no added salt, other sodium salts, or ingredients that contain sodium that functionally substitute for added salt.
- *Lightly salted:* The food contains at least 50% less added sodium than the sodium added to a similar reference food.

Sugars

- *Free of sugars:* The food contains less than 0.5 milligrams of sugars per reference amount and serving of stated size.
- *Reduced in sugars:* The food is processed, formulated, reformulated, or otherwise modified so that it contains at least 25% less sugars, totalling at least 5 grams less, per reference amount of the food.

- *Lower in sugars:* The food contains at least 25% less sugars, totalling at least 5 grams less, per reference amount of the food.
- *No added sugars:* The food contains no added sugars, no ingredients containing added sugars or ingredients that contain sugars that functionally substitute for added sugars.

Fibre

- *Source of fibre:* The food contains 2 grams or more (*a*) of fibre per reference amount and serving of stated size, if no fibre or fibre source is identified in the statement or claim; or (*b*) of each identified fibre or fibre from an identified fibre source per reference amount and serving of stated size, if a fibre or fibre source is identified in the statement or claim.
- *High source of fibre:* The food contains 4 grams or more (*a*) of fibre per reference amount and serving of stated size, if no fibre or fibre source is identified in the statement or claim; or (*b*) of each identified fibre or fibre from an identified fibre source per reference amount and serving of stated size, if a fibre or fibre source is identified in the statement or claim.
- *Very high source of fibre:* The food contains 6 grams or more (*a*) of fibre per reference amount and serving of stated size, if no fibre or fibre source is identified in the statement or claim; or (*b*) of each identified fibre or fibre from an identified fibre source per reference amount and serving of stated size, if a fibre or fibre source is identified in the statement or claim.
- *More fibre:* The food contains at least 25% more fibre, totalling at least 1 gram more, if no fibre or fibre source is identified in the statement or claim, or at least 25% more of an identified fibre or fibre from an identified fibre source, totalling at least 1 gram more, if a fibre or fibre source is identified in the statement or claim compared to reference amount of a similar food.

Light and Lean

- *Light in energy or fat:* The food meets the conditions set out for the subject "reduced in energy" or "reduced in fat."
- *Lean:* The food (*a*) is meat or poultry that has not been ground, a marine or fresh water animal or a product of any of these; and (*b*) contains 10% or less fat.
- *Extra lean:* The food (*a*) is meat or poultry that has not been ground, a marine or fresh water animal or a product of any of these; and (*b*) contains 7.5% or less fat.

Approved Health Claims for Nutrition Labels

If a manufacturer follows specific guidelines addressing both the nutrients noted in the claim as well as guidelines pertaining to other nutrients in a food, the following health claims can be made.

- A healthy diet containing foods high in potassium and low in sodium may reduce the risk of high blood pressure, a risk factor for stroke and heart disease.
- A healthy diet with adequate calcium and vitamin D, and regular physical activity, may help to achieve strong bones and may reduce the risk of osteoporosis.
- A healthy diet low in saturated and *trans* fats may reduce the risk of heart disease.
- A healthy diet rich in a variety of vegetables and fruit may help reduce the risk of some types of cancer.
- Foods very low in starch and fermentable sugars can make the following health claims:
  - Won't cause cavities;
  - Does not promote tooth decay;
  - Does not promote dental caries; or is
  - Non-cariogenic.

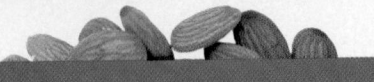

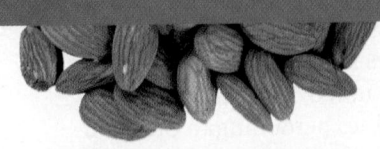

Exchange System A system for classifying foods into numerous lists based on the foods' macronutrient composition and establishing serving sizes, so that one serving of each food on a list contains the same amount of carbohydrate, protein, fat, and calorie content.

exchange The serving size of a food on a specific exchange list.

THE EXCHANGE SYSTEM

The **Exchange System** is a valuable tool for roughly estimating the calorie, protein, carbohydrate, and fat content of a food or meal. This tool organizes many details of the nutrient composition of foods into a manageable framework. By using the Exchange System, you can plan daily menus to fall roughly within specific percentages of macronutrients without having to look up or memorize the nutrient values of numerous foods, so the time you spend now becoming familiar with the Exchange System will pay off in the future.

In the Exchange System, individual foods are placed into three broad groups: carbohydrate, meat and meat substitutes, and fat. Within these groups are lists that contain foods of similar macronutrient composition: various types of milk, fruit, vegetables, starch, other carbohydrates, meat and meat substitutes, and fat. These lists are designed so that, when the proper serving size is observed, each food on a list provides about the same amount of carbohydrate, protein, fat, and calories. This equality allows the exchange of foods on each list, hence the term *Exchange System*.

The Exchange System was originally developed for planning diabetic diets. Diabetes is easier to control if the person's diet has about the same composition day after day. If a certain number of **exchanges** from each of the various lists is eaten each day, that regularity is easier to achieve. However, because the Exchange System provides a quick way to estimate the calorie, carbohydrate, protein, and fat content in any food or meal, it is a valuable menu-planning tool for people without diabetes, as well.

Becoming Familiar with the Exchange System

To use the Exchange System, you must know which foods are on each list and the serving sizes for each food.

Table D-1 gives the serving sizes for foods on each exchange list, as well as the carbohydrate, protein, fat, and calorie content per exchange. The meat and milk lists are divided into subclasses, which vary in fat content and, hence, in the amount of calories they provide. Foods on the meat and fat lists contain essentially no carbohydrate; those on the fruit and fat lists lack appreciable amounts of protein; and those on the vegetable, fruit, and other carbohydrates lists contain essentially no fat. You need to study Table D-1 and Figure D-1 to become familiar with the exchange lists, the sizes of the exchanges (that is, serving sizes) on each list, and the amounts of carbohydrate, protein, fat, and calories per exchange.

Before you can turn a group of exchanges into a daily meal plan, you must be aware of which foods are on each exchange list (Fig. D-1). The entire Exchange Lists for Diabetes (2008) is presented in Appendix D, which you should consult frequently while exploring the system to discover its various peculiarities. For example, the starch list includes not only bread, dry cereal, cooked cereal, rice, and pasta, but also baked beans, corn on the cob, and potatoes. These foods are not identical to those composing the grains group from MyPlate. The Exchange System is not concerned with the origin of a food, whether animal or vegetable. It is primarily concerned with the macronutrients carbohydrate, protein, and fat in each food on a specific list. For example, the carbohydrate composition of potatoes resembles that of bread more than that of broccoli, although potatoes are vegetables. In addition, several foods on the meat and meat substitutes list are not meats. The list of other carbohydrates includes jam, angel food cake, fat-free frozen yogurt, and foods such as frosted cake that count as both other carbohydrate exchanges and fat exchanges. Bacon appears in the fat list, rather than the high-fat meat category.

TABLE D-1   Nutrient Composition of Exchange System Lists (Based on *Choose Your Foods: Exchange Lists for Diabetes*, 2007)

Groups/Lists	Household Measures*	Carbohydrate (g)	Protein (g)	Fat (g)	Energy (kcal)
Carbohydrate Group					
Starch	1 slice, ¾ cup raw, or ½ cup cooked	15	3	1 or less†	80
Fruit	1 small/medium piece	15	—	—	60
Milk	1 cup				
Fat-free/very low-fat		12	8	0–3†	90
Reduced-fat		12	8	5	120
Whole		12	8	8	150
Other carbohydrates	Varies	15	Varies	Varies	Varies
Nonstarchy vegetables	1 cup raw or ½ cup cooked	5	2	—	25
Meat and Meat Substitutes Group	1 ounce				
Very lean		—	7	0–1	35
Lean		—	7	3	55
Medium-fat		—	7	5	75
High-fat		—	7	8	100
Fat Group	1 teaspoon	—	—	5	45

*An estimate; see exchange lists for actual amounts.
†Calculated as 1 gram for purposes of calorie contribution.

Reproduction of the exchange lists in whole or in part, without permission of The American Dietetic Association or the American Diabetes Association, Inc. is a violation of federal law. This material has been modified from *Choose Your Foods: Exchange Lists for Diabetes*, 2007 which is the basis of a meal planning system designed by a committee of the American Diabetes Association and The American Dietetic Association. While designed primarily for people with diabetes and others who must follow special diets, the exchange lists are based on principles of good nutrition that apply to everyone. © 2008 by the American Diabetes Association and the American Dietetic Association.

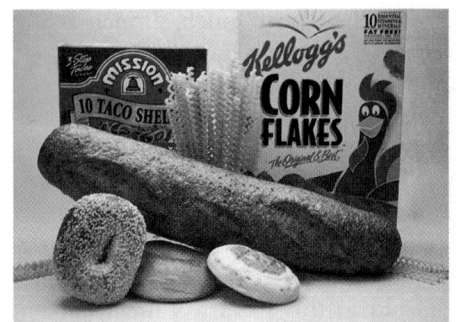

Starch exchange choices

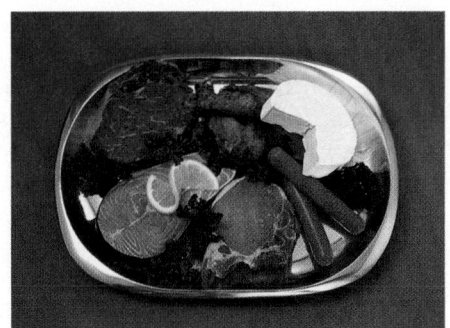

Meat and meat substitutes exchange choices

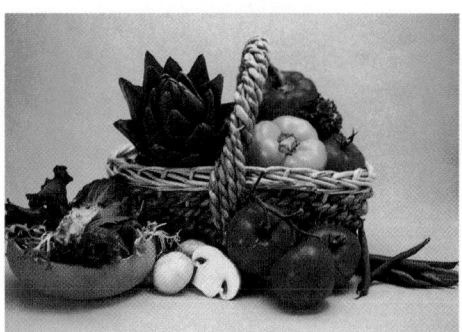

Vegetable exchange choices

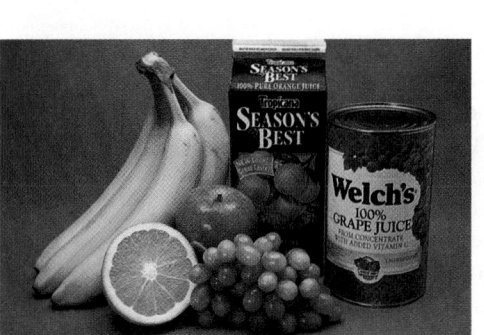

Fruit exchange choices

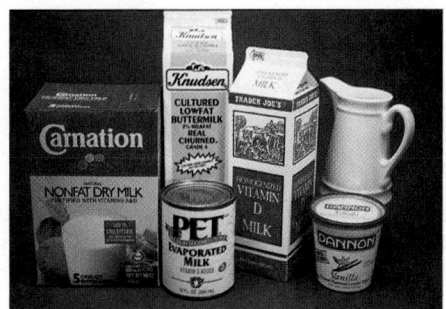

Milk exchange choices

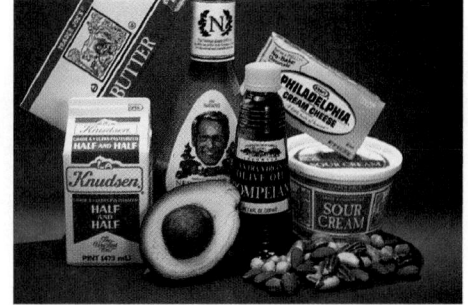

Fat exchange choices

FIGURE D-1 ▶ Foods arranged according to the Exchange Lists for Diabetes.

TABLE D-2 Possible Exchange Patterns That Yield 55% of Calories as Carbohydrate, 30% as Fat, and 15% as Protein

Exchange List	kcal/Day						
	1200*	1600*	2000	2400	2800	3200	3600
Milk (reduced-fat)	2	2	2	2	2	2	2
Vegetable	3	3	3	4	4	4	4
Fruit	3	4	5	6	8	9	9
Starch	5	8	11	13	15	18	21
Meat (lean)	4	4	4	5	6	7	8
Fat	2	4	6	8	10	11	13

This is just one set of options. More meat could be included if less milk were used, for example.

*Calorie intakes of 1200 and 1600 kcal contain 20% of calories as protein and 50% of calories as carbohydrate to allow for greater flexibility in diet planning.

Free foods (essentially calorie-free) include bouillon, diet soda, coffee, tea, dill pickles, and vinegar, as well as herbs and spices. Many vegetables, such as cabbage, celery, mushrooms, lettuce, and zucchini, also can be considered free foods; their minimal energy contribution need not count in the calculations when they are eaten in moderation (1 to 2 servings per meal or snack).

Using the Exchange System to Develop Daily Menus

Now let's use the Exchange System to plan a 1-day menu. Let's target a calorie content of 2000 kcal, with 55% derived from carbohydrates (1100 kcal), 15% from protein (300 kcal), and 30% from fat (600 kcal). This can be translated into 2 reduced-fat milk exchanges, 3 vegetable exchanges, 5 fruit exchanges, 11 starch exchanges, 4 lean meat exchanges, and 6 fat exchanges (Table D-2). This is only one of many possible combinations; the Exchange System offers great flexibility.

Table D-3 arbitrarily separates these exchanges into breakfast, lunch, dinner, and a snack. Breakfast includes 1 reduced-fat milk exchange, 2 fruit exchanges, 2 starch exchanges, and 1 fat exchange. This total corresponds to ¾ cup of a ready-to-eat breakfast cereal, 1 cup of reduced-fat milk, 1 slice of bread with 1 teaspoon margarine, and 1 cup of orange juice.

Lunch consists of 2 fat exchanges, 4 starch exchanges, 1 vegetable exchange, 1 reduced-fat milk exchange, and 2 fruit exchanges. This translates into one slice of bacon with 1 teaspoon mayonnaise on two slices of bread, with tomato—in other words, a bacon and tomato sandwich. You can also add lettuce to the sandwich. This can be considered a free vegetable choice. Add to this meal a 9-inch banana (1 exchange = 1 small banana), 1 cup of reduced-fat milk, and 6 graham crackers (2½ inches by 2½ inches). Later add a snack of ¾ ounce of pretzels for another starch exchange.

Dinner consists of 4 lean meat exchanges, 1 fruit exchange, 2 vegetable exchanges, 1 fat exchange, and 2 starch exchanges. This total corresponds to a 4-ounce broiled steak (meat only, no bone), 1 medium baked potato (1 exchange = 1 small baked potato) with 1 teaspoon of margarine, 1 cup of broccoli, and 1 kiwi fruit. Coffee (if desired) is not counted, because it contains no appreciable calories.

Finally, we have a snack containing 2 starch exchanges and 2 fat exchanges. This translates into 1 bagel with 2 tablespoons of regular cream cheese.

This 1-day menu is only one of many possible with the exchange lists. Apple juice could replace the orange juice; two apples could be exchanged for the banana. The choices are endless. An exchange diet is much easier to plan if you use individual foods, as was done here; however, the Exchange System tables list some combination foods to help you. Using combination foods, such as pizza or lasagna, however, makes it more difficult to calculate the number of exchanges in a serving. For

TABLE D-3 Sample 1-Day 2000-kcal Menu Based on the Exchange Lists for
Diabetes Plan*

Breakfast

1 reduced-fat milk exchange	1 cup reduced-fat milk (some on cereal)
2 fruit exchanges	1 cup orange juice
2 starch exchanges	¾ cup ready-to-eat breakfast cereal, 1 piece whole-wheat toast
1 fat exchange	1 teaspoon soft margarine on toast

Lunch

4 starch exchanges	2 slices whole-wheat bread, 6 graham crackers (2½ inches by 2½ inches)
2 fat exchanges	1 slice bacon, 1 teaspoon mayonnaise
1 vegetable exchange	1 sliced tomato
2 fruit exchanges	1 banana (9 inches)
1 reduced-fat milk exchange	1 cup reduced-fat milk

Snack

| 1 starch exchange | ¾ ounce pretzels |

Dinner

4 lean meat exchanges	4 ounces lean steak (well trimmed)
2 starch exchanges	1 medium baked potato
1 fat exchange	1 tsp soft margarine
2 vegetable exchanges	1 cup cooked broccoli
1 fruit exchange	1 kiwi fruit
	Coffee (if desired)

Snack

| 2 starch exchanges | 1 bagel |
| 2 fat exchanges | 2 tablespoons regular cream cheese |

*The target plan was a 2000 kcal intake, with 55% of calories from carbohydrate, 15% from protein, and 30% from fat. Computer analysis indicates that this menu yielded 2040 kcal, with 53% of calories from carbohydrate, 16% from protein, and 31% from fat—in close agreement with the targeted goals.

instance, lasagna typically has meat exchanges, vegetable exchanges, and starch exchanges. With practice, you will be able to tackle such complex foods (Fig. D-2). For now, using individual foods makes learning the Exchange System much easier. Finally, you might want to prove to yourself that the food choices listed in Table D-3 really meet the Exchange plan. This demonstration will give you practice turning exchanges into food servings.

FIGURE D-2 ► Record the Exchange Lists for Diabetes pattern you have chosen in the left-hand column. Then distribute the exchanges throughout the day, noting the food to be used and the serving size.

Exchange List	Total Exchanges to be Consumed Daily	Exchanges Consumed at Each Meal		
		Breakfast	Lunch	Dinner
MILK				
VEGETABLE				
FRUIT				
STARCH				
MEAT AND SUBSTITUTES				
FAT				

EXCHANGE FOR DIABETES LISTS

The exchange lists are the basis of a meal planning system designed by a committee of the American Diabetes Association and the American Dietetic Association. While designed primarily for people with diabetes and others who must follow special diets, the exchange lists are based on principles of good nutrition that apply to everyone.

© 2008 by the American Diabetes Association and the American Dietetic Association.

MILK EXCHANGE LIST

Fat-Free and Low-Fat Milk

(12 g carbohydrate, 8 g protein, 0–3 g fat, 100 kcal)

Serving Size	Food
1 cup	fat-free, ½%, and 1% milk, and buttermilk
½ cup	canned, evaporated fat-free milk
1 cup	soy milk (light or regular)
⅔ cup (6 oz)	yogurt with fruit, low-fat
⅔ cup (6 oz)	yogurt, low carbohydrate (less than 6 grams), sweetened with nonnutritive sweetener and fructose

Reduced-Fat Milk

(12 g carbohydrate, 8 g protein, 5 g fat, 120 kcal)

Serving Size	Food
1 cup	2% milk, acidophilus milk, kefir
⅔ cup (6 oz)	yogurt plain, low-fat (added milk solids)
1 cup	whole milk, buttermilk, goat's milk

Whole Milk

(12 g carbohydrate, 8 g protein, 8 g fat, 160 kcal)

Serving Size	Food
½ cup	evaporated whole milk
1 cup	yogurt, plain (made from whole milk)

NON-STARCHY VEGETABLE EXCHANGE LIST

(5 g carbohydrate, 2 g protein, 0 g fat, 25 kcal)
Vegetables with small amounts of carbohydrate and calories are on the Nonstarchy Vegetables list. 1 vegetable exchange equals:
½ cup cooked vegetables or vegetable juice or 1 cup raw vegetables

artichoke
artichoke hearts
asparagus
beans (green, wax, Italian)
bean sprouts
beets
broccoli
brussels sprouts
cabbage (green, bok choy, Chinese)
carrots
cauliflower
celery

cucumber
eggplant
green onions or scallions
greens (e.g., collard, kale, mustard, turnip)
kohlrabi
leeks
mixed vegetables (without corn, peas, or pasta)
mushrooms, all kinds, fresh
okra
onions
pea pods

peppers (all varieties)
radishes
rutabaga
sauerkraut
spinach
squash (summer, zucchini)
Sugar pea snaps
Swiss chard
tomato (fresh, canned, sauce)
tomato/vegetable juice
turnips
water chestnuts

FRUIT EXCHANGE LIST

Fruit

(15 g carbohydrate, 0 g protein, 0 g fat, 60 kcal)
In general, 1 fruit choice is ½ cup of canned or fresh fruit or unsweetened fruit juice, 1 small fresh fruit (4 oz) or 2 tablespoons of dried fruit. 1 fruit exchange equals:

Serving Size	Food	Serving size	Food
1 (4 oz)	apple, unpeeled (small)	17 (3 oz)	grapes (small)
4 rings	apple, dried	1 slice (10 oz)	honeydew melon (or 1 cup cubes)
½ cup	applesauce (unsweetened)	1 (3½ oz)	kiwi
4 (5½ oz)	apricots, fresh	¾ cup	mandarin orange sections
8 halves	apricots, dried	½ (5½ oz)	mango (or ½ cup)
½ cup	apricots, canned	1 (5 oz)	nectarine (small)
1 (4 oz)	banana (small)	1 (6½ oz)	orange (small)
¾ cup	blackberries	½ (8 oz)	papaya (or 1 cup cubes)
¾ cup	blueberries	1 (4–6 oz)	peach, fresh (medium)
⅓ melon (11 oz)	cantaloupe (small)	½ cup	peaches, canned
1 cup cubes	cantaloupe	1 (4 oz)	pear, fresh
12 (3 oz)	cherries	½ cup	pear, canned
½ cup	cherries, sweet canned	¾ cup	pineapple, fresh
3	dates	½ cup	pineapple, canned
2 tbsp	Dried fruits (blueberries, cherries, cranberries, mixed fruit, raisins)	2 (5 oz)	plums (small)
		½ cup	plums, canned
2 (3½ oz)	figs, fresh (large)	3	plums dried (prunes)
1½	figs, dried	1 cup	raspberries
½ cup	fruit cocktail	1¼ cup	strawberries (raw, whole)
½ (11 oz)	grapefruit (large)	2 (8 oz)	tangerines (small)
¾ cup	grapefruit sections, canned	1 slice (13½ oz)	watermelon (or 1¼ cups cubes)

Fruit Juice

Serving Size	Food	Serving Size	Food
½ cup	apple juice/cider	½ cup	orange juice
⅓ cup	fruit juice blends, 100% juice	½ cup	pineapple juice
⅓ cup	grape juice	⅓ cup	prune juice
½ cup	grapefruit juice		

STARCH EXCHANGE LIST

(15 g carbohydrate, 0–3 g protein, 0–1 g fat, 80 kcal)
In general, 1 starch is ½ cup of cooked cereal, grain, or starchy vegetable, ⅓ cup of cooked rice or pasta, 1 oz of a bread product, such as 1 slice of bread, or ¾ oz to 1 oz of most snack foods. 1 starch exchange equals:

Bread

Serving Size	Food	Serving Size	Food
¼ (1 oz)	bagel, large (about 4 oz)	1	pancake, 4 inch across × ¼ inch thick
2 slices (1½ oz)	bread, reduced-calorie	½	pita, 6 inches across
1 slice (1 oz)	bread, white, whole-wheat, pumpernickel, grain or rye, or unfrosted raisin	1 slice (1 oz)	raisin bread, unfrosted
		1 (1 oz)	roll, plain (small)
4 (⅔ oz)	bread sticks, crisp, 4 inch × ½ inch	1	tortilla, corn, 6 inches across
½	English muffin	1	tortilla, flour, 6 inches across
½ (1 oz)	hot dog or hamburger bun	⅓	tortilla, flour, 10 inches across
¼	naan, 8 inch × 2 inch	1	waffle, 4 inches square or across, reduced-fat

Cereals and Grains

Serving Size	Food	Serving Size	Food
½ cup	bran cereal, bran	3 tbsp	cornmeal (dry)
½ cup	bulgur	⅓ cup	couscous
½ cup	cereal, cooked (oats, oatmeal)	3 tbsp	flour (dry)
¾ cup	cereal, unsweetened, ready-to-eat	¼ cup	granola, low-fat

Serving Size	Food	Serving Size	Food
½ cup	grits	⅓ cup	quinoa, cooked
½ cup	kasha	⅓ cup	rice, white or brown
⅓ cup	millet, cooked	½ cup	tabbouleh (tabouli), prepared
¼ cup	muesli	3 tbsp	wheat germ
⅓ cup	pasta, cooked	½ cup	wild rice, cooked
⅓ cup	polenta, cooked		

Starchy Vegetables

Serving Size	Food	Serving Size	Food
⅓ cup	cassava	½ cup or ½ medium (3 oz)	potato, boiled
½ cup	corn	¼ large (3 oz)	potato, baked with skin
½ (5 oz)	corn on the cob (large)	½ cup	potato, mashed with milk and fat
1 cup	mixed vegetables with corn, peas, or pasta	½ cup	spaghetti or pasta sauce, canned
½ cup	peas, green	1 cup	squash, winter (acorn, butternut, pumpkin)
½ cup	plantain, ripe	½ cup	yam, sweet potato, plain

Crackers and Snacks

Serving Size	Food	Serving Size	Food
8	animal crackers	¾ oz	pretzels
3	graham crackers, 2½-inch square	2	rice cakes, 4 inches across
¾ oz	matzoh	6	saltine-type crackers
4 slices	melba toast	15–20 (¾ oz)	snack chips, fat-free (tortilla, potato)
20	oyster crackers	2–5 (¾ oz)	whole-wheat crackers, no fat added
3 cups	popcorn (no fat added or lower-fat microwave)		

Dried Beans, Peas, and Lentils

(Counts as 1 starch exchange plus 1 very lean meat exchange)

Serving Size	Food	Serving Size	Food
⅓ cup	baked beans	½ cup	lentils
½ cup	beans and peas (garbanzo, pinto, kidney, white, split, black-eyed)	⅔ cup	lima beans
		3 tbsp	miso

Starchy Foods Prepared with Fat

(Counts as 1 starch exchange, plus 1 fat exchange)

Serving Size	Food	Serving Size	Food
1	biscuit, 2½ inches across	3 cups	popcorn, with butter
½ cup	chow mein noodles	3	sandwich crackers, cheese or peanut butter filling
1 piece (2 oz)	corn bread, 2-inch cube	9–13 (3/4 oz)	snack chips (potato, tortilla)
6	crackers, round butter type	⅓ cup	stuffing, bread
1 cup	croutons	2	taco shells, 6 inches across
1 cup (2 oz)	French-fried potatoes (oven-baked) (see also the fast-foods list)	1	waffle, 4-inch square or across
¼ cup	granola	4–6 (1 oz)	whole-wheat crackers, fat added
⅓ cup	hummus		

SWEETS, DESSERTS AND OTHER CARBOHYDRATES EXCHANGE LIST

One exchange equals 15 g carbohydrate, protein, fat and kcal vary.

Exchanges per Serving

Serving Size	Food	
1/12 cake (about 2 oz)	angel food cake, unfrosted	2 carbohydrates
2-inch square (about 1 oz)	brownie, unfrosted (small)	1 carbohydrate, 1 fat
2-inch square (about 1 oz)	cake, unfrosted	1 carbohydrate, 1 fat
2-inch square (about 2 oz)	cake, frosted	2 carbohydrates, 1 fat
2	cookies, fat-free (small)	1 carbohydrate
2 (about ⅔ oz)	cookies or sandwich cookies with creme filling (small)	1 carbohydrate, 1 fat
¼ cup	cranberry sauce, jellied	1½ carbohydrates
1 (about 2 oz)	cupcake, frosted (small)	2 carbohydrates, 1 fat
1 (1½ oz)	doughnut, plain cake (medium)	1½ carbohydrates, 2 fats
3¾ inches across (2 oz)	doughnuts, glazed	2 carbohydrates, 2 fats
1 bar (1⅓ oz)	Energy, sport, or breakfast bar	2 carbohydrates, 1 fat
1 bar (2 oz)	Energy, sport, or breakfast bar	3 carbohydrates, 1 fat
½ cup (3 ½ oz)	fruit cobbler	3 carbohydrates, 1 fat
1 bar (3 oz)	fruit juice bars, frozen, 100% juice	1 carbohydrate
1 roll (¾ oz)	fruit snacks, chewy (puréed fruit concentrate)	1 carbohydrate
1½ tbsp	fruit spread, 100% fruit	1 carbohydrate
½ cup	gelatin, regular	1 carbohydrate
3	gingersnaps	1 carbohydrate
1 bar (1 oz)	granola or snack bar (regular and low-fat)	1½ carbohydrates
1 tbsp	honey	1 carbohydrate
½ cup	ice cream, low-fat	1½ carbohydrates
½ cup	ice cream	1 carbohydrate, 2 fats
½ cup	ice cream, light	1 carbohydrate, 1 fat
½ cup	ice cream, fat-free, no sugar added	1 carbohydrate
1 tbsp	jam or jelly, regular	1 carbohydrate
1 cup	milk, chocolate, whole	2 carbohydrates, 1 fat
¼ (1 oz)	muffin, 5 oz	1 carbohydrate, ½ fat
⅙ pie	pie, fruit, 2 crusts (8 inches across)	3 carbohydrates, 2 fats
⅛ pie	pie, pumpkin or custard (8 inches across)	2 carbohydrates, 2 fats
½ cup	pudding, regular (made with reduced-fat milk)	2 carbohydrates
½ cup	pudding, sugar-free (made with fat-free milk)	1 carbohydrate
1 can (10–11 oz)	reduced-calorie meal replacement (shake)	1½ carbohydrates, 0–1 fat
1 cup	rice milk, low-fat or fat-free, plain	1 carbohydrate
1 cup	rice milk, low-fat, flavored	1½ carbohydrates
¼ cup	salad dressing, fat-free	1 carbohydrate
½ cup	sherbet, sorbet	2 carbohydrates
1 cup (8 oz)	sports drinks	1 carbohydrate
1 tbsp	sugar	1 carbohydrate
1 (2½ oz)	sweet roll or Danish	2½ carbohydrates, 2 fats
2 tbsp	syrup, light	1 carbohydrate
1 tbsp	syrup, regular	1 carbohydrate
5	vanilla wafers	1 carbohydrate, 1 fat
⅓ cup	yogurt, frozen, fat-free	1 carbohydrate
1 cup	yogurt, low-fat with fruit	3 carbohydrates, 0–1 fat

MEAT AND MEAT SUBSTITUTES EXCHANGE LIST

Lean Meat and Substitutes List

(0 g carbohydrate, 7 g protein, 0–3 g fat, and 45 kcal)
One lean meat exchange equals:

Serving Size	Food	Serving Size	Food
1 oz	Beef: USDA Select or Choice grades of lean beef trimmed of fat: round, sirloin, and flank steak; tenderloin; roast (rib, chuck, rump); steak (T-bone, porterhouse, cubed), ground round	1 oz 6	Fish, smoked: herring or salmon (lox) oysters (medium)
1 oz	Pork, lean: ham; Canadian bacon; tenderloin, center loin chop	1 oz	Fish, fresh or frozen, plain: catfish, cod, flounder, haddock, halibut, orange roughy, salmon, tilapia, trout, tune
1 oz	Lamb: roast, chop, leg	1 oz ¼ cup	Game: buffalo, ostrich, rabbit, venison cottage cheese
1 oz	Veal, lean chop, roast	1 oz	cheeses with 3 g or less fat per oz
1 oz	Poultry, without skin: chicken, turkey, domestic duck or goose (well drained of fat, no skin)	¼ cup 2 1½ oz 1 oz	egg substitute, plain egg whites hot dogs with 3 g or less fat per oz Shellfish: clams, crab, lobster, scallops, shrimp, imitation shellfish
1 oz	processed sandwich meats with 1 g or less fat per oz, such as deli thin, shaved meats, chipped beef, turkey, ham	1 oz	sausage with 1 g or less fat per os

Medium-Fat Meat and Substitutes List

(0 g carbohydrate, 7 g protein, 4–7 g fat, and 75 kcal)
One medium-fat meat exchange equals:

Serving Size	Food	Serving Size	Food
1 oz	Beef: (ground beef; meatloaf; corned beef; short ribs; prime grades of meat trimmed (prime rib)	1 oz 1 oz	Fish: any fish product Cheese with 4–7 grams pf fat per oz: feta, mozzarella, pasteurized processed cheese spread, reduced-fat cheeses, string
1 oz	Pork: top loin, chop, Boston butt, cutlet, shoulder roast	¼ cup (2 oz)	ricotta cheese
1 oz	Lamb: rib roast, ground		**Other**
1 oz	Veal, cutlet (no breading) cubed, unbreaded	1	egg (high in cholesterol, limit to 3 per week)
1 oz	Poultry: chicken (with skin), dove, pheasant, wild duck or goose, ground turkey, fried chicken	1 oz	sausage with 4–7 grams of fat per oz

Plant-Based Proteins

(each exchange provides 7 g protein, carbohydrate, fat, and kcal vary)

Serving Size	Food	
3 strips	"bacon" strips, soy-based	1 medium-fat meat
⅓ cup	baked beans	1 starch + 1 lean meat
½ cup	beans, cooked: black, garbanzo, kidney, lima, navy, pinto, white	1 starch + 1 lean meat
2 oz	"beef" or "sausage" crumbles, soy-based	½ carbohydrate + 1 lean meat
2 nuggets (1½ oz)	"chicken" nuggets, soy-based	½ carbohydrate + 1 medium-fat meat
½ cup	edamame	½ carbohydrate + 1 lean meat
3 patties	falafel (spiced chickpea and wheat patties about 2 inches across)	1 carbohydrate + 1 high-fat meat
1 (1½ oz)	hot dog, soy-based	½ carbohydrate + 1 lean meat
⅓ cup	hummus	1 carbohydrate + 1 high-fat meat

Serving Size	Food	
½ cup	lentils, brown, green or yellow	1 carbohydrate + 1 lean meat
3 oz	meatless burger, soy-based	½ carbohydrate + 2 lean meats
1 tbsp	nut spreads: almond butter, cashew butter, peanut butter, soy nut butter	1 high-fat meat
½ cup	peas, cooked: black-eyed and split peas	1 starch + 1 lean meat
½ cup	refried beans, canned	1 starch + 1 lean meat
1 (1½ oz)	"sausage" patties, soy-based	1 medium-fat meat
¾ oz	soy nuts, unsalted	½ carbohydrate + 1 medium-fat meat
¼ cup	tempeh	1 medium-fat meat
4 oz (½ cup)	tofu	1 medium-fat meat
4 oz (½ cup)	tofu, light	1 lean meat

High-Fat Meat and Substitutes List

(0 g carbohydrate, 7 g protein, 8+ g fat, and 100 kcal)
One high-fat meat exchange equals:

Serving Size	Food
1 oz	Pork: spareribs, ground sausage
1 oz	Cheese: regular: American, bleu, brie, cheddar, hard goat, Monterey jack, queso, Swiss
1 oz	processed sandwich meats with 8 grams or more per oz, such as bologna, pastrami, hard salami
1 oz	sausage with 8 grams of fat or more per oz: such as bratwurst, chorizo, Italian, knockwurst, Polish, smoked, summer

Serving Size	Food
1	hot dog (turkey or chicken) (10 per pound)
2 slices	pork bacon (16 slices per pound)
3 slices	turkey bacon (½ oz each before cooking) bacon (20 slices per pound)
Counts as one high-fat meat plus one fat exchange:	
1	hot dog (beef, pork, or combination; turkey or chicken) (10 per pound-sized package)

FAT EXCHANGE LIST

Monounsaturated Fats List

(5 g fat and 45 kcal)
One exchange equals:

Serving Size	Food
2 tbsp (1 oz)	avocado (medium)
1 tsp	oil (canola, olive, peanut)
	olives:
8	ripe, black (large)
10	green, stuffed (large)
6 nuts	almonds, cashews
6 nuts	mixed (50% peanuts)

Serving Size	Food
10 nuts	peanuts
16 nuts	pistachios
4 halves	pecans
1 tbsp	nut butters (**trans** fat-free): almond butter, cashew butter, peanut butter, smooth or crunchy

Polyunsaturated Fats List

(5 g fat and 45 kcal)
One exchange equals:

Serving Size	Food
	margarine:
1 tsp	stick, tub, or squeeze (**trans** fat-free)
1 tbsp	lower-fat (30% to 50% vegetable oil) (**trans** fat-free)
	mayonnaise:
1 tsp	regular
1 tbsp	reduced-fat
4 halves	nuts, walnuts, English
1 tbsp	nuts, pignolia (pine nuts)

Serving Size	Food
1 tsp	oil (corn, cottonseed, flaxseed, grape seed, safflower, soybean, sunflower)
	salad dressing:
1 tbsp	regular
2 tbsp	reduced-fat
1 tbsp	seeds: flaxseed (whole), pumpkin, sesame, sunflower
2 tsp	tahini or sesame paste

Saturated Fats List

(5 g fat and 45 kcal)
One exchange equals:

Serving Size	Food	Serving Size	Food
1 slice	bacon, cooked, regular or turkey	1 tsp	shortening or lard
2 tbsp (½ oz)	chitterlings, boiled		butter blends made with oil:
2 tbsp	coconut, sweetened, shredded cream	1½ tsp	regular
2 tbsp	half and half	1 tbsp	reduced-fat or light
1 tbsp	heavy		butter:
1½ tbsp	light	1 tsp	stick
2 tbsp	whipped	2 tsp	whipped
¼ cup	whipped, pressurized	1 tbsp	reduced-fat
	cream cheese:		sour cream:
1 tbsp (½ oz)	regular	2 tbsp	regular
1½ tbsp (¾ oz)	reduced-fat	3 tbsp	reduced-fat

FREE FOODS LIST

A *free food* is any food or drink that contains less than 20 kcal or less than 5 g of carbohydrate per serving. Foods with a serving size listed should be limited to three servings per day. Foods listed without a serving size can be eaten as often as you like.

Modified Fat Foods with Carbohydrate

Serving Size	Food	Serving Size	Food
1 tbsp (½ oz)	cream cheese, fat-free	1 tsp	mayonnaise, reduced-fat
1 tbsp	creamers, nondairy, liquid	1 tbsp	salad dressing, fat-free or low-fat, Italian
2 tsp	creamers, nondairy, powdered	2 tbsp	salad dressing, fat-free, Italian
1 tbsp	margarine, fat-free	1 tbsp	sour cream, fat-free, reduced-fat
1 tsp	margarine, reduced-fat	1 tbsp	whipped topping, regular
1 tbsp	mayonnaise, fat-free	2 tbsp	whipped topping, light or fat-free

Low Carbohydrate Foods

Serving Size	Food	Serving Size	Food
1 candy	candy, hard, (regular or sugar-free)		salad greens
2 tsp	jam or jelly, light or no sugar added*		sugar substitutes
		2 tbsp	syrup, sugar-free

Drinks

Serving Size	Food	Serving Size	Food
	bouillon, broth, consommé		diet soft drinks, sugar-free
	bouillon or broth, low-sodium		drink mixes, sugar-free
	carbonated or mineral water		tea, unsweetened or with sugar substitute
	club soda		tonic water, sugar-free
1 tbsp	cocoa powder, unsweetened		water
	coffee, unsweetened or with sugar substitute		water, flavored, carbohydrate free

Condiments

Serving Size	Food	Serving Size	Food
2 tsp	barbecue sauce	2 slices	pickles, sweet (bread and butter)
1 tbsp	catsup	¾ oz	pickles, sweet (gherkin)
	horseradish	¼ cup	salsa
	lemon juice	1 tbsp	soy sauce, regular or light
	mustard	1 tbsp	taco sauce
1½ tsp	miso		vinegar
1 tbsp	pickle relish	2 tbsp	yogurt, any type
1½	pickles, dill (medium)		

Seasonings

flavoring extracts
garlic
herbs, fresh or dried
nonstick cooking spray
pimento

spices
hot pepper sauce
wine, used in cooking
Worcestershire sauce

COMBINATION FOODS LIST

Serving Size	Food Desription	Exchanges per Serving
	Entrées	
1 cup (8 oz)	Casserole type (tuna noodle), lasagna, spaghetti with meatballs, chili with beans, macaroni and cheese	2 carbohydrates, 2 medium-fat meats
1 cup (8 oz)	stews (beef/other meats and vegetables)	1 carbohydrate, 1 medium-fat meat, 0–3 fats
½ cup (3½ oz)	tuna or chicken salad	½ carbohydrate, 2 lean meats, 1 fat
	Frozen Entrées and Meals	
1 (5 oz)	burrito (beef and bean)	
generally 14–17 oz	dinner-type meal	3 carbohydrates, 1 lean meat, 2 fats
¼ of 12-inch (6 oz)	pizza, cheese, thin crust	2 carbohydrates, 2 medium-fat meats, 1½ fats
¼ of 12-inch (6 oz)	pizza, meat topping, thin crust	2 carbohydrates, 2 medium-fat meats, 1½ fats
1 (4½ oz)	pocket sandwich	
1 (7 oz)	pot pie	2½ carbohydrates, 1 medium-fat meat, 3 fats
8–11 oz	entrée or meal with less than 340 kcal	2–3 carbohydrates, 1–2 lean meats
	Soups	
1 cup	bean	1 carbohydrate, 1 very lean meat
1 cup (8 oz)	cream (made with water)	1 carbohydrate, 1 fat
6 oz prepared	instant	1 carbohydrate
8 oz prepared	instant with beans/lentils	2½ carbohydrates, 1 very lean meat
½ cup (4 oz)	split pea (made with water)	1 carbohydrate
1 cup (8 oz)	tomato (made with water)	1 carbohydrate
1 cup (8 oz)	vegetable beef, chicken noodle, or other broth-type	1 carbohydrate

Fast-Foods

Serving Size	Food Description	Exchanges per Serving
1 (about 8 oz)	burritos beef and beans	3 carbohydrates, 3 medium-fat meat, 3 fat
6	chicken nuggets	1 carbohydrate, 2 medium-fat meats, 1 fat
1 each	chicken breast, breaded and fried	1 carbohydrate, 4 medium-fat meats
1	chicken sandwich, grilled	2 carbohydrates, 3 very lean meats
6 (5 oz)	chicken wings, hot	5 high-fat meats, 1½ fats
1	fish sandwich/tartar sauce	2½ carbohydrates, 2 medium-fat meats, 2 fats
1 medium serving (5 oz)	French fries	4 carbohydrates, 4 fats
1	hamburger (regular)	2 carbohydrates, 1 medium-fat, 1 fat
1	hamburger (large)	2 carbohydrates, 3 medium-fat meats, 1 fat
1	hot dog with bun	1 carbohydrate, 1 high-fat meat, 1 fat
¼ 12-inch (about 6 oz)	pizza, cheese, thin crust	2½ carbohydrates, 2 medium-fat meats, 1½ fat
⅛ 14-inch (about 4 oz)	pizza, meat, thin crust	2½ carbohydrates, 1 medium-fat meat, 1½ fat
1 (5 oz)	soft-serve cone (small)	2½ carbohydrates, 1 fat
1 sub (6 inches)	submarine sandwich	3½ carbohydrates, 2 medium-fat meats, 1 fat
1 (3–3½ oz)	taco, hard or soft shell	1 carbohydrate, 1 medium-fat meat, 1½ fat

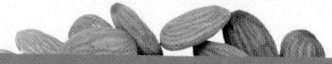

APPENDIX E Dietary Intake and Energy Expenditure Assessment

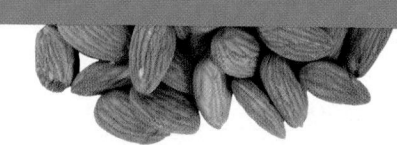

Although it may seem overwhelming at first, it is easy to track the foods you eat. One tip is to record foods and beverages consumed as soon as possible after consumption.

I. **Fill in the food record form that follows.** Appendix E contains a blank copy (see the completed example in Table E-1). Then, to estimate the nutrient values of the foods you are eating, consult food labels and use the NutritionCalc Plus software (CD or online) available with this book. If these resources do not have the serving size you need, adjust the value. If you drink ½ cup of orange juice, for example, but a table has values only for 1 cup, halve all values before you record them. Then, consider pooling all the same food to save time; if you drink a cup of 1% milk three times throughout the day, enter your milk consumption only once as 3 cups. As you record your intake for use on the nutrient analysis form that follows, consider the following tips:

- Measure and record the amounts of foods eaten in portion sizes of cups, teaspoons, tablespoons, ounces, slices, or inches (or convert metric units to these units).
- Record brand names of all food products, such as "Quick Quaker Oats."
- Measure and record all those little extras, such as gravies, salad dressings, taco sauces, pickles, jelly, sugar, catsup, and margarine.
- For beverages
  - List the type of milk, such as whole, fat-free, 1%, evaporated, chocolate, or reconstituted dry.
  - Indicate whether fruit juice is fresh, frozen, or canned.
  - Indicate type for other beverages, such as fruit drink, fruit-flavored drink, Kool-Aid, and hot chocolate made with water or milk.
- For fruits
  - Indicate whether fresh, frozen, dried, or canned.
  - If whole, record number eaten and size with approximate measurements (such as 1 apple—3 in. in diameter).
  - Indicate whether processed in water, light syrup, or heavy syrup.
- For vegetables
  - Indicate whether fresh, frozen, dried, or canned.
  - Record as portion of cup, teaspoon, or tablespoon, or as pieces (such as carrot sticks—4 in. long, ½ in. thick).
  - Record preparation method.
- For cereals
  - Record cooked cereals in portions of tablespoon or cup (a level measurement after cooking).
  - Record dry cereal in level portions of tablespoon or cup.
  - If margarine, milk, sugar, fruit, or something else is added, measure and record amount and type.
- For breads
  - Indicate whether whole wheat, rye, white, and so on.
  - Measure and record number and size of portion (biscuit—2 in. across, 1 in. thick; slice of homemade rye bread—3 in. by 4 in., ¼ in. thick).
  - Sandwiches: list all ingredients (lettuce, mayonnaise, tomato, and so on).

- For meat, fish, poultry, and cheese
  - Give size (length, width, thickness) in inches or weight in ounces after cooking for meat, fish, and poultry (such as cooked hamburger patty—3 in. across, ½ in. thick).
  - Give size (length, width, thickness) in inches or weight in ounces for cheese.
  - Record measurements only for the cooked, edible part—without bone or fat left on the plate.
  - Describe how meat, poultry, or fish was prepared.
- For eggs
  - Record as soft or hard cooked, fried, scrambled, poached, or omelet.
  - If milk, butter, or drippings are used, specify types and amount.
- For desserts
  - List commercial brand or "homemade" or "bakery" under brand.
  - Purchased candies, cookies, and cakes: specify kind and size.
  - Measure and record portion size of cakes, pies, and cookies by specifying thickness, diameter, and width or length, depending on the item.

TABLE E-1 One Day's Food Record—This Activity Can Help You Understand More About Your Food Habits

Time	Minutes Spent Eating	M or S*	H† (0–3)	Activity While Eating	Place of Eating	Food and Quantity	Others Present	Reason for Choice
7:10 a.m.	15	M	2	Standing, fixing lunch	Kitchen	Orange juice, 1 cup Crispix, 1 cup Non-fat milk, ½ cup Sugar, 2 tsp Black coffee	—	Health Habit Health Taste Habit
10:00 a.m.	4	S	1	Sitting, taking notes	Classroom	Diet cola, 12 oz	Class	Weight control
12:15 p.m.	40	M	2	Sitting, talking	Student union	Chicken sandwich with lettuce and mayonnaise (3 oz chicken, 2 slices of white bread, 2 tsp mayonnaise) Pear, 1 medium Non-fat milk, 1 cup	Friends	Taste Health Health
2:30 p.m.	10	S	1	Sitting, studying	Library	Regular cola, 12 oz	Friend	Hunger
6:30 p.m.	35	M	3	Sitting, talking	Kitchen	Pork chop, 1 Baked potato, 1 Margarine, 2 tbsp Lettuce and tomato salad, 1 cup Ranch dressing, 2 tbsp Peas, ½ cup Whole milk, 1 cup Cherry pie, 1 piece Iced tea, 12 oz	Boyfriend	Convenience Health Taste Health Taste Health Habit Taste Health
9:10 p.m.	10	S	2	Sitting, studying	Living room	Apple, 1 medium Glass mineral water, 1	—	Weight control Weight control

*M or S: Meal or snack
†H: Degree of hunger (0 = none; 3 = maximum)

Time	Minutes Spent Eating	M or S*	H† (0–3)	Activity While Eating	Place of Eating	Food and Quantity	Others Present	Reason for Choice

*M or S: Meal or snack
†H: Degree of hunger (0 = none; 3 = maximum)

II. **Now complete the nutrient analysis form as shown, using your food record.**
A blank copy of this form for your use is on pages A-41 and A-42. NutritionCalc Plus will create such a table for you if you enter all food eaten.

Nutrient Analysis Form (Sample)

Name	Quantity	kcal	Protein (g)	Carbohydrates (g)	Fiber (g)	Total fat (g)	Monounsaturated fat (g)	Polyunsaturated fat (g)	Saturated fat (g)	Cholesterol (g)	Calcium (mg)	Iron (mg)
Egg bagel, 3.5-in. diameter	1 ea.	180	7.45	34.7	0.748	1.00	0.286	0.400	0.171	44.0	20.0	2.10
Jelly	1 tbsp	49.0	0.018	12.7	—	0.018	0.005	0.005	0.005	—	2.00	0.120
Orange juice, prepared fresh or frozen	1½ cup	165	2.52	40.2	1.49	0.210	0.037	0.045	0.025	—	33.0	0.411
Cheeseburger, McDonald's	2 ea.	636	30.2	57.0	0.460	32.0	12.2	2.18	13.3	80.0	338	5.68
French fries, McDonald's	1 order	220	3.00	26.1	4.19	11.5	4.37	0.570	4.61	8.57	9.10	0.605
Cola beverage, regular	1½ cup	151	—	38.5	—	—	—	—	—	—	9.00	0.120
Pork loin chop, broiled, lean	4 oz	261	36.2	—	—	11.9	5.35	1.43	4.09	112	5.67	1.04
Baked potato with skin	1 ea.	220	4.65	51.0	3.90	0.200	0.004	0.087	0.052	—	20.0	2.75
Peas, frozen, cooked	½ cup	63.0	4.12	11.4	3.61	0.220	0.019	0.103	0.039	—	19.0	1.25
Margarine, regular or soft, 80% fat	20 g	143	0.160	0.100	—	16.1	5.70	6.92	2.76	—	5.29	—
Iceberg lettuce, chopped	2 cup	14.6	1.13	2.34	1.68	0.212	0.008	0.112	0.028	—	21.2	0.560
French dressing	2 oz	300	0.318	3.63	0.431	32.0	14.2	12.4	4.94	—	7.10	0.227
Reduced-fat (i.e., 2%) milk	1 cup	121	8.12	11.7	—	4.78	1.35	0.170	2.92	22.0	297	0.120
Graham crackers	2 ea.	60.0	1.04	10.8	1.40	1.46	0.600	0.400	0.400	—	6.00	0.367
Totals		2584	99.0	300	17.9	112	44.1	24.8	33.4	266	792	15.4
RDA or related nutrient standard*		2900	58	130	38						1000	8
% of nutrient needs		89	170	230	47						79	193

Abbreviations: g = grams, mg = milligrams, µg = micrograms

*Values from inside cover. The values listed are for a male age 19 years. The number of kcal is a rough estimate. It is better to base energy needs on actual energy output.

†In RAE units. Table values generally are in RE units because the food values have not been updated to reflect the latest vitamin A standards. RAE equals RE for foods with preformed vitamin A, such as for the pork chop, but RAE are only about half the RE listed for foods with provitamin A carotenoids, such as for the peas (see Chapter 8 for details).

‡Amounts refer to actual folate content, rather than dietary folate equivalents (DFE). This difference is important to consider if the food contains added synthetic folic acid as part of enrichment or fortification. Any such folic acid is absorbed about twice as much as the folate present naturally in foods. So the total contribution of folate in the food in comparison to human needs will be greater than if all the folate was naturally in the food product. Nutrient analysis tables have yet to be updated to reflect the dietary folate equivalents of products (see Chapter 8 for more details).

Nutrient Analysis Form (Sample) Cont'd

Magnesium (mg)	Phosphorus (mg)	Potassium (mg)	Sodium (mg)	Zinc (mg)	Vitamin A (RE)	Vitamin C (mg)	Vitamin E (mg)	Thiamin (mg)	Riboflavin (mg)	Niacin (mg)	Vitamin B-6 (mg)	Folate (µg)	Vitamin B-12 (µg)
18.0	61.0	65.0	300	0.612	7.00	—	1.80	2.58	0.197	2.40	0.030	16.3	0.065
0.720	1.00	16.0	4.00	—	0.200	0.710	0.016	0.002	0.005	0.036	0.005	2.00	—
36.0	60.0	711	3.00	0.192	28.5	145	0.714	0.300	0.060	0.750	0.165	163	
45.8	410	314	1460	5.20	134	4.10	0.560	0.600	0.480	8.66	0.230	42.0	1.82
26.7	101	564	109	0.320	5.00	12.5	0.203	0.122	0.020	2.26	0.218	19.0	0.027
3.00	46.0	4.00	15.0	0.049	—	—	—	—	—	—	—	—	—
34.0	277	476	88.2	2.54	3.15	0.454	0.405	1.30	0.350	6.28	0.535	6.77	0.839
55.0	115	844	16.0	0.650	—	26.1	0.100	0.216	0.067	3.32	0.701	22.2	—
23.0	72.0	134	70.0	0.750	53.4	7.90	0.400	0.226	0.140	1.18	0.090	46.9	—
0.467	4.06	7.54	216	0.041	199	0.028	2.19	0.002	0.006	0.004	0.002	0.211	0.017
10.1	22.4	177	10.1	0.246	37.0	4.36	0.120	0.052	0.034	0.210	0.044	62.8	—
5.81	3.63	7.03	666	0.045	0.023	—	15.9	—	—	—	0.006	—	—
33.0	232	377	122	0.963	140	2.32	0.080	0.095	0.403	0.210	0.105	12.0	0.888
6.00	20.0	36.0	86.0	0.113	—	—	—	0.020	0.030	0.600	0.011	1.80	—
298	1425	3732	3165	11.7	607	204	22.5	5.52	1.79	25.9	2.14	395	3.65
400	700	4700	1500	11	900†	90	15	1.2	1.3	16	1.3	400‡	2.4
75	204	80	210	106	67	226	150	450	138	162	160	99	152

Nutrient Analysis Form

Name	Quantity	kcal	Protein (g)	Carbohydrates (g)	Fiber (g)	Total fat (g)	Monounsaturated fat (g)	Polyunsaturated fat (g)	Saturated fat (g)	Cholesterol (g)	Calcium (mg)	Iron (mg)
Totals												
RDA or related nutrient standard*												
% of nutrient needs												

*Values from inside cover. The number of kcals is a rough estimate. It is better to base energy needs on actual energy output.

†Use RAE values.

‡Use DFE values.

Nutrient Analysis Form cont'd

Magnesium (mg)	Phosphorous (mg)	Potassium (mg)	Sodium (mg)	Zinc (mg)	Vitamin A (RE)	Vitamin C (mg)	Vitamin E (mg)	Thiamin (mg)	Riboflavin (mg)	Niacin (mg)	Vitamin B-6 (mg)	Folate (µg)	Vitamin B-12 (µg)

III. **Complete the following table as you summarize your dietary intake.**

Percentage of kcal from Protein, Fat, Carbohydrate, and Alcohol

Intake

Protein (P):   ____g/day × 4 kcal per gram   = (P)____kcal per day
Fat (F):   ____g/day × 9 kcal per gram   = (F)____kcal per day
Carbohydrate (C):   ____g/day × 4 kcal per gram   = (C)____kcal per day
Alcohol (A):   = (A)____kcal per day*
                          Total kcal (T)/day   = (T)____kcal per day

Percentage of kcal from protein:

$$\frac{(P)}{(T)} \times 100 = \text{____}\%$$

Percentage of kcal from fat:

$$\frac{(F)}{(T)} \times 100 = \text{____}\%$$

Percentage of kcal from carbohydrate:

$$\frac{(C)}{(T)} \times 100 = \text{____}\%$$

Percentage of kcal from alcohol:

$$\frac{(A)}{(T)} \times 100 = \text{____}\%$$

Note: The four percentages can total 99, 100, or 101, depending on the way in which figures were rounded off earlier.

*To calculate how many kcal in a beverage are from alcohol, first look up the beverage using the Nutrition Calc software. Then determine how many kcal are from carbohydrate (multiply carbohydrate grams times 4), fat (fat grams times 9), and protein (protein grams times 4). The remaining kcal are from alcohol.

IV. **Use the table on the following page to again record your food intake for one day, placing each food item in the correct category of MyPlate, with the correct number of servings (see Chapter 2).** A food such as a turkey and cheese sandwich contributes to three categories: grains, protein foods, and dairy. You can expect that many food choices will contribute to more than one group. Indicate the number of servings from MyPlate that each food yields.

Indicate the Number of Servings from MyPlate That Each Food Yields

Food or Beverage	Amount Eaten	Dairy	Protein	Fruits	Vegetables	Grains	SoFAS*
Group totals							
Recommended servings from www.Choose MyPlate.gov's Daily Food Plan							
Overages/Shortages in numbers of servings							

*SoFAS: solid fats and added sugars

V. **Evaluation.** Are there weaknesses suggested in your nutrient intake that correspond to missing servings in MyPlate? Consider adjusting your food choices to comply with MyPlate standards to improve your nutrient intake.

VI. **For the same day you keep your food record, also keep a 24-hour record of your activities.** Include sleeping, sitting, and walking, as well as the obvious forms of exercise. Calculate your energy expenditure for these activities using Table 7-4 in Chapter 7 or the diet analysis software available with this book. Try to substitute a similar activity if your particular activity is not listed. Calculate the total kcal you used for the day (total for column 3). Following is an example of an activity record. A blank form follows for your use. Ask your professor whether you are to turn in the form or the activity printout from NutritionCalc Plus.

Weight (kg)*: 70 kg

Activity	Time (Minutes): Convert to Hours	Energy Cost		
		Column 1 kcal/kg/hr (from Table 7-4)	Column 2 (Column 1 × Time)	Column 3 (Column 2 × Weight in kg)
Brisk walking	(60 min) 1 hr	4.4	(× 1) = 4.4	(× 70) = 308

*lb/2.2

Weight (kg)*:

Activity	Time (Minutes): Convert to Hours	Energy Cost		
		Column 1 kcal/kg/hr (from Table 7-4)	Column 2 (Column 1 × Time)	Column 3 (Column 2 × Weight in kg)

Total kcal used (from adding all of column 3)
*lb/2.2

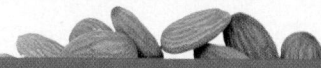

APPENDIX F Chemical Structures Important in Nutrition

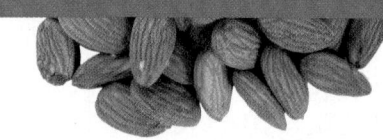

AMINO ACIDS

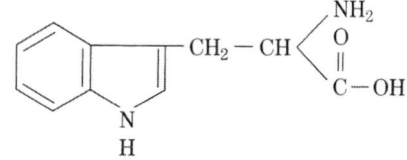

Histidine (His)
(essential)

Tryptophan (Trp)
(essential)

Glycine (Gly)

Methionine (Met)
(essential)

Leucine (Leu)
(essential)

Alanine (Ala)

Arginine (Arg)
(essential in infancy)

Lysine (Lys)
(essential)

Proline (Pro)

Glutamic Acid (Glu)

Aspartic Acid (Asp)

Serine (Ser)

Phenylalanine (Phe)
(essential)

Isoleucine (Ile)
(essential)

Tyrosine (Tyr)

Glutamine (Gln)

Asparagine (Asn)

Threonine (Thr)
(essential)

Valine (Val)
(essential)

Cysteine (Cys)

VITAMINS

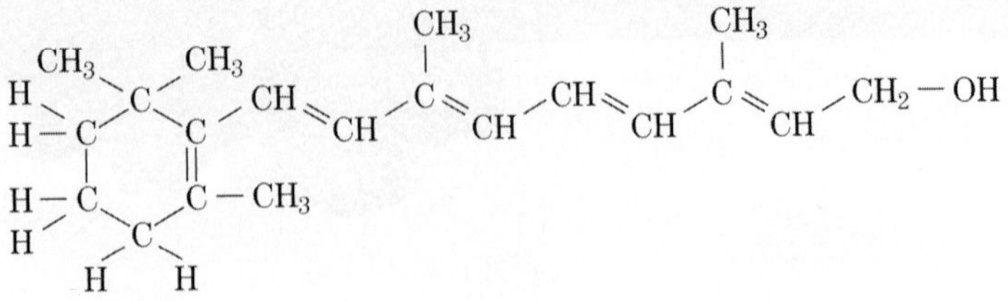

Vitamin A: retinol

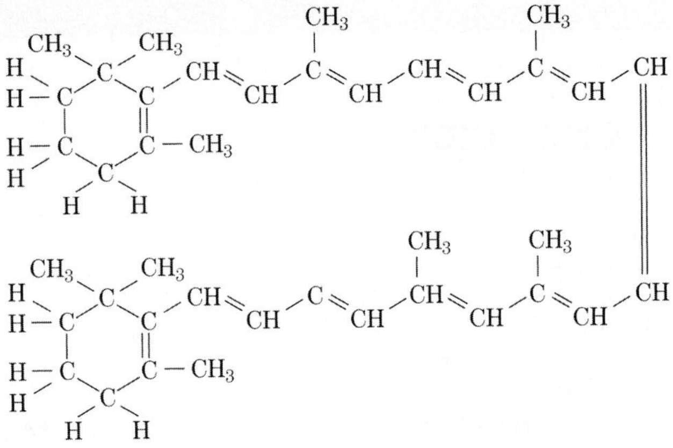

Beta-carotene

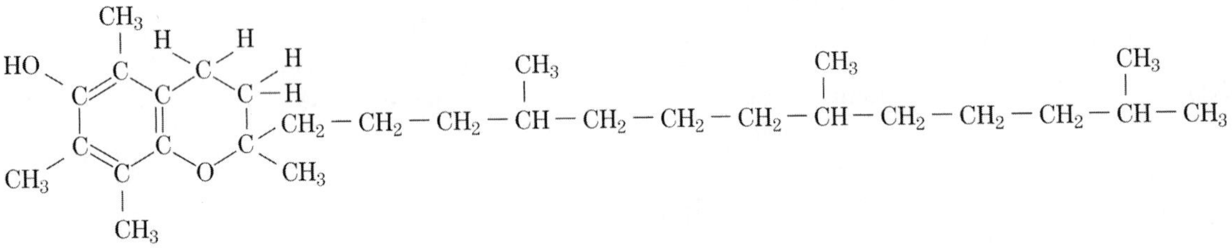

Vitamin E

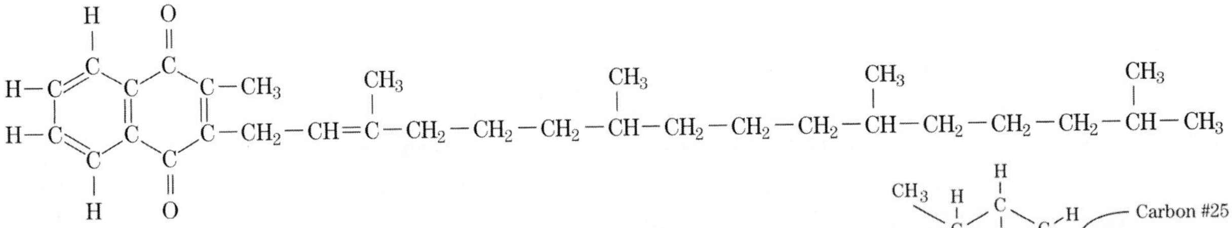

Vitamin K

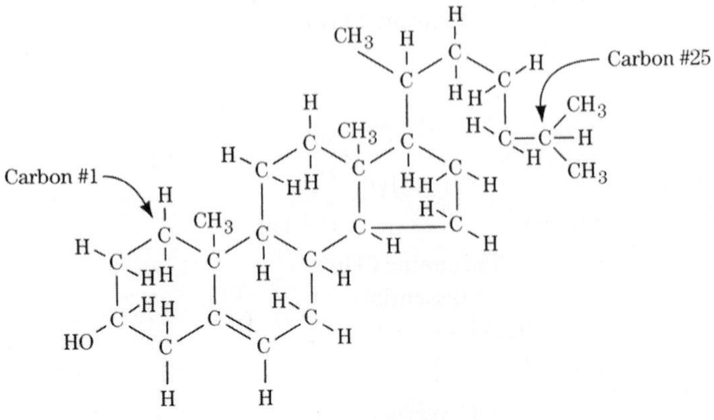

7-dehydrocholesterol

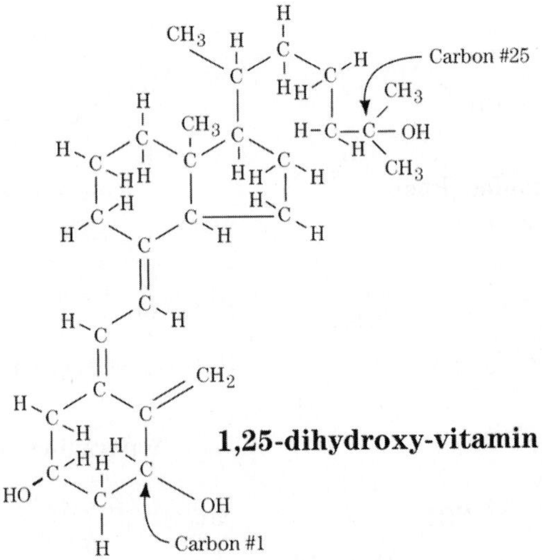

1,25-dihydroxy-vitamin D₃ (calcitriol)

Active vitamin D (calcitriol) and its precursor 7-dehydrocholesterol

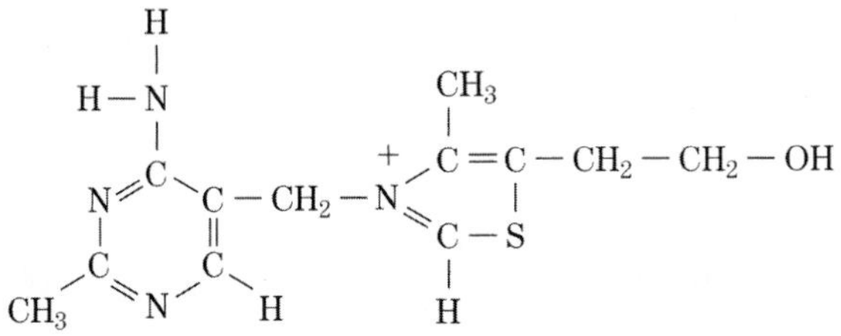

Thiamin

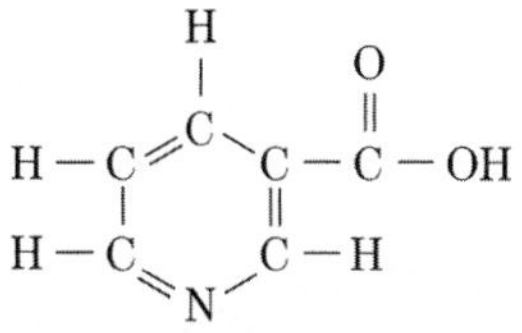

Nicotinic acid 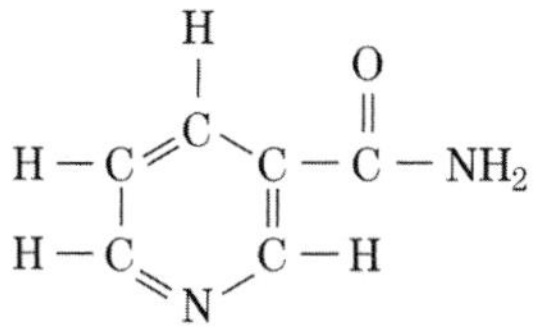   Nicotinamide

Niacin (nicotinic acid and nicotinamide)

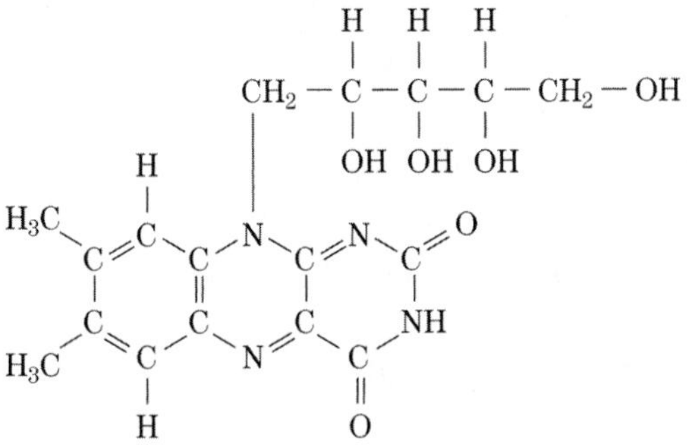

Riboflavin

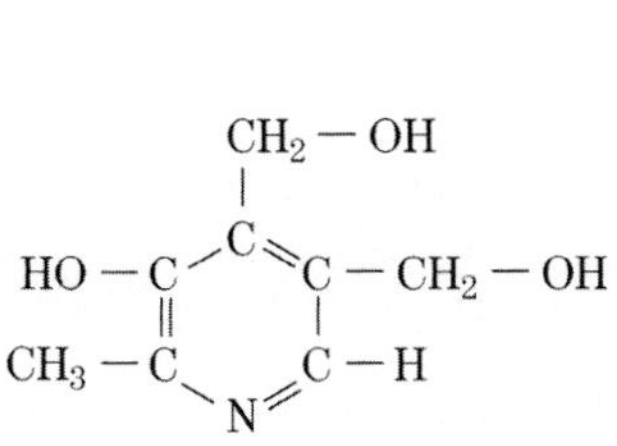

Pyridoxine 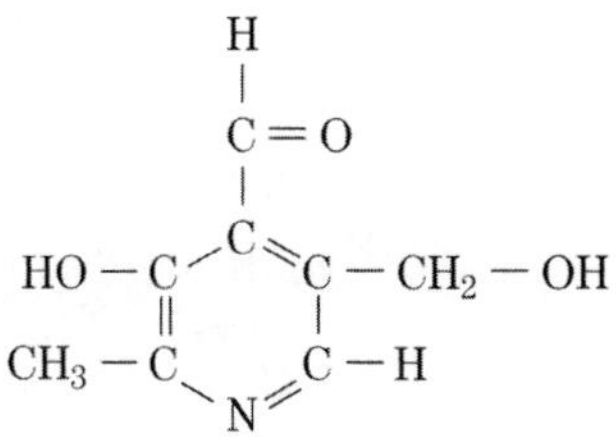   Pyridoxal 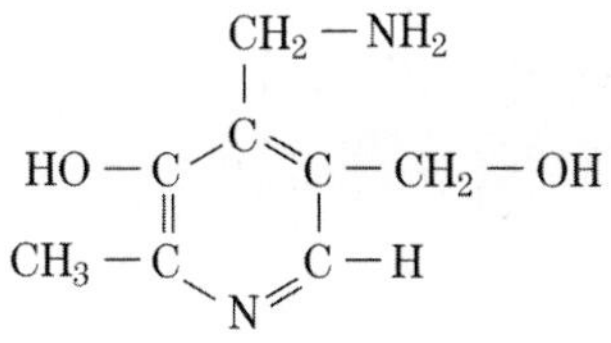   Pyridoxamine

**Vitamin B-6 (a general name for three compounds—
pyridoxine, pyridoxal, and pyridoxamine)**

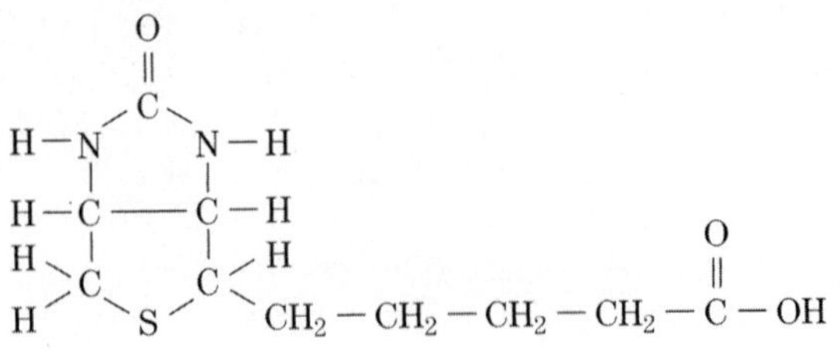

Biotin

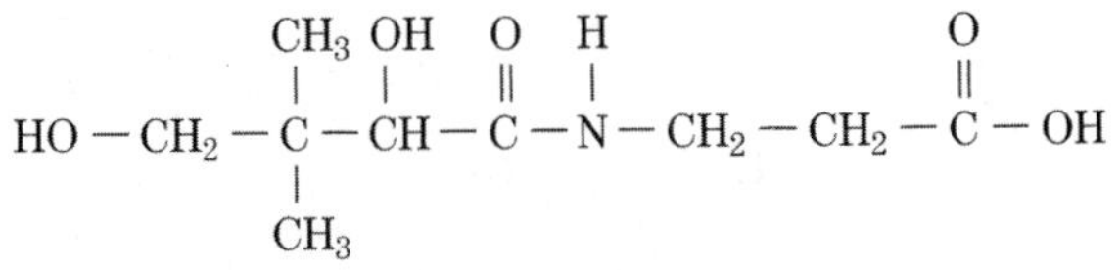

Pantothenic acid

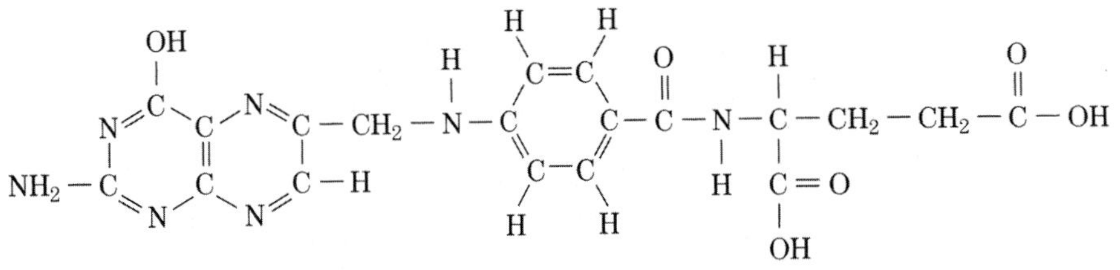

Folate (folic acid form)

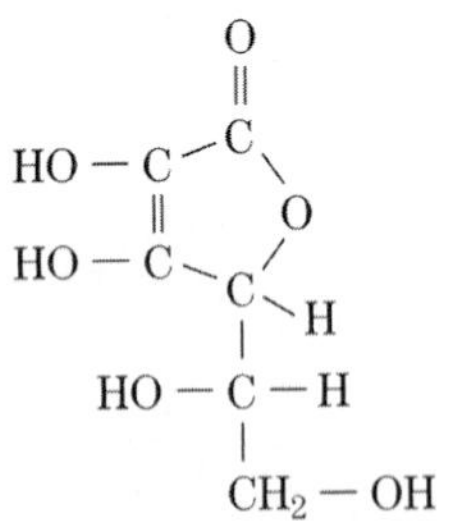

Vitamin C (ascorbic acid)

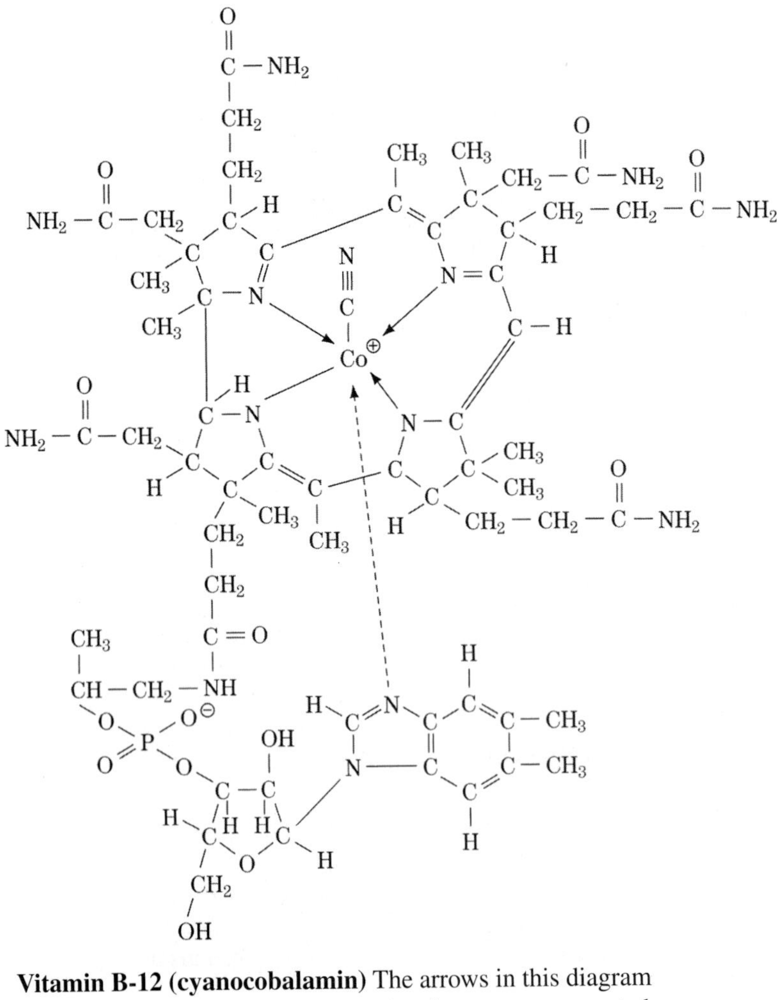

Vitamin B-12 (cyanocobalamin) The arrows in this diagram indicate that the spare electrons on the nitrogens are attracted to the cobalt atom.

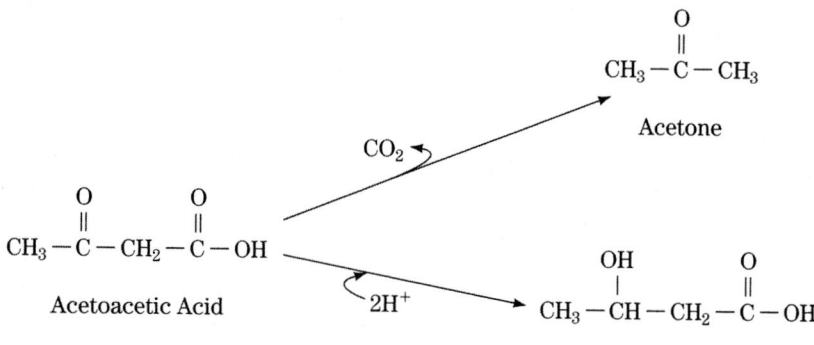

Ketone Bodies

Acetone

Acetoacetic Acid

ß-Hydroxybutyric Acid

Triphosphate

Point of cleavage to yield
ADP and energy release

Adenine

Ribose
(a sugar)

**Adenosine Triphosphate
(ATP)**

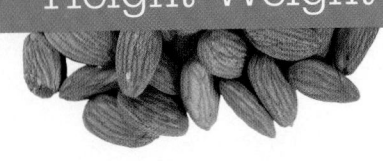
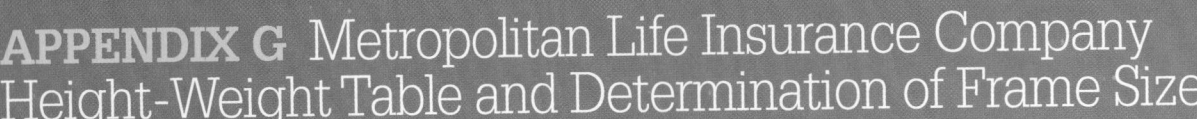

1983 Metropolitan Life Insurance Company Height-Weight Table* †

Women					Men				
Height		Frame			Height		Frame		
Ft.	In.	Small	Medium	Large	Ft.	In.	Small	Medium	Large
4	10	102–111	109–121	118–131	5	2	128–134	131–141	138–150
4	11	103–113	111–123	120–134	5	3	130–136	133–143	140–153
5	0	104–115	113–126	122–137	5	4	132–138	135–145	142–156
5	1	106–118	115–129	125–140	5	5	134–140	137–148	144–160
5	2	108–121	118–132	128–143	5	6	136–142	139–151	146–164
5	3	111–124	121–135	131–147	5	7	138–145	142–154	149–168
5	4	114–127	124–138	134–151	5	8	140–148	145–157	152–172
5	5	117–130	127–141	137–155	5	9	142–151	148–160	155–176
5	6	120–133	130–144	140–159	5	10	144–154	151–163	158–180
5	7	123–136	133–147	143–163	5	11	146–157	154–166	161–184
5	8	126–139	136–150	146–167	6	0	149–160	157–170	164–188
5	9	129–142	139–153	149–170	6	1	152–164	160–174	168–192
5	10	132–145	142–156	152–173	6	2	155–168	164–178	172–197
5	11	135–148	145–159	155–176	6	3	158–172	167–182	176–202
6	0	138–151	148–162	158–179	6	4	162–176	171–187	181–207

*Based on a weight-height mortality study conducted by the Society of Actuaries and the Association of Life Insurance Medical Directors of America, Metropolitan Life Insurance Medical Directors of America, Metropolitan Life Insurance Company, revised 1983.
†Weights in pounds (lb) at ages 25 to 59 based on lowest mortality. Height includes 1-in. heel. Weight for women includes 3 lb for indoor clothing. Weight for men includes 5 lb for indoor clothing.

Reprinted courtesy of Metropolitan Life Insurance Company, *Statistical Bulletin*.

Permission granted courtesy of Metropolitan Life Insurance Company, *Statistical Bulletin*.

USING THE METROPOLITAN LIFE INSURANCE TABLE TO ESTIMATE HEALTHY WEIGHT

The Metropolitan Life Insurance table is a common method for estimating healthy weight. The table lists, for any height, the weight that is associated with a maximum life span. The table does not tell the healthiest weight for a living person; it lists the weight associated with longevity.

There are many criticisms of this table. These stem from the inclusion of some people and the exclusion of others. For example, only policyholders of life insurance are included. In addition, smokers are included, but anyone over the age of 60 is excluded. Weight is only measured at the time of purchase of insurance, and there is no follow-up. All of these factors contribute to the fact that this table is to be used only as a rough screening tool; not meeting the exact recommendations should not be cause for alarm.

To diagnose overweight or obesity using the table, calculate the percentage of the Metropolitan Life Insurance table weight. Use the midpoint of a weight range for a specific height.

Equation:
$$\frac{(\text{Current wt.} - \text{wt. from table})}{\text{Weight from table}} \times 100$$

Example: $$\frac{140 - 120}{120} \times 100 = 17\% \text{ over standard}$$

Overweight can be defined as weighing at least 10% more than the weight listed on the table. Determination of obesity is 20% more than that listed on the table. Moreover, this measure of obesity comes in degrees. Whereas mild obesity carries little health risk, severe obesity raises overall health risk twelvefold.

Degrees of Obesity	
% Over Healthy Body Weight	**Form of Obesity**
20–40%	Mild
41–99%	Moderate
100%+	Severe

DETERMINING FRAME SIZE

Method 1

Height is recorded without shoes.

Wrist circumference is measured just beyond (toward the hand) the bony (styloid) process at the wrist joint on the right arm, using a tape measure.

The following formula is used:

$$r = \frac{\text{Height (cm)}}{\text{Wrist circumference (cm)}}$$

Frame size can be determined as follows:[†]

Males	Females
$r > 10.4$ small	$r > 11$ small
$r = 9.6–10.4$ medium	$r = 10.1–11$ medium
$r < 9.6$ large	$r < 10.1$ large

[†]From Grant JP: *Handbook of Total Parenteral Nutrition*. Philadelphia: WB Saunders, 1980.

Method 2

The person's right arm is extended forward, perpendicular to the body, with the arm bent so the angle at the elbow forms 90 degrees, with the fingers pointing up and the palm turned away from the body. The greatest breadth across the elbow joint is measured with a sliding caliper along the axis of the upper arm, on the two prominent bones on either side of the elbow. This is recorded as the elbow breadth. The following tables give elbow breadth measurements for medium-framed men and women of various heights. Measurements lower than those listed indicate a small frame size; higher measurements indicate a large frame size.[‡]

Men		Women	
Height in 1″ Heels	**Elbow Breadth**	**Height in 1″ Heels**	**Elbow Breadth**
5′2″–5′3″	2½–2⅞″	4′10″–4′11″	2¼–2½″
5′4″–5′7″	2⅝–2⅞″	5′0″–5′3″	2¼–2½″
5′8″–5′11″	2¾–3″	5′4″–5′7″	2⅜–2⅝″
6′0″–6′3″	2¾–3¼″	5′8″–5′11″	2⅜–2⅝″
6′4″ and over	2⅞–3¾″	6′0″ and over	2½–2¾″

[‡]From Metropolitan Life Insurance Co., 1983.

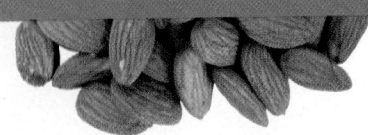

Consider the following reliable sources of food and nutrition information:

Journals That Regularly Cover Nutrition Topics

American Family Physician*
American Journal of Clinical Nutrition
American Journal of Epidemiology
American Journal of Medicine
American Journal of Nursing
*American Journal of Obstetrics and
    Gynecology*
American Journal of Physiology
American Journal of Public Health
American Scientist
Annals of Internal Medicine
Annual Review of Medicine
Annual Review of Nutrition
Archives of Disease in Childhood
Archives of Internal Medicine
British Journal of Nutrition
BMJ (British Medical Journal)
*Canadian Journal of Dietetic Practice and
    Research*
Cancer

Cancer Research
Circulation
Diabetes
Diabetes Care
Disease-a-Month
FASEB Journal
FDA Consumer*
Food and Chemical Toxicology
Food Engineering
Food Technology
Gastroenterology
Geriatrics
Gut
*Journal of the American College of
    Nutrition**
*Journal of the American Dietetic
    Association**
Journal of the American Geriatrics Society
*JAMA (Journal of the American Medical
    Association)*
Journal of Applied Physiology
Journal of Clinical Investigation
Journal of Food Science

*JNCI (Journal of the National Cancer
    Institute)*
Journal of Nutrition
*Journal of Nutrition Education and
    Behavior**
Journal of Nutrition for the Elderly
Journal of Pediatrics
Lancet
Mayo Clinic Proceedings
Medicine & Science in Sports & Exercise
Nature
The New England Journal of Medicine
Nutrition
Nutrition Reviews
Nutrition in Clinical Practice*
Nutrition Today*
Pediatrics
The Physician and Sports Medicine
Postgraduate Medicine*
Proceedings of the Nutrition Society
Science
Science News*
Scientific American*

The majority of these journals are available in college and university libraries or in a specialty library on campus, such as one designated for health services or home economics. As indicated, a few journals will be filed under their abbreviations, rather than the first word in their full name. A reference librarian can help you locate any of these sources. The journals with an asterisk (*) are ones you may find especially interesting and useful because of the number of nutrition articles presented each month or the less technical nature of the presentation.

Magazines for the Consumer That Cover Nutrition Topics

Better Homes and Gardens
Good Housekeeping

Health
Men's Health

Parents
Self

Textbooks and Other Sources for Advanced Study of Nutrition Topics

Bowman BA, Russell RM: *Present knowledge in nutrition.* Vol. I and II. 9th ed. Washington DC: International Life Sciences Institute, 2006.

Brody T: *Nutritional biochemistry.* 2nd ed. San Diego: Academic Press, 1999.

Gropper SS, Smith JL: *Advanced nutrition and human metabolism.* 5th ed. Florence, KY: Wadsworth, Cengage 2009.

Mahan LK, Escott-Stump S: *Krause's food, and nutrition, therapy.* 12th ed. St. Louis: W.B. Saunders, 2008.

Murray RK and others: *Harper's illustrated biochemistry.* 28th ed. New York: McGraw-Hill, 2009.

Schils ME, Shike M, Ross AC, Caballero B, Cousins RJ: *Modern nutrition in health and disease.* 10th ed. Philadelphia: Lippincott, Williams & Wilkins, 2005.

Stipanuk MH: *Biochemical, physiological, & molecular aspects of human nutrition.* 2nd ed. Philadelphia: Elsevier Health Sciences, 2006.

Newsletters That Cover Nutrition Issues on a Regular Basis

American Institute for Cancer Research e.Newsletter
American Institute for Cancer Research
www.aicr.org

Consumer Health Digest
National Council Against Health Fraud
www.ncahf.org

The Dairy Download
National Dairy Council
www.nationaldairycouncil.org

Diabetes E-News (and others)
American Diabetes Association
www.diabetes.org

Environmental Nutrition
www.environmentalnutrition.com

Harvard Health Letter (and others)
Harvard Medical School
www.health.harvard.edu/newsletters

Health and Nutrition Letter
Tufts University
www.healthletter.tufts.edu

In-Touch
Heinz Infant Nutrition Institute
www.hini.org

Mayo Clinic House call
Mayo Clinic
www.mayoclinic.com

Nutrition Action Healthletter
Center for Science in the Public Interest
www.cspinet.org

Nutrition CloseUp
Egg Nutrition Center
www.enc-online.org

Soy Connection
United Soybean Board
www.soyconnection.com

U-Mail: Everyday Nutrition Solutions You Can Use
National Cattlemen's Beef Association
www.beefnutrition.org

Wellness Letter
University of California at Berkeley
www.wellnessletter.com

Professional Organizations

American Academy of Pediatrics
141 Northwest Point Boulevard
Elk Grove Village, IL 60007-1098
www.aap.org

American Cancer Society
1599 Clifton Road, NE
Atlanta, GA 30329
www.cancer.org

American College of Sports Medicine
PO Box 1440
Indianapolis, IN 46206-1440
www.acsm.org

American Dental Association
211 East Chicago Avenue
Chicago, IL 60611-2678
www.ada.org

American Diabetes Association
1701 North Beauregard Street
Alexandria, VA 22311
www.diabetes.org

American Dietetic Association
120 South Riverside Plaza #2000
Chicago, IL 60606-6995
www.eatright.org

American Geriatrics Society
40 Fulton Street, 18th Floor
New York, NY 10038
www.americangeriatrics.org

American Heart Association
7272 Greenville Avenue
Dallas, TX 75231
www.americanheart.org

American Medical Association
515 North State Street
Chicago, IL 60610
www.ama-assn.org

American Public Health Association
800 I Street, NW
Washington, DC 20001-3710
www.apha.org

American Society for Nutrition
9650 Rockville Pike #L-4500
Bethesda, MD 20814
www.nutrition.org

Canadian Council of Food and Nutrition
2810 Matheson Boulevard East, 1st Floor
Mississaugo, Ontario L4W 4X7
http://www.ccfn.ca/

Canadian Diabetes Association
1400-522 University Avenue
Toronto, ON M5G 2R5
www.diabetes.ca

Canadian Nutrition Society
310-2175 Sheppard Avenue East
Toronto, Ontario M2J 1W8
www.cns-scn.ca

Dietitians of Canada
480 University Avenue #604
Toronto, ON M5G 1V2
www.dietitians.ca

Environmental Working Group
1436 U Street, NW #100
Washington, DC 20009
www.ewg.org

Food and Nutrition Board
Institute of Medicine
The National Academies
500 Fifth Street, NW
Washington, DC 20001
www.iom.edu/cMs/3788.aspx

Institute of Food Technologists
525 West Van Buren #1000
Chicago, IL 60607
www.ift.org

National Council on Aging
1901 L Street, NW, 4th floor
Washington, DC 20036
www.ncoa.org

National Osteoporosis Foundation
1150 17th Street, NW #850
Washington, DC 20036
www.nof.org

Society for Nutrition Education
9100 Purdue Road, Suite 200
Indianapolis, IN 46268
www.sne.org

Professional Organizations with a Commitment to Nutrition Issues

Bread for the World Institute
425 3rd Street SW #1200
Washington, DC 20024
www.bread.org

Food Research and Action Center
1875 Connecticut Avenue, NW #540
Washington, DC 20009 http://frac.org/

Institute for Food and Development Policy
398 60th Street
Oakland, CA 94618
www.foodfirst.org

La Leche League International
957 N. Plum Grove Road
Schaumburg, IL 60173
www.llli.org

March of Dimes
1275 Mamaroneck Avenue
White Plains, NY 10605
www.marchofdimes.com

National Council Against Health Fraud
119 Foster Street
Peabody, MA 01960
www.ncahf.org

National WIC Association
2001 S Street, NW #580
Washington, DC 20009
www.nwica.org

Overeaters Anonymous
PO Box 44020
Rio Rancho, NM 87174-4020
www.oa.org

Oxfam America
226 Causeway Street, 5th floor
Boston, MA 02114-2206
www.oxfamamerica.org

Local Resources for Advice on Nutrition Issues

Registered dietitians (RDs or in Canada also RDNs) in health care, city, county, or state agencies, as well as in private practice
Cooperative extension agents in county extension offices
Nutrition faculty affiliated with departments of food and nutrition, home economics, and dietetics

Government Agencies Concerned with Nutrition Issues or That Distribute Nutrition Information

United States

Agricultural Research Service
United States Department of Agriculture
Jamie L. Whitten Building
1400 Independence Avenue, SW
Washington, DC 20250
www.ars.usda.gov

Federal Citizen Information Center
31201 Bryan Circle
Pueblo, CO 81001
www.pueblo.gsa.gov

Food and Drug Administration
10903 New Hampshire Avenue
Silver Spring, MD 20993
www.fda.gov

Food Safety & Inspection Service
United States Department of Agriculture
331-E Jamie L. Whitten Building
1400 Independence Avenue, SW
Washington, DC 20250-3700
www.fsis.usda.gov

MyPlate
USDA Center for Nutrition Policy and Promotion
3101 Park Center Drive #1034
Alexandria, VA 22302-1594
www.choosemyplate.gov

National Agricultural Library
Abraham Lincoln Building
10301 Baltimore Avenue
Beltsville, MD 20705-2351
www.nal.usda.gov

National Cancer Institute
6116 Executive Boulevard #3036A
Bethesda, MD 20892-8322
www.cancer.gov

National Center for Health Statistics
1600 Clifton Road
Atlanta, GA 30333
www.cdc.gov/nchs

National Heart, Lung, and Blood Institute
Building 31, Room 5A52
31 Center Drive, MSC 2486
Bethesda, MD 20892
www.nhlbi.nih.gov

National Institute on Aging
Building 31, Room 5C27
31 Center Drive, MSC 2292
Bethesda, MD 20892
www.nia.nih.gov

U.S. Government Printing Office
710 North Capitol Street, NW
Washington, DC 20401
www.gpo.gov

Canada

Canadian Food Inspection Agency
1400 Merivale Road
Ottawa, Ontario K1A 0Y9
www.inspection.gc.ca

Health Canada
Brooke Claxton Building
Ottawa, Ontario K1A 0K9
www.hc-sc.gc.ca

United Nations

Food and Agriculture Organization
Liaison Office with North America
1 United Nations Plaza #DC1 - 1125
New York, NY 10017
www.fao.org

World Health Organization
Avenue Appia 20
1211 Geneva 27
Switzerland
www.who.int

Trade Organizations and Companies That Distribute Nutrition Information

Abbott Nutrition
625 Cleveland Avenue
Columbus, OH 43215-1724
www.abbottnutrition.com

American Institute of Baking
1213 Bakers Way
PO Box 3999
Manhattan, Kansas 66505-3999
www.aibonline.org

American Meat Institute
1150 Connecticut Avenue, NW, 12th floor
Washington, DC 20036
www.meatami.com

Beech-Nut Nutrition
13023 Tesson Ferry Road
St. Louis, MO 63128
www.beechnut.com

Campbell Soup Company
1 Campbell Place
Camden, NJ 08103-1701
www.campbellsoup.com

Dannon Company
P.O. Box 90296
Allentown, PA 18109-0296
www.dannon.com

Del Monte Foods
One Maritime Plaza
San Francisco, CA 94111
www.delmonte.com

DSM Nutritional Products
45 Waterview Boulevard
Parsippany, NJ 07054-1298
www.dsm.com

General Mills/Pillsbury
PO Box 9452
Minneapolis, MN 55440
www.generalmills.com

Gerber Products Company
445 State Street
Fremont, MI 49413-0001
www.gerber.com

H.J. Heinz
90 Sheppard Avenue East #400
Toronto, ON M2N 7K5
www.heinzbaby.com

Idaho Potato Commission
661 South Rivershore Lane
Eagle, ID 83616
www.idahopotatoes.com

Kellogg Company
One Kellogg Square
Battle Creek, MI 49016
www.kelloggs.com/us/

Kraft Foods Global
1 Kraft Court
Glenview, IL 60025
www.kraftrecipes.com

Mead Johnson Nutritionals
2400 West Lloyd Expressway
Evansville, IN 47721-0001
www.meadjohnson.com

National Dairy Council
10255 West Higgins Road #900
Des Plaines, IL 60018
www.nationaldairycouncil.org

NutraSweet Company
222 Merchandise Mart Plaza
Chicago, IL 60654
www.nutrasweet.com

Sunkist Growers
14130 Riverside Drive
Sherman Oaks, CA 91423
www.sunkist.com

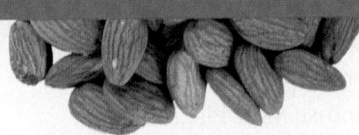

APPENDIX I English-Metric Conversions and Metric Units

METRIC-ENGLISH CONVERSIONS

Length

English (USA)	Metric
inch (in)	= 2.54 cm, 25.4 mm
foot (ft)	= 0.30 m, 30.48 cm
yard (yd)	= 0.91 m, 91.4 cm
mile (statute) (5280 ft)	= 1.61 km, 1609 m
mile (nautical) (6077 ft, 1.15 statute mi)	= 1.85 km, 1850 m

Metric	English (USA)
millimeter (mm)	= 0.039 in (thickness of a dime)
centimeter (cm)	= 0.39 in
meter (m)	= 3.28 ft, 39.37 in
kilometer (km)	= 0.62 mi, 1091 yd, 3273 ft

Weight

English (USA)	Metric
grain	= 64.80 mg
ounce (oz)	= 28.35 g
pound (lb)	= 453.60 g, 0.45 kg
ton (short—2000 lb)	= 0.91 metric ton (907 kg)

Metric	English (USA)
milligram (mg)	= 0.002 grain (0.000035 oz)
gram (g)	= 0.04 oz ($^1/_{28}$ of an oz)
kilogram (kg)	= 35.27 oz, 2.20 lb
metric ton (1000 kg)	= 1.10 tons

Volume

English (USA)	Metric
cubic inch	= 16.39 cc
cubic foot	= 0.03 m³
cubic yard	= 0.765 m³
teaspoon (tsp)	= 5 ml
tablespoon (tbsp)	= 15 ml
fluid ounce	= 0.03 liter (30 ml)*
cup (c)	= 237 ml
pint (pt)	= 0.47 liter
quart (qt)	= 0.95 liter
gallon (gal)	= 3.79 liters

Metric	English (USA)
milliliter (ml)	= 0.03 oz
liter (L)	= 2.12 pt
liter	= 1.06 qt
liter	= 0.27 gal

1 liter ÷ 1000 = 1 milliliter or 1 cubic centimeter (10^{-3} liter)
1 liter ÷ 1,000,000 = 1 microliter (10^{-6} liter)
*Note: 1 ml = 1 cc

METRIC AND OTHER COMMON UNITS

Unit/Abbreviation	Other Equivalent Measure
milligram/mg	$^1/_{1000}$ of a gram
microgram/μg	$^1/_{1,000,000}$ of a gram
deciliter/dl	$^1/_{10}$ of a liter (about ½ cup)
milliliter/ml	$^1/_{1000}$ of a liter (5 ml is about 1 tsp)
International Unit/IU	Crude measure of vitamin activity generally based on growth rate seen in animals

FAHRENHEIT-CELSIUS CONVERSION SCALE

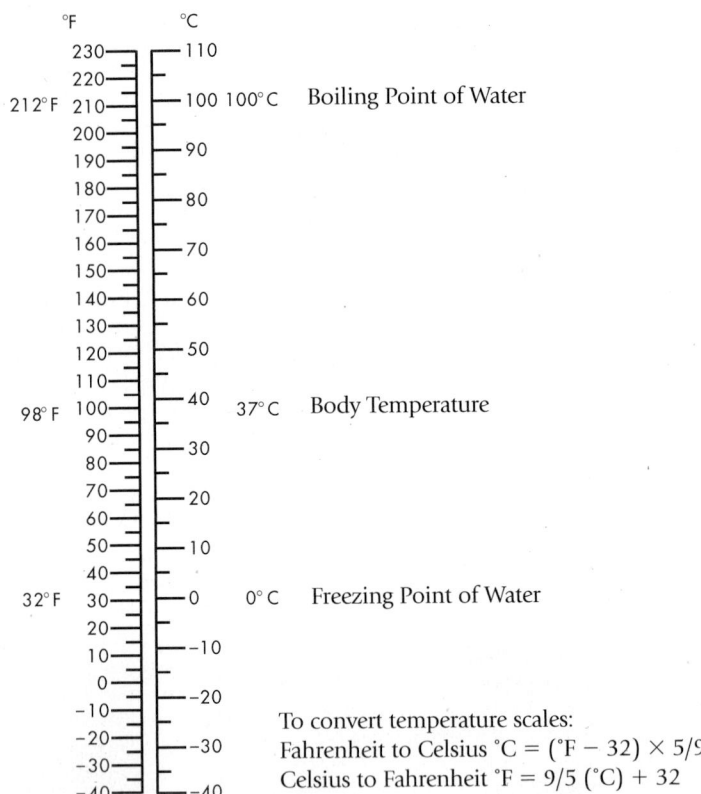

To convert temperature scales:
Fahrenheit to Celsius $°C = (°F - 32) \times 5/9$
Celsius to Fahrenheit $°F = 9/5 (°C) + 32$

HOUSEHOLD UNITS

3 teaspoons	= 1 tablespoon	= 15 grams
4 tablespoons	= ¼ cup	= 60 grams
5⅓ tablespoons	= ⅓ cup	= 80 grams
8 tablespoons	= ½ cup	= 120 grams
10⅔ tablespoons	= ⅔ cup	= 160 grams
16 tablespoons	= 1 cup	= 240 grams
1 tablespoon	= ½ fluid ounce	= 15 milliliters
1 cup	= 8 fluid ounces	= 15 milliliters
1 cup	= ½ pint	= 240 grams
2 cups	= 1 pint	= 480 grams
4 cups	= 1 quart	= 960 grams = 1 liter
2 pints	= 1 quart	= 960 grams = 1 liter
4 quarts	= 1 gallon	= 3840 grams = 4 liters

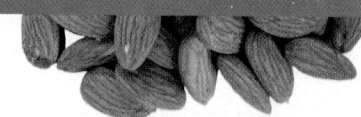

absorption The process by which substances are taken up from the GI tract and enter the bloodstream or the lymph.

absorptive cells The intestinal cells that line the villi; these cells participate in nutrient absorption.

Acceptable Daily Intake (ADI) Estimate of the amount of a sweetener that an individual can safely consume daily over a lifetime. ADIs are given as mg per kg of body weight per day.

acesulfame K Alternative sweetener that yields no energy.

acetaldehyde dehydrogenase An enzyme used in ethanol metabolism that eventually converts acetaldehyde into carbon dioxide and water.

acquired immune deficiency syndrome (AIDS) A disorder in which a virus (human immunodeficiency virus [HIV]) infects specific types of immune system cells. This leaves the person with reduced immune function and, in turn, defenseless against numerous infectious agents; typically contributes to the person's death.

added sugars Sugars or syrups that are added to foods during processing or preparation.

additives Substances added to foods, such as preservatives.

adenosine diphosphate (ADP) A breakdown product of ATP. ADP is synthesized into ATP using energy from foodstuffs and a phosphate group (abbreviated P_i).

adenosine triphosphate (ATP) The main energy currency for cells. ATP energy is used to promote ion pumping, enzyme activity, and muscular contraction.

Adequate Intake (AI) Nutrient intake amount set for any nutrient for which insufficient research is available to establish an RDA. AIs are based on estimates of intakes that appear to maintain a defined nutritional state in a specific life stage.

adipose tissue A group of fat storing cells.

adjustable gastric banding A restrictive procedure in which the opening from the esophagus to the stomach is reduced by a hollow gastric band.

aerobic Requiring oxygen.

aging Time-dependent physical and physiological changes in body structure and function that occur normally and progressively throughout adulthood as humans mature and become older.

air displacement A method for estimating body composition that makes use of the volume of space taken up by a body inside a small chamber.

alcohol Ethyl alcohol or ethanol (CH_3CH_2OH) is the compound in alcoholic beverages.

alcohol abuse Excessive alcohol consumption that leads to severe alcohol-related health and other problems, such as recurrent sickness, inability to fulfill major obligations, use in hazardous situations (e.g., driving), related legal problems, or use despite social and interpersonal difficulties.

alcohol dehydrogenase An enzyme used in alcohol (ethanol) metabolism that converts alcohol into acetaldehyde.

alcohol dependence The person experiences repeated alcohol-related difficulties, such as an inability to control use, spending a great deal of time associated with alcohol use, continued use of alcohol despite physical or psychological consequences, persistent desire or unsuccessful efforts to cut down or control alcohol use, and withdrawal symptoms. Tolerance is also seen.

alcoholism As defined by the American Medical Association, an illness characterized by significant impairment directly related to persistent and excessive use of alcohol.

alcohol-related birth defects (ARBDs) One or more birth defects (e.g., malformations of the heart, bones, kidneys, eyes, or ears) related to confirmed alcohol exposure during gestation.

alcohol-related neurodevelopmental disorders (ARNDs) One or more abnormalities of the central nervous system (e.g., small head size, impaired motor skills, hearing loss, or poor hand-eye coordination) related to confirmed alcohol exposure during gestation.

aldosterone A hormone produced by the adrenal glands that acts on the kidneys to conserve sodium (and therefore water).

allergen A foreign protein, or antigen, that induces excess production of certain immune system antibodies; subsequent exposure to the same protein leads to allergic symptoms. Whereas all allergens are antigens, not all antigens are allergens.

allergy A hypersensitive immune response that occurs when immune bodies produced by us react with a protein we sense as foreign (an antigen).

alpha-linolenic acid An essential omega-3 fatty acid with 18 carbons and three double bonds.

amino acid The building block for proteins containing a central carbon atom with nitrogen and other atoms attached.

amniotic fluid Fluid contained in a sac within the uterus. This fluid surrounds and protects the fetus during development.

amphetamine A group of medications that induce stimulation of the central nervous system and have other effects in the body. Abuse is linked to physical and psychological dependence.

amylase Starch-digesting enzyme produced by the salivary glands or pancreas.

amylopectin A digestible branched-chain type of starch composed of glucose units.

amylose A digestible straight-chain type of starch composed of glucose units.

anaerobic Not requiring oxygen.

anal sphincters A group of two sphincters (inner and outer) that help control expulsion of feces from the body.

analog A chemical compound that differs slightly from another, usually natural, compound. Analogs generally contain extra or altered chemical groups and may have similar or opposite metabolic effects compared with the native compound. Also spelled *analogue*.

anaphylactic shock A severe allergic response that results in lowered blood pressure and respiratory and gastrointestinal distress. This can be fatal.

anemia Generally refers to a decreased oxygen-carrying capacity of the blood. This can be caused by many factors, such as iron deficiency or blood loss.

animal model Use of animals to study disease to understand more about human disease.

anorexia nervosa An eating disorder involving a psychological loss or denial of appetite, followed by self-starvation; related in part to a distorted body image and to various social pressures commonly associated with puberty.

anthropometric assessment Measurement of body weight and the lengths, circumferences, and thicknesses of parts of the body.

antibody Blood protein (immunoglobulin) that binds foreign proteins found in the body. This helps to prevent and control infections.

antidiuretic hormone A hormone that is secreted by the pituitary gland and that acts on the kidneys to decrease water excretion.

antigen Any substance that induces a state of sensitivity and/or resistance to microorganisms or toxic substances after a lag period; foreign substance that stimulates a specific aspect of the immune system.

antioxidant Generally a compound that stops the damaging effects of reactive substances seeking an electron (i.e., oxidizing agents). This prevents breakdown (oxidizing) of substances in foods or the body, particularly lipids.

anus Last portion of the GI tract; serves as an outlet for that organ.

appetite The primarily psychological (external) influences that encourage us to find and eat food, often in the absence of obvious hunger.

arachidonic acid An omega-6 fatty acid made from linoleic acid with 20 carbon atoms and four carbon-carbon double bonds.

artery A blood vessel that carries blood away from the heart.

aseptic processing A method by which food and container are separately and simultaneously sterilized; it allows manufacturers to produce boxes of milk that can be stored at room temperature.

aspartame Alternative sweetener made of 2 amino acids and methanol; about 200 times sweeter than sucrose.

atherosclerosis A buildup of fatty material (plaque) in the arteries, including those surrounding the heart.

atom Smallest combining unit of an element, such as iron or calcium. Atoms consist of protons, neutrons, and electrons.

bacteria Single-cell microorganisms; some produce poisonous substances, which cause illness in humans. Bacteria can be carried by water, animals, and people. They survive on skin, clothes, and hair and thrive in foods at room temperature. Some can live without oxygen and survive by means of spore formation.

bariatrics The medical specialty focusing on the treatment of obesity.

basal metabolism The minimal amount of calories the body uses to support itself in a fasting state when resting (e.g., 12 hours for both) and awake in a warm, quiet environment. It amounts to roughly 1 kcal per kilogram per hour for men and 0.9 kcal per kilogram per hour for women; these values are often referred to as *basal metabolic rate (BMR)*.

benign Noncancerous; tumors that do not spread.

beriberi The thiamin deficiency disorder characterized by muscle weakness, loss of appetite, nerve degeneration, and sometimes edema.

BHA, BHT Butylated hydroxyanisole and butylated hydroxytoluene—two common synthetic antioxidants added to foods.

bile A liver secretion stored in the gallbladder and released through the common bile duct into the first segment of the small intestine. It is essential for the digestion and absorption of fat.

binge-eating disorder An eating disorder characterized by recurrent binge eating and feelings of loss of control over eating that have lasted at least 6 months. Binge episodes can be triggered by frustration, anger, depression, anxiety, permission to eat forbidden foods, and excessive hunger.

bioavailability The degree to which an ingested nutrient is absorbed and thus is available to the body.

biochemical assessment Measurement of biochemical functions (e.g., concentrations of nutrient by-products or enzyme activities in the blood or urine) related to a nutrient's function.

bioelectrical impedance The method to estimate total body fat that uses a low-energy electrical current. The more fat storage a person has, the more impedance (resistance) to electrical flow will be exhibited.

biological pest management Control of agricultural pests by using natural predators, parasites, or pathogens. For example, ladybugs can be used to control an aphid infestation.

biotechnology A collection of processes that involves the use of biological systems for altering and, ideally, improving the characteristics of plants, animals, and other forms of life.

bisphosphonates Compounds primarily composed of carbon and phosphorus that bind to bone mineral and in turn reduce bone breakdown. Examples are alendronate (Fosamax), risedronate (Actonel), and ibandronate (Boniva).

body mass index (BMI) Weight (in kilograms) divided by height (in meters) squared; a value of 25 and above indicates overweight and a value of 30 and above indicates obesity.

bolus A moistened mass of food swallowed from the oral cavity into the pharynx.

bomb colorimeter An instrument used to determine the calorie content of a food.

bond A linkage between two atoms formed by the sharing of electrons, or attractions.

bone mass Total mineral substance (such as calcium or phosphorus) in a cross section of bone, generally expressed as grams per centimeter of length.

bone mineral density Total mineral content of bone at a specific bone site divided by the width of the bone at that site, generally expressed as grams per cubic centimeter.

branched-chain amino acids Amino acids with a branching carbon backbone; these are leucine, isoleucine, and valine. All are essential amino acids.

brown adipose tissue A specialized form of adipose tissue that produces large amounts of heat by metabolizing energy-yielding nutrients without synthesizing much useful energy for the body. The unused energy is released as heat.

buffers Compounds that cause a solution to resist changes in acid-base conditions.

bulimia nervosa An eating disorder in which large quantities of food are eaten at one time (binge eating) and then purged from the body by vomiting, or misuse of laxatives, diuretics, or enemas. Alternate means to counteract the binge behavior are fasting and excessive exercise.

capillary A microscopic blood vessel that connects the smallest arteries and veins; site of nutrient, oxygen, and waste exchange between body cells and the blood.

capillary bed Network of one-cell-thick vessels that create a junction between arterial and venous circulation. It is here that gas and nutrient exchange occurs between body cells and the blood.

carbohydrate A compound containing carbon, hydrogen, and oxygen atoms. Most are known as *sugars*, *starches*, and *fibers*.

carbohydrate loading A process in which a high carbohydrate intake is consumed for 6 days before an athletic event while tapering exercise duration in an attempt to increase muscle glycogen stores.

carbon skeleton Amino-acid structure that remains after the amino group ($-NH_2$) has been removed.

cardiovascular system The body system consisting of the heart, blood vessels, and blood. This system transports nutrients, waste products, gases, and hormones throughout the body and plays an important role in immune responses and regulation of body temperature.

carotenoids Pigment materials in fruits and vegetables that range in color from yellow to orange to red; three of the various carotenoids yield vitamin A. Many are antioxidants.

case-control study A study in which individuals who have a disease or condition, such as lung cancer, are compared with individuals who do not have the condition.

celiac disease Immunological or allergic reaction to the protein gluten in certain grains, such as wheat and rye. The effect is to destroy the intestinal enterocytes, resulting in a much reduced surface area due to flattening of the villi. Elimination of wheat, rye, and certain other grains from the diet restores the intestinal surface.

cell The structural basis of plant and animal organization. In animals it is bounded by a cell membrane. Cells contain both genetic material and systems for synthesizing energy-yielding compounds. Cells have the ability to take up compounds from and excrete compounds into their surroundings.

cell-mediated immunity A process in which certain white blood cells come in contact with the invading cells to destroy them.

cell nucleus An organelle bound by its own double membrane and containing chromosomes, the genetic information for cell protein synthesis and cell replication.

cellulose An undigestible nonfermentable straight-chain polysaccharide made of glucose molecules.

cerebrovascular accident (CVA) Death of part of the brain tissue due typically to a blood clot. Also termed a *stroke*.

chain-breaking Breaking the link between two or more behaviors that encourage overeating, such as snacking while watching television.

chemical reaction An interaction between two chemicals that changes both chemicals.

cholecystokinin (CCK) A hormone that participates in enzyme release from the pancreas, bile release from the gallbladder, and hunger regulation.

cholesterol A waxy lipid found in all body cells. It has a structure containing multiple chemical rings that is found only in foods that contain animal products.

chromosome A single, large DNA molecule and its associated proteins; contains many genes to store and transmit genetic information.

chylomicron Lipoprotein made of dietary fats surrounded by a shell of cholesterol, phospholipids, and protein. Chylomicrons are formed in the absorptive cells of the small intestine after fat absorption and travel through the lymphatic system to the bloodstream.

chyme A mixture of stomach secretions and partially digested food.

cirrhosis A loss of functioning liver cells, which are replaced by nonfunctioning connective tissue. Any substance that poisons liver cells can lead to cirrhosis. The most common cause is a chronic, excessive alcohol intake. Exposure to certain industrial chemicals also can lead to cirrhosis.

cis fatty acid A form of an unsaturated fatty acid that has the hydrogens lying on the same side of the carbon-carbon double bond.

clinical assessment Examination of general appearance of skin, eyes, and tongue; evidence of rapid hair loss; sense of touch; and ability to cough and walk.

coagulation Blood clotting; essentially a transition of blood from a liquid cell suspension into a solid, gel-like form.

coenzyme A compound that combines with an inactive enzyme to form a catalytically active form. In this manner, coenzymes aid in enzyme function.

cofactor A mineral or other substance that binds to a specific region on a protein, such as an enzyme, and is necessary for the protein's function.

cognitive behavior therapy Psychological therapy in which the person's assumptions about dieting, body weight, and related issues are confronted. New ways of thinking are explored and then practiced by the person. In this way, an individual can learn new ways to control disordered eating behaviors and related life stress.

cognitive restructuring Changing one's frame of mind regarding eating—for example, instead of using a difficult day as an excuse to overeat, substituting other pleasures for rewards, such as a relaxing walk with a friend.

colostrum The first fluid secreted by the breast during late pregnancy and the first few days after birth. This thick fluid is rich in immune factors and protein.

Community-supported agriculture (CSA) Farms that are supported by a community of growers and consumers who provide mutual support and share the risks and benefits of food production, usually including a system of weekly delivery or pick-up of vegetables and fruit, sometimes dairy products and meat.

complementary proteins Two food protein sources that make up for each other's inadequate supply of specific essential amino acids; together they yield a sufficient amount of all nine and, so provide high-quality (complete) protein for the diet.

complex carbohydrate Carbohydrate composed of many monosaccharide molecules. Examples include glycogen, starch, and fiber.

compound A group of different types of atoms bonded together in definite proportion.

compression of morbidity Delay of the onset of disabilities caused by chronic disease.

connective tissue Protein tissue that holds different structures in the body together. Some body structures are made up of connective tissue— notably, tendons and cartilage. Connective tissue also forms part of bone and the nonmuscular structures of arteries and veins.

constipation A condition characterized by infrequent bowel movements.

contingency management Forming a plan of action to respond to a situation in which overeating is likely, such as when snacks are within arm's reach at a party.

control group Participants in an experiment who are not given the treatment being tested.

cortical bone Dense, compact bone that comprises the outer surface and shafts of bone; also called compact bone.

creatine An organic (i.e., carbon-containing) molecule in muscle cells that serves as a part of a high-energy compound (termed creatine phosphate or phosphocreatine) capable of synthesizing ATP from ADP.

cretinism The stunting of body growth and poor mental development in the offspring that results from inadequate maternal intake of iodide during pregnancy.

cystic fibrosis Inherited disease that can cause overproduction of mucus. Mucus can block the pancreatic duct, decreasing enzyme output.

cytoplasm The fluid and organelles (except the nucleus) in a cell.

Delaney Clause A clause to the 1958 Food Additives Amendment of the Pure Food and Drug Act in the United States that prevents the intentional (direct) addition to foods of a compound shown to cause cancer in laboratory animals or humans.

dementia A general loss or decrease in mental function.

denaturation Alteration of a protein's three-dimensional structure, usually because of treatment by heat, enzymes, acid or alkaline solutions, or agitation.

dental caries Erosions in the surface of a tooth caused by acids made by bacteria as they metabolize sugars.

deoxyribonucleic acid (DNA) The site of hereditary information in cells; DNA directs the synthesis of cell proteins.

diastolic blood pressure The pressure in the arterial blood vessels when the heart is between beats.

dietary assessment Estimation of typical food choices relying mostly on the recounting of one's usual intake or a record of one's previous days' intake.

dietary fiber Fiber found in food.

Dietary Guidelines for Americans General goals for nutrient intakes and diet composition set by the USDA and the U.S. Department of Health and Human Services.

Dietary Reference Intakes (DRIs) Term used to encompass nutrient recommendations made by the Food and Nutrition Board of the National Academy of Sciences. These include RDAs, EARs, AIs, EERs, and ULs.

digestion The process by which large ingested molecules are mechanically and chemically broken down to produce basic nutrients that can be absorbed across the wall of the GI tract.

digestive system The body system consisting of the gastrointestinal tract and accessory structures such as the liver, gallbladder, and pancreas. This system performs the mechanical and chemical processes of digestion, absorption of nutrients, and elimination of wastes.

diglyceride A breakdown product of a triglyceride consisting of two fatty acids bonded to a glycerol backbone.

direct calorimetry A method of determining a body's energy use by measuring heat released from the body. An insulated chamber is usually used.

disaccharide Class of sugars formed by the chemical bonding of two monosaccharides.

discretionary calories The calories allowed in a diet after the person has met overall nutrition needs. This generally small amount of calories gives individuals the flexibility to consume some foods and beverages that may contain alcohol (e.g., beer and wine), added sugars (e.g., soft drinks, candy, and desserts), or added fats that are part of moderate- or high-fat foods (e.g., many snack foods).

disordered eating Mild and short-term changes in eating patterns that occur in relation to a stressful event, an illness, or a desire to modify one's diet for a variety of health and personal appearance reasons.

diuretic A substance that increases the volume of urine.

diverticula Pouches that protrude through the exterior wall of the large intestine.

diverticulitis An inflammation of the diverticula caused by acids produced by bacterial metabolism inside the diverticula.

diverticulosis The condition of having many diverticula in the large intestine.

docosahexaenoic acid (DHA) An omega-3 fatty acid with 22 carbons and six carbon-carbon double bonds. It is present in large amounts in fatty fish and is slowly synthesized in the body from alpha-linolenic acid. DHA is especially present in the retina and brain.

double-blind study An experimental design in which neither the participants nor the researchers are aware of each participant's assignment (test or placebo) or the outcome of the study until it is completed. An independent third party holds the code and the data until the study has been completed.

dual energy X-ray absorptiometry (DEXA) A highly accurate method of measuring body composition and bone mass and density using multiple low-energy X rays.

early childhood caries Tooth decay that results from formula or juice (and even human milk) bathing the teeth as the child sleeps with a bottle in his or her mouth. The upper teeth are mostly affected as the lower teeth are protected by the tongue; formerly called *nursing bottle syndrome* and *baby bottle tooth decay*.

eating disorder Severe alterations in eating patterns linked to physiological changes. The alterations are associated with food restriction, binge eating, purging, and fluctuations in weight. They also involve a number of emotional and cognitive changes that affect the way a person perceives and experiences his or her body.

eating pattern A combination of foods and beverages that constitute an individual's complete dietary intake over time.

edema The buildup of excess fluid in extracellular spaces.

eicosapentaenoic acid (EPA) An omega-3 fatty acid with 20 carbons and five carbon-carbon double bonds. It is present in large amounts in fatty fish and is slowly synthesized in the body from alpha-linolenic acid.

electrolytes Substances that separate into ions in water and, in turn, are able to conduct an electrical current. These include sodium, chloride, and potassium.

element A substance that cannot be separated into simpler substances by chemical processes. Common elements in nutrition include carbon, oxygen, hydrogen, nitrogen, calcium, phosphorus, and iron.

elimination diet A restrictive diet that systematically tests foods that may cause an allergic response by first eliminating them for 1 to 2 weeks and then adding them back, one at a time.

embryo In humans, the developing offspring in utero from about the beginning of the third week to the end of the eighth week after conception.

empty calories Calories from solid fats and/or added sugars. Foods with empty calories supply energy but few or no other nutrients.

emulsifier A compound that can suspend fat in water by isolating individual fat droplets, using a shell of water molecules or other substances to prevent the fat from coalescing.

endocrine gland A hormone-producing gland.

endocrine system The body system consisting of the various glands and the hormones these glands secrete. This system has major regulatory functions in the body, such as reproduction and cell metabolism.

endometrium The membrane that lines the inside of the uterus. It increases in thickness during the menstrual cycle until ovulation occurs. The surface layers are shed during menstruation if conception does not take place.

endoplasmic reticulum (ER) An organelle in the cytoplasm composed of a network of canals running through the cytoplasm. Part of the endoplasmic reticulum contains ribosomes.

endorphins Natural body tranquilizers that may be involved in the feeding response and function in pain reduction.

energy balance The state in which energy intake, in the form of food and beverages, matches the energy expended, primarily through basal metabolism and physical activity.

energy density A comparison of the calorie (kcal) content of a food with the weight of the food. An energy-dense food is high in calories but weighs very little (e.g., potato chips), whereas a food low in energy density has few calories but weighs a lot, such as an orange.

enterohepatic circulation A continual recycling of compounds such as bile acids between the small intestine and the liver.

environmental assessment Includes details about living conditions, education level, and the ability of the person to purchase, transport, and cook food. The person's weekly budget for food purchases is also a key factor to consider.

enzyme A compound that speeds the rate of a chemical reaction but is not altered by the reaction. Almost all enzymes are proteins (some are made of genetic material).

epidemiology The study of how disease rates vary among different population groups.

epiglottis The flap that folds down over the trachea during swallowing.

epigenetics Inherited changes in gene expression caused by mechanisms other than changes in the DNA sequence.

epigenome The way that the genome is marked and packaged inside the cell nucleus.

epinephrine A hormone also known as *adrenaline*; it is released by the adrenal glands (located on each kidney) and various nerve endings in the body. It acts to increase glycogen breakdown in the liver, among other functions.

epithelial cells The cells that line the outside of the body and the inside of all external passages within it, such as the GI tract.

epithelial tissue The surface cells that line the outside of the body and all external passages within it.

ergogenic Work-producing. An ergogenic aid is a mechanical, nutritional, psychological, pharmacological, or physiological substance or treatment intended to directly improve exercise performance.

erythrocytes Mature red blood cells. These have no nucleus and a life span of about 120 days; they contain hemoglobin, which transports oxygen and carbon dioxide.

erythropoietin A hormone secreted mostly by the kidneys that enhances red blood cell synthesis and stimulates red blood cell release from bone marrow.

esophagus A tube in the GI tract that connects the pharynx with the stomach.

essential amino acids The amino acids that cannot be synthesized by humans in sufficient amounts or at all and therefore must be included in the diet; there are nine essential amino acids. These are also called *indispensable amino acids*.

essential fatty acids Fatty acids that must be supplied by the diet to maintain health. Currently, only linoleic acid and alpha-linolenic acid are classified as essential.

essential nutrient In nutritional terms, a substance that, when left out of a diet, leads to signs of poor health. The body either cannot produce this nutrient or cannot produce enough of it to meet its needs. Then, if added back to a diet before permanent damage occurs, the affected aspects of health are restored.

estimated Energy Requirement (EER) Estimate of the energy (kcal) intake needed to match the energy use of an average person in a specific life stage.

ethanol Chemical term for the form of alcohol found in alcoholic beverages.

extracellular fluid Fluid present outside the cells; represents about one-third of body fluid.

extracellular space The space outside cells; represents one-third of body fluid.

famine An extreme shortage of food, which leads to massive starvation in a population; often associated with crop failures, war, and political unrest.

fasting hypoglycemia Low blood glucose that follows about a day of fasting.

fat-soluble vitamins Vitamins that dissolve in fat and such substances as ether and benzene but not readily in water. These vitamins are A, D, E, and K.

fatty acid Major part of most lipids; primarily composed of a chain of carbons flanked by hydrogen.

female athlete triad A condition characterized by disordered eating, lack of menstrual periods (amenorrhea), and osteoporosis.

fermentation The conversion of carbohydrates to alcohols, acids, and carbon dioxide without the use of oxygen.

fetal alcohol effects (FAE) Hyperactivity, attention deficit disorder, poor judgment, sleep disorders, and delayed learning as a result of prenatal exposure to alcohol.

fetal alcohol spectrum disorders (FASDs) A group of irreversible physical and mental abnormalities in the infant that result from the mother's consuming alcohol during pregnancy. [NOTE: This is previous definition for *fetal alcohol syndrome (FAS)*.]

fetal alcohol syndrome (FAS) Severe form of FASD that involves abnormal facial features and problems with development of the nervous system and overall growth as a result of maternal alcohol consumption during pregnancy.

fetus The developing human life form from 8 weeks after conception until birth.

fiber Substances in plant foods not digested by the processes that take place in the human stomach or small intestine. These add bulk to feces. Fiber naturally found in foods is also called dietary fiber.

food desert An area where 33% or 500 people, whichever is less, live more than a mile from a grocery store in an urban area or more than 10 miles away in a rural area.

food insecure Condition in which the quality, variety, and/or desirability of the diet is reduced and there is difficulty at times providing enough food for everyone in the household.

food insecurity A condition of anxiety regarding running out of either food or money to buy more food.

food intolerance An adverse reaction to food that does not involve an allergic reaction.

food sensitivity A mild reaction to a substance in a food that might be expressed as slight itching or redness of the skin.

foodborne illness Sickness caused by the ingestion of food containing harmful substances.

fructose A six-carbon monosaccharide that usually exists in a ring form; found in fruits and honey; also known as *fruit sugar.*

fruitarian A person who primarily eats fruits, nuts, honey, and vegetable oils.

functional fiber Fiber added to foods that has been shown to provide health benefits.

functional foods Foods that provide health benefits beyond those supplied by the traditional nutrients they contain. For example, a tomato contains the phytochemical lycopene, so it can be called a functional food.

fungi Simple parasitic life forms, including molds, mildews, yeasts, and mushrooms. They live on dead or decaying organic matter. Fungi can grow as single cells, like yeast, or as a multicellular colony, as seen with molds.

galactose A six-carbon monosaccharide that usually exists in a ring form; closely related to glucose.

gallbladder An organ attached to the underside of the liver; site of bile storage, concentration, and eventual secretion.

gastroesophageal reflux disease (GERD) Disease that results from stomach acid backing up into the esophagus. The acid irritates the lining of the esophagus, causing pain.

gastrointestinal (GI) tract The main sites in the body used for digestion and absorption of nutrients. It consists of the mouth, esophagus, stomach, small intestine, large intestine, rectum, and anus. Also called the digestive tract.

gastroplasty Gastric bypass surgery performed on the stomach to limit its volume to approximately 30 milliliters. Also referred to as stomach stapling.

gender and development (GAD) approach Understanding the roles and responsibilities of both men and women in the process of sustainable development.

gene A specific segment on a chromosome. Genes provide the blueprint for the production of cell proteins.

gene expression Use of DNA information on a gene to produce a protein. Thought to be a major determination of cell development.

generally recognized as safe (GRAS) A list of food additives that in 1958 were considered safe for consumption. Manufacturers were allowed to continue to use these additives, without special clearance, when needed for food products. FDA bears responsibility for proving they are not safe, but can remove unsafe products from the list.

genetic engineering Manipulation of the genetic makeup of any organism with recombinant DNA technology.

genetically modified organism (GMO) Any organism created by genetic engineering.

gestation The period of intrauterine development of offspring, from conception to birth; in humans, gestation lasts for about 40 weeks after the woman's previous menstrual period.

gestational diabetes A high blood glucose concentration that develops during pregnancy and returns to normal after birth; one cause is the placental production of hormones that antagonize the regulation of blood glucose by insulin.

ghrelin A hormone made by the stomach that increases the desire to eat.

glucagon A hormone made by the pancreas that stimulates the breakdown of glycogen in the liver into glucose; this ends up increasing blood glucose. Glucagon also performs other functions.

glucose A six-carbon sugar that exists in a ring form; found as such in blood, and in table sugar bound to fructose; also known as *dextrose,* it is one of the simple sugars.

glycemic index (GI) The blood glucose response of a given food, compared to a standard (typically, glucose or white bread). Glycemic index is influenced by starch structure; fiber content; food processing; physical structure; and macronutrients in the meal, such as fat.

glycemic load (GL) The amount of carbohydrate in a serving of food multiplied by the glycemic index of that carbohydrate. The result is then divided by 100.

glycerol A three-carbon alcohol used to form triglycerides.

glycogen A carbohydrate made of multiple units of glucose with a highly branched structure. It is the storage form of glucose in humans and is synthesized (and stored) in the liver and muscles.

glycosylation The process by which glucose attaches to (glycates) other compounds, such as proteins.

goiter An enlargement of the thyroid gland; this is often caused by insufficient iodide in the diet.

Golgi complex The cell organelle near the nucleus that processes newly synthesized protein for secretion or distribution to other organelles.

green revolution This refers to increases in crop yields that accompanied the introduction of new agricultural technologies in less-developed countries, beginning in the 1960s. The key technologies were high-yielding, disease-resistant strains of rice, wheat, and corn; greater use of fertilizer and water; and improved cultivation practices.

gruels A thin mixture of grains or legumes in milk or water.

gums A viscous fiber containing chains of galactose, glucuronic acid, and other monosaccharides; characteristically found in exudates from plant stems.

H2 blocker Medication, such as cimetidine (Tagamet®), that blocks the increase of stomach acid production caused by histamine.

heart attack Rapid fall in heart function caused by reduced blood flow through the heart's blood vessels. Often part of the heart dies in the process. Technically called a myocardial infarction.

heat cramps A frequent complication of heat exhaustion. They usually occur in people who have experienced large sweat losses from exercising for several hours in a hot climate and have consumed a large volume of water. The cramps occur in skeletal muscles and consist of contractions for 1 to 3 minutes at a time.

heat exhaustion The first stage of heat-related illness that occurs because of depletion of blood volume from fluid loss by the body. This increases body temperature and can lead to headache, dizziness, muscle weakness, and visual disturbances, among other effects.

heatstroke Heatstroke can occur when internal body temperature reaches 104°F. Sweating generally ceases if left untreated, and blood circulation is greatly reduced. Nervous system damage may ensue, and death is likely. Often the skin of individuals who suffer heatstroke is hot and dry.

helminth Parasitic worm that can contaminate food, water, feces, animals, and other substances.

hematocrit The percentage of blood made up of red blood cells.

heme iron Iron provided from animal tissues in the form of hemoglobin and myoglobin. Approximately 40% of the iron in meat is heme iron; it is readily absorbed.

hemicellulose A nonfermentable fiber containing xylose, galactose, glucose, and other monosaccharides bonded together.

hemochromatosis A disorder of iron metabolism characterized by increased iron absorption and deposition in the liver and heart tissue. This eventually poisons the cells in those organs.

hemoglobin The iron-containing part of the red blood cell that carries oxygen to the cells and some carbon dioxide away from the cells. The heme iron portion is also responsible for the red color of blood.

hemolysis Destruction of red blood cells. The red blood cell membrane breaks down, allowing cell contents to leak into the fluid portion of the blood.

hemorrhage An escape of blood from blood vessels.

hemorrhagic stroke Damage to part of the brain resulting from rupture of a blood vessel and subsequent bleeding within or over the internal surface of the brain.

hemorrhoid A pronounced swelling of a large vein, particularly veins found in the anal region.

high-density lipoprotein (HDL) The lipoprotein in the blood that picks up cholesterol from dying cells and other sources and transfers it to the other lipoproteins in the bloodstream, as well as directly to the liver; low HDL increases the risk for cardiovascular disease.

high-quality (complete) proteins Dietary proteins that contain ample amounts of all nine essential amino acids.

histamine A breakdown product of the amino acid histidine that stimulates acid secretion by the stomach and has other effects on the body, such as contraction of smooth muscles, increased nasal secretions, relaxation of blood vessels, and changes in relaxation of airways.

hormone A compound secreted into the bloodstream by one type of cell that acts to control the function of another type of cell. For example, certain cells in the pancreas produce insulin, which in turn acts on muscle and other types of cells to promote uptake of nutrients from the blood.

hospice care A facility offering care that emphasizes comfort and dignity in death.

human immunodeficiency virus (HIV) The virus that leads to acquired immune deficiency syndrome (AIDS).

hunger The primarily physiological (internal) drive to find and eat food, mostly regulated by internal cues to eating.

hydrogenation The addition of hydrogen to a carbon-carbon double bond, producing a single carbon-carbon bond with two hydrogens attached to each carbon. Hydrogenation of unsaturated fatty acids in a vegetable oil increases its hardness, so this process is used to convert liquid oils into more solid fats, used in making margarine and shortening. *Trans* fatty acids are a by-product of hydrogenation of vegetable oils.

hyperglycemia High blood glucose, above 125 milligrams per 100 milliliters of blood.

hypoglycemia Low blood glucose, below 40 to 50 milligrams per 100 milliliters of blood.

hypothalamus A region at the base of the brain that contains cells that play a role in the regulation of hunger, respiration, body temperature, and other body functions.

hypotheses Tentative explanations by a scientist to explain a phenomenon.

identical twins Two offspring that develop from a single ovum and sperm and, consequently, have the same genetic makeup.

ileocecal sphincter The ring of smooth muscle between the end of the small intestine and the large intestine.

immune system The body system consisting of white blood cells, lymph glands and vessels, and various other body tissues. The immune system provides defense against foreign invaders, primarily due to the action of various types of white blood cells.

immunoglobulins Proteins found in the blood that bind to specific antigens; also called antibodies. The five major classes of immunoglobulins play different roles in antibody-mediated immunity.

incidental food additives Additives that appear in food products indirectly, from environmental contamination of food ingredients or during the manufacturing process.

indirect calorimetry A method to measure energy use by the body by measuring oxygen uptake. Formulas are then used to convert this gas exchange value into energy use.

infrastructure The basic framework of a system of organization. For a society, this includes roads, bridges, telephones, and other basic technologies.

inorganic Any substance lacking carbon atoms bonded to hydrogen atoms in the chemical structure.

insulin A hormone produced by the pancreas. Among other processes, insulin increases the synthesis of glycogen in the liver and the movement of glucose from the bloodstream into body cells.

intentional food additives Additives knowingly (directly) incorporated into food products by manufacturers.

international unit (IU) A crude measure of vitamin activity, often based on the growth rate of animals in response to the vitamin. Today IUs have largely been replaced by more precise milligram or microgram measures.

intracellular fluid Fluid contained within a cell; it represents about two-thirds of body fluid.

intrinsic factor A proteinlike compound produced by the stomach that enhances vitamin B-12 absorption.

ion An atom with an unequal number of electrons and protons. Negative ions have more electrons than protons; positive ions have more protons than electrons.

irradiation A process in which radiation energy is applied to foods, creating compounds (free radicals) within the food that destroy cell membranes, break down DNA, link proteins together, limit enzyme activity, and alter a variety of other proteins and cell functions of microorganisms that can lead to food spoilage. This process does not make the food radioactive.

isomers Different chemical structures for compounds that share the same chemical formula.

ketone bodies Partial breakdown products of fat that contain three or four carbons.

ketosis The condition of having a high concentration of ketone bodies and related breakdown products in the bloodstream and tissues.

kidney nephrons The units of kidney cells that filter wastes from the bloodstream and deposit them into the urine.

kilocalorie (kcal) Heat energy needed to raise the temperature of 1000 grams (1 L) of water 1 degree Celsius; also written as *Calories*.

kwashiorkor A disease occurring primarily in young children who have an existing disease and consume a marginal amount of calories and insufficient protein in relation to needs. The child generally suffers from infections and exhibits edema, poor growth, weakness, and an increased susceptibility to further illness.

lactase An enzyme made by absorptive cells of the small intestine; this enzyme digests lactose to glucose and galactose.

lactation The period of milk secretion following pregnancy; typically called *breast-feeding*.

lactic acid A three-carbon acid formed during anaerobic cell metabolism; a partial breakdown product of glucose; also called *lactate*.

***Lactobacillus bifidus* factor** A protective factor secreted in the colostrum that encourages growth of beneficial bacteria in the newborn's intestines.

lactoovovegetarian A person who consumes plant products, dairy products, and eggs.

lactose intolerance A condition in which symptoms such as abdominal gas and bloating appear as a result of severe lactose maldigestion.

lactose maldigestion (primary and secondary) Primary lactose maldigestion occurs when production of the enzyme lactase declines for no apparent reason. Secondary lactose maldigestion occurs when a specific cause, such as long-standing diarrhea, results in a decline in lactase production. When significant symptoms develop after lactose intake, it is then called lactose intolerance.

lactose Glucose bonded to galactose; also known as *milk sugar*.

lactovegetarian A person who consumes plant products and dairy products.

lanugo Down-like hair that appears after a person has lost much body fat through semi-starvation. The hair stands erect and traps air, acting as insulation for the body to compensate for the relative lack of body fat, which usually functions as insulation.

laxative A medication or other substance that stimulates evacuation of the intestinal tract.

lean body mass Body weight minus fat storage weight equals lean body mass. This includes organs such as the brain, muscles, and liver, as well as bone and blood and other body fluids.

lecithin A group of phospholipid compounds that are major components of cell membranes.

leptin A hormone made by adipose tissue in proportion to total fat stores in the body that influences long-term regulation of fat mass. Leptin also influences reproductive functions, as well as other body processes, such as release of the hormone insulin.

let-down reflex A reflex stimulated by infant suckling that causes the release (ejection) of milk from milk ducts in the mother's breasts; also called *milk ejection reflex.*

life expectancy The average length of life for a given group of people born in a specific year (such as this year).

life span The potential oldest age a person can reach.

lignins A nonfermentable fiber made up of a multiringed alcohol (noncarbohydrate) structure.

limiting amino acid The essential amino acid in lowest concentration in a food or diet relative to body needs.

linoleic acid An essential omega-6 fatty acid with 18 carbons and two double bonds.

lipase Fat-digesting enzyme produced by the salivary glands, stomach, and pancreas.

lipid A compound containing much carbon and hydrogen, little oxygen, and sometimes other atoms. Lipids do not dissolve in water, and include fats, oils, and cholesterol.

lipoprotein A compound found in the bloodstream containing a core of lipids with a shell composed of protein, phospholipid, and cholesterol.

lipoprotein lipase An enzyme attached to the cells that form the inner lining of blood vessels; it breaks down triglycerides into free fatty acids and glycerol.

lobules Saclike structures in the breast that store milk.

locavore Someone who eats food grown or produced locally or within a certain radius such as 50, 100, or 500 miles.

long-chain fatty acid A fatty acid that contains 12 or more carbons.

low birth weight (LBW) Referring to any infant weighing less than 2.5 kilograms (5.5 pounds) at birth; most commonly results from preterm birth.

low-density lipoprotein (LDL) The lipoprotein in the blood containing primarily cholesterol; elevated LDL is strongly linked to cardiovascular disease risk.

lower esophageal sphincter A circular muscle that constricts the opening of the esophagus to the stomach. Also called the *gastroesophageal sphincter.*

lower-body obesity The type of obesity in which fat storage is primarily located in the buttocks and thigh area. Also known as gynoid or gynecoid obesity.

lower-quality (incomplete) proteins Dietary proteins that are low in or lack one or more essential amino acids.

lymph A clear fluid that flows through lymph vessels; carries most forms of fat after their absorption by the small intestine.

lymphatic system A system of vessels and lymph that accepts fluid surrounding cells and large particles, such as products of fat absorption. Lymph eventually passes into the bloodstream from the lymphatic system.

lysosome A cellular organelle that contains digestive enzymes for use inside the cell for turnover of cell parts.

lysozyme An enzyme produced by a variety of cells; it can destroy bacteria by rupturing their cell membranes.

macronutrient A nutrient needed in gram quantities in a diet.

macular degeneration A painless condition leading to disruption of the central part of the retina (in the eye) and, in turn, blurred vision.

major mineral A mineral vital to health that is required in the diet in amounts greater than 100 milligrams per day.

malignant Malicious; in reference to a tumor, the property of spreading locally and to distant sites.

malnutrition Failing health that results from long-standing dietary practices that do not coincide with nutritional needs.

maltase An enzyme made by absorptive cells of the small intestine; this enzyme digests maltose to two glucoses.

maltose Glucose bonded to glucose.

marasmus A disease resulting from consuming a grossly insufficient amount of protein and calories; one of the diseases classed as protein-calorie malnutrition. Victims have little or no fat stores, little muscle mass, and poor strength. Death from infections is common.

megadose Intake of a nutrient beyond estimates of needs to prevent a deficiency or what would be found in a balanced diet; 2 to 10 times human needs is a starting point for such a pharmacological dosage.

megaloblast A large, immature red blood cell that results from the particular cell's inability to divide normally.

megaloblastic anemia Anemia characterized by the presence of abnormally large red blood cells.

menarche The onset of menstruation. Menarche usually occurs around age 13, 2 or 3 years after the first signs of puberty start to appear.

menopause The cessation of the menstrual cycle in women, usually beginning at about 50 years of age.

metabolic syndrome A condition in which a person has poor blood glucose regulation, hypertension, increased blood triglycerides, and other health problems. This condition is usually accompanied by obesity, lack of physical activity, and a diet high in refined carbohydrates. Also called Syndrome X.

metabolism Chemical processes in the body by which energy is provided in useful forms and vital activities are sustained.

metastasize The spreading of disease from one part of the body to another, even to parts of the body that are remote from the site of the original tumor. Cancer cells can spread via blood vessels, the lymphatic system, or direct growth of the tumor.

methyl group CH_3

micronutrient A nutrient needed in milligram or microgram quantities in a diet.

microorganism Bacteria, virus, or other organism invisible to the naked eye, some of which cause diseases. Also called *microbes.*

mineral Element used in the body to promote chemical reactions and to form body structures.

mitochondria The main sites of energy production in a cell. They contain the pathway for oxidizing fat for fuel, among other metabolic pathways.

moderate-intensity aerobic physical activity Aerobic activity that increases a person's heart rate and breathing to some extent (5–6 on RPE scale). Examples include brisk walking, dancing, swimming, or bicycling on level terrain.

monoglyceride A breakdown product of a triglyceride consisting of one fatty acid attached to a glycerol backbone.

monosaccharide Simple sugar, such as glucose, that is not broken down further during digestion.

monounsaturated fatty acid A fatty acid containing one carbon-carbon double bond.

motility Generally, the ability to move spontaneously. It also refers to movement of food through the GI tract.

mottling The discoloration or marking of the surface of teeth from fluorosis.

mucilages A viscous fiber consisting of chains of galactose, mannose, and other monosaccharides; characteristically found in seaweed.

mucus A thick fluid secreted by many cells throughout the body. It contains a compound that has both carbohydrate and protein parts. It acts as a lubricant and means of protection for cells.

muscle dysmorphia psychological condition in which a person preceives him-or herself as too thin or small, despite normal or above-average muscularity. People with this condition engage in disordered eating and extreme exercise practices in the pursuit of hypermuscularity.

muscle tissue A type of tissue adapted to contract to cause movement.

muscle-strengthening activity Physical activity, including exercise, that increases skeletal muscle strength, power, endurance, and mass. Examples include strength training, resistance training, and muscle strength and endurance exercises.

myelin sheath A lipid and protein combination (lipoprotein) that covers nerve fibers.

myocardial infarction Death of part of the heart muscle. Also termed a *heart attack.*

myoglobin Iron-containing protein that binds oxygen in muscle tissue.

negative energy balance The state in which energy intake is less than energy expended, resulting in weight loss.

negative protein balance A state in which protein intake is less than related protein losses, such as often seen during acute illness.

neotame General-purpose, non-nutritive sweetener that is approximately 7000 to 13,000 times sweeter than table sugar. It has a chemical structure similar to aspartame's.

nervous system The body system consisting of the brain, spinal cord, nerves, and sensory receptors. This system detects sensations, directs movements, and controls physiological and intellectual functions.

nervous tissue Tissue composed of highly branched, elongated cells, which transport nerve impulses from one part of the body to another.

neural tube defect A defect in the formation of the neural tube occurring during early fetal development. This type of defect results in various nervous system disorders, such as spina bifida. Folate deficiency in the pregnant woman increases the risk that the fetus will develop this disorder.

neuron The structural and functional unit of the nervous system. Consists of a **cell body, dendrites,** and an **axon.**

neuropeptide Y A chemical substance made in the hypothalamus that stimulates food intake. The hormone leptin inhibits neuropeptide Y production.

neurotransmitter A compound made by a nerve cell that allows for communication between it and other cells.

night blindness A vitamin A deficiency condition in which the retina (in the eye) cannot adjust to low amounts of light.

night eating syndrome Eating a lot of food in the late evening and nocturnal awakenings with ingestion of food.

nitrosamine A carcinogen formed from nitrates and breakdown products of amino acids; can lead to stomach cancer.

non-specific immunity Defenses that stop the invasion of pathogens; requires no previous encounter with a pathogen.

nonessential amino acids Amino acids that can be synthesized by a healthy body in sufficient amounts; there are 11 nonessential amino acids. These are also called *dispensable amino acids.*

nonfermentable fiber A fiber that is not easily metabolized by intestinal bacteria.

nonheme iron Iron provided from plant sources and animal tissues other than in the forms of hemoglobin and myoglobin. Nonheme iron is less efficiently absorbed than heme iron; absorption is closely dependent on body needs.

norepinephrine A neurotransmitter from nerve endings and a hormone from the adrenal gland. It is released in times of stress and is involved in hunger regulation, blood glucose regulation, and other body processes.

NSAIDs Nonsteroidal anti-inflammatory drugs; includes aspirin, ibuprofen (Advil®), and naproxen (Aleve®).

nutrient density The ratio derived by dividing a food's nutrient content by its calorie content. When the food's contribution to our nutrient need for that nutrient exceeds its contribution to our calorie need, the food is considered to have a favorable nutrient density.

nutrients Chemical substances in food that contribute to health, many of which are essential parts of a diet. Nutrients nourish us by providing calories to fulfill energy needs, materials for building body parts, and factors to regulate necessary chemical processes in the body.

nutrigenomics Study of how food impacts health through its interaction with our genes and its subsequent effect on gene expression.

nutritional state The nutritional health of a person as determined by anthropometric measurements (height, weight, circumferences, and so on), biochemical measurements of nutrients or their by-products in blood and urine, a clinical (physical) examination, a dietary analysis, and economic evaluation; also called nutritional status.

obesogenic Tending to promote obesity by encouraging excessive calorie intake and/or discouraging physical activity.

oleic acid An omega-9 fatty acid with 18 carbons and one double bond.

omega-3 (ω-3) fatty acid An unsaturated fatty acid with the first double bond on the third carbon from the methyl end (CH_3).

omega-6 (ω-6) fatty acid An unsaturated fatty acid with the first double bond on the sixth carbon from the methyl end (CH_3).

organ A group of tissues designed to perform a specific function—for example, the heart, which contains muscle tissue, nerve tissue, and so on.

organ system A collection of organs that work together to perform an overall function.

organelles Compartments, particles, or filaments that perform specialized functions within a cell.

organic Any substance that contains carbon atoms bonded to hydrogen atoms in the chemical structure.

osmosis The passage of a solvent such as water through a semipermeable membrane from a less concentrated compartment to a more concentrated compartment.

osteomalacia Adult form of rickets. The weakening of the bones seen in this disease is caused by low calcium content. A reduction in the amount of the vitamin D hormone in the body is one cause.

osteoporosis Decreased bone mass related to the effects of aging, genetic background, and poor diet in both genders, and hormonal changes at menopause in women.

ostomy Surgically created short circuit in intestinal flow where the end point usually opens from the abdominal cavity rather than the anus—for example, a colostomy. Short circuiting the intestinal flow means more water is lost in fecal matter than would be if the intestinal tract were intact.

overnutrition A state in which nutritional intake greatly exceeds the body's needs.

ovum The egg cell from which a fetus eventually develops if the egg is fertilized by a sperm cell.

oxalic acid (oxalate) An organic acid found in spinach, rhubarb, and other leafy green vegetables that can depress the absorption of certain minerals present in the food, such as calcium.

oxidize In the most basic sense, the loss of an electron or gain of an oxygen by a chemical substance. This change typically alters the shape and/or function of the substance.

oxytocin A hormone secreted by the pituitary gland. It causes contraction of the musclelike cells surrounding the ducts of the breasts and the smooth muscle of the uterus.

parasite An organism that lives in or on another organism and derives nourishment from it.

parathyroid hormone (PTH) A hormone made by the parathyroid glands that increases synthesis of the vitamin D hormone and aids calcium release from bone and calcium conservation by the kidneys, among other functions.

pasteurizing The process of heating food products to kill pathogenic microorganisms and reduce the total number of bacteria.

pectin A viscous fiber containing chains of galacturonic acid and other monosaccharides; characteristically found between plant cell walls.

pepsin A protein-digesting enzyme produced by the stomach.

peptide bond A chemical bond formed between amino acids in a protein.

percentile Classification of a measurement of a unit into divisions of 100 units.

peristalsis A coordinated muscular contraction used to propel food down the gastrointestinal tract.

pernicious anemia The anemia that results from a lack of vitamin B-12 absorption; it is pernicious because of associated nerve degeneration that can result in eventual paralysis and death.

peroxisome A cell organelle that destroys toxic products within the cell.

pH A measure of relative acidity or alkalinity of a solution. The pH scale is 0 to 14. A pH of 7 is netural; a pH below 7 is acidic; a pH above 7 is alkaline.

phagocytes Cells that engulf substances; include neutrophils and macrophages.

phagocytosis A process in which a cell forms an indentation, and particles or fluids entering the indentation are then engulfed by the cell.

pharynx The organ of the digestive tract and respiratory tract located at the back of the oral and nasal cavities, commonly known as the throat.

phenylketonuria (PKU) Disease caused by a defect in the liver's ability to metabolize the amino acid phenylalanine into the amino acid tyrosine; untreated, toxic by-products of phenylalanine build up in the body and lead to mental retardation.

phosphocreatine (PCr) A high-energy compound that can be used to re-form ATP. It is used primarily during bursts of activity, such as lifting and jumping.

phospholipid Any of a class of fat-related substances that contain phosphorus, fatty acids, and a nitrogen-containing component. Phospholipids are an essential part of every cell.

photosynthesis Process by which plants use energy from the sun to synthesize energy-yielding compounds, such as glucose.

physical fitness The ability to perform moderate to vigorous activity without undue fatigue.

physiological anemia The normal increase in blood volume in pregnancy that dilutes the concentration of red blood cells, resulting in anemia; also called *hemodilution.*

phytic acid (phytate) A constituent of plant fibers that binds positive ions to its multiple phosphate groups.

phytochemical A chemical found in plants. Some phytochemicals may contribute to a reduced risk of cancer or cardiovascular disease in people who consume them regularly.

pica The practice of eating nonfood items, such as dirt, laundry starch, or clay.

placebo Generally a fake medicine or treatment used to disguise the treatments given to the participants in an experiment.

placenta An organ that forms in the uterus in pregnant women. Through this organ, oxygen and nutrients from the mother's blood are transferred to the fetus, and fetal wastes are removed. The placenta also releases hormones that maintain the state of pregnancy.

plaque A cholesterol-rich substance deposited in the blood vessels; it contains various white blood cells, smooth muscle cells, various proteins, cholesterol and other lipids, and eventually calcium.

plasma The fluid, extracellular portion of the circulating blood. This includes the blood serum plus all blood-clotting factors. In contrast, serum is the fluid that remains after clotting factors have been removed from plasma.

polypeptide A group of amino acids bonded together, from 50 to 2000 or more.

polysaccharide Class of complex carbohydrates containing many glucose units, from 10 to 1000 or more.

polyunsaturated fatty acid A fatty acid containing two or more carbon-carbon double bonds.

pool The amount of a nutrient stored within the body that can be mobilized when needed.

portal circulation The portion of the circulatory system that uses a large vein (portal vein) to carry nutrient-rich blood from capillaries in the intestines and portions of the stomach to the liver.

portal vein Large vein leaving the intestine and stomach and connecting to the liver.

positive energy balance The state in which energy intake is greater than energy expended, generally resulting in weight gain.

positive protein balance A state in which protein intake exceeds related protein losses, as is needed during times of growth.

prebiotic Substance that stimulates bacterial growth in the large intestines.

pregnancy-induced hypertension A serious disorder that can include high blood pressure, kidney failure, convulsions, and even death of the mother and fetus. Although its exact cause is not known, an adequate diet (especially adequate calcium intake) and prenatal care may prevent this disorder or limit its severity. Mild cases are known as *preeclampsia;* more severe cases are called *eclampsia* (formerly called *toxemia*).

preservatives Compounds that extend the shelf life of foods by inhibiting microbial growth or minimizing the destructive effect of oxygen and metals.

preterm An infant born before 37 weeks of gestation; also referred to as *premature* .

probiotic Product that contains specific types of bacteria. Use is intended to colonize the large intestine with the specific bacteria in the product. An example is yogurt.

prolactin A hormone secreted by the pituitary gland that stimulates the synthesis of milk in the breast.

prostate gland A solid, chestnut-shaped organ surrounding the first part of the urinary tract in the male. The prostate gland secretes substances into the semen.

protease Protein-digesting enzyme produced by the stomach, small intestine, and pancreas.

protein equilibrium A state in which protein intake is equal to related protein losses; the person is said to be in protein balance.

protein turnover The process by which cells break down old proteins and resynthesize new proteins. In this way the cell will have the proteins it needs to function at that time.

protein-calorie malnutrition (PCM) A condition resulting from regularly consuming insufficient amounts of calories and protein. The deficiency eventually results in body wasting, primarily of lean tissue, and an increased susceptibility to infections.

protein Food and body compounds made of amino acids; proteins contain carbon, hydrogen, oxygen, nitrogen, and sometimes other atoms, in a specific configuration. Proteins contain the form of nitrogen most easily used by the human body.

proton pump inhibitor A medication that inhibits the ability of gastric cells to secrete hydrogen ions. Low doses of this class of medications are also available without prescription (e.g., omeprazole [Prilosec]).

protozoa One-celled animals that are more complex than bacteria. Disease-causing protozoa can be spread through food and water.

provitamin/precursor A substance that can be made into a vitamin, if the body needs it.

pyloric sphincter The ring of smooth muscle between the stomach and the small intestine.

pyruvic acid A three-carbon compound formed during glucose metabolism; also called *pyruvate.*

radiation Literally, energy that is emitted from a center in all directions. Various forms of radiation energy include X-rays and ultra-violet rays from the sun.

rancid Containing products of decomposed fatty acids that have an unpleasant flavor and odor.

reactive hypoglycemia Low blood glucose that follows a meal high in simple sugars, with corresponding symptoms of irritability, headache, nervousness, sweating, and confusion; also called *postprandial hypoglycemia.*

receptor A site in a cell at which compounds (such as hormones) bind. Cells that contain receptors for a specific compound are partially controlled by that compound.

recombinant DNA technology A test tube technology that rearranges DNA sequences in an organism by cutting the DNA, adding or deleting a DNA sequence, and rejoining DNA molecules with a series of enzymes.

Recommended Dietary Allowance (RDA) Nutrient intake amount sufficient to meet the needs of 97% to 98% of the individuals in a specific life stage.

rectum Terminal portion of the large intestine.

registered dietitian (R.D.) A person who has completed a baccalaureate degree program approved by the American Dietetic Association, performed at least 1200 hours of supervised professional practice, passed a registration examination, and complies with continuing education requirements.

relapse prevention A series of strategies used to help prevent and cope with weight-control lapses, such as recognizing high-risk situations and deciding beforehand on appropriate responses.

reserve capacity The extent to which an organ can preserve essentially normal function despite decreasing cell number or cell activity.

resting metabolism The amount of calories the body uses when the person has not eaten in 4 hours and is resting (e.g., 15 to 30 minutes) and awake in a warm, quiet environment. It is roughly 6% higher than basal metabolism due to the less strict criteria for the test; often referred to as *resting metabolic rate (RMR)*.

retinoids Chemical forms of preformed vitamin A; one source is animal foods.

ribonucleic acid (RNA) The single-stranded nucleic acid involved in the transcription of genetic information and translation of that information into protein structure.

ribosomes Cytoplasmic particles that mediate the linking together of amino acids to form proteins; may exist freely in the cytoplasm or attached to endoplasmic reticulum.

rickets A disease characterized by poor mineralization of newly synthesized bones because of low calcium content. This deficiency disease arises in infants and children from insufficient amounts of the vitamin D hormone in the body.

saccharin Alternative sweetener that yields no energy to the body; 300 times sweeter than sucrose.

saliva Watery fluid, produced by the salivary glands in the mouth, that contains lubricants, enzymes, and other substances.

salivary amylase A starch-digesting enzyme produced by salivary glands.

salt Compound of sodium and chloride in a 40:60 ratio.

sarcopenia In general, loss of muscle tissue. Among older adults this loss of lean mass greatly increases their risk of illness and death.

sarcopenic obesity Loss of muscle mass accompanied by gains in fat mass.

satiety A state in which there is no longer a desire to eat; a feeling of satisfaction.

saturated fatty acid A fatty acid containing no carbon-carbon double bonds.

scavenger cells Specific form of white blood cells that can bury themselves in the artery wall and accumulate LDL. As these cells take up LDL, they contribute to the development of atherosclerosis.

scurvy The deficiency disease that results after a few weeks to months of consuming a diet that lacks vitamin C; pinpoint sites of bleeding on the skin are an early sign.

secretory vesicles Membrane-bound vesicles produced by the Golgi apparatus; contain protein and other compounds to be secreted by the cell.

self-monitoring Tracking foods eaten and conditions affecting eating; actions are usually recorded in a diary, along with location, time, and state of mind. This is a tool to help people understand more about their eating habits.

sequestrants Compounds that bind free metal ions. By so doing, they reduce the ability of ions to cause rancidity in foods containing fat.

serotonin A neurotransmitter synthesized from the amino acid tryptophan that affects mood (sense of calmness), behavior, and appetite, and induces sleep.

set point Often refers to the close regulation of body weight. It is not known what cells control this set point or how it functions in weight regulation. There is evidence, however, that mechanisms exist that help regulate weight.

sickle cell disease (sickle cell anemia) An illness that results from a malformation of the red blood cell because of an incorrect structure in part of its hemoglobin protein chains. The disease can lead to episodes of severe bone and joint pain, abdominal pain, headache, convulsions, paralysis, and even death.

simple sugar Monosaccharide or disaccharide in the diet.

small for gestational age (SGA) Referring to infants who weigh less than the expected weight for their length of gestation. This corresponds to less than 2.5 kilograms (5.5 pounds) in a full-term newborn. A preterm infant who is also SGA will most likely develop some medical complications.

solid fats Fats that are solid at room temperature, such as butter and margarine. Foods containing solid fats tend to be high in saturated fatty acids or *trans* fatty acids.

solvent A liquid substance in which other substances dissolve.

sorbitol Alcohol derivative of glucose that yields about 3 kcal/g but is slowly absorbed from the small intestine; used in some sugarless gums and dietetic foods.

specific immunity Function of lymphocytes directed at specific antigens.

spontaneous abortion Cessation of pregnancy and expulsion of the embryo or nonviable fetus prior to 20 weeks gestation. This is the result of natural causes, such as a genetic defect or developmental problem; also called *miscarriage* .

spores Dormant reproductive cells capable of turning into adult organisms without the help of another cell. Various bacteria and fungi form spores.

starch A carbohydrate made of multiple units of glucose attached together in a form the body can digest; also known as *complex carbohydrate*.

sterol A compound containing a multi-ring (steroid) structure and a hydroxyl group (–OH). Cholesterol is a typical example.

stevia Alternative sweetener derived from South American shrub; 100 to 300 times sweeter than sucrose.

stimulus control Altering the environment to minimize the stimuli for eating—for example, removing foods from sight and storing them in kitchen cabinets.

stress fracture A fracture that occurs from repeated jarring of a bone. Common sites include bones of the foot.

stroke A decrease or loss in blood flow to the brain that results from a blood clot or other change in arteries in the brain. This in turn causes the death of brain tissue. Also called a *cerebrovascular accident*.

subclinical Stage of a disease or disorder not severe enough to produce symptoms that can be detected or diagnosed.

sucralose Alternative sweetener that has chlorines in place of 3 hydroxyl (–OH) groups on sucrose; 600 times sweeter than sucrose.

sucrase An enzyme made by absorptive cells of the small intestine; this enzyme digests sucrose to glucose and fructose.

sucrose Fructose bonded to glucose; table sugar.

sugar A simple carbohydrate with the chemical composition $(CH_2O)_n$. The basic unit of all sugars is glucose, a six-carbon ring structure. The primary sugar in the diet is sucrose, which is made up of glucose and fructose.

sustainable agriculture Agricultural system that provides a secure living for farm families; maintains the natural environment and resources; supports the rural community; and offers respect and fair treatment to all involved, from farm workers to consumers to the animals raised for food.

sustainable development Economic growth that will simultaneously reduce poverty, protect the environment, and preserve natural capital.

symptom A change in health status noted by the person with the problem, such as stomach pain.

synapse The space between one neuron and another neuron (or cell).

systolic blood pressure The pressure in the arterial blood vessels associated with the pumping of blood from the heart.

teratogen A substance that may cause or increase the risk of a birth defect. Exposure to a teratogen does not always lead to a birth defect; its effects on the fetus depend on the dose, timing, and duration of exposure.

tetany A body condition marked by sharp contraction of muscles and failure to relax afterward; usually caused by abnormal calcium metabolism.

theory An explanation for a phenomenon that has numerous lines of evidence to support it.

thermic effect of food (TEF) The increase in metabolism that occurs during the digestion, absorption, and metabolism of energy-yielding nutrients. This represents 5% to 10% of calories consumed.

thermogenesis This term encompasses the ability of humans to regulate body temperature within narrow limits (thermoregulation). Two visible examples of thermogenesis are fidgeting and shivering when cold.

thyroid hormones Hormones produced by the thyroid gland that among their functions increase the rate of overall metabolism in the body.

tissues Collections of cells adapted to perform a specific function.

tocopherols The chemical name for some forms of vitamin E. The alpha form is the most potent.

Tolerable Upper Intake Level (UL) Maximum chronic daily intake level of a nutrient that is unlikely to cause adverse health effects in almost all people in a specific life stage.

total fiber Combination of dietary fiber and functional fiber in a food. Also just called *fiber*.

total parenteral nutrition The intravenous feeding of all necessary nutrients, including the most basic forms of protein, carbohydrates, lipids, vitamins, minerals, and electrolytes.

toxins Poisonous compounds produced by an organism that can cause disease.

trabecular bone The spongy, inner matrix of bone, found primarily in the spine, pelvis, and ends of bones; also called spongy or cancellous bone.

trace mineral A mineral vital to health that is required in the diet in amounts less than 100 milligrams per day.

trans fatty acids A form of an unsaturated fatty acid, usually a monounsaturated one when found in food, in which the hydrogens on both carbons forming that double bond lie on opposite sides of that bond, rather than on the same side, as in most natural fats. Stick margarine, shortenings, and deep fat-fried foods in general are rich sources.

transcription Information on DNA needed to make a protein is copied onto RNA.

transgenic Organism that contains genes originally present in another organism.

translation The information contained in RNA is used to determine the amino acids in a protein.

triglyceride The major form of lipid in the body and in food. It is composed of three fatty acids bonded to glycerol.

trimesters Three 13- to 14-week periods into which the normal pregnancy (the length of a normal pregnancy is about 40 weeks, measured from the first day of the woman's last menstrual period) is divided somewhat arbitrarily for purposes of discussion and analysis. Development of the offspring, however, is continuous throughout pregnancy, with no specific physiological markers demarcating the transition from one trimester to the next.

trypsin A protein-digesting enzyme secreted by the pancreas to act in the small intestine.

tumor Mass of cells; may be cancerous (malignant) or noncancerous (benign).

type 1 diabetes A form of diabetes prone to ketosis and that requires insulin therapy.

type 2 diabetes A form of diabetes characterized by insulin resistance and often associated with obesity. Insulin therapy can be used but is often not required.

ulcer Erosion of the tissue lining, usually in the stomach (gastric ulcer) or the upper small intestine (duodenal ulcer). As a group these are generally referred to as peptic ulcers.

umami A brothy, meaty, savory flavor in some foods. Monosodium glutamate enhances this flavor when added to foods.

undernutrition Failing health that results from a long-standing dietary intake that is not enough to meet nutritional needs.

underwater weighing A method of estimating total body fat by weighing the individual on a standard scale and then weighing him or her again submerged in water. The difference between the two weights is used to estimate total body volume.

underweight A body mass index below 18.5. The cutoff is less precise than for obesity because this condition has been less studied.

unsaturated fatty acid A fatty acid containing one or more carbon-carbon double bonds.

upper-body obesity The type of obesity in which fat is stored primarily in the abdominal area; defined as a waist circumference more than 40 inches (102 centimeters) in men and more than 35 inches (89 centimeters) in women; closely associated with a high risk for cardiovascular disease, hypertension, and type 2 diabetes. Also known as android obesity.

urea Nitrogenous waste product of protein metabolism; major source of nitrogen in the urine.

ureter Tube that transports urine from the kidney to the urinary bladder.

urethra Tube that transports urine from the urinary bladder to the outside of the body.

urinary system The body system consisting of the kidneys, urinary bladder, and the ducts that carry urine. This system removes waste products from the circulatory system and regulates blood acid-base balance, overall chemical balance, and water balance in the body.

vegan A person who eats only plant foods.

vein A blood vessel that carries blood to the heart.

very-low-calorie diet (VLCD) Known also as *protein-sparing modified fast (PSMF)*, this diet allows a person 400 to 800 kcal per day, often in liquid form. Of this, 120 to 480 kcal is carbohydrate, and the rest is mostly high-quality protein.

very-low-density lipoprotein (VLDL) The lipoprotein created in the liver that carries cholesterol and lipids that have been taken up or newly synthesized by the liver.

vigorous-intensity aerobic physical activity Aerobic activity that greatly increases a person's heart rate and breathing (7–8 on RPE scale). Examples include jogging, singles tennis, swimming continuous laps, or bicycling uphill.

villi (singular, **villus**) The fingerlike protrusions into the small intestine that participate in digestion and absorption of food.

virus The smallest known type of infectious agent, many of which cause disease in humans. A virus is essentially a piece of genetic material surrounded by a coat of protein. They do not metabolize, grow, or move by themselves. They reproduce only with the aid of a living cellular host.

viscous fiber A fiber that is readily fermented by bacteria in the large intestine.

vitamin Compound needed in small amounts in the diet to help regulate and support chemical reactions and processes in the body.

water The universal solvent; chemically, H_2O. The body is composed of about 60% water. Water (fluid) needs are about 9 (women) or 13 (men) cups per day; needs are greater if one exercises heavily.

water-soluble vitamins Vitamins that dissolve in water. These vitamins are the B vitamins and vitamin C.

white blood cells One of the formed elements of the circulating blood system; also called *leukocytes*. White blood cells are able to squeeze through intracellular spaces and migrate. They phagocytize bacteria, fungi, and viruses, as well as detoxify proteins that may result from allergic reactions, cellular injury, and other immune system cells.

whole grains Grains containing the entire seed of the plant, including the bran, germ, and endosperm (starchy interior). Examples are whole-wheat and brown rice.

xerophthalmia Literally "dry eye." This is a cause of blindness that results from a vitamin A deficiency. A lack of mucus production by the eye, which leaves it at a greater risk of damage from surface dirt and bacteria.

xylitol Alcohol derivative of the 5-carbon monosaccharide xylose.

zygote The fertilized ovum; the cell resulting from the union of an egg cell (ovum) and sperm until it divides.

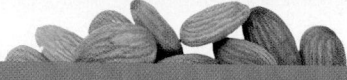

PHOTO CREDITS

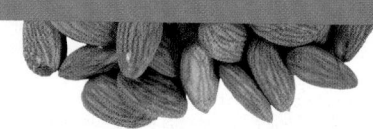

Design Elements

Part One(apple): © Ingram Publishing/SuperStock/RF; Two(yellow pepper): © Getty Images/Stockbyte RF; Three(Onions): © Dynamic Graphics/PunchStock/RF; Four(Tomatoes): © Getty Images/Stockbyte/RF; Part Five(Pear): © Getty Images/Stockbyte/RF; "Nutrition and your Health"(banner of berries): © David Cook/blueshiftstudios/Alamy RFJ; "Rate your Plate"(Choose Your Plate.gov): Courtesy USDA; (soup bowl): © Burke/Triolo Productions/Getty Images RF.

Front Matter

(kebab): © The McGraw-Hill Companies, Inc., Kevin May Photography; (tomato): © Burke Triolo Productions/Getty Images RF; (radishes): © C Squared Studios/Getty Images RF; (cherries): © Burke Triolo Productions/Getty Images RF; (title page): © The McGraw-Hill Companies, Inc., Kevin May Photography.

Chapter 1

Opener: © Corbis/Punchstock RF; 1-1: © BananaStock/PunchStock RF; p. 5: © Stockbyte/PunchStock; p. 8: Reproduction with permission. © Culinary Hearts Kitchen; p. 9: © Photodisc/Getty Images RF; p. 12: © Royalty Free/Corbis; p. 13: © Lifesize/Getty Images RF; p. 15 (both): Brand X RF; p. 19: Steve Cole/Getty Images RF; p. 20: U.S. Department of Health and Human Services. Office of Disease Prevention and Health Promotion. Healthy People 2020. Washington, DC; p. 22: RF/Getty Images; p. 23: © Digital Vision/PunchStock RF; p. 24: © Stockbyte/Punchstock RF; p. 25 (bottom): Punchstock RF; p. 26: © BananaStock/PunchStock RF; p. 27: © Blue Moon Stock/PunchStock RF; p. 28: © Image 100/Corbis RF; p. 30: © Stockbyte/Getty Images RF.

Chapter 2

Opener: © Plush Studios/Blend Images LLC RF; p. 36: © The McGraw-Hill Companies, Inc./Ken Karp, photographer; p. 38: Courtesy of U.S. Rice Federation; p. 39: © Comstock/PunchStock RF; p. 40: © Steve Allen/Getty Images RF; p. 41: © Photodisc/Vol. 67 RF; p. 42: © The McGraw-Hill Companies, Inc./Lars A. Niki, photographer; 2-3(Anthropometric): © The McGraw-Hill Companies, Inc./Lars A. Niki, photographer; (Biochemical): © Photodisc/Vol. 29 RF; (Clinical): © Photodisc Website RF; (Dietary): © Mike Kemp/Rubberball/Getty Images RF; (Environmental): © Comstock/PunchStock RF; p. 45: © Comstock/PunchStock RF; p. 49: © Corbis/Vol. 130 RF; 2-7 (women on scale): © David Buffington/Getty Images RF; (salt shaker): © Photodisc/Getty Images RF; (women w/ child in cart): © RF Getty Images; p. 53: © Karl Weatherly/Getty Images RF; 2-9: © JGI/Blend Images LLC RF; p. 55 (top): © Peter Cade/Getty Images RF; (bottom): © Comstock/PunchStock RF; p. 56: Canada's Food Guide. Health Canada, 2007. Reproduced with the permission of the Minister of Health, 2011; 2-11: USDA; 2-12 (golf ball): © Corbis/Vol. 127 RF; (tennis ball): © PhotoDisc/OS25 RF; (cards): © The McGraw-Hill Companies, Inc./Jacques Cornell photographer; (baseball): © PhotoDisc/OS25 RF; p. 60: © Imagestate Media (John Foxx)/Imagestate RF; p. 61 (cereal): © Mitch Hrdlicka/Getty Images RF; (apple/sandwich): © Getty Images RF; (salmon): © C Squared Studios/Getty Images RF; p. 62: Office of Disease Prevention and Health Promotion, U.S. Department of Health and Human Services; p. 64: Steve Cole/Getty Images RF; p. 66: © Ryan

McVay/Getty Images RF; p. 69, 70: © The McGraw-Hill Companies, Inc./Jill Braaten, photographer; p. 73 (dietitian): © liquidlibrary/PictureQuest RF; (pill): © Royalty Free/Corbis; p. 75: © Ingram Publishing RF.

Chapter 3

Opener: © Getty Images/Jonelle Weaver RF; 3-1: © Dynamic Graphics/JupiterImages RF; p. 86: © Photodisc RF; p. 99: © Ingram Publishing/SuperStock RF; p. 107: © PhotoDisc/Vol. 83 RF; p. 109: © Royalty Free/Corbis; p. 110: © Rob Meinychuk/Getty Images RF; 3-22b: © J. James/Photo Researchers, Inc.; p. 115: © C Squared Studios/Getty Images RF; p. 117 (top): © Gladden Willis, M.D./Visuals Unlimited; (bottom): © Stockdisc/Becky Denzin RF; p. 119 (top): © Getty Images/Jonelle Weaver RF; (bottom): © Royalty Free/Corbis.

Chapter 4

Opener: © Getty Images/Jonelle Weaver RF; p. 125: © Imagestate media (John Foxx)/Imagestate RF; p. 128: © C Squared Studios/Getty Images RF; p. 131: © Jupiterimages/ImageSource RF; 4-7(grains): Keith Weller/USDA; (vegetables): © Mitch Hrdlicka/Getty Images RF; (fruits): © Ingram Publishing/SuperStock RF; p. 132: Ken Karp/McGraw-Hill Companies; p. 133: © BananaStock/PunchStock RF; p. 134(top): © BananaStock/PunchStock RF; (bottom): © Ryan McVay/Getty Images RF; p. 135: © Nancy R. Cohen/Getty Images RF; p. 136(top): © The McGraw-Hill Companies, Inc./Jill Braaten, photographer; (bottom): © Burke/Triolo Productions/Getty Images RF; p. 138: © Ingram Publishing/SuperStock RF; p. 139: Beano is a registered trademark of AkPharma Inc.; p. 140: © PhotoDisc/Getty Images RF; p. 142: Royalty Free/Corbis; p. 143: © BananaStock/PunchStock RF; p. 145 (top): © John A. Rizzo/Getty Images RF; (bottom): © Nancy R. Cohen/Getty Images RF; p. 146: © Getty Images; p. 147: © Nancy R. Cohen/Getty Images RF; p. 148: © Brand X/Punchstock RF; p. 149: © BananaStock/PunchStock RF; Table 4-5(cart): © Photodisc/Getty Images RF; (kitchen utensils): © CMCD/Getty Images RF; (silverware): © The McGraw-Hill Companies, Inc./Jack Holtel photographer; p. 153: © Stockdisc/PunchStock RF; p. 154: © Ariel Skelley/Blend Images LLC RF; p. 155: Dynamic Graphics/JupiterImages RF; p. 157: © Getty Images/Eyewire RF; p. 159: © Real Food by Warren Diggles/Alamy RF; Table 4-7(Breakfast): © Image Source/Corbis RF; (Lunch): © BananaStock/PunchStock RF; (Dinner): © Getty Images/Jonelle Weaver RF; p. 162: © Kevin Sanchez/Cole Group/Getty Images RF.

Chapter 5

Opener: © Ingram Publishing/SuperStock RF; p. 167: © Tetra Images/Getty Images RF; p. 169: © The McGraw-Hill Companies, Inc./Elite Images; 5-5 (Avocado): © Ingram Publishing/SuperStock RF; (chicken & fries): © BananaStock/PunchStock RF; (cheese): © Pixtal/age fotostock RF; p. 172 (bottom): © Jamie Grill/Corbis RF; p. 173: © Burke/Tiolo Productions/Getty Images RF; p. 174: © Allan Rosenberg/Cole Group/Getty Images RF; p. 176(top): © D. Hurst/Alamy RF; (bottom): © The McGraw-Hill Companies Inc./Ken Cavanagh Photographer; p. 177: © Ingram Publishing/Alamy RF; p. 178: © The McGraw-Hill Companies, Inc./Eilte Images; p. 179: © Getty Images/Digital Vision RF; p. 186: Courtesy National Fisheries Institute; p. 187: © Jack Star/PhotoLink/Getty Images RF; p. 188: © SW Productions/Getty Images RF; p. 190: Royalty

Free/Corbis; p. 192: © Digital Vision/Getty Images RF; p. 193: RF/Getty Images; p. 194 (top): © John A. Rizzo/Getty Images RF; (bottom): Royalty Free/Corbis; p. 196: © image100/PunchStock RF; p. 197: © The McGraw-Hill Companies, Inc./Photo by Erick Misko, Elite Images Photography; p. 198: © The McGraw-Hill Companies, Inc./Gary He, photographer; p. 200: © The McGraw-Hill Companies, Inc./Mark Dierker, photographer; p. 201, 203: © trbfoto/Brand X Pictures/Jupiterimages RF; p. 206(donut): © Jules Frazier/Getty Images RF; (bagel): © Ingram Publishing/Alamy RF.

Chapter 6

Opener: © The McGraw-Hill Companies; p. 212: © PhotoLink/Getty Images RF; p. 213: © Corbis/PictureQuest RF; p. 214: © Comstock/Jupiterimages RF; 6.3: © Dr. Stanley Flegler/Visuals Unlimited; p. 216(Panini): © Ingram Publishing/SuperStock RF; (eggs): © IT Stock/PunchStock RF; (milk): © Ingram Publishing/SuperStock RF : (beans): © IT Stock/PunchStock RF; p. 217: © Creatas/Punchstock RF; 6.6: © Corbis/Vol. 130 RF; p. 221: © Dynamic Graphics/JupiterImages RF; 6-11a: © Photodisc RF; 6-11b: © Stockbyte/Punchstock Images RF; 6-11c: © Dynamic Graphics/JupiterImages RF; Table 6.2(breakfast): © Image Source/Corbis RF; (lunch): © John A. Rizzo/Getty Images RF; (dinner): © Kevin Sanchez/Cole Group/Getty Images RF; (snack): © Comstock/Punchstock RF; p. 227: © Ingram Publishing/SuperStock RF; 6-12(left): © Kevin Fleming/Corbis; (right): © Peter Turnley/Corbis; p. 230: © The McGraw-Hill Companies/Barr Barker, photographer; p. 231: © Getty Images/Jonelle Weaver RF; p. 233(top): Walnut Marketing Board; (bottom): © Getty Images/Vol. 49 RF; p. 234: © Comstock/PunchStock RF; p. 235: © Getty Images/Jonelle Weaver RF; p. 236: © Image Source/JupiterImages RF; p. 238: © Ingram Publishing/SuperStock RF; p. 241: © Ryan McVay/Getty Images RF.

Chapter 7

Opener: © Ingram Publishing/SuperStock RF; p. 247: © Mitch Hrdlicka/Getty Images RF; p. 249: © Corbis/Vol. 130 RF; 7-5: © Samuel Ashfield/SPL/Photo Researchers, Inc.; p. 252: © Steve Mason/Getty Images RF; p. 254: © The McGraw-Hill Companies/Jill Braaton, photographer; 7-9: © Paul Efland University of Georgia; 7-10: Courtesy of Life Measurement Inc.; 7-11: © FotoSearch Stock Photography RF; 7-12: Maltron International Ltd; 7-13: Custom Medical Stock Photo; p. 258: © Corbis/RF website; p. 260(top): © Ingram Publishing/SuperStock RF; (bottom): © Jack Hollingsworth/Getty Images RF; p. 261: © Getty Images/SW Productions RF; p. 262: © PhotoDisc/Getty Images RF; 7-16(1): © Jon Feingersh/Blend Images LLC; (2): © Jose Luis Pelaez Inc/Blend Images LLC; (3): © Picture Net/Getty Images RF; p. 263: © Jose Luis Pelaez Inc/Blend Images/Jupiter Images RF; p. 265: © Zefa RF/Alamy; p. 266: © PhotoDisc/Vol. 20 RF; p. 268: © PhotoDisc/Vol. 20 RF; p. 269: © Royalty Free/Corbis Vol. 306; p. 270: © Dynamic Graphics/JupiterImages RF; p. 274: © Dynamic Graphics Group/Creatas/Alamy RF; p. 277: © Ernie Friedlander/Cole Group/Getty Images RF; p. 278: © Ryan McVay/Getty Images RF; p. 280(top): © Ingram Publishing/SuperStock RF; (bottom): © Comstock Images RF.

Chapter 8

Opener: © Royalty Free/Corbis; p. 291: © Liquid library/Picture Quest RF; p. 292: © PhotoLink/Getty Images RF; p. 293: © PhotoDisc/OS49 RF; 8-1: A Colour Atlas and Text of Nutritional Disorders by Dr. Donald D. McLaren/Mosby-Wolfe Europe Ltd.; 8-2: National Eye Institute, National Institute of Health; p. 295: © Kevin Sanchez/Cole Group/Getty Images RF; p. 297(broccoli): © Image Source/PunchStock RF; (cantaloupe): © Jupiterimages/ImageSource RF; (eggs): © IT Stock/PunchStock RF; p. 297: © Kevin Sanchez/Cole Group/Getty Images RF; p. 298: © Royalty Free/Corbis; 8-6: © Jeffrey L. Rotman/Corbis; p. 301: © Gregg Kidd and Joanne Scott; p. 303: © C Squared Studios/Getty Images RF; p. 304(cabbage): © Isabelle Rozenbaum & Frederic Cirou/PhotoAlto/PunchStock RF; (apple): © Photodisc/Getty Images RF; (nuts): © Stockbyte/Corbis RF; p. 304: © Banana Stock/PunchStock RF; p. 305: Visuals Unlimited; p. 306, 309: © Royalty Free/Corbis; p. 310: © Blue Moon Stock/PunchStock RF; 8-18a: A Colour Atlas and Text of Nutritional Disorders by Dr. Donald D. McLaren/Mosby-Wolfe Europe Ltd.; 8-18b: © Dr. P. Marazzi/Science Photo Library/Photo Researchers, Inc.; 8-20a: © Dr. M.A. Ansary/Photo Researchers, Inc.; 8-20b: © Lester V. Bergman/Corbis; p. 314: © Getty Images/Jonelle Weaver RF; p. 318: © Corbis/Vol. 130 RF; p. 319(potatoes): © Ingram Publishing/SuperStock RF; (watermelon): © Siede Preis/Getty Images RF; (raw chicken): © Ingram Publishing/SuperStock RF; p. 319: © Getty Images/Jonelle Weaver RF; p. 320: © C Squared Studios/Getty Images RF.

Chapter 9

Opener: © Burke Triolo Productions/Getty Images RF; p. 350: © Royalty-Free/Corbis; 9.3(tomato): © Getty Images/Stockbyte RF; p. 352: © Royalty-Free/Corbis; p. 355(top): © Getty Images RF; (bottom): © Corbis/Vol. 83 RF; p. 357: © Burke Triolo Productions/Getty Images RF; p. 358: MHHE Image Library; p. 359: © Royalty Free/Corbis; p. 360: © Corbis/Vol. 43 RF; p. 362: © C Squared Studios/Getty Images RF; p. 363(tomatoes) © Brand X Pictures/PunchStock RF; (Pears) © Corbis RF; (Shrimp) © Comstock Images/Jupiterimages RF; p. 364: © Stockdisc/PunchStock RF; p. 365: MHHE Image Library; p. 366: © Getty Images/PhotoDisc RF; p. 367(reading milk label): McGraw-Hill Companies/Andrew Resek, photographer; p. 367(beans): © Image Source/PunchStock RF; (yogurt): © Mitch Hrdlicka/Getty Images RF; (nuts): © Image Source/PunchStock RF; p. 368: © The McGraw-Hill Companies, Inc./Jill Braaten; p. 369: © Corbis/Vol. 43 RF; p. 371(gourds): © Burke/Triolo/Getty Images RF; (peaches): © Jupiterimages/ImageSource RF; (beans): © Image Source/PunchStock RF; p. 372(top): © Corbis/RF website; (bottom): © Michael Lamotte/Cole Group/Getty Images RF; p. 374: © Royalty Free/Corbis; p. 376(peas): © Ingram Publishing/SuperStock RF; (apricots): © Image Source/PunchStock RF; (meats): © Brand X Pictures/PunchStock RF; p. 377: Courtesy National Cattlemen's Beef Associations; p. 378(top): © Keith Brofsky/Getty Images RF; (bottom): Photo courtesy of Harold H. Sandstead, M.D.; p. 379: © Corbis/Vol. 130 RF; p. 380(milk): © Pixtal/SuperStock RF; (asparagus): © Brand X Pictures/PunchStock RF; (chicken): © Ernie Friedlander/Cole Group/Getty Images RF; p. 381: © Ingram Publishing/SuperStock RF; p. 382: © Scott Camazine/Photo Researchers, Inc.; p. 384: Courtesy of Fishery Products International, Denver, MA; p. 386(top): © Paul Casamassimo, DDS, MS; (bottom): © PhotoDisc/Vol. 02 RF; p. 387(top): © Corbis/RF website; (bottom): © C Squared Studios/Getty Images RF; 9-23: © Ryan McVay/Getty Images RF; p. 392(left): © PhotoDisc/Vol. 40 RF; (right): © Rob Melnychuk/Getty Images RF; p. 393: © Ryan McVay/Getty Images RF; p. 396: © Yoav Levy/Phototake; p. 398: © Royalty Free/Corbis; p. 399: © Royalty Free/Corbis; p. 401(top): © Comstock Images RF; (bottom): © JGI Blend Images LLC RF.

Chapter 10

Opener: © Getty Images; 10.1: © Rubberball/Getty Images RF; 10.2: © John Lund/Sam Diephuis/Blend Images LLC RF; 10.2: © Tetra Images/SuperStock RF; p. 413: © PhotoDisc/Sports Metaphors RF; p. 414: © Royalty Free/Corbis; p. 416: © JupiterImages RF; p. 417: © Corbis/Vol. 20 RF; p. 418: © James Mulligan; p. 419: © Corbis/RF website; p. 422(top): © IngramPublishing/SuperStock RF; (bottom): © Royalty Free/Corbis, p. 423(top): © Gordon Wardlaw; (bottom): © Royalty Free/Corbis; p. 425: © PhotoDisc/Vol. 51 RF; p. 428(top): © Getty Images/Jonelle Weaver RF; (bottom): © John A. Rizzo/Getty Images RF; p. 429: © PhotoDisc/Vol. 51 RF; p. 434 (top): © Corbis/Vol. 20 RF; (bottom): © Comstock Images RF; p. 436: © Stockbyte/Getty Images RF; p. 438: © JupiterImages RF.

Chapter 11

Opener: © Corbis/Vol. 75 RF; p. 447: © The McGraw-Hill Companies, Inc./Lars A. Niki, photographer; p. 448: © Photodisc website RF; p. 449: © Royalty Free/Corbis; p. 450: © Mark Andersen/Getty Images RF; p. 451: © Stockbyte/PunchStock RF; p. 452: © PhotoDisc website RF; p. 455: © Tom Stewart Photography/Corbis; p. 456: © Comstock Images RF; 11-2: © Brand X Pictures/PunchStock RF; p. 458: © Royalty Free/Corbis; p. 459: © PhotoDisc Website RF; p. 460: © Jack Star/PhotoLink/Getty Images RF; p. 462: © BananaStock/PunchStock RF; 11-3: © Photodisc/Vol. 45 RF; p. 463: © The McGraw-Hill Companies, Inc./Lars A. Niki, photographer; p. 464: © PhotoDisc website RF; p. 465: © Digital Vision/Getty Images RF; p. 466: © Corbis/RF website; p. 467: © BananaStock/PunchStock RF; p. 469: © Don Manson/Blend Images LLC RF; p. 471: © Digital Vision/PunchStock RF.

Chapter 12

Opener: © Nicholas Pitt/Digital Vision/Getty Images RF; p. 474: © Corbis/RF website; p. 478: USDA photo by Peter Manzelli; p. 480: © Royalty Free/Corbis; p. 481: © PhotoDisc/Vol. 25 RF; p. 483: © The McGraw-Hill Companies, Inc./Barry Barker, photographer, p. 484: © Getty Images/Digital Vision RF; p. 485: © The McGraw-Hill Companies, Inc./Barry Barker, photographer; p. 486(both): © The Ohio State University Communications Photo Service; p. 487: © Corbis/RF website; p. 489: © Corbis/Vol. 25 RF; p. 491: © Erin Koran RF; p. 494: © Corbis/Vol. 609 RF; p. 495: © The Ohio State University Communications Photo Service, Jodi Miller; 12-7(child mortality): © Corbis/RF website; (human suffering, loss of parents, exploitation of women): AP Wide World Photos; p. 498: © Corbis/RF website; p. 499: © Digital Vision/PunchStock RF; p. 501: © Getty Images RF.

Chapter 13

Opener: © Lifesize/Getty Images RF; p. 507: © Royalty Free/Corbis; p. 508: © The Ohio State University Communications Photo Service; p. 511: © John A. Rizzo/Getty Images RF; Table 13-3(Salmonella species): © Photodisc/Getty Images RF; (Campylobacter jejuni): © I. Rozenbaum/F. Cirou/Photo Alto RF; (Escherichia coli): © John A. Rizzo/Getty Images RF; (Shigella species): © Comstock Images/PictureQuest RF; (Staphylococcus aureus): © Michael Lamotte/Cole Group/Getty Images RF; (Clostridium perfringens): © Ingram Publishing/Fotosearch RF; (Listeria monocytogenes): © Digital Vision/Getty Images RF; (Clostridium botulinum): Photo provided by Jarden Home Brands, marketers of Ball® and Kerr® fresh preserving products. Jarden Home Brands is a division of Jarden Corporation (NYSE: JAH); (Vibrio): © I. Rozenbaum/F. Cirou/Photo Alto RF; (Yersinia enterocolitica): © Foodcollection/Getty Images RF; p. 514(top): © Royalty Free/Corbis; (bottom): © Image Source/Corbis RF; Table 13-5(Trichinella spiralis): © Ingram Publishing/Alamy RF; (Anisakis): © Image Source/Corbis RF; (Tapeworms):

© I. Rozenbaum/F. Cirou/Photo Alto RF; (Toxoplasma gondii): © The Ohio State University Communications Photo Service; (Cyclospora cayetenensis): © Don Farrall/Getty Images RF; (Cryptosporidium): © John A. Rizzo/Getty Images RF; p. 517: © Corbis/Vol. 83 RF; p. 518: © Corbis/Vol. 192 RF; p. 520: © Bob Montesciaros/Cole Group/Getty Images RF; p. 521(top): © Rob Melnychuk/Getty Images RF; (bottom): © The Ohio State University Communications Photo Service; p. 522: © Image Source/Corbis RF; p. 523: © Corbis/Vol. 43 RF; p. 525: © The Ohio State University Communications Photo Service; p. 526: © PhotoDisc website RF; p. 527(basket): © Corbis/Vol. 49 RF; (facet): © Comstock Images/PictureQuest RF; (USDA seal): USDA; p. 528: © C Squared Studios/Getty Images RF; p. 529: © The McGraw-Hill Companies, Inc./Christopher Kerrigan, photographer; p. 530: © Iconotec.com RF; p. 532(top): USDA; (bottom): © Greg Wolff; p. 533: © PhotoDisc/Vol. 48 RF; p. 535: © PhotoDisc/Vol. 58 RF; p. 537: © The McGraw Hill Companies, Inc.; p. 538: © Jess Alford/Getty Images RF; p. 539(top): © Digital Vision/Getty Images RF; (bottom): © David Buffington/Getty Images RF.

Chapter 14

Opener: © Getty Images RF; p. 543: © BananaStock/PunchStock RF; p. 546: © Gordon Wardlaw, photographer Greg Wolff; p. 547: © Blend Images/Getty Images RF; p. 549: USDA; p. 550: © Tanya Constantine/Blend Images LLC RF; p. 552: © Getty Images RF; p. 555: © Photodisc Collection/Getty Images RF; p. 556: © Getty Images/Jonelle Weaver RF; p. 558: © Corbis/Vol. 83 RF; p. 560: © Getty Images RF; p. 563: © Scott T. Baxter/Getty Images RF; p. 564: © PhotoDisc/Vol. 192 RF; p. 565: © PhotoDisc/EP039 RF; p. 566: © 2008 Medela AG; p. 567: © Corbis/Vol. 52 RF; p. 569: © Getty Images RF; p. 572: © Digital Vision/PunchStock RF; p. 574: © Hill Street Studios/Blend Images LLC RF; p. 577: © Andersen Ross/Getty Images RF.

Chapter 15

Opener: © Banana Stock/PunchStock RF; p. 583(top): World Health Organization; (bottom): © PhotoDisc/Vol. 113 RF; p. 584: © PhotoAlto/PictureQuest RF; p. 589(top): © PhotoDisc/Vol. 58 RF; (bottom): © Corbis/PictureQuest RF; p. 591: © PhotoDisc/Vol. 113 RF; p. 592(top): © Corbis/PictureQuest RF; (bottom): © Paul Casamassimo, DDS, MS; p. 593: © Corbis/Vol. 9 RF; p. 594: © Digital Vision/Getty Images RF; p. 595: Joanne Scott; p. 596: © Banana Stock/PunchStock RF; p. 597: USDA Photo by Ken Hammond; p. 598: © Ablestock/Alamy RF; p. 600: © Banana Stock/PunchStock RF; p. 602: © Corbis/Vol. 552 RF; p. 603: © Ingram Publishing/SuperStock RF; p. 604: © Stockbyte/PunchStock; p. 605: © Corbis/RF website; p. 606: © PhotoDisc/Vol. 95 RF; p. 607: © Corbis/Vol. 124 RF; p. 609: © The McGraw-Hill Companies, Inc./Ken Karp photographer; p. 611: © PhotoDisc/Vol. 61 RF; p. 613: © Dynamic Graphics/JupiterImages RF; p. 615: © The McGraw-Hill Companies, Inc./Jill Braaten, photographer.

Chapter 16

Opener: © Digital Vision/PunchStock RF; p. 621: © Royalty Free/Corbis; p. 622: © Corbis/RF website; p. 628: © Blend Images/Getty Images RF; p. 629: © Image Source/Corbis RF; p. 632: © PhotoDisc Vol. 15 RF; p. 633: © Stockbyte/Punchstock RF; p. 635: © Ingram Publishing RF; p. 638(top): © PhotoDisc/Vol. 20 RF; (bottom): © Corbis/Vol. 192 RF; p. 640: © PhotoDisc website RF; p. 642(both): © Arthur Glauberman/Photo Researchers, Inc.; p. 643: © PhotoDisc/Vol. 48 RF; p. 644: © RF/Corbis; p. 646(both): © PhotoDisc/OS49 RF; p. 650: © PhotoDisc website RF; p. 652: © Ingram Publishing RF; p. 654: © RF/Corbis; p. 655: © PhotoDisc/SS45 RF.

Appendix

Figure D-1(all): © Greg Kidd & Joanne Scott.
Appendix, Glossary, Index (Almonds): © Getty Images/Stockbyte

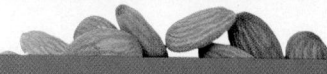
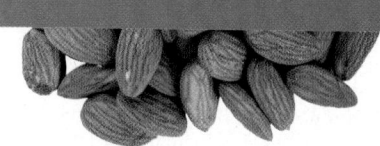

INDEX

A

ABCDE. *See* Anthropometric, Biochemical, Clinical, Dietary, and Environmental
Absorption, 82, 96
   processes, 96–97
   sites, 105t
Absorptive cells, 100, 101
Absorptive processes, types, 103f
Acceptable Daily Intake (ADI), 136
Accessory organs, 106
Acesulfame-K, 135, 136
Acetaldehyde dehydrogenase, 639
Acid-base balance (pH), 107
   proteins, impact, 222
Acid group, 167
Acne
   nutrition, relationship, 606
   vitamin A analogs, usage, 295–296
Acquired immunodeficiency syndrome
     (AIDS), 484
   nutrition, relationship, 489
   Vitamin B-12 deficiency, 327
   worldwide impact, 488–489
Actionable health messages, usage, 56
Active absorption, 103
Activities, calorie cost approximation, 266t
Added sugars, 53, 59f, 564
   intake, limitation, 20
   sources, 149f
Additives, 515
Adenosine diphosphate (ADP), 412
Adenosine triphosphate (ATP), 86, 412
   energy form, 418
   formation, 416f
   yield, 414f
Adequate intake (AI), 48, 50f
Adipose cell, 188
Adipose tissue growth, 583
Adjustable gastric banding, 272
Adolescents (weight gain), food advertising/
     marketing (impact), 5
Adulthood
   Alzheimer's disease, 637
   body composition, 630
   calcium/vitamin D, impact, 628
   calories, requirement, 626–627
   carbohydrate intake, 627
   carotenoid, dietary intakes, 629
   chronic disease, 633
   depression, 636–637
   dietary recommendations, 629
   diet quality, 643–645
   diet recommendations, 631t
   digestive system, 632–633
   eating, guidelines, 644t
   economic factors, 637–638
   endocrine system, 633
   environment, impact, 624–625
   exercise guidelines, 632
   fat intake, 627
   folate/Vitamins B-6/B-12, role, 628

immune system, 633
iron, impact, 628
lifestyle, 624
   responses, 631t
magnesium intake, 628
medications, 634
minerals/vitamins, usage, 627–628
nervous system, 633
nutrient needs, 625–638
nutrition checklist, 626f
physiological changes, 621–625, 631t
physiological factors, 630–634
protein intake, 627
psychosocial factors, 636–638
relative nutrient requirements, 627f
skeletal system, 630, 632
Vitamin E, dietary intake, 628
water consumption, 627
zinc intake, 628
Adult obesity
   percentage, 18f
   trends, 245
Adult physical activity/exercise, *Healthy People
     2010* objectives, 409
Adult zinc deficiency, symptoms, 379
Advanced glycation endproducts (AGEs), 152
Advertising, media tool, 6
Aerobic, term (usage), 414
Aerobic glucose use, ATP yield, 414f
Aerobic process, 84
Aerobic workout, 411–412
Age
   bone, relationship, 395–396
   groups, MyPlate calorie guidelines, 251f
Age-related macular degeneration, impact, 295
Aging, 621
   alternative medicine, relationship, 634–635
   causes, 622
   nutritional deficiencies, 643
   physiological function, declines, 621
   process, health rating, 654
   rate, factors, 623
   success, 623
Air displacement, 254
Alcohol, 15
   absorption/metabolism, 639–640
   abuse, 639
     risks, 640, 642
   calorie content/source, 15
   consumption, nutrition implications,
     638–643
   dehydrogenase, 639
   dependence, 640
   drinking, 26
   intake, limitation, 20
   proof, representation, 639
   release, 15
   thiamin, relationship, 312
Alcoholic beverages
   alcohol/carbohydrate/calorie content, 638t
   production process, 639
Alcoholism, 640

Alcohol-related birth defects (ARBDs), 570
Alcohol-related neurodevelopmental disorders
     (ARNDs), 570
Alcohol use
   benefits/risks, 641t
   guidance, 642–643
   moderation, benefits, 640
Aldosterone, 353
Allergen, 608
Allergies, 585
   prevention, 590–591
   types, 608
Alpha-linolenic acid, 169
   DRI, 187
Alternative sweeteners, 133t, 135–136
Alzheimer's disease, 637
American Heart Association (AHA), 2006 Diet
    and Lifestyle Goals/Recommendations
    for Cardiovascular Disease Risk
    Reduction, 191t
Amino acids, 12, 211–213
   bonding, 12, 213–216
   B vitamin input, 308
   classification, 212t
   metabolism, 224f
     Vitamin B-6, impact, 318
   R group, 211
   supplements, 227–228, 238
Amniotic fluid, 351
Amphetamines, 270
Amylase, 99
Amylopectin, 128, 129f
Amylose, 128, 129f
Anaerobic, term (usage), 84, 414
Anaerobic glucose breakdown
   advantage, 414
   energy, 414–416
Anaerobic glucose use, ATP yield, 414f
Anaerobic metabolism, 84
Anaerobic process, disadvantages, 414
Anal canal, moisture (presence), 115
Analog, 295
Anal sphincters, 105
Anaphylactic shock, 609
Anemia, 375. *See also* Iron-deficiency anemia;
    Pernicious anemia; Physiological anemia
Angular cheilitis (angular stomatitis), 312f
Animal cell, 84f
Animal food, cholesterol (presence), 173–174
Animal model, 47
Animal sources, protein supply, 19
Anorexia nervosa, 447–451
   characteristics, 449t, 465–466
   cognitive behavior therapy, 455
   early warning signs, 451–452
   examination, 450–455

A

Dietary Reference Intakes (DRIs): Recommended Intakes for Individuals, Vitamins
Food and Nutrition Board, Institute of Medicine, National Academies

Life Stage Group	Vitamin A (μg/d)[a]	Vitamin C (mg/d)	Vitamin D (μg/d)[b,c]	Vitamin E (mg/d)[d]	Vitamin K (μg/d)	Thiamin (mg/d)	Riboflavin (mg/d)	Niacin (mg/d)[e]	Vitamin B-6 (mg/d)	Folate (μg/d)[f]	Vitamin B-12 (μg/d)	Pantothenic Acid (mg/d)	Biotin (μg/d)	Choline (mg/d)[g]
Infants														
0–6 mo	400*	40*	10	4*	2.0*	0.2*	0.3*	2*	0.1*	65*	0.4*	1.7*	5*	125*
7–12 mo	500*	50*	10	5*	2.5*	0.3*	0.4*	4*	0.3*	80*	0.5*	1.8*	6*	150*
Children														
1–3 y	300	15	15	6	30*	0.5	0.5	6	0.5	150	0.9	2*	8*	200*
4–8 y	400	25	15	7	55*	0.6	0.6	8	0.6	200	1.2	3*	12*	250*
Males														
9–13 y	600	45	15	11	60*	0.9	0.9	12	1.0	300	1.8	4*	20*	375*
14–18 y	900	75	15	15	75*	1.2	1.3	16	1.3	400	2.4	5*	25*	550*
19–30 y	900	90	15	15	120*	1.2	1.3	16	1.3	400	2.4	5*	30*	550*
31–50 y	900	90	15	15	120*	1.2	1.3	16	1.3	400	2.4	5*	30*	550*
51–70 y	900	90	15	15	120*	1.2	1.3	16	1.7	400	2.4[h]	5*	30*	550*
>70 y	900	90	20	15	120*	1.2	1.3	16	1.7	400	2.4[h]	5*	30*	550*
Females														
9–13 y	600	45	15	11	60*	0.9	0.9	12	1.0	300	1.8	4*	20*	375*
14–18 y	700	65	15	15	75*	1.0	1.0	14	1.2	400[i]	2.4	5*	25*	400*
19–30 y	700	75	15	15	90*	1.1	1.1	14	1.3	400[i]	2.4	5*	30*	425*
31–50 y	700	75	15	15	90*	1.1	1.1	14	1.3	400[i]	2.4	5*	30*	425*
51–70 y	700	75	15	15	90*	1.1	1.1	14	1.5	400	2.4[h]	5*	30*	425*
>70 y	700	75	20	15	90*	1.1	1.1	14	1.5	400	2.4[h]	5*	30*	425*
Pregnancy														
≤18 y	750	80	15	15	75*	1.4	1.4	18	1.9	600[j]	2.6	6*	30*	450*
19–30 y	770	85	15	15	90*	1.4	1.4	18	1.9	600[j]	2.6	6*	30*	450*
31–50 y	770	85	15	15	90*	1.4	1.4	18	1.9	600[j]	2.6	6*	30*	450*
Lactation														
≤18 y	1200	115	15	19	75*	1.4	1.6	17	2.0	500	2.8	7*	35*	550*
19–30 y	1300	120	15	19	90*	1.4	1.6	17	2.0	500	2.8	7*	35*	550*
31–50 y	1300	120	15	19	90*	1.4	1.6	17	2.0	500	2.8	7*	35*	550*

mg = milligram, mg = microgram

NOTE: This table (taken from the DRI reports; see www.nap.edu) presents Recommended Dietary Allowances (RDAs) in **bold type** and Adequate Intakes (AIs) in ordinary type followed by an asterisk (*). RDAs and AIs may both be used as goals for individual intake. RDAs are set to meet the needs of almost all (97 to 98%) individuals in a group. For healthy breastfed infants, the AI is the mean intake. The AI for other life stage and gender groups is believed to cover needs of all individuals in the group, but lack of data or uncertainty in the data prevents being able to specify with confidence the percentage of individuals covered by this intake.

[a] As retinol activity equivalents (RAEs). 1 RAE = 1 μg retinol, 12 μg β-carotene, 24 μg α-carotene, or 24 μg β-cryptoxanthin. To calculate RAEs from REs of provitamin A carotenoids in foods, divide the REs by 2. For preformed vitamin A in foods or supplements and for provitamin A carotenoids in supplements, 1 RE = 1 RAE.

[b] cholecalciferol. 1 μg cholecalciferol = 40 IU vitamin D.

[c] In the absence of adequate exposure to sunlight.

[d] As α-tocopherol. α-Tocopherol includes RRR-α-tocopherol, the only form of α-tocopherol that occurs naturally in foods, and the 2R-stereoisomeric forms of α-tocopherol (RRR-, RSR-, RRS-, and RSS-α-tocopherol) that occur in fortified foods and supplements. It does not include the 2S-stereoisomeric forms of α-tocopherol (SRR-, SSR-, SRS-, and SSS-α-tocopherol), also found in fortified foods and supplements.

[e] As niacin equivalents (NE). 1 mg of niacin = 60 mg of tryptophan; 0–6 months = preformed niacin (not NE).

[f] As dietary folate equivalents (DFE). 1 DFE = 1 μg food folate = 0.6 μg of folic acid from fortified food or as a supplement consumed with food = 0.5 μg of a supplement taken on an empty stomach.

[g] Although AIs have been set for choline, there are few data to assess whether a dietary supply of choline is needed at all stages of the life cycle, and it may be that the choline requirement can be met by endogenous synthesis at some of these stages.

[h] Because 10 to 30% of older people may malabsorb food-bound B-12, it is advisable for those older than 50 years to meet their RDA mainly by consuming foods fortified with B-12 or a supplement containing B-12.

[i] In view of evidence linking folate intake with neural tube defects in the fetus, it is recommended that all women capable of becoming pregnant consume 400 μg from supplements or fortified foods in addition to intake of food folate from a varied diet.

[j] It is assumed that women will continue consuming 400 μg from supplements or fortified food until their pregnancy is confirmed and they enter prenatal care, which ordinarily occurs after the end of the periconceptional period—the critical time for formation of the neural tube.

Adapted from the Dietary Reference Intakes series, National Academies Press. Copyright 1997, 1998, 2000, 2001, 2011, by the National Academy of Sciences. The full reports are available from the National Academies Press at www.nap.edu.

Dietary Reference Intakes (DRIs): Recommended Intakes for Individuals, Elements
Food and Nutrition Board, Institute of Medicine, National Academies

Life Stage Group	Calcium (mg/d)	Chromium (µg/d)	Copper (µg/d)	Fluoride (mg/d)	Iodine (µg/d)	Iron (mg/d)	Magnesium (mg/d)	Manganese (mg/d)	Molybdenum (µg/d)	Phosphorus (mg/d)	Selenium (µg/d)	Zinc (mg/d)
Infants												
0–6 mo	200*	0.2*	200*	0.01*	110*	0.27*	30*	0.003*	2*	100*	15*	2*
7–12 mo	260*	5.5*	220*	0.5*	130*	11	75*	0.6*	3*	275*	20*	3
Children												
1–3 y	700	11*	340	0.7*	90	7	80	1.2*	17	460	20	3
4–8 y	1000	15*	440	1*	90	10	130	1.5*	22	500	30	5
Males												
9–13 y	1300	25*	700	2*	120	8	240	1.9*	34	1250	40	8
14–18 y	1300	35*	890	3*	150	11	410	2.2*	43	1250	55	11
19–30 y	1000	35*	900	4*	150	8	400	2.3*	45	700	55	11
31–50 y	1000	35*	900	4*	150	8	420	2.3*	45	700	55	11
51–70 y	1000	30*	900	4*	150	8	420	2.3*	45	700	55	11
>70 y	1200	30*	900	4*	150	8	420	2.3*	45	700	55	11
Females												
9–13 y	1300	21*	700	2*	120	8	240	1.6*	34	1250	40	8
14–18 y	1300	24*	890	3*	150	15	360	1.6*	43	1250	55	9
19–30 y	1000	25*	900	3*	150	18	310	1.8*	45	700	55	8
31–50 y	1000	25*	900	3*	150	18	320	1.8*	45	700	55	8
51–70 y	1200	20*	900	3*	150	8	320	1.8*	45	700	55	8
>70 y	1200	20*	900	3*	150	8	320	1.8*	45	700	55	8
Pregnancy												
≤18 y	1300	29*	1000	3*	220	27	400	2.0*	50	1250	60	12
19–30 y	1000	30*	1000	3*	220	27	350	2.0*	50	700	60	11
31–50 y	1000	30*	1000	3*	220	27	360	2.0*	50	700	60	11
Lactation												
≤18 y	1300	44*	1300	3*	290	10	360	2.6*	50	1250	70	13
19–30 y	1000	45*	1300	3*	290	9	310	2.6*	50	700	70	12
31–50 y	1000	45*	1300	3*	290	9	320	2.6*	50	700	70	12

NOTE: This table presents Recommended Dietary Allowances (RDAs) in **bold type** and Adequate Intakes (AIs) in ordinary type followed by an asterisk (*). RDAs and AIs may both be used as goals for individual intake. RDAs are set to meet the needs of almost all (97 to 98%) individuals in a group. For healthy breastfed infants, the AI is the mean intake. The AI for other life stage and gender groups is believed to cover needs of all individuals in the group, but lack of data or uncertainty in the data prevents being able to specify with confidence the percentage of individuals covered by this intake.

Sources: Dietary Reference Intakes for Calcium, Phosphorus, Magnesium, Vitamin D, and Fluoride (1997); Dietary Reference Intakes for Thiamin, Riboflavin, Niacin, Vitamin B-6, Folate, Vitamin B-12, Pantothenic Acid, Biotin, and Choline (1998); Dietary Reference Intakes for Vitamin C, Vitamin E, Selenium, and Carotenoids (2000); Dietary Reference Intakes for Vitamin A, Vitamin K, Arsenic, Boron, Chromium, Copper, Iodine, Iron, Manganese, Molybdenum, Nickel, Silicon, Vanadium, and Zinc (2001); and Dietary Reference Intakes for Calcium and Vitamin D (2011). These reports may be accessed via www.nap.edu. Copyright 1997, 1998, 2000, 2001, and 2011 by the National Academy of Sciences. The full reports are available from the National Academies Press at www.nap.edu.

Adapted from the Dietary Reference Intake series, National Academies Press.

B

Dietary Reference Intakes (DRIs): Recommended Intakes for Individuals, Macronutrients
Food and Nutrition Board, Institute of Medicine, National Academies

Life Stage Group	Carbohydrate (g/d)	Total Fiber (g/d)	Fat (g/d)	Linoleic Acid (g/d)	α-Linolenic Acid (g/d)	Protein[a] (g/d)
Infants						
0–6 mo	60*	ND	31*	4.4*	0.5*	9.1*
7–12 mo	95*	ND	30*	4.6*	0.5*	11.0
Children						
1–3 y	130	19*	ND[b]	7*	0.7*	13
4–8 y	130	25*	ND	10*	0.9*	19
Males						
9–13 y	130	31*	ND	12*	1.2*	34
14–18 y	130	38*	ND	16*	1.6*	52
19–30 y	130	38*	ND	17*	1.6*	56
31–50 y	130	38*	ND	17*	1.6*	56
51–70 y	130	30*	ND	14*	1.6*	56
>70 y	130	30*	ND	14*	1.6*	56
Females						
9–13 y	130	26*	ND	10*	1.0*	34
14–18 y	130	26*	ND	11*	1.1*	46
19–30 y	130	25*	ND	12*	1.1*	46
31–50 y	130	25*	ND	12*	1.1*	46
51–70 y	130	21*	ND	11*	1.1*	46
>70 y	130	21*	ND	11*	1.1*	46
Pregnancy						
14–18 y	175	28*	ND	13*	1.4*	71
19–30 y	175	28*	ND	13*	1.4*	71
31–50 y	175	28*	ND	13*	1.4*	71
Lactation						
14–18 y	210	29*	ND	13*	1.3*	71
19–30 y	210	29*	ND	13*	1.3*	71
31–50 y	210	29*	ND	13*	1.3*	71

NOTE: This table presents Recommended Dietary Allowances (RDAs) in **bold type** and Adequate Intakes (AIs) in ordinary type followed by an asterisk (*). RDAs and AIs may both be used as goals for individual intake. RDAs are set to meet the needs of almost all (97 to 98%) individuals in a group. For healthy breastfed infants, the AI is the mean intake. The AI for other life stage and gender groups is believed to cover needs of all individuals in the group, but lack of data or uncertainty in the data prevents being able to specify with confidence the percentage of individuals covered by this intake.

[a]Based on 0.8 g protein/kg body weight for reference body weight.

[b]ND = not determinable at this time.

Sources: Dietary Reference Intakes for Energy, Carbohydrate, Fiber, Fat, Fatty Acids, Cholesterol, Protein, and Amino Acids (2002). This report may be accessed via www.nap.edu.
Reprinted with permission from the Dietary Reference Intake series, National Academies Press. Copyright 1997, 1998, 2000, 2001, by the National Academy of Sciences. The full reports are available from the National Academies Press at www.nap.edu.
Adapted from the Dietary Reference Intake series, National Academies Press.

Dietary Reference Intakes (DRIs): Recommended Intakes for Individuals, Electrolytes and Water
Food and Nutrition Board, Institute of Medicine, National Academies

Life Stage Group	Sodium (mg/d)	Potassium (mg/d)	Chloride (mg/d)	Water (L/d)
Infants				
0–6 mo	120*	400*	180*	0.7*
7–12 mo	370*	700*	570*	0.8*
Children				
1–3 y	1000*	3000*	1500*	1.3*
4–8 y	1200*	3800*	1900*	1.7*
Males				
9–13 y	1500*	4500*	2300*	2.4*
14–18 y	1500*	4700*	2300*	3.3*
19–30 y	1500*	4700*	2300*	3.7*
31–50 y	1500*	4700*	2300*	3.7*
51–70 y	1300*	4700*	2000*	3.7*
> 70 y	1200*	4700*	1800*	3.7*
Females				
9–13 y	1500*	4500*	2300*	2.1*
14–18 y	1500*	4700*	2300*	2.3*
19–30 y	1500*	4700*	2300*	2.7*
31–50 y	1500*	4700*	2300*	2.7*
51–70 y	1300*	4700*	2000*	2.7*
> 70 y	1200*	4700*	1800*	2.7*
Pregnancy				
14–18 y	1500*	4700*	2300*	3.0*
19–50 y	1500*	4700*	2300*	3.0*
Lactation				
14–18 y	1500*	5100*	2300*	3.8*
19–50 y	1500*	5100*	2300*	3.8*

NOTE: The table is adapted from the DRI reports. See www.nap.edu. Adequate Intakes (AIs) are followed by an asterisk (*). These may be used as a goal for individual intake. For healthy breastfed infants, the AI is the average intake. The AI for other life stage and gender groups is believed to cover the needs of all individuals in the group, but lack of data prevent being able to specify with confidence the percentage of individuals covered by this intake; therefore, no Recommended Dietary Allowance (RDA) was set.

Source: *Dietary Reference Intakes for Water, Potassium, Sodium, Chloride, and Sulfate* (2005). This report may be accessed via www.nap.edu.

Acceptable Macronutrient Distribution Ranges

Macronutrient	Range (percent of energy)		
	Children, 1–3 y	Children, 4–18 y	Adults
Fat	30–40	25–35	20–35
omega-6 polyunsaturated fats (linoleic acid)	5–10	5–10	5–10
omega-3 polyunsaturated fats[a] (α-linolenic acid)	0.6–1.2	0.6–1.2	0.6–1.2
Carbohydrate	45–65	45–65	45–65
Protein	5–20	10–30	10–35

[a]Approximately 10% of the total can come from longer-chain n-3 fatty acids.

SOURCE: *Dietary Reference Intakes for Energy, Carbohydrate, Fiber, Fat, Fatty Acids, Cholesterol, Protein, and Amino Acids* (2002). The report may be accessed via www.nap.edu.

Adapted from the Dietary Reference Intakes series, National Academies Press. Copyright 1997, 1998, 2000, 2001, 2011, by the National Academy of Sciences. The full reports are available from the National Academies Press at www.nap.edu.

Dietary Reference Intakes (DRIs): Tolerable Upper Intake Levels (UL[a]), Vitamins

Food and Nutrition Board, Institute of Medicine, National Academies

Life Stage Group	Vitamin A (μg/d)[b]	Vitamin C (mg/d)	Vitamin D (μg/d)	Vitamin E (mg/d)[c,d]	Vitamin K	Thiamin	Riboflavin	Niacin (mg/d)[d]	Vitamin B-6 (mg/d)	Folate (μg/d)[d]	Vitamin B-12	Pantothenic Acid	Biotin	Choline (g/d)	Carotenoids[e]
Infants															
0–6 mo	600	ND	25	ND	ND	ND	ND	ND	ND	ND	ND	ND	ND	ND	ND
7–12 mo	600	ND	38	ND	ND	ND	ND	ND	ND	ND	ND	ND	ND	ND	ND
Children															
1–3 y	600	400	63	200	ND	ND	ND	10	30	300	ND	ND	ND	1.0	ND
4–8 y	900	650	75	300	ND	ND	ND	15	40	400	ND	ND	ND	1.0	ND
Males, Females															
9–13 y	1700	1200	100	600	ND	ND	ND	20	60	600	ND	ND	ND	2.0	ND
14–18 y	2800	1800	100	800	ND	ND	ND	30	80	800	ND	ND	ND	3.0	ND
19–70 y	3000	2000	100	1000	ND	ND	ND	35	100	1000	ND	ND	ND	3.5	ND
>70 y	3000	2000	100	1000	ND	ND	ND	35	100	1000	ND	ND	ND	3.5	ND
Pregnancy															
≤18 y	2800	1800	100	800	ND	ND	ND	30	80	800	ND	ND	ND	3.0	ND
19–50 y	3000	2000	100	1000	ND	ND	ND	35	100	1000	ND	ND	ND	3.5	ND
Lactation															
≤18 y	2800	1800	100	800	ND	ND	ND	30	80	800	ND	ND	ND	3.0	ND
19–50 y	3000	2000	100	1000	ND	ND	ND	35	100	1000	ND	ND	ND	3.5	ND

[a] UL = The maximum level of daily nutrient intake likely to pose no risk of adverse effects. Unless otherwise specified, the UL represents total intake from food, water, and supplements. Due to lack of suitable data, ULs could not be established for vitamin K, thiamin, riboflavin, vitamin B-12, pantothenic acid, biotin, or carotenoids. In the absence of ULs, extra caution may be warranted in consuming levels above recommended intakes.

[b] As preformed vitamin A only.

[c] As α-tocopherol; applies to any form of supplemental α-tocopherol.

[d] The ULs for vitamin E, niacin, and folate apply to synthetic forms obtained from supplements, fortified foods, or a combination of the two.

[e] β-Carotene supplements are advised only to serve as a provitamin A source for individuals at risk of vitamin A deficiency.

ND = Not determinable due to lack of data of adverse effects in this age group and concern with regard to lack of ability to handle excess amounts. Source of intake should be from food only to prevent high levels of intake.

SOURCES: Dietary Reference Intakes for Calcium and Vitamin D (2011); Dietary Reference Intakes for Thiamin, Riboflavin, Niacin, Vitamin B-6, Folate, Vitamin B-12, Pantothenic Acid, Biotin, and Choline (1998); Dietary Reference Intakes for Vitamin C, Vitamin E, Selenium, and Carotenoids (2000); Dietary Reference Intakes for Calcium, Phosphorus, Magnesium, Vitamin D, and Fluoride (1997); Dietary Reference Intakes for Vitamin A, Vitamin K, Arsenic, Boron, Chromium, Copper, Iodine, Iron, Manganese, Molybdenum, Nickel, Silicon, Vanadium, and Zinc (2001). These reports may be accessed via www.nap.edu.

Adapted from the Dietary Reference Intakes series, National Academies Press. Copyright 1997, 1998, 2000, 2001, 2011, by the National Academy of Sciences. The full reports are available from the National Academies Press at www.nap.edu.

E

CONTEMPORARY *Nutrition*

W9-BKO-280

Ninth Edition

Gordon M. Wardlaw PH.D.
Formerly of Department of Human Nutrition,
College of Education and Human Ecology
The Ohio State University

Anne M. Smith PH.D., R.D., L.D.
Department of Human Nutrition,
College of Education and Human Ecology
The Ohio State University

With contributions by
Angela L. Collene M.S., R.D., L.D.
Dietetics Program
Department of Family and Consumer Sciences
Ashland University

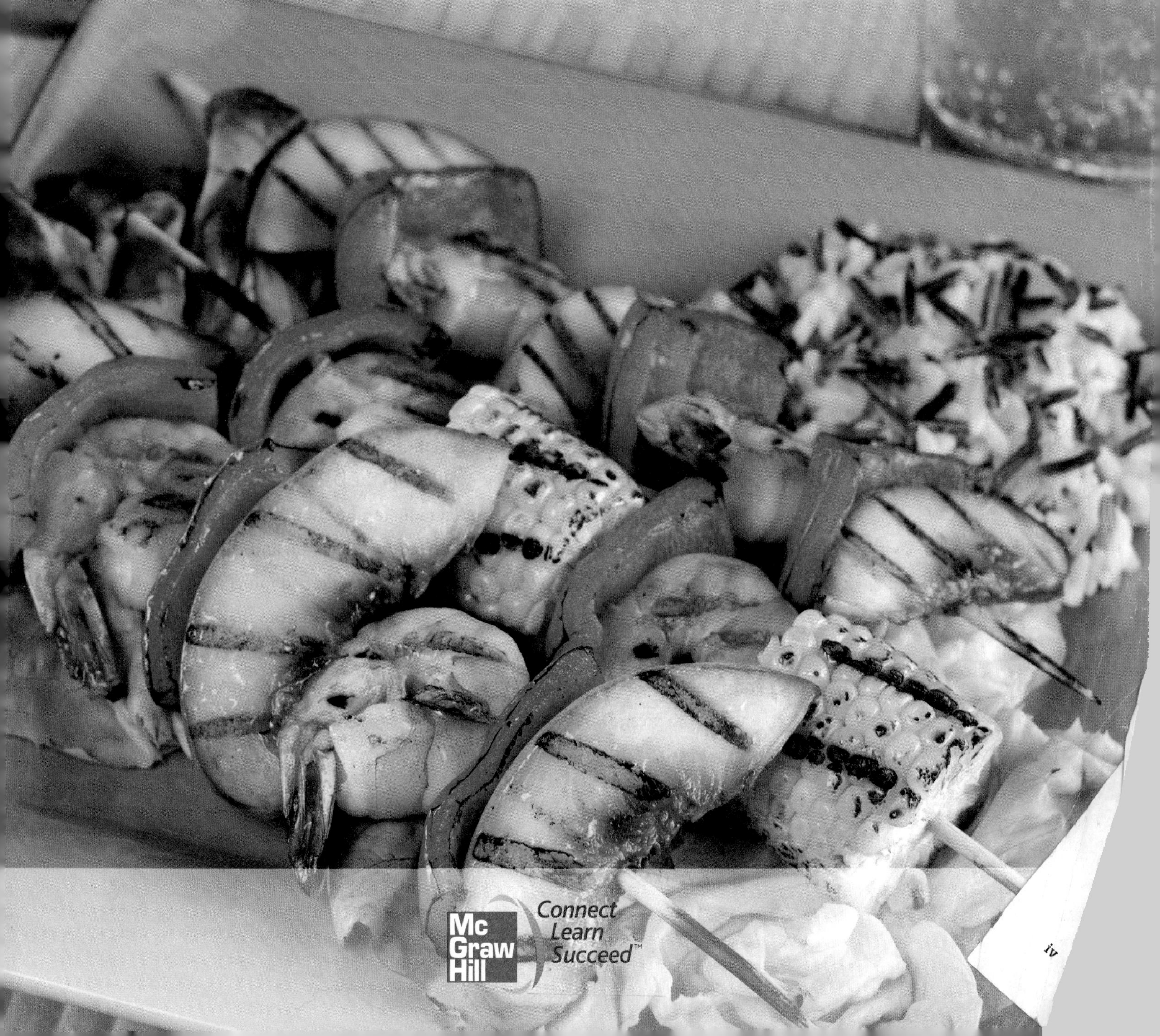

McGraw Hill

Connect
Learn
Succeed™

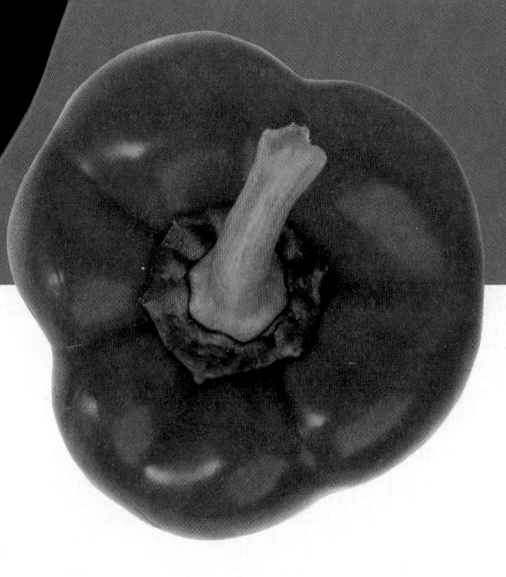

About the Authors

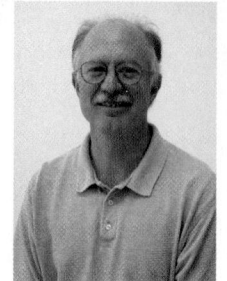

GORDON M. WARDLAW, Ph.D., has taught introductory nutrition courses to students in the Department of Human Nutrition at The Ohio State University and at other colleges and universities. Dr. Wardlaw is the author of many articles that have appeared in prominent nutrition, biology, physiology, and biochemistry journals and was the 1985 recipient of the American Dietetic Association's Mary P. Huddleson Award. Dr. Wardlaw is a member of the American Society for Nutritional Sciences and is certified as a Specialist in Human Nutrition by the American Board of Nutrition. Dr. Wardlaw is currently retired from academia.

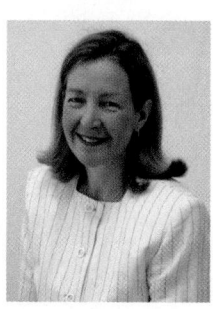

ANNE M. SMITH, Ph.D., R.D., L.D., currently teaches nutrition majors and nonmajors at The Ohio State University and was the recipient of the 1995 Outstanding Teacher Award from the College of Human Ecology. Dr. Smith is the Director of the Didactic Program in Dietetics in the Department of Human Nutrition, College of Education and Human Ecology, of The Ohio State University and received the 2008 Outstanding Dietetic Educator Award from the Ohio Dietetic Association and the 1998 Emerging Dietetic Leader Award from the American Dietetic Association. She also was the recipient of the 2006 Outstanding Faculty Member Award from the Department of Human Nutrition for her commitment to undergraduate education in nutrition and the 2011 Distinquished Service Award from the College of Education and Human Ecology. Dr. Smith has conducted research in the area of vitamin and mineral metabolism and was awarded the 1996 Departmental Research Award from the Ohio Agricultural Research and Development Center. Dr. Smith's research articles have appeared in prominent nutrition journals. She is a member of the American Nutrition Society and the American Dietetic Association.

BLACKBOARD®

The next big thing in digital education!

Ingredients

1 Single sign-on with Blackboard Learn

1 Deeply integrated McGraw-Hill content and tools

1 Automatic Roster/Gradebook synchronization

1 Company—first to use Learning Technology Interoperability (LTI) Standards

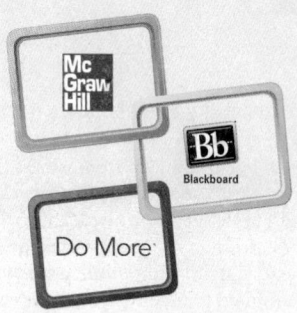

Directions

1. Go to **www.domorenow.com**.

2. Customize and integrate McGraw-Hill content and ground-breaking learning tools into your Bb courses.

3. Increase student retention and satisfaction.

4. Less building and managing. More teaching!

5. More integration on the way—ask us about the LMS used on your campus.

McGRAW-HILL CREATE™

Customize your perfect course solution!

Ingredients

1 New, self-service website that allows you to quickly and easily create custom course materials with McGraw-Hill's comprehensive, cross-disciplinary content and other third party resources

1 Place to create, edit, view, and purchase customized products

1 eBook or print text—you choose the best format for your students

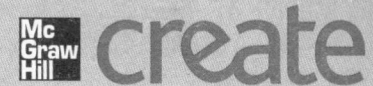

Directions

1. Go to **www.mcgrawhillcreate.com**.

2. Select, then arrange the content in a way that makes sense for your course.

3. Combine material from different sources and even upload your own content.

4. Edit and update your course materials as often as you'd like.

5. Receive your pdf review copy in minutes!

6. Create what you've only imagined!

McGRAW-HILL TEGRITY®

Students can focus on your lectures with digital lecture capture!

Ingredients

1 Ability to record from anywhere, anytime, with or without an Internet connection

1 Key word search allows students to search for exactly what they need to review

1 Highly personalized learning environment makes study time incredibly efficient

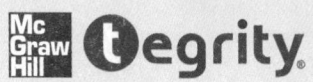

Directions

1. You need nothing more than a computer and microphone to quickly and easily record lectures.

2. Tegrity captures synchronized audio, video, and computer screen activity with the click of a button.

3. View recordings on a PC, Mac, or mobile device 24/7. Tegrity's intuitive interface with a detailed timeline and associated thumbnails makes it easy to find exactly what you're looking for.

4. Help students retain more and achieve higher levels of performance!

Tip: Learn more at **www.tegrity.com**

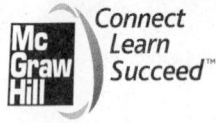

The McGraw·Hill Companies

Connect
Learn
Succeed™

CONTEMPORARY NUTRITION, NINTH EDITION

Published by McGraw-Hill, a business unit of The McGraw-Hill Companies, Inc., 1221 Avenue of the Americas, New York, NY 10020. Copyright © 2013 by The McGraw-Hill Companies, Inc. All rights reserved. Printed in the United States of America. Previous editions © 2011, 2009, and 2006. No part of this publication may be reproduced or distributed in any form or by any means, or stored in a database or retrieval system, without the prior written consent of The McGraw-Hill Companies, Inc., including, but not limited to, in any network or other electronic storage or transmission, or broadcast for distance learning.

Some ancillaries, including electronic and print components, may not be available to customers outside the United States.

This book is printed on acid-free paper.

4 5 6 7 8 9 0 RMN/RMN 1 0 9 8 7 6 5 4

ISBN 978–0–07–340254–3
MHID 0–07–340254–0

Vice President, Editor-in-Chief: *Marty Lange*
Vice President, EDP: *Kimberly Meriwether David*
Senior Director of Development: *Kristine Tibbetts*
Publisher: *Michael S. Hackett*
Sponsoring Editor: *Lynn M. Breithaupt*
Director of Digital Content Development: *Barbekka Hurtt, Ph.D.*
Senior Developmental Editor: *Lynne M. Meyers*
Marketing Manager: *Amy L. Reed*
Lead Project Manager: *Sheila M. Frank*
Senior Buyer: *Kara Kudronowicz*
Senior Media Project Manager: *Tammy Juran*
Manager, Creative Services: *Michelle D. Whitaker*
Cover/Interior Designer: *Ellen Pettengell*
Cover Image: *© The McGraw-Hill Companies, Inc., Kevin May Photography*
Senior Photo Research Coordinator: *John C. Leland*
Photo Research: *Mary Reeg*
Compositor: *Laserwords Private Limited*
Typeface: *10/12 Giovanni Book*
Printer: *RR Donnelley*

All credits appearing on page or at the end of the book are considered to be an extension of the copyright page.

Library of Congress Cataloging-in-Publication Data
Wardlaw, Gordon M.
  Contemporary nutrition / Gordon M. Wardlaw, Anne M. Smith, Angela Collene.—9th ed.
    p. cm.
  Includes index.
  ISBN 978–0–07–340254–3 — ISBN 0–07–340254–0 (hard copy : alk. paper) 1. Nutrition—Textbooks.
  I. Smith, Anne M., 1955– II. Collene, Angela. III. Title.
  QP141.W378 2013
  612.3—dc23
                                                                    2011036913

Brief Contents

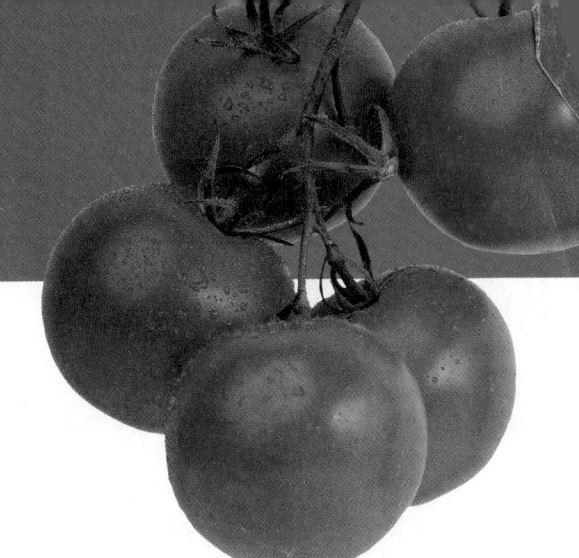

Preface

Dear Students,

Welcome to the fascinating world of nutrition! We are all nutrition experts, in a sense, because we all eat—several times a day. At the same time, though, nutrition can seem a bit confusing. One reason for all the confusion is that it seems like "good nutrition" is a moving target: different authorities have different ideas of how we should eat and nutrition recommendations are subject to change! Are eggs good for us or not? Should we model our diets after a pyramid or a plate? Second, there are so many choices. Did you know that the average supermarket carries about 40,000 food and beverage products? Food manufacturers and grocery chains have one purpose—to make as large a profit as possible. Typically, the most aggressively marketed items are not the healthiest. This has made shopping very complicated. In addition, as a nation, we eat out a lot. When we eat foods that someone else has prepared for us, we surrender control over how much salt and fat is in our food and how much food goes on our plates. There is a lot yet to learn, and you are undoubtedly interested in what you personally should be eating and how the food you eat affects you.

Contemporary Nutrition is designed to accurately convey changing and seemingly conflicting messages to all kinds of students. Our students commonly have misconceptions about nutrition, and many have a limited background in biology or chemistry. Contemporary Nutrition teaches complex scientific concepts at a level that will enable you to meaningfully apply the material to your own life.

We have written Contemporary Nutrition to help you make informed choices about the food you eat. We will take you through explanations of the nutrients in food and their relationship to health, but will also make you aware of the multitude of other factors that drive food choices. To guide you, we refer to many reputable research studies, books, policies, and web sites throughout the book. With this information at your fingertips, you will be well equipped to make your own informed choices about what and how much to eat. There is much to learn, so let's get started!

-Anne Smith

Connecting Students to Course Concepts

Introducing McGraw-Hill ConnectPlus™ Nutrition

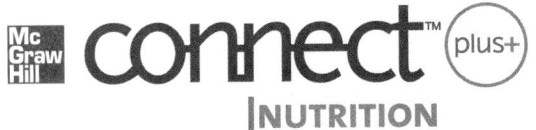

McGraw-Hill Connect® is a web-based assignment and assessment platform that gives students the means to better connect with coursework, instructors, and important concepts that they will need to know for success now and in the future. Connect Nutrition includes high quality interactive questions and tutorials, LearnSmart, digital lecture capture, eBook, and more!

Save time with auto-graded assessments and tutorials.

You can easily create customized assessments that will be automatically graded. All Connect content is created by nutrition instructors so it is pedagogical, instructional, and at the appropriate level. Interactive questions using high-quality art from the textbook, animations and videos from a variety of sources, take you way beyond multiple choice.

Connect Assessment: Classification Interactive

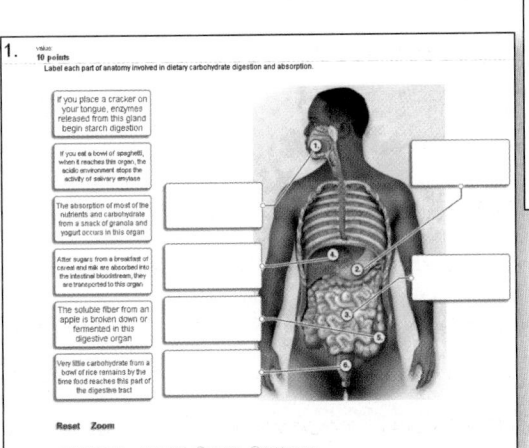

Connect Assessment: Labeling Interactive

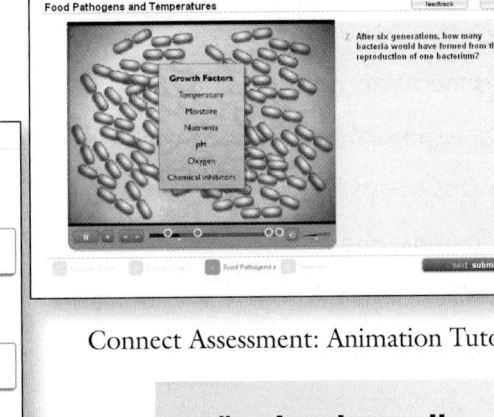

Connect Assessment: Animation Tutorial

> "... I and my adjuncts have reduced the time we spend on grading by 90 percent and student test scores have risen, on average, 10 points since we began using Connect!"
>
> —William Hoover, Bunker Hill Community College

Gather assessment information

All Connect questions are tagged to learning outcome, specific topics, level of difficulty, and allow you to tag your own learning outcomes—so you can easily track assessment data!

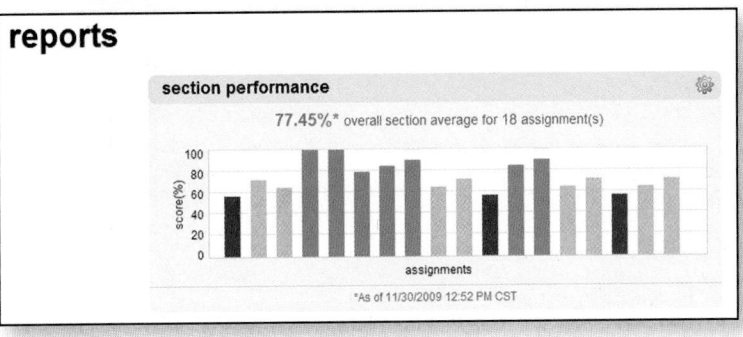

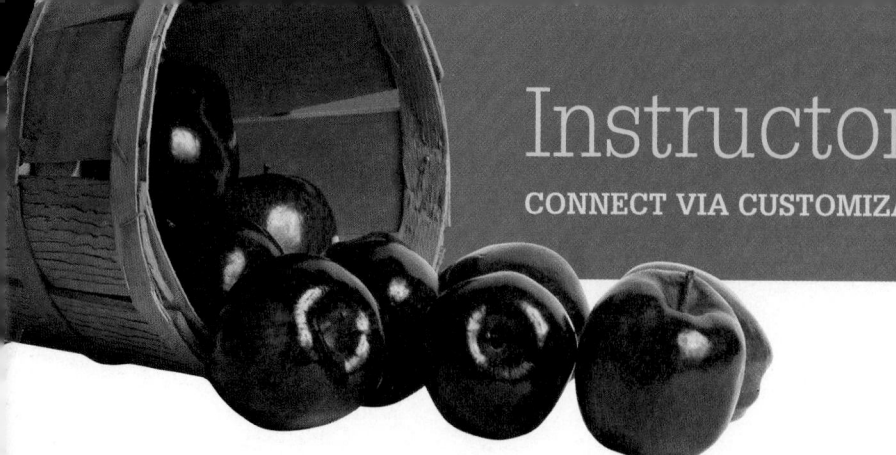

Instructors
CONNECT VIA CUSTOMIZATION

Presentation Tools allow you to customize your lectures.

Enhanced Lecture Presentations contain lecture outlines, art, photos, tables, and animations embedded where appropriate. Fully customizable, complete and ready to use, these presentations will streamline your work and let you spend less time preparing for lecture!

Editable Art   Fully editable (labels and leaders) line art from the text.

Animations   Over 50 animations bringing key concepts to life, available for instructors *and* students.

Animation PPTs   Animations are truly embedded in PowerPoint® for ultimate ease of use! Just copy and paste into your custom slideshow and you're done!

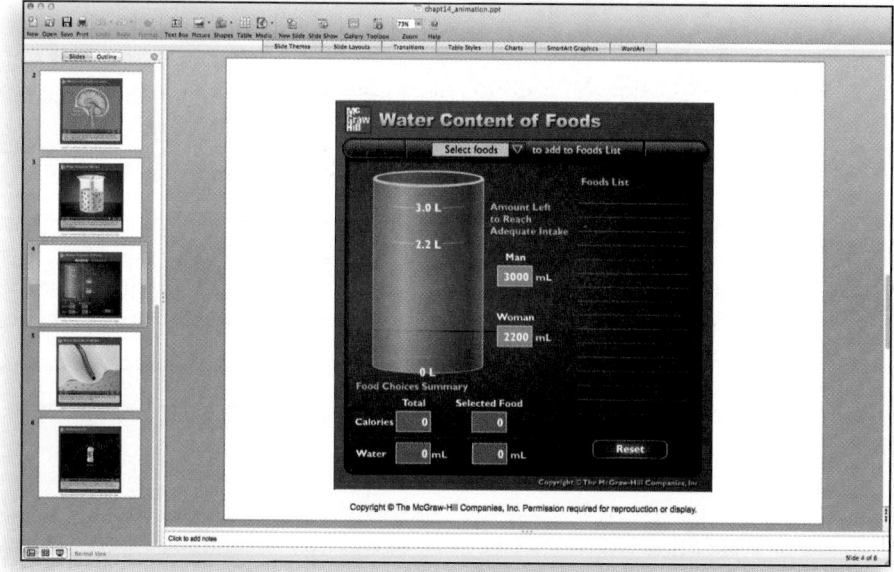

Take your course online—*easily and quickly* with one-click Digital Lecture Capture.

McGraw-Hill Tegrity® records and distributes your lectures with just a click of a button. Students can view them anytime/anywhere via computer, iPod, or mobile device. Tegrity® indexes and records your slideshow presentations, and anything shown on your computer, so **students can use keywords to find exactly what they want to study.**

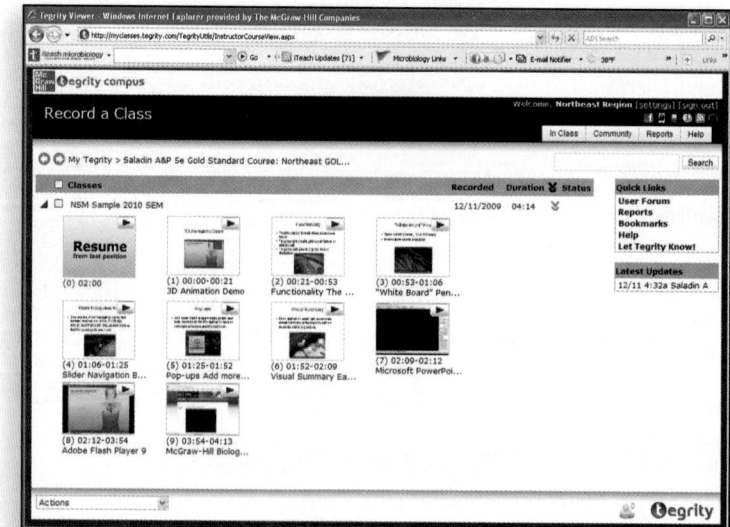

Students

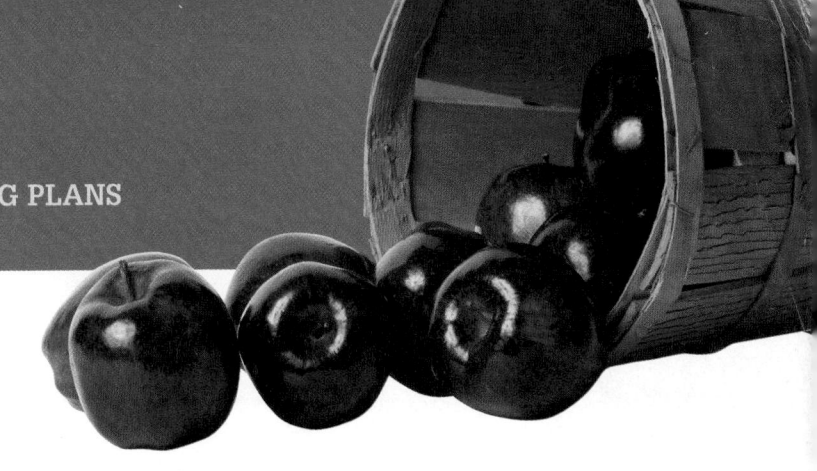

Access content anywhere, any time, with a customizable, interactive eBook.

McGraw-Hill ConnectPlus eBook takes digital texts beyond a simple PDF. With the same content as the printed book, but optimized for the screen, ConnectPlus has embedded animations and videos, which bring concepts to life and provide "just in time" learning for students. Fully integrated self-study questions allow students to interact with the questions in the text and determine if they're gaining mastery of the content.

> "Use of technology, especially LEARNSMART, assisted greatly in keeping on track and keeping up with the material."
>
> —student, Triton College

McGraw-Hill LearnSmart™
A Diagnostic, Adaptive Learning System

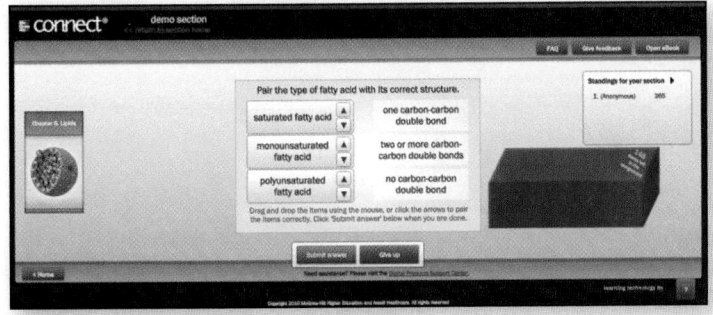

McGraw-Hill *LearnSmart* is an adaptive learning system designed to help students learn faster, study more efficiently, and retain more knowledge for greater success.

LearnSmart effectively assesses students' skill levels to determine which topics students have mastered and which require further practice. A personalized learning path based upon student strengths and weaknesses gives students exactly the help they need, when they need it.

Self-study resources are also available at www.mhhe.com/wardlawcont9.

> "I love LearnSmart. Without it, I would not be doing as well."
>
> —student, Triton College

ix

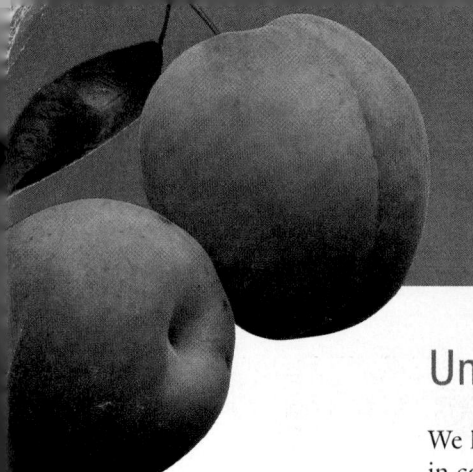

Connecting Today's Students to Today's Nutrition

Understanding Our Audience

We have written *Contemporary Nutrition* assuming that our students have a limited background in college-level biology, chemistry, or physiology. We have been careful to include the essential science foundation needed to adequately comprehend certain topics in nutrition, such as protein synthesis in Chapter 6. The science in this text has been presented in a simple, straightforward manner so that undergraduate students can master the material and apply it to their own lives. The Concept Maps that provide a visual depiction of macronutrient functions and characteristics are an additional aid to help students grasp nutrition science.

Featuring the Latest Guidelines and Research

The vast amount of published research is constantly reshaping our knowledge of nutritional science. The ninth edition has been carefully updated to reflect current scientific understanding, as well as the latest health and nutrition guidelines. Students will learn about the Dietary Guidelines for Americans, 2010, MyPlate, and Healthy People 2020.

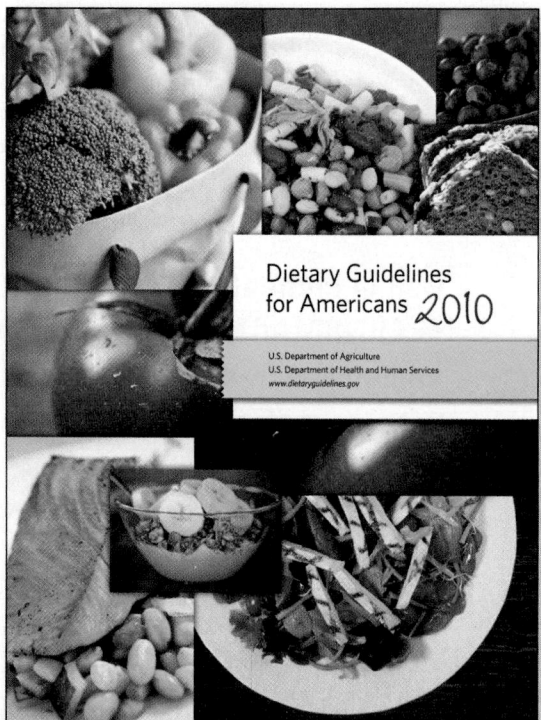

Dietary Guidelines
for Americans 2010

U.S. Department of Agriculture
U.S. Department of Health and Human Services
www.dietaryguidelines.gov

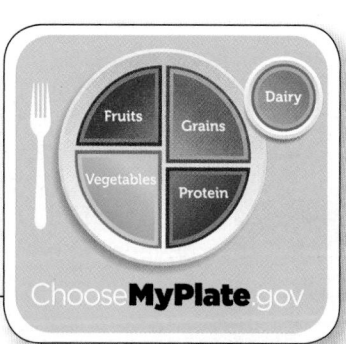

ChooseMyPlate.gov

Healthy People 2020

Connecting with a Personal Focus

Applying Nutrition on a Personal Level

Throughout the ninth edition we reinforce the fact that each person responds differently to nutrients. To further convey the importance of applying nutrition to their personal lives, we include many examples of people and situations that resonate with college students. We also stress the importance of learning to intelligently sort through the seemingly endless range of nutrition messages to recognize reliable information and to sensibly apply it to their own lives. Our goal is to provide students the tools they need to eat healthy and make informed nutrition decisions after they leave this course.

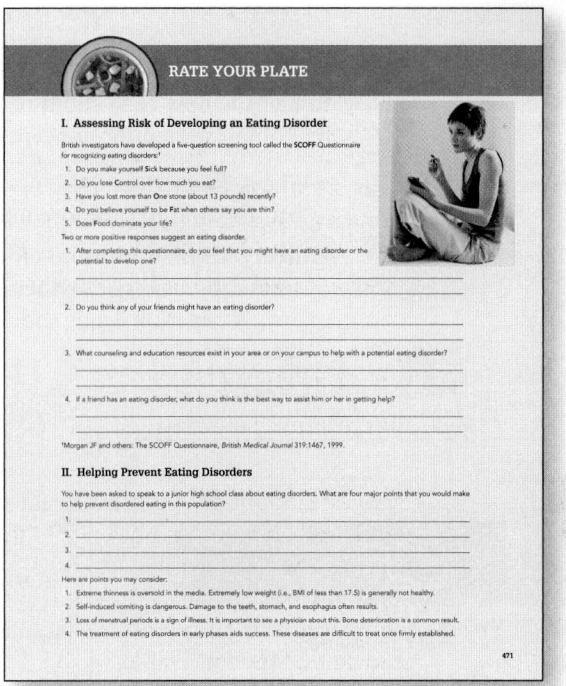

RATE YOUR PLATE

I. Assessing Risk of Developing an Eating Disorder

British investigators have developed a five-question screening tool called the **SCOFF** Questionnaire for recognizing eating disorders:[1]

1. Do you make yourself **S**ick because you feel full?
2. Do you lose **C**ontrol over how much you eat?
3. Have you lost more than **O**ne stone (about 13 pounds) recently?
4. Do you believe yourself to be **F**at when others say you are thin?
5. Does **F**ood dominate your life?

Two or more positive responses suggest an eating disorder.

1. After completing this questionnaire, do you feel that you might have an eating disorder or the potential to develop one?

2. Do you think any of your friends might have an eating disorder?

3. What counseling and education resources exist in your area or on your campus to help with a potential eating disorder?

4. If a friend has an eating disorder, what do you think is the best way to assist him or her in getting help?

[1]Morgan JF and others: The SCOFF Questionnaire, British Medical Journal 319:1467, 1999.

II. Helping Prevent Eating Disorders

You have been asked to speak to a junior high school class about eating disorders. What are four major points that you would make to help prevent disordered eating in this population?

1.
2.
3.
4.

Here are points you may consider:

1. Extreme thinness is oversold in the media. Extremely low weight (i.e., BMI of less than 17.5) is generally not healthy.
2. Self-induced vomiting is dangerous. Damage to the teeth, stomach, and esophagus often results.
3. Loss of menstrual periods is a sign of illness. It is important to see a physician about this. Bone deterioration is a common result.
4. The treatment of eating disorders in early phases aids success. These diseases are difficult to treat once firmly established.

471

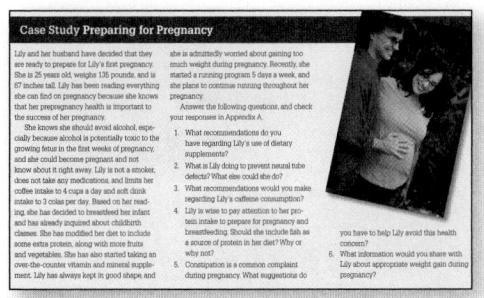

Case Study Preparing for Pregnancy

Lily and her husband have decided that they are ready to prepare for Lily's first pregnancy. She is 25 years old, weighs 135 pounds, and is 67 inches tall. Lily has been reading everything she can find on pregnancy because she knows that her prepregnancy health is important to the success of her pregnancy.

She knows she should avoid alcohol especially because alcohol is potentially toxic to the growing fetus in the first weeks of pregnancy, and she could become pregnant and not know about it right away. Lily is not a smoker, does not take any medications, and limits her coffee intake to 4 cups a day and soft drink intake to 3 colas per day. Based on her reading, she has decided to breastfeed her infant and has already inquired about childbirth classes. She has modified her diet to include some extra protein, along with more fruits and vegetables. She has also started taking an over-the-counter vitamin and mineral supplement. Lily has always kept in good shape, and

she is admittedly worried about gaining too much weight during pregnancy. Recently, she started a running program 5 days a week, and she plans to continue running throughout her pregnancy.

Answer the following questions, and check your responses in Appendix A.

1. What recommendations do you have regarding Lily's use of dietary supplements?
2. What is Lily doing to prevent neural tube defects? What else could she do?
3. What recommendations would you make regarding Lily's caffeine consumption?
4. Lily is wise to pay attention to her protein intake to prepare for pregnancy and breastfeeding. Should she include fish as a source of protein in her diet? Why or why not?
5. Constipation is a common complaint during pregnancy. What suggestions do

you have to help Lily avoid this health concern?
6. What information would you share with Lily about appropriate weight gain during pregnancy?

Challenging Students to Think Critically

The pages of *Contemporary Nutrition* contain numerous opportunities for students to learn more about themselves and their diet and to use their new knowledge of nutrition to improve their health. In the ninth edition, pedagogical elements, such as Making Decisions, Critical Thinking, Case Studies, and Nutrition and Your Health, are further enhanced by the addition of What Would You Choose? and Newsworthy Nutrition. Many of the thought-provoking topics highlighted in these features are expanded upon in the online resources found in Connect Nutrition.

	Men (grams per day)	Women (grams per day)
Linoleic acid (omega-6)	17	12
Alpha-linolenic acid (omega-3)	1.6	1.1

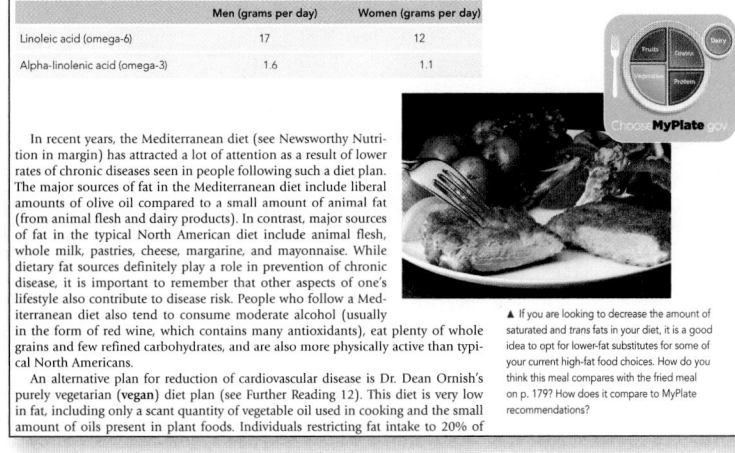

In recent years, the Mediterranean diet (see Newsworthy Nutrition in margin) has attracted a lot of attention as a result of lower rates of chronic diseases seen in people following such a diet plan. The major sources of fat in the Mediterranean diet include liberal amounts of olive oil compared to a small amount of animal fat (from animal flesh and dairy products). In contrast, major sources of fat in the typical North American diet include animal flesh, whole milk, pastries, cheese, margarine, and mayonnaise. While dietary fat sources definitely play a role in prevention of chronic disease, it is important to remember that other aspects of one's lifestyle also contribute to disease risk. People who follow a Mediterranean diet also tend to consume moderate alcohol (usually in the form of red wine, which contains many antioxidants), eat plenty of whole grains and few refined carbohydrates, and are also more physically active than typical North Americans.

An alternative plan for reduction of cardiovascular disease is Dr. Dean Ornish's purely vegetarian (**vegan**) diet plan (see Further Reading 12). This diet is very low in fat, including only a scant quantity of vegetable oil used in cooking and the small amount of oils present in plant foods. Individuals restricting fat intake to 20% of

▲ If you are looking to decrease the amount of saturated and trans fats in your diet, it is a good idea to opt for lower-fat substitutes for some of your current high-fat food choices. How do you think this meal compares with the fried meal on p. 179? How does it compare to MyPlate recommendations?

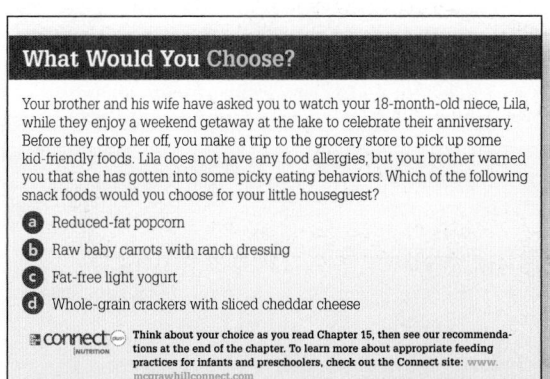

What Would You Choose?

Your brother and his wife have asked you to watch your 18-month-old niece, Lila, while they enjoy a weekend getaway at the lake to celebrate their anniversary. Before they drop her off, you make a trip to the grocery store to pick up some kid-friendly foods. Lila does not have any food allergies, but your brother warned you that she has gotten into some picky eating behaviors. Which of the following snack foods would you choose for your little houseguest?

a Reduced-fat popcorn

b Raw baby carrots with ranch dressing

c Fat-free light yogurt

d Whole-grain crackers with sliced cheddar cheese

connect NUTRITION Think about your choice as you read Chapter 15, then see our recommendations at the end of the chapter. To learn more about appropriate feeding practices for infants and preschoolers, check out the Connect site: www.mcgrawhillconnect.com

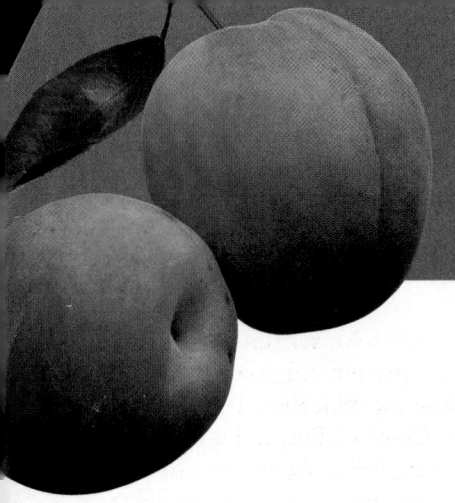

Making Visual Connections

Attractive, Accurate Artwork

More than 1000 drawings, photographs, and tables in the text were critically analyzed to identify how each could be enhanced and refined to help students more easily master complex scientific concepts.

- Many illustrations were updated or replaced to inspire student inquiry and comprehension and to promote interest and retention of information.
- Many illustrations were redesigned to use brighter colors and a more attractive, contemporary style. Others were fine-tuned to make them clearer and easier to follow. Navigational aids show where a function occurs and put it in perspective of the whole body.

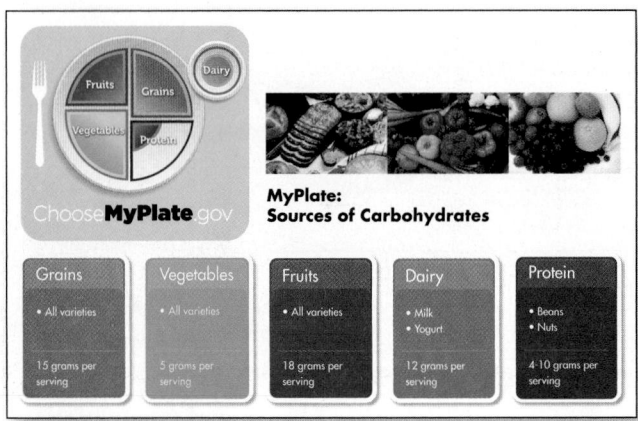

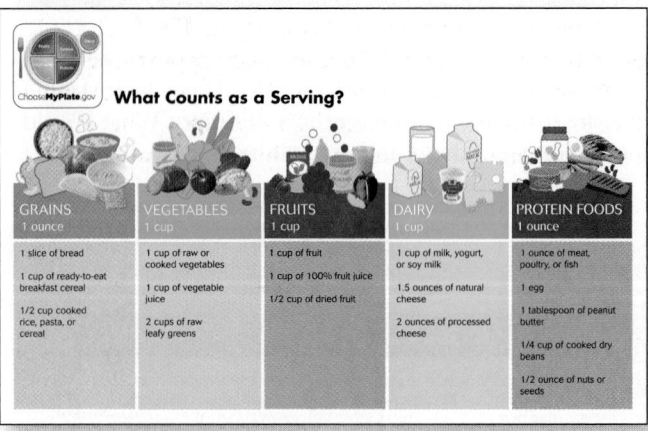

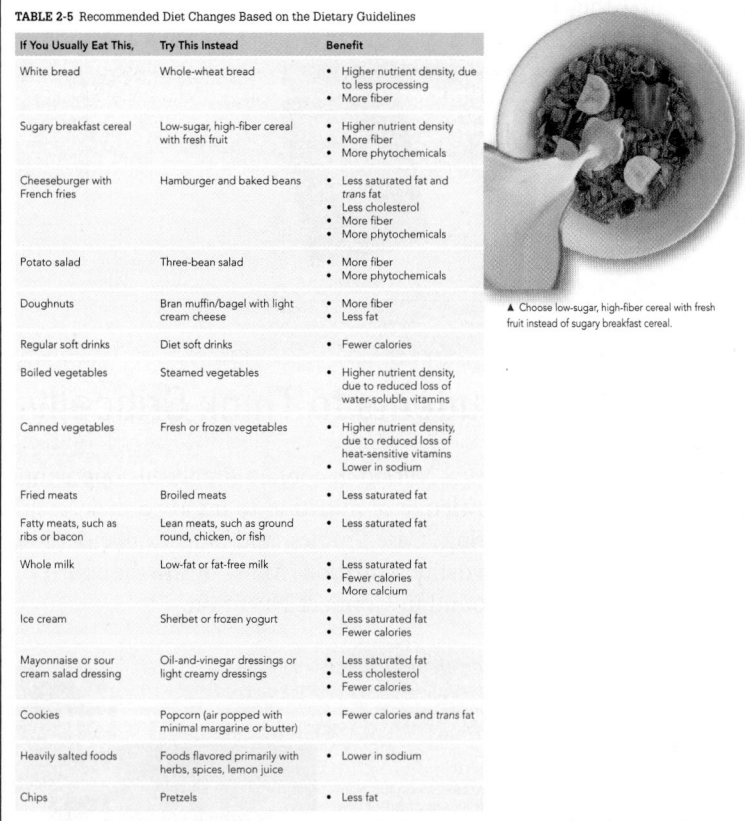

TABLE 2-5 Recommended Diet Changes Based on the Dietary Guidelines

If You Usually Eat This,	Try This Instead	Benefit
White bread	Whole-wheat bread	• Higher nutrient density, due to less processing • More fiber
Sugary breakfast cereal	Low-sugar, high-fiber cereal with fresh fruit	• Higher nutrient density • More fiber • More phytochemicals
Cheeseburger with French fries	Hamburger and baked beans	• Less saturated fat and trans fat • Less cholesterol • More fiber • More phytochemicals
Potato salad	Three-bean salad	• More fiber • More phytochemicals
Doughnuts	Bran muffin/bagel with light cream cheese	• More fiber • Less fat
Regular soft drinks	Diet soft drinks	• Fewer calories
Boiled vegetables	Steamed vegetables	• Higher nutrient density, due to reduced loss of water-soluble vitamins
Canned vegetables	Fresh or frozen vegetables	• Higher nutrient density, due to reduced loss of heat-sensitive vitamins • Lower in sodium
Fried meats	Broiled meats	• Less saturated fat
Fatty meats, such as ribs or bacon	Lean meats, such as ground round, chicken, or fish	• Less saturated fat
Whole milk	Low-fat or fat-free milk	• Less saturated fat • Fewer calories • More calcium
Ice cream	Sherbet or frozen yogurt	• Less saturated fat • Fewer calories
Mayonnaise or sour cream salad dressing	Oil-and-vinegar dressings or light creamy dressings	• Less saturated fat • Less cholesterol • Fewer calories
Cookies	Popcorn (air popped with minimal margarine or butter)	• Fewer calories and trans fat
Heavily salted foods	Foods flavored primarily with herbs, spices, lemon juice	• Lower in sodium
Chips	Pretzels	• Less fat

▲ Choose low-sugar, high-fiber cereal with fresh fruit instead of sugary breakfast cereal.

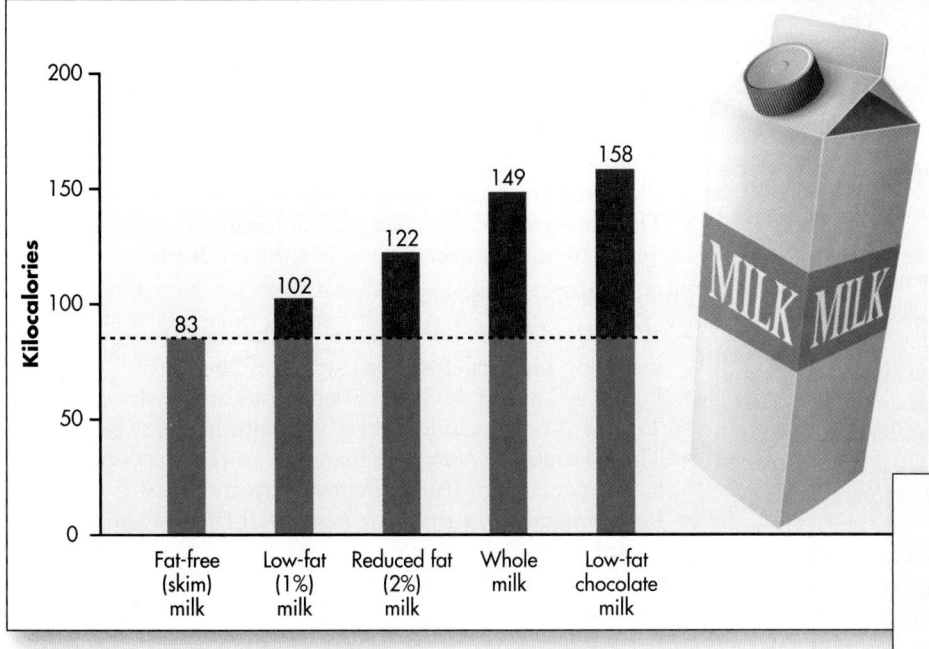

- Coordinated color schemes and drawing styles keep presentations consistent and strengthen the educational value of the artwork. Color-coding and directional arrows in figures make it easier to follow events and reinforce interrelationships.

- In many figures, process descriptions appear in the body of the figures. This pairing of the action and an explanation walks students step-by-step through the process and increases the teaching effectiveness of these figures.

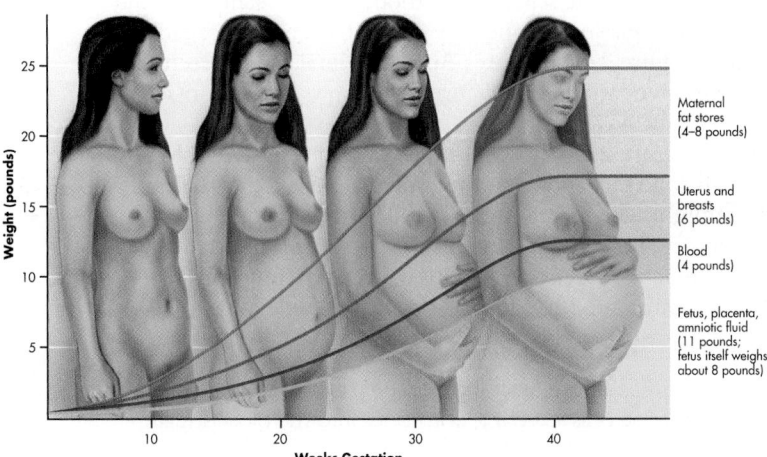

Finally, a careful comparison of artwork with its corresponding text was done to ensure that they are completely coordinated and consistent. The final result is a striking visual program that holds readers' attention and supports the goals of clarity, ease of comprehension, and critical thinking. The attractive layout and design of this edition are clean, bright, and inviting. This creative presentation of the material is geared toward engaging today's visually oriented students.

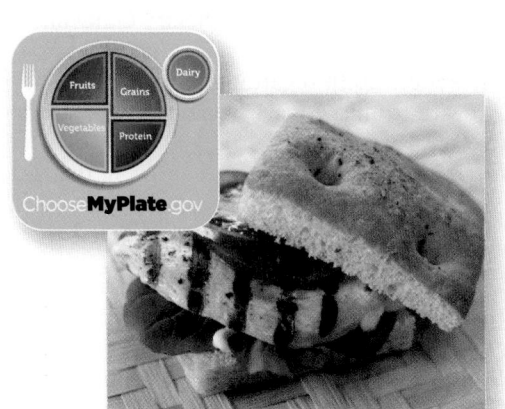

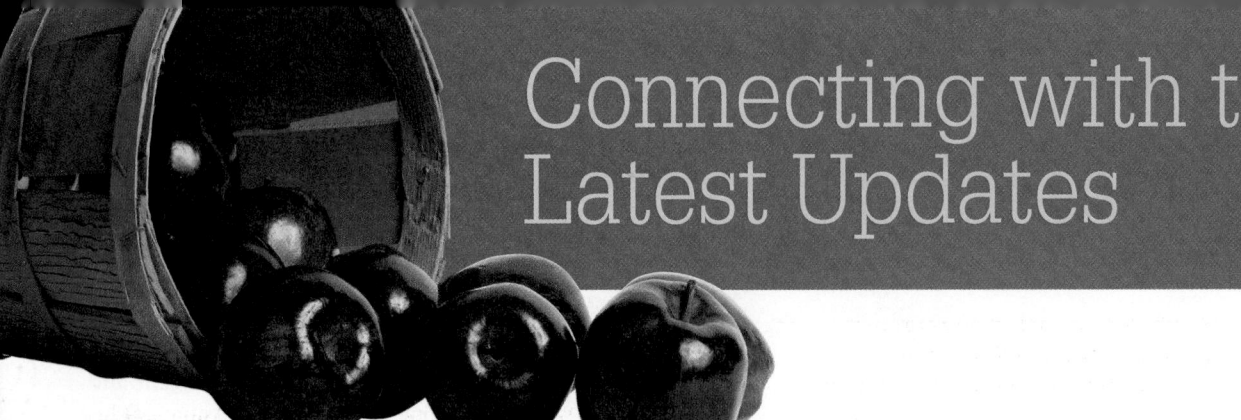

Chapter-by-Chapter Revisions

Chapter 1: *Choosing What You Eat and Why*

- Chapter 1 has been reorganized beginning with a discussion of factors that influence our food choices and ending with a conversation about eating well in college.
- Chemical details of nutrients (e.g., dissacharides) have been moved to chapters on specific nutrients. Details on the hormonal control of appetite have been moved to Chapter 7.
- The newly released *Healthy People 2020* (HP2020) report is discussed, including its key "Nutrition and Weight Status" objectives.
- The new *What Would You Choose* feature focuses on time-saving breakfast options, especially for college students.
- Two *Newsworthy Nutrition* margin features are included in Chapter 1. One describes the link between TV food ads and childhood obesity and the other the link between a healthy diet and risk of sudden cardiac death.
- Causes of Death have been updated in Table 1-2.
- Added Figure 1-4 to illustrate the percentage of adults who are obese by state in 2009.

Chapter 2: *Guidelines for Designing a Healthy Diet*

- The *What Would You Choose* feature illustrates nutrient density and energy density.
- The new USDA food guide, MyPlate, released in June 2011, has been included with references to www.Choose MyPlate.gov and the Daily Food Plans that accompany MyPlate.
- The new Dietary Guidelines for Americans, 2010, released in January 2011, are fully discussed.
- Discussion of the scientific method, nutrient standards, and recommendations for healthy eating have been reorganized.
- New Figure 2-8 compares American intakes to current recommendations and Figure 2-11 shows what counts as a serving with MyPlate.
- New Figure 2-26 illustrates the concept of empty calories from solid fats and/or added sugars. *Newsworthy Nutrition* highlights the increasing costs of healthy eating.
- The new Rate Your Plate, "Are you putting health advice into practice?" reflects the 2010 Dietary Guidelines for Americans and 2008 Physical Activity Guidelines.

Chapter 3: *The Human Body: A Nutrition Perspective*

- Figure 3-7 is a new illustration of the pancreas and the function of endocrine cells secreting hormones into the bloodstream.

- *What Would You Choose* focuses on the best menu options to alleviate gastrointestinal complaints such as constipation.
- The *Newsworthy Nutrition* margin feature focuses on the link between gut bacteria and health and disease.

Chapter 4: *Carbohydrates*

- *What Would You Choose* focuses on the sugar content, including high-fructose corn syrup, of beverages.
- Figure 4-7 is now MyPlate: Sources of Carbohydrates.
- Table 4-2 now includes Stevia as an alternative sweetener.
- The *Newsworthy Nutrition* margin feature focuses on the link between high-fructose corn syrup and obesity.
- Recommendations from the new 2010 Dietary Guidelines regarding carbohydrate intake have been added.
- Figure 4-12 is a new illustration from the 2010 Dietary Guidelines of the sources of added sugars in U.S. diets.

Chapter 5: *Lipids*

- The new *What Would You Choose* feature focuses on the fat content of ground beef.
- Figure 5-5 has been revised to MyPlate: Sources of Fats.
- Peanut Butter: Is it "good fat?," has been included.
- Recommendations from the new 2010 Dietary Guidelines regarding fat intake have been added.
- Goals of Healthy People 2020 regarding reducing saturated fat intake, death from coronary heart disease, and total blood cholesterol are included.
- *Newsworthy Nutrition* focuses on research showing that a low-fat diet is not necessary for weight loss.

Chapter 6: *Proteins*

- The new *What Would You Choose* feature focuses on protein and amino acid intake and weight training.
- Figure 6-4 is now MyPlate: Sources of Protein.
- Recommendations from the new 2010 Dietary Guidelines regarding protein intake have been added.
- *Newsworthy Nutrition* focuses on the link between colon cancer and recent fat, protein, and red meat consumption.

Chapter 7: *Energy Balance and Weight Control*

- The new *What Would You Choose* feature focuses on the calorie content of frozen desserts.
- Figure 7-1 has been updated with obesity trends for 2009.
- New Weight Status Objectives from Healthy People 2020 are included.
- Recommendations from the new 2010 Dietary Guidelines regarding "Balancing Calories to Manage Weight," have been added.

- Two *Newsworthy Nutrition* features are included. One focuses on research indicating that small changes result in large weight changes and the other on a popular weight loss drug that has been withdrawn from the market.

Chapter 8: *Vitamins*

- The new *What Would You Choose* feature focuses on rich sources of folic acid, especially for pregnant women.
- Food group sources of the vitamins are now illustrated using the MyPlate graphic.
- The new Recommended Dietary Allowances for vitamin D, released in 2010, are discussed.
- Recommendations from the new 2010 Dietary Guidelines regarding vitamin intake have been added.
- Figure 8-27, Supplement Sales, has been updated to include sales for 2009 and 2010, and the Top Five Dietary Supplements have been updated for 2010.
- *Newsworthy Nutrition* focuses on research showing that folic acid added to cereal reduces neural-tube defects.

Chapter 9: *Water and Minerals*

- The new *What Would You Choose* feature focuses on the best choice of bottled water, especially when working out.
- Food group sources of the vitamins are now illustrated using the MyPlate graphic.
- *Newsworthy Nutrition* focuses on research indicating that lower sodium and higher potassium intakes reduce risk of cardiovascular disease.

Chapter 10: *Nutrition: Fitness and Sports*

- The *What Would You Choose* feature compares and contrasts some popular sports nutrition products.
- Discussion of the 2008 Physical Activity Guidelines for Americans has been expanded.
- Table 10-5 has been updated with protein needs of athletes.
- New products have been added to Table 10-6, Popular Energy Drinks and Table 10-8, Popular Energy Bars and Gels. Table 10-6 now includes caffeine, energy, and sugar content of energy drinks.
- The *Newsworthy Nutrition* feature distinguishes between sports drinks and energy drinks for athletic performance.

Chapter 11: *Eating Disorders*

- The *What Would You Choose* feature addresses how to approach a friend with a suspected eating disorder.
- The upcoming revisions to the *Diagnostic and Statistical Manual of Mental Disorders* related to eating disorders have been discussed, including the probable reclassification of Binge-Eating Disorder as an eating disorder.
- Discussion of genetics and eating disorders has been enhanced.
- Information on Muscle Dysmorphia has been included.
- The *Newsworthy Nutrition* feature points out common threads between binge eating and binge drinking.

Chapter 12: *Undernutrition Throughout the World*

- The new *What Would You Choose* feature focuses on choices to help put an end to world hunger.
- The content has been updated with current statistics on food insecurity, homelessness, hunger, and malnutrition.
- Table 12-2 has been updated to include new federally subsidized programs that supply food for people in the U.S.

- A New section, "Access to Healthy Food," includes discussion of food deserts in low income neighborhoods.
- The global impact of HIV/AIDS has been updated and illustrated in Figure 12-4.
- The *Newsworthy Nutrition* margin feature focuses on whether HIV-positive women should choose to breastfeed.
- Prevalence of genetically modified crops is updated.

Chapter 13: *Safety of Our Food Supply*

- *What Would You Choose* focuses on choosing fruits and vegetables with the best nutritional value, fewest preservatives and pesticides, and lowest risk for foodborne illness.
- The content has been updated with information about the most recent outbreaks of foodborne illnesses.
- Discussion of the new FDA Food Safety Modernization Act, signed into law in 2011 is included.
- The Food Safety Danger Zone has been updated.
- *Newsworthy Nutrition* focuses on the *E. coli* outbreak that was linked to German organic sprouts.

Chapter 14: *Pregnancy and Breastfeeding*

- The *What Would You Choose* feature addresses food choices to meet the needs of a pregnant vegetarian.
- Physical Activity Guidelines for pregnancy are included.
- New figures have been added to illustrate how nutrient requirements for pregnancy and breastfeeding differ from those of the RDAs/AIs of adult women.
- The *Newsworthy Nutrition* feature explores a proposed increase in vitamin D recommendations during pregnancy.
- Recommendations from the new 2010 Dietary Guidelines pertinent to pregnancy and breastfeeding have been added.
- Advice on maternal dietary restrictions to prevent food allergies has been updated to reflect the updated position of the American Academy of Pediatrics.
- Discussion of Fetal Alcohol Syndrome has been updated with the updated Fetal Alcohol Spectrum Disorders.

Chapter 15: *Nutrition from Infancy through Adolescence*

- The *What Would You Choose* feature looks into healthy and age-appropriate food choices for children.
- Throughout the chapter, including the *Newsworthy Nutrition* feature, the importance of family meals is emphasized.
- The latest American Academy of Pediatrics (AAP) recommendations on infant feeding have been included.
- Revised recommendations from the AAP and National Institute of Allergy and Infectious Disease for preventing food allergies and atopic disease have been included.
- New Figure 15-3 shows examples of meals that comply with MyPlate for children, ages 2, 4, 8, and 16.

Chapter 16: *Nutrition During Adulthood*

- The *What Would You Choose* feature explores nutritional approaches for reducing cancer risk.
- Recommendations from the new 2010 Dietary Guidelines and the 2008 Physical Activity Guidelines pertaining to older adults have been included.
- Figures have been added comparing nutrient requirements for older adults with those of the young adults.
- The *Newsworthy Nutrition* feature focuses on research regarding caloric restriction and longevity.

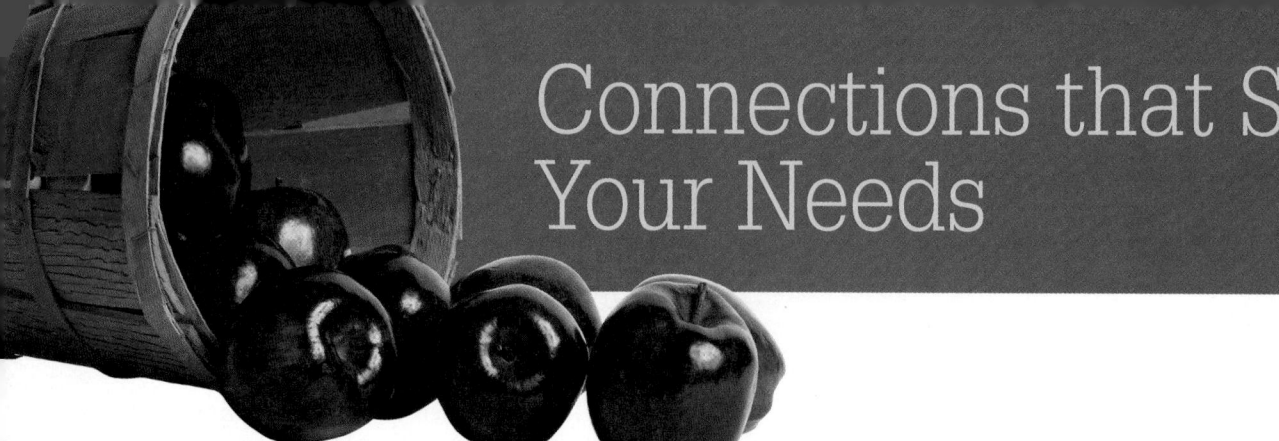

Connections that Suit Your Needs

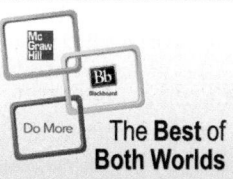

The **Best** of Both Worlds

McGraw-Hill Higher Education and Blackboard® have teamed up!

What does this mean for you?

- **Life simplified.** Now, all McGraw-Hill content (text, tools, & homework) can be accessed directly from within your Blackboard course. All with one sign-on.

- **Deep integration.** McGraw-Hill's content and content engines are seamlessly woven within your Blackboard course.

- **No more manual synching!** Connect® assignments within Blackboard automatically (and instantly) feed grades directly to your Blackboard grade center. No more keeping track of two gradebooks!

- **A solution for everyone.** Even if your institution is not currently using Blackboard, we have a solution for you. Ask your McGraw-Hill representative for details.

Customize your course materials to your learning outcomes!

Create what you've only imagined.

Introducing McGraw-Hill Create™—a new, self-service website that allows you to create custom course materials—print and eBooks—by drawing upon McGraw-Hill's comprehensive, cross-disciplinary content. Add your own content quickly and easily. Tap into other rights-secured third-party sources as well. Then, arrange the content in a way that makes the most sense for your course. Even personalize your book with your course name and information! Choose the best format for your course: color print, black-and-white print, or eBook. The eBook is now even viewable on an iPad! And, when you are done, you will receive a free PDF review copy in just minutes!

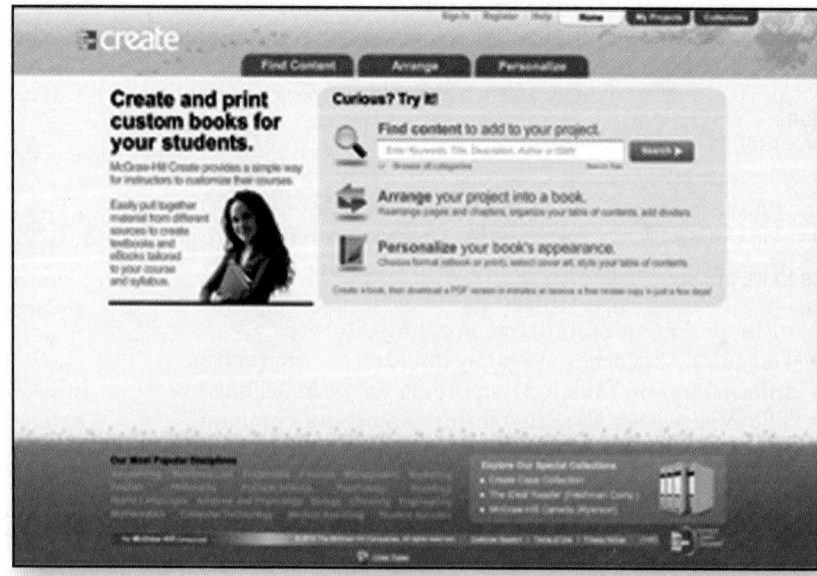

Finally, a way to quickly and easily create the course materials you've always wanted.

Imagine that.

Visit McGraw-Hill Create—www.mcgrawhillcreate.com—today and begin building your perfect book.

Acknowledgments

Special Acknowledgements

Writing a textbook requires much energy and constant support. We are indebted to several individuals for their creative abilities and generous interest in the production of this book. First, our deepest gratitude to our long-time editor Lynne Meyers, whose commitment, patience and encouragement has been extraordinary. She and her staff at McGraw-Hill have guided and assisted us through every phase of this and several previous revisions of Contemporary Nutrition. This edition is also much improved by the written contributions of Angela Collene, M.S., R.D. We thank her for always being ready at a moment's notice, especially with the recent updates to the Dietary Guidelines, MyPlate, and Healthy People 2020. Finally, we are grateful to Sheila Frank and her staff for the meticulous coordination of the many production efforts needed to produce the very appealing yet accurate ninth edition.

Thank you to reviewers

Our goal is to provide students and educators with the most accurate, up-to-date, and useful textbook possible. As with earlier editions, the quality of the ninth edition of *Contemporary Nutrition* is largely dependent on the thorough, professional assistance of nutrition educators from academic institutions across the nation. We are indebted to these colleagues who reviewed the eighth edition, evaluated new material for the ninth edition, participated in instructional symposia, and responded to surveys. The advice and suggestions from these colleagues have been used in every chapter and have resulted in a textbook that is current and inviting.

Gregory Avellana
Ohio University

Alena Clark
University of Northern Colorado

Robert DiSilvestro
The Ohio State University

Mary Jeanne Doyle
The University of Montana Missoula College of Technology

Keith M. Erikson
The University of North Carolina, Greensboro

Leslie Sisson Goudarzi
Kilgore College

Megan Govindan
West Virginia University

Charlene Harkins
University of Minnesota, Duluth

Maureen Baun Jamgochian
College of the Canyons

Gail L. Kaye
The Ohio State University

Molly Michelman
University of Nevada

Maria Montemagni
College of the Sequoias

Cheryl Neudauer
Minneapolis Community and Technical College

Janet Tou
West Virginia University

Ann M. Volk
Antelope Valley College

Mary Watson
University of Nebraska, Omaha

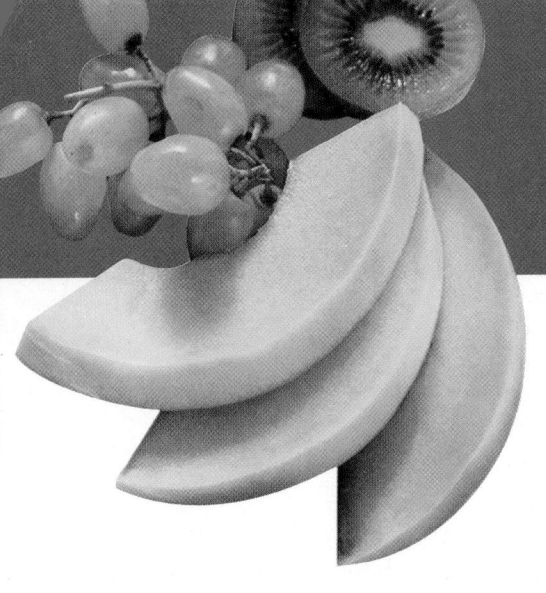

Contents

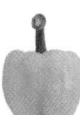

Part Two Energy Nutrients and Energy Balance 122

Chapter 4 Carbohydrates 122

Chapter 5 Lipids 164

Chapter 6 Proteins 208

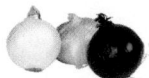

Part Three Vitamins, Minerals, and Water 288

Part Four Nutrition: Beyond
the Nutrients 406

Part Five   Nutrition: A Focus on Life Stages 540

Chapter 14   Pregnancy and Breastfeeding 540

Chapter 1 Choosing What You Eat and Why

Rate Your Plate: We begin each chapter with a "What Would You Choose?" activity to get you thinking. We hope you will be able to make a choice that is right for you using the concepts discussed in the chapter. At the end of each chapter, we provide a discussion and summary of the logic behind what we would recommend. The "choice" aspect of this activity fits well with the new food guide tool, ChooseMy-Plate. You will learn more about this new tool in Chapter 2, and we will reinforce its guidelines in our "What Would You Choose?" activities.

Student Learning Outcomes

Chapter 1 is designed to allow you to:

1.1 Describe how our food habits are affected by the flavor, texture, and appearance of food; routines and habits; early experiences and customs; advertising; nutrition and health concerns; restaurants; social changes; and economic, as well as physiological processes affected by meal size and composition.

1.2 Identify diet and lifestyle factors that contribute to the 15 leading causes of death in North America.

1.3 Define the terms *nutrition, carbohydrate, protein, lipid (fat), alcohol, vitamin, mineral, water, kilocalorie (kcal)*, and *fiber*.

1.4 Determine the total calories (kcal) of a food or diet using the weight and calorie content of the energy-yielding nutrients and use the basic units of the metric system to calculate percentages, such as percent of calories from fat in a diet.

1.5 List the major characteristics of the North American diet, the food habits that often need improvement, and the key "Nutrition and Weight Status" objectives of the *Healthy People 2020* report.

1.6 Describe a basic plan for health promotion and disease prevention and what to expect from good nutrition and a healthy lifestyle.

1.7 Identify food and nutrition issues relevant to college students.

What Would You Choose?

You were awake last night until 2:30 A.M. finishing a group project. Unfortunately, your Psychology 101 class meets at 9:00 this morning. When your alarm goes off at 7:30 A.M., you decide to sleep those extra 20 minutes it would take to sit down and enjoy breakfast at the dining hall. What's your best time-saving breakfast option?

a Skip breakfast, but plan to consume a few extra calories at lunch and dinner.

b Eat a low-fat granola bar and iced coffee from the vending machines in your dorm.

c Fix yourself a quick bowl of Wheaties with a banana and low-fat milk along with a yogurt, all from your dorm room "pantry."

d Pick up a ham, egg, and cheese bagel.

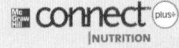 **NUTRITION** **Think about your choice as you read Chapter 1, then see our recommendations at the end of the chapter. To learn more about breakfast choices, check out the Connect site: www.mcgrawhillconnect.com**

Part One
Nutrition: A Key to Health

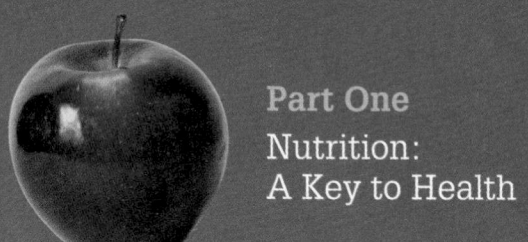

Research has clearly shown that a lifestyle that includes a diet rich in fruits, vegetables, and whole grains, coupled with regular exercise, can enhance our quality of life in the short term and keep us healthy for many years to come. Unfortunately, this healthy lifestyle is not always easy to follow. When it comes to "nutrition," it is clear that some of our diets are out of balance with our metabolism, physiology, and physical activity level.

We begin Chapter 1 with some questions. What influences your daily food choices? How important are factors such as taste, appearance, convenience, cost or value? Is nutrition one of the factors you consider? Are your food choices influencing your quality of life and long-term health? By making optimal dietary choices, we can bring the goal of a long, healthy life within reach. This is the primary theme of Chapter 1 and throughout this book.

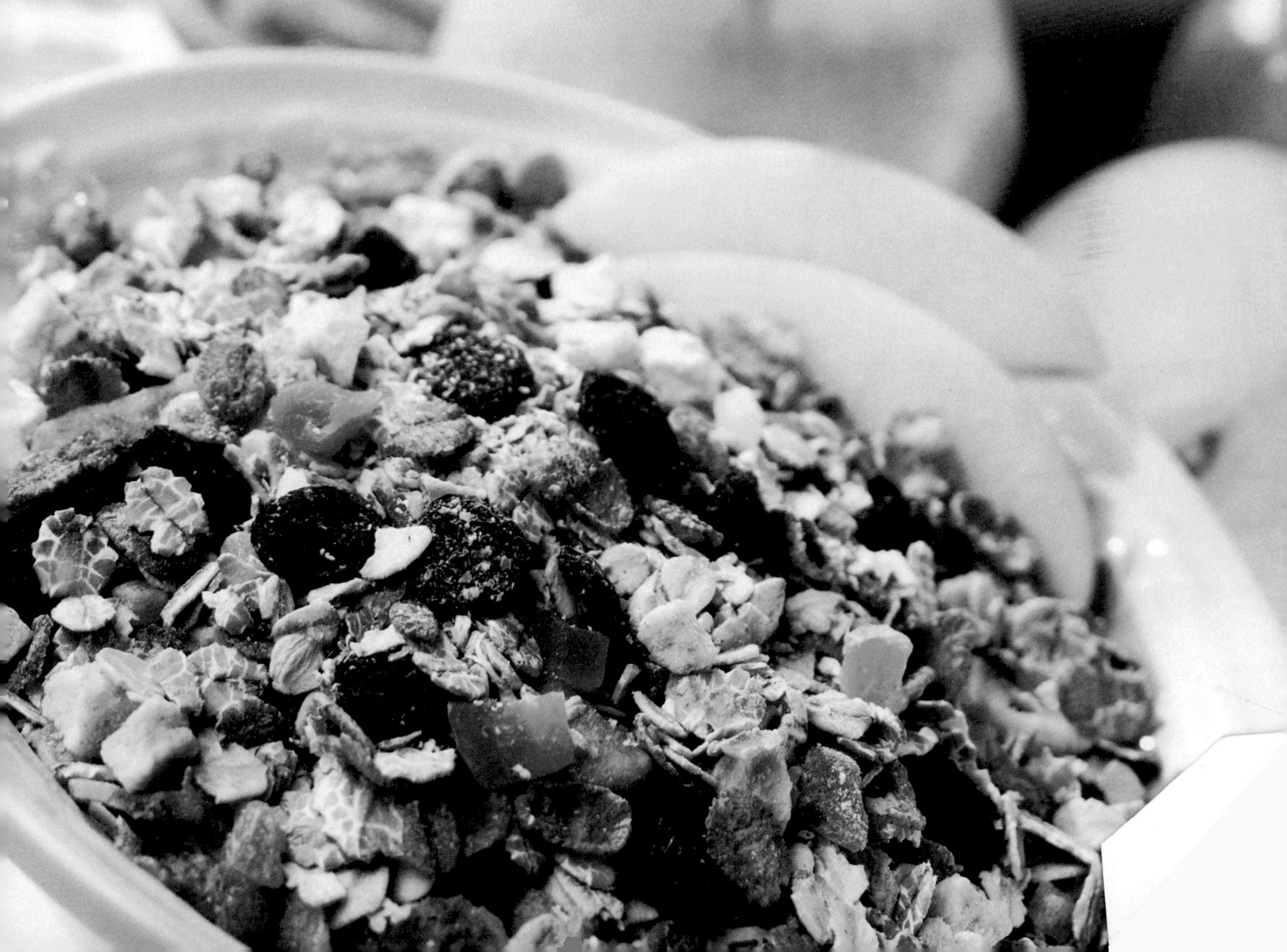

The ultimate goal of this book is to help you find the best path to good nutrition. The information presented is based on emerging science that is translated into everyday actions that improve health. After completion of your nutrition course you should understand the knowledge behind the food choices you make and recommend to others. We call this achievement of making food choices that are right for you "nutrition literacy."

 Refresh Your Memory

As you begin your study of choosing what you eat and why in Chapter 1, you may want to review:

- The metric system in Appendix I.

1.1 Why Do You Choose the Food You Eat?

In your lifetime, you will eat about 70,000 meals and 60 tons of food. Many factors influence our food choices including celebrations (see the comic below). Chapter 1 begins with a discussion of these factors and ends with a conversation specifically about eating well as a college student. In between, we examine the powerful effect of dietary habits in determining overall health and take a close look at the general classes of nutrients—as well as the calories—supplied by the food we eat, the major characteristics of the North American diet, the food habits that often need improvement, and the key "Nutrition and Weight Status" objectives in the *Healthy People 2020* report.

Understanding what drives us to eat and what affects food choice will help you understand the complexity of factors that influence eating, especially the effects of our routines and food advertising (Fig. 1-1). You can then appreciate why foods may have different meanings to different people and thus why food habits and preferences of others may differ from yours.

What Influences Your Food Choices?

Food means so much more to us than nourishment—it reflects much of what we think about ourselves. In the course of our lives, we spend the equivalent of 3 to 4 years eating. Yes, the Bureau of Labor Statistics estimated that in 2010 Americans spent the equivalent of 17 days eating and drinking. If we live to be 80 years old, that will add up to 3.7 years of eating and drinking. Overall, our daily food choices stem

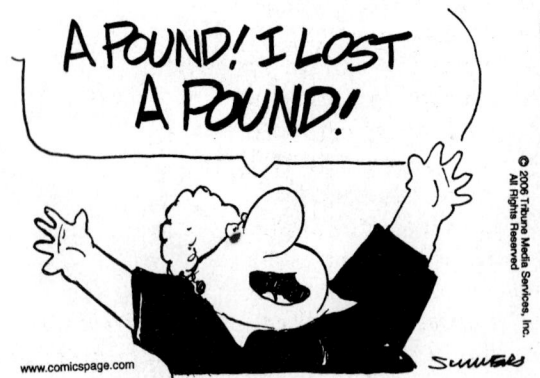
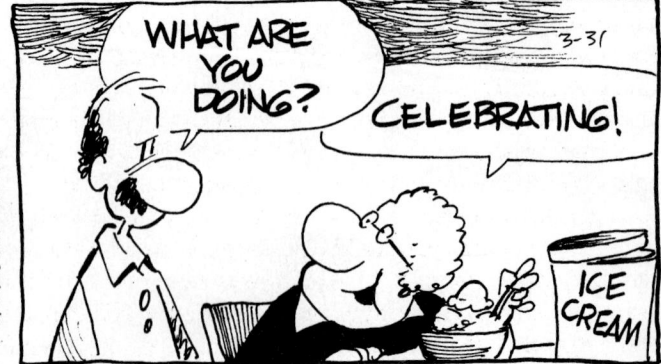

Copyright, 2002, Tribune Media Services. Reprinted with permission.

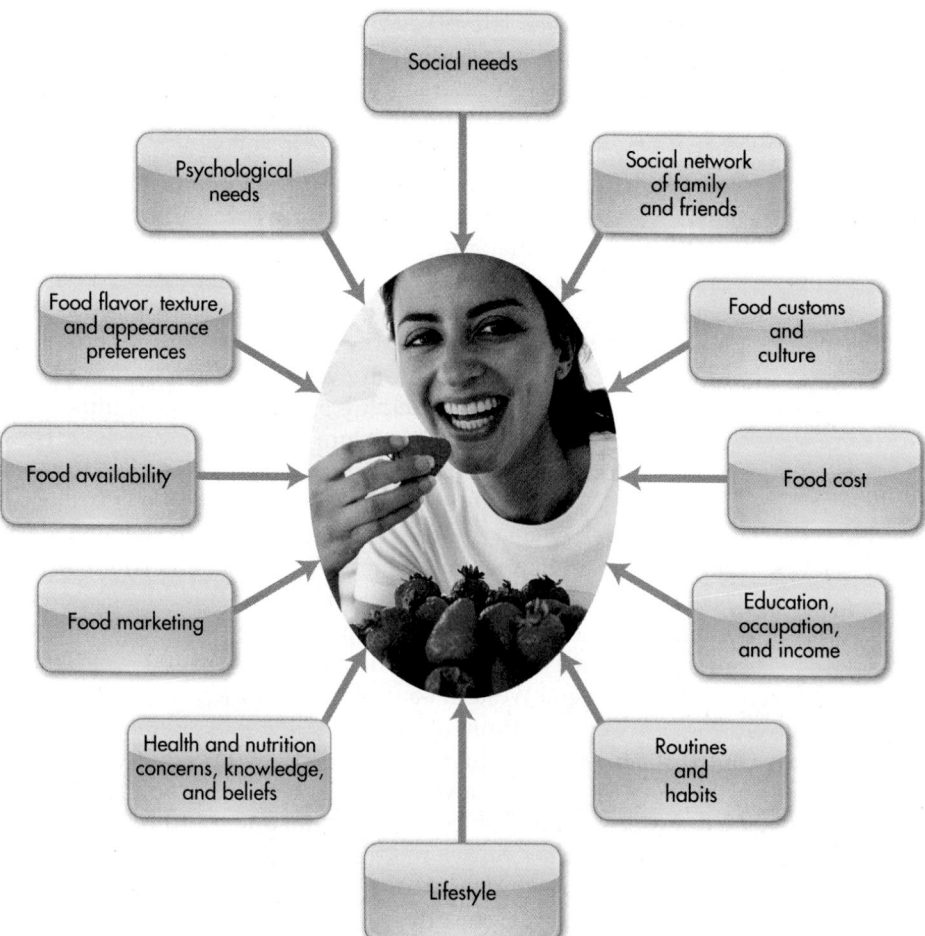

FIGURE 1-1 ▶ Food choices are affected by many factors. Which have the greatest impact on your food choices?

from a complicated mix of biological and social influences (see Fig. 1-1). Let's examine some of the key reasons we choose what we eat.

Flavor, texture, and *appearance* are the most important factors determining our food choices. Creating more flavorful foods that are both healthy and profitable is a major focus of the food industry. These foods are often referred to as "healthy" choices or "better for you" products. The challenge to the food industry is to match the "taste" of the foods we prefer with the nutrition and health characteristics of these products.

Early influences that expose us to various people, places, and events have a continuing impact on our food choices. Many ethnic diet patterns begin as we are introduced to foods during childhood. Developing healthy patterns during childhood, therefore, will go a long way to ensuring healthy preferences and choices when we are teenagers and adults. Food advertising and marketing have been shown to have a definite effect on weight gain in children and adolescents. Read more about the effect of television advertising and the development of obesity in childhood in the Newsworthy Nutrition margin note.

Routines and habits are tied to some food choices. Food habits, food availability, and convenience strongly influence choices. Most of us eat from a core group of foods with about 100 basic items accounting for 75% of an individual's total food intake. Recent surveys indicate that the most commonly purchased foods in America are milk (about 30 gallons yearly), ready-to-eat cereal, bottled water (about 25 gallons per year), soft drinks (nearly 50 gallons per year), and bread. It is no surprise that milk and cereal are both on the top-five list because they are eaten together as the daily breakfast for many Americans. Bottled water has become the drink of choice for business meetings and other large-group gatherings, including outdoor activities. Despite the

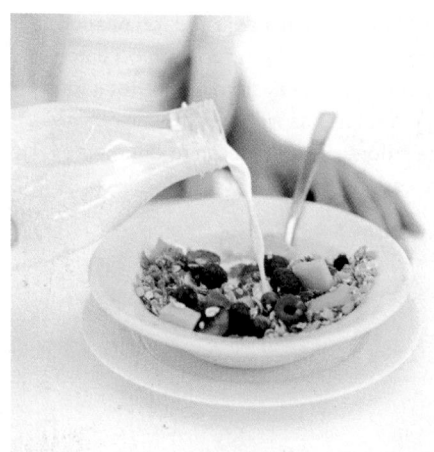

▲ Cereal and milk are two of the most commonly purchased foods in America largely because they are eaten together for breakfast every day by many.

NEWSWORTHY NUTRITION | Link found between TV food ads and childhood obesity

The higher prevalence of childhood obesity in the United States compared to other countries could be explained by greater exposure to TV food advertising. Scientists estimated the exposure of children ages 6 to 11 years in six countries to TV food advertising and its connection with obesity. The contribution of TV food ads to the occurrence of childhood obesity was greatest for the United States at 16% to 40%; lower in Australia and Italy at 10% to 28%; and lowest in Great Britain, Sweden, and the Netherlands at 4% to 18%. Children in the United States were exposed to 11.5 min/day of TV food ads compared to only 1.8 min/day in the Netherlands. Conclusions are that the contribution of TV food ads to the prevalence of childhood obesity is significant in some countries and greatest in the United States.

Source: Goris JM and others: Television food advertising and the prevalence of childhood overweight and obesity: A multicountry comparison. *Public Health Nutrition* 13: 1003, July 2010 (see Further Reading 7).

connect Check out the Connect site www.mcgrawhillconnect.com to further explore TV food ads and childhood obesity.

popularity of water and milk, Americans still drink nearly twice as many carbonated soft drinks per year as either water or milk. The large amount of sugar in many soft drinks is of particular concern because studies have found an association between consumption of sugar-sweetened drinks and obesity in children. Bread is also on the list because it is typically consumed at every meal in America, making it one of the most common forms of grain eaten.

Advertising is a major media tool for capturing the food interest of the consumer. Consumers have more food choices than ever and these choices are well advertised in newspapers, magazines, billboards, radio, television, and now the Internet. The food industry in the United States spends well over $33 billion on advertising. Some of this advertising is helpful, as it promotes the importance of food components such as calcium and fiber in our diets. However, the food industry also advertises highly sweetened cereals, cookies, cakes, and soft drinks because they bring in the greatest profits. It is estimated that as much as $10 billion is spent on advertising food and beverages to America's children and youth. A 2008 Federal Trade Commission survey of 44 major food and beverage marketers in the United States found that they spent $1.6 billion to promote products to children and adolescents in 2006 (see Further Reading 6). Recent studies in several Western countries clearly indicate an association between TV advertising of foods and drinks and the prevalence of childhood obesity, especially in the United States. (Read about one of these studies in Newsworthy Nutrition.) Concern for the negative effect of advertising and marketing on the diets and health of children led the Center for Science in the Public Interest to publish *Guidelines for Responsible Food Marketing to Children* in 2005 (see Further Reading 2). These guidelines provide criteria for marketing food to children in a manner that does not undermine children's diets or harm their health.

Restaurant dining plays a significant role in our food choices, although the recession caused a 11.5 percent decline in food eaten away from home between 2006 and 2009 (Fig 1-2). Restaurant food is often calorie-dense, in large portions, and of poorer nutritional quality compared to foods made at home. Fast-food and pizza restaurant menus typically emphasize meat, cheese, fried foods, and carbonated beverages. I response to recent consumer demands, restaurants have placed healthier items on

FIGURE 1-2 ▶ This chart shows the total food expenditures adjusted for inflation from 1990 to 2009 including food eaten at home and away from home. Total food expenditures as well as food eaten away from home dipped declined during the recession from 2006 to 2009.

Source: http://www.ers.usda.gov/AmberWaves/September11/Features/FoodSpending.htm

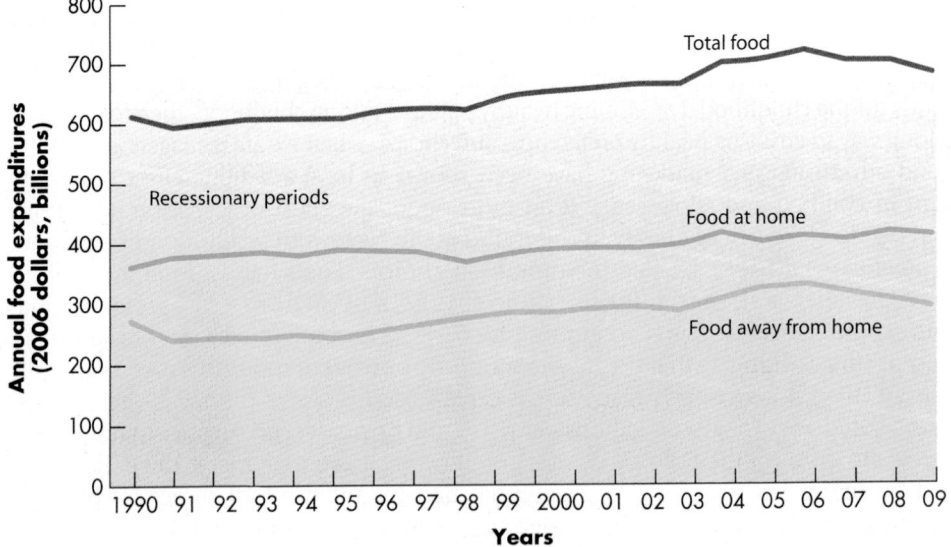

Total food expenditures adjusted for inflation dipped during the 2007–09 recession

their menus and many are listing nutritional content on their menus. Mandatory posting of the calorie content of restaurant items is expected to go into effect soon as a result of the health care reform bill that President Obama signed into law in March 2010. The law requires that chain restaurants with 20 or more locations post the calorie content of their offerings on menus or menu boards with other nutritional information available upon request.

Social changes are leading to a general time shortage for many of us. This creates the need for *convenience.* Supermarkets now supply prepared meals, microwavable entrees, and various quick-prep frozen products.

Economics play a minor role in our food choices. Increases in personal income have exceeded increases in dollars spent for food. This has resulted in the average North American spending only about 12% of after-tax income on food (greater for low-income people). However, as income increases, so do meals eaten away from home and preferences for foods such as cookies, chocolate, cheese, and meat. Also keep in mind that as calorie intake increases so does the food bill.

Last but not least, *nutrition*—or what we think of as "healthy foods"—also directs our food purchases. North Americans who tend to make health-related food choices are often well-educated, middle-class professionals. These same people are generally health-oriented, have active lifestyles, and focus on weight control. In the 2008 Health and Diet Survey (a snapshot of the nation's dietary habits), the Food and Drug Administration (FDA) found that more than half (54%) of consumers in the United States read the food label when buying a product for the first time. This number was an increase since 2002. Among those who are reading the Nutrition Facts, 67% use the label "often" to check how high or low a food is in calories and in substances such as salt, vitamins, and fat; 55% "often" use the label to get a general idea of the food's nutritional content; and 46% "often" use the calorie information on the label. Their key findings also indicate that consumers are increasingly aware of the link between diet and heart disease. Of those surveyed, 91% knew of this link, 81% knew that certain foods or drinks may help prevent heart disease or heart attacks, and 62% mentioned fats as a factor related to heart disease (see Further Reading 4).

Why Are You So Hungry?

Two drives, **hunger** and **appetite,** influence our desire to eat. These drives differ dramatically. Hunger is primarily our physical biological drive to eat and is controlled by internal body mechanisms. For example, as foods are digested and absorbed by the stomach and small intestine, these organs send signals to the liver and brain to reduce further food intake.

Appetite, our primarily psychological drive to eat, is affected by many of the external food choice mechanisms we discussed in the last section, such as environmental and psychological factors and social customs (see Fig. 1-1). Appetite can be triggered simply by seeing a tempting dessert or smelling popcorn popping at the movie theater. Fulfilling either or both drives by eating sufficient food normally brings a state of **satiety,** a feeling of satisfaction that temporarily halts our desire to continue eating.

A region of the brain helps regulate satiety. Imagine a game of tug-of-war in the brain. The *feeding center* and the *satiety center* work in opposite ways to promote adequate availability of nutrients at all times. When stimulated, cells in the feeding center signal us to eat. As we eat, cells in the satiety center are stimulated and we stop eating. For example, when we haven't eaten for a while, stimulation of the feeding center signals

hunger The primarily physiological (internal) drive to find and eat food, mostly regulated by internal cues to eating.

appetite The primarily psychological (external) influences that encourage us to find and eat food, often in the absence of obvious hunger.

satiety State in which there is no longer a desire to eat; a feeling of satisfaction.

MAKING DECISIONS

Putting Our Food Choices into Perspective

The next time you pick up a candy bar or reach for a second helping, remember the internal and external influences on eating behavior. You should now understand that daily food intake is a complicated mix of biological and social influences. Body cells, nutrients in the blood, hormones, brain chemicals, and our social and family customs all influence food choices. When food is abundant, appetite—not hunger—most likely triggers eating. Satiety associated with consuming a meal may reside primarily in our psychological frame of mind. Also, because satiety regulation is not perfect, body weight can fluctuate. We become accustomed to a certain amount of food at a meal. Providing less than that amount leaves us wanting more. One way to use this observation for weight-loss purposes is to train your eye to expect less food by slowly decreasing serving sizes to more appropriate amounts. Your appetite then readjusts as you expect less food. Keep track of what triggers your eating for a few days. Is it primarily hunger or appetite? The Rate Your Plate activity in this chapter also asks you to keep track of what influences your food intake on a daily basis.

CRITICAL THINKING

Sarah is majoring in nutrition and is well aware of the importance of a healthy diet. She has recently been analyzing her diet and is confused. She notices that she eats a great deal of high-fat foods, such as peanut butter, cheese, chips, ice cream, and chocolate, and few fruits, vegetables, and whole grains. She also has become hooked on her daily cappuccino with lots of whipped cream. What three factors may be influencing Sarah's food choices? What advice would you give her on how to have her diet match her needs?

nutrients   Chemical substances in food that contribute to health, many of which are essential parts of a diet. Nutrients nourish us by providing calories to fulfill energy needs, materials for building body parts, and factors to regulate necessary chemical processes in the body.

essential nutrient   In nutritional terms, a substance that, when left out of a diet, leads to signs of poor health. The body either cannot produce this nutrient or cannot produce enough of it to meet its needs. Then, if added back to a diet before permanent damage occurs, the affected aspects of health are restored.

us to eat. When the nutrient content in the blood rises after a meal, the satiety center is stimulated and we no longer have a strong desire to seek food. Admittedly, this concept of a tug-of-war between the feeding and satiety centers is an oversimplification of a complex process. The various feeding and satiety messages from body cells to the brain do not single-handedly determine what we eat. We often eat because food confronts us (see Further Reading 17). Almost everyone has encountered a mouthwatering dessert and devoured it, even on a full stomach. It smells, tastes, and looks good. We might eat because it is the right time of day, we are celebrating (see the cartoon in this section), or we are seeking emotional comfort to overcome the blues. After a meal, memories of pleasant tastes and feelings reinforce appetite. If stress or depression sends you to the refrigerator, you are mostly seeking comfort, not food calories. Appetite may not be a physical process, but it does influence food intake. We will discuss more about this mechanism, including the effect of meal size and composition on satiety, in Chapter 7 on energy balance and weight control.

CONCEPT CHECK

Hunger is the primarily physical or internal desire to find and eat food. Fulfilling it creates satiety—no further desire to eat exists. Satiety is influenced by hunger-related (internal) signals from the brain and other organs, as well as the content of the foods in the meal. Food intake is also affected by appetite-related (external) forces like social customs, time of day, and being with others. Factors such as flavor, appearance, and texture; early influences, routines, and habits; advertising and restaurant menus; economics and convenience; seeking emotional comfort; social changes; and hopefully, nutrition and health concerns, also greatly influence our food choices. North Americans probably respond more to external, appetite-related forces than to hunger-related ones in choosing when and what to eat.

1.2 How Is Nutrition Connected to Good Health?

Fortunately the foods we eat can support good health in many ways depending on their components. You just learned, however, that lifestyle habits and other factors may have a bigger impact on our food choices than the food components themselves. Unfortunately many North Americans suffer from diseases that could have been prevented if they had known more about the foods and, more importantly, had applied this knowledge to planning meals and designing their diet. We will now look at the effect these choices are having on our health both today and in the future.

What Is Nutrition?

Nutrition is the science that links foods to health and disease. It includes the processes by which the human organism ingests, digests, absorbs, transports, and excretes food substances.

Nutrients Come from Food

What is the difference between food and **nutrients**? Food provides the energy (in the form of calories) as well as the materials needed to build and maintain all body cells. Nutrients are the substances obtained from food that are vital for growth and maintenance of a healthy body throughout life. For a substance to be considered an **essential nutrient**, three characteristics are needed:

- First, at least one specific biological function of the nutrient in the body must be identified.

▲ Many foods are rich sources of nutrients.

- Second, omission of the nutrient from the diet must lead to a decline in certain biological functions, such as production of blood cells.
- Third, replacing the omitted nutrient in the diet before permanent damage occurs will restore those normal biological functions.

Why Study Nutrition?

Nutrition is a lifestyle factor that is a key to developing and maintaining an optimal state of health for you. A poor diet and a sedentary lifestyle are known to be **risk factors** for life-threatening **chronic** diseases such as **cardiovascular (heart) disease, hypertension, diabetes,** and some forms of **cancer** (Table 1-1). Together, these and related disorders account for two-thirds of all deaths in North America (Table 1-2)

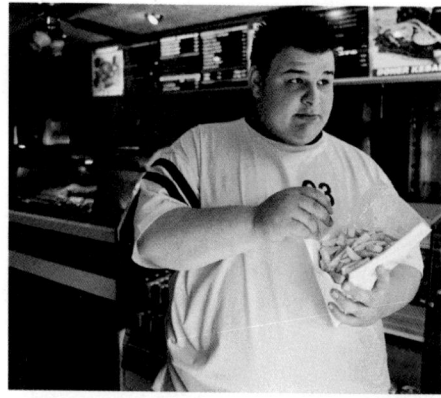

▲ Major health problems are largely caused by a poor diet, excessive calorie intake, and not enough physical activity.

TABLE 1-1 Glossary Terms to Aid Your Introduction to Nutrition*

Cancer	A condition characterized by uncontrolled growth of abnormal cells.
Cardiovascular (heart) disease	A general term that refers to any disease of the heart and circulatory system. This disease is generally characterized by the deposition of fatty material in the blood vessels (hardening of the arteries), which in turn can lead to organ damage and death. Also termed coronary heart disease (CHD), as the vessels of the heart are the primary sites of the disease.
Cholesterol	A waxy lipid found in all body cells; it has a structure containing multiple chemical rings. Cholesterol is found only in foods of animal origin.
Chronic	Long-standing, developing over time. When referring to disease, this term indicates that the disease process, once developed, is slow and lasting. A good example is cardiovascular disease.
Diabetes	A group of diseases characterized by high blood **glucose.** Type 1 diabetes involves insufficient or no release of the hormone insulin by the pancreas and therefore requires daily insulin therapy. Type 2 diabetes results from either insufficient release of insulin or general inability of insulin to act on certain body cells, such as muscle cells. Persons with type 2 diabetes may or may not require insulin therapy.
Hypertension	A condition in which blood pressure remains persistently elevated. Obesity, inactivity, alcohol intake, excess salt intake, and genetics may each contribute to the problem.
Kilocalorie (kcal)	Unit that describes the energy content of food. Specifically, a kilocalorie (kcal) is the heat energy needed to raise the temperature of 1000 grams (1 liter) of water 1° Celsius. Kcal refers to a 1000 calorie unit of measurement, but is commonly referred to as calories. It is a familiar term for the energy content of a food, so we will use it in this book.
Obesity	A condition characterized by excess body fat.
Osteoporosis	Decreased bone mass related to the effects of aging (including estrogen loss during menopause in women), genetic background, and poor diet.
Risk factor	A term used frequently when discussing the factors contributing to the development of a disease. A risk factor is an aspect of our lives—such as heredity, lifestyle choices (e.g., smoking), or nutritional habits.

glucose A six-carbon sugar that exists in a ring form; found as such in blood, and in table sugar bound to fructose; also known as *dextrose*, it is one of the simple sugars.

*Many bold terms are also defined in the page margins within each chapter and in the glossary at the end of this book.

stroke A decrease or loss in blood flow to the brain that results from a blood clot or other change in arteries in the brain. This in turn causes the death of brain tissue. Also called a *cerebrovascular accident.*

TABLE 1-2 Fifteen Leading Causes of Death in the United States

Rank	Cause of Death	Percent of Total Deaths
	All causes	100
1	Heart disease[*†#]	24.6
2	Cancer[*‡]	23.3
3	Chronic lower respiratory diseases[‡]	5.6
4	Stroke (cerebrovascular diseases)[*†‡#]	5.3
5	Accidents (unintentional injuries)	4.8
6	Alzheimer's disease[*]	3.2
7	Diabetes mellitus[*]	2.8
8	Influenza and pneumonia	2.2
9	Kidney disease[*‡]	2.0
10	Intentional self harm (suicide)	1.5
11	Blood-borne infections (septicemia)	1.4
12	Chronic liver disease and cirrhosis[†]	1.2
13	Essential hypertension[*]	1.1
14	Parkinson's disease	0.8
15	Assault (homicide)	0.7

From Centers for Disease Control and Prevention, *National Vital Statistics Report,* Preliminary Data for 2009, March 16, 2011. Canadian statistics are quite similar.

*Causes of death in which diet plays a part.

†Causes of death in which excessive alcohol consumption plays a part.

‡Causes of death in which tobacco use plays a part.

#Diseases of the heart and cerebrovascular disease are included in the more global term "cardiovascular disease."

NEWSWORTHY NUTRITION

Healthy diet lowers women's risk of sudden cardiac death

Sudden cardiac death (death occurring within 1 hour after symptom onset) is the cause of more than half of all heart-related deaths and usually occurs as the first sign of heart disease, especially in women. Lifestyle information from the Nurses' Health Study (81,722 women) was used to determine if adherence to a healthy lifestyle lowers the risk of sudden cardiac death among women. Low-risk lifestyle was considered as not smoking, not overweight, exercising 30 minutes/day or longer, and following the Mediterranean Diet. Risk of sudden cardiac death dropped by 92% with a combination of the four healthy lifestyles; and women who ate a diet most similar to the Mediterranean Diet with a high proportion of vegetables, fruits, nuts, omega-3 fats, and fish, along with moderate amounts of alcohol and small amounts of red meat, had a 40% less risk than women whose diets least resembled this diet. The conclusion is that a healthy diet along with other healthy lifestyle factors can protect women from sudden cardiac death.

Source: Chiuve SE, and others: Adherence to a low-risk, healthy lifestyle and risk of sudden cardiac death among women. *Journal of the American Medical Association,* 306:62, 2011 (see Further Reading 3).

connect NUTRITION **Check out the Connect site** www.mcgrawhillconnect.com **to further explore women's risk of sudden cardiac death.**

(see Further Reading 9). Not meeting nutrient needs in younger years makes us more likely to suffer health consequences, such as bone fractures from the disease **osteoporosis,** in later years. At the same time, taking too much of a nutrient—such as a vitamin A supplement—can be harmful. Another dietary problem, drinking too much alcohol, is associated with many health problems.

U.S. government scientists have calculated that a poor diet combined with a lack of sufficient physical activity contributes to hundreds of thousands of fatal cases of cardiovascular disease, cancer, and diabetes each year among adults in the United States. Thus, the combination of poor diet and too little physical activity may be the second leading cause of death in the United States. In addition, **obesity** is considered the second leading cause of preventable death in North America (smoking is the first). When they occur together, obesity and smoking cause even more health problems. Obesity and chronic diseases are often preventable. An important key to good health and more health care dollars in your pocket, is to realize that the cost of prevention, usually when we are children and young adults, is a small fraction of the cost of treating these diseases when we are older.

The good news is that the increased interest in health, fitness, and nutrition shown by Americans has been associated with long-term decreasing trends for heart disease, cancer, and stroke (the three leading causes of death) that continued in 2009. Mortality from heart disease, the leading cause of death, has been declining steadily since 1980. As you gain understanding about your nutritional habits and increase your knowledge about optimal nutrition, you will have the opportunity to dramatically reduce your risk for many common health problems. Read more about research on the link between eating a healthy diet and protection against death from heart disease in Newsworthy Nutrition. For additional help, the U.S. federal government provides two websites that contain links to many sources of health and nutrition information (www.healthfinder.gov and www.nutrition.gov). Other useful sites are www.webmd.com and www.eatright.org.

1.3 What Are the Classes and Sources of Nutrients?

To begin the study of nutrition, let's start with an overview of the six classes of nutrients. You are probably already familiar with the terms **carbohydrates, lipids** (fats and oils), **proteins, vitamins,** and **minerals.** These, plus **water,** make up the six classes of nutrients found in food.

Nutrients can then be assigned to three functional categories: (1) those that primarily provide us with calories to meet energy needs (expressed in **kilocalories [kcal]**); (2) those important for growth, development, and maintenance; and (3) those that act to keep body functions running smoothly. Some function overlap exists among these categories. The energy-yielding nutrients, carbohydrate, fat, and protein, make up a major portion of most foods (Table 1-3).

Let's now look more closely at these six classes of nutrients.

Carbohydrates

Chemically, carbohydrates can exist in foods as simple sugars and complex carbohydrates. **Simple sugars,** frequently referred to as *sugars,* are relatively small molecules. These sugars are found naturally in fruits, vegetables, and dairy products. Table sugar, sucrose, is an example of a simple sugar that is added to many foods we eat. Glucose, also known as blood sugar or dextrose, is an example of a simple sugar in your blood. **Complex carbohydrates** are formed when many simple sugars are joined together. For example, plants store carbohydrates in the form of **starch,** a complex carbohydrate made up of hundreds of sugar units. Breads, cereals, grains, and starchy vegetables are the main sources of complex carbohydrates.

carbohydrate A compound containing carbon, hydrogen, and oxygen atoms. Most are known as *sugars, starches,* and *fibers.*

lipid A compound containing much carbon and hydrogen, little oxygen, and sometimes other atoms. Lipids do not dissolve in water, and include fats, oils, and cholesterol.

protein Food and body compounds made of amino acids; proteins contain carbon, hydrogen, oxygen, nitrogen, and sometimes other atoms, in a specific configuration. Proteins contain the form of nitrogen most easily used by the human body.

vitamin Compound needed in very small amounts in the diet to help regulate and support chemical reactions in the body.

mineral Element used to promote chemical reactions and to form body structures.

water The universal solvent; chemically, H_2O. The body is composed of about 60% water. Water (fluid) needs are about 9 (women) or 13 (men) cups per day; needs are greater if one exercises heavily.

kilocalorie (kcal) Heat energy needed to raise the temperature of 1000 grams (1 L) of water 1 degree Celsius; also written as *Calories.*

simple sugar Monosaccharide or disaccharide in the diet.

complex carbohydrate Carbohydrate composed of many monosaccharide molecules. Examples include glycogen, starch, and fiber.

macronutrient A nutrient needed in gram quantities in a diet.

micronutrient A nutrient needed in milligram or microgram quantities in a diet.

TABLE 1-3 Major Functions of the Various Classes of Nutrients

Nutrient Classes That Provide Energy	Nutrient Classes That Promote Growth, Development, and Maintenance	Nutrient Classes That Regulate Body Processes
Most carbohydrates	Proteins	Proteins
Proteins	Lipids	Some lipids
Most lipids	Some vitamins	Some vitamins
	Some minerals	Some minerals
	Water	Water

Carbohydrates, proteins, lipids, and water are needed in relatively large amounts, so they are called **macronutrients.** Vitamins and minerals are needed in such small amounts in the diet that they are called **micronutrients.**

During digestion, complex carbohydrates are broken down into single sugar molecules (such as glucose), and absorbed via **cells** lining the small intestine into the bloodstream (see Chapter 3 for more on digestion and absorption). However, the **bonds** between the sugar molecules in certain complex carbohydrates, called **fiber,** cannot be broken down by human digestive processes. Fiber passes through the small intestine undigested to provide bulk for the stool (feces) formed in the large intestine (colon).

Aside from enjoying their taste, we need sugars and other carbohydrates in our diets primarily to help satisfy the calorie needs of our body cells. Carbohydrates provide a major source of calories for the body, on average 4 kcal per gram. Glucose, a simple sugar that the body can derive from most carbohydrates, is a major source of calories for most cells. When not enough carbohydrate is consumed to supply sufficient glucose, the body is forced to make glucose from proteins—not a healthy change. Chapter 4 focuses on carbohydrates.

Lipids

Lipids (mostly fats and oils) in the foods we eat also provide energy. Lipids yield more calories per gram than do carbohydrates—on the average, 9 kcal per gram—because of differences in their chemical composition. They are also the main form for energy storage in the body.

Lipids dissolve in certain chemical solvents (e.g., ether and benzene) but not in water. In this book, the more familiar terms *fats* and *oils* will generally be used, rather than lipids or triglycerides. Generally, fats are lipids that are solid at room temperature and oils are lipids that are liquid at room temperature. We obtain fats and oils from animal and plant sources. Animal fats, such as butter or lard, are solid at room temperature. Plant oils, such as corn or olive oil, tend to be liquid at room temperature. Solid fat should be limited in our diet because it can raise blood **cholesterol.** High blood cholesterol leads to clogged arteries and can eventually lead to cardiovascular disease (see Chapter 5).

Certain fats are essential nutrients that must come from our diet. These key fats that the body cannot produce, called essential fatty acids, perform several important functions in the body: they help regulate blood pressure and play a role in the synthesis and repair of vital cell parts. However, we need only about 4 tablespoons of a common plant oil (such as the canola or soybean oil) each day to supply these essential fatty acids. A serving of fatty fish, such as salmon or tuna, at least twice a week is another healthy source of essential fatty acids. The unique fatty acids in these fish complement the healthy aspects of common vegetable oils. This will be explained in greater detail in Chapter 5, which focuses on lipids.

Proteins

Proteins are the main structural material in the body. For example, proteins constitute a major part of bone and muscle; they are also important components in blood, body cells, **enzymes,** and immune factors. Proteins can also provide calories for the body—on average, 4 kcal per gram. Typically, however, the body uses little protein for the purpose of meeting daily calorie needs. Proteins are formed when **amino acids** are bonded together. Some of these are essential nutrients.

Protein in our diet also comes from animal and plant sources. The animal products meat, poultry, fish, dairy products, and eggs are significant sources of protein in most diets. Beans, grains, and some vegetables are good plant protein sources. Plant protein is important to include in vegetarian diets.

Most North Americans eat up to two times as much protein as the body needs to maintain health. This amount of extra protein in the diet reflects the standard of living and the dietary habits of most North Americans and is generally not harmful for healthy persons with no evidence of heart or kidney disease, diabetes, or family history of colon cancer or kidney stones. The excess is used for calorie needs and carbohydrate production but ultimately can contribute to storage of fat. Chapter 6 focuses on proteins.

cell The structural basis of plant and animal organization. Cells contain genetic material and systems for synthesizing energy-yielding compounds. Cells have the ability to take up compounds from and excrete compounds into their surroundings.

bond A linkage between two atoms formed by the sharing of electrons, or attractions.

fiber Substances in plant foods not digested by the processes that take place in the human stomach or small intestine. These add bulk to feces. Fiber naturally found in foods is also called dietary fiber.

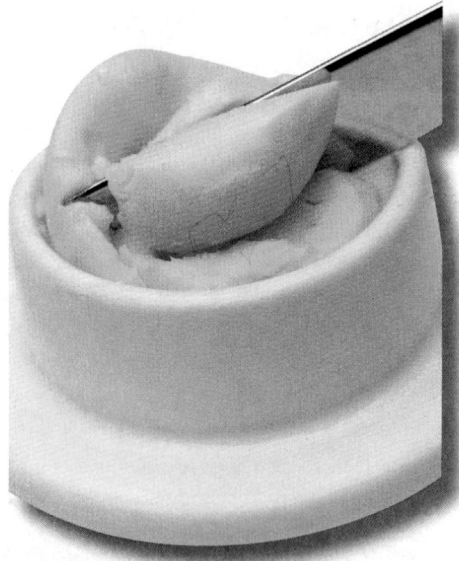

▲ Butter is an animal fat made from milk fat and is solid at room temperature.

enzyme A compound that speeds the rate of a chemical reaction but is not altered by the reaction. Almost all enzymes are proteins (some are made of genetic material).

amino acid The building block for proteins containing a central carbon atom with nitrogen and other atoms attached.

Vitamins

The main function of vitamins is to enable many <u>chemical reactions</u> to occur in the body. Some of these reactions help release the energy trapped in carbohydrates, lipids, and proteins. Remember, however, that vitamins themselves contain no usable calories for the body.

The 13 vitamins are divided into two groups: four are **fat-soluble** because they dissolve in fat (vitamins A, D, E, and K); nine are **water-soluble** because they dissolve in water (the B vitamins and vitamin C). The two groups of vitamins have different sources, functions, and characteristics. Water-soluble vitamins are found mainly in fruits and vegetables, whereas dairy products, nuts, seeds, oils, and breakfast cereals are good sources of fat-soluble vitamins. Cooking destroys water-soluble vitamins much more readily than it does fat-soluble vitamins. Water-soluble vitamins are also excreted from the body much more readily than are fat-soluble vitamins. Thus, the fat-soluble vitamins, especially vitamin A, are much more likely to accumulate in excessive amounts in the body, which then can lead to toxicity. Vitamins are the focus of Chapter 8.

Minerals

Minerals are structurally simple, **inorganic** substances, which do not contain carbon atoms. Minerals such as sodium and potassium typically function independently in the body, whereas minerals such as calcium and phosphorus function as parts of simple mineral combinations, such as bone mineral. Because of their simple structure, minerals are not destroyed during cooking, but they can still be lost if they dissolve in the water used for cooking and that water is then discarded. Minerals are critical players in nervous system functioning, water balance, structural (e.g., skeletal) systems, and many other cellular processes, but produce no calories as such for the body.

The 16 or more essential minerals required in the diet for good health are divided into two groups: **major minerals** and **trace minerals** because dietary needs vary enormously. If daily needs are less than 100 milligrams, the mineral is classified as a trace mineral; otherwise, it is a major mineral. Minerals that function based on their electrical charge when dissolved in water are also called **electrolytes;** these include sodium, potassium, and chloride. Many major minerals are found naturally in dairy products and fruits, whereas many trace minerals are found in meats, poultry, fish, and nuts. Minerals are the focus of Chapter 9.

Water

Water makes up the sixth class of nutrients. Although sometimes overlooked as a nutrient, water (chemically, H_2O) has numerous vital functions in the body. It acts as a **solvent** and lubricant, as a vehicle for transporting nutrients and waste, and as a medium for temperature regulation and chemical processes. For these reasons, and because the human body is approximately 60% water, the average man should consume about 3 liters—equivalent to 3000 grams or about 13 cups—of water and/or other fluids containing water every day. Women need closer to 2200 grams or about 9 cups per day.

Water is not only available from the obvious sources, but it is also the major component in some foods, such as many fruits and vegetables (e.g., lettuce, grapes, and melons). The body even makes some water as a by-product of **metabolism.** Water is examined in detail in Chapter 2.

Other Important Components in Food

Another group of compounds in foods from plant sources, especially within the fruit and vegetable groups, is what scientists call **phytochemicals.** Although these plant components are not considered essential nutrients in the diet, many of these substances provide significant health benefits. Considerable research attention is focused on various phytochemicals in reducing the risk for certain diseases. For example, evidence from animal and laboratory studies indicate that compounds in blueberries and

chemical reaction An interaction between two chemicals that changes both chemicals.

inorganic Any substance lacking carbon atoms bonded to hydrogen atoms in the chemical structure.

electrolytes Substances that separate into ions in water and, in turn, are able to conduct an electrical current. These include sodium, chloride, and potassium.

solvent A liquid substance in which other substances dissolve.-

metabolism Chemical processes in the body by which energy is provided in useful forms and vital activities are sustained.

phytochemical A chemical found in plants. Some phytochemicals may contribute to a reduced risk of cancer or cardiovascular disease in people who consume them regularly.

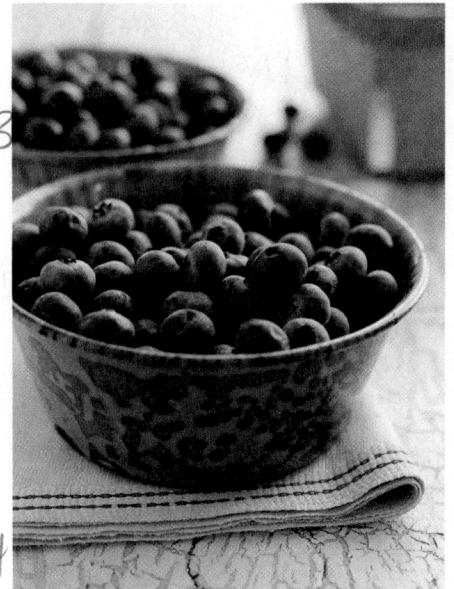

▲ Blueberries are among the fruits, vegetables, beans, and whole-grain breads and cereals that are typically rich in phytochemicals.

TABLE 1-4 Food Sources of Some Phytochemical Compounds under Study

Phytochemical	Food Sources
Allyl sulfides/organosulfurs	Garlic, onions, leeks
Saponins	Garlic, onions, licorice, legumes
Carotenoids (e.g., lycopene)	Orange, red, yellow fruits and vegetables (egg yolks are a source as well)
Monoterpenes	Oranges, lemons, grapefruit
Capsaicin	Chili peppers
Lignans	Flaxseed, berries, whole grains
Indoles	Cruciferous vegetables (broccoli, cabbage, kale)
Isothiocyanates	Cruciferous vegetables, especially broccoli
Phytosterols	Soybeans, other legumes, cucumbers, other fruits and vegetables
Flavonoids	Citrus fruit, onions, apples, grapes, red wine, tea, chocolate, tomatoes
Isoflavones	Soybeans, other legumes
Catechins	Tea
Polyphenols	Blueberries, strawberries, raspberries, grapes, apples, bananas, nuts
Anthocyanosides	Red, blue, and purple plants (blueberries, eggplant)
Fructooligosaccharides	Onions, bananas, oranges (small amounts)
Resveratrol	Grapes, peanuts, red wine

Some related compounds under study are found in animal products, such as sphingolipids (meat and dairy products) and conjugated linoleic acid (meat and cheese). These are not phytochemicals per se because they are not from plant sources, but they have been shown to have health benefits.

strawberries prevent the growth of certain cancer cells. Although certain phytochemicals are available as dietary supplements, research suggests that their health benefits are best obtained through the consumption of whole foods. Foods with high phytochemical content are sometimes called "superfoods" because of the health benefits they are thought to confer. There is no legal definition of the term superfood, however, and there is concern that it is being over-used in marketing certain foods. Table 1-4 lists some noteworthy phytochemicals with their common food sources. Tips for boosting the phytochemical content of your diet will be discussed in Chapter 2.

Sources of Nutrients

Now that we know the six classes of nutrients, it is important to understand that the quantities of the various nutrients that people consume in different foods vary widely. On a daily basis we consume about 500 grams, or about 1 pound, of protein, fat, and carbohydrate. In contrast, the typical daily mineral intake totals about 20 grams (about 4 teaspoons), and the daily vitamin intake totals less than 300 milligrams (1/15 of a teaspoon). Although we require a gram or so of some minerals, such as calcium and phosphorus, we need only a few milligrams or less of other minerals each day. For example, we need about 10 milligrams of zinc per day, which is just a few specks of the mineral.

 The nutrient content of the foods we eat also differs from the nutrient composition of the human body. This is because growth, development, and later maintenance of the human body are directed by the genetic material (DNA) inside body cells. This genetic blueprint determines how each cell uses the essential nutrients to perform body functions. These nutrients can come from a variety of sources. Cells are not concerned about whether available amino acids come from animal or plant sources. The carbohydrate glucose can come from sugars or starches. The food that you eat provides cells with basic materials to function according to the directions supplied by the genetic material (**genes**) housed in body cells. Genetics and nutrition will be discussed in Chapter 3.

1.4 What Are Your Sources of Energy?

Calories

Humans obtain the energy we need for involuntary body functions and voluntary physical activity from various calorie sources: carbohydrates (4 kcal per gram), fats (9 kcal per gram), and proteins (4 kcal per gram). Foods generally provide more than one calorie source. Plant oils, such as soybean or canola oil are one exception; these are 100% fat at 9 kcal per gram.

Alcohol is also a source of calories for some of us, supplying about 7 kcal per gram. It is not considered an essential nutrient, however, because it has no required function. Still, alcoholic beverages, such as beer—also rich in carbohydrate—are a contributor of calories to the diet of many adults.

The body releases the energy from the chemical bonds in carbohydrate, protein, and fat (and alcohol) into other forms of energy in order to:

- Build new **compounds.**
- Perform muscular movements.
- Promote nerve transmissions.
- Maintain electrolyte balance within cells.

Chapters 7 and 12 describe how that energy is released from the chemical bonds in energy-yielding nutrients and then used by body cells to support the processes just described.

The energy in food is often expressed in terms of calories on food labels. As defined earlier, a calorie is the amount of heat energy it takes to raise the temperature of 1 gram of water 1 degree Celsius (1°C, centigrade scale). (Chapter 7 has a diagram of the bomb calorimeter that can be used to measure calories in foods.) A calorie is a tiny measure of heat, so food energy is more conveniently expressed in terms of the kilocalorie (kcal), which equals 1000 calories. (If the "c" in calories is capitalized, this also signifies kilocalories.) A kcal is the amount of heat energy it takes to raise the temperature of 1000 grams (1 liter) of water 1°C. The abbreviation *kcal* is used throughout this book. On food labels, the word *calorie* (without a capital "C") is also used loosely to mean *kilocalorie.* Any values given on food labels in calories are actually in kilocalories (Fig. 1-3). A suggested intake of 2000 calories per day on a food label is technically 2000 kcal.

genes A specific segment on a chromosome. Genes provide the blueprints for the production of all body proteins.

alcohol Ethyl alcohol or ethanol (CH_3CH_2OH) is the compound in alcoholic beverages.

compound A group of different types of atoms bonded together in definite proportion.

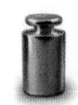 Carbohydrate
4 kcal per gram

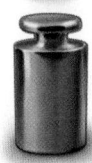 Fat
9 kcal per gram

 Protein
4 kcal per gram

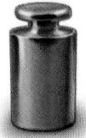 Alcohol
7 kcal per gram

▲ Calorie content of energy nutrients and alcohol.

Nutrition Facts			
Serving Size 1 slice (36g)		Servings Per Container 19	
Amount Per Serving			
Calories 80		Calories from Fat 10	
% Daily Value*		**% Daily Value***	
Total Fat 1g	**2%**	**Total Carbohydrate** 15g	**5%**
Saturated Fat 0g	**0%**	Dietary Fiber 2g	**8%**
Trans Fat less than 1g	**		
Cholesterol 0mg	**0%**	Sugars less than 1g	
Sodium 200mg	**8%**	**Protein** 3g	
Vitamin A 0%	Vitamin C 0%	Calcium 0%	Iron 4%

HONEY WHEAT BREAD

*Percent Daily Values (DV) are based on a 2,000 calorie diet. Your daily values may be higher or lower depending on your calorie needs:

	Calories:	2,000	2,500
Total Fat	Less than	65g	80g
Sat Fat	Less than	20g	25g
Cholesterol	Less than	300mg	300mg
Sodium	Less than	2,400mg	2,400mg
Total Carbohydrate		300g	375g
Dietary Fiber		25g	30g

** Intake of *trans* fat should be as low as possible.

INGREDIENTS: WHOLE WHEAT, WATER, ENRICHED WHEAT FLOUR [FLOUR, MALTED BARLEY, NIACIN, REDUCED IRON, THIAMINE MONONITRATE (VITAMIN B1) AND RIBOFLAVIN (VITAMIN B2)], CORN SYRUP, PARTIALLY HYDROGENATED COTTONSEED OIL, SALT, YEAST.

FIGURE 1-3 ▶ Use the nutrient values on the Nutrition Facts label to calculate calorie content of a food. Based on carbohydrate, fat, and protein content, a serving of this food (Honey Wheat Bread) contains 81 kcal ([15 × 4] + [1 × 9] + [3 × 4] = 81). The label lists 80, suggesting that the calorie value was rounded down.

Calculating Calories

Use the 4-9-4 estimates for the calorie content of carbohydrate, fat, and protein introduced over the last few pages to determine calorie content of a food. Consider these foods:

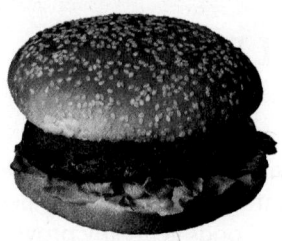

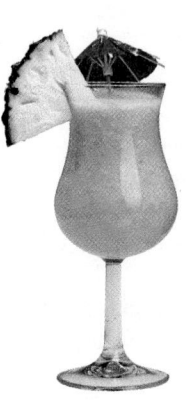

1 Large Hamburger

Carbohydrate	39 grams × 4 =	156 kcal
Fat	32 grams × 9 =	288 kcal
Protein	30 grams × 4 =	120 kcal
Alcohol	0 grams × 7 =	0 kcal
Total		**564 kcal**

8-ounce Piña Colada

Carbohydrate	57 grams × 4 =	228 kcal
Fat	5 grams × 9 =	45 kcal
Protein	1 gram × 4 =	4 kcal
Alcohol	23 grams × 7 =	161 kcal
Total		**438 kcal**

You can also use the 4-9-4 estimates to determine what portion of total calorie intake is contributed by the various calorie-yielding nutrients. Assume that one day you consume 290 grams of carbohydrates, 60 grams of fat, and 70 grams of protein. This consumption yields a total of 1980 kcal ([290 × 4] + [60 × 9] + [70 × 4]5 = 1980). The percentage of your total calorie intake derived from each nutrient can then be determined:

$$\% \text{ of kcal as carbohydrate} = (290 \times 4) \div 1980 = 0.59 \ (\times 100 = 59\%)$$
$$\% \text{ of kcal as fat} = (\ 60 \times 9) \div 1980 = 0.27 \ (\times 100 = 27\%)$$
$$\% \text{ of kcal as protein} = (\ 70 \times 4) \div 1980 = 0.14 \ (\times 100 = 14\%)$$

Check your calculations by adding the percentages together. Do they total 100?

MAKING DECISIONS

Percentages and the Metric System

You will use a few mathematical concepts in studying nutrition. Besides performing addition, subtraction, multiplication, and division, you need to know how to calculate percentages and convert English units of measurement to metric units.

Percentages

The term percent (%) refers to a part of the total when the total represents 100 parts. For example, if you earn 80% on your first nutrition examination, you will have answered the equivalent of 80 out of 100 questions correctly. This equivalent could be 8 correct answers out of 10; 80% also describes 16 of 20 (16/20 = 0.80 or 80%). The decimal form of percents is based on 100% being equal to 1.00. It is difficult to succeed in a nutrition course unless you know what a percentage means and how to calculate one. Percentages are used frequently when referring to menus and nutrient composition. The best way to master this concept is to calculate some percentages. Some examples follow:

Question	Answer
What is 6% of 45?	6% = 0.06 or 0.06 × 45 = 2.7
What percent of 99 is 3?	3/99 = 0.03 or 3% (0.03 × 100)

Joe ate 15% of the adult Recommended Dietary Allowance (RDA = 8 milligrams) for iron at lunch. How many milligrams did he eat?

$$0.15 \times 8 \text{ milligrams} = 1.2 \text{ milligrams}$$

The Metric System

The basic units of the metric system are the meter, which indicates length; the gram, which indicates weight; and the liter, which indicates volume. Appendix I in this textbook lists conversions from the metric system to the English system (pounds, feet, cups) and vice versa. Here is a brief summary:

A gram (g) is about 1/30 of an ounce (28 grams to the ounce).
5 grams of sugar or salt is about 1 teaspoon.
A pound (lb) weighs 454 grams.
A kilogram (kg) is 1000 grams, equivalent to 2.2 pounds.
To convert your weight to kilograms, divide it by 2.2.
A 154-pound man weighs 70 kilograms (154/2.2 = 70).
A gram can be divided into 1000 milligrams (mg) or 1,000,000 micrograms (μg or mcg).
    10 milligrams of zinc (approximate adult needs) would be a few grains of zinc.
Liters are divided into 1000 units called milliliters (ml).
One teaspoon equals about 5 milliliters (ml), 1 cup is about 240 milliliters, and 1 quart
    (4 cups) equals almost 1 liter (L) (0.946 liter to be exact).

If you plan to work in any scientific field, you will need to learn the metric system. *For now, remember that a kilogram equals 2.2 pounds, an ounce weighs 28 grams, 2.54 centimeters equals 1 inch, and a liter is almost the same as a quart.* In addition, know the fractions that the following prefixes represent: micro (1/1,000,000), milli (1/1000), centi (1/100), and kilo (1000).

CONCEPT CHECK

Nutrition is the study of food and nutrients—their digestion, absorption, and metabolism, and their effect on health and disease. Food contains the vital nutrients essential for good health: carbohydrates, lipids (fats and oils), proteins, vitamins, minerals, and water. Nutrients have three general functions in the body: (1) to provide materials for building and maintaining the body; (2) to act as regulators for key metabolic reactions; and (3) to participate in metabolic reactions that provide the energy necessary to sustain life. A common unit of measurement for this energy is the kilocalorie (kcal). On average, carbohydrates and protein provide 4 kcal per gram of energy to the body, while lipids provide 9 kcal per gram. Although not considered a nutrient, alcohol provides about 7 kcal per gram. The other classes of nutrients (vitamins, minerals, and water) do not supply calories but are essential for proper body functioning.

1.5 What Is the Current State of the North American Diet and Health?

Does Obesity Threaten Our Future?

In 2001, the U.S. Surgeon General issued a Call to Action about the obesity epidemic in America. Over the past 10 years, however, the problem has worsened. Whereas in 2001 61% of U.S. adults were overweight or obese, in 2010 the rates were even higher with 68%, or 190 million people, overweight or obese. A recent report from the Trust for America's Health and the Robert Wood Johnson Foundation indicated that between 2009 and 2010 the percentage of obese adults increased in 16 states and did not decline in any states. Their report, "F as in Fat: How Obesity Threatens America's Future 2011" (July 2011), also revealed that 12 states now have obesity rates above 30%, compared to 2006, when only one state was above 30%. This recent report (Fig. 1-4) is based on self-reported state-by-state obesity data from the Centers for Disease Control and Prevention (CDC) (see Further Reading 16). Because we tend to underreport our

FIGURE 1-4 ▶ Percentage of adults who are obese,* by state, 2009.

*Body mass index (BMI) ≥ 30, or about 30 pounds overweight for a 5′ 4″ person, based on self-reported weight and height.

Source: CDC, Behavioral Risk Factor Surveillance System.

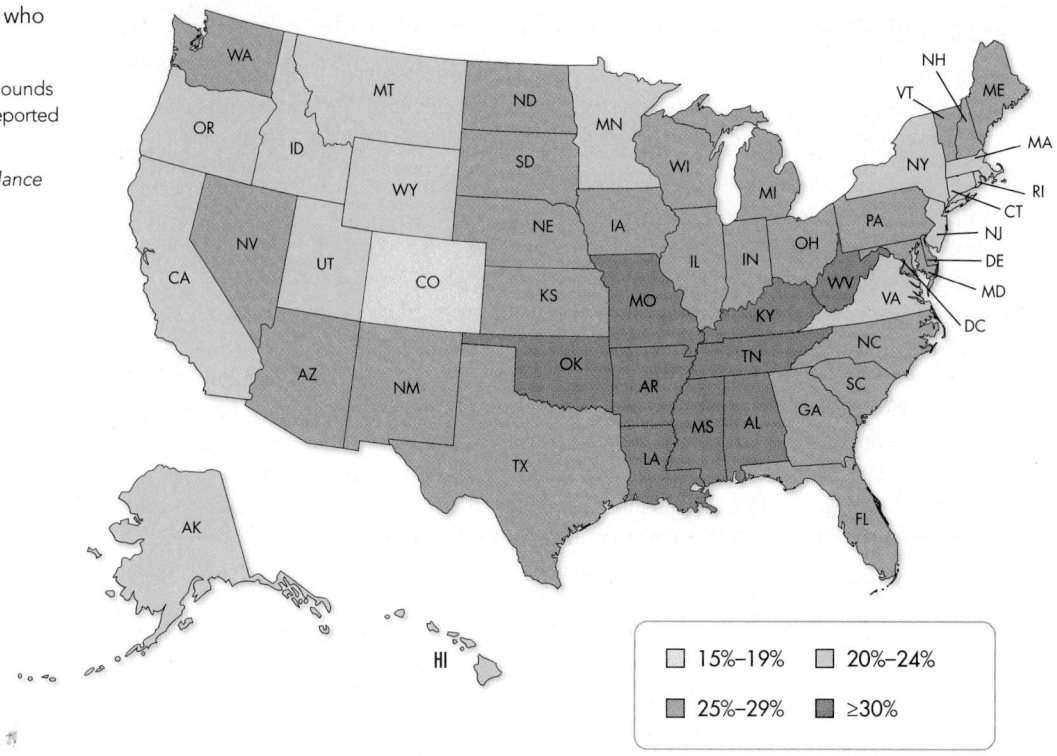

☐ 15%–19%   ☐ 20%–24%
■ 25%–29%   ■ ≥30%

weight, the percentage of Americans who are obese is probably greater than reported. Even more alarming are the statistics for children. In 2001 nearly 12% of children and adolescents were overweight, whereas in 2010 nearly one-third of children and teens fell into these categories.

It is well documented that this extra weight of more than 4.5 billion extra pounds has and will continue to have dangerous consequences. In an earlier section of this chapter, we already pointed out that obesity plays a role in chronic illness, including heart disease, stroke, high blood pressure, high cholesterol, diabetes, arthritis, and certain cancers. It is estimated that obesity kills more than 110,000 Americans a year. Because of its role in so many chronic disorders, obesity is also an expensive condition. More than $150 billion is spent annually on health care related to obesity, and obesity costs U.S. employers $73 billion in lost productivity every year. It has become obvious that the answers to the obesity crisis are not simple. From a nutrition perspective, however, the problem can be clearly stated. Most of us continue to eat too much, especially foods with a high number of calories and a low number of nutrients, and we do not engage in enough physical activity.

Assessing the Current North American Diet

With the aim of finding out what North Americans eat, federal agencies conduct surveys to collect data about food and nutrient consumption, as well as connections between diet and health. In the United States, the U.S. Department of Health and Human Services monitors food consumption with the National Health and Nutrition Examination Survey (NHANES). In Canada, this information is gathered by Health Canada in conjunction with Agriculture and Agrifood Canada. Survey data indicate that North American adults consume about 15% of their calorie intake as proteins, 52% as carbohydrates, and 33% as fats. These percentages, which do not consider alcohol, fall within the ranges recommended by the Food and Nutrition Board (FNB) of the National Academy of Sciences. The FNB advocates that 10%

to 35% of calories come from protein, 45% to 65% from carbohydrate, and 20% to 35% from fat. These standards apply to people in both the United States and Canada.

Food-consumption data also indicate that animal sources supply about two-thirds of protein intake for most North Americans, whereas plant sources supply only about one-third. In many other parts of the world, it is just the opposite: plant proteins—from rice, beans, corn, and other grains and vegetables—dominate protein intake. About half the carbohydrate in North American diets comes from simple sugars; the other half comes from starches (such as in pastas, breads, and potatoes). About 60% of dietary fat comes from animal sources and 40% from plant sources.

Results from national nutrition surveys and other studies show that North Americans consume more calories than ever before and from a wide variety of foods. Individuals, however, often do not choose the foods that will meet all their nutrient needs. Food availability data from 1909 to 2007 confirm that the major contributors to increased energy intake over the last century are oils, shortening, meat, cheese, and frozen desserts. Since 1970 there has been an increase in added sweeteners, and carbonated beverage availability has increased at the expense of milk.

In the next section, we discuss recommendations to consume a variety of nutrient-dense foods within and across the food groups, especially whole grains, fruits, vegetables, low-fat or fat-free milk or milk products, and lean meats and other protein sources. These foods will provide nutrients that are often overlooked, including various B vitamins, vitamin C (especially for smokers), vitamin D, vitamin E, calcium, potassium, magnesium, iron, fiber, and many phytonutrients. Daily intake of a balanced multivitamin and mineral supplement is another strategy to help meet nutrient needs but does not make up for a poor diet, particularly for calcium, potassium, and fiber intake. Also keep in mind that taking numerous dietary supplements can lead to health problems (see Chapter 8).

Routinely, experts also recommend that we pay more attention to balancing calorie intake with needs. An excess intake of calories is usually tied to overindulgence in sugar, fat, and alcoholic beverages. African-Americans and Hispanics have a greater chance of developing hypertension than do other ethnic groups in North America and therefore may need to decrease the amount of **salt** (sodium chloride) and alcohol in their diets. These substances are two of the many factors linked to hypertension. Moderation of salt and alcohol intake—along with certain fats, cholesterol, and total calorie intake—is a recommended practice for all adults.

Many North Americans would benefit from a healthier balance of food in their diets. Moderation is the key for some foods, such as sugared soft drinks and fried foods. For other foods, such as fruits and vegetables, increased quantity and variety are warranted. Few adults currently meet the new recommendation to "fill half your plate with fruits and vegetables" promoted in the new USDA MyPlate guidelines for total servings of vegetables and fruits.

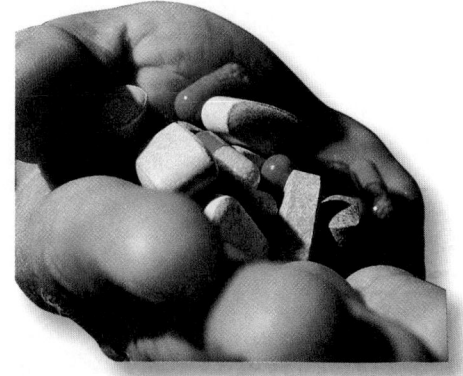

▲ Taking numerous nutrient supplements can lead to health problems. Chapter 8 will explore the appropriate and safe use of nutrient supplements in detail.

salt Compound of sodium and chloride in a 40:60 ratio.

Health Objectives for the United States for the Year 2020

Health promotion and disease prevention have been public health strategies in North America for the past three decades. One part of this strategy is *Healthy People 2020*, a report issued in December 2010 by the U.S. Department of Health and Human Services' (DHHS) Public Health Service. Every 10 years, DHHS issues a collection of health objectives for the nation. These objectives are developed by experts in federal agencies and target major public health concerns, setting goals for the coming decade. *Healthy People 2020* sets forth more than 600 health objectives across 42 topic areas and outlines national standards to eliminate health disparities, improve access to health education and quality health care, and strengthen public health services. The vision for 2020 is a society in which all people live long, healthy lives. Important new features of *Healthy People 2020* include a focus on health equity and

social determinants of health, and a move to an interactive, personalized website at
www.HealthyPeople.gov.

The overarching goals of *Healthy People 2020* aim to:

- Attain high-quality, longer lives free of preventable disease, disability, injury, and premature death.
- Achieve health equity, eliminate disparities, and improve health of all groups.
- Create social and physical environments that promote good health for all.
- Promote quality of life, healthy development, and healthy behaviors across all life stages.

Healthy People 2020, like earlier versions, includes a topic area specific to nutrition. This topic is called Nutrition and Weight Status, and its objectives target individual behaviors, as well as the policies and environments that support these behaviors. Nutrition and weight status is important because a healthful diet helps us reduce our risks for numerous health conditions that burden the public health system, including heart disease, high blood pressure, diabetes, osteoporosis, and some cancers. Good nutrition for children is also emphasized in this report because of its importance for growth and development. The goal of this topic is to promote health and reduce chronic disease risk through the consumption of healthful diets and achievement and maintenance of healthy body weights. This goal also includes increasing household food security and eliminating hunger.

The Nutrition and Weight Status objectives are based on strong science that supports the health benefits of eating a healthful diet and maintaining a healthy body weight. A healthful diet is described as one that includes:

- Consuming a variety of nutrient-dense foods within and across the food groups, especially whole grains, fruits, vegetables, low-fat or fat-free milk or milk products, and lean meats and other protein sources
- Limiting intake of solid fats, cholesterol, added sugars, sodium (salt), and alcohol
- Limiting intake of calories to meet needs for calories

The objectives also emphasize that individual behaviors, as well as the policies and environments that support these behaviors in settings such as schools, worksites, health care organizations, and communities, should be addressed in any efforts to change diet and weight.

Table 1-5 is a list of the six categories of objectives for the Nutrition and Weight Status topic, along with the the 22 specific objectives. Table 1-6 provides a more detailed sample of nine of the specific Nutrition and Weight Status objectives along with the current status of these objectives and their targets for 2020.

Other new topic areas highlight changes in the health needs of specific segments of the population: Early and Middle Childhood, Adolescence, and Older Adults. Because young people develop habits, including eating and physical activity behaviors, which are likely to persist throughout life, new objectives promote strengthened health education in schools and communities and fostering an environment in which young people can develop healthy habits. Older adults are the fastest-growing segment of the American population and are at high risk for experiencing the chronic health problems that so severely impact our health care system. The objectives for Older Adults include improving access to health care, helping older adults to manage their own health conditions, and ensuring proper training and support of professionals and nonprofessionals who care for this population.

A scientifically exciting new topic area is **Genomics.** Nine of the ten leading causes of death have a strong genetic component. Genetic testing is becoming a

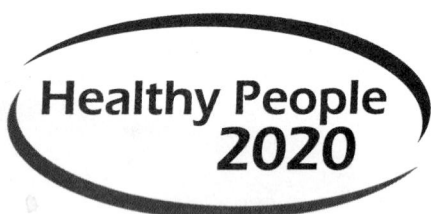

▲ Many nutrition-related objectives are part of the *Healthy People 2020* report. The report outlines health promotion and disease prevention objectives for the United States for the year 2020.

TABLE 1-5 *Healthy People 2020*: Nutrition and Weight Status Objectives

Category 1: Healthier Food Access

1. Increase the number of states with nutrition standards for child care.

2. Increase the proportion of schools that offer nutritious foods and beverages outside of school meals.

3. Increase the number of states that have incentive policies for food retail to provide foods that are encouraged by the 2010 Dietary Guidelines for Americans.

4. Increase the proportion of Americans who have retail access to foods recommended by the 2010 Dietary Guidelines for Americans.

Category 2: Health Care and Worksite Settings

5. Increase the proportion of primary care physicians who measure patients' body mass index (BMI).

6. Increase the proportion of physician office visits that include nutrition or weight counseling or education.

7. Increase the proportion of worksites that offer nutrition and weight-management classes and counseling.

Category 3: Weight Status

8. Increase the proportion of adults who are at a healthy weight.

9. Reduce the proportion of adults who are obese.

10. Reduce the proportion of children and adolescents who are considered obese.

11. Prevent inappropriate weight gain in youth and adults.

Category 4: Food Insecurity

12. Eliminate very low food security among children.

13. Reduce household food insecurity and in so doing reduce hunger.

Category 5: Food and Nutrient Consumption

14. Increase the contribution of fruits to the diets of the population ages 2 years and older.

15. Increase the variety and contribution of vegetables to the diets of the population ages 2 years and older.

16. Increase the contribution of whole grains to the diets of the population ages 2 years and older.

17. Reduce consumption of calories from solid fats and added sugars in the population ages 2 years and older.

18. Reduce consumption of saturated fat in the population ages 2 years and older.

19. Reduce consumption of sodium in the population ages 2 years and older.

Category 6: Iron Deficiency

20. Increase consumption of calcium in the population ages 2 years and older.

21. Reduce iron deficiency among young children and females of childbearing age.

22. Reduce iron deficiency among pregnant females.

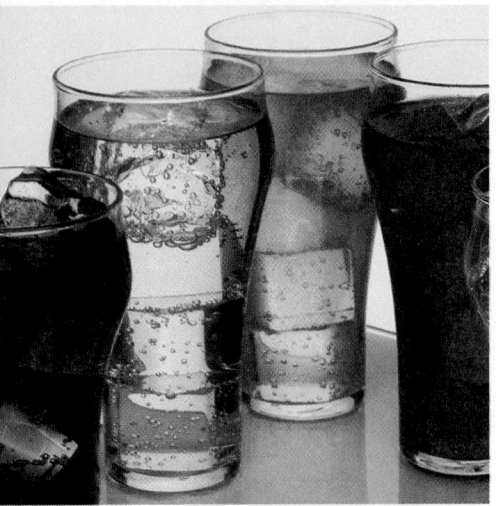

▲ Moderation in the intake of some foods, such as sugared soft drinks and fried foods, can lead to a healthier balance of food in the North American diet.

TABLE 1-6 A Sample of Nutrition and Weight Status Objectives from *Healthy People 2020* along with Details about the Current Status and Targets for 2020

	Target	Current Estimate
Increase the proportion of adults at a healthy weight.	33.9%	30.8%
Reduce the proportion of overweight or obese children and adolescents.	14.6%	16.2%
Increase the contribution of the following to the diets of the population ages 2 years and older (per 1000 calories).		
• Fruits	0.9 cup	0.5 cup
• Total vegetables	1.1 cups	0.8 cup
• Whole grains	0.6 ounce	0.3 ounce
Reduce consumption of calories from solid fats (of total calorie intake).	16.7%	18.9%
Reduce consumption of calories from added sugars (of total calorie intake).	10.8%	15.7%
Increase consumption of calcium in the population ages 2 years and older.	1300 mg	1118 mg
Reduce iron deficiency among females of childbearing age.	9.4%	10.4%

Note: In later chapters, we will explore additional nutrition-related objectives, such as those addressing osteoporosis, various forms of cancer, diabetes prevention and treatment, food allergies, cardiovascular disease, low birth weight, nutrition during pregnancy, breastfeeding, eating disorders, physical activity, and alcohol use.

valuable tool for improving diagnosis and treatment of chronic diseases, especially for cancers of the breast and colon. In combination with family history, genetic testing can help health care professionals guide patients in treatment options, including lifestyle changes. The relationship between genetics and nutrition will be discussed in Chapter 3.

1.6 What Can You Expect from Good Nutrition and a Healthy Lifestyle?

The obesity epidemic in the United States illustrates that something is not right with many of our diets and/or lifestyles. The strong association between obesity and poor health is clear. The reverse is also well documented—when an obese or overweight person loses just 5% to 10% of body weight, that person's risks of many chronic diseases are greatly reduced.

Because weight gain is one of the greatest lifelong nutrition challenges we face, we encourage you to seek a lifestyle that will make gaining weight more difficult and maintaining a healthy weight easier. Believe it or not, preventing obesity in the first place is the easiest approach. Unfortunately, many aspects of our society make it hard for us not to gain weight. The earlier (preferably in childhood) we develop lifestyle habits of good nutrition, regular physical activity, and the avoidance of addictions to salt, fat, sweets, high-calorie foods, and sedentary lifestyles, the better (see

Further Readings 14 and 15). As you enter the workforce, seek out employers who offer wellness programs that encourage weight management and weight loss among their employees. Aim to live in a city or town that has opportunities for physical activity such as bike paths, walking trails, and parks, as well as access to fresh fruits and vegetables through farmers' markets and community gardens. Seek out organizations that offer running or walking clubs. Make a habit of shopping at grocery stores that offer a good selection of fruits, vegetables, and other healthy foods. When dining out, choose restaurants that have tasty but healthy options on their menu. While we still are choosing foods with too many calories, many other dietary habits have improved during the past decade. Today we can choose from a tremendous variety of food products, the result of continual innovation by food manufacturers. We are eating more breakfast cereals, pizza, pasta entrees, stir-fried meats and vegetables served on rice, salads, tacos, burritos, and fajitas than ever before. Sales of whole milk are down, and sales of fat-free and 1% low-fat milk have increased. Consumption of frozen vegetables rather than canned vegetables is also on the rise. Despite the alarming problem of overweight and obesity, our cultural diversity, varied cuisines, and general lack of nutrient deficiencies should be points of pride for North Americans.

Today, North Americans live longer than ever and enjoy better general health. Many also have more money and more diverse food and lifestyle choices to consider. The nutritional consequences of these trends are varied. Deaths from cardiovascular disease, for example, have dropped dramatically since the late 1960s, partly because of better medical care and diets. Affluence, however, has also led to sedentary lifestyles and high intakes of animal fat, cholesterol, salt, and alcohol. This lifestyle pattern has led to problems such as cardiovascular disease, hypertension, diabetes, and, of course, obesity. Greater efforts are needed by the general public to lower intake of animal fat and cholesterol and to improve variety in our diets, especially from fruits, vegetables, and whole grains. With better technology and greater choices, we can have a much better diet today than ever before—if we know what choices to make.

Nutrition experts generally agree that there are no "good" or "bad" foods, but some foods provide relatively few nutrients in comparison to calorie content. In Chapter 2, you will learn that an individual's total diet is the proper focus in a nutritional evaluation. Health experts have prepared many reports and outlined numerous objectives to get us closer to being a *Healthy People* as soon as 2020. In Chapter 2, we will discuss the new "Dietary Guidelines" that were published in 2010, and the new interactive program called "ChooseMyPlate.gov" that was unveiled in 2011. As you reexamine your nutritional habits, remember your health is largely your responsibility. Your body has a natural ability to heal itself. Offer it what it needs, and it will serve you well. Confusing and conflicting health messages hinder diet change. Nutrition science does not have all the answers, but as you will see, enough is known to help you set a path to good health and put diet-related recommendations you hear in the future into perspective. Table 1-7 summarizes several diet, physical activity, and general lifestyle recommendations to promote your health and prevent chronic diseases in the future. In total, these contribute to maximal health and prevention of the diseases listed. The final section in Chapter 1, Nutrition and Your Health: Eating Well in College, elaborates on several nutrition issues very relevant to most college students, including the "freshman 15," vegetarianism, fuel for athletes, eating disorders, and alcohol and binge drinking. This section gives you a "sneak peek" at issues that will be covered more fully later in the book.

▼ A healthy diet benefits people of all ages.

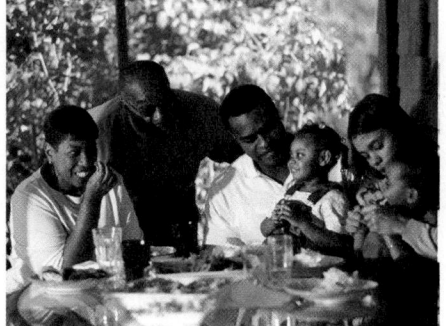

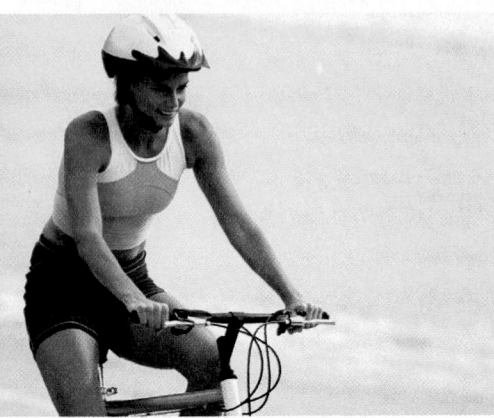

▲ Regular physical activity complements a healthy diet. Whether it is all at once or in segments throughout the day, incorporate 30 to 60 minutes or more of such activity into your daily routine.

TABLE 1-7 Recommendations for Health Promotion and Disease Prevention

Diet

Consuming enough essential nutrients, including fiber, while moderating energy, solid fat, cholesterol, added sugar, and alcohol intake can result in:

- Increased bone mass during childhood and adolescence
- Prevention of some adult bone loss and osteoporosis, especially in older adults
- Fewer dental caries
- Prevention of digestive problems, such as constipation
- Decreased susceptibility to some cancers
- Decreased degradation of the retina (intake of green and orange vegetables, in particular)
- Lower risk of obesity and related diseases, such as type 2 diabetes and cardiovascular disease
- Reduced risk for deficiency diseases, such as cretinism (lack of iodide), scurvy (lack of vitamin C), and anemia (lack of iron, folate, or other nutrients)

Physical Activity

Adequate, regular physical activity (at least 30 minutes on most or all days) helps reduce the risk of:

- Obesity
- Type 2 diabetes
- Cardiovascular disease
- Some adult bone loss and loss of muscle tone
- Premature aging
- Certain cancers

Lifestyle

Minimizing alcohol intake (no more than two drinks per day for men and one drink for both women and all adults age 65 years and older) helps prevent:

- Liver disease
- Accidents

Not smoking cigarettes or cigars helps prevent:

- Lung cancer, other lung disease, kidney disease, cardiovascular disease, and degenerative eye diseases

In addition, minimum use of medication, no illicit drug use, adequate sleep (7 to 8 hours), adequate water and related fluid intake (9 to 13 cups per day), and a reduction in stress (practice better time management, relax, listen to music, have a massage, and stay physically active) provide a more complete approach to good nutrition and health. Add to this maintaining close relationships with others and a positive outlook on life. Finally, consultation with health care professionals on a regular basis is important. This is because early diagnosis is especially useful for controlling the damaging effects of many diseases. Prevention of disease is an important investment of one's time, including during the college years.

CONCEPT CHECK

Surveys in the United States and Canada show that we generally have a variety of foods available to us. However, some of us could improve our diets by focusing on food sources rich in various vitamins, minerals, and fiber. In addition, many of us should reduce our consumption of calories, added sugar, protein, solid fat, cholesterol, salt, and alcoholic beverages. These recommendations are consistent with an overall goal to attain and maintain good health.

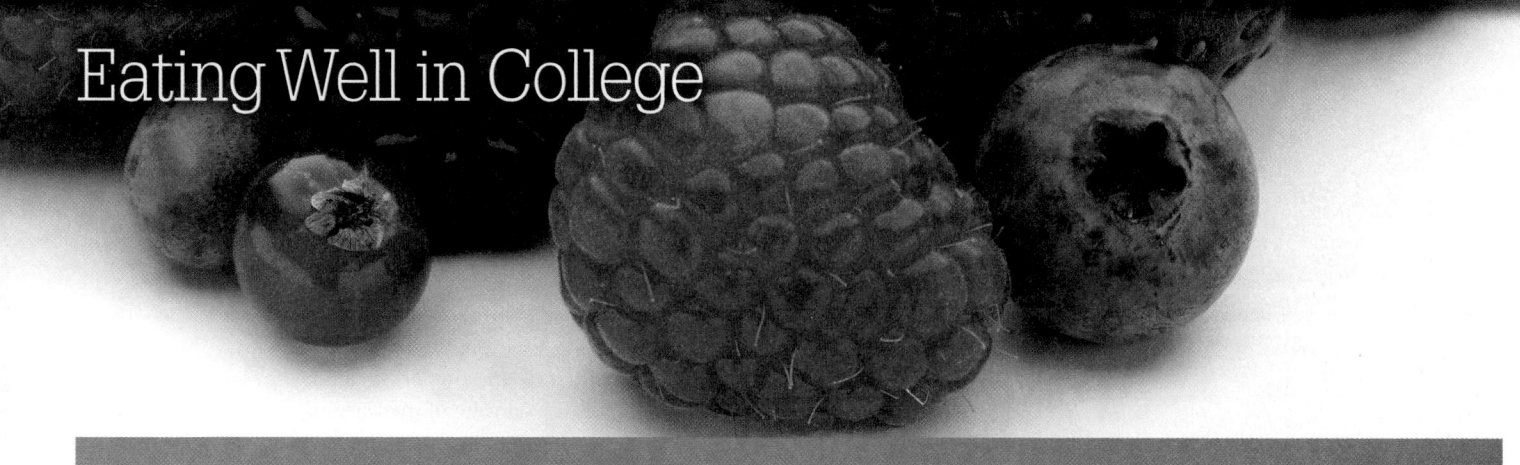

Eating Well in College

The college years are a time for freedom and a chance to make personal lifestyle decisions. Studies show that the diets of college students are not optimal. Typically, students fall short of diet recommendations for whole grains, vegetables, fruits, milk, and meat, opting instead to max out on fats, sweets, and alcohol. This information is disturbing because young adulthood is the time when many health behaviors are formed that will persist throughout life.

What is it about the college lifestyle that makes it so difficult to build healthy habits? In this section we will discuss several topics and provide possible solutions.

Food Choices

College students face changes in academic requirements, interpersonal relationships, and living environment. These stressful situations contribute to poor health behaviors. For example, when writing papers and cramming for exams, balanced meals are all-too-easily replaced by high-fat and

▼ Late-night pizza can add extra calories to the college student's daily intake.

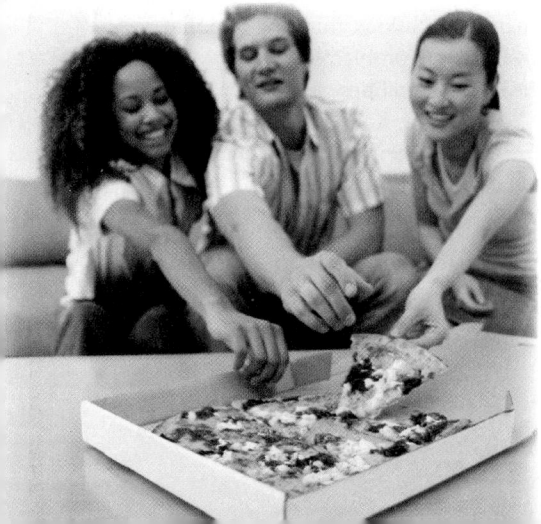

high-calorie fast-foods; convenience items; and sugary, caffeinated beverages. Physical activity is sacrificed in favor of study time.

Also consider that on campus, you are faced with a wide variety of dining choices. Dining halls, fast-food establishments, bars, and vending machines combine to offer food 24 hours per day. While it is certainly possible to make wise food choices at each of these outlets, the temptations of convenience, taste, and value (i.e., inexpensive, oversized portions) may persuade the college student to select unhealthy options.

Meals and snacks are also times to socialize. You may feel pressured to eat a big lunch at noon without regard to hunger if your peers are meeting in the dining hall to catch up. While chatting, it is easy to lose track of portions and to overeat. In addition, food may be a source of familiarity and comfort in a new and stressful place.

Weight Control and the "Freshman Fifteen"

Studies show that most college students gain weight during their first year (see Further Reading 5). The "freshman fifteen" is a term used to describe the weight gained by students during their first year of college. Although most freshman do not gain the fifteen pounds, a recent study of U.S. and Canadian college students found that students pack on 6 to 9 pounds their first year away from home. Although calorie intake does not increase significantly, dramatic increases in beer drinking and significant decreases in physical activity are key reasons for the weight gain (see Further Reading 8).

There are several reasons to maintain a healthy weight. Over the long term, risk of chronic diseases goes up as weight increases. In the short term, losing excess weight can improve how you feel and perform. Detecting "flab" around your midsection or feeling that your clothes are getting tighter are two good indicators that you are carrying excess weight. If weight loss is necessary, with some knowledge and perseverance, you can safely lose excess pounds.

Behavioral research clearly demonstrates that setting several small, achievable goals will spur motivation. As you will learn in Chapter 7, body weight is a balancing act between calories in and calories burned. Try keeping track of your calorie consumption for several days and comparing that to your energy needs, based on your age, gender, and activity level. You can use one of the equations presented in Chapter 7 or take advantage of the interactive tools on www.Choose MyPlate.gov to estimate your energy needs.

A healthy rate of weight loss is one to two pounds per week. Greater rates of weight loss will not likely be sustained over time. Remember that the numbers on the scale are not as important as your body composition—the amount of fat in relation to lean mass. One pound of weight loss requires a deficit of 3500 kilocalories. Thus, to lose one pound per week, you will need to cut back on food intake and/or increase your exercise routine to shift the energy balance equation by 500 kilocalories per day.

Although many students skip breakfast, breakfast is the *most* important meal of the day. Starting the day off with a fortified,

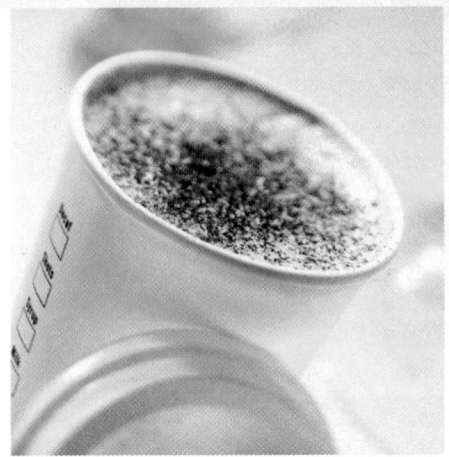

▲ Research (see Further Reading 13) has shown that gourmet coffee beverages, such as lattes and cappuccinos, can increase calorie consumption by about 200 kcal per day.

whole-grain breakfast cereal, skim milk, and a serving of fruit puts you on the right path for meeting recommendations for fiber, calcium, and fruit intake. Even though it may seem that coffee gets your brain going in the morning, your brain is fueled best by carbohydrates, not caffeine. Studies also show that eating breakfast prevents overeating later in the day. Read more about breakfast choices in the *What Would You Choose* recommendations at the end of this chapter.

One of the biggest contributors to weight gain for college students is consuming several hundred calories per day

▶ **Five Simple Tips to Avert Weight Gain**

- **Eat breakfast.** Rev up your metabolism with a protein source such as an egg or low-fat yogurt, at least one serving of whole grains such as a breakfast cereal, and a fruit such as a banana.

- **Plan ahead.** Eat a balanced meal or snack every 3 to 4 hours.

- **Limit liquid calories.** Drink water instead of high-calorie soft drinks, fruit juice, alcohol, or coffee; if you drink alcohol, limit it to 1 or 2 drinks per day.

- **Stock the fridge.** Keep a stash of low-calorie, nutritious snacks, such as pretzels, light microwave popcorn, fruit (fresh, canned, or dried).

- **Exercise regularly.** Find a friend to work out with you. Experts recommend 30 minutes of moderate exercise at least 5 days a week.

in sugary or alcoholic beverages. One 12-ounce can of regular cola contains about 140 kcal. A 12-ounce can of regular beer has 150 kcal. Consuming gourmet coffee beverages, such as lattes and cappuccinos can increase average calorie consumption by about 200 kilocalories per day (see Further Reading 13). Even fruit juices have at least 100 kcal per 8-ounce glass. Furthermore, a 24-ounce mug of a soft drink makes you feel no fuller than an equal volume of water, yet the soft drink adds 300 kcal more. A convenient stash of water is the best way to quench your thirst.

Exercise is very important to any weight loss and weight maintenance plan but sticking with it is hard to do. When you find yourself short on time, exercise is often the first thing we sacrifice. To ensure your success at boosting daily activity, choose activities you enjoy such as working out with friends at the campus recreation center, participating in intramural sports, or taking an activity class like dancing. Don't forget the brisk walking to and from classes. For more information on planning an exercise program, see Chapter 10.

Alcohol and Binge Drinking

Excessive alcohol consumption is a big problem on college campuses. Legal or not, many college students consider drinking alcohol to be a "rite of passage" into adulthood. On campuses, binge drinking—consuming five or more drinks in a row for men, or four drinks or more for women—has become an epidemic. A new level of "extreme drinking" goes far beyond binge drinking. For example, recent studies indicate that college students celebrate twenty-first birthdays with an average of 12 drinks for men and nine for women (see Further Reading 12).

The statistics on the impact of binge drinking on college campuses are sobering. An estimated two of every five students on college campuses participates in binge drinking. Each year, 1400 college students between the ages of 18 and 24 die from alcohol-related unintentional injuries, including motor vehicle crashes. In addition to deaths and injuries, other problems stemming from binge drinking include unsafe sex and its consequences, long-term health problems, suicides, academic problems, legal troubles, and

alcohol abuse or dependence. Thirty-one percent of college students meet the criteria for a diagnosis of alcohol abuse.

In addition alcohol consumption definitely contributes to weight gain—by virtue of its own calories and the increased food consumption at events where drinking occurs. If you choose to drink alcohol, do so in moderation—no more than two drinks per day for men and one drink per day for women. Be aware of the warning signs and dangers of alcohol poisoning shown in the margin. Excessive alcohol intake, has many long-term health and nutrition implications that are covered in Chapter 16.

Eating Disorders

As many as 30% of college students are at risk of developing an eating disorder. As you will learn in Chapter 13, disordered eating is a mild and short-term change in eating patterns that typically occurs in response to life stress, a desire to change appearance, or a bad habit. Sometimes, disordered eating habits may lead to an eating disorder, such as anorexia nervosa, bulimia nervosa, or binge-eating disorder. Chapter 13 includes advice on what to do if you suspect that your roommate or friend is suffering from an eating disorder.

Starving the body also starves the brain, limiting performance in academics and beyond, and the negative consequences of disordered eating may last a lifetime. Ultimately, eating disorders do not arise from problems with food but rather from problems with self-esteem, control, and abusive relationships. Frequently, what begins as a diet spirals into a much larger problem. Eating disorders are not just diets gone bad—they require professional intervention. Left unchecked, eating disorders lead to serious adverse effects, such as loss of menstrual periods, thinning of bones, gastrointestinal problems, kidney problems, heart abnormalities, and eventually death.

Choosing a Vegetarian Lifestyle

Many college students experiment with or adopt a vegetarian eating pattern. Plant-based diets can meet nutrition needs and decrease risk of many chronic diseases, but they require appropriate planning at all life stages.

Protein is not typically deficient, even with a vegan diet, which contains no animal products. However, vegetarians, and especially vegans, may be at risk for deficiencies of several vitamins and minerals. Consuming a ready-to-eat breakfast cereal is an easy and inexpensive way to obtain these nutrients. See Chapter 6 for more information on vegetarian food planning.

Restaurants and campus dining services have responded to the growing interest in vegetarian meals by offering a variety of vegetarian options. For optimal health benefits, choose foods that are baked, steamed, or stir-fried rather than deep-fried; select whole grains rather than refined carbohydrates; and consume food fortified with vitamins and minerals. Even if you do not follow a plant-based diet all the time, choosing several plant-based meals each week can help with weight control and boost intake of fiber and healthy phytochemicals. You will learn in Chapter 2 that the new ChooseMyPlate program recommends that the largest portion of your plate be filled with plant foods, including whole grains, fruits and vegetables.

Fuel for Competition: Student Athletes

Students who compete in sports such as intramural and intercollegiate athletics need to consume more calories and nutrients. Despite an emphasis on a lean physique athletes at all levels must take care not to severely restrict calories, as this could impact performance and health. Muscles require adequate carbohydrates for fuel and protein for growth and repair. Fat, as well, is an important source of stored energy for use during exercise. Low levels of body fat in women may lead to amenorrhea (cease menstruating), a condition costly to long-term bone health.

In addition to fueling the body with calories, fluids are essential for health and performance. While water is adequate for events lasting less than 60 minutes, sports drinks are ideal for longer events because they supply carbohydrates to fuel fatigued muscles as well as electrolytes to replenish those lost in perspiration. Intentional fluid losses to "make weight" for a competition are detrimental to health and performance.

Athletes also should take care not to be wooed by the supplement industry.

Increasing food intake to meet the energy demands of athletic training is usually sufficient to also meet vitamin and mineral needs. As an exception, athletes may be at risk for iron-deficiency anemia. Consuming a balanced multivitamin and mineral supplement is adequate for most people. Individual vitamin, mineral, amino acid, or herbal supplements are not advised, in spite of the hype of supplement makers.

Tips for Eating Well on a College Student's Budget

Because higher education can be hard on the wallet it is good to know that it is possible to eat well on campus on a budget. If you live on campus, participate in a prepaid campus meal plan (see Further Reading 1). These are generally designed to offer great food value with a variety of healthy foods. If you live off campus or have your own kitchen, plan ahead. Packing a lunch from home will save a lot of cash compared to grabbing lunch on the run and puts you more in control of healthy choices. For example, preparing a sandwich at home costs less than half as much as purchasing one at a fast-food restaurant or deli.

Never go grocery shopping on an empty stomach—everything will look good and you'll buy more. Also, go to the store with a list in hand and stick to it, because impulse buys tend to drain your wallet. Buy store-brand foods rather than name-brand items. Make use of canned and frozen fruits and vegetables—they are just as nutritious as fresh fruits and vegetables, particularly if you choose low-sodium and low-sugar varieties. Rather than buying cartons of fruit juice, select cans of fruit juice concentrate and mix with water at home. Likewise, preparing other drinks, such as iced tea, from store-brand powder (look for sugar-free) will save over gallon jugs or vending machine containers of drinks. Canned (fruits, tuna) and dry (oatmeal) foods can be nutritious and last a long time, so you can avoid throwing out spoiled items. Finally, eggs and peanut butter are inexpensive and simple sources of protein.

In conclusion, *The College Student's Guide to Eating Well on Campus* (see Further Reading 10) and *The Dorm Room Diet* (see Further Reading 11) are excellent books with more details on ways college students can plan a healthy diet and stay fit.

► **The warning signs and symptoms of alcohol poisoning**

- Semiconsciousness or unconsciousness
- Slow respiration of eight or fewer breaths per minute or lapses between breaths of more than 8 seconds
- Cold, clammy, pale, or bluish skin
- Strong odor of alcohol, which usually accompanies these symptoms

Some calorie traps for college students:

Number of Calories	
Six-pack of regular beer	900
Two handfuls of almonds	500
Two handfuls of granola	330
Personal-size pizza	500 to 600
1 cup of ice cream	300
Two handfuls of frosted cereal	250

Source: Ann Litt, *The College Student's Guide to Eating Well on Campus*

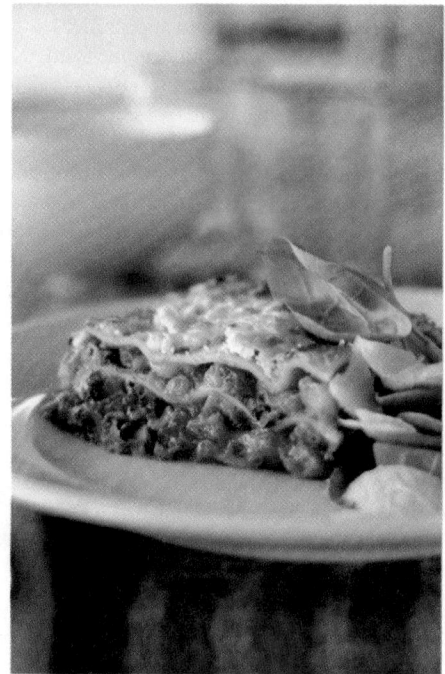

▲ Many students adopt a vegetarian diet during college. Guidelines for planning a nutritious vegetarian diet, with items such as this veggie lasagna, and spinach salad are presented in Chapter 6.

Case Study Typical College Student

Andy is like many other college students. He grew up on a quick bowl of cereal and milk for breakfast and a hamburger, French fries, and cola for lunch, either in the school cafeteria or at a local fast-food restaurant. At dinner, he generally avoided eating any of his salad or vegetables, and by 9 o'clock he was deep into bags of chips and cookies. Andy has taken most of these habits to college. He prefers coffee for breakfast and possibly a chocolate bar. Lunch is still mainly a hamburger, French fries, and cola, but pizza and tacos now alternate more frequently than when he was in high school. One thing Andy really likes about the restaurants surrounding campus is that, for less than a dollar more, he can make his hamburger a double or get extra cheese and pepperoni on his pizza. This helps him stretch his food dollar; searching out large-portion value meals for lunch and dinner now has become part of a typical day.

Provide some dietary advice for Andy. Start with his positive habits and then provide some constructive criticism, based on what you now know.

Answer the following questions, and check your responses in Appendix A.

1. **Start with Andy's positive habits:** What healthy choices are being made when Andy eats at local restaurants?

2. **Now provide some constructive criticisms:**

   a. What are some of the negative aspects of items available at fast-food restaurants?

   b. Why is ordering the "value meals" a dangerous habit?

   c. What healthier substitutions could he make at each meal?

   d. List some healthier choices he could make at fast-food restaurants on campus.

Summary (Numbers refer to numbered sections in the chapter.)

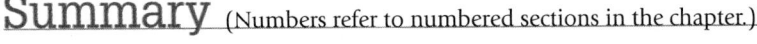

1. The flavor, texture, and appearance of foods primarily influence our food choices. Several other factors also help determine food habits and choices: food availability and convenience; early childhood experiences and ethnic customs; nutrition and health concerns; advertising; restaurants; social changes; and economics. A variety of external (appetite-related) forces affect satiety (feeling of satisfaction that halts our desire to continue eating). Hunger cues combine with appetite cues, such as easy availability of food, to promote food intake.

2. Nutrition is a lifestyle factor that is a key to developing and maintaining an optimal state of health. A poor diet and a sedentary lifestyle are known to be risk factors for life-threatening chronic diseases such as heart disease, hypertension, diabetes, and cancer. Not meeting nutrient needs in younger years makes us more likely to suffer health consequences in later years. Too much of a nutrient also can be harmful. Drinking too much alcohol is another dietary problem associated with many health problems.

3. Nutrition is the study of the food substances vital for health and the study of how the body uses these substances to promote and support growth, maintenance, and reproduction of cells. Nutrients in foods fall into six classes: (1) carbohydrates, (2) lipids (mostly fats and oils), (3) proteins, (4) vitamins, (5) minerals, and (6) water. The first three, along with alcohol, provide calories for the body to use.

4. The body transforms the energy contained in carbohydrate, protein, and fat into other forms of energy that in turn allow the body to function. Fat provides, on average, 9 kcal per gram, whereas both protein and carbohydrate provide, on average, 4 kcal per gram. Vitamins, minerals, and water do not supply calories to the body but are essential for proper body function.

5. The overweight and obesity problem has worsened with 68% of people in the United States (190 million people) reported to be overweight or obese in 2010. This increase is a result of eating too much, especially foods with a high number of calories and a low number of nutrients, and not engaging in enough physical activity. Results from large nutrition surveys in the United States and Canada suggest that some of us need to concentrate on consuming foods that supply more of certain vitamins, minerals, and fiber. *Healthy People 2020* is a national initiative that includes Nutrition and Weight Status objectives related to eating a healthful diet and maintaining a healthy body weight. A healthful diet includes consuming a variety of nutrient-dense foods within and across the food groups, especially whole grains, fruits, vegetables, low-fat or fat-free milk or milk products, and lean meats and other protein sources; limiting intake of solid fats, cholesterol, added sugars, sodium (salt), and alcohol; and limiting intake of calories to meet energy needs.

6. A basic plan for health promotion and disease prevention includes eating a varied diet, performing regular physical activity, not smoking, not abusing nutrient supplements (if used), consuming adequate water and other fluids, getting enough sleep, limiting alcohol intake (if consumed), and limiting or appropriately coping with stress. The primary focus of nutrition planning should be on food, not on dietary supplements. The focus on foods to supply nutrient needs avoids the possibility of severe nutrient imbalances.

7. Studies show that the diets and other health habits of college students are not optimal. Students fall short of recommendations for servings of grains, vegetables, fruits, milk, and meat, opting instead for fats, sweets, and alcohol. This information is disturbing from a public health

standpoint, because young adulthood is the time when many health behaviors are formed and will likely persist throughout life. Issues of particular importance on college campuses are weight control, making healthy meal choices, alcohol and binge drinking, and eating disorders.

Check Your Knowledge (Answers to the following multiple choice questions are below.)

1. Our primary psychological drive to eat that is affected by many external food-choice mechanisms is called
   a. hunger.   c. satiety.
   b. appetite.   d. feeding.

2. Energy-yielding nutrients include
   a. vitamins, minerals, and water.
   b. carbohydrates, proteins, and fats.
   c. trace minerals and fat-soluble vitamins.
   d. iron, vitamin C, and potassium.

3. The *essential* nutrients
   a. must be consumed at every meal.
   b. are required for infants but not adults.
   c. can be made in the body when they are needed.
   d. cannot be made by the body and therefore must be consumed to maintain health.

4. Sugars, starches, and dietary fibers are examples of
   a. proteins.   c. carbohydrates.
   b. vitamins.   d. minerals.

5. Which nutrient classes are most important in the regulation of body processes?
   a. vitamins
   b. carbohydrates
   c. minerals
   d. lipids
   e. Both a and c.

6. A kcal is a
   a. measure of heat energy.
   b. measure of fat in food.
   c. heating device.
   d. term used to describe the amount of sugar and fat in foods.

7. A food that contains 10 grams of fat would yield _____ kcal.
   a. 40   c. 90
   b. 70   d. 120

8. If you consume 300 grams of carbohydrate in a day that you consume 2400 kcal, the carbohydrates will provide _____% of your total energy intake.
   a. 12.5   c. 50
   b. 30   d. 60

9. Which of the following is true about the North American diet?
   a. Most of our protein comes from plant sources.
   b. About half of the carbohydrates come from simple sugars.
   c. Most of our fats come from plant sources.
   d. Most of our carbohydrates come from starches.

10. The _____ is a term used to describe the amount of weight college students gain during the first year of college.
    a. varsity 8
    b. stadium 7
    c. dormitory 12
    d. freshman 15

Answer Key: 1. b (LO 1.1), 2. b (LO 1.3), 3. d (LO 1.3), 4. c (LO 1.3), 5. e (LO 1.3), 6. a (LO 1.4), 7. c (LO 1.4), 8. c (LO 1.4), 9. b (LO 1.5), 10. d (LO 1.7)

Study Questions (Numbers refer to Learning Outcomes)

1. Describe the process that controls hunger and satiety in the body. List other factors that influence our food choices. **(LO 1.1)**

2. Describe how your food preferences have been shaped by the following factors:
   a. Exposure to foods at an early age
   b. Advertising (what is the newest food you have tried?)
   c. Eating out
   d. Peer pressure
   e. Economic factors **(LO 1.1)**

3. What products in your supermarket reflect the consumer demand for healthier foods? For convenience? **(LO 1.1)**

4. Name one chronic disease associated with poor nutrition habits. Now list a few corresponding risk factors. **(LO 1.2)**

5. Describe two sources of fat and explain why the differences are important in terms of overall health. **(LO 1.3)**

6. Identify three ways that water is used in the body. **(LO 1.3)**

7. Explain the concept of calories as it relates to foods. What are the values used to calculate kcals from grams of carbohydrate, fat, protein, and alcohol? **(LO 1.4)**

8. Wendy's Big Bacon Classic contains 44 grams carbohydrate, 36 grams fat, and 37 grams protein. Calculate the percentage of calories derived from fat. **(LO 1.4)**

9. According to national nutrition surveys, which nutrients tend to be underconsumed by many North Americans? Why do you think this is the case? **(LO 1.5)**

10. List four *Healthy People 2020* objectives for the United States. How would you rate yourself in each area? Why? **(LO 1.5 & 1.6)**

11. List five strategies to avoid weight gain during college. **(LO 1.7)**

What Would You Choose Recommendations

Even bleary-eyed procrastinators can fuel their bodies for a new day of higher education! *Skipping breakfast is not a smart plan.* After a period of fasting (i.e., overnight), the body and the brain need fuel to operate at peak efficiency. In addition, many research studies demonstrate that eating a sensible breakfast is a good way to control weight. Compared to those who eat breakfast, people who skip breakfast tend to crave higher-calorie foods, snack more throughout the day, and eat more at subsequent meals. Consider eating breakfast each day as part of your plan to fend off the freshman fifteen.

Grab-and-go food options, such as those available in vending machines or from fast-food establishments, are often high in calories but low in nutrients. For example, a low-fat granola bar has only 100 kcal and 3 grams of fat but offers little else in terms of nutrition. Also, a granola bar is not likely to stave off hunger for very long.

On the other hand, a fast-food breakfast sandwich will probably promote satiety but its calorie, fat, and sodium contents are too high. This type of sandwich provides 550 kcal, 23 grams of fat (38% of a day's total kcal in the sandwich and 35% of the whole day's limit for fat), and 1490 mg sodium (just under the 1500 mg Adequate Intake for this nutrient). A fast-food breakfast sandwich can fit into an otherwise healthy diet on occasion but should not be part of your normal routine.

Keeping nutritious but convenient breakfast options accessible is a good strategy for any time-pressed college student. Whole-grain, fortified, ready-to-eat breakfast cereal with fat-free milk is a great choice: it is quick, provides a wide variety of vitamins and minerals, and boosts fiber intake. Adding a source of protein will help to support body processes and make you feel full for a longer time. Hard-boiled eggs or a handful of dry-roasted nuts provide protein in ready-to-eat form. A cup of low-fat yogurt offers protein with the added benefit of calcium. Fresh and dried fruit are portable and nutritious options for breakfast. Many fruit choices are loaded with potassium and vitamin C, plus they provide fiber. A 1.5-ounce box of raisins, which can be stored for months without a refrigerator, provides about 130 kcal, no fat or cholesterol, very little sodium, 2 grams of fiber, and 320 mg potassium.

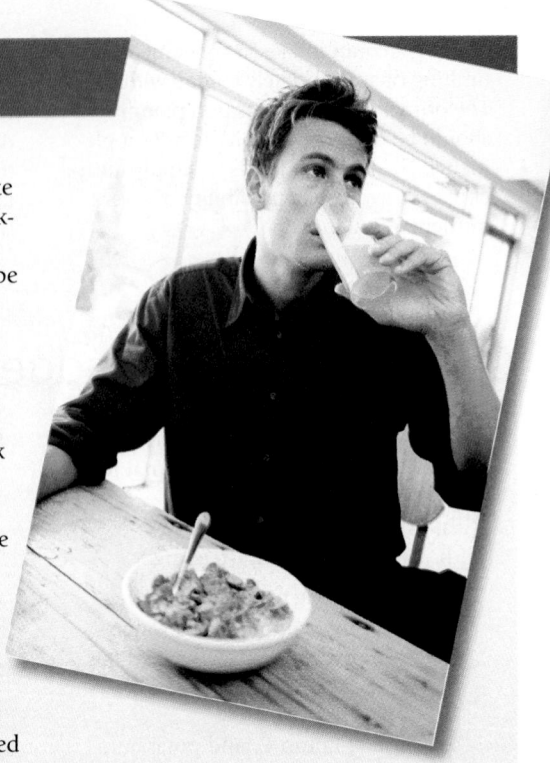

▲ With a little bit of planning, breakfast can be both quick and healthy.

So, the bowl of Wheaties with a banana and low-fat milk along with a yogurt, all from your dorm room "pantry," would be the healthiest choice for most.

Further Readings

1. Brown LB and others: College students can benefit by participating in a prepaid meal plan. *Journal of the American Dietetic Association* 105:445, 2005.

   Participation in a prepaid campus meal plan resulted in modest nutritional benefits to students through an increase in servings of foods from fruit, vegetable, and meat groups.

2. Center for Science in the Public Interest: *Guidelines for Responsible Food Marketing to Children.* Washington, DC, 2005. *www.cspinet.org/marketingguidelines.pdf.*

   These guidelines are written for all companies or organizations who manufacture, sell, market, advertise, or promote food to children. Criteria are provided for marketing food to children in a manner that does not undermine children's diets or harm their health. The guidelines address not only how food is marketed but also which foods are marketed to children.

3. Chiuve SE and others: Adherence to a low-risk, healthy lifestyle and risk of sudden cardiac death among women. *Journal of the American Medical Association* 306: 62, 2011.

   Sudden cardiac death causes more than half of all heart-related deaths and usually occurs as the first sign of heart disease, especially in women. Adherence to a healthy lifestyle and the risk of sudden cardiac death was studied in women from the Nurses' Health Study. Risk of sudden cardiac death dropped by 92% with a combination of the four healthy lifestyles (not smoking, not overweight, exercising 30 minutes/day or longer, and following the Mediterranean Diet). Women who ate a high proportion of vegetables, fruits, nuts, omega-3 fats, and fish, along with moderate amounts of alcohol and small amounts of red meat, had a 40% less risk than women whose diets least resembled this diet. Therefore, a healthy diet along with other healthy lifestyle factors appears to protect women from sudden cardiac death.

4. Choinière CJ, Lando A: *2008 Health and Diet Survey,* Food and Drug Administration, March 2010. *www.fda.gov/Food/Science-Research/ResearchAreas/ConsumerResearch/ucm193895.htm.*

   This report is a snapshot of the nations dietary habits based on the FDA 2008 telephone survey of more than 2500 adults in every state and the District of Columbia. One of the key findings was that more than half of consumers in the United States often read the food label when buying a product for the first time, and they are increasingly aware of the link between diet and heart disease..

5. Edmonds MJ and others: Body weight and percent body fat increase during the transition from high school to university in females. *Journal of the American Dietetic Association* 108:1033, 2008.

   The notion that weight gain occurs during the first year of university was studied in Canadian females making the transition from high school to university. There was a significant increase in body weight of 2.4 kg (5.28 pounds) during the first 6 to 7 months of university. Percent body fat also increased from 23.8% to 25.6%. Although dietary energy (calorie) intake did not increase, a decrease in moderate physical activity was an important predictor of weight. Body weight, therefore, may be modified by lifestyle factors during this formative period.

6. Federal Trade Commission: Marketing food to children and adolescents: A review of industry expenditures, activities, and self-regulation, a report to Congress. July 2008. *http://www.ftc.gov/opa/2008/07/foodmkting .shtm.*

   This study by the Federal Trade Commission found that 44 major food and beverage marketers spent $1.6 billion to promote their products to children under 12 and adolescents ages 12 to 17 in the United States in 2006. The report states that food advertising to youth is dominated by advertising campaigns that combine traditional media, such as television, with previously unmeasured forms of marketing, such as packaging, in-store advertising, sweepstakes, and Internet. This advertising often involves cross-promotion with a new movie or popular television program. The report calls for all food companies "to adopt and adhere to meaningful, nutrition-based standards for marketing their products to children under 12."

7. Goris JM and others: Television food advertising and the prevalence of childhood overweight and obesity: A multicountry comparison. *Public Health Nutrition* 13:1003, 2010.

   The higher prevalence of childhood obesity in the United States compared to other countries could be explained by greater exposure to TV food advertising. In a study of children ages 6 to 11 years in six countries, the contribution of TV food ads to the occurrence of childhood obesity was greatest for the United States at 16% to 40% and lowest in Great Britain, Sweden, and the Netherlands at 4% to 18%. Children in the United States were exposed to 11.5 minutes/day of TV food ads compared to only 1.8 minutes/day in the Netherlands. The authors conclude that the contribution of TV food ads to the prevalence of childhood obesity is significant in some countries and greatest in the United States.

8. Hoffman DY and others: Changes in body weight and fat mass of men and women in the first year of college: A study of the "freshman 15." *Journal of American College of Health* 55:41, 2006.

It is commonly thought that there is a high risk of gaining 15 pounds of weight during freshman year of college. In this study, changes in body weight and percentage of body fat were measured in first-year college students. Body weight increased by an average of almost 3 pounds (1.3 kilograms) and body fat increased an average of 0.7%. This study, therefore, found that weight and fat gain may occur during the first year of college.

9. Kochanek KD and others: *National Vital Statistics Reports*, Deaths: Preliminary Data for 2009: 59, 2011.

   Preliminary U.S. data on deaths, death rates, life expectancy, leading causes of death, and infant mortality for 2009 are presented. Death rates decreased significantly from 2008 to 2009 for 10 of the 15 leading causes of death: heart diseases, cancer, chronic lower respiratory diseases, cerebrovascular diseases, accidents (unintentional injuries), Alzheimer's disease, diabetes mellitus, influenza and pneumonia, septicemia, and assault (homicide).

10. Litt, AS: *The College Student's Guide to Eating Well on Campus.* Tulip Hill Press, Glen Echo, MD, 2005.

    This book provides important information on how to survive and eat well during your college years and covers how to avoid and spot eating disorders.

11. Oz D: *The Dorm Room Diet: The 10-Step Program for Creating a Healthy Lifestyle Plan That Really Works.* Newmarket Press, 2010.

    This book is written to help students stay fit while at college. The 10-step program shows students how to stop eating out of emotional need; navigate the most common danger zones at school for unhealthy eating; get the exercise you need, even in your small dorm room; choose vitamins and supplements wisely; and relax and rejuvenate amid the stress of college life.

12. Rutledge PC and others: 21st birthday drinking: Extremely extreme. *Journal of Consulting and Clinical Psychology* 76:511, 2008.

    A new level of extreme drinking goes beyond the four or five drinks in one sitting defined as "bingeing." At the University of Missouri, a study of 2518 students found 34% of men and 24% of women who imbibed on their 21st birthdays drank 21 alcoholic drinks or more. The authors conclude that interventions shown to be effective with general risky drinking may prove effective in reducing 21st birthday excess.

13. Shields DH and others: Gourmet coffee beverage consumption among college women. *Journal of the American Dietetic Association* 104:650, 2004.

    A significant percentage of college women were shown to consume gourmet coffee beverages,

which contributed additional calories and fat to their daily dietary intake.

14. Woolf K and others: Physical activity is associated with risk factors for chronic disease across adult women's life cycle. *Journal of the American Dietetic Association* 108:948, 2008.

    The results of this study confirm that younger age and greater physical activity across the adult women's life cycle are associated with more favorable serum lipid levels; less inflammation; lower concentrations of insulin, glucose, and leptin in serum; and more favorable body composition. These factors are associated with reduced risk for several chronic diseases including cardiovascular disease, type 2 diabetes, and obesity.

15. U.S. Department of Health and Human Services. 2008 Physical Activity Guidelines for Americans. *www.health.gov/paguidelines.*

    Inactivity remains relatively high among American children, adolescents, and adults. These science-based guidelines are designed to help Americans aged six and older use appropriate physical activity to improve their health. The guidelines include information about the health benefits of physical activity; how to do physical activity in a manner that meets the guidelines; how to reduce the risks of activity-related injury; and how to assist others in participating regularly in physical activity.

16. Vital Signs: State-Specific Obesity Prevalence Among Adults—United States, 2009. *Morbidity and Mortality Weekly Report* 59(30), 2010.

    Each year state health departments collect obesity data through a series of telephone interviews with U.S. adults. Obesity is defined as body mass index (BMI) of 30 or higher. Prevalence of obesity has increased significantly since 1985. In 2009, nine of these states (Alabama, Arkansas, Kentucky, Louisiana, Mississippi, Missouri, Oklahoma, Tennessee, and West Virginia) had a prevalence of obesity equal to or greater than 30%; 33 states had a prevalence equal to or greater than 25%; only Colorado and the District of Columbia had a prevalence of obesity less than 20%.

17. Yanover T, Sacco WP: Eating beyond satiety and body mass index. *Eating and Weight Disorders* 13:119, 2008.

    Eating beyond satiety (EBS), snacking, night eating, and hunger were examined in undergraduate females. EBS was the strongest predictor of body mass and therefore may be a variable to target in interventions to prevent and treat overweight and obesity.

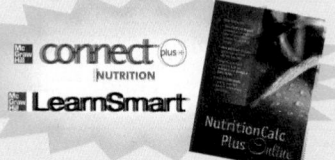

To get the most out of your study of nutrition, go to McGraw-Hill's online resources: Connect www.mcgrawhillconnect.com, where you will find NutritionCalc Plus, LearnSmart, and many other dynamic tools.

I. Examine Your Eating Habits More Closely

Choose one day of the week that is typical of your eating pattern. Using the first table found in Appendix E, list all foods and drinks you consumed for 24 hours. In addition, write down the approximate amounts of food you ate in units, such as cups, ounces, teaspoons, and tablespoons. After you record the amount of each food and drink consumed, indicate in the table why you chose to consume the item. Place the corresponding abbreviation in the space provided to indicate why you picked that food or drink.

FLVR	Flavor/texture	ADV	Advertisement	PEER	Peers
CONV	Convenience	WTCL	Weight control	NUTR	Nutritive value
EMO	Emotions	HUNG	Hunger	$	Cost
AVA	Availability	FAM	Family/cultural	HLTH	Health

There can be more than one reason for choosing a particular food or drink.

Application

Ask yourself what your most frequent reason is for eating or drinking. To what degree is health or nutritive value a reason for your food choices? Should you make these higher priorities?

II. Observe the Supermarket Explosion

Today's supermarkets carry up to 60,000 items, compared to 20,000 items 10 years ago. Think about your last grocery shopping trip and the items you purchased to eat. Following is a list of 20 newer food products added to supermarket shelves. Check the items that you have tried. Then use the key from Part I of the Rate Your Plate exercise to identify why you might have chosen these products.

_____ Prepackaged salad greens (variety packs other than iceberg lettuce) _____

_____ Gourmet or sprayable salad oils (e.g., walnut, almond, olive, or sesame oil) _____

_____ Gourmet vinegars (e.g., balsamic or rice) _____

_____ Prepackaged lunch products (e.g., nacho, pizza, taco, and tortilla Lunchables) _____

_____ Precooked frozen turkey patties, precooked bacon _____

_____ Bean soup mixes (e.g., lentil, black bean, combination bean soups) _____

_____ Microwavable sandwiches (e.g., Hotpockets, frozen sandwiches) _____

_____ Microwavable meals in a bowl (e.g., mac and cheese, soup) _____

_____ Refrigerated, precooked pasta (e.g., tortellini, fettucini) and accompanying sauces (e.g., pesto, tomato basil) _____

_____ Imported grain products (e.g., risotto, farfalline, gnocchi, fusilli) _____

_____ Whole-grain pasta or rice _____

_____ Frozen dinners (list your favorite of any of the wide variety) _____

_____ Imported sauces for food preparation (e.g., hoisin or brown bean sauce; mandarin marinade, sesame, curry, or fire oils) _____

_____ Bottled waters (flavored or unflavored) _____

_____ Trendy juices (e.g., draft apple cider, acai, pomegranate) _____

_____ Roasted and/or flavored coffees (e.g., beans, ground, instant, or k-cups) _____

_____ Gourmet jelly beans and candies (e.g., gummi coca-colas or imported chocolates) _____

_____ Instant hot cereal in a bowl (add water and go!) _____

_____ "Fast-shake" pancake mix (add water, shake, and ready to cook) _____

_____ Breakfast bars or cookies (e.g., granola or fruit-flavored bars) _____

_____ Meal replacement/fitness products (e.g., "energy" bars, high-protein bars, sports drinks) _____

_____ Low-carbohydrate meat and pasta dishes _____

_____ Low-calorie muffin tops, bagel thins _____

_____ Packaged yogurt smoothies _____

_____ Milk substitutes (e.g., rice milk, soy milk) _____

Finally, identify three new food products not on this list that you have seen in the past year. Discuss the appeal of these products to the North American consumer.

Chapter 2 Guidelines for Designing a Healthy Diet

Chapter Outline

Student Learning Outcomes

Chapter 2 is designed to allow you to:

2.1 Develop a healthy eating plan.

2.2 Outline the measurements used (ABCDEs) in nutrition assessment: **A**nthropometric, **B**iochemical, **C**linical, **D**ietary, and **E**nvironmental status.

2.3 Understand the basis of the scientific method as it is used in developing hypotheses and theories in the field of nutrition, including the determination of nutrient needs.

2.4 Describe what the Recommended Dietary Allowances (RDAs) and other dietary standards represent.

2.5 List the purpose and key recommendations of the Dietary Guidelines and the 2008 Physical Activity Guidelines for Americans.

2.6 Exemplify a meal that conforms to MyPlate recommendations.

2.7 Describe the components of the Nutrition Facts panel and the various health claims and label descriptors that are allowed.

2.8 Identify reliable sources of nutrition information.

What Would You Choose?

Living and learning in close quarters make it easy to share germs when flu season rolls around. You have heard that vitamin C supports the immune system, helping your body to fight infections. Many varieties of fruit juice and other beverages contain 100% of the Daily Value of vitamin C. In terms of nutrient density, is it better to get your vitamin C from a glass of orange juice or by eating a whole orange? How do oranges compare to orange juice in terms of energy density?

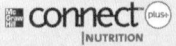 **Think about your choice as you read chapter 2, then see our recommendations at the end of the chapter. To learn more about nutrient density and energy density, check out the Connect site:** www.mcgrawhillconnect.com

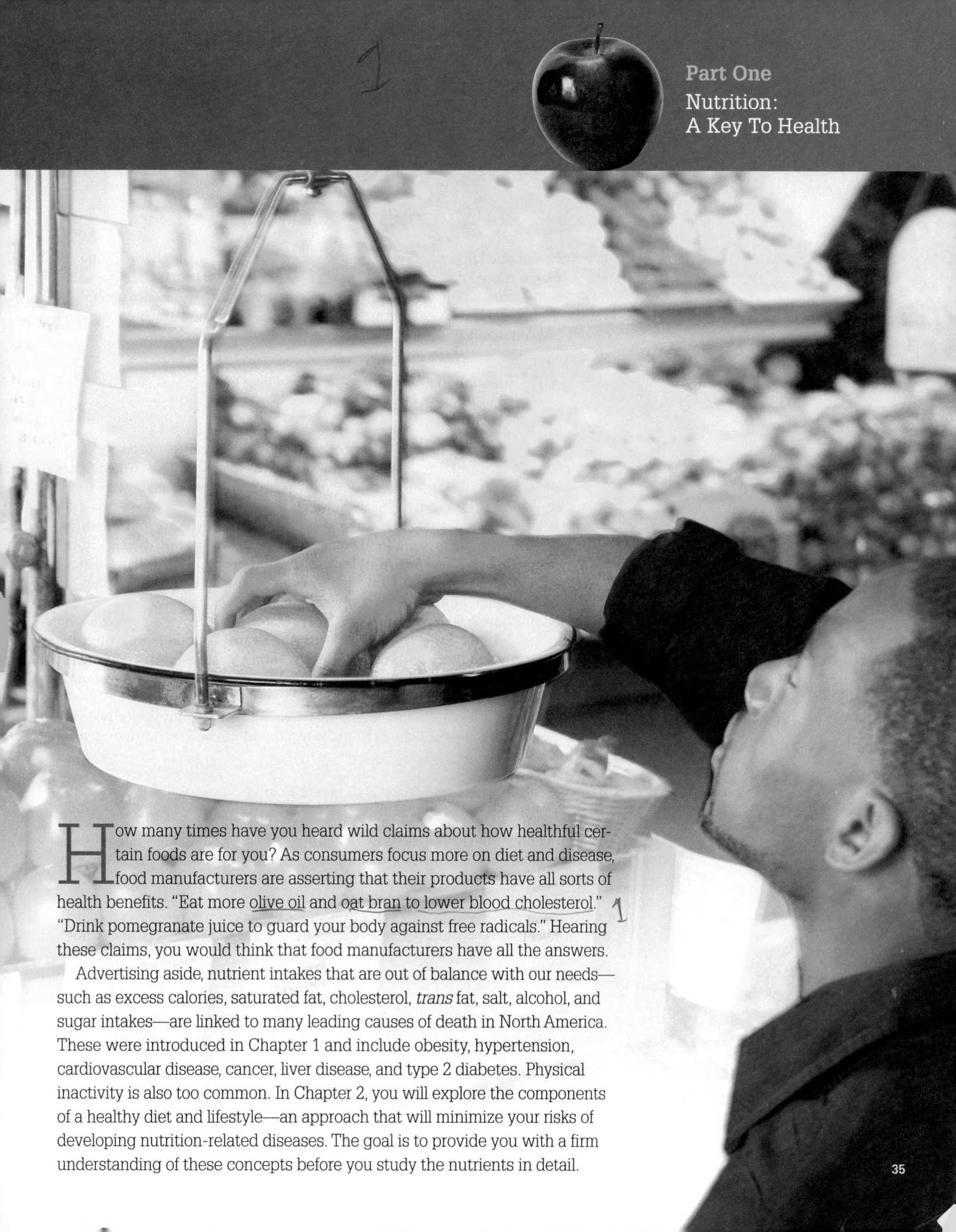

How many times have you heard wild claims about how healthful certain foods are for you? As consumers focus more on diet and disease, food manufacturers are asserting that their products have all sorts of health benefits. "Eat more <u>olive oil</u> and <u>oat bran</u> to lower blood cholesterol." "Drink pomegranate juice to guard your body against free radicals." Hearing these claims, you would think that food manufacturers have all the answers.

Advertising aside, nutrient intakes that are out of balance with our needs—such as excess calories, saturated fat, cholesterol, *trans* fat, salt, alcohol, and sugar intakes—are linked to many leading causes of death in North America. These were introduced in Chapter 1 and include obesity, hypertension, cardiovascular disease, cancer, liver disease, and type 2 diabetes. Physical inactivity is also too common. In Chapter 2, you will explore the components of a healthy diet and lifestyle—an approach that will minimize your risks of developing nutrition-related diseases. The goal is to provide you with a firm understanding of these concepts before you study the nutrients in detail.

Refresh Your Memory

As you begin your study of diet planning in Chapter 2, you may want to review:

▪ The terms in the margin in Chapter 1 and Table 1-1.

2.1 A Food Philosophy That Works

You may be surprised that what you should eat to minimize the risk of developing the nutrition-related diseases seen in North America is exactly what you have heard many times before: *Consume a variety of foods balanced by a moderate intake of each food.* Health professionals have recommended the same basic diet and health plan for the past 50 years:

• Control *how much* you eat.
• Pay attention to *what* you eat—choose whole grains, fruits, and vegetables.
• Stay physically active.

It is disappointing, however, that according to a recent survey conducted by the American Dietetic Association, two of five people in the United States believe that following a healthful diet means completely giving up foods they enjoy. To the contrary, a healthful diet does not have to mean deprivation and misery; it simply requires some basic nutrition know-how and planning. Besides, eliminating favorite foods typically does not work for "dieters" in the long run. The best plan consists of learning the basics of a healthful diet: variety, balance, and moderation. Monitoring total calorie intake is also important for many of us, especially if unwanted weight gain is taking place.

As noted in Chapter 1, many nutrition experts agree that there are no exclusively "good" or "bad" foods. Even so, many North Americans have diets that miss the mark when it comes to the foundations of healthy eating. Diets overloaded with fatty meats, fried foods, sugared soft drinks, and refined starches can result in substantial risk for nutrition-related chronic diseases.

Let's now define *variety, balance,* and *moderation.* We will also introduce two very important concepts that will help us to make healthy food choices: nutrient density and energy density.

Variety Means Eating Many Different Foods

Variety in your diet means choosing a number of different foods within any given food group rather than eating the "same old thing" day after day. Variety makes meals more interesting and helps ensure that a diet contains sufficient nutrients. A variety of foods is best because no one food meets all your nutrient needs. For example, meat provides protein and iron but little calcium and no vitamin C. Eggs are a source of protein, but they provide little calcium because the calcium is mostly in the shell. Cow's milk contains calcium but very little iron. None of these foods contains fiber.

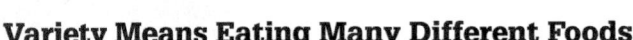

▲ A plate mostly full of fruits, vegetables, and whole-grain breads and cereals will help ward off disease and control body weight.

What do nutrition experts recommend for a healthy diet? Why are whole grains, fruits, and vegetables so important? How many servings do we need from each food group? How big is a serving? Are North Americans generally following the advice of the Dietary Guidelines? Chapter 2 provides some answers.

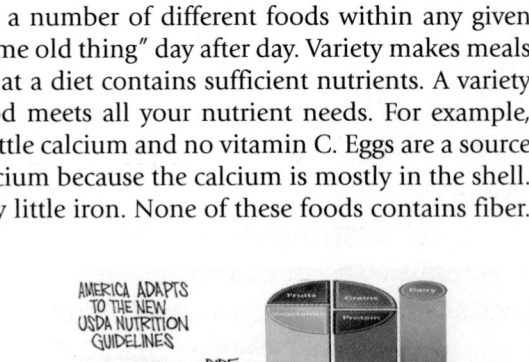

Carrots—a source of fiber and a pigment that forms vitamin A—may be your favorite vegetable. However, if you choose carrots every day as your only vegetable source, you may miss out on the vitamin folate. Other vegetables, such as broccoli and asparagus, are rich sources of this nutrient. Hopefully, you're beginning to get a sense of how different foods and food groups vary in the nutrients they contain. You'll learn much more about this in Chapters 8 and 9. For now, just recognize that you need a variety of foods in your diet because the required nutrients are scattered among many foods.

An added bonus of variety in the diet, especially within the fruit and vegetable groups, is the inclusion of a rich supply of **phytochemicals.** Recall from Chapter 1 that phytochemicals were discussed along with the nutrient classes. Many of these substances provide significant health benefits. Considerable research attention is focused on various phytochemicals in reducing the risk for certain diseases (e.g., cancer). You can't just buy a bottle of phytochemicals—they are generally available only within whole foods. Current multivitamin and mineral supplements contain few or none of these beneficial plant chemicals.

Numerous population studies show reduced cancer risk among people who regularly consume fruits and vegetables (see Further Reading 9). Researchers suspect that some phytochemicals present in the fruits and vegetables block the cancer process. Links between cancer and nutrition are described more thoroughly in the Nutrition and Your Health section in Chapter 16. Some phytochemicals also have been linked to a reduced risk of cardiovascular disease. Could it be that, because humans evolved eating a wide variety of plant-based foods, the body developed with a need for these phytochemicals, along with the various nutrients present, to maintain optimal health?

Foods rich in phytochemicals are now part of a family of foods referred to as **functional foods.** A functional food provides health benefits beyond those supplied by the traditional nutrients it contains. For example, a tomato contains the phytochemical lycopene, so it can be called a functional food. You may hear this term more from the food industry in the future.

It will likely take many years for scientists to unravel all of the important effects of the myriad of phytochemicals in foods, and it is unlikely that all will ever be available or effective in supplement form. For this reason, leading nutrition and medical experts suggest that a diet rich in fruits, vegetables, and whole-grain breads and cereals is the most reliable way to obtain the potential benefits of phytochemicals.

A note of caution: Some research suggests that increasing dietary variety can lead to overeating. Thus, as one incorporates a wide variety of foods in a diet, attention to total calorie intake is also important to consider. Table 2-1 provides a number of suggestions for including more phytochemicals in your diet, as do the websites www.fruitsandveggiesmorematters.org and www.fruitsandveggiesmatter.gov.

functional foods Foods that provide health benefits beyond those supplied by the traditional nutrients they contain. For example, a tomato contains the phytochemical lycopene, so it can be called a functional food.

Balance Means Consuming Food from Each Group

One way to balance your diet as you consume a variety of foods is to select foods from each of these five major food groups every day:

- Grains
- Vegetables
- Fruits
- Dairy
- Protein

MyPlate, a food guide plan discussed later in this chapter, offers a visual reminder and advice to help you make smart choices from each of these food groups. A dinner consisting of a bean burrito, lettuce and tomato salad with oil-and-vinegar dressing, a glass of milk, and an apple covers all groups.

Balance also refers to matching your energy intake (how many total calories you consume) with energy expenditure (calories burned by metabolism and physical activity) over time. As you will see in Chapter 7, a prolonged imbalance between energy intake and energy expenditure leads to fluctuations in body weight.

CRITICAL THINKING

Andy would benefit from more variety in his diet. What are some practical tips he can use to increase his fruit and vegetable intake?

TABLE 2-1 Tips for Boosting the Phytochemical Content of a Diet

- Include vegetables in main and side dishes. Add these to rice, omelets, potato salad, and pastas. Try broccoli or cauliflower florets, mushrooms, peas, carrots, corn, or peppers.

- Look for quick-to-fix grain side dishes in the supermarket. Pilafs, couscous, rice mixes, and tabbouleh are just a few that you'll find.

- Choose fruit-filled cookies, such as fig bars, instead of sugar-rich cookies. Use fresh or canned fruit as a topping for pudding, hot or cold cereal, pancakes, and frozen desserts.

- Put raisins, grapes, apple chunks, pineapples, grated carrots, zucchini, or cucumber into coleslaw, chicken salad, or tuna salad.

- Be creative at the salad bar: Try fresh spinach, leaf lettuce, red cabbage, zucchini, yellow squash, cauliflower, peas, mushrooms, or red or yellow peppers.

- Pack fresh or dried fruit for snacks away from home instead of grabbing a candy bar or going hungry.

- Add slices of cucumber, zucchini, spinach, or carrot slivers to the lettuce and tomato on your sandwiches.

- Each week try one or two vegetarian meals, such as beans and rice or pasta; vegetable stir fry; or spaghetti and tomato sauce.

- If your daily protein intake exceeds the recommended amounts, reduce the meat, fish, or poultry in casseroles, stews, and soups by one-third to one-half and add more vegetables and legumes.

- Keep a container of fresh vegetables in the refrigerator for snacks.

- Choose fruit or vegetable juices (preferably 100% juice varieties) instead of soft drinks.

- Substitute tea for coffee or soft drinks on a regular basis.

- Have a bowl of fresh fruit on hand.

- Switch from crisp head lettuce to leaf lettuce, such as romaine.

- Use salsa as a dip for chips in place of creamy dips.

- Choose whole-grain breakfast cereals, breads, and crackers.

- Add flavor to your plate with ginger, rosemary, basil, thyme, garlic, onions, parsley, and chives in place of salt.

- Incorporate soy products, such as tofu, soy milk, soy protein isolate, and roasted soybeans into your meals (see Chapter 6).

Moderation Refers Mostly to Portion Size

Eating in moderation requires paying attention to portion sizes and planning your day's diet so that you do not overconsume any nutrients. This is especially important for fat, salt, and sugar because Americans typically consume too much of these food components—and too many calories overall. For example, if you plan to eat a bacon cheeseburger (relatively high in fat, salt, and calories) at lunch, you should eat foods such as fruits and salad greens (less concentrated sources of these nutrients) at other meals that same day. If you prefer whole milk to low-fat or fat-free milk, reduce the fat elsewhere in your meals. Try low-fat salad dressings, or use jam rather than butter or margarine on toast. Overall, it is more feasible to consume moderate portions of foods that supply lots of fat, salt, and sugar than to try to eliminate these foods altogether.

Let's be clear that moderation is important for all food components, not just fat, salt, and sugar. For example, many North Americans do not consume enough

nutrient density The ratio derived by dividing a food's nutrient content by its calorie content. When the food's contribution to our nutrient need for that nutrient exceeds its contribution to our calorie need, the food is considered to have a favorable nutrient density.

4

vitamin E, which is found in plant oils, nuts, and some fruits and vegetables. However, taking large doses of vitamin E (e.g., from supplements) can lead to excessive bleeding because of its effects on blood clotting. You *can* get too much of a good thing!

Nutrient Density Focuses on Nutrient Content

The **nutrient density** of a food is a characteristic used to determine its nutritional quality. Nutrient density of a food is determined by comparing its protein, vitamin, or mineral content with the amount of calories it provides. A food is deemed nutrient dense if it provides a large amount of a nutrient for a relatively small amount of calories when compared with other food sources. The higher a food's nutrient density, the better it is as a nutrient source. Comparing the nutrient density of different foods is an easy way to estimate their relative nutritional quality.

Generally, nutrient density is determined with respect to individual nutrients (see Further Reading 4). For example, many fruits and vegetables have a high content of vitamin C compared with their modest calorie content; that is, they are nutrient-dense foods for vitamin C. Figure 2-1 shows that fat-free milk is much more nutrient dense than sugared soft drinks for many nutrients, especially protein, vitamin A, riboflavin, and calcium.

As noted previously, menu planning should focus mainly on the total diet—not on the selection of one critical food as the key to an adequate diet. Nutrient-dense foods—such as fat-free and low-fat milk, lean meats, legumes (beans), oranges, carrots, broccoli, whole-wheat bread, and whole-grain breakfast cereals—do help balance less nutrient-dense foods—such as cookies and potato chips, which many people like to eat. The latter are often called empty-calorie foods because they tend to be high in sugar and/or fat but provide few other nutrients.

Eating nutrient-dense foods is especially important for people who consume diets relatively low in calories. This includes some older people and those following weight-loss diets. This is because nutrient needs remain high even though calorie needs may be diminished.

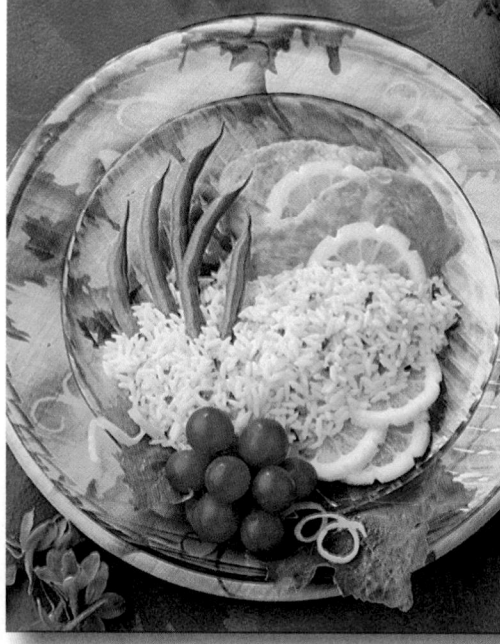

▲ Focus on nutrient-rich foods as you strive to meet your nutrient needs. The more colorful the food on your plate, the greater the content of nutrients and phytochemicals.

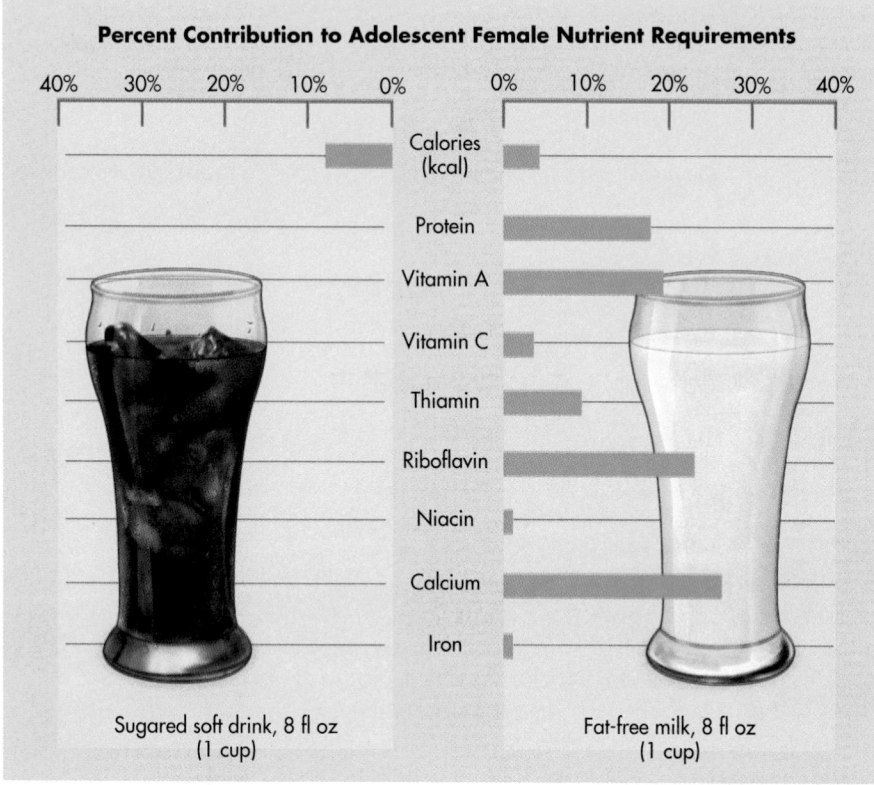

Percent Contribution to Adolescent Female Nutrient Requirements

Sugared soft drink, 8 fl oz
(1 cup)

Fat-free milk, 8 fl oz
(1 cup)

Calories (kcal)
Protein
Vitamin A
Vitamin C
Thiamin
Riboflavin
Niacin
Calcium
Iron

FIGURE 2-1 ▶ Comparison of the nutrient contributions of a sugared soft drink with that of fat-free (i.e., nonfat or skim) milk. Choosing a glass of fat-free milk makes a significantly greater contribution to nutrient intake than does a sugared soft drink. An easy way to determine nutrient density from this chart is to compare the lengths of the bars indicating vitamin or mineral contribution with the bar that represents calorie contribution. For the soft drink, no nutrient surpasses calorie content. Fat-free milk, in contrast, has longer nutrient bars for protein, vitamin A, the vitamins thiamin and riboflavin, and the mineral calcium than it does for calories. Including many nutrient-dense foods in your diet is a good way to meet nutrient needs without exceeding calorie needs.

energy density A comparison of the calorie (kcal) content of a food with the weight of the food. An energy-dense food is high in calories but weighs very little (e.g., potato chips), whereas a food low in energy density has few calories but weighs a lot, such as an orange.

Energy (kcal) Density Affects Calorie Intake

Energy density is a measurement that best describes the calorie content of a food. Energy density of a food is determined by comparing the calorie (kcal) content with the weight of food. A food that is rich in calories but weighs relatively little is considered energy dense. Examples include nuts; cookies; fried foods in general; and even fat-free snacks, such as fat-free pretzels. Foods with low energy density include fruits, vegetables, and any food that incorporates lots of water during cooking, such as oatmeal (Table 2-2).

Researchers have shown that eating a meal with many foods of low energy density promotes satiety without contributing many calories (see Further Reading 6). This is probably because we typically consume a constant weight of food at a meal rather than a constant number of calories. How this constant weight of food is regulated is not known, but careful laboratory studies show that people consume fewer calories in a meal if most of the food choices are low in energy density, compared with foods high in energy density. Eating a diet low in energy density can aid in losing (or maintaining) weight.

Overall, foods with lots of water and fiber (i.e., low-energy-density foods) contribute few calories even though they help one feel full. Alternatively, foods with high energy density must be eaten in greater amounts to promote fullness. This is one more reason to eat a diet rich in fruits, vegetables, and whole-grain breads and cereals, a pattern that is typical of many ethnic diets throughout rural areas of the world.

Still, favorite foods, even if they are high in energy density, can have a place in your dietary pattern, but you will have to plan for them. For example, chocolate is a very energy-dense food, but a small portion at the end of a meal can supply a satisfying finale. In addition, foods with high energy density can help people with poor appetites, such as some older people, to maintain or gain weight.

The following sections of Chapter 2 describe various states of nutritional health and provide tools and nutrient guidelines for planning healthy diets to support overall health.

TABLE 2-2 Energy Density of Common Foods (Listed in Relative Order)

Very Low Energy Density (less than 0.6 kcal per gram)	Low Energy Density (0.6 to 1.5 kcal per gram)	Medium Energy Density (1.5 to 4 kcal per gram)	High Energy Density (greater than 4 kcal per gram)
Lettuce	Whole milk	Eggs	Graham crackers
Tomatoes	Oatmeal	Ham	Fat-free sandwich cookies
Strawberries	Cottage cheese	Pumpkin pie	Chocolate
Broccoli	Beans	Whole-wheat bread	Chocolate chip cookies
Salsa	Bananas	Bagels	Tortilla chips
Grapefruit	Broiled fish	White bread	Bacon
Fat-free milk	Fat-free yogurt	Raisins	Potato chips
Carrots	Ready-to-eat breakfast cereals with 1% low-fat milk	Cream cheese	Peanuts
Vegetable soup		Cake with frosting	Peanut butter
		Pretzels	Mayonnaise
	Plain baked potato	Rice cakes	Butter or margarine
	Cooked rice		Vegetable oils
	Spaghetti noodles		

Data adapted from Rolls B, *The Volumetrics Eating Plan.* New York: HarperCollins, 2005.

▲ Salads are low in energy density if we limit additional calories from salad dressing, bacon bits, cheese crumbles or cubes, and croutons.

CONCEPT CHECK

Healthy diet planning requires variety, balance, and moderation. Variety involves choosing different foods within each food group. Balance refers to consuming foods from each of the five food groups, as well as balancing calorie intake with calorie expenditure. Moderation implies limiting portion sizes with each food choice, so that the diet is not excessive in calories or any particular nutrient. Nutrient-dense foods, such as fat-free milk, fruits, vegetables, and whole-grain breads and cereals, supply many nutrients without contributing excessive calories. Consuming foods of low energy density, such as fruits and vegetables, may also help in weight control, because they promote satiety with relatively few calories.

MAKING DECISIONS

Some people frequently choose French fries as their vegetable. What is the nutrient content of French fries? Check the food composition supplement for the vitamin C content of French fries. How many servings would you need to eat to meet vitamin C needs (75 to 95 milligrams)?

(Answer: 4 to 5 servings)

2.2 States of Nutritional Health

The body's nutritional health is determined by considering the **nutritional state** of each needed nutrient. Three general categories of nutritional status are recognized: desirable nutrition, undernutrition, and overnutrition. The common term **malnutrition** can refer to either **overnutrition** or **undernutrition.** Neither state is conducive to good health. Furthermore, it is possible to be both overnourished (e.g., consume excess calories) and undernourished (e.g., consume too few essential vitamins and minerals) at the same time.

The amount of each nutrient needed to maintain a state of desirable nutrition is the basis for published dietary intake recommendations. Diet plans to meet those needs are discussed later in this chapter.

Desirable Nutrition

The **nutritional state** for a particular nutrient is desirable when body tissues have enough of the nutrient to support normal metabolic functions as well as surplus stores that can be used in times of increased need. A desirable nutritional state can be achieved by obtaining essential nutrients from a variety of foods.

Undernutrition

Undernutrition occurs when nutrient intake does not meet nutrient needs. At first, any surpluses are put to use; then, as stores are exhausted, health begins to decline. Many nutrients are in high demand due to constant cell loss and regeneration in the body, such as in the gastrointestinal tract. For this reason, the stores of certain nutrients, including many of the B vitamins, are exhausted rapidly and therefore require a regular intake. In addition, some women in North America do not consume sufficient iron to meet monthly losses and eventually deplete their iron stores (Fig. 2-2).

Once availability of a nutrient falls sufficiently low, biochemical evidence indicates that the body's metabolic processes have slowed or stopped. At this state of deficiency, there are no outward **symptoms;** thus, it is termed a **subclinical** deficiency. A subclinical deficiency can go on for some time before clinicians are able to detect its effects.

Eventually, clinical symptoms will develop. Clinical evidence of a nutritional deficiency—perhaps in the skin, hair, nails, tongue, or eyes—can occur within months but may take years to develop. Often, clinicians do not detect a problem until a deficiency produces outward symptoms, such as small areas of bruising on the skin from a vitamin C deficiency.

Overnutrition

Prolonged consumption of more nutrients than the body needs can lead to overnutrition. In the short run (e.g., 1 to 2 weeks), overnutrition may cause only a few symptoms, such as stomach distress from excess iron intake. If an excess intake continues, however, some nutrients may accumulate to toxic amounts, which can lead to serious disease. For example, too much vitamin A during pregnancy can cause birth defects.

nutritional state The nutritional health of a person as determined by anthropometric measurements (height, weight, circumferences, and so on), biochemical measurements of nutrients or their by-products in blood and urine, a clinical (physical) examination, a dietary analysis, and economic evaluation; also called nutritional status.

malnutrition Failing health that results from long-standing dietary practices that do not coincide with nutritional needs.

overnutrition A state in which nutritional intake greatly exceeds the body's needs.

undernutrition Failing health that results from a long-standing dietary intake that is not enough to meet nutritional needs.

symptom A change in health status noted by the person with the problem, such as stomach pain.

subclinical Stage of a disease or disorder not severe enough to produce symptoms that can be detected or diagnosed.

FIGURE 2-2 ▶ The general scheme of nutritional status. Green reflects good status, yellow marginal status, and red poor status (undernutrition or overnutrition). This general concept can be applied to all nutrients. Iron was chosen as an example because iron deficiency is the most common nutrient deficiency worldwide.

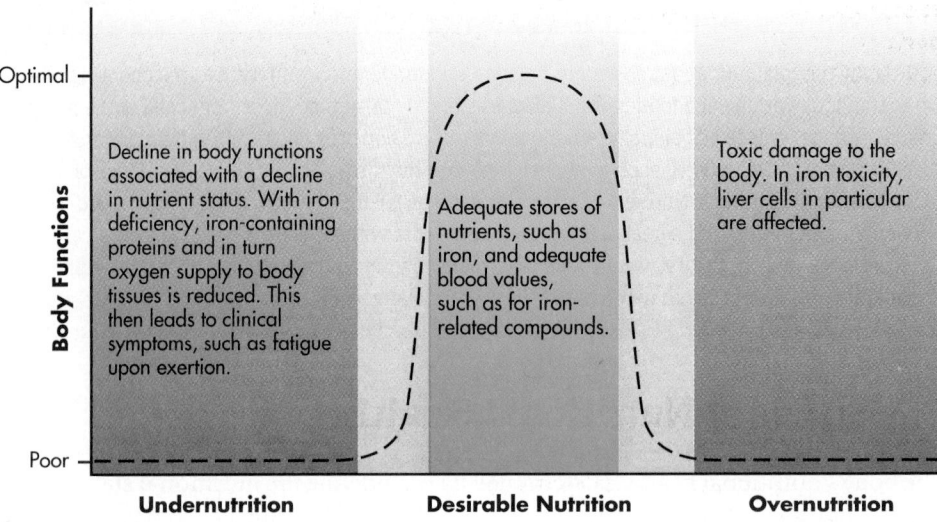

Body Functions

Optimal

Poor

Decline in body functions associated with a decline in nutrient status. With iron deficiency, iron-containing proteins and in turn oxygen supply to body tissues is reduced. This then leads to clinical symptoms, such as fatigue upon exertion.

Adequate stores of nutrients, such as iron, and adequate blood values, such as for iron-related compounds.

Toxic damage to the body. In iron toxicity, liver cells in particular are affected.

Undernutrition   **Desirable Nutrition**   **Overnutrition**

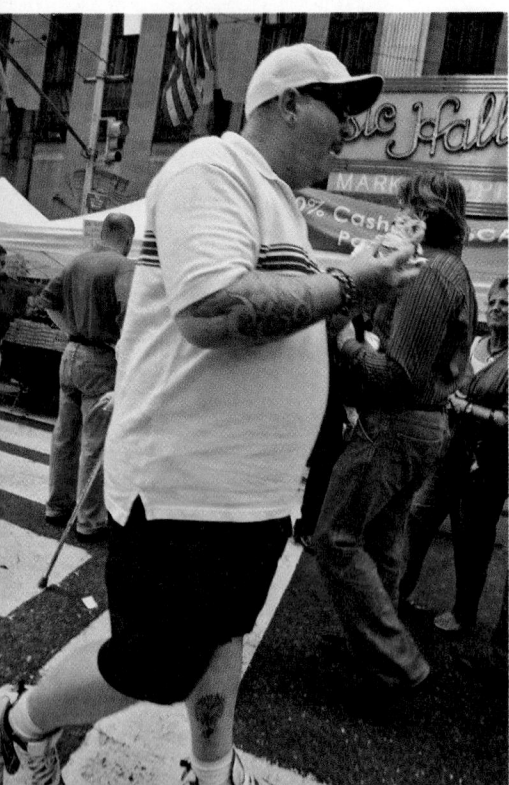

▲ The most common type of overnutrition in North America is the excess intake of calories, which often leads to obesity.

anthropometric assessment Measurement of body weight and the lengths, circumferences, and thicknesses of parts of the body.

biochemical assessment Measurement of biochemical functions (e.g., concentrations of nutrient by-products or enzyme activities in the blood or urine) related to a nutrient's function.

The most common form of overnutrition in developed nations is an excess intake of calories that leads to obesity. In the long run, outcomes of obesity include other serious diseases, such as type 2 diabetes and certain forms of cancer. Use the website www.shapeup.org to learn more about the importance of lifelong weight control.

For most vitamins and minerals, the gap between desirable intake and overnutrition is wide. Therefore, even if people take a typical balanced multivitamin and mineral supplement daily, they probably will not receive a harmful dose of any nutrient. The gap between desirable intake and overnutrition is smallest for vitamin A and the minerals calcium, iron, and copper. Thus, if you take nutrient supplements, keep a close eye on your total vitamin and mineral intake from both food and supplements to avoid toxicity (see Chapter 8 for further advice on use of nutrient supplements).

2.3 How Can Your Nutritional State Be Measured?

To find out how nutritionally fit *you* are, a nutritional assessment—either whole or in part—needs to be performed (Table 2-3). Generally, this is performed by a physician, often with the aid of a registered dietitian.

Analyzing Background Factors

Because family health history plays an important role in determining nutritional and health status, it must be carefully recorded and critically analyzed as part of a nutritional assessment. Other related background information includes: (1) a medical history, especially for any disease states or treatments that could decrease nutrient absorption or ultimate use; (2) a list of medications taken; (3) a social history (e.g., marital status, living conditions); (4) level of education to determine the degree of complexity that can be used in written materials and oral discussions; and (5) economic status to determine the ability to purchase, transport, and cook food.

Assessing Nutritional Status Using the ABCDEs

In addition to background factors, four nutritional-assessment categories complete the picture of nutritional status. **Anthropometric** measurements of height, weight (and weight changes), skinfold thicknesses, and body circumferences provide information about the current state of nutrition. Most measures of body composition are easy to obtain and are generally reliable. However, an in-depth examination of nutritional health is impossible without the more expensive process of **biochemical assessment.** This involves the measurement of the concentrations of nutrients and nutrient by-products in the blood, urine, and feces and of specific blood enzyme activities.

TABLE 2-3 Conducting an Evaluation of Nutritional Health

Parameters	Example
Background	Medical history (e.g., current diseases, past surgeries, current weight, weight history, and current medications)
	Social history (marital status, living conditions)
	Family health history
	Education level
	Economic status
Nutritional	Anthropometric assessment: height, weight, skinfold thickness, arm muscle circumference, and other parameters
	Biochemical (laboratory) assessment of blood and urine: enzyme activities, concentrations of nutrients or their by-products
	Clinical assessment (physical examination): general appearance of skin, eyes, and tongue; rapid hair loss; sense of touch; ability to walk
	Dietary assessment: usual intake or record of previous days' meals

A **clinical assessment** would follow, during which a health professional would search for any physical evidence (e.g., high blood pressure) of diet-related diseases or deficiencies. Then, a close look at the person's diet (**dietary assessment**), including a record of at least the previous few days' food intake, would help to determine any possible problem areas.

Finally, adding the **environmental assessment** (from the background analysis) provides further details about the living conditions, education level, and ability to purchase and prepare foods needed to maintain health. Now the true nutritional state of a person emerges. Taken together, these five assessments form the ABCDEs of nutritional assessment: anthropometric, biochemical, clinical, dietary, and environmental (Fig. 2-3).

MAKING DECISIONS

Nutritional Assessment

A practical example using the ABCDEs for evaluating nutritional status can be illustrated in a person who chronically abuses alcohol. Upon evaluation, the physician notes:

(A) Low weight for height, recent 10-pound weight loss, muscle wasting in the upper body
(B) Low amounts of the vitamins thiamin and folate in the blood
(C) Psychological confusion, facial sores, and uncoordinated movement
(D) Dietary intake of little more than wine and hamburgers for the last week
(E) Currently residing in a homeless shelter; $35.00 in wallet; unemployed

Evaluation: This person needs medical attention, including nutrient repletion.

clinical assessment Examination of general appearance of skin, eyes, and tongue; evidence of rapid hair loss; sense of touch; and ability to cough and walk.

dietary assessment Estimation of typical food choices relying mostly on the recounting of one's usual intake or a record of one's previous days' intake.

environmental assessment Includes details about living conditions, education level, and the ability of the person to purchase, transport, and cook food. The person's weekly budget for food purchases is also a key factor to consider.

heart attack Rapid fall in heart function caused by reduced blood flow through the heart's blood vessels. Often part of the heart dies in the process. Technically called a myocardial infarction.

Recognizing the Limitations of Nutritional Assessment

A long time may elapse between the initial development of poor nutritional health and the first clinical evidence of a problem. A diet high in saturated (typically solid) fat often increases blood cholesterol but without producing any clinical evidence for years. However, when the blood vessels become sufficiently blocked by cholesterol and other materials, chest pain during physical activity or a **heart attack** may occur. An active area of nutrition research is the development of better methods for early detection of nutrition-related problems such as heart attack risk.

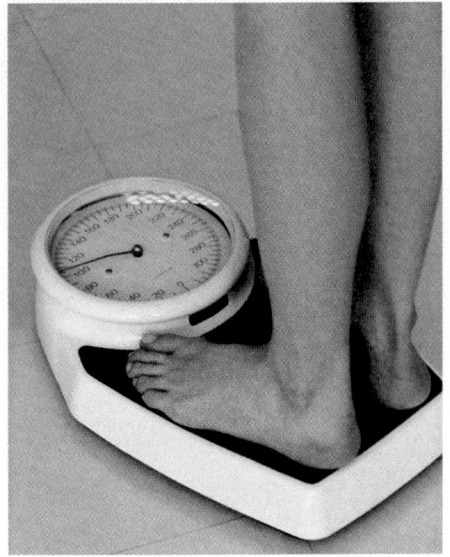

Anthropometric

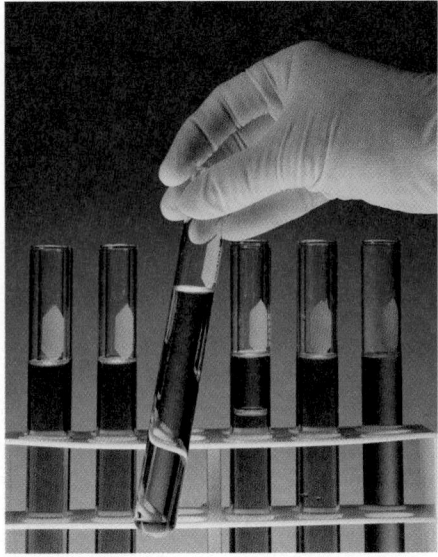

Biochemical

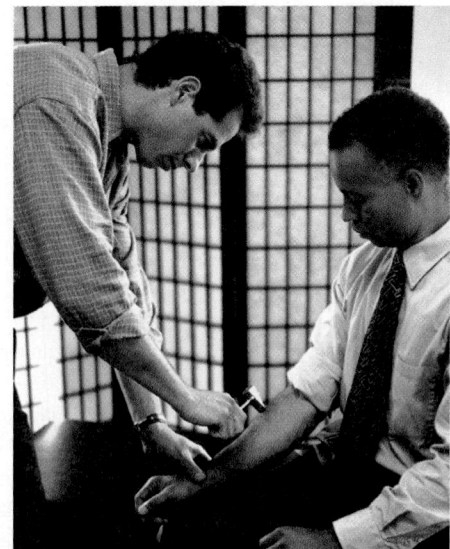

Clinical

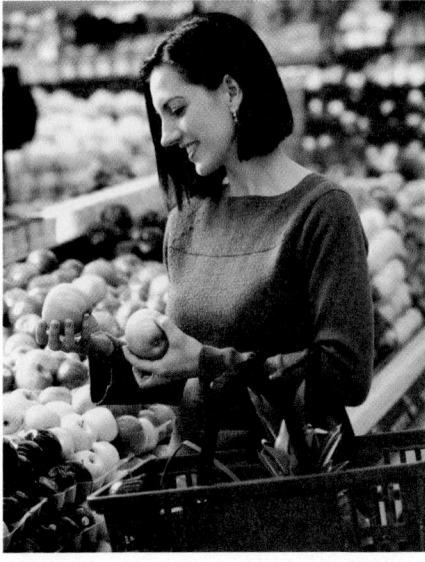

Dietary

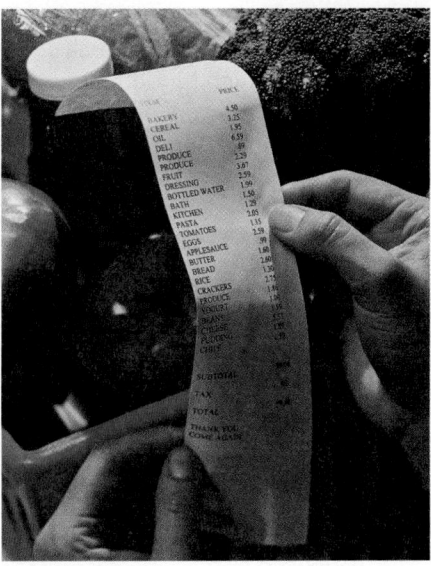

Environmental

FIGURE 2-3 ▶ A complete nutritional assessment includes anthropometric, biochemical, clinical, and dietary information. Environmental status adds further information, rounding out the ABCDEs of nutritional assessment.

Another example of a serious health condition with delayed symptoms is low bone density resulting from a calcium deficiency—a particularly relevant issue for adolescent and young adult females. Many young women do not consume the needed amount of calcium but suffer no obvious effects in their younger years. However, the bone structures of these women with low calcium intakes do not reach full potential during the years of growth, making osteoporosis more likely later in life.

Furthermore, clinical symptoms of some nutritional deficiencies (e.g., diarrhea, inability to walk normally, and facial sores) are not very specific. These may have causes other than poor nutrition. The long time it takes for symptoms to develop and their potential to be vague often make it difficult to establish a link between an individual's current diet and nutritional state.

Concern About the State of Your Nutritional Health Is Important

Table 1-7 in Chapter 1 portrayed the close relationship between nutrition and health. The good news is that people who focus on maintaining nutritional health are apt to enjoy a long, vigorous life. For example, a recent study found that women with a healthy lifestyle had a decreased risk for heart attacks (80% reduction) compared to women without such healthy practices. The healthy habits included:

- Consumed a healthy diet
  - Varied
  - Rich in fiber
  - Included some fish
  - Low in animal fat and *trans* fat
- Maintained a healthy weight
- Occasionally consumed alcohol in small amounts
- Exercised for at least 30 minutes daily
- Avoided use of tobacco

Should all adults follow this example (with optional use of alcohol)?

CONCEPT CHECK

A desirable nutritional state results when the body has enough nutrients to function fully and contains stores to use in times of increased needs. When nutrient intake fails to meet body needs, undernutrition develops. Symptoms of such an inadequate nutrient intake can take months or years to develop. Overloading the body with nutrients, leading to overnutrition, is another potential problem to avoid. Nutritional state can be assessed by using anthropometric, biochemical, clinical, dietary, and economic assessments (ABCDEs).

2.4 Using the Scientific Method to Determine Nutrient Needs

How do we know what we know about nutrient needs? In a word, research. Like other sciences, the research that sets the foundation for nutrition knowledge has developed through the use of the *scientific method*, a testing procedure designed to detect and eliminate error.

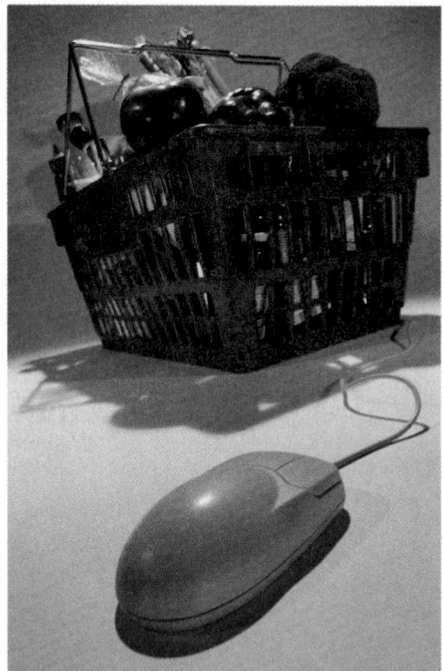

▲ Is there an app for that? Yes, there is! Health-conscious consumers can tap into a growing number of smartphone applications to help them stay on track with a healthy lifestyle. From calorie counters to pedometers to gentle reminders to get up and stretch, smartphone users have access to a virtual arsenal against diet-related disease. Log onto the Connect site to find links to apps from reputable sources.

MAKING DECISIONS

Research on Stomach Ulcers

Overall, the scientific method requires a skeptical attitude. A recent example of this need for skepticism involves stomach **ulcers.** Not so many years ago, everyone "knew" that stomach ulcers were caused by a stressful lifestyle and a poor diet. Then, in 1983, an Australian physician, Dr. Barry Marshall, reported in a respected medical journal that ulcers are usually caused by a common **microorganism** called *Helicobacter pylori*. Furthermore, he stated that a cure is possible using antibiotics. At first, other physicians were skeptical about this finding and continued to prescribe medications such as antacids that reduce stomach acid. But, as more studies were published demonstrating that patients using antibiotics were cured of ulcers, the medical profession eventually accepted the findings. Today, ulcers are managed for the most part by medications that destroy the microorganism. (We will discuss the treatment of stomach ulcers in more detail in Chapter 3.) Sound scientific discoveries will always be subject to challenge and change.

ulcer Erosion of the tissue lining, usually in the stomach (gastric ulcer) or the upper small intestine (duodenal ulcer). As a group these are generally referred to as peptic ulcers.

microorganism Bacterium virus, or other organism invisible to the naked eye, some of which cause diseases. Also called *microbe*.

hypotheses Tentative explanations by a scientist to explain a phenomenon.

scurvy The deficiency disease that results after a few weeks to months of consuming a diet that lacks vitamin C; pinpoint sites of bleeding on the skin are an early sign.

epidemiology The study of how disease rates vary among different population groups.

The first step of the scientific method is the observation of a natural phenomenon. Scientists then suggest possible explanations, called **hypotheses,** about its cause. At times, historical events can provide clues to important relationships in nutrition science, such as the link between vitamin C and **scurvy** (see Chapter 8). In a related approach, scientists may study diet and disease patterns among various populations, a research method called **epidemiology**.

Historical and epidemiological findings can *suggest* hypotheses about the role of diet in various health problems. *Proving* the role of particular dietary components, however, requires controlled experiments. The data gathered from experiments may either support or refute each hypothesis. If the results of many experiments support a hypothesis, scientists accept the hypothesis as a **theory** (such as the theory of gravity). Often, the results from one experiment suggest a new set of questions (Fig. 2-4).

The most rigorous type of controlled experiment follows a randomized, double-blind, placebo-controlled study design. In this type of study, a group of participants—the experimental group—follows a specific protocol (e.g., consuming a certain food or nutrient), and participants in a corresponding **control group** follow their normal habits or consume a **placebo**. People are randomly assigned to each group, such as by the flip of a coin. Scientists then observe the experimental group over time to see if there is any effect not found in the control group.

theory An explanation for a phenomenon that has numerous lines of evidence to support it.

control group Participants in an experiment who are not given the treatment being tested.

placebo Generally a fake medicine or treatment used to disguise the treatments given to the participants in an experiment.

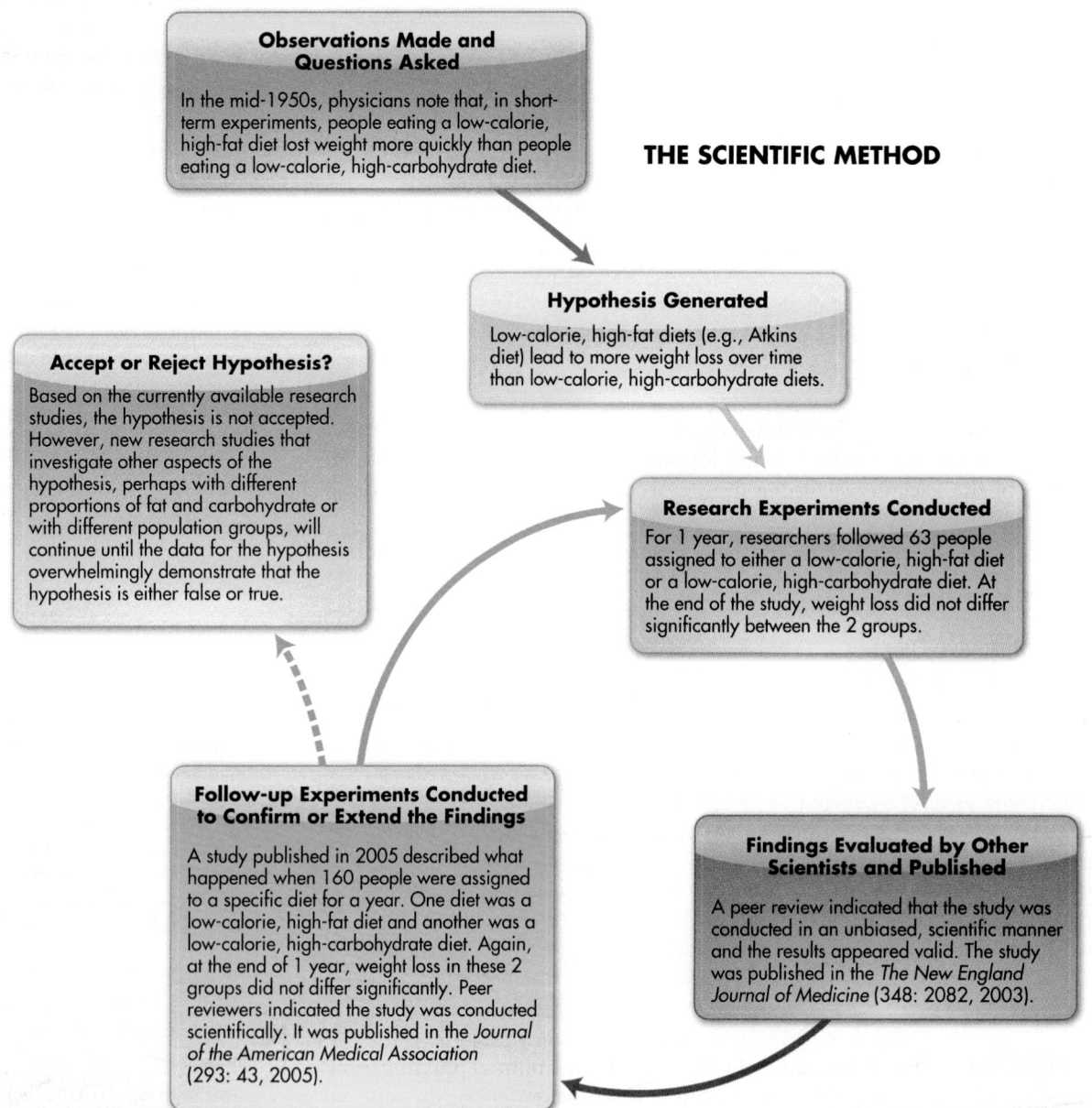

THE SCIENTIFIC METHOD

Observations Made and Questions Asked

In the mid-1950s, physicians note that, in short-term experiments, people eating a low-calorie, high-fat diet lost weight more quickly than people eating a low-calorie, high-carbohydrate diet.

Hypothesis Generated

Low-calorie, high-fat diets (e.g., Atkins diet) lead to more weight loss over time than low-calorie, high-carbohydrate diets.

Accept or Reject Hypothesis?

Based on the currently available research studies, the hypothesis is not accepted. However, new research studies that investigate other aspects of the hypothesis, perhaps with different proportions of fat and carbohydrate or with different population groups, will continue until the data for the hypothesis overwhelmingly demonstrate that the hypothesis is either false or true.

Research Experiments Conducted

For 1 year, researchers followed 63 people assigned to either a low-calorie, high-fat diet or a low-calorie, high-carbohydrate diet. At the end of the study, weight loss did not differ significantly between the 2 groups.

Follow-up Experiments Conducted to Confirm or Extend the Findings

A study published in 2005 described what happened when 160 people were assigned to a specific diet for a year. One diet was a low-calorie, high-fat diet and another was a low-calorie, high-carbohydrate diet. Again, at the end of 1 year, weight loss in these 2 groups did not differ significantly. Peer reviewers indicated the study was conducted scientifically. It was published in the *Journal of the American Medical Association* (293: 43, 2005).

Findings Evaluated by Other Scientists and Published

A peer review indicated that the study was conducted in an unbiased, scientific manner and the results appeared valid. The study was published in the *The New England Journal of Medicine* (348: 2082, 2003).

FIGURE 2-4 ▶ This example shows how the scientific method was used to test a hypothesis about the effects of low-calorie, high-fat diets on weight loss. Scientists consistently follow these steps when testing all types of hypotheses. Scientists do not accept a nutrition or another scientific hypothesis until it has been thoroughly tested using the scientific method.

Human experiments provide the most convincing evidence about relationships between nutrients and health, but they are often not practical or ethical. Thus, much of what we know about human nutritional needs and functions has been gleaned from animal experiments. The use of animal experiments to study the role of nutrition in certain human diseases depends on the availability of an **animal model**—a disease in laboratory animals that closely mimics a particular human disease. Often, however, if no animal model is available and human experiments are ruled out, scientific knowledge cannot advance beyond what can be learned from epidemiological studies.

Once an experiment is complete, scientists summarize the findings and seek to publish the results in scientific journals. Generally, before articles are published in scientific journals, they are critically reviewed by other scientists familiar with the subject, which helps to ensure that only high-quality, objective research findings are published.

Keep in mind, one experiment is never enough to prove a particular hypothesis or provide a basis for nutritional recommendations. Rather, through follow-up studies, the results obtained in one laboratory must be confirmed by experiments conducted in other laboratories and, possibly, under varying circumstances. Only then can we really trust and use the results. The more lines of evidence available to support an idea, the more likely it is to be true (Fig. 2-5).

Epidemiological studies may suggest hypotheses, but controlled experiments are needed to rigorously test hypotheses before nutrition recommendations can be made. For example, epidemiologists found that smokers who regularly consumed fruits and vegetables had a lower risk for lung cancer than smokers who ate few fruits and vegetables. Some scientists proposed that beta-carotene, a pigment present in many fruits and vegetables, may be responsible for reducing the damage that tobacco smoke creates in the lungs. However, in **double-blind studies** involving heavy smokers, the risk of lung cancer was found to be *higher* for those who took beta-carotene supplements than for those who did not (this is not true for the small amount of beta-carotene found naturally in foods). Soon after these results were reported, the U.S. federal agency supporting two other large ongoing studies that employed beta-carotene supplements called a halt to the research, stating that these supplements are ineffective in preventing both lung cancer and cardiovascular disease.

animal model Use of animals to study disease to understand more about human disease.

case-control study A study in which individuals who have a disease or condition, such as lung cancer, are compared with individuals who do not have the condition.

double-blind study An experimental design in which neither the participants nor the researchers are aware of each participant's assignment (test or placebo) or the outcome of the study until it is completed. An independent third party holds the code and the data until the study has been completed.

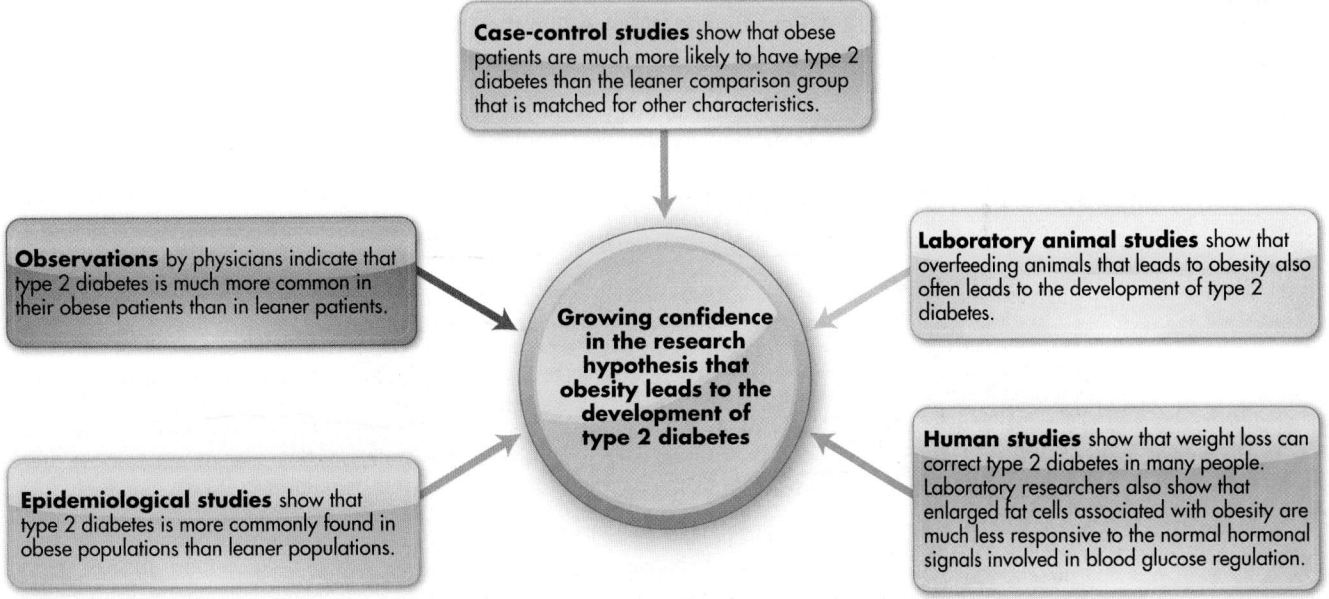

FIGURE 2-5 ▶ Data from a variety of sources can come together to support a research hypothesis. This diagram shows how various types of research data support the hypothesis that obesity leads to the development of type 2 diabetes (see Chapter 4).

2.5 Specific Nutrient Standards and Recommendations

The overarching goal of any healthy diet plan is to meet nutrient needs. To begin, we must determine what amount of each essential nutrient is necessary to maintain health. Most of the terms that describe nutrient needs fall under one umbrella term—**Dietary Reference Intakes (DRIs)**. The development of DRIs is an ongoing, collaborative effort between the Food and Nutrition Board of the Institute of Medicine in the United States and Health Canada (see Further Reading 2). Included under the DRI umbrella are **Recommended Dietary Allowances (RDAs)**, **Adequate Intakes (AIs)**, **Estimated Energy Requirements (EERs)**, and **Tolerable Upper Intake Levels (Upper Levels or ULs)**.

As you begin your study of nutrition, all these acronyms can seem like an alphabet soup of abbreviations! However, you can more easily sift through these nutrient standards if you have some basic knowledge about their development and use (summarized in Table 2-4).

Recommended Dietary Allowance

A Recommended Dietary Allowance (RDA) is the amount of a nutrient that will meet the needs of nearly all individuals (about 97%) in a particular age and gender group. A person can compare his or her individual intake of specific nutrients to the RDA. Although an intake slightly above or below the RDA for a particular nutrient is no reason for concern, a significant deviation below (about 70%) or above (about three times or more for some nutrients) the RDA for an extended time can eventually result in a deficiency or toxicity of that nutrient, respectively.

Adequate Intake

An RDA can be set for a nutrient only if there is sufficient information on the human needs for that particular nutrient. Today, there is not enough information on some nutrients, such as chromium, to set such a precise standard as an RDA. For this and other nutrients, the DRIs include a category called an Adequate Intake (AI). This standard is based on the dietary intakes of people that appear to be maintaining nutritional health. That amount of intake is assumed to be adequate, as no evidence of a nutritional deficiency is apparent.

TABLE 2-4 Recommendations within the Dietary Reference Intakes

RDA	Recommended Dietary Allowance. Use to evaluate your current intake for a specific nutrient. The further you stray above or below this value, the greater your chances of developing nutritional problems.
AI	Adequate Intake. Use to evaluate your current intake of nutrients, but realize that an AI designation implies that further research is required before scientists can establish a more definitive recommendation.
EER	Estimated Energy Requirement. Use to estimate calorie needs of the average person within a specific height, weight, gender, age, and physical activity pattern.
UL	Upper Level. Use to evaluate the highest amount of daily nutrient intake unlikely to cause adverse health effects in the long run in almost all people (97% to 98%) in a population. This number applies to chronic use and is set to protect even very susceptible people in the healthy general population. As intake increases above the Upper Level, the potential for adverse effects generally increases.
DV	Daily Value. Use as a rough guide for comparing the nutrient content of a food to approximate human needs. Typically, the Daily Value used on food labels refers to ages 4 years through adulthood. It is based on a 2000 kcal diet. Some Daily Values also increase slightly with higher calorie intakes (see Fig. 2-16 in the section on food labeling).

Although nutrition recommendations are often made for the entire healthy population, each of us have individual needs based on our particular health status and genetic background. It would be more appropriate, but also more expensive, if recommendations were made on an individual basis once a person's health status is known.

Dietary Reference Intakes (DRIs) Term used to encompass nutrient recommendations made by the Food and Nutrition Board of the National Academy of Sciences. These include RDAs, EARs, AIs, EERs, and ULs.

Recommended Dietary Allowance (RDA) Nutrient intake amount sufficient to meet the needs of 97% to 98% of the individuals in a specific life stage.

Adequate Intake (AI) Nutrient intake amount set for any nutrient for which insufficient research is available to establish an RDA. AIs are based on estimates of intakes that appear to maintain a defined nutritional state in a specific life stage.

Estimated Energy Requirement (EER) Estimate of the energy (kcal) intake needed to match the energy use of an average person in a specific life stage.

Tolerable Upper Intake Level (UL) Maximum chronic daily intake level of a nutrient that is unlikely to cause adverse health effects in almost all people in a specific life stage.

Estimated Energy Requirement

For calorie needs, we use the Estimated Energy Requirement (EER) instead of an RDA or AI. As described, the RDAs are set somewhat higher than the average needs for nutrients. This is fine for nutrients other than calories because a slight excess of vitamins and minerals is not harmful. However, a long-term excess of even a small amount of calories will lead to weight gain. Therefore, the calculation of EER needs to be more specific, taking into account age, gender, height, weight, and physical activity (e.g., sedentary or moderately active). In some cases, the additional calorie needs for growth and lactation are also included (see Chapters 7, 14, and 15 for the specific formulas used). Note that the EER is based on the "average" person. Thus, it can only serve as a starting point for estimating calorie needs.

Tolerable Upper Intake Level

A Tolerable Upper Intake Level (Upper Level or UL) has been set for some vitamins and minerals (see the inside cover). The UL is the highest amount of a nutrient unlikely to cause adverse health effects in the long run. As intake exceeds the UL, the risk of ill effects increases. These amounts generally should not be exceeded day after day, as toxicity could develop. For people eating a varied diet and/or using a balanced multivitamin and mineral supplement, exceeding the UL is unusual. Problems are more likely to arise with diets that promote excessive intakes of a limited variety of foods, with the use of many fortified foods, or with excessive doses of individual vitamins or minerals.

Daily Value

A nutrition standard more relevant to everyday life is the Daily Value (DV). This is a generic standard used on food labels. It is applicable to both genders from 4 years of age through adulthood, and is based on consuming a 2000 kcal diet. DVs are mostly set at or close to the highest RDA value or related nutrient standard seen in the various age and gender categories for a specific nutrient (see Appendix B). DVs have been set for vitamins, minerals, protein, and other dietary components. For fat and cholesterol, the DVs represent a maximum level, not a goal one should strive to reach. DVs allow consumers to compare their intake from a specific food to desirable (or maximum) intakes.

How Should These Nutrient Standards Be Used?

To sum up the acronyms described so far, the type of standard set for nutrients depends on the quality of available evidence. A nutrient recommendation backed by lots of experimental research will have an RDA. For a nutrient that still requires more research, only an AI is presented. We use the EER as a starting point for determining calorie needs. Some nutrients also have a UL if information on toxicity or adverse health effects is available. Periodically, new DRIs become available as expert committees review and interpret the available research.

RDAs and related standards are intended mainly for diet planning. Specifically, a diet plan should aim to meet the RDA or AI as appropriate and not to exceed the UL over the long term (Fig. 2-6). Specific RDA, AI, EER, and UL standards are printed on the inside cover of this book. To learn more about these nutrient standards, visit the link for Food and Nutrition on the Institute of Medicine's website (www.iom.edu).

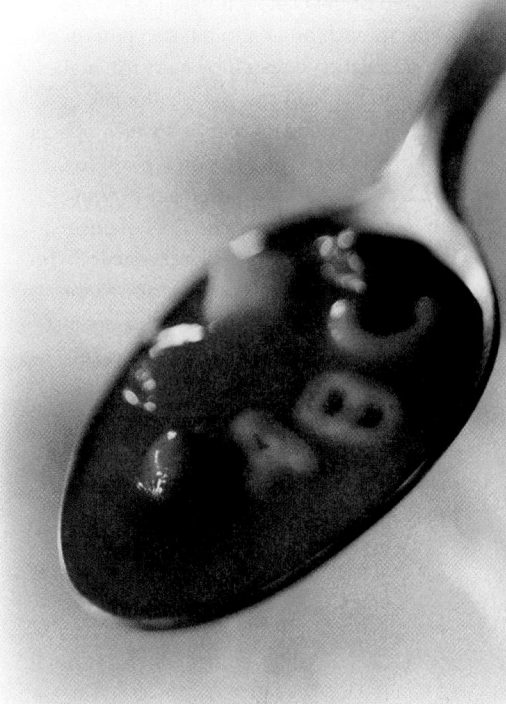

▲ With a little bit of study, you can master the alphabet soup of nutrition recommendations.

MAKING DECISIONS

Using Nutrient Recommendations

As nutrient intake increases, the Recommended Dietary Allowance (RDA) for the nutrient, if set, is eventually met and a deficient state is no longer present. An individual's needs most likely will be met since RDAs are set high to include almost all people. Related to the RDA concept of meeting an individual's needs are the standards of Adequate Intake (AI) and the Estimated Energy Requirement (EER). These can be used to estimate an individual's needs for some nutrients and calories, respectively. Still, keep in mind that these standards do not share the same degree of accuracy as the RDA. For example, EER may have to be adjusted upward if the individual is very physically active. Finally, as nutrient intake increases above the Upper Level (UL), poor nutritional health is again likely. However, this poor health is due now to the toxic effects of a nutrient, rather than those of a deficiency.

CONCEPT CHECK

Standards for nutrient intake are included in the broad category of Dietary Reference Intakes (DRIs). The Recommended Dietary Allowances (RDAs) are the amounts of each nutrient that will meet the needs of healthy individuals within specific gender and age categories. If not enough information is available to set an RDA, an Adequate Intake (AI) value is used. Tolerable Upper Intake Levels (ULs) are the highest amounts of a nutrient unlikely to cause adverse health effects. ULs have been set for some vitamins and minerals.

FIGURE 2-6 ▶ This figure shows the relationship of the Dietary Reference Intakes (DRIs) to each other and the percentage of the population covered by each. At intakes between the RDA and the UL, the risk of either an inadequate diet or adverse effects from the nutrient in question is close to 0. The UL is then the highest level of nutrient intake likely to pose no risks of adverse health effects to almost all individuals in the general population. At intakes above the UL, the margin of safety to protect against adverse effects is reduced. The AI is set for some nutrients instead of an RDA. The Food and Nutrition Board states that there is no established benefit for healthy individuals if they consume nutrient intakes above the RDA or AI.

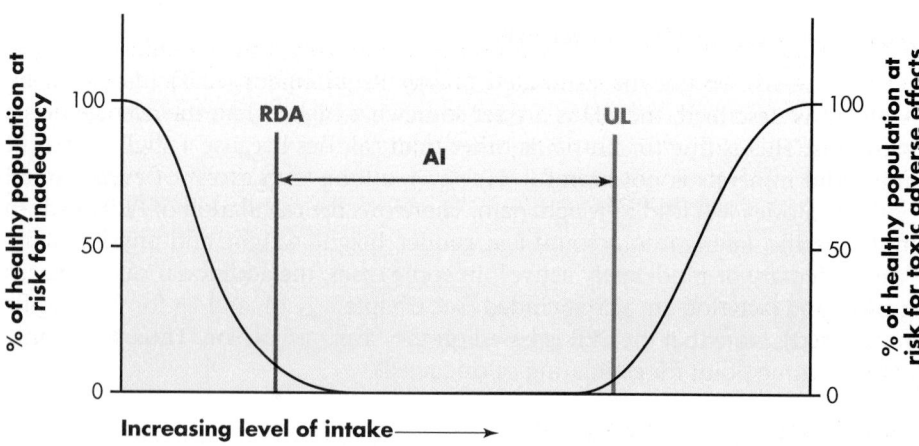

Recommended Dietary Allowance (RDA): The dietary intake level that is sufficient to meet the nutrient requirement of nearly all (97% to 98%) healthy individuals in a particular life stage and gender group. When set for a nutrient, aim for this intake.

Adequate Intake (AI): A recommended intake value based on observed or experimentally determined approximations or estimates of nutrient intake by a group (or groups) of healthy people that is assumed to be adequate—used when an RDA cannot be determined. When set for a nutrient, aim for this intake.

Tolerable Upper Intake Level (Upper Level or UL): The highest level of nutrient intake that is likely to pose no risk of adverse health effects for almost all individuals in the general population. As intake increases above the Upper Level, the risk of adverse effects increases.

2.6 Recommendations for Healthy Living

Since the early twentieth century, researchers have worked to translate the science of nutrition into practical terms so that people with no special training could estimate whether their nutritional needs were being met. Early food guidance systems aimed to reduce risk for nutrient deficiencies, but severe deficiency diseases are no longer common. Marginal deficiencies of calcium, iron, folate and other B vitamins, vitamin C, vitamin D, vitamin E, potassium, magnesium, and fiber are still a problem; but for many North Americans, major health problems stem from overconsumption of one or more of the following: calories, saturated fat, cholesterol, *trans* fat, alcohol, and sodium (see Further Reading 18).

The following sections of Chapter 2 will describe guidelines and tools for planning healthy lifestyles. You will notice how those core concepts of variety, balance, and moderation keep showing up throughout our discussions of the Dietary Guidelines, MyPlate, and the Physical Activity Guidelines.

Dietary Guidelines—The Basis for Menu Planning

The 2010 **Dietary Guidelines for Americans** provide nutrition and physical activity advice based on the latest and strongest scientific information to improve the health of all Americans age 2 and older (see Further Readings 12 and 14). The USDA and U.S. Department of Health and Human Services (DHHS) have published Dietary Guidelines since 1980 to aid diet planning. In light of the current epidemic of overweight and obesity—pressing health issues that now affect two-thirds of adults and one-third of children and adolescents—the message of calorie balance is woven throughout this seventh edition of the Dietary Guidelines.

The most important changes from the 2005 edition of the Dietary Guidelines include powerful emphases on reduction of total calories, sugar-sweetened beverages, saturated fat, and sodium. In addition, the report calls for a much-needed increase in physical activity among all population groups. Previous editions of the Dietary Guidelines have targeted healthy Americans, but these latest recommendations also include those at risk of developing chronic diseases. The health of children is highlighted. The new recommendations are also more culturally sensitive to reflect the

Dietary Guidelines for Americans General goals for nutrient intakes and diet composition set by the USDA and the U.S. Department of Health and Human Services.

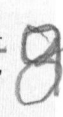

Losing weight is a challenge that takes time and continual awareness of calorie balance. We live in an *obesogenic* environment. With around-the-clock access to an increasing variety of super-sized, energy-dense foods, the typical American consumes about 600 more kilocalories per day than in 1970. Furthermore, out of convenience or necessity, our work, school, and home lives are dominated by sedentary activities.

growing diversity and varied health concerns of the American population. Finally, the new Dietary Guidelines recognize the prevalence of food insecurity (see Chapter 12), aiming to help populations with limited access to food optimize the nutritional content of meals within their resource constraints.

The Dietary Guidelines give direction for the development of educational materials, aid policy makers, and serve as the basis for consumer nutrition messages (see Further Reading 7). Overall, Americans should use this information along with related tools, such as MyPlate and the Physical Activity Guidelines for Americans, to form lifestyle patterns that optimize health.

The report identifies 29 key recommendations (outlined in Figure 2-7) to support three major goals:

- Balance calories with physical activity to manage weight. ✓
- Consume more of certain foods and nutrients, such as fruits, vegetables, whole grains, fat-free and low-fat dairy products, and seafood. ✓
- Consume fewer foods with sodium (salt), saturated fats, *trans* fats, cholesterol, added sugars, and refined grains.

Appendix C contains nutrient guidelines for Canadians.

CRITICAL THINKING

Shannon has grown up eating the typical American diet. Having recently read and heard many media reports about the relationship between nutrition and health, she is beginning to look critically at her diet and is considering making changes. However, she doesn't know where to begin. What advice would you give her?

FIGURE 2-7 ▶ Key Recommendations from the 2010 Dietary Guidelines for Americans

BALANCING CALORIES TO MANAGE WEIGHT

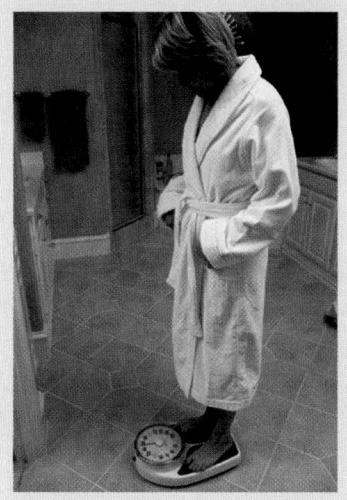

- Prevent and/or reduce overweight and obesity through improved eating and physical activity behaviors.
- Control total calorie intake to manage body weight. For people who are overweight or obese, this will mean consuming fewer calories from foods and beverages.
- Increase physical activity and reduce time spent in sedentary behaviors.
- Maintain appropriate calorie balance during each stage of life—childhood, adolescence, adulthood, pregnancy and breastfeeding, and older age.

Key Recommendations for Specific Population Groups

- Women of childbearing age: Achieve and maintain a healthy weight before becoming pregnant.
- *Pregnant women*: Gain weight within the 2009 Institute of Medicine gestational weight-gain guidelines.
- Adults ages 65 years and older: If overweight, avoid additional weight gain. For those with cardiovascular disease risk factors, lose weight to improve quality of life and reduce risk of chronic diseases and associated disabilities.

FOODS AND FOOD COMPONENTS TO REDUCE

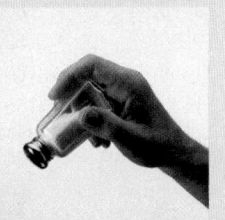

- Reduce daily sodium intake to less than 2300 mg and further reduce intake to 1500 mg among persons who are 51 and older and those of any age who are African-American or have hypertension, diabetes, or chronic kidney disease. The 1500-mg recommendation applies to about half of the U.S. population, including children, and the majority of adults.
- Consume less than 10% of calories from saturated fatty acids by replacing them with monounsaturated and polyunsaturated fatty acids.
- Consume less than 300 mg per day of dietary cholesterol.
- Keep *trans* fatty acid consumption as low as possible by limiting foods that contain synthetic sources of *trans* fats, such as partially hydrogenated oils, and by limiting other solid fats.
- Reduce the intake of calories from solid fats and added sugars.
- Limit the consumption of foods that contain refined grains, especially refined grain foods that contain solid fats, added sugars, and sodium.
- If alcohol is consumed, it should be consumed in moderation—up to one drink per day for women and two drinks per day for men—and only by adults of legal drinking age.

continued on next page

10, 11, 12, 13, 14

FIGURE 2-7 ▶ continued

FOODS AND NUTRIENTS TO INCREASE

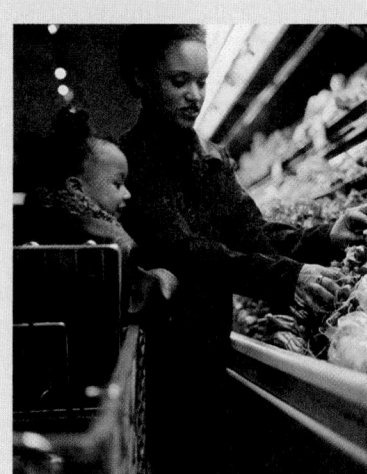

- Increase vegetable and fruit intake.

- Eat a variety of vegetables, especially dark-green and red and orange vegetables and beans and peas.

- Consume at least half of all grains as whole gains. Increase whole-grain intake by replacing refined grains with whole grains.

- Increase intake of fat-free or low-fat milk and milk products, such as milk, yogurt, cheese, or fortified soy beverages.

- Choose a variety of protein foods, which include seafood, lean meat and poultry, eggs, beans and peas, soy products, and unsalted nuts and seeds.

- Increase the amount and variety of seafood consumed by choosing seafood in place of some meat and poultry.

- Replace protein foods that are higher in solid fats with choices that are lower in solid fat and calories and/or sources of oils.

- Use oils to replace solid fats where possible.

10
- Choose foods that provide more potassium, dietary fiber, calcium, and vitamin D, which are nutrients of concern in American diets. These foods include vegetables, fruits, whole grains, and milk and milk products.

For women capable of becoming pregnant:

11
- Choose foods that supply heme iron (e.g., lean red meat), which is more readily absorbed by the body, additional iron sources, and enhancers of iron absorption, such as vitamin C-rich foods.

12
- Consume 400 micrograms per day of synthetic folic acid (from fortified foods and/or supplements) in addition to food forms of folate from a varied diet.

For women who are pregnant or breastfeeding:

13
- Consume 8 to 12 ounces of seafood per week from a variety of seafood types.

- Due to their high methyl mercury content, limit white (albacore) tuna to 6 ounces per week and do not eat the following four types of fish: tilefish, shark, swordfish, and king mackerel.

14
- If pregnant, take an iron supplement, as recommended by an obstetrician or other health care provider.

For individuals ages 50 years and older:

- Consume foods fortified with vitamin B-12, such as fortified cereals, or dietary supplements.

	Calorie Range (kcal)	
Children	Sedentary ⟶	Active
2–3 years	1000 ⟶	1400
Females		
4–8 years	1200 ⟶	1800
9–13	1400 ⟶	2200
14–18	1800 ⟶	2400
19–30	1800 ⟶	2400
31–50	1800 ⟶	2200
51+	1600 ⟶	2200
Males		
4–8 years	1200 ⟶	2000
9–13	1600 ⟶	2600
14–18	2000 ⟶	3200
19–30	2400 ⟶	3000
31–50	2200 ⟶	3000
51+	2000 ⟶	2800

The full report contains background on the development of the Dietary Guidelines, many informative tables and charts to support the recommendations, and a comprehensive list of consumer behaviors and key strategies for achieving each recommendation. This information is available at www.health .gov/dietaryguidelines.

Balancing Calories to Manage Weight. As you will see in Chapter 7, the balance between calories consumed (from foods and beverages) and calories expended (through physical activity and metabolic processes) determines body weight. Consuming too many calories without increasing physical activity will inevitably lead to weight gain, which exacts an enormous toll on individuals and communities. Many chronic diseases, especially cardiovascular disease, type 2 diabetes, and osteoporosis, could be alleviated by meeting nutrient needs within calorie limits.

The Dietary Guidelines encourage all Americans to achieve and maintain a healthy body weight. Knowing how many calories you need each day is a good place to start (Fig. 2-8). You can calculate your EER on your own (see Chapter 7) or use an online calculator such as the one at www.ChooseMyPlate.gov. Once calorie needs are known, the next step is to become familiar with the calorie

FIGURE 2-8 ▶ Estimates of calorie needs (kcals).

content of foods and beverages. Chapters 4, 5, and 6 will cover sources of calories in the diet. Finally, monitoring weight over time will allow you to see how your food and physical activity choices are balancing out.

Foods and Food Components to Reduce. Typical American diets contain too much sodium (salt), **solid fats** (e.g., butter), **added sugars,** and refined grains. Diets predominated by these food components especially increase risk for obesity, type 2 diabetes, hypertension, cardiovascular disease, and cancer.

Moderate alcohol consumption is associated with reduced risk of cardiovascular disease, deaths, and cognitive decline. However, those who do not drink should not begin drinking to attain these health benefits, because there are risks associated with even moderate alcohol consumption, including increased risk of breast cancer, violence, drowning, and injuries from falls and motor vehicle crashes. Heavy drinking is inherently risky and should be avoided altogether. More information about alcohol is presented in Chapter 16.

Foods and Nutrients to Increase. The Dietary Guidelines urge Americans to replace the problem foods we have discussed with nutrient-dense foods. Emphasize vegetables, fruits, whole grains, fat-free or low-fat milk and milk products, seafood, lean meats and poultry, eggs, beans and peas, and nuts and seeds. Instead of solid fats, choose foods made with vegetable oils.

These recommendations reflect the nutrient inadequacies of greatest public health concern: potassium, dietary fiber, calcium, and vitamin D. Individuals should strive to meet these goals without exceeding their calorie needs. Focusing on vegetables, fruits, whole grains, lean sources of protein, and low-fat or fat-free dairy products will not only contribute to nutrient adequacy but will also lower intake of problem nutrients, improve gastrointestinal function, aid in weight management, and decrease risk for a variety of chronic diseases.

A basic premise of the Dietary Guidelines is that nutrient needs should be met primarily through consuming foods. Foods provide an array of nutrients and other compounds that may benefit health. In certain cases, fortified foods and dietary supplements may be useful sources of one or more nutrients that otherwise might be consumed in less than recommended amounts. These are especially important for people whose typical food choices lead to a diet that cannot meet one or more nutrient recommendations, such as for vitamin D, vitamin E, or calcium. However, dietary supplements cannot and should not replace a healthy diet.

Building Healthy Eating Patterns. The Dietary Guidelines steer clear of a rigid prescription and, instead, promote an array of healthful options that can accommodate cultural, ethnic, traditional, and personal preferences, as well as food cost and availability factors. Well-studied examples of **eating patterns** consistent with the Dietary Guidelines include Dietary Approaches to Stop Hypertension (DASH), the USDA Food Patterns that accompanied MyPyramid (now MyPlate), vegetarian eating patterns, and Mediterranean-style eating patterns (see Further Reading 5). Common among these patterns are an abundance of vegetables and fruits, emphasis on whole grains, moderate amounts and varied sources of protein-rich foods, limited added sugars and solid fats, a high proportion of unsaturated fats compared to saturated fats, high potassium, and lower sodium.

The Dietary Guidelines and You. When applying the Dietary Guidelines, you need to consider your own state of health. Make specific changes and see whether they are effective for you. Note that results do not occur overnight and may not meet your expectations. Even when carefully following a diet low in saturated fat, some people continue to have high blood cholesterol. Other people can eat greater amounts of saturated fats and keep their blood cholesterol under control. Differences in genetic background are a key reason for these different responses, as you will learn in Chapter 3. Each of us must take into consideration our individual nutritional needs and

solid fats Fats that are solid at room temperature, such as butter and margarine. Foods containing solid fats tend to be high in saturated fatty acids or *trans* fatty acids.

added sugars Sugars or syrups that are added to foods during processing or preparation.

eating pattern A combination of foods and beverages that constitute an individual's complete dietary intake over time.

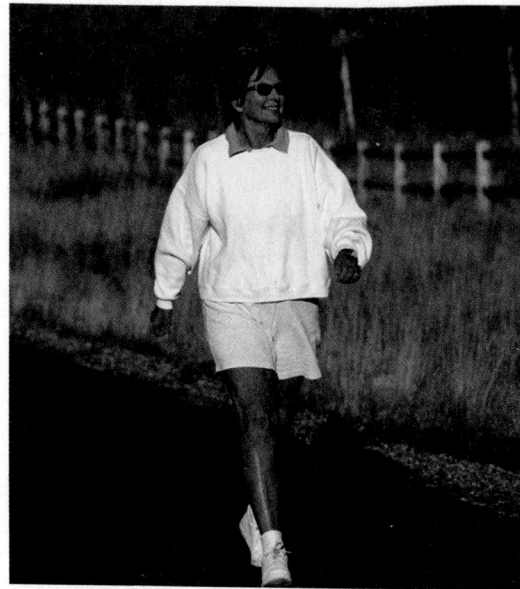

▲ Active means a lifestyle that includes physical activity equivalent to walking more than 3 miles per day at 3 to 4 miles per hour, in addition to the light physical activity associated with typical day-to-day life.

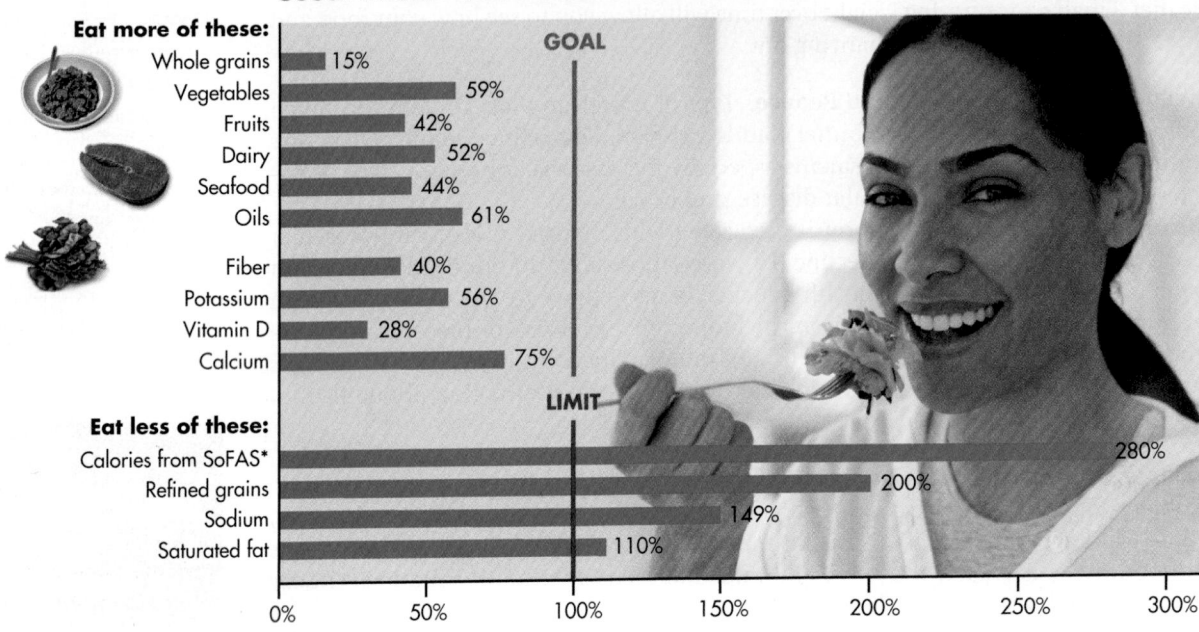

Usual Intake as a Percent of Goal or Limit

Eat more of these:

Whole grains	15%
Vegetables	59%
Fruits	42%
Dairy	52%
Seafood	44%
Oils	61%
Fiber	40%
Potassium	56%
Vitamin D	28%
Calcium	75%

Eat less of these:

Calories from SoFAS*	280%
Refined grains	200%
Sodium	149%
Saturated fat	110%

Percent of goal or limit

FIGURE 2-9 ▶

Comparing American Dietary habits to the Dietary Guidelines.

Source: Based on data from: U.S. Department of Agriculture, Agricultural Research Service and U.S. Department of Health and Human Services, Centers for Disease Control and Prevention. What We Eat in America, NHANES 2001–2004 or 2005–2006.

*SoFAS = solid fats and added sugars.
Note: Bars show average intakes for all individuals (ages 1 or 2 years or older, depending on the data source) as a percent of the recommended intake level or limit. Recommended intakes for food groups and limits for refined grains and solid fats and added sugars are based on amounts in the USDA 2000-calorie food pattern. Recommended intakes for fiber, potassium, vitamin D, and calcium are based on the highest AI or RDA for age 14 to 70 years. Limits for sodium are based on the UL and for saturated fat on 10% of calories. The protein foods group is not shown here because, on average, intake is close to recommended levels.

our risks of developing certain diseases (see Further Reading 3). Plan your diet with your specific needs in mind, taking into account your current health status and family history.

Whereas the Dietary Guidelines are not able to tailor a unique nutrition program for every North American citizen, they do provide adults with simple nutritional advice, which can be implemented by anyone willing to take a step toward good health. Table 2-5 provides examples of recommended diet changes based on the Dietary Guidelines. Although the cost of healthy eating is on the rise, you can make good choices and stay within your budget—canned or frozen fruits and vegetables and non-fat dry milk are a few of the available lower-cost foods.

Diet recommendations for adults have been issued by other scientific groups, such as the American Heart Association, U.S. Surgeon General, National Academy of Sciences, American Cancer Society, Canadian Ministries of Health (see Appendix C), and World Health Organization. All are consistent with the spirit of the Dietary Guidelines. These groups encourage people to modify their eating behaviors in ways that are both healthful and pleasurable.

MyPlate—A Menu-Planning Tool

The titles, food groupings, and shapes of food guides have evolved since the first edition published by the U.S. Department of Agriculture (USDA) nearly a century ago. The most recent food-guidance systems have incorporated physical activity and provided a means for individualization of dietary advice via interactive technology available on the Internet.

To keep pace with updated nutrition advice presented by the 2010 Dietary Guidelines for Americans and *Healthy People 2020* (see Chapter 1), MyPlate was released in 2011 as the leading depiction of healthy eating for Americans (Fig. 2-10). MyPlate,

FIGURE 2-10 ▶ MyPlate is a visual representation of the advice contained in the 2010 Dietary Guidelines for Americans.

TABLE 2-5 Recommended Diet Changes Based on the Dietary Guidelines

If You Usually Eat This,	Try This Instead	Benefit
White bread	Whole-wheat bread	• Higher nutrient density, due to less processing • More fiber
Sugary breakfast cereal	Low-sugar, high-fiber cereal with fresh fruit	• Higher nutrient density • More fiber • More phytochemicals
Cheeseburger with French fries	Hamburger and baked beans	• Less saturated fat and *trans* fat • Less cholesterol • More fiber • More phytochemicals
Potato salad	Three-bean salad	• More fiber • More phytochemicals
Doughnuts	Bran muffin/bagel with light cream cheese	• More fiber • Less fat
Regular soft drinks	Diet soft drinks	• Fewer calories
Boiled vegetables	Steamed vegetables	• Higher nutrient density, due to reduced loss of water-soluble vitamins
Canned vegetables	Fresh or frozen vegetables	• Higher nutrient density, due to reduced loss of heat-sensitive vitamins • Lower in sodium
Fried meats	Broiled meats	• Less saturated fat
Fatty meats, such as ribs or bacon	Lean meats, such as ground round, chicken, or fish	• Less saturated fat
Whole milk	Low-fat or fat-free milk	• Less saturated fat • Fewer calories • More calcium
Ice cream	Sherbet or frozen yogurt	• Less saturated fat • Fewer calories
Mayonnaise or sour cream salad dressing	Oil-and-vinegar dressings or light creamy dressings	• Less saturated fat • Less cholesterol • Fewer calories
Cookies	Popcorn (air popped with minimal margarine or butter)	• Fewer calories and *trans* fat
Heavily salted foods	Foods flavored primarily with herbs, spices, lemon juice	• Lower in sodium
Chips	Pretzels	• Less fat

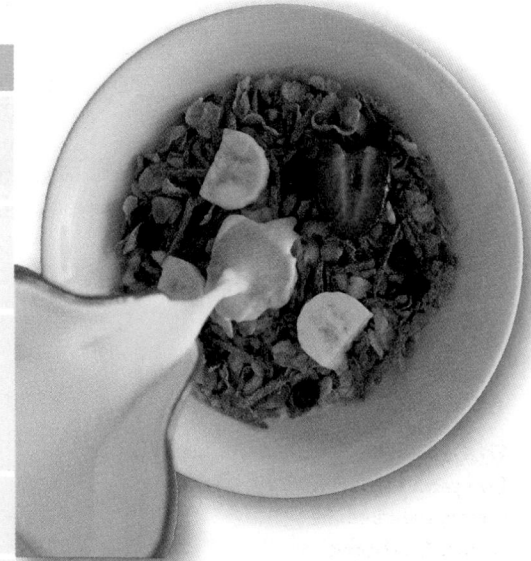

▲ Choose low-sugar, high-fiber cereal with fresh fruit instead of sugary breakfast cereal.

which replaces the familiar MyPyramid, shapes the key recommendations from the Dietary Guidelines into an easily recognizable and universally applicable visual: a place setting.

empty calories Calories from solid fats and/or added sugars. Foods with empty calories supply energy but few or no other nutrients.

NEWSWORTHY NUTRITION

Diet quality impacts waistlines and wallets

Diets with low energy density are associated with higher intakes of nutrients but also with higher food costs. Researchers used food-frequency questionnaires to assess dietary intake and food costs among 164 men and women in Seattle, Washington. Dietary data were compared with components of socioeconomic status. Household income and especially education were strong predictors of dietary energy density. The association between food spending and energy density was particularly strong for women. Nutrition advice to consume foods with lower energy density may be difficult to follow with limited financial resources. The increasing cost of consuming foods with low energy density and high nutrient density may play a role in the correlations between socioeconomic status (e.g., income and education) and rates of obesity and diet-related chronic diseases.

Source: Monsivais P, Drewnowski A. Lower-energy-density diets are associated with higher monetary costs per kilocalorie and are consumed by women of higher socioeconomic status. *Journal of the American Dietetic Association* 109:804, 2009.

connect NUTRITION

Check out the Connect site www.mcgrawhillconnect.com **to further explore energy density and food costs.**

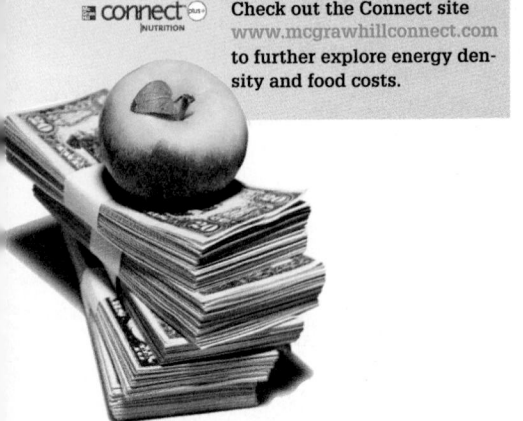

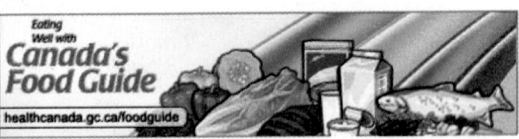

▲ In 1942, Canada released its first set of Official Food Rules. Since then, food guidance has evolved based on nutrition research and the changing needs of the population. Now, Health Canada publishes *Canada's Food Guide to Healthy Eating*, available in Appendix C.

Dishing Up MyPlate. Although it is not intended to stand alone as a source of dietary advice, MyPlate serves as a reminder of how to build a healthy plate at mealtimes (see Further Reading 13). It emphasizes important areas of the American diet that are in need of improvement. Recall from the discussion of the Dietary Guidelines that Americans need to increase the relative proportions of fruits, vegetables, whole grains, and fat-free or low-fat dairy products while simultaneously decreasing consumption of refined grains and high-fat meats.

The new MyPlate icon emphasizes five food groups:

- **Fruits** and **vegetables** cover half of the plate. These foods are dense sources of nutrients and health-promoting phytochemicals despite their low calorie contents.
- **Grains** occupy slightly more than one-fourth of the plate. The message to make half your grains whole is stressed throughout accompanying consumer-education materials.
- The remaining space on the plate is reserved for sources of **protein**. Specifically, the Dietary Guidelines recommend lean meats and poultry, plant sources of protein, and inclusion of fish twice a week.
- A cup of **dairy** appears next to the plate. Depending on personalized calorie recommendations, users should have 2 to 3 cups per day of low-fat or fat-free dairy products or other rich sources of calcium.

Unlike MyPyramid, MyPlate does not display a separate group for fats and oils, as they are mostly incorporated into other foods. Consumer messages tied to the MyPlate campaign reinforce recommendations to limit solid fats and focus instead on plant oils, which are sources of essential fatty acids and vitamin E.

Actionable Health Messages. Consumer research points to the need for simple, actionable health messages to capture the attention of the public and achieve successful behavior change. Accordingly, ChooseMyPlate.gov provides a series of succinct imperatives to help Americans make healthier food choices. Consumer messages include:

Balancing Calories

- Enjoy your food, but eat less.
- Avoid oversized portions.

Foods to Increase

- Make half your plate fruits and vegetables.
- Make at least half your grains whole.
- Switch to skim or 1% milk.

Foods to Reduce

- Compare sodium in foods like soup, bread, and frozen meals—and choose the foods with lower numbers.
- Drink water instead of sugary drinks.

Daily Food Plan. The Daily Food Plan is an interactive tool that estimates your calorie needs and suggests a food pattern based on your age, gender, height, and weight (Table 2-6). The Daily Food Plan provides useful information for each food group, including recommended daily amounts in common household measures, suggested oil intake, limits for **empty calories** and sodium, as well as advice for physical activity.

The recommended numbers of servings are given in cups for vegetables, fruits, and dairy foods. Grains and protein foods are listed in ounces. See Figure 2-11 for a description of what counts as a MyPlate serving. Pay close attention to the stated serving size for each choice when following your Daily Food Plan to help control calorie intake. Figure 2-12 provides a convenient guide to estimating common serving size measurements.

Modified daily food plans are also available for preschoolers, pregnant or breastfeeding mothers, and those interested in losing weight. Be sure to visit www.ChooseMyPlate.gov to generate your own Daily Food Plan.

TABLE 2-6 MyPlate Food-Intake Patterns Based on Calorie Needs

Daily Amount of Food from Each Group

Calorie Level	1000	1200	1400	1600	1800	2000	2200	2400	2600	2800	3000	3200
Fruits	1 cup	1 cup	1.5 cups	1.5 cups	1.5 cups	2 cups	2 cups	2 cups	2 cups	2.5 cups	2.5 cups	2.5 cups
Vegetables[1,2]	1 cup	1.5 cups	1.5 cups	2 cups	2.5 cups	2.5 cups	3 cups	3 cups	3.5 cups	3.5 cups	4 cups	4 cups
Grains[3]	3 oz-eq	4 oz-eq	5 oz-eq	5 oz-eq	6 oz-eq	6 oz-eq	7 oz-eq	8 oz-eq	9 oz-eq	10 oz-eq	10 oz-eq	10 oz-eq
Protein Foods	2 oz-eq	3 oz-eq	4 oz-eq	5 oz-eq	5 oz-eq	5.5 oz-eq	6 oz-eq	6.5 oz-eq	6.5 oz-eq	7 oz-eq	7 oz-eq	7 oz-eq
Dairy[4]	2 cups	2 cups	2 cups	3 cups	3 cups	3 cups	3 cups	3 cups	3 cups	3 cups	3 cups	3 cups
Oils[5]	3 tsp	4 tsp	4 tsp	5 tsp	5 tsp	6 tsp	6 tsp	7 tsp	8 tsp	8 tsp	10 tsp	11 tsp
Empty Calorie Limit[6]	140	120	120	120	160	260	270	330	360	400	460	600

oz-eq stands for ounce equivalent; tsp stands for teaspoon.

[1]Vegetables are divided into five subgroups (dark green, orange, legumes, starchy, and other). Over a week's time, a variety of vegetables should be eaten, especially green and orange vegetables.

[2]Dry beans and peas can be counted *either* as vegetables (dry beans and peas subgroup), *or* in the protein foods group. Generally, individuals who regularly eat meat, poultry, and fish would count dry beans and peas in the vegetable group. Individuals who seldom eat meat, poultry, or fish (vegetarians) would consume more dry beans and peas and count some of them in the protein foods group until enough servings from that group are chosen for the day.

[3]At least half of the grain servings should be whole-grain varieties.

[4]Most of the dairy servings should be fat-free or low-fat.

[5]Limit solid fats such as butter, stick margarine, shortening, and meat fat, as well as foods that contain these.

[6]Empty calories refers to added sugars and/or solid fats.

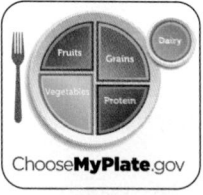

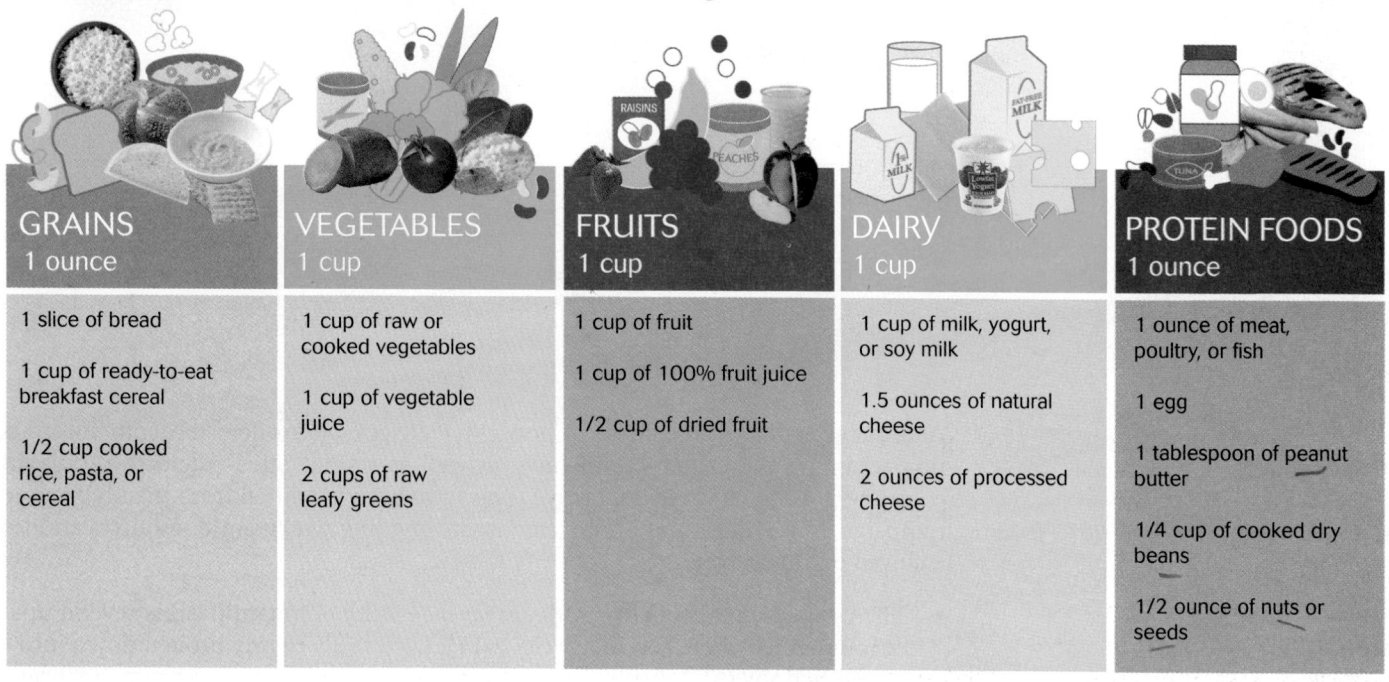

FIGURE 2-11 ▶ MyPlate: What counts as a serving?

Portion sizes

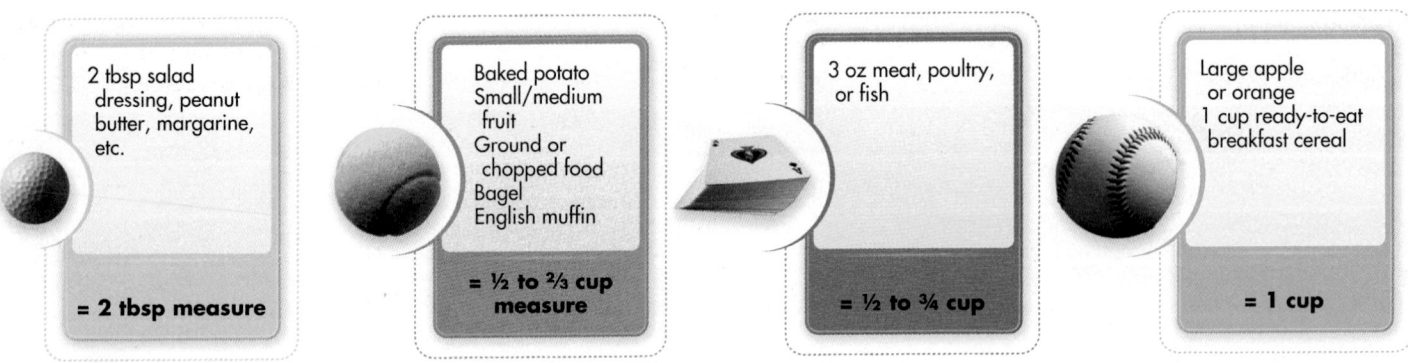

2 tbsp salad dressing, peanut butter, margarine, etc.	Baked potato Small/medium fruit Ground or chopped food Bagel English muffin	3 oz meat, poultry, or fish	Large apple or orange 1 cup ready-to-eat breakfast cereal
= 2 tbsp measure	= ½ to ⅔ cup measure	= ½ to ¾ cup	= 1 cup

FIGURE 2-12 ▶ A golf ball, tennis ball, deck of cards, and baseball are standard-size objects that make convenient guides for judging serving sizes. Your hand provides an additional handy guide (for the greatest accuracy, compare your fist with a baseball, and adjust the following guides accordingly).

Fist = 1 cup
Thumb = 1 oz of cheese
Thumb tip to first joint = 1 tsp

Palm of hand = 3 oz
Handful = 1 or 2 oz of a snack food

MAKING DECISIONS

Measuring Your Portion Size

How familiar are you with serving size measurements? Common household units are listed in Appendix I with their metric equivalents. Ounces and fluid ounces differ. Ounces are a measure of weight, while fluid ounces are a measure of volume. Fluid ounces are based on the corresponding volume of water as the standard; 1 ounce of water by weight equals 1 fluid ounce. Any fluid more or less dense than water will yield a different number of fluid ounces per ounce of material.

MAKING DECISIONS

Empty Calories

MyPlate sets limits for empty calories, which come from solid fats and/or added sugars (Fig. 2-13). Solid fats and added sugars add calories to the diet but contribute few nutrients. Solid fats are solid at room temperature and include butter, beef fat, and shortening. Some solid fats, such as the marbling in a cut of ribeye steak, are naturally present in foods. Others, such as the shortening used to make a flaky croissant, are added during food processing or preparation. Added sugars include sugars and syrups that are added to foods during processing or preparation. Examples of foods that are major contributors of empty calories in the American diet are cakes, cookies, pastries, soft drinks, energy drinks, cheese, pizza, ice cream, and processed meats. The Daily Food Plans available on www.ChooseMyPlate.gov allow for 120 to 600 empty calories per day, depending on total energy needs:

Calorie Intake (kcal)	Empty Calories (kcal)	Calorie Intake (kcal)	Empty Calories (kcal)
1000*	140	2200	270
1200*	120	2400	330
1400*	120	2600	360
1600	120	2800	400
1800	160	3000	460
2000	260	3200	600

*Calorie intakes below 1600 kcal per day are generally intended for children 2 to 8 years of age. Unless under the guidance of a physician or registered dietitian, adults should consume at least 1600 kcal per day.

The International Food Information Council, available online at www.ific.org, is another great resource for current nutrition information.

Additional MyPlate Resources. ChooseMyPlate.gov also offers in-depth information regarding the Dietary Guidelines, as well as several other interactive tools for consumers. Many of these interactive tools have been modified from the MyPyramid campaign, but updates and improvements are ongoing. MyPyramid resources are also archived on the website.

- USDA's consumer brochure, *Let's Eat for the Health of It,* emphasizes several tips for improving Americans' diets (Fig. 2-14). Each tip is clearly broken down into specific actions the consumer can take. For example, one key recommendation

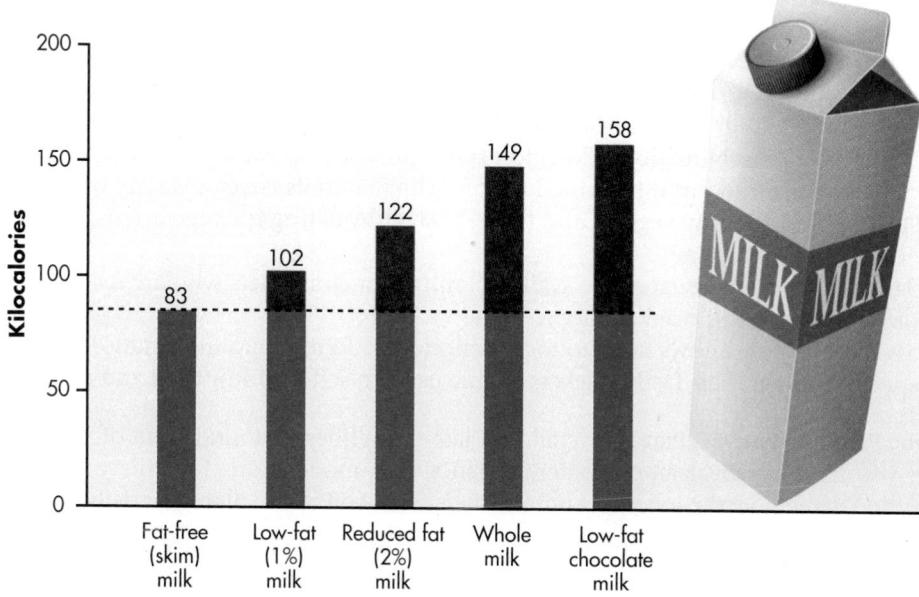

FIGURE 2-13 ▶ Empty calories come from solid fats and/or added sugars. This bar graph compares the amounts of empty calories in various types of milk.

Grains
Make half your grains whole grains

Use whole grains in mixed dishes, such as barley in vegetable soup or stews and bulgur wheat in casseroles or stir-fries.

Add whole-grain flour or oatmeal when making cookies or other baked treats.

Use the Nutrition Facts label and choose whole-grain products with a higher % Daily Value (%DV) for fiber. Many, but not all, whole-grain products are good or excellent sources of fiber.

Vegetables
Vary your veggies

Buy fresh vegetables in season. They cost less and are likely to be at their peak flavor.

Include chopped vegetables in pasta sauce or lasagna.

Allow children to pick a new vegetable to try while shopping.

Fruits
Focus on fruits

Make most of your choices whole or cut-up fruit rather than fruit juice, for the benefits dietary fiber provides.

Select fruits with more potassium often, such as bananas, prunes and prune juice, dried peaches and apricots, and orange juice.

Add fruits like pineapple or peaches to kabobs as part of a barbeque meal.

Dairy
Get your calcium-rich foods

Include milk or calcium-fortified soymilk as a beverage at meals. Choose fat-free or low-fat milk.

If you avoid milk because of lactose intolerance, the most reliable way to get the health benefits of dairy products is to choose lactose-free alternatives within the Dairy Group, such as cheese, yogurt, lactose-free milk, or calcium-fortified soy milk or to consume the enzyme lactase before consuming milk.

Protein
Go lean with protein

The leanest beef cuts include round steaks and roasts (eye of round, top round, bottom round, round tip), top loin, sirloin, and chuck shoulder and arm roasts.

Trim away all of the visible fat from meats and poultry before cooking.

Choose beans, peas, or soy products as a main dish or part of a meal often.

Physical Activity

Find your balance between food and physical activity
- Do stretches, exercises, or pedal a stationary bike while watching television.
- Replace a coffee break with a brisk 10-minute walk. Ask a friend to go with you.
- Get the whole family involved—enjoy an afternoon bike ride with your kids.

Food Safety

Keep food safe to eat
- Wash your hands with warm water and soap for at least 20 seconds before and after handling food and after using the bathroom or changing diapers.
- Separate raw meat, poultry, seafood, and eggs from other foods in your grocery shopping cart, grocery bags, and in your refrigerator.
- Use a food thermometer, which measures the internal temperature of cooked meat, poultry, and egg dishes, to make sure that the food is cooked to a safe internal temperature.

FIGURE 2-14 ▶ These consumer tips have been developed by the USDA to help you build healthy meals with MyPlate. Many more tips are available at www.ChooseMyPlate.gov.

is "Cut back on foods high in solid fats, added sugars, and salt." One way a consumer can put this message into practice is to choose foods and drinks with little or no added sugars. Specific techniques associated with this recommendation include "Drink water instead of sugary drinks," "Select fruit for dessert," and "Choose 100% fruit juice instead of fruit-flavored drinks."

- USDA's Ten Tips Nutrition Education series provides access to one-page handouts for consumers and health educators. The materials cover a variety of topics, such as "Kid-friendly veggies and fruits," "Healthy eating for vegetarians," and "Got your dairy today?"
- Sample menus and recipes are available online for consumers who are ready to make a change and need a place to start.
- MyFood-a-Pedia allows users to locate calorie and food group information for specific food entries. Daily trackers enable users to self-monitor food and activity.

Menu Planning with MyPlate. Overall, MyPlate exemplifies the foundations of a healthy diet you have already learned: variety, balance, and moderation. To achieve optimal nutrition, remember the following points when using MyPlate to plan your daily menus:

- The guide does not apply to infants or children under 2 years of age. Daily Food Plans for children from ages 2 to 8 are based on average height and weight for age and gender.
- Variety is key to successful implementation of MyPlate. There is no single, perfect food that is absolutely essential to good nutrition. Each food is rich in some nutrients but deficient in at least one essential nutrient. Likewise, no food group is more important than another; each food group makes an important, distinctive contribution to nutritional intake (Table 2-7). Choose foods from each food group and also choose different foods within each food group. For a sample meal plan, see Table 2-8.
- The foods within a group may vary widely with respect to nutrients and calories. For example, the calorie content of 3 ounces of baked potato is 98 kcal, whereas that of 3 ounces of potato chips is 470 kcal. With respect to vitamin C, an orange has 70 mg and an apple has 10 mg.

Solid fats contribute almost 20% of total calories in typical American diets, but they have little to offer in terms of essential nutrients and dietary fiber. Instead of solid fats, choose foods containing plant oils.

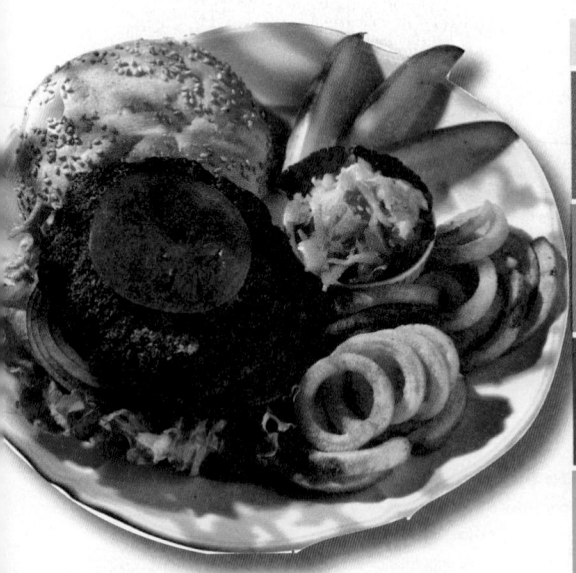

▲ Typical restaurant meals contain oversized portions that do not align with MyPlate.

TABLE 2-7 Nutrient Contributions of MyPlate Food Groups

Food Category	Major Nutrient Contributions
Grains	Carbohydrate Vitamins such as thiamin Minerals such as iron Fiber*
Vegetables	Carbohydrate Vitamins such as plant pigments that form vitamin A Minerals such as magnesium Fiber
Fruits	Carbohydrate Vitamins such as folate and vitamin C Minerals such as potassium Fiber
Dairy	Carbohydrate Protein Vitamins such as vitamin D Minerals such as calcium and phosphorus
Protein Foods	Protein Vitamins such as vitamin B-6 Minerals such as iron and zinc

*Whole-grain varieties

TABLE 2-8 Putting MyPlate into Practice.

Meal	Food Group
Breakfast	
1 small orange	Fruits
¾ cup Healthy Choice Low-fat Granola	Grains
with ½ cup fat-free milk	Dairy
½ toasted, small raisin bagel	Grains
with 1 tsp soft margarine	Oils
Optional: coffee or tea	
Lunch	
Turkey sandwich	
2 slices whole-wheat bread	Grains
2 oz turkey	Protein Foods
2 tsp mustard	
1 small apple	Fruits
2 oatmeal-raisin cookies (small)	Empty Calories
Optional: diet soft drink	
3 P.M. Study Break	
6 whole-wheat crackers	Grains
1 tbsp peanut butter	Protein Foods
½ cup fat-free milk	Dairy
Dinner	
Tossed salad	
1 cup romaine lettuce	Vegetables
½ cup sliced tomatoes	Vegetables
1½ tbsp Italian dressing	Oils
½ carrot, grated	Vegetables
3 oz broiled salmon	Protein Foods
½ cup rice	Grains
½ cup green beans	Vegetables
with 1 tsp soft margarine	Oils
Optional: coffee or tea	
Late-Night Snack	
1 cup "light" fruit yogurt	Dairy
Nutrient Breakdown	
1800 kcal	
Carbohydrate	56% of kcal
Protein	18% of kcal
Fat	26% of kcal

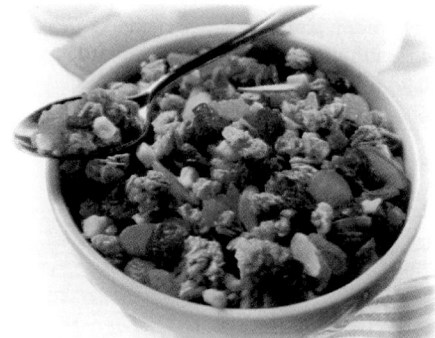
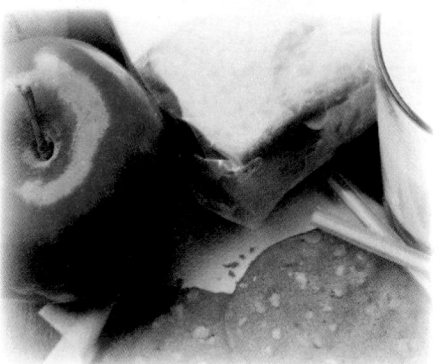
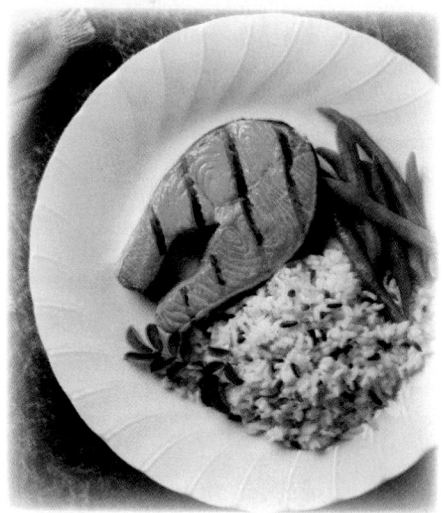

This menu meets nutrient needs for all vitamins and minerals for an average adult who needs 1800 kcal. For adolescents, teenagers, and older adults, add one additional serving of milk or other calcium-rich sources.

- •Choose primarily low-fat and fat-free items from the dairy group. By reducing calorie intake in this way, you can select more items from other food groups. If milk causes intestinal gas and bloating, emphasize yogurt and cheese (see Chapter 4 for details on the problem of lactose maldigestion and lactose intolerance).

Check out CONNECT for links to alternative menu planning tools, such as the Healthy Eating Plate from Harvard School of Public Health. ☰connect NUTRITION

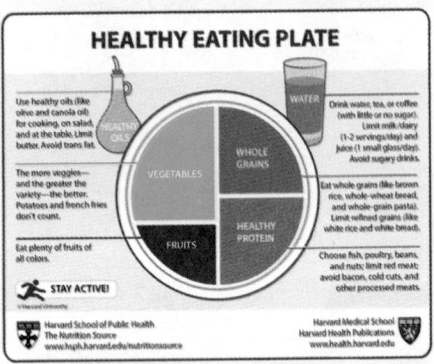

The **Exchange System** is an alternative menu-planning tool. This tool organizes foods based on calorie, protein, carbohydrate, and fat content. The result is a manageable framework for designing diets, especially for treatment of diabetes. For more information on the Exchange System, see Appendix D.

2008 Physical Activity Guidelines for Americans

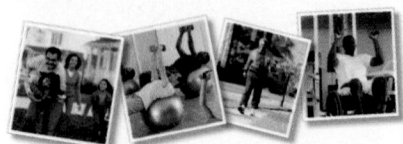

Be Active, Healthy, and Happy!

www.health.gov/paguidelines

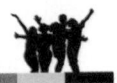

▲ http://www.health.gov/PAGuidelines/.

- Include plant foods that are good sources of proteins, such as beans and nuts, at least several times a week because many are rich in vitamins (such as vitamin E), minerals (such as magnesium), and fiber.
- For vegetables and fruits, try to include a dark-green or orange vegetable for vitamin A and a vitamin-C rich fruit, such as an orange, every day. Do not focus primarily on potatoes (e.g., French fries) for your vegetable choices. Surveys show that fewer than 5% of adults eat a full serving of a dark-green vegetable on any given day. Increased consumption of these foods is important because they contribute vitamins, minerals, fiber, and phytochemicals.
- Choose whole-grain varieties of breads, cereals, rice, and pasta because they contribute vitamin E and fiber. A daily serving of a whole-grain, ready-to-eat breakfast cereal is an excellent choice because the vitamins (such as vitamin B-6) and minerals (such as zinc) typically added to it, along with fiber, help fill in common nutritional gaps.
- Include some plant oils on a daily basis, such as those in salad dressing, and eat fish at least twice a week. This supplies you with health-promoting essential fatty acids.

Reviews of MyPlate. Although MyPlate will promote important changes in American diets, it does have some limitations. Some critics say that the new icon is too simple. For example, it does not immediately provide information about overall calories, serving sizes, or number of servings to choose from each food group (recall the comic at the beginning of this chapter). However, many of these details will vary by person. Users will need to access the accompanying materials available on www.ChooseMyPlate.gov to obtain a personally tailored Daily Food Plan.

Food *quality* is just as important as food *quantity* when it comes to good nutrition. Consider the difference in calorie contents of the following two meals, both of which fit the proportions suggested by MyPlate:

Fried chicken fillet sandwich with mayonnaise on a white sandwich roll, 1 each	Skinless grilled chicken breast, 3 ounces
French fries, 1 medium order	Brown rice, prepared with reduced-fat tub margarine, 1 cup
Apple-filled pastry, 1 each	Steamed green beans, 1 cup
Whole milk, 1 cup	Cubed watermelon, 1 cup
1293 kcal	Skim milk, 1 cup
	513 kcal

The MyPlate icon does not address the types of foods to choose within each food group. Making appropriate food choices for weight management and prevention of diet-related chronic diseases requires consumers to have some nutrition knowledge. Fortunately, public health messages and online content related to MyPlate are available to educate Americans.

MyPlate shows how to build a healthy plate at mealtimes, but it does not adequately address the total diet, which, in reality, includes many snacks between meals. Consumer messages about healthy snacking will be a part of the consumer communications initiative over the next few years.

As with any public health campaign, it is possible that the people who need it most will overlook the MyPlate message. Educated consumers with access to interactive MyPlate tools likely already comply with many of the Dietary Guidelines. Populations with poor diets may be unlikely or unable to click through to find a personalized Daily Food Plan. The USDA's best response is to rely on the coordinated partnership of the National Communicator's Network to spread those actionable MyPlate messages, such as "Switch to fat-free or low-fat (1%) milk."

Overall, the new MyPlate icon is an attractive and relevant tool that immediately shows us how to build a healthy plate at meals. The strength of MyPlate lies in its simplicity. It conveys the major messages that are needed when shopping, cooking, and eating and can be enhanced with the details provided on www.ChooseMyPlate.gov and in forthcoming materials.

MAKING DECISIONS

The Mediterranean Diet Pyramid

Recently updated in 2009, the Mediterranean Diet Pyramid (Fig. 2-15) is a useful alternative to MyPlate. It is based on the dietary patterns of the southern Mediterranean region, which has enjoyed the lowest recorded rates of chronic diseases and the highest adult life expectancy. An abundance of research supports the health benefits of following the Mediterranean Diet (see Further Reading 9). Characteristics include:

- Foods from plant sources form the foundation of every meal.
- A variety of minimally processed and, wherever possible, seasonally fresh and locally grown foods are emphasized.
- Olive oil is the principal fat.
- Total fat ranges from less than 25% to over 35% of energy, with saturated fat no more than 7% to 8% of calories.
- Fish and seafood are consumed at least twice weekly.
- Lean or low-fat sources of protein, such as cheese, yogurt, poultry, and eggs, should be consumed in moderation.
- Red meats and sweet desserts are consumed less often.
- Regular physical activity is performed at a level that promotes a healthy weight, fitness, and well-being.
- Moderate wine drinking has health benefits.
- Water is the beverage of choice.

Oldways—a respected, international, nonprofit culinary think tank—also publishes the Latin-American Diet Pyramid and was the force behind development of the Whole Grain stamp seen on food packages.

Source: Oldways Food Issues Think Tank, 266 Beacon St., Boston, MA 02116, www.oldwayspt.org.

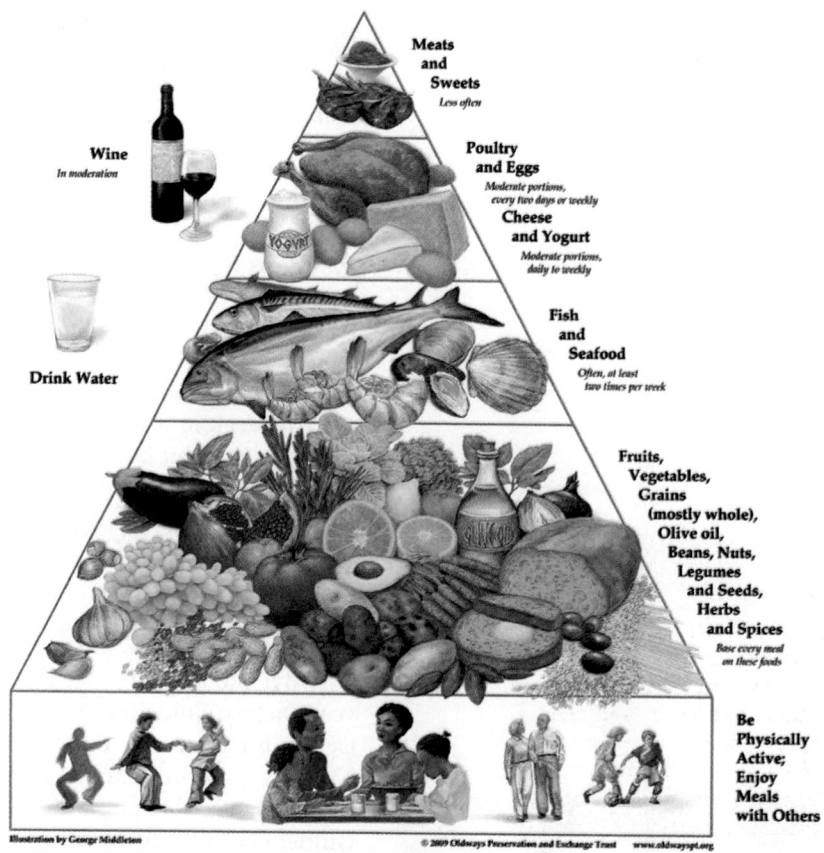

FIGURE 2-15 ▶ The Mediterranean Diet Pyramid is based on dietary patterns from the Mediterranean region, which has low rates of chronic diseases and high life expectancy.

How Does Your Plate Rate? Regularly comparing your daily food intake with your personalized Daily Food Plan recommendations is a relatively simple way to evaluate the quality of your overall diet. Identify the nutrients that are low in your diet based on the nutrients found in each food group (review Table 2-7). For example, if you do not consume enough servings from the milk group, your calcium intake is most likely too low. Look for foods that you enjoy that supply calcium, such as calcium-fortified orange juice.

For a more detailed analysis of your current diet, use the Food Tracker tool on www.ChooseMyPlate.gov. Your NutritionCalc software also helps you compare your food choices to MyPlate. With a detailed dietary analysis, you can compare your intakes of individual nutrients to the DRI standards and clearly see the areas that need improvement. Even small diet and exercise changes can have positive results.

Physical Activity Guidelines for Americans

In line with its goal for all Americans to live healthier, more prosperous, and more productive lives, the U.S. Department of Health and Human Services issued its first Physical Activity Guidelines for Americans in 2008 as a complement to the Dietary Guidelines (see Further Reading 11). The overarching idea is that regular physical activity—for people of all ages, races, ethnicities, and physical abilities—produces long-term health benefits. The guidelines are truly meant to inform the work of health professionals and policy makers, but consumer materials are available. *Be Active Your Way: A Guide for Adults*, available at www.health.gov, translates the guidelines into consumer-friendly, practical advice.

The key guidelines, listed in Table 2-9, provide measurable physical activity standards for Americans age 6 and older. Specific recommendations (not listed in Table 2-9) also apply to special population groups, including pregnant women, adults with disabilities, and people with chronic medical conditions. For adults, the guidelines emphasize that health benefits occur with at least 150 minutes per week of moderate-intensity physical activity. Adults may accumulate activity throughout the week in a variety of ways—extended sessions (e.g., 50 minutes on 3 days a week) or in short bursts throughout the week that amount to at least 150 minutes. Children and adolescents should strive to include 60 minutes of physical activity per day. For optimum benefits, include both aerobic and muscle-strengthening activities. Overall, physical activity should be enjoyable and safe for each individual.

A Coordinated Effort

The MyPlate icon fits together with a variety of educational tools as part of a multiyear Dietary Guidelines for Americans consumer communications initiative. USDA's Center for Nutrition Policy and Promotion heads up a National Communicator's Network to coordinate the efforts of public and private organizations, including the Department of Health and Human Services (sponsors of the 2008 Physical Activity Guidelines) as well as city governments, educational institutions, health networks, fitness centers, grocery chains, and a growing list of other organizations throughout the nation.

The Partnership program promotes a series of nutrition messages, starting with "Make half your plate fruits and vegetables." The campaign also incorporates the physical activity theme, "Be Active Your Way." The Dietary Guidelines Communications Message Calendar is available at http://www.choosemyplate.gov/downloads/MyPlate/DGCommunicationsMessageCalendar.pdf. Through a multifaceted media approach, this coordinated effort will help to expand the reach of the Dietary Guidelines, MyPlate, and Physical Activity Guidelines to individuals who, despite needing health improvements, may not be likely to access these tools.

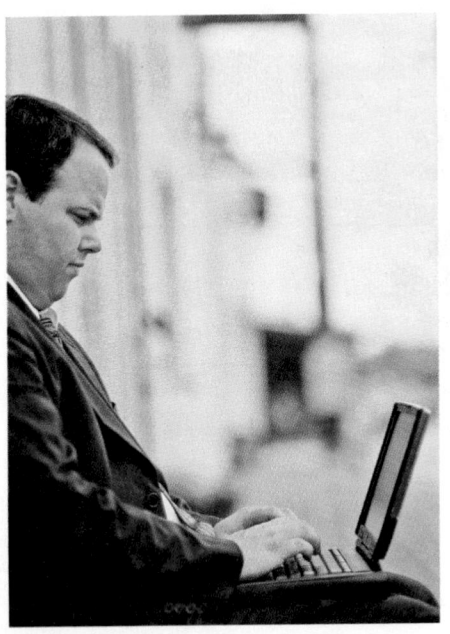

▲ Americans of all ages should limit screen time—hours spent watching TV, at the computer, or playing video games.

CONCEPT CHECK

The 2010 Dietary Guidelines for Americans aim to improve the health of all Americans, ages 2 and older. Three major goals include: (1) balancing calories with physical activity to manage weight; (2) increasing intake of fruits, vegetables, whole grains, fat-free and low-fat dairy products, and seafood; and (3) reducing intake of foods with sodium, saturated fats, *trans* fats, cholesterol, added sugars, and refined grains. MyPlate and associated tools found at www.ChooseMyPlate.gov embody the Dietary Guidelines with a plate icon that serves as a reminder for healthy eating. Grains, fruits, vegetables, protein, and dairy are the five major food groups represented on MyPlate. The 2008 Physical Activity Guidelines for Americans advise a minimum of 150 minutes per week of moderate-intensity physical activity for adults or at least 60 minutes daily for children and adolescents.

TABLE 2-9 Selected Recommendations of the 2008 Physical Activity Guidelines for Americans*

Key Guidelines for Children and Adolescents

- Children and adolescents should do 60 minutes or more of physical activity daily.

  - Aerobic: Most of the 60 or more minutes a day should be either moderate- or vigorous-intensity aerobic physical activity and should include vigorous-intensity activity at least 3 days a week.

  - Muscle-strengthening: As part of their 60 or more minutes of daily physical activity, children and adolescents should include muscle-strengthening physical activity on at least 3 days of the week.

  - Bone-strengthening: As part of their 60 or more minutes of daily physical activity, children and adolescents should include bone-strengthening physical activity on at least 3 days of the week.

- It is important to encourage young people to participate in physical activities that are appropriate for their age, that are enjoyable, and that offer variety.

Key Guidelines for Adults

- All adults should avoid inactivity. Some physical activity is better than none, and adults who participate in any amount of physical activity gain some health benefits.

- For substantial health benefits, adults should do at least 150 minutes a week of moderate-intensity, or 75 minutes a week of vigorous-intensity aerobic physical activity, or an equivalent combination of moderate- and vigorous-intensity aerobic activity. Aerobic activity should be performed in episodes of at least 10 minutes, and preferably, it should be spread throughout the week.

- For additional and more extensive health benefits, adults should increase their aerobic physical activity to 300 minutes a week of moderate-intensity, or 150 minutes a week of vigorous-intensity aerobic physical activity, or an equivalent combination of moderate- and vigorous-intensity activity. Additional health benefits are gained by engaging in physical activity beyond this amount.

- Adults should also do muscle-strengthening activities that are moderate or high intensity and involve all major muscle groups on 2 or more days a week, as these activities provide additional health benefits.

Key Guidelines for Older Adults

- When older adults cannot do 150 minutes of moderate-intensity aerobic activity a week because of chronic conditions, they should be as physically active as their abilities and conditions allow.

- Older adults should do exercises that maintain or improve balance if they are at risk of falling.

- Older adults should determine their level of effort for physical activity relative to their level of fitness.

- Older adults with chronic conditions should understand whether and how their conditions affect their ability to do regular physical activity safely.

Key Guidelines for Safe Physical Activity

To do physical activity safely and reduce the risk of injuries and other adverse events, people should:

- Understand the risks and yet be confident that physical activity is safe for almost everyone.

- Choose to do types of physical activity that are appropriate for their current fitness level and health goals, because some activities are safer than others.

- Increase physical activity gradually over time whenever more activity is necessary to meet guidelines or health goals. Inactive people should "start low and go slow" by gradually increasing how often and how long activities are done.

- Protect themselves by using appropriate gear and sports equipment; looking for safe environments; following rules and policies; and making sensible choices about when, where, and how to be active.

- Be under the care of a health care provider if they have chronic conditions or symptoms. People with chronic conditions and symptoms should consult their health care provider about the types and amounts of activity appropriate for them.

*The 2008 Physical Activity Guidelines for Americans also include recommendations for pregnant women, adults with disabilities, and people with chronic medical conditions. These are available at www.health.gov.

2.7 Food Labels and Diet Planning

Today, nearly all foods sold in stores must be in a package that has a label containing the following information: the product name, name and address of the manufacturer, amount of product in the package, and ingredients listed in descending order by weight. This food and beverage labeling is monitored in North America by government agencies such as the Food and Drug Administration (FDA) in the United States (see Further Reading 10). The listing of certain food constituents also is required—specifically, on a Nutrition Facts panel (Fig. 2-16). Use the information in the Nutrition Facts panel to learn more about what you eat. The following components must be listed: total calories (kcal), calories from fat, total fat, saturated fat, *trans* fat, cholesterol, sodium, total carbohydrate, fiber, sugars, protein, vitamin A, vitamin C, calcium, and iron. In addition to these required components, manufacturers can choose to list polyunsaturated and monounsaturated fat, potassium, and others. Listing these components becomes *required* if the food is fortified with that nutrient or if a claim is made about the health benefits of the specific nutrient (see the upcoming section in Chapter 2 entitled "Health Claims on Food Labels").

Remember that the Daily Value is a generic standard used on the food label. The percentage of the Daily Value (% Daily Value or % DV) is usually given for each nutrient per serving. These percentages are based on a 2000 kcal diet. In other words, they are not as applicable to people who require considerably more or less than 2000 kcal per day with respect to fat and carbohydrate intake. DVs are mostly set at or close to the highest RDA value or related nutrient standard seen in the various age and gender categories for a specific nutrient.

Serving sizes on the Nutrition Facts panel must be consistent among similar foods. This means that all brands of ice cream, for example, must use the same serving size on their label. (These serving sizes may differ from those of MyPlate because those on food labels are based on typical serving sizes.) In addition, food claims made on packages must follow legal definitions (Table 2-10). For example, if a product claims to be "low sodium," it must have 140 milligrams of sodium or less per serving.

Many manufacturers list the Daily Values set for dietary components such as fat, cholesterol, and carbohydrate on the Nutrition Facts panel. This can be useful as a reference point. As noted, they are based on 2000 kcal; if the label is large enough, amounts based on 2500 kcal are listed as well for total fat, saturated fat, carbohydrate, and other components. As mentioned, DVs allow consumers to compare their intake from a specific food to desirable (or maximum) intakes.

Exceptions to Food Labeling

Foods such as fresh fruits and vegetables and fish currently are not required to have Nutrition Facts labels. However, many grocers have voluntarily chosen to provide their customers with information about these products. The next time you are at the grocery store, ask where you might find information on the fresh products that do not have a Nutrition Facts panel. You will likely find a poster or pamphlet near the product; often, these pamphlets contain recipes that use your favorite fruit, vegetable, or fish fillet. They may even assist you in your endeavor to improve your diet.

Protein deficiency is not a public health concern in the United States, so declaration of the % Daily Value for protein is not mandatory on foods for people over 4 years of age. If the % Daily Value for protein is given on a label, FDA requires that the product be analyzed for protein quality. This procedure is expensive and time-consuming, so many companies opt not to list a % Daily Value for protein. However, labels on food for infants and children under 4 years of age must

The Nutrition Facts label uses the term "calorie" to express energy content in some cases, but kilocalorie (kcal) values are actually listed.

Nutrient and herbal supplement labels have a different layout with a "Supplement Facts" heading. The Nutrition and Your Health section at the end of this chapter and Chapter 8 show examples of these labels.

▼ Use the Nutrition Facts label to learn more about the nutrient content of the foods you eat. Nutrient content is expressed as a percent of Daily Value. Canadian food laws and related food labels have a slightly different format (review Appendix C).

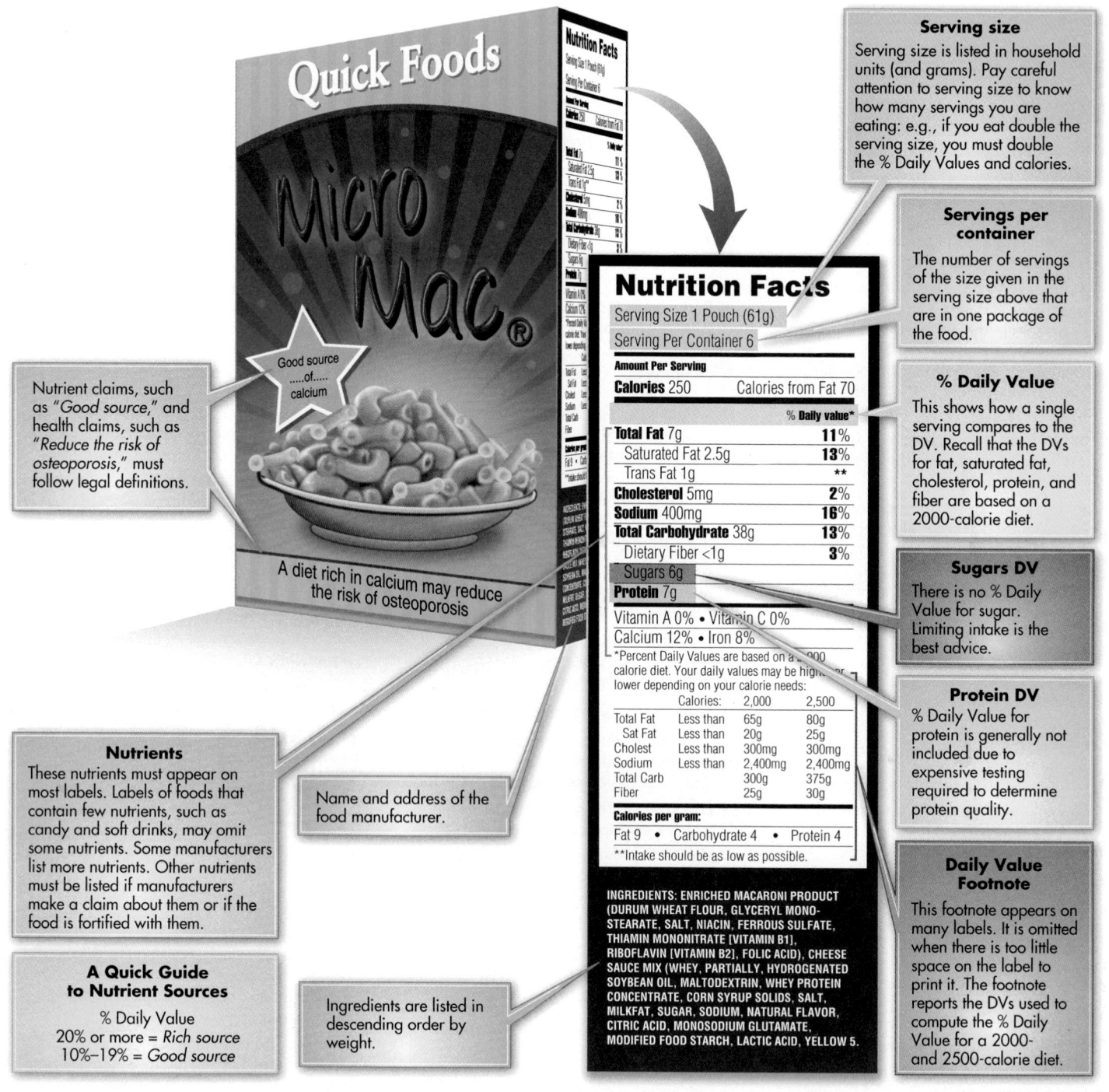

Serving size

Serving size is listed in household units (and grams). Pay careful attention to serving size to know how many servings you are eating: e.g., if you eat double the serving size, you must double the % Daily Values and calories.

Servings per container

The number of servings of the size given in the serving size above that are in one package of the food.

% Daily Value

This shows how a single serving compares to the DV. Recall that the DVs for fat, saturated fat, cholesterol, protein, and fiber are based on a 2000-calorie diet.

Sugars DV

There is no % Daily Value for sugar. Limiting intake is the best advice.

Protein DV

% Daily Value for protein is generally not included due to expensive testing required to determine protein quality.

Daily Value Footnote

This footnote appears on many labels. It is omitted when there is too little space on the label to print it. The footnote reports the DVs used to compute the % Daily Value for a 2000- and 2500-calorie diet.

Nutrient claims, such as "Good source," and health claims, such as "Reduce the risk of osteoporosis," must follow legal definitions.

Nutrients

These nutrients must appear on most labels. Labels of foods that contain few nutrients, such as candy and soft drinks, may omit some nutrients. Some manufacturers list more nutrients. Other nutrients must be listed if manufacturers make a claim about them or if the food is fortified with them.

Name and address of the food manufacturer.

A Quick Guide to Nutrient Sources

% Daily Value
20% or more = *Rich source*
10%–19% = *Good source*

Ingredients are listed in descending order by weight.

Nutrition Facts

Serving Size 1 Pouch (61g)

Serving Per Container 6

Amount Per Serving

Calories 250 Calories from Fat 70

	% Daily value*
Total Fat 7g	**11**%
Saturated Fat 2.5g	**13**%
Trans Fat 1g	**
Cholesterol 5mg	**2**%
Sodium 400mg	**16**%
Total Carbohydrate 38g	**13**%
Dietary Fiber <1g	**3**%
Sugars 6g	
Protein 7g	

Vitamin A 0% • Vitamin C 0%

Calcium 12% • Iron 8%

*Percent Daily Values are based on a 2,000 calorie diet. Your daily values may be higher or lower depending on your calorie needs:

	Calories:	2,000	2,500
Total Fat	Less than	65g	80g
Sat Fat	Less than	20g	25g
Cholest	Less than	300mg	300mg
Sodium	Less than	2,400mg	2,400mg
Total Carb		300g	375g
Fiber		25g	30g

Calories per gram:

Fat 9 • Carbohydrate 4 • Protein 4

**Intake should be as low as possible.

INGREDIENTS: ENRICHED MACARONI PRODUCT (DURUM WHEAT FLOUR, GLYCERYL MONO-STEARATE, SALT, NIACIN, FERROUS SULFATE, THIAMIN MONONITRATE [VITAMIN B1], RIBOFLAVIN [VITAMIN B2], FOLIC ACID), CHEESE SAUCE MIX (WHEY, PARTIALLY, HYDROGENATED SOYBEAN OIL, MALTODEXTRIN, WHEY PROTEIN CONCENTRATE, CORN SYRUP SOLIDS, SALT, MILKFAT, SUGAR, SODIUM, NATURAL FLAVOR, CITRIC ACID, MONOSODIUM GLUTAMATE, MODIFIED FOOD STARCH, LACTIC ACID, YELLOW 5.

FIGURE 2-16 ▶ Food packages must list product name, name and address of the manufacturer, amount of product in the package, and ingredients. The Nutrition Facts panel is required on virtually all packaged food products. The % Daily Value listed on the label is the percent of the amount of a nutrient needed daily that is provided by a single serving of the product. Canadian food labels use a slightly different group of health claims and label descriptors (see Appendix C).

include the % Daily Value for protein, as must the labels on any food carrying a claim about protein content (see Chapter 15).

Health Claims on Food Labels

As a marketing tool directed toward the health-conscious consumer, food manufacturers like to claim that their products have all sorts of health benefits. The FDA has

TABLE 2-10 Definitions for Nutrient Claims Allowed on Food Labels

Sugar

- **Sugar free:** less than 0.5 grams (g) per serving.
- **No added sugar; without added sugar; no sugar added:**
  - No sugars were added during processing or packing, including ingredients that contain sugars (for example, fruit juices, applesauce, or jam).
  - Processing does not increase the sugar content above the amount naturally present in the ingredients. (A functionally insignificant increase in sugars is acceptable for processes used for purposes other than increasing sugar content.)
  - The food that it resembles and for which it substitutes normally contains added sugars.
  - If the food doesn't meet the requirements for a low- or reduced-calorie food, the product bears a statement that the food is not low calorie or calorie reduced and directs consumers' attention to the Nutrition Facts panel for further information on sugars and calorie content.
- **Reduced sugar:** at least 25% less sugar per serving than reference food

Calories

- **Calorie free:** fewer than 5 kcal per serving
- **Low calorie:** 40 kcal or less per serving and, if the serving is 30 g or less or 2 tablespoons or less, per 50 g of the food
- **Reduced or fewer calories:** at least 25% fewer kcal per serving than reference food

Fiber

- **High fiber:** 5 g or more per serving. (Foods making high-fiber claims must meet the definition for low fat, or the level of total fat must appear next to the high-fiber claim.)
- **Good source of fiber:** 2.5 to 4.9 g per serving
- **More or added fiber:** at least 2.5 g more per serving than reference food

Fat

- **Fat free:** less than 0.5 g of fat per serving
- **Saturated fat free:** less than 0.5 g per serving, and the level of *trans* fatty acids does not exceed 0.5 g per serving

- **Low fat:** 3 g or less per serving and, if the serving is 30 g or less or 2 tablespoons or less, per 50 g of the food. 2% milk can no longer be labeled low fat, as it exceeds 3 g per serving. *Reduced fat* will be the term used instead.
- **Low saturated fat:** 1 g or less per serving and not more than 15% of kcal from saturated fatty acids
- **Reduced or less fat:** at least 25% less per serving than reference food
- **Reduced or less saturated fat:** at least 25% less per serving than reference food

Cholesterol

- **Cholesterol free:** less than 2 milligrams (mg) of cholesterol and 2 g or less of saturated fat per serving
- **Low cholesterol:** 20 mg or less of cholesterol and 2 g or less of saturated fat per serving or, if the serving is 30 g or less or 2 tablespoons or less, per 50 g of the food
- **Reduced or less cholesterol:** at least 25% less cholesterol than reference food and 2 g or less of saturated fat per serving

Sodium

- **Sodium free:** less than 5 mg per serving
- **Very low sodium:** 35 mg or less per serving and, if the serving is 30 g or less or 2 tablespoons or less, per 50 g of the food
- **Low sodium:** 140 mg or less per serving or, if the serving is 30 g or less or 2 tablespoons or less, per 50 g of the food
- **Light in sodium:** at least 50% less per serving than reference food
- **Reduced or less sodium:** at least 25% less per serving than reference food

Other Terms

- **Fortified or enriched:** Vitamins and/or minerals have been added to the product in amounts in excess of at least 10% of that normally present in the usual product. Enriched generally refers to replacing nutrients lost in processing, whereas fortified refers to adding nutrients not originally present in the specific food.
- **Healthy:** An individual food that is low fat and low saturated fat and has no more than 360 to 480 mg of sodium or 60 mg of cholesterol per serving can be labeled "healthy" if it provides at least 10% of the Daily Value for vitamin A, vitamin C, protein, calcium, iron, or fiber.

- **Light or lite:** The descriptor *light* or *lite* can mean two things: first, that a nutritionally altered product contains one-third fewer kcal or half the fat of reference food (if the food derives 50% or more of its kcal from fat, the reduction must be 50% of the fat) and, second, that the sodium content of a low-calorie, low-fat food has been reduced by 50%. In addition, "light in sodium" may be used for foods in which the sodium content has been reduced by at least 50%. The term *light* may still be used to describe such properties as texture and color, as long as the label explains the intent—for example, "light brown sugar" and "light and fluffy."

Diet: A food may be labeled with terms such as *diet, dietetic, artificially sweetened,* or *sweetened with nonnutritive sweetener* only if the claim is not false or misleading. The food can also be labeled *low calorie* or *reduced calorie.*

Good source: *Good source* means that a serving of the food contains 10% to 19% of the Daily Value for a particular nutrient. If 5% or less, it is a *low source.*

High: *High* means that a serving of the food contains 20% or more of the Daily Value for a particular nutrient.

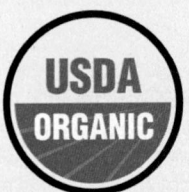

Organic: Federal standards for organic foods allow claims when much of the ingredients do not use chemical fertilizers or pesticides, genetic engineering, sewage sludge, antibiotics, or irradiation in their production. At least 95% of ingredients (by weight) must meet these guidelines to be labeled "organic" on the front of the package. If the front label instead says "made with organic ingredients," only 70% of the ingredients must be organic. For animal products, the animals must graze outdoors, be fed organic feed, and cannot be exposed to large amounts of antibiotics or growth hormones.

Natural: The food must be free of food colors, synthetic flavors, or any other synthetic substance.

The following terms apply only to meat and poultry products regulated by USDA.

Extra lean: less than 5 g of fat, 2 g of saturated fat, and 95 mg of cholesterol per serving (or 100 g of an individual food)

Lean: less than 10 g of fat, 4.5 g of saturated fat, and 95 mg of cholesterol per serving (or 100 g of an individual food)

Many definitions are from FDA's *Dictionary of Terms*, as established in conjunction with the 1990 Nutrition Labeling and Education Act (NLEA).
g = grams; mg = milligrams

legal oversight over most food products and permits some health claims with certain restrictions.

Overall, claims on foods fall into one of four categories:

- Health claims—closely regulated by FDA
- Preliminary health claims—regulated by FDA but evidence may be scant for the claim
- Nutrient claims—closely regulated by FDA (review Table 2-10)
- Structure/function claims—as discussed in the Nutrition and Your Health section at the end of this chapter, these are not FDA-approved or necessarily valid

Table 2-10 lists the definitions for nutrient claims on food labels. Currently, FDA limits the use of health messages to specific instances in which there is significant scientific agreement that a relationship exists between a nutrient, food, or food constituent and the disease. The claims allowed at this time may show a link between the following:

- A diet with enough calcium and vitamin D and a reduced risk of osteoporosis
- A diet low in total fat and a reduced risk of some cancers
- A diet low in saturated fat and cholesterol and a reduced risk of cardiovascular disease (typically referred to as heart disease on the label)
- A diet rich in fiber—containing grain products, fruits, and vegetables—and a reduced risk of some cancers
- A diet low in sodium and high in potassium and a reduced risk of hypertension and stroke
- A diet rich in fruits and vegetables and a reduced risk of some cancers
- A diet adequate in the synthetic form of the vitamin folate (called folic acid) and a reduced risk of neural tube defects (a type of birth defect) (see Chapter 8)
- Use of sugarless gum and a reduced risk of tooth decay, especially when compared with foods high in sugars and starches
- A diet rich in fruits, vegetables, and grain products that contain fiber and a reduced risk of cardiovascular disease. Oats (oatmeal, oat bran, and oat flour) and psyllium are two fiber-rich ingredients that can be singled out in reducing the risk of cardiovascular disease, as long as the statement also says the diet should also be low in saturated fat and cholesterol.
- A diet rich in whole-grain foods and other plant foods, as well as low in total fat, saturated fat, and cholesterol, and a reduced risk of cardiovascular disease and certain cancers
- A diet low in saturated fat and cholesterol that also includes 25 grams of soy protein and a reduced risk of cardiovascular disease. The statement "one serving of the (name of food) provides _____ grams of soy protein" must also appear as part of the health claim.
- Fatty acids from oils present in fish and a reduced risk of cardiovascular disease
- Margarines containing plant stanols and sterols and a reduced risk of cardiovascular disease (see Chapter 5 for more details on plant stanols and sterols)

A "may" or "might" qualifier must be used in the statement.

In addition, before a health claim can be made for a food product, it must meet two general requirements. First, the food must be a "good source" (before any fortification) of fiber, protein, vitamin A, vitamin C, calcium, or iron. The legal definition of "good source" appears in Table 2-10. Second, a single serving of the food product cannot contain more than 13 grams of fat, 4 grams of saturated fat, 60 milligrams of cholesterol, or 480 milligrams of sodium. If a food exceeds any one of these requirements, no health claim can be made for it, despite its other nutritional qualities. For example, even though whole milk is high in calcium, its label can't make the health

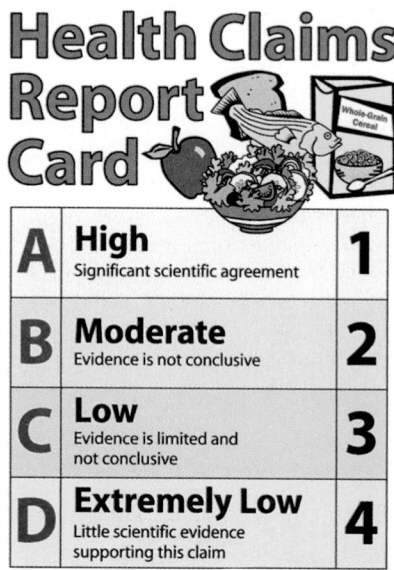

A	**High** Significant scientific agreement	**1**
B	**Moderate** Evidence is not conclusive	**2**
C	**Low** Evidence is limited and not conclusive	**3**
D	**Extremely Low** Little scientific evidence supporting this claim	**4**

▲ In 2003, FDA unveiled a new process, including the Health Claims Report card, to provide more science-based, FDA-regulated health information on food product labels. This process is used to rank the claim based on the amount of scientific evidence and agreement. Only the first three classes are allowed.

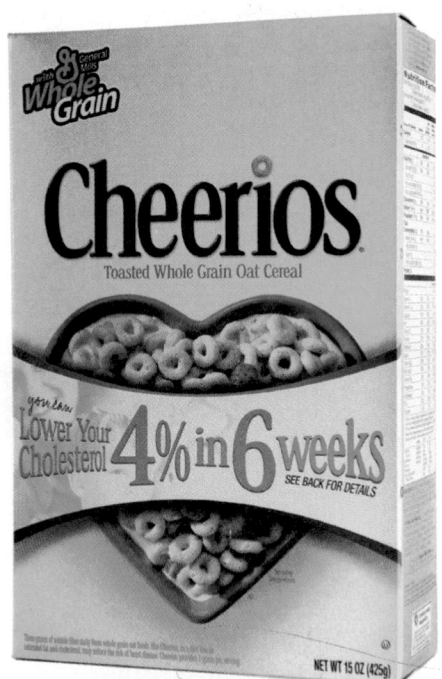

▲ Specific health claims can be made on food labels for whole-grain cereals.

claim about calcium and osteoporosis because whole milk contains 5 grams of saturated fat per serving. In another example, a health claim regarding fat and cancer can be made only if the product contains 3 grams or less of fat per serving, the standard for low-fat foods.

MAKING DECISIONS

Health Claims

FDA allows the three preliminary classes of health claims shown in the preceding section as long as the label qualifies the food with a disclaimer such as "this evidence is not conclusive." These preliminary health claims haven't shown up on many foods at this time (nuts, such as walnuts, and fish have been some of the first examples). These claims also cannot be used on foods considered unhealthy (review Table 2-10 for the definition of healthy with regard to a food).

CONCEPT CHECK

The Nutrition Facts panel on a food label provides key information for helping track one's food intake. Nutrient quantities are compared with the Daily Values and expressed on a percentage basis (% Daily Value). This information can be used to either increase or reduce intake of specific nutrients. Health and nutrient claims on food labels are closely regulated by FDA. Fruits, vegetables, whole-grain breads and cereals, soy, and good sources of calcium are prominent among the foods that can make specific health claims.

2.8 Epilogue

The tools discussed in Chapter 2 greatly aid in menu planning. Menu planning can start with MyPlate. The totality of choices made within the groups can then be evaluated using the Dietary Guidelines. Individual foods that make up a diet can be examined more closely using the Daily Values listed on the Nutrition Facts panel of the product. For the most part, these Daily Values are in line with the Recommended Dietary Allowances and related nutrient standards. The Nutrition Facts panel is especially useful in identifying nutrient-dense foods—foods high in a specific nutrient, such as the vitamin folate, but low in the relative amount of calories provided—and the energy-dense foods—foods that fill you up without providing a lot of calories. Generally speaking, the more you learn about and use these tools, the more they will benefit your diet.

Evaluating Nutrition Claims and Dietary Supplements

The following suggestions should help you make healthful and logical nutrition decisions:

1. Apply the basic principles of nutrition as outlined in this chapter (along with the 2010 Dietary Guidelines for Americans and related resources in Chapter 2) to any nutrition claim including those on websites. Do you note any inconsistencies? Do reliable references support the claims? Beware of the following:
   - Testimonials about personal experience
   - Disreputable publication sources
   - Promises of dramatic results (rarely true)
   - Lack of evidence from other scientific studies

2. Examine the background and scientific credentials of the individual, organizations, or publication making the nutritional claim. Usually, a reputable author is one whose educational background or present affiliation is with a nationally recognized university or medical center that offers programs or courses in the field of nutrition, medicine, or a closely allied specialty.

3. Be wary if the answer is "Yes" to any of the following questions about a health-related nutrition claim:
   - Are only advantages discussed and possible disadvantages ignored?
   - Are claims made about "curing" disease? Do they sound too good to be true?
   - Is extreme bias against the medical community or traditional medical treatments evident? Physicians as a group strive to cure diseases in their patients, using what proven techniques are available. They do not ignore reliable cures.
   - Is the claim touted as a new or secret scientific breakthrough?

4. Note the size and duration of any study cited in support of a nutrition claim. The larger it is and the longer it went on, the more dependable its findings. Also consider the type of study: epidemiology versus case-control versus double-blind. Check out the group studied; a study of men or women in Sweden may be less relevant than one of men or women of Southern European, African, or Hispanic descent, for example. Keep in mind that "contributes to," "is linked to," or "is associated with" does not mean "causes."

5. Beware of press conferences and other hype regarding the latest findings. Much of this will not survive more detailed scientific evaluation.

6. When you meet with a nutrition professional, you should expect that he or she will do the following:
   - Ask questions about your medical history, lifestyle, and current eating habits.
   - Formulate a diet plan tailored to your needs, as opposed to simply tearing a form from a tablet that could apply to almost anyone.
   - Schedule follow-up visits to track your progress, answer any questions, and help keep you motivated.
   - Involve family members in the diet plan, when appropriate.
   - Consult directly with your physician and readily refer you back to your physician for those health problems a nutrition professional is not trained to treat.

7. Avoid practitioners who prescribe **megadoses** of vitamin and mineral supplements for everyone.

8. Examine product labels carefully. Be skeptical of any promotional information about a product that is not clearly stated on the label. A product is not likely to do something not specifically claimed on its label or package insert (legally part of the label).

Dietary Supplements

A cautious approach to nutrition-related advice and products is even more important today because of broad changes in U.S. federal law passed in 1994.

The Dietary Supplement Health and Education Act (DSHEA) of 1994 classified vitamins, minerals, amino acids, and herbal remedies as "foods," which restrains the U.S. Food and Drug Administration (FDA) from regulating them as tightly as drugs and food additives. According to this act, rather than the manufacturer having to prove a dietary supplement is safe, FDA must prove it is unsafe before preventing its sale. In contrast, the safety of food additives and drugs must be demonstrated to FDA's satisfaction before they are marketed.

megadose Large intake of a nutrient beyond estimates of needs or what would be found in a balanced diet; 2 to 10 times human needs is a starting point.

▶ Recently, major nutrition organizations put together 10 red flags that they consider signals for poor nutrition advice:

1. Recommendations that promise a quick fix
2. Dire warnings of dangers from a single product or regimen
3. Claims that sound too good to be true
4. Simplistic conclusions drawn from a complex study
5. Recommendations based on a single study
6. Dramatic statements refuted by reputable scientific organizations
7. Lists of "good" and "bad" foods
8. Recommendations made to help sell a product
9. Recommendations based on studies published without peer review
10. Recommendations from studies that ignore differences among individuals or groups

▶ The FDA can act if evidence accumulates showing that a product is harmful. This has been true for some herbal remedies marketed as dietary supplements, such as ephedra.

Currently, a dietary supplement (or herbal product) can be marketed in the United States without FDA approval if (1) there is a history of its use or other evidence that it is expected to be reasonably safe when used under the conditions recommended or suggested in its labeling, and (2) the product is labeled as a dietary supplement. The Supplement Facts panel resembles the Nutrition Facts panel on foods and is required on all dietary supplements. It is permissible for the labels on such products to claim a benefit related to a classic nutrient-deficiency disease, describe how a nutrient affects human body structure or function (called structure/function claims), and claim that general well-being results from consumption of the ingredient(s). Examples could be "maintains bone health" or "improves blood circulation." However, the label of products bearing such claims also must prominently display in boldface type the following disclaimer: "This statement has not been evaluated by the Food and Drug Administration. This product is not intended to diagnose, treat, cure, or prevent disease" (Fig. 2-17). Despite this warning, when consumers find these products on the shelves of supermarkets,

health-food stores, and pharmacies, they may mistakenly assume FDA has carefully evaluated the products.

Many of us are willing to try untested nutrition products and believe in their miraculous actions. Popular products claim to increase muscle growth, enhance sexuality, boost energy, reduce body fat, increase strength, supply missing nutrients, increase longevity, and even improve brain function. Clearly, many nutritional products commonly found in stores are not strictly regulated in terms of effectiveness and safety (see Further Reading 8). The amount and potency of dietary supplements have also been in question. In June 2007, FDA issued long-awaited standards that require supplement manufacturers to test the purity, strength, and composition of all their products. The usefulness of supplements is discussed further in the Nutrition and Your Health section in Chapter 8, "Dietary Supplements—Who Needs Them?"

If you embark on a self-cure by means of such products, you will probably waste money and possibly risk ill health. A better approach is to consult a physician or **registered dietitian** first (see Further Reading 1). You can find a registered dietitian in North America by consulting the Yellow Pages in the telephone directory, contacting the local dietetic association, calling the dietary department of a local hospital, or visiting www.eatright.org/ or www.dietitians.ca. Make sure the person has the credentials "R.D." after his/her name ("R.D.N." is also used in Canada). This indicates the person has completed rigorous classroom and clinical training in nutrition and participates in continuing education. Appendix H also lists many reputable sources of nutrition advice for your use. Finally, the following websites can help you evaluate ongoing nutrition and health claims:

Supplement Facts

Serving Size 1 Softgel

Each Softgel Contains | % DV
Ginseng Extract *(Panax ginseng)* (root) 100 mg *
(Standardized to 4% Ginsenosides)

*Daily Value (DV) not established.

INGREDIENTS: Gelatin, Soybean Oil, Panax Ginseng Extract, Vegetable Oil, Lecithin, Palm Oil, Glycerin, Sorbitol, Yellow Beeswax, Hydrogenated Coconut Oil, Titanium Dioxide, Yellow 5, Blue 1, Red 40, Green 3, Chlorophyll.

DIST. BY NUTRA ASSOC., INC.
4411 WHITE POINT RD., SPRING CITY, IL 12345

Suggested use: Adults- 1 to 2 capsules daily taken with a full glass of water, or as a tea, add one to two capsules to a cup of hot water.

When you need to perform your best, take ginseng.

This statement has not been evaluated by the Food and Drug Administration. This product is not intended to diagnose, treat, cure, or prevent disease.

- Suggested serving size
- Product and amount
- Name and address of manufacturer
- Suggested use
- Structure/function claim
- Standard FDA disclaimer

FIGURE 2-17 ▶ Supplement Facts label on an herbal product. Note the structure/function claim and the FDA disclaimer. Any nutrients or other food constituents would also be listed if contained in the product.

registered dietitian (R.D.) A person who has completed a baccalaureate degree program approved by the American Dietetic Association, performed at least 1200 hours of supervised professional practice, passed a registration examination, and complies with continuing education requirements.

www.acsh.org/
American Council on Science and Health

www.quackwatch.org/
Quackwatch: Your Guide to Quackery,
Health Fraud, and Intelligent Decisions

www.ncahf.org/
National Council Against Health Fraud

http://dietary-supplements.info.nih.gov/
National Institutes of Health, Office
of Dietary Supplements

www.fda.gov/
U.S. Food and Drug Administration

Overall, nutrition is a rapidly advancing field and there are always new findings.

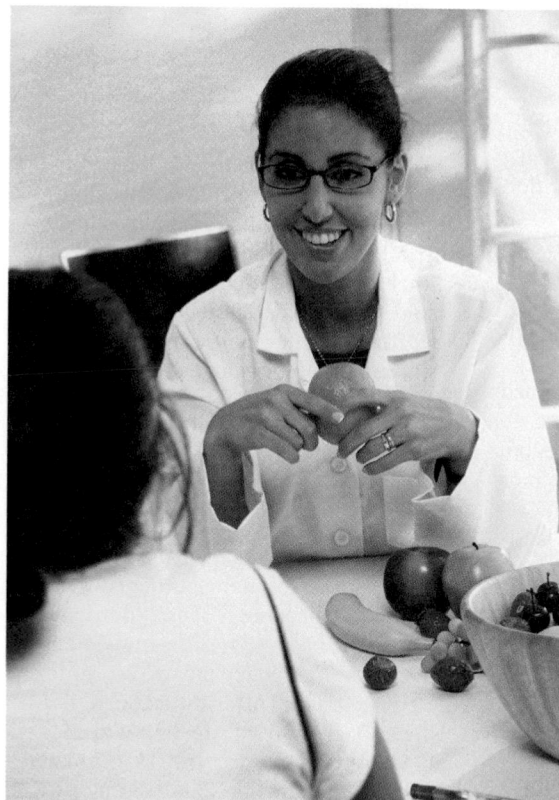

◀ Registered dietitians are a reliable source of nutrition advice.

Case Study Dietary Supplements

While Whitney was driving to campus last week, she heard an advertisement for a supplement containing a plant substance recently imported from China. It supposedly gives people more energy and helps one cope with the stress of daily life. This advertisement caught Whitney's attention because she has been feeling run-down lately. She is taking a full-course load and has been working 30 hours a week at a local restaurant to try to make ends meet. Whitney doesn't have a lot of extra money. Still, she likes to try new things and this recent breakthrough from China sounded almost too good to be true. After searching for more information about this supplement on the Internet, she discovered that the recommended dose would cost $60 per month. Because Whitney is looking for some help with her low energy level, she decides to order a 1-month supply.

Answer the following questions, and check your response in Appendix A.

1. Is the advertised supplement regulated by the FDA or other government agency?

2. What type of label claim is the phrase "increases energy," and does it require government approval?

3. Can Whitney feel confident that the supplement is safe and effective?

4. Is the amount of active ingredients in supplements tightly controlled?

5. Does it make sense for Whitney to spend the extra $60 per month for this supplement?

6. What advice would you give Whitney about the fact that she has been feeling run-down lately?

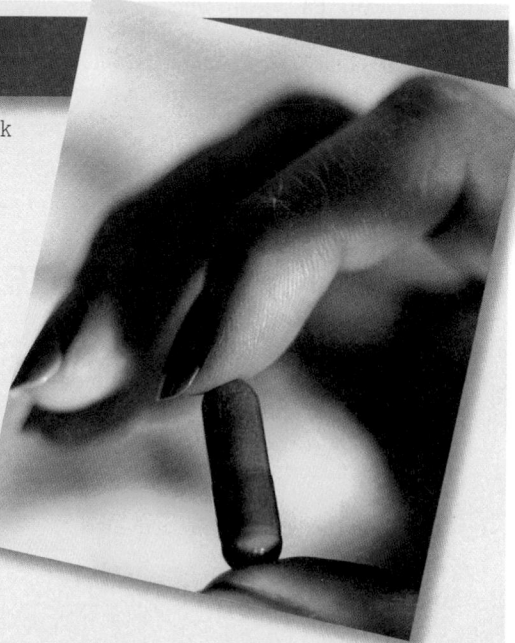

▲ Do you agree with Whitney's decision to try this supplement?

Summary (Numbers refer to numbered sections in the chapter.)

2.1 A healthy eating plan is based on consuming a *variety* of foods *balanced* by a moderate intake of each food and will minimize the risk of developing nutrition-related diseases.

Nutrient density reflects the nutrient content of a food in relation to its calorie content. Nutrient-dense foods are relatively rich in nutrients, in comparison with calorie content.

Energy density of a food is determined by comparing calorie content with the weight of food. A food rich in calories but weighing relatively very little, such as nuts, cookies, fried foods in general, and most snack foods (including fat-free brands), is considered energy dense. Foods with low energy density include fruits, vegetables, and any food that incorporates lots of water during cooking, such as oatmeal.

2.2 A person's nutritional state can be categorized as *desirable nutrition*, in which the body has adequate stores for times of increased needs; *undernutrition*, which may be present with or without clinical symptoms; and *overnutrition*, which can lead to vitamin and mineral toxicities and various chronic diseases.

2.3 Evaluation of nutritional state involves analyzing background factors, as well as anthropometric, biochemical, clinical, dietary, and environmental assessments. It is not always possible to detect nutritional inadequacies via nutrition assessment because symptoms of deficien-

cies are often nonspecific and may not appear for many years.

2.4 The scientific method is the procedure for testing the validity of possible explanations of a phenomenon, called hypotheses. Experiments are conducted to either support or refute a specific hypothesis. Once we have enough experimental information to support a specific hypothesis, it then can be called a theory. All of us need to be skeptical of new ideas in the nutrition field, waiting until many lines of experimental evidence support a concept before adopting any suggested dietary practice.

2.5 Recommended Dietary Allowances (RDAs) are set for many nutrients. These amounts yield enough of each nutrient to meet the needs of healthy individuals within specific gender and age categories. Adequate Intake (AI) is the standard used when not enough information is available to set a more specific RDA. Estimated Energy Requirements (EERs) set calorie needs for both genders at various ages and physical activity patterns. Tolerable Upper Intake Levels (Upper Levels or ULs) for nutrient intake have been set for some vitamins and minerals.

All of the many dietary standards fall under the term *Dietary Reference Intakes (DRIs)*. Daily Values are used as a basis for expressing the nutrient content of foods on the Nutrition Facts panel and are based for the most part on the RDAs.

2.6 Dietary Guidelines for Americans have been issued to help improve the health of all Americans ages 2 and older. The guidelines emphasize balancing calories to manange weight; performing regular physical activity; moderating consumption of fat, *trans* fat, cholesterol, sugar, salt, and alcohol; eating plenty of whole-grain products, fruits, and vegetables; and safely preparing and storing foods, especially perishable foods.

MyPlate and accompanying online tools are designed to translate nutrient recommendations into a food plan that exhibits variety, balance, and moderation. The best results are obtained by using low-fat or fat-free dairy products; incorporating some vegetable proteins in the diet in addition to animal-protein foods; including citrus fruits and dark-green vegetables; and emphasizing whole-grain breads and cereals.

2.7 Food labels, especially the Nutrition Facts panels, are a useful tool to track your nutrient intake and learn more about the nutritional characteristics of the foods you eat. Any health claims listed must follow criteria set by FDA.

N&YH Apply the basic principles of nutrition to evaluate any nutrition claim. Dietary supplements can be marketed in the United States without FDA approval. Certain health claims can be made on supplement labels, although few have been thoroughly evaluated by reputable scientists.

Check Your Knowledge (Answers to the following questions are below.)

1. Anthropometric measurements include
   a. height, weight, skinfolds, and body circumferences.
   b. blood concentrations of nutrients.
   c. a diet history of the previous days' intake.
   d. blood levels of enzyme activities.

2. Foods with *high* nutrient density offer the _____ nutrients for the _____ calories.
   a. least, lowest
   b. least, most
   c. most, lowest
   d. most, most

3. A meal of a bean burrito, tossed salad, and glass of milk represents foods from all MyPlate food groups except
   a. dairy.   c. vegetables.
   b. protein.   d. fruits.

4. The Dietary Guidelines for Americans were recently revised in
   a. 2000   c. 2008
   b. 2005   d. 2010

5. The term Daily Value is used on
   a. restaurant menus.
   b. food labels.
   c. medical charts.
   d. None of the above.

6. The Tolerable Upper Intake Level, or UL, is used to
   a. estimate calorie needs of the average person.
   b. evaluate the highest amount of daily nutrient intake unlikely to cause adverse health effects.
   c. evaluate your current intake for a specific nutrient.
   d. compare the nutrient content of a food to approximate human needs.

7. The current food label must list
   a. a picture of the product.
   b. a uniform and realistic serving size.

  c. the RDA for each age group.
  d. ingredients alphabetically.

8. Dietary supplements are tightly regulated by the
  a. FDA.
  b. USDA.
  c. FTC.
  d. None of the above.

9. The scientific method begins with
  a. a hypothesis.
  b. research experiments.
  c. publication of research findings.
  d. observations made and questions asked.

10. The most common type of undernutrition in industrialized nations, such as the United States, is
  a. anorexia.
  b. protein deficiency.
  c. obesity.
  d. iron deficiency.

Answer Key: 1. a (LO 2.2), 2. c (LO 2.1), 3. d (LO 2.6), 4. d (LO 2.5), 5. b (LO 2.4), 6. b (LO 2.4), 7. b (LO 2.7), 8. d (LO 2.8), 9. d (LO 2.3), 10. d (LO 2.2)

Study Questions (Numbers refer to Learning Outcomes)

1. Among your classmates, you observe that students who consume coffee get better grades. Provide an example of how you could use the scientific method to examine the effects of coffee consumption on academic performance (LO 2.3).

2. How would you explain the concepts of nutrient density and energy density to a fourth-grade class (LO 2.1)?

3. Trace the progression, in terms of physical results, of a person who went from an overnourished to an undernourished state (LO 2.2).

4. How could the nutritional state of the person at each state in question 3 be evaluated (LO 2.2)?

5. Describe the philosophy underlying the creation of MyPlate. What dietary changes would you need to make to comply with the healthy eating guidelines exemplified by MyPlate on a regular basis (LO 2.6)?

6. Describe the intent of the Dietary Guidelines for Americans. Point out one criticism for their general application to all North American adults (LO 2.5).

7. Based on the discussion of the Dietary Guidelines for Americans, suggest two key dietary changes the typical North American adult should consider making (LO 2.5).

8. How do RDAs and AIs differ from Daily Values in intention and application (LO 2.4)?

9. Dietitians encourage all people to read labels on food packages to learn more about what they eat. What four nutrients could easily be tracked in your diet if you read the Nutrition Facts panels regularly on food products (LO 2.7)?

10. What would you list as the top five sources of reliable nutrition information? What makes these sources reliable (LO 2.8)?

What Would You Choose Recommendations

An 8-ounce glass of orange juice provides 114 kcal, 24 grams of sugar, 0 grams of fiber, and 72 mg of vitamin C. The weight of this serving of orange juice is about 250 grams, or almost 9 ounces (there are about 28 grams in 1 ounce). To estimate energy density, compare the calorie content of this food to its weight: 114 kcal/250 grams = 0.456 kcal/gram. To find nutrient density for vitamin C, calculate a ratio of vitamin C content to the calorie content of the food: 72 milligrams of vitamin C/114 kcal = 0.63 mg vitamin C/kcal.

A whole, fresh, medium orange has about 60 kcal, 12 grams of sugar, 3 grams of fiber, and 70 mg of vitamin C. The weight of an orange is about 130 grams. Comparing calorie content to weight of the food results in 60 kcal/130 grams = 0.462 kcal/gram for energy density. Nutrient density for vitamin C is calculated as 70 milligrams of vitamin C/60 kcal = 1.17 mg vitamin C/kcal.

Oranges and orange juice have about the same energy density, but the nutrient density for vitamin C is almost twice as high as that for orange juice. Oranges and 100% orange juice are both good choices in terms of energy density, and both are rich sources of vitamin C. The RDA for vitamin C is 75 mg/day for women and 90 mg/day for men. A person who is trying to restrict calorie intake while still consuming adequate nutrients should choose the whole, fresh orange instead of the orange juice as a source of vitamin C because it has higher nutrient density—it provides excellent nutrition in fewer calories than the serving of orange juice. Whole fruits also provide more fiber and phytochemicals than juice. Be assured that 100% fruit juice is still a healthy choice. When choosing your servings of fruit, choose whole fruits more often than fruit juice to get the best nutrition in the fewest calories.

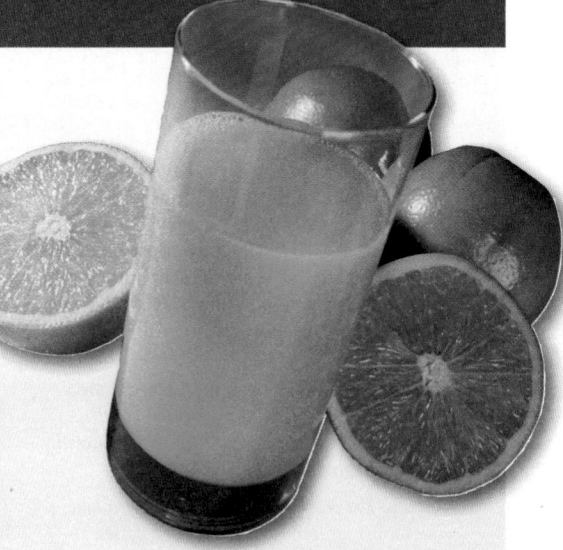

▲ The nutrient density of whole oranges surpasses that of orange juice.

Further Readings

1. ADA Reports: Position of the American Dietetic Association: Food and nutrition misinformation. *Journal of the American Dietetic Association* 106:601, 2006.

   Much food and nutrition misinformation pervades North American society. Individuals should carefully consider the training of those who give advice and be assured that registered dietitians are credible and reliable resources.

2. Barr SI: Introduction to dietary reference intakes. *Applied Physiology, Nutrition, and Metabolism* 31:61, 2006.

   The development of the Dietary Reference Intakes (DRIs) was a joint initiative by the United States and Canada to update and replace the former Recommended Nutrient Intakes for Canadians and the Recommended Dietary Allowances for Americans. The new DRIs are described.

3. Kennedy ET: Evidence for nutritional benefits in prolonging wellness. *American Journal of Clinical Nutrition* 83:410S, 2006.

   The interaction between genes; the environment; and lifestyle factors, especially diet and physical activity, are involved in healthy aging. The need to consider all the lifestyle and environmental factors contributing to suboptimal eating and lifestyle patterns is discussed.

4. Mobley AR and others: Putting the nutrient-rich foods index into practice. *Journal of the American College of Nutrition* 28:427S, 2009.

   In response to a need for a standardized definition of nutrient density as well as a growing interest among consumers and food manufacturers in front-of-pack labeling to convey nutrient information in a glance, the Nutrient Rich Foods Coalition formulated a Nutrient-Rich Foods educational tool and a symbol, called My5, which conveys nutrient content of a food within the context of a healthy diet.

5. Reedy J, Krebs-Smith SM: A comparison of food-based recommendations and nutrient values of three food guides: USDA's MyPyramid, NHLBI's dietary approaches to stop hypertension eating plan, and Harvard's healthy eating pyramid. *Journal of the American Dietetic Association* 108: 522, 2008.

   The three food guides share consistent messages to eat more fruits, vegetables, legumes, and whole grains; eat less added sugar and saturated fat; and emphasize plant oils.

6. Rolls B: *The volumetric eating plan: Techniques and recipes for feeling full on fewer calories.* Harper, New York, 2005.

   Energy density of food choices strongly affects total calories consumed at a meal and throughout the day. The volumetric eating plan includes techniques and recipes that decrease energy density of the diet—incorporating more fiber and water—which helps people lower their calories without feeling deprived.

7. Rowe S and others: Translating the Dietary Guidelines for Americans 2010 to bring about real behavior change. *Journal of the American Dietetic Association* 111:28, 2011.

   Nutition experts devised a set of recommendations to assist health professionals, government authorities, and food manufacturers in implementing the Dietary Guidelines for Americans, 2010. The coordination of efforts of educators, health care providers, policy makers, and industry leaders is needed to reach the public. Nutrition messages should be simple and targeted. Along with efforts to encourage people to want to change their habits, food manufacturers should make gradual changes in food composition to better align products with the goals of the Dietary Guidelines. Education efforts should begin at an early age and should be sensitive to differences in culure and ethnic background.

8. Sheth A and others: Potential liver damage associated with over-the-counter vitamin supplements. *Journal of the American Dietetic Association* 108:1536, 2008.

   This case report provides an example of the potential for liver damage associated with long-term intakes of megadose dietary supplements. In this case, a patient developed liver cirrhosis after long-term (2 years) daily ingestion of over-the-counter dietary supplements containing 13,000 micrograms of vitamin A. Such adverse effects indicate the need for medical supervision of use of these products.

9. Sofi F and others: Adherence to Mediterranean Diet and health status: Meta-analysis. *British Medical Journal* 337:a1344, 2008.

   A systematic review found that greater adherence to a Mediterranean Diet is associated with a significant reduction in overall mortality (9%), mortality from cardiovascular diseases (9%), incidence of mortality from cancer (6%), and incidence of Parkinson's disease and Alzheimer's disease (13%). These results indicate that a Mediterranean-like dietary pattern should be encouraged for primary prevention of major chronic diseases.

10. Taylor CL, Wilkening VL: How the nutrition food label was developed, Part 1: The nutrition facts panel. Part 2: The purpose and promise of nutrition claims. *The Journal of the American Dietetic Association* 108: 437, 618, 2008.

    These articles offer insight into the development of the nutrition label and discuss its role in improving the diet and health of Americans. The issues discussed highlight the fact that the nutrition label is a "work in progress."

11. U.S. Department of Health and Human Services. *2008 Physical Activity Guidelines for Americans.* 2008. www.health.gov/ PAGuidelines/.

    Inactivity remains high among American children, adolescents, and adults, putting Americans at unnecessary risk of disease. The Guidelines provide science-based guidance to help Americans aged six and older improve their health through appropriate physical activity.

12. U.S. Department of Health and Human Services. *Dietary Guidelines for Americans, 2010.* 2011. www.health.gov/ dietaryguidelines/2010.

    The most recent Dietary Guidelines have three overarching goals. 1.) balance calories with physical activity to manage weight; 2.) consume more fruits, vegetables, whole grains, fat-free and low-fat dairy products, and seafoods; and 3.) consume fewer foods with sodium, saturated fats, trans fats, cholesterol, added sugars, and refined grains.

13. United States Department of Agriculture. *USDA's MyPlate.* 2011. www.choosemyplate .gov.

    MyPlate replaces MyPyramid as the icon depicting healthy eating for Americans. In addition to the graphic representations of MyPlate, www. ChooseMyPlate.gov. provides Daily Food Plans specific to individual energy needs, several interactive tools for consumers, and resources for health educators. Building a healthy meal with balanced proportions of fruits, vegetables, grains, protein, and dairy will help Americans reach the goals set forth by the Dietary Guidelines.

14. Watts ML and others: The art of translating nutritional science into dietary guidance: History and evolution of the Dietary Guidelines for Americans. *Nutrition Reviews* 69:404, 2011.

    The U.S. government has issued dietary guidance for more than 100 years. Over time, the guidelines have become more firmly rooted in scientific evidence and more specific to the target audience. There is widespread recognition that successful implementation of dietary guidance requires the coordination of stakeholders at all levels—policy makers, health care providers, educators, industry, and consumers.

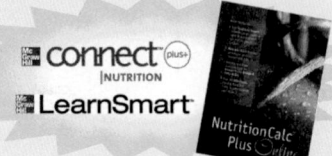

To get the most out of your study of nutrition, go to McGraw-Hill's online resources: Connect www.mcgrawhillconnect.com, **where you will find NutritionCalc Plus, LearnSmart, and many other dynamic tools.**

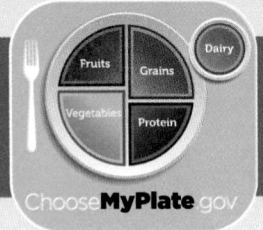

RATE YOUR PLATE

I. Does your Diet Compare to MyPlate?

Using your food-intake record from Chapter 1, place each food item in the appropriate group of the accompanying MyPlate chart. That is, for each food item, indicate how many servings it contributes to each group based on the amount you ate (see Food Composition Table Supplement for serving sizes). Many of your food choices may contribute to more than one group. For example, spaghetti with meat sauce contributes to three categories; grains, vegetables, and protein. After entering all the values, add the number of servings consumed in each group. Finally, compare your total in each food group with the recommended number of servings shown in Table 2-6 or obtained from the www.ChooseMyPlate.gov website. Enter a minus sign (−) if your total falls below the recommendation or a plus sign (+) if it equals or exceeds the recommendation.

Indicate the number of servings from MyPlate that each food yields:

Food or Beverage	Amount Eaten	Grains	Vegetables	Fruits	Dairy	Protein	Oils
Group totals							
Recommended servings							
Shortages/overages in numbers of servings							

II. Are You Putting Health Advice into Practice?

The broad range of diet and physical activity advice provided by the 2010 Dietary Guidelines for Americans, 2008 Physical Activity Guidelines for Americans, and MyPlate can seem overwhelming. Fill out the following inventory to see how well you comply with the basic intent of these consumer health guidelines and identify areas in which you need improvement.

Build a Healthy Plate

Y	N	Do fruits and vegetables cover at least half of your plate at meal times?
Y	N	Do you use fruits, vegetables, or unsalted nuts as snacks?
Y	N	Do you use either skim or 1% milk?
Y	N	Do you consume at least three servings of whole grains per day?
Y	N	Do you include seafood as your source of protein at least twice per week?
Y	N	Do you include beans as your source of protein at least once per week?
Y	N	Do you consume alcohol in moderation (≤1 drink/day for women; ≤2 drinks/day for men)?
Y	N	Do you use a meat thermometer to determine if your foods are thoroughly cooked?
Y	N	Do you clean hands, food contact surfaces, and fruits and vegetables before preparation?

Cut Back on Foods High in Solid Fats, Added Sugars, and Salt

Y	N	Do you choose water or other calorie-free beverages to drink most of the time?
Y	N	When you drink juice, do you choose 100% fruit juice?
Y	N	Do you use the Nutrition Facts panel to select foods low in sodium?
Y	N	Do you use spices and herbs instead of salt to season your food?
Y	N	Do you use vegetable oils rather than butter, lard, or shortening when preparing foods?
Y	N	Do you select foods that are reduced-fat, low-fat, or fat-free?

Eat the Right Amount of Calories for You

Y	N	Is your weight within a healthy range?
Y	N	Do you know how many calories you need per day?
Y	N	Do you limit your portions to one serving (i.e., as listed on food labels) of most foods?
Y	N	Do you stop eating when you are satisfied rather than uncomfortably full?
Y	N	Do you prepare most of your own foods?
Y	N	When eating out, do you seek out nutrition information on menu items?
Y	N	Do you take home leftovers or share meals with a friend when dining out?

Be Physically Active Your Way

Y	N	
		Do you exercise at least 150 minutes per week?
Y	N	Do you include aerobic and muscle-strengthening activities into your exercise routine?
Y	N	Do you protect yourself from injury when participating in physical activity?
Y	N	Does your exercise routine match your current level of fitness, ability, and health?

III. Applying the Nutrition Facts Label to Your Daily Food Choices

Imagine that you are at the supermarket looking for a quick meal before a busy evening. In the frozen food section, you find two brands of frozen cheese manicotti (see labels a and b). Which of the two brands would you choose? What information on the Nutrition Facts label in the figure contributed to this decision?

_____

_____

_____

_____

Nutrition Facts
Serving Size 1 Package (260g)
Servings Per Container 1

Amount Per Serving

Calories 390   Calories from Fat 160

	% Daily Value*
Total Fat 18g	**27**%
Saturated Fat 9g	**45**%
Trans Fat 2g	**
Cholesterol 45mg	**14**%
Sodium 880mg	**36**%
Total Carbohydrate 38g	**13**%
Dietary Fiber 4g	**15**%
Sugars 12g	
Protein 17g	

Vitamin A 10%   •   Vitamin C 4%

Calcium 40%   •   Iron 8%

*Percent Daily Values are based on a 2,000 calorie diet. Your daily values may be higher or lower depending on your calorie needs:

		Calories:	2,000	2,500
Total Fat	Less than		65g	80g
Sat Fat	Less than		20g	25g
Cholesterol	Less than		300mg	300mg
Sodium	Less than		2,400mg	2,400mg
Total Carbohydrate			300g	375g
Dietary Fiber			25g	30g

Calories per gram:
Fat 9 • Carbohydrate 4 • Protein 4

**Intake of _trans_ fat should be as low as possible.

(a)

Nutrition Facts
Serving Size 1 Package (260g)
Servings Per Container 1

Amount Per Serving

Calories 230   Calories from Fat 35

	% Daily Value*
Total Fat 4g	**6**%
Saturated Fat 2g	**10**%
Trans Fat 1g	**
Cholesterol 15mg	**4**%
Sodium 590mg	**24**%
Total Carbohydrate 28g	**9**%
Dietary Fiber 3g	**12**%
Sugars 10g	
Protein 19g	

Vitamin A 10%   •   Vitamin C 10%

Calcium 35%   •   Iron 4%

*Percent Daily Values are based on a 2,000 calorie diet. Your daily values may be higher or lower depending on your calorie needs:

		Calories:	2,000	2,500
Total Fat	Less than		65g	80g
Sat Fat	Less than		20g	25g
Cholesterol	Less than		300mg	300mg
Sodium	Less than		2,400mg	2,400mg
Potassium			3,500mg	3,500mg
Total Carbohydrate			300g	375g
Dietary Fiber			25g	30g

Calories per gram:
Fat 9 • Carbohydrate 4 • Protein 4

**Intake of _trans_ fat should be as low as possible.

(b)

Chapter 3 The Human Body: A Nutrition Perspective

Student Learning Outcomes

Chapter 3 is designed to allow you to:

3.1 Understand some basic roles of nutrients in human physiology.

3.2 Identify the functions of the common cellular components.

3.3 Define tissue, organ, and organ system.

3.4 Identify the role of the cardiovascular and lymphatic systems in nutrition.

3.5 List basic characteristics of the nervous system and its role in nutrition.

3.6 List basic characteristics of the endocrine system, especially the pancreas, and its role in nutrition.

3.7 List basic characteristics of the immune system and its role in nutrition.

3.8 Outline the overall processes of digestion and absorption in the mouth, stomach, small intestine, and large intestine, as well as the roles played by the liver, gallbladder, and pancreas.

3.9 List basic characteristics of the urinary system and its role in nutrition.

3.10 Understand the importance of the body storage areas for nutrients.

3.11 Understand the emerging field of nutrigenomics.

3.12 Identify the major nutrition-related gastrointestinal health problems and approaches to treatment.

What Would You Choose?

For spring break, you are volunteering to help build a house with Habitat for Humanity. You are carpooling with some friends and staying in a retreat house. Unfortunately, the travel, budget, living accommodations, and your building schedule won't allow for home-cooked meals this week. Being out of your normal routine and relying on fast-food sandwiches and pizza have left you feeling constipated. This reminds you that you will need to make smarter choices at fast-food establishments. To decrease your constipation which menu combination would you choose from a pizza buffet?

a 2 slices of pepperoni pizza, 2 cups of tossed salad

b 2 slices of veggie pizza, 1 cup of bean and pasta soup

c 2 slices of ham and pineapple pizza, 1 cup of pasta with Alfredo sauce

d 2 slices of cheese pizza, 1 garlic breadstick with marinara sauce

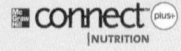 **connect** plus+ |NUTRITION

Think about your choices as you read Chapter 3, then see our recommendations at the end of the chapter. To learn more about the connection between our diets and our bodies, check out the Connect site: www.mcgrawhillconnect.com

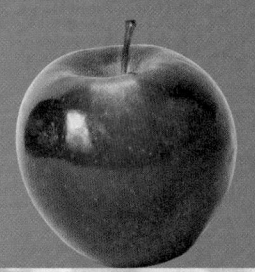

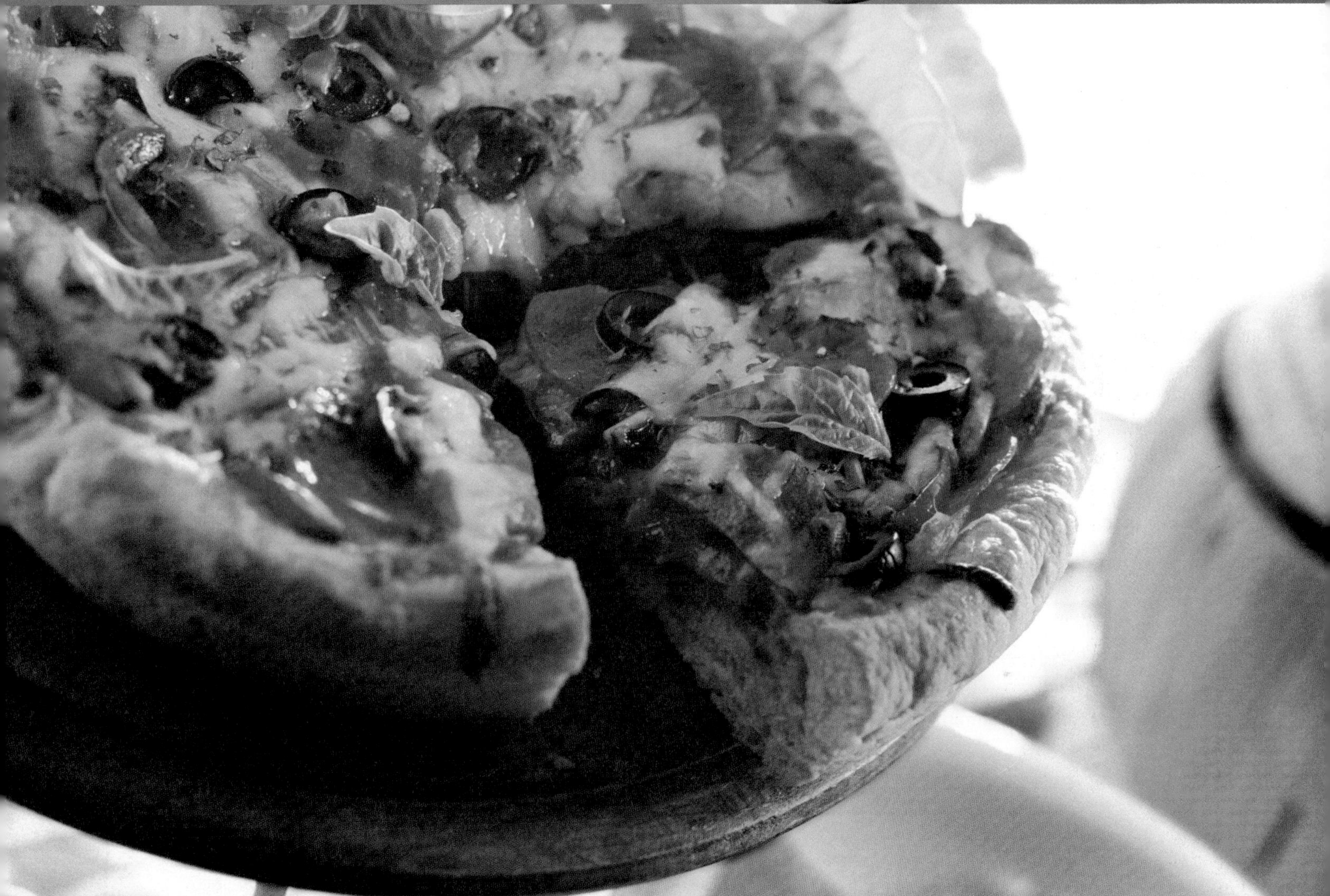

Merely eating food won't nourish you. You must first digest the food by breaking it down into usable forms of the essential nutrients that can be absorbed into the bloodstream. Once nutrients are taken up by the bloodstream, they can be distributed to and used by body cells.

We rarely think about, let alone control, digesting and absorbing foods. Except for a few voluntary responses—such as deciding what and when to eat, how well to chew food, and when to eliminate the remains—most digestion and absorption processes control themselves. As suggested in the comic in this chapter, we don't consciously decide when the pancreas will secrete digestive substances into the small intestine or how quickly foodstuffs will be propelled down the intestinal tract. Various hormones and the nervous system mostly control these functions. Your only awareness of these involuntary responses may be a hunger pang right before lunch or a "full" feeling after eating that last slice of pizza.

Let's examine digestion and absorption as well as other aspects of human physiology that support nutritional health. In the process you will become acquainted with the basic anatomy (structure) and physiology (function) of the circulatory system, nervous system, endocrine system, immune system, digestive system, urinary system, and storage capabilities of the human body.

Refresh Your Memory

As you begin your study of human physiology in Chapter 3, you may want to review:

- Cell structure and function from previous coursework in university-level biology courses
- Each of the body's organ systems from any previous biology training

3.1 Nutrition's Role in Human Physiology

Overall, the human body is a coordinated unit of many highly structured organ systems (Fig. 3-1). Together, these system are composed of trillions of cells. Each cell is a self-contained, living entity. Cells of the same type normally join together, using intercellular substances to form **tissues,** such as muscle tissue. One, two, or more tissues then combine in a particular way to form more complex structures, called **organs.** All organs contribute to nutritional health, and a person's overall nutritional state determines how well each organ functions. At a still higher level of coordination, several organs can cooperate for a common purpose to form an **organ system,** such as the digestive system.

Chemical processes (reactions) occur constantly in every living cell: The production of new substances is balanced by the breaking down of older ones. An example is the constant formation and degradation of bone. For this turnover of substances to occur, cells require a continuous supply of energy in the form of dietary carbohydrate, protein, and/or fat. Cells also need water; building supplies, especially protein and minerals; and chemical regulators, such as the vitamins. Almost all cells also need a steady supply of oxygen. These substances enable the tissues, made from individual cells, to function properly.

Getting an adequate supply of all nutrients to the body's cells begins with a healthy diet. To assure optimal use of nutrients, the body's cells, tissues, organs, and organ systems also must work efficiently.

tissues Collections of cells adapted to perform a specific function.

organ A group of tissues designed to perform a specific function—for example, the heart, which contains muscle tissue, nerve tissue, and so on.

organ system A collection of organs that work together to perform an overall function.

FRANK & ERNEST® by Bob Thaves

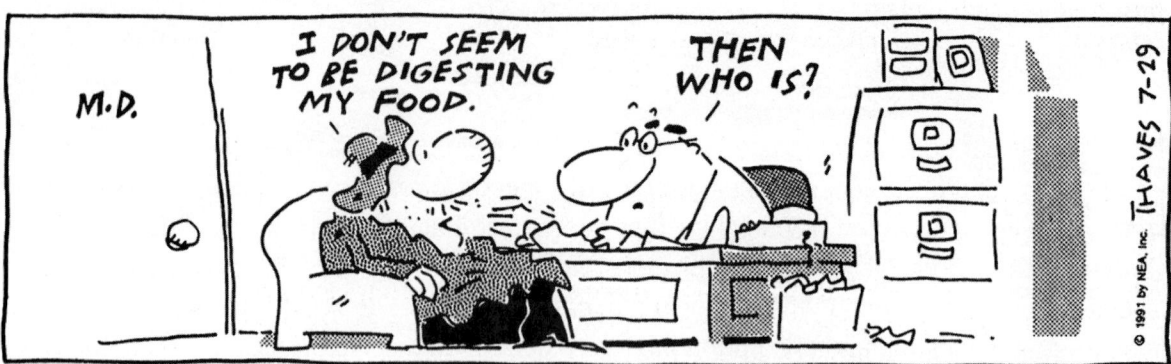

Some popular (fad) diets suggest not combining meat and potatoes to improve digestion and that fruit should only be eaten before noon. These diets might also claim that foods get stuck in the body and in turn putrefy and create toxins. Are there any scientific reasons to suggest that the timing of our food intake should optimize digestion? Do certain food practices improve digestion and subsequent absorption? This chapter provides some answers.

FRANK AND ERNEST reprinted by permission of Newspaper Enterprise Association, Inc.

1 **Chemical level.** Atoms combine to form molecules.

2 **Cell level.** Molecules form organelles, such as the nucleus and mitochondria, which make up cells.

3 **Tissue level.** Similar cells and surrounding materials make up tissues.

4 **Organ level.** Different tissues combine to form organs, such as the stomach.

5 **Organ system level.** Organs such as the stomach and intestines make up an organ system.

6 **Organism level.** Organ systems make up an organism.

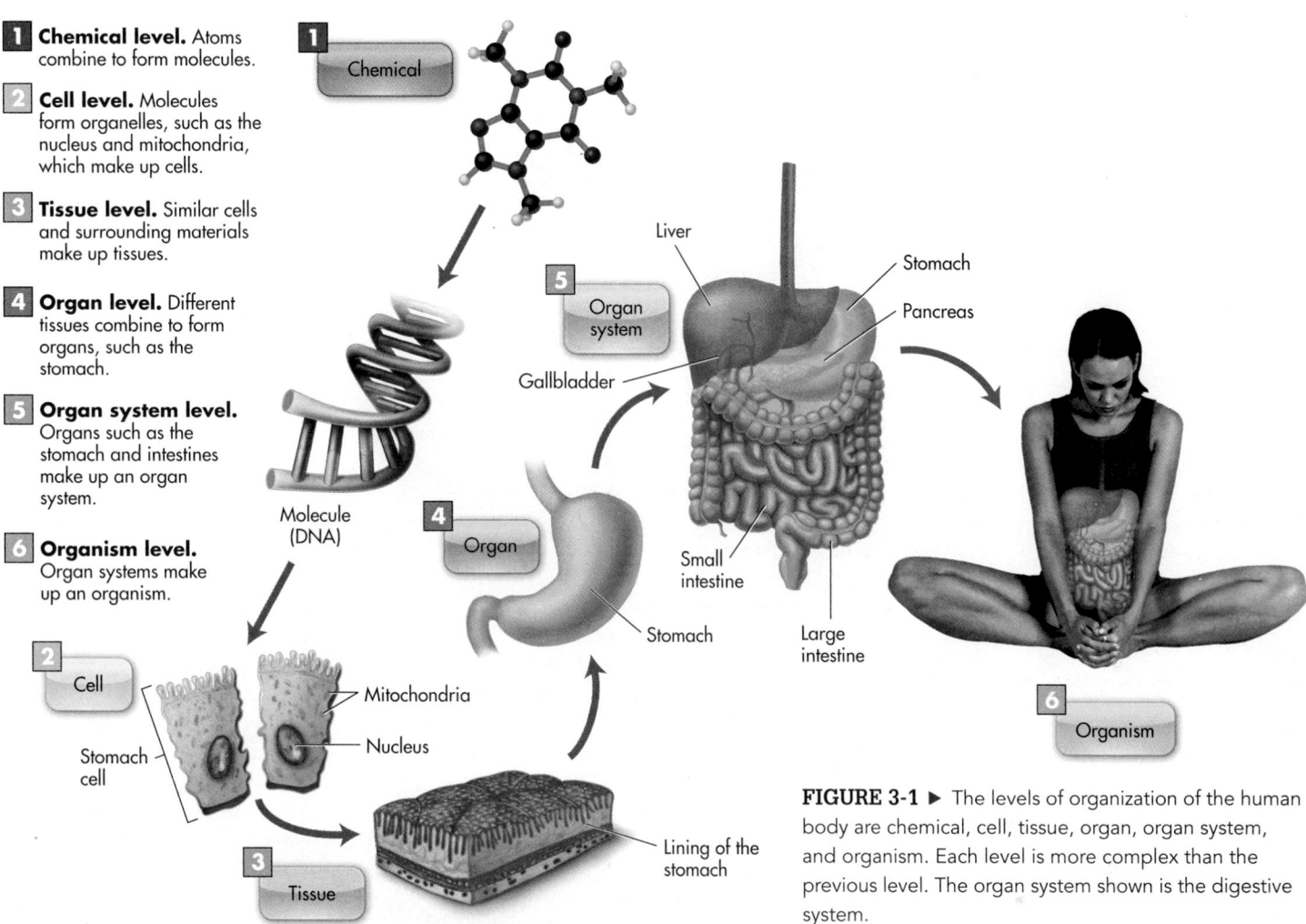

FIGURE 3-1 ▶ The levels of organization of the human body are chemical, cell, tissue, organ, organ system, and organism. Each level is more complex than the previous level. The organ system shown is the digestive system.

Chapter 3 covers the anatomy and physiology of the cell and major organ systems, especially as they relate to human nutrition. The information you are about to study is limited to the components of the various organ systems specifically influenced by the more than 45 essential nutrients discussed in this text.

3.2 The Cell: Structure, Function, and Metabolism

The cell is the basic structural and functional component of life. Living organisms are made of many different kinds of cells specialized to perform particular functions, and all cells are derived from preexisting cells. In the human body, all cells have certain common features. These cells have compartments and specialized structures that perform particular functions; these components are called **organelles** (Fig. 3-2). There are at least 15 different organelles. Eight of the most important organelles will be discussed. The numbers following the names of the cell structures correspond to the structures illustrated in Figure 3-2. Metabolism, the chemical processes that take place in body cells, will also be discussed.

organelles Compartments, particles, or filaments that perform specialized functions within a cell.

Cell (Plasma) Membrane 1

There is an outside and inside to every cell, separated by the cell (plasma) membrane. This membrane holds the cellular contents together and regulates the direction and flow of substances into and out of the cell. Cell-to-cell communication also occurs by way of this membrane.

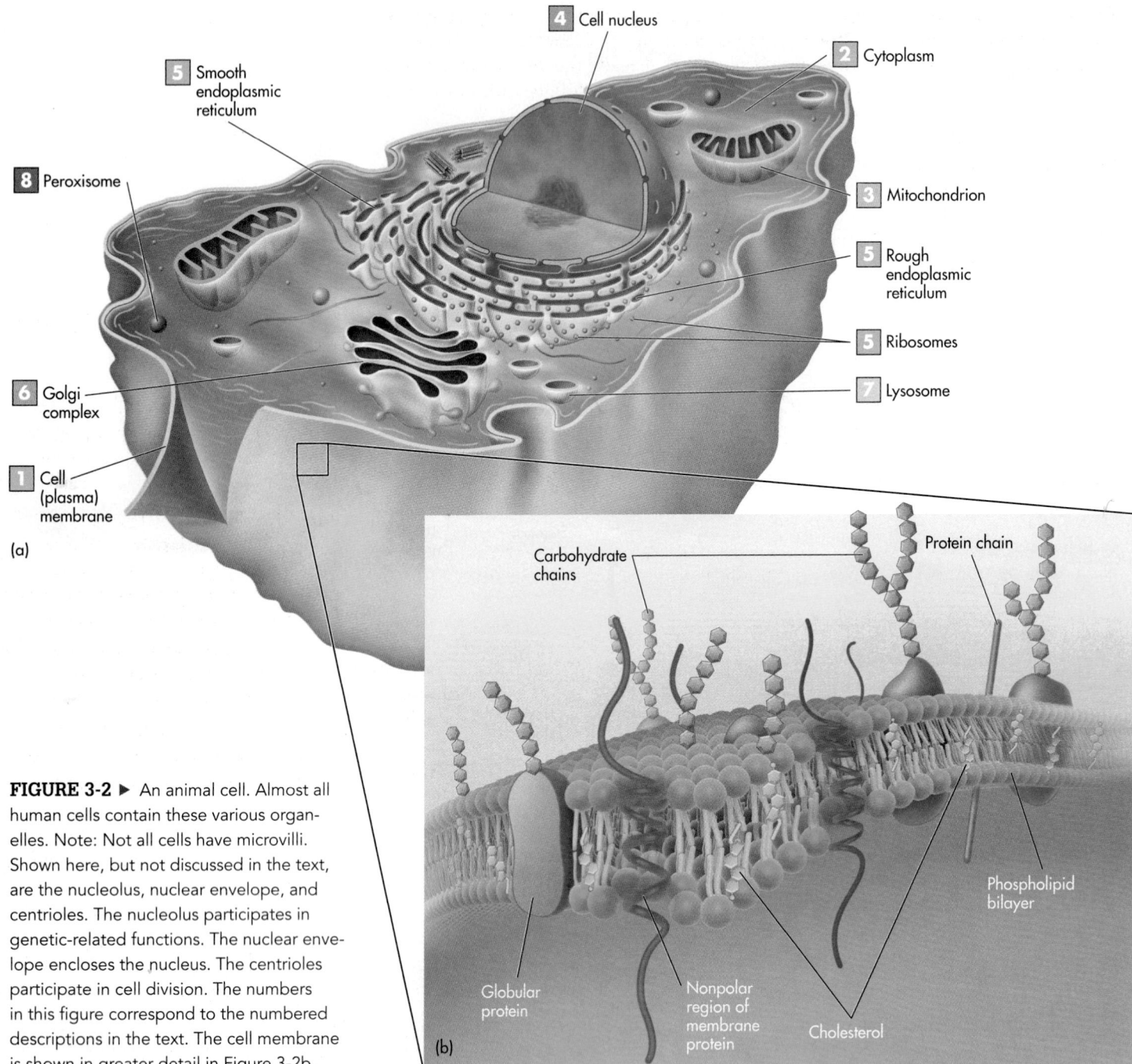

FIGURE 3-2 ▶ An animal cell. Almost all human cells contain these various organelles. Note: Not all cells have microvilli. Shown here, but not discussed in the text, are the nucleolus, nuclear envelope, and centrioles. The nucleolus participates in genetic-related functions. The nuclear envelope encloses the nucleus. The centrioles participate in cell division. The numbers in this figure correspond to the numbered descriptions in the text. The cell membrane is shown in greater detail in Figure 3-2b.

phospholipid Any of a class of fat-related substances that contain phosphorus, fatty acids, and a nitrogen-containing component. Phospholipids are an essential part of every cell.

enzyme A compound that speeds the rate of a chemical process but is not altered by that process. Almost all enzymes are proteins.

The cell membrane, illustrated in Figure 3-2(b), is a lipid bilayer (or double membrane) of **phospholipids** with their water-soluble heads facing both the interior of the cell and the exterior of the cell. Their water-insoluble tails are tucked into the center portion of the cell membrane.

Cholesterol is another component of the cell membrane. It is fat soluble, so it is embedded within the bilayer. This cholesterol provides rigidity and thus stability to the membrane.

There are also various proteins embedded in the cell membrane. Proteins provide structural support, act as transport vehicles, and function as **enzymes** that affect chemical processes within the membrane (see the later section on digestion for more about enzymes). Some proteins form open channels that allow water-soluble substances to pass into and out of the cell. Proteins on the outside surface of the membrane act as receptors, snagging essential substances that the cell needs and drawing them into the cell. Other proteins act as gates that open and close to control the flow of various particles into and out of the cell.

In addition to the lipid and protein, the membrane also contains carbohydrates that mark the exterior of the cell. These carbohydrates are combined either with protein or fat, and they help send messages to the cell's organelles and act as identification markers for the cell. In addition, they detect invaders and initiate defensive actions. In sum, these carbohydrates provide tags that are important to cellular identity and interaction.

Cytoplasm 2

The **cytoplasm** is the combination of fluid material and organelles within the cell, not including the nucleus. A small amount of energy for use by the cell can be produced by chemical processes that occur in the cytoplasm. This contributes to the survival of all cells and is the sole source of energy production in red blood cells. This energy production is called **anaerobic** metabolism because it doesn't require oxygen.

Organelles. Included within the cytoplasm are organelles. As described in the next two pages, they carry out vital roles in cell functions.

Mitochondria 3

Mitochondria are sometimes called the "power plants," or the powerhouse of the cell. These organelles are capable of converting the food energy in energy-yielding nutrients (carbohydrate, protein, and fat) to a form of energy that cells can use. This is an **aerobic** process that uses the oxygen we inhale, as well as water, enzymes, and other compounds (see Chapter 10 for details). With the exception of red blood cells, all cells contain mitochondria; only the size, shape, and quantity vary.

Cell Nucleus 4

With the exception of the red blood cell, all cells have one or more nuclei. The **cell nucleus** is bounded by its own double membrane. The nucleus contains the genetic material responsible for controlling actions that occur in the cell. The genetic material consists of **genes** on **chromosomes** made up of **deoxyribonucleic acid (DNA).** DNA is the "code book" that contains directions for making substances, specifically proteins, the cell needs. This code book remains in the nucleus of the cell, but sends its information to other cell organelles by way of a similar "messenger" molecule called **ribonucleic acid (RNA).** The information on the DNA is copied onto the RNA through the process of **transcription** and then moves out to the cytoplasm through pores in the nuclear membrane. The RNA carries the transcribed DNA code to protein-synthesizing sites called **ribosomes.** There, the RNA code is used in the process of **translation** to make a specific protein (see Chapter 6 for details on protein synthesis). This process is also known as **gene expression.**

All of the DNA in a cell is copied during cell replication. DNA is a double-stranded molecule, and when the cell begins to divide, each strand is separated and an identical copy of each is made. Thus, each new DNA contains one new strand of DNA and one strand from the original DNA. In this way, the genetic code is preserved from one cell generation to the next. (The mitochondria contain their own DNA, so they reproduce themselves within a cell independent of action in the cell's nucleus.)

cytoplasm The fluid and organelles (except the nucleus) in a cell.

anaerobic Not requiring oxygen.

mitochondria The main sites of energy production in a cell. They contain the pathway for oxidizing fat for fuel, among other metabolic pathways.

aerobic Requiring oxygen.

cell nucleus An organelle bound by its own double membrane and containing chromosomes, the genetic information for cell protein synthesis and cell replication.

gene A specific segment on a chromosome. Genes provide the blueprint for the production of cell proteins.

chromosome A single, large DNA molecule and its associated proteins; contains many genes to store and transmit genetic information.

deoxyribonucleic acid (DNA) The site of hereditary information in cells; DNA directs the synthesis of cell proteins.

ribonucleic acid (RNA) The single-stranded nucleic acid involved in the transcription of genetic information and translation of that information into protein structure.

transcription Information on DNA needed to make a protein is copied onto RNA.

ribosomes Cytoplasmic particles that mediate the linking together of amino acids to form proteins; may exist freely in the cytoplasm or attached to endoplasmic reticulum.

translation The information contained in RNA is used to determine the amino acids in a protein.

gene expression Use of DNA information on a gene to produce a protein. Thought to be a major determination of cell development.

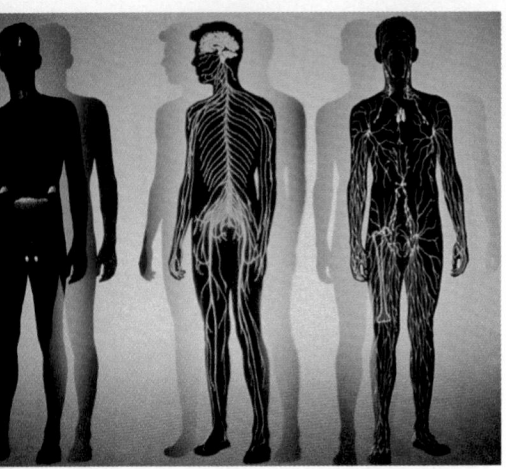

▲ The body is made up of numerous organ systems including the endocrine, nervous, and circulatory systems shown here.

endoplasmic reticulum (ER) An organelle in the cytoplasm composed of a network of canals running through the cytoplasm. Part of the endoplasmic reticulum contains ribosomes.

Golgi complex The cell organelle near the nucleus that processes newly synthesized protein for secretion or distribution to other organelles.

secretory vesicles Membrane-bound vesicles produced by the Golgi apparatus; contain protein and other compounds to be secreted by the cell.

lysosome A cellular organelle that contains digestive enzymes for use inside the cell for turnover of cell parts.

peroxisome A cell organelle that destroys toxic products within the cell.

adenosine triphosphate (ATP) The main energy currency for cells. ATP energy is used to promote ion pumping, enzyme activity, and muscular contraction.

Endoplasmic Reticulum (ER) 5

The outer membrane of the cell nucleus is continuous with a network of tubes called the **endoplasmic reticulum (ER)**. Part of the endoplasmic reticulum (termed the rough [as opposed to smooth] endoplasmic reticulum) contains the ribosomes, where the RNA code is translated into proteins during protein synthesis. Many of these proteins play a central role in human nutrition. Parts of the endoplasmic reticulum also are involved in lipid synthesis, detoxification of toxic substances, and calcium storage and release in the cell.

Golgi Complex 6

The **Golgi complex** is a packaging site for proteins used in the cytoplasm or exported from the cell. It consists of sacs within the cytoplasm in which proteins are "packaged" as **secretory vesicles** for secretion by the cell.

Lysosomes 7

Lysosomes are the cell's digestive system. They are sacs that contain enzymes for the digestion of foreign material. Sometimes known as "suicide bags," they are responsible for digesting worn-out or damaged cell components. Certain cells associated with immune functions contain many lysosomes (see the later section on the immune system).

Peroxisomes 8

Peroxisomes contain enzymes that detoxify harmful chemicals. Peroxisomes get their name from the fact that hydrogen peroxide (H_2O_2) is formed as a result of such enzyme action. Peroxisomes also contain a protective enzyme called *catalase*, which prevents excessive accumulation of hydrogen peroxide in the cell, which would be very damaging. Peroxisomes also play a minor role in metabolizing one possible source of energy for cells—alcohol.

Cell Metabolism

Metabolism refers to the entire network of chemical processes involved in maintaining life. It encompasses all the sequences of chemical reactions that occur in the body's cells. These biochemical reactions take place in the cell cytoplasm and organelles that we have just discussed. They enable us to release and use energy from foods, synthesize one substance from another, and prepare waste products for excretion.

The reactions of metabolism that take place within your body can be categorized into one of two types. One type of reaction, anabolic, puts different molecules together and, therefore, requires energy. The other type of reaction, catabolic, takes molecules apart and, therefore, releases energy. The metabolism of the nutrients, carbohydrates, proteins, and fats are interrelated and yield energy. The other nutrients, vitamins and minerals, contribute to the enzyme activity that supports metabolic reactions in the cell.

The metabolism of energy production begins in the cytoplasm with the initial anaerobic breakdown of glucose. The remaining aerobic steps of energy production take place in the mitochondria. Ultimately, the cells of the body use these interconnected processes to convert the energy found in food to energy stored in the high-energy compound, **adenosine triphosphate (ATP)**. You will learn more about the metabolism of energy sources in Chapter 10, "Nutrition: Fitness and Sports."

CONCEPT CHECK

In Chapter 1, you learned that fat (lipids), protein, and carbohydrate function as fuels. Now you recognize that these nutrients also serve as structural materials in the cell membrane. This is typical of many nutrients; they can carry out multiple functions. The cell receives nutrients and other substances through the cell membrane by using various transport systems.

The basic structural unit in the body is the cell. Within the cell are a variety of organelles with unique functions to perform. Although there is no typical cell, virtually all cells have the same organelles, each performing the same essential task.

3.3 Body Systems

As noted earlier, when groups of similar cells work together to accomplish a specialized task, the arrangement is referred to as a tissue. Humans are composed of four primary types of tissue: **epithelial, connective, muscle,** and **nervous.** Epithelial tissue is composed of cells that cover surfaces both inside and outside the body. For example, the lining of the respiratory tract is made up of epithelial cells. These cells of epithelial tissue secrete important substances, absorb nutrients, and excrete waste. Connective tissue supports and protects the body, stores fat, and produces blood cells. Muscle tissue is designed for movement. Nervous tissue found in the brain and spinal cord is designed for communication. These four types of tissues then go on to form various organs, and ultimately, organ systems (Table 3-1).

We will focus primarily on the digestive system in Chapter 3. The nutrients we consume in food are unavailable until such time as they have been processed by the digestive system. This employs chemical and mechanical means to alter food so that the nutrients can be released and absorbed into the body for distribution to body tissues.

Sometimes organs within a system can serve another system. For example, the basic function of the digestive system is to convert the food we eat into absorbable nutrients. At the same time, the digestive system serves the immune system by preventing dangerous pathogens from invading the body and causing illness. As you study nutrition, you will note the multiple roles played by many organs (Fig. 3-3).

The overriding theme of human nutrition is to understand the actions of nutrients as they affect different cells, tissues, organs, and organ systems. Each type of organ system is impacted by nutrient intake and simultaneously determines how each nutrient is used.

Our task now is to explore the key systems in the body as they specifically relate to the study of human nutrition: circulatory (cardiovascular and lymphatic), nervous, endocrine, immune, digestive, and urinary systems. This part of Chapter 3 will set the stage for a more detailed look at these and other organ systems in later chapters covering various aspects of human nutrition.

Also in this chapter, we will introduce the emerging area of genetics and nutrition. Throughout this book, discussions will point out how you can personalize nutrition advice based on your genetic background. In this way, you can identify and avoid the "controllable" risk factors that would contribute to development of genetically linked diseases present in your family.

epithelial tissue The surface cells that line the outside of the body and all external passages within it.

connective tissue Protein tissue that holds different structures in the body together. Some body structures are made up of connective tissue—notably, tendons and cartilage. Connective tissue also forms part of bone and the nonmuscular structures of arteries and veins.

muscle tissue A type of tissue adapted to contract to cause movement.

nervous tissue Tissue composed of highly branched, elongated cells, which transport nerve impulses from one part of the body to another.

cardiovascular system The body system consisting of the heart, blood vessels, and blood. This system transports nutrients, waste products, gases, and hormones throughout the body and plays an important role in immune responses and regulation of body temperature.

lymphatic system A system of vessels and lymph that accepts fluid surrounding cells and large particles, such as products of fat absorption. Lymph eventually passes into the bloodstream from the lymphatic system.

3.4 Cardiovascular System and Lymphatic System

The body has two separate organ systems that circulate fluids in the body: the **cardiovascular system** and the **lymphatic system.** The cardiovascular system consists of the heart and blood vessels. The lymphatic system consists of lymphatic vessels and

TABLE 3-1 Organ Systems of the Body

System	Major Components	Functions Related to Nutrition
Cardiovascular	Heart, blood vessels, and blood	Transports nutrients, waste products, gases, and hormones throughout the body and plays a role in the immune response and the regulation of body temperature
Lymphatic	Lymph vessels, lymph nodes, and other lymph organs	Removes foreign substances from the blood and lymph, combats disease, maintains tissue fluid balance, and aids in fat absorption
Nervous	Brain, spinal cord, nerves, and sensory receptors	A major regulatory system: detects sensation, controls movements, and controls physiological and intellectual functions
Endocrine	Endocrine glands, such as the pituitary, thyroid, and adrenal glands	A major regulatory system: participates in the regulation of metabolism, reproduction, and many other functions through the action of hormones
Immune	White blood cells, lymph vessels and nodes, spleen, thymus gland, and other lymph tissues	Provides defense against foreign invaders; formation of white blood cells
Digestive	Mouth, esophagus, stomach, intestines, and accessory structures (liver, gallbladder, and pancreas)	Performs the mechanical and chemical processes of digestion, absorption of nutrients, and elimination of wastes
Urinary	Kidneys, urinary bladder, and the ducts that carry urine	Removes waste products from the circulatory system and regulates the acidity, chemical composition, and water content of the blood
Integumentary	Skin, hair, nails, and sweat glands	Protects the body, regulates temperature, prevents water loss, and produces a substance that converts to vitamin D upon sun exposure
Skeletal	Bones, associated cartilage, and joints	Supports the body, and allows for body movement, produces blood cells, and stores minerals
Muscular	Smooth, cardiac, and skeletal muscle	Produces body movement, maintains posture, and produces body heat
Respiratory	Lungs and respiratory passages	Exchanges gases (oxygen and carbon dioxide) between the blood and the atmosphere and regulates blood acid-base (pH) balance
Reproductive	Gonads, accessory structures, and genitals of males and females	Performs the processes of reproduction and influences sexual functions and behaviors

lymph A clear fluid that flows through lymph vessels; carries most forms of fat after their absorption by the small intestine.

plasma The fluid, extracellular portion of the circulating blood. This includes the blood serum plus all blood-clotting factors. In contrast, serum is the fluid that remains after clotting factors have been removed from plasma.

a number of lymph tissues. Blood flows through the cardiovascular system, while **lymph** flows through the lymphatic system.

Cardiovascular System

The heart is a muscular pump that normally contracts and relaxes 50 to 90 times per minute when the body is at rest. This continual pumping, measured by taking your pulse, keeps blood moving through the blood vessels. The blood that flows through the cardiovascular system is composed of **plasma,** red blood cells, white blood cells, platelets, and many other substances. It travels two basic routes. In the first route, blood circulates from the right side of the heart, through the lungs, and then back to the heart. In the lungs, blood picks up oxygen and releases carbon dioxide. After this exchange of gases has taken place, blood is said to be *oxygenated* and returns to the left side of your heart. In the second route, the oxygenated blood circulates from the left side of the heart to all other body cells, eventually returning back to the right side of the heart (Fig. 3-4). After blood has circulated throughout the body, it is *deoxygenated*. (As you review the cardiovascular system, recall from your previous studies of biology that *left* and *right* designations of the heart refer to the left and right sides of your body, not of the page in your textbook.)

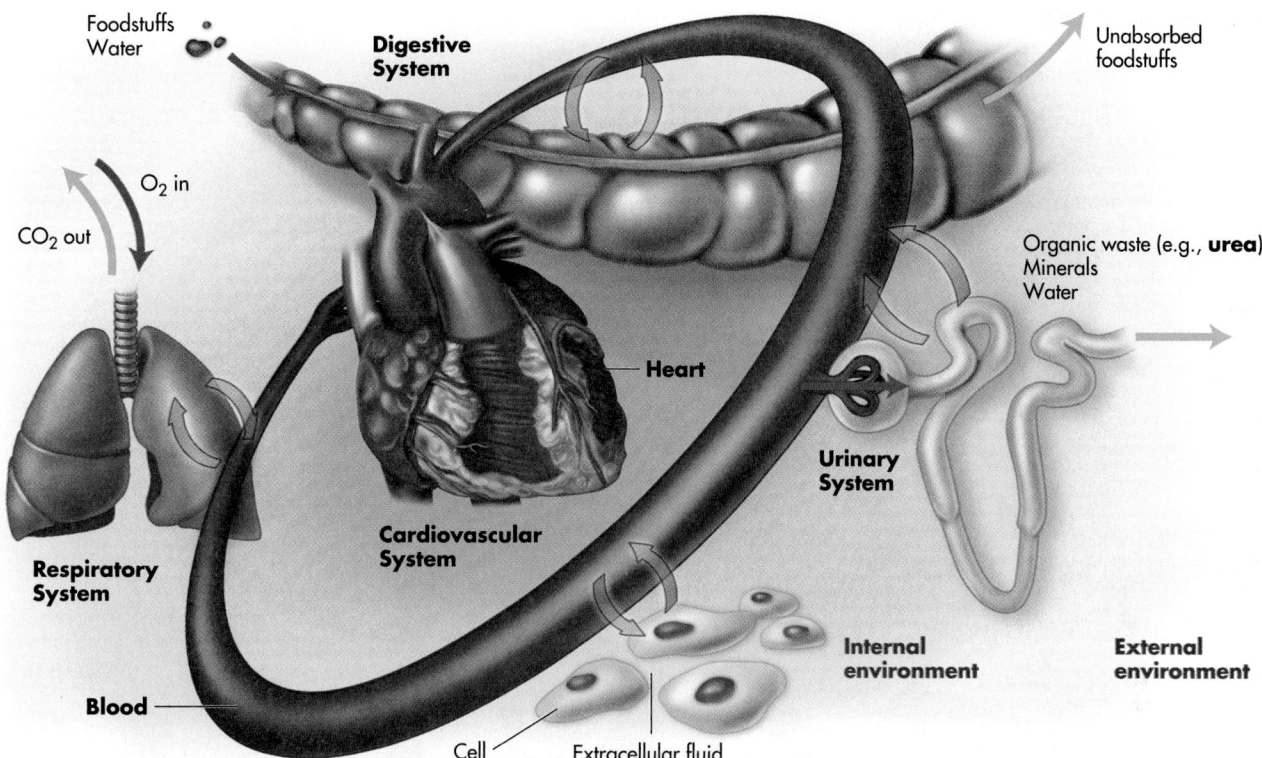

FIGURE 3-3 ▶ Exchanges of nutrients occur between our external environment and the internal environment of the circulatory system via the digestive, respiratory, and urinary systems. Overall, the human body is a combination of 12 systems working together to support cell needs.

In the cardiovascular system, blood leaves the heart via **arteries,** which branch into **capillaries,** a network of tiny blood vessels. Exchange of nutrients, oxygen, and waste products between the blood and cells occurs through the minute, web-like pores of the capillaries (Fig. 3-5). Capillaries service every region of the body via individual capillary beds only one cell layer thick. The blood then returns to the heart via the **veins.**

The cardiovascular system distributes nutrients absorbed from food and oxygen from the air to all body cells (review Fig. 3-3). Other functions include delivery of hormones to their target cells, maintenance of a constant body temperature, and distribution of white blood cells throughout the body to protect against pathogens as part of the immune system (see the later section, "Immune System").

Portal Circulation in the Gastrointestinal Tract. Water and nutrients are transferred to the circulatory system through capillary beds. Once absorbed through the stomach or intestinal wall, nutrients reach one of two destinations. Some nutrients are taken up by cells in the intestines and portions of the stomach to nourish those organs. Most of the nutrients from recently eaten foods, however, are transferred into **portal circulation.** To enter portal circulation, the nutrients pass from the intestinal capillaries into veins that eventually merge into a very large vein called a **portal vein.** Unlike most veins in the body—which carry blood back to the heart—this portal vein leads directly to the liver. This enables the liver to process absorbed nutrients before they enter the general circulation of the bloodstream. Overall, portal circulation represents a special form of circulation in the cardiovascular system.

Lymphatic System

The **lymphatic system** is also a circulatory system. It consists of a network of lymphatic vessels and the fluid (lymph) that moves through them. Lymph is similar to

artery A blood vessel that carries blood away from the heart.

capillary A microscopic blood vessel that connects the smallest arteries and veins; site of nutrient, oxygen, and waste exchange between body cells and the blood.

vein A blood vessel that carries blood to the heart.

portal circulation The portion of the circulatory system that uses a large vein (portal vein) to carry nutrient-rich blood from capillaries in the intestines and portions of the stomach to the liver.

urea Nitrogenous waste product of protein metabolism; major source of nitrogen in the urine.

portal vein Large vein leaving the intestine and stomach and connecting to the liver.

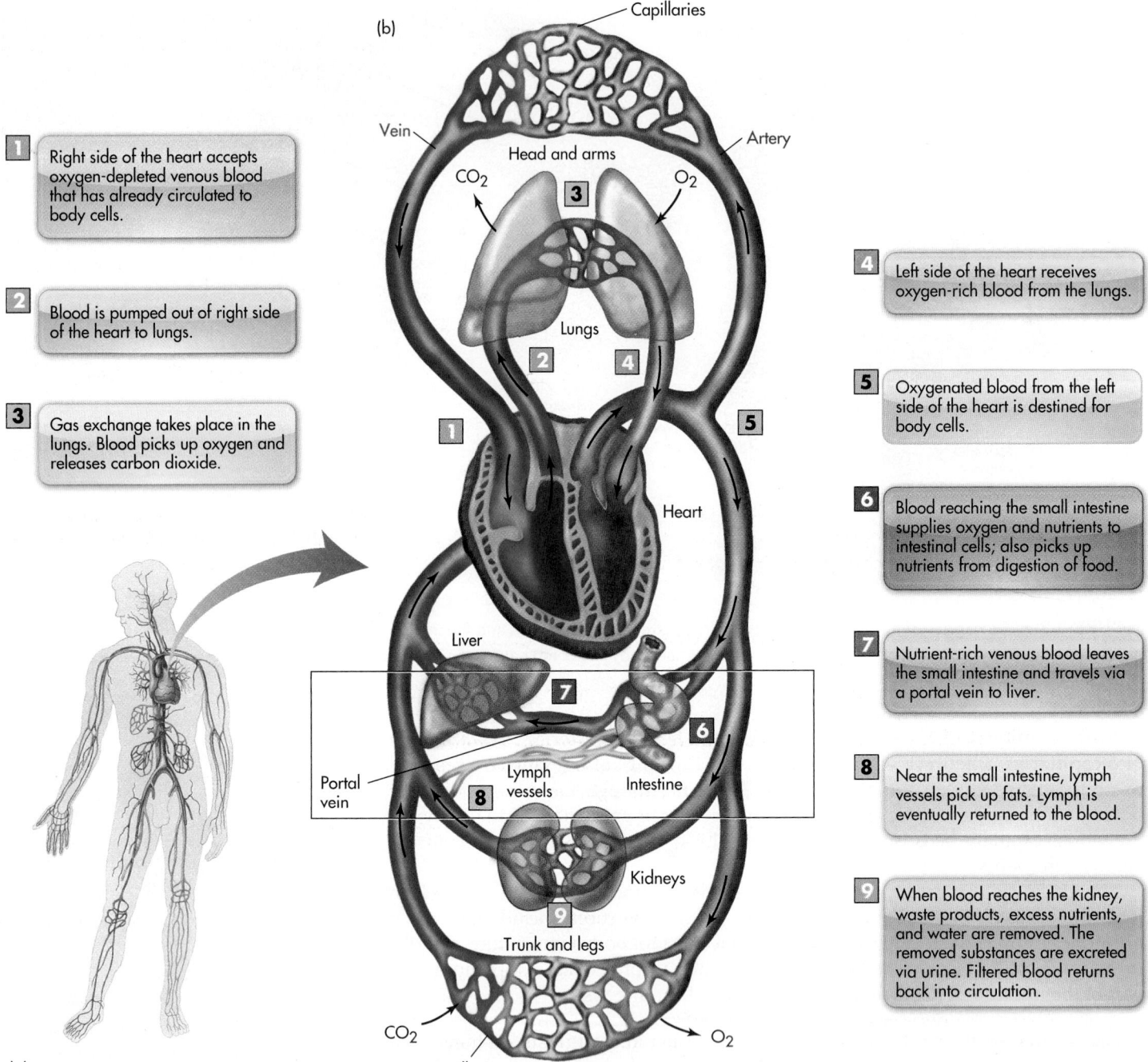

(b)

1 Right side of the heart accepts oxygen-depleted venous blood that has already circulated to body cells.

2 Blood is pumped out of right side of the heart to lungs.

3 Gas exchange takes place in the lungs. Blood picks up oxygen and releases carbon dioxide.

4 Left side of the heart receives oxygen-rich blood from the lungs.

5 Oxygenated blood from the left side of the heart is destined for body cells.

6 Blood reaching the small intestine supplies oxygen and nutrients to intestinal cells; also picks up nutrients from digestion of food.

7 Nutrient-rich venous blood leaves the small intestine and travels via a portal vein to liver.

8 Near the small intestine, lymph vessels pick up fats. Lymph is eventually returned to the blood.

9 When blood reaches the kidney, waste products, excess nutrients, and water are removed. The removed substances are excreted via urine. Filtered blood returns back into circulation.

(a)

FIGURE 3-4 ▶ Blood circulation through the body. Figure (a) shows the heart and some examples of the major arteries and veins of the cardio-vascular system. Figure (b) shows the paths that blood takes from the heart to the lungs (1–3), back to the heart (4), and through the rest of the body (5–9). The red color indicates blood richer in oxygen; blue is for blood carrying more carbon dioxide. Keep in mind that arteries and veins go to all parts of the body.

blood, consisting largely of blood plasma that has found its way out of capillaries and into the spaces between cells. It contains a full array of the various white blood cells that play an important role in the immune system. However, neither red blood cells nor platelets are present. Lymph is collected in tiny lymph vessels all over the body and moves through even larger vessels until it eventually enters the cardiovascular system through major veins near the heart. This flow is driven by muscle contractions arising from normal body movements.

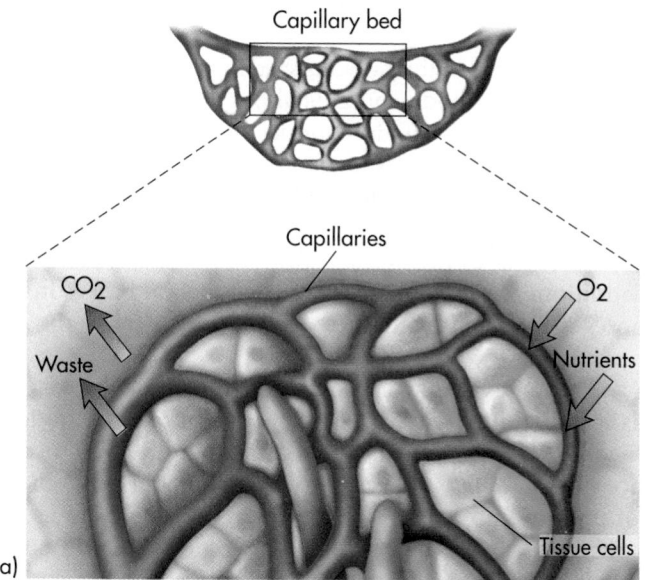

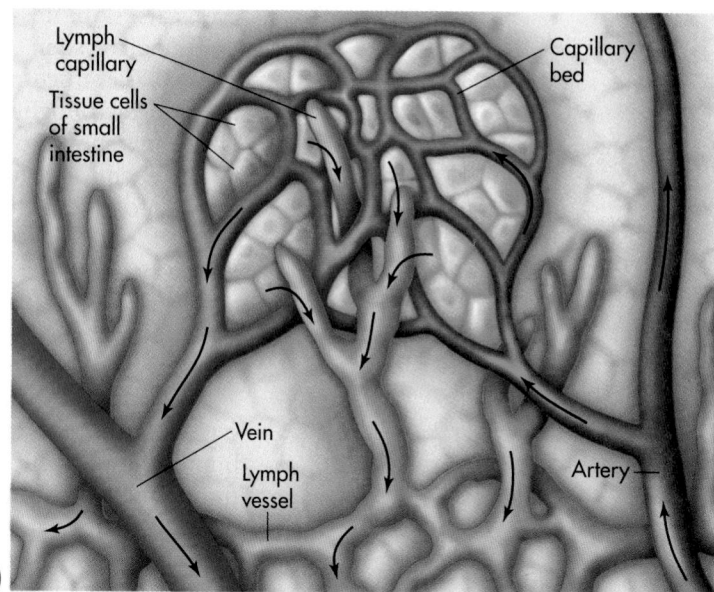

FIGURE 3-5 ▶ Capillary and lymph vessels. (a) Exchange of oxygen (O_2) and nutrients for carbon dioxide (CO_2) and waste products occurs between the capillaries and the surrounding tissue cells. (b) Lymph vessels are also present in capillary beds, such as in the small intestine. Lymph vessels in the small intestine are also called lacteals. The lymph vessels have closed ends and are important for fat absorption.

Lymphatic Circulation in the Gastrointestinal Tract. Besides contributing to the defense of the body against invading pathogens, lymphatic vessels that serve the small intestine play an important role in nutrition. These vessels pick up and transport the majority of products of fat digestion and fat absorption. These fat-related products are too large to enter the bloodstream directly and therefore are generally emptied into the bloodstream only after passing through the lymphatic system. The lymph vessels also take up excess fluid that collects between cells and returns it to the bloodstream.

CONCEPT CHECK

Blood is transported from the right side of the heart to the capillaries in the lungs. Carbon dioxide is removed and oxygen is taken up by red blood cells. The oxygenated blood returns to the left side of the heart. Here it is pumped into general circulation. In the capillaries, oxygen is released from the red blood cells and delivered through pores in the capillaries to the surrounding cells. Nutrients also are distributed from the bloodstream to body cells via the capillaries. Carbon dioxide released from cells travels through the capillary pores to the blood.

The lymph system serves several purposes: the transport of absorbed dietary fats, the uptake and return to the bloodstream of excess fluid that collects between cells, and the defense of the body against invading pathogens.

3.5 Nervous System

The **nervous system** is a regulatory system that centrally controls most body functions. The nervous system can detect changes occurring in various organs and the external environment and initiate corrective action when needed to maintain a constant internal body environment. The nervous system also regulates activities that change almost instantly, such as muscle contractions and perception of danger. The body has many receptors that receive information about what is happening within the body and in the outside environment. For the most part these receptors are found in our

nervous system The body system consisting of the brain, spinal cord, nerves, and sensory receptors. This system detects sensations, directs movements, and controls physiological and intellectual functions.

neuron The structural and functional unit of the nervous system. Consists of a cell body, dendrites, and an axon.

synapse The space between one neuron and another neuron (or cell).

neurotransmitter A compound made by a nerve cell that allows for communication between it and other cells.

eyes, ears, skin, nose, and stomach. We act on information from these receptors via the nervous system.

The basic structural and functional unit of the nervous system is the **neuron.** These are elongated, highly branched cells. The body contains about 100 billion neurons. Neurons respond to electrical and chemical signals, conduct electrical impulses, and release chemical regulators. Overall, neurons allow us to perceive what is occurring in our environment, engage in learning, store vital information in memory, and control the body's voluntary (and involuntary) actions.

The brain stores information, reacts to incoming information, solves problems, and generates thoughts. In addition, the brain plans a course of action based on the other sensory inputs. Responses to the stimuli are carried out mostly through the rest of the nervous system.

Simply put, the nervous system receives information through stimulation of various receptors, processes this information, and sends out signals through its various branches for an action that needs to be taken. Actual transmission of the signal occurs through a change in the concentration of two nutrients, sodium and potassium, in the neuron. There is an influx of sodium into the neuron and a loss of potassium as the message is sent. Concentrations of these minerals are then restored to normal amounts in the neuron after the signal passes, making it ready to conduct another message.

When the signal must bridge a gap **(synapse)** between the branches of different neurons, the message is generally converted to a chemical signal called a **neurotransmitter.** The neurotransmitter is then released into the gap, and its target may be another neuron or another type of cell, such as a muscle cell (Fig. 3-6). If the signal is sent to another neuron, this allows it to continue on to its final destination. The neurotransmitters

FIGURE 3-6 ▶ Transmission of a message from one neuron to another neuron or to another type of cell that relies on neurotransmitters. Vesicles containing neurotransmitters, formed within the neuron, fuse with the membrane of the neuron and the neurotransmitter is released into the synapse. The neurotransmitter then binds to the receptors on the nearby neuron (or cell). In this way, the message is transmitted from one neuron to another or to the cell that ultimately performs the action directed by the message.

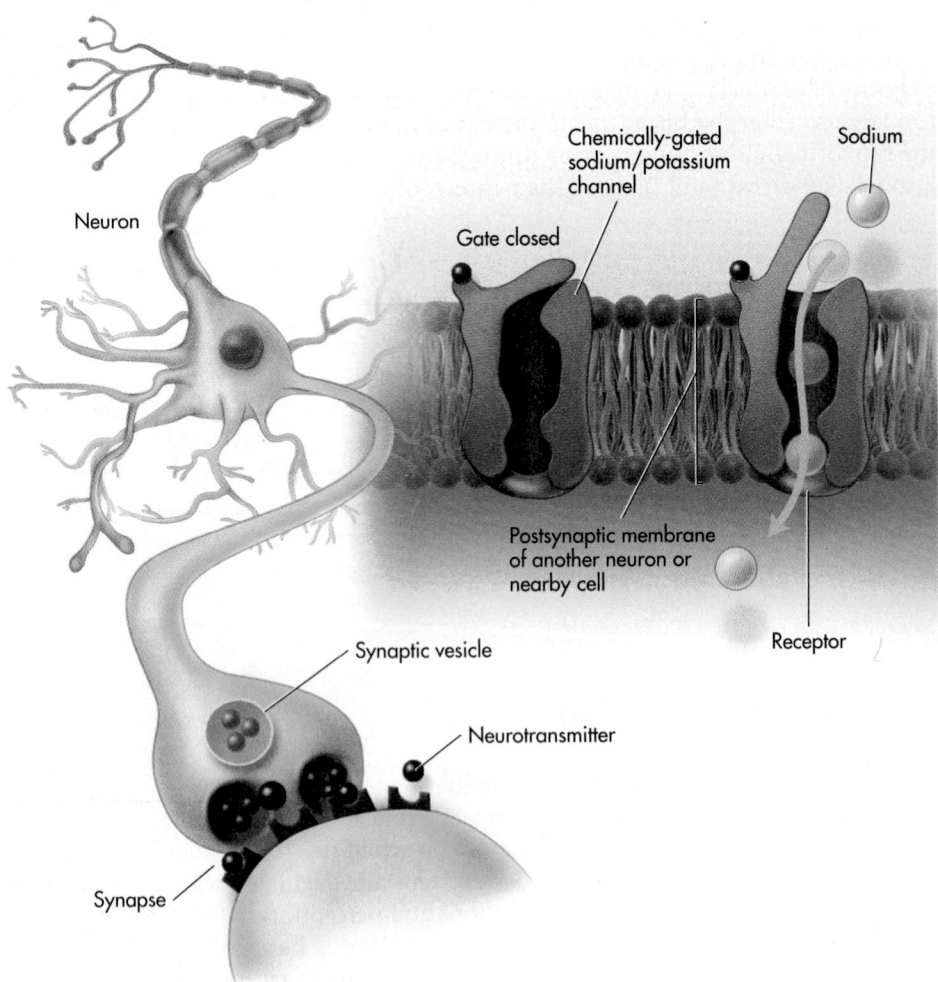

Neuron

Chemically-gated sodium/potassium channel

Sodium

Gate closed

Postsynaptic membrane of another neuron or nearby cell

Receptor

Synaptic vesicle

Neurotransmitter

Synapse

used in this process are often made from common nutrients found in foods, such as amino acids. The amino acid tryptophan is converted to the neurotransmitter serotonin, and the amino acid tyrosine is converted to the neurotransmitters **norepinephrine** and **epinephrine** (also called adrenaline).

Other nutrients also play a role in the nervous system. Calcium is needed for the release of neurotransmitters from neurons. Vitamin B-12 plays a role in the formation of the **myelin sheath,** which provides insulation around specific parts of most neurons. Finally, a regular supply of carbohydrate in the form of glucose is important for supplying fuel for the brain. The brain can use other calorie sources, but generally relies on glucose.

3.6 Endocrine System

The **endocrine system** plays a major role in the regulation of metabolism, reproduction, water balance, and many other functions by producing hormones in the **endocrine glands** of the body and subsequently releasing them into the blood (Table 3-2). The term *hormone* comes from the Greek word for "to stir or excite." A true hormone is a regulatory compound that has a specific site of synthesis from which it then enters the bloodstream to reach target cells. Hormones are the messengers of the body. They can be permissive (turn on), antagonistic (turn off), or synergistic (work in cooperation with another hormone) in performing a task. Some compounds must undergo chemical changes before they can function as hormones. For example, vitamin D, synthesized in the skin or obtained from food, is converted into an active hormone by chemical changes made in the liver and kidneys.

The hormone **insulin,** synthesized in and released from the pancreas, helps control the amount of glucose in the blood (Fig. 3-7). Insulin is mostly produced when glucose in the blood rises to a certain level, usually after a meal. At this point, insulin is released and it travels to the muscle, adipose, and liver cells of the body. Among its many functions, insulin allows for the movement of glucose from the blood into muscle and adipose cells. In the liver cells, insulin causes an increase in stored glycogen by stimulating the synthesis of glycogen from glucose. Once a sufficient amount of glucose has been cleared from the blood, the production of insulin lessens. The hormones epinephrine, norepinephrine, glucagon, and growth hormone have just the opposite effect on blood glucose. They all cause an increase in blood glucose through a variety of actions (Table 3-2). **Thyroid hormones,** synthesized in and released from the thyroid gland

norepinephrine A neurotransmitter from nerve endings and a hormone from the adrenal gland. It is released in times of stress and is involved in hunger regulation, blood glucose regulation, and other body processes.

epinephrine A hormone also known as *adrenaline;* it is released by the adrenal glands (located on each kidney) at times of stress. It acts to increase glycogen breakdown in the liver, among other functions.

myelin sheath A lipid and protein combination (lipoprotein) that covers nerve fibers.

endocrine system The body system consisting of the various glands and the hormones these glands secrete. This system has major regulatory functions in the body, such as reproduction and cell metabolism.

endocrine gland A hormone-producing gland.

thyroid hormones Hormones produced by the thyroid gland that among their functions increase the rate of overall metabolism in the body.

TABLE 3-2 Some Hormones of the Endocrine System with Nutritional Significance

Hormone	Gland/Organ	Target	Effect	Role in Nutrition
Insulin	Pancreas	Adipose (fat) and muscle cells	Decreased blood glucose	Uptake and storage of glucose, fat, and amino acids by cells
Glucagon	Pancreas	Liver	Increased blood glucose	Release of glucose from liver stores, release of fat from adipose tissue
Epinephrine, Norepinephrine	Adrenal glands	Heart, blood vessels, brain, lungs	Increased body metabolism and blood glucose	Release of glucose and fat into the blood
Growth hormone	Pituitary gland	Most cells	Promotion of amino acid uptake by cells, increased blood glucose	Promotion of protein synthesis and growth, increased fat use for energy
Thyroid hormones	Thyroid gland	Most organs	Increased oxygen consumption, overall growth, brain development of the nervous system	Protein synthesis, increased body metabolism

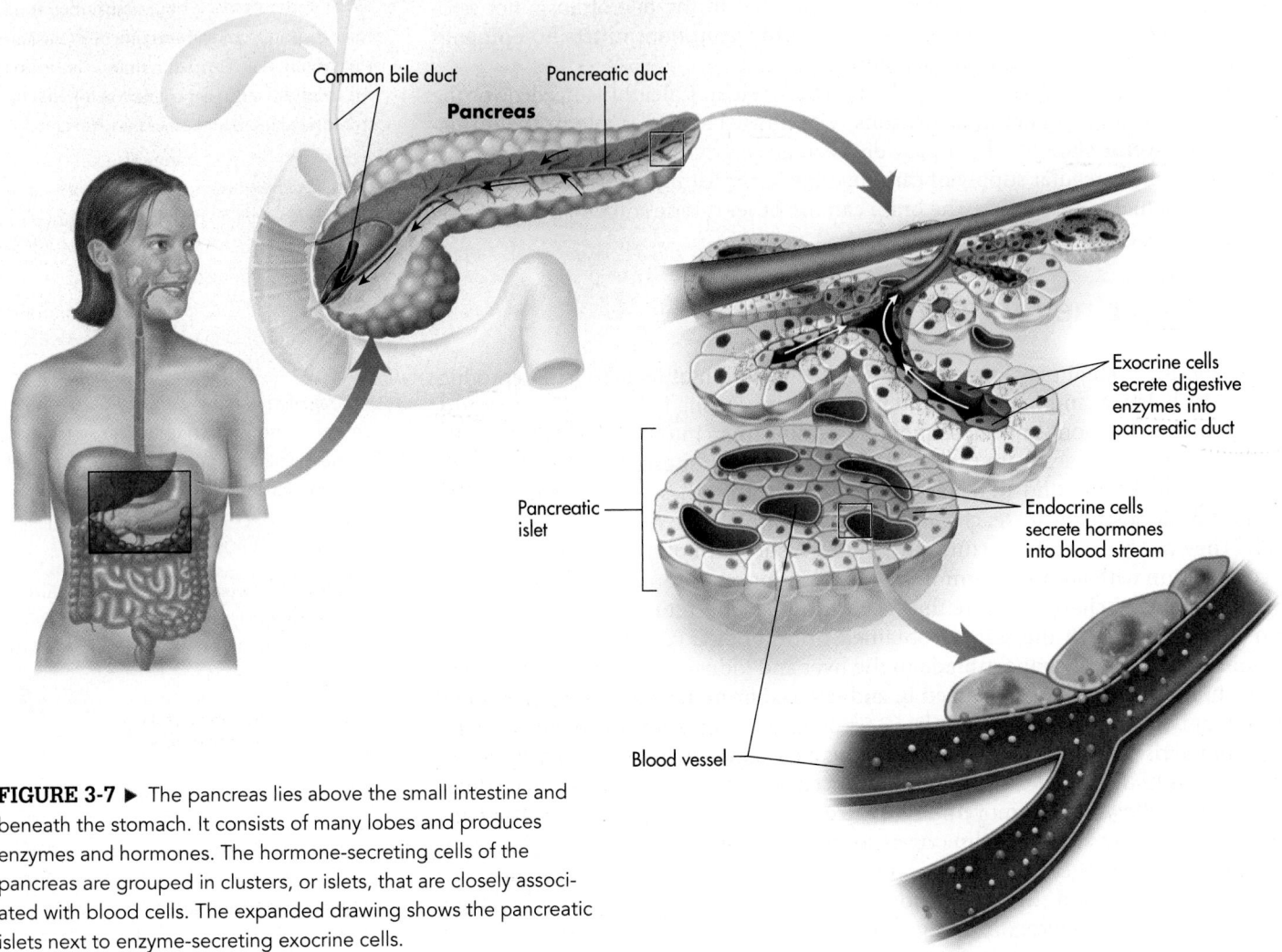

FIGURE 3-7 ▶ The pancreas lies above the small intestine and beneath the stomach. It consists of many lobes and produces enzymes and hormones. The hormone-secreting cells of the pancreas are grouped in clusters, or islets, that are closely associated with blood cells. The expanded drawing shows the pancreatic islets next to enzyme-secreting exocrine cells.

help to control the body's rate of metabolism. Other hormones are especially important in regulating digestive processes (see the later section, "Digestive System").

Hormones are not taken up by all cells in the body, but only those with the correct **receptor** protein. These binding sites are highly specific for a certain hormone. They are generally found on the cell membrane. The hormone attaches to its receptor on the cell membrane. This binding activates additional compounds called second messengers within the cell to carry out the assigned task. This is true of insulin. A few hormones can penetrate the cell membrane and eventually bind to receptors on the DNA in the nucleus (e.g., thyroid hormone and estrogen).

receptor A site in a cell at which compounds (such as hormones) bind. Cells that contain receptors for a specific compound are partially controlled by that compound.

CONCEPT CHECK

The functional unit of the nervous system is the neuron. Communication between neurons themselves, and other types of cells, is via neurotransmitters released into the synapse between the cells.

In the endocrine system, hormones are produced by glands in response to a change in the internal or external environment of the body. The gland secretes the hormone into the blood, and the blood delivers it to target cells. The hormone either attaches to receptors in the cell membrane and, through the action of second messengers, causes changes within the cell, or enters the cell and binds to the DNA in the cell to cause changes within the cell.

3.7 Immune System

Many types of body cells and body components work in cooperation as part of the **immune system** to maintain a defense against infection (Fig. 3-8). The components that work as part of the immune system include the skin, intestinal cells, and white blood cells. Several nutrients, including protein; minerals iron, copper, and zinc; and vitamins A, B-6, B-12, C, and folate have important roles in the immune system. These nutrients are key factors in the synthesis, growth, development, and activity of immune cells and additional factors that kill pathogens. It is easy to demonstrate the importance of nutritional health for immune function. Early humans were plagued by famine and thus, malnutrition; this contributed to infections, often leading to death. Today, largely because of better nutrition, most of the world avoids that cycle.

We are born with most aspects of immune function; these are termed **non-specific** (or innate) because the targets are a variety of microorganisms. In contrast, white blood cells produce **immunoglobulins,** also called **antibodies,** that target specific organisms or foreign proteins called **antigens.** These immunoglobulins constitute **specific** (or adaptive) immune function. Once exposed, a memory is created such that a second exposure to the substance will produce a more vigorous and rapid attack.

Skin

The skin is a large component of the immune system, forming an almost continuous barrier surrounding the body. Invading microorganisms have difficulty penetrating the skin. However, if the skin is split by lesions, bacteria can easily penetrate this barrier. Skin health is poor during deficiencies of such nutrients as essential fatty acids, vitamin A, niacin, and zinc. Vitamin A deficiency also decreases gland secretions in the skin that contain the enzyme **lysozyme,** capable of killing bacteria. Bacterial eye infections are common in developing countries, often as a result of a vitamin A deficiency.

Intestinal Cells

The cells of the intestines form an important barrier to invading microorganisms. The cells are packed closely together, producing a physical barrier to microorganisms. In addition, specialized cells that produce immune factors—such as immunoglobulins—are scattered throughout the intestinal tract. These immune factors bind to the invading microorganisms, preventing them from entering the bloodstream. These factors are part of the mucosal membrane aspect of immunity.

Nutrient deficiencies can cause the intestinal cells to break down weakening the mucosal membrane so that microorganisms more easily enter the body and cause infections. Thus, two common results of undernutrition related to an impaired immune system are diarrhea and bacterial infections of the bloodstream. To protect the health of the intestinal tract, an adequate nutrient intake is necessary—especially of protein, vitamin A, vitamin B-6, vitamin B-12, vitamin C, folate, and zinc.

MAKING DECISIONS

Immune Status

Although many studies show that a healthy nutritional state is associated with good immune status, other studies show that an overabundance of certain nutrients can harm the immune system. For example, taking too much zinc may decrease immune function (see Chapter 9).

FIGURE 3-8 ▶ Just as the roof and other external structures of a house protect the inside environment from outside elements, host protective factors (shown on the bricks) of the immune system "shelter" humans from threats such as diseases and toxins (shown in the rain).

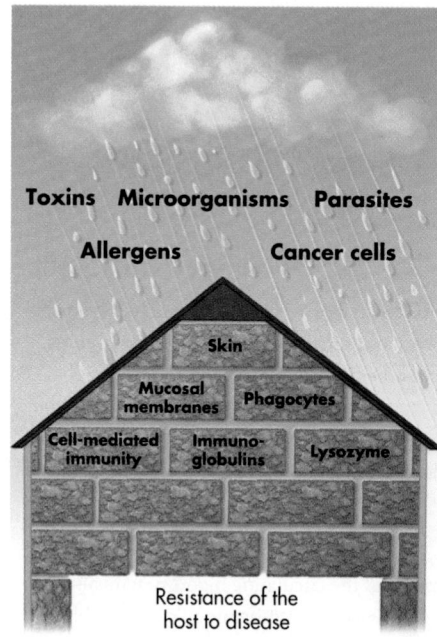

immune system The body system consisting of white blood cells, lymph glands and vessels, and various other body tissues. The immune system provides defense against foreign invaders, primarily due to the action of various types of white blood cells.

non-specific immunity Defenses that stop the invasion of pathogens; requires no previous encounter with a pathogen.

immunoglobulins Proteins found in the blood that bind to specific antigens; also called antibodies. The five major classes of immunoglobulins play different roles in antibody-mediated immunity.

antigen Any substance that induces a state of sensitivity and/or resistance to microorganisms or toxic substances after a lag period; foreign substance that stimulates a specific aspect of the immune system.

antibody Blood protein (immunoglobulin) that binds foreign proteins found in the body. This helps to prevent and control infections.

specific immunity Function of lymphocytes directed at specific antigens.

lysozyme An enzyme produced by a variety of cells; it can destroy bacteria by rupturing their cell membranes.

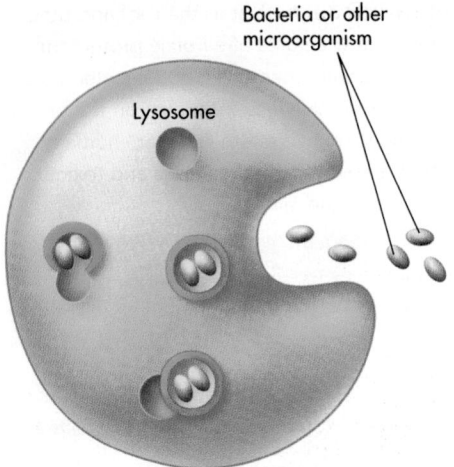

Bacteria or other microorganism

Lysosome

Phagocyte

FIGURE 3-9 ▶ One class of white blood cell, phagocytes, can ingest bacteria, fungi, viruses, and other foreign particles in the process of phagocytosis. An indentation is formed and the particle is engulfed by the cell. The foreign material is eventually digested by lysosomes in the cell.

white blood cells One of the formed elements of the circulating blood system; also called *leukocytes*. White blood cells are able to squeeze through intracellular spaces and migrate. They phagocytize bacteria, fungi, and viruses, as well as detoxify proteins that may result from allergic reactions, cellular injury, and other immune system cells.

phagocytes Cells that engulf substances; include neutrophils and macrophages.

phagocytosis Process in which a cell forms an indentation, and particles or fluids enter the indentation and are engulfed by the cell.

cell-mediated immunity A process in which certain white blood cells come in contact with the invading cells to destroy them.

digestive system System consisting of the gastrointestinal tract and accessory structures (liver, gallbladder, and pancreas). This system performs the mechanical and chemical processes of digestion, absorption of nutrients, and elimination of wastes.

digestion Process by which large ingested molecules are mechanically and chemically broken down to produce basic nutrients that can be absorbed across the wall of the GI tract.

absorption The process by which substances are taken up from the GI tract and enter the bloodstream or the lymph.

White Blood Cells

Once a microorganism enters the bloodstream, **white blood cells** move in to attack it. Several types of white blood cells participate in this response and function in unique ways. For example, a class called **phagocytes** circulates throughout the circulatory system and ingests and sometimes digests microorganisms and foreign particles (via lysosomes present in the cells) in a process called **phagocytosis** (Fig. 3-9). Other white blood cells participate in **cell-mediated immunity**, achieved when certain immune cells recognize foreign cells or proteins and directly attack and destroy them. Immunoglobulins, also known as antibodies and made by these cells, elicit an antibody-antigen response that binds microorganisms and proteins that are foreign to the body and destroys them, and then creates a template (memory) that allows future recognition of the microorganism or foreign protein. Recognition allows more rapid attacks in the future.

Some white blood cells live only a few days. Their constant resynthesis requires steady nutrient intake. The immune system needs the following nutrients: (1) iron to produce an important killing factor; (2) copper for synthesis of a specific type of white blood cell; and (3) protein, vitamin B-6, vitamin B-12, vitamin C, and folate for general cell synthesis and, later, cell activity. Zinc and vitamin A are also needed for the overall growth and development of immune cells.

CONCEPT CHECK

Many types of body cells and body components work in cooperation as part of the immune system to maintain a defense against infection. The skin forms an almost continuous barrier surrounding the body. Cell secretions contain the enzyme lysozyme. Specialized cells in the intestines and certain white blood cells secrete antibodies (immunoglobulins). Phagocytes roam throughout the circulatory system and ingest and sometimes digest microorganisms and foreign particles. Other white blood cells participate in cell-mediated immunity. This occurs when certain immune cells recognize foreign cells and directly attack them. Many nutrients, including protein, iron, copper, zinc, vitamin B-6, B-12, C, and folate, are needed for the overall growth and development of immune cells.

3.8 Digestive System

The foods and beverages we consume, for the most part, must undergo extensive alteration by the **digestive system** to provide us with usable nutrients. The processes of **digestion** and **absorption** take place in a long tube that is open at both ends and extends from the mouth to the anus. This tube is called the **gastrointestinal (GI) tract** (Fig. 3-10). Nutrients from the food we eat must pass through the walls of the GI tract—from the inside to the outside—to be absorbed into the bloodstream. The organs that make up the GI tract, as well as some additional accessory organs located nearby, are collectively known as the digestive system.

In the digestive system, food is broken down mechanically and chemically. Mechanical digestion takes place as soon as you begin chewing your food and continues as muscular contractions simultaneously mix and move food through the length of the GI tract (as part of a process known as **motility**). Chemical digestion refers to the chemical breakdown of foods by substances secreted into the GI tract. Finally, the digestive system eliminates wastes. In addition to nutrients that arise from digestion of food, the bacteria that live in the large intestine produce vitamin K and the vitamin biotin, some of which we can absorb and use.

Most of the processes of digestion and absorption are under autonomic control; that is, they are involuntary. Almost all of the functions involved in digestion and absorption are controlled by signals from the nervous system, hormones from the

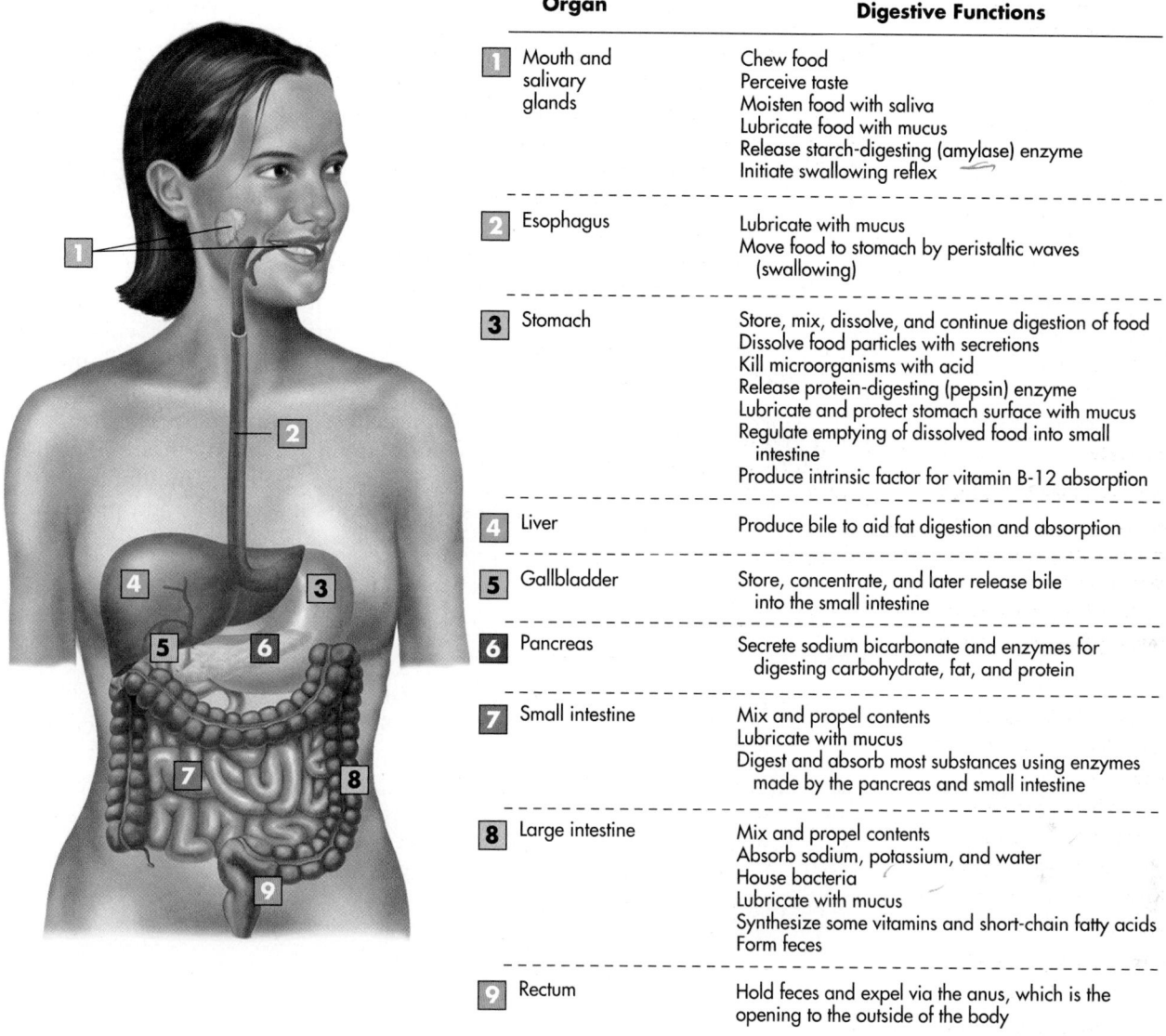

Organ	Digestive Functions
1 Mouth and salivary glands	Chew food Perceive taste Moisten food with saliva Lubricate food with mucus Release starch-digesting (amylase) enzyme Initiate swallowing reflex
2 Esophagus	Lubricate with mucus Move food to stomach by peristaltic waves (swallowing)
3 Stomach	Store, mix, dissolve, and continue digestion of food Dissolve food particles with secretions Kill microorganisms with acid Release protein-digesting (pepsin) enzyme Lubricate and protect stomach surface with mucus Regulate emptying of dissolved food into small intestine Produce intrinsic factor for vitamin B-12 absorption
4 Liver	Produce bile to aid fat digestion and absorption
5 Gallbladder	Store, concentrate, and later release bile into the small intestine
6 Pancreas	Secrete sodium bicarbonate and enzymes for digesting carbohydrate, fat, and protein
7 Small intestine	Mix and propel contents Lubricate with mucus Digest and absorb most substances using enzymes made by the pancreas and small intestine
8 Large intestine	Mix and propel contents Absorb sodium, potassium, and water House bacteria Lubricate with mucus Synthesize some vitamins and short-chain fatty acids Form feces
9 Rectum	Hold feces and expel via the anus, which is the opening to the outside of the body

FIGURE 3-10 ▶ Physiology of the GI tract. Many organs cooperate in a regulated fashion to allow the digestion and absorption of nutrients in foods.

endocrine system, and hormone-like compounds. Many common ailments arise from problems with the digestive system. Several of these digestive problems are discussed in the "Nutrition and Your Health" section at the end of this chapter.

The digestive system is composed of six separate organs; each organ performs one, or more, specific job(s). Let's look briefly at the role of each organ. These organs are listed in Figure 3-10 and in the flowchart on the next page. More detailed descriptions of digestive processes will be explained in later chapters as each nutrient is introduced.

Mouth

The mouth performs many functions in the digestion of food. Besides chewing food to reduce it to smaller particles, the mouth also senses the taste of the foods we consume. The tongue, through the use of its taste buds, identifies foods on the basis of their specific flavor(s). Sweet, sour, salty, bitter, and **umami** comprise the primary taste sensations we experience. Surprisingly, the nose and our sense of smell greatly contribute to our ability to sense the taste of food. When we chew a food, chemicals are released that stimulate the nasal passages. Thus, it makes perfect sense that when

gastrointestinal (GI) tract The main sites in the body used for digestion and absorption of nutrients. It consists of the mouth, esophagus, stomach, small intestine, large intestine, rectum, and anus. Also called the *digestive tract*.

motility Generally, the ability to move spontaneously. It also refers to movement of food through the GI tract.

umami A brothy, meaty, savory flavor in some foods. Monosodium glutamate enhances this flavor when added to foods.

GI Tract Components and Flow

Mouth
↓
Esophagus (10 inches long)
↓
Stomach—4-cup (1-liter) capacity. Food remains about 2 to 3 hours, or longer for large meals.
↓
Small intestine—duodenum (10 in long), jejunum (4 ft long), ileum (5 ft long)— about 10 ft (3.1 meters) in total length. Food remains about 3 to 10 hours.
↓
Large intestine (colon)—cecum, ascending colon, transverse colon, descending colon, sigmoid colon—3½ ft (1.1 meters) in total length. Food can remain up to 72 hours.
↓
Rectum
↓
Anus

saliva Watery fluid, produced by the salivary glands in the mouth, that contains lubricants, enzymes, and other substances.

salivary amylase A starch-digesting enzyme produced by salivary glands.

we have a cold and our noses are stuffed up and congested, even our most favorite foods will not taste as good as they normally do.

The taste of food, or the anticipation of it, signals the rest of the GI tract to prepare for the digestion of food. Once in the mouth, mechanical and chemical digestion begins. Salivary glands produce **saliva,** which functions as a solvent so that food particles can be further separated and tasted. In addition, saliva contains a starch-digesting enzyme, **salivary amylase** (see Chapter 4 for more on starch-digesting enzymes).

Enzymes are a key part of digestion. Each enzyme is specific to one type of chemical process. For example, enzymes that recognize and digest table sugar (sucrose) ignore milk sugar (lactose). Besides working on only specific types of chemicals, enzymes are sensitive to acidic and alkaline conditions, temperature, and the types of vitamins and minerals they require. Digestive enzymes that work in the acidic environment of the stomach do not work well in the alkaline environment of the small intestine. Overall, enzymes work to hasten certain events that take place in the body (Fig. 3-11).

The pancreas and the small intestine produce most of the digestive enzymes; however, the mouth and the stomach also contribute their own enzymes to digestion. **Mucus,** another component of saliva, makes it easy to swallow a mouthful of food. The food then travels to the esophagus. The important secretions and products of digestion are listed in Table 3-3.

MAKING DECISIONS

Enzymes and Digestion

The authors of some popular (fad) diet books contend that eating certain combinations of foods, such as meats and fruits together, hinders the digestive process. However, does this make sense in light of our newly gained knowledge about GI tract physiology? The body is able to increase the production of certain digestive enzymes in response to the type of diet consumed. The GI tract can respond to the nutritional makeup and amount of food consumed because of this fine-tuning. Once consumed, foods are attacked by multiple enzymes to release nutrients and other compounds for absorption.

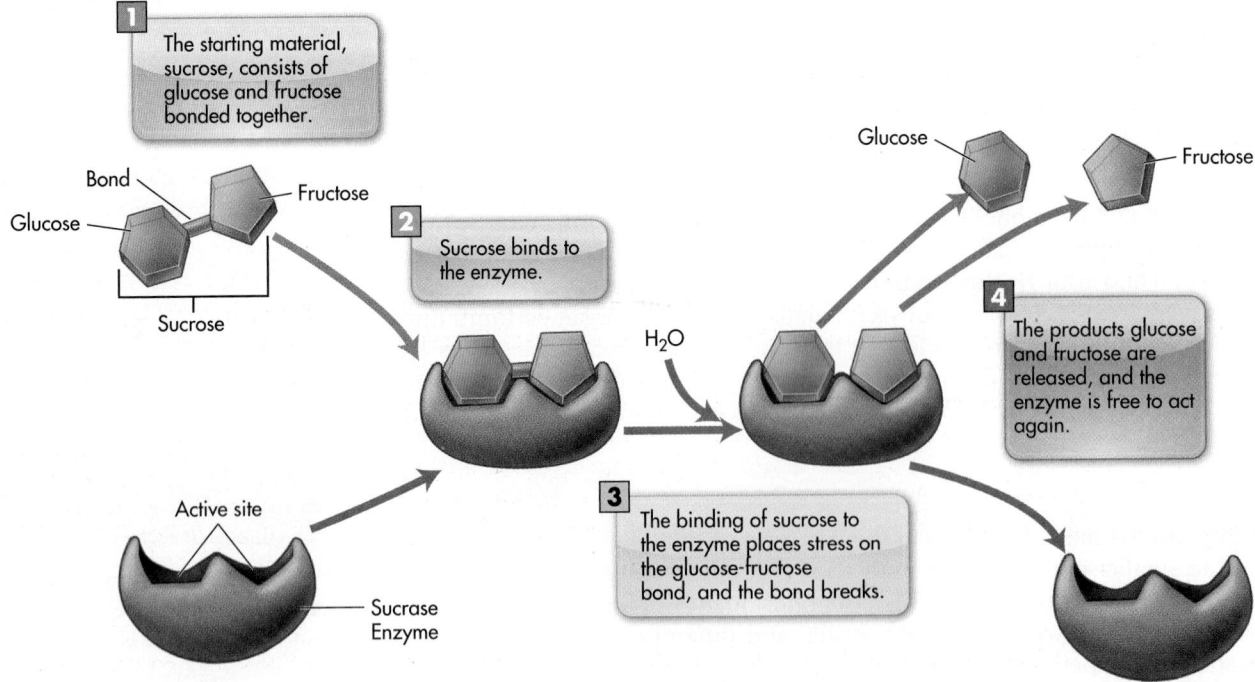

FIGURE 3-11 ▶ A model of enzyme action. The enzyme sucrase splits the sugar sucrose into two simpler sugars; glucose and fructose. [Note that sometimes energy input is needed to make reactions occur.]

TABLE 3-3 Important Secretions and Products of the Digestive Tract

Secretion	Site of Production	Purpose
Saliva	Mouth	Partial starch digestion using **salivary amylase,** lubrication of food for swallowing
Mucus	Mouth, stomach, small intestine, large intestine	Protects GI tract cells, lubricates food as it travels through the GI tract
Enzymes	Mouth, stomach, small intestine, pancreas	Promote digestion of carbohydrates, fats, and proteins into forms small enough for absorption (Examples: **amylases, lipases, proteases)**
Acid	Stomach	Promotes digestion of protein among other functions
Bile	Liver (stored in gallbladder)	Aids fat digestion in the small intestine by suspending fat in water using **bile acids, cholesterol,** and **lecithin**
Bicarbonate	Pancreas, small intestine	Neutralizes stomach acid when it reaches the small intestine
Hormones	Stomach, small intestine, pancreas	Stimulate production and/or release of acid, enzymes, bile, and bicarbonate; help regulate peristalsis and overall GI tract flow (Examples: gastrin, secretin, insulin, cholecystokinin, glucagon)

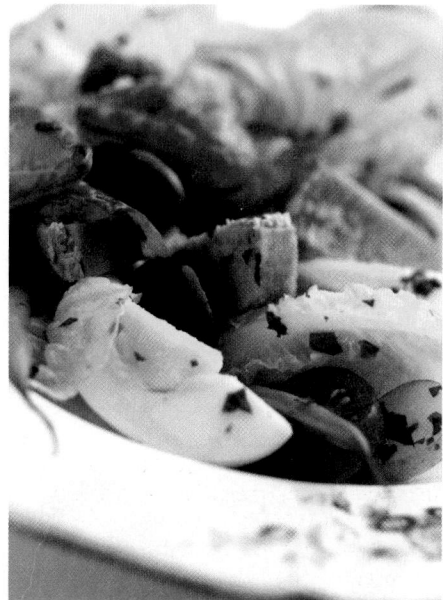

▲ The body digests the foods as they are presented—the order in which foods are eaten plays no role in digestion.

Esophagus

The **esophagus** is a long tube that connects the **pharynx** with the stomach. Near the pharynx is a flap of tissue (called the **epiglottis**) that prevents the **bolus** of swallowed food from entering the trachea (wind pipe) (Fig. 3-12). During swallowing, food lands on the epiglottis, folding it down to cover the opening of the trachea. Breathing also stops automatically. These responses ensure that swallowed food will only travel down the esophagus. If food instead travels down the trachea, choking may occur (the victim will not be able to speak or breathe). A group of techniques to treat such a person are called the Heimlich maneuver (see www.heimlichinstitute.org for details).

At the top of the esophagus, nerve fibers release signals to tell the GI tract that food has been consumed. This results in an increase in gastrointestinal muscle action, called **peristalsis.** These continual waves of muscle contractions, followed by muscle relaxation, force the food down the digestive tract from the esophagus onward (Fig. 3-13).

At the end of the esophagus is the **lower esophageal sphincter,** a muscle that constricts (closes) after food enters the stomach. The main function of sphincters is to prevent the backflow of GI tract contents. Sphincters respond to various stimuli, such as signals from the nervous system, hormones, acidic versus alkaline conditions, and pressure that builds up around the sphincter. The primary function of the lower esophageal sphincter is to prevent the acidic contents of the stomach from flowing back up into the esophagus—which can cause some of the health problems we will discuss in the "Nutrition and Your Health" section at the end of Chapter 3.

Stomach

The stomach is a large sac that can hold up to 4 cups (or 1 quart) of food for several hours until all of the food is able to enter the small intestine. Stomach size varies individually and can be reduced surgically as a radical treatment for obesity (more on this in Chapter 7). While in the stomach, the food is mixed with gastric juice,

mucus A thick fluid secreted by many cells throughout the body. It contains a compound that has both carbohydrate and protein parts. It acts as a lubricant and means of protection for cells.

amylase Starch-digesting enzyme produced by the salivary glands and pancreas.

lipase Fat-digesting enzyme produced by the salivary glands, stomach, and pancreas.

protease Protein-digesting enzyme produced by the stomach, small intestine, and pancreas.

esophagus A tube in the GI tract that connects the pharynx with the stomach.

pharynx The organ of the digestive tract and respiratory tract located at the back of the oral and nasal cavities, commonly known as the throat.

epiglottis The flap that folds down over the trachea during swallowing.

bolus A moistened mass of food swallowed from the oral cavity into the pharynx.

peristalsis A coordinated muscular contraction used to propel food down the gastrointestinal tract.

lower esophageal sphincter A circular muscle that constricts the opening of the esophagus to the stomach. Also called the *gastroesophageal sphincter.*

FIGURE 3-12 ▶ The process of swallowing. (a) During swallowing, food does not normally enter the trachea because the epiglottis closes over the larynx. (b) The closed epiglottis allows food to proceed down the esophagus. When a person chokes, food becomes lodged in the trachea, blocking air flow to the lungs. (c) The food should move down the esophagus.

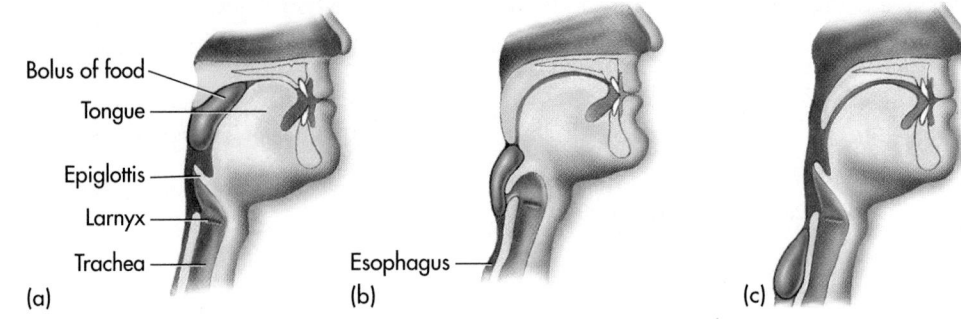

Bolus of food
Tongue
Epiglottis
Larnyx
Trachea
(a)

Esophagus
(b)

(c)

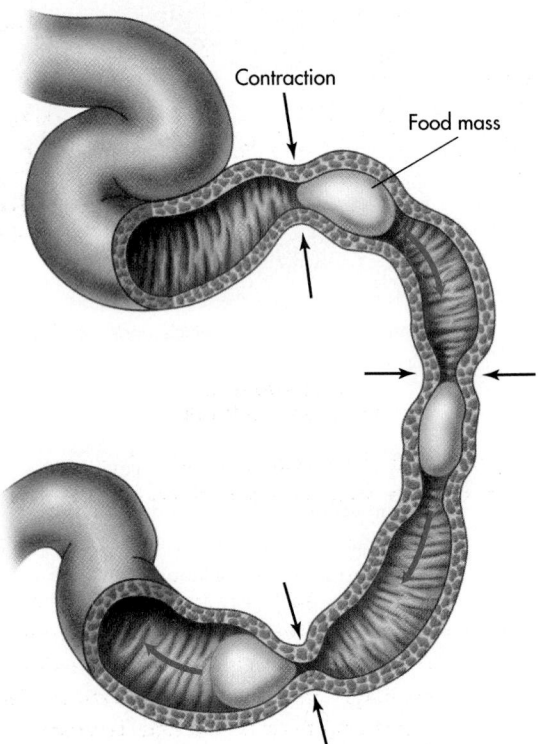

Contraction
Food mass

FIGURE 3-13 ▶ Peristalsis. Peristalsis is a progressive type of movement, propelling material from point to point along the GI tract. To begin this, a ring of contraction occurs where the GI wall is stretched, passing the food mass forward. The moving food mass triggers a ring of contraction in the next region, which pushes the food mass even farther along. The result is a ring of contraction that moves like a wave along the GI tract, pushing the food mass down the tract.

chyme A mixture of stomach secretions and partially digested food.

pyloric sphincter Ring of smooth muscle between stomach and small intestine.

intrinsic factor A proteinlike compound produced by the stomach that enhances vitamin B-12 absorption.

villi (singular, **villus**) The fingerlike protrusions into the small intestine that participate in digestion and absorption of food.

which contains water, a very strong acid, and enzymes. (Gastric is a term pertaining to the stomach.) The acid in the gastric juice maintains the acidity of the stomach contents and, thereby destroys the biological activity of proteins, converts inactive digestive enzymes to their active form, partially digests food protein, and makes dietary minerals soluble so that they can be absorbed. The mixing that takes place in the stomach produces a watery food mixture, called **chyme,** which slowly leaves the stomach a teaspoon (5 milliliters) at a time and enters the small intestine. Following a meal, the stomach contents are emptied into the small intestine over the course of 1 to 4 hours. The **pyloric sphincter,** located at the base of the stomach, controls the rate at which the chyme is released into the small intestine (Fig. 3-14). There is very little absorption of nutrients from the stomach, except for some alcohol.

You might wonder how the stomach prevents itself from being digested by the acid and enzymes it produces. First, the stomach has a thick layer of mucus that lines and protects it. The production of acid and enzymes also requires the release of a specific hormone (gastrin). This release happens primarily when we are eating or thinking about eating. Last, as the concentration of acid in the stomach increases, hormonal control causes acid production to taper off.

One other important function of the stomach is the production of a substance called **intrinsic factor.** This vital proteinlike compound is essential for the absorption of vitamin B-12.

Small Intestine

The small intestine is about 10 feet (3 meters) long, beginning at the stomach and ending at the large intestine (colon) (Fig. 3-15). The small intestine is considered "small" because of its narrow (1 inch [2.5 centimeters]) diameter. Most of the digestion and absorption of food occurs in the small intestine. The chyme secreted from the stomach is moved through the small intestine by peristaltic contractions so that it can be well mixed with the digestive juices of the small intestine (review Fig. 3-13). These juices contain many enzymes that function in the breakdown of carbohydrates, protein, and fat, as well as in the preparation of vitamins and minerals for absorption.

The physical structure of the small intestine is very important to the body's ability to digest and absorb the nutrients it needs. The lining of the small intestine is called the mucosa and is folded many times; within these folds are fingerlike projections called **villi.** These "fingers" are constantly moving, which helps them trap food to enhance absorption. Each individual villus (singular) is made up of many **absorptive cells,** and each of these cells has a highly folded cap. The combined folds, villi, and caps in the small intestine increase its surface area 600 times beyond that of a simple tube (Fig. 3-16).

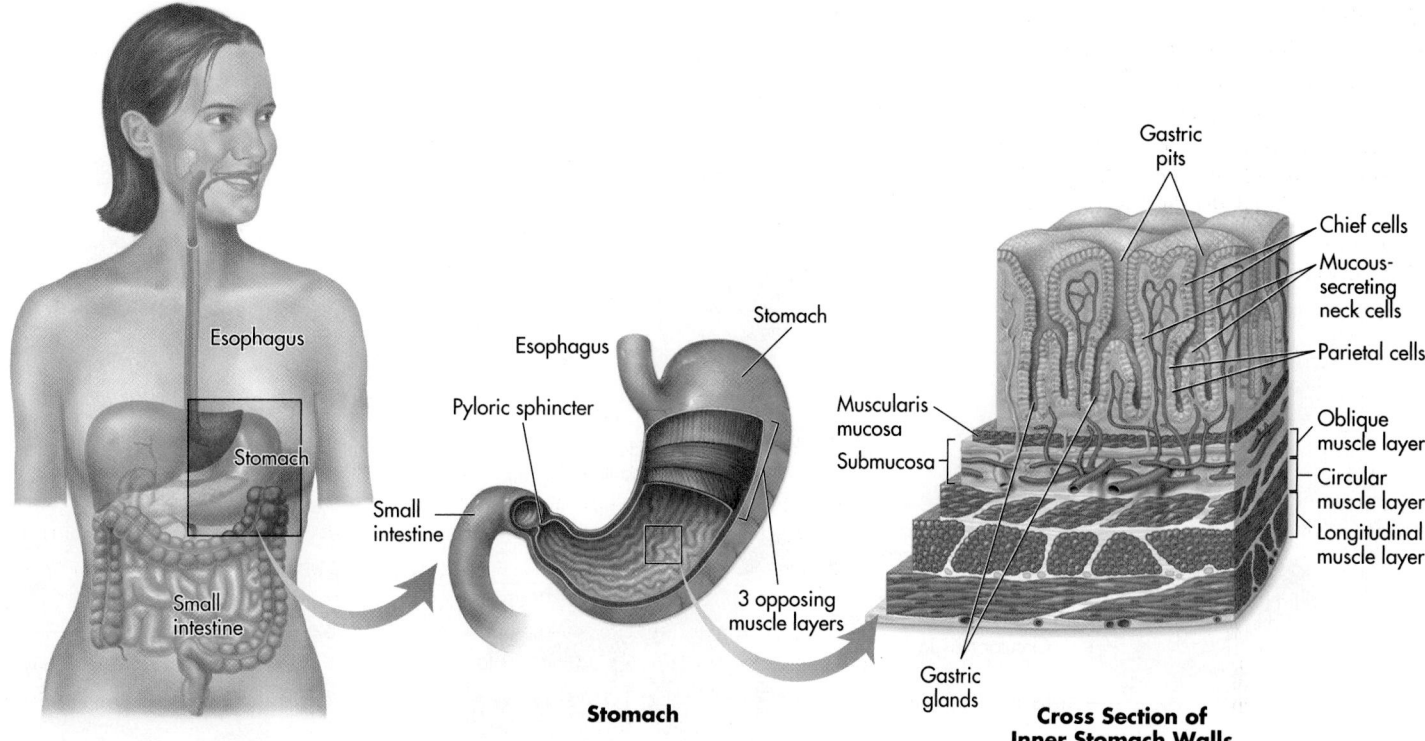

FIGURE 3-14 ▶ Physiology of the stomach. The interior surface mucous cells produce mucus for protection from stomach acid and enzymes. Parietal cells produce the hydrochloric acid (HCL), and chief cells produce the enzymes. Mucous neck cells, scattered among the cells in the gastric pits, also produce mucus. The exterior surface is made up of three types of muscle layers.

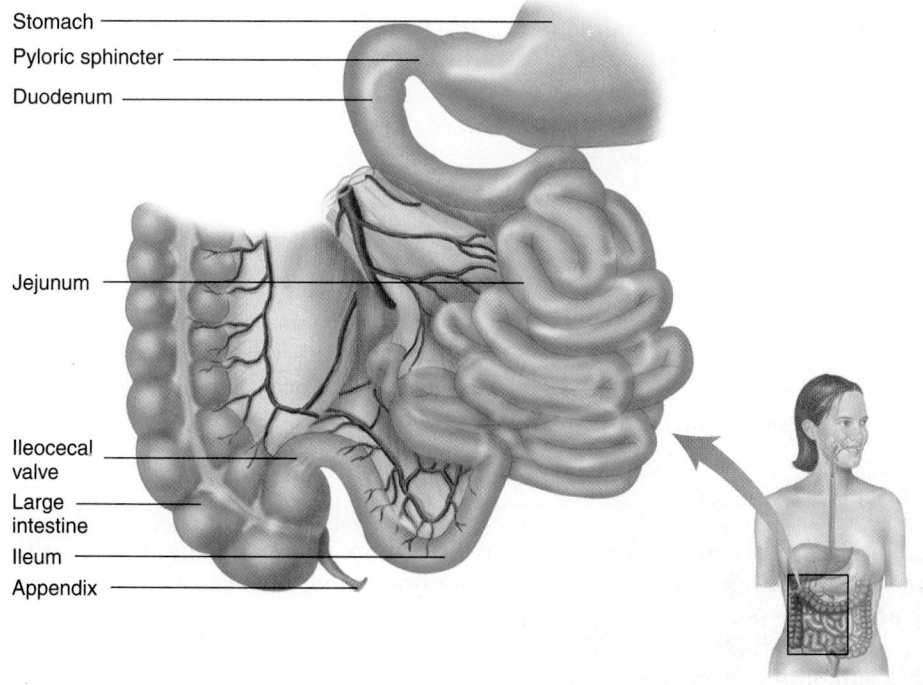

FIGURE 3-15 ▶ The small intestine and beginning of the large intestine. The three parts of the small intestine are the duodenum, jejunum, and ileum. Notice the smaller diameter of the small intestine, compared with the large intestine.

The absorptive cells have a short life. New intestinal absorptive cells are constantly produced in the crypts of the small intestine (Fig. 3-16) and appear daily along the surface of each villus "finger." This is probably because absorptive cells are subjected to a harsh environment, so renewal of the intestinal cell lining is necessary. This rapid cell turnover leads to high nutrient needs for the small intestine. Fortunately, many of

absorptive cells Intestinal cells that line the villi; and participate in nutrient absorption.

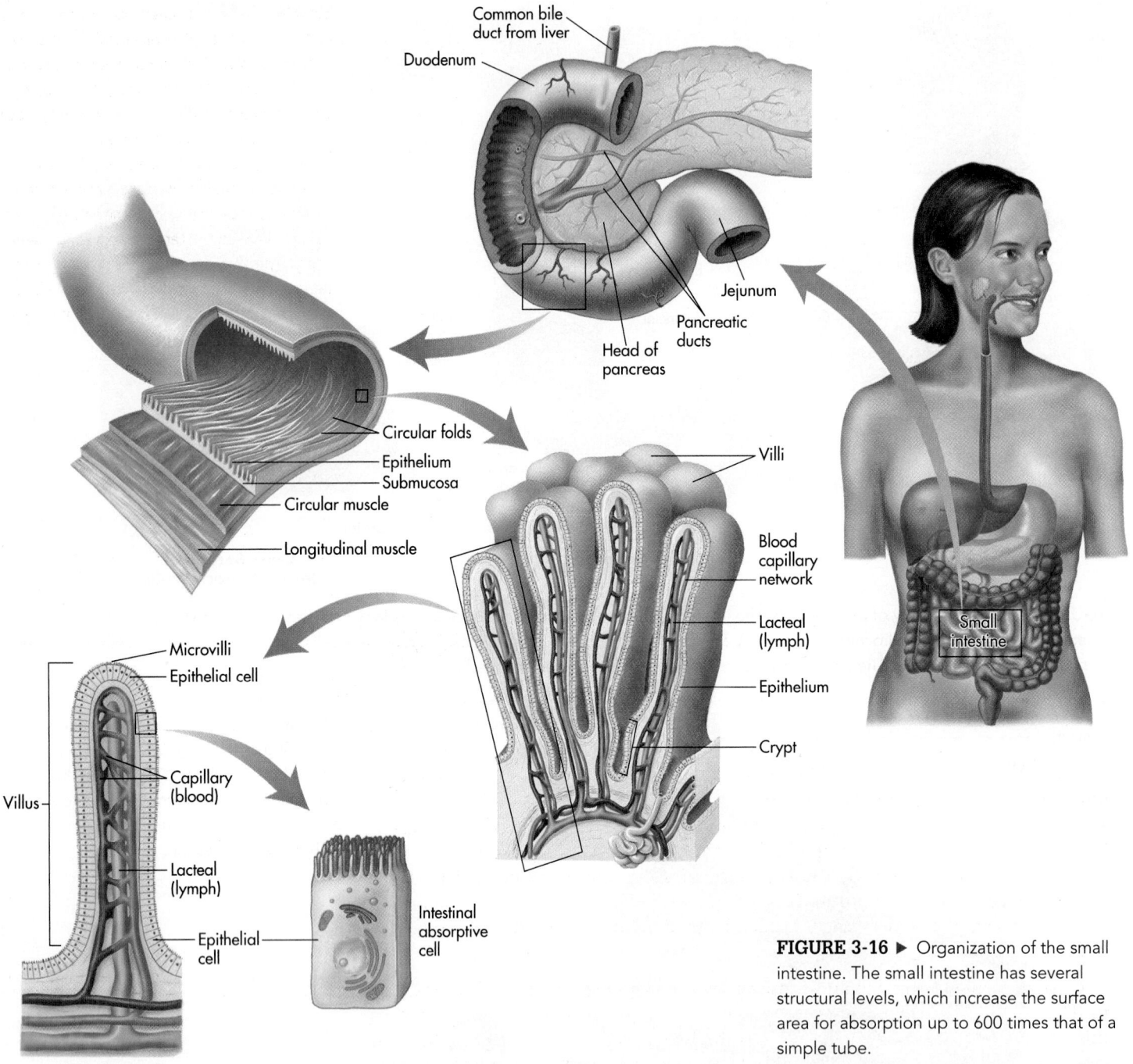

FIGURE 3-16 ▶ Organization of the small intestine. The small intestine has several structural levels, which increase the surface area for absorption up to 600 times that of a simple tube.

the old cells can be broken down and have their component parts reused. The health of the cells is further enhanced by various hormones and other substances that participate in or are produced as part of the digestive process.

The small intestine absorbs nutrients through the intestinal wall through various means and processes, as illustrated in Figure 3-17:

- **Passive diffusion:** When the nutrient concentration is higher in the cavity (lumen) of the small intestine than in the absorptive cells, the difference in nutrient concentration drives the nutrient into the absorptive cells by diffusion. Fats, water, and some minerals are absorbed by passive diffusion.

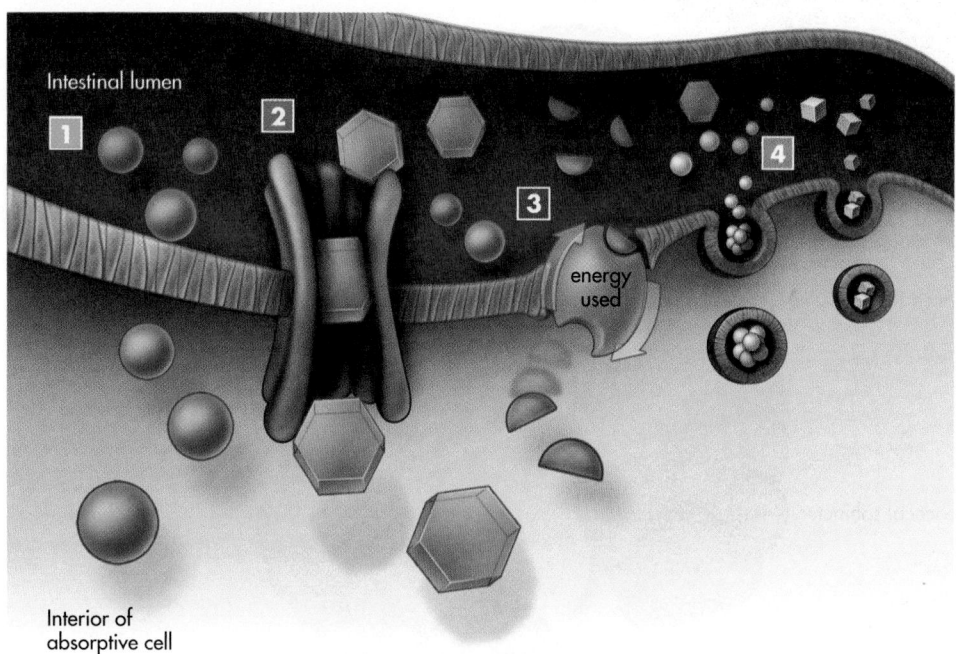

Intestinal lumen

energy used

Interior of absorptive cell

FIGURE 3-17 ▶ Nutrient absorption relies on four major absorptive processes. **1** Passive diffusion (in blue) is diffusion of nutrients across the absorptive cell membranes. **2** Facilitated diffusion (in green) uses a carrier protein to move nutrients down a concentration gradient. **3** Active absorption (in purple) involves a carrier protein as well as energy to move nutrients (against a concentration gradient) into absorptive cells. **4** Phagocytosis and pinocytosis (in green and brown) are forms of active transport in which the absorptive cell membrane forms an indentation that engulfs a nutrient to bring it into the cell.

- **Facilitated diffusion:** Some compounds require a carrier protein to drive them into absorptive cells. This type of absorption is called faciliated diffusion. Fructose is one example of a compound that makes use of such a carrier to allow for facilitated diffusion.
- **Active absorption:** In addition to the need for a carrier protein, some nutrients also require energy input to move from the lumen of the small intestine into the absorptive cells. This mechanism makes it possible for cells to take up nutrients even when they are consumed in low concentrations. Some sugars, such as glucose, are actively absorbed, as are amino acids.
- **Phagocytosis** and **pinocytosis:** In a further means of active absorption, absorptive cells literally engulf compounds (phagocytosis) or liquids (pinocytosis). As described earlier, a cell membrane can form an indentation of itself so that when particles or fluids move into the indentation, the cell membrane surrounds and engulfs them. This process is used when an infant absorbs immune substances from human milk (see Chapter 14).

Once absorbed, water-soluble compounds such as glucose and amino acids go to the capillaries and then on to the portal vein. Recall that the liver is the end of this process. Most fats eventually go into the lymph vessels. In doing so, they can eventually enter the bloodstream (see the earlier section on the circulatory system for details; and review Figs. 3-4 and 3-5).

Undigested food cannot be absorbed into cells of the small intestine. Any undigested food that reaches the end of the small intestine must pass through the **ileocecal sphincter** on the way to the large intestine (Fig. 3-18). This sphincter prevents the contents of the large intestine from reentering the small intestine.

ileocecal sphincter The ring of smooth muscle between the end of the small intestine and the large intestine.

Large Intestine

When the contents of the small intestine enter the large intestine, the material left bears little resemblance to the food originally eaten. Under normal circumstances, only a minor amount (5%) of carbohydrate, protein, and fat escape absorption to reach the large intestine (Table 3-4).

FIGURE 3-18 ▶ The parts of the colon: cecum ascending colon, transverse colon, descending colon, and sigmoid colon.

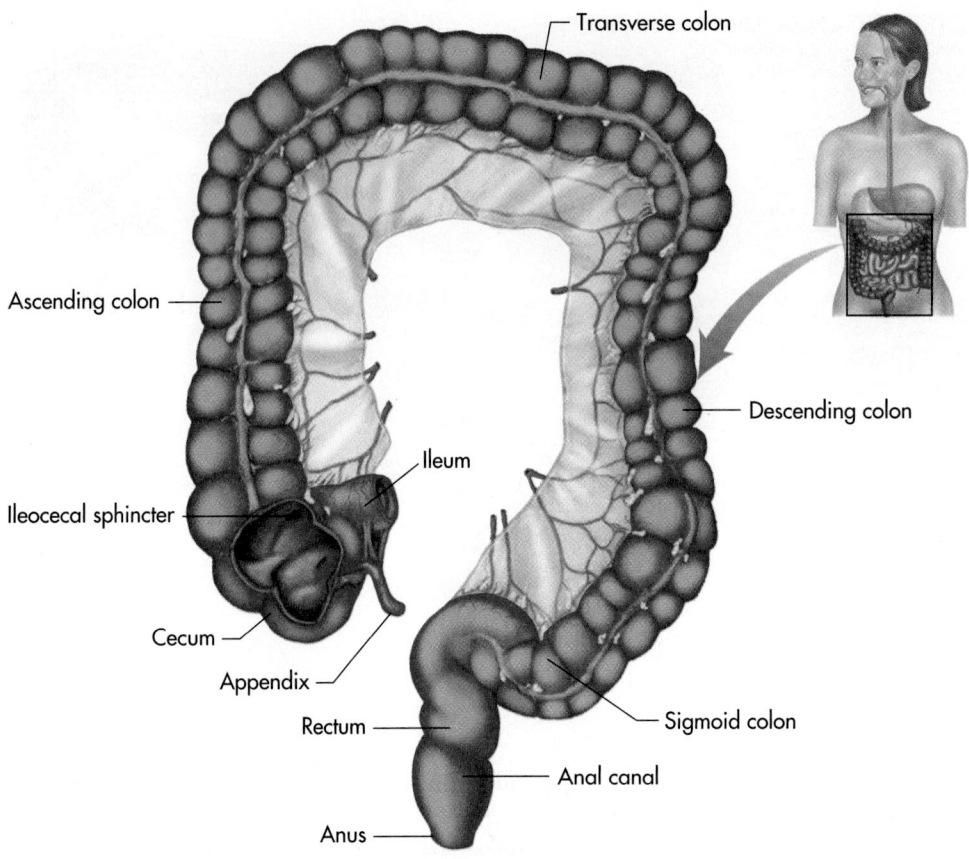

Transverse colon

Ascending colon

Descending colon

Ileum

Ileocecal sphincter

Cecum

Appendix

Rectum

Sigmoid colon

Anal canal

Anus

Physiologically, the large intestine differs from the small intestine in that there are no villi or digestive enzymes. The absence of villi means that little absorption takes place in the large intestine in comparison to the small intestine. Nutrients absorbed from the large intestine include water, some vitamins, some fatty acids, and the minerals sodium and potassium. Unlike the small intestine, the large intestine has a number of mucus-producing cells. The mucus secreted by these cells functions to hold the feces together and to protect the large intestine from the bacterial activity within it. The large intestine is home to a large population of bacteria (over 500 different species). Whereas the stomach and small intestine have some bacterial activity, the large intestine is the organ most heavily colonized with bacteria. Starting at infancy, the diet plays a major part in determining the type of bacteria in our digestive tracts. The number and type of bacteria in the human colon recently has become of great interest. Research has shown that intestinal bacteria play a significant role in the maintenance of health, especially health of the colon. It is speculated that higher levels of beneficial organisms can reduce the activity of disease-causing bacteria. This is another illustration of the intestinal tract working as an important immune organ. The strains *bifidobacteria* and *lactobacilli* are typically associated with health, whereas *clostridia* are considered problematic. These bacteria are able to break down some of the remaining food products that enter the large intestine, such as the milk sugar lactose (in lactose intolerant people), and some components of fiber. The products of bacterial metabolism in the large intestine, which include various acids, can then be absorbed.

Foods containing certain live microorganisms such as lactobacilli have been linked to some health benefits, such as improving intestinal tract health. These microorganisms are called **probiotics** because once consumed, they take up residence in the large

probiotic Product that contains specific types of bacteria. Use is intended to colonize the large intestine with the specific bacteria in the product. An example is yogurt.

TABLE 3-4 Major Sites of Absorption Along the GI Tract

Organ	Primary Nutrients Absorbed
Stomach	Alcohol (20% of total)
	Water (minor amount)
Small intestine	Calcium, magnesium, iron, and other minerals
	Glucose
	Amino acids
	Fats
	Vitamins
	Water (70% to 90% of total)
	Alcohol (80% of total)
	Bile acids
Large intestine	Sodium
	Potassium
	Some fatty acids
	Gases
	Water (10% to 30% of total)

NEWSWORTHY NUTRITION

Link between gut bacteria and health and disease

The benefits of probiotics and prebiotics have been confirmed in over 700 research studies. Probiotics, especially, are now recommended for the prevention and treatment of gastrointestinal tract disorders including inflammation, infections, and allergy. Evidence is available to support the growing interest in these microorganisms and to aid the development of intervention strategies and practical guidelines for their use.

Source: Wallace TC and others al. Human gut microbiota and its relationship to health and disease. *Nutrition Reviews* 69(7):392 2011 (see Further Reading 16).

connect NUTRITION   **Check out the Connect site** www.mcgrawhillconnect.com **to further explore probiotics.**

intestine and confer a health benefit. You can find these probiotic microorganisms in certain forms of fluid milk, fermented milk, yogurt, and in pill form (see Further Reading 13). A related term is **prebiotic.** These are substances that increase growth of probiotic microorganisms. One example is fructooligosaccharides (see Table 1-5 in Chapter 1 for dietary sources). The beneficial organisms of the large intestine and their use as probiotics are highlighted in "Newsworthy Nutrition" and will be discussed further in Chapter 4 when we explore their use as probiotics.

Some water remains in the material that enters the large intestine because the small intestine absorbs only 70% to 90% of the fluid it receives, which includes large amounts of GI-tract secretions produced during digestion. The remnants of a meal also contain some minerals and some fiber. Because water is removed from the large intestine, its contents become semisolid by the time they have passed through the first two-thirds of it. What remains in the **feces,** besides water and undigested fiber, is tough connective tissues (from animal foods); bacteria from the large intestine; and some body wastes, such as parts of dead intestinal cells.

Rectum

The feces or stool remains in the last portion of the large intestine, the **rectum,** until muscular movements push it into the **anus** to be eliminated. The presence of feces in the rectum stimulates elimination. The anus contains two **anal sphincters** (internal and external), one of which is under voluntary control (external sphincter). Relaxation of this sphincter allows for elimination.

prebiotic Substance that stimulates bacterial growth in the large intestines.

rectum Terminal portion of the large intestine.

anus Last portion of the GI tract; serves as an outlet for that organ.

anal sphincters A group of two sphincters (inner and outer) that help control expulsion of feces from the body.

gallbladder An organ attached to the underside of the liver; site of bile storage, concentration, and eventual secretion.

bile A liver secretion stored in the gallbladder and released through the common bile duct into the first segment of the small intestine. It is essential for the digestion and absorption of fat.

See Nutrition and Your Health: Common Problems with Digestion at the end of Chapter 3.

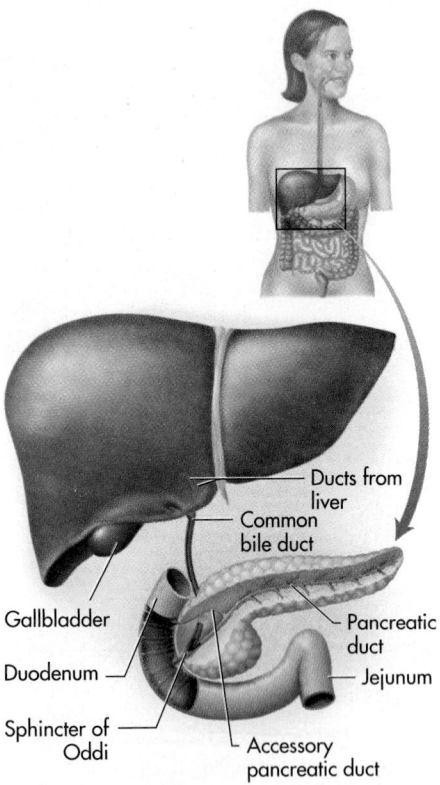

FIGURE 3-19 ► The liver, gallbladder, and pancreas are accessory organs that work with the GI tract. The liver produces bile, stored in the gallbladder and released into the duodenum portion of the small intestine, via the common bile duct, to help digest fat. The pancreas secretes pancreatic juice containing water, bicarbonate, and digestive enzymes into the duodenum via the common bile duct. The common bile duct from the liver and gallbladder and the pancreatic duct join together at the sphincter of Oddi to deliver bile, pancreatic enzymes, and bicarbonate to the duodenum.

Accessory Organs

The liver, **gallbladder,** and pancreas work with the GI tract and are considered accessory organs to the process of digestion (review Fig. 3-10). These accessory organs are not part of the GI tract through which food passes, but they play necessary roles in the process of digestion. These organs secrete digestive fluids into the GI tract and enable the process of converting food into absorbable nutrients.

The liver produces a substance called **bile.** The bile is stored and concentrated in the gallbladder until the gallbladder receives a hormonal signal to release the bile. This signal is induced by the presence of fat in the small intestine. Bile is released and delivered to the small intestine via a tube called the bile duct (Fig. 3-19).

In action, bile is like soap. Components of the bile enable large portions of fat to break into smaller bits so that they can be suspended in water (Chapter 5 will cover this process in detail). Interestingly, some of the bile constituents can be "recycled" in a process known as **enterohepatic circulation.** These components of bile are reabsorbed from the small intestine, returned to the liver via the portal vein, and reused.

In addition to bile, the liver releases a number of other unwanted substances that travel with the bile to the gallbladder and end up in the small intestine and eventually in the large intestine for excretion. The liver functions in this manner to remove unwanted substances from the blood. (Other byproducts are excreted via the urine; see the next section, "Urinary System.")

The pancreas manufactures hormones and pancreatic juice. The hormones include glucagon and insulin, which as noted earlier function in glucose regulation (review Fig. 3-7). Pancreatic juice contains water, bicarbonate, and a variety of digestive enzymes capable of breaking apart carbohydrates, proteins, and fats into small fragments. Bicarbonate is a base that neutralizes the acidity of chyme as it moves from the stomach into the small intestine. In contrast to the stomach, the small intestine, does not have a protective layer of mucus, because mucus would impede nutrient absorption. Instead, the neutralizing capacity of bicarbonate from the pancreas protects the walls of the small intestine from erosion by acid, which would otherwise lead to formation of an ulcer (see the "Nutrition and Your Health" section at the end of Chapter 3).

CONCEPT CHECK

Digestion is a mechanical and chemical process mediated by enzymes and coordinated by hormones and nerves. Whereas swallowing and ultimate elimination of feces from the anus are voluntary, the majority of the digestive processes are involuntary. The stomach initiates the process of digestion by mixing food with gastric juice and converting this partially digested food into chyme. The products of digestion are molecules of the original food or beverage small enough to be absorbed into the villi of the small intestine and transferred to the blood or lymph. For the most part, nutrients are absorbed in the small intestine; only a few are absorbed in the large intestine. Any dietary component that escapes digestion by human or bacterial enzymes exits the body as feces.

3.9 Urinary System

The **urinary system** is composed of two kidneys, one on each side of the spinal column. Each kidney is connected to the bladder by a **ureter.** The bladder is emptied by way of the **urethra** (Fig. 3-20). The main function of the kidneys is to remove waste from the body. The kidneys are constantly filtering blood to control its composition. This results in the formation of urine, mostly water, along with dissolved waste products of metabolism such as urea, and excess and unneeded water-soluble vitamins and various minerals.

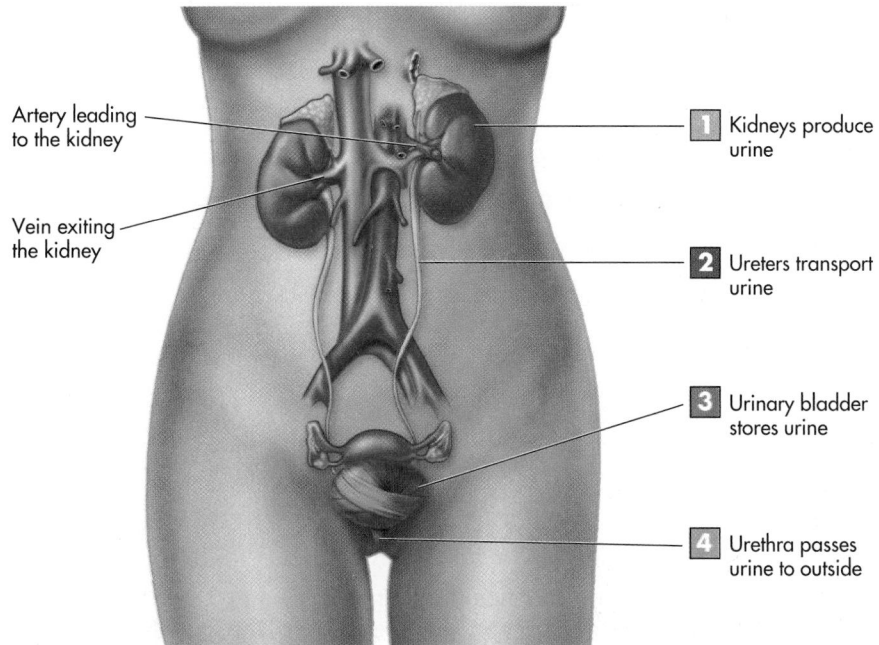

Artery leading
to the kidney

Vein exiting
the kidney

1 Kidneys produce
urine

2 Ureters transport
urine

3 Urinary bladder
stores urine

4 Urethra passes
urine to outside

FIGURE 3-20 ▶ Organs of the urinary system. The kidneys, 1 bean-shaped organs located on either side of the spinal column, filter waste from the blood and form urine, which is transported to the bladder by the ureters 2 and stored in the bladder 3 as urine. The urethra 4 transports the urine to outside the body. The urinary system of the female is shown. The male's urinary system is the same, except that the urethra extends through the penis.

enterohepatic circulation A continual recycling of compounds such as bile acid between the small intestine and the liver.

urinary system The body system consisting of the kidneys, urinary bladder, and the ducts that carry urine. This system removes waste products from the circulatory system and regulates blood acid-base balance, overall chemical balance, and water balance in the body.

ureter Tube that transports urine from the kidney to the urinary bladder.

urethra Tube that transports urine from the urinary bladder to the outside of the body.

pH A measure of relative acidity or alkalinity of a solution. The pH scale is 0 to 14. A pH of 7 is neutral; A pH below 7 is acidic; a pH above 7 is alkaline.

erythropoietin A hormone secreted mostly by the kidneys that enhances red blood cell synthesis and stimulates red blood cell release from bone marrow.

Together with the lungs, the kidneys also maintain the acid-base balance **(pH)** of the blood. The kidneys also convert a form of vitamin D into its active hormone form and produce a hormone that stimulates red blood cell synthesis (**erythropoietin;** see Chapter 12 for information on misuse of this hormone by some athletes). During times of fasting, the kidneys even produce glucose from certain amino acids. Thus, the kidneys perform many important functions related to nutrition and are a vital component of the body.

The proper function of the kidneys is closely tied to the strength of the cardiovascular system, particularly its ability to maintain adequate blood pressure, and the consumption of sufficient fluid. Uncontrolled diabetes, hypertension, and drug abuse are harmful to the kidneys.

3.10 Nutrient Storage Capabilities

The human body must maintain reserves of nutrients, otherwise we would need to eat continuously. Storage capacity varies for each different nutrient. Most fat is stored in adipose tissue, made up of cells designed specifically for this. Short-term storage of carbohydrate occurs in muscle and liver in the form of glycogen. The blood maintains a small reserve of glucose and amino acids. Many vitamins and minerals are stored in the liver, while other nutrient stores are found in other sites in the body.

When people do not meet certain nutrient needs, these nutrients are obtained by breaking down a tissue that contains high concentrations of the nutrient. For example, calcium is taken from bone and protein is taken from muscle. In cases of long-term deficiency, these nutrient losses weaken and harm these tissues.

Many people believe that if too much of a nutrient is obtained—for example, from a vitamin or mineral supplement—only what is needed is stored and the rest is excreted by the body. Though true for some nutrients, such as vitamin C, the large dosages of other nutrients frequently found in supplements, such as vitamin A and iron, can cause harmful side effects because they are not readily excreted. This is one reason why obtaining your nutrients primarily (or exclusively) from a balanced diet is the safest means to acquire the building blocks you need to maintain the good health of all organ systems.

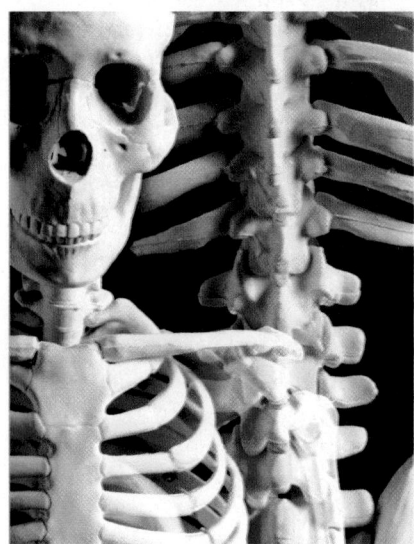

▲ The skeletal system provides a reserve of calcium for day-to-day needs when dietary intake is inadequate. Long-term use of this reserve, however, reduces bone strength.

CONCEPT CHECK

The urinary system removes the wastes produced by the body and many nutrients ingested in excess of storage capacity and need. The kidneys maintain the chemical composition and acidity of the blood. In addition, the kidneys help convert vitamin D to its active form and produce a hormone needed for red blood cell synthesis.

In well-nourished individuals, nutrients are constantly present in the blood for immediate use and are stored in the body tissues for later use when sufficient amounts are not consumed from food. However, when the body suffers a nutrient deficiency after an inadequate diet is consumed over a long period, vital tissues will be broken down for their nutrients, which can lead to ill health. Additionally, too much of any nutrient can be detrimental. It's best to focus primarily (or exclusively) on obtaining all essential nutrients from a balanced diet rather than mostly from dietary supplements.

3.11 Nutrition and Genetics

epigenome The way that the genome is marked and packaged inside the cell nucleus.

epigenetics Inherited changes in gene expression caused by mechanisms other than changes in the DNA sequence.

Once nutrients and other dietary components are taken up by cells, they may interact with our genes and have an effect on gene expression. The growth, development, and maintenance of cells, and ultimately of the entire organism, are directed by genes present in the cells. Each gene essentially represents a recipe, noting the ingredients (amino acids) and how those ingredients should be put together (to make proteins). The products (proteins) of all the recipes in the cookbook (the human genome) would then make up the human organism. The genome and the **epigenome**, the way the genome is marked and packaged inside a cell's nucleus, control the expression of individual traits, such as height, eye color, and susceptibility to many diseases. **Epigenetics** refers to inherited changes in gene expression caused by mechanisms other than changes in the underlying DNA sequence. While our genome contains the code for the proteins that can be made by our bodies, our epigenome is an extra layer of instructions that influences gene activity. In many cases it is the epigenome that can be repaired by treatments, or affected by diet, rather than the genetics.

A genetic variation can directly affect the proteins encoded by our genes and result in different:

- nutrient requirements among individuals.
- susceptibilities to diseases.
- effects of environmental factors (such as our diet) on our genes and their proteins.

The causes of chronic diseases are complex and include a significant genetic component. Fortunately, the science of genetics is moving swiftly such that medical breakthroughs are beginning to touch our lives. Genetic discoveries are leading to new drugs that disrupt disease processes at the molecular level and to tests that predict our risk for disease. In 2008, scientists discovered more than 100 genetic variations associated with many medical conditions associated with aging, including type 2 diabetes, Alzheimer's disease, osteoporosis, high blood pressure, and heart disease.

The Emerging Field of Nutrigenomics

nutrigenomics Study of how food impacts health through its interaction with our genes and its subsequent effect on gene expression.

In the near future, genetic information will enhance the ability of health professionals to help individuals manage diseases and optimize health. Nutritional genomics or **nutrigenomics** is the study of how food impacts health through its interaction with our genes and its subsequent effect on gene expression. Nutrigenomics also includes the study of how genes determine our nutritional requirements. Research in this area highlights the fallacy of a "one-size-fits-all" approach to nutrition interventions for disease prevention and management. It is becoming clear that the general nutrient requirements do not apply to certain genetic subgroups. Research is very active in identifying these subgroups and classifying the human genetic variation that may affect nutrient utilization and physiological function and therefore their unique nutrient requirements (see Further Readings 5, 14, and 15).

In addition to the direct effect of genes on disease risk, in many cases, genes influence the effect of diet and nutrition on disease development and progression. In some cases, a food component can cause a gene to be turned on or off, thus manipulating the production of proteins that can affect—positively or negatively—development or progression of diseases. With a better understanding of the interactions between genes and our diet, it will not be long before dietary recommendations may be personalized to help those with various genetically-linked diseases (see Further Reading 7).

Nutritional Diseases with a Genetic Link

Studies of families, including those with twins and adopted children, provide strong support for the effects of genetics in various disorders. In fact, family history is considered to be an important risk factor in the development of many nutrition-related diseases.

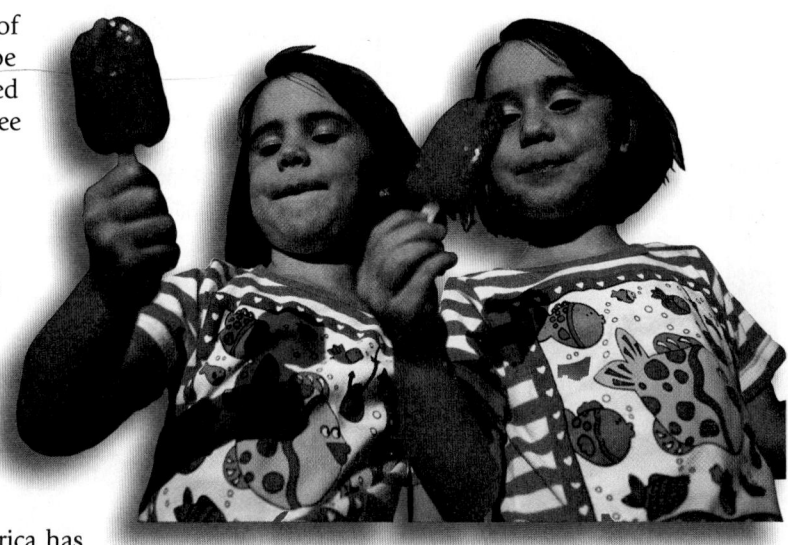

▲ Studies of twins have provided strong evidence for the interaction between genes and diet and their combined effects on disease risk.

Cardiovascular Disease. There is strong evidence that cardiovascular disease is the result of gene-environment interactions. About 1 of every 500 people in North America has a defective gene that greatly delays cholesterol removal from the bloodstream. As discussed in Chapter 1, elevated blood cholesterol is one major risk factor for development of cardiovascular disease. The gene-diet interactions being discovered for cardiovascular disease, particularly the cases of high blood lipid levels, will likely be the first to lead to nutrition plans personalized to decrease cardiovascular disease risk. Another genetic variation can cause abnormally high levels of an amino acid called homocysteine, which increases cardiovascular disease risk. Diet changes can help these people, but medications and even surgery are needed to address these problems.

Obesity. Most obese North Americans have at least one obese parent. This strongly suggests a genetic link. Findings from many human studies suggest that a variety of genes (likely 60 or more) are involved in the regulation of body weight. Little is known, however, about the specific nature of these genes in humans or how the actual changes in body metabolism (such as lower calorie-burning in general or fat use in particular) are produced.

Still, although some individuals may be genetically predisposed to store body fat, whether they do so depends on how many calories they consume relative to their needs. A common concept in nutrition is that *nurture*—how people live and the environmental factors that influence them—allows *nature*—each person's genetic potential—to be expressed. Although not every person with a genetic tendency toward obesity becomes obese, those genetically predisposed to weight gain have a higher lifetime risk than individuals without a genetic predisposition to obesity.

Diabetes. Both of the two common types of diabetes—type 1 and type 2—have genetic links. Evidence for these genetic links comes from studies of families, including twins, and from the high incidence of diabetes among certain population groups (e.g., South Asians or Pima Indians). Diabetes, in fact, is a complex disease with more than 200 genes identified as possible causes. Only sensitive and expensive testing can determine who is at risk. Type 2 diabetes is the most common form of diabetes (90% of all cases), and also has a strong link to obesity. Typically a genetic tendency for type 2 diabetes is expressed once a person becomes obese but often not before, again illustrating that nurture affects nature.

Cancer. A few types of cancer (e.g., some forms of colon [large intestine] and breast cancer) have a strong genetic link, and genetics may play a role in others, such as **prostate cancer.** Because obesity increases the risk of several forms of cancer, a long-standing excess calorie intake is also a risk factor. Although genes are an important determinant in the development of cancer, environmental and lifestyle factors, such as excessive sun exposure and a poor diet, also contribute significantly to the risk profile.

CRITICAL THINKING

Wesley notices that at family gatherings his parents, uncles, aunts, and older siblings typically drink excessive amounts of alcohol. His father has been arrested for driving while intoxicated, as has one of his aunts. Two of his uncles died before the age of 60 from alcohol abuse. As Wesley approaches the age of legal drinking, he wonders if he is destined to fall into the pattern of alcohol abuse. What advice would you give to Wesley concerning his future use of alcohol?

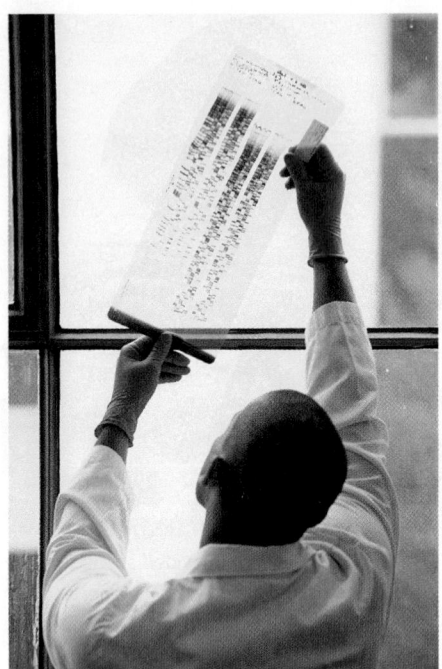

▲ Genetic testing for disease susceptibility will be more common in the future as the genes that increase the risk of developing various diseases are isolated and decoded.

The following weblinks will help you gather more information about genetic conditions and testing:

http://nutrigenomics.ucdavis.edu/
Center for Excellence for Nutritional Genomics. Website dedicated to promoting the new science of nutritional genomics

www.geneticalliance.org
Alliance of Genetic Support Groups

www.kumc.edu/gec/support
Information on genetic and rare conditions

www.cancer.gov/cancertopics/
prevention-genetics-causes
Genetics information from the National Cancer Institute

http://www.genome.gov/
National Human Genome Research Institute (at the National Institutes of Health) website. Describes the latest research finding, discusses some ethical issues, and provides a talking glossary.

http://history.nih.gov/exhibits/genetics/
Revolution in Progress: Human Genetics and Medical Research

MAKING DECISIONS

Research is opening the way for "personalized nutrition" that uses the results of genetic testing to determine which diet will work most effectively with the person's genetic makeup. There are genetic tests available for at least 1500 diseases and conditions, but mechanisms are not in place to ensure that the tests are based on adequate evidence or that marketing claims are truthful. Many companies are already tailoring genetic testing services and products for certain genetic profiles even though there are insufficient data on which to base genotype-specific recommendations. Most of these offers are online. As we discussed in Chapter 2, caution is always needed when evaluating nutrition information and claims. Genetic testing is no exception. Some DNA-testing companies are responsible organizations, and some are not. Some are offering DNA tests to determine the best weight-loss diets or the best supplements. These marketing schemes belittle the science of genetics to consumers. Use the principles outlined in Chapter 2 to evaluate any genetic testing services or products.

Your Genetic Profile

From this discussion, you can see that your genes can greatly influence your risk of developing certain diseases. By recognizing your potential for developing a particular disease, you can avoid behavior that further raises your risk. How can you figure out your genetic profile? Genetic testing can be valuable if it confirms that you carry a gene for a disease that you can do something about in terms of protecting against it. Testing is also of interest when you do not know your family medical history or there are gaps in your family tree. About 1000 genetic tests have become available in recent years. It typically costs about $1000 to have your DNA read to reveal the diseases to which you are most susceptible. Many tests are covered by health insurance plans. The Genetic Information Nondiscrimination Act (GINA) became a law in May 2008, and prohibits health insurers from raising premiums or denying coverage based on genetic information and applies to people who have genes that carry the risk of disease. DNA testing includes providing a saliva sample from which your DNA will be separated. Certain areas of the genome are then read and measured in the process known as genotyping. After this 1-to 2-month process, you receive your DNA profile, which will supplement what you already know about your family history. You can also compare your DNA profile to future findings from DNA research.

Many of the genes involved in common diseases, such as diabetes, are still unknown. Although there are genetic tests available for some diseases, your family history of certain diseases is still a much better indicator of your genetic profile and risk of disease. Put together a family tree of illnesses and deaths by compiling a few key facts on your primary relatives: siblings, parents, aunts and uncles, and grandparents, as suggested in the "Rate Your Plate" section. In general, the greater number of your relatives who had a genetically transmitted disease and the closer they are related to you, the greater your risk. If there is a significant family history of a certain disease, lifestyle changes may be appropriate. For example, women with a family history of breast cancer should avoid becoming obese, should minimize alcohol use, and should obtain mammograms regularly.

Figure 3-22 shows an example of a family tree (also called a *genogram*). High-risk conditions include two or more first-degree relatives in a family with a specific disease (first-degree relatives include one's parents, siblings, and offspring). Another sign of risk of inherited disease is development of the disease in a first-degree relative before the age of 50 to 60 years. In the family depicted in Figure 3-21, prostate cancer killed the man's father. Knowing this, the man should be tested regularly for prostate cancer. His sisters should have frequent mammograms and other preventive practices because their mother died of breast cancer. Because heart attack and stroke are also common in the family, all the children should adopt a lifestyle that minimizes the risk of developing these conditions, such as avoiding excessive animal fat and salt intake. Colon cancer is also evident, so careful screening throughout life is important.

Information about our genetic makeup will increasingly influence our dietary and lifestyle choices. Throughout this book we will discuss "controllable" risk factors that could contribute to development of genetically linked diseases present in your family. This information will help you personalize nutrition advice based on your genetic background and identify and avoid the risk factors that could lead to the diseases present in your family.

This review of human anatomy, physiology, and genetics from a nutrition perspective sets the stage for developing a more detailed understanding of the nutrients. Chapters 4, 5, and 6 will build on this information.

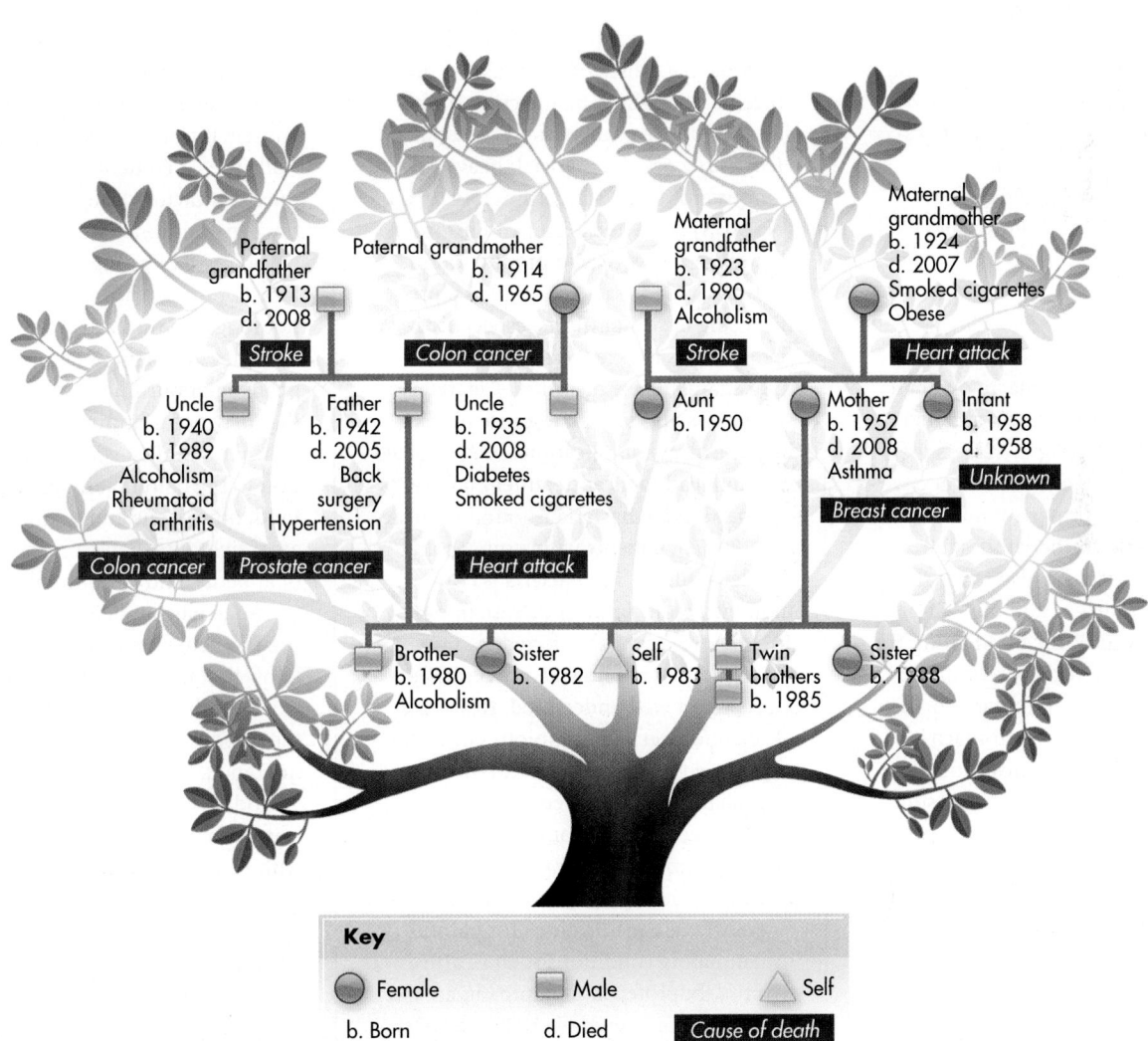

FIGURE 3-21 ▶ Example of a family tree for Justin, designated as "Self" at the trunk of the tree. The gender of each family member is identified by color (blue squares for males, orange circles for females). Dates of birth (b) and death (d) are listed below each family member. If deceased, the cause of death is highlighted using white text against a red background. Other medical conditions the family members experienced are noted beneath each name. Create your own family tree of frequent diseases using the diagram in "Rate Your Plate" and this figure as a guide. Then show your family tree to your physician to get a more complete picture of what the information means for your health.

Common Problems with Digestion

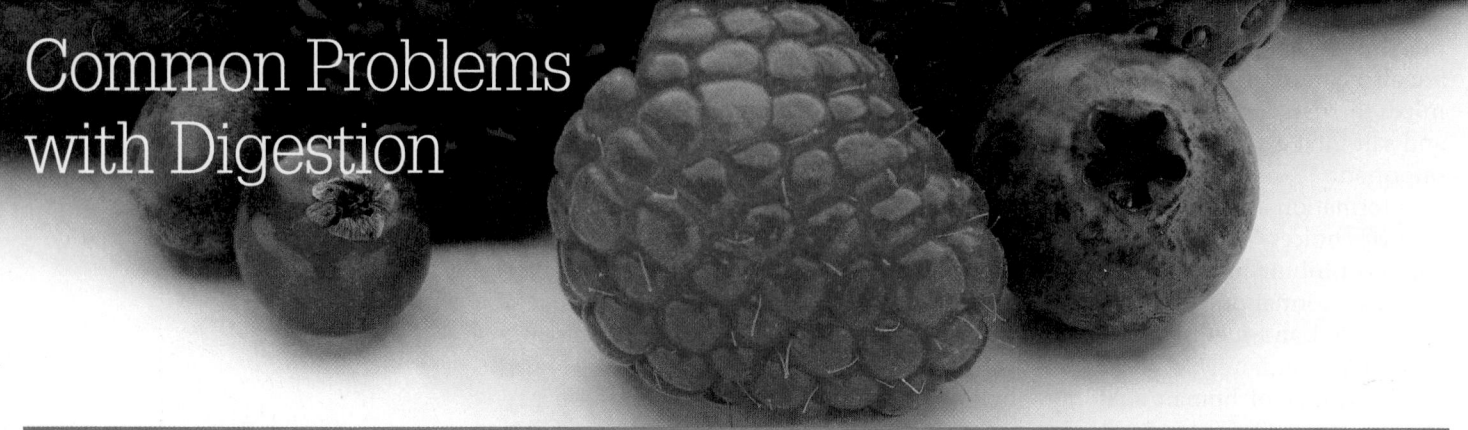

The fine-tuned organ system we call the digestive system can develop problems. Knowing about these common problems can help you avoid or lessen them. Two common GI tract-related problems are diverticulosis and lactose maldigestion and intolerance. These disorders will be discussed in Chapter 4 after you learn more about carbohydrates.

Ulcers

A peptic **ulcer** can occur when the lining of the esophagus, stomach, or small intestine is eroded by the acid secreted by the stomach cells (Fig. 3-22). As the stomach lining deteriorates in ulcer development, it loses its protective mucus layer, and the acid further erodes the stomach tissue. Acid can also erode the lining of the esophagus and the first part of the small intestine, the duodenum. In young people, most ulcers occur in the small intestine, wheras in older people they occur primarily in the stomach.

Millions of North Americans develop ulcers during their lifetimes. As a result, billions of healthcare dollars are spent annually on the treatment of peptic ulcers and their complications. Fortunately, our understanding of ulcer formation has increased, resulting in a variety of improved treatment options. The typical symptom of an ulcer is pain about 2 hours after eating. Stomach acid acting on a meal irritates the ulcer after most of the meal has moved from the site of the ulcer.

Not long ago, the major cause of ulcer disease was thought to be excess acid. Therefore, neutralizing and curtailing the secretion of stomach acid were the logical treatment choices. Although acid is still a significant player in ulcer formation, the principal causes of ulcer disease are currently thought to be infection of the stomach by the acid-resistant bacteria, *Helicobacter pylori (H. pylori);* heavy use of nonsteroidal anti-inflammatory drugs **(NSAIDS),** such as aspirin; and disorders that cause excessive acid production in the stomach. Stress is regarded as a predisposing factor for ulcers, especially if the person is infected with *H. pylori* or has certain anxiety disorders. Cigarette smoking is also known to cause ulcers, increase ulcer complications such as bleeding, and lead to ulcer treatment failure.

The *H. pylori* bacteria is found in more than 80% of patients with stomach and duodenal ulcers. The bacteria is common but results in ulcer disease in only 10% to 15% of those infected. Although the mechanism of how *H. pylori* causes ulcers is not well understood, treatment of the infection with antibiotics heals the ulcers and prevents their recurrence. Two Australian physicians were awarded the Nobel Prize in 2005 "for their discovery of the bacterium *Helicobacter pylori* and its role in gastritis and peptic ulcer disease."

NSAIDs are medications for painful inflammatory conditions such as arthritis. Aspirin, ibuprofen, and naproxen are the most commonly used NSAIDs. NSAIDs reduce the mucus secreted by the stomach. Newer medications, called "Cox-2 inhibitors" (e.g., celecoxib [Celebrex]), have been used as a replacement for NSAIDs because they are less likely to cause stomach ulcers. They do offer some advantages over NSAIDs, but they may not be totally safe for some people, especially those with a history of cardiovascular disease or strokes.

The primary risk associated with an ulcer is the possibility that it will erode entirely through the stomach or intestinal wall. The GI contents could then spill into the body cavities, causing a massive infection. In addition, an ulcer may erode a blood vessel, leading to substantial blood loss. For these reasons, it is important not to ignore the early warning signs of ulcer development, including a persistent gnawing or burning near the stomach that may occur immediately following a meal or awaken you at night. In addition to the pain that may improve with food, other signs and symptoms of ulcers are weight loss, nausea, vomiting, loss of appetite, and abdominal bloating.

In the past, milk and cream therapy was used to help cure ulcers. Clinicians now know that milk and cream are two of the worst foods for an ulcer. The calcium in these foods stimulates stomach acid secretion and actually inhibits ulcer healing.

Today, a combination of approaches is used for ulcer therapy. People infected with *H. pylori* are given antibiotics as well as stomach acid-blocking medica-

---

ulcer Erosion of the tissue lining, usually in the stomach or the upper small intestine. As a group these are generally referred to as *peptic ulcers.*

NSAIDs Nonsteroidal anti-inflammatory drugs; includes aspirin, ibuprofen (Advil®), and naproxen (Aleve®).

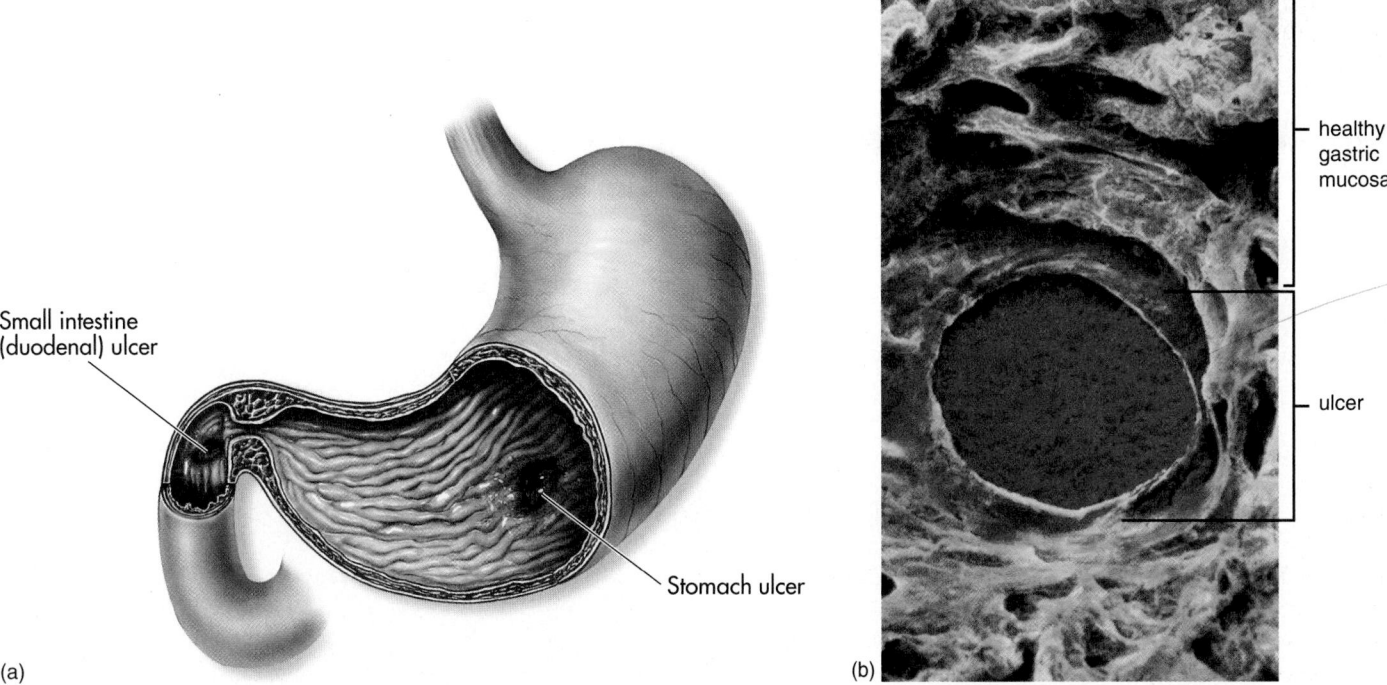

FIGURE 3-22 ▶ (a) A peptic ulcer in the stomach or small intestine. *H. pylori* bacteria and NSAIDs (e.g., aspirin) cause ulcers by impairing mucosal defense, especially in the stomach. In the same way, smoking, genetics, and stress can impair mucosal defense, as well as cause an increase in the release of pepsin and stomach acid. All of these factors can contribute to ulcers. (b) Close-up of a stomach ulcer. This needs to be treated or eventual perforation of the stomach is possible.

▶ When suffering from persistent heartburn or GERD, see a doctor if you have:

- Difficulty swallowing or pain when swallowing
- Heartburn that has persisted for more than 10 years
- Initial onset of heartburn after age 50
- Heartburn that resists treatment with medications
- Sudden, unexplained weight loss
- Chest pain
- Blood loss or anemia
- Blood in stool or vomit

tions called **proton** (proton is another name for the hydrogen ion that creates acidity) **pump inhibitors** (e.g., omeprazole [Prilosec], esomeprazole [Nexium], and lansoprazole [Prevacid]). In many cases, there is a 90% cure rate for *H. pylori* infections in the first week of this treatment. Recurrence is unlikely if the infection is cured, but an incomplete cure almost certainly leads to repeated ulcer formation (see Further Reading 2).

Antacid medications may also be part of ulcer care, as is a class of medicines called **H2 blockers**. These include cimetidine (Tagamet), ranitidine (Zantac), nizatidine (Axid), and famotidine (Pepcid), all of which prevent **histamine**-related acid secretion in the stomach. Medications that coat the ulcer, such as sucralfate (Carafate), are also commonly used.

People with ulcers should refrain from smoking and minimize the use of NSAIDs. These practices reduce the mucus secreted by the stomach. Overall, a combination of lifestyle therapy and medical treatment has so revolutionized ulcer

therapy that dietary changes are of minor importance today. Current diet-therapy approaches recommend avoiding foods that increase ulcer symptoms (Table 3-5).

proton pump inhibitor A medication that inhibits the ability of gastric cells to secrete hydrogen ions. Low doses of this class of medications are also available without prescription (e.g., omeprazole [Prilosec]).

H_2 blocker Medication, such as cimetidine (Tagamet®), that blocks the increase of stomach acid production caused by histamine.

histamine A breakdown product of the amino acid histidine that stimulates acid secretion by the stomach and has other effects on the body, such as contraction of smooth muscles, increased nasal secretions, relaxation of blood vessels, and changes in relaxation of airways.

TABLE 3-5 Recommendations to Prevent Ulcers and Heartburn from Occurring or Recurring

Ulcers
1. Stop smoking if you are now a smoker.
2. Avoid large doses of aspirin, ibuprofen, and other NSAID compounds unless a physician advises otherwise. For people who must use these medications, FDA has approved an NSAID combined with a medication to reduce gastric damage. The medication reduces gastric acid production and enhances mucus secretion.
3. Limit consumption of coffee, tea, and alcohol (especially wine), if this helps.
4. Limit consumption of pepper, chili powder, and other strong spices, if this helps.
5. Eat nutritious meals on a regular schedule; include enough fiber (see Chapter 4 for sources of fiber).
6. Chew foods well.
7. Lose weight if you are currently overweight.

Heartburn
1. Follow ulcer prevention recommendations.
2. Wait about 2 hours after a meal before lying down.
3. Don't overeat. Eat smaller meals that are low in fat.
4. Elevate the head of the bed at least 6 inches.

Heartburn

About half of North American adults experience occasional heartburn, also known as acid reflux (Fig. 3-23). This gnawing pain in the upper chest is caused by the movement of acid from the stomach into the esophagus. The recurrent and therefore more serious form of the problem is called **gastroesophageal reflux disease (GERD)**. Unlike the stomach, the esophagus has very little mucus lining to protect it, so acid quickly erodes the lining of the esophagus, causing pain. Symptoms may also include nausea, gagging, cough, or hoarseness. GERD is characterized by the occurrence of such symptoms of acid reflux two or more times per week. People who have GERD experience occasional relaxation of the gastroesophageal sphincter. Typically it should be relaxed only during swallowing, but in individuals with GERD it is relaxed at other times as well.

The majority of heartburn sufferers say it significantly affects their quality of life, particularly their enjoyment of many favorite foods. On a more serious note, however, if left untreated, heartburn can, over time, damage the lining of the esophagus, leading to chronic esophageal inflammation and an increased risk of esophageal cancer (see Further Reading 8). Heartburn sufferers should follow the general recommendations given in Table 3-5. For occasional heartburn, quick relief can be found with over-the-counter (OTC) antacids. Taking antacids will reduce the acid in the stomach but will not stop the acid reflux. For more persistent (few days a week or everyday) heartburn or GERD, the H2 blockers or PPIs, discussed in the previous section on ulcers, may be needed. PPIs provide long-lasting relief by reducing stomach acid production and should be taken before the first meal of the day because they take longer to work. If the proper medications are not effective at controlling GERD, surgery may be

gastroesophageal reflux disease (GERD) Disease that results from stomach acid backing up into the esophagus. The acid irritates the lining of the esophagus, causing pain.

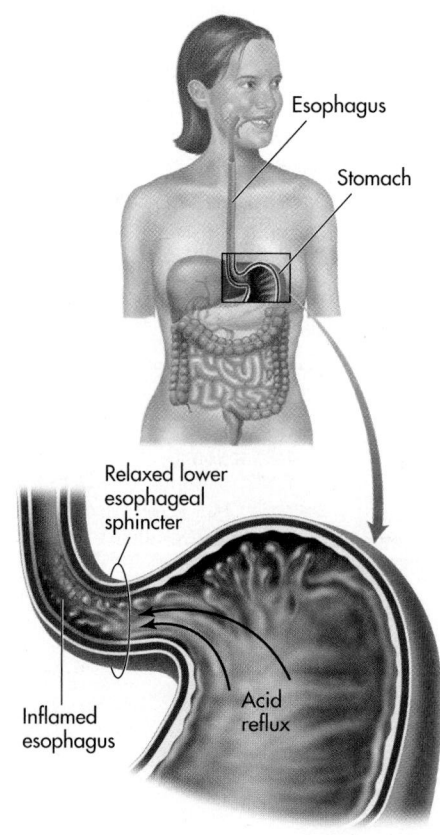

FIGURE 3-23 ▶ Heartburn results from stomach acid refluxing into the esophagus.

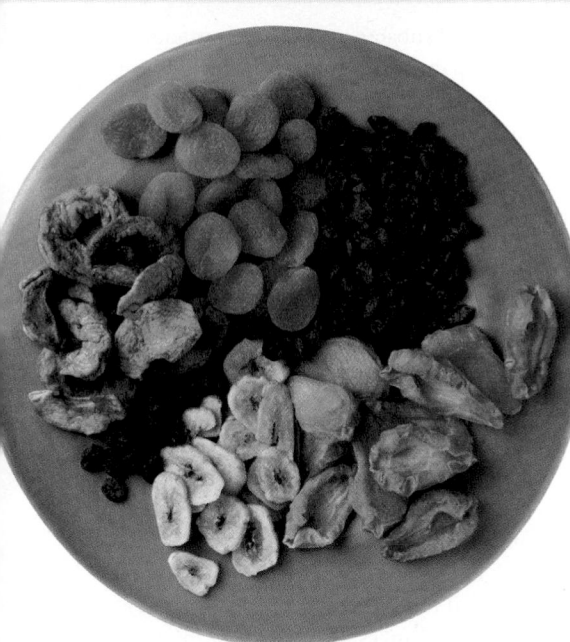

▲ Dried fruits are a natural source of fiber and can help prevent constipation when consumed with an adequate amount of fluid.

MAKING DECISIONS

Use of Laxatives

Perhaps you have heard that taking laxatives after overeating prevents deposition of body fat from excess calorie intake. This erroneous and dangerous premise has gained popularity among followers of numerous fad diets. You may temporarily feel less full after using a laxative because laxatives hasten emptying of the large intestine and increase fluid loss. Most laxatives, however, do not speed the passage of food through the small intestine, where digestion and most nutrient absorption take place. As a result, do you think you can count on laxatives to prevent fat gain from excess calorie intake?

needed to strengthen the weakened esophageal sphincter (see Further Reading 3). A popular theory is that relaxation of the lower esophageal sphincter allows acid and stomach contents to flow back into the esophagus. This situation will be more of a problem when lying down.

Both pregnancy and obesity can lead to heartburn (see Further Reading 6). These conditions result in increased production of estrogen and progesterone, which relax the lower esophageal sphincter, making heartburn more likely. In obesity, adipose tissue turns certain circulating hormones into estrogen; thus, the more adipose tissue one has, the more estrogen produced.

Constipation and Laxatives

Constipation, difficult or infrequent evacuation of the bowels, is commonly reported by adults. Slow movement of fecal material through the large intestine causes constipation. As more fluid is absorbed during the extended time the feces stay in the large intestine, they become dry and hard.

Constipation can result when people regularly ignore their normal bowel reflexes for long periods. People may ignore normal urges when it is inconvenient to interrupt occupational or social activities. Muscle spasms of an irritated large intestine can also slow the movement of feces and contribute to constipation. Calcium, iron supplements, and medications such as antacids can also cause constipation.

Eating foods with plenty of fiber, such as whole-grain breads, cereals, and beans, along with drinking adequate fluid to avoid dehydration, is the best method for treating mild cases of constipation. Fiber stimulates peristalsis by drawing water into the large intestine and helping form a bulky, soft fecal output. Dried fruits are a good source of fiber and therefore can also help stimulate the bowel. Additional fluid should be consumed to facilitate fiber's action in the large intestine. In addition, people with constipation may need to develop more regular bowel habits; allowing the same time each day for a bowel move-

ment can help train the large intestine to respond routinely. Finally, relaxation facilitates regular bowel movements, as does regular physical activity.

Laxatives, as well as various other medications, can also lessen constipation. Some laxatives work by irritating the intestinal nerve junctions to stimulate the peristaltic muscles, while others that contain fiber draw water into the intestine to enlarge fecal output. The larger output stretches the peristaltic muscles, making them rebound and then constrict. Regular use of laxatives, however, should be supervised by a physician. Overall the bulk-forming fiber laxatives are the safest to use.

Hemorrhoids

Hemorrhoids, also called *piles,* are swollen veins of the rectum and anus. The blood vessels in this area are subject to intense pressure, especially during bowel movements. Added stress to the vessels from pregnancy, obesity, prolonged sitting, violent coughing or sneezing, or straining during bowel movements, particularly with constipation, can lead to a hemorrhoid. Hemorrhoids can develop unnoticed until a strained bowel movement precipitates symptoms, which may include pain, itching, and bleeding.

Itching, caused by moisture in the anal canal, swelling, or other irritation, is perhaps the most common symptom. Pain, if present, is usually aching and steady. Bleeding may result from a hemorrhoid and appear in the toilet as a bright red streak in the feces. The sensation of a mass in the anal canal after a bowel movement is symptomatic of an internal hemorrhoid that protrudes through the anus.

Anyone can develop a hemorrhoid, and about half of adults over age 50 do. Diet, lifestyle, and possibly heredity play

constipation A condition characterized by infrequent bowel movements.

laxative A medication or other substance that stimulates evacuation of the intestinal tract.

a role. For example, a low-fiber diet can lead to hemorrhoids as a result of straining during bowel movements. If you think you have a hemorrhoid, you should consult your physician. Rectal bleeding, although usually caused by hemorrhoids, may also indicate other problems, such as cancer.

A physician may suggest a variety of self-care measures for hemorrhoids. Pain can be lessened by applying warm, soft compresses or sitting in a tub of warm water for 15 to 20 minutes. Dietary recommendations are the same as those for treating constipation, emphasizing the need to consume adequate fiber and fluid. Over-the-counter remedies, such as Preparation H, can also offer relief of symptoms.

Irritable Bowel Syndrome

Many adults (25 million or more in the United States alone) have irritable bowel syndrome, noted as a combination of cramps, gassiness, bloating, and irregular bowel function (diarrhea, constipation, or alternating episodes of both). It is more common in younger women than in younger men. In older adults the ratio is closer to 50:50. The disease leads to about 3.5 million visits to physicians in the United States each year.

Symptoms associated with irritable bowel syndrome include visible abdominal distention, pain relief after a bowel movement, increased stool frequency, loose stools with pain onset, mucus in stool, and a feeling of incomplete elimination even after a bowel movement.

The cause is thought to be altered intestinal peristalsis coupled with a decreased pain threshold for abdominal distension—in other words, a minor amount of abdominal bloating causes pain that the average person would not sense. It is also noteworthy that up to 50% of sufferers report a history of verbal or sexual abuse.

Therapy is individualized and can include a trial of high-fiber foods (soluble fiber is more effective than insoluble fiber) or elimination diets that focus on avoiding dairy products and gas-forming foods, such as legumes, certain vegetables (cabbage, beans, and broccoli), and some fruits (grapes, raisins, cherries, and cantaloupe). Herbal formulations, certain probiotics, and cognitive behavioral therapy have been shown to decrease symptoms of irritable bowel syndrome and improve overall quality of life (see Further Reading 1). The patient should moderate or eliminate caffeine-containing foods/beverages altogether. Low-fat and more frequent, small meals may help because large meals can trigger contractions of the large intestine. Other strategies include a reduction in stress, psychological counseling, and certain antidepressant and other medications. Hypnosis has been shown to relieve symptoms in severe cases.

Referral to a registered dietitian can be beneficial, as many patients experience improvement with the elimination of specific problem foods. A good patient/physician relationship is also necessary for the treatment of irritable bowel syndrome; however, before any single treatment is applauded, note that response to placebos alone has been as high as 70% in this population. Although irritable bowel syndrome can be uncomfortable and upsetting, it is harmless as it carries no risk for cancer or other serious digestive problems. The website www.ibsgroup.org provides further information.

Diarrhea

Diarrhea, a GI tract disease that generally lasts only a few days, is defined as increased fluidity, frequency, or amount of bowel movements compared to a person's usual pattern. Most cases of diarrhea result from infections in the intestines, with bacteria and viruses the usual offending agents. They produce substances that cause the intestinal cells to secrete fluid rather than absorb fluid. Another form of diarrhea can be caused by consumption of substances not readily absorbed, such as the sugar alcohol sorbitol found in sugarless gum (see Chapter 4) or large amounts of a high-fiber source such as bran. When consumed in large amounts, the unabsorbed substance draws much water into the intestines, in turn leading to diarrhea. Treatment of diarrhea generally requires drinking lots of fluid during the affected stage; reduced intake of the poorly absorbed substance also is important if that is a cause. Prompt treatment—within 24 to 48 hours—is especially important for infants and older people, as they are more susceptible to the effects of dehydration associated with diarrhea (see Chapters 15 and 16). Diarrhea that lasts more than 7 days in adults should be investigated by a physician as it can be a symptom of more serious intestinal disease, especially if there is also blood in the stool.

Gallstones

Gallstones are a major cause of illness and surgery, affecting 10% to 20% of U.S. adults. Gallstones are pieces of solid material that develop in the gallbladder when substances in the bile—primarily cholesterol (80% of gallstones)—form crystal-like particles. They may be as small as a grain of sand or as large as a golf ball. These stones are caused by a combination of factors, with excess weight being the primary modifiable factor, especially in women 20 to 60 years old. Other factors include genetic background (e.g., Native Americans), advanced age (> 60 years for both women and men), reduced activity of the gallbladder (contracts less than normal), altered bile composition (e.g., too much cholesterol or not enough bile salts), diabetes, and diet (e.g., low-fiber diets). In addition, gallstones may develop during rapid weight loss or prolonged fasting (as the liver metabolizes more fat, it secretes more cholesterol into the bile).

Attacks due to gallstones include intermittent pain in the upper right abdomen, gas and bloating, nausea or vomiting, or other health problems. Surgical removal of the gallbladder is the most common method for treating gallstones (500,000 surgeries per year in the United States).

Prevention of gallstones revolves around avoiding becoming overweight, especially for women. Avoiding rapid weight loss (> 3 pounds per week), limiting animal protein and focusing more on plant protein intake (especially some nut intake), and following a high-fiber diet can help as well. Regular physical activity is also recommended, as is moderate to no caffeine and alcohol intake.

Less Common Digestive Disorders

In **cystic fibrosis**—an inherited disease of infants, children, and sometimes adults—the pancreas often develops thick mucus that blocks its ducts, and active cells then die. As a result, the pancreas is not able to effectively deliver its digestive enzymes into the small intestine. Digestion of carbohydrate, protein, and—most notably—fat then is impaired. Often the missing enzymes must be ingested in capsule form with meals to aid in digestion. Another intestinal problem gaining attention is **celiac disease.** People with this disease experience an allergic reaction to the protein gluten in certain cereals, such as wheat and rye. This reaction damages the absorptive cells, resulting in a much-reduced surface area due to flattening of the villi. Elimination of wheat, rye, and certain other grains from the diet typically cures the problem.

Summary

Overall, typical medical disorders of the GI tract arise from differences in anatomical features and lifestyle habits among individuals. Because of the importance of various nutrition and lifestyle habits, such as adequate fiber and fluid intake, as well as not smoking or abusing NSAID medications, nutrition and lifestyle therapy is often effective in helping treat GI tract disorders.

cystic fibrosis Inherited disease that can cause overproduction of mucus. Mucus can block the pancreatic duct, decreasing enzyme output.

celiac disease Immunological or allergic reaction to the protein gluten in certain grains, such as wheat and rye. The effect is to destroy the intestinal enterocytes, resulting in a much reduced surface area due to flattening of the villi. Elimination of wheat, rye, and certain other grains from the diet restores the intestinal surface.

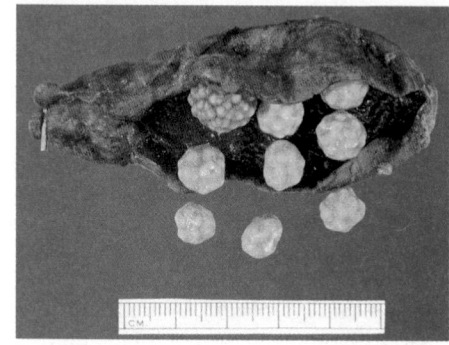

▲ Gallbladder and gallstones seen after surgical removal from the body. Size and composition of the stones vary from one case to another.

Case Study Gastroesophageal Reflux Disease

Caitlin is a 20-year-old college sophomore. Over the last few months, she has been experiencing regular bouts of heartburn. This usually happens after a large lunch or dinner. Occasionally she has even bent down after dinner to pick up something and had some stomach contents travel back up her esophagus and into her mouth. This especially frightened Caitlin, so she visited the University Health Center.

The nurse practitioner at the Center told Caitlin it was good that she came in for a checkup because she suspects Caitlin has a disease called gastroesophageal reflux disease (GERD). She tells Caitlin that this can lead to serious problems, such as a rare form of cancer if not controlled. She provides Caitlin with a pamphlet describing GERD and schedules an appointment with a physician for further evaluation.

Answer the following questions, and check your response in Appendix A.

1. What dietary and lifestyle habits likely contribute to Caitlin's symptoms of GERD?

2. What is the dietary and lifestyle management advice that will help Caitlin cope with this health problem?

3. What types of medications have been especially useful for treating this problem?

4. Overall, how will Caitlin cope with this health problem, and will it ever go away?

5. Why is management of GERD so important?

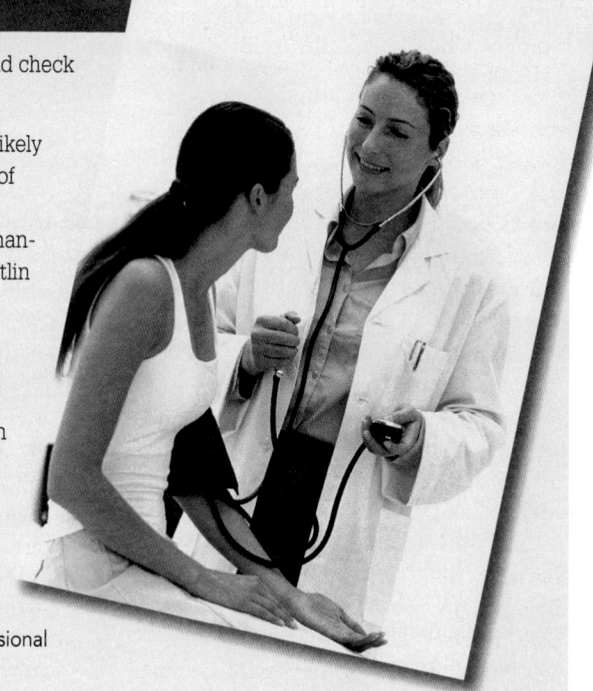

▶ Caitlin was wise to see a health professional about her persistent heartburn.

Summary (Numbers refer to numbered sections in the chapter.)

3.1 Cells join together to make up tissues, tissues unite to form organs, and organs work together as an organ system.

3.2 The basic structural unit of the human body is the cell. A most all cells contain the same organelles (nucleus, mitochondria, endoplasmic reticulum, lysosomes, peroxisomes, and cytoplasm), but cell structure varies according to the type of job they must perform.

3.3 Epithelial, connective, muscle, and nervous, are the four primary types of tissues in the human body. Each type of organ system is affected by nutrient intake.

3.4 Blood is pumped from the heart to the lungs, picking up oxygen. Blood delivers essential nutrients, oxygen, and water to all body cells. Nutrients and wastes are exchanged between blood and cells across the cell membrane. This exchange occurs in the capillaries. Water-soluble compounds absorbed by the small intestine cells enter the portal vein and travel to the liver. Fat-soluble compounds enter the lymphatic system, which eventually connects to the bloodstream.

3.5 The nervous system's neurons are the body's communication network. They control and manage all other organ systems of the body. Neurotransmitters are used to carry the message from one neuron to another (or to another cell).

3.6 The endocrine system produces hormones, which chemically regulate almost all other cells.

3.7 The immune system protects the body from invading pathogens. We activate immunity, such as production of antibodies (immunoglobulins), when we come in contact with a pathogen.

3.8 The gastrointestinal (GI) tract consists of the mouth, esophagus, stomach, small intestine, large intestine (colon), rectum, and anus.

Spaced along the GI tract are ring-like valves (sphincters) that regulate the flow of foodstuffs. Muscular contractions, called *peristalsis*, move the foodstuffs down the GI tract. A variety of nerves, hormones, and other substances control the activity of sphincters and peristaltic muscles.

Digestive enzymes are secreted by the mouth, stomach, wall of the small intestine, and pancreas. The presence of food in the small intestine stimulates the release of pancreatic enzymes.

The major absorptive sites consist of fingerlike projections called *villi*, located in the small intestine. Absorptive cells cover the villi. This intestinal lining is continually renewed. Absorptive cells can perform various forms of passive diffusion and active absorption.

Little digestion and absorption occur in the stomach or large intestine, but some protein is digested in the stomach. Some constituents of fiber and undigested starch are broken down by bacteria in the large intestine and some of the products are absorbed; any undigested fiber that remains is eliminated in the feces.

Final water and mineral absorption takes place in the large intestine. Products from bacterial breakdown of some fibers and other substances are also absorbed here. The presence of feces in the rectum provides the impetus for elimination.

The liver, gallbladder, and pancreas participate in digestion and absorption. Products from these organs, such as enzymes and bile, enter the small intestine help in digesting protein, fat, and carbohydrate.

3.9 The urinary system, including the kidneys, is responsible for filtering the blood, removing body wastes, and maintaining the chemical composition of the blood.

3.10 Limited stores of nutrients are present in the blood for immediate use and stored to a greater or lesser extent in body tissues for later use when sufficient food is unavailable. When the body suffers a nutrient deficiency caused by a poor diet, it breaks down vital tissues for their nutrients, which can lead to ill health. Additionally, too much of any nutrient can be detrimental.

3.11 Genetic background influences the risk for many health-related diseases. Examining one's family tree provides clues for an individual to such risks. Preventative measures are then import ant to implement, especially with respect to diet.

N&YH Common GI-tract diseases, such as heartburn, constipation, and irritable bowel syndrome, can be treated with diet changes. These can include increasing fiber intake and avoiding large meals high in fat. Medications are also very helpful in many cases.

Check Your Knowledge (Answers to the following questions are below.)

1. The stomach is protected from digesting itself by producing
   a. bicarbonate.
   b. a thick layer of mucus.
   c. hydroxyl ions to neutralize acid.
   d. antipepsin that destroys enzymes.

2. The lower esophageal sphincter is located between the
   a. stomach and esophagus.
   b. stomach and duodenum.
   c. ileum and the cecum.
   d. colon and the anus.

3. A muscular contraction that propels food down the GI tract is called
   a. a sphincter.
   b. enterohepatic circulation.
   c. gravitational pull.
   d. peristalsis.

4. Bicarbonate ions (HCO_3-) from the pancreas
   a. neutralize acid in the stomach.
   b. are synthesized in the pyloric sphincter.
   c. neutralize bile in the duodenum.
   d. neutralize the acid in the duodenum.

5. Most digestive processes occur in the
   a. mouth.
   b. stomach.
   c. small intestine.
   d. large intestine.
   e. colon.

6. Bile is formed in the _____ and stored in the _____.
   a. stomach, pancreas
   b. duodenum, kidney
   c. liver, gallbladder
   d. gallbladder, liver

7. Much of the digestion that occurs in the large intestine is caused by
   a. lipase.
   b. pepsin.
   c. saliva.
   d. bacteria.

8. Nexium ("the purple pill") acts as a(n)
   a. H₂ blocker.
   b. laxative.
   c. analgesic.
   d. proton pump inhibitor.

9. The study of how food impacts health through interaction with genes is
   a. nutrigenomics.
   b. epidemiology.
   c. immunology.
   d. genetics.

10. Energy production that takes place in the cytoplasm is anaerobic metabolism because it does not require
   a. water.
   b. oxygen.
   c. anabolic steroids.
   d. anaerobic bacteria.

Answer Keys: 1. b (LO 3.11), 2. a (LO 3.8), 3. d (LO 3.8), 4. d (LO 3.8), 5. c (LO 3.8), 6. c (LO 3.8), 7. d, 8. d (LO 3.12), 9. a, 10. b (LO 3.2)

Study Questions (Numbers refer to Learning Outcomes)

1. Identify at least one function of the 12 organ systems related to nutrition (**LO 3.3**)

2. Draw and label parts of the cell, and explain the function of each organelle as it relates to human nutrition. (**LO 3.2**)

3. Trace the flow of blood from the right side of the heart and back to the same site. How is blood routed through the small intestine? Which class of nutrients enters the body via the blood? Via the lymph? (**LO 3.4**)

4. Explain why the small intestine is better suited than the other GI tract organs to carry out the absorptive process. (**LO 3.8**)

5. Identify the four basic tastes. Give an example of one food that exemplifies each of these basic taste sensations. (**LO 3.8**)

6. What is one role of acid in the process of digestion? Where is it secreted? (**LO 3.8**)

7. Contrast the processes of active absorption and passive diffusion of nutrients. (**LO 3.8**)

8. Identify two accessory organs that empty their contents into the small intestine. How do the digestive substances secreted by these organs contribute to the digestion of food? (**LO 3.8**)

9. In which organ systems would the following substances be found?
   chyme (**LO 3.8**), plasma (**LO 3.4**), lymph (**LO 3.4**), urine (**LO 3.9**)

10. Describe the nutrition-related diseases for which genetics or family history is considered to be an important risk factor. (**LO 3.11**)

What Would You Choose Recommendations

Constipation results from slow movement of fecal material through the large intestine. Increasing fiber and water in your diet can often relieve constipation without the aid of an over-the-counter laxative. To boost your fiber intake, choose whole grains, fruits, vegetables, and legumes (beans). This can be a tough task when most of the menu options you will find in fast-food restaurants and convenience stores are low in fiber.

As you select your pizza, look for slices with extra vegetables or fruit. This will increase the fiber content by about 1 gram per slice. Pizza with whole-grain crust, would add another 1 gram of fiber per slice. These are small improvements, so you will probably still need to look for additional fiber sources.

What about your side dish? Unless they are made with whole grains, the pasta and breadsticks will not add much fiber to your meal. A breadstick and a cup of pasta with Alfredo sauce provide about 1 and 2 grams of fiber, respectively. These carbohydrate-rich add-ons are supplying extra calories and would be better off skipped. The salad provides about 1 to 3 grams of fiber, depending on its size and ingredients. The core ingredients of tossed salad—lettuce, cucumbers, tomato—are mostly water and not particularly high in fiber. Toppings such as cheese, egg, or diced meat will not help relieve constipation. Instead, dried fruit (e.g., dried cranberries or raisins) and nuts supply some additional fiber.

An even better choice, however, is the soup! A cup of bean and pasta soup is just what the doctor ordered to help relieve constipation. It provides about 6 grams of fiber and some extra water, as well.

Lastly, be sure to drink plenty of water. Dehydration is an often overlooked cause of constipation. Water helps lubricate the digestive tract and adds bulk to the feces when absorbed by fiber in the large intestine.

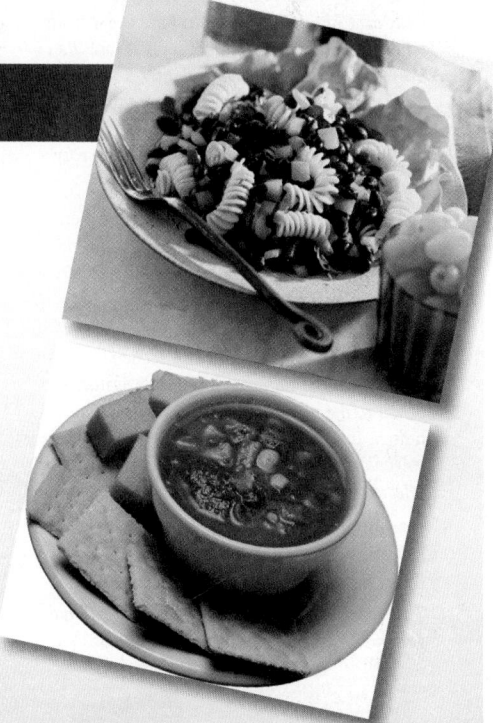

▶ Whole-grain pasta and beans used in salads and soups are good sources of fiber that can prevent intestinal issues such as constipation.

Further Readings

1. Camilleri M: Probiotics and irritable bowel syndrome: Rationale, putative mechanisms, and evidence of clinical efficacy. *Journal of Clinical Gastroenterology* 40:264, 2006.

   The evidence that Bifidobacteria or Lactobacilli species alone or in the specific probiotic combination of VSL#3 are beneficial for treatment of symptoms in IBS is discussed.

2. Consumers Union : Drugs to treat heartburn and stomach acid reflux: The proton pump inhibitors—comparing effectiveness, safety, and price ConsumerReportHealth.org/Best Buy Drugs, 16 pp. May 2010. www.consumer reports.org/health/resources/pdf/best-buy-drugs/PPlsUpdate-FINAL.pdf

   PPIs are the most widely prescribed medicines in the United States to treat heartburn and GERD in individuals who have symptoms that persist, are chronic or severe, or are unrelieved by antacids or H2 blockers. The seven available PPI medicines were found to be roughly equal in effectiveness and safety but differed in cost. The report recommended three of the less expensive drugs that are available without a prescription.

3. Galmiche J-P, Deshpande AR: Laparoscopic antireflux surgery versus esomeprazole treatment for chronic GERD: The LOTUS Randomized Clinical Trial. *Journal of the American Medical Association* 305(19): 1969, 2011.

   Study Taking daily medication (Nexium) or undergoing a minimally invasive surgery to treat acid reflux disease control the worst symptoms of the disease in many people. More than 500 persons were studied and after 5 years, 92% of people in the medication group and 85% in the surgery group reported having no GERD symptoms, or symptoms that were easy to live with.

4. Gosden RG, Feinberg AP: Genetics and epigenetics, Nature's pen-and-pencil set. *New England Journal of Medicine* 356:731; 2007.

   Epigenetics refers to inherited changes in gene expression caused by mechanisms other than changes in the underlying DNA sequence. Epigenetic information is like a code written in pencil in the margins around the DNA, which is written in indelible ink. In many cases it is the epigenome that can be repaired by treatments, or affected by diet.

5. Institute of Medicine: *Nutrigenomics and beyond: Informing the future.* Washington, DC: The National Academy Press, 2007.

   This report summarizes the state of nutritional genomics research and policy. It includes guidance for further development and translation of this knowledge into nutrition practice and policy.

6. Jacobson BC and others: Body mass index and symptoms of gastroesophageal reflux in women. *New England Journal of Medicine* 354:2340, 2006.

   BMI was associated with symptoms of GERD in 10,545 participants in the Nurses' Health Study. Even moderate weight gain caused or exacerbated symptoms of reflux.

7. Katsanis SH and others: A case study of personalized medicine. *Science* 320:53, 2008.

   Personalized medicine promises to revolutionize health care by tailoring treatments based on individual genetic information. The need for regulating personalized genomic medicine in a manner beneficial to public health is discussed. Currently, in most states companies are not required to demonstrate clinical validity before offering new genetic tests.

8. Layke JC, Lopez PP: Esophageal cancer. A review and update. *American Family Physician* 73:2187, 2006.

   Esophageal cancer is aggressive and is commonly diagnosed at an advanced stage with a poor prognosis. Associations among the development of esophageal cancer, Helicobacter pylori infection and GERD are discussed. Despite increased use of proton pump inhibitors and eradication of H. pylori, the number of new cases of esophageal cancer continues to grow.

9. Lynch A, Webb C: What are the most effective nonpharmacologic therapies for irritable bowel syndrome? *Journal of Family Practice* 57:57, 2008.

   Herbal formulations, certain probiotics, elimination diets based on immunoglobulin G antibodies, cognitive behavioral therapy, and self-help books are discussed because they have been shown to decrease global symptoms of irritable bowel syndrome (IBS) and improve overall quality of life. Soluble fiber is more effective than insoluble fiber at improving IBS symptoms.

10. Muller-Lisser and others: Myths and misconceptions about constipation. *American Journal of Gastroenterology* 100:232, 2005.

    Increasing fiber intake and avoiding dehydration help in mild cases of constipation. More difficult cases require physician evaluation and likely the use of laxatives and other medications.

11. Niewinski MM: Advances in celiac disease and gluten-free diet. *Journal of the American Dietetic Association* 108:661, 2008.

    Recognition of celiac disease as a disorder, is increasing. This review focuses on the gluten-free diet and the importance for all patients with celiac disease to receive expert dietary counseling. Recent advances in the gluten-free diet are discussed.

12. Omoruyi O, Holten KB: How should we manage GERD? *Journal of Family Practice* 55:410, 2006.

    Guidelines for the use of proton pump inhibitors, H2 blockers, and surgery for the treatment of GERD are presented.

13. Santosa S and others: Probiotics and their potential health claims. *Nutrition Reviews* 64:265, 2006.

    This paper provides strong evidence of the ability of different probiotic strains to prevent and treat diarrhea, and some forms of irritable bowel syndrome.

14. Stover PJ: Influence of human genetic variation on nutritional requirements. *American Journal of Clinical Nutrition* 83:436S, 2006.

    The complexity of the interaction between genes and diet is discussed as well as the reevaluation of criteria used to determine RDAs relative to the contribution of genetic variation to optimal nutrition for individuals.

15. Stover PJ, Caudill MA: Genetic and epigenetic contributions to human nutrition and health: Managing genome-diet interactions. *Journal of the American Dietetic Association* 108:1480, 2008.

    This article discusses ways that nutritional genomics will facilitate the establishment of genome-informed nutrient and food-based dietary guidelines for disease prevention and healthful aging, individualized medical nutrition therapy for disease management, and targeted public health nutrition interventions that maximize benefits and minimize adverse outcomes within genetically diverse human populations.

16. Wallace TC and others: Human gut microbiota and its relationship to health and disease. *Nutrition Review* 69 (7): 392, 2011.

    Evidence is available from over 700 research studies to support the growing interest in the benefits of probiotics and prebiotics and to aid the development of intervention strategies and practical guidelines for their use in the prevention and treatment of gastrointestinal tract disorders.

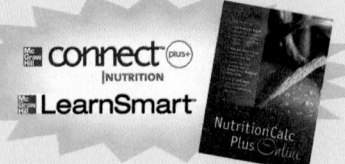

To get the most out of your study of nutrition, go to McGraw-Hill's online resources: Connect www.mcgrawhillconnect.com, **where you will find NutritionCalc Plus, LearnSmart, and many other dynamic tools.**

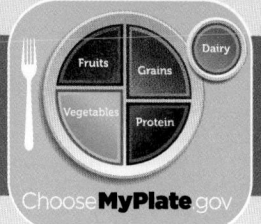

RATE YOUR PLATE

I. Are You Taking Care of Your Digestive Tract?

People need to think about the health of their digestive tracts. There are symptoms we need to notice, as well as habits we need to practice to protect it. The following assessment is designed to help you examine your habits and symptoms associated with the health of your digestive tract. Put a *Y* in the blank to the left of the question to indicate yes and an *N* to indicate no.

_____ 1. Are you currently experiencing greater than normal stress and tension?

_____ 2. Do you have a family history of digestive tract problems (e.g., ulcers, hemorrhoids, recurrent heartburn, constipation)?

_____ 3. Do you experience pain in your stomach region about 2 hours after you eat?

_____ 4. Do you smoke cigarettes?

_____ 5. Do you take aspirin frequently?

_____ 6. Do you have heartburn at least once per week?

_____ 7. Do you commonly lie down after eating a large meal?

_____ 8. Do you drink alcoholic beverages more than two or three times per day?

_____ 9. Do you experience abdominal pain, bloating, or gas 1½ to 2 hours after consuming milk products?

_____ 10. Do you often have to strain while having a bowel movement?

_____ 11. Do you consume less than 9 (women) or 13 (men) cups of a combination of water and other fluids per day?

_____ 12. Do you perform physical activity for less than 60 minutes on most or all days of the week (e.g., jog, swim, walk briskly, row, stair climb)?

_____ 13. Do you eat a diet relatively low in fiber (recall that significant fiber is found in whole fruits, vegetables, legumes, nuts and seeds, whole-grain breads, and whole-grain cereals)?

_____ 14. Do you frequently have diarrhea?

_____ 15. Do you frequently use laxatives or antacids?

Add up the number of yes answers and record the total. If your score is from 8 to 15, your habits and symptoms put you at risk for experiencing future digestive tract problems. Take particular note of the habits to which you answered yes. Consider trying to cooperate more with your digestive tract.

II. Create Your Family Tree for Health-Related Concerns

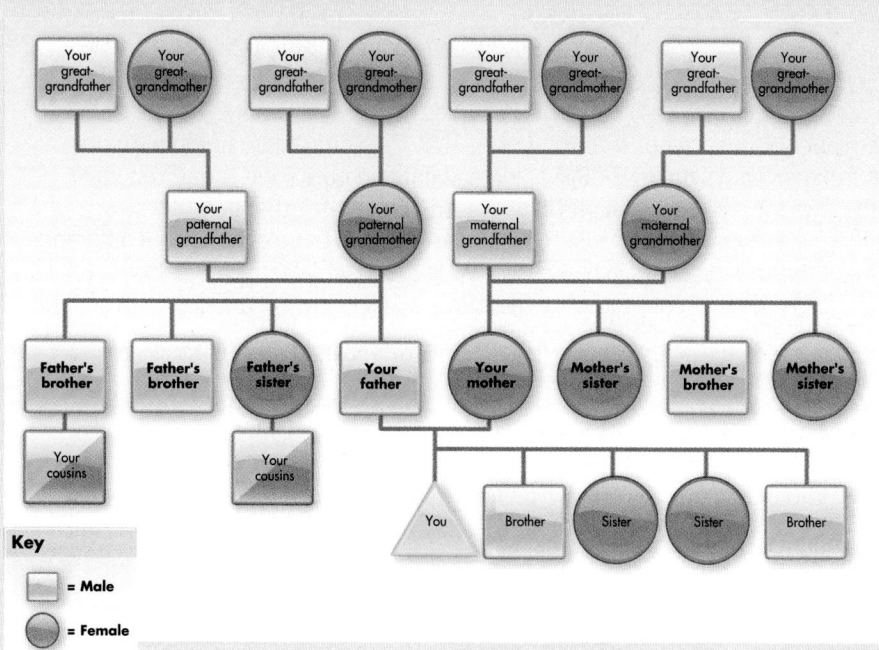

Adapt this diagram to your family tree. Under each heading, list year born, year died (if applicable), major diseases that developed during the person's lifetime, and cause of death (if applicable). Figure 3-21 provides one such example.

You are likely to be at risk for any diseases listed. Creating a plan for preventing such diseases when possible, especially those that developed in your family members before age 50 to 60 years, is advised. Speak with your physician about any concerns arising from this exercise.

Chapter 4 Carbohydrates

Student Learning Outcomes

Chapter 4 is designed to allow you to:

4.1 Identify the basic structures and food sources of the major carbohydrates—monosaccharides, disaccharides, polysaccharides (e.g., starches), and fiber.

4.2 Describe food sources of carbohydrate and list some alternative sweeteners.

4.3 Explain how carbohydrates are digested and absorbed, including the consequences of lactose maldigestion (and lactose intolerance).

4.4 List the functions of carbohydrate in the body and the problems that result from not eating enough carbohydrate.

4.5 Describe the regulation of blood glucose and discuss how other nutrients can be converted to blood glucose.

4.6 Outline the beneficial effects of fiber on the body.

4.7 State the RDA for carbohydrate and various guidelines for carbohydrate intake.

4.8 Identify the consequences of diabetes, and explain appropriate dietary measures that will reduce the adverse effects of this health problem.

What Would You Choose?

In between classes, you stop at a nearby convenience store to pick up a cold drink that will quench your thirst and fill your growling stomach. Immediately, you reach for your favorite cola but the Jones Soda Co.® display with its personalized labels catches your eye. You notice that these sodas are made with no high-fructose corn syrup (HFCS) but instead contain pure cane sugar. You have heard news reports that liken HFCS to poison, but on the other hand, there are commercials saying HFCS is just the same as sugar. Is there a nutritional difference between the added sugars in these two types of sodas? What is the better beverage choice that could provide the calories and energy of an afternoon snack?

a 20-ounce bottle of regular cola (e.g., Coca-Cola®) containing high-fructose corn syrup

b 20-ounce bottle of diet cola (e.g., Coke Zero®) containing aspartame

c 12-ounce bottle of Jones Soda Co.® Pure Cane Root Beer Soda

d ½ pint (8 fluid ounces) of low-fat (1%) chocolate milk

e 16-ounce bottle of water

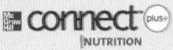 **CONNECT** PLUS+ |NUTRITION **Think about your choice as you read Chapter 4, then see our recommendations at the end of the chapter. To learn more about various sweeteners, including how HFCS is made and arguments for and against use of HFCS, check out the Connect site:** www.mcgrawhillconnect.com

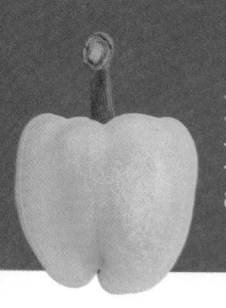

Part Two
Energy Nutrients and Energy Balance

hat did you eat to obtain the energy you are using right now? Chapters 4, 5, and 6 will examine this question by focusing on the main nutrients the human body uses for fuel. These nutrients are carbohydrates (on average, 4 kcal per gram) and fats and oils (on average, 9 kcal per gram). Although protein (on average, 4 kcal per gram) *can* be used for energy needs, the body typically reserves this nutrient for other processes.

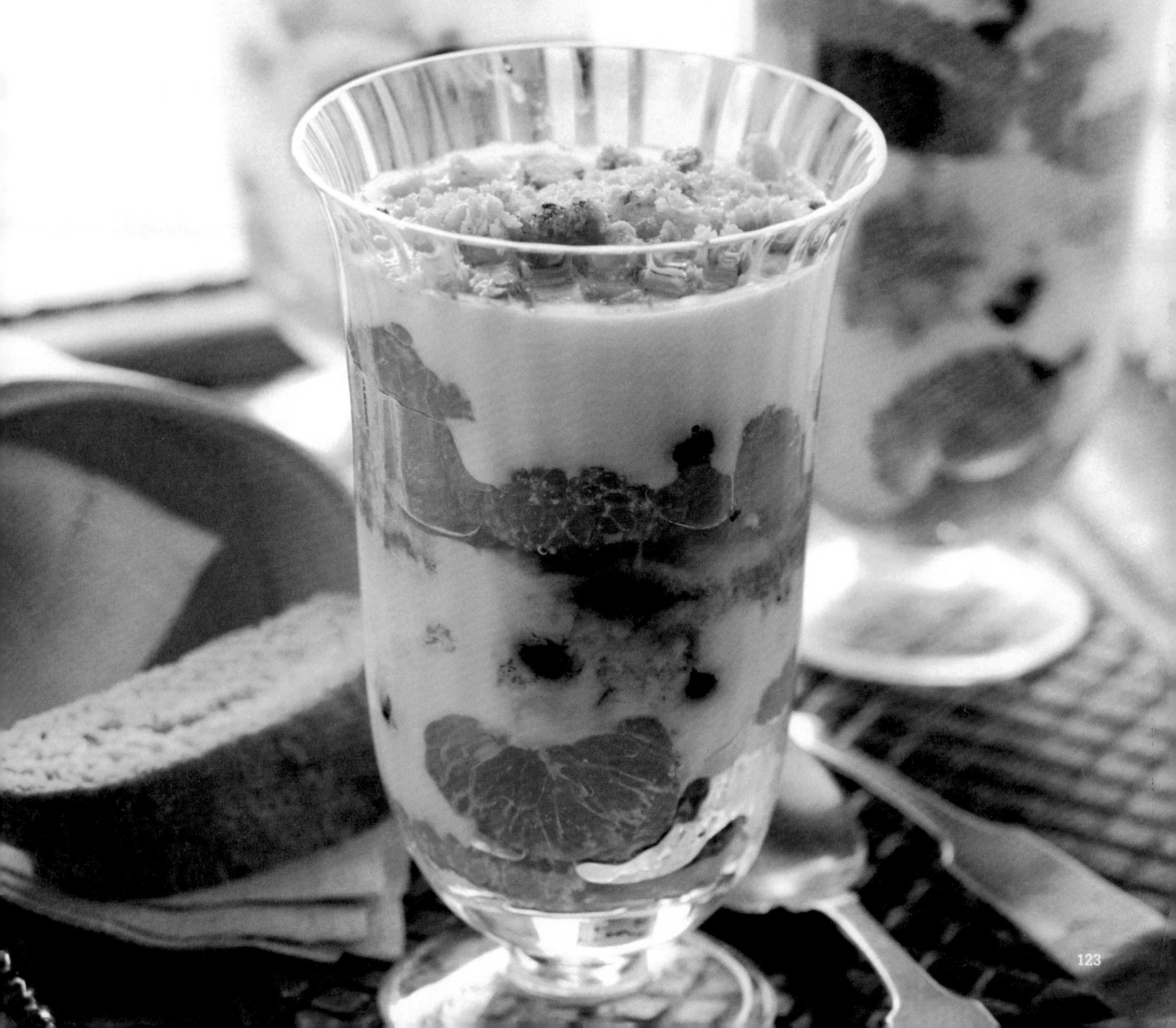

It is likely that you have recently consumed fruits, vegetables, dairy products, cereal, breads, and pasta. These foods supply carbohydrates. Although some carbohydrate sources are more beneficial than others (for example, whole-grain bread compared to white bread, as suggested in the Ziggy comic in this chapter), carbohydrates should be a major part of our diets. Many people think carbohydrate-rich foods cause weight gain but they do not any more so than fat or protein. In fact, pound for pound, carbohydrates are much less fattening than fats and oils. Furthermore, high-carbohydrate foods, especially fiber-rich foods such as fruits, vegetables, whole-grain breads and cereals, and legumes, provide many important health benefits in addition to the calories they contain. Almost all carbohydrate-rich foods, except pure sugars, provide several essential nutrients and should generally constitute 45% to 65% of our daily calorie intake. Let's take a closer look at carbohydrates.

Refresh Your Memory

As you begin your study of carbohydrates in Chapter 4, you may want to review:

- The concept of energy density and the health claims for various carbohydrates in Chapter 2
- The processes of digestion and absorption in Chapter 3
- The hormones that regulate blood glucose in Chapter 3

4.1 Carbohydrates—An Introduction

Carbohydrates are a main fuel source for some cells, especially those in the brain, nervous system, and red blood cells. Muscles also rely on a dependable supply of carbohydrates to fuel intense physical activity. Carbohydrates provide on average 4 kcal per gram and are a readily available fuel for all cells, both in the form of blood glucose and **glycogen** stored in the liver and muscles. The glycogen stored in the liver can be used to maintain blood glucose concentrations in times when you have not eaten for several hours or the diet does not supply enough carbohydrates. Regular intake of carbohydrates is important, because liver glycogen stores are depleted in about 18 hours if no carbohydrate is consumed. After that point, the body is forced to produce carbohydrates, largely from breakdown of proteins in the body. This eventually leads

glycogen A carbohydrate made of multiple units of glucose with a highly branched structure. It is the storage form of glucose in humans and is synthesized (and stored) in the liver and muscles.

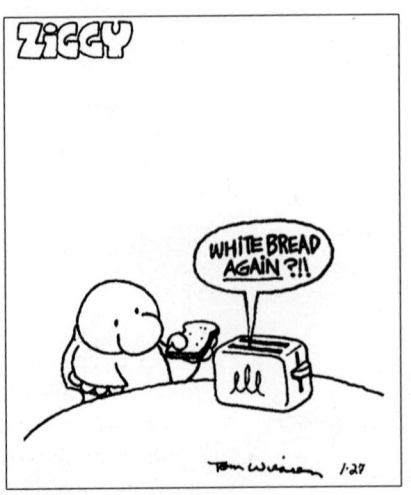

A class of carbohydrate that needs more attention in our diet is fiber. Why is this so? As Ziggy is reminded, white bread is a poor source of fiber. Which health problems typically result from a limited intake of fiber? Which foods are good sources of fiber? How much fiber is enough? Too much? Chapter 4 provides some answers.

ZIGGY © ZIGGY AND FRIENDS, INC. Reprinted with permission of UNIVERSAL PRESS SYNDICATE. All rights reserved.

to health problems including the loss of muscle tissue. To obtain adequate energy, the Food and Nutrition Board recommends that 45% to 65% of the calories we consume each day be from carbohydrates. (See the Acceptable Macronutrient Distribution Range table in the DRI charts in the back pages of this book.)

Despite their important role as a calorie source, some forms of carbohydrate promote health more than others. As you will see in this chapter, whole-grain breads and cereals have greater health benefits than refined and processed forms of carbohydrate. Choosing the healthiest carbohydrate sources most often, while moderating intake of less healthful sources, contributes to a healthy diet. It is difficult to eat so little carbohydrate that body fuel needs are not met, but it is easy to overconsume the simple carbohydrates that can contribute to health problems. Let's explore this concept further as we look at carbohydrates in detail.

Green plants create the carbohydrates in our foods. Leaves capture the sun's solar energy in their cells and transform it to chemical energy. This energy is then stored in the chemical bonds of the carbohydrate glucose as it is produced from carbon dioxide from the air and water from the soil. This complex process is called **photosynthesis** (Fig. 4-1).

$$6 \text{ carbon dioxide} + 6 \text{ water (solar energy)} \rightarrow \text{glucose} + 6 \text{ oxygen}$$
$$(CO_2) \qquad\qquad (H_2O) \qquad\qquad (C_6H_{12}O_6) \qquad (O_2)$$

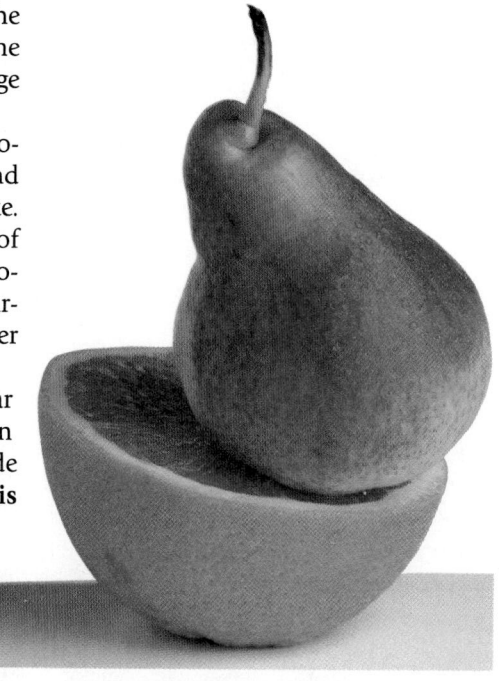

▲ Fruits such as oranges and pears are an excellent source of carbohydrate, including sugar, starch, and fiber.

Translated into English, this reads: 6 molecules of carbon dioxide combine with 6 molecules of water to form one molecule of **glucose**. Converting solar energy into chemical bonds in the sugar is a key part of the process. Six molecules of oxygen are then released into the air.

4.2 Simple Carbohydrates

As the name suggests, most carbohydrate molecules are composed of carbon, hydrogen, and oxygen atoms. Simple forms of carbohydrates are called **sugars**. Larger, more complex forms are primarily called either **starches** or **fibers**, depending on their digestibility by human GI tract enzymes. Starches are the digestible form. The Concept Map on page 127 summarizes the forms and characteristics of carbohydrates.

Monosaccharides and disaccharides are often referred to as *simple sugars* because they contain only one or two sugar units. Food labels lump all of these sugars under one category, listing them as "sugars."

photosynthesis Process by which plants use energy from the sun to synthesize energy-yielding compounds, such as glucose.

glucose A six-carbon monosaccharide that usually exists in a ring form; found as such in blood, and in table sugar bonded to fructose; also known as *dextrose*.

sugar A simple carbohydrate with the chemical composition $(CH_2O)_n$. The basic unit of all sugars is glucose, a six-carbon ring structure. The primary sugar in the diet is sucrose, which is made up of glucose and fructose.

starch A carbohydrate made of multiple units of glucose attached together in a form the body can digest; also known as *complex carbohydrate*.

fiber Substances in plant foods not digested by the processes that take place in the stomach or small intestine. These add bulk to feces. Fibers naturally found in foods are also called dietary fiber.

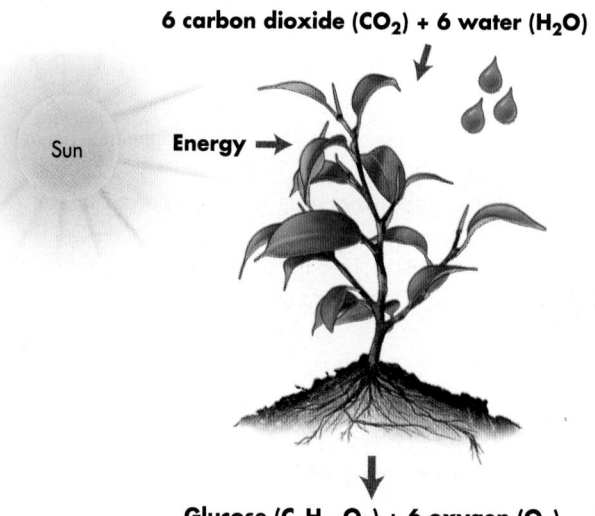

6 carbon dioxide (CO₂) + 6 water (H₂O)

Sun

Energy →

Glucose (C₆H₁₂O₆) + 6 oxygen (O₂)

FIGURE 4-1 ▶ A summary of photosynthesis. Plants use carbon dioxide, water, and energy to produce glucose. Glucose is then stored in the leaf but can also undergo further metabolism to form starch and fiber in the plant. With the addition of nitrogen from soil or air, glucose also can be transformed into protein.

FIGURE 4-2 ▶ Chemical forms of the important monosaccharides.

Monosaccharides

Glucose   Fructose   Galactose

Monosaccharides—Glucose, Fructose, and Galactose

monosaccharide Simple sugar, such as glucose, that is not broken down further during digestion.

simple sugar Monosaccharide or disaccharide in the diet.

sucrose Fructose bonded to glucose; table sugar.

fructose A six-carbon monosaccharide that usually exists in a ring form; found in fruits and honey; also known as *fruit sugar*.

high-fructose corn syrup Corn syrup that has been manufactured to contain 42 and 90% fructose.

galactose A six-carbon monosaccharide that usually exists in a ring form; closely related to glucose.

lactose Glucose bonded to galactose; also known as *milk sugar*.

disaccharide Class of sugars formed by the chemical bonding of two monosaccharides.

maltose Glucose bonded to glucose.

Monosaccharides are the **simple sugar** units (*mono* means one) that serve as the basic unit of all carbohydrate structures. The most common monosaccharides in foods are glucose, fructose, and galactose (Fig. 4-2).

Glucose is the major monosaccharide found in the body. Glucose is also known as *dextrose*, and glucose in the bloodstream may be called blood sugar. Glucose is an important source of energy for human cells, although foods contain very little carbohydrate as this single sugar. Most glucose comes from the digestion of starches and **sucrose** (common table sugar) from our food. The latter is made up of the monosaccharides glucose and fructose. For the most part, sugars and other carbohydrates in foods are eventually converted to glucose in the liver. This glucose then goes on to serve as a source of fuel for cells.

Fructose, also called *fruit sugar*, is another common monosaccharide. After it is consumed, fructose is absorbed by the small intestine and then transported to the liver, where it is quickly metabolized. Much is converted to glucose, but the rest goes on to form other compounds, such as fat, if fructose is consumed in very high amounts. Most of the free fructose in our diets comes from the use of **high-fructose corn syrup** in soft drinks, candies, jams, jellies, and many other fruit products and desserts (see the later discussion on nutritive sweeteners and in What Would You Choose?). Fructose also is found naturally in fruits and forms half of each sucrose molecule.

The sugar **galactose** has nearly the same structure as glucose. Large quantities of pure galactose do not exist in nature. Instead, galactose is usually found bonded to glucose in **lactose**, a sugar found in milk and other milk products. After lactose is digested and absorbed, galactose arrives in the liver. There it is either transformed into glucose or further metabolized into glycogen.

MAKING **DECISIONS**

Nutrient Metabolism

Now is a good time to begin emphasizing a key concept in nutrition: the difference between *intake* of a substance and the body's *use* of that substance. The body often does not use all nutrients in their original states. Some of these substances are broken down and later reassembled into the same or a different substance when and where they are needed. For example, much of the galactose in the diet is metabolized to glucose. When later required for the production of milk in the mammary gland of a lactating female, galactose is resynthesized from glucose to help form the milk sugar lactose. Knowing this, do you think it is necessary for a lactating women to drink milk to make milk?

Disaccharides—Sucrose, Lactose, and Maltose

Disaccharides are formed when two monosaccharides combine (*di* means two). The disaccharides in food are sucrose, lactose, and **maltose**. All contain glucose.

Disaccharides

Sucrose: glucose + fructose
Lactose: glucose + galactose
Maltose: glucose + glucose

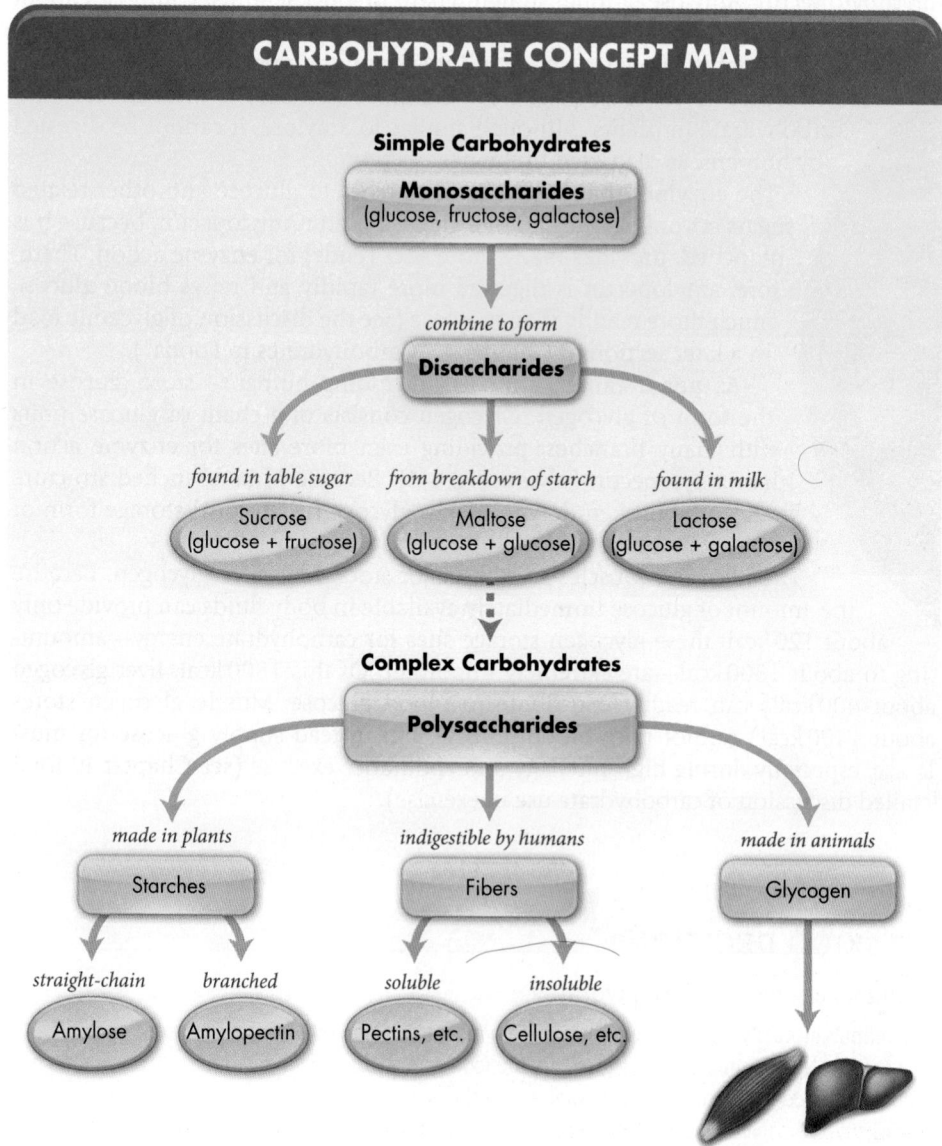

FIGURE 4-3 ▶ Chemical form of the disaccharide sucrose.

Sucrose

Sucrose forms when the two sugars glucose and fructose bond together (Fig. 4-3). Sucrose is found naturally in sugarcane, sugar beets, honey, and maple sugar. These products are processed to varying degrees to make brown, white, and powdered sugars. Animals do not produce sucrose or much of any carbohydrate except glycogen.

Lactose forms when glucose bonds with galactose during the synthesis of milk. Again, our major food source for lactose is milk products. A later section on lactose maldigestion and lactose intolerance discusses the problems that result when a person can't readily digest lactose.

◀ This Concept Map summarizes the various forms and characteristics of the simple and complex carbohydrates.

CARBOHYDRATE CONCEPT MAP

Simple Carbohydrates

Monosaccharides
(glucose, fructose, galactose)

combine to form

Disaccharides

found in table sugar
Sucrose
(glucose + fructose)

from breakdown of starch
Maltose
(glucose + glucose)

found in milk
Lactose
(glucose + galactose)

Complex Carbohydrates

Polysaccharides

made in plants
Starches

indigestible by humans
Fibers

made in animals
Glycogen

straight-chain
Amylose

branched
Amylopectin

soluble
Pectins, etc.

insoluble
Cellulose, etc.

stored in muscle and liver

Maltose results when starch is broken down to just two glucose molecules bonded together. Maltose plays an important role in the beer and liquor industry. In the production of alcoholic beverages, starches in various cereal grains are first converted to simpler carbohydrates by enzymes present in the grains. The products of this step—maltose, glucose, and other sugars—are then mixed with yeast cells in the absence of oxygen. The yeast cells convert most of the sugars to alcohol (ethanol) and carbon dioxide, a process called **fermentation**. Little maltose remains in the final product. Few other food products or beverages contain maltose. In fact, most maltose that we ultimately digest in the small intestine is produced during our own digestion of starch.

4.3 Complex Carbohydrates

In many foods, single-sugar units are bonded together to form a chain, known as a polysaccharide (*poly* means many). **Polysaccharides**, also called *complex carbohydrates* or *starch*, may contain 1000 or more glucose units and are found chiefly in grains, vegetables, and fruits. When food labels list "Other Carbohydrates," this primarily refers to starch content.

Plants store carbohydrate in two forms of starch digestible by humans: **amylose** and **amylopectin**. Amylose, a long, straight chain of glucose units, comprises about 20% of the digestible starch found in vegetables, beans, breads, pasta, and rice. Amylopectin is a highly branched chain and makes up the remaining 80% of digestible starches in the diet (Fig. 4-4). Cellulose (a fiber) is another complex carbohydrate in plants. Although similar to amylose, it cannot be digested by humans, as discussed in the next section.

The enzymes that break down starches to glucose and other related sugars act only at the end of a glucose chain. Amylopectin, because it is branched, provides many more sites (ends) for enzyme action. Therefore, amylopectin is digested more rapidly and raises blood glucose much more readily than amylose (see the discussion of glycemic load in a later section of Chapter 4, "Carbohydrates in Foods").

As noted earlier, animals—including humans—store glucose in the form of glycogen. Glycogen consists of a chain of glucose units with many branches, providing even more sites for enzyme action than amylopectin (review Fig. 4-4). Because of its branched structure that can be broken down quickly, glycogen is an ideal storage form of carbohydrate in the body.

The liver and muscles are the major storage sites for glycogen. Because the amount of glucose immediately available in body fluids can provide only about 120 kcal, these glycogen storage sites for carbohydrate energy—amounting to about 1800 kcal—are extremely important. Of this 1800 kcal, liver glycogen (about 400 kcal) can readily contribute to blood glucose. Muscle glycogen stores (about 1400 kcal) cannot raise blood glucose, but instead supply glucose for muscle use, especially during high-intensity and endurance exercise (see Chapter 10 for a detailed discussion of carbohydrate use in exercise).

fermentation The conversion of carbohydrates to alcohols, acids, and carbon dioxide without the use of oxygen.

polysaccharides Carbohydrates containing many glucose units, from 10 to 1000 or more.

amylose A digestible straight-chain type of starch composed of glucose units.

amylopectin A digestible branched-chain type of starch composed of glucose units.

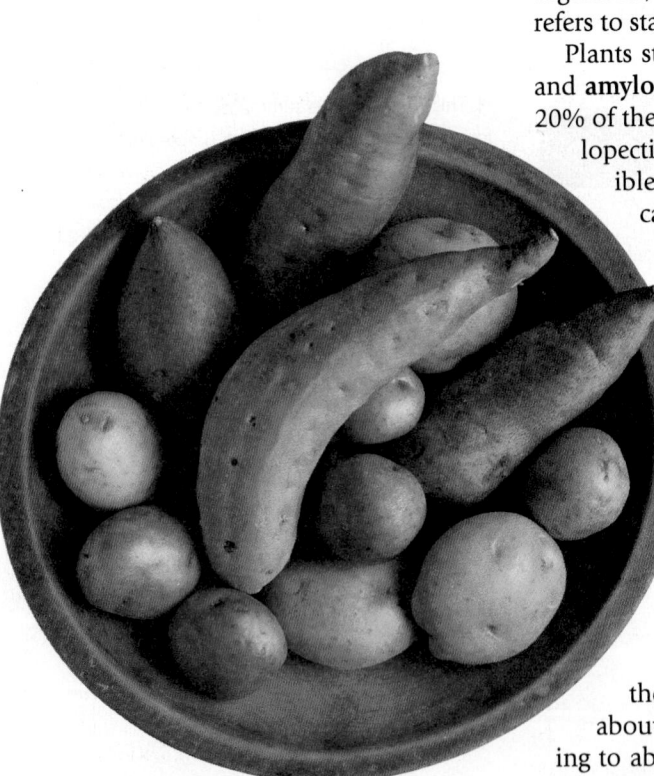

▲ Root vegetables such as potato, yams, and tapioca are high in amylopectin starch.

MAKING DECISIONS

Animal Sources of Carbohydrates

If animals store glycogen in their muscles, are meats, fish, and poultry a good source of carbohydrates? No—animal products are not good food sources of this (or any other) carbohydrate because glycogen stores quickly degrade after the animal dies.

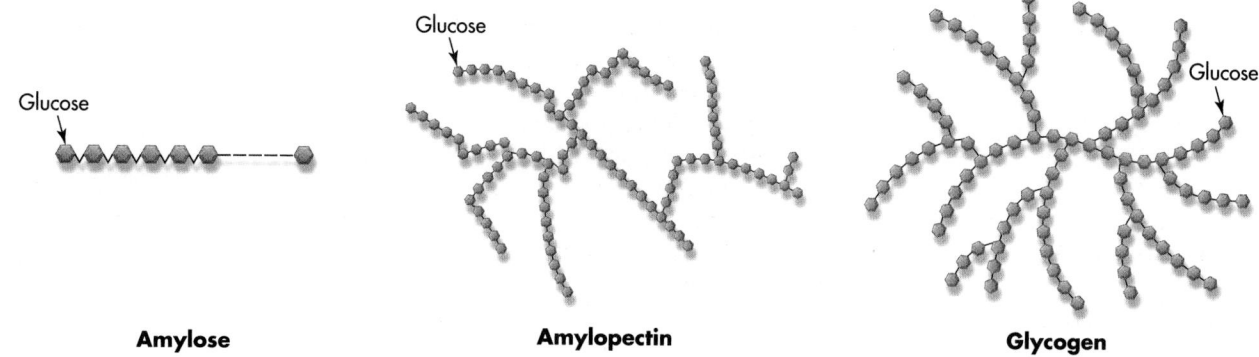

Glucose

Glucose

Glucose

Amylose

Amylopectin

Glycogen

FIGURE 4-4 ▶ Some common starches, amylose and amylopectin, and glycogen. We consume essentially no glycogen. All glycogen found in the body is made by our cells, primarily in the liver and muscles.

4.4 Fiber

Fiber as a class is mostly made up of polysaccharides, but they differ from starches insofar as the chemical links that join the individual sugar units cannot be digested by human enzymes in the GI tract. This prevents the small intestine from absorbing the sugars that make up the various fibers. Fiber is not a single substance but a group of substances with similar characteristics (Table 4-1). The group is comprised of the carbohydrates **cellulose**, **hemicelluloses**, **pectins**, **gums**, and **mucilages**, as well as the noncarbohydrate, **lignin**. In total, these constitute all the nonstarch polysaccharides in foods. Nutrition Facts labels generally do not list these individual forms of fiber, but instead lump them together under the term **dietary fiber**.

Cellulose, hemicelluloses, and lignin form the structural parts of plants. Bran fiber is rich in hemicelluloses and lignin. (The woody fibers in broccoli are partly lignin.) Bran layers form the outer covering of all grains, so **whole grains** (i.e., unrefined) are good sources of bran fiber (Fig. 4-5). Because the majority of these fibers neither readily dissolve in water nor are easily metabolized by intestinal bacteria, they are called **nonfermentable** or insoluble fibers.

Pectins, gums, and mucilages are contained around and inside plant cells. These fibers either dissolve or swell when put into water and are therefore called **viscous** or soluble fibers. They also are readily fermented by bacteria in the large intestine. These fibers are found in salad dressings, some frozen desserts, jams, and jellies as gum arabic, guar gum, locust bean gum, and various pectin forms. Some forms of hemicelluloses also fall into the soluble category.

Most foods contain mixtures of soluble and insoluble fibers. Food labels do not generally distinguish between the two types, but, manufacturers have the option to do so. Often, if food is listed as a good source of one type of fiber, it usually contains some

cellulose An undigestible nonfermentable straight-chain polysaccharide made of glucose molecules.

hemicellulose A nonfermentable fiber containing xylose, galactose, glucose, and other monosaccharides bonded together.

pectin A viscous fiber containing chains of galacturonic acid and other monosaccharides; characteristically found between plant cell walls.

mucilages A viscous fiber consisting of chains of galactose, mannose, and other monosaccharides; characteristically found in seaweed.

lignins A nonfermentable fiber made up of a multiringed alcohol (noncarbohydrate) structure.

dietary fiber Fiber found in food.

whole grains Grains containing the entire seed of the plant, including the bran, germ, and endosperm (starchy interior). Examples are whole wheat and brown rice.

nonfermentable fiber A fiber that is not easily metabolized by intestinal bacteria.

TABLE 4-1 Classification of Fibers

Type	Component(s)	Physiological Effects	Major Food Sources
Nonfermentable or Insoluble			
Noncarbohydrate form	Lignin	Increases fecal bulk	Whole grains, wheat bran
Carbohydrate form	Cellulose, hemicelluloses	Increases fecal bulk Decreases intestinal transit time	All plants, wheat products Wheat, rye, rice, vegetables
Viscous or Soluble			
Carbohydrate form	Pectins, gums, mucilages, some hemicelluloses	Delays stomach emptying; slows glucose absorption; can lower blood cholesterol	Citrus fruits, apples, bananas, oat products, carrots, barley, beans, thickeners added to foods

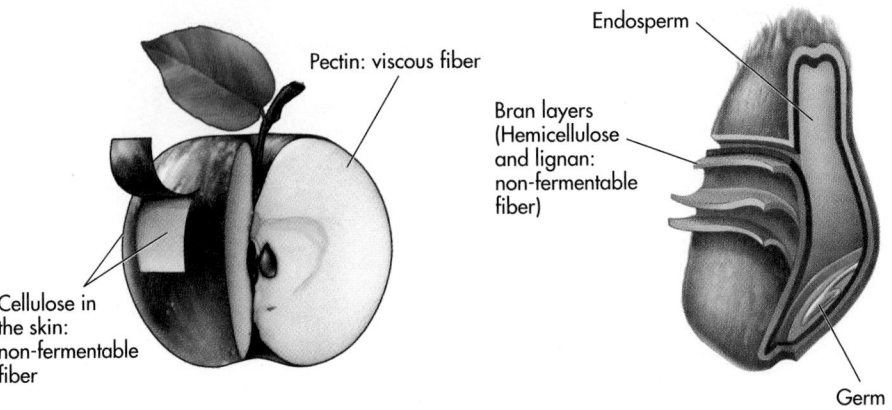

FIGURE 4-5 ▶ Viscous and nonfermentable fiber. (a) The skin of an apple consists of the nonfermentable fiber cellulose, which provides structure for the fruit. The viscous fiber pectin "glues" the fruit cells together. (b) The outside layer of a wheat kernel is made of layers of bran—primarily hemicellulose, a nonfermentable fiber—making this whole grain a good source of fiber. Overall, fruits, vegetables, whole-grain breads and cereals, and beans are rich in fiber.

viscous fiber A fiber that is readily fermented by bacteria in the large intestine.

functional fiber Fiber added to foods that has been shown to provide health benefits.

total fiber Combination of dietary fiber and functional fiber in a food. Also just called *fiber*.

of the other type of fiber as well. The definition of fiber has recently been expanded to include both the dietary fiber found naturally in foods and additional fiber that is added to foods. This second category is called **functional fiber;** a fiber of this type must show beneficial effects in humans to be included in the category. **Total fiber** (or just the term *fiber*) is then the combination of dietary fiber and functional fiber in the food product. Currently the Nutrition Facts label only includes the category dietary fiber; the label has yet to be updated to reflect the latest definition of fiber.

A newly studied category of functional fiber are the prebiotics. Prebiotics include a group of short-chain carbohydrates or oligosaccharides, resistant to digestion, but fermented by bacteria in the colon. They are thought to stimulate the growth or activity of beneficial bacteria in the large intestine and therefore promote the host's health.

CONCEPT CHECK

Important monosaccharides in nutrition are glucose, fructose, and galactose. Glucose is a primary energy source for body cells. Disaccharides form when two monosaccharides bond together. Important disaccharides in nutrition are sucrose (glucose + fructose), maltose (glucose + glucose), and lactose (glucose + galactose). Once digested into monosaccharides and absorbed, most carbohydrates are transformed into glucose by the liver.

Amylose, amylopectin, and glycogen are all polysaccharides, which function as storage forms of glucose. Amylose and amylopectin are the major digestible plant polysaccharides and contain multiple glucose units bonded together. Glycogen is a storage form of glucose in our liver and muscle cells.

Fiber is essentially the portion of plant food that remains undigested as it enters the large intestine. There are two general classes of fiber: nonfermentable and viscous. Nonfermentable (insoluble) fibers are mostly made up of cellulose, hemicelluloses, and lignins. Viscous (soluble) fibers are made up mostly of pectins, gums, and mucilages. Both nonfermentable and viscous fibers are resistant to human digestive enzymes, but bacteria in the large intestine can break down viscous fibers.

4.5 Carbohydrates in Foods

The food components that yield the highest percentage of calories from carbohydrates are table sugar, honey, jam, jelly, fruit, and plain baked potatoes (Fig. 4-6). Corn flakes, rice, bread, and noodles all contain at least 75% of calories as carbohydrates. Foods with moderate amounts of carbohydrate calories are peas, broccoli, oatmeal, dry beans and other legumes, cream pies, French fries, and fat-free milk. In these foods, the carbohydrate content is diluted either by protein, as in the case of fat-free milk, or by fat, as in the case of a cream pie. Foods with essentially no carbohydrates include beef, eggs, chicken, fish, vegetable oils, butter, and margarine.

Food Sources of Carbohydrate

Food Item	Carbohydrate (grams)	% RDA
RDA	130	100%
Baked potato, 1 each	51	39%
Cola drink, 12 fluid oz	39	30%
Plain M&M's, ½ oz	30	23%
Banana, 1 each	28	22%
Cooked rice, ½ cup	22	17%
Cooked corn, ½ cup	21	16%
Light yogurt, 1 cup	19	15%
Kidney beans, ½ cup	19	15%
Spaghetti noodles, ½ cup	19	15%
Orange, 1 each	16	12%
Seven grain bread, 1 slice	12	9%
Fat-free milk, 1 cup	12	9%
Pineapple chunks, ½ cup	10	8%
Cooked carrots, ½ cup	8	6%
Peanuts, 1 ounce	6	5%

Key:
- Grains
- Vegetables
- Fruits
- Dairy
- Protein
- Empty calories
- Oils

FIGURE 4-6 ▶ Food sources of carbohydrates compared to the RDA of 130 grams for carbohydrate.

The percentage of calories from carbohydrate is more important than the total amount of carbohydrate in a food when planning a healthy high-carbohydrate diet. Figure 4-7 shows that the grain, vegetable, fruit, and dairy groups contain the most nutrient-dense sources of carbohydrate. In planning a healthy high-carbohydrate diet, you need to emphasize whole grains, fruits, and vegetables, rather than potato chips and French fries, because these foods contain too much fat. Currently, the top five carbohydrate sources for U.S. adults are white bread, soft drinks, cookies and cakes (including doughnuts), sugars/syrups/jams, and potatoes. Clearly, many North Americans (teenagers included) should take a closer look at their main carbohydrate sources and strive to improve them from a nutritional standpoint by including more whole-grain versions of breads, pasta, rice, and cereals, as well as fruits and vegetables.

Starch

Starches contribute much of the carbohydrate in our diets. Recall that plants store glucose as polysaccharides in the form of starches. Thus, plant-based foods, such as beans, potatos, and the grains (wheat, rye, corn, oats, barley, and rice) used to make breads, cereals, and pasta, are the best sources of starch. A diet rich in these starches provides ample carbohydrate, as well as many micronutrients.

Fiber

Fiber can be found in many of the same foods as starch, so a diet rich in grains, beans, and potatoes also can provide significant amounts of dietary fiber (especially insoluble cellulose, hemicellulose, and lignins). Because much of the fiber in whole grains

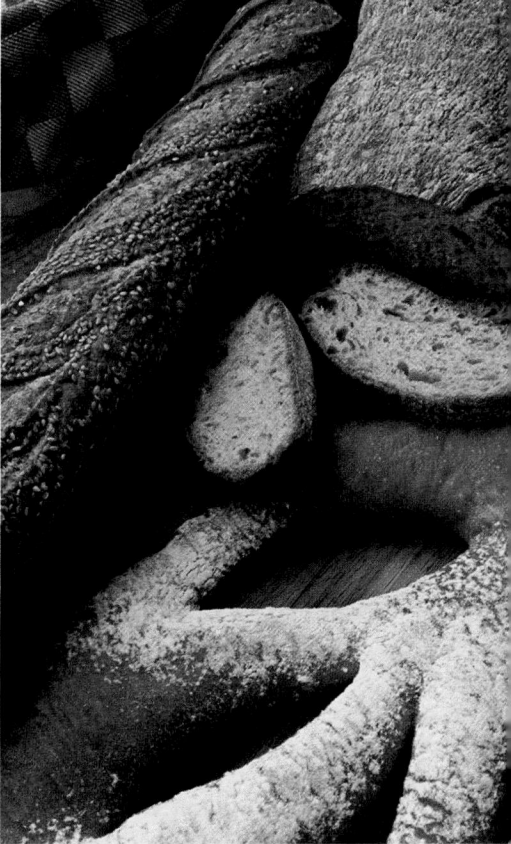

▲ Breads are a rich source of carbohydrate, especially starch and fiber.

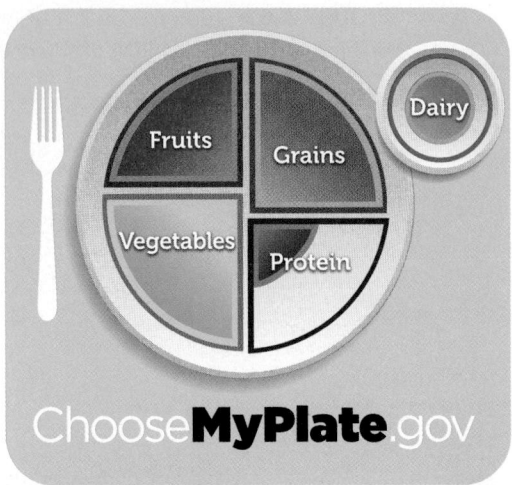

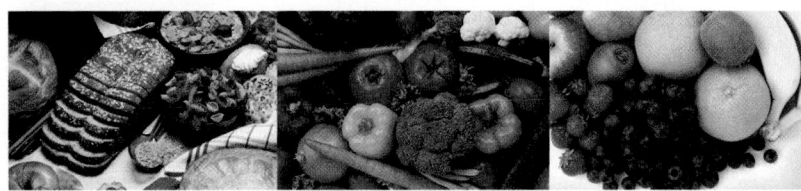

MyPlate:
Sources of Carbohydrates

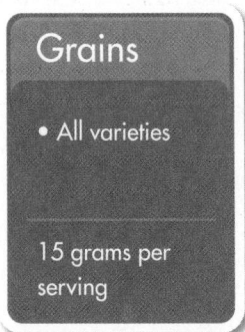

Grains

• All varieties

15 grams per serving

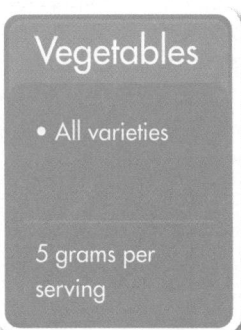

Vegetables

• All varieties

5 grams per serving

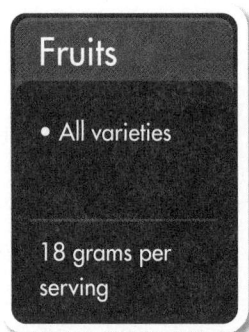

Fruits

• All varieties

18 grams per serving

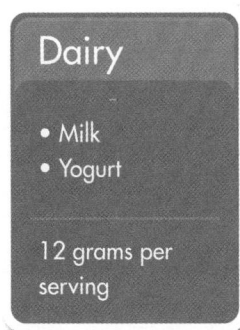

Dairy

• Milk
• Yogurt

12 grams per serving

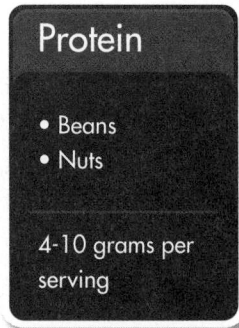

Protein

• Beans
• Nuts

4-10 grams per serving

FIGURE 4-7 ▶ Sources of carbohydrates from MyPlate. The fill of the background color (none, 1/3, 2/3, or completely covered) within each group in the plate indicates the average nutrient density for carbohydrate in that group. Overall, the grain group, vegetable group, fruit group, and dairy group contain many foods that are nutrient-dense sources of carbohydrate. With regard to physical activity, carbohydrates are a key fuel in most endeavors.

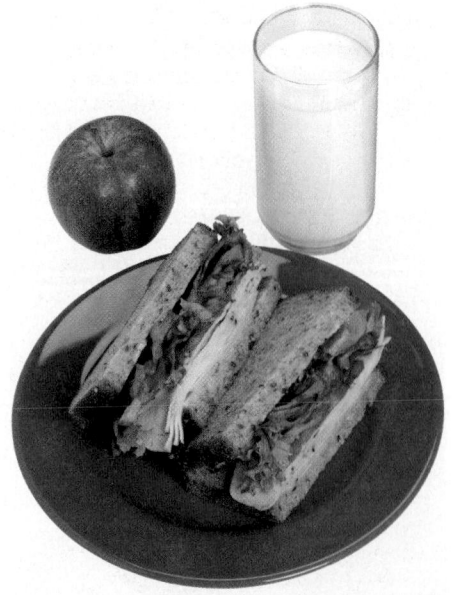

▲ This turkey, cheese, lettuce, and tomato sandwich on whole-grain bread with an apple and glass of low-fat milk fits on **MyPlate** in the right proportions and offers excellent carbohydrate sources of fruits, vegetables, whole grains, and low-fat dairy.

is found in the outer layers, which are removed in processing, highly processed grains are low in fiber. Soluble fibers (pectin, gums, mucilages) are found in the skins and flesh of many fruits and berries; as thickeners and stabilizers in jams, yogurts, sauces, and fillings; and in products that contain psyllium and seaweed.

For individuals who have difficulties consuming adequate dietary fiber, fiber is available as a supplement or as an additive to certain foods (functional fiber). In this way, individuals with relatively low dietary fiber intakes can still obtain the health benefits of fiber.

Nutritive Sweeteners

The various substances that impart sweetness to foods fall into two broad classes: nutritive sweeteners, which can provide calories for the body; and alternative sweeteners, which for the most part provide no calories. As shown in Table 4-2, the alternative sweeteners are much sweeter on a per-gram basis than the nutritive sweeteners. The taste and sweetness of sucrose make it the benchmark against which all other sweeteners are measured. Sucrose is obtained from sugar cane and sugar beet plants. Both sugars and sugar alcohols provide calories along with sweetness. Sugars are found in many different food products, whereas sugar alcohols have rather limited uses.

Sugars. All of the monosaccharides (glucose, fructose, and galactose) and disaccharides (sucrose, lactose, and maltose) discussed earlier are designated *nutritive sweeteners* (Table 4-3). Many forms of sugar are used in food products and result in an intake of about 82 grams or 16 teaspoons of sugar per day.

TABLE 4-2 The Sweetness of Sugars (Nutritive) and Alternative Sweeteners

Type of Sweetener	Relative Sweetness* (Sucrose = 1)	Typical Sources
Sugars		
Lactose	0.2	Dairy products
Maltose	0.4	Sprouted seeds
Glucose	0.7	Corn syrup
Sucrose	1.0	Table sugar, most sweets
Invert sugar[†]	1.3	Some candies, honey
Fructose	1.2–1.8	Fruit, honey, some soft drinks
Sugar Alcohols		
Sorbitol	0.6	Dietetic candies, sugarless gum
Mannitol	0.7	Dietetic candies
Xylitol	0.9	Sugarless gum
Maltitol	0.9	Baked goods, chocolate, candies
Alternative Sweeteners		
Tagatose (Naturlose™)	0.9	Ready-to-eat breakfast cereals, diet soft drinks, meal replacement bars, frozen desserts, candy, frosting
Cyclamate[‡]	30	Tabletop sweetener, medicines
Stevia (Truvia®)	100–300	Tabletop sweetener, food ingredient
Aspartame (Equal®)	180	Diet soft drinks, diet fruit drinks, sugarless gum, tabletop sweetener
Acesulfame-K (Sunette®)	200	Sugarless gum, diet drink mixes, tabletop sweetener, puddings, gelatin desserts
Saccharin (Sweet'N Low®)	300	Diet soft drinks, tabletop sweetener
Sucralose (Splenda®)	600	Diet soft drinks, tabletop sweetener, sugarless gums, jams, frozen desserts
Neotame	7000 to 13,000	Tabletop sweetener, baked goods, frozen desserts, jams

*On a per gram basis.

[†]Sucrose broken down into glucose and fructose.

[‡]Not available in the United States, but available in Canada.

From the *American Dietetic Association*, 2004, and other sources (see Further Reading 1).

High-fructose corn syrup (HFCS) is made by an enzymatic process that converts some of the glucose in cornstarch into fructose, which tastes sweeter than glucose. It is called "high-fructose" corn syrup because it contains 55% fructose, compared to sucrose, which contains only 50% fructose. In the United States, corn is abundant and inexpensive compared to sugar cane or sugar beets, much of which is imported. Food manufacturers prefer HFCS because it is easy to transport, has better shelf-stability, and improves food properties. Because of its low cost and broad range of food-processing applications, HFCS is now used in all kinds of foods, from soft drinks to barbecue sauce. An average American consumes about 60 pounds of HFCS each year. The dramatic rise in obesity has paralleled the increase in HFCS consumption over the past 40 years, and some researchers speculate that properties of the HFCS are to blame. Read more about this in the Newsworthy Nutrition column in the margin and in our recommendations for What Would You Choose?

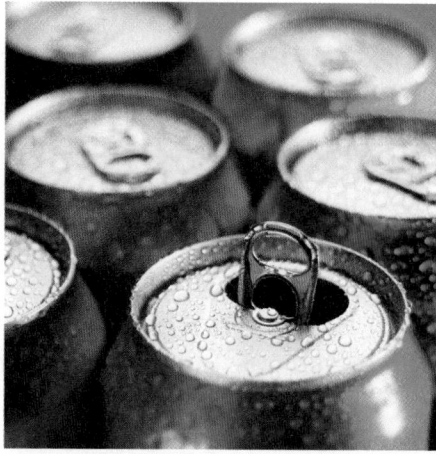

▲ Soft drinks are typical sources of either sugars or alternative sweeteners, depending on the type of soft drink chosen.

NEWSWORTHY NUTRITION

Link between high-fructose corn syrup and obesity

The intake of high-fructose corn syrup (HFCS) from 1967 to 2000 was studied and compared to the development of obesity. HFCS consumption increased >1000% between 1970 and 1990. It was estimated that Americans consume 132 to 316 kcal daily from HFCS. The increase in HFCS use has paralleled the increase in obesity. Differences in the digestion, absorption, and metabolism of fructose compared to glucose have been suggested as explanations for the relationship between HFCS and obesity. Studies of HFCS in humans, however, have been unable to separate the effects of the widely consumed sweetener from the impact of physical inactivity, large portion sizes, smoking cessation, increased consumption of foods prepared outside the home, and other environmental factors.

Source: Bray GA and others. Consumption of high-fructose corn syrup in beverages may play a role in the epidemic of obesity. *American Journal of Clinical Nutrition*, 79(4):537, 2004 (see Further Reading 4).

connect **Check out the Connect site** www.mcgrawhillconnect.com **to further explore HFCS and obesity.**

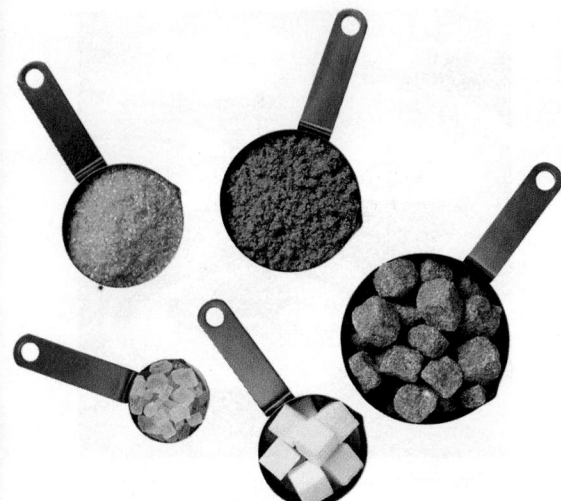

TABLE 4-3 Names of Sugars Used in Foods

Sugar	Invert sugar	Honey	Maple syrup
Sucrose	Glucose	Corn syrup or sweeteners	Dextrose
Brown sugar	Sorbitol	High-fructose corn syrup	Fructose
Confectioner's sugar (powdered sugar)	Levulose		Maltodextrins
	Polydextrose	Molasses	Caramel
Turbinado sugar	Lactose	Date sugar	Fruit sugar

▲ There are many forms of sugar on the market. Used in many foods, together they contribute to our daily intake of approximately 82 grams (16 teaspoons) of sugars in our diets.

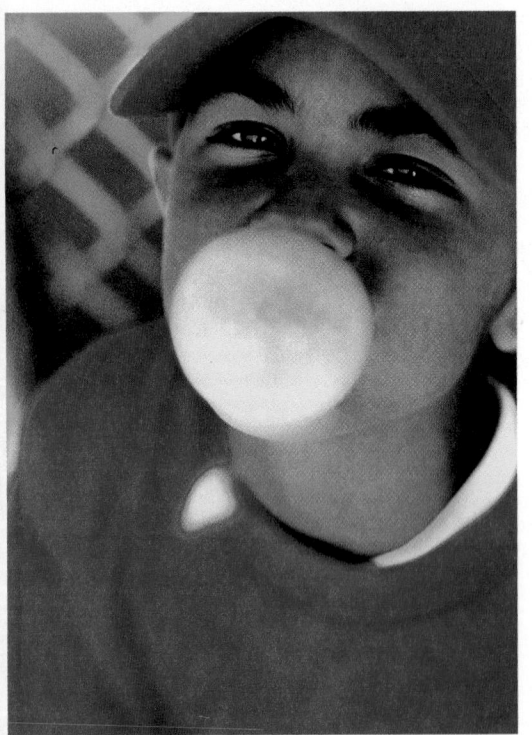

▲ Sugarless gum is typically sweetened with sugar alcohols.

sorbitol Alcohol derivative of glucose that yields about 3 kcal/g but is slowly absorbed from the small intestine; used in some sugarless gums and dietetic foods.

xylitol Alcohol derivative of the 5-carbon monosaccharide xylose.

In addition to sucrose and high-fructose corn syrup, brown sugar, turbinado sugar (sold as raw sugar), honey, maple syrup, and other sugars are also added to foods. Brown sugar is essentially sucrose containing some molasses that is not totally removed from the sucrose during processing or is added to the sucrose crystals. Turbinado sugar is a partially refined version of raw sucrose. Maple syrup is made by boiling down and concentrating the sap that runs during the late winter in sugar maple trees. Because pure maple syrup is expensive, most pancake syrup is primarily corn syrup and high-fructose corn syrup with maple flavor added.

Honey is a product of plant nectar that has been altered by bee enzymes. The enzymes break down much of the nectar's sucrose into fructose and glucose. Honey offers essentially the same nutritional value as other simple sugars—a source of energy and little else. However, honey is not safe to feed to infants because it can contain spores of the bacterium *Clostridium botulinum* that causes fatal food-borne illness. Unlike the acidic environment of an adult's stomach, which inhibits the growth of the bacteria, an infant's stomach does not produce much acid, making infants susceptible to the threat that this bacterium poses.

Sugar Alcohols. Food manufacturers and consumers have numerous options for obtaining sweetness while consuming less sugar and calories. Overall, sugar alcohols and alternative sweeteners enable people with diabetes to enjoy the flavor of sweetness while controlling sugars in their diets; they also provide noncaloric or very-low-calorie sugar substitutes for persons trying to lose (or control) body weight.

Sugar alcohols such as **sorbitol** and **xylitol** are used as nutritive sweeteners. Sugar alcohols contribute fewer calories (about 2.6 kcal per gram) than sugars. They also are absorbed and metabolized to glucose more slowly than are simple sugars. Because of this, they remain in the intestinal tract for a longer time and in large quantities can cause diarrhea. In fact, any products that may be consumed in amounts that may result in a daily ingestion of 50 grams of sugar alcohols, must bear this labeling statement: "Excess consumption may have a laxative effect."

Sugar alcohols are used in sugarless gum, breath mints, and candy. Unlike sucrose, sugar alcohols are not readily metabolized by bacteria to acids in the mouth and thus do not promote tooth decay (see the later section on problems linked to carbohydrate intake).

Sugar alcohols must be listed on labels. If only one sugar alcohol is used in a product, its name must be listed. However, if two or more are used in one product, they are grouped together under the heading "sugar alcohols." The caloric value of each sugar alcohol used in a food product is calculated so that when one reads the total amount of calories a product provides, it includes the sugar alcohols in the overall amount.

Alternative Sweeteners

Alternative sweeteners in increasing order of sweetness include **tagatose**, **cyclamate**, **stevia**, **aspartame**, **acesulfame-K**, **saccharin**, **sucralose**,and **neotame**. Unlike sugar alcohols, alternative sweeteners yield little or no calories when consumed in amounts typically used in food products. All except cyclamate are currently available in the United States. Cyclamate was banned for use in the United States in 1970, although it has never been conclusively proven to cause health problems when used appropriately. Cyclamate is used in Canada as a sweetener in medicines and as a tabletop sweetener.

The safety of sweeteners is determined by the FDA and is indicated by an **Acceptable Daily Intake (ADI)** guideline. The ADI is the amount of alternative sweetener considered safe for daily use over one's lifetime. ADIs are based on studies in laboratory animals and are set at a level 100 times less than the level at which no harmful effects were noted in animal studies. Alternative sweeteners can be used safely by adults and children. Although general use is considered safe during pregnancy, pregnant women may want to discuss this issue with their health-care providers.

Saccharin. The oldest alternative sweetener, saccharin, was first produced in 1879 and is currently approved for use in more than 90 countries. It represents about half of the alternative sweetener market in North America (typically packaged in pink packets, including Sweet 'N Low®). Based on laboratory animal studies, saccharin was once thought to increase the risk of bladder cancer but it is no longer listed as a potential cause of cancer.

Aspartame. Aspartame is in widespread use throughout the world (typically packaged in blue packets, including Equal®). It has been approved for use by more than 90 countries, and its use has been endorsed by the World Health Organization, the American Medical Association, the American Diabetes Association, and other groups.

The components of aspartame are the amino acids phenylalanine and aspartic acid, along with methanol. Recall that amino acids are the building blocks of proteins, so aspartame is more of a protein than a carbohydrate. Aspartame yields about 4 kcal per gram, but it is about 200 times sweeter than sucrose. Thus, only a small amount of aspartame is needed to obtain the desired sweetness, and the amount of calories added is insignificant unless the product is consumed in unusually high amounts. Aspartame is used in beverages, gelatin desserts, chewing gum, toppings and fillings in precooked bakery goods, and cookies. Aspartame does not cause tooth decay. Like other proteins, however, aspartame is damaged when heated for a long time and thus would lose its sweetness if used in products requiring cooking.

Some complaints have been filed with FDA by people claiming to have had adverse reactions to aspartame: headaches, dizziness, seizures, nausea, and other side effects. It is important for people who are sensitive to aspartame to avoid it, but the percentage of sensitive people is likely to be extremely small.

The acceptable daily intake of aspartame set by FDA is 50 milligrams per kilogram of body weight. This is equivalent to the aspartame in about 14 cans of diet soft drink for an adult or about 80 packets of Equal®. Aspartame appears to be safe for pregnant women and children, but some scientists suggest cautious use by these groups, especially young children, who need ample calories to grow.

Sucralose. Sucralose (Splenda®) is 600 times sweeter than sucrose. It is made by adding three chlorines to sucrose. Sucralose is approved for use as an additive to foods such as soft drinks, gum, baked goods, syrups, gelatins, frozen dairy desserts such as ice cream, jams, processed fruits and fruit juices, and for tabletop use. Sucralose doesn't break down under high heat conditions and can be used in cooking and baking. It is also excreted as such in the feces. The small amount absorbed is excreted in the urine.

Sugar alcohols as a class are also called polyols.

---

stevia Alternative sweetener derived from South American shrub; 100 to 300 times sweeter than sucrose.

aspartame Alternative sweetener made of 2 amino acids and methanol; about 200 times sweeter than sucrose.

sucralose Alternative sweetener that has chlorines in place of 3 hydroxyl (—OH) groups on sucrose; 600 times sweeter than sucrose.

acesulfame K Alternative sweetener that yields no energy to the body; 200 times sweeter than sucrose.

saccharin Alternative sweetener that yields no energy to the body; 300 times sweeter than sucrose.

neotame General-purpose, nonnutritive sweetener that is approximately 7000 to 13,000 times sweeter than table sugar. It has a chemical structure similar to aspartame's.

Persons with an uncommon disease called **phenylketonuria (PKU),** which interferes with the metabolism of phenylalanine, should avoid aspartame because of its high phenylalanine content. A warning label is required on products containing aspartame, alerting people with PKU that a product with aspartame contains phenylalanine.

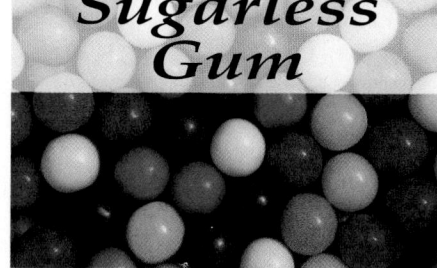

INGREDIENTS: SORBITOL, GUM BASE, MANNITOL, GLYCEROL, HYDROGENATED GLUCOSE SYRUP, XYLITOL, ARTIFICIAL AND NATURAL FLAVORS, ASPARTAME, RED 40, YELLOW 6 AND BHT (TO MAINTAIN FRESHNESS). PHENYLKETONURICS: CONTAINS PHENYLALANINE.

Sugarless Gum

▲ Sugar alcohols and the alternative sweetener aspartame are used to sweeten this product. Note the warning for people with phenylketonuria PKU that this product is made with aspartame and, thus, contains phenylalanine.

Acceptable Daily Intake (ADI) Estimate of the amount of a sweetener that an individual can safely consume daily over a lifetime. ADIs are given as mg per kg of body weight per day.

phenylketonuria (PKU) Disease caused by a defect in the liver's ability to metabolize the amino acid phenylalanine into the amino acid tyrosine; untreated, toxic by-products of phenylalanine build up in the body and lead to mental retardation.

Neotame. Neotame was recently approved by FDA for use as a general-purpose sweetener in a wide variety of food products, other than meat and poultry. Neotame is a nonnutritive, high-intensity sweetener that, depending on its food application, is approximately 7000 to 13,000 times sweeter than table sugar. It has a chemical structure similar to aspartame. Neotame is heat stable and can be used as a tabletop sweetener as well as in cooking applications. Examples of uses for which it has been approved include baked goods, nonalcoholic beverages (including soft drinks), chewing gum, confections and frostings, frozen desserts, gelatins and puddings, jams and jellies, processed fruits and fruit juices, toppings, and syrups. Neotame is safe for use by the general population, including children, pregnant and lactating women, and people with diabetes. In addition, no special labeling for people with phenylketonuria is needed because neotame is not broken down in the body to its amino acid components.

Acesulfame-K. The alternative sweetener acesulfame-K (the *K* stands for potassium; Sunette®) was approved by the FDA in July 1988. It is approved for use in more than 40 countries and has been in use in Europe since 1983. Acesulfame-K is 200 times sweeter than sucrose. It contributes no calories to the diet because it is not digested by the body, and it does not cause dental caries.

Unlike aspartame, acesulfame-K can be used in baking because it does not lose its sweetness when heated. In the United States, it is currently approved for use in chewing gum, powdered drink mixes, gelatins, puddings, baked goods, tabletop sweeteners, candy, throat lozenges, yogurt, and nondairy creamers; additional uses may soon be approved. One recent trend is to combine it with aspartame in soft drinks.

Tagatose. Tagatose, sold as Naturlose,® is a slightly altered form of the simple sugar fructose. It is approved for use in ready-to-eat breakfast cereals, diet soft drinks, meal replacement bars, frozen desserts, candy, frosting, and chewing gum. Tagatose is poorly absorbed, so it yields only 1.5 kcal per gram to the body. Use also does not raise the risk for dental caries, nor does it increase blood glucose. Eventual fermentation in the large intestine may even lead to a beneficial effect on that organ (i.e., a prebiotic effect, covered in Chapter 3).

Stevia. Stevia, sold as the dietary supplement Sweet Leaf®, is an alternative sweetener derived from a South American shrub. Stevia extracts are 100 to 300 times sweeter than sucrose but provide no energy. It has been used in teas and as a sweetener in Japan since the 1970s, and the FDA recently (December 2008) stated that stevia is considered generally recognized as safe (GRAS) for use in foods. Stevia can be purchased as a dietary supplement in natural and health food stores and as an alternative sweetener in grocery stores.

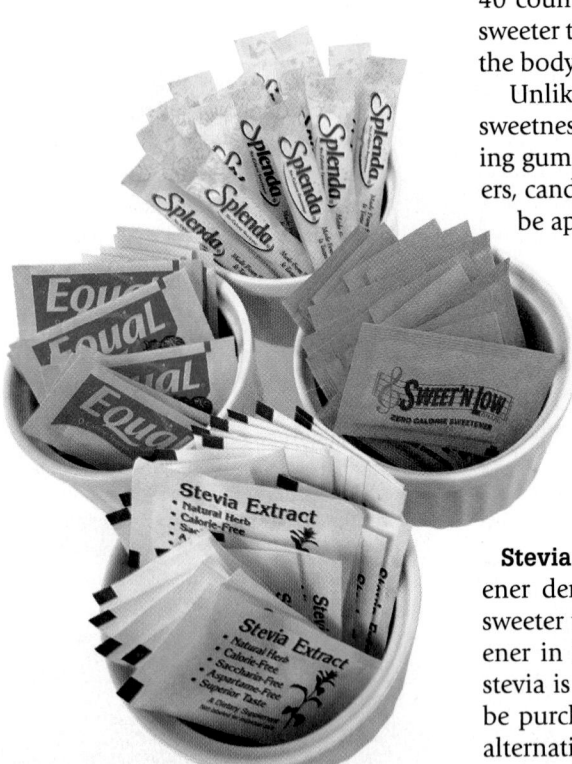

▲ A variety of alternative sweeteners are available.

CONCEPT CHECK

Table sugar, honey, jam, fruit, and plain baked potatoes contain the highest percentage of calories from carbohydrates. Foods such as cream pies, potato chips, whole milk, and oatmeal contain moderate amounts of carbohydrate. Common nutritive sweeteners added to foods include sucrose, maple sugar, honey, brown sugar, and high-fructose corn syrup. For people who want to limit calories from sugar intake, other sweeteners are available and include the sugar alcohols, saccharin, aspartame, sucralose, neotame, acesulfame-K, tagatose, and stevia. Of these, aspartame is the most common alternative sweetener in use.

4.6 Making Carbohydrates Available for Body Use

As discussed in Chapter 3, simply eating a food does not supply nutrients to body cells. Digestion and absorption must occur first.

Digestion

Food preparation can be viewed as the start of carbohydrate digestion because cooking softens tough connective structures in the fibrous parts of plants, such as broccoli stalks. When starches are heated, the starch granules swell as they soak up water, making them much easier to digest. All of these effects of cooking generally make carbohydrate-containing foods easier to chew, swallow, and break down during digestion.

The enzymatic digestion of starch begins in the mouth, when the saliva, which contains an enzyme called salivary **amylase**, mixes with the starchy products during the chewing of the food. This amylase breaks down starch into many smaller units, primarily disaccharides, such as maltose (Fig. 4-8). You can taste this conversion while chewing a saltine cracker. Prolonged chewing of the cracker causes it to taste sweeter as some starch breaks down into the sweeter disaccharides, such as maltose. Still, food is in the mouth for such a short amount of time that this phase of digestion is negligible. In addition, once the food moves down the esophagus and reaches the stomach, the acidic environment inactivates salivary amylase.

amylase Starch-digesting enzyme from the salivary glands or pancreas.

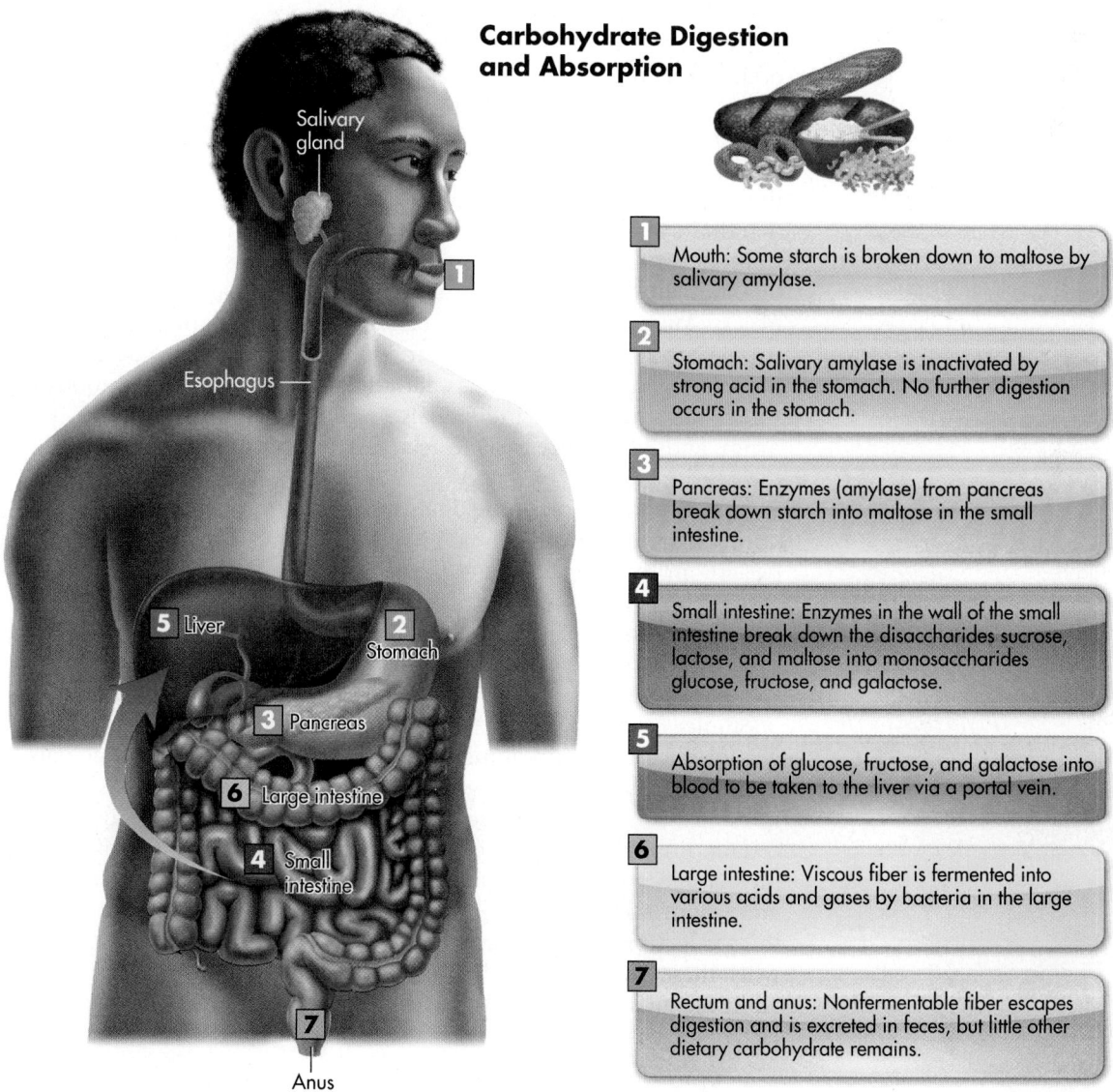

Carbohydrate Digestion and Absorption

1. Mouth: Some starch is broken down to maltose by salivary amylase.

2. Stomach: Salivary amylase is inactivated by strong acid in the stomach. No further digestion occurs in the stomach.

3. Pancreas: Enzymes (amylase) from pancreas break down starch into maltose in the small intestine.

4. Small intestine: Enzymes in the wall of the small intestine break down the disaccharides sucrose, lactose, and maltose into monosaccharides glucose, fructose, and galactose.

5. Absorption of glucose, fructose, and galactose into blood to be taken to the liver via a portal vein.

6. Large intestine: Viscous fiber is fermented into various acids and gases by bacteria in the large intestine.

7. Rectum and anus: Nonfermentable fiber escapes digestion and is excreted in feces, but little other dietary carbohydrate remains.

FIGURE 4-8 ▶ Carbohydrate digestion and absorption. Enzymes made by the mouth, pancreas, and small intestine participate in the process of digestion. Most carbohydrate digestion and absorption take place in the small intestine. Chapter 3 covered the physiology of digestion and absorption in detail.

When the carbohydrates reach the small intestine, the more alkaline environment of the intestine is better suited for further carbohydrate digestion. The pancreas releases enzymes, such as pancreatic amylase, to aid the last stage of starch digestion. After amylase action, the original carbohydrates in a food are now present in the small intestine as the monosaccharides glucose and fructose, originally present as such in food, and disaccharides (maltose from starch breakdown, lactose mainly from dairy products, and sucrose from food and that added at the table).

The disaccharides are digested to their monosaccharide units once they reach the wall of the small intestine, where the specialized enzymes on the absorptive cells digest each disaccharide into monosaccharides. The enzyme **maltase** acts on maltose to produce two glucose molecules. **Sucrase** acts on sucrose to produce glucose and fructose. **Lactase** acts on lactose to produce glucose and galactose.

Lactose Maldigestion and Lactose Intolerance. Lactose maldigestion is a normal pattern of physiology that often begins to develop after early childhood, at about ages 3 to 5 years. It can lead to symptoms of abdominal pain, gas, and diarrhea after consuming lactose, generally when eaten in large amounts. This *primary* form of lactose maldigestion is estimated to be present in about 75% of the world's population, although not all of these individuals experience symptoms. (When significant symptoms develop after lactose intake, it is then called **lactose intolerance**.) Another form of the problem, *secondary* lactose maldigestion, is a temporary condition in which lactase production is decreased in response to another condition, such as intestinal diarrhea. The symptoms of lactose intolerance include gas, abdominal bloating, cramps, and diarrhea. The bloating and gas are caused by bacterial fermentation of lactose in the large intestine. The diarrhea is caused by undigested lactose in the large intestine as it draws water from the circulatory system into the large intestine.

In North America, approximately 25% of adults show signs of decreased lactose digestion in the small intestine. Many lactose maldigesters are Asian Americans, African Americans, and Latino/Hispanic Americans, and the occurrence increases as people age. It is hypothesized that approximately 3000 to 5000 years ago, a genetic mutation occurred in regions that relied on milk and dairy foods as a main food source, allowing those individuals (mostly in northern Europe, pastoral tribes in Africa, and the Middle East) to retain the ability to maintain high lactase output for their entire lifetime.

Still, many of these individuals can consume moderate amounts of lactose with minimal or no gastrointestinal discomfort because of eventual lactose breakdown by bacteria in the large intestine (see Further Reading 12). Thus, it is unnecessary for these people to greatly restrict their intake of lactose-containing foods, such as milk and milk products. These calcium-rich food products are important for maintaining bone health. Obtaining enough calcium and vitamin D from the diet is much easier if milk and milk products are included in a diet.

Studies have shown that nearly all individuals with decreased lactase production can tolerate ½ to 1 cup of milk with meals, and that most individuals adapt to intestinal gas production resulting from the fermentation of lactose by bacteria in the large intestine. Combining lactose-containing foods with other foods also helps because certain properties of foods can have positive effects on rates of digestion. For example, fat in a meal slows digestion, leaving more time for lactase action. Hard cheese and yogurt also are more easily tolerated than milk. Much of the lactose is lost in the production of cheese, and the active bacteria cultures in yogurt digest the lactose when these bacteria are broken apart in the small intestine and release their lactase. In addition, an array of products, such as low-lactose milk (Lactaid®, Dairy Ease®) and lactase pills, is available to assist lactose maldigesters when needed.

Absorption

Monosaccharides found naturally in foods and those formed as by-products of starch and disaccharide digestion in the mouth and small intestine generally follow an

maltase An enzyme made by absorptive cells of the small intestine; this enzyme digests maltose to two glucoses.

sucrase An enzyme made by absorptive cells of the small intestine; this enzyme digests sucrose to glucose and fructose.

lactase An enzyme made by absorptive cells of the small intestine; this enzyme digests lactose to glucose and galactose.

lactose maldigestion (primary and secondary) Primary lactose maldigestion occurs when production of the enzyme lactase declines for no apparent reason. Secondary lactose maldigestion occurs when a specific cause, such as long-standing diarrhea, results in a decline in lactase production. When significant symptoms develop after lactose intake, it is then called lactose intolerance.

lactose intolerance A condition in which symptoms such as abdominal gas and bloating appear as a result of severe lactose maldigestion.

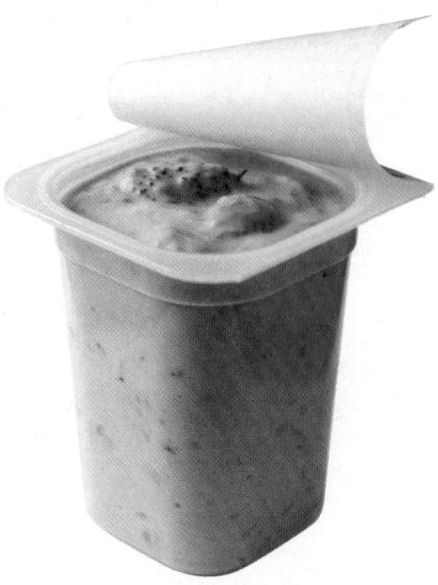
▲ Use of yogurt helps lactose maldigesters meet calcium needs.

active absorption process. Recall from Chapter 3 that this is a process that requires a specific carrier and energy input for the substance to be taken up by the absorptive cells in the small intestine. Glucose and its close relative, galactose, undergo active absorption. They are pumped into the absorptive cells along with sodium.

Fructose is taken up by the absorptive cells via facilitated diffusion. In this case, a carrier is used, but no energy input is needed. This absorptive process is thus slower than that seen with glucose or galactose. So, large doses of fructose are not readily absorbed and can contribute to diarrhea as the monosaccharide remains in the small intestine and attracts water.

Once glucose, galactose, and fructose enter the absorptive cells, some fructose is metabolized into glucose. The single sugars in the absorptive cells are then transferred to the portal vein that goes directly to the liver. The liver then metabolizes those sugars by transforming the monosaccharides galactose and fructose into glucose and:

- Releasing it directly into the bloodstream for transport to organs such as the brain, muscles, kidneys, and adipose tissues
- Producing glycogen for storage of carbohydrate
- Producing fat (minor amount, if any)

Of these three options, producing fat is the least likely, except when carbohydrates are consumed in high amounts and overall calorie needs are exceeded.

Unless an individual has a disease that causes malabsorption, or an intolerance to a carbohydrate such as lactose (or fructose), only a minor amount of some sugars (about 10%) escapes digestion. Any undigested carbohydrate travels to the large intestine and is fermented there by bacteria. The acids and gases produced by bacterial metabolism of the undigested carbohydrate are absorbed into the bloodstream. Scientists suspect that some of these products of bacterial metabolism promote the health of the large intestine by providing it with a source of calories.

MAKING DECISIONS

Fermentable Fiber

Bacteria in the large intestine ferment soluble fibers into such products as acids and gases. The acids, once absorbed, also provide calories for the body. In this way, soluble fibers provide about 1.5 to 2.5 kcal per gram. Although the intestinal gas (flatulence) produced by this bacterial fermentation is not harmful, it can be painful and sometimes embarrassing. Over time, however, the body tends to adapt to a high-fiber intake, eventually producing less gas.

Name some potentially gas-forming foods. Are these foods good sources of soluble fiber?

CONCEPT CHECK

Carbohydrate digestion is the process of breaking down larger carbohydrates into smaller units, and eventually to monosaccharide forms. The enzymatic digestion of starches in the body begins in the mouth with salivary amylase. Enzymes made by the pancreas and small intestine complete the digestion of carbohydrates to single sugars in the small intestine. Lactose maldigestion is a condition that results when cells of the intestine do not make sufficient lactase, the enzyme necessary to digest lactose, resulting in symptoms such as abdominal gas, pain, and diarrhea. Most people with lactose maldigestion can tolerate cheeses and yogurt, as well as moderate amounts of milk. When significant symptoms develop after lactose intake, it is called lactose intolerance. Following primarily an active absorption process, glucose and galactose (resulting from the digestive process or present in the meal) are taken up by absorptive cells in the intestine. Fructose undergoes facilitated absorption. All of the monosaccharides then enter the portal vein that goes directly to the liver. The liver finally exercises its metabolic options, producing glucose, glycogen, and even fat if carbohydrates are consumed in great excess and overall calorie needs are exceeded.

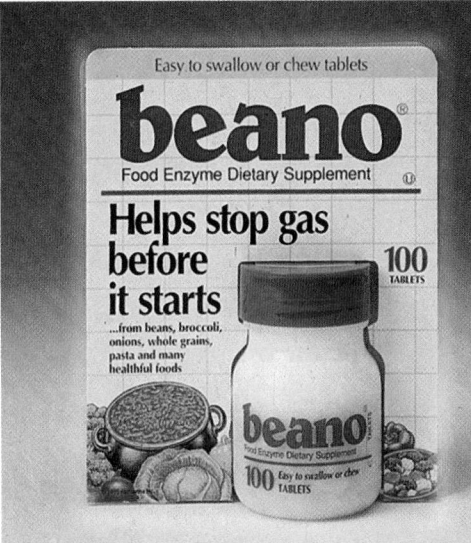

▲ Beano® is a dietary supplement that contains natural digestive enzymes. Such products can be used to reduce intestinal gas produced by bacterial metabolism of undigested sugars in beans and some vegetables in the large intestine.

4.7 Putting Simple Carbohydrates to Work in the Body

As just discussed, all of the digestible carbohydrate that we eat is eventually converted to glucose. Glucose then is the form of carbohydrate that goes on to function in body metabolism. The other sugars can generally be converted to glucose and the starches are broken down to yield glucose, so the functions described here apply to most carbohydrates. The functions of glucose in the body start with supplying calories to fuel the body.

Yielding Energy

The main function of glucose is to supply calories for use by the body. Certain tissues in the body, such as red blood cells, can use only glucose and other simple carbohydrate forms for fuel. Most parts of the brain and central nervous system also derive energy only from glucose, unless the diet contains almost none. In that case, much of the brain can use partial breakdown products of fat—called **ketone bodies**—for energy needs. Other body cells, including muscle cells, can use simple carbohydrates as fuel but many of these cells can also use fat or protein for energy needs.

ketone bodies Partial breakdown products of fat that contain three or four carbons.

ketosis The condition of having a high concentration of ketone bodies and related breakdown products in the bloodstream and tissues.

Sparing Protein from Use as an Energy Source and Preventing Ketosis

A diet that supplies enough digestible carbohydrates to prevent breakdown of proteins for energy needs is considered *protein sparing*. Under normal circumstances, digestible carbohydrates in the diet mostly end up as blood glucose, and protein is reserved for functions such as building and maintaining muscles and vital organs. However, if you don't eat enough carbohydrates, your body is forced to make glucose from body proteins, draining the pool of amino acids available in cells for other critical functions. During long-term starvation, the continuous withdrawal of proteins from the muscles, heart, liver, kidneys, and other vital organs can result in weakness, poor function, and even failure of body systems.

In addition to the loss of protein, when you don't eat enough carbohydrates, the metabolism of fats is inefficient. In the absence of adequate carbohydrate, fats don't break down completely in metabolism and instead form ketone bodies. This condition, known as **ketosis**, should be avoided because it disturbs the body's normal acid-base balance and leads to other health problems. This is a good reason to question the long-term safety of the low-carbohydrate diets that have been popular.

MAKING DECISIONS

Carbohydrates and Protein Sparing

The wasting of protein that occurs during long-term fasting can be life threatening. This has prompted companies that make formulas for rapid weight loss to include sufficient carbohydrate in the products to decrease protein breakdown and thereby protect vital tissues and organs, including the heart. Most of these very low-calorie products are powders that can be mixed with different types of fluids and are consumed five or six times per day. When considering any weight-loss products, be sure that your total diet provides at least the RDA for carbohydrate.

▲ When following a weight-loss diet, be sure that your diet provides at least the RDA for carbohydrate.

Regulating Glucose

Under normal circumstances, a person's blood glucose concentration is regulated within a narrow range. Recall from Chapter 3 that when carbohydrates are digested and taken up by the absorptive cells of the small intestine, the resulting monosaccharides are transported directly to the liver. One of the liver's roles, then, is to guard against excess glucose entering the bloodstream after a meal. The liver works in concert with the pancreas to regulate blood glucose.

When the concentration of glucose in the blood is high, such as during and immediately after a meal, the pancreas releases the hormone **insulin** into the bloodstream. Insulin delivers two different messages to various body cells to cause the level of glucose in the blood to fall. First, insulin directs the liver to store the glucose as glycogen. Second, insulin directs muscle, adipose, and other cells to remove glucose from the bloodstream by taking it into those cells. By triggering both glycogen synthesis in the liver and glucose movement out of the bloodstream into certain cells, insulin keeps the concentration of glucose from rising too high in the blood (Fig. 4-9).

On the other hand, when a person has not eaten for a few hours and blood glucose begins to fall, the pancreas releases the hormone **glucagon**. This hormone has the opposite effect of insulin. It prompts the breakdown of liver glycogen into glucose, which is then released into the bloodstream. In this way, glucagon keeps blood glucose from falling too low.

A different mechanism increases blood glucose during times of stress. **Epinephrine** (adrenaline) is the hormone responsible for the "flight or fight" reaction. Epinephrine and a related compound are released in large amounts from the adrenal glands (located on each kidney) and various nerve endings in response to a perceived threat, such as a car approaching head-on. These hormones cause glycogen in the liver to be quickly broken down into glucose. The resulting rapid flood of glucose from the liver into the bloodstream helps promote quick mental and physical reactions.

In essence, the actions of insulin on blood glucose are balanced by the actions of glucagon, epinephrine, and other hormones. If hormonal balance is not maintained, such as during over- or underproduction of insulin or glucagon, major changes in blood glucose concentrations occur. The disease, type 1 diabetes, is an example of the underproduction of insulin. To maintain blood glucose within an acceptable range, the body relies on a complex regulatory system. This provides a safeguard against extremely high blood glucose (**hyperglycemia**) or low blood glucose (**hypoglycemia**). The failure of blood glucose regulation will be discussed in the Nutrition and Your Health section at the end of this chapter.

insulin A hormone produced by the pancreas. Among other processes, insulin increases the synthesis of glycogen in the liver and the movement of glucose from the bloodstream into body cells.

glucagon A hormone made by the pancreas that stimulates the breakdown of glycogen in the liver into glucose; this ends up increasing blood glucose. Glucagon also performs other functions.

epinephrine A hormone also known as *adrenaline*; it is released by the adrenal glands (located on each kidney) and various nerve endings in the body. It acts to increase glycogen breakdown in the liver, among other functions.

hyperglycemia High blood glucose, above 125 milligrams per 100 milliliters of blood.

hypoglycemia Low blood glucose, below 40 to 50 milligrams per 100 milliliters of blood.

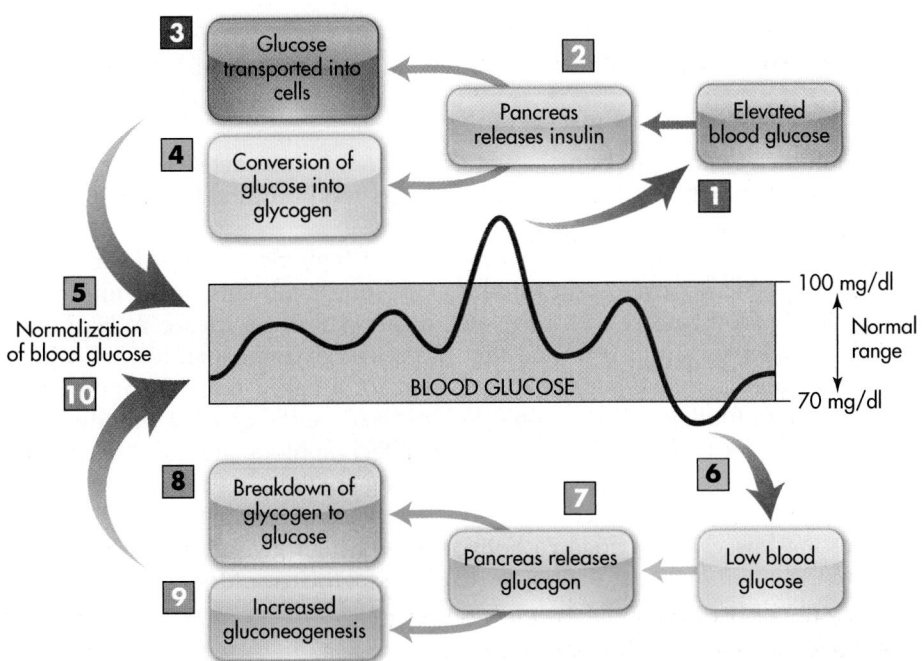

FIGURE 4-9 ▶ Regulation of blood glucose. Insulin and glucagon are key factors in controlling blood glucose. When blood glucose rises above the normal range of 70 to 90 milligrams per deciliter (mg/dl) **1**, insulin is released **2** to lower it **3** and **4** blood glucose then falls back into the normal range **5**. When blood glucose falls below the normal range **6**, glucagon is released **7**, which has the opposite effect of insulin **8**, and **9** this then restores blood glucose to the normal range **10**. Other hormones, such as epinephrine, norepinephrine, cortisol, and growth hormone, also contribute to blood glucose regulation.

See Nutrition and Your Health: Diabetes—When Blood Glucose Regulation Fails at the end of Chapter 4.

A term you might see on food labels is *net carbs*. Although this term is not FDA-approved, sometimes it is used to describe the carbohydrates that increase blood glucose. Fiber and sugar alcohol content are subtracted from the total carbohydrate content to yield net carbs because they have a negligible effect on blood glucose.

glycemic index (GI) The blood glucose response of a given food, compared to a standard (typically, glucose or white bread). Glycemic index is influenced by starch structure; fiber content; food processing; physical structure; and macronutrients in the meal, such as fat.

glycemic load (GL) The amount of carbohydrate in a serving of food multiplied by the glycemic index of that carbohydrate. The result is then divided by 100.

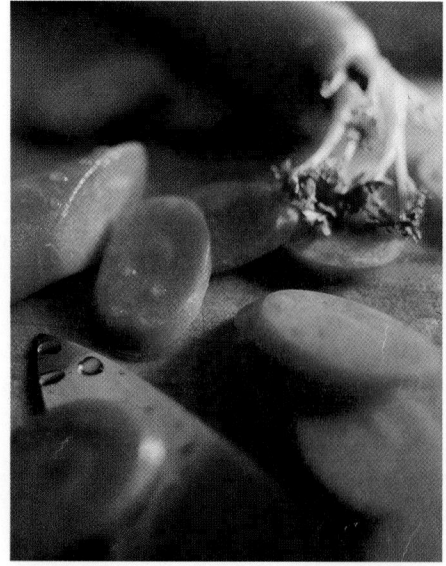

▲ Carrots, criticized in the popular press for having a high glycemic index (which isn't even true), actually contribute a low glycemic load to a diet.

The Glycemic Index and Glycemic Load of Carbohydrate Sources

Our bodies react uniquely to different sources of carbohydrates, such that a serving of a high-fiber food, such as baked beans, results in lower blood glucose levels compared to the same size serving of mashed potatoes. Why are we concerned with the effects of various foods on blood glucose? Foods that result in a high blood glucose elicit a large release of insulin from the pancreas. Chronically high insulin output leads to many deleterious effects on the body: high blood triglycerides, increased fat deposition in the adipose tissue, increased tendency for blood to clot, increased fat synthesis in the liver, and a more rapid return of hunger after a meal (insulin rapidly lowers the macronutrients in the blood as it stimulates their storage, signaling hunger). Over time, this increase in insulin output may cause the muscles to become resistant to the action of insulin, and eventually lead to type 2 diabetes in some people. Two food measurements have been developed that are useful in predicting the blood sugar response to various foods and for planning a diet to avoid hyperglycemia (high blood glucose).

The first of these tools is **glycemic index (GI)**. Glycemic index is a ratio of the blood glucose response to a given food compared to a standard (typically, glucose or white bread) (Table 4-4). Glycemic index is influenced by starch structure, fiber content, food processing, physical structure, and other macronutrients in the meal, such as fat. Foods with particularly high glycemic index values are potatoes, especially baking potatoes (due to higher amylopectin content compared to red potatoes), mashed potatoes (due to greater surface area exposed), short-grain white rice, honey, and jelly beans. A major shortcoming of glycemic index is that the measurement is based on a serving of food that would provide 50 grams of carbohydrate. As you can imagine, this amount of food may not reflect the amount typically consumed.

Another way of describing how different foods affect blood glucose (and insulin) levels is **glycemic load (GL)**. The glycemic load is more useful because it takes into account the glycemic index and the amount of carbohydrate consumed. Glycemic load, therefore, better reflects a food's effect on one's blood glucose than either number alone. To calculate the glycemic load of a food, the amount (in grams) of carbohydrate in a serving of the food is multiplied by the glycemic index of that food, and then divided by 100 (because glycemic index is a percentage). For example, vanilla wafers have a glycemic index of 77, and a small serving contains 15 grams of carbohydrate:

$$(\text{Glycemic Index} \times \text{Grams of Carbohydrate}) \div 100 = \text{Glycemic Load}$$
$$(77 \times 15) \div 100 = 12$$

Even though the glycemic index of vanilla wafers (77) is considered high, the glycemic load calculation shows that the impact of this food on blood glucose levels is fairly low (review Table 4-4).

There are many ways to address this problem of high glycemic load foods. The most important is to not overeat these foods at any one meal. This greatly minimizes their effects on blood glucose and the related increased insulin release. At least once per meal, consider substituting a food that has a low glycemic load for one with a higher value, such as long-grain rice or spaghetti for a baked potato. Combining a low glycemic load food, such as an apple, kidney beans, milk, or salad with dressing, with a high glycemic load food also reduces the effect on blood glucose. In addition, maintaining a healthy body weight and performing regular physical activity further reduces the effects of a high glycemic load diet (see Further Reading 9).

Substituting low glycemic load carbohydrates for high glycemic load foods can help in the treatment of diabetes; Chapter 10 discusses the use of foods with different glycemic load values in planning diets for athletes.

TABLE 4-4 Glycemic Index (GI) and Glycemic Load (GL) of Common Foods

Reference food glucose = 100
Low GI foods—below 55
Intermediate GI foods—between 55 and 70
High GI foods—more than 70

Low GL foods—below 15
Intermediate GL foods—between 15 and 20
High GL foods—more than 20

	Serving Size (grams)	Glycemic Index (GI)	Carbohydrate (grams)	Glycemic Load (GL)
Pastas/Grains				
White, long grain	1 cup	56	45	25
White, short grain	1 cup	72	53	38
Spaghetti	1 cup	41	40	16
Vegetables				
Carrots, boiled	1 cup	49	16	8
Sweet corn	1 cup	55	39	21
Potato, baked	1 cup	85	57	48
Dairy Foods				
Milk, skim	1 cup	32	12	4
Yogurt, low-fat	1 cup	33	17	6
Ice cream	1 cup	61	31	19
Legumes				
Baked beans	1 cup	48	54	26
Kidney beans	1 cup	27	38	10
Navy beans	1 cup	38	54	21
Sugars				
Honey	1 tsp	73	6	4
Sucrose	1 tsp	65	5	3
Fructose	1 tsp	23	5	1
Breads and Muffins				
Bagel	1 small	72	30	22
Whole-wheat bread	1 slice	69	13	9
White bread	1 slice	70	10	7
Fruits				
Apple	1 medium	38	22	8
Banana	1 medium	55	29	16
Orange	1 medium	44	15	7
Beverages				
Orange juice	1 cup	46	26	13
Gatorade	1 cup	78	15	12
Coca-Cola	1 cup	63	26	16
Snack Foods				
Potato chips	1 oz	54	15	8
Vanilla wafers	5 cookies	77	15	12
Jelly beans	1 oz	80	26	21

Source: Foster-Powell K. and others: International table of glycemic index and glycemic load. *American Journal of Clinical Nutrition* 76:5, 2002.

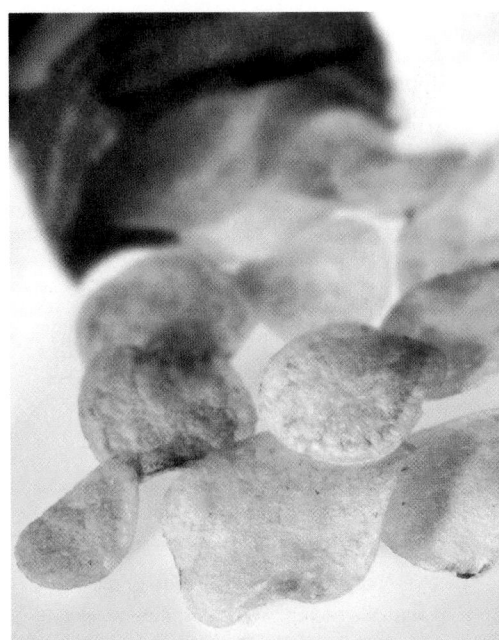

▲ A food such as potato chips, with a low glycemic index, can still have a high glycemic load if eaten in large portions.

You might wonder why the glycemic index and glycemic load of white bread and whole wheat are similar. This is because whole-wheat flour is typically so finely ground that it is quickly digested. Thus the effect of fiber in slowing digestion and related absorption of glucose is no longer present. Some experts suggest we focus more on minimally processed (e.g., coarsely ground, steel cut, or rolled) grains, such as with whole-wheat flour and oatmeal, to get the full benefits of these fiber sources in reducing blood glucose levels.

Recall from Chapter 2 that FDA has approved the following claim: "Diets rich in whole-grain foods and other plant foods and low in total fat, saturated fat, and cholesterol may decrease the risk for cardiovascular (heart) disease and certain cancers."

diverticula Pouches that protrude through the exterior wall of the large intestine.

hemorrhoid A pronounced swelling of a large vein, particularly veins found in the anal region.

diverticulosis The condition of having many diverticula in the large intestine.

diverticulitis An inflammation of the diverticula caused by acids produced by bacterial metabolism inside the diverticula.

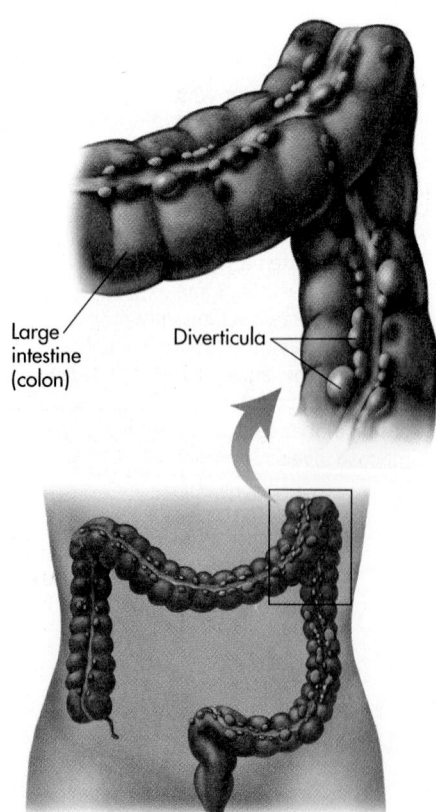

FIGURE 4-10 ▶ Diverticula in the large intestine. A low-fiber diet increases the risk of developing diverticula. About one-third of people over age 45 have diverticulosis, while two-thirds of people over 85 do.

CONCEPT CHECK

Carbohydrates provide glucose for the energy needs of red blood cells and parts of the brain and nervous system. Eating too little carbohydrates forces the body to make glucose using primarily amino acids from proteins found in muscles and other vital organs. A low glucose supply in cells also inhibits efficient metabolism of fats. Ketosis can then result.

Blood glucose concentration is maintained within a narrow range. When blood glucose rises after a meal, the hormone insulin is released in great amounts from the pancreas. Insulin acts to lower blood glucose by increasing glucose storage in the liver and glucose up-take by other body cells. If blood glucose falls during fasting, glucagon and other hormones increase the liver's release of glucose into the bloodstream to restore normal blood glucose concentrations. In a similar way, the hormone epinephrine can make more glucose available in response to stress. This balance in hormone activity helps maintain blood glucose within a healthy range.

4.8 Putting Fiber to Work

Promoting Bowel Health

Fiber supplies mass to the feces, making elimination much easier. This is especially true for insoluble fibers. When enough fiber is consumed, the stool is large and soft because many types of plant fibers attract water. The larger size stimulates the intestinal muscles to contract, which aids elimination. Consequently, less pressure is necessary to expel the stool.

When too little fiber is eaten, the opposite can occur: very little water is present in the feces, making it small and hard. Constipation may result, which forces one to exert excessive pressure in the large intestine during defecation. This high pressure can force parts of the large intestine (colon) wall out from between the surrounding bands of muscle, forming many small pouches called **diverticula** (Fig. 4-10). **Hemorrhoids** may also result from excessive straining during defecation (review Chapter 3).

Diverticula are asymptomatic in about 80% of affected people; that is, they are not noticeable. The asymptomatic form of this disease is called **diverticulosis**. If the diverticula become filled with food particles, such as hulls and seeds, they may eventually become inflamed and painful, a condition known as **diverticulitis**. Surprisingly, intake of fiber then should be reduced to limit further bacterial activity. Once the inflammation subsides, a high-fiber diet is resumed to ease stool elimination and reduce the risk of a future attack.

Over the past 30 years, many population studies have shown a link between increased fiber intake and a decrease in colon cancer development (see Further Reading 10). Most of the research on diet and colon cancer is focusing on the potential preventive effects of fruits, vegetables, whole-grain breads and cereals, and beans (rather than just fiber). Smoking, obesity in men, excessive alcohol use, starch- and sugar-rich foods, and processed meat intake are under study as potential causes of colon cancer. Overall, the health benefits to the colon that stem from a high-fiber diet are partially due to the nutrients that are commonly present in most high-fiber foods, such as vitamins, minerals, phytochemicals, and in some cases essential fatty acids. Thus it is more advisable to increase fiber intake using fiber-rich foods, rather than mostly relying on fiber supplements.

Reducing Obesity Risk

Aside from its role in maintaining bowel regularity, the consumption of fiber has many additional health benefits. A diet high in fiber likely controls weight and reduces the risk of developing obesity (see Further Reading 13). The bulky nature of high-fiber foods requires more time to chew and fills us up without yielding many calories. Increasing intake of foods rich in fiber is one strategy for feeling satisfied or full after a meal (review the discussion of energy density in Chapter 2). This is still another reason to question the low-carbohydrate diets—where is the whole-grain fiber going to come from?

Enhancing Blood Glucose Control

Consuming large amounts of viscous fibers, such as oat fiber, slows glucose absorption from the small intestine, and so contributes to better blood glucose regulation. This effect can be helpful in the treatment of diabetes. In fact, adults whose main carbohydrate source is low-fiber foods are much more likely to develop diabetes than those who have high-fiber diets.

Reducing Cholesterol Absorption

Recall that good sources of viscous fiber are apples, bananas, oranges, carrots, barley, oats, and kidney beans. A high intake of viscous fiber also inhibits absorption of cholesterol and cholesterol-rich bile acids from the small intestine, thereby reducing blood cholesterol and possibly reducing the risk of cardiovascular disease and gallstones. The beneficial bacteria in the large intestine degrade soluble fiber and produce certain fatty acids that probably also reduce cholesterol synthesis in the liver. In addition, the slower glucose absorption that occurs with diets high in viscous fiber is linked to a decrease in insulin release. One of the effects of insulin is to stimulate cholesterol synthesis in the liver, so this reduction in insulin may contribute to the ability of viscous fiber to lower blood cholesterol. Overall, a fiber-rich diet containing fruits, vegetables, beans, and whole-grain breads and cereals (including whole-grain breakfast cereals) is advocated as part of a strategy to reduce cardiovascular disease (coronary heart disease and stroke) risk. And again, this is something that a low-carbohydrate diet can't promise.

▲ Oatmeal is a rich source of viscous fiber. FDA allows a health claim for the benefits of oatmeal to lower blood cholesterol that arise from the effects of this viscous fiber.

CONCEPT CHECK

Fiber forms a vital part of the diet by adding mass to the stool, which eases elimination. Fiber-rich foods also help in weight control and reduce the risk of developing obesity and cardiovascular disease, and possibly colon cancer. Soluble fiber can also be useful for controlling blood glucose in patients with diabetes and in lowering blood cholesterol. Whole-grain breads and cereals, vegetables, beans, and fruits are excellent sources of fiber.

4.9 Carbohydrate Needs

Currently, recommendations for carbohydrate intake vary widely in the scientific literature and popular press. The RDA for carbohydrates is 130 grams per day for adults (see Further Reading 6). This is based on the amount needed to supply adequate glucose for the brain and nervous system, without having to rely on ketone bodies from incomplete fat breakdown as a calorie source. Somewhat exceeding this amount is fine; the Food and Nutrition Board recommends that carbohydrate intake should range from 45% to 65% of total calorie intake. The Nutrition Facts panel on food labels uses 60% of calorie intake as the standard for recommended carbohydrate intake. This would be 300 grams of carbohydrate when consuming a 2000-calorie diet.

North American adults consume about 180 to 330 grams of carbohydrates per day, which supply about 50% of calorie intake. Worldwide, however, carbohydrates account for about 70% of all calories consumed, and in some countries, up to 80% of the calories consumed. One recommendation on which almost all experts agree is that one's carbohydrate intake should be based primarily on fruits, vegetables, whole-grain breads and cereals, and beans, rather than on refined grains, potatoes, and sugar.

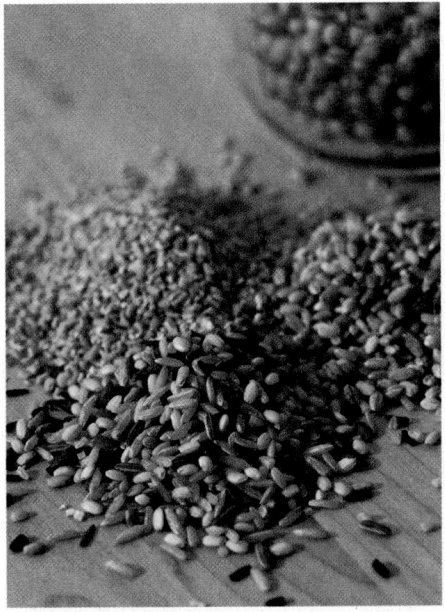

▲ The 2010 Dietary Guidelines define whole grain as the entire grain seed or kernel made of three components: bran, germ, and endosperm.

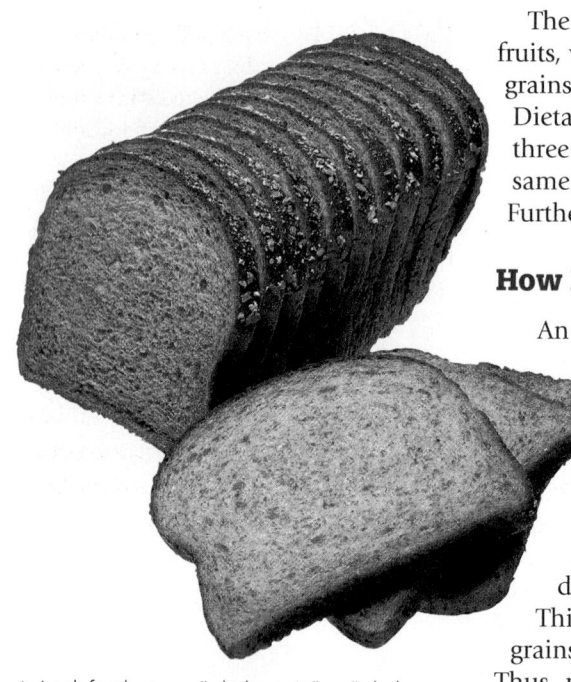

▲ Look for the term "whole-grain" or "whole-wheat" flour on the label for breads that are an excellent source of fiber.

The 2010 Dietary Guidelines for Americans recommend that we choose fiber-rich fruits, vegetables, and whole grains often. More specifically, three or more ounces of grains, roughly one-half of one's grains, should be whole. Remember that the 2010 Dietary Guidelines define whole grain as the entire grain seed or kernel made of three components: the bran, germ, and endosperm, which must be in nearly the same relative proportions as the original grain if cracked, crushed, or flaked (see Further Reading 14).

How Much Fiber Do We Need?

An Adequate Intake for fiber has been set based on the ability of fiber to reduce risk of cardiovascular disease (and likely many cases of diabetes). The Adequate Intake for fiber for adults is 25 grams per day for women and 38 grams per day for men. The goal is to provide at least 14 grams per 1000 kcal in a diet. After age 50, the Adequate Intake falls to 21 grams per day and 30 grams per day, respectively. The Daily Value used for fiber on food and supplement labels is 25 grams for a 2000 kcal diet. In North America, fiber intake averages 13 grams per day for women and 17 grams per day for men and the average whole-grain intake is less than one serving per day. This low intake is attributed to the lack of knowledge on the benefits of whole grains, and the inability to recognize whole-grain products at the time of purchase. Thus, most of us should increase our fiber intake. At least three servings of whole grains per day is recommended. Eating a high-fiber cereal (at least 3 grams of fiber per serving) for breakfast is one easy way to increase fiber intake (Fig. 4-11).

The "Rate Your Plate" exercise shows a diet containing 25 or 38 grams of fiber within moderate calorie intakes. Diets to meet the fiber recommendations are possible and enjoyable if you incorporate plenty of whole-wheat bread, fruits, vegetables, and beans. Use the "Rate Your Plate" exercise to estimate the fiber content of your diet. What is *your* fiber score?

The 2010 Dietary Guidelines for Americans provide the following recommendations regarding carbohydrate intake as part of a healthy eating pattern while staying within their calorie needs:

- Limit the consumption of foods that contain refined grains, especially refined grain foods that contain solid fats, added sugars, and sodium.

- Increase vegetable and fruit intake.

- Eat a variety of vegetables, especially dark-green and red and orange vegetables and beans and peas.

- Consume at least half of all grains as whole grains. Increase whole-grain intake by replacing refined grains with whole grains.

- Choose foods that provide more potassium, dietary fiber, calcium, and vitamin D, which are nutrients of concern in American diets. These foods include vegetables, fruits, whole grains, and milk and milk products.

MAKING DECISIONS

Whole Grains

When buying bread, if you see the name "wheat bread" on the label, do you think you are buying a whole-wheat product? Most people do. The flour is from the wheat plant, so manufacturers correctly list enriched white (refined) flour as wheat flour on food labels. However, if the label does not list "whole-wheat flour" first, then the product is not primarily a whole-wheat bread and thus does not contain as much fiber as it could. Careful reading of labels is important in the search for more fiber. Look especially for the term whole grains on the food label to ensure that you are getting a good source of natural fiber.

In the final analysis, keep in mind that any nutrient can lead to health problems when consumed in excess. High carbohydrate, high fiber, and low fat do not mean zero calories. Carbohydrates help moderate calorie intake in comparison with fats, but high-carbohydrate foods also contribute to total calorie intake.

4.10 Health Concerns Related to Carbohydrate Intake

Aside from the health risks related to ketosis, both excessive fiber and sugar intakes can pose health problems. Too much lactose in the diet is also a problem for some people.

Problems with High-Fiber Diets

Very high intakes of fiber—for example, 60 grams per day—can pose some health risks and therefore should be followed only under the guidance of a physician. Increased

Nutrition Facts

Serving Size   1 cup (55g/2.0 oz.)
Servings Per Container   10

Amount Per Serving	Cereal	Cereal with ½ Cup Vitamins A & D Skim Milk
Calories	170	210
Calories from Fat	10	10
	% Daily Value**	
Total Fat 1.0g*	2%	2%
Sat. Fat 0g	0%	0%
Trans Fat 0g		*
Cholesterol 0mg	0%	0%
Sodium 300mg	13%	15%
Potassium 340mg	10%	16%
Total Carbohydrate 43g	14%	16%
Dietary Fiber 7g	**28%**	**28%**
Sugars 16g		
Other Carbohydrate 20g		
Protein 4g		
Vitamin A	15%	20%
Vitamin C	20%	22%
Calcium	2%	15%
Iron	65%	65%
Vitamin D	10%	25%
Thiamin	25%	30%
Riboflavin	25%	35%
Niacin	25%	25%
Vitamin B_6	25%	25%
Folic acid	30%	30%
Vitamin B_{12}	25%	35%
Phosphorus	20%	30%
Magnesium	20%	25%
Zinc	25%	25%
Copper	10%	10%

*Amount in cereal. One half cup skim milk contributes an additional 40 calories, 65mg sodium, 6g total carbohydrate (6g sugars), and 4g protein.
**Percent Daily Values are based on a 2,000 calorie diet. Your daily values may be higher or lower depending on your calorie needs:

	Calories:	2,000	2,500
Total Fat	Less than	65g	80g
Sat Fat	Less than	20g	25g
Cholesterol	Less than	300mg	300mg
Sodium	Less than	2,400mg	2,400mg
Potassium		3,500mg	3,500mg
Total Carbohydrate		300g	375g
Dietary Fiber		25g	30g

Calories per gram:
Fat 9 • Carbohydrate 4 • Protein 4

*Intake of *trans* fat should be as low as possible.

Ingredients: Wheat bran with other parts of wheat, raisins, sugar, corn syrup, salt, malt flavoring, glycerin, iron, niacinamide, zinc oxide, pyridoxine hydrochloride (vitamin B_6), riboflavin (vitamin B_2), vitamin A palmitate, thiamin hydrochloride (vitamin B_1), folic acid, vitamin B_{12}, and vitamin D.

Nutrition Facts

Serving Size: ¾ Cup (30g)
Servings Per Package: About 17

Amount Per Serving	Cereal	Cereal With ½ Cup Skim Milk
Calories	170	210
Calories from Fat	0	5
	%Daily Value**	
Total Fat 0g*	0%	1%
Saturated Fat 0g	0%	1%
Trans Fat 0g		*
Cholesterol 0mg	0%	1%
Sodium 60mg	2%	4%
Potassium 80mg	2%	8%
Total Carbohydrate 35g	9%	11%
Dietary Fiber 1g	4%	4%
Sugars 20g		
Other Carbohydrate 13g		
Protein 3g		
Vitamin A	25%	30%
Vitamin C	0%	2%
Calcium	0%	15%
Iron	10%	10%
Vitamin D	10%	20%
Thiamin	25%	25%
Riboflavin	25%	35%
Niacin	25%	25%
Vitamin B_6	25%	25%
Folic acid	25%	25%
Vitamin B_{12}	25%	30%
Phosphorus	4%	15%
Magnesium	4%	8%
Zinc	10%	10%
Copper	2%	2%

*Amount in Cereal. One-half cup skim milk contributes an additional 65mg sodium, 6g total carbohydrate (6g sugars), and 4g protein.
**Percent Daily Values are based on a 2,000 calorie diet. Your daily values may be higher or lower depending on your calorie needs:

	Calories:	2,000	2,500
Total Fat	Less than	65g	80g
Sat. Fat	Less than	20g	25g
Cholesterol	Less than	300mg	300mg
Sodium	Less than	2,400mg	2,400mg
Potassium		3,500mg	3,500mg
Total Carbohydrate		300g	375g
Dietary Fiber		25g	30g

Calories per gram:
Fat 9 • Carbohydrate 4 • Protein 4

*Intake of *trans* fat should be as low as possible.

Ingredients: Wheat, Sugar, Corn Syrup, Honey, Caramel Color, Partially Hydrogenated Soybean Oil, Salt, Ferric Phosphate, Niacinamide (Niacin), Zinc Oxide, Vitamin A (Palmitate), Pyridoxine Hydrochloride (Vitamin B6), Riboflavin, Thiamin Mononitrate, Folic Acid (Folate),Vitamin B12 and Vitamin D.

FIGURE 4-11 ▶ Reading the Nutrition Facts on food labels helps us choose more nutritious foods. Based on the information from these nutrition labels, which cereal is the better choice for breakfast? Consider the amount of fiber in each cereal. Did the ingredient lists give you any clues? (Note: Ingredients are always listed in descending order by weight on a label.) When choosing a breakfast cereal, it is generally wise to focus on those that are rich sources of fiber. Sugar content can also be used for evaluation. However, sometimes this number does not reflect added sugar but simply the addition of fruits, such as raisins, complicating the evaluation.

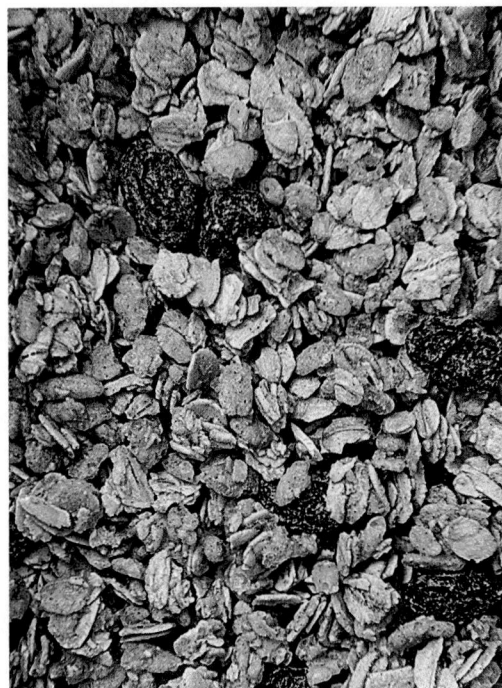

▲ Whole-grain foods, such as granola, are excellent sources of fiber.

fluid intake is extremely important with a high-fiber diet. Inadequate fluid intake can leave the stool very hard and painful to eliminate. In more severe cases, the combination of excess fiber and insufficient fluid may contribute to blockages in the intestine, which may require surgery.

Aside from problems with the passage of materials through the GI tract, a high-fiber diet may also decrease the availability of nutrients. Certain components of fiber may bind to essential minerals, keeping them from being absorbed. For example, when fiber is consumed in large amounts, zinc and iron absorption may be hindered. In children, a very high fiber intake may reduce overall calorie intake, because fiber can quickly fill a child's small stomach before food intake meets energy needs.

Problems with High-Sugar Diets

The main problems with consuming an excess amount of sugar are that it provides empty calories and increases the risk for dental decay.

Diet Quality Declines When Sugar Intake Is Excessive. Overcrowding the diet with sweet treats can leave little room for important, nutrient-dense foods, such as fruits and vegetables. Children and teenagers are at the highest risk for overconsuming empty calories in place of nutrients essential for growth. Many children and teenagers are drinking an excess of sugared soft drinks and other sugar-containing beverages and much less milk than ever before. This exchange of soft drinks for milk can compromise bone health because milk contains calcium and vitamin D, both essential for bone health.

Supersizing sugar-rich beverages is also a growing problem; for example, in the 1950s a typical serving size of a soft drink was a 6½-ounce bottle, and now a 20-ounce plastic bottle is a typical serving. This one change in serving size contributes 170 extra kcal of sugars to the diet. Most convenience stores now offer cups that will hold 64 ounces of soft drinks. Filling up on sugared soft drinks in place of foods is not a healthy practice, but enjoying an occasional soft drink or limiting intake to one 12-ounce serving a day is generally fine. Switching to diet soft drinks would spare the simple sugar calories but still lacks nutritional value except for the fluid.

The sugar found in cakes, cookies, and ice cream also supplies many extra calories that promote weight gain, unless an individual is physically active. Today's low-fat and fat-free snack products usually contain lots of added sugar to produce a product with an acceptable taste. The result is to produce a high-calorie food equal to or greater in calorie content than the high-fat food product it was designed to replace.

With regard to sugar intake, an upper limit of 25% of total calorie intake from "added sugars" has been set by the Food and Nutrition Board (sugars added to foods during processing and preparation). Diets that go beyond this upper limit are likely to be deficient in vitamins and minerals. The World Health Organization suggests that added sugars provide no more than 10% of total daily calorie intake.

A moderate intake of about 10% of calorie intake corresponds to a maximum of approximately 50 grams (or 12 tsp) of sugars per day, based on a 2000 kcal diet. Most of the sugars we eat come from foods and beverages to which sugar has been added during processing and/or manufacture. On average, North Americans eat about 82 grams of added sugars daily, amounting to about 16% of calorie intake. Major sources of added sugars include soft drinks; cakes; cookies; fruit drinks; and dairy desserts, such as ice cream (Fig. 4-12). Following the recommendation of having no more than 10% of added calories from sugars is easier if sweet desserts such as cakes, cookies, and ice cream (full and reduced fat) are consumed sparingly (Table 4-5).

An excess intake of sugared soft drinks has recently been linked to a risk for both weight gain and type 2 diabetes in adults.

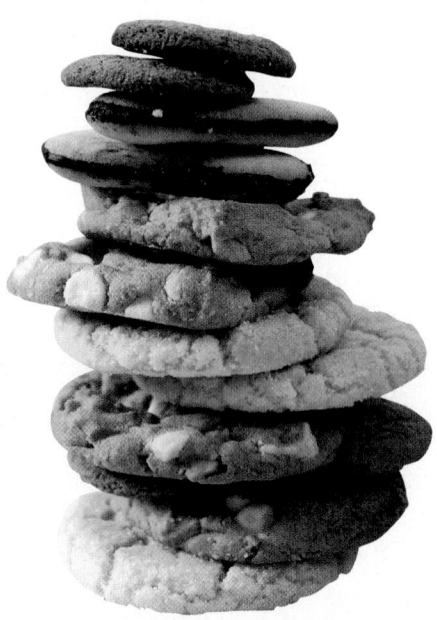

▲ Cookies and cakes are one of the top five carbohydrate sources for U.S. adults.

MAKING DECISIONS

Sugar and Hyperactivity

There is a widespread notion that high sugar intake by children causes hyperactivity, typically part of the syndrome called *attention deficit hyperactivity disorder (ADHD)*. However, most researchers find that sucrose may have the opposite effect. A high-carbohydrate meal, if also low in protein and fat, has a calming effect and induces sleep; this effect may be linked to changes in the synthesis of certain neurotransmitters in the brain, such as serotonin. If there is a problem, it is probably the excitement or tension in situations in which sugar-rich foods are served, such as at birthday parties and on Halloween.

TABLE 4-5 Suggestions for Reducing Simple-Sugar Intake

Many foods we enjoy are sweet. These should be eaten in moderation.

At the Supermarket

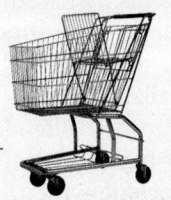

- Read ingredient labels. Identify all the added sugars in a product. Select items lower in total sugar when possible.
- Buy fresh fruits or fruits packed in water, juice, or light syrup rather than those packed in heavy syrup.
- Buy fewer foods that are high in sugar, such as prepared baked goods, candies, sugared cereals, sweet desserts, soft drinks, and fruit-flavored punches. Substitute vanilla wafers, graham crackers, bagels, English muffins, diet soft drinks, and other low-sugar alternatives.
- Buy reduced-fat microwave popcorn to replace candy for snacks.

In the Kitchen

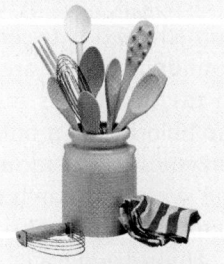

- Reduce the sugar in foods prepared at home. Try new low-sugar recipes or adjust your own. Start by reducing the sugar gradually until you've decreased it by one-third or more.
- Experiment with spices, such as cinnamon, cardamom, coriander, nutmeg, ginger, and mace, to enhance the flavor of foods.
- Use home-prepared items with less sugar instead of commercially prepared ones that are higher in sugar.

At the Table

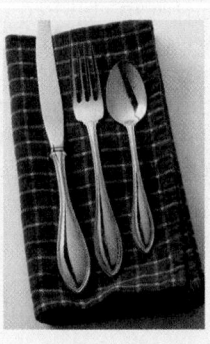

- Reduce your use of white and brown sugars, honey, molasses, syrups, jams, and jellies.
- Choose fewer foods high in sugar, such as prepared baked goods, candies, and sweet desserts.
- Reach for fresh fruit instead of cookies or candy for dessert and between-meal snacks.
- Add less sugar to foods—coffee, tea, cereal, and fruit. Cut back gradually to a quarter or half the amount. Consider using sugar alternatives to substitute for some sugar.
- Reduce the number of sugared soft drinks, punches, and fruit juices you drink. Substitute water, diet soft drinks, and whole fruits.

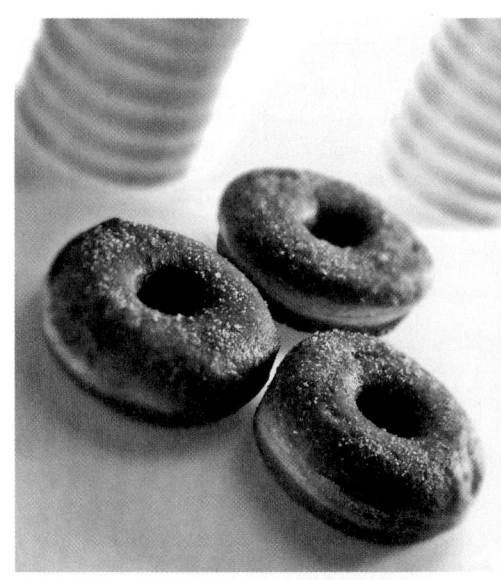

▲ Many foods we enjoy are sweet. These should be eaten in moderation.

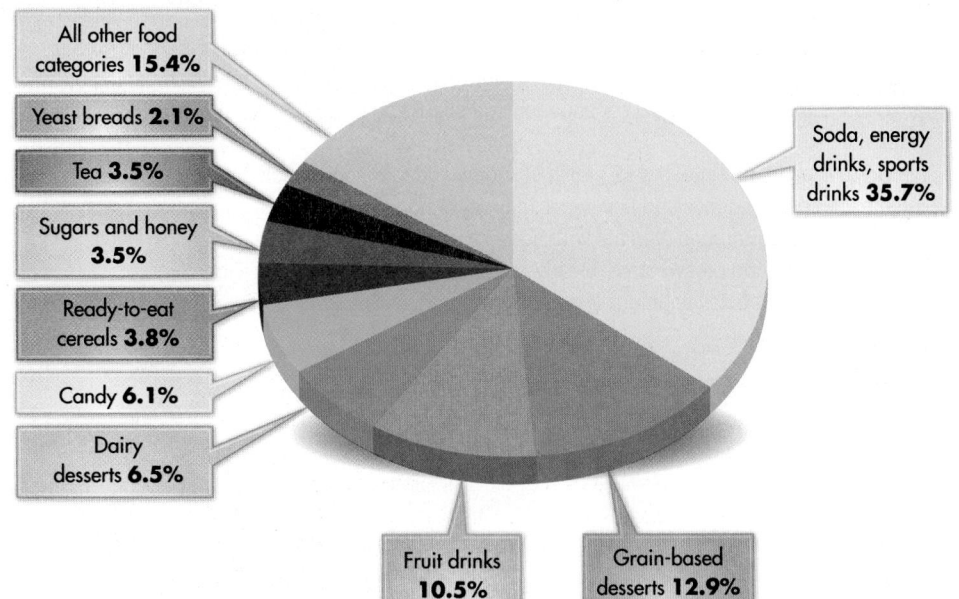

All other food categories **15.4%**

Yeast breads **2.1%**

Tea **3.5%**

Sugars and honey **3.5%**

Ready-to-eat cereals **3.8%**

Candy **6.1%**

Dairy desserts **6.5%**

Fruit drinks **10.5%**

Grain-based desserts **12.9%**

Soda, energy drinks, sports drinks **35.7%**

FIGURE 4-12 ▶ Sources of added sugars in the diets of the U.S. population ages 2 years and olders.

Sources: Dietary Guidelines for Americans Chapter Three.

National Cancer Institute. Sources of added sugars in the diets of the U.S. population ages 2 years and older, NHANES 2005–2006. Risk Factor Monitoring and Methods. Cancer Control and Population Sciences. http://riskfactor.cancer.gov/diet/foodsources/added_sugars/table5a.html. Accessed Auguest 11, 2010.

dental caries Erosions in the surface of a tooth caused by acids made by bacteria as they metabolize sugars.

Dental Caries

Sugars in the diet (and starches readily fermented in the mouth, such as crackers and white bread) also increase the risk of developing **dental caries**. Recall that caries, also known as cavities, are formed when sugars and other carbohydrates are metabolized into acids by bacteria that live in the mouth. These acids dissolve the tooth enamel and underlying structure. Bacteria also use the sugars to make plaque, a sticky substance that both adheres acid-producing bacteria to teeth and diminishes the acid-neutralizing effect of saliva.

The worst offenders in terms of promoting dental caries are sticky and gummy foods high in sugars, such as caramel, because they stick to the teeth and supply the bacteria with a long-lived carbohydrate source. Frequent consumption of liquid sugar sources (e.g., fruit juices) can also cause dental caries. Snacking regularly on sugary foods is also likely to cause caries because it gives the bacteria on the teeth a steady source of carbohydrate from which to continually make acid. Sugared gum chewed between meals is a prime example of a poor dental habit. Still, sugar-containing foods are not the only foods that promote acid production by bacteria in the mouth. As mentioned, if starch-containing foods (e.g., crackers and bread) are held in the mouth for a long time, the starch will be broken down to sugars by enzymes in the mouth; bacteria can then produce acid from these sugars. Overall, the sugar and starch content of a food and its ability to remain in the mouth largely determine its potential to cause caries.

Fluoridated water and toothpaste have contributed to fewer dental caries in North American children over the past 20 years due to fluoride's tooth-strengthening effect (see Chapter 10). Research has also indicated that certain foods—such as cheese, peanuts, and sugar-free chewing gum—can help reduce the amount of acid on teeth. In addition, rinsing the mouth after meals and snacks reduces the acidity in the mouth. Certainly, good nutrition, habits that do not present an overwhelming challenge to oral health (e.g., chewing sugar-free gum), and routine visits to the dentist all contribute to improved dental health.

CRITICAL THINKING

John and Mike are identical twins who like the same games, sports, and foods. However, John likes to chew sugar-free gum and Mike doesn't. At their last dental visit, John had no cavities but Mike had two. Mike wants to know why John, who chews gum after eating, doesn't have cavities and he does. How would you explain this to him?

CONCEPT CHECK

The RDA for carbohydrate is 130 grams per day. The typical North American diet provides 180 to 330 grams per day. A reasonable goal is to have about half of our calorie intake coming from starch and our total carbohydrate intake making up about 60% of our calorie intake, with a range of 45% to 65%. This should allow for the recommended intake of 25 to 38 grams of fiber per day for women and men, respectively. High-fiber diets must be accompanied by adequate fluid intakes to avoid constipation and should be followed only under a physician's guidance.

North Americans eat about 82 grams of sugars added to foods each day. Most of these sugars are added to foods and beverages in processing. To reduce consumption of sugars, one must reduce consumption of items with added sugars, such as some baked goods, sweetened beverages, and presweetened ready-to-eat breakfast cereals. This is one practice that can help reduce the development of dental caries and likely improve diet quality and various aspects of health.

Diabetes—When Blood Glucose Regulation Fails

Improper regulation of blood glucose results in either hyperglycemia (high blood glucose) or hypoglycemia (low blood glucose) as noted in this chapter. High blood glucose is most commonly associated with diabetes (technically, *diabetes mellitus*), a disease that affects 6.5% of the North American population (see Further Reading 5). Of these, it is estimated one-third to one-half of these people do not know that they have the disease. Diabetes leads to about 200,000 deaths each year in North America. Diabetes is currently increasing in epidemic proportions in North America. New recommendations promote testing fasting blood glucose in adults over age 45 every 3 years to help diagnose the problem. Diabetes is diagnosed when one's fasting blood glucose is 126 milligrams per 100 milliliters of blood or greater. In contrast, low blood glucose is a much rarer condition.

Diabetes

There are two major forms of diabetes: **type 1** (formerly called insulin-dependent or juvenile-onset diabetes), and **type 2 diabetes** (formerly called non–insulin-dependent or adult-onset diabetes) (Table 4-6). The change in names to type 1 and type 2 diabetes stems from the fact that many type 2 diabetics eventually must also rely on insulin injections as a part of their treatment. In addition, many children today have type 2 diabetes. A third form, called gestational diabetes, occurs in some pregnant women (see Chapter 16). It is usually treated with an insulin regimen and diet and resolves after delivery of the baby. However, women who have gestational diabetes during pregnancy are at high risk for developing type 2 diabetes later in life.

Traditional symptoms of diabetes are excessive urination, excessive thirst, and excessive hunger. No one symptom is diagnostic of diabetes, and other

TABLE 4-6 Comparison of Type 1 and Type 2 Diabetes

	Type 1 Diabetes	Type 2 Diabetes
Occurrence	5%–10% of cases of diabetes	90% of cases of diabetes
Cause	Autoimmune attack on the pancreas	Insulin resistance
Risk Factors	Moderate genetic predisposition	Strong genetic predisposition Obesity and physical inactivity Ethnicity Metabolic Syndrome Pre-diabetes
Characteristics	Distinct symptoms (frequent thirst, hunger, and urination) Ketosis Weight loss	Mild symptoms, especially in early phases of the disease (fatigue and nighttime urination) Ketosis does not generally occur.
Treatment	Insulin Diet Exercise	Diet Exercise Oral medications to lower blood glucose Insulin (in advanced cases)
Complications	Cardiovascular disease Kidney disease Nerve disease Blindness Infections	Cardiovascular disease Kidney disease Nerve damage Blindness Infections
Monitoring	Blood glucose Urine ketones HbA1c*	Blood glucose HbA1c

*Hemoglobin Alc.

type 1 diabetes A form of diabetes prone to ketosis and that requires insulin therapy.

type 2 diabetes A form of diabetes characterized by insulin resistance and often associated with obesity. Insulin therapy can be used but is often not required.

symptoms—such as unexplained weight loss, exhaustion, blurred vision, tingling in hands and feet, frequent infections, poor wound healing, and impotence—often accompany traditional symptoms.

Type 1 Diabetes

Type 1 diabetes often begins in late childhood, around the age of 8 to 12 years, but can occur at any age. The disease runs in certain families, indicating a clear genetic link. Children usually are admitted to the hospital with abnormally high blood glucose after eating, as well as evidence of ketosis.

The onset of type 1 diabetes is generally associated with decreased release of insulin from the pancreas. As insulin in the blood declines, blood glucose increases, especially after eating. Figure 4-13 shows a typical glucose tolerance curve observed in a patient with this form of diabetes after consuming about 75 grams of glucose. When blood glucose levels are high, the kidneys let excess glucose spill into the urine, resulting in frequent urination of urine high in sugar.

A common clinical method to determine a person's success in controlling blood glucose is to measure glycated (also termed glycosylated) hemoglobin (hemoglobin A1c). Over time, blood glucose attaches to (glycates) hemoglobin in red blood cells and more so when blood glucose remains elevated. A hemoglobin A1c value of over 7% indicates poor blood glucose control. Maintaining near-normal hemoglobin A1c levels (6% or less) greatly reduces the risk of death and developing other diseases in people with diabetes. Elevated blood glucose also leads to glycation of other proteins and fats in the body, forming what are called advanced glycation endproducts (AGEs). These have been shown to be toxic to cells, especially those of the immune system and kidneys.

Most cases of type 1 diabetes begin with an immune system disorder, which causes destruction of the insulin-producing cells in the pancreas. Most likely, a virus or protein foreign to the body sets off the destruction. In response to their damage, the affected pancreatic cells release other proteins, which stimulate a more furious

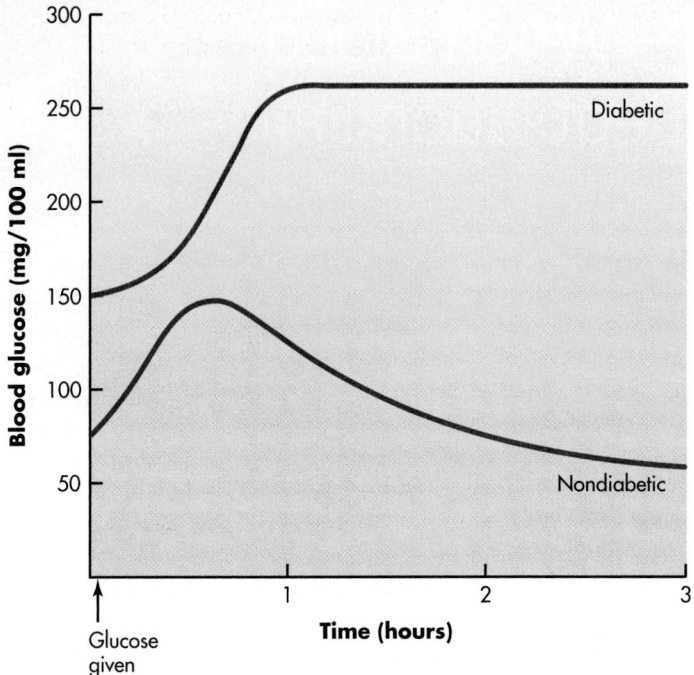

FIGURE 4-13 ▶ Glucose tolerance test. A comparison of blood glucose concentrations in untreated diabetic and healthy nondiabetic persons after consuming a 75 g test load of glucose.

attack. Eventually, the pancreas loses its ability to synthesize insulin, and the clinical stage of the disease begins. Consequently, early treatment to stop the immune-linked destruction in children may be important. Research into this area is ongoing.

Type 1 diabetes is treated primarily by insulin therapy, either with injections two to six times per day or with an insulin pump. The pump dispenses insulin at a steady rate into the body, with greater amounts delivered after each meal. Inhaled forms of insulin also are available. Dietary therapy includes three regular meals and one or more snacks (including one at bedtime) and having a regulated ratio of carbohydrate:protein:fat to maximize insulin action and minimize swings in blood glucose (see Further Reading 2 and 3 for more information on nutrition treatment of diabetes). If one does not eat often enough, the injected insulin can cause a severe drop in blood glucose or hypoglycemia, because it acts on whatever glucose is available. The diet should be moderate in simple carbohydrates, include ample fiber and polyunsaturated fat, but be low in both animal and *trans* fats, supply an amount of calories in balance with needs, and include fish twice a week.

▶ **Symptoms of Diabetes**

The symptoms of diabetes may occur suddenly, and include one or more of the following:

- Extreme thirst
- Frequent urination
- Drowsiness, lethargy
- Sudden vision changes
- Increased appetite
- Sudden weight loss
- Sugar in urine
- Fruity, sweet, or winelike odor on breath
- Heavy, labored breathing
- Stupor, unconsciousness

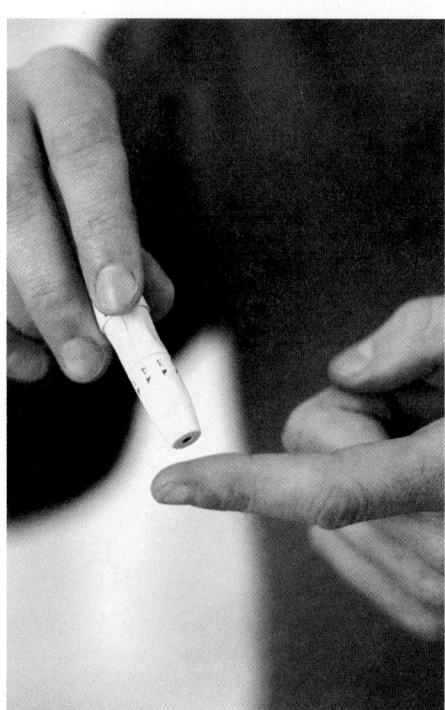

▲ Regularly checking blood glucose is part of diabetes therapy.

MAKING DECISIONS

Are You Prediabetic?

Often people with type 2 diabetes did not develop the disease suddenly. It may develop for years before symptoms are noticed. Prediabetes is a condition in which the concentration of blood glucose has drifts up higher than normal. By the time symptoms are noticeable, organs and tissues may be damaged. Simple tests of your fasting blood glucose level can determine if you are prediabetic. Early detection of diabetes risk can help prevent diabetes if you make lifestyle changes. If you have a family history of diabetes or if your habits (being physically inactive and overweight, and having a poor diet) put you at risk, it is fortunate to discover if your blood glucose is still in the prediabetic stage. Prediabetes, also called impaired fasting glucose, is diagnosed if the fasting blood glucose is 100–125 mg/dL.

Meeting magnesium needs is also helpful, as well as a moderate intake of coffee.

If a high carbohydrate intake raises triglycerides and cholesterol in the blood beyond desired ranges, carbohydrate intake can be reduced and replaced with unsaturated fat. Surprisingly, this change tends to reduce blood triglycerides and cholesterol. Chapter 5 discusses how to implement such a diet (as well as when certain related medications may be beneficial). Some consumption of sugars with meals is fine, as long as blood glucose regulation is preserved and the sugars replace other carbohydrates in the meal, so that undesirable weight gain does not take place.

The latest evidence suggests that diabetes essentially guarantees development of cardiovascular disease. Because people with diabetes (type 1, as well as type 2) are at a high risk for cardiovascular disease and related heart attacks, they should take an aspirin each day (generally 80 to 160 milligrams per day) if their physicians find no reason not to do so. Blood cholesterol lowering medications also may be prescribed. As discussed in Chapter 5, these practices reduce the risk of heart attack.

The hormone imbalances that occur in people with untreated type 1 diabetes—chiefly, not enough insulin—lead to mobilization of body fat, taken up by liver cells. Ketosis is the result because the fat is partially broken down to ketone bodies. Ketone bodies can rise excessively in the blood, eventually forcing ketone bodies into the urine. These pull sodium and potassium ions and water with them into the urine. This series of events also causes frequent urination and can contribute to a chain reaction that eventually leads to dehydration; ion imbalance; coma; and even death, especially in patients with poorly controlled type 1 diabetes. Treatment includes provision of insulin, fluids, and minerals such as sodium and potassium.

In addition to cardiovascular disease, other degenerative complications that result from poor blood glucose regulation, specifically long-term hyperglycemia, include blindness, kidney disease, and deterioration of nerves. The high blood sugar concentration physically deteriorates small blood vessels (capillaries) and nerves. When improper nerve stimulation

occurs in the intestinal tract, intermittent diarrhea and constipation result. Because of nerve deterioration in the extremities, many people with diabetes lose the sensation of pain associated with injuries or infections. They do not have as much pain, so they often delay treatment of hand or foot problems. This delay, combined with a rich environment for bacterial growth (bacteria thrive on glucose) sets the stage for damage and death of tissues in the extremities, sometimes leading to the need for amputation of feet and legs. Current research has shown that the development of blood vessel and nerve complications of diabetes can be slowed with aggressive treatment directed at keeping blood glucose within the normal range. The therapy poses some risks of its own, such as hypoglycemia, so it must be implemented under the close supervision of a physician.

A person with diabetes generally must work closely with a physician and registered dietitian to make the correct alterations in diet and medications and to perform physical activity safely. Physical activity enhances glucose uptake by muscles independent of insulin action, which in turn can lower blood glucose. This outcome is beneficial, but people with type 1 diabetes need to be aware of their blood glucose response to physical activity and compensate appropriately.

Type 2 Diabetes

Type 2 diabetes usually begins after age 40. This is the most common type of diabetes, accounting for about 90% of the cases diagnosed in North America. Minority populations such as Latino/Hispanic Americans, African Americans, Asian Americans, Native Americans, and those from Pacific Islands are at particular risk. As noted in the introduction, the overall number of people affected also is on the rise, primarily because of widespread inactivity and obesity in our population. There has been a substantial increase in type 2 diabetes in children, due mostly to an increase in overweight in this population (coupled with limited physical activity). Type 2 diabetes is also genetically linked, so family history is an important risk factor. However, the initial problem is not with the insulin-secreting cells of the pancreas. Instead, type 2 diabetes arises when the insulin receptors on the cell surfaces of certain body tissues, especially muscle tissue, become insulin resistant. In this case, blood glucose is not readily transferred into cells, so the person develops high blood glucose as a result of the glucose remaining in the bloodstream. The pancreas attempts to increase insulin output to compensate, but there is a limit to its ability to do this. Thus, rather than insufficient insulin production, there is an abundance of insulin, particularly during the onset of the disease. As the disease develops, pancreatic function can fail, leading to reduced insulin output. Because of the genetic link for type 2 diabetes, those who have a family history should schedule regular blood glucose tests and be careful to avoid risk factors such as obesity, inactivity, a diet rich in animal and *trans* fats, and simple carbohydrates.

Many cases of type 2 diabetes (about 80%) are associated with obesity (especially with fat located in the abdominal region), but high blood glucose is not directly caused by the obesity. In fact, some lean people also develop this type of diabetes. Obesity associated with oversized adipose cells increases the risk for insulin resistance by the body as more fat is added to these cells during weight gain.

Type 2 diabetes linked to obesity often disappears if the obesity is corrected. Achieving a healthy weight therefore should be a primary goal of treatment, but even limited weight loss can lead to better blood glucose regulation. Although many cases of type 2 diabetes can be relieved by reducing excess adipose tissue stores, many people are not able to lose weight. They remain affected with diabetes and may experience the degenerative complications seen in the type 1 form of the disease. Ketosis, however, is not usually seen in type 2 diabetes. Certain oral medications can also help control blood glucose. Adequate chromium intake is also important for blood glucose regulation (see Chapter 11). Patients with type 2 diabetes may experience decreased effectiveness of their treatments over time resulting in spikes in blood glucose after meals and weight gain. New classes of drugs that mimic gut hormones are helping diabetic patients overcome the chronic

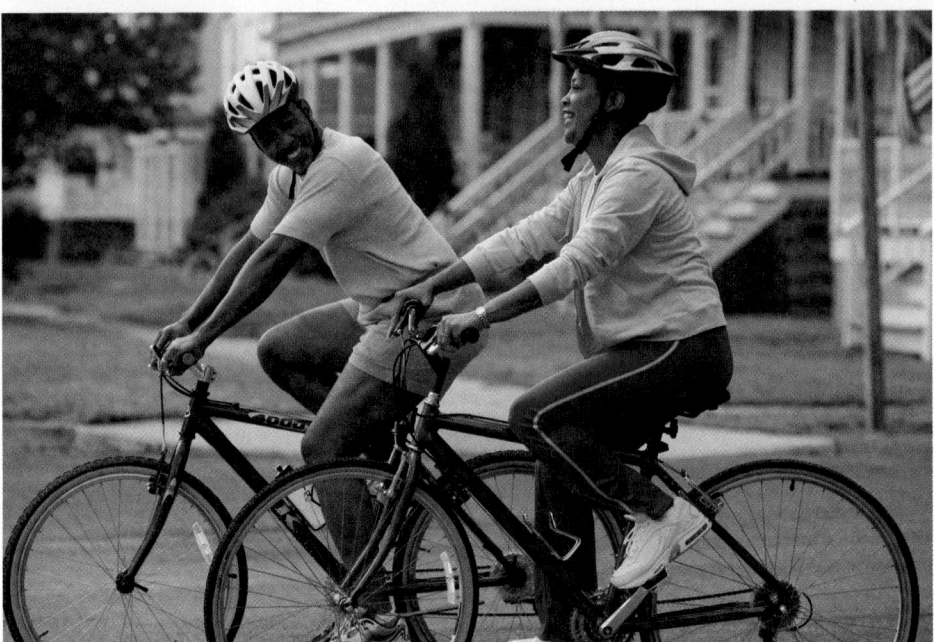

▲ Regular exercise is a key part of a plan to prevent (and control) type 2 diabetes (see Further Reading 8).

problems that conventional treatments alone have been unable to control.

Sometimes it may be necessary to provide insulin injections in type 2 diabetes because nothing else is able to control the disease. (This eventually becomes true in about half of all cases of type 2 diabetes.) Regular physical activity also helps the muscles take up more glucose. And regular meal patterns, with an emphasis on control of calorie intake and consumption of mostly fiber-rich carbohydrates, as well as regular fish intake, is important therapy. Nuts help fulfill the goal of increased fiber consumption. (An almost daily intake of nuts was even shown to reduce the risk of developing type 2 diabetes in one study.) Some sugar consumption is fine with meals, but again these must be substituted for other carbohydrates, not simply added to the meal plan. Distributing carbohydrates throughout the day is also important, as this helps minimize the high and low swings in blood glucose concentrations. Moderate alcohol use is acceptable (1 serving per day) and has been shown to substantially reduce heart attack risk in people with type 2 diabetes. Still, the person must be warned that alcohol can lead to hypoglycemia and that regular testing for this possibility is necessary. And, as mentioned

before, meeting magnesium needs and moderate coffee intake are also helpful.

People with type 2 diabetes who have high blood triglycerides should moderate their carbohydrate intake and increase their intake of unsaturated fat and fiber, as noted earlier for people with type 1 diabetes.

Hypoglycemia

As noted earlier, people with diabetes who are taking insulin sometimes have hypoglycemia if they do not eat frequently enough. Hypoglycemia can also develop in nondiabetic individuals. The two common forms of nondiabetic hypoglycemia are termed *reactive* and *fasting*.

Reactive hypoglycemia occurs 2 to 4 hours after eating a meal, especially a meal high in simple sugars. It results

▶ For more information on diabetes, consult the following websites: **www.diabetes.org** and **www.ndep.nih.gov**.

reactive hypoglycemia Low blood glucose that follows a meal high in simple sugars, with corresponding symptoms of irritability, headache, nervousness, sweating, and confusion; also called *postprandial hypoglycemia*.

in irritability, nervousness, headache, sweating, and confusion. The cause of reactive hypoglycemia is unclear, but it may be overproduction of insulin by the pancreas in response to rising blood glucose. In **fasting hypoglycemia**, blood glucose falls to low concentrations after fasting for about 8 hours to 1 day. It usually is caused by pancreatic cancer, which may lead to excessive insulin secretion. This form of hypoglycemia is rare.

The diagnosis of hypoglycemia requires the simultaneous presence of low blood glucose and the typical hypoglycemic symptoms. Blood glucose of 40 to

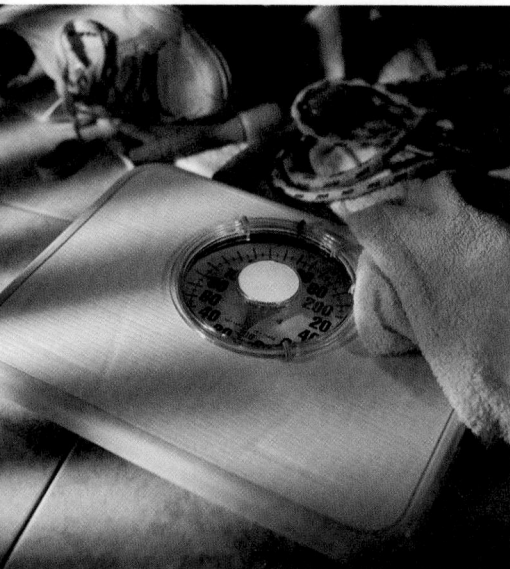

▲ Decreasing body weight and increasing physical activity are interventions to help prevent metabolic syndrome.

fasting hypoglycemia Low blood glucose that follows about a day of fasting.

metabolic syndrome A condition in which a person has poor blood glucose regulation, hypertension, increased blood triglycerides, and other health problems. This condition is usually accompanied by obesity, lack of physical activity, and a diet high in refined carbohydrates. Also called Syndrome X.

50 milligrams per 100 milliliters is suggestive, but just having low blood glucose after eating is not enough evidence to make the diagnosis of hypoglycemia. Although many people think they have hypoglycemia, few actually do.

It is normal for healthy people to have some hypoglycemic symptoms, such as irritability, headache, and shakiness, if they have not eaten for a prolonged period. If you sometimes have symptoms of hypoglycemia, you need to eat regular meals, make sure you have some protein and fat in each meal, and eat complex carbohydrates with ample soluble fiber. Avoid meals or snacks that contain little more than simple carbohydrates. This standard nutrition therapy is one we all could follow. If symptoms continue, try small protein-containing snacks or fruits and juice between meals. Fat, protein, and viscous fiber in the diet tend to moderate swings in blood glucose. Last, moderate caffeine and alcohol intake.

Metabolic Syndrome

Metabolic syndrome, also known as Syndrome X, is characterized by the occurrence of several risk factors for diabetes and cardiovascular disease. The precise definition and criteria for diagnosis have recently been debated by health scholars (see Further Readings 7 and 11). A person with metabolic syndrome has several or all of the following conditions: abdominal obesity (accumulation of fat around and within the midsection), high blood triglycerides, low HDL or "good" cholesterol, hypertension, high fasting blood glucose, increased blood clotting, and increased inflammation (Fig. 4-14). Each aspect of metabolic syndrome is a unique health problem with its own treatment. In metabolic syndrome, however, these risk factors are clustered together, making a person twice as likely to develop cardiovascular disease and five times more likely to develop diabetes.

It is generally accepted that one key element unifies all the aspects of metabolic syndrome: *insulin resistance*. As you learned in this chapter, insulin is a hormone that directs tissues to pull glucose out of the blood and into cells for storage or fuel. With insulin resistance, the pancreas

produces plenty of insulin, but the cells of the body do not respond to it effectively. Instead, excess glucose stays in the bloodstream. For a while the pancreas may be able to compensate for the resistance of cells to insulin by overproducing insulin. Over time, however, the pancreas is unable to keep up the accelerated insulin production and blood glucose levels remain elevated. With metabolic syndrome, blood glucose is not high enough to be classified as diabetes ($\geq$ 126 milligrams per deciliter), but without intervention, it is likely to get worse and eventually lead to diabetes.

Genetics and aging contribute to the development of insulin resistance and the other elements of metabolic syndrome, but environmental factors such as diet and activity play an important role. Obesity, particularly abdominal obesity, is highly related to insulin resistance. More than half of adults in the United States are overweight, 30% are obese, and these numbers continue to climb year after year. Increases in body weight among children and adolescents are of great concern because it places them at high risk for these health problems. This increase in body weight has precipitated a dramatic surge in cardiovascular disease and diabetes risk—an estimated 50 million Americans now have metabolic syndrome.

There is controversy among health professionals over whether to treat each risk factor uniquely or to attempt to integrate therapies to treat all the risk factors simultaneously. For example, the chief culprits contributing to the high blood triglycerides of metabolic syndrome are excessively large meals full of foods rich in simple sugars and refined starches and low in fiber, coupled with little physical activity. Nutrition and lifestyle changes are key strategies in addressing all of the unhealthy conditions of metabolic syndrome as a whole. Suggested interventions include:

- Decrease body weight. Even small improvements (e.g., 5% weight loss) for overweight and obese individuals can lessen disease risk. The most successful weight-loss and weight-maintenance programs include moderate dietary restriction combined with physical activity.

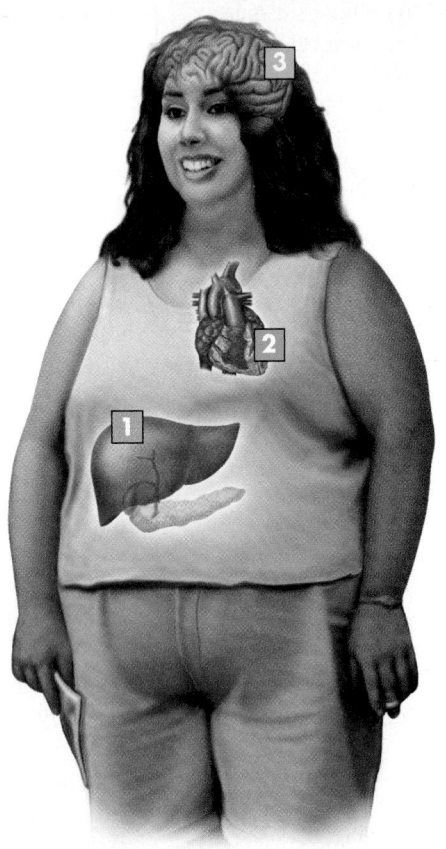

Metabolic Syndrome Risk Indicators

- **High blood pressure**
  130/85 mmHg or higher

- **Low HDL cholesterol**
  - Men with HDL level less than 40 mg/dl
  - Women with HDL level less than 50 mg/dl

- **Elevated glucose**
  Fasting level of 100 mg/dl or higher

- **Elevated triglycerides (blood fat)**
  150 mg/dl or higher

- **Abdominal obesity**
  - Men with waist circumference greater than 40 inches
  - Women with waist circumference greater than 35 inches

Medical Conditions Related to Metabolic Syndrome

1 Type 2 diabetes
Over time, insulin resistance can increase blood glucose levels, which can lead to type 2 diabetes.

2 Coronary artery disease
Elevated blood pressure and cholesterol levels can cause plaque to build up inside coronary arteries, which may eventually lead to a heart attack.

3 Stroke
Plaque buildup in arteries can lead to blood clots that prevent blood flow to the brain, causing damage to brain tissue.

FIGURE 4-14 ▶ For a patient to be diagnosed with metabolic syndrome, he or she must have three of the five risk factors listed above.

- Increase physical activity. To alleviate risks for chronic diseases, the 2010 Dietary Guidelines for Americans include a recommendation to do the equivalent of 150 minutes of moderate-intensity physical activity each week.
- Choose healthy fats. Limiting intakes of total fat, saturated fat, and *trans* fat are generally recommended for improving blood lipids. Including omega-3 fats, such as those found in fish and nuts, is another way to combat chronic disease.
- For those with particularly high risk for cardiovascular disease, medications may be warranted.

Case Study Problems with Milk Intake

Myeshia is a 19-year-old African-American female who recently read about the health benefits of calcium and decided to increase her intake of dairy products. To start, she drank a cup of 1% milk at lunch. Not long afterward, she experienced bloating, cramping, and increased gas production. She suspected that the culprit of this pain was the milk she consumed, especially because her parents and her sister complain of the same problem. She wanted to determine if other milk products were, in fact, the cause of her discomfort so the next day she substituted a cup of yogurt for the glass of milk at lunch. Subsequently, she did not have any pain.

Answer the following questions, and check your response in Appendix A.

1. Why did Myeshia believe that she was sensitive to milk?
2. What component of milk is likely causing the problems that Myeshia experiences after drinking milk?
3. Why does this component cause intestinal discomfort in some individuals?
4. What is the name of this condition?
5. What groups of people are most likely to experience this condition?
6. Why did consuming yogurt not cause the same effects for Myeshia?
7. Are there any other products on the market that can replace regular milk or otherwise alleviate symptoms for individuals with this problem?
8. Can people with this condition ever drink regular milk?
9. What nutrients may be inadequate in the diet if dairy products are not consumed?
10. Why do some individuals have trouble tolerating milk products during or immediately after an intestinal viral infection?

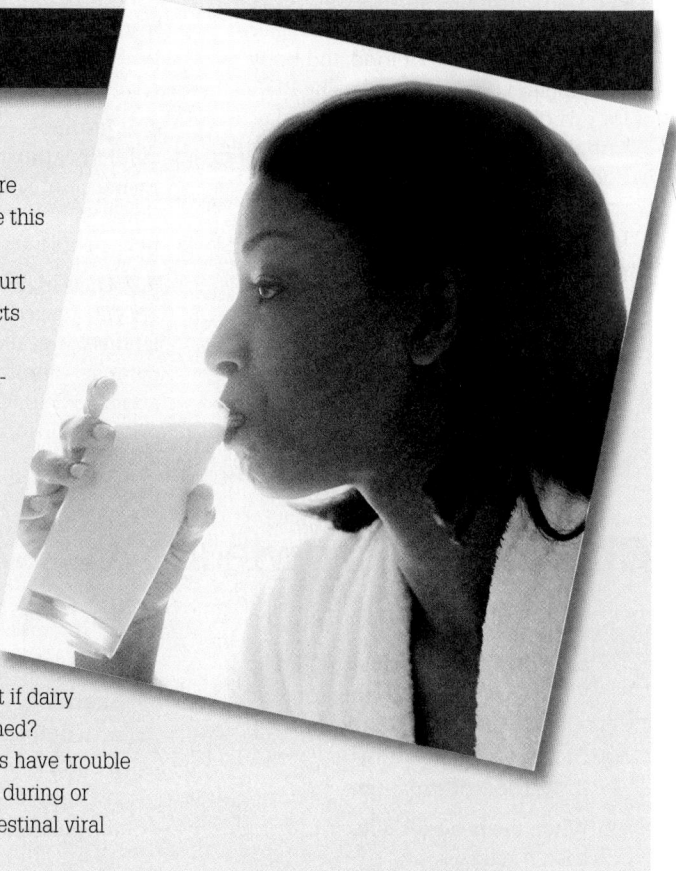

Summary (Numbers refer to numbered sections in the chapter.)

4.1. Carbohydrates are created in plants through photosynthesis. They are our main fuel source for body cells. Some carbohydrates promote health more than others.

4.2 The common monosaccharides in food are glucose, fructose, and galactose. Once these are absorbed from the small intestine and delivered to the liver, much of the fructose and galactose is converted to glucose.

The major disaccharides are sucrose (glucose + fructose), maltose (glucose + glucose), and lactose (glucose + galactose). When digested, these yield their component monosaccharides.

4.3 One major group of polysaccharides consists of storage forms of glucose: starches in plants and glycogen in humans. These can be broken down by human digestive enzymes, releasing the glucose units. The main plant starches—straight-chain amylose and branched-chain amylopectin—are digested by enzymes in the mouth and small intestine. In humans, glycogen is synthesized in the liver and muscle tissue from glucose. Under the influence of hormones, liver glycogen is readily broken down to glucose, which can enter the bloodstream.

4.4 Fiber is composed primarily of the polysaccharides cellulose, hemicellulose, pectin, gum, and mucilage, as well as the noncarbohydrate lignins. These substances are not broken down by human digestive enzymes. However, soluble (also called viscous) fiber is fermented by bacteria in the large intestine.

4.5 Table sugar, honey, jelly, fruit, and plain baked potatoes are some of the most concentrated sources of carbohydrates. Other high-carbohydrate foods, such as pie and fat-free milk, are diluted by either fat or protein. Nutritive sweeteners in food include sucrose, high-fructose corn syrup, brown sugar, and maple syrup. Several alternative sweeteners are approved for use by FDA: saccharin, aspartame, sucralose, neotame, acesulfame-K, and tagatose.

4.6 Some starch digestion occurs in the mouth. Carbohydrate digestion is completed in the small intestine. Some plant fibers are digested by the bacteria present in the large intestine; undigested plant fibers become part of the feces. Monosaccharides in the intestinal contents mostly follow an active absorption process. They are then transported via the portal vein that leads directly to the liver.

The ability to digest large amounts of lactose often diminishes with age. People in some ethnic groups are especially affected. This condition often develops early in childhood and is referred to as *lactose maldigestion*. Undigested lactose travels to the large intestine, resulting in such symptoms as abdominal gas, pain, and diarrhea. Most people with lactose maldigestion can tolerate cheese, yogurt, and moderate amounts of milk.

4.7 Carbohydrates provide calories (on average, 4 kcal per gram), protect against wasteful breakdown of food and body protein, and prevent ketosis. The RDA for carbohydrate is 130 grams per day. If carbohydrate intake is inadequate for the body's needs, protein is metabolized to provide glucose for energy needs. However, the price is loss of body protein, ketosis, and eventually a general body weakening. For this reason, low-carbohydrate diets are not recommended for extended periods.

Blood glucose concentration is regulated within a narrow range of 70 to 99 mg/dl. Insulin and glucagon are hormones that control blood glucose concentration. When we eat a meal, insulin promotes glucose uptake by cells. When fasting, glucagon promotes glucose release from glycogen stores in the liver.

4.8 Insoluble (also called nonfermentable) fiber provides mass to the feces, thus easing elimination. In high doses, soluble fiber can help control blood glucose in diabetic people and lower blood cholesterol.

4.9 Diets high in complex carbohydrates are encouraged as a replacement for high-fat diets. A goal of about half of calories as complex carbohydrates is a good one, with about 45% to 65% of total calories coming from carbohydrates in general. Foods to consume are whole-grain cereal products, pasta, legumes, fruits, and vegetables. Many of these foods are rich in fiber.

4.10 Moderating sugar intake, especially between meals, reduces the risk of dental caries. Alternative sweeteners, such as aspartame, aid in reducing intake of sugars.

N&YH Diabetes is characterized by a persistent high blood glucose concentration. A healthy diet and regular physical activity are helpful in treating both type 1 and type 2 diabetes. Insulin is the main medication employed—it is required in type 1 diabetes and may be used in type 2 diabetes.

Check Your Knowledge (Answers to the following questions are below.)

1. Dietary fiber
   a. raises blood cholesterol levels.
   b. speeds up transit time for food through the digestive tract.
   c. causes diverticulosis.
   d. causes constipation.

2. When the pancreas detects excess glucose, it releases the
   a. enzyme amylase.
   b. monosaccharide glucose.
   c. hormone insulin.
   d. hormone glucagon.

3. Cellulose is a(n)
   a. indigestible fiber.
   b. simple carbohydrate.
   c. energy-yielding nutrient.
   d. animal polysaccharide.

4. Digested white sugar is broken into _____ and _____.
   a. glucose, lactose
   b. glucose, fructose

   c. sucrose, maltose
   d. fructose, sucrose

5. Starch is a
   a. complex carbohydrate.
   b. fiber.
   c. simple carbohydrate.
   d. gluten.

6. Fiber content of the diet can be increased by adding
   a. fresh fruits.
   b. fish and poultry.
   c. eggs.
   d. whole grains and cereals.
   e. Both a and d.

7. Which form of diabetes is most common?
   a. type 1
   b. type 2
   c. type 3
   d. gestational

8. The recommended daily intake for fiber is approximately _____ grams.
   a. 5   c. 100
   b. 30   d. 450

9. Glucose, galactose, and fructose are
   a. disaccharides.
   b. sugar alcohols.
   c. monosaccharides.
   d. polysaccharides.

10. One of the components of metabolic syndrome is
   a. obesity.
   b. diabetes.
   c. low blood sugar.
   d. low blood pressure.

Answer Key: 1. b (LO 4.6), 2. c (LO 4.5), 3. a (LO 4.1), 4. b (LO 4.1), 5. a (LO 4.1), 6. e (LO 4.2), 7. b (LO 4.8), 8. b (LO 4.7), 9. c (LO 4.1), 10. b (LO 4.8)

Study Questions (Numbers refer to Learning Outcomes)

1. Why do we need carbohydrates in the diet? (LO 4.3)
2. What are the three major monosaccharides and the three major disaccharides? Describe how each plays a part in the human diet. (LO 4.3)
3. Why are some foods that are high in carbohydrates, such as cookies and fat-free milk, not considered to be concentrated sources of carbohydrates? (LO 4.3)
4. Describe the digestion of the various types of carbohydrates in the body. (LO 4.3)
5. Describe the reason why some people are unable to tolerate high intakes of milk. (LO 4.3)
6. List three alternatives to simple sugars for adding sweetness to the diet. (LO 4.3)
7. Outline the basic steps in blood glucose regulation, including the roles of insulin and glucagon. (LO 4.3)
8. What are the important roles that fiber plays in the diet? (LO 4.3)
9. Summarize current carbohydrate intake recommendations. (LO 4.3)
10. What, if any, are the proven ill effects of sugar in the diet? (LO 4.3)

What Would You Choose Recommendations

It is smart to reach for a carbohydrate-containing beverage when needing quick energy. Some of us also rely on caffeine in drinks to give us a boost. Many beverages on the market contain high concentrations of carbohydrate as "added sugar." This added sugar has recently been the subject of many debates because the consumption of added sugars, especially high-fructose corn syrup (HFCS), has been on the rise since 1970 and excessive sugar intake has been linked to several adverse health conditions. The major sources of added sugars are sodas, energy drinks, and sports drinks (review Fig. 4-12). Sugar intake has been of concern based on total consumption and source of the sugar.

Does the source of the added sugar matter? As we discussed in Chapter 4, the glucose and fructose in HFCS exist in free form, compared to their bound form in cane sugar, sucrose. Sucrose is quickly and completely digested to glucose and fructose in the small intestine so that nearly equal amounts of glucose and fructose are being absorbed from beverages containing HFCS and pure cane sugar. Once absorbed, fructose is more easily converted to and stored as fat than glucose. Researchers speculate that the extra 5% of fructose in HFCS may be responsible for increased body fatness. Also, fructose does not stimulate the release of chemical signals that help to regulate appetite, in the same way glucose does. Changes in appetite can dramatically affect how much of a particular sweetener is consumed. It is still unclear whether altering the type of sweetener in soft drinks will impact our nation's obesity epidemic.

The larger issue here is the abundance of empty calories supplied by soft drinks—regardless of whether these calories come

from HFCS or pure cane sugar (sucrose). HFCS represents nearly 100% of sweeteners in all soft drinks, and since soft drink consumption has skyrocketed, so has HFCS consumption. Studies show that liquid calories do not promote satiety in the same way that food calories do. In other words, consuming 250 kcal of cola does not mean that you will feel full enough to eat one less slice of pizza to compensate for those extra kcal. Excess calories from any source will lead to weight gain over time.

Clearly, portion size is an issue. A 20-ounce bottle of regular cola contains about 68 grams (about 15 teaspoons) of sweeteners. This means that a soft drink sweetened with HFCS has 37 grams of fructose compared to 34 grams in a 20-ounce soft drink made with pure cane sugar. Both types of soft drink provide about 250 kcal. Is 3 grams of fructose a big deal? In terms of a soft drink, a 12-ounce soda, such as the Jones Root Beer Soda, will have proportionally less sugar (48 grams) due to its smaller volume. If you consume one soft drink per day or less, the type of sweetener is not likely to make a big difference. If you consume several soft drinks per day, you would be better off choosing a beverage that does not contain calories, such as diet cola or water.

Beverages, such as Coke Zero®, with artificial sweeteners such as aspartame, typically are calorie-free and therefore provide you with no energy when you need a boost. You may feel a temporary lift from the caffeine in some of these products. Water is the perfect drink to restore fluid losses and prevent dehydration but also contains no calories for energy.

Your best choice when needing a quick energy boost in this case is the low-fat chocolate milk. The chocolate milk not only

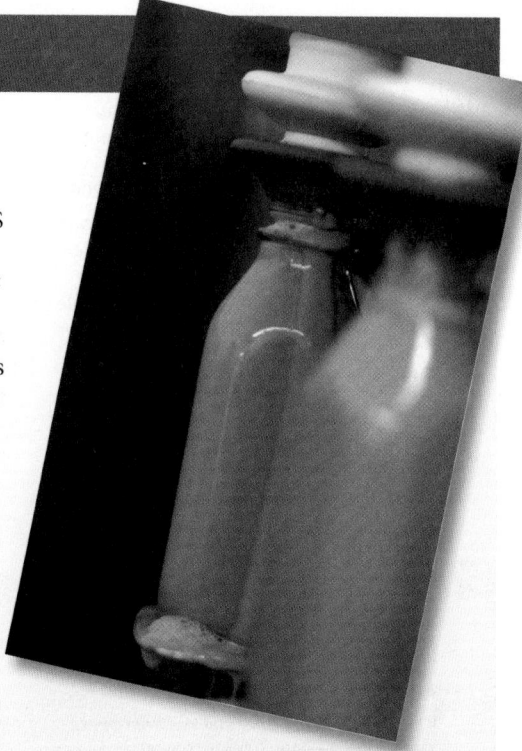

▲ Chocolate milk is a very nutritious beverage that provides protein, vitamins, and minerals, along with calories.

provides less sugar than the sodas on our list but is also the best source of total nutrition. Most convenience stores sell chocolate milk in pint bottles or ½-pint (8-ounce) cartons (similar to those served in school cafeterias). The 8-ounce carton of chocolate milk provides a good amount of calories (150 kcal) as well as 8 grams of protein, 2.5 grams of fat, and 25 grams of sugar. It also provides calcium (290 mg), vitamin A (490 IU), and vitamin D (2.8 micrograms), as well as other vitamins and minerals. A pint bottle (16 ounces) would provide twice the amount of calories and other nutrients. In addition, the chocolate provides a source of caffeine that you may be looking for.

Further Readings

1. ADA Reports: Position of the American Dietetic Association: Use of nutritive and nonnutritive sweeteners. *Journal of the American Dietetic Association* 104:225, 2004.

   When currently recommended diet practices are met, such as the Dietary Guidelines for Americans, use of some nutritive and nonnutritive sweeteners is acceptable. The text of the article explores in detail both classes of sweeteners, in turn supporting this overall conclusion.

2. American Diabetes Association: Nutrition recommendations and interventions for diabetes: A position statement of the American Diabetes Association. *Diabetes Care* 31 (suppl 1):S61, 2008.

   This article provides a comprehensive look at the treatment of diabetes. Goals for therapy and medical tools to help reach those goals are highlighted.

3. American Diabetes Association and American Dietetic Association: *Choose your foods: Exchange lists for diabetes.* 2008.

   This update of a booklet that has been in existence for more than 50 years is used as the basis for nutrition education for diabetes meal planning. Foods are grouped into general categories (or lists) that, per serving size, are similar in macronutrients and calories. Changes have been made so they are easier to use and foods within the lists have been updated.

4. Bray GA and others: Consumption of high-fructose corn syrup in beverages may play a role in the epidemic of obesity. *American Journal of Clinical Nutrition,* 79(4):537, 2004.

   The intake of high-fructose corn syrup (HFCS) was studied and compared to the development of obesity. The increase in HFCS use has paralleled the increase in obesity. Although differences in the digestion, absorption, and metabolism of fructose compared to glucose have been suggested as explanations for the relationship between HFCS and obesity, studies have been unable to separate the effects of the widely consumed sweetener from the impact of other environmental factors.

5. Cowie CC and others: Prevalence of diabetes and impaired fasting glucose in adults in the U.S. population. *Diabetes Care* 29:1263, 2006.

   The results of this study of the National Health And Nutrition Examination Survey (NHANES) suggest that 73 million Americans have diabetes or are at risk based on higher-than-normal blood glucose levels. The prevalence of diagnosed diabetes increased significantly over the last decade, and minority groups remain disproportionately affected. The overall prevalence of total diabetes in 1999–2002 was 9.3% (19.3 million), consisting of 6.5% diagnosed and 2.8% undiagnosed.

   The prevalence of diagnosed diabetes rose from 5.1% in 1988–1994 to 6.5% in 1999–2002. The prevalence of total diabetes was much greater (21.6%) in older individuals aged ≥ 65 years. Diagnosed diabetes was twice as prevalent in non-Hispanic blacks and Mexican-Americans compared with non-Hispanic whites.

6. Food and Nutrition Board: *Dietary reference intakes for energy, carbohydrate, fiber, fat, fatty acids, cholesterol, protein, and amino acids.* Washington, DC: National Academy Press, 2005.

   This report provides the latest guidance for macronutrient intakes. With regard to carbohydrate, the RDA has been set at 130 grams per day. Carbohydrate intake should range from 45% to 65% of calorie intake. Sugars added to foods should constitute no more than 25% of calorie intake.

7. Grundy SM: Does a diagnosis of metabolic syndrome have a value in clinical practice? *American Journal of Clinical Nutrition* 83:1248, 2006.

   The metabolic syndrome concept has led to the development of clinical guidelines by the World Health Organization and the National Cholesterol Education Program. These guidelines have been well accepted by medical professionals. This article reviews the new diagnosis of metabolic syndrome and discusses why organizations including the American Diabetes Association and many diabetes specialists have not embraced the clustering of its risk factors.

8. Hayes C, Kriska A: Role of physical activity in diabetes management and prevention. *Journal of the American Dietetic Association* 108:S19, 2008.

   Evidence supporting the important role of physical activity in the prevention and treatment of diabetes has accumulated. Despite the benefits of physical activity, many people are physically inactive. As the prevalence of overweight and obesity, prediabetes, and type 2 diabetes rises, physical inactivity has become an urgent public health concern. This article reviews research about physical activity/exercise in diabetes and summarizes the current exercise recommendations. This information can be used by health professionals to make safe and effective recommendations for integrating physical activity/exercise into plans for individuals with or at risk of developing diabetes.

9. McMillan-Price J and others: Comparison of 4 diets of varying glycemic load on weight loss and cardiovascular risk reduction in overweight and obese young adults. *Archives of Internal Medicine* 166:1466, 2006.

   In this study of 128 overweight or obese young adults, both high-protein and low-glycemic

   index diets increased body fat loss. Cardiovascular disease risk was decreased best with a high-carbohydrate, low-glycemic index diet.

10. Park Y and others: Dietary fiber intake and risk of colorectal cancer. *Journal of the American Medical Association* 294:2849, 2005.

    In this large analysis of pooled data from 13 prospective studies, dietary fiber was inversely associated with risk of colorectal cancer when data were adjusted for age. However, when other dietary risk factors (red meat, total milk, and alcohol intake) were accounted for, high-dietary fiber intake was not associated with a decreased risk of colorectal cancer. The authors conclude that a diet high in dietary fiber from whole plant foods can still be advised because this has been related to lower risks of other chronic conditions, including heart disease and diabetes.

11. Pastors JG: Metabolic syndrome—is obesity the culprit? *Today's Dietitian* 8(3):12, 2006.

    Metabolic syndrome, especially its link to obesity, has become better understood in recent years. This article reviews the role of obesity, the dilemmas of diagnosis, new diet and activity guidelines, and the need for a combination of therapeutic approaches for metabolic syndrome.

12. Savaiano DA and others: Lactose intolerance symptoms assessed by meta-analysis: A grain of truth that leads to exaggeration. *Journal of Nutrition* 136:1107, 2006.

    An analysis of the results of 21 studies of lactose intolerance revealed that lactose is not a major cause of symptoms for lactose maldigesters after a moderate intake of dairy foods equaling about 1 cup.

13. Slavin J and others: How fiber affects weight regulation. *Food Technology,* p. 34, February 2008.

    High-fiber diets are linked to lower body weight. This article discusses the effect of different fibers on satiety and food intake. Dietary fiber has intrinsic, hormonal, and intestinal effects that decrease food intake by promoting satiety. Examples of these effects include decreased gastric emptying and/or slowed energy and nutrient absorption.

14. Swann L: Educate your brain about whole grain. *Today's Dietitian* 8(6):36, 2006.

    The 2005 Dietary Guidelines recommend 3 or more ounces of whole-grain products per day. This equals about one-half of one's intake from the grain group. Recent surveys, however, have found that only 5% of American adults eat one-half of their grains as whole grains. This article discusses the need to better educate consumers about whole grain including better definitions and ways of measuring these foods.

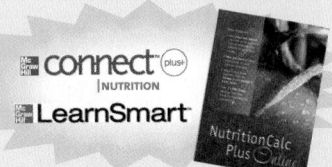

To get the most out of your study of nutrition, go to McGraw-Hill's online resources: Connect www.mcgrawhillconnect.com, **where you will find NutritionCalc Plus, LearnSmart, and many other dynamic tools.**

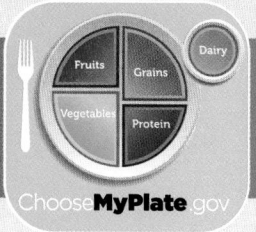

I. Estimate Your Fiber Intake

Review the sample menus shown in Table 4-7. The first menu contains 1600 kcal and 25 grams of fiber (AI for women); the second menu contains 2100 kcal and 38 grams of fiber (AI for men).

TABLE 4-7 Sample Menus Containing 1600 kcal with 25 g of Fiber and 2000 kcal with 38 g of Fiber*

Menu	25 g Fiber			38 g Fiber		
	Serving Size	Carbohydrate Content (g)	Fiber Content (g)	Serving Size	Carbohydrate Content (g)	Fiber Content (g)
Breakfast						
Muesli cereal	1 cup	60	6	1 cup	60	6
Raspberries	½ cup	11	2	½ cup	11	2
Whole-wheat toast	1 slice	13	2	2 slices	26	4
Margarine	1 tsp	0	0	1 tsp	0	0
Orange juice	1 cup	28	0	1 cup	28	0
1% milk	1 cup	24	0	1 cup	24	0
Coffee	1 cup	0	0	1 cup	0	0
Lunch						
Bean and vegetable burrito	2 small	50	4.5	3 small	75	7
Guacamole	¼ cup	5	4	¼ cup	5	4
Monterey Jack cheese	1 oz	0	0	1 oz	0	0
Pear (with skin)	1	25	4	1	25	4
Carrot sticks	—	—	—	¾ cup	6	3
Sparkling water	2 cups	0	0	2 cups	0	0
Dinner						
Grilled chicken (no skin)	3 oz	0	0	3 oz	0	0
Salad	½ cup red cabbage ½ cup romaine ¼ cup peach slices	7	3	½ cup red cabbage ½ cup romaine 1 cup peach slices	19	6
Toasted almonds	—	—	—	½ oz	3	2
Fat-free salad dressing	2 tbsp	0	0	2 tbsp	0	0
1% milk	1 cup	24	0	1 cup	24	0
Total		247	25		306	38

*The overall diet is based on MyPlate Breakdown of approximate energy content: carbohydrate 58%; protein 12%; fat 30%.

To roughly estimate your daily fiber consumption, determine the number of servings that you ate yesterday from each food category listed here. If you are not meeting your needs, how could you do so? Multiply the serving amount by the value listed and then add up the total amount of fiber.

Food	Servings	Grams
Vegetables (serving size: 1 cup raw leafy greens or 1/2 cup other vegetables)	_____ × 2	_____
Fruits (serving size: 1 whole fruit; 1/2 grapefruit; 1/2 cup berries or cubed fruit; 1/4 cup dried fruit)	_____ × 2.5	_____
Beans, lentils, split peas (serving size: 1/2 cup cooked)	_____ × 7	_____
Nuts, seeds (serving size: 1/4 cup; 2 tbsp peanut butter)	_____ × 2.5	_____
Whole grains (serving size: 1 slice whole-wheat bread; 1/2 cup whole-wheat pasta, brown rice, or other whole grain; 1/2 each bran or whole-grain muffin)	_____ × 2.5	_____
Refined grains (serving size: 1 slice bread, 1/2 cup pasta, rice, or other processed grains; and 1/2 each refined bagels or muffins)	_____ × 1	_____
Breakfast cereals (serving size: check package for serving size and amount of fiber per serving)	_____ × grams of fiber per serving	_____
Total Grams of Fiber =		_____

Adapted from Fiber: Strands of protection. *Consumer Reports on Health*, p. 1, August 1999.

How does your total fiber intake for yesterday compare with the general recommendation of 25 to 38 g of fiber per day for women and men, respectively? If you are not meeting your needs, how could you do so?

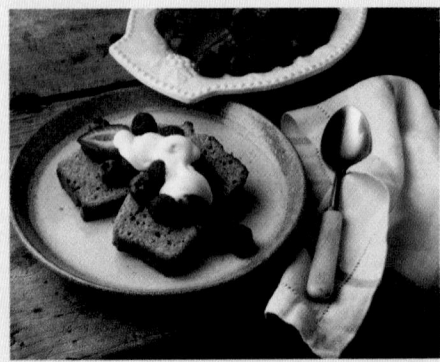

▲ This dessert is an excellent source of fiber from
2 slices of whole-wheat banana bread (7 grams)
with ½ cup of berries (1.8 grams) and 2 ounces
of yogurt for a total of 8.8 grams of fiber.

II. Can You Choose the Sandwich with the Most Fiber?

Assume the sandwiches on this blackboard are available at your local deli and sandwich shop. All of the sandwiches provide about 350 kcal. The fiber content ranges from about 1 gram to about 7.5 grams. Rank the sandwiches from highest amount of fiber to lowest amount; then check your answers at the bottom of the page.

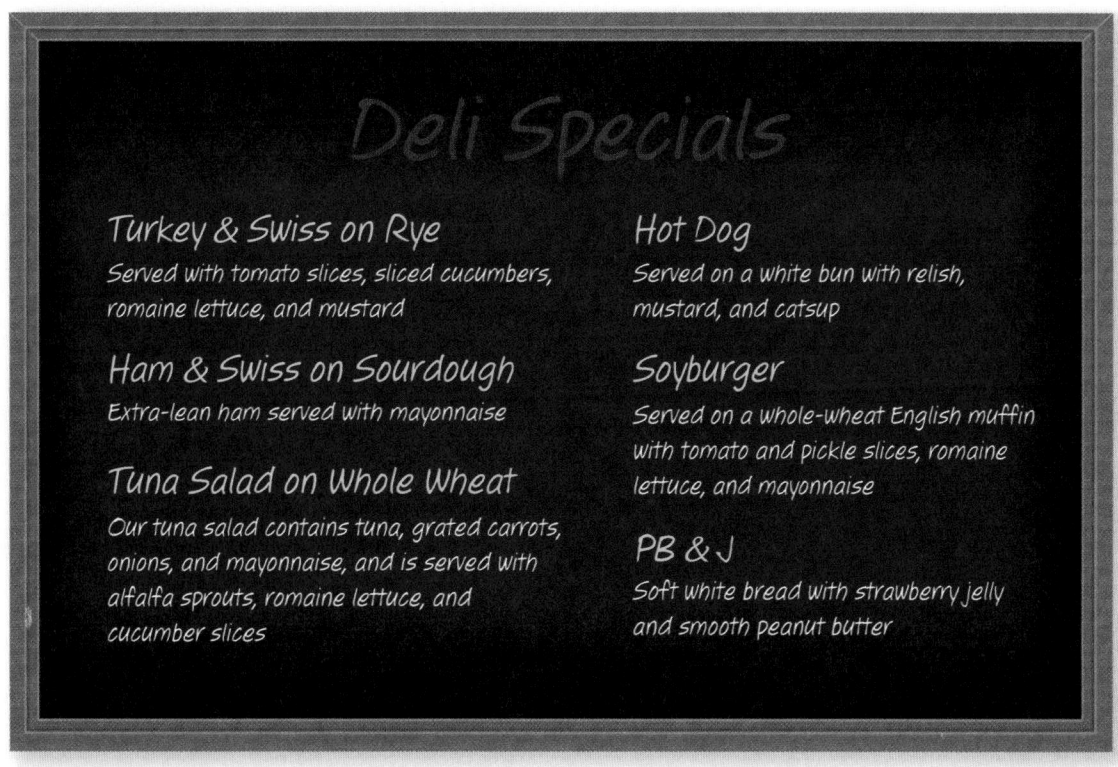

Deli Specials

Turkey & Swiss on Rye
Served with tomato slices, sliced cucumbers, romaine lettuce, and mustard

Ham & Swiss on Sourdough
Extra-lean ham served with mayonnaise

Tuna Salad on Whole Wheat
Our tuna salad contains tuna, grated carrots, onions, and mayonnaise, and is served with alfalfa sprouts, romaine lettuce, and cucumber slices

Hot Dog
Served on a white bun with relish, mustard, and catsup

Soyburger
Served on a whole-wheat English muffin with tomato and pickle slices, romaine lettuce, and mayonnaise

PB & J
Soft white bread with strawberry jelly and smooth peanut butter

Answer Key:
1. Soyburger: 7.5 grams
2. Tuna Salad on Whole Wheat: 7 grams
3. Turkey & Swiss on Rye: 4 grams
4. PB & J: 3 grams
5. Ham & Swiss on Sourdough: 1.5 grams
6. Hot Dog: 1 gram

Chapter 5 Lipids

Student Learning Outcomes

Chapter 5 is designed to allow you to:

5.1 Understand the common properties of lipids.

5.2 List four classes of lipids (fats) and the role of each in nutritional health. Distinguish between fatty acids and triglycerides.

5.3 Differentiate among saturated, monounsaturated, and polyunsaturated fatty acids in terms of structure and food sources.

5.4 Explain how lipids are digested and absorbed.

5.5 Name the classes of lipoproteins and classify them according to their functions.

5.6 Discuss the implications of various fats, including omega-3 fatty acids, with respect to cardiovascular disease.

5.7 List the function of lipids, including the two essential fatty acids.

5.8 Explain the roles of phospholipids in the body.

5.9 Discuss the functions of cholesterol in the body.

5.10 Explain the recommendations for fat intake.

5.11 Characterize the symptoms of cardiovascular disease and highlight some known risk factors.

What Would You Choose?

Several of your friends are getting together for a cookout and you have volunteered to be the grill master. Hamburgers will be the main "protein" portion of your meal. (Remember the size of that group on MyPlate?) You have heard that eating red meat is bad for your heart. Is all red meat bad for your heart? In the meat section of the grocery store, you see several varieties of ground beef. Which of the following types of ground beef would you choose for heart health?

a Ground round

b Ground chuck

c Ground sirloin

d Ground beef

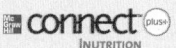 **Think about your choice as you read Chapter 5, then see our recommendations at the end of the chapter. To learn more about ground beef choices, check out the Connect site:** www.mcgrawhillconnect.com

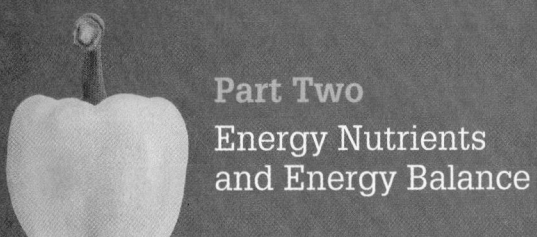
L ipids contain more than twice the calories per gram (on average, 9 kcal) as proteins and carbohydrates (on average, 4 kcal each). Consumption of common solid fats also contributes to the risk of cardiovascular disease. As the comic in this chapter suggests, for these reasons, some concern about certain lipids is warranted, but lipids also play vital roles both in the body and in foods. Their presence in the diet is essential to good health, and in general, lipids such as those found in plant oils and fish, such as the salmon pictured here, should comprise 20% to 35% of an adult's total calorie intake.

Let's look at lipids in detail—their forms, functions, metabolism, and food sources. Chapter 5 will also look at the link between various lipids and the major "killer" disease in North America: cardiovascular disease, which involves the heart, including the coronary arteries (coronary heart disease), as well as other arteries in the body.

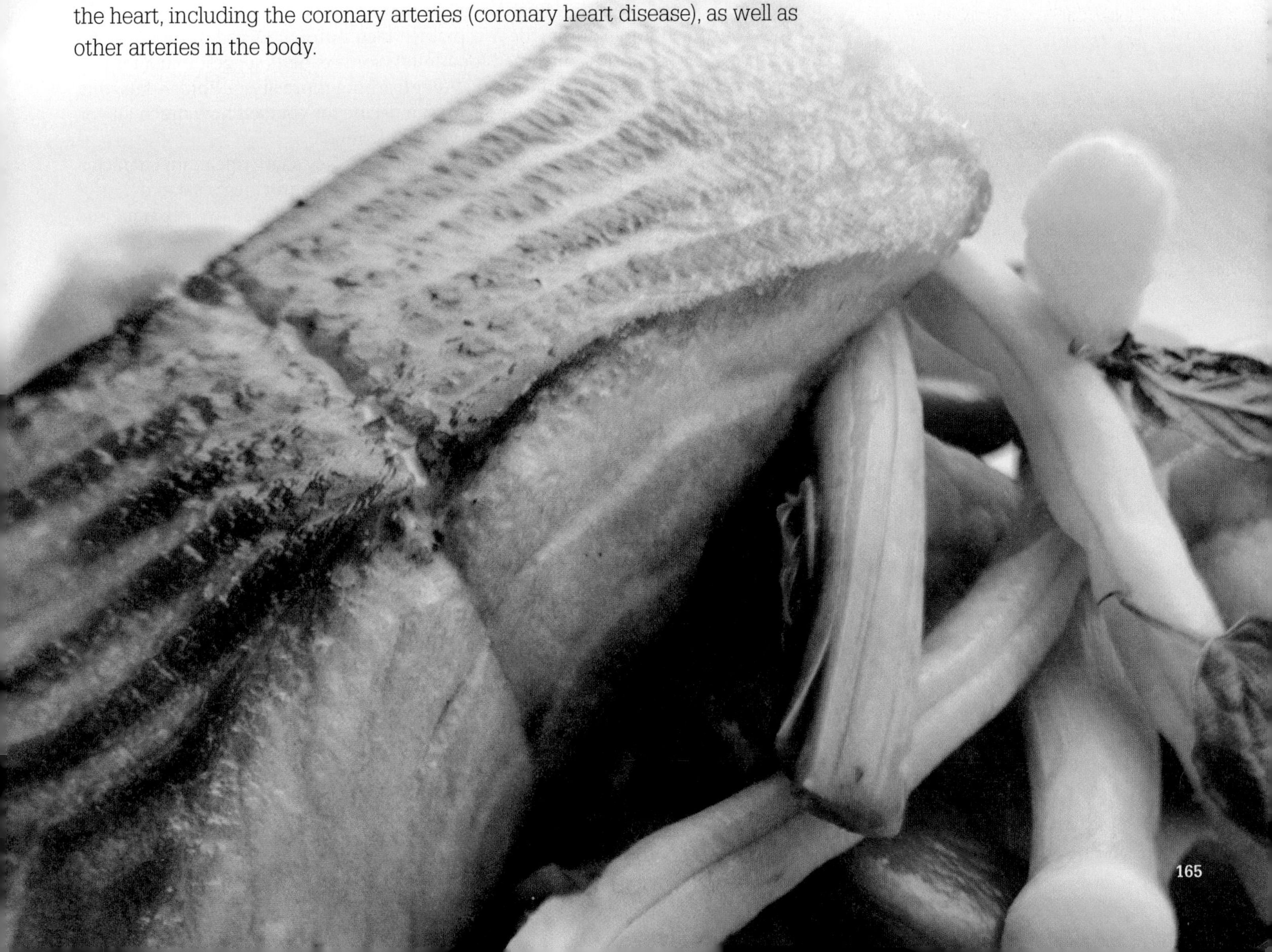

Refresh Your Memory

As you begin your study of lipids in Chapter 5, you may want to review:

- Legal definitions for various label descriptors, such as low fat and fat free in Chapter 2
- The concept of energy density in Chapter 2
- The processes of digestion and absorption in Chapter 3
- The metabolic syndrome in Chapter 4

5.1 Lipids: Common Properties

Humans need very little fat in their diet to maintain health. In fact, the body's need for the essential fatty acids can be met by daily consumption of about 2 to 4 tablespoons of plant oil incorporated into foods and consumption of fatty fish such as salmon or tuna at least twice weekly. If fish is not consumed, the essential fatty acids in canola oil, soybean oil, and walnuts contribute much of the same health benefits as those found in fish. Thus, one could follow a purely vegetarian diet containing about 10% of calories from fat and still maintain health. However, as long as animal fat, cholesterol, and other solid fat are minimized, fat intake can safely be higher than that 10% allotment. The Food and Nutrition Board suggests that fat intake can be as high as 35% of calories consumed for an adult (the Acceptable Macronutrient Distribution Range for fat is 20%–35% of calories consumed for adults). Some experts suggest that an intake as high as 40% of calories is appropriate. After learning more about lipids—fats, oils, and related compounds—in Chapter 5, you can decide for yourself how much fat you want to consume, as well as how to track your daily intake.

Lipids are a diverse group of chemical compounds. They share one main characteristic: They do not readily dissolve in water. Think of an oil and vinegar salad dressing. The oil is not soluble in the water-based vinegar; on standing, the two separate into distinct layers, with oil on top and vinegar on the bottom.

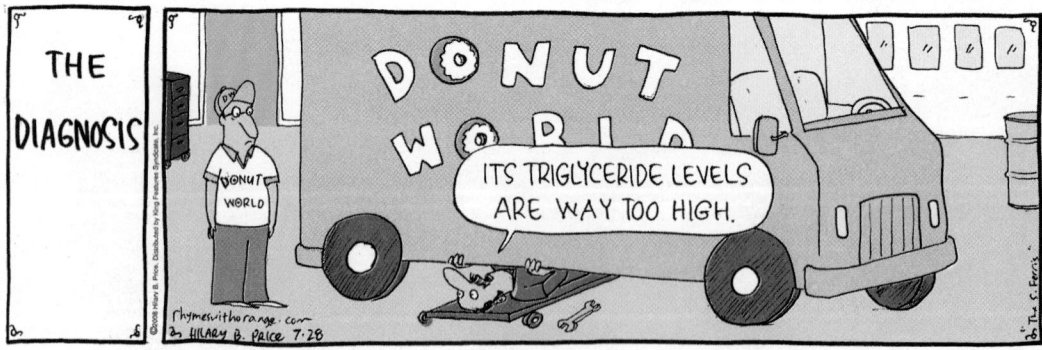

High fat, low fat, no fat—which is best? And why is there such a debate? Would it be easier just to avoid fat altogether? Doesn't a high-fat diet lead to obesity? To cardiovascular disease? Overall, which are the "best" fats, and why are French fries, "donuts," stick margarine, and crackers getting such a bad rap? Chapter 5 provides some answers.

© 2001 Batiuk, Inc. Distributed by North American Syndicates, Inc. All rights reserved.

5.2 Lipids: Main Types

The chemical structure of lipids is diverse. Lipids (mostly fats and oils) are composed primarily of the elements carbon and hydrogen; they contain fewer oxygen **atoms** than do carbohydrates. Lipids yield more calories per gram than do carbohydrates—on the average, 9 kcal per gram—because of this difference in composition. **Triglycerides** are the most common type of lipid found in the body and in foods. Each triglyceride molecule consists of three fatty acids bonded to **glycerol. Phospholipids** and **sterols,** including **cholesterol,** are also classified as lipids, although their structures can be quite different from the structure of triglycerides. All of these lipid compounds are described in Chapter 5.

Food experts, such as chefs, call lipids that are solid at room temperature *fats,* and lipids that are liquid *oils.* Most people use the word *fat* to refer to all lipids because they don't realize there is a difference. However, *lipid* is a generic term that includes triglycerides and many other substances. To simplify our discussion, Chapter 5 primarily uses the term *fat.* When necessary for clarity, the name of a specific lipid, such as cholesterol, will be used. This word use is consistent with the way many people use these terms.

Fatty Acids: The Simplest Form of Lipids

In the body and in foods, fatty acids are found in the main form of lipids, triglycerides. A fatty acid is basically a long chain of carbons bonded together and flanked by hydrogens. At one end of the molecule (the alpha end), is an **acid group.** At the other end (the omega end) is a **methyl group** (Fig. 5-1).

Fats in foods are not composed of a single type of fatty acid. Rather, each dietary fat, or triglyceride, is a complex mixture of many different fatty acids, the combination of which provides each food its unique taste and smell.

Fatty acids can be saturated or unsaturated. Chemically speaking, a carbon atom can form four bonds. Within the carbon chain of a fatty acid, the carbons bond to other carbons and to hydrogens. The carbons that make up the chain of a **saturated fatty acid** are all connected to each other by single bonds. This allows for the maximum number of hydrogens to be bound. Just as a sponge can be saturated (full) with water, a saturated fatty acid such as stearic acid is saturated with hydrogen (Fig. 5-1a).

Most fats high in saturated fatty acids, such as animal fats, remain solid at room temperature. A good example is the solid fat surrounding a piece of uncooked steak. Chicken fat, semisolid at room temperature, contains less saturated fat than beef fat. However, in some foods, saturated fats are suspended in liquid, such as the butterfat in whole milk, so the solid nature of these fats at room temperature is less apparent.

If the carbon chain of a fatty acid contains a double bond, those carbons in the chain have fewer bonds to share with hydrogen, and the chain is said to be *unsaturated.* A fatty acid with only one double bond is **monounsaturated** (Fig. 5-1b). Canola and olive oils contain a high percentage of monounsaturated fatty acids. Likewise, if two or more of the bonds between the carbons are double bonds, the fatty acid is even less saturated with hydrogens, and so it is **polyunsaturated** (Fig. 5-1c, d). Corn, soybean, sunflower, and safflower oils are rich in polyunsaturated fatty acids.

Unsaturated fatty acids can exist in two different structural forms, the *cis* and *trans* forms. In their natural form, monounsaturated and polyunsaturated fatty acids usually are in the *cis* form (Fig. 5-2). By definition, the resulting *cis* **fatty acid** has the hydrogens on the same side of the carbon-carbon double bond. During certain types of food processing (discussed later in this chapter), some hydrogens are

triglyceride The major form of lipid in the body and in food. It is composed of three fatty acids bonded to glycerol, an alcohol.

glycerol A three-carbon alcohol used to form triglycerides.

phospholipid Any of a class of fat-related substances that contain phosphorus, fatty acids, and a nitrogen-containing base. The phospholipids are an essential part of every cell.

sterol A compound containing a multi-ring (steroid) structure and a hydroxyl group (–OH). Cholesterol is a typical example.

cholesterol A waxy lipid found in all body cells. It has a structure containing multiple chemical rings that is found only in foods that contain animal products.

saturated fatty acid A fatty acid containing no carbon-carbon double bonds.

monounsaturated fatty acid A fatty acid containing one carbon-carbon double bond.

polyunsaturated fatty acid A fatty acid containing two or more carbon-carbon double bonds.

cis **fatty acid** A form of an unsaturated fatty acid that has the hydrogens lying on the same side of the carbon-carbon double bond.

acid group
$$-\overset{\overset{\textstyle O}{\|}}{\underset{|}{C}}-OH$$

methyl group $-CH_3$

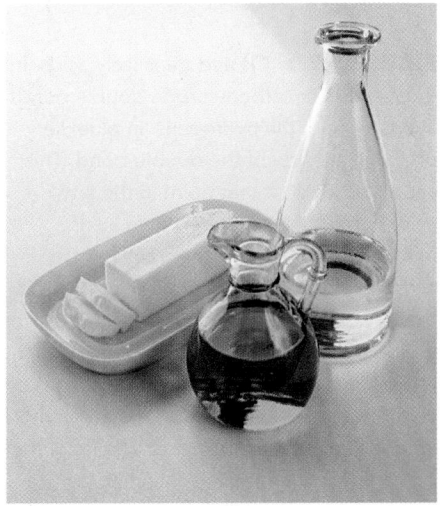

▲ Saturated fats, such as butter, are solid at room temperature, whereas unsaturated fats, such as olive and corn oil, are liquid at room temperature.

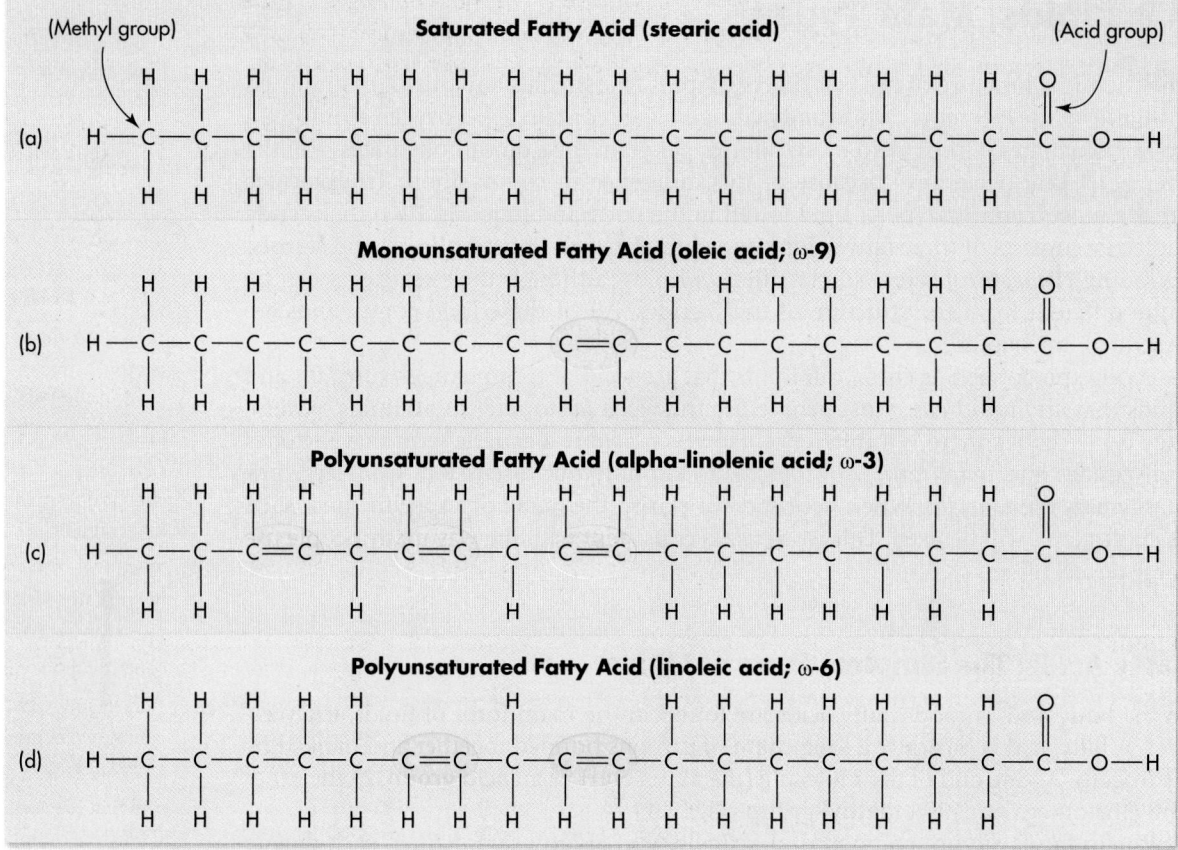

FIGURE 5-1 ▶ Chemical forms of saturated, monounsaturated, and polyunsaturated fatty acids. Each of the depicted fatty acids contains 18 carbons, but they differ from each other in the number and location of double bonds. The double bonds are shaded. The linear shape of saturated fatty acids, as shown in (a), allows them to pack tightly together and so form a solid at room temperature. In contrast, unsaturated fatty acids have "kinks" where double bonds interrupt the carbon chain (see Figure 5-2). Thus, unsaturated fatty acids pack together only loosely, and are usually liquid at room temperature.

FIGURE 5-2 ▶ *Cis* and *trans* fatty acids. In the *cis* form at carbon-carbon double bonds in a fatty acid, the hydrogens (in blue) lie on the same side of the double bond. This causes a "kink" at that point in the fatty acid, typical of unsaturated fatty acids in foods. In contrast, in the *trans* form at carbon-carbon double bonds in a fatty acid, the hydrogens lie across from each other at the double bond. This causes the fatty acid to exist in a linear form, like a saturated fatty acid. *Cis* fatty acids are much more common in foods than *trans* fatty acids. The latter are primarily found in foods containing partially-hydrogenated fats, notably stick margarine, shortening, and deep-fat fried foods.

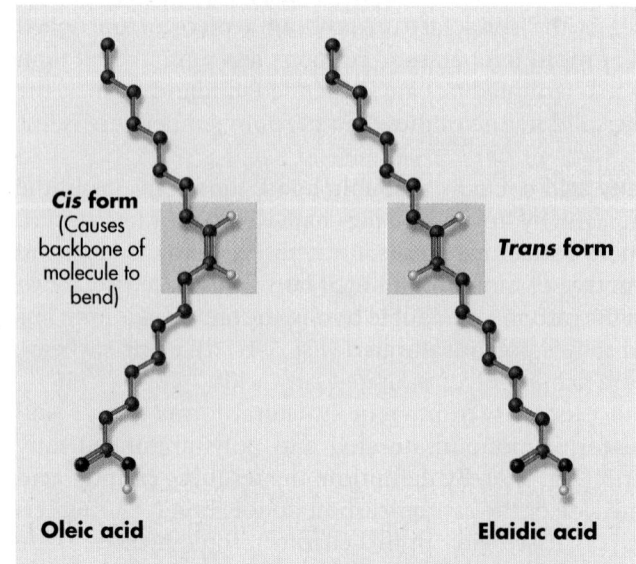

transferred to opposite sides of the carbon-carbon double bond, creating the *trans* form, or a ***trans* fatty acid**. As seen in Figure 5-2, the *cis* bond causes the fatty acid backbone to bend, whereas the *trans* bond allows the backbone to remain straighter. This makes it similar to the shape of a saturated fatty acid. The Food and Nutrition Board suggests limiting intake of *trans* fatty acids in processed foods (also referred to as *trans* fats) as much as possible. Later you will see why.

You may be surprised to learn that some *trans* fatty acids, known as conjugated linoleic acid (CLA), occur naturally. CLA is a family of derivatives of the fatty acid linoleic acid. The bacteria that live in the rumens of some animals (cows, sheep, and goats, for example) produce *trans* fatty acids that eventually appear in foods such as beef, milk, and butter. These naturally occurring *trans* fats are currently under study for possible health benefits, including prevention of cancer, decreasing body fat, and improvement in insulin levels in diabetics. About 20% of *trans* fatty acids in our diets come from this source. Dietary supplements of CLA are available but are highly variable in their quality.

Overall, a fat or an oil is classified as saturated, monounsaturated, or polyunsaturated based on the type of fatty acids present in the greatest concentration (Fig. 5-3). Fats in foods that contain primarily saturated fatty acids are solid at room temperature, especially if the fatty acids have long carbon chains (i.e., a **long-chain fatty acid**), as opposed to shorter versions. In contrast, fats containing primarily polyunsaturated or monounsaturated fatty acids (long chain or shorter) are usually liquid at room temperature. Almost all fatty acids in the body and in foods are long-chain varieties.

An important characteristic of unsaturated fatty acids is the location of the double bonds. If the first double bond starts three carbons from the methyl (omega) end of the fatty acid, it is an **omega-3 (ω-3) fatty acid** (review Fig. 5-1c). If the first double bond is located six carbons from the omega end, it is an **omega-6 (ω-6) fatty acid** (review Fig. 5-1d). Following this scheme, an omega-9 fatty acid has its first double bond starting at the ninth carbon from the methyl end (review Fig. 5-1b). In foods, **alpha-linolenic acid** is the major omega-3 fatty acid; **linoleic acid** is the major omega-6 fatty acid. These are also the **essential fatty acids** we need to consume (more on this in the later section about putting lipids to work in the body). **Oleic acid** is the major omega-9 fatty acid.

Triglycerides

Fats and oils in foods are mostly in the form of triglycerides. The same is true for fats found in body structures. Although some fatty acids are transported in the bloodstream attached to proteins, most fatty acids are formed into triglycerides by cells in the body.

As noted before, triglycerides contain a simple three-carbon alcohol, glycerol, which serves as a backbone for the three attached fatty acids (Fig. 5-4a). Removing one fatty acid from a triglyceride forms a **diglyceride**. Removing two fatty acids from a triglyceride forms a **monoglyceride**. Later you will see that before most dietary fats are absorbed in the small intestine, the two outer fatty acids are typically removed from the triglyceride. This produces a mixture of fatty acids and monoglycerides, absorbed into the intestinal cells. After absorption, the fatty acids and monoglycerides are mostly re-formed into triglycerides.

Phospholipids

Phospholipids are another class of lipid. Like triglycerides, they are built on a backbone of glycerol. However, at least one fatty acid is replaced with a compound containing phosphorus (and often other elements, such as nitrogen) (Fig. 5-4b).

trans **fatty acid** A form of an unsaturated fatty acid, usually a monounsaturated one when found in food, in which the hydrogens on both carbons forming the double bond lie on opposite sides of that bond.

long-chain fatty acid A fatty acid that contains 12 or more carbons.

omega-3 (ω-3) fatty acid An unsaturated fatty acid with the first double bond on the third carbon from the methyl end (—CH₃).

omega-6 (ω-6) fatty acid An unsaturated fatty acid with the first double bond on the sixth carbon from the methyl end (—CH₃).

alpha-linolenic acid An essential omega-3 fatty acid with 18 carbons and three double bonds.

linoleic acid An essential omega-6 fatty acid with 18 carbons and two double bonds.

essential fatty acids Fatty acids that must be supplied by the diet to maintain health. Currently, only linoleic acid and alpha-linolenic acid are classified as essential.

oleic acid An omega-9 fatty acid with 18 carbons and one double bond.

diglyceride A breakdown product of a triglyceride consisting of two fatty acids bonded to a glycerol backbone.

monoglyceride A breakdown product of a triglyceride consisting of one fatty acid attached to a glycerol backbone.

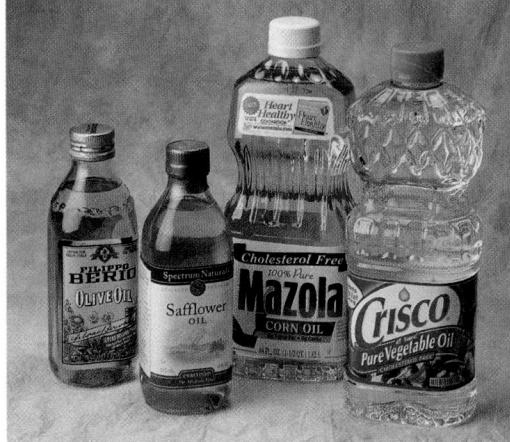

▲ Plant oils vary in their content of specific fatty acids. Oils similar in appearance may vary significantly in fatty acid composition. Olive and canola oils are rich in monounsaturated fat; olive oil has been awarded much attention in recent years. Canola oil, however, is a much less expensive choice of monounsaturated fat. Safflower oil is rich in polyunsaturated fat.

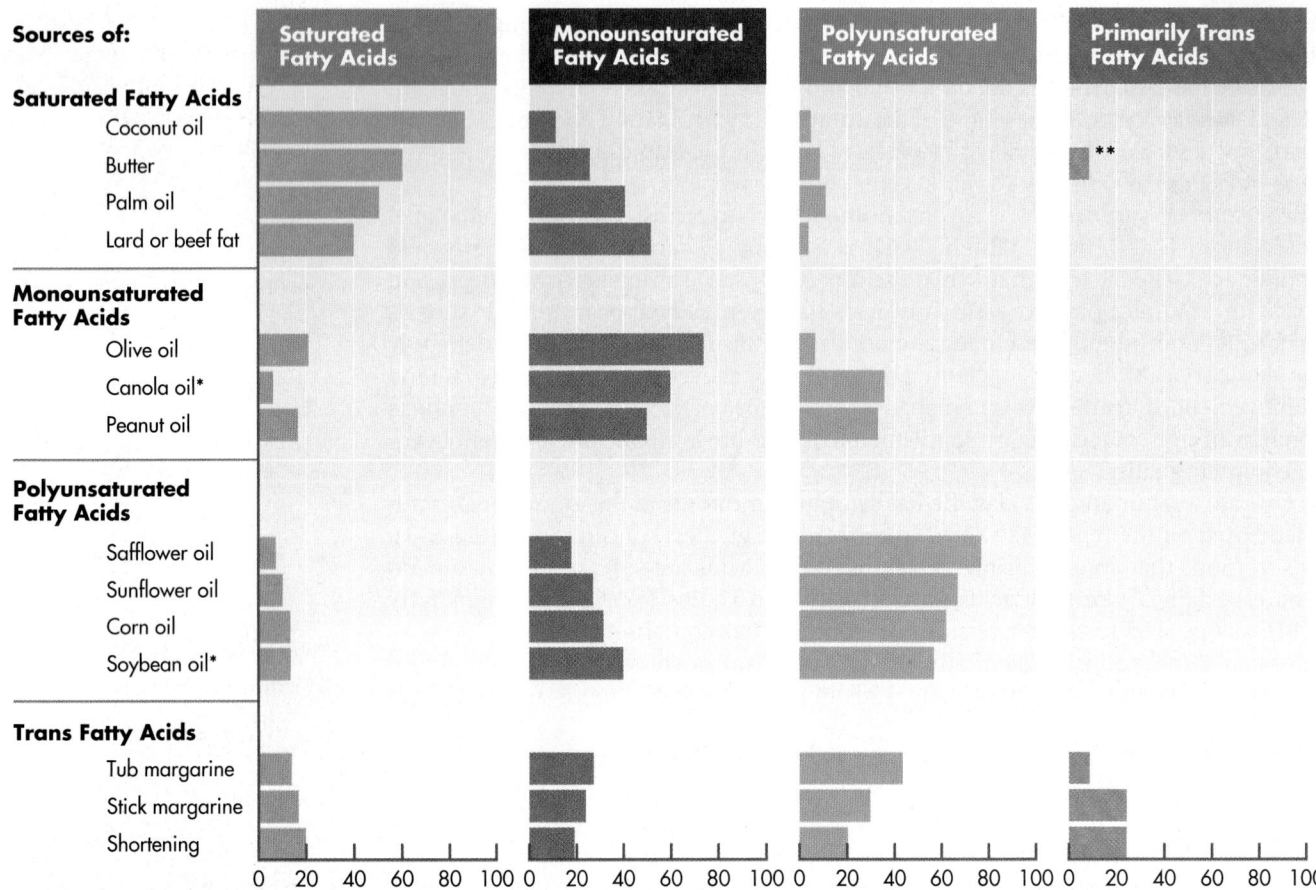

*Rich source of the omega-3 fatty acid alpha-linolenic acid (7% and 12% of total fatty acid content for soybean oil and canola oil, respectively).

**The natural *trans* fatty acids in butter are not harmful and may even have health-promoting properties, such as preventing certain forms of cancer.

FIGURE 5-3 ▶ Saturated, monounsaturated, polyunsaturated, and *trans* fatty acid composition of common fats and oils (expressed as % of all fatty acids in the product).

lecithin A group of compounds that are major components of cell membranes.

Many types of phospholipids exist in the body, especially in the brain. They form important parts of cell membranes. **Lecithin** is a common example of a phospholipid. Various forms are found in body cells and they participate in fat digestion, absorption, and transport. The body is able to produce all the phospholipids it needs. Even though lecithin is sold as a dietary supplement and is present as an additive in many foods, phospholipids such as this one are not essential components of the diet.

Sterols

Sterols are a class of lipids with a characteristic multi-ringed structure that makes them different from the other lipids already discussed (Fig. 5-4c). The most common example of a sterol is cholesterol. This waxy substance doesn't look like a triglyceride—it doesn't have a glycerol backbone or any fatty acids. Still, because it doesn't readily dissolve in water, it is a lipid. Among other functions, cholesterol is used to form certain hormones and bile acids and is incorporated into cell structures. The body can make all the cholesterol it needs.

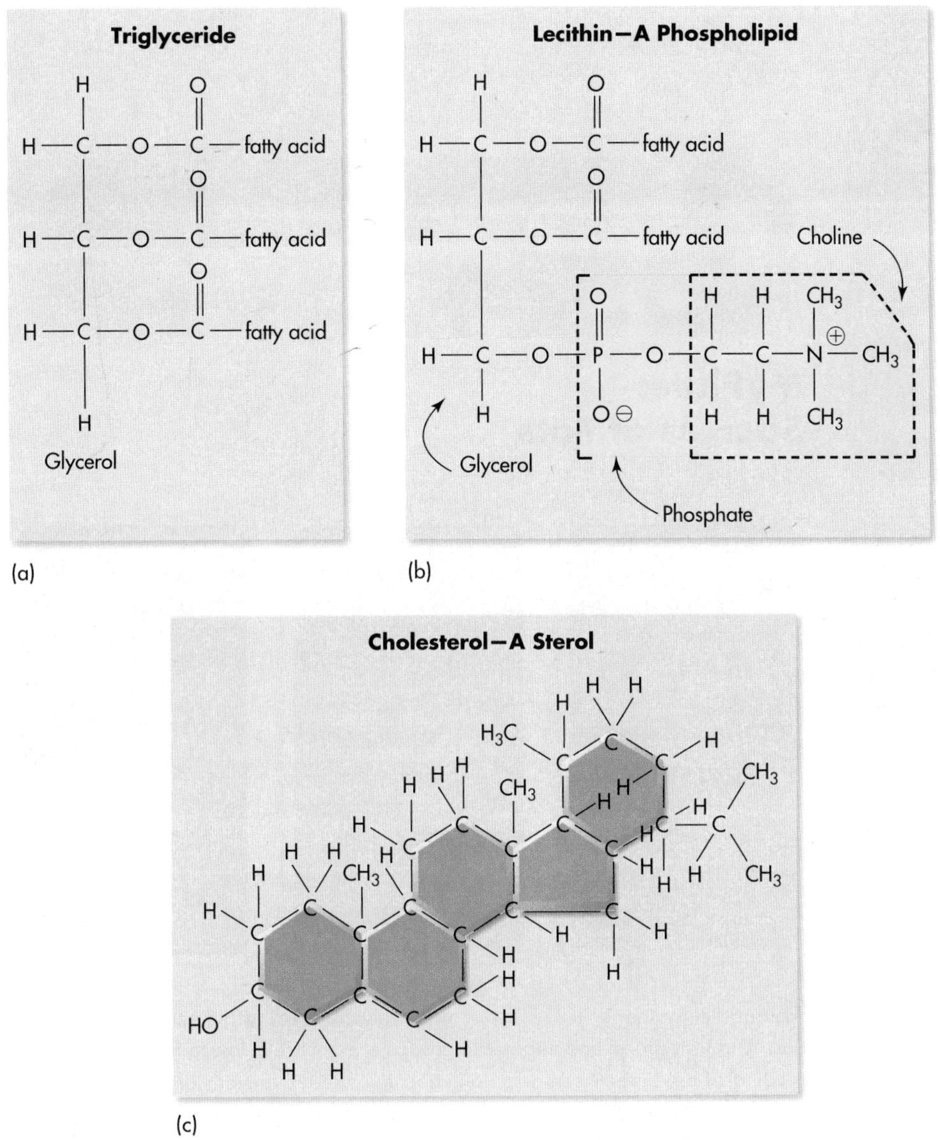

Triglyceride (a)

Lecithin—A Phospholipid (b)

Cholesterol—A Sterol (c)

FIGURE 5-4 ▶ Chemical forms of common lipids: (a) triglyceride, (b) phospholipid (in this case, lecithin), and (c) sterol (in this case, cholesterol).

CONCEPT CHECK

Lipids are a group of compounds that do not dissolve readily in water. Included in this group are fatty acids, triglycerides, phospholipids, and sterols. Fatty acids can be distinguished from one another by the length of the carbon skeleton and the number and position of double bonds along that skeleton. Saturated fatty acids contain no double bonds within their carbon skeleton; that is, they are fully saturated with hydrogens. Monounsaturated fatty acids contain one carbon-carbon double bond, and polyunsaturated fatty acids contain two or more of these bonds. Certain omega-3 and omega-6 fatty acids are essential in the human diet.

Triglycerides are the major form of fat in the body and in foods. These consist of three fatty acids bonded to a glycerol backbone. Phospholipids are similar to triglycerides in structure, but at least one fatty acid is replaced by another compound containing phosphorus. Phospholipids play an important structural role in cell membranes. Sterols, another class of lipids, do not resemble either triglycerides or phospholipids, but instead have a multi-ringed structure. Cholesterol, one example of a sterol, forms parts of cells, some hormones, and bile acids. Whereas certain essential fatty acids (as components of triglycerides) are needed in the diet, the body produces all the triglycerides, phospholipids, and cholesterol it needs. Next we will discuss the sources of fat in foods (Fig. 5-5).

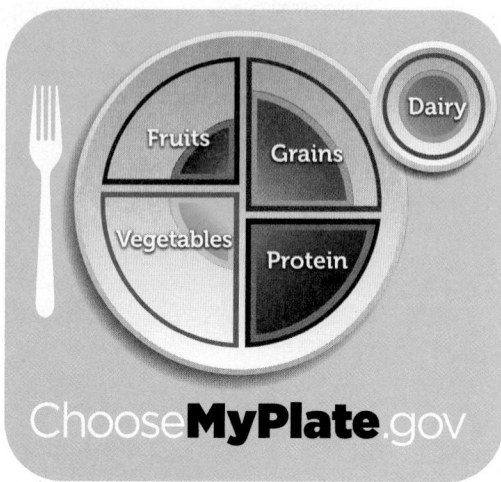

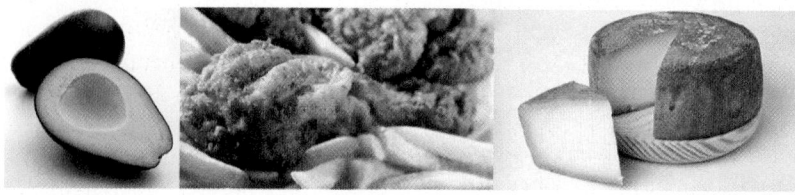

MyPlate: Sources of Fats

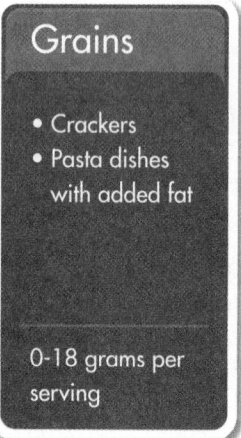

Grains

• Crackers
• Pasta dishes with added fat

0-18 grams per serving

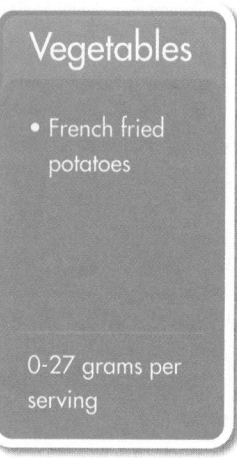

Vegetables

• French fried potatoes

0-27 grams per serving

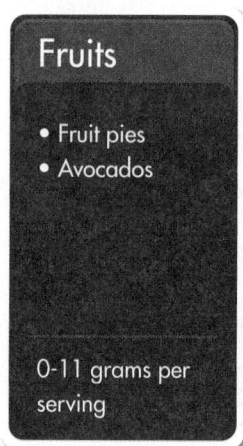

Fruits

• Fruit pies
• Avocados

0-11 grams per serving

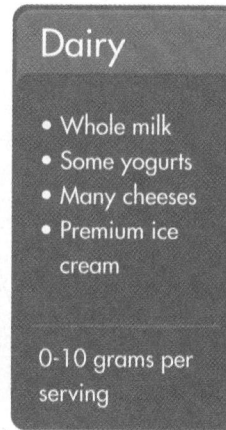

Dairy

• Whole milk
• Some yogurts
• Many cheeses
• Premium ice cream

0-10 grams per serving

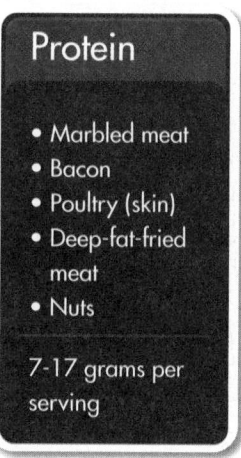

Protein

• Marbled meat
• Bacon
• Poultry (skin)
• Deep-fat-fried meat
• Nuts

7-17 grams per serving

FIGURE 5-5 ▶ Sources of fats from MyPlate. The fill of the background color (none, 1/3, 2/3, or completely covered) within each group in the plate indicates the average nutrient density for fat in that group. The fruit group and vegetable groups are generally low in fat. In the other groups, both high-fat and low-fat choices are available. Careful reading of food labels can help you choose lower-fat versions of some foods. In general, any type of frying adds significant amounts of fat to a product, as with French fries and fried chicken. With regard to physical activity, fats are a key fuel in prolonged events, such as long-distance cycling, long-distance running, and prolonged slow to brisk walking.

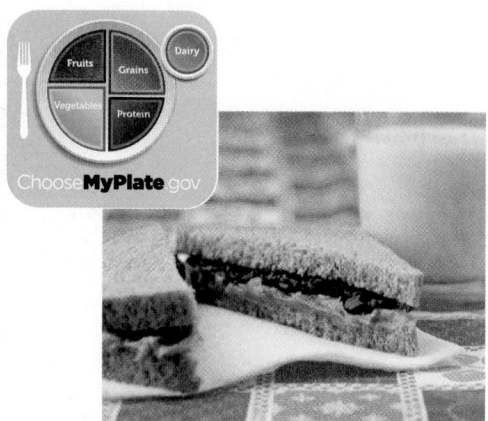

▲ This peanut butter (**protein**) and jelly (**fruit**) sandwich on whole-grain bread (**grain**) with low-fat milk (**dairy**) follows **MyPlate** guidelines well and provides a healthy source of plant fat from the peanut butter. Which section are we missing?

5.3 Fats and Oils in Foods

Lipids in the form of triglycerides are abundant in the North American diet. The foods highest in fat (and therefore energy dense) include salad oils and spreads such as butter, margarine, and mayonnaise. All of these foods contain close to 100% of calories as fat. In reduced-fat margarines, water replaces some of the fat. Whereas regular margarines are 80% fat by weight (11 grams per tablespoon), some reduced-fat margarines are as low as 30% fat by weight (4 grams per tablespoon). When used in recipes, the extra water added to these margarines can cause texture and volume changes in the finished product. Cookbooks can suggest alterations in recipes to compensate for the increased water content of these products.

Still considering the overall fat content, whole foods highest in fat include nuts, bologna, avocados, and bacon, which have about 80% of calories as fat. Next, peanut butter and cheddar cheese have about 75%. Marbled steak and hamburgers (ground chuck) have about 60%, and chocolate bars, ice cream, doughnuts, and whole milk have about 50% of calories as fat. Eggs, pumpkin pie, and cupcakes have 35%, as do lean cuts of meat, such as top round (and ground round) and sirloin. Bread contains about 15%. Finally, foods such as cornflakes, sugar, and fat-free milk have essentially no fat. Figure 5-6 shows examples of food sources of fat. Label reading is necessary to determine the true fat content of food.

The type of fat in food is important to consider along with the total amount of fat. Animal fats are the chief contributors of saturated fatty acids to the North American diet. About 40% to 60% of total fat in dairy and meat products is in the form of saturated fatty acids. In contrast, plant oils contain mostly unsaturated fatty acids, ranging from 73% to 94% of total fat. A moderate to high proportion of total fat (49% to 77%) is supplied by monounsaturated fatty acids in canola oil, olive oil, and peanut oil. Some animal fats are also good sources of monounsaturated fatty acids (30% to 47%) (review Fig. 5-3). Corn, cottonseed, sunflower, soybean, and safflower oils contain mostly polyunsaturated fatty acids (54% to 77%). These plant oils supply the majority of the linoleic and alpha-linolenic acid in the North American food supply.

Wheat germ, peanuts, egg yolk, soy beans, and organ meats are rich sources of phospholipids. Phospholipids such as lecithin, a component of egg yolks, are often added to salad dressing. Lecithin is used as an **emulsifier** in these and other products because of its ability to keep mixtures of lipids and water from separating (see Fig. 5-7). Emulsifiers are added to salad dressings to keep the vegetable oil suspended in water. Eggs added to cake batters likewise emulsify the fat with the milk.

Cholesterol is found only in animal foods. An egg yolk contains about 210 milligrams of cholesterol. Eggs are our main dietary source of cholesterol, along with

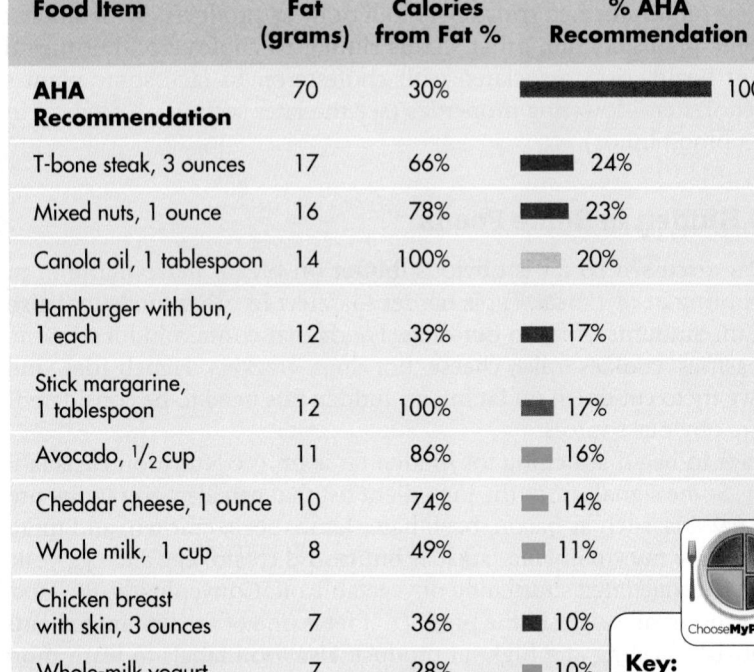

▲ Peanuts are a source of lecithins, as are wheat germ and egg yolks.

emulsifier A compound that can suspend fat in water by isolating individual fat droplets, using a shell of water molecules or other substances to prevent the fat from coalescing.

FIGURE 5-6 ▶ Food sources of fat compared to the American Heart Association (AHA) recommendation of 70 grams per day, or 30% of calories from fat for a 2100 kcal diet.

Food Sources of Fat

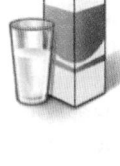
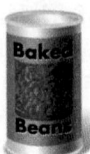

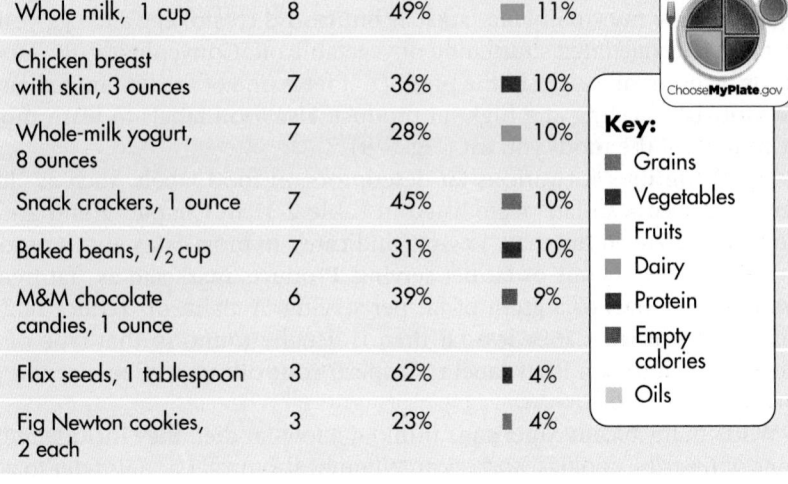

Food Item	Fat (grams)	Calories from Fat %	% AHA Recommendation
AHA Recommendation	70	30%	100%
T-bone steak, 3 ounces	17	66%	24%
Mixed nuts, 1 ounce	16	78%	23%
Canola oil, 1 tablespoon	14	100%	20%
Hamburger with bun, 1 each	12	39%	17%
Stick margarine, 1 tablespoon	12	100%	17%
Avocado, 1/2 cup	11	86%	16%
Cheddar cheese, 1 ounce	10	74%	14%
Whole milk, 1 cup	8	49%	11%
Chicken breast with skin, 3 ounces	7	36%	10%
Whole-milk yogurt, 8 ounces	7	28%	10%
Snack crackers, 1 ounce	7	45%	10%
Baked beans, 1/2 cup	7	31%	10%
M&M chocolate candies, 1 ounce	6	39%	9%
Flax seeds, 1 tablespoon	3	62%	4%
Fig Newton cookies, 2 each	3	23%	4%

ChooseMyPlate.gov

Key:
■ Grains
■ Vegetables
■ Fruits
■ Dairy
■ Protein
■ Empty calories
■ Oils

FIGURE 5-7 ▶ Emulsifiers in action. Emulsifiers prevent many brands of salad dressings and other condiments from separating into layers of water and fat. Emulsifiers attract fatty acids inside and have a water-attracting group on the outside. Add them to salad dressing, shake well, and they hold the oil in the dressing away from the water. Emulsification is important in both food production and fat digestion/absorption.

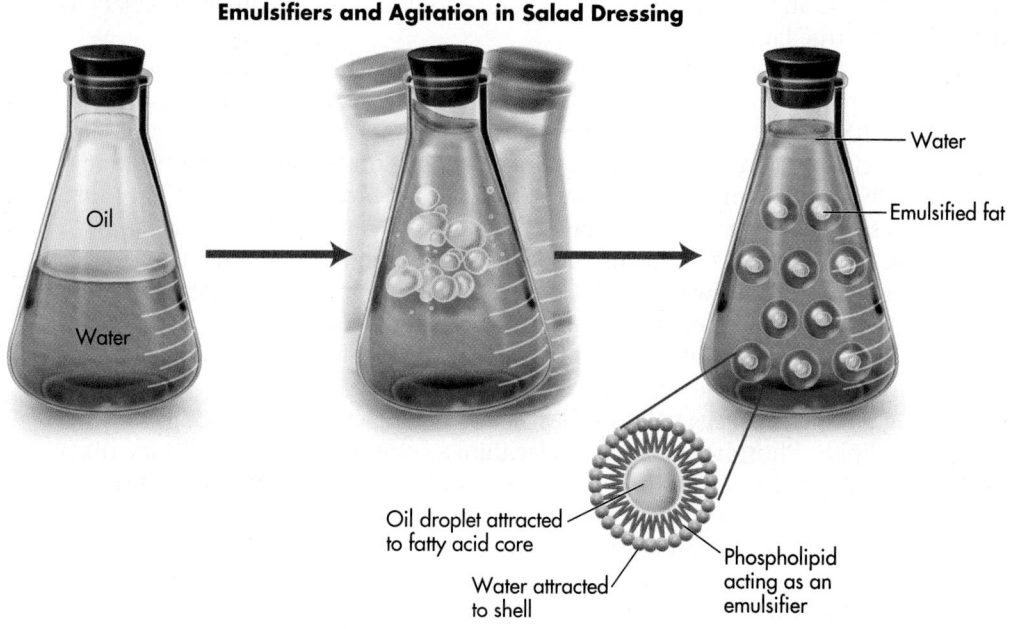

Emulsifiers and Agitation in Salad Dressing

Water
Emulsified fat

Oil droplet attracted to fatty acid core
Water attracted to shell
Phospholipid acting as an emulsifier

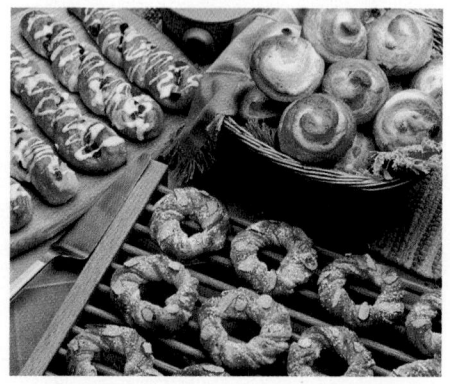

▲ The North American diet contains many high-fat foods—including typical pastry choices. Portion control with these foods is thus important, especially if one is trying to control calorie intake.

meats and whole milk. Manufacturers who advertise their brand of peanut butter, vegetable shortening, margarines, and vegetable oils as "cholesterol-free" are taking advantage of uninformed consumers—all of these products are naturally cholesterol-free. Some plants contain other sterols similar to cholesterol, but they do not pose the heart health risks associated with cholesterol. In fact, some plant sterols have blood cholesterol-lowering properties (see the later section on medical interventions to lower blood lipids).

Fat Is Hidden in Some Foods

Some fat discussed so far is obvious: butter on bread, mayonnaise in potato salad, and marbling in raw meat. Fat is harder to detect in other foods that also contribute significant amounts of fat to our diets. Foods that contain hidden fat include whole milk, pastries, cookies, cake, cheese, hot dogs, crackers, French fries, and ice cream. When we try to cut down on fat intake, hidden fats need to be considered, along with the more obvious sources.

A place to begin searching for hidden fat is on the Nutrition Facts labels of foods you buy. Some signals from the ingredient list that can alert you to the presence of fat are animal fats, such as bacon, beef, ham, lamb, pork, chicken, and turkey fats; lard; vegetable oils; nuts; dairy fats, such as butter and cream; egg and egg-yolk solids; and partially-hydrogenated shortening or vegetable oil. Conveniently, the label lists ingredients by order of weight in the product. If fat is one of the first ingredients listed, you are probably looking at a high-fat product. Use food labels to learn more about the fat content of the foods you eat (Fig. 5-8).

The definitions for various fat descriptors on food labels, such as "low-fat," "fat-free," and "reduced-fat," were listed in Table 2-11 in Chapter 2 and are reprinted in the margin here. Recall that "low-fat" indicates, in most cases, that a product contains no more than 3 grams of fat per serving. Products marketed as "fat-free" must have less than one-half of a gram of fat per serving. A claim of "reduced-fat" means the product has at least 25% less fat than is usually found in that type of food. When there is no Nutrition Facts label to inspect, controlling portion size is a good way to control fat intake.

When many North Americans think of a low-fat diet, they include reduced-fat versions of pastries, cookies, and cakes. When health professionals refer to a low-fat diet,

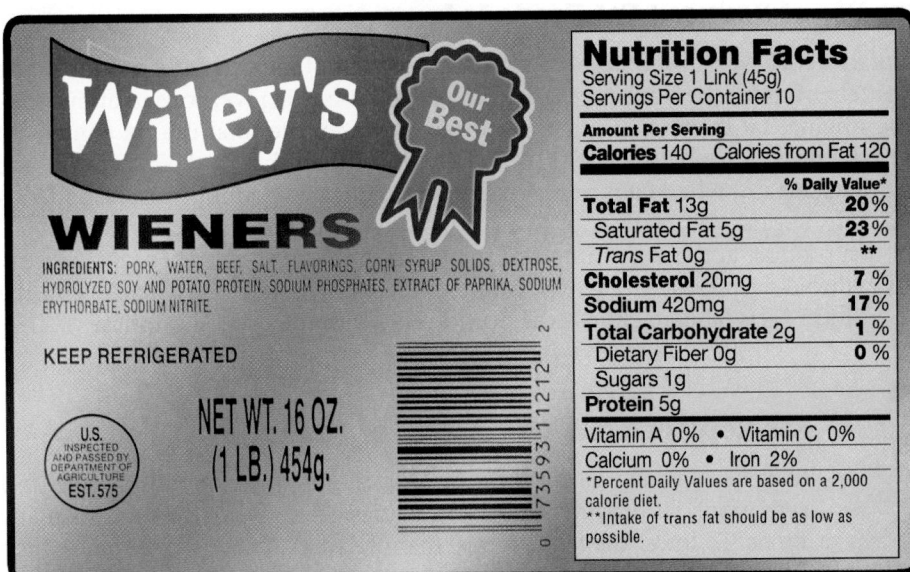

INGREDIENTS: PORK, WATER, BEEF, SALT, FLAVORINGS, CORN SYRUP SOLIDS, DEXTROSE, HYDROLYZED SOY AND POTATO PROTEIN, SODIUM PHOSPHATES, EXTRACT OF PAPRIKA, SODIUM ERYTHORBATE, SODIUM NITRITE.

KEEP REFRIGERATED

NET WT. 16 OZ. (1 LB.) 454g.

U.S. INSPECTED AND PASSED BY DEPARTMENT OF AGRICULTURE EST. 575

Nutrition Facts

Serving Size 1 Link (45g)
Servings Per Container 10

Amount Per Serving

Calories 140   Calories from Fat 120

	% Daily Value*
Total Fat 13g	**20**%
Saturated Fat 5g	**23**%
Trans Fat 0g	**
Cholesterol 20mg	**7** %
Sodium 420mg	**17**%
Total Carbohydrate 2g	**1** %
Dietary Fiber 0g	**0** %
Sugars 1g	
Protein 5g	

Vitamin A 0%	•	Vitamin C 0%
Calcium 0%	•	Iron 2%

*Percent Daily Values are based on a 2,000 calorie diet.
**Intake of trans fat should be as low as possible.

FIGURE 5-8 ▶ Reading labels helps locate hidden fat. Who would think that wieners (hot dogs) can contain about 85% of food calories as fat? Looking at the hot dog does not suggest that almost all of its food calories come from fat, but the label shows otherwise. Let's do the math: 13 grams total fat × 9 kcal per gram of fat = 120 kcal from fat; 120 kcal/140 kcal per link = 0.86 or 86% kcal from fat.

they often have a different plan in mind: focusing primarily on fruits, vegetables, and whole-grain breads and cereals. Whether to choose a fat-rich food should depend on how much fat you have eaten or will eat during that particular day. So, if you plan to eat high-fat foods at your evening meal, you could reduce your fat intake at a previous meal to balance overall fat intake for the day.

Fat in Food Provides Some Satiety, Flavor, and Texture

Fat in foods has generally been considered to be the most satiating of all the macronutrients. However, studies show that protein and carbohydrate probably lead to the most satiety (gram for gram). High-fat meals do provide satiety, but primarily because one consumes a lot of calories in the process. A high-fat meal is likely to be a high-calorie meal.

Various fats play important roles in foods, so much ingenuity must go into the production of reduced-fat products to preserve flavor and texture. In some cases, "fat-free" also means tasteless. Fat components in foods provide important textures and carry flavors. If you've ever eaten a high-fat yellow cheese or cream cheese, you probably agree that fat melting on the tongue feels good. The fat in reduced-fat and whole milk also gives body, which fat-free milk lacks. The most tender cuts of meat are high in fat, visible as the marbling of meat. In addition, many flavorings dissolve in fat. Heating spices in oil intensifies the flavors of an Indian curry or a Mexican dish, carried to the sensory cells that discriminate taste and smell in the mouth.

MAKING DECISIONS

Low-Fat Diets

A person who has been following a typical North American diet will probably need some time to adjust to the taste of a lower-fat diet. Emphasizing flavorful fruits, vegetables, and whole grains will help one to adapt to a low-fat diet. Interestingly, after an adjustment period, higher-fat foods may not be as palatable or may lead to gastrointestinal discomfort. For example, after switching from whole to 1% low-fat milk for a few weeks, whole milk begins to taste more like cream than milk. It is certainly possible to make the change from a higher-fat diet to a lower-fat diet. The benefits of weight control and reduced risk for several chronic diseases make the adjustment worth the effort.

▶ **Definitions for Nutrient Claims About Fat and Cholesterol on Food Labels**

Fat

- **Fat free:** less than 0.5g of fat per serving

- **Saturated fat free:** less than 0.5g per serving, and the level of *trans* fatty acids does not exceed 0.5g per serving

- **Low fat:** 3g or less per serving and, if the serving is 30g or less or 2 tablespoons or less, per 50g of the food. 2% milk can no longer be labeled low fat, as it exceeds 3g per serving. *Reduced fat* will be the term used instead.

- **Low saturated fat:** 1g or less per serving and not more than 15% of kcal from saturated fatty acids

- **Reduced or less fat:** at least 25% less per serving than reference food

- **Reduced or less saturated fat:** at least 25% less per serving than reference food

Cholesterol

- **Cholesterol free:** less than 2 milligrams (mg) of cholesterol and 2g or less of saturated fat per serving

- **Low cholesterol:** 20mg or less cholesterol and 2g or less of saturated fat per serving and, if the serving is 30g or less or 2 tablespoons or less, per 50g of the food

- **Reduced or less cholesterol:** at least 25% less cholesterol and 2g or less of saturated fat per serving than reference food

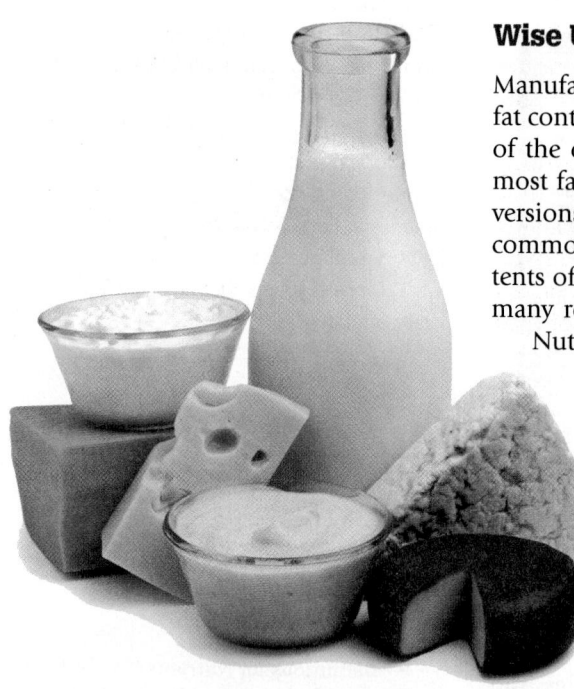

▲ Dairy products are a primary contributor of saturated fat to our diets.

Wise Use of Reduced-Fat Foods Is Important

Manufacturers have introduced reduced-fat versions of numerous food products. The fat content of these alternatives ranges from 0% in fat-free Fig Newtons to about 75% of the original fat content in other products. However, the total calorie content of most fat-reduced products is not substantially lower than that of their conventional versions. Generally, when fat is removed from a product, something must be added—commonly, sugars—in its place. It is difficult to reduce both the fat and sugar contents of a product at the same time and maintain flavor and texture. For this reason, many reduced-fat products (e.g., cakes and cookies) are still energy dense. Use the Nutrition Facts label to choose the portion size with the desired calories.

Fat-Replacement Strategies for Foods

To help consumers trim their fat intake and still enjoy the mouth feel sensations fat provides, food companies offer low-fat versions of many foods. To lower the fat in foods, manufacturers may replace some of the fat with water, protein (Dairy-Lo®), or forms of carbohydrates such as starch derivatives (Z-trim®), fiber (Maltrin®, Stellar™, Oatrim), and gums. Manufacturers also may use engineered fats, such as olestra (Olean®) and salatrim (Benefat®), that are made with fat and sucrose (table sugar) but that provide few or no calories because they cannot be digested and/or absorbed well.

So far, fat replacements have had little impact on our diets, partly because the currently approved forms are either not very versatile or not used extensively by manufacturers. In addition, fat replacements are not practical for use in the foods that provide the most fat in our diets—beef, cheese, whole milk, and pastries.

CONCEPT CHECK

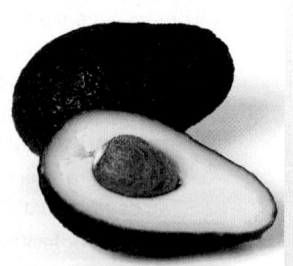

Fat-dense foods—those with more than 60% of total calories as fat—include plant oils, butter, margarine, mayonnaise, nuts, bacon, avocados, peanut butter, cheddar cheese, steak, and hamburger. Of the foods we typically eat, cholesterol is found naturally only in those of animal origin, with eggs being a primary source. Emulsifiers, such as the phospholipids, lecithins, are added to salad dressings and other fat-rich products to keep the vegetable oils and other fats suspended in the water. Hidden fat exists in foods such as whole milk, pastries, cookies, cake, cheese, hot dogs, crackers, French fries, and ice cream. Fat has a variety of roles in foods, including that of contributing to flavor and texture. Fat also provides the pleasurable mouth feel of many of our favorite foods, intensifies the taste of many spices, and tenderizes many popular cuts of meat. Fat free doesn't mean calorie free; moderation in the use of reduced-fat products is still important.

Fat Rancidity Limits Shelf Life of Foods

CRITICAL THINKING

Allison has decided to start eating a low-fat diet. Allison has mentioned to you that all she needs to do is add less butter, oil, or margarine to her foods and she will dramatically lower her fat intake. How can you explain to Allison that she needs to be aware of the hidden fats in her diet as well?

Decomposing oils emit a disagreeable odor and taste sour and stale. Stale potato chips are a good example. The double bonds in unsaturated fatty acids break down, producing rancid by-products. Ultraviolet light, oxygen, and certain procedures can break double bonds and, in turn, destroy the structure of polyunsaturated fatty acids. Saturated fats and *trans* fats can much more readily resist these effects because they contain fewer carbon-carbon double bonds.

Rancidity is not a major problem for consumers because the odor and taste generally discourage us from eating enough to become sick. However, rancidity is a problem for manufacturers because it reduces a product's shelf life. To increase shelf life, manufacturers often add partially-hydrogenated plant oils to products. Foods most likely to become rancid are deep-fried foods and foods with a large amount of exposed surface. The fat in fish is also susceptible to rancidity because it is highly polyunsaturated.

Antioxidants such as vitamin E help protect foods against rancidity by guarding against fat breakdown. The vitamin E naturally occurring in plant oils reduces the breakdown of double bonds in fatty acids. When food manufacturers want to prevent rancidity in polyunsaturated fats, they often add the synthetic antioxidants **BHA** and **BHT** or vitamin C to products that contain fat such as salad dressings and cake mixes. Manufacturers also tightly seal products and use other methods to reduce oxygen levels inside packages.

Hydrogenation of Fatty Acids in Food Production Increases *Trans* Fatty Acid Content

As mentioned previously, most fats with long-chain saturated fatty acids are solid at room temperature, and those with unsaturated fatty acids are liquid at room temperature. In some kinds of food production, solid fats work better than liquid oils. In pie crust, for example, solid fats yield a flaky product, whereas crusts made with liquid oils tend to be greasy and more crumbly. If oils with unsaturated fatty acids are used to replace solid fats, they often must be made more saturated (with hydrogen), as this solidifies the vegetable oils into shortenings and margarines. Hydrogen is added by bubbling hydrogen gas under pressure into liquid vegetable oils in a process called **hydrogenation** (Fig. 5-9). The fatty acids aren't fully hydrogenated to the saturated fatty acid form, as this would make the product too hard and brittle. Partial hydrogenation—leaving some monounsaturated fatty acids—creates a semi-solid product.

The process of hydrogenation produces *trans* fatty acids as was described earlier in this chapter. Most natural monounsaturated and polyunsaturated fatty acids exist in the *cis* form, causing a bend in the carbon chain, whereas the straighter carbon forms of *trans* fat more closely resemble saturated fatty acids. This may be the mechanism

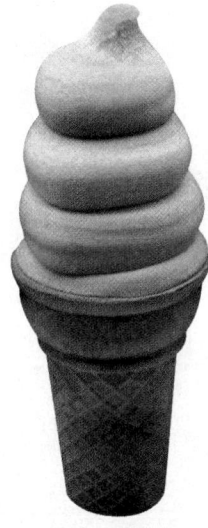

▲ Fat replacements such as gum fiber are typically seen in soft serve ice cream.

Canada has not approved the use of olestra in food products; the United States is the sole country that permits the use of this fat substitute in foods.

BHA, BHT Butylated hydroxyanisole and butylated hydroxytoluene—two common synthetic antioxidants added to foods.

hydrogenation The addition of hydrogen to a carbon-carbon double bond, producing a single carbon-carbon bond with two hydrogens attached to each carbon. Hydrogenation of unsaturated fatty acids in a vegetable oil increases its hardness, so this process is used to convert liquid oils into more solid fats, used in making margarine and shortening. *Trans* fatty acids are a by-product of hydrogenation of vegetable oils.

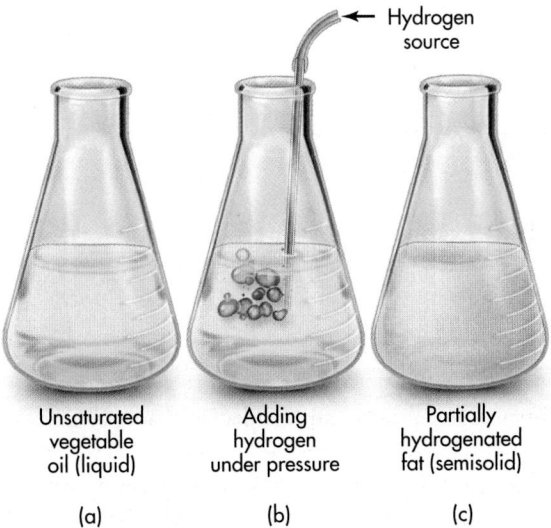

Unsaturated vegetable oil (liquid)

(a)

← Hydrogen source

Adding hydrogen under pressure

(b)

Partially hydrogenated fat (semisolid)

(c)

FIGURE 5-9 ▶ How liquid oils become solid fats. (a) Unsaturated fatty acids are present in liquid form. (b) Hydrogens are added (hydrogenation), changing some carbon-carbon double bonds to single bonds and producing some *trans* fatty acids. (c) The partially hydrogenated product is likely to be used in margarine, shortening, or for deep-fat frying.

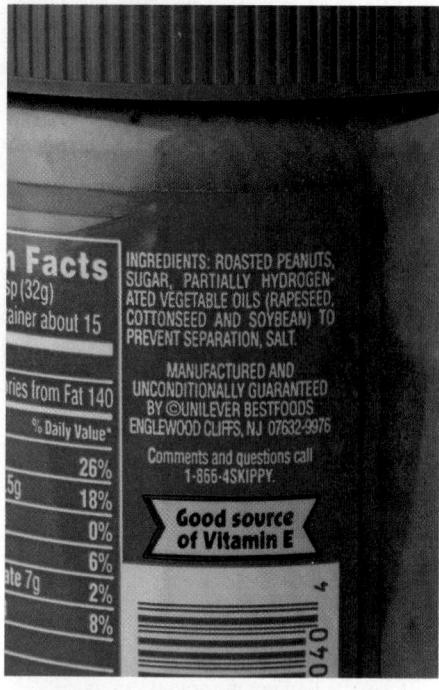

Peanut Butter: Is It "Good" Fat?

At the grocery store, there are several brands of peanut butter on the shelf. The label on one brand of peanut butter indicates that the product is "cholesterol free," whereas none of the other brands make the same claim. A jar of "natural" peanut butter claims to have no hydrogenated fats. Which jar of peanut butter is best for heart health?

Cholesterol is a type of lipid that is only found in animal products. Therefore, all peanut butter is cholesterol free! Hydrogenated oils are used to increase shelf life of many products, including peanut butter. The process of hydrogenation can produce *trans* fats, which have many of the same detrimental health effects as saturated fat. *Trans* fats increase levels of "bad" blood cholesterol (LDL) and decrease "good" blood cholesterol (HDL). If hydrogenated oils appear in the list of ingredients as in the label shown here, there is a good chance the product contains *trans* fats. As you learned in Chapter 2, a product may claim to be free of *trans* fats as long as the product contains no more than 0.5 g of *trans* fats per serving. Therefore, the only guarantee to avoiding *trans* fat in peanut butter is to buy the "natural" peanut butter made from only peanuts.

whereby *trans* fat increases the risk for heart disease. Studies also indicate that *trans* fats increase overall inflammation in the body, which is not healthful. Thus, people should limit intake of partially-hydrogenated fat and thus *trans* fat. This may not be such a concern for the average person, as long as *trans* fat intake is not excessive and the diet is adequate in polyunsaturated fat. However, because *trans* fatty acids serve no particular role in maintaining body health, the latest Dietary Guidelines for Americans, the American Heart Association, and the Food and Nutrition Board each recommend minimal *trans* fat intake.

Not so long ago, public pressure persuaded manufacturers to eliminate the tropical oils rich in saturated fat (palm, palm olein, and coconut) from food processing. Partially-hydrogenated soybean oil—rich in *trans* fat—became the major replacement. Currently, *trans* fat intake in North America is estimated to contribute about 3% to 4% of total calories, amounting to 10 grams per day, on average. Table 5-1 lists typical sources.

FDA is now requiring the *trans* fat content of foods on food labels (review Fig. 5-8). The food labels in Canada also must list *trans* fat content. FDA hopes to make consumers more aware of the amounts of *trans* fat in foods as well as the negative health consequences associated with their excessive consumption. North American companies are already responding to this issue by creating products free of *trans* fat. For example, Promise, Smart Beat, and some Fleischmann's margarines are lower in or free of *trans* fat (less than 0.5 grams per serving) compared to typical margarines.

This addition of the *trans* fat listing on labels helps consumers at the supermarket, but when dining out, consumers are "left in the dark" as to which foods contain *trans* fat. Knowing which foods are low in *trans* fat when ordering at a restaurant is difficult because information about preparation methods and precise fat

TABLE 5-1 Main Sources of Fatty acids and Their State at Room Temperature

Type and Health Effects	Main Sources	State at Room Temperature
Saturated Fatty Acids Increase blood levels of cholesterol		
Long Chain	Lard; fat in beef, pork, and lamb	Solid
Medium and Short Chain	Milk fat (butter), coconut oil, palm oil, palm kernel oil	Soft or liquid
Monounsaturated Fatty Acids Decrease blood levels of cholesterol	Olive oil, canola oil, peanut oil	Liquid
Polyunsaturated Fatty Acids Decrease blood levels of cholesterol	Sunflower oil, corn oil, safflower oil, fish oil	Liquid
Essential Fatty Acids Omega 3: alpha–linolenic acid Reduces inflammation responses, blood clotting, and plasma triglycerides	Cold-water fish (salmon, tuna, sardines, mackerel), walnuts, flaxseed, hemp oil, canola oil, soybean oil	Liquid
Omega 6: Linoleic Acid Regulates blood pressure and increases blood clotting	Beef, poultry, safflower oil, sunflower oil, corn oil	Solid to liquid
***Trans* Fatty Acids** Increase blood cholesterol more than saturated fat	Margarine (squeeze, tub, stick), shortening	Soft to very solid

composition is rarely available. Many cities, including New York, Philadelphia, and Boston, have banned *trans* fat use in restaurants (see Further Reading 2). To minimize *trans* fat intake, a general guideline is to limit consumption of fried (especially deep-fat fried) food items, any pastries or flaky bread products (such as pie crusts, crackers, croissants, and biscuits), and cookies.

Until all foods are labeled with *trans* fat content, consumers can also make educated guesses on the *trans* fat content of foods by examining the list of ingredients on the food label. If partially-hydrogenated vegetable oil is one of the first three ingredients on the label, you can assume there is a significant amount of *trans* fat in the product.

Limiting *trans* fat at home is a much easier task. Most importantly, use little or no stick margarine or shortening. Instead, substitute vegetable oils and softer tub margarines (whose labels list vegetable oil or water as the first ingredient). Avoid deep-fat frying any food in shortening. Substitute baking, panfrying, broiling, steaming, grilling, or deep-fat frying in unhydrogenated vegetable oils. Replace nondairy creamers with reduced-fat or fat-free milk, since most nondairy creamers are rich in partially-hydrogenated vegetable oils. Finally, read the ingredients on food labels, using the previous tips to estimate *trans* fat content.

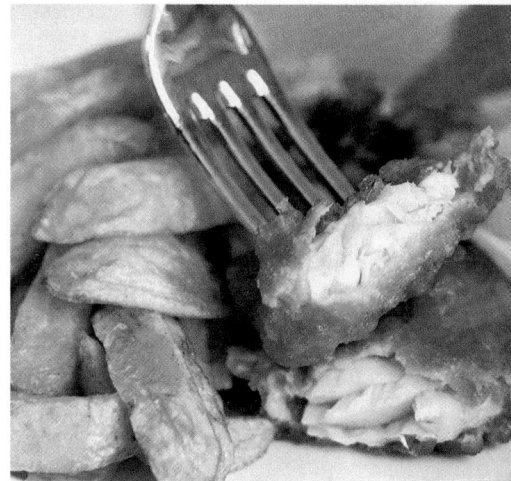

▲ Fried foods are a rich source of fat and *trans* fats. Reducing the intake of these foods can help lower blood lipid levels.

CONCEPT CHECK

Hydrogenation of unsaturated fatty acids is the process of adding hydrogen to carbon-carbon double bonds to produce single bonds. This results in the creation of some *trans* fatty acids. Hydrogenation changes vegetable oil to solid fat. It is wise to monitor *trans* fat intake, as this form of fat increases the risk for heart disease.

The carbon-carbon double bonds in polyunsaturated fatty acids are easily broken, yielding products responsible for rancidity. The presence of antioxidants, such as vitamin E in oils, naturally protects unsaturated fatty acids against oxidative destruction. Manufacturers can use hydrogenated fats and add natural or synthetic antioxidants to reduce the likelihood of rancidity.

5.4 Making Lipids Available for Body Use

It's no secret that fats and oils make foods more appealing. Their presence in foods adds flavor, lubrication, and texture. What happens to lipids once they are eaten? Let's take a closer look at the digestion, absorption, and physiological roles of lipids in the body.

Digestion

In the first phase of fat digestion, the stomach (and salivary glands to some extent) secretes **lipase.** This enzyme acts primarily on triglycerides that have fatty acids with short chain lengths, such as those found in butterfat. The action of salivary and stomach lipase, however, is usually dwarfed by that of the lipase enzyme released from the pancreas and active in the small intestine. Triglycerides and other lipids found in common vegetable oils and meats have longer chain lengths and are generally not digested until they reach the small intestine (Fig. 5-10).

In the small intestine, triglycerides are broken down by lipase into smaller products, namely monoglycerides (glycerol backbones with a single fatty acid attached) and fatty acids. Under the right circumstances, digestion is rapid and thorough. The "right" circumstances include the presence of bile from the gallbladder. Bile acids present in the bile act as emulsifiers on the digestive products of lipase action, suspending the monoglycerides and fatty acids in the watery digestive juices. This emulsification improves digestion and absorption because as large fat globules are broken down into smaller ones, the total surface area for lipase action increases (Fig. 5-11).

lipase Fat-digesting enzyme produced by the salivary glands, stomach, and pancreas.

FIGURE 5-10 ▶ A summary of fat digestion and absorption. Chapter 3 covered general aspects of this process.

Fat Digestion and Absorption

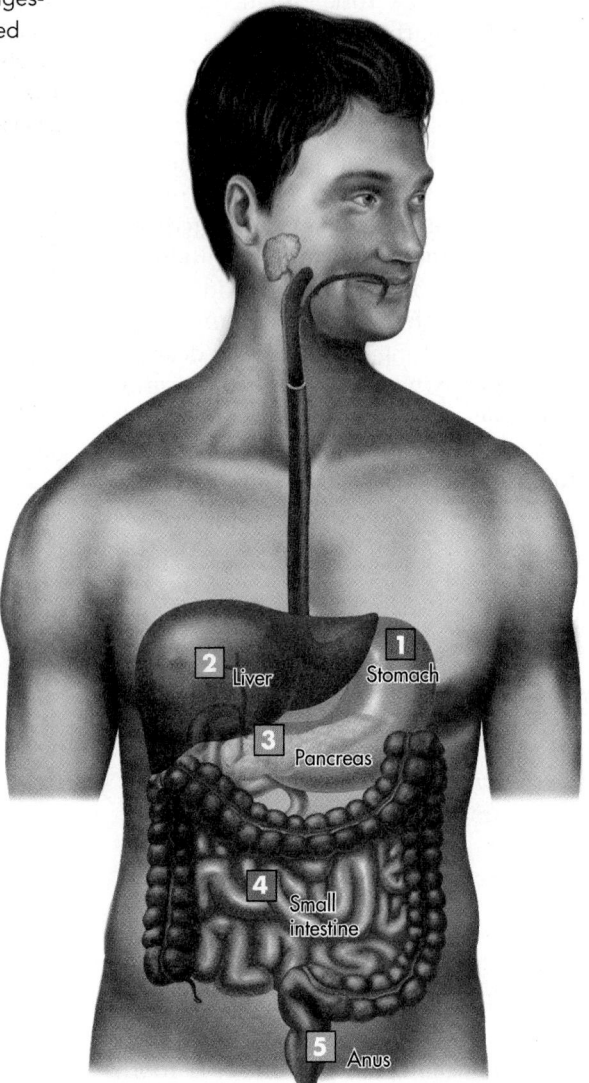

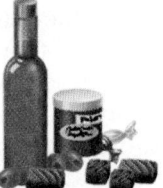

1 Stomach: Only minor digestion of fat takes place in the stomach through the action of lipase enzymes.

2 Liver: The liver produces bile, stored in the gallbladder and released through the bile duct into the small intestine. Bile aids in fat digestion and absorption by emulsifying lipids in the digestive juices.

3 Pancreas: The pancreas secretes a mixture of enzymes, including lipase, into the small intestine.

4 Small intestine: The small intestine is the primary site for digestion and absorption of lipids. Once absorbed, long-chain fatty acids are packaged for transport through the lymph and bloodstream. (Shorter-chain fatty acids are absorbed directly into portal circulation.)

5 Large intestine: Less than 5% of ingested fat is normally excreted in the feces.

If the gallbladder is surgically removed (e.g., in cases of gallstone formation), bile will enter the small intestine directly from the liver.

With regard to phospholipid digestion, certain enzymes from the pancreas and cells in the wall of the small intestine digest phospholipids. The eventual products are glycerol, fatty acids, and remaining parts. With regard to cholesterol digestion, any cholesterol with a fatty acid attached is broken down to free cholesterol and fatty acids by certain enzymes released from the pancreas.

MAKING DECISIONS

Bile Acids

During meals, bile acids circulate in a path that begins in the liver, goes on to the gallbladder, and then moves to the small intestine. After participating in fat digestion, most bile acids are absorbed and end up back at the liver. Approximately 98% of the bile acids are recycled. Only 1% to 2% ends up in the large intestine to be eliminated in the feces. Using medicines that block some of this reabsorption of bile acids is one way to treat high blood cholesterol. The liver takes cholesterol from the bloodstream to form replacement bile acids. Viscous fiber in the diet can also bind to bile acids to produce the same effect (see a later section on medical interventions related to cardiovascular disease for details).

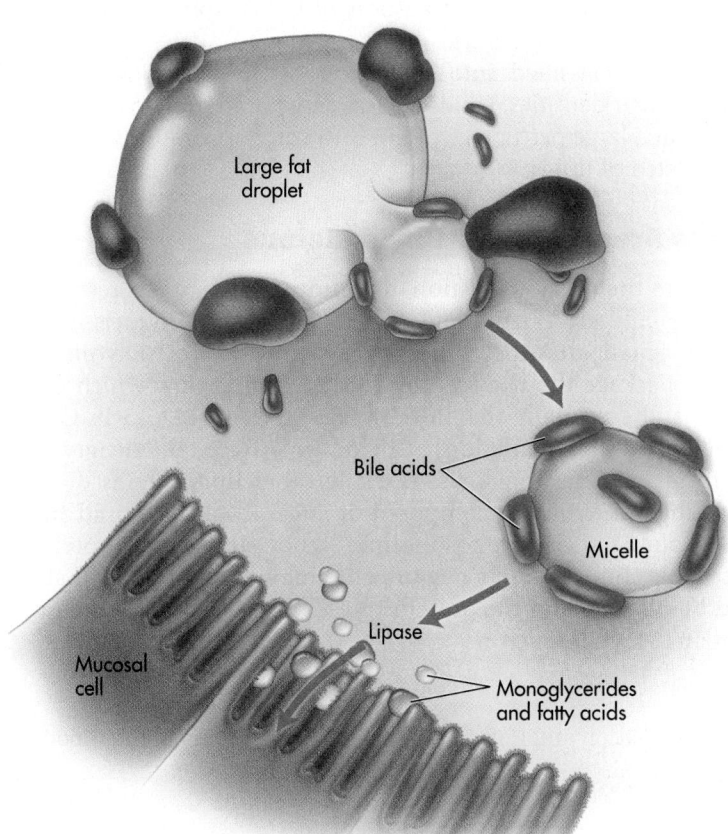

FIGURE 5-11 ▶ Bile acids mix with fats to form small droplets called micelles that facilitate the absorption of monoglycerides and fatty acids into the mucosal cells of the small intestine.

Absorption

The products of fat digestion in the small intestine are fatty acids and monoglycerides. These products diffuse into the absorptive cells of the small intestine. About 95% of dietary fat is absorbed in this way. The chain length of fatty acids affects the ultimate fate of fatty acids and monoglycerides after absorption. If the chain length of a fatty acid is less than 12 carbon atoms, it is water soluble and will therefore probably travel as such through the portal vein that connects directly to the liver. If the fatty acid is a more typical long-chain variety, it must be reformed into a triglyceride in the intestinal absorptive cell and eventually enter circulation via the lymphatic system (review Chapter 3 for an overview of this process).

CONCEPT CHECK

In the small intestine, a lipase enzyme released from the pancreas digests dietary triglycerides into monoglycerides (glycerol backbones with single fatty acids attached) and fatty acids. These breakdown products then diffuse into the absorptive cells of the small intestine. Long-chain fatty acids are transported through the lymphatic system, whereas fatty acids with shorter carbon chains are absorbed directly into the portal vein that connects directly to the liver. Other lipids are prepared for absorption by different enzymes.

5.5 Carrying Lipids in the Bloodstream

As noted earlier, fat and water don't mix easily. This incompatibility presents a challenge for the transport of fats through the watery media of the blood and lymph.

lipoprotein A compound found in the bloodstream containing a core of lipids with a shell composed of protein, phospholipid, and cholesterol.

chylomicron Lipoprotein made of dietary fats surrounded by a shell of cholesterol, phospholipids, and protein. Chylomicrons are formed in the absorptive cells of the small intestine after fat absorption and travel through the lymphatic system to the bloodstream.

Lipoproteins serve as vehicles for transport of lipids from the small intestine and liver to the body tissues (Table 5-2).

Lipoproteins are classified into four groups—chylomicrons, VLDL, LDL, and HDL—based on their densities. Lipids are less dense than proteins. Therefore, lipoproteins that contain a large percentage of lipids in comparison to protein are less dense than those depleted of lipids.

Dietary Fats Are Carried by Chylomicrons

As you learned in the previous section, digestion of dietary fats results in a mixture of glycerol, monoglycerides, and fatty acids. Once these products are absorbed by the cells of the small intestine, they are reassembled into triglycerides. Then, the intestinal cells package the triglycerides into **chylomicrons,** which enter the lymphatic system and eventually the bloodstream (review Fig. 3-5 in Chapter 3 for a depiction of lymphatic circulation). Chylomicrons contain dietary fat and originate only from the intestinal cells. Like the other lipoproteins described in the next section, chylomicrons are composed of large droplets of lipid surrounded by a thin, water-soluble shell of phospholipids, cholesterol, and protein (Fig. 5-12). The water-soluble shell around a chylomicron allows the lipid to float freely in the water-based blood. Some of the proteins present may also help other cells identify the lipoprotein as a chylomicron.

TABLE 5-2 Composition and Roles of the Major Lipoproteins in the Blood

Lipoprotein	Primary Component	Key Role
Chylomicron	Triglyceride	Carries dietary fat from the small intestine to cells
VLDL	Triglyceride	Carries lipids made and taken up by the liver to cells
LDL	Cholesterol	Carries cholesterol made by the liver and from other sources to cells
HDL	Protein	Contributes to cholesterol removal from cells and, in turn, excretion of it from the body

FIGURE 5-12 ▶ The structure of a lipoprotein, in this case an LDL. This structure allows fats to circulate in the water-based bloodstream. Various lipoproteins are found in the bloodstream. The primary component of LDL is cholesterol.

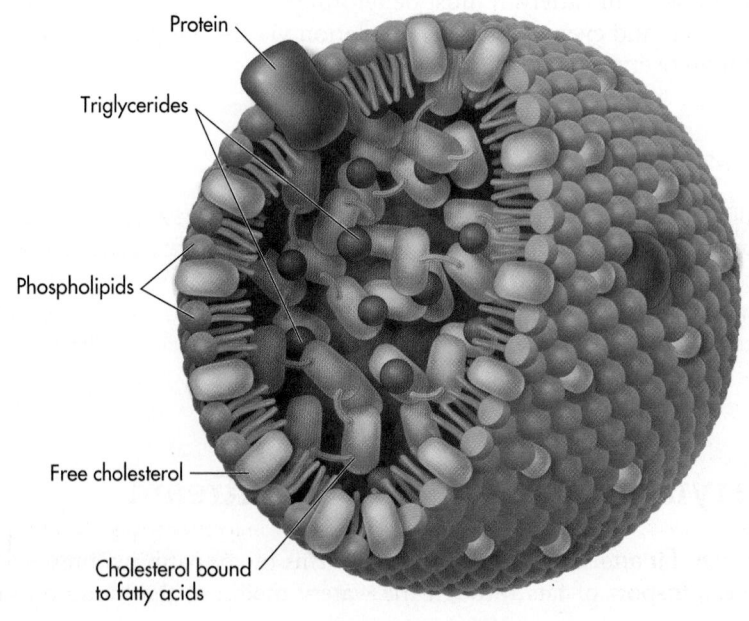

Protein

Triglycerides

Phospholipids

Free cholesterol

Cholesterol bound to fatty acids

Once a chylomicron enters the bloodstream, the triglycerides in its core are broken down into fatty acids and glycerol by an enzyme called **lipoprotein lipase,** attached to the inside walls of the blood vessels (Fig. 5-13). As soon as the fatty acids are released to the bloodstream, they are absorbed by cells in the vicinity, while much of the glycerol circulates back to the liver. Muscle cells can immediately use the absorbed fatty acids for fuel. Adipose cells, on the other hand, tend to re-form the fatty acids into triglycerides for storage. After triglycerides have been removed, a chylomicron remnant remains. Chylomicron remnants are removed from circulation by the liver and their components are recycled to make other lipoproteins and bile acids.

lipoprotein lipase An enzyme attached to the cells that form the inner lining of blood vessels; it breaks down triglycerides into free fatty acids and glycerol.

Other Lipoproteins Transport Lipids from the Liver to the Body Cells

The liver takes up various lipids from the blood. The liver also is the manufacturing site for lipids and cholesterol. The raw materials for lipid and cholesterol synthesis include free fatty acids taken up from the bloodstream, as well as carbon and hydrogen derived from carbohydrates, protein, and alcohol. The liver then must package these synthesized lipids as lipoproteins for transport in the blood to body tissues.

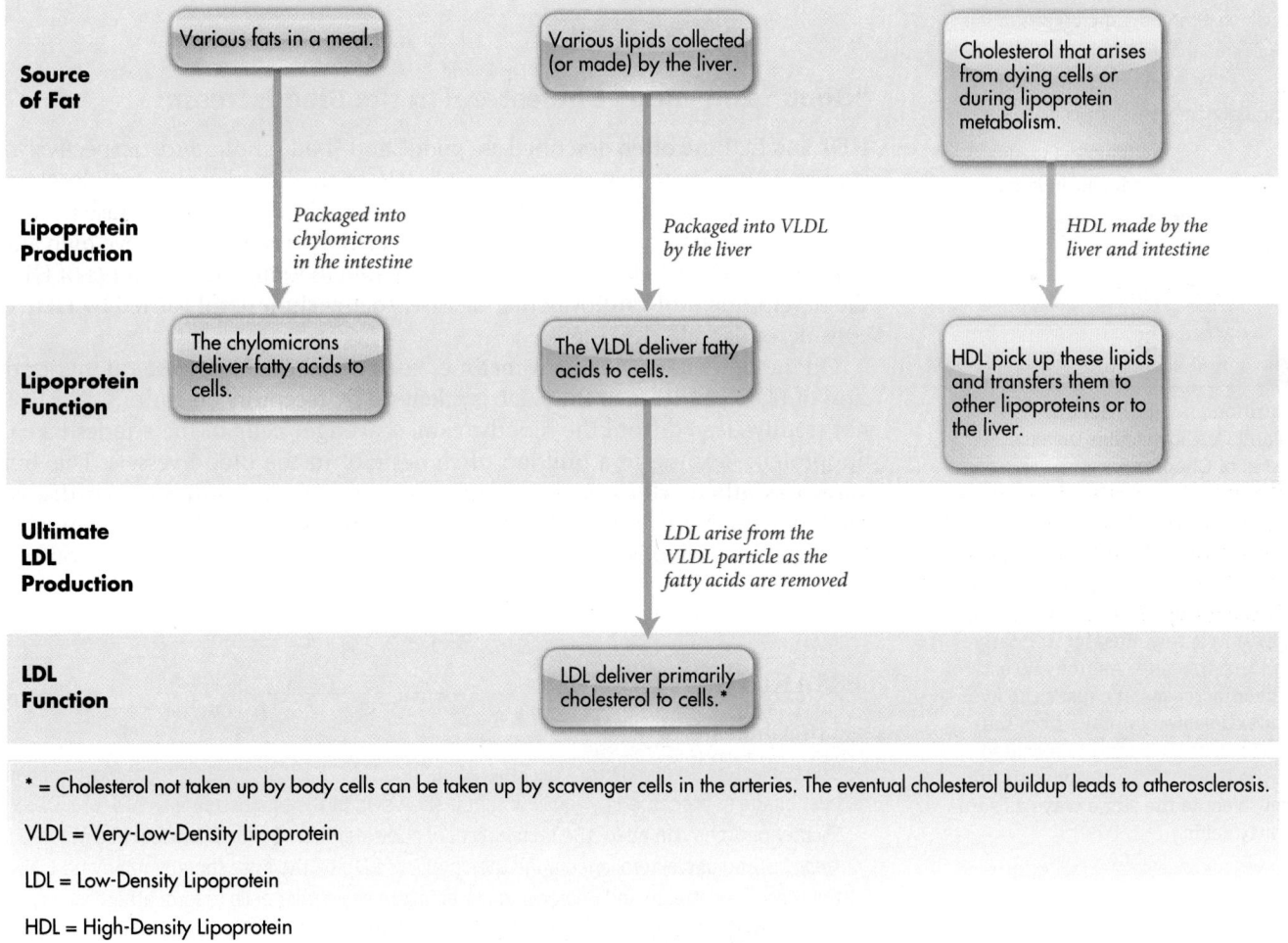

* = Cholesterol not taken up by body cells can be taken up by scavenger cells in the arteries. The eventual cholesterol buildup leads to atherosclerosis.

VLDL = Very-Low-Density Lipoprotein

LDL = Low-Density Lipoprotein

HDL = High-Density Lipoprotein

FIGURE 5-13 ▶ Lipoprotein production and function. Chylomicrons carry absorbed fat to body cells. VLDL carries fat taken up from the bloodstream by the liver, as well as any fat made by the liver, to body cells. LDL arises from VLDL and carries mostly cholesterol to cells. HDL arises mostly from the liver and intestine. HDL carries cholesterol from cells to other lipoproteins and to the liver for excretion.

very-low-density lipoprotein (VLDL) The lipoprotein created in the liver that carries cholesterol and lipids that have been taken up or newly synthesized by the liver.

low-density lipoprotein (LDL) The lipoprotein in the blood containing primarily cholesterol; elevated LDL is strongly linked to cardiovascular disease risk.

high-density lipoprotein (HDL) The lipoprotein in the blood that picks up cholesterol from dying cells and other sources and transfers it to the other lipoproteins in the bloodstream, as well as directly to the liver; low HDL increases the risk for cardiovascular disease.

menopause The cessation of the menstrual cycle in women, usually beginning at about 50 years of age.

scavenger cells Specific form of white blood cells that can bury themselves in the artery wall and accumulate LDL. As these cells take up LDL, they contribute to the development of atherosclerosis.

atherosclerosis A buildup of fatty material (plaque) in the arteries, including those surrounding the heart.

See Nutrition and Your Health: Lipids and Cardiovascular Disease at the end of Chapter 5.

It appears that saturated fatty acids promote an increase in the amount of free cholesterol (not attached to fatty acids) in the liver, whereas unsaturated fatty acids do the opposite. As free cholesterol in the liver increases, it causes the liver to reduce cholesterol uptake from the bloodstream, contributing to elevated LDL in the blood. (*Trans* fatty acids are thought to act in the same ways as saturated fatty acids.)

First in our discussion of lipoproteins made by the liver are **very-low-density lipoproteins (VLDL).** These particles are composed of cholesterol and triglycerides surrounded by a water-soluble shell. VLDLs are rich in triglycerides and thus are very low in density. Once in the bloodstream, lipoprotein lipase on the inner surface of the blood vessels breaks down the triglyceride in the VLDL into fatty acids and glycerol. Fatty acids and glycerol are released into the bloodstream and taken up by the body cells.

As its triglycerides are released, the VLDL becomes proportionately denser. Much of what eventually remains of the VLDL fraction is then called **low-density lipoprotein (LDL);** this is composed primarily of the remaining cholesterol. The primary function of LDL is to transport cholesterol to tissues. LDL particles are taken up from the bloodstream by specific receptors on cells, especially liver cells, and are then broken down. The cholesterol and protein components of LDL provide some of the building blocks necessary for cell growth and development, such as synthesis of cell membranes and hormones.

The final group of lipoproteins, **high-density lipoproteins (HDL),** is a critical and beneficial participant in this process of lipid transport. Its high proportion of protein makes it the densest lipoprotein. The liver and intestine produce most of the HDL in the blood. It roams the bloodstream, picking up cholesterol from dying cells and other sources. HDL donates the cholesterol primarily to other lipoproteins for transport back to the liver to be excreted. Some HDL travels directly back to the liver.

"Good" and "Bad" Cholesterol in the Bloodstream

HDL and LDL are often described as "good" and "bad" cholesterol, respectively. Many studies demonstrate that the amount of HDL in the bloodstream can closely predict the risk for cardiovascular disease. Risk increases with low HDL because little cholesterol is transported back to the liver and excreted. Women tend to have high amounts of HDL, especially before **menopause,** compared to men. High amounts of HDL slow the development of cardiovascular disease, so any cholesterol carried by HDL can be considered "good" cholesterol.

On the other hand, LDL is sometimes considered "bad" cholesterol. In our discussion of LDL, you learned that LDL is taken up by receptors on various cells. If LDL is not readily cleared from the bloodstream, **scavenger cells** in the arteries take up the lipoprotein, leading to a buildup of cholesterol in the blood vessels. This buildup, known as **atherosclerosis,** greatly increases the risk for cardiovascular disease (see the following Nutrition and Your Health section). LDL is only a problem when it is too high in the bloodstream because low amounts are needed as part of routine body functions.

MAKING DECISIONS

LDL Cholesterol

The cholesterol in foods is not designated as "good" or "bad." It is only after cholesterol has been made or processed by the liver that it shows up in the bloodstream as LDL or HDL. Dietary patterns can affect the metabolism of cholesterol, however. Diets low in saturated fat, *trans* fat, and cholesterol encourage the uptake of LDL by the liver, thereby removing LDL from the bloodstream and decreasing the ability of scavenger cells to form atherosclerotic plaques in the blood vessels. Likewise, diets high in saturated fat, *trans* fat, and cholesterol reduce the uptake of LDL by the liver, increasing cholesterol in the blood and the risk for cardiovascular disease. What foods in your diet are high in saturated fat, *trans* fat, or cholesterol?

CONCEPT CHECK

Lipids generally move through the bloodstream as part of lipoproteins. Dietary fats absorbed from the small intestine are packaged and transported as chylomicrons, whereas lipids synthesized in the liver are packaged as very-low-density lipoproteins (VLDL). Lipoprotein lipase removes triglycerides from the interiors of both chylomicrons and VLDL, breaking the triglycerides down into glycerol and fatty acids, which are taken up by tissues for energy needs or storage. What remains after the action of lipoprotein lipase are chylomicron remnants (from chylomicrons), the components of which are recycled by the liver, or low-density lipoproteins (LDL, from VLDL), rich in cholesterol. LDL is picked up by receptors on body cells, especially liver cells. Scavenger cells in the arteries may do the same, speeding the development of atherosclerosis. High-density lipoprotein (HDL), also produced in part by the liver, picks up cholesterol from cells and transports it primarily to other lipoproteins for eventual transport back to the liver. Risk factors for cardiovascular disease include an elevated level of LDL and/or low amounts of HDL in the blood.

5.6 Essential Functions of Fatty Acids

The various classes of lipids have diverse functions in the body. All are necessary for health, but, as mentioned earlier, many can be made by the body and therefore are not needed in our diet. Of all the classes of lipids, only certain polyunsaturated fatty acids are essential parts of a diet.

The Essential Fatty Acids

We must obtain linoleic acid (an omega-6 fatty acid) and alpha-linolenic acid (an omega-3 fatty acid) from foods to maintain health, so they are called *essential* fatty acids (Fig. 5-14). These omega-6 and omega-3 fatty acids form parts of vital body structures, perform important roles in immune system function and vision, help form cell membranes, and produce hormonelike compounds. Omega-6 and omega-3 fatty acids must be obtained through the diet because human cells lack the enzymes needed to produce these fatty acids. Other fatty acids, such as omega-9 fatty acids, can be synthesized in the body, and therefore are not essential components of the diet.

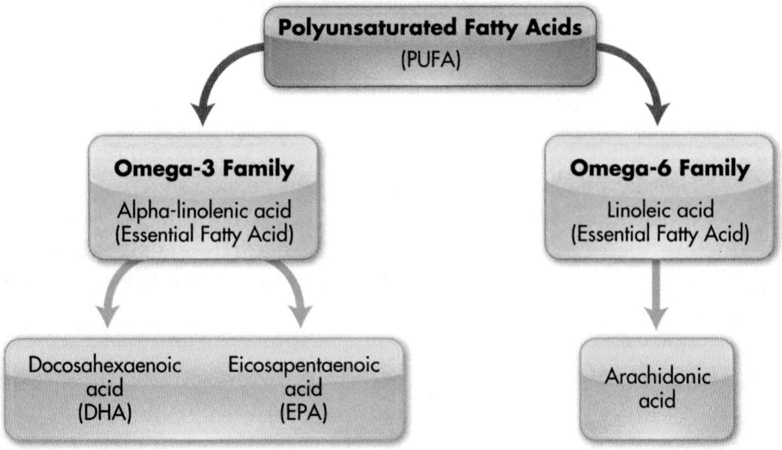

Omega-3 Fatty Acids in Fish (grams per 3 ounce serving)	
Atlantic salmon	1.8
Anchovy	1.7
Sardines	1.4
Rainbow trout	1.0
Coho salmon	0.9
Bluefish	0.8
Striped bass	0.8
Tuna, white, canned	0.7
Halibut	0.4
Catfish, channel	0.2

Recommended omega-3 fatty acid (alpha-linolenic acid) intake per day:	
Men	1.6 grams
Women	1.1 grams

FIGURE 5-14 ▶ The essential fatty acid (EFA) family. Linoleic acid and alpha-linolenic acid are available from dietary sources, and must be consumed as body synthesis does not take place. These are the essential fatty acids. The other fatty acids in this figure can be synthesized from the essential fatty acids.

eicosapentaenoic acid (EPA) An omega-3 fatty acid with 20 carbons and five carbon-carbon double bonds. It is present in large amounts in fatty fish and is slowly synthesized in the body from alpha-linolenic acid.

docosahexaenoic acid (DHA) An omega-3 fatty acid with 22 carbons and six carbon-carbon double bonds. It is present in large amounts in fatty fish and is slowly synthesized in the body from alpha-linolenic acid. DHA is especially present in the retina and brain.

arachidonic acid An omega-6 fatty acid made from linoleic acid with 20 carbon atoms and four carbon-carbon double bonds.

hemorrhagic stroke Damage to part of the brain resulting from rupture of a blood vessel and subsequent bleeding within or over the internal surface of the brain.

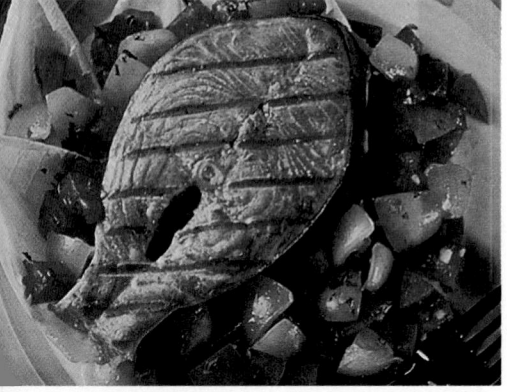

▲ The American Heart Association recommends eating fatty fish such as salmon at least twice a week. As a source of omega-3 fatty acids, fish is a heart-healthy alternative to other animal sources of protein, which can be high in saturated fat and cholesterol.

See Nutrition and Your Health:
Lipids and Cardiovascular Disease
at the end of Chapter 5.

Still, we need to consume only about 5% of our total calories per day from essential fatty acids. That corresponds to about 2 to 4 tablespoons of plant oil each day. We can easily get that much—from mayonnaise, salad dressings, and other foods—without much effort. Regular consumption of vegetables and whole-grain breads and cereals also helps to supply enough essential fatty acids.

Research also suggests that we include a regular intake of the omega-3 fatty acids, **eicosapentaenoic acid (EPA)** and **docosahexaenoic acid (DHA),** which can be made from alpha-linolenic acid. EPA and DHA are naturally high in fatty fish such as salmon, tuna, sardines, anchovies, striped bass, catfish, herring, mackerel, trout, or halibut. Consumption of one or more of these fish at least twice a week is recommended to obtain EPA and DHA. Additional sources of omega-3 fatty acids include canola and soybean oils, walnuts, flax seeds, mussels, crab, and shrimp (see Further Readings 4, 5, and 15).

MAKING DECISIONS

Mercury in Fish

Consumption of fatty fish at least twice a week is recommended as a good source of the omega-3 fatty acids. Some fish can be a source of mercury, toxic in high amounts, especially swordfish, shark, king mackerel, and tile fish (see Chapter 13). Albacore tuna also is a potential source, while other forms of tuna are much lower in mercury. Those fish low in mercury are salmon, sardines, bluefish, and herring. Shrimp is also low in mercury. For others, varying your choices rather than always eating the same species of fish and limiting overall intake to 12 ounces per week (on average 2 to 3 meals of fish or shellfish per week) is recommended to reduce mercury exposure, especially for pregnant women and children. Existing research indicates that the benefits of fish intake, especially in reducing the risk of cardiovascular disease, outweigh the possible risks of mercury contamination.

The recommendation to consume omega-3 fatty acids stems from the observation that compounds made from omega-3 fatty acids tend to decrease blood clotting and inflammatory processes in the body. The omega-6 fatty acids, notably **arachidonic acid** made from linoleic acid, generally increase clotting and inflammation, and saturated fatty acids also increase blood clotting.

Some studies show that people who eat fish at least twice a week (total weekly intake: 8 ounces [240 grams]) run lower risks for heart attack than do people who rarely eat fish. In these cases, the omega-3 fatty acids in fish oil are probably acting to reduce blood clotting. As will be covered in detail in the "Nutrition and Your Health" section, blood clots are part of the heart attack process. In addition, these omega-3 fatty acids have a favorable effect on heart rhythm. Consequently, the risk of heart attack decreases with the consumption of omega-3 fatty acids from fish, especially for people already at high risk.

We need to remember, however, that blood clotting is a normal body process. Certain groups of people, such as Eskimos in Greenland, eat so much seafood that their normal blood-clotting ability can be impaired. An excess of omega-3 fatty acid intake can allow uncontrolled bleeding and may cause **hemorrhagic stroke.** However, no increase in risk of stroke has been observed in studies using moderate amounts of omega-3 fatty acids.

Studies also have shown that large amounts of omega-3 fatty acids from fish (2 to 4 grams per day) can lower blood triglycerides in people with high triglyceride concentrations. In addition, these omega-3 fatty acids are suspected to be helpful in managing the pain of inflammation associated with rheumatoid arthritis by suppressing immune system responses. This may also help with certain behavioral disorders and cases of mild depression.

In some instances, fish oil capsules can be safely substituted for fish consumption if a person does not like fish. Generally, about 1 gram of omega-3 fatty acids (about three capsules) from fish oil per day is recommended, especially for people with evidence of cardiovascular disease. (Freezing fish oil capsules before consumption or using enteric coated capsules will reduce the fishy aftertaste.) The American Heart Association also recently suggested that fish oil supplements (providing 2 to 4 grams of omega-3 fatty acids per day) could be employed to treat elevated blood triglycerides, as previously noted. However, fish oil capsules should be limited for individuals who have bleeding disorders, take anticoagulant medications, or anticipate surgery, because they may increase risk of uncontrollable bleeding and hemorrhagic stroke. Thus for fish oil capsules, as well as other dietary supplements, it is important to follow a physician's recommendations. Remember that fish oil supplements are not regulated by the FDA. The quality of these supplements, therefore, is not standardized, and contaminants naturally present in the fish oil may not have been removed.

In summary, the regular consumption of fatty fish is advised. Consuming whole fish is thought to have greater benefits and be safer than using fish oil supplements. Fish is not only a rich source of omega-3 fatty acids, but is also a valuable source of protein and trace elements that may also provide protective effects for the cardiovascular system. Broiled or baked fish is recommended rather than fried fish because frying may decrease the ratio of omega-3 to omega-6 fatty acids and may produce *trans* fatty acids and oxidized lipid products that may increase cardiovascular disease risk.

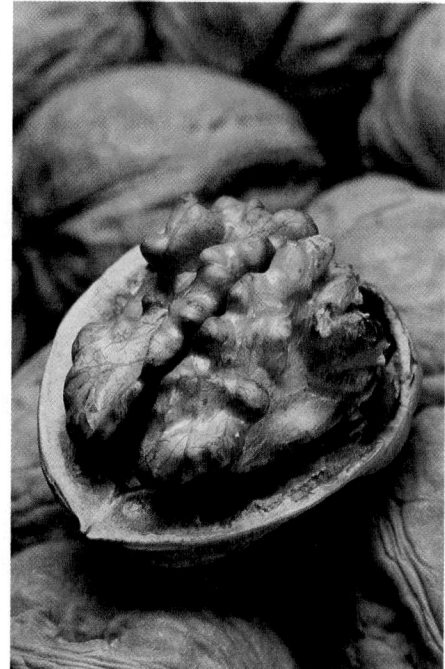

▲ Walnuts are one of the richest plant sources of the omega-3 fatty acid, alpha-linolenic acid, and are also a good source of plant sterols (see Further Reading 8).

MAKING DECISIONS

Flax Seeds or Walnuts?

Flax seeds and walnuts are getting attention today because they are rich vegetable sources of the omega-3 alpha-linolenic acid. About 2 tablespoons of flax seed per day is typically recommended if used as an omega-3 fatty acid source. Flax seeds can be purchased in many natural food stores rather inexpensively. These need to be chewed thoroughly or they will pass through the GI tract undigested. Many people find it easier to grind them in a coffee grinder before eating them. Flax seed oil is also available, but it turns **rancid** very quickly, especially if not refrigerated. Compared to other nuts and seeds, walnuts are one of the richest sources of alpha-linolenic acid (2.6 grams per 1-ounce serving or 14 walnut halves). The DRI for alpha-linolenic acid is 1.6 grams/day for men and 1.1 grams/day for women. In addition, walnuts are a rich source of plant sterols known to inhibit intestinal absorption of cholesterol.

CRITICAL THINKING

Advertisements often claim that fats are bad. Your classmate Mike asks, "If fats are so bad for us, why do we need to have any in our diets?" How would you answer him?

rancid Containing products of decomposed fatty acids that have an unpleasant flavor and odor.

total parenteral nutrition The intravenous feeding of all necessary nutrients, including the most basic forms of protein, carbohydrates, lipids, vitamins, minerals, and electrolytes.

Effects of a Deficiency of Essential Fatty Acids

If humans fail to consume enough essential fatty acids, their skin becomes flaky and itchy, and diarrhea and other symptoms such as infections often are seen. Growth and wound healing may be restricted. These signs of deficiency have been seen in people fed intravenously by **total parenteral nutrition** containing little or no fat for 2 to 3 weeks, as well as in infants receiving formulas low in fat. However, because our bodies need the equivalent of only about 2 to 4 tablespoons of plant oils a day, even a low fat diet will provide enough essential fatty acids if it follows a balanced plan such as MyPyramid and includes a serving of fatty fish at least twice a week.

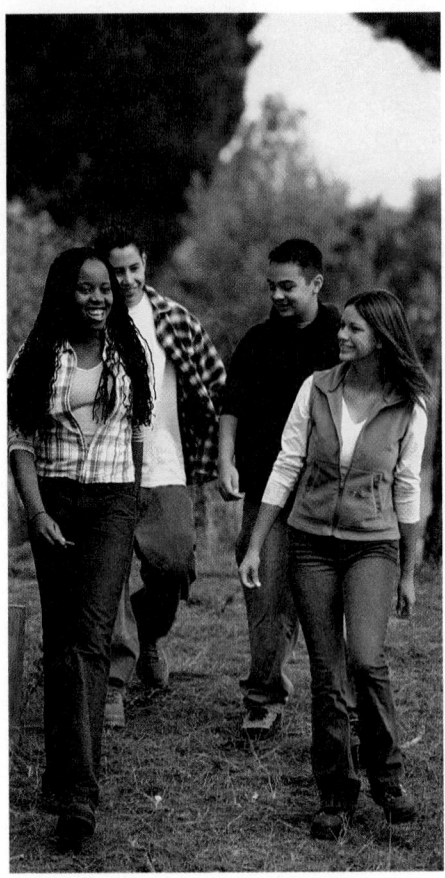

▲ When at rest or during light activity, the body uses mostly fatty acids for fuel.

CONCEPT CHECK

Because humans can't make either omega-3 or omega-6 fatty acids, which perform vital functions in the body, they must be obtained from the diet and therefore are called essential fatty acids. Plant oils are generally rich in omega-6 fatty acids. Eating fatty fish at least twice a week is a good way to meet omega-3 fatty acid needs. Fish oil supplementation (about 1 gram per day of the related omega-3 fatty acids) is generally acceptable under a physician's guidance if a person does not like fish; however, people with certain medical conditions (e.g., taking anti-coagulant medications) should be cautious with use of fish oil supplements due to increased risk of hemorrhagic stroke. Essential fatty acid deficiency can occur after 2 to 3 weeks if fat is omitted from total parenteral nutrition solutions, which in turn can lead to skin disorders, diarrhea, and other health problems.

5.7 Broader Roles for Fatty Acids and Triglycerides in the Body

Many key functions of fat in the body require the use of fatty acids in the form of triglycerides. Triglycerides are used for energy storage, insulation, and transportation of fat-soluble vitamins.

Providing Energy

Triglycerides contained in the diet and stored in adipose tissue provide the fatty acids that are the main fuel for muscles while at rest and during light activity. Muscles use carbohydrate for fuel in addition to fatty acids supplied by triglycerides only in endurance exercise, such as long-distance running and cycling, or in short bursts of intense activity, such as a 200-meter run. Other body tissues also use fatty acids for energy needs. Overall, about half of the energy used by the entire body at rest and during light activity comes from fatty acids. When considering the whole-body, the use of fatty acids by skeletal and heart muscle is balanced by the use of glucose by the nervous system and red blood cells. Recall from Chapter 4 that cells need a supply of carbohydrate to efficiently process fatty acids for fuel. The details about how we burn fat as a fuel will be discussed in Chapter 7.

Storing Energy for Later Use

We store energy mainly in the form of triglycerides. The body's ability to store fat is essentially limitless. Its fat storage sites, adipose cells, can increase about 50 times in weight. If the amount of fat to be stored exceeds the ability of the existing cells to expand, the body can form new adipose cells.

An important advantage of using triglycerides to store energy in the body is that they are energy dense. Recall that these yield, on average, 9 kcal per gram, whereas proteins and carbohydrates yield only about 4 kcal per gram. In addition, triglycerides are chemically stable, so they are not likely to react with other cell constituents, making them a safe form for storing energy. Finally, when we store triglycerides in adipose cells, we store little else, especially water. Adipose cells contain about 80% lipid and only 20% water and protein. In contrast, imagine if we were to store energy as muscle tissue, which is about 73% water. Body weight linked to energy storage would increase dramatically. The same would be true if we stored energy primarily as glycogen, as about 3 grams of water are stored for every gram of glycogen.

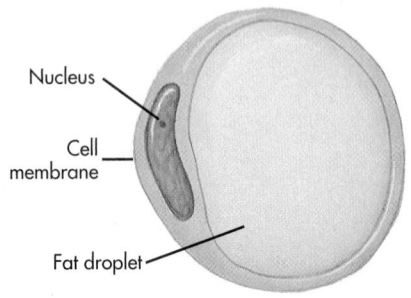

Nucleus

Cell membrane

Fat droplet

Adipose cell

Insulating and Protecting the Body

The insulating layer of fat just beneath the skin is made mostly of triglycerides. Fat tissue also surrounds and protects some organs—kidneys, for example—from injury. We usually don't notice the important insulating function of fat tissue, because we wear clothes and add more as needed. A layer of insulating fat is important in animals living in cold climates. Polar bears, walruses, and whales all build a thick layer of fat tissue around themselves to insulate against cold-weather environments. The extra fat also provides energy storage for times when food is scarce.

Transporting Fat-Soluble Vitamins

Triglycerides and other fats in food carry fat-soluble vitamins to the small intestine and aid their absorption. People who absorb fat poorly, such as those with the disease cystic fibrosis, are at risk for deficiencies of fat-soluble vitamins, especially vitamin K. A similar risk comes from taking mineral oil as a laxative at mealtimes. The body cannot digest or absorb mineral oil, so the undigested oil carries the fat-soluble vitamins from the meal into the feces, where they are eliminated. Unabsorbed fatty acids can bind minerals, such as calcium and magnesium, and draw them into the stool for elimination. This can harm mineral status (see Chapter 9). Recall that the main problem with the fat replacer, olestra, is that it can bind the fat-soluble vitamins and reduce their absorption.

5.8 Phospholipids in the Body

Many types of phospholipids exist in the body, especially in the brain. They form important parts of cell membranes. Phospholipids are found in body cells, and they participate in fat digestion in the intestine. Recall that the various forms of lecithin (discussed earlier) are common examples of phospholipids (review Fig. 5-4b).

Cell membranes are composed primarily of phospholipids. A cell membrane looks much like a sea of phospholipids with protein "islands" (Fig. 5-15). The proteins

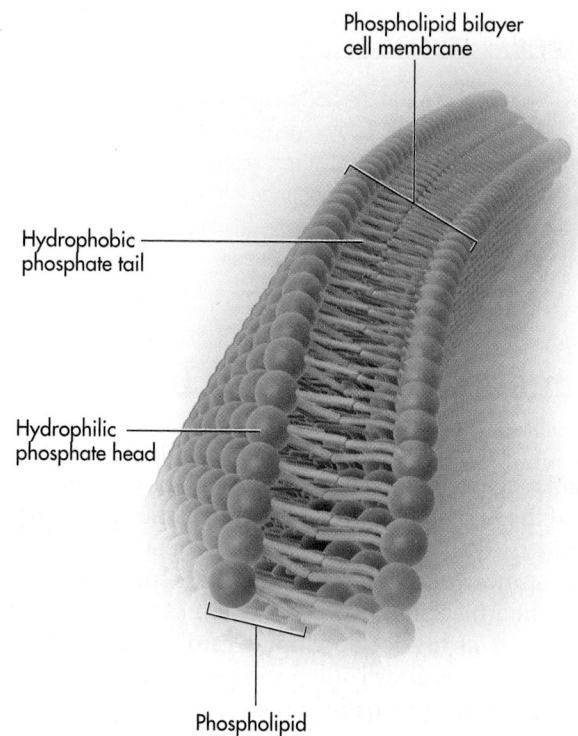

Phospholipid bilayer cell membrane

Hydrophobic phosphate tail

Hydrophilic phosphate head

Phospholipid

FIGURE 5-15 ▶ Phospholipids are the main components of cell membranes, forming a double or bilayer of lipid.

form receptors for hormones, function as enzymes, and act as transporters for nutrients. The fatty acids on the phospholipids serve as a source of essential fatty acids for the cell. Some cholesterol is also present in the membrane.

In some foods, phospholipids function as emulsifiers (as covered earlier) allowing fat and water to mix. By breaking fat globules into small droplets, emulsifiers enable a fat to be suspended in water. They act as bridges between the oil and water that in turn lead to the formation of tiny oil droplets surrounded by thin shells of water. In an emulsified solution, such as salad dressing or mayonnaise, millions of tiny oil droplets are separated by shells of water (review Fig. 5-7).

The body's main emulsifiers are the lecithins and bile acids, produced by the liver and released into the small intestine via the gallbladder during digestion.

5.9 Cholesterol in the Body

Cholesterol plays many vital roles in the body. It forms part of some important hormones, such as estrogen, testosterone, and a form of the active vitamin D hormone. Cholesterol is also the building block of bile acids, needed for fat digestion. Finally, cholesterol is an essential structural component of cells and the outer layer of the lipoprotein particles that transport lipids in the blood. The cholesterol content of the heart, liver, kidney, and brain is high, reflecting its critical role in these organs.

About two-thirds of the cholesterol circulating through your body is made by body cells; the remaining one-third is consumed in the diet. Each day, our cells produce approximately 875 milligrams of cholesterol. Of the 875 milligrams of cholesterol made by the body, about 400 milligrams are used to make new bile acids to replenish those lost in the feces, and about 50 milligrams are used to make hormones. In addition to all the cholesterol cells make, we consume about 180 to 325 milligrams of cholesterol per day from animal-derived food products, with men consuming the higher amount compared to women. Absorption of cholesterol from food ranges from about 40% to 65%. The effect of blood cholesterol, especially LDL cholesterol, on cardiovascular disease risk will be discussed in the "Nutrition and Your Health" section.

See Nutrition and Your Health: Lipids and Cardiovascular Disease at the end of Chapter 5.

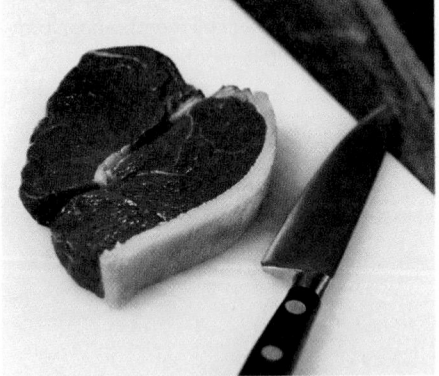

▲ Trimming the fat off meats can help reduce saturated fat intake. Limiting intake of meat that is highly marbled with fat (streaks of fat running through the lean) helps, too.

CONCEPT CHECK

Triglycerides are the major form of fat in the body. They are used for energy and stored in adipose tissue, they insulate and protect body organs, and they transport fat-soluble vitamins. Phospholipids are emulsifiers—compounds that can suspend fat in water. Phospholipids also form parts of cell membranes and various compounds in the body. Cholesterol, a sterol, forms part of cell membranes, hormones, and bile acids. If sufficient amounts are not consumed, the body makes what phospholipids and cholesterol it needs.

5.10 Recommendations for Fat Intake

There is no RDA for total fat intake for adults, although there is an Adequate Intake set for total fat for infants (see Chapter 15). The 2010 Dietary Guidelines for Americans recommendation and the Acceptable Macronutrient Distribution Range is that total fat intake should be 20% to 35% of total calories, which equates to 44 to 78 grams per day for a person who consumes 2000 kcal daily. The most specific recommendations for fat intake come from the American Heart Association (AHA) (see Further Reading 9). Many North Americans are at risk for developing cardiovascular disease, so AHA promotes dietary and lifestyle goals aimed at reducing this risk. The AHA diet and lifestyle goals for cardiovascular disease risk reduction for the general public are presented in Table 5-3. These goals include aiming for an overall healthy eating pattern; appropriate

TABLE 5-3 American Heart Association 2006 Diet and Lifestyle Goals for Cardiovascular Disease Risk Reduction

- Consume an overall healthy diet.

- Aim for a healthy body weight.

- Aim for recommended levels of low-density lipoprotein (LDL) cholesterol, high-density lipoprotein (HDL) cholesterol, and triglycerides.

- Aim for a normal blood pressure.

- Aim for a normal blood glucose level.

- Be physically active.

- Avoid use of and exposure to tobacco products.

From: Lichtenstein AH and others: Diet and lifestyle recommendations revision 2006. A scientific statement from the American Heart Association Nutrition Committee. *Circulation* 114:82, 2006.

body weight; and a desirable blood cholesterol profile, blood pressure, and blood glucose level. In Table 5-4, a more detailed list of recommendations is provided for those who currently are at high risk or have cardiovascular disease.

To reduce risk for cardiovascular disease, the AHA recommends that no more than 7% of total calories come from saturated fat and no more than 1% from *trans* fat. These are the primary fatty acids that raise LDL. In addition, cholesterol should amount to a maximum of 300 mg per day. Table 5-5 lists the cholesterol content of some foods. This often happens along with the reduction in saturated fat and *trans* fat intake. Table 5-6 is an example of a diet that adheres to 20% or 30% of calories as fat. Compare these recommendations to the actual dietary intake patterns of these fats by North Americans: 33% of calories from total fat, about 13% of calories from saturated fat, and 180 to 320 milligrams of cholesterol each day.

TABLE 5-4 American Heart Association 2006 Diet and Lifestyle Recommendations for Cardiovascular Disease Risk Reduction

- Balance calorie intake and physical activity to achieve or maintain a healthy body weight.

- Consume a diet rich in vegetables and fruits.

- Choose whole-grain, high-fiber foods.

- Consume fish, especially oily fish, at least twice a week.

- Limit your intake of saturated fat to less than 7% of energy, *trans* fat to less than 1% of energy, and cholesterol to less than 300 milligrams per day by
  — choosing lean meats and vegetable alternatives;
  — selecting fat-free (skim), 1%-fat, and low-fat dairy products; and
  — minimizing intake of partially-hydrogenated fats.

- Minimize your intake of beverages and foods with added sugars.

- Choose and prepare foods with little or no salt.

- If you consume alcohol, do so in moderation.

- When you eat food prepared outside of the home, follow the AHA Diet and Lifestyle Recommendations.

From: Lichtenstein AH and others: Diet and lifestyle recommendations revision 2006. A scientific statement from the American Heart Association Nutrition Committee. *Circulation* 114:82, 2006.

One goal of *Healthy People 2020* is to reduce consumption of saturated fat in the population ages 2 years and older to 9.5% of total calorie intake.

TABLE 5-5 Cholesterol Content of Foods

3 oz beef brains	2635 mg
3 oz beef liver	337 mg
1 large egg yolk*	209 mg
3 oz shrimp	166 mg
3 oz beef*	75 mg
3 oz pork	75 mg
3 oz chicken or turkey (white meat)*	75 mg
1 cup ice cream	63 mg
3 oz trout	60 mg
3 oz tuna	45 mg
3 oz hot dog	38 mg
1 oz cheddar cheese*	30 mg
1 cup whole milk*	24 mg
1 cup 1% milk	12 mg
1 cup fat-free milk	5 mg
1 large egg white	0 mg

*Leading dietary sources of cholesterol in American diets.

Some advice regarding fat intake from the 2010 Dietary Guidelines:

- Consume less than 10% of calories from saturated fatty acids by replacing them with monounsaturated and polyunsaturated fatty acids.

- Consume less than 300 mg per day of dietary cholesterol.

- Keep *trans* fatty acid consumption as low as possible by limiting foods that contain synthetic sources of *trans* fats, such as partially hydrogenated oils, and by limiting other solid fats.

- Reduce the intake of calories from solid fats and added sugars.

Continued

- Use oils to replace solid fats where possible.
- Limit the consumption of foods that contain refined grains, especially refined grain foods that contain solid fats, added sugars, and sodium.
- Replace protein foods that are higher in solid fats with choices that are lower in solid fats and calories and/or are sources of oils.
- Increase the amount and variety of seafood in place of same meat and poultry.
- Increase intake of fat-free or low-fat milk and milk products, such as milk, yogurt, cheese, or fortified soy beverages.

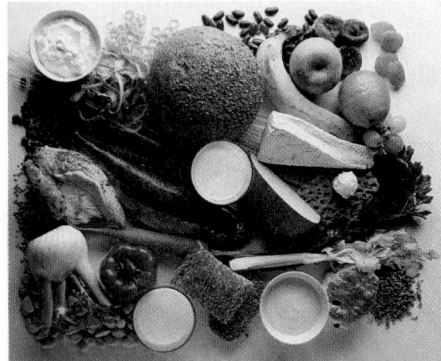

▲ **Whole grains** (shredded wheat, whole-wheat bread, oatmeal cookies, popcorn), **fruits** (orange juice, apple, banana, raisins), **vegetables** (carrots, lettuce, tomato), **lean meats** (roast beef, turkey, chicken), and **fat-free milk** are the primary components of the low-fat menus in Table 5-6.

The advice to consume 20% to 35% of calories as fat does not apply to infants and toddlers below the age of 2 years. These youngsters are forming new tissue that requires fat, especially in the brain, so their intake of fat and cholesterol should not be greatly restricted.

TABLE 5-6 Daily Menu Examples Containing 2000 kcal and 30% or 20% of Calories as Fat

30% of Calories as Fat		20% of Calories as Fat	
Food	Fat (grams)	Food	Fat (grams)
Breakfast			
Orange juice, 1 cup	0.5	Same	0.5
Shredded wheat, ¾ cup	0.5	Shredded wheat, 1 cup	0.7
Toasted bagel	1.1	Same	1.1
Tub margarine, 3 teaspoons	11.4	Tub margarine, 2 teaspoons	7.6
1% low-fat milk, 1 cup	2.5	Fat-free milk, 1 cup	0.6
Lunch			
Whole-wheat bread, 2 slices	2.4	Same	2.4
Roast beef, 2 ounces	4.9	Light turkey roll, 2 ounces	0.9
Mayonnaise, 3 teaspoons	11.0	Mayonnaise, 2 teaspoons	7.3
Lettuce	—	Same	—
Tomato	—	Same	—
Oatmeal cookie, 1	3.3	Oatmeal cookie, 2	6.6
Snack			
Apple	—	Same	—
Dinner			
Chicken tenders frozen meal	18.0	Fat-free chicken tenders	—
Carrots, ½ cup	—	Same	—
Dinner roll, 1	2.0	Same	2.0
Margarine, 1 teaspoon	3.8	Same	3.8
Banana	0.6	Same	0.6
1% low-fat milk, 1 cup	2.5	Fat-free milk, 1 cup	0.6
Snack			
Raisins, 2 teaspoons	—	Raisins, ½ cup	—
Air-popped popcorn, 3 cups	1.0	Air-popped popcorn, 6 cups	2.0
Margarine, 2 teaspoons	7.6	Same	7.6
Totals	**73.1**		**44.3**

The American Dietetic Association, the Dietitians of Canada (see Further Reading 1), the National Cholesterol Education Program (NCEP), and the Food and Nutrition Board are in agreement with the advice of the AHA. The 2010 Dietary Guidelines also support this advice. In addition to fat intake, controlling total calorie intake is also significant, as weight control is a vital component of cardiovascular disease prevention.

Regarding essential fatty acids, the Food and Nutrition Board has issued recommendations for both omega-6 and omega-3 fatty acids. The amounts listed in Table 5-7 work out to about 5% of calorie in-take for the total of both essential fatty acids. Infants and children have lower needs (again, see Chapter 15). Consumption of fish at least twice a week is one step toward meeting requirements for essential fatty acids.

The typical North American diet derives about 7% of calories from polyunsaturated fatty acids, and thus meets essential fatty acid needs. An upper limit of 10% of calorie intake as polyunsaturated fatty acids is often recommended, in part because the breakdown (oxidation) of those present in lipoproteins is linked to increased cholesterol deposition in the arteries (see the Nutrition and Your Health section in this chapter). Depression of immune function is also suspected to be caused by an excessive intake of polyunsaturated fatty acids.

TABLE 5-7 Food and Nutrition Board Recommendations for Omega-6 and Omega-3 Fatty Acids per Day

	Men (grams per day)	Women (grams per day)
Linoleic acid (omega-6)	17	12
Alpha-linolenic acid (omega-3)	1.6	1.1

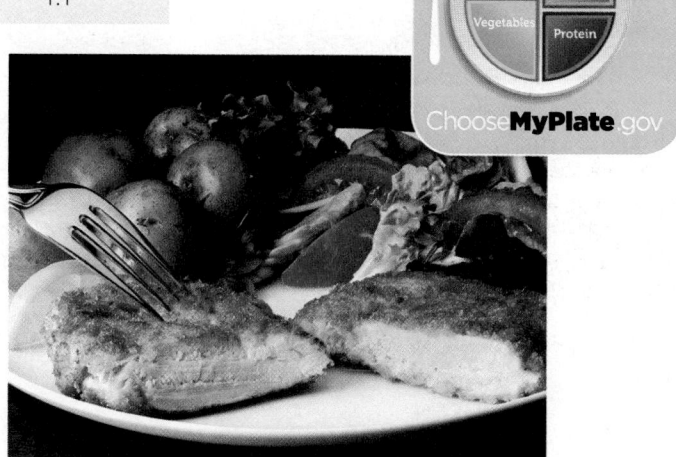

In recent years, the Mediterranean diet (see Newsworthy Nutrition in margin) has attracted a lot of attention as a result of lower rates of chronic diseases seen in people following such a diet plan. The major sources of fat in the Mediterranean diet include liberal amounts of olive oil compared to a small amount of animal fat (from animal flesh and dairy products). In contrast, major sources of fat in the typical North American diet include animal flesh, whole milk, pastries, cheese, margarine, and mayonnaise. While dietary fat sources definitely play a role in prevention of chronic disease, it is important to remember that other aspects of one's lifestyle also contribute to disease risk. People who follow a Mediterranean diet also tend to consume moderate alcohol (usually in the form of red wine, which contains many antioxidants), eat plenty of whole grains and few refined carbohydrates, and are also more physically active than typical North Americans.

An alternative plan for reduction of cardiovascular disease is Dr. Dean Ornish's purely vegetarian (**vegan**) diet plan (see Further Reading 12). This diet is very low in fat, including only a scant quantity of vegetable oil used in cooking and the small amount of oils present in plant foods. Individuals restricting fat intake to 20% of calories should be monitored by a physician, as the resulting increase in carbohydrate intake can increase blood triglycerides in some people, which is not a healthful change. Over time, however, the initial problem of high blood triglycerides on a low-fat diet may self-correct. Among people following the Ornish plan, blood triglycerides initially increased, but within a year, fell to normal values as long as they emphasized high-fiber carbohydrate sources, controlled (or improved) body weight, and followed a regular exercise program.

In summary, the general consensus among nutrition experts suggests that limitation of saturated fat, cholesterol, and *trans* fat intake should be the primary focus, and that the diet needs to contain some omega-3 and omega-6 fatty acids (Table 5-8). Furthermore, if fat intake exceeds 30% of total calories, the extra fat should come from monounsaturated fat.

▲ If you are looking to decrease the amount of saturated and *trans* fats in your diet, it is a good idea to opt for lower-fat substitutes for some of your current high-fat food choices. How do you think this meal compares with the fried meal on p. 179? How does it compare to MyPlate recommendations?

vegan A person who eats only plant foods.

NEWSWORTHY NUTRITION

Low-fat diet not necessary for weight loss

A low-fat; Mediterranean, or low-carbohydrate diet, was studied in moderately obese adults. Weight loss on the Mediterranean Diet (4.6 kg) and low-carbohydrate diet (5.5 kg) was greater than weight loss on the low-fat diet. This, along with the more favorable effects on lipids (low-carbohydrate diet) and on glycemic control (Mediterranean Diet), indicates they may be effective alternatives to low-fat diets.

Source: Shai I and others: Weight loss with a low-carbohydrate, Mediterranean, or low-fat diet. *New England Journal of Medicine* 359:229, 2008 (see Further Reading 14).

connect NUTRITION **Check out the Connect site www.mcgrawhillconnect.com to further explore weight-loss diets.**

CONCEPT CHECK

There is no RDA for fat. We need about 5% of total calorie intake from plant oils to obtain the needed essential fatty acids. Eating fatty fish at least twice a week is also advised to supply omega-3 fatty acids. Many health-related agencies recommend a diet containing no more than 35% of calorie intake as fat, with no more than 7% to 10% of calorie intake as a combination of saturated fat and *trans* fat for the general public. Cholesterol intake should be limited to 200 to 300 milligrams per day. These practices help maintain a normal LDL value in the blood. The North American diet contains about 33% of calories as fat, with about 13% of calories as saturated fat and about 3% as *trans* fatty acids. Cholesterol intake varies from about 200 to 400 milligrams per day.

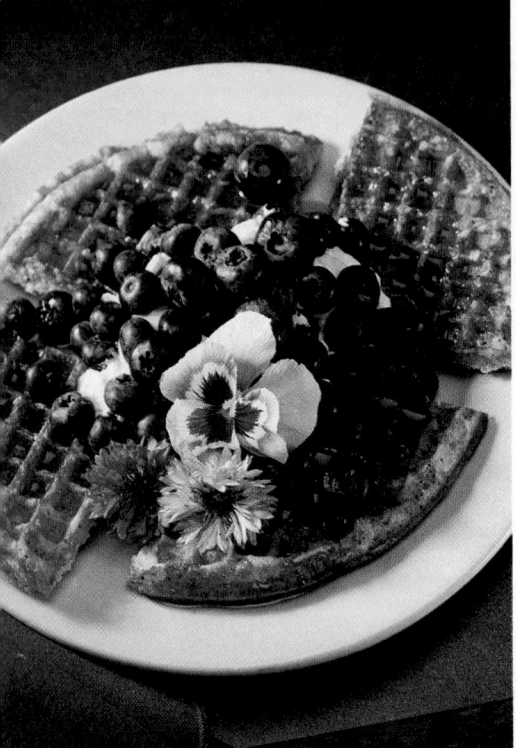

TABLE 5-8 Tips for Avoiding Too Much Fat, Saturated Fat, Cholesterol, and *Trans* Fat

	Eat Less of These Foods	Eat More of These Foods
Grains	• Pasta dishes with cheese or cream sauces • Croissants • Pastries • Doughnuts • Pie crust	• Whole-grain breads • Whole-grain pasta • Brown rice • Angel food cake • Animal or graham crackers • Air-popped popcorn
Vegetables	• French fries • Potato chips • Vegetables cooked in butter, cheese, or cream sauces	• Fresh, frozen, baked, or steamed vegetables
Fruit	• Fruit pies	• Fresh, frozen, or canned fruits
Dairy	• Whole milk • Ice cream • High-fat cheese • Cheesecake	• Fat-free and reduced-fat milk • Low-fat frozen desserts (e.g., yogurt, sherbet, ice milk) • Reduced-fat/part-skim cheese
Protein	• Bacon • Sausage • Organ meats (e.g., liver) • Egg yolks	• Fish • Skinless poultry • Lean cuts of meat (with fat trimmed away) • Soy products • Egg whites/egg substitutes
Oils	• Butter and stick margarine	• Canola oil or olive oil • Tub or liquid margarine (in small amounts)

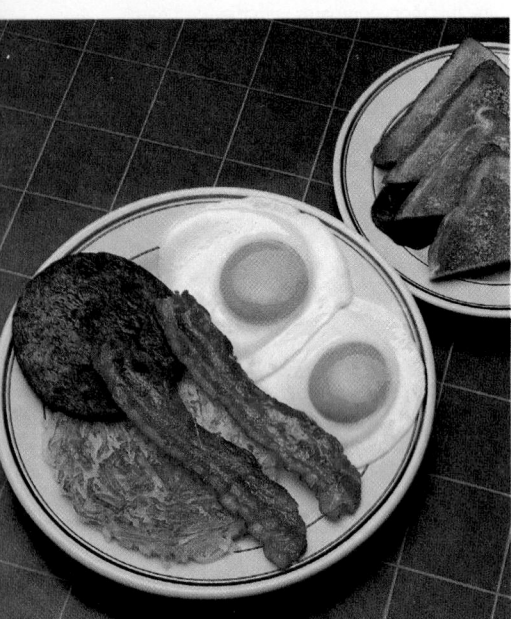

▲ To avoid too much saturated fat and cholesterol, for breakfast eat fewer foods like bacon, sausage, hash browns and whole eggs and more foods like whole-grain waffles and fresh fruit.

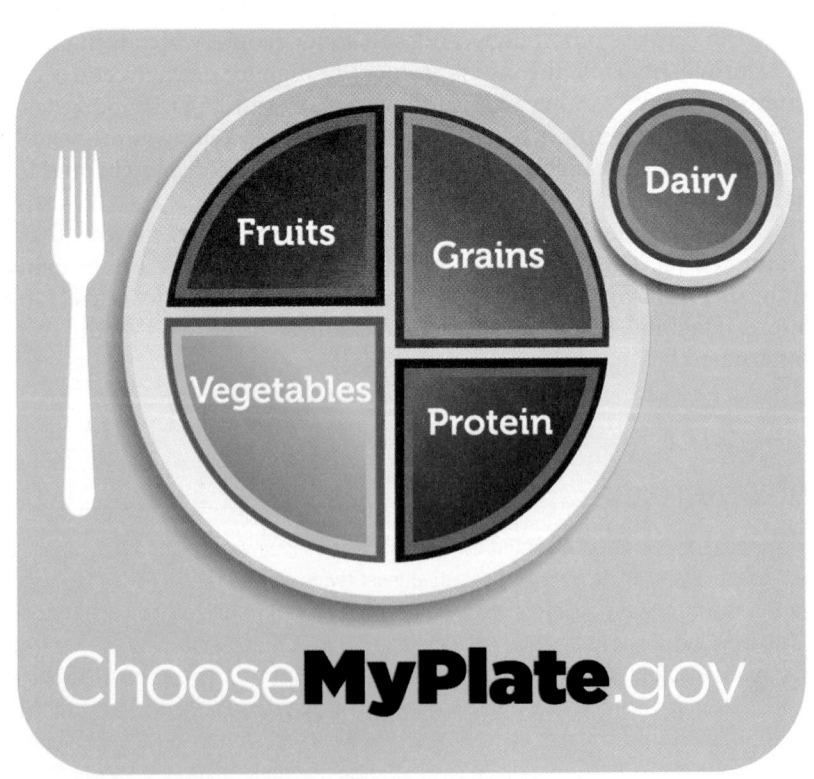

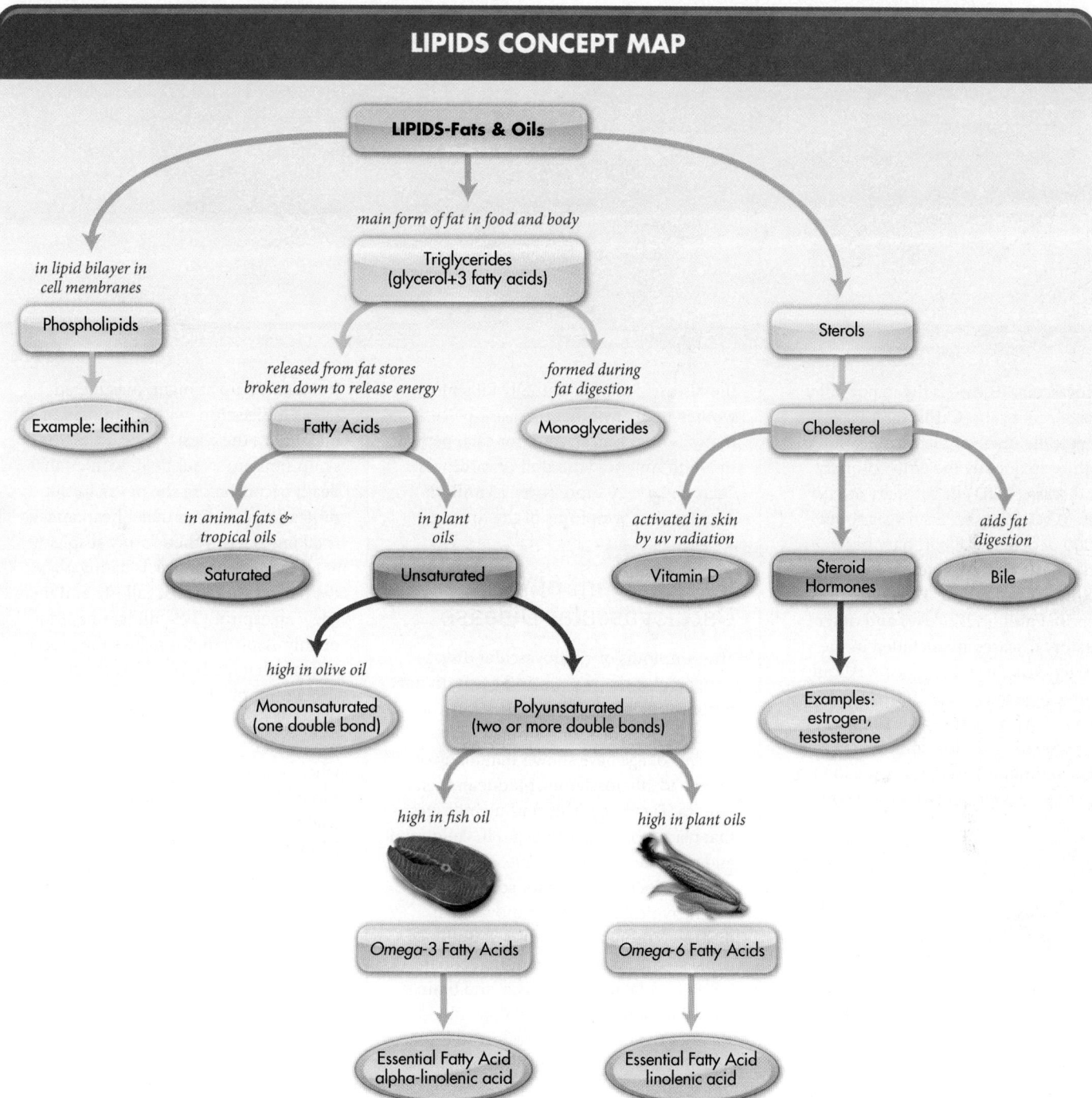

LIPIDS CONCEPT MAP

LIPIDS-Fats & Oils

main form of fat in food and body

Triglycerides
(glycerol+3 fatty acids)

in lipid bilayer in cell membranes

Phospholipids

Example: lecithin

released from fat stores broken down to release energy

Fatty Acids

formed during fat digestion

Monoglycerides

Sterols

Cholesterol

in animal fats & tropical oils

Saturated

in plant oils

Unsaturated

activated in skin by uv radiation

Vitamin D

Steroid Hormones

aids fat digestion

Bile

high in olive oil

Monounsaturated
(one double bond)

Polyunsaturated
(two or more double bonds)

Examples:
estrogen,
testosterone

high in fish oil

high in plant oils

Omega-3 Fatty Acids

Omega-6 Fatty Acids

Essential Fatty Acid
alpha-linolenic acid

Essential Fatty Acid
linolenic acid

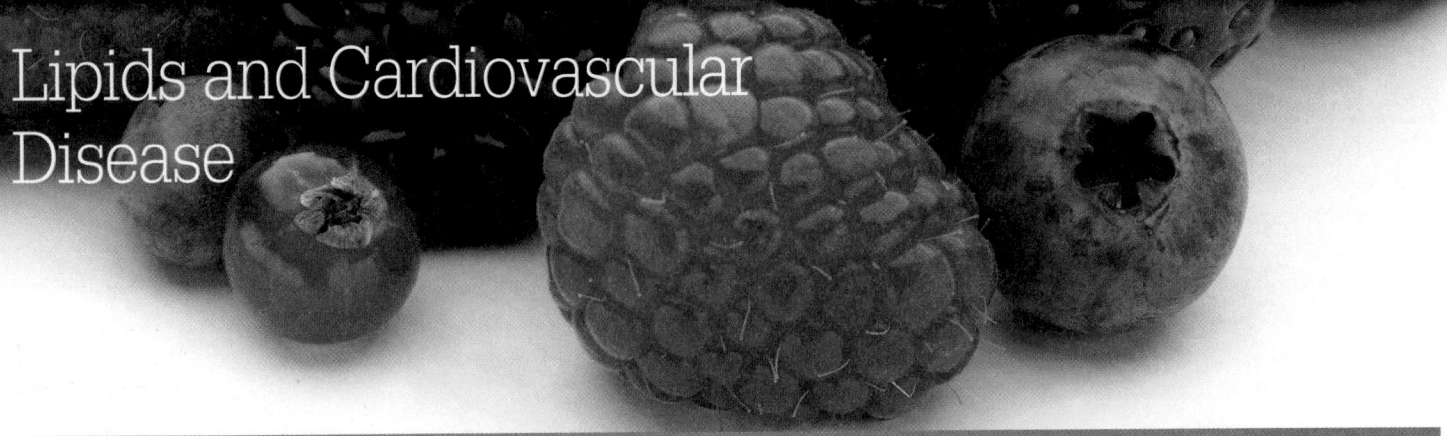

Lipids and Cardiovascular Disease

Cardiovascular disease is the major killer of North Americans. Cardiovascular disease typically involves the coronary arteries and, thus, frequently the term coronary heart disease (CHD) or coronary artery disease (CAD) is used. Each year about 500,000 people die of coronary heart disease in the United States, about 60% more than die of cancer. The figure rises to almost 1 million if strokes and other circulatory diseases are included in the global term *cardiovascular disease*. About 1.5 million people in the United States each year have a heart attack. The overall male-to-female ratio for cardiovascular disease is about 2:1. Women generally lag about 10 years behind men in developing

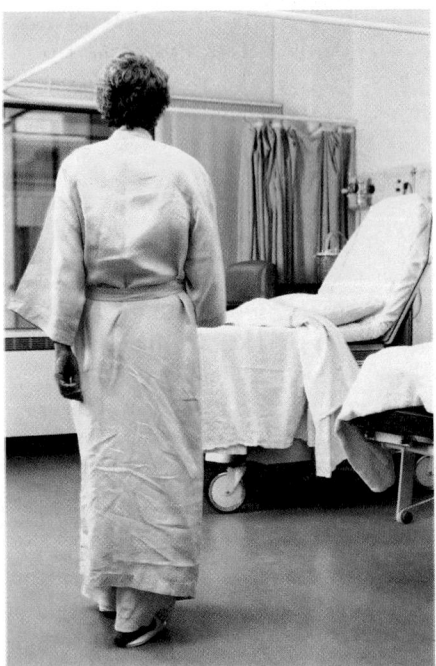

▲ Cardiovascular disease kills more women than any other disease—twice as many as does cancer.

the disease. Still, it eventually kills more women than any other disease—twice as many as does cancer. And, for each person in North America who dies of cardiovascular disease, 20 more (over 13 million people) have symptoms of the disease.

Development of Cardiovascular Disease

The symptoms of cardiovascular disease develop over many years and often do not become obvious until old age. Nonetheless, autopsies of young adults under 20 years of age have shown that many of them had atherosclerotic **plaque** in their arteries (Fig. 5-16). This finding indicates that plaque buildup can begin in childhood and continue throughout life, although it usually goes undetected for some time.

The typical forms of cardiovascular disease—coronary heart disease and strokes—are associated with inadequate blood circulation in the heart and brain related to buildup of this plaque. Blood supplies the heart muscle, brain, and other body organs with oxygen and nutrients. When blood flow via the coronary arteries surrounding the heart is interrupted, the heart muscle can be damaged. A heart attack, or **myocardial infarction,** may result (review Fig. 5-16). This may cause the heart to beat irregularly or to stop. About 25% of people do not survive their first heart attack. If blood flow to parts of the brain is interrupted long enough, part of the brain dies, causing a **cerebrovascular accident,** or stroke.

A heart attack can strike with the sudden force of a sledgehammer, with pain radiating up the neck or down the arm.

It can sneak up at night, masquerading as indigestion, with slight pain or pressure in the chest. Many times, the symptoms are so subtle in women that death occurs before she or the health professional realizes that a heart attack is taking place. If there is any suspicion at all that a heart attack is taking place, the person should first call 911 and then chew an aspirin (325 milligrams) thoroughly. Aspirin helps reduce the blood clotting that leads to a heart attack.

Continuous formation and breakdown of blood clots in the blood vessels is a normal process. However, in areas where plaques build up, blood clots are more likely to remain intact and then lead to a blockage, cutting off or diminishing the supply of blood to the heart (via the coronary arteries) or brain (via the carotid arteries). More than 95% of heart attacks are caused by such blood clots. Heart attacks generally are caused by total blockage of the coronary arteries due to a blood clot forming in an area of the artery already partially blocked by plaque. Disruption of the plaque may even lead to eventual clot formation.

plaque A cholesterol-rich substance deposited in the blood vessels; it contains various white blood cells, smooth muscle cells, various proteins, cholesterol and other lipids, and eventually calcium.

myocardial infarction Death of part of the heart muscle. Also termed a *heart attack.*

cerebrovascular accident (CVA) Death of part of the brain tissue due typically to a blood clot. Also termed a *stroke.*

► Typical warning signs of a heart attack are:

- Intense, prolonged chest pain or pressure, sometimes radiating to other parts of the upper body (men and women)
- Shortness of breath (men and women)
- Sweating (men and women)
- Nausea and vomiting (especially women)
- Dizziness (especially women)
- Weakness (men and women)
- Jaw, neck, and shoulder pain (especially women)
- Irregular heartbeat (men and women)

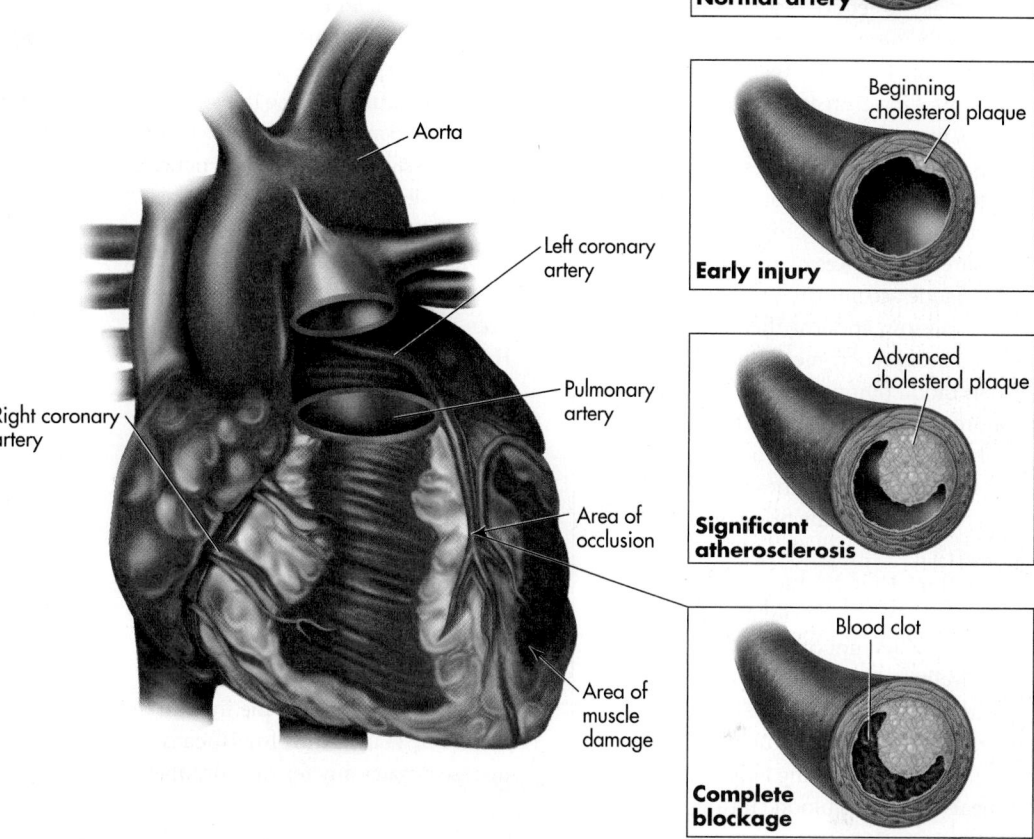

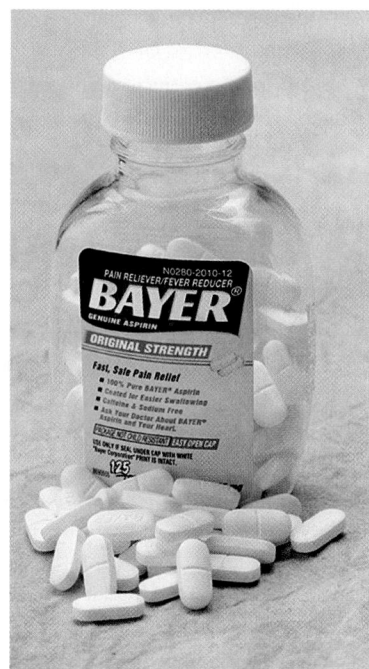

▲ At the first sign of a possible heart attack, the person should first call 911 and then thoroughly chew an aspirin.

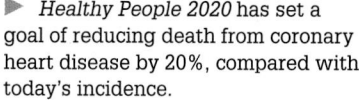

► *Healthy People 2020* has set a goal of reducing death from coronary heart disease by 20%, compared with today's incidence.

FIGURE 5-16 ► The road to a heart attack. Injury to an artery wall begins the process. This is followed by a progressive buildup of plaque in the artery walls. The heart attack represents the terminal phase of the process. Blockage of the left coronary artery by a blood clot is evident. The heart muscle served by the portion of the coronary artery beyond the point of blockage lacks oxygen and nutrients and is damaged and may die. This damage can lead to a significant drop in heart function and often total heart failure.

Atherosclerosis probably first develops to repair damage in a vessel lining. The damage that starts this process can be caused by smoking, diabetes, hypertension, LDL, and viral and bacterial infection. Ongoing inflammation in the blood vessel is also suspected to cause blood vessel damage. (A laboratory test for c-reactive protein in the blood is used to assess if inflammation is present.) (see Further Reading 3). Atherosclerosis can be seen in arteries throughout the body. The damage develops especially at points where an artery branches into two smaller vessels. A great deal of stress is placed on the vessel walls at these points due to changes in blood flow.

Once blood vessel damage has occurred, the next step in the development of atherosclerosis is the progression phase. This step is characterized by deposition of plaque at the site of initial damage. The rate of plaque buildup during the progression phase is directly related to the amount of LDL in the blood. The form of LDL that contributes to atherosclerosis is **oxidized** LDL (see Further Readings 6 and 10). This

oxidize In the most basic sense, the loss of an electron or gain of an oxygen by a chemical substance. This change typically alters the shape and/or function of the substance.

form is preferentially taken up by scavenger cells in the arterial wall. Nutrients and phytochemicals that have **antioxidant** properties may reduce LDL oxidation. Fruits and vegetables are particularly rich in these compounds. Eating fruits and vegetables regularly is one positive step we can make to reduce plaque buildup and slow the progression of cardiovascular disease. Some fruits and vegetables particularly helpful in this regard include legumes (beans), nuts, dried plums (prunes), raisins, berries, plums, apples, cherries, oranges, grapes, spinach, broccoli, red bell peppers, potatoes, and onions. Tea and coffee are also sources of antioxidants.

As plaque accumulates, arteries harden, narrow, and lose their elasticity. Affected arteries become further damaged as blood pumps through them and pressure increases. Finally, in the terminal phase, a clot or spasm in a plaque-clogged artery leads to a heart attack.

Factors that typically bring on a heart attack in a person already at risk include dehydration; acute emotional stress (such as firing an employee); strenuous physical activity when not otherwise physically fit (shoveling snow, for example); waking during the night or getting up in the morning (linked to an abrupt increase in stress); and consuming large, high-fat meals (increases blood clotting).

Risk Factors for Cardiovascular Disease

Many of us are free of the risk factors that contribute to rapid development of atherosclerosis. If so, the advice of health experts is to consume a balanced diet, perform regular physical activity, have a complete fasting lipoprotein analysis performed at age 20 or beyond, and reevaluate risk factors every 5 years.

For most people, however, the most likely risk factors are:

- **Total blood cholesterol over 200 milligrams per 100 milliliters of blood** (mg/dl; dl is short for deciliter or 100 milliliters). Risk is especially high when total cholesterol is at or over 240 mg/dl and LDL-cholesterol readings are over 130 to 160 mg/dl. (The terms LDL-cholesterol and HDL-cholesterol

are used when expressing the blood concentration because it is the cholesterol content of these lipoproteins that is measured.)

- **Smoking.** Smoking is the main cause of about 20% of cardiovascular disease deaths and generally negates the female advantage of later occurrence of the disease. A combination of smoking and oral contraceptive use increases the risk of cardiovascular disease in women even more. Smoking greatly increases the expression of a person's genetically linked risk for cardiovascular disease, even if one's blood lipids are low. Smoking also makes blood more likely to clot. Even secondhand smoke has been implicated as a risk factor.
- **Hypertension. Systolic blood pressure** over 139 (millimeters of mercury) and **diastolic blood pressure** over 89 indicate hypertension. Healthy blood pressure values are less than 120 and 80, respectively. (Treatment of hypertension is reviewed in Chapter 9.)
- **Diabetes.** Diabetes virtually guarantees development of cardiovascular disease and so puts a person with diabetes in the high-risk group. Insulin increases cholesterol synthesis in the liver, in turn increasing LDL in the bloodstream. This disease negates any female advantage.

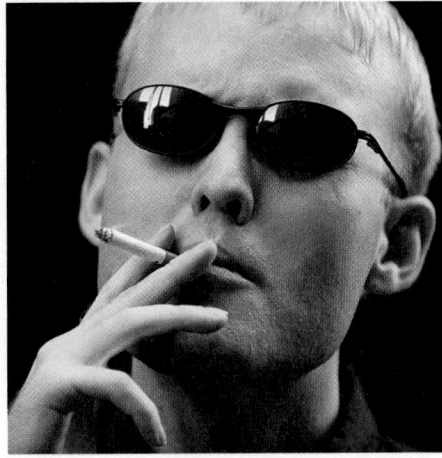

▲ Smoking is one of the four major risk factors for developing cardiovascular disease.

antioxidant Generally a compound that stops the damaging effects of reactive substances seeking an electron (i.e., oxidizing agents). This prevents breakdown (oxidizing) of substances in foods or the body, particularly lipids.

systolic blood pressure The pressure in the arterial blood vessels associated with the pumping of blood from the heart.

diastolic blood pressure The pressure in the arterial blood vessels when the heart is between beats.

MAKING DECISIONS

Antioxidant Supplements and Cardiovascular Disease

Are large doses of antioxidant vitamin supplements a reliable way to reduce LDL oxidation, and thereby prevent cardiovascular disease? Controversy about such dietary supplementation exists among the experts, as will be detailed in Chapter 8. The American Heart Association does not support use of antioxidant supplements (such as vitamin E) to reduce cardiovascular disease risk. This is because large-scale studies have shown no decrease in cardiovascular disease risk with use of antioxidant supplements. One study even showed a modest increase for heart failure in people with diabetes or otherwise at high risk for cardiovascular disease after taking antioxidant supplements. However, further trials of antioxidant supplementation (e.g., 600 IU of vitamin E every other day) for prevention of heart disease in men are ongoing. With regard to women, 600 IU of natural-source vitamin E taken every other day provided no overall benefit for major cardiovascular events (or cancer). More research is warranted, however, as a decrease in sudden cardiac death was seen in a subset of older women in this study. Some experts suggest daily vitamin E supplementation (100 IU to 400 IU) may be helpful for *preventing* cardiovascular disease, while other experts recommend against the practice. One thing is certain: any supplementation of vitamin E should be taken only under the guidance of a physician, because of interactions with vitamin K and anticlotting medications (and possibly high-dose aspirin use).

For more information on cardiovascular disease, see the website of the American Heart Association at www.americanheart.org or the heart disease section of Healthfinder at www.healthfinder.gov/tours/heart.htm. This is a site created by the U.S. government for consumers. In addition, visit the website www.nhlbi.nih.gov/.

Healthy People 2020 has set a goal of reducing total blood cholesterol among adults from the average of 198 mg/dl to 178 mg/dl, as well as reducing the percentage of adults with high blood cholesterol from 15% to 13.5%.

Cardiovascular Disease Risk Factors

- Total blood cholesterol > 200 mg/dl
- Smoking
- Hypertension
- Diabetes
- HDL cholesterol < 40 mg/dl
- Age: Men > 45 yr; Women > 55 yr
- Family history of cardiovascular disease
- Blood triglycerides > 200 mg/dl
- Obesity
- Inactivity

Two approaches have been shown to cause reversal of atherosclerosis in the body. One employs a vegan diet and other lifestyle changes that are part of the Dr. Dean Ornish program. The other employs aggressive LDL lowering with medications.

As noted earlier, aspirin in small doses reduces blood clotting. It is often used under a physician's guidance to treat people at risk for heart attack or stroke, especially if one has already occurred. About 80 to 160 milligrams per day is needed for such benefits. Individuals who may especially benefit from aspirin therapy are men over 40, smokers, postmenopausal women, and people with diabetes, hypertension, or a family history of cardiovascular disease.

Together, the previous four risk factors explain most cases of cardiovascular disease.

Other risk factors to consider:

- HDL-cholesterol under 40 mg/dl, especially when the ratio of total cholesterol to HDL-cholesterol is greater than 4:1 (3.5:1 or less is optimal). Women often have high values for HDL-cholesterol, and therefore it is important for this to be measured in women to establish cardiovascular disease risk. A value of 60 mg/dl or more is especially protective. Exercising for at least 45 minutes four times a week can increase HDL by about 5 mg/dl. Losing excess weight (especially around the waist) and avoiding smoking and overeating also help maintain or raise HDL, as does moderate alcohol consumption.
- Age. Men over 45 years and women over 55 years.
- Family history of cardiovascular disease, especially before age 50.
- Blood triglycerides 200 mg/dl or greater in the fasting state (less than 100 mg/dl is optimal).
- Obesity (especially fat accumulation in the waist). Typical weight gain seen in adults is a chief contributor to the increase in LDL seen with aging. Obesity also typically leads to insulin resistance, creating a diabetes-like state, and ultimately the disease itself. It also increases overall inflamation throughout the body.
- Inactivity. Exercise conditions the arteries to adapt to physical stress. Regular exercise also improves insulin action in the body. The corresponding reduction in insulin output leads to a reduction in lipoprotein synthesis in the liver. Both regular aerobic exercise and resistance exercise are recommended. A person with existing cardiovascular disease should seek physician approval before starting such a program, as should older adults.

Researchers are trying to unravel and quantify numerous other factors that may be linked to premature cardiovascular disease, such as the connection between inadequate intake of vitamin B-6, folate, and vitamin B-12, which can lead to increased homocysteine in the blood. As noted, homocysteine may damage the cells lining the blood vessels, in turn promoting atherosclerosis. Studies show that supplementation with folic acid and B vitamins does not reduce risk of recurrent cardiovascular disease in patients that had previous heart attacks or had existing vascular diseases.

The term *risk factor* is not equivalent to cause of disease; nevertheless, the more of these risk factors one has, the greater the chances of ultimately developing cardiovascular disease. A good example is the **metabolic syndrome** (also called *Syndrome X)* discussed in Chapter 4. A person with the metabolic syndrome would have abdominal obesity, high blood triglycerides, low HDL-cholesterol, hypertension, poor blood glucose regulation (i.e., high fasting blood glucose), and increased blood clotting. This profile raises the risk for cardiovascular disease considerably. On a positive note, cardiovascular disease is rare in populations who have low LDL-cholesterol, normal blood pressure, and do not smoke or have diabetes. By minimizing these risk factors, as well as following the dietary recommendations of the American Heart Association on page 193 and staying physically active, one will most likely reduce many of the other controllable risk factors listed. In other words, develop and follow a total lifestyle plan. Medications may also be added to lower blood lipids, as discussed next. Finally, if a person has a family history of cardiovascular disease but the usual risk factors aren't present, a rarer defect might be the cause. In this case, having a detailed physical examination for other potential causes is advised.

Medical Interventions to Lower Blood Lipids

Some people need even more aggressive therapy added to their regimen of a diet and lifestyle overhaul to treat elevated blood lipids. The clearest indication for this more aggressive approach is in people who already have had a heart attack or have cardiovascular disease symptoms or diabetes.

Medications are the cornerstone of this more aggressive therapy. The National

Cholesterol Education Program in the United States has developed a formula based on age, total blood cholesterol, HDL-cholesterol, smoking history, and blood pressure to determine who needs such medications. Check out this formula at http://hp2010.nhlbihin.net/atpiii/calculator.asp?usertype=pub. This formula provides an estimate for having a heart attack in the next 10 years.

Medications work to lower LDL in one of two ways. Some reduce cholesterol synthesis in the liver. Such medicines are known as "statins" (e.g., atorvistatin [Lipitor]). The cost of treatment with one of these drugs can be from $1,600 or more per year, depending on the dose needed. These medications lead to problems in some people, and so require physician monitoring, especially of liver function. Another group of medications binds bile acids or the cholesterol that is part of bile secreted into the small intestine. This binding leads to their elimination in the feces and so requires the liver to synthesize new bile acids and/or cholesterol. The liver removes LDL from the blood to do this. Some of these medications taste gritty and therefore are not popular.

The current therapeutic goal for people with (or at high risk for) cardiovascular disease (Table 5-9) is to drive LDL down to less than 70 mg/dl.

The statin drug simvastatin (Zocor) has been combined with another drug (ezetimibe) and is marketed as Vytorin, a drug that will treat the two sources of cholesterol, "food and family." While the statin reduces the cholesterol made by the liver, the ezetimibe helps block the absorption of cholesterol from food.

A third group of drugs can be used to lower blood triglycerides by decreasing the triglyceride production of the liver. These include gemfibrozil (Lopid) and megadoses of the vitamin nicotinic acid. The use of nicotinic acid does result in pesky side effects, however, but these are typically manageable.

Other Possible Medical Therapies for Cardiovascular Disease

FDA has approved two margarines that have positive effects on blood cholesterol levels—Benecol and Take Control. These margarines contain plant stanols/sterols.

The plant stanols/sterols, also called phytosterols, work by reducing cholesterol absorption in the small intestine and lowering its return to the liver. The liver responds by taking up more cholesterol from the blood so it can continue to make bile acids. The studies done on the cholesterol-lowering effect of these margarines have found that 2 to 5 grams of plant stanols/sterols per day reduces total blood cholesterol by 8% to 10% and LDL-cholesterol by 9% to 14% (similar to what is seen with some cholesterol-lowering drugs). (see Further Readings 7, 11, and 13.)

Benecol is made from plant stanols extracted from wood pulp. It is sold as margarine and has been added to salad dressings. Take Control is made from plant sterols isolated from soybeans. The recommended amount for both is about 2 to 3 grams per day as part of at least two meals; this works out to about 1 or 2 tablespoons per day. Use would cost about $1.00 per day, as these margarines are more expensive than regular margarines.

In people who have borderline high total blood cholesterol (between 200 and 239 mg/dl), these margarines can be helpful in avoiding future drug therapy. Plant stanols/sterols have been made available in pill form as well. Remember that plant sterols are naturally present in nuts in high concentrations. Wheat germ, sesame seeds, pistachios, and sunflower seeds are some of the richest sources.

The two most common surgical treatments for coronary artery blockage are percutaneous transluminal coronary angioplasty (PTCA) and coronary artery bypass graft (CABG). PTCA involves the insertion of a balloon catheter into an artery. Once it is advanced to the area of the lesion, the balloon is expanded to crush the lesion. This method works best when only one vessel is blocked, and it may be held open with metal mesh, called a stent. CABG involves the removal and use of a saphenous vein, a large vein in the leg, or use of a mammary artery. The relocated vein is sewn to the main heart vessel (aorta) and then used to bypass the blocked artery. The procedure can be performed on one or more blockages.

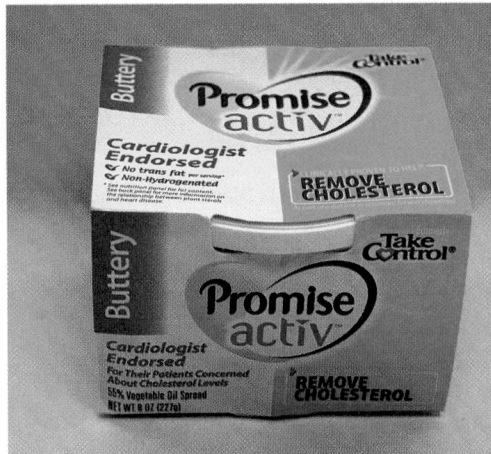

▲ Benecol and Take Control are margarines that are examples of "functional foods" because they contain added cholesterol-lowering plant stanols/sterols.

TABLE 5-9 Sorting Out One's Goals for Cardiovascular Disease Prevention/Treatment

Risk Class	This Is You If . . .	Your LDL (mg/dl) Goal
Very high	You have cardiovascular disease *and* other risk factors such as diabetes, obesity, smoking	Below 70
High	You have cardiovascular disease *or* diabetes *or* two or more risk factors for cardiovascular disease (e.g., smoking, hypertension)	Below 100
Moderately high	You have cardiovascular disease risks and an increased 10-year risk of developing a heart attack	100–130
Moderate	You have two or more risk factors and a marginal chance of developing cardiovascular disease in the next 10 years.	Below 130
Low	You have few or no cardiovascular disease risk factors	Below 160

Case Study Planning a Heart-Healthy Diet

Jackie is a 21-year-old health-conscious individual majoring in business. She recently learned that a diet high in saturated fat can contribute to high blood cholesterol and that exercise is beneficial for the heart. Jackie now takes a brisk 30-minute walk each morning before going to class, and she has started to cut as much fat out of her diet as she can, replacing it mostly with carbohydrates. A typical day for Jackie now begins with a bowl of Fruity Pebbles with 1 cup of skim milk and ½ cup of apple juice. For lunch, she might pack a turkey sandwich on white bread with lettuce, tomato, and mustard; a small package of fat-free pretzels; and a handful of reduced-fat vanilla wafers. Dinner could be a large portion of pasta with some olive oil and garlic mixed in, and a small iceberg lettuce salad with lemon juice squeezed over it. Her snacks are usually baked chips, low-fat cookies, fat-free frozen yogurt, or fat-free pretzels. She drinks diet soft drinks throughout the day as her main beverage.

Answer the following questions, and check your response in Appendix A.

1. Has Jackie made the best diet changes with regard to lowering blood cholesterol and maintaining heart health?
2. Is there much fat left in Jackie's new diet plan? Is it necessary for her to drastically lower her fat intake?
3. What types of fat should Jackie try to consume? Why are these types of fat the most desirable?
4. What types of foods has Jackie used to replace the fat in her diet?
5. What food groups are missing from her new diet plan? How many servings should she be including from these food groups?
6. Is Jackie's new exercise routine appropriate?

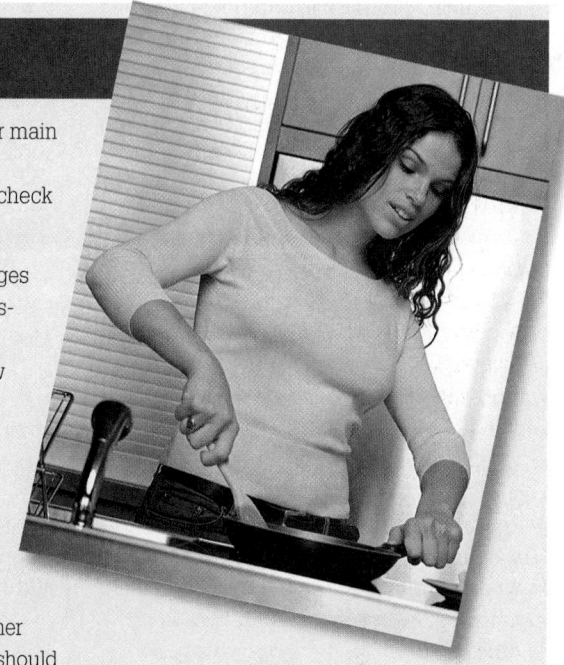

▲ Are there important food groups missing from Jackie's new diet plan?

Summary (Numbers refer to numbered sections in the chapter.)

5.1 Lipids are a group of compounds that do not dissolve in water. Fatty acids are the simplest form of lipid. There are three fatty acids on every triglyceride, the most common type of lipid found in the body and foods. Phospholipids and sterols are two other classes of lipids in food and our bodies.

5.2 Saturated fatty acids contain no carbon-carbon double bonds, monounsaturated fatty acids contain one carbon-carbon double bond, and polyunsaturated fatty acids contain two or more carbon-carbon double bonds in the carbon chain. In omega-3 polyunsaturated fatty acids, the first of the carbon-carbon double bonds is located three carbons from the methyl end of the carbon chain. In omega-6 polyunsaturated fatty acids, the first carbon-carbon double bond counting from the methyl end occurs at the sixth carbon. Both omega-3 and omega-6 fatty acids are essential fatty acids; these must be included in the diet to maintain health.

Triglycerides are formed from a glycerol backbone with three fatty acids.

Triglycerides rich in long-chain saturated fatty acids tend to be solid at room temperature, whereas those rich in monounsaturated and polyunsaturated fatty acids are liquid at room temperature. Triglyceride is the major form of fat in both food and the body. It allows for efficient energy storage, protects certain organs, transports fat-soluble vitamins, and helps insulate the body.

5.3 Foods rich in fat include salad oils, butter, margarine, and mayonnaise. Nuts, bologna, avocados, and bacon are also high in fat, as are peanut butter and cheddar cheese. Steak and hamburger are moderate in fat content, as is whole milk. Many grain products, and fruits and vegetables in general, are low in fat.

Fats and oils have several functions as components of foods. Fats add flavor and texture to foods and provide some satiety after meals. Some phospholipids are used in foods as emulsifiers, which suspend fat in water. When fatty acids break down, food becomes rancid, resulting in a foul odor and unpleasant flavor.

Hydrogenation is the process of converting carbon-carbon double bonds into single bonds by adding hydrogen at the point of unsaturation. The partial-hydrogenation of fatty acids in vegetable oils changes the oils to semisolid fats and helps in food formulation and reduces rancidity. Hydrogenation also increases *trans* fatty acid content. High amounts of *trans* fat in the diet are discouraged, as these increase LDL and reduce HDL.

5.4 Fat digestion takes place primarily in the small intestine. Lipase enzyme released from the pancreas digests long-chain triglycerides into smaller breakdown products—namely, monoglycerides (glycerol backbones with single fatty acids attached) and fatty acids. The breakdown products are then taken up by the absorptive cells of the small intestine. These products are mostly remade into triglycerides and eventually enter the lymphatic system, in turn passing into the bloodstream.

5.5 Lipids are carried in the bloodstream by various lipoproteins, which consist of a central triglyceride core encased in a shell of protein, cholesterol, and phospholipid. Chylomicrons are released from intestinal cells and carry lipids arising from dietary intake. Very-low-density lipoprotein (VLDL) and low-density lipoprotein (LDL) carry lipids both taken up by and synthesized in the liver. High-density lipoprotein (HDL) picks up cholesterol from cells and facilitates its transport back to the liver.

5.6 The essential fatty acids are linoleic acid (an omega-6 fatty acid) and alpha-linolenic acid (on omega-3 fatty acid). Body cells can synthesize hormone-like compounds from both omega-3 and omega-6 fatty acids.

5.7 The compounds produced from omega-3 fatty acids tend to reduce blood clotting, blood pressure, and inflammatory responses in the body. Those produced from omega-6 fatty acids tend to increase blood clotting.

5.8 Phospholipids are derivatives of triglycerides in which one or two of the fatty acids are replaced by phosphorus-containing compounds. Phospholipids are important parts of cell membranes, and some act as efficient emulsifiers.

5.9 Cholesterol forms vital biological compounds, such as hormones, components of cell membranes, and bile acids. Cells in the body make cholesterol whether we eat it or not. It is not a necessary part of an adult's diet.

5.10 There is currently no RDA for fat for adults. Plant oils should contribute about 5% of total calories to achieve the Adequate Intakes proposed for essential fatty acids (linoleic acid and alpha-linolenic acid). Fatty fish are a rich source of omega-3 fatty acids and should be consumed at least twice a week.

Many health agencies and scientific groups suggest a fat intake of no more than 30% to 35% of total calories. Some health experts advocate an even further reduction to 20% of calorie intake for some people to maintain a normal LDL value, but such a diet requires professional guidance. Medications such as "statins" may be added also to lower LDL. If fat intake exceeds 30% of total calories, the diet should emphasize monounsaturated fat. The typical North American diet contains about 33% of total calories as fat.

N&YH In the blood, elevated amounts of LDL and low amounts of HDL are strong predictors of the risk for cardiovascular disease. Additional risk factors for the disease are smoking, hypertension, diabetes, obesity, and inactivity.

Check Your Knowledge (Answers to the following questions are below.)

1. Margarine usually is made by a process called _____, in which hydrogen atoms are added to carbon-carbon double bonds in the polyunsaturated fatty acids found in vegetable oils.
   a. saturation
   b. esterification
   c. isomerization
   d. hydrogenation

2. Essential fatty acids that cause a decrease in blood clotting are
   a. omega-3. c. omega-9.
   b. omega-6. d. prostacyclins.

3. Cholesterol is
   a. a dietary essential; the human body cannot synthesize it.
   b. found in foods of plant origin.
   c. an important part of human cell membranes and necessary to make some hormones.
   d. All of the above.

4. Which of the following groups of foods would be important sources of saturated fatty acids?
   a. olive oil, peanut oil, canola oil
   b. palm oil, palm kernel oil, coconut oil
   c. safflower oil, corn oil, soybean oil
   d. All of the above.

5. Lipoproteins are important for
   a. transport of fats in the blood and lymphatic system.
   b. synthesis of triglycerides.
   c. synthesis of adipose tissue.
   d. enzyme production.

6. Which of the following foods is the best source of omega-3 fatty acids?
   a. fatty fish
   b. peanut butter and jelly
   c. lard and shortenings
   d. beef and other red meats

7. Immediately after a meal, newly digested and absorbed dietary fats appear in the lymph, and then blood, as part of which of the following?
   a. LDL
   b. HDL
   c. chylomicrons
   d. cholesterol

8. High blood concentrations of _____ decrease the risk for cardiovascular disease.

   a. low-density lipoproteins
   b. chylomicrons
   c. high-density lipoproteins
   d. cholesterol

9. Phospholipids such as lecithin are used extensively in food preparation because they
   a. provide the agreeable feel of fat melting on the tongue.
   b. are excellent emulsifiers.
   c. provide important textural features.
   d. impart delicate flavors.

10. The main form of lipid found in the food we eat is
   a. cholesterol.
   b. phospholipids.
   c. triglycerides.
   d. plant sterols

Answers: 1. d (LO 5.3), 2. a (LO 5.6), 3. c (LO 5.9), 4. b (LO 5.3), 5. a (LO 5.5), 6. a (LO 5.6), 7. c (LO 5.5), 8. c (LO 5.5), 9. b (LO 5.8), 10. c (LO 5.2)

Study Questions (Numbers refer to Learning Outcomes)

1. Describe the chemical structures of saturated and polyunsaturated fatty acids and their different effects in both food and the human body. **(LO 5.3)**

2. Relate the need for omega-3 fatty acids in the diet to the recommendation to consume fatty fish at least twice a week. **(LO 5.7)**

3. Describe the structures, origins, and roles of the four major blood lipoproteins. **(LO 5.5)**

4. What are the recommendations from various health-care organizations regarding fat intake? What does this mean in terms of food choices? **(LO 5.10)**

5. What are two important attributes of fat in food? How are these different from the general functions of lipids in the human body? **(LO 5.3)**

6. Describe the significance of and possible uses for reduced-fat foods. **(LO 5.10)**

7. Does the total cholesterol concentration in the bloodstream tell the whole story with respect to cardiovascular disease risk? **(LO 5.9)**

8. List the four main risk factors for the development of cardiovascular disease. **(LO 5.11)**

9. What three lifestyle factors decrease the risk of cardiovascular disease development? **(LO 5.11)**

10. When are medications most needed in cardiovascular disease therapy, and how in general do the various classes of medications operate to reduce risk? **(LO 5.11)**

What Would You Choose Recommendations

With heart health in mind you will want to choose the ground meat with the lowest fat, saturated fat, and cholesterol. Check the Nutrition Facts label to compare the lipid content of various products. Look for cuts of meat with "round " or "loin" in the name for lowest fat content.

The USDA allows up to 30% fat (by weight) in raw ground beef, so the cut of beef makes a difference. Regular ground beef typically contains the most fat (about 20% to 30% fat). Next comes ground chuck (about 15% fat), followed by ground round (about 10% fat), and ground sirloin (about 3% fat). Table 5-10 shows a further breakdown of the fat content of varieties of ground beef. Based on this information, you can see that the ground sirloin will give you the leanest burgers.

The ground sirloin, however, will also be the most expensive variety of ground beef. You may, therefore, want to take advantage of the fact that ground beef loses a lot of fat during cooking—as much as 50% for the highest fat products. Typically, regular ground beef is the least expensive product. As the % lean increases, so does price. You can purchase the higher-fat regular ground beef and reduce the amount of fat in the final product by draining, blotting with paper towels, or rinsing under warm water.

For foods in which the ground beef will be shaped then cooked (e.g., hamburger patties, meatballs, or meatloaf), bake, grill, or broil the ground meat on a rack so that fat will drain from the product as it cooks, then let the cooked product rest on paper

TABLE 5-10 Calorie, Fat and Cholesterol Content of Types of Ground Beef

	Energy (kcal)	Total Fat(g)	Saturated Fat (g)	Cholesterol (mg)
Regular ground beef, 3.5 oz cooked	273	18	7	82
Ground chuck, 3.5 oz cooked	232	14	5	86
Ground round, 3.5 oz cooked	204	11	4	82
Ground sirloin, 3.5 oz cooked	164	6	3	76

towels for 1 minute after cooking. For recipes that incorporate browned ground beef into a mixed dish (e.g., casseroles or spaghetti sauce), brown ground beef, crumbling as you cook, then blot with paper towels or rinse under warm water to achieve a final cooked product with nearly the same fat content as the ground round. Using the rinsing method, 100 grams (about 3.5 ounces) of ground beef yields a final product with just 4 grams of fat. Because a greater percentage of the starting product is lost during cooking, you will

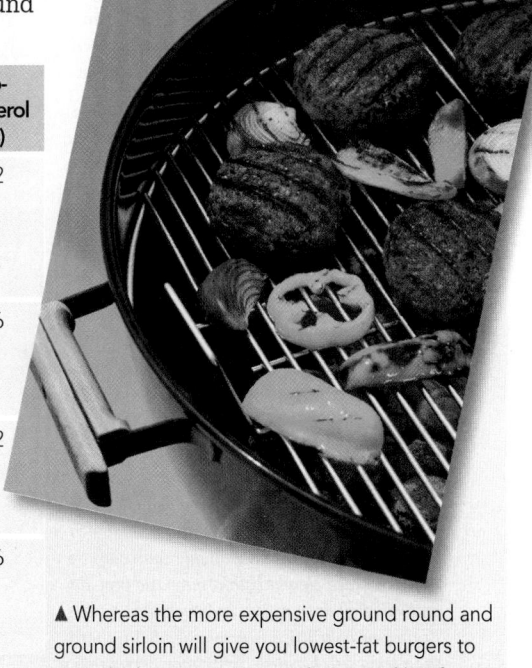

▲ Whereas the more expensive ground round and ground sirloin will give you lowest-fat burgers to start, the less expensive regular ground beef or ground chuck burgers will lose fat while cooking. You will therefore want to consider both fat content and cost when making your choice.

end up with less meat in the final product. However, this is not such a big deal because most Americans consume two to three times as much protein as they need. To further enhance the heart-healthiness of mixed dishes, replace some of that lost product with beans, Chili or tacos would be excellent recipes to try with this method.

Further Readings

1. ADA Reports: Position of the American Dietetic Association and Dietitians of Canada: Dietary fatty acids. *Journal of the American Dietetic Association* 107:1599, 2007.

   A diet is recommended that reduces fatty acids that increase risk of disease, while promoting fatty acids that benefit health. Dietary fat should provide 20% to 35% of energy and emphasize a reduction in saturated fatty acids and trans fatty acids and an increase in n-3 polyunsaturated fatty acids. A food-based approach should be used that includes fruits and vegetables, whole grains, legumes, nuts and seeds, lean protein, and fish. Nonhydrogenated margarines and oils are recommended such that unsaturated fatty acids are the predominant fat source in the diet.

2. Getz L: A burger and fries (hold the *trans* fats). *Today's Dietitian* 11(2):35, 2009.

   Several cities across the United States, including New York, Philadelphia, and Boston, have banned trans fat use in restaurants. Most eating establishments have willingly responded to the demand for healthier oils. It is important to remember that choosing trans fat-free foods does not necessarily make it a healthy choice.

3. Hansson GK: Inflammation, atherosclerosis, and coronary artery disease. *The New England Journal of Medicine* 352:1685, 2005.

   Excellent review of the role of inflammation in causing cardiovascular disease. Identifying atherosclerosis as an inflammatory disease offers new opportunities for the prevention and treatment of coronary artery disease.

4. He KA, Daviglus ML: A few more thoughts about fish and fish oil. *Journal of the American Dietetic Association* 105:428, 2005.

   Fish consumption has been shown to have beneficial effects on cardiovascular disease. Consuming whole fish is thought to have greater benefits and be safer than using fish oil supplements. Fish is not only a rich source of omega-3 fatty acids, but is also a valuable source of protein and trace elements that may also provide protective effects for the cardiovascular system. Broiled or baked fish is recommended rather than fried fish because frying may decrease the ratio of omega-3 to omega-6 fatty acids and may produce trans fatty acids and oxidized lipid products that may increase cardiovascular disease risk.

5. Kris-Etherton PM, Hill AM: n-3 fatty acids: Food or supplements? *Journal of the American Dietetic Association* 108:1125, 2008.

   A food-based approach is recommended for all fatty acids including the n-3 fatty acids. If an individual does not eat fish, the richest source of n-3 fatty acids, other options such as "designer" foods high in n-3 fatty acids, foods fortified with these fatty acids, or even supplements can be used. For vegans, algal supplements are an alternative source of DHA instead of fish or fish oil.

6. Kuller LH: Nutrition, lipids, and cardiovascular disease. *Nutrition Reviews* 64:S15, 2006.

   The development of coronary heart disease is discussed as an epidemic due to increased consumption of saturated fat and cholesterol, low intakes of polyunsaturated fat, and obesity. The risk of the disease is increased by hypertension, smoking, and diabetes. The careful monitoring and prevention of this disease beginning in young adults is important but expensive.

7. Lau VWY and others: Plant sterols are efficacious in lowering plasma LDL and non-HDL cholesterol in hypercholesterolemic type 2 diabetic and nondiabetic persons. *American Journal of Clinical Nutrition* 81:1351, 2005.

   Incorporation of plant sterols into a low-saturated-fat and low-cholesterol diet for persons at increased risk of CVD mortality could have a positive effect on reducing the mortality rate, including in those people with type 2 diabetes.

8. Lewis NM and others: The walnut: A nutritional nut case. *Today's Dietitian* 6(8):36, 2004.

   Compared to other nuts and seeds, walnuts are one of the richest sources of alpha-linolenic acid (2.6 grams per 1-ounce serving or 14 walnut halves). The DRI for alpha-linolenic acid is 1.6 grams/day for men and 1.1 grams/day for women. In addition, walnuts are a rich source of plant sterols known to inhibit intestinal absorption of cholesterol.

9. Lichtenstein AH and others: Diet and lifestyle recommendations revision 2006. A scientific statement from the American Heart Association Nutrition Committee. *Circulation* 114:82, 2006.

   The American Heart Association presents recommendations designed to reduce the risk of cardiovascular disease in the general population. Specific goals are presented and include consuming an overall healthy diet; to aim for a healthy body weight, recommended levels of low-density lipoprotein cholesterol, high-density lipoprotein cholesterol, and triglycerides; normal blood pressure; normal blood glucose level; being physically active; and avoiding the use of and exposure to tobacco products.

10. Meisinger C and others: Plasma oxidized low-density lipoprotein, a strong predictor for acute coronary heart disease events in apparently healthy, middle-aged men from the general population. *Circulation* 112:651, 2005.

    Elevated concentrations of oxidized low-density lipoprotein are predictive of future coronary heart disease events in apparently healthy men. Thus, oxidized LDL may represent a promising risk marker for clinical coronary heart disease complications and should be evaluated in further studies.

11. Micallef MA, Garg ML: The lipid-lowering effects of phytosterols and (n-3) polyunsaturated fatty acids are synergistic and complementary in hyperlipidemic men and women. *Journal of Nutrition* 138:1086, 2008.

    Phytosterols are plant compounds with structures similar to cholesterol. Some margarines and other products are enriched with phytosterols. Consuming phytosterols can reduce the intestinal absorption of cholesterol by 30% to 40%. Fish oils are rich in omega-3 polyunsaturated fatty acids (PUFA) and can reduce blood triglycerides and raise HDL-cholesterol. The combined effect of phytosterols and omega-3 PUFA on blood lipid profiles was studied in individuals with high blood lipids. The combined supplementation with phytosterols and omega-3 PUFA had synergistic and complementary lipid-lowering effects in men and women with high blood lipids, resulting in a reduction in plasma total and LDL-cholesterol concentrations, an increase in HDL-cholesterol concentration, and a decrease in plasma triglyceride concentration.

12. Palmer S: Fighting heart disease the Dean Ornish way. *Today's Dietitian* 2:48, 2009.

    The Ornish diet has been proven to prevent as well as reverse heart disease. Diet guidelines include eating no more than 10% of calories from fat from mostly a plant-based diet; consuming no more than 10 milligrams of cholesterol per day; and eating one serving of soy foods each day. Omega-3 fatty acids are recommended from supplements.

13. Phillips KM and others: Phytosterol composition of nuts and seeds commonly consumed in the United States. *Journal of Agriculture and Food Chemistry* 53:9436, 2005.

    This study set out to find the nuts and seeds that could provide the most heart-protective benefits. Of the 27 nuts and seeds analyzed, wheat germ and sesame seeds had the greatest concentration of phytosterols and Brazil nuts and walnuts ranked the lowest. Pistachio and sunflower seeds were the richest sources of phytosterols for products typically consumed as snack foods.

14. Shai I and others: Weight loss with a low-carbohydrate, Mediterranean, or low-fat diet. *The New England Journal of Medicine* 359:229, 2008.

Moderately obese adults (mean age, 52 years) were assigned to one of three diets: low-fat, restricted-calorie; Mediterranean, restricted-calorie; or low-carbohydrate, non-restricted-calorie, and studied for two years. The diet was monitored for various components, including amount and type of carbohydrates, fat, protein, and cholesterol. The mean weight loss among the 272 participants who remained on their diets was 3.3 kg for the low-fat group, 4.6 kg for the Mediterranean-diet group, and 5.5 kg for

the low-carbohydrate group. The results indicate that Mediterranean and low-carbohydrate diets may be effective alternatives to low-fat diets. The more favorable effects on lipids (with the low-carbohydrate diet) and on glycemic control (with the Mediterranean diet) suggest that personal preferences and metabolic considerations might inform individualized tailoring of dietary interventions.

15. Wang C and others: n-3 fatty acids from fish or fish oil supplements, but not

alpha-linolenic acid, benefit cardiovascular disease outcomes in primary- and secondary-prevention studies: A systematic review. *American Journal of Clinical Nutrition* 84:5, 2006.

This review of previous studies found that consumption of omega-3 fatty acids from fish or fish oil but not alpha-linolenic acid, significantly reduced all-cause mortality, myocardial infarction, cardiac and sudden death, or stroke.

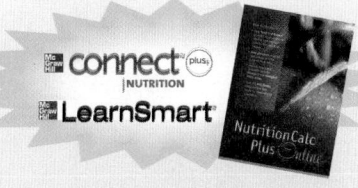

To get the most out of your study of nutrition, go to McGraw-Hill's online resources: Connect www.mcgrawhillconnect.com, **where you will find NutritionCalc Plus, LearnSmart, and many other dynamic tools.**

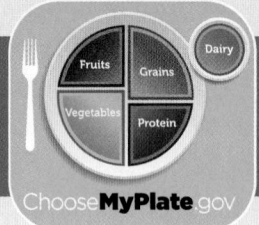
I. Is Your Diet High in Saturated and *Trans* Fat?

Instructions: In each row of the following list, circle your typical food selection from column A or B.

Column A		Column B
Bacon and eggs	or	Ready-to-eat whole-grain breakfast cereal
Doughnut or sweet roll	or	Whole-wheat roll, bagel, or bread
Breakfast sausage	or	Fruit
Whole milk	or	Reduced-fat, low-fat, or fat-free milk
Cheeseburger	or	Turkey sandwich, no cheese
French fries	or	Plain baked potato with salsa
Ground chuck	or	Ground round
Soup with cream base	or	Soup with broth base
Macaroni and cheese	or	Macaroni with marinara sauce
Cream/fruit pie	or	Graham crackers
Cream-filled cookies	or	Granola bar
Ice cream	or	Frozen yogurt, sherbet, or reduced-fat ice cream
Butter or stick margarine	or	Vegetable oils or soft margarine in a tub

Interpretation

The foods listed in column A tend to be high in saturated fat, *trans* fatty acids, cholesterol, and total fat. Those in column B generally are low in these dietary components. If you want to help reduce your risk of cardiovascular disease, choose more foods from column B and fewer from column A.

II. Applying the Nutrition Facts Label to Your Daily Food Choices

Imagine that you are at the supermarket looking for a quick snack to help you keep your energy up during afternoons. In the snack section, you settle on two choices (see labels a and b). Evaluate the products using the table on the left.

Compare the nutrients in each product by completing this list. For each serving, which product is lower in each of the following?

Calories	(a)	(b)	no difference
Calories from Fat	(a)	(b)	no difference
Total Fat	(a)	(b)	no difference
Saturated Fat	(a)	(b)	no difference
Trans Fat	(a)	(b)	no difference
Cholesterol	(a)	(b)	no difference
Sodium	(a)	(b)	no difference
Total Carbohydrates	(a)	(b)	no difference
Dietary Fiber	(a)	(b)	no difference
Sugars	(a)	(b)	no difference
Protein	(a)	(b)	no difference
Iron	(a)	(b)	no difference

Which package has more servings per container?
(a)   (b)   no difference

Which of the two brands would you choose?
(a)   (b)   no difference

What information on the Nutrition Facts labels contributed to your decision?

(a)

Nutrition Facts

Serving Size: 2 bars (42g)
Servings Per Container: 6

Amount Per Serving   2 bars
Calories 180   Calories from Fat 50

	% Daily Value*
Total Fat 6g	**9**%
Saturated Fat 0.5g	**3**%
Trans fat 0g	**
Cholesterol 0mg	**0**%
Sodium 160mg	**7**%
Total Carbohydrates 29g	**10**%
Dietary Fiber 2g	**8**%
Sugars 11g	
Protein 4g	
Iron	6%

Not a significant source of Vitamin A, Vitamin C, and calcium.

** Intake of trans fat should be as low as possible.

* Daily values are based on a 2,000 calorie diet. Your daily values may be higher or lower depending on your calorie needs:

** Intake should be as low as possible.

		Calories	2,000	2,500
Total Fat	Less than		65g	80g
Saturated Fat	Less than		20g	25g
Cholesterol	Less than		300mg	300mg
Sodium	Less than		2,400mg	2,400mg
Total Carbohydrates			300g	375g
Dietary Fiber			25g	30g

INGREDIENTS: WHOLE GRAIN ROLLED OATS, SUGAR, CANOLA OIL, CRISP RICE WITH SOY PROTEIN (RICE FLOUR, SOY PROTEIN CONCENTRATE, SUGAR, MALT, SALT), HONEY, BROWN SUGAR SYRUP, HIGH FRUCTOSE CORN SYRUP, SALT, SOY LECITHIN, BAKING SODA, NATURAL FLAVOR, PEANUT FLOUR, ALMOND FLOUR, HAZELNUT FLOUR, WALNUT FLOUR, PECAN FLOUR.

(b)

Nutrition Facts

Serving Size: 2 cookies (38g)
Servings Per Container: about 12

Amount Per Serving
Calories 180   Calories from Fat 70

	% Daily Value*
Total Fat 7g	**11**%
Saturated Fat 2g	**10**%
Trans fat 2g	**
Cholesterol 0mg	**0**%
Sodium 100mg	**4**%
Total Carbohydrate 26g	**9**%
Dietary Fiber 1g	**4**%
Sugars 12g	
Protein 2g	

Vitamin A 0% • Vitamin C 0%
Calcium 0% • Iron 2%

** Intake of trans fat should be as low as possible.

* Daily values are based on a 2,000 calorie diet. Your daily values may be higher or lower depending on your calorie needs:

** Intake should be as low as possible.

		Calories	2,000	2,500
Total Fat	Less than		65g	80g
Saturated Fat	Less than		20g	25g
Cholesterol	Less than		300mg	300mg
Sodium	Less than		2,400mg	2,400mg
Total Carbohydrates			300g	375g
Dietary Fiber			25g	30g

Calories per gram: • Fat 9 • Carbohydrate 4
• Protein 4

INGREDIENTS: ENRICHED FLOUR (WHEAT FLOUR, NIACIN, REDUCED IRON, THIAMINE MONONITRATE, RIBOFLAVIN, FOLIC ACID), SUGAR, VEGETABLE OIL SHORTENING (PARTIALLY HYDROGENATED SOYBEAN, COCONUT, COTTONSEED, CORN AND/OR SAFFLOWER AND/OR CANOLA OIL), CORN SYRUP, HIGH FRUCTOSE CORN SYRUP, WHEY (A MILK INGREDIENT), CORN STARCH, SALT, SKIM MILK, LEAVENING (BAKING SODA, AMMONIUM BICARBONATE), ARTIFICIAL FLAVOR, SOYBEAN LECITHIN, COLOR (CONTAINING FD&C YELLOW #5 LAKE).

Chapter 6 Proteins

Student Learning Outcomes

Chapter 6 is designed to allow you to:

6.1 Distinguish between essential and nonessential amino acids and explain why adequate amounts of each of the essential amino acids are required for protein synthesis.

6.2 Describe how amino acids form proteins.

6.3 Distinguish between high-quality and lower-quality proteins, identify examples of each, and describe the concept of complementary proteins.

6.4 Describe how protein is digested and absorbed in the body.

6.5 List the primary functions of protein in the body.

6.6 Calculate the RDA for protein for an adult when a healthy weight is given.

6.7 Describe what is meant by positive protein balance, negative protein balance, and protein equilibrium.

6.8 Describe how protein-calorie malnutrition eventually can lead to disease in the body.

6.9 Develop vegetarian diet plans that meet the body's nutritional needs.

What Would You Choose?

About 3 weeks ago, you started lifting weights at the student recreation center. You are disappointed that you have not seen the results you were anticipating. You can lift more now than you could when you started, but you were hoping to tone and define the muscles in your arms, back, and abs. Perhaps you need more protein. Bodybuilding magazines have numerous advertisements for protein and amino-acid supplements, but they are expensive. What would you choose as optimal nutrition to support your weight-training regimen?

a Take whey protein supplements.

b Take individual amino-acid supplements.

c Increase your consumption of animal protein.

d Consume a diet that provides 10% to 35% of calories from a variety of sources of protein.

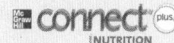 Think about your choice as you read Chapter 6, then see our recommendations at the end of the chapter. To learn more about supplements and diet, check out the Connect site: www.mcgrawhillconnect.com

Part Two

Energy Nutrients and Energy Balance

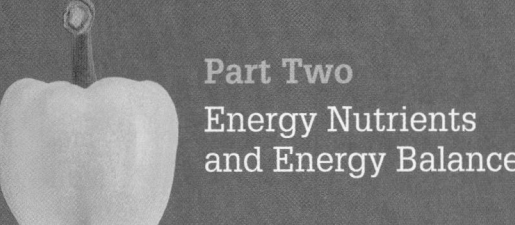

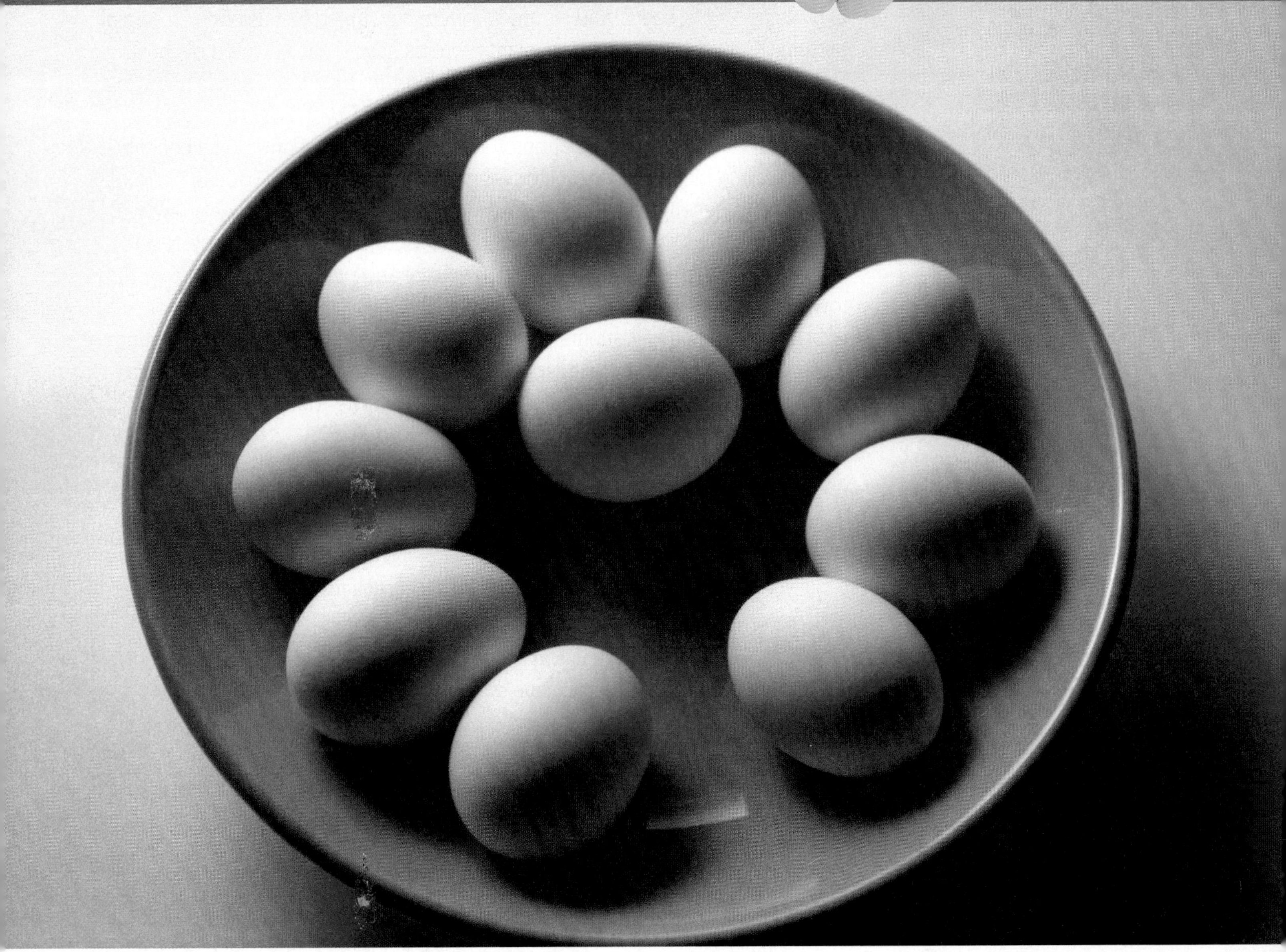

Consuming enough protein is vital for maintaining health. Proteins form important structures in the body, make up a key part of the blood, help regulate many body functions, and can fuel body cells.

North Americans generally eat more protein than is needed to maintain health. High-protein weight-loss diets have come and gone over the past 30 years. Our daily protein intake comes mostly from animal sources such as meat, poultry, fish, eggs, milk, and cheese. In contrast, in the developing world, diets can be deficient in protein.

Diets that are mostly vegetarian still predominate in much of Asia and areas of Africa, and, as suggested in the comic on the next page, some North Americans are currently adopting the practice. Plant sources of protein are worthy of more attention from North Americans. In the early 1900s, plant sources of proteins—nuts, seeds, and legumes—were consumed just as often as animal proteins. Over the years, though, plant proteins have been sidelined by meats. During this time, nuts have been viewed as high-fat foods, and beans have gotten the inferior reputation of "the poor man's meat." Contrary to these popular misconceptions, sources of plant proteins offer a wealth of nutritional benefits—from lowering blood cholesterol to preventing certain forms of cancer.

We could benefit from eating more plant sources of proteins. As shown in the comic in this chapter, it takes some knowledge to do so. It is possible—and desirable—to enjoy the benefits of animal and plant protein as we work toward the goal of meeting protein needs. This chapter takes a close look at protein, including the benefits of plant proteins in a diet. It will also examine vegetarian diets: their benefits and their risks, if not properly planned. Let's see why a detailed study of protein is worth your attention.

Refresh Your Memory

As you begin your study of proteins in Chapter 6, you may want to review:

- Organization of the cell in Chapter 3
- The processes of digestion and absorption in Chapter 3
- The nervous system and immune system in Chapter 3
- The role of carbohydrates in sparing protein for energy in Chapter 4

FRANK & ERNEST® by Bob Thaves

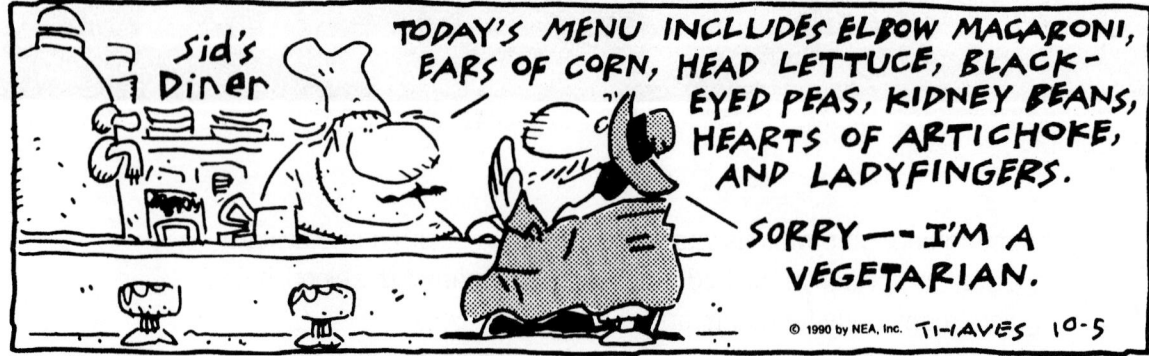

Can a vegetarian diet provide enough protein? What is prompting the growing interest in various forms of vegetarian diets? Why are plant protein sources, especially soy and nuts, gaining more attention? Should meat-eaters abandon that dietary practice? Chapter 6 provides some answers.

FRANK & ERNEST © United Features Syndicate. Reprinted by Permission.

6.1 Protein—An Introduction

Diets in the developed parts of the world, such as the United States and Canada, are typically rich in protein, and therefore a specific focus on eating enough protein is generally not needed. In the developing world, however, it is important to focus on protein in diet planning because diets in those areas of the world can be deficient in protein.

Thousands of substances in the body are made of proteins. Aside from water, proteins form the major part of lean body tissue, totaling about 17% of body weight. Amino acids—the building blocks for proteins—are unique in that they contain nitrogen along with carbon, oxygen, and hydrogen. Plants combine nitrogen from the soil with carbon and other elements to form amino acids. They then link these amino acids together to make proteins. We get the nitrogen we need by consuming dietary proteins. Proteins are thus an essential part of a diet because they supply nitrogen in a form we can readily use—namely, amino acids. Using simpler forms of nitrogen is, for the most part, impossible for humans.

Proteins are crucial to the regulation and maintenance of the body. Body functions such as blood clotting, fluid balance, hormone and enzyme production, visual processes, transport of many substances in the bloodstream, and cell repair require specific proteins. The body makes proteins in many configurations and sizes so that they can serve these greatly varied functions. Formation of these body proteins begins with amino acids from both the protein-containing foods we eat and those synthesized from other compounds within the body. Proteins can also be broken down to supply energy for the body—on average, 4 kcal per gram.

If you fail to consume an adequate amount of protein for weeks at a time, many metabolic processes slow down. This is because the body does not have enough amino acids available to build the proteins it needs. For example, the immune system no longer functions efficiently when it lacks key proteins, thereby increasing the risk of infections, disease, and death.

Amino Acids

Amino acids—the building blocks of proteins—are formed mostly of carbon, hydrogen, oxygen, and nitrogen. The following diagram shows the structure of a generic amino acid and also what one of the specific amino acids, glutamic acid, looks like. The amino acids have different chemical makeups, but all are slight variations of the generic amino acid pictured (see Appendix F). Each amino acid has an "acid" group; an "amino" group; and a "side" or R group specific to the amino acid.

The R group on some amino acids has a branched shape, like a tree. These so-called **branched-chain amino acids** are leucine, isoleucine, and valine (see Appendix F for the chemical structures of the amino acids). The branched-chain amino acids are the primary amino acids used by muscles for energy needs. This is one reason why proteins from milk (e.g., whey proteins) are popular with strength-training athletes (see Chapter 10 for details).

branched-chain amino acids Amino acids with a branching carbon backbone; these are leucine, isoleucine, and valine. All are essential amino acids.

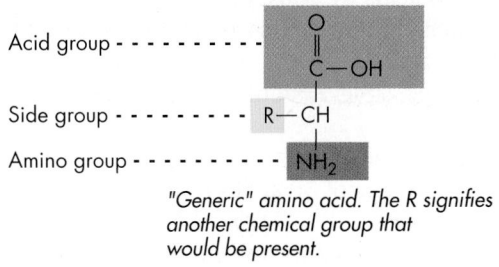

Acid group - - - - - - - - -

Side group - - - - - - - -

Amino group - - - - - - - -

"Generic" amino acid. The R signifies another chemical group that would be present.

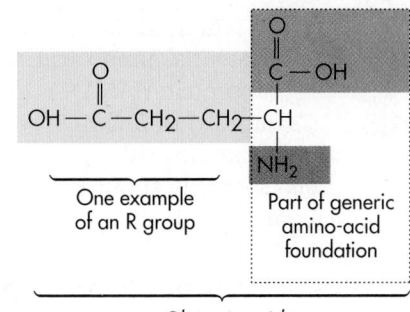

One example of an R group

Part of generic amino-acid foundation

Glutamic acid

nonessential amino acids Amino acids that can be synthesized by a healthy body in sufficient amounts; there are 11 nonessential amino acids. These are also called *dispensable amino acids.*

essential amino acids The amino acids that cannot be synthesized by humans in sufficient amounts or at all and therefore must be included in the diet; there are nine essential amino acids. These are also called *indispensable amino acids.*

limiting amino acid The essential amino acid in lowest concentration in a food or diet relative to body needs.

TABLE 6-1 Classification of Amino Acids

Essential Amino Acids	Nonessential Amino Acids
Histidine	Alanine
Isoleucine*	Arginine
Leucine*	Asparagine
Lysine	Aspartic acid
Methionine	Cysteine
Phenylalanine	Glutamic acid
Threonine	Glutamine
Tryptophan	Glycine
Valine*	Proline
	Serine
	Tyrosine

*A branched-chain amino acid.

Your body needs to use 20 different amino acids to function (Table 6-1). Although all these commonly found amino acids are important, 11 are considered **nonessential** (also called *dispensable*) with respect to our diets. Human cells can produce these certain amino acids as long as the right ingredients are present—the key factor being nitrogen that is already part of another amino acid. Therefore it is not essential that these amino acids be in our diet.

The nine amino acids the body cannot make in sufficient amounts or at all are known as **essential** (also called *indispensable*)—they must be obtained from foods. This is because body cells either cannot make the needed carbon-based foundation of the amino acid, cannot put a nitrogen group on the needed carbon-based foundation, or just cannot do the whole process fast enough to meet body needs.

Eating a balanced diet can supply us with both the essential and nonessential amino-acid building blocks needed to maintain good health. Both nonessential and essential amino acids are present in foods that contain protein. If you don't eat enough essential amino acids, your body first struggles to conserve what essential amino acids it can. However, eventually your body progressively slows production of new proteins until at some point you will break protein down faster than you can make it. When that happens, health deteriorates.

The essential amino acid in smallest supply in a food or diet in relation to body needs becomes the limiting factor (called the **limiting amino acid**) because it limits the amount of protein the body can synthesize. For example, assume the letters of the alphabet represent the 20 or so different amino acids we consume. If *A* represents an essential amino acid, we need three of these letters to spell the hypothetical protein *BANANA*. If the body had a *B*, two *N*s, but only two *A*s, the "synthesis" of *BANANA* would not be possible. *A* would then be seen as the limiting amino acid.

Adults need only about 11% of their total protein requirement to be supplied by essential amino acids. Typical diets supply an average of 50% of protein as essential amino acids.

The estimated needs for essential amino acids for infants and preschool children are 40% of total protein intake; however, in later childhood the need drops to 20%.

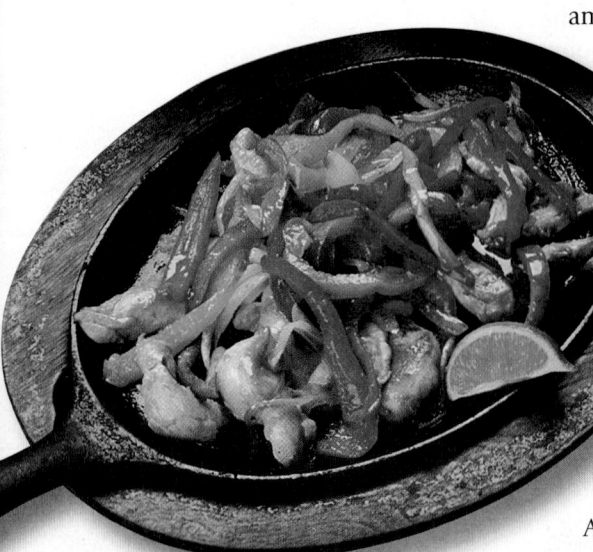

▲ When combined with vegetables, high-protein foods such as meats also help balance the amino-acid content of the diet.

MAKING DECISIONS

Phenylketonuria

Some of the nonessential amino acids are also classed as conditionally essential. This means they must be made from essential amino acids if insufficient amounts are eaten. When that occurs, the body's supply of certain essential amino acids is depleted. Tyrosine is an example of a conditionally essential amino acid that can be made from the essential amino-acid phenylalanine.

The disease phenylketonuria (PKU) illustrates the importance of phenylalanine to make tyrosine. Recall from Chapter 4 that a person with PKU has a limited ability to metabolize the essential amino-acid phenylalanine. Normally, the body uses an enzyme to convert much of our dietary phenylalanine intake into tyrosine.

In PKU-diagnosed persons, the activity of the enzyme used in processing phenylalanine to tyrosine is insufficient. When the enzyme cannot synthesize enough tyrosine, both amino acids must be derived from foods. The point is that phenylalanine and tyrosine become *essential* in terms of dietary needs because the body can't produce enough tyrosine from phenylalanine. Phenylalanine levels in the blood increase because it is not converted to tyrosine. PKU is treated by limiting the consumption of phenylalanine with a special diet so that phenylalanine and its by-products do not rise to toxic concentrations in the body and cause the severe mental retardation seen in untreated PKU cases.

Rina is 7 months pregnant and has read about various tests that her baby will undergo when he or she is born. How can you explain to Rina the purpose and significance of one of those tests, the one that screens for PKU?

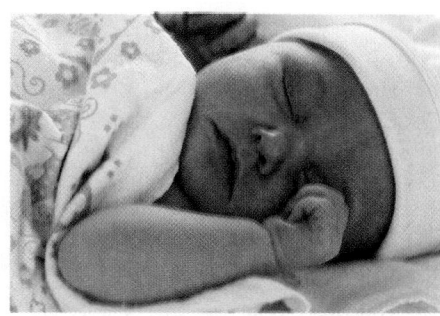

▲ Within the first few days of life all newborns are tested for phenylketonuria.

Diets designed for infants and young children need to take this into account to make sure enough proteins are present to yield a high-quality protein intake. Including some animal products in the diet, such as human milk or formula for infants, or cow's milk for children, helps ensure this. Otherwise, complementary amino acids from plant proteins should be consumed in each meal or within two subsequent meals. A major health risk for infants and children occurs in famine situations in which only one type of cereal grain is available, increasing the probability that one or more of the nine essential amino acids is lacking in the total diet. This is discussed further in a later section on protein-calorie malnutrition.

CONCEPT CHECK

The human body uses 20 different amino acids from protein-containing foods. A healthy body can synthesize 11 of the amino acids, so it is not necessary to obtain all amino acids from foods—only nine of these must come from the diet and are therefore termed *essential (indispensable) amino acids*. The essential amino acid in smallest supply in a food in relation to body needs is called the limiting amino acid because it limits the amount of protein the body can synthesize.

6.2 Proteins—Amino Acids Bonded Together

Amino acids are linked together by chemical bonds—technically called **peptide bonds**—to form proteins. Although these bonds are difficult to break, acids, enzymes, and other agents are able to do so—for example, during digestion.

The body can synthesize many different proteins by linking together the 20 common types of amino acids with peptide bonds.

peptide bond A chemical bond formed between amino acids in a protein.

polypeptide A group of amino acids bonded together, from 50 to 2000 or more.

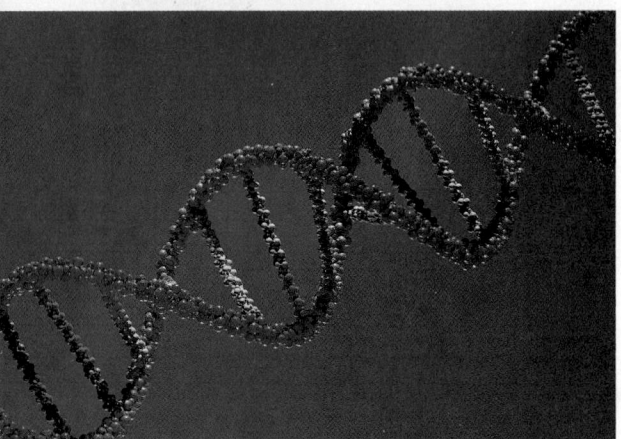

▲ Genes are present on DNA—a double-stranded helix. The cell nucleus contains most of the DNA in the body.

Protein Synthesis

Our discussion of protein synthesis, begins with DNA. DNA is present in the nucleus of the cell and contains coded instructions for protein synthesis (i.e., which specific amino acids are to be placed in a protein and in which order). Recall from Chapter 3 that DNA is a double-stranded molecule.

Protein synthesis in a cell, however, takes place in the cytoplasm, not in the nucleus. Thus, the DNA code used for synthesis of a specific protein must be transferred from the nucleus to the cytoplasm to allow for protein synthesis. This transfer is the job of messenger RNA (mRNA). Enzymes in the nucleus read the code on one segment (a gene) of one strand of the DNA and *transcribe* that information into a single-stranded mRNA molecule (Fig. 6-1). This mRNA undergoes processing and then it is ready to leave the nucleus.

Once in the cytoplasm, mRNA travels to the ribosomes. The ribosomes read the mRNA code and *translate* those instructions to produce a specific protein. Amino acids are added one at a time to the growing **polypeptide** chain according to the instructions on the mRNA. Another key participant in protein synthesis, transfer RNA (tRNA), is responsible for bringing the specific amino acids to the ribosomes as needed during protein synthesis (review Fig. 6-1). Energy input is required to add each amino acid to the chain, making protein synthesis "costly" in terms of calorie use.

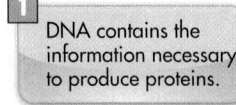

1 DNA contains the information necessary to produce proteins.

2 Transcription or copying of a segment of DNA results in mRNA, a copy of the information in DNA needed to make a protein.

3 The mRNA leaves the nucleus and goes to a ribosome.

4 Amino acids, the building blocks of proteins, are carried to the ribosome by tRNAs containing the code that matches that on the mRNA.

5 In the process of translation, the information contained in mRNA is used to determine the number, types, and arrangement of amino acids in the protein.

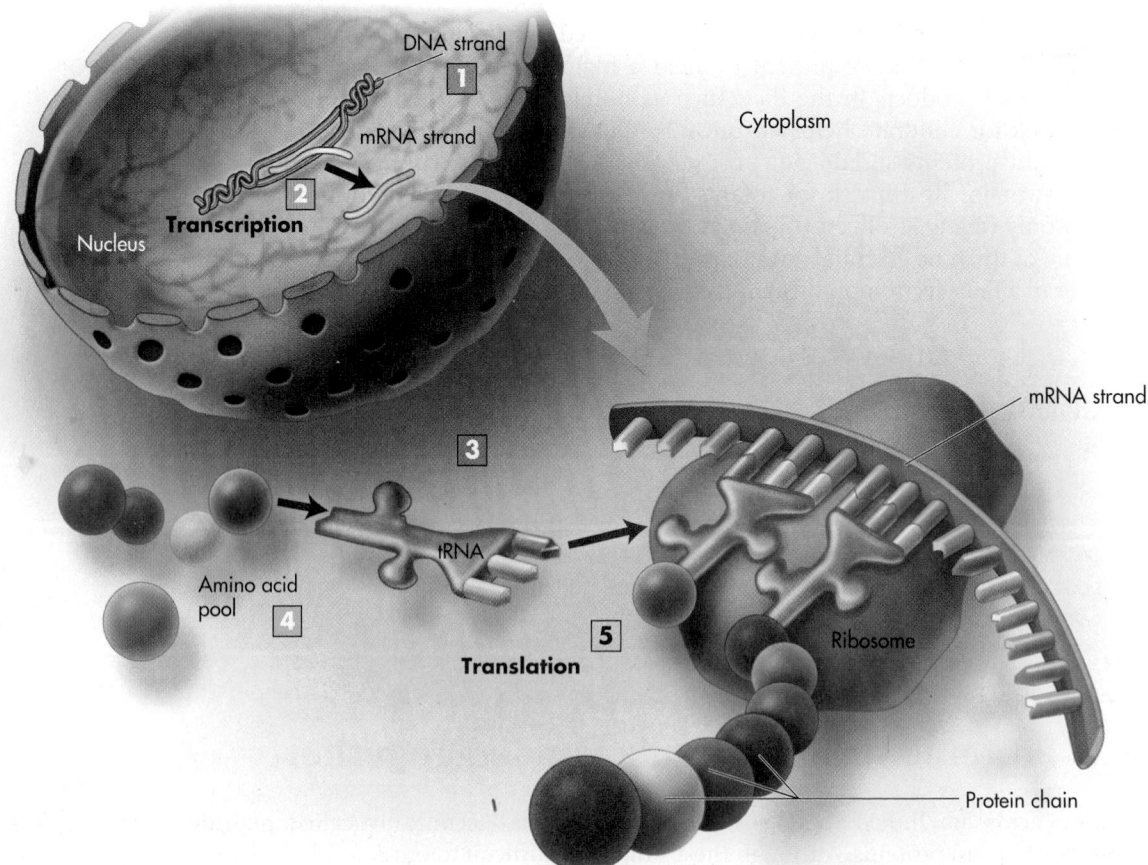

FIGURE 6-1 ▶ Protein synthesis (simplified). Once the mRNA is fully read, the amino acids have been connected into the polypeptide, which is released into the cytoplasm. It generally is then processed further to become a cell protein.

Once synthesis of a polypeptide is complete, it twists and folds into the appropriate three-dimensional structure of the intended protein. These structural changes occur based on specific interactions between the amino acids that make up the polypeptide chain (see the next section on protein organization for details). Some polypeptides, such as the hormone insulin, also undergo further changes in the cell before they are functional.

The important message in this discussion is the relationship between DNA and the proteins eventually produced by a cell. If the DNA code contains errors, an incorrect mRNA will be produced. The ribosomes will then read this incorrect message and an incorrect amino acid will be added and an incorrect polypeptide chain will be produced. As discussed in Chapter 3, genetic engineering may ultimately be able to correct many gene defects in humans, by placing the correct DNA code in the nucleus, so that the correct protein can be made by the ribosomes.

Protein Organization

As noted before, by bonding together various combinations of the 20 common types of amino acids, the body synthesizes thousands of different proteins. The sequential order of the amino acids then ultimately determines the protein's shape. The main point is that only correctly positioned amino acids can interact and fold properly to form the intended shape for the protein. The resulting unique, three-dimensional form goes on to dictate the function of each particular protein (Fig. 6-2). If it lacks the proper structure, a protein cannot function.

Sickle cell disease (also called **sickle cell anemia**) is one example of what happens when amino acids are out of order on a protein. North Americans of African descent are especially prone to this genetic disease. It occurs because of defects in the structure of the protein chains of hemoglobin, a protein that carries oxygen in red blood cells. In two of its four protein chains, an error in the amino-acid order occurs. This error produces a profound change in hemoglobin structure. It can no longer form the shape needed to carry oxygen efficiently inside the red blood cell. Instead of forming normal circular disks, the red blood cells collapse into crescent (or sickle) shapes (Fig. 6-3). Health deteriorates, and eventually episodes of severe pain in the bones and joints, abdominal pain, headaches, convulsions, and paralysis may occur.

These life-threatening symptoms are caused by a minute, but critical, error in the hemoglobin amino-acid order. Why does this error happen? It results from a defect in a person's genetic blueprint, DNA, inherited through one's parents. A defect in the DNA can dictate that a wrong amino acid will be built into the sequence of the body proteins. Many diseases, including cancer, stem from errors in the DNA code.

Denaturation of Proteins

Exposure to acid or alkaline substances, heat, or agitation can alter a protein's structure, leaving it uncoiled or otherwise deformed. This process of altering the three-dimensional structure of a protein is called **denaturation** (see Fig. 6-7 on p. 219). Changing a protein's shape often destroys its ability to function normally, such that it loses its biological activity.

Denaturation of proteins is useful for some body processes, especially digestion. The heat produced during cooking denatures some proteins. After food is ingested, the secretion of stomach acid denatures some bacterial proteins, plant hormones, many active enzymes, and other forms of proteins in foods, making it safer to eat. Digestion is also enhanced by denaturation because the unraveling increases exposure of the polypeptide chain to digestive enzymes. Denaturing proteins in some foods can also reduce their tendencies to cause allergic reactions.

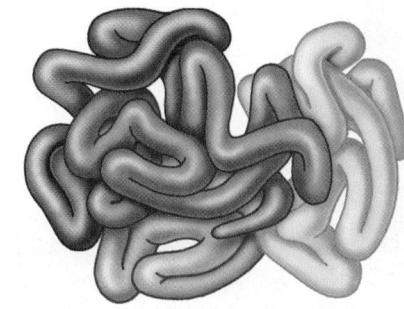

FIGURE 6-2 ▶ Protein organization. Proteins often form a coiled shape, as shown by this drawing of the blood protein hemoglobin. This shape is dictated by the order of the amino acids in the protein chain. To get an idea of its size, consider that each teaspoon (5 milliliters) of blood contains about 10^{18} hemoglobin molecules. One billion is 10^9.

sickle cell disease (sickle cell anemia) An illness that results from a malformation of the red blood cell because of an incorrect structure in part of its hemoglobin protein chains. The disease can lead to episodes of severe bone and joint pain, abdominal pain, headache, convulsions, paralysis, and even death.

denaturation Alteration of a protein's three-dimensional structure, usually because of treatment by heat, enzymes, acid or alkaline solutions, or agitation.

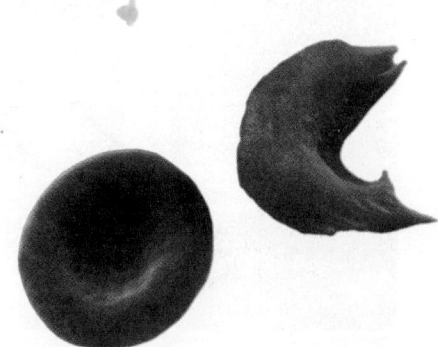

FIGURE 6-3 ▶ An example of the consequences of errors in DNA coding of proteins. (*a*) Normal red blood cell; (*b*) red blood cell from a person with sickle cell anemia—note its abnormal crescent (sicklelike) shape.

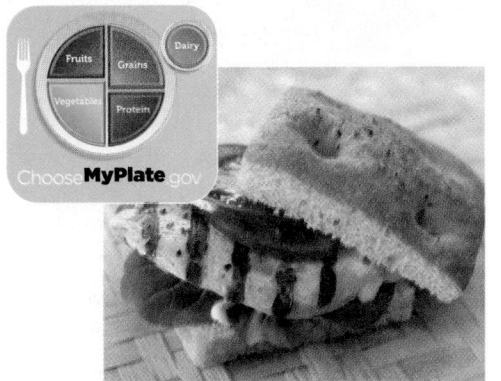

▲ This grilled chicken (protein) sandwich with lettuce and tomato (vegetables) on foccacia bread (grains) completes three section of MyPlate and provides a good source of protein. Which sections are missing?

Recall that we need the essential amino acids that the proteins in the diet supply—not the proteins themselves. We dismantle ingested dietary proteins and use the amino-acid building blocks to assemble the proteins we need.

CONCEPT CHECK

Amino acids are bonded together in specific sequences to form distinct proteins. DNA provides the directions for synthesizing these new proteins. Specifically, DNA directs the order of the amino acids on the protein. The amino-acid order within a protein determines its ultimate shape and function. Destroying the shape of a protein denatures it. Stomach acid, heat, and other factors can denature proteins, causing them to lose their biological activity. Proteins must be denatured during digestion so that amino acids are available for absorption.

6.3 Protein in Foods

Of the typical foods we eat, about 70% of our protein comes from animal sources (Fig. 6-4). The most nutrient-dense source of protein is water-packed tuna, which has 87% of calories as protein (Fig. 6-5). The top five contributors of protein to the North

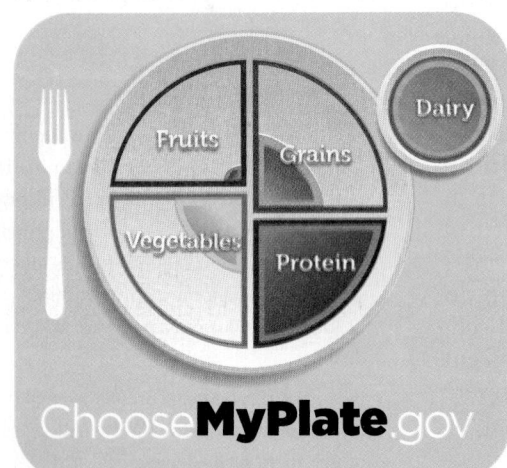

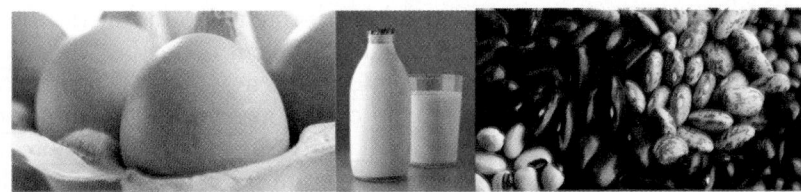

MyPlate: Sources of Protein

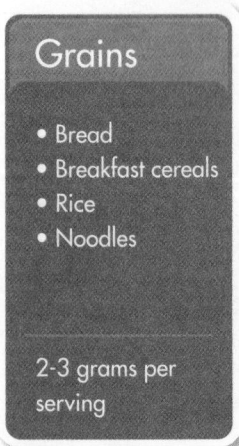
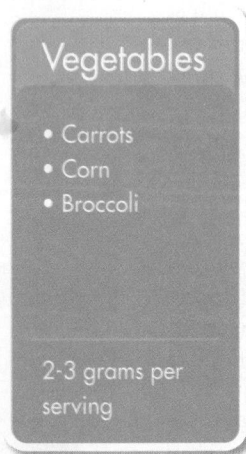
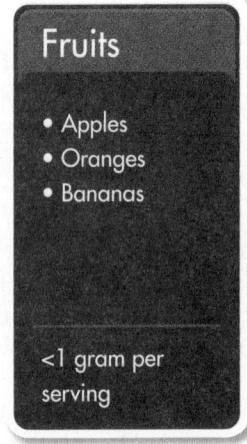
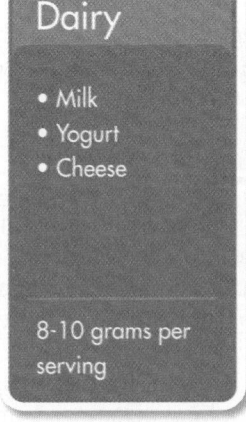
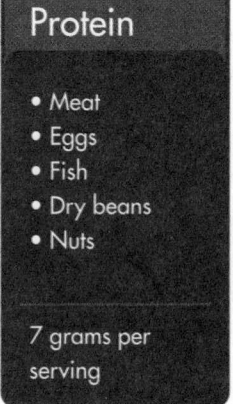

Grains	Vegetables	Fruits	Dairy	Protein
• Bread • Breakfast cereals • Rice • Noodles	• Carrots • Corn • Broccoli	• Apples • Oranges • Bananas	• Milk • Yogurt • Cheese	• Meat • Eggs • Fish • Dry beans • Nuts
2-3 grams per serving	2-3 grams per serving	<1 gram per serving	8-10 grams per serving	7 grams per serving

FIGURE 6-4 ▶ Sources of protein from MyPlate. The fill of the background color (none, 1/3, 2/3, or completely covered) within each group on the plate indicates the average nutrient density for protein in that group. Overall, the dairy group and the protein group contain many foods that are nutrient-dense sources of protein. Based on serving sizes listed for MyPlate, the fruits group provides little or no protein (less than 1 gram per serving). Food choices from the vegetables group and grains group provide moderate amounts of protein (2 to 3 grams per serving). The dairy group provides much protein (8 to 10 grams per serving), as does the protein group (7 grams per serving).

American diet are beef, poultry, milk, white bread, and cheese. In North America, meat and poultry consumption amounts to about 150 pounds per person per year. Worldwide, 35% of protein comes from animal sources. In Africa and East Asia, only about 20% of the protein eaten comes from animal sources.

Protein Quality of Foods

Animal and plant proteins can differ greatly in their proportions of essential and non-essential amino acids. Animal proteins contain ample amounts of all nine essential amino acids. (Gelatin—made from the animal protein collagen—is an exception because it loses one essential amino acid during processing and is low in other essential amino acids.) With the exception of soy protein, plant proteins don't match our need for essential amino acids as precisely as animal proteins. Many plant proteins, especially those found in grains, are low in one or more of the nine essential amino acids.

As you might expect, human tissue composition resembles animal tissue more than it does plant tissue. The similarities enable us to use proteins from any single animal source more efficiently to support human growth and maintenance than we do those from any single plant source. For this reason, animal proteins, except gelatin, are considered **high-quality** (also called **complete**) **proteins,** which contain the nine essential amino acids we need in sufficient amounts. Individual plant sources of proteins, except for soy beans, are considered **lower-quality** (also called **incomplete**) **proteins** because their amino-acid patterns can be quite different from ours. Thus, a single plant protein source, such as corn alone, cannot easily support body growth and maintenance. To obtain a sufficient amount of essential amino acids, a variety of plant proteins need to be consumed because each plant protein lacks adequate amounts of one or more essential amino acids.

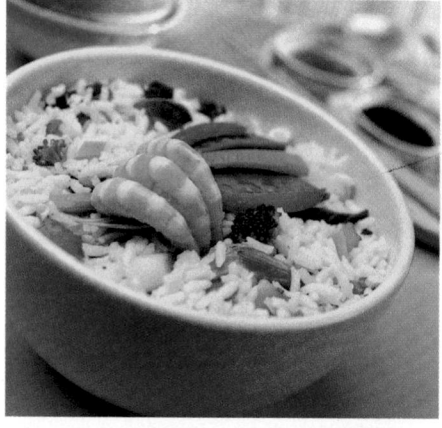

▲ Small amounts of animal protein in a meal easily add up to meet daily protein needs when mixed with grains and vegetables.

high-quality (complete) proteins
Dietary proteins that contain ample amounts of all nine essential amino acids.

lower-quality (incomplete) proteins
Dietary proteins that are low in or lack one or more essential amino acids.

Food Sources of Protein

FIGURE 6-5 ▶ Food sources of protein compared to the RDA of 56 grams for a 70 kg man.

Food Item and Amount	Protein (grams)	% RDA
RDA	56*	100%
Canned tuna, 3 ounces	21.6	38.6%
Broiled chicken, 3 ounces	21.3	38%
Beef chuck, 3 ounces	15.3	27%
Yogurt, 1 cup	10.6	19%
Kidney beans, 1/2 cup	8.1	14.5%
1% low-fat milk, 1 cup	8.0	14%
Peanuts, 1 ounce	7.3	13%
Cheddar cheese, 1 ounce	7.0	12.5%
Egg, 1	5.5	10%
Cooked corn, 1/2 cup	2.7	5%
Seven grain bread, 1 slice	2.6	4.6%
White rice, 1/2 cup	2.1	4%
Pasta, 1 ounce	1.2	2%
Banana, 1	1.2	2%
* for 70 kg man		

Key:
- Grains
- Vegetables
- Fruits
- Dairy
- Protein

ChooseMyPlate.gov

complementary proteins Two food protein sources that make up for each other's inadequate supply of specific essential amino acids; together they yield a sufficient amount of all nine and, so provide high-quality (complete) protein for the diet.

When only lower-quality protein foods are consumed, enough of the essential amino acids needed for protein synthesis may not be obtained. Therefore, when compared to high-quality proteins, a greater amount of lower-quality protein is needed to meet the needs of protein synthesis. Moreover, once any of the nine essential amino acids in the plant protein we have eaten is used up, further protein synthesis becomes impossible. Because the depletion of just one of the essential amino acids prevents protein synthesis, the process illustrates the *all-or-none principle*: Either all essential amino acids are available or none can be used. The remaining amino acids would then be used for energy needs, or converted to carbohydrate or fat.

When two or more proteins combine to compensate for deficiencies in essential amino acid content in each protein, the proteins are called **complementary proteins.** Mixed diets generally provide high-quality protein because a complementary protein pattern results. Therefore, healthy adults should have little concern about balancing foods to yield the proteins needed to obtain enough of all nine essential amino acids. Even on plant-based diets, complementary proteins need not be consumed at the same meal by adults. Meeting amino-acid needs over the course of a day is a reasonable goal because there is a ready supply of amino acids from those present in body cells and in the blood (see Fig. 6-10 on page 224).

In general, plant sources of protein deserve more attention and use than they currently receive from many North Americans. Plant foods contribute fewer calories to the diet than most animal products and they supply an ample amount of protein, plus magnesium, plenty of fiber, and several other nutritional benefits (Fig. 6-6). The vegetable proteins we eat are a heart-healthy alternative to animal proteins because they contain no cholesterol and little saturated fat, aside from that added during processing or cooking. Legumes and nut sources of protein especially have received a lot of recent attention.

CRITICAL THINKING

Evan, a vegetarian, has heard of the "all-or-none principle" of protein synthesis but doesn't understand how this principle applies to protein synthesis in the body. He asks you, "How important is this nutritional concept for diet planning?" How would you answer his question?

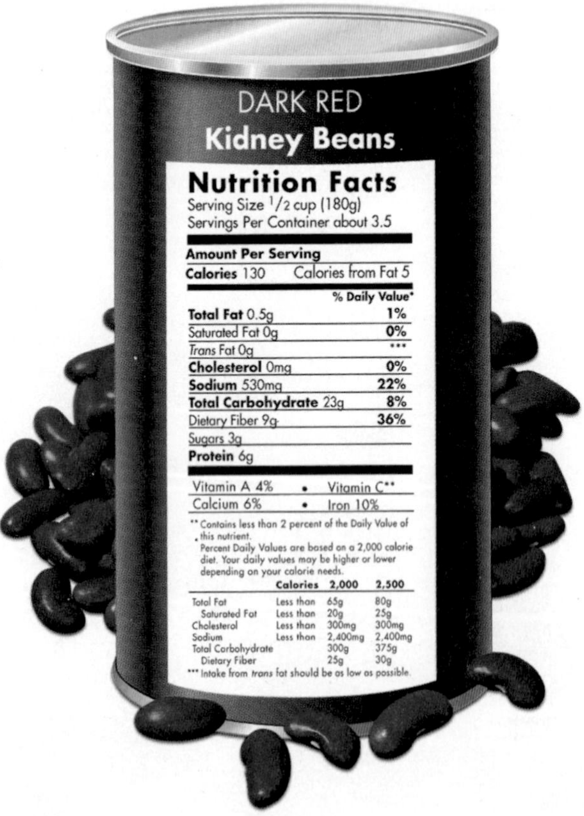

A Closer Look at Plant Sources of Proteins

In proportion to the amount of calories they supply, plant foods provide not only protein, but also magnesium, fiber, folate, vitamin E, iron (absorption is increased by the vitamin C also present), zinc, and some calcium. In addition, phytochemicals from these foods are implicated in prevention of a wide variety of chronic diseases.

Nuts have a hard shell surrounding an edible kernel. Almonds, pistachios, walnuts, and pecans are some common examples. The defining characteristic of a nut is that it grows on a tree. (Peanuts, because they grow underground, are legumes.) Seeds (such as pumpkin, sesame, and sunflower seeds) differ from nuts in that seeds grow on vegetable or flowering plants, but they are similar to nuts in nutrient composition. In general, nuts and seeds supply 160 to 190 kcal, 6 to 10 grams of protein, and 14 to 19 grams of fat per 1 ounce serving. Although they are a dense source of calories, nuts and seeds make a powerful contribution to health when consumed in moderation.

Legumes are a plant family with pods that contain a single row of seeds. Besides peanuts, examples include garden and black-eyed peas, kidney beans, great northern beans, lentils, and soy beans. Dried varieties of the mature legume seeds—what we know as beans—also make an impressive contribution to the protein, vitamin, mineral, and fiber content of a meal. A one-half cup serving of legumes provides 100 to 150 kcal, 5 to 10 grams of protein, less than one gram of fat, and about 5 grams of fiber. Recall from Chapter 4 that consumption of beans can lead to intestinal gas because our bodies lack the enzymes to break down certain carbohydrates that beans contain. An over-the counter preparation called Beano® can greatly lessen symptoms if taken right before the meal. It is also helpful to soak dry beans in water, which

DARK RED
Kidney Beans

Nutrition Facts
Serving Size 1/2 cup (180g)
Servings Per Container about 3.5

Amount Per Serving
Calories 130   Calories from Fat 5

	% Daily Value*
Total Fat 0.5g	1%
Saturated Fat 0g	0%
Trans Fat 0g	***
Cholesterol 0mg	0%
Sodium 530mg	22%
Total Carbohydrate 23g	8%
Dietary Fiber 9g	36%
Sugars 3g	
Protein 6g	

Vitamin A 4%	•	Vitamin C**
Calcium 6%	•	Iron 10%

** Contains less than 2 percent of the Daily Value of this nutrient.
* Percent Daily Values are based on a 2,000 calorie diet. Your daily values may be higher or lower depending on your calorie needs.

	Calories	2,000	2,500
Total Fat	Less than	65g	80g
Saturated Fat	Less than	20g	25g
Cholesterol	Less than	300mg	300mg
Sodium	Less than	2,400mg	2,400mg
Total Carbohydrate		300g	375g
Dietary Fiber		25g	30g

*** Intake from trans fat should be as low as possible.

FIGURE 6-6 ▶ Legumes are rich sources of protein. One-half cup of these kidney beans has 6 grams of protein and meets about 10% of protein needs but contributes only about 5% of energy needs.

leaches the indigestible carbohydrates into the water so they can be disposed. However, intestinal gas is not harmful. In fact, fermentation products of ingestible carbohydrates promote the health of your colon (review Chapter 3 for more information on probiotics and prebiotics).

The impact of plant proteins on health will be discussed in the Nutrition and Your Health section at the end of this chapter.

MAKING DECISIONS

Soy and Nut Allergies

For some of us, food allergies from soy, peanuts and tree nuts (e.g., almonds and walnuts), and wheat are a concern. Overall, food allergies occur in up to 8% of children 4 years of age or younger and in up to 2% of adults. Eight foods account for 90% of food-related allergies; soy, peanuts, tree nuts, and wheat are four of these foods (see Further Reading 11). (The other foods are milk, egg, fish, and shellfish.) The allergic reactions can range from a mild intolerance to fatal allergic reactions (see Nutrition and Your Health in Chapter 15 for details). For prevention of food allergies, exclusive breastfeeding for the first six months of life is the best strategy. Although experts no longer recommend delaying introduction of potentially allergenic foods past six months of age, for those people with allergies to specific proteins, such as wheat, soy, peanuts, and tree nuts, strict avoidance of these foods is the only proven treatment.

In sum, plant proteins are a nutritious alternative to animal proteins. They are inexpensive, versatile, tasty, add color to your plate, and benefit health beyond their contribution of protein to the diet. Simply adding these foods to your diet can lead to weight gain, but learning to substitute plant proteins in place of other less healthy foods is one way to reduce your risk for many diseases. Watch for news about additional research progress into this area.

6.4 Protein Digestion and Absorption

As with carbohydrate digestion, protein digestion begins with the cooking of food. Cooking unfolds (denatures) proteins (Fig. 6-7) and softens tough connective tissue in meat. Cooking also makes many protein-rich foods easier to chew and swallow and facilitates their breakdown during later digestion and absorption. As you will see in Chapter 13, cooking also makes many protein-rich foods, such as meats, eggs, fish, and poultry, much safer to eat.

Digestion

The enzymatic digestion of protein begins in the stomach (Fig. 6-8). Proteins are first denatured by stomach acid. **Pepsin,** a major stomach enzyme for digesting proteins, then goes to work on the unraveled polypeptide chains. Pepsin breaks the polypeptide into shorter chains of amino acids because it can break only a few of the many peptide bonds found in these large molecules. The release of pepsin is controlled by the hormone gastrin. Thinking about food or chewing food stimulates gastrin release in the stomach. Gastrin also strongly stimulates the stomach to produce acid.

The partially digested proteins move from the stomach into the small intestine along with the rest of the nutrients and other substances in a meal (chyme). Once in the small intestine, the partially digested proteins (and any fats accompanying them) trigger the release of the hormone cholecystokinin (CCK) from the walls of the small intestine. CCK, in turn, travels through the bloodstream to the pancreas where it causes the pancreas to release protein-splitting enzymes, such as **trypsin.** These digestive enzymes further divide the chains of amino acids into segments of two to three amino acids and some individual amino acids. Eventually, this mixture is digested

See Nutrition and Your Health: Vegetarian and Plant-Based Diets at the end of Chapter 6.

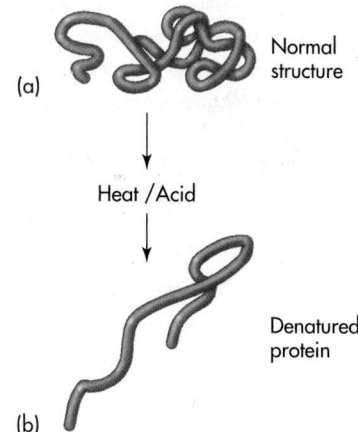

FIGURE 6-7 ▶ Denaturation. (a) Protein showing typical coiled state. (b) Protein is now partly uncoiled. This uncoiling can reduce biological activity and allow digestive enzymes to act on peptide bonds.

pepsin A protein-digesting enzyme produced by the stomach.

trypsin A protein-digesting enzyme secreted by the pancreas to act in the small intestine.

into amino acids, using other enzymes from the lining of the small intestine and enzymes present in the absorptive cells themselves.

Absorption

The short chains of amino acids and any individual amino acids in the small intestine are taken up by active transport into the absorptive cells lining the small intestine. Any remaining peptide bonds are broken down to yield individual amino acids inside the intestinal cells. They are water-soluble, so the amino acids travel to the liver via the portal vein, which drains absorbed nutrients from the intestinal tract. In the liver, individual amino acids can undergo several modifications, depending on the needs of the body. Individual amino acids may be combined into the proteins needed by the body; broken down for energy needs; released into the bloodstream; or converted to nonessential amino acids, glucose, or fat. With excess protein intake, amino acids are converted to fat as a last resort.

Except during infancy, it is uncommon for intact proteins to be absorbed from the digestive tract. In infants up to 4 to 5 months of age, the gastrointestinal tract is somewhat permeable to small proteins, so some whole proteins can be absorbed. Because proteins from some foods (e.g., cow's milk and egg whites) may predispose an infant to food allergies, pediatricians and registered dietitians recommend waiting until an infant is at least 6 to 12 months of age before introducing commonly allergenic foods (see Chapter 15 for details).

FIGURE 6-8 ▶ A summary of protein digestion and absorption. Enzymatic protein digestion begins in the stomach and ends in the absorptive cells of the small intestine, where any remaining short groupings of amino acids are broken down into single amino acids. Stomach acid and enzymes contribute to protein digestion. Absorption from the intestinal lumen into the absorptive cells requires energy input.

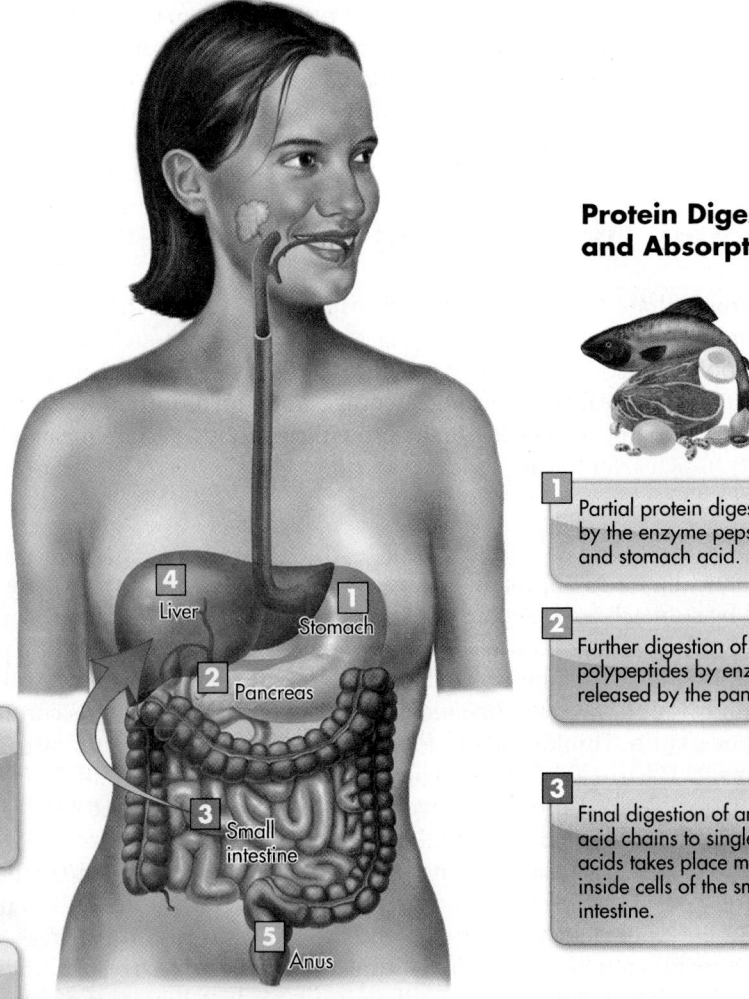

Protein Digestion and Absorption

4 | Liver

1 | Stomach

2 | Pancreas

3 | Small intestine

5 | Anus

4 | Amino acids absorbed into the portal vein and transported to the liver. From there they enter the general bloodstream.

5 | Little dietary protein is present in feces.

1 | Partial protein digestion by the enzyme pepsin and stomach acid.

2 | Further digestion of polypeptides by enzymes released by the pancreas.

3 | Final digestion of amino acid chains to single amino acids takes place mostly inside cells of the small intestine.

CONCEPT CHECK

Protein digestion begins with cooking, as proteins are denatured by heat. Once protein reaches the stomach, enzymes cleave proteins into smaller segments of amino acids. As food travels through the small intestine, protein breakdown products formed in the stomach are broken down further to individual amino acids or short segments of amino acids and taken up into the absorptive cells of the small intestine where final breakdown into amino acids occurs. The amino acids then travel to the liver via the portal vein.

6.5 Putting Proteins to Work in the Body

Proteins function in many crucial ways in human metabolism and in the formation of body structures. We rely on foods to supply the amino acids needed to form these proteins. However, only when we also eat enough carbohydrate and fat can food proteins be used most efficiently. If we don't consume enough calories to meet needs, some amino acids from proteins are broken down to produce energy, rendering them unavailable to build body proteins.

Producing Vital Body Structures

Every cell contains protein. Muscles, connective tissue, mucus, blood-clotting factors, transport proteins in the bloodstream, lipoproteins, enzymes, immune antibodies, some hormones, visual pigments, and the support structure inside bones are primarily made of protein. Excess protein in the diet doesn't enhance the synthesis of these body components, but eating too little protein can prevent it.

Most vital body proteins are in a constant state of breakdown, rebuilding, and repair. For example, the intestinal tract lining is constantly sloughed off. The digestive tract treats sloughed cells just like food particles, digesting them and absorbing their amino acids. In fact, most of the amino acids released throughout the body can be recycled to become part of the pool of amino acids available for synthesis of future proteins. Overall, **protein turnover** is a process by which a cell can respond to its changing environment by producing proteins that are needed and disassembling proteins that are not needed.

During any day, an adult makes and degrades about 250 grams of protein, recycling many of the amino acids. Relative to the 65 to 100 grams of protein typically consumed by adults in North America, recycled amino acids make an important contribution to total protein metabolism.

If a person's diet is low in protein for a long period, the processes of rebuilding and repairing body proteins will slow down. Over time, skeletal muscles; blood proteins; and vital organs, such as the heart and liver, will decrease in size or volume. Only the brain resists protein breakdown.

Maintaining Fluid Balance

Blood proteins help maintain body fluid balance. Normal blood pressure in the arteries forces blood into capillary beds. The blood fluid then moves from the **capillary beds** into the spaces between nearby cells (**extracellular spaces**) to provide nutrients to those cells (Fig. 6-9). Proteins in the bloodstream are too large however, to move out of the capillary beds into the tissues. The presence of these proteins in the capillary beds attracts the proper amount of fluid back to the blood, partially counteracting the force of blood pressure.

With an inadequate consumption of protein, the concentration of proteins in the bloodstream drops below normal. Excessive fluid then builds up in the surrounding tissues because the counteracting force produced by the smaller amount of blood proteins is too weak to pull enough of the fluid back from the tissues into the bloodstream. As

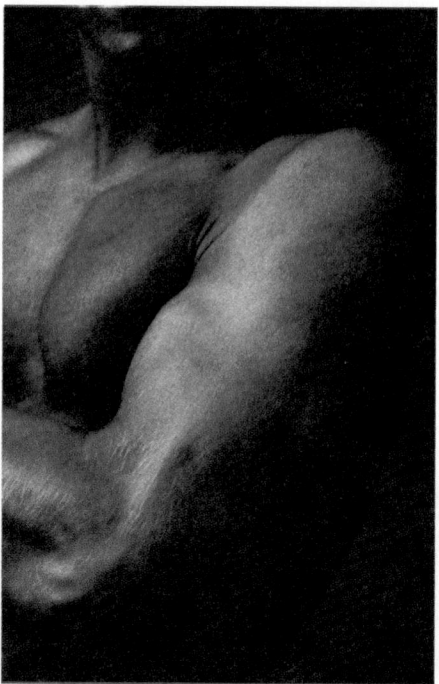

▲ Protein contributes to the structure and function of muscle.

protein turnover The process by which cells break down old proteins and resynthesize new proteins. In this way the cell will have the proteins it needs to function at that time.

capillary bed Network of one-cell-thick vessels that create a junction between arterial and venous circulation. It is here that gas and nutrient exchange occurs between body cells and the blood.

extracellular space The space outside cells; represents one-third of body fluid.

FIGURE 6-9 ▶ Blood proteins in relation to fluid balance. (a) Blood proteins are important for maintaining the body's fluid balance. (b) Without sufficient protein in the bloodstream, edema develops.

Arterial end of a capillary bed

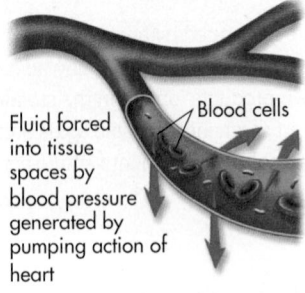

Fluid forced into tissue spaces by blood pressure generated by pumping action of heart

Blood cells

(a)

Venous end of a capillary bed

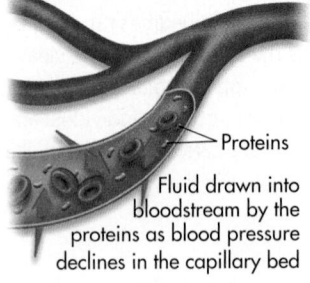

Proteins

Fluid drawn into bloodstream by the proteins as blood pressure declines in the capillary bed

Normal tissue

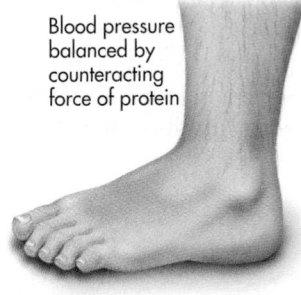

Blood pressure balanced by counteracting force of protein

Swollen tissue (edema)

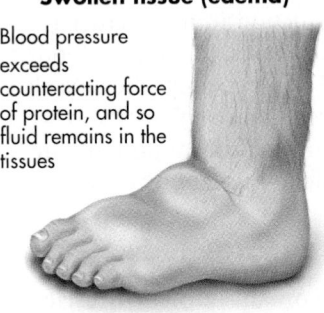

Blood pressure exceeds counteracting force of protein, and so fluid remains in the tissues

(b)

edema The buildup of excess fluid in extracellular spaces.

buffers Compounds that cause a solution to resist changes in acid-base conditions.

fluids accumulate in the tissues, the tissues swell, causing **edema.** Edema may be a symptom of a variety of medical problems, so its cause must be identified. An important step in diagnosing the cause is to measure the concentration of blood proteins.

Contributing to Acid-Base Balance

Proteins help regulate acid-base balance in the blood. Proteins located in cell membranes pump chemical ions in and out of cells. The ion concentration that results from the pumping action, among other factors, keeps the blood slightly alkaline. In addition, some blood proteins are especially good **buffers** for the body. Buffers are compounds that maintain acid-base conditions within a narrow range.

Forming Hormones and Enzymes

Amino acids are required for the synthesis of many hormones—our internal body messengers. Some hormones, such as the thyroid hormones, are made from only one type of amino acid, tyrosine. Insulin, on the other hand, is a hormone composed of 51 total amino acids. Almost all enzymes are proteins or have a protein component.

Neurotransmitters, released by nerve endings, are often derivatives of amino acids. This is true for dopamine and norepinephrine (both synthesized from the amino-acid tyrosine), and serotonin (synthesized from the amino-acid tryptophan).

Contributing to Immune Function

Proteins are a key component of the cells within the immune system. An example is the antibodies, proteins produced by one type of white blood cell. These antibodies can bind to foreign proteins in the body, an important step in removing invaders from the body. Without sufficient dietary protein, the immune system lacks the materials needed to function properly. For example, a low protein status can turn measles into a fatal disease for a malnourished child.

The vitamin niacin can be made from the amino-acid tryptophan, illustrating another role of proteins.

Forming Glucose

In Chapter 4 you learned that the body must maintain a fairly constant concentration of blood glucose to supply energy for the brain, red blood cells, and nervous tissue. At rest, the brain uses about 19% of the body's energy requirements, and it gets most

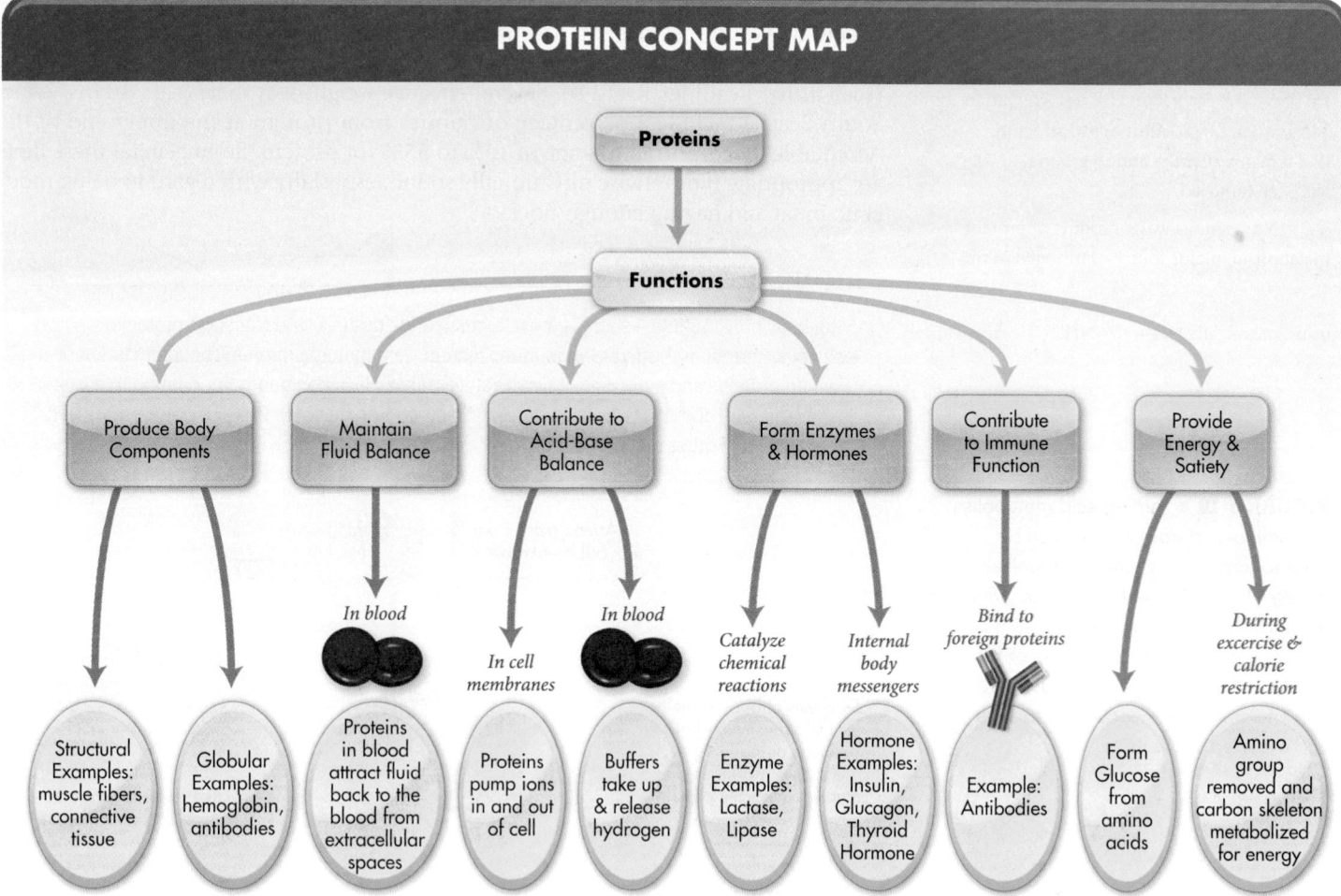

PROTEIN CONCEPT MAP

Proteins

Functions

Produce Body Components
- *Structural Examples:* muscle fibers, connective tissue
- *Globular Examples:* hemoglobin, antibodies

Maintain Fluid Balance
- *In blood* — Proteins in blood attract fluid back to the blood from extracellular spaces

Contribute to Acid-Base Balance
- *In cell membranes* — Proteins pump ions in and out of cell
- *In blood* — Buffers take up & release hydrogen

Form Enzymes & Hormones
- *Catalyze chemical reactions* — Enzyme Examples: Lactase, Lipase
- *Internal body messengers* — Hormone Examples: Insulin, Glucagon, Thyroid Hormone

Contribute to Immune Function
- *Bind to foreign proteins* — Example: Antibodies

Provide Energy & Satiety
- Form Glucose from amino acids
- *During exercise & calorie restriction* — Amino group removed and carbon skeleton metabolized for energy

of that energy from glucose. If you don't consume enough carbohydrate to supply the glucose, your liver (and kidneys, to a lesser extent) will be forced to make glucose from amino acids present in body tissues (Fig. 6-10).

Making some glucose from amino acids is normal. For example, when you skip breakfast and haven't eaten since 7 P.M. the preceding evening, glucose must be manufactured. In an extreme situation, however, such as in starvation, amino acids from muscle tissue are converted into glucose, which wastes muscle tissue and can produce edema.

Providing Energy

Proteins supply little energy for a weight-stable person. Two situations in which a person does use protein to meet energy needs are during prolonged exercise (see Chapter 10 for information about the use of amino acids for energy needs during exercise) and during calorie restriction, as with a weight-loss diet. In these cases, the amino group ($-NH_2$) from the amino acid is removed and the remaining carbon skeleton is metabolized for energy needs (Fig. 6-10). Still, under most conditions, cells primarily use fats and carbohydrates for energy needs. Although proteins contain the same amount of calories (on average, 4 kcal per gram) as carbohydrates, proteins are a costly source of calories, considering the amount of processing the liver and kidneys must perform to use this calorie source.

Contributing to Satiety

Compared to the other macronutrients, proteins provide the highest feeling of **satiety** after a meal. Thus, including some protein with each meal helps control overall

satiety A state in which there is no longer a desire to eat; a feeling of satisfaction.

pool The amount of a nutrient stored within the body that can be mobilized when needed.

carbon skeleton Amino-acid structure that remains after the amino group (—NH$_2$) has been removed.

urea Nitrogenous waste product of protein metabolism; major source of nitrogen in the urine, chemically NH$_2$—$\overset{\overset{\displaystyle O}{\|}}{C}$—NH$_2$.

food intake. Many experts warn against skimping on protein when trying to reduce energy intake to lose weight. Meeting protein needs is still important and exceeding needs somewhat may provide an additional benefit when dieting to lose weight (see Further Readings 7 and 8). Several effective weight-loss diets (e.g., Atkins, Zone, South Beach) include a percentage of calories from protein at the upper end of the Acceptable Macronutrient Range of 10% to 35% for protein. So in general these diets are appropriate if otherwise nutritionally sound, especially with regard to being moderate in fat and having enough fiber.

CONCEPT CHECK

Vital body constituents—such as muscle, connective tissue, blood transport proteins, enzymes, hormones, buffers, and immune factors—are mainly proteins. The degradation of existing proteins and synthesis of new proteins takes place constantly, amounting to a turnover rate of about 250 grams a day for the entire human body. Proteins can also be used for glucose and other fuel production and contributes to satiety.

FIGURE 6-10 ▶ Amino-acid metabolism. The amino-acid **pool** in a cell can be used to form body proteins, as well as a variety of other possible products. When the **carbon skeletons** of amino acids are metabolized to produce glucose or fat, ammonia (NH$_3$) is a resulting waste product. The ammonia is converted to **urea** and excreted in the urine.

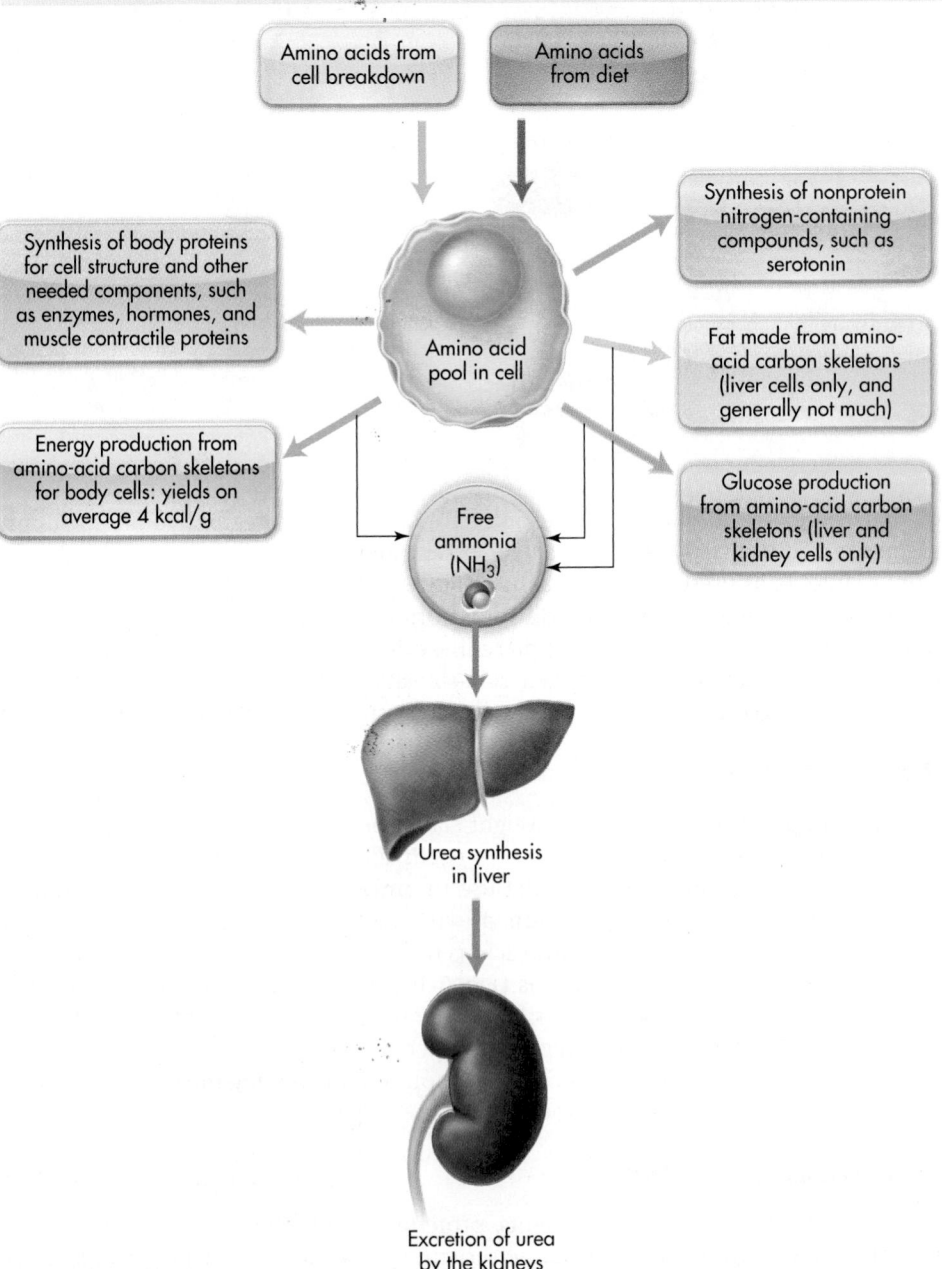

Amino acids from cell breakdown

Amino acids from diet

Synthesis of body proteins for cell structure and other needed components, such as enzymes, hormones, and muscle contractile proteins

Amino acid pool in cell

Synthesis of nonprotein nitrogen-containing compounds, such as serotonin

Fat made from amino-acid carbon skeletons (liver cells only, and generally not much)

Energy production from amino-acid carbon skeletons for body cells: yields on average 4 kcal/g

Free ammonia (NH$_3$)

Glucose production from amino-acid carbon skeletons (liver and kidney cells only)

Urea synthesis in liver

Excretion of urea by the kidneys

6.6 Protein Needs

How much protein (actually, amino acids) do we need to eat each day? People who aren't growing need to eat only enough protein to match whatever they lose daily from protein breakdown. The amount of breakdown can be determined by measuring the amount of urea and other nitrogen-containing compounds in the urine, as well as losses of protein from feces, skin, hair, nails, and so on. In short, people need to balance protein intake with such losses to maintain a state of **protein equilibrium,** also called *protein balance* (Fig. 6-11).

When a body is growing or recovering from an illness or injury, it needs a **positive protein balance** to supply the raw materials required to build new tissues. To achieve this, a person must eat more protein daily than he or she loses. In addition, the hormones insulin, growth hormone, and testosterone all stimulate positive protein balance. Resistance exercise (weight training) also enhances positive protein balance. Consuming less protein than needed leads to **negative protein balance,** such as when acute illness reduces the desire to eat and so one loses more protein than consumed.

For healthy people, the amount of dietary protein needed to maintain protein equilibrium (wherein intake equals losses) can be determined by increasing protein intake until it equals losses of protein and its related breakdown products (e.g., urea). Calorie needs must also be met so that amino acids are not diverted for such use.

Today, the best estimate for the amount of protein required for nearly all adults to maintain protein equilibrium is 0.8 grams of protein per kilogram of healthy

protein equilibrium A state in which protein intake is equal to related protein losses; the person is said to be in protein balance.

positive protein balance A state in which protein intake exceeds related protein losses, as is needed during times of growth.

negative protein balance A state in which protein intake is less than related protein losses, as is often seen during acute illness.

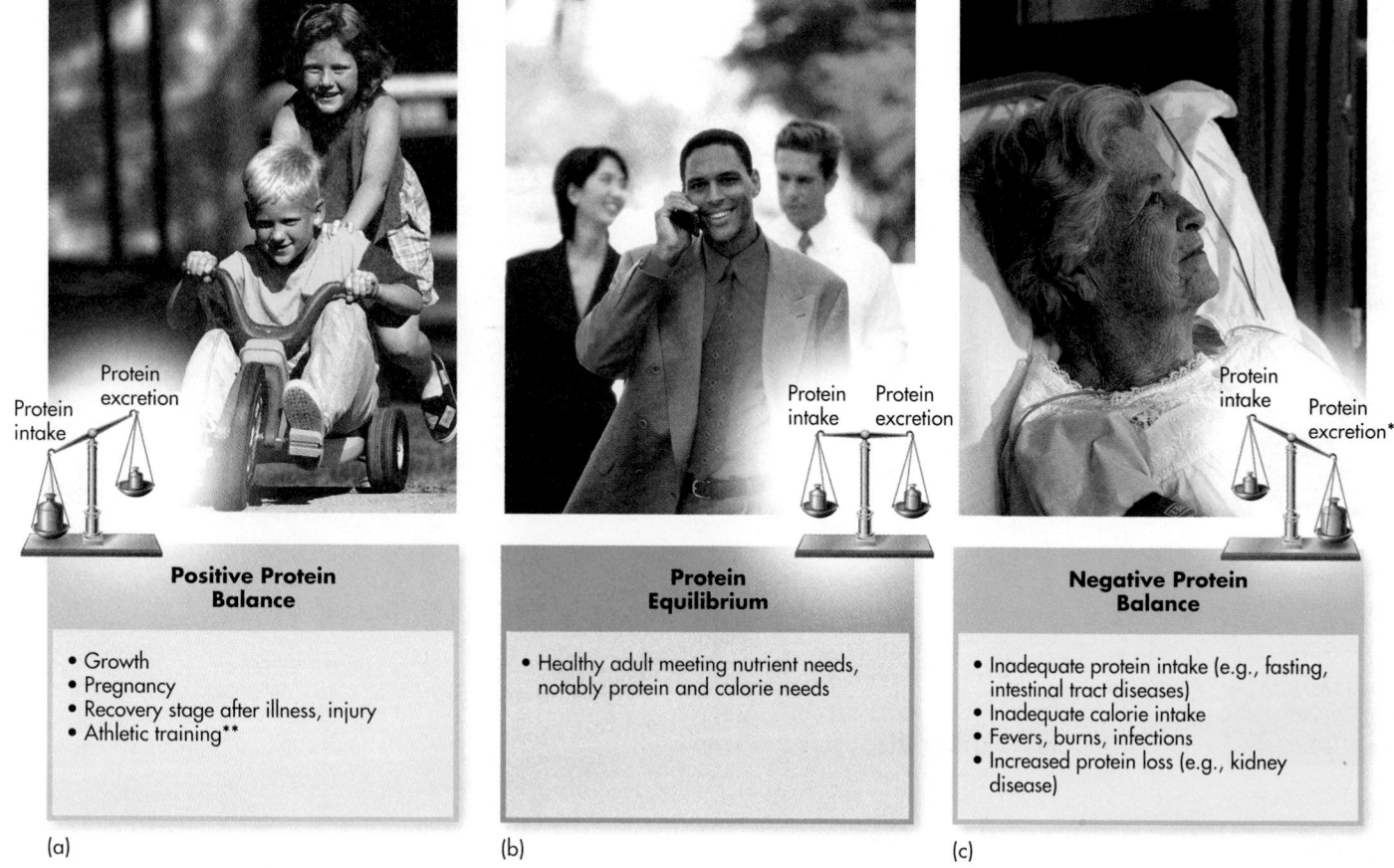

Positive Protein Balance

- Growth
- Pregnancy
- Recovery stage after illness, injury
- Athletic training**

Protein Equilibrium

- Healthy adult meeting nutrient needs, notably protein and calorie needs

Negative Protein Balance

- Inadequate protein intake (e.g., fasting, intestinal tract diseases)
- Inadequate calorie intake
- Fevers, burns, infections
- Increased protein loss (e.g., kidney disease)

(a)　　　　　　　　　(b)　　　　　　　　　(c)

*Based on losses of urea and other nitrogen-containing compounds in the urine, as well as protein lost from feces, skin, hair, nails, and other minor routes.
**Only when additional lean body mass is being gained. Nevertheless, the athlete is probably already eating enough protein to support this extra protein synthesis; protein supplements are not needed.

FIGURE 6-11 ▶ Protein balance in practical terms: (a) positive protein balance; (b) protein equilibrium; (c) negative protein balance.

The 2010 Dietary Guidlines for Americans in "**Food and Nutrients to Increase**," provide the following recommendatins regarding protein intake as part of healthy eating pattern and while staying within their calorie needs:

- Increase intake of fat-free or low-fat milk and milk product, such as milk, yogurt, cheese, or fortified soy beverages.
- Choose a variety of protein foods, which include seafood, lean meat and poultry, eggs, beans and peas, soy products, and unsalted nuts and seeds.
- Increase the amount and variety of seafood consumed by choosing seafood in place of some meat and poultry.
- Replace protein foods that are higher in solid fats with choices that are lower in solid fats and calories and/or are sources of oils.

body weight. This is the RDA for protein. Requirements are higher during periods of growth, such as pregnancy and infancy (see Chapters 14 and 15 for specific values for pregnant women, infants, and children). Healthy weight is used as a reference in the determination of protein needs because excess fat storage doesn't contribute much to protein needs (see Chapter 7 for insight into the concept of healthy weight). Calculations using this RDA are shown in the margin and estimate a requirement of about 56 grams of protein daily for a typical 70-kilogram (154-pound) man and about 46 grams of protein daily for a typical 57-kilogram (125-pound) woman.

The RDA for protein translates into about 10% of total calories. Many experts recommend up to 15% of total calories to provide more flexibility in diet planning, in turn allowing for the variety of protein-rich foods North Americans typically consume. Protein-rich foods are also part of the "Food and Nutrients to increase" in the 2010 Dietary Guidelines. As noted earlier, the Food and Nutrition Board has set an upper range for protein intake at 35% of calories consumed. It is easy to meet currently suggested daily protein needs (Table 6-2). On a daily basis, typical North American protein intakes are about 100 grams of protein for men and 65 grams for women. Thus, most of us consume much more protein than the RDA recommends because we like many high-protein foods and can afford to buy them. Our bodies cannot store excess protein once it is consumed, so the excess amino acids are converted to carbon skeletons that are turned into glucose or fat and then stored as fat or metabolized for energy needs (review Fig. 6-10).

TABLE 6-2 Protein Content of Sample Menus Containing 1600 kcal and 2000 kcal

Menu	1600 kcal		2000 kcal	
	Serving Size	Protein (g)	Serving Size	Protein (g)
Breakfast				
Low-fat granola	²/₃ cup	5	²/₃ cup	5
Blueberries	1 cup	1	1 cup	1
Fat-free (skim) milk	1 cup	8.5	1 cup	8.5
Coffee	1 cup	0	1 cup	0
Lunch				
Broiled chicken breast	3 oz	25	4 oz	33
Salad greens	3 cups	5	3 cups	5
Baked taco shell strips	½ cup	2	½ cup	2
Low-fat salad dressing	2 tbsp	0	2 tbsp	0
Fat-free (skim) milk	1 cup	8.5	1 cup	8.5
Dinner				
Yellow rice	1¼ cups	5	2½ cups	10
Shrimp	4 large	5	6 large	7
Mussels	4 medium	8	6 medium	12
Clams	5 small	12	10 small	24
Peas	¼ cup	4	½ cup	4
Sweet red pepper	¼ cup	0	½ cup	0
Snack				
Muffin	1 small	4	1 small	4
Swiss cheese	1 oz	7.5	1 oz	7.5
Banana	½ small	0.5	½ small	0.5
Total		101		132

Mental stress, physical labor, and recreational weekend sports activities do not require an increase in the protein RDA. For some highly trained athletes, such as those participating in endurance or strength training, protein consumption may need to exceed the RDA. This is an area of debate in sports nutrition: the Food and Nutrition Board does not support an increased need, but some experts suggest an increase to about 1.7 grams per kilogram. Many North Americans already consume that much protein, especially men.

6.7 Does Eating a High-Protein Diet Harm You?

People frequently ask about the potential harm of protein intakes in excess of the RDA. Problems with diets that are high in protein foods primarily stem from the fact that they typically rely on animal sources of protein. Diets rich in animal products will most likely be simultaneously low in the beneficial substances found in plant sources, including fiber, some vitamins (e.g., folate), some minerals (e.g., magnesium), as well as phytochemicals, and high in substances such as saturated fat and cholesterol. A high animal-protein diet, therefore, is unlikely to follow the recommendations of the Dietary Guidelines for Americans or the Food and Nutrition Board in terms of reducing risk for cardiovascular disease.

Some, but not all, studies show that high-protein diets can increase calcium losses in urine. For people with adequate calcium intakes, little concern about this relationship is warranted, but keep in mind that calcium is commonly deficient in North American diets.

Meat is one of the richest sources of protein. Excessive intake of red meat, however, especially processed forms, is linked to colon cancer in population studies (see Further Reading 3). This association is still being studied (see Newsworthy Nutrition in margin), and there are several possible explanations for this connection. The curing agents used to process meats such as ham and salami may cause cancer. Substances that form during cooking of red meat at high temperatures may also cause cancer. The excessive fat or low-fiber contents of diets rich in red meat may also be a contributing factor. Because of these concerns, some nutrition experts suggest we focus more on poultry, fish, nuts, legumes, and seeds to meet protein needs. In addition, any red or other type of meat should be trimmed of all visible fat before grilling.

Some researchers have expressed concern that a high-protein intake may overburden the kidneys by forcing them to excrete the extra nitrogen as urea. Additionally, animal proteins may contribute to kidney stone formation in certain individuals. There is some support for limiting protein intake for people in the early stages of kidney disease, because low-protein diets somewhat slow the decline in kidney function. Laboratory animal studies show that moderate protein intakes that just meet nutritional needs preserve kidney function over time better than high-protein diets. Preserving kidney function is especially important for those who have diabetes, early signs of kidney disease, or only one functioning kidney, so a high-protein diet is not recommended for these people. High-protein diets increase urine output, in turn posing a risk for dehydration. This is a special concern for athletes (see Chapter 10).

Convert weight from pounds to kilograms:	154 pounds
	2.2 pounds/kilogram
	= 70 kilograms
	125 pounds
	2.2 pounds/kilogram
	= 57 kilograms

Calculate protein RDA:

$$70 \text{ kilograms} \times \frac{0.8 \text{ grams protein}}{\text{kilogram body weight}}$$
$$= 56 \text{ grams}$$

$$57 \text{ kilograms} \times \frac{0.8 \text{ grams protein}}{\text{kilogram body weight}}$$
$$= 46 \text{ grams}$$

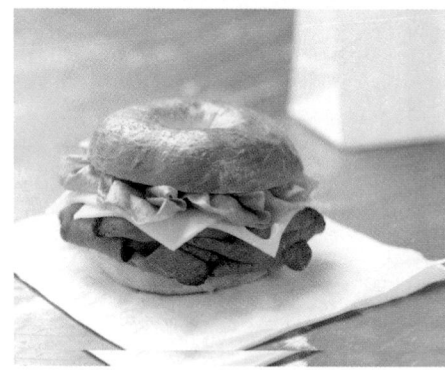

▲ Animal protein foods, such as the roast beef and swiss cheese on this bagel, are typically our main sources of protein in the North American diet.

NEWSWORTHY NUTRITION | **Link between colon cancer and recent fat, protein, and red meat consumption not supported**

The risk of distal colorectal cancer and the consumption of fat, protein, and red and processed meat was determined in whites and African-Americans. The diet was assessed for the previous 12 months in the 945 cases of colon cancer and 959 controls. No association was found between total, saturated, or monounsaturated fat intake and colon cancer risk; the percentages of calories from protein and red meat intake were both associated with a reduction (rather than increase) in risk of colon cancer, in whites. Although these results do not support the general hypotheses that fat, protein and red meat increase the risk of colon cancer, we must remember that the diet was only measured for 12 months prior to the study. A more long-term effect of these dietary factors, therefore, cannot be ruled out.

Source: Williams CD and others: Associations of red meat, fat, and protein intake with distal colorectal cancer risk. *Nutrition and Cancer* 62(6): 701, 2010 (see Further Reading 14).

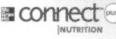 **Check out the Connect site** www.mcgrawhillconnect .com **to further explore diet and colorectal cancer.**

MAKING DECISIONS

Amino-Acid Supplements

Protein and amino-acid supplements are used primarily by athletes and dieters. Athletes use them hoping they will help build muscle. The branched-chain amino acids described earlier are especially popular with athletes looking to enhance their performance. Dieters have turned to these supplements hoping they will increase their weight loss. Although the right amount of protein in the diet will aid athletic performance and help in weight control, consuming this protein in the form of amino-acid supplements cannot be considered safe.

Earlier in this chapter, you learned that the body is designed to handle whole proteins as a dietary source of amino acids. When individual amino-acid supplements are taken, they can overwhelm the absorptive mechanisms in the small intestine, triggering amino-acid imbalances in the body. Imbalances occur because groups of chemically similar amino acids compete for absorption sites in the absorptive cells. For example, lysine and arginine are absorbed by the same transporter, so an excess of lysine can impair absorption of arginine. The amino acids most likely to cause toxicity when consumed in large amounts are methionine, cysteine, and histidine. Due to the potential for imbalances and toxicities of individual amino acids, the best advice to ensure adequacy is to stick to whole foods rather than supplements as sources of amino acids. Amino acids as such also have a disagreeable odor and flavor and are also much more expensive than food protein. In Canada the sale of individual amino acids to consumers is banned. Read more about this issue in the What Would You Choose Recommendations at the end of this chapter.

CONCEPT CHECK

The Recommended Dietary Allowance (RDA) for adults is 0.8 grams of protein per kilogram of healthy body weight. This is approximately 56 grams of protein daily for a 70-kilogram (156-pound) person. The average North American man consumes about 100 grams of protein daily, and a woman consumes about 65 grams. Thus, typically we eat more than enough protein to meet our needs. This even includes well-balanced vegetarian diets. Diets high in protein can compromise kidney health in people with diabetes and those with kidney disease, and animal protein sources likely increase cardiovascular disease and kidney stone risk when consumed in high amounts.

protein-calorie malnutrition (PCM)
A condition resulting from regularly consuming insufficient amounts of calories and protein. The deficiency eventually results in body wasting, primarily of lean tissue, and an increased susceptibility to infections.

kwashiorkor A disease occurring primarily in young children who have an existing disease and consume a marginal amount of calories and insufficient protein in relation to needs. The child generally suffers from infections and exhibits edema, poor growth, weakness, and an increased susceptibility to further illness.

marasmus A disease resulting from consuming a grossly insufficient amount of protein and calories; one of the diseases classed as protein-calorie malnutrition. Victims have little or no fat stores, little muscle mass, and poor strength. Death from infections is common.

6.8 Protein-Calorie Malnutrition

Protein deficiency is rarely an isolated condition and usually accompanies a deficiency of calories and other nutrients resulting from insufficient food intake. In the developed world, alcoholism can lead to cases of protein deficiency because of the low protein content of alcoholic beverages. Protein and calorie malnutrition is a significant problem in hospitals worldwide, affecting patients of all ages from infants to geriatric patients. Malnutrition can be caused by the illnesses or injuries for which the patients are admitted to the hospital and by the hospitalization itself (see Further Reading 4). In developing areas of the world, people often have diets low in calories and also in protein. This state of undernutrition stunts the growth of children and makes them more susceptible to disease throughout life. (Undernutrition is a main focus of Chapter 12.) People who consume too little protein calories can eventually develop **protein-calorie malnutrition (PCM),** also referred to as *protein-energy malnutrition (PEM)*. In its milder form, it is difficult to tell if a person with PCM is consuming too little calories or protein, or both. When an inadequate intake of nutrients, including protein, is combined with an already existing disease, especially an infection, a form of malnutrition called **kwashiorkor** can develop. But if the nutrient deficiency—especially for calories—becomes severe, a deficiency disease called **marasmus** can result. Both conditions are seen primarily in children but also may develop in adults, even in those hospitalized in North America. These two conditions form the tip of the iceberg with respect to states of undernutrition, and symptoms of these two conditions can even be present in the same person (Fig. 6-12).

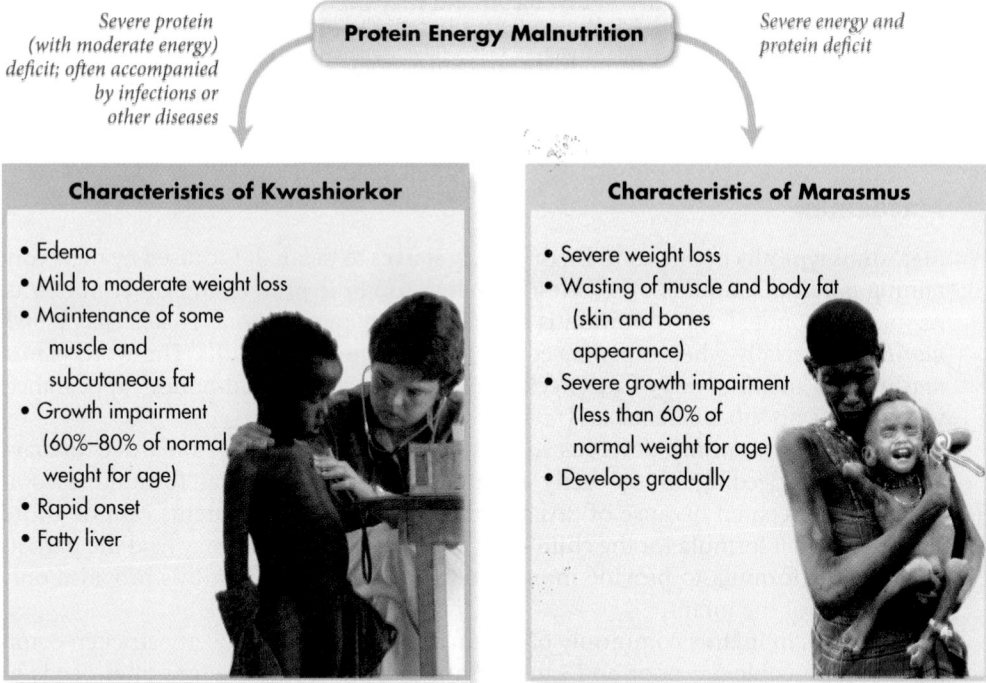

Severe protein (with moderate energy) deficit; often accompanied by infections or other diseases

Protein Energy Malnutrition

Severe energy and protein deficit

FIGURE 6-12 ▶ Classification of undernutrition in children.

Characteristics of Kwashiorkor

- Edema
- Mild to moderate weight loss
- Maintenance of some muscle and subcutaneous fat
- Growth impairment (60%–80% of normal weight for age)
- Rapid onset
- Fatty liver

Characteristics of Marasmus

- Severe weight loss
- Wasting of muscle and body fat (skin and bones appearance)
- Severe growth impairment (less than 60% of normal weight for age)
- Develops gradually

Kwashiorkor

Kwashiorkor is a word from Ghana that means "the disease that the first child gets when the new child comes." From birth, an infant in developing areas of the world is usually breastfed. Often by the time the child reaches 1 to 1.5 years of age, the mother is pregnant or has already given birth again, and the new child gets preference for breastfeeding. The older child's diet then abruptly changes from nutritious human milk to starchy roots and **gruels.** These foods have low-protein densities, compared with total energy. Additionally, the foods are usually full of plant fibers, often bulky, making it difficult for the child to consume enough to meet calorie needs. The child generally also has infections, which acutely raise calorie and protein needs. For these reasons, calorie needs of these children are met just barely, at best, and their protein consumption is grossly inadequate, especially in view of the increased amount needed to combat infections. Many vitamin and mineral needs are also far from being fulfilled. Famine victims face similar problems.

The major symptoms of kwashiorkor are apathy, diarrhea, listlessness, failure to grow and gain weight, and withdrawal from the environment. These symptoms complicate other diseases present. For example, a condition such as measles, a disease that normally makes a healthy child ill for only a week or so, can become severely debilitating and even fatal. Further symptoms of kwashiorkor are changes in hair color, potassium deficiency, flaky skin, fatty liver, reduced muscle mass, and massive edema in the abdomen and legs. The presence of edema in a child who has some subcutaneous fat (i.e., directly under the skin) is the hallmark of kwashiorkor (review Fig. 6-12). In addition, these children seldom move. If you pick them up, they don't cry. When you hold them, you feel the plumpness of edema, not muscle and fat tissue.

Many symptoms of kwashiorkor can be explained based on what we know about proteins. Proteins play important roles in fluid balance, lipoprotein transport, immune function, and production of tissues, such as skin, cells lining the GI tract, and hair. Children with an insufficient protein intake do not grow and mature normally.

If children with kwashiorkor are helped in time—if infections are treated and a diet ample in protein, calories, and other essential nutrients is provided—the disease

gruels A thin mixture of grains or legumes in milk or water.

Toxic products in moldy grains may also contribute to kwashiorkor.

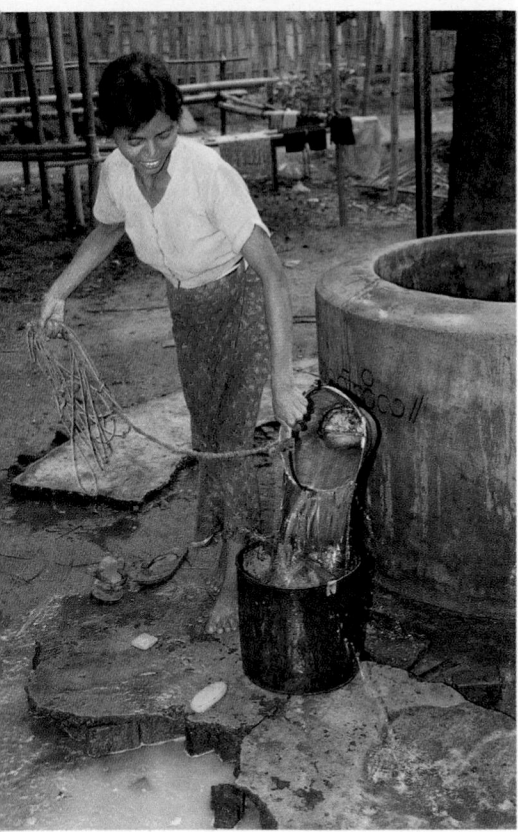

▲ Unsafe water supplies in developing countries contribute to the incidence of marasmus, particularly in bottle-fed infants.

preterm An infant born before 37 weeks of gestation; also referred to as premature.

process reverses. They begin to grow again and may even show no signs of their previous condition, except perhaps shortness of stature. Unfortunately, by the time many of these children reach a hospital or care center, they already have severe infections. Despite the best care, they still die. Or, if they survive, they return home only to become ill again.

Marasmus

Marasmus typically occurs as an infant slowly starves to death. It is caused by diets containing minimal amounts of calories, as well as too little protein and other nutrients. As previously noted, the condition is also commonly referred to as *protein-calorie malnutrition*, especially when experienced by older children and adults. The word *marasmus* means "to waste away," in Greek. Victims have a "skin-and-bones" appearance, with little or no subcutaneous fat (review Fig. 6-12).

Marasmus commonly develops in infants who either are not breastfed or have stopped breastfeeding in the early months. Often the weaning formula used is improperly prepared because of unsafe water and because the parents cannot afford sufficient infant formula for the child's needs. The latter problem may lead the parents to dilute the formula to provide more feedings, not realizing that this provides only more water for the infant.

Marasmus in infants commonly occurs in the large cities of poverty-stricken countries. When people are poor and sanitation is lacking, bottle feeding often leads to marasmus. In the cities, bottle feeding is often necessary because the infant must be cared for by others when the mother is working or away from home. An infant with marasmus requires large amounts of calories and protein—like a **preterm** infant—and, unless the child receives them, full recovery from the disease may never occur. The majority of brain growth occurs between conception and the child's first birthday. In fact, the brain is growing at its highest rate after birth. If the diet does not support brain growth during the first months of life, the brain may not grow to its full adult size. This reduced or retarded brain growth may lead to diminished intellectual function. Both kwashiorkor and marasmus plague infants and children; mortality rates in developing countries are often 10 to 20 times higher than in North America.

CONCEPT CHECK

Most undernutrition consists of mild deficits in calories, protein, and often other nutrients. If a person needs more nutrients because of disease and infection but does not consume enough calories and protein, a condition known as kwashiorkor can develop. The person suffers from edema and weakness. Children around age 2 are especially susceptible to kwashiorkor, particularly if they already have other diseases. Famine situations in which only starchy root products are available to eat contribute to this problem. Marasmus is a condition wherein people—infants, especially—starve to death. Symptoms include muscle wasting, absence of fat stores, and weakness. Both an adequate diet and the treatment of concurrent diseases must be promoted to regain and then maintain nutritional health.

Vegetarian and Plant-Based Diets

Vegetarianism has evolved over the centuries from a necessity into an option. Historically, vegetarianism was linked with specific philosophies and religions or with science. Today, about 1 in 40 adults in the United States (and about 1 in 25 in Canada) is a vegetarian. Vegetarian diets have evolved to include such new products as soy-based sloppy joes, chili, tacos, burgers, and more. In addition, cookbooks that feature the use of a variety of fruits, vegetables, and seasonings are enhancing food selection for vegetarians of all degrees.

Vegetarianism is popular among college students. Fifteen percent of college students in one survey said they select vegetarian options at lunch or dinner on any given day. In response, dining services offer vegetarian options at every meal, such as pastas with meatless sauce and pizza. Many teenagers are also turning to vegetarianism. Many restaurants offer vegetarian meals in response to the growing number of its customers who want a vegetarian option when they eat out (see Further Reading 13). Many customers cite health and taste as reasons for choosing vegetarian meals.

As nutrition science has grown, new information has enabled the design of nutritionally adequate vegetarian diets. It is important for vegetarians to take advantage of this information because a diet of only plant-based foods has the potential to promote various nutrient deficiencies and substantial growth retardation in infants and children. People who choose a vegetarian diet can meet their nutritional needs by following a few basic rules and knowledgeably planning their diets.

Studies show that death rates from some chronic diseases, such as certain forms of cardiovascular disease, hypertention, many forms of cancer, type 2 diabetes, and obesity, are lower for vegetarians than for non-vegetarians. Vegetarians often live longer, as shown in

religious groups that practice vegetarianism. Other aspects of healthful lifestyles, such as not smoking, abstaining from alcohol and drugs, and regular physical activity often go along with vegetarianism and probably partially account for the lower risks of chronic disease and longer lives seen in this population.

As you learned in Chapter 2, MyPlate and the 2010 Dietary Guidelines for Americans emphasize a plant-based diet of whole-grain breads and cereals, fruits, and vegetables. In addition, the American Institute for Cancer Research promotes "The New American Plate," which includes plant-based foods covering two-thirds (or more) of the plate and meat, fish, poultry, or lowfat dairy covering only one-third (or less) of the plate. Although these recommendations do allow the inclusion of animal products, they are definitely more "vegetarian-like" than typical North American diets.

Why Do People Become Vegetarians?

People choose vegetarianism for a variety of reasons including ethics, religion, economics, and health. Some believe that killing animals for food is unethical. Hindus and Trappist monks eat vegetarian meals as a practice of their religion. In North America, many Seventh Day Adventists base their practice of vegetarianism on biblical texts and believe it is a more healthful way to live.

Some advocates of vegetarianism base their food preference upon the inefficient use of animals as a source of protein. Forty percent of the world's grain production is used to raise meat-producing animals.

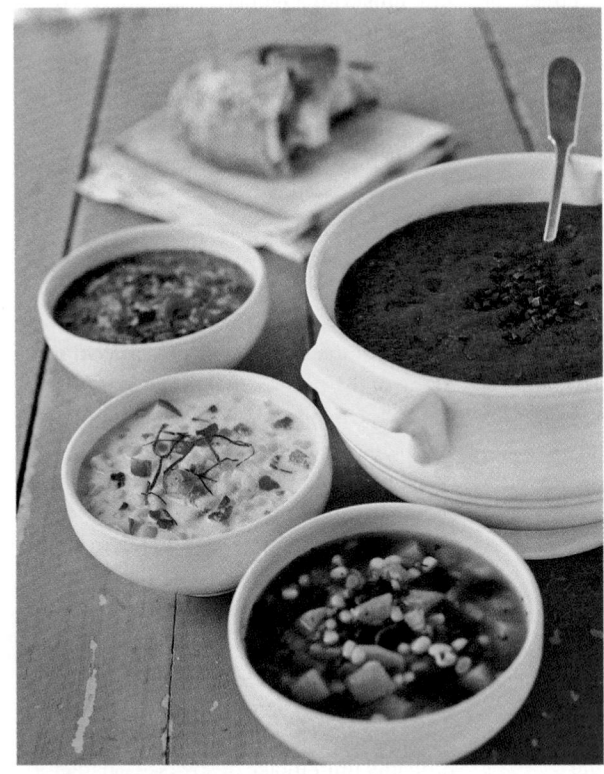

▲ Recipes for vegetarian and plant-based foods are widely available today. Soups are an excellent way to combine complementary plant proteins.

The New American Plate

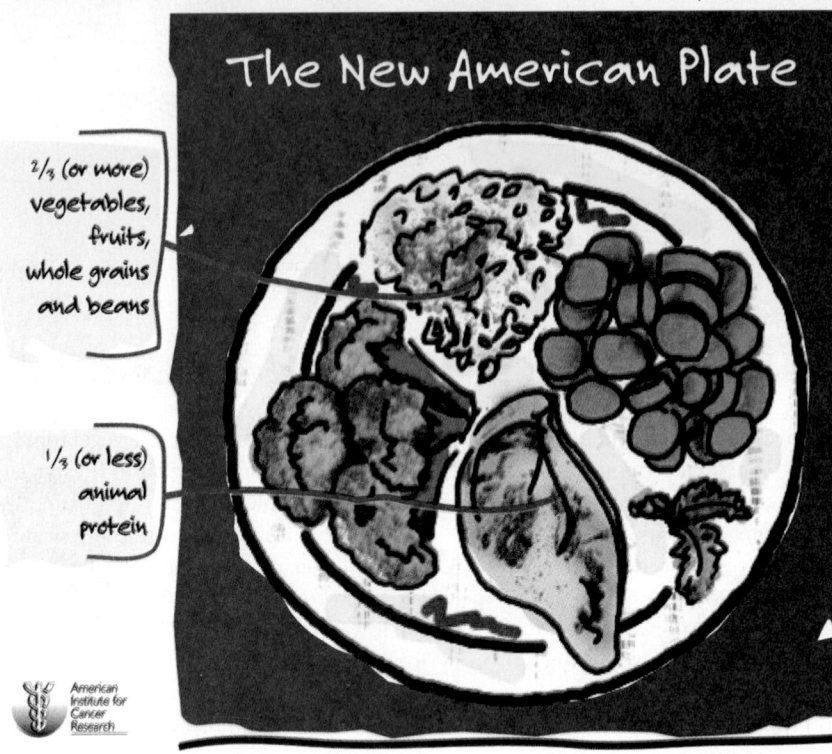

The New American Plate

²/₃ (or more) vegetables, fruits, whole grains and beans

¹/₃ (or less) animal protein

American Institute for Cancer Research

▶ American Institute for Cancer Research Diet and Health Guidelines for Cancer Prevention

1. Choose a diet rich in a variety of plant-based foods.

2. Eat plenty of vegetables and fruit.

3. Maintain a healthy weight and be physically active

4. Drink alcohol only in moderation, if at all.

5. Select foods low in fat and salt.

6. Prepare and store food safely.

And always remember. . .

Do not use tobacco in any form.

▶ "The New American Plate" published by the Amercian Institute for Cancer Research, was a forerunner of and embodies the same concepts as the new ChooseMyPlate program.

Although animals that humans eat sometimes eat grasses that humans cannot digest, many also eat grains that humans can eat.

People might also practice vegetarianism because it limits saturated fat and cholesterol intake, while encouraging a high intake of complex carbohydrates, vitamins A, E, and C, carotenoids, magnesium, and fiber.

Good for Disease Prevention

Plant sources of proteins can positively impact heart health in several ways (see Further Readings 5, 6, 9, and 10). First, the plant foods we eat contain no cholesterol nor *trans* fat and little saturated fat. The major type of fats in plant foods are monounsaturated and polyunsaturated fats. Nuts in particular are high in monounsaturated fat, which helps to keep blood cholesterol low.

Beans and nuts contain soluble fiber, which binds to cholesterol in the small intestine and prevents it from being absorbed by the body. Also, due to the activity of some phytochemicals, foods made from soybeans can lower production of cholesterol by the body. The effect is modest (about a 2% to 6% drop). In 1999, the Food and Drug Administration allowed health claims for the cholesterol-lowering properties of soy foods, and in 2000, the American Heart Association recommended inclusion of some soy protein in the diets of people with high blood cholesterol. As noted in Chapter 2, to list a health claim for soy on the label, a food product must have at least 6.25 grams of soy protein and less than 3 grams of fat, 1 gram of saturated fat, and 20 milligrams of cholesterol per serving.

There are several other compounds in plant foods under study for their heart-protective roles. Some of the phytochemicals may help to prevent blood clots and relax the blood vessels. Nuts are an especially good source of nutrients implicated in heart health, including vitamin E, folate, magnesium, and copper. Frequent consumption of nuts (about 1 ounce of nuts five times per week) is associated with a decreased risk of cardiovascular disease. Recall from Chapter 2 that FDA also allows a provisional health claim to link nuts with a reduced risk of developing cardiovascular disease. As noted in Chapter 5, a vegan diet coupled with regular exercise and other lifestyle changes can lead to a reversal of atherosclerotic plaque in various arteries in the body.

Cancer-Fighting Agents

The numerous phytochemicals in plant foods are thought to aid in preventing cancers of the breast, prostate, and colon. Many of the proposed anticancer effects of foods containing plant protein are through antioxidant mechanisms.

Consumption of plant sources of proteins can aid in prevention of cardiovascular disease and cancer, but there are also other areas for future study. Some studies show that replacing animal proteins with plant proteins is beneficial for kidney health. However, because plant foods such as soy are high in oxalates, people with a history of kidney stones should probably limit intake of soy (see Chapter 9 for more about oxalates). Plants may be particularly good sources of protein for people with diabetes or impaired glucose tolerance because the high fiber content of plant foods leads to a slower increase in blood glucose (review Chapter 4 for a discussion of glycemic load). Frequent nut consumption may even reduce the risk of developing gallstones, obesity, and type 2 diabetes. A recent review of 18 studies concluded that soy consumption was associated with a 14% reduction in breast cancer risk, but several other studies have shown little benefit of soy in preventing many forms of cancer, in lowering blood cholesterol, contributing to bone maintenance in women after menopause, and in treating menopausal symptoms in women (see Further Readings 12 and 15).

Increasing Plant Proteins in Your Diet

Now that you've seen how much you can benefit from including plant proteins in your diet, here are some suggestions for putting the theory onto your plate:

- At your next cookout, try a veggie burger instead of a hamburger. These are usually made from beans and are available in the frozen foods section of the grocery store and come in a variety of delicious flavors. Many restaurants have added veggie burgers to their menus.
- Sprinkle sunflower seeds or chopped almonds on top of your salad to add taste and texture.
- Mix chopped walnuts into the batter of your banana bread to boost your intake of monounsaturated fats.
- Eat soy nuts (oil-roasted soybeans) as a great snack.
- Spread some peanut butter on your bagel instead of butter or cream cheese.
- Instead of having beef or chicken tacos for dinner, heat up a can of great northern beans in your skillet with one half of a packet of taco seasoning and chopped tomatoes. Use this as a filling in a tortilla shell.
- Consider using soy milk, especially if you have lactose malabsorption or lactose intolerance. Look for varieties fortified with calcium.

Food Planning for Vegetarians

There are a variety of vegetarian diet styles. **Vegans,** or "total vegetarians," eat only plant foods (and do not use animal products for other purposes, such as leather shoes or feather pillows). **Fruitarians** primarily eat fruits, nuts, honey, and vegetable oils. This plan is not recommended because it can lead to nutrient deficiencies in people of all ages. **Lactovegetarians** modify vegetarianism a bit—they include dairy products in their plant-based diet. **Lactoovovegetarians** modify the diet even further and eat dairy products and eggs, as well as plant foods. Including these animal products makes food planning easier because they are rich in some nutrients that are missing or minimal in plants, such as vitamin B-12 and calcium. The more variety in the diet, the easier it is to meet nutritional needs. Thus, the practice of eating no animal sources of food signif cantly separates the vegans and fruitaria from all other semivegetarian styles.

Most people who call themselves vegetarians consume at least some dairy products, if not all dairy products and eggs. A food-group plan has been developed for lactovegetarians and vegans (Table 6-3). This plan includes servings of nuts, grains, legumes, and seeds to help meet protein needs. There is also a vegetable group, a fruit group, and a milk group.

Vegan Diet Planning

Planning a vegan diet requires knowled and creativity to yield high-quality protein and other key nutrients without animal products. Earlier in this chapter, you learned about complementing proteins, whereby the essential amino acids deficient in one protein source are supplied by those of another consumed at the same meal or the next (Fig. 6-13). Many legumes are deficient in the essential amino-acid methionine, while cereals are limited in lysine. Eating a combination of legumes and cereals, such as beans and rice, will supply the body with adequate amounts of all essential amino acids (Fig. 6-13). As for

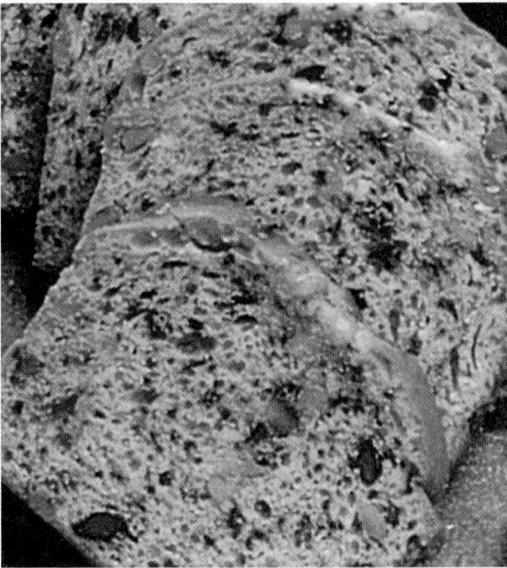

▲ Plant proteins, like those in walnuts, can be incorporated into one's diet in numerous ways, such as adding them to banana bread.

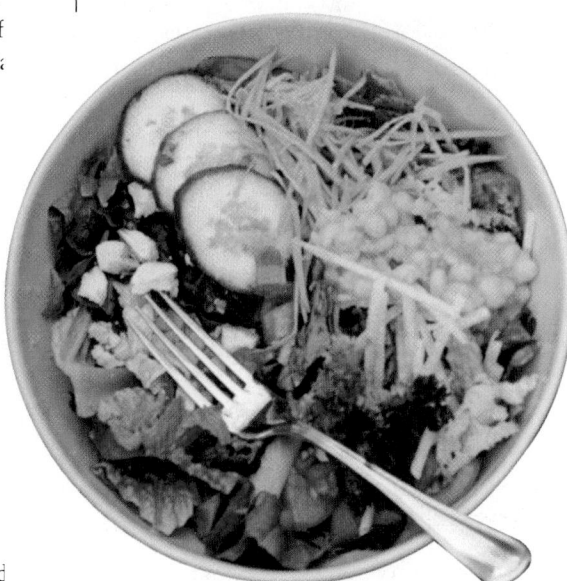

▲ A salad containing numerous types of vegetables and legumes is a healthy vegetarian choice.

vegan A person who eats only plant foods.

fruitarian A person who primarily eats fruits, nuts, honey, and vegetable oils.

lactovegetarian A person who consumes plant products and dairy products.

lactoovovegetarian A person who consumes plant products, dairy products, and eggs.

TABLE 6-3 Food Plan for Vegetarians Based on MyPlate

Food Group	MyPlate Servings Lactovegetarian[a]	Vegan[b]	Key Nutrients Supplied[c]
Grains	6–11	8–11	Protein, thiamin, niacin, folate, vitamin E, zinc, magnesium, iron, and fiber
Beans and other legumes	2–3	3	Protein, vitamin B-6, zinc, magnesium, and fiber
Nuts, seeds	2–3	3	Protein, vitamin E, and magnesium
Vegetables	3–5 (include 1 dark-green or leafy variety daily)	4–6 (include 1 dark-green or leafy variety daily)	Vitamin A, vitamin C, folate, vitamin K, potassium, and magnesium
Fruits	2–4	4	Vitamin A, vitamin C, and folate
Milk	3	_____	Protein, riboflavin, vitamin D, vitamin B-12, and calcium
Fortified soy milk	_____	3	Protein, riboflavin, vitamin D, vitamin B-12, and calcium

[a]This plan contains about 75 grams of protein in 1650 kcal.

[b]This plan contains about 79 grams of protein in 1800 kcal.

[c]One serving of vitamin- and mineral-enriched ready-to-eat breakfast cereal is recommended to meet possible nutrient gaps. Alternatively, a balanced multivitamin and mineral supplement can be used. Vegans also may benefit from the use of fortified soy milk to provide calcium, vitamin D, and vitamin B-12.

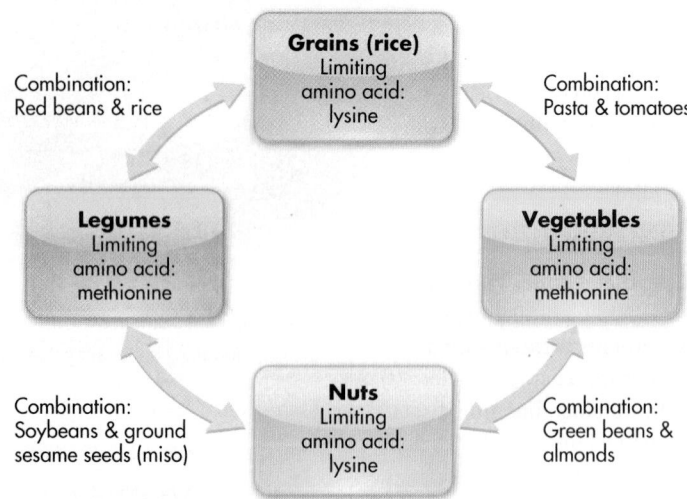

FIGURE 6-13 ▶ Plant group combinations in which the proteins complement each other in a meal based on their limiting amino acids.

any diet, variety is an especially important characteristic of a nutritious vegan diet.

Aside from amino acids, low intakes of certain micronutrients can be a problem for the vegan. At the forefront of nutritional concerns are riboflavin, vitamins D and B-12, iron, zinc, iodide, and calcium. The following dietary advice should be implemented. In addition, use of a balanced multivitamin and mineral supplement can help as well.

Riboflavin can be obtained from green leafy vegetables, whole grains, yeast, and legumes—components of most vegan diets. Alternate sources of vitamin D include fortified foods (e.g., margarine), as well as regular sun exposure (see Chapter 8).

Vitamin B-12 only occurs naturally in animal foods. Plants can contain soil or microbial contaminants that provide trace amounts of vitamin B-12, but these are negligible sources of the vitamin. Because the body can store vitamin B-12 for about 4 years, it may take a long time after removal of animal foods from the diet for a vitamin B-12 deficiency to surface. If dietary B-12 inadequacy persists, deficiency can lead to a form of anemia, nerve damage, and mental dysfunction. These deficiency consequences have been noted in the infants of vegetarian mothers whose breast milk was low in vitamin B-12. Vegans can prevent a vitamin B-12 deficiency by finding a reliable source of vitamin B-12,

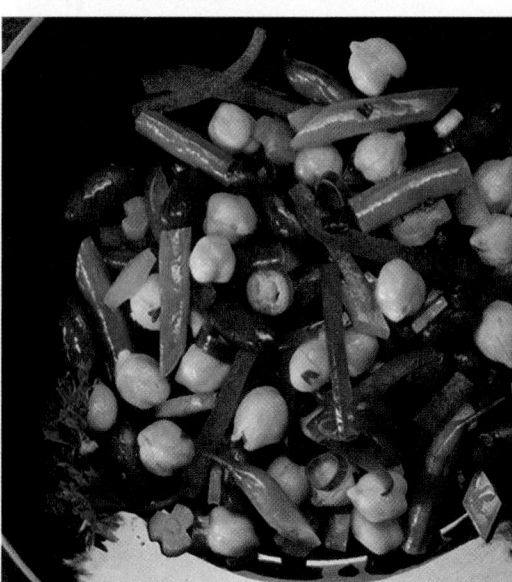

▲ Keep in mind that amino acids in vegetables are best used when a combination of sources is consumed.

such as fortified soybean milk, ready-to-eat breakfast cereals, and special yeast grown on media rich in vitamin B-12.

For iron, the vegan can consume whole grains (especially ready-to-eat breakfast cereals), dried fruits and nuts, and legumes. The iron in these foods is not absorbed as well as iron in animal foods. A good source of vitamin C helps with the absorption of iron so it is recommended that vitamin C be consumed with every meal that contains iron-rich plant foods. Cooking in iron pots and skillets can also add iron to the diet (see Chapter 9).

The vegan can find zinc in whole grains (especially ready-to-eat breakfast cereals), nuts, and legumes, but phytic acid and other substances in these foods limit zinc absorption. Breads are a good source of zinc because the leavening process (rising of the bread dough) reduces the influence of phytic acid. Iodized salt is a reliable source of iodide. It should be used instead of plain salt, both of which are found in U.S. supermarkets.

Of all nutrients, calcium is the most difficult to consume in sufficient quantities for vegans. Fortified foods including fortified soy milk, fortified orange juice, calcium-rich tofu (check the label), as well as certain ready-to-eat breakfast cereals and snacks are the vegan's best option for obtaining calcium. Green leafy vegetables and nuts also contain calcium, but the mineral is either not well absorbed or not very plentiful from these sources. Calcium supplements are another option (see Chapter 9). Special diet planning is always required, because even a multivitamin and mineral supplement will not supply enough calcium to meet the needs of the body.

Consuming adequate quantities of omega-3 fatty acids is yet another nutritional concern for vegetarians, especially vegans. Fish and fish oils, abundant sources of these

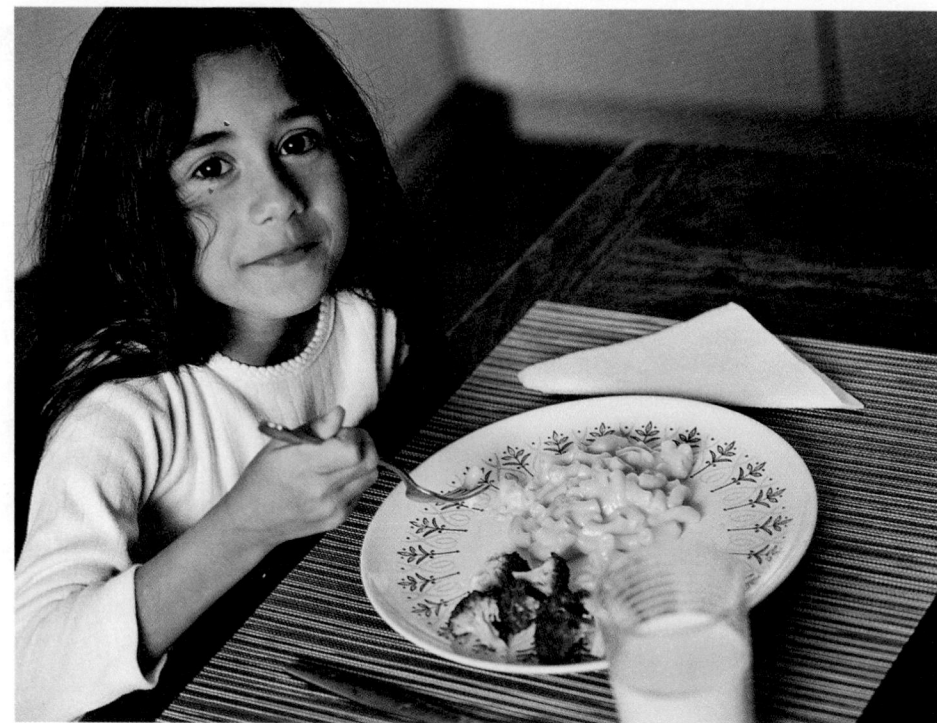

▲ Children can safely enjoy vegetarian and vegan diets as long as certain adjustments are made to meet their age-specific nutritional needs.

heart-healthy fats, are omitted from many types of vegetarian diets. Alternative plant sources of omega-3 fatty acids include canola oil, soybean oil, seaweed, microalgae, flax seeds, and walnuts.

Special Concerns for Infants and Children

Infants and children, notoriously picky eaters in the first place, are at highest risk for nutrient deficiencies as a result of improperly planned vegetarian and vegan diets. With the use of complementary proteins and good sources of problem nutrients just discussed, the calorie, protein, vitamin, and mineral needs of vegetarian and vegan infants and children can be met (see Further Reading 1). The most common nutritional concerns

for infants and children following vegetarian and vegan diets are deficiencies of iron, vitamin B-12, vitamin D, and calcium.

Vegetarian and vegan diets tend to be high in bulky, high-fiber, low-calorie foods that cause a feeling of fullness. While this is a welcome advantage for adults, children have small stomach volume and relatively high nutrient needs compared to their size, and therefore may feel full before their calorie needs are met. For this reason, the fiber content of a child's diet may need to be decreased by replacing high-fiber sources with some refined grain products, fruit juices, and peeled fruit. Other concentrated sources of calories for vegetarian and vegan children include fortified soy milk, nuts, dried fruits, avocados, and cookies made with vegetable oils or tub margarine.

Case Study Planning a Vegetarian Diet

Jordan is a freshman in college. He lives in a campus residence hall and teaches martial arts in the afternoon. He eats two or three meals a day at the residence hall cafeteria and snacks between meals. Jordan and his roommate both decided to become vegetarians because they recently read a magazine article describing the health benefits of a vegetarian diet. Yesterday Jordan's vegetarian diet consisted of a Danish pastry for breakfast and a tomato-rice dish (no meat) with pretzels and a diet soft drink for lunch. In the afternoon, after his martial arts class, he had a milk shake and two cookies. At dinnertime he had a vegetarian sub sandwich consisting of lettuce, sprouts, tomatoes, cucumbers, and cheese, with two glasses of fruit punch. In the evening, he had a bowl of popcorn.

Answer the following questions, and check your response in Appendix A.

1. What type of health benefits can Jordan expect from following a well-planned vegetarian diet?
2. What is missing from Jordan's current diet plan in terms of foods that should be emphasized in a vegetarian diet?
3. Which nutrients are missing in this current diet plan?
4. Are there any food components in the current diet plan that should be minimized or avoided?
5. How could he improve his new diet at each meal and snack to meet his nutritional needs and avoid undesirable food components?

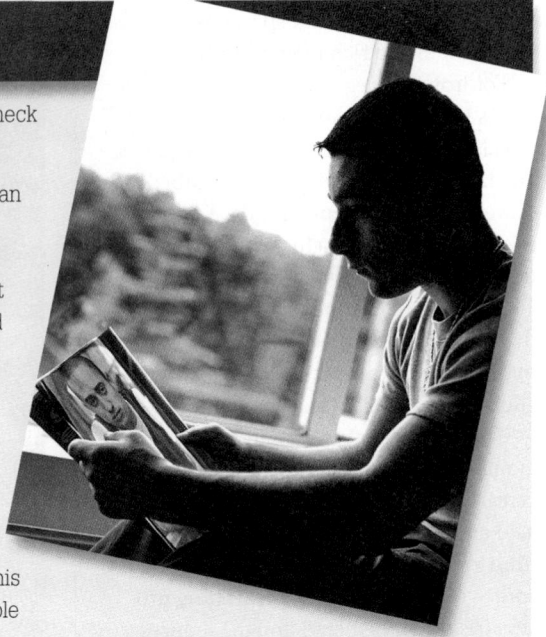

▲ Has Jordan planned a healthy and nutritious vegetarian diet?

Summary (Numbers refer to numbered sections in the chapter.)

6.1 Amino acids, the building blocks of proteins, contain a very usable form of nitrogen for humans. Of the 20 common types of amino acids found in food, nine must be consumed in food (essential) and the rest can be synthesized by the body (nonessential).

6.2 Individual amino acids are bonded together to form proteins. The sequential order of amino acids determines the protein's ultimate shape and function. This order is directed by DNA in the cell nucleus. Diseases such as sickle cell anemia can occur if the amino acids are incorrect on a polypeptide chain. When the three-dimensional shape of a protein is unfolded—denatured—by treatment with heat, acid or alkaline solutions, or other processes, the protein also loses its biological activity.

6.3 Almost all animal products are nutrient-dense sources of protein. The high quality of these proteins means that they can be easily converted into body proteins. Rich plant sources of protein, such as beans, are also available.

High-quality (complete) protein foods contain ample amounts of all nine essential amino acids. Furthermore, foods derived from animal sources provide high biological value protein. Lower-quality (incomplete) protein foods lack sufficient amounts of one or more essential amino acids. This is typical of plant foods, especially cereal grains. Different types of plant foods eaten together often complement each other's amino-acid deficits, thereby providing high-quality protein in the diet.

6.4 Protein digestion begins in the stomach, dividing the proteins into breakdown products containing shorter polypeptide chains of amino acids. In the small intestine, these polypeptide chains eventually separate into amino acids in the absorptive cells. The free amino acids then travel via the portal vein that connects to the liver. Some then enter the bloodstream.

6.5 Important body components—such as muscles, connective tissue, transport proteins in the bloodstream, visual pigments, enzymes, some hormones, and immune cells—are made of proteins. These proteins are in a state of constant turnover. The carbon chains of proteins may be used to produce glucose (or fat) when necessary.

6.6 The protein RDA for adults is 0.8 grams per kilogram of healthy body weight. For a typical 70-kilogram (154-pound) person, this corresponds to 56 grams of protein daily; for a 57-kilogram (125-pound) person, this corresponds to 46 grams per day. The North American diet generally supplies plenty of protein. Men typically consume about 100 grams of protein daily, and women consume closer to 65 grams. These usual protein intakes are also of sufficient quality to support body functions. This is even true for well-balanced vegetarian diets.

6.7 People need to balance protein intake with such losses to maintain a state of protein equilibrium, also called *protein balance.*

When a body is growing or recovering from an illness or injury, it needs a positive protein balance to supply the raw materials required to build new tissues. To achieve this, a person must eat more protein daily than he or she loses. Consuming less protein than needed leads to negative protein balance, such as when acute illness reduces the desire to eat and so one loses more protein than consumed.

6.8 Undernutrition can lead to protein-calorie malnutrition in the form of kwashiorkor or marasmus. Kwashiorkor results primarily from an inadequate calorie and protein intake in comparison with body needs, which often increase with concurrent disease and infection. Kwashiorkor often occurs when a child is weaned from human milk and fed mostly starchy gruels. Marasmus results from extreme starvation—a negligible intake of both protein and calories. Marasmus commonly occurs during famine, especially in infants.

N&YH Consumption of vegetarian and other plant-based diets provides many health benefits, including lower risks of chronic diseases including cardiovascular disease, diabetes, and certain cancers. The benefits associated with the plant-based diets appear to stem from the lower content of saturated fat and cholesterol and the higher amount of fiber, vitamins, minerals, and phytochemicals.

Check Your Knowledge (Answers to the following questions are below.)

1. The "instructions" for making proteins are located in the
   a. cell membrane.
   b. DNA and RNA genetic material.
   c. stomach.
   d. small intestine.

2. A nutrient that could easily be deficient in the diet of a vegan would be
   a. vitamin C.
   b. folic acid.
   c. calcium.
   d. All of the above.

3. If an essential amino acid is unavailable for protein synthesis, the
   a. cell will make the amino acid.
   b. synthesis of the protein will stop.
   c. cell will continue to attach amino acids to the protein.
   d. partially completed protein will be stored for later completion.

4. An example of protein complementation used in vegetarian diet planning would be the combination of
   a. cereal and milk.
   b. bacon and eggs.
   c. rice and beans.
   d. macaroni and cheese.

5. An individual who eats only plant food is referred to as a
   a. planetarium.
   b. vegan.
   c. lactovegetarian.
   d. ovovegetarian.

6. Which of the following groups accounts for the differences among amino acids?
   a. amine group
   b. side chain
   c. acid group
   d. keto group

7. Absorption of amino acids takes place in the
   a. stomach.
   b. liver.
   c. small intestine.
   d. large intestine.

8. Jack is not an athlete and weighs 176 pounds (80 kilograms). His RDA for protein would be _____ grams.
   a. 32
   b. 40
   c. 64
   d. 80

9. Which of the following is true about protein intake of people in the United States?
   a. Most do not consume enough protein.
   b. Most consume approximately the amount needed to balance losses.
   c. Athletes generally do not get enough protein without supplementation.
   d. Most consume more than is needed.

10. The basic building block of a protein is called a(n)
    a. fatty acid.
    b. monosaccharide.
    c. amino acid.
    d. gene.

Answers Key: 1. b (LO 6.2), 2. c (LO 6.3), 3. b (LO 6.2), 4. c (LO 6.9), 5. b (LO 6.9), 6. b (LO 6.1), 7. c (LO 6.4), 8. c (LO 6.6), 9. d (LO 6.7), 10. c (LO 6.1)

Study Questions (Numbers refer to Learning Outcomes)

1. Discuss the relative importance of essential and nonessential amino acids in the diet. Why is it important for essential amino acids lost from the body to be replaced in the diet? **(LO 6.1)**

2. Describe the concept of complementary proteins. **(LO 6.3)**

3. What is a limiting amino acid? Explain why this concept is a concern in a vegetarian diet. How can a vegetarian compensate for limiting amino acids in specific foods? **(LO 6.9)**

4. Briefly describe the organization of proteins. How can this organization be altered or damaged? What might be a result of damaged protein organization? **(LO 6.2)**

5. Describe four functions of proteins. Provide an example of how the structure of a protein relates to its function. **(LO 6.5)**

6. How are DNA and protein synthesis related? **(LO 6.2)**

7. What would be one health benefit of reducing high-protein intake(s) to RDA amounts for some people? **(LO 6.6)**

8. What characteristics of vegetable proteins could improve the North American diet? What foods would you include to provide a diet that has ample protein from both plant and animal sources but is moderate in fat? **(LO 6.9)**

9. Outline the major differences between kwashiorkor and marasmus. **(LO 6.8)**

10. What are the possible long-term effects of an inadequate intake of dietary protein among children between the ages of 6 months and 4 years? **(LO 6.8)**

What Would You Choose Recommendations

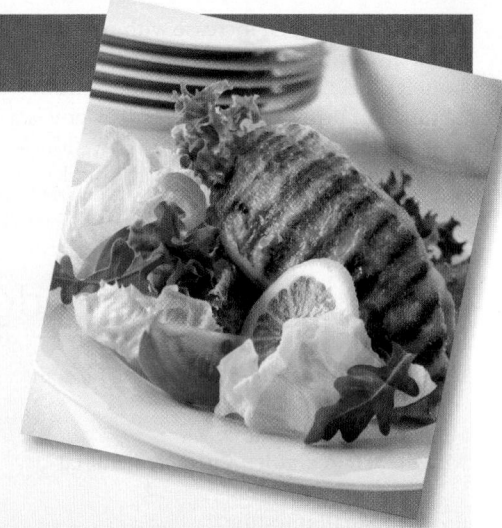

It is not a good idea to take individual amino-acid supplements. Your digestive tract is made to handle whole proteins—hydrochloric acid and enzymes break polypeptides into amino acids that can be absorbed by the cells of the small intestine. Taking large doses of one amino acid can impair the absorption and/or metabolism of other amino acids.

Whey protein, a by-product of cheese production from cow's milk, is considered to be a high-quality protein because it is easily digested and contains all of the essential amino acids. It is a source of the branched-chain amino acids, valine, leucine, and isoleucine. BCAAs can be used for fuel by exercising muscles and are particularly important for synthesizing muscle tissue. The rationale is that whey protein supports muscle recovery and anabolism after exercise.

Consuming adequate protein is important for muscle repair and synthesis, but consuming excessive protein from any source provides no advantage. Excess protein will be metabolized as fuel or stored as fat, not muscle. In fact, some excess subcutaneous fat is probably the reason you have not seen your toned muscles yet. Cutting back on calories or including more endurance exercise in your routine can help to reduce body weight and body fat as you tone your muscles. Animal protein, in particular, is often a source of excess total fat, saturated fat, and cholesterol. Not only will this hinder efforts at weight loss, but it is detrimental to heart health.

Americans typically consume two to three times as much protein as they actually need. The average American intake of 100 grams per day for men or 65 grams per day for women easily meets even the highest protein recommendations for resistance exercise (1.7 grams of protein per kilogram). Also, omnivorous diets and even appropriately planned vegan diets can supply ample amino acids to support muscle recovery and synthesis. Protein and amino

▲ This 4-ounce grilled chicken breast is an excellent choice, providing 38 grams of high-quality yet inexpensive lean protein.

acid supplements are expensive and may be detrimental to health. It is safer and more economical to focus on a diet that provides 10% to 35% of calories from a variety of lean sources of protein.

Further Readings

1. ADA Reports: Position of the American Dietetic Association and Dietitians of Canada: Vegetarian diets. *Journal of the American Dietetic Association* 109:1266, 2009.

   It is the position of the American Dietetic Association and Dietitians of Canada that appropriately planned vegetarian diets are healthful, nutritionally adequate, and provide health benefits in the prevention and treatment of certain diseases. Vegetarian diets are appropriate for all stages of the life cycle.

2. Barnard ND and others: A low-fat vegan diet improves glycemic control and cardiovascular risk factors in a randomized clinical trial in individuals with type 2 diabetes. *Diabetes Care* 29:1777, 2006.

   Improvements in glycemic (decreased hemoglobin A1C) and lipid (decreased LDL cholesterol) control were greater in type 2 diabetic patients that followed a low-fat vegan diet compared to a diet based on American Diabetes Association guidelines. In the vegan group, 43% of the subjects reduced their diabetes medications compared to 26% of the subjects on the ADA diet.

3. Chao A and others: Meat consumption and colorectal cancer. *Journal of the American Medical Association* 293:172, 2005.

   Diets rich in red meat, especially processed meat, increase the risk of colon cancer. Protein from poultry and fish, in contrast, does not pose the same risk.

4. Fessler TA: Malnutrition: A serious concern for hospitalized patients. *Today's Dietitian* 10(7): 44, 2008.

   Malnutrition continues to be a significant problem in hospitals worldwide, affecting patients of all ages from infants to geriatric patients. Malnutrition can be caused by the illnesses or injuries for which the patients are admitted to the hospital and by the hospitalization itself. This article outlines the need for prompt identification, treatment, and monitoring of malnourished patients among healthcare professionals.

5. Gardner CD and others: The effect of a plant-based diet on plasma lipids in hypercholesterolemic adults. *Annals of Internal Medicine* 142:725, 2005.

   Adding plant proteins to a diet already low in saturated fat and cholesterol provides additional benefits regarding lowering blood cholesterol. The authors emphasize the importance of including fruits, vegetables, legumes, and whole grains in a diet.

6. Key TJ and others: Health effects of vegetarian and vegan diets. *Proceedings of the Nutrition Society* 65:35, 2006.

   This study reviewed recent findings from large studies and summarizes the latest understanding of the health effects of vegetarian and vegan diets. Results indicated that vegetarians have a lower BMI and lower obesity rates than comparable nonvegetarians; total plasma cholesterol is lower in vegetarians that nonvegetarians; between vegetarians and nonvegetarians there is no significant differences in blood pressure; studies of vegetarians indicate a moderate reduction in mortality from ischemic heart disease; and studies showed no differences between vegetarians and nonvegetarians for colorectal cancer, breast cancer, prostate cancer, or total mortality.

7. Lejeune MP and others: Additional protein intake limits weight regain after weight loss in humans. *British Journal of Nutrition* 93:281, 2005.

   Adding 30 grams of protein per day to their usual diets helped people in this study limit weight regain after weight loss. The diet ended up 18% of calorie intake as protein, compared to 15% in the control group. This protein intake in the experimental group would not be considered excessive given an upper limit of 35% of calorie intake set by the Food and Nutrition Board.

8. Mangels R: Weight control the vegan way. *Vegetarian Journal* XXV(1), 2006.

   This article provides suggestions for vegans, or people interested in following a vegan diet, who want to lose weight. Two eating plans are included that were developed for people who are moderately active, spending 30 to 60 minutes daily in moderate physical activity. The first eating plan has approximately 1500 calories and is designed for women who want to lose 1 to 2 pounds per week. The second has about 1900 calories and is designed for men who want to lose 1 to 2 pounds per week. Protein foods include kidney beans, chickpeas, and other beans; tofu; lite or plain soymilk; nuts and nut butters; seitan (say-than, wheat meat); and meat analogs. Recipes are also included.

9. Newby PK: Risk of overweight and obesity among semivegetarian, lactovegetarian, and vegan women. *American Journal of Clinical Nutrition* 81:1267, 2005.

   Semivegetarian women in this study were less likely to be overweight and obese compared to omnivorous women. Consuming more plant foods and less animal products may help individuals control their weight.

10. Sacks FM and others: Soy protein, isoflavones, and cardiovascular health. An American Heart Association Science Advisory for Professionals From the Nutrition Committee. *Circulation* 113:1034, 2006.

    This scientific advisory evaluates recent work published on soy protein and its component isoflavones and their potential role in improving risk factors for cardiovascular disease. In the majority of studies, soy protein with isoflavones, as compared with milk or other proteins, decreased LDL cholesterol concentrations; the average effect was ~ 3% and no significant effects on HDL cholesterol, triglycerides, lipoprotein(a), or blood pressure were evident. The authors conclude that soy products should be beneficial to cardiovascular and overall health because of their high content of polyunsaturated fats, fiber, vitamins, and minerals and low content of saturated fat.

11. Taylor SL: Estimating prevalence of soy protein allergy. *The Soy Connection* 14(2):1, 2006.

    This article discusses the issue of soy protein allergy. Although soy protein has been designated one of the major allergens by the U.S. Food and Drug Administration, rigorous prevalence data for this allergy are not available, and indirect evidence suggests it occurs less frequently than other common allergens including shellfish, peanuts, tree nuts, and fish.

12. Trock BJ and others: Meta-analysis of soy intake and breast cancer risk. *Journal of the National Cancer Institute* 98(7):459, 2006.

    This study analyzed data from 18 previously published studies and concludes that consumption of soy foods among healthy women was associated with a significant reduction (14%) in breast cancer risk.

13. Who's the veggie-friendliest of them all? *Vegetarian Journal* XXVII, p. 14, 2008.

    The Vegetarian Resource Group evaluated the menus of the 400 largest restaurant chains in the United States. This article highlights the establishments that appeared to make the best effort at serving vegetarians of diverse needs. You can find more than 2000 veggie-friendly restaurants at their website *www.vrg.org*.

14. Williams CD and other: Associations of red meat, fat, and protein intake with distal colorectal cancer risk. *Nutrition and Cancer* 62(6):701, 2010.

    Studies suggest that red and processed meat consumption increase the risk of colon cancer. The risk of distal colorectal cancer (CRC) associated with red and processed meat, fat, and protein intakes was determined in whites and African-Americans. Dietary intake was assessed in 945 cases of distal CRC and in 959 controls in the previous 12 months. The results did not support the hypothesis that fat, protein, and red meat increase the risk of distal CRC. There was no association between total, saturated, or monounsaturated fat and distal CRC risk, and the percentages of energy from protein and red meat consumption were associated with a risk reduction (rather than increase).

15. Xiao CW: Health effects of soy protein and isoflavones in humans. *Journal of Nutrition* 138:1244S, 2008.

    The results of epidemiological and clinical studies have suggested that soy consumption may be associated with a lower incidence of certain chronic diseases and a reduction in the risk factors for cardiovascular disease. These results led to an FDA-approved food-labeling health claim for soy proteins in the prevention of coronary heart disease. This article reviews the evidence for health claims on the effects of soy protein and isoflavones in humans and concludes that the existing data are inconsistent or inadequate to support most of the suggested health benefits of consuming soy protein or ISF.

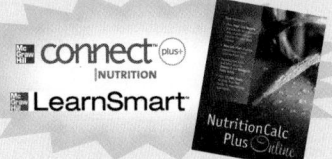

To get the most out of your study of nutrition, go to McGraw-Hill's online resources: Connect www.mcgrawhillconnect.com, **where you will find NutritionCalc Plus, LearnSmart, and many other dynamic tools.**

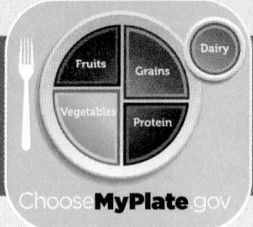

RATE YOUR PLATE

ChooseMyPlate.gov

I. Protein and the Vegetarian

Alana is excited about all the health benefits that might accompany a vegetarian diet. However, she is concerned that she will not consume enough protein to meet her needs. She is also concerned about possible vitamin and mineral deficiencies. Use NutritionCalc Plus or a food composition table to calculate her protein intake and see if her concerns are valid.

	Protein (g)
Breakfast Calcium fortified orange juice, 1 cup Soy milk, 1 cup Fortified bran flakes, 1 cup Banana, medium	
Snack Calcium-enriched granola bar	
Lunch GardenBurger, 4 oz Whole-wheat bun Mustard, 1 tbsp Soy cheese, 1 oz Apple, medium Green leaf lettuce, 1 ½ cups Peanuts, 1 oz Sunflower seeds, 1/4 cup Tomato slices, 2 Mushrooms, 3 Vinaigrette salad dressing, 2 tbsp Iced tea	
Dinner Kidney beans, ½ cup Brown rice, 3/4 cup Fortified margarine, 2 tbsp Mixed vegetables, 1/4 cup Hot tea	
Dessert Strawberries, ½ cup Angel food cake, 1 small slice Soy milk, ½ cup	
	TOTAL PROTEIN (grams) _____

Alana's diet contained 2150 kcal, with _____ grams (you fill in) of protein (Is this plenty for her?), 360 grams of carbohydrate, 57 grams of total dietary fat (only 9 grams of which came from saturated fat), and 50 grams of fiber. Her vitamin and mineral intake with respect to those of concern to vegetarians—vitamin B-12, vitamin D, calcium, iron, and zinc—met her needs.

II. Meeting Protein Needs When Dieting to Lose Weight

Your father has been steadily gaining weight for the last 30 years and now has developed hypertension and type 2 diabetes as a result. His physician recommends that he lose some weight by following an 1800 kcal diet. You know that it will be important for your father to meet protein needs as he tries to lose weight. Design a 1-day diet for him that contains about 20% of calorie intake as protein. Table 6-2 will provide some help. Will this diet meet his protein RDA? Does the diet look like a plan you could also follow?

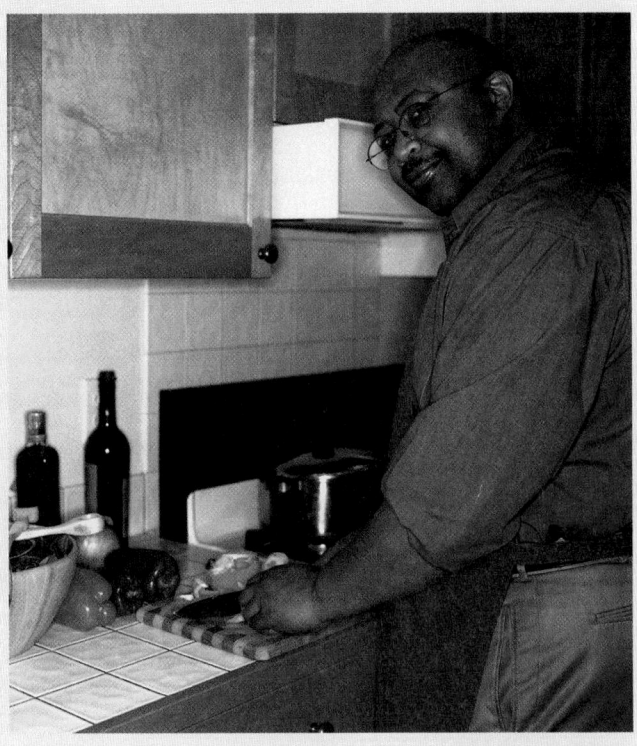

Chapter 7 Energy Balance and Weight Control

Student Learning Outcomes

Chapter 7 is designed to allow you to:

7.1 Describe energy balance and the uses of energy by the body.

7.2 Compare methods to determine energy use by the body.

7.3 Discuss methods for assessing body composition and determining whether body weight and composition are healthy.

7.4 Outline the risks to health posed by overweight and obesity.

7.5 Explain factors associated with the development of obesity.

7.6 List and discuss characteristics of a sound weight-loss program

7.7 Describe why reduced calorie intake is the main key to weight loss and maintenance.

7.8 Discuss why physical activity is a key to weight loss and especially important for later weight maintenance.

7.9 Describe why and how behavior modification fits into a weight-less program.

7.10 Outline the benefits and hazards of various weight-loss methods for severe obesity.

7.11 Discuss the causes and treatment of underweight.

7.12 Evaluate popular weight-reduction diets and determine which are unsafe, doomed to fail, or both.

What Would You Choose?

There are so many choices when it comes to controlling calorie intake. Is it possible to have dessert and still manage your weight? Consider the following frozen treats: regular ice cream, light ice cream, and frozen yogurt. Which of these desserts would you choose to cut back on calories? What information from the Nutrition Facts label is most helpful when it comes to weight management?

a Regular ice cream

b Light ice cream

c Frozen yogurt

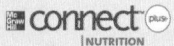 **connect** NUTRITION

Think about your choice as you read Chapter 7, then see our recommendations at the end of the chapter. To learn more about controlling calorie intake, check out the Connect site: www.mcgrawhillconnect.com

Part Two
Energy Nutrients and Energy Balance

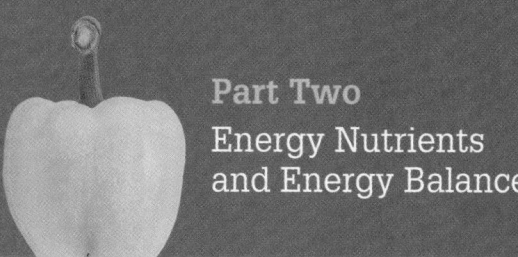

In the last 25 years (the years since most college students were born), there has been a dramatic increase in the percentage of individuals who are overweight or obese. The ranks of the obese are growing in North America and worldwide. Recall from Chapter 1 that an estimated 1 billion people in the world are overweight. This problem is increasing not only in the United States but also globally among affluent peoples and in developing countries where Westernized diets (high-fat, high-calorie) are increasing in popularity. Excess weight increases the likelihood of many health problems, such as cardiovascular disease, cancer, hypertension, strokes, certain bone and joint disorders, and type 2 diabetes, especially if a person performs minimal physical activity.

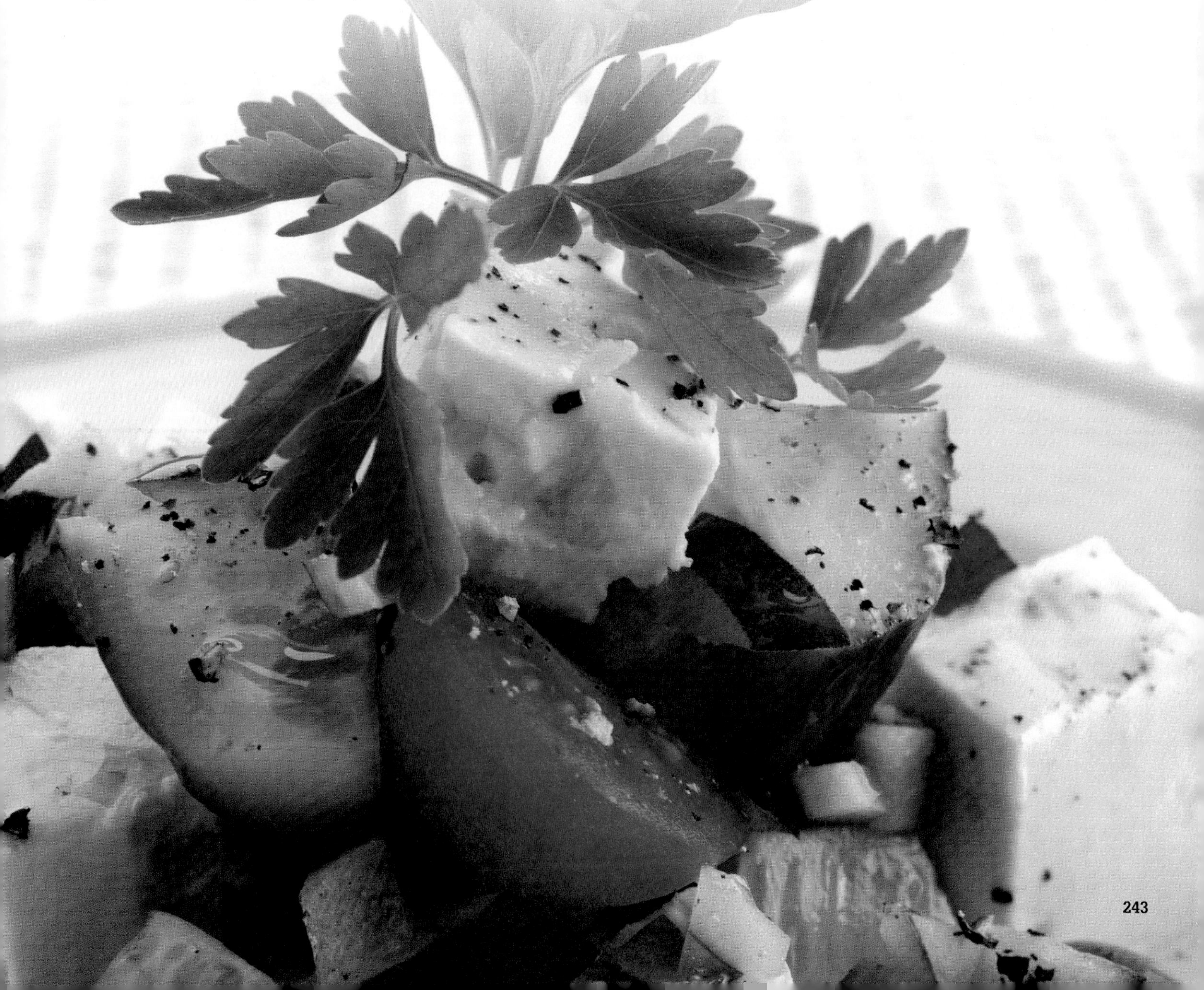

Currently, most weight-reduction efforts fizzle before bodies fall into a healthy weight range. As suggested in this chapter's comic, typical popular ("fad") diets are generally monotonous, ineffective, and confusing. They may even endanger some populations, such as children, teenagers, pregnant women, and people with various health disorders. A more logical approach to weight loss is straightforward: (1) eat less; (2) increase physical activity; and (3) change problematic eating behaviors.

A national commitment has begun from a variety of groups, including government agencies, the food industry, health professionals, and communities, to address the growing weight problem in North America. It has become obvious that, without this national effort to promote weight maintenance and effective new approaches to making our social environment more favorable to maintaining healthy weight, the current trends will not be reversed (Fig. 7-1) (see Futher Readings 3 and 9). Chapter 7 discusses these recommendations to help you understand obesity's causes, consequences, and potential treatments.

Refresh Your Memory

As you begin your study of weight control in Chapter 7, you may want to review:

- Biological and social influences of food intake in Chapter 1
- The concept of energy density and appropriate serving sizes for foods in Chapter 2
- The role of fiber in weight regulation in Chapter 4
- The fat content of various foods in Chapter 5
- The long-term risks of high-protein diets in Chapter 6

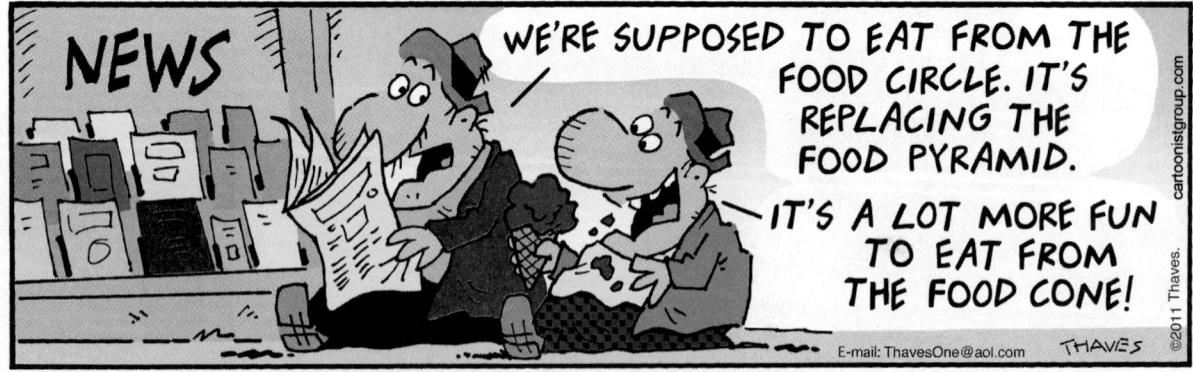

What components make up a successful diet plan? What constitutes a "fad" diet? Why are overweight and obesity growing problems worldwide? What might be the future consequences of this trend? Chapter 7 provides some answers.

"Frank and Ernest" used with the permission of the Thaves and the Cartoonist Group. All rights reserved. 2/28/1997

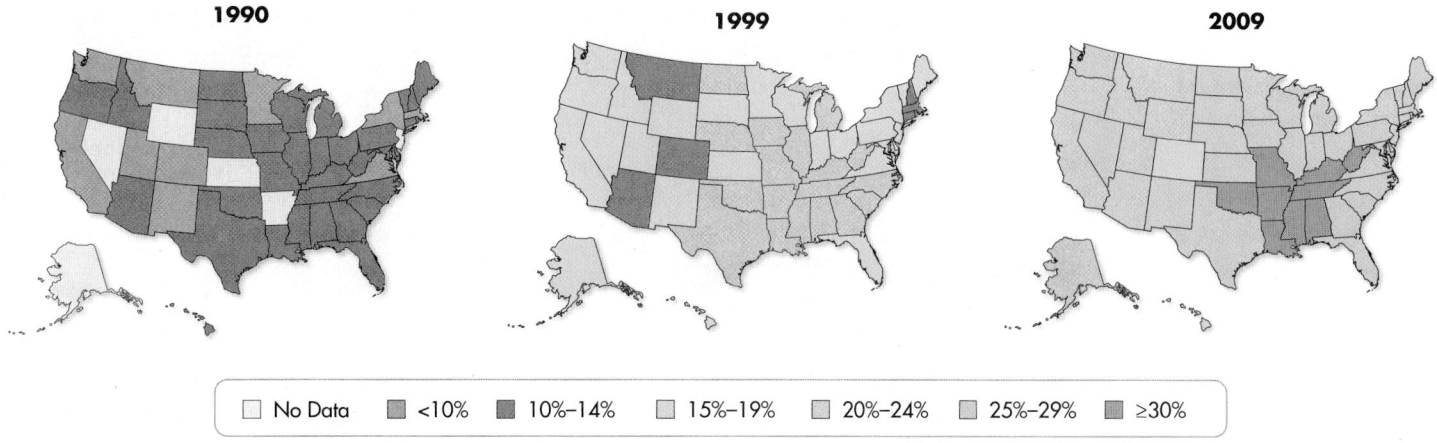

1990   **1999**   **2009**

☐ No Data   ■ <10%   ■ 10%–14%   ☐ 15%–19%   ■ 20%–24%   ■ 25%–29%   ■ ≥30%

FIGURE 7-1 ▶ Obesity trends among U.S. adults: 1990, 1999, 2009 (BMI ≥ 30, or about 30 pounds overweight for 5′4″ person).
Source: CDC Behavioral Risk Factor Surveillance System.

7.1 Energy Balance

We begin this chapter with some good news and some bad news. The good news is that if you stay at a healthy body weight, you increase your chances of living a long and healthy life. The bad news is that currently 68% of all North American adults are overweight, significantly more than in the 1980s. Of those, about 50% (34% of the total population) are obese. There is a good chance that any of us could become part of those statistics if we do not pay attention to the prevention of significant weight gain in adulthood. Gaining more than 10 pounds or 2 inches in waist circumference are signals that a reevaluation of diet and lifestyle is in order.

There is no quick cure for overweight, despite what the advertisements claim. Successful weight loss comes from hard work and commitment. A combination of decreased calorie intake, increased physical activity, and behavior modification is considered to be the most reliable treatment for the overweight condition. And without a doubt, the prevention of the overweight condition in the first place is the most successful approach.

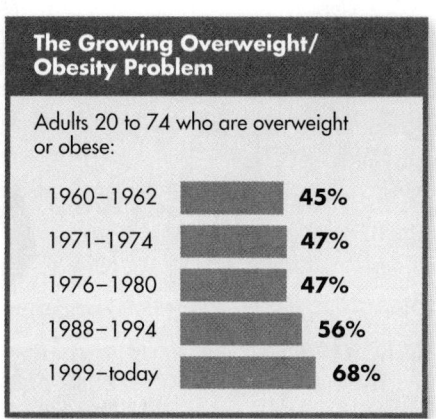

The Growing Overweight/ Obesity Problem

Adults 20 to 74 who are overweight or obese:

1960–1962	**45%**
1971–1974	**47%**
1976–1980	**47%**
1988–1994	**56%**
1999–today	**68%**

Positive and Negative Energy Balance

A healthy weight can result from paying more attention to the important concept of **energy balance.** Think of energy balance as an equation:

Energy Input (calories from food intake) = Energy Output (metabolism; digestion, absorption, and transport of nutrients; physical activity)

The balance of calories (measured in kcals) on the two sides of this equation can influence energy stores, especially the amount of triglyceride stored in adipose tissue (Fig. 7-2). Fat tissue contains about 3500 calories per pound. Therefore to lose 1 pound of fat per week, calorie intake must be decreased by about 500 calories per day. When energy input is greater than energy output, the result is **positive energy balance.** The excess calories consumed are stored, which results in weight gain. There are some situations in which positive energy balance is normal and healthy. During pregnancy, a surplus of calories supports the developing fetus. Infants and children require a positive energy balance for growth and development. In adults, however, even a small positive energy balance is usually in the form of fat storage rather than muscle and bone and, over time, can cause body weight to climb.

energy balance The state in which energy intake, in the form of food and beverages, matches the energy expended, primarily through basal metabolism and physical activity.

positive energy balance The state in which energy intake is greater than energy expended, generally resulting in weight gain.

FIGURE 7-2 ▶ A model for energy balance—input versus output. This figure depicts energy balance in practical terms.

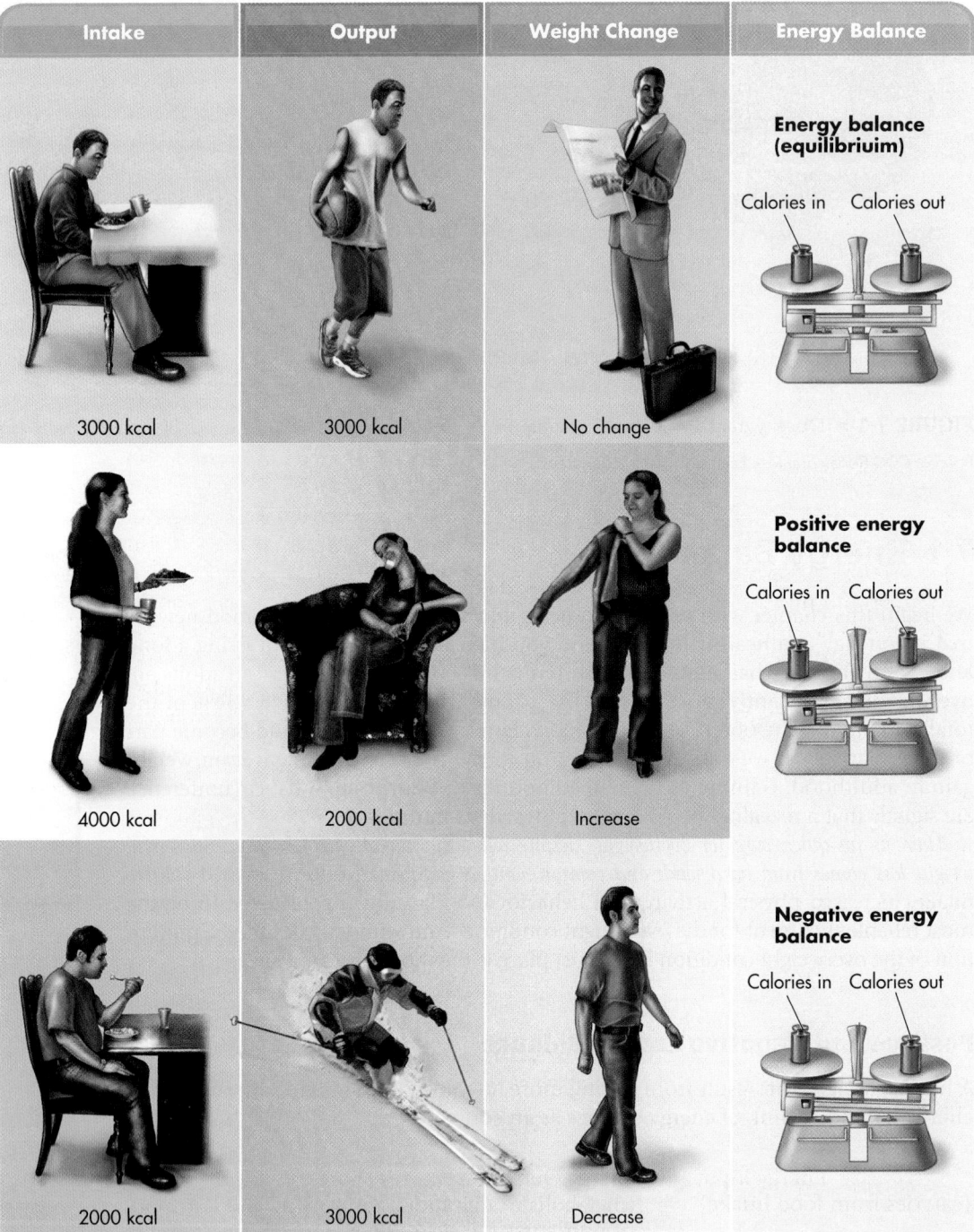

Intake	Output	Weight Change	Energy Balance
3000 kcal	3000 kcal	No change	**Energy balance (equilibriuim)** — Calories in Calories out
4000 kcal	2000 kcal	Increase	**Positive energy balance** — Calories in Calories out
2000 kcal	3000 kcal	Decrease	**Negative energy balance** — Calories in Calories out

CRITICAL THINKING

As she gets closer to age 30, a 28-year-old classmate of yours has been thinking about the process of aging. One of the things she fears most as she gets older is gaining weight. How would you explain energy balance to her?

negative energy balance The state in which energy intake is less than energy expended, resulting in weight loss.

On the other hand, if energy input is less than energy output, there is a calorie deficit and **negative energy balance** results. A negative energy balance is necessary for successful weight loss. It is important to realize that during negative energy balance, weight loss involves a reduction in both lean and adipose tissue, not just "fat."

The maintenance of energy balance substantially contributes to health and well-being in adults by minimizing the risk of developing many common health problems. Adulthood is often a time of subtle increases in weight gain, which eventually turns into obesity if left unchecked. The process of aging does not cause weight gain; rather the problem stems from a pattern of excess food intake coupled with limited physical activity and slower metabolism. Let's look in detail at the factors that affect the energy balance equation.

Energy Intake

Energy needs are met by food intake, represented by the number of calories eaten each day. Determining the appropriate amount and type of food to match our energy needs is a challenge for many of us. Our desire to consume food and the ability of our bodies to use it efficiently are survival mechanisms that have evolved with humans. However, because of current North American food supplies and accessibility, many of us are now too successful in obtaining food energy. The abundant food supply has essentially replaced the need to store body fat. Given the wide availability of food in vending machines, drive-up windows, social gatherings, and fast-food restaurants—combined with *supersized* portions—it is no wonder that the average adult is 8 pounds heavier than just 10 years ago. In response to this cultural trend of food being widely available, "defensive eating" (i.e., making careful and conscious food choices, especially in regard to portion size) on a continual basis is important for many of us.

The number of calories in a food is determined with an instrument called a **bomb calorimeter.** This calorie determination is described in Figure 7-3. The bomb calorimeter measures the amount of calories coming from carbohydrate, fat, protein, and alcohol. Recall that carbohydrates yield about 4 kcal per gram, proteins yield about 4 kcal per gram, fats yield about 9 kcal per gram, and alcohol yields 7 kcal per gram. These energy figures have been adjusted for (1) our ability to digest the food and (2) substances in food, such as fibrous plant parts that burn in the bomb calorimeter but do not provide calories to the human body. The figures are then rounded to whole numbers. However, today it is also possible and more common to determine the calorie content of a food by quantifying its carbohydrate, protein, and fat (and possibly alcohol) content. Then the kcal per gram factors listed previously are used to calculate the total kcals. (Recall that Chapter 1 showed how to do this calculation.)

Energy Output

So far, some factors concerning energy intake have been discussed. Now let's look at the other side of the equation—energy output.

The body uses energy for three general purposes: basal metabolism; physical activity; and digestion, absorption, and processing of ingested nutrients. A fourth minor form of energy output, known as thermogenesis, refers to energy expended during fidgeting or shivering in response to cold (Fig. 7-4).

bomb calorimeter An instrument used to determine the calorie content of a food.

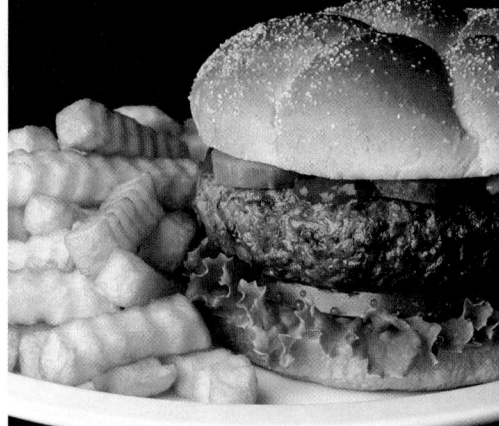

▲ The cultural trend of serving large quantities can easily lead to positive energy balance. Sharing your meal with another person is a good way to avoid overeating when served large portions.

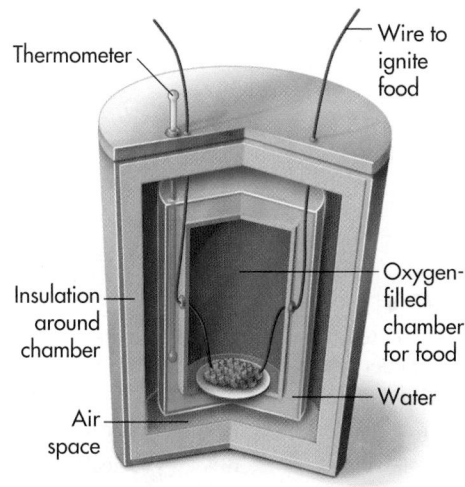

FIGURE 7-3 ▶ Bomb calorimeters measure calorie content by igniting and burning a dried portion of food. The burning food raises the temperature of the water surrounding the chamber holding the food. The increase in water temperature indicates the number of kilocalories in the food because 1 kilocalorie equals the amount of heat needed to raise the temperature of 1 kg of water by 1°C.

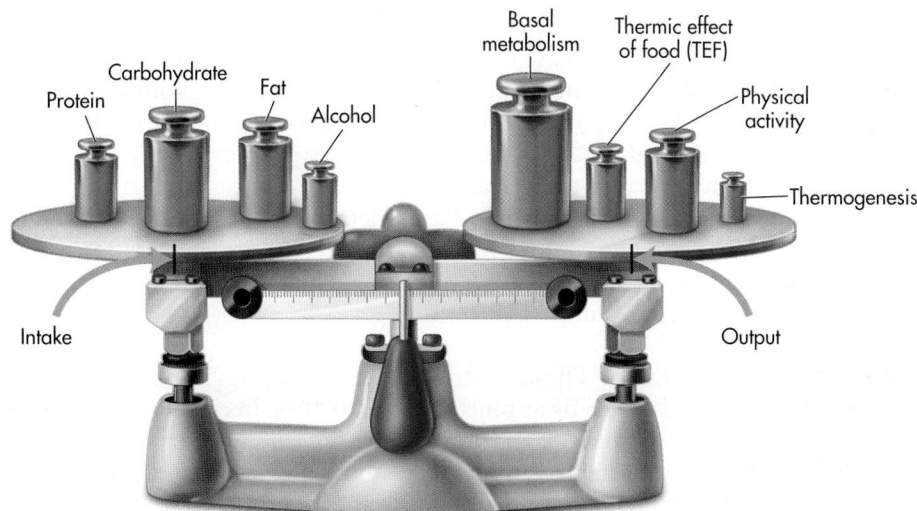

FIGURE 7-4 ▶ The components of energy intake and expenditure. This figure incorporates the major variables that influence energy balance. *Remember that alcohol is an additional source of energy for some of us.* The size of each component shows the relative contribution of that component to energy balance.

basal metabolism The minimal amount of calories the body uses to support itself in a fasting state when resting (e.g., 12 hours for both) and awake in a warm, quiet environment. It amounts to roughly 1 kcal per kilogram per hour for men and 0.9 kcal per kilogram per hour for women; these values are often referred to as *basal metabolic rate (BMR)*.

resting metabolism The amount of calories the body uses when the person has not eaten in 4 hours and is resting (e.g., 15 to 30 minutes) and awake in a warm, quiet environment. It is roughly 6% higher than basal metabolism due to the less strict criteria for the test; often referred to as *resting metabolic rate (RMR)*.

lean body mass Body weight minus fat storage weight equals lean body mass. This includes organs such as the brain, muscles, and liver, as well as bone and blood and other body fluids.

Basal Metabolism. **Basal metabolism** is expressed as basal metabolic rate (BMR) and represents the minimal amount of calories expended in a fasting state (for 12 hours or more) to keep a resting, awake body alive in a warm, quiet environment. For a sedentary person, basal metabolism accounts for about 60% to 70% of total energy use by the body. Some of the processes involved include the beating of the heart, respiration by the lungs, and the activity of other organs such as the liver, brain, and kidney. It does not include energy used for physical activity or digestion, absorption, and processing of recently consumed nutrients. If the person is not fasting or completely rested, the term **resting metabolism** is used and expressed as resting metabolic rate (RMR). An individual's RMR is typically 6% higher than his or her BMR.

To see how basal metabolism contributes to energy needs, consider a 130-pound woman. First, knowing that there are 2.2 pounds for every kilogram, convert her weight into metric units:

$$130 \text{ lbs} \div 2.2 \text{ lbs/kilograms} = 59 \text{ kilograms}$$

Then, using a rough estimate of basal metabolic rate of 0.9 kcal per kilogram per hour for an average female (1.0 kcal per kilogram per hour is used for an average male), calculate her basal metabolic rate:

$$59 \text{ kg} \times 0.9 \text{ kcal/kg} = 53 \text{ kcal per hour}$$

Finally, use this hourly basal metabolic rate to find her basal metabolic rate for an entire day:

$$53 \text{ kcal/hr} \times 24 \text{ hrs} = 1272 \text{ kcal}$$

These calculations give only an estimate of basal metabolism, as it can vary 25% to 30% among individuals. Factors that increase basal metabolism include:

- Greater **lean body mass**
- Larger body surface area per body volume
- Male gender (caused by greater lean body mass)
- Body temperature (fever or cold environmental conditions)
- Thyroid hormones
- Aspects of nervous system activity (release of norepinephrine)
- Pregnancy
- Caffeine and tobacco use (Using the practice of smoking to control body weight is not recommended as too many health risks are increased.)

Of those factors, the amount of lean body mass a person has is the most important one.

In contrast to factors that increase basal metabolism, a low calorie intake, such as that during an extreme diet regime, decreases basal metabolism by about 10% to 20% (about 150 to 300 kcal per day) as the body shifts into a conservation mode. This is a barrier to sustained weight loss during dieting that involves extremely low calorie diets. In addition, the effects of aging make weight maintenance a challenge. As lean body mass slowly and steadily decreases, basal metabolism declines 1% to 2% for each decade past the age of 30. However, because physical activity aids in maintenance of lean body mass, remaining active as one ages helps to preserve a high basal metabolism and, in turn, aids in weight control.

While a person is resting, the percentage of total energy use and corresponding energy use by various organs is approximately as follows:

Brain	19%	265 kcal/day
Skeletal muscle	18%	250 kcal/day
Liver	27%	380 kcal/day
Kidney	10%	140 kcal/day
Heart	7%	100 kcal/day
Other	19%	265 kcal/day

Energy for Physical Activity. Physical activity increases energy expenditure above and beyond basal energy needs by as much as 25% to 40%. In choosing to be active or inactive, we determine much of our total calorie expenditure for a day. Calorie expenditure from physical activity varies widely among people. For example, climbing stairs rather than riding the elevator, walking rather than driving to the store, and standing in a bus rather than sitting increase physical activity and, hence, energy use. The alarming incidence of and recent increase in obesity in North America are partially the result of our inactivity. Jobs demand less physical activity, and leisure time is often spent in front of a television or computer.

Thermic Effect of Food (TEF). In addition to basal metabolism and physical activity, the body uses energy to digest food, and absorb and further process the nutrients recently consumed. Energy used for these tasks is referred to as the **thermic effect of food (TEF).** TEF is similar to a sales tax—it is like being charged about 5% to 10% for the total amount of calories you eat to cover the cost of processing that food eaten. We may even recognize this increase in metabolism as a warming of the body during and right after a meal. Because of this "tax," you must eat between 105 and 110 kcal (5 to 10 kcal extra) for every 100 kcal needed for basal metabolism and physical activity. If your daily calorie intake was 3000 kcal, TEF would account for 150 to 300 kcal. As with other components of energy output, the total amount can vary somewhat among individuals.

Food composition influences TEF. For example, the TEF value for a protein-rich meal is 20% to 30% of the calories consumed and is higher than that of a carbohydrate-rich (5% to 10%) or fat-rich (0% to 3%) meal. This is because it takes more energy to metabolize amino acids into fat than to convert glucose into glycogen or transfer absorbed fat into adipose stores. In addition, large meals result in higher TEF values than the same amount of food eaten over many hours.

Thermogenesis. Thermogenesis represents the increase in nonvoluntary physical activity triggered by cold conditions or overeating. Some examples of nonvoluntary activities include shivering when cold, fidgeting, maintenance of muscle tone, and maintaining body posture when not lying down. Studies have shown that some people are able to resist weight gain from overfeeding by inducing thermogenesis, while others are not able to do so to a great extent.

The contribution of thermogenesis to overall calorie output is fairly small. The combination of basal metabolism and TEF accounts for 70% to 80% of energy used by a sedentary person. The remaining 20% to 30% is used mostly for physical activity, with a small amount used for thermogenesis.

Brown adipose tissue is a specialized form of adipose tissue that participates in thermogenesis. It is found in small amounts in infants. The brown appearance results from its rich blood flow. Brown adipose tissue contributes to thermogenesis by releasing some of the energy from energy-yielding nutrients into the environment as heat. In infants, brown adipose tissue contributes as much as 5% of body weight and is thought to be important for heat regulation. Hibernating animals also use brown adipose tissue to generate heat to withstand a long winter. Adults have very little brown adipose tissue, and its role in adulthood is unknown.

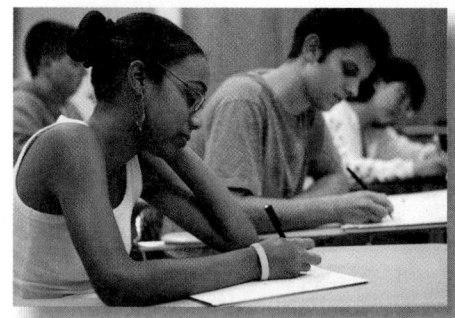

▲ Classwork leads to mental stress but puts little physical stress on the body. Hence, energy needs are only about 1.5 kcal per minute.

The TEF value for alcohol is 20%.

thermic effect of food (TEF) The increase in metabolism that occurs during the digestion, absorption, and metabolism of energy-yielding nutrients. This represents 5% to 10% of calories consumed.

thermogenesis This term encompasses the ability of humans to regulate body temperature within narrow limits (thermoregulation). Two visible examples of thermogenesis are fidgeting and shivering when cold.

brown adipose tissue A specialized form of adipose tissue that produces large amounts of heat by metabolizing energy-yielding nutrients without synthesizing much useful energy for the body. The unused energy is released as heat.

CONCEPT CHECK

Energy balance involves matching energy intake with energy output. Energy content of food is expressed in kcals and can be determined using a bomb calorimeter. This analysis yields the 4-9-4-7 estimates for the kcals in a gram of carbohydrate, fat, protein, and alcohol, respectively.

The body uses energy for four main purposes:

1. Basal metabolism (60% to 70% of total energy output) represents the minimal amount of calories needed to maintain the body at rest. Primary determinants of basal metabolic rate include quantity of lean body mass, amount of body surface, and thyroid hormone concentrations in the bloodstream.
2. Physical activity calorie expenditure (20% to 30% of total energy output) represents calorie use for total body cell metabolism above what is needed during rest.
3. Thermic effect of food (5% to 10% of total energy output) represents the calories needed to digest food and absorb and process nutrients recently consumed.
4. Thermogenesis (small, variable percentage of total energy output) includes nonvoluntary, heat-producing activities, such as fidgeting, as well as shivering when cold.

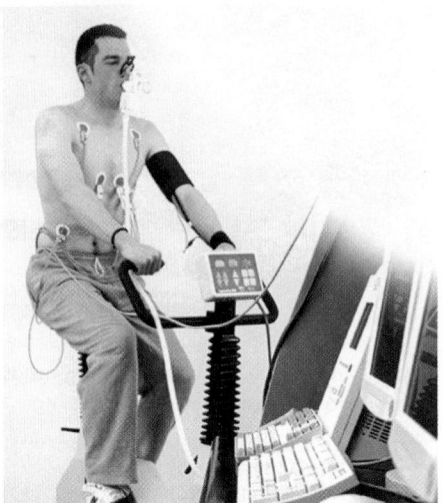

FIGURE 7-5 ▶ Indirect calorimetry measures oxygen intake and carbon dioxide output to determine energy expended during daily activities.

direct calorimetry A method of determining a body's energy use by measuring heat released from the body. An insulated chamber is usually used.

indirect calorimetry A method to measure energy use by the body by measuring oxygen uptake. Formulas are then used to convert this gas exchange value into energy use.

7.2 Determination of Energy Use by the Body

The amount of energy a body uses can be measured by both direct and indirect calorimetry or can be estimated based on height, weight, degree of physical activity, and age.

Direct and Indirect Calorimetry

Direct calorimetry measures the amount of body heat released by a person. The subject is put into an insulated chamber, often the size of a small bedroom, and body heat released raises the temperature of a layer of water surrounding the chamber. A kcal, as you recall, is related to the amount of heat required to raise the temperature of water. By measuring the water temperature in the direct calorimeter before and after the body releases heat, scientists can determine the energy expended.

Direct calorimetry works because almost all the energy used by the body eventually leaves as heat. However, few studies use direct calorimetry, mostly because of its expense and complexity.

The most commonly used method of **indirect calorimetry** measures the amount of oxygen a person consumes instead of measuring heat output (Fig. 7-5). A predictable relationship exists between the body's use of energy and oxygen. For example, when metabolizing a typical mixed diet of the energy-yielding nutrients, carbohydrate, fat, and protein, the human body uses 1 liter of oxygen to yield about 4.85 kcal of energy.

Instruments to measure oxygen consumption for indirect calorimetry are widely used. They can be mounted on carts and rolled up to a hospital bed or carried in backpacks while a person plays tennis or jogs. There are even newly developed handheld instruments (Body Gem). Tables showing energy costs of various forms of exercises rely on information gained from indirect calorimetry studies.

Estimates of Energy Needs

As covered in Chapter 2, the Food and Nutrition Board has published a number of formulas to estimate energy needs, called Estimated Energy Requirements (EERs). Those for adults are shown here (remember to do multiplication and division before addition and subtraction). (Formulas for pregnant women, lactating women, children, and teenagers, are listed in Chapters 14 and 15.) The calories used for basal metabolism are already factored into these formulas.

Estimated Energy Requirement Calculation for Men 19 Years and Older

$$EER = 662 - (9.53 \times AGE) + PA \times (15.91 \times WT + 539.6 \times HT)$$

Estimated Energy Requirement Calculation for Women 19 Years and Older

$$EER = 354 - (6.91 \times AGE) + PA \times (9.36 \times WT + 726 \times HT)$$

The variables in the formulas correspond to the following:

$$EER = \text{Estimated Energy Requirement}$$
$$AGE = \text{age in years}$$
$$PA = \text{Physical Activity Estimate (see following table)}$$
$$WT = \text{weight in kilograms (pounds} \div 2.2)$$
$$HT = \text{height in meters (inches} \div 39.4)$$

Physical Activity (PA) Estimates

Activity Level	PA (Men)	PA (Women)
Sedentary (e.g., no exercise)	1.00	1.00
Low activity (e.g., walks the equivalent of 2 miles per day at 3 to 4 mph)	1.11	1.12
Active (e.g., walks the equivalent of 7 miles per day at 3 to 4 mph)	1.25	1.27
Very active (e.g., walks the equivalent of 17 miles per day at 3 to 4 mph)	1.48	1.45

The following is a sample calculation for a man who is 25 years old, 5 feet, 9 inches (1.75 meters), 154 pounds (70 kilograms), and has an active lifestyle. His EER is:

$$EER = 662 - (9.53 \times 25) + 1.25 \times (15.91 \times 70 + 539.6 \times 1.75) = 2997 \text{ kcal}$$

The next equation is a sample calculation for a woman who is 25 years old, 5 feet, 4 inches (1.62 meters), 120 pounds (54.5 kilograms), and has an active lifestyle. Her EER is:

$$EER = 354 - (6.91 \times 25) + 1.27 \times (9.36 \times 54.5 + 726 \times 1.62) = 2323 \text{ kcal}$$

You have determined the man's EER to be about 3000 kcal and the woman's EER to be about 2300 kcal per day. Remember that this is only an estimate; many other factors, such as genetics and hormones, can affect actual energy needs.

A simple method of tracking your energy expenditure, and thus your energy needs, is to use the forms in Appendix E. Begin by taking an entire 24-hour period and listing all activities performed, including sleep. Record the number of minutes spent in each activity; the total should equal 1440 minutes (24 hours). Next record the energy cost for each activity in kcal per minute following the directions in Appendix E. Multiply the energy cost by the minutes. This gives the energy expended for each activity. Total all the kcal values. This gives your estimated energy expenditure for the day.

The www.ChooseMyPlate.gov website provides an interactive tool to estimate your calorie needs called Daily Food Plan. Figure 7-6 shows the range of activity levels and calorie recommendations for age and gender groups.

MyPlate Calorie Guidelines

Children	Sedentary →	Active
2–3 years	1000 →	1400

Females	Sedentary →	Active
4–8 years	1200 →	1800
9–13	1400 →	2200
14–18	1800 →	2400
19–30	1800 →	2400
31–50	1800 →	2200
51+	1600 →	2200

Males	Sedentary →	Active
4–8 years	1200 →	2000
9–13	1600 →	2600
14–18	2000 →	3200
19–30	2400 →	3000
31–50	2200 →	3000
51+	2000 →	2800

FIGURE 7-6 ▶ MyPlate Calorie Guidelines for age and gender groups.

CONCEPT CHECK

Energy use by the body can be measured as heat given off by direct calorimetry or as oxygen used by indirect calorimetry. A person's Estimated Energy Requirement can be calculated based on the following factors: gender, height, weight, age, and amount of physical activity.

7.3 Estimation of a Healthy Weight

Numerous methods are used to establish what body weight should be, typically called *healthy weight*. Healthy weight is currently the preferred term to use for weight recommendations. Older terms, such as *ideal weight* and *desirable weight*, are subjective and are no longer used in medical literature. Several tables exist, generally based on weight for height. These tables arise from studies of large population groups. When applied to a population, they provide good estimates of weight associated with health and longevity. However, they do not necessarily indicate the healthiest body weight

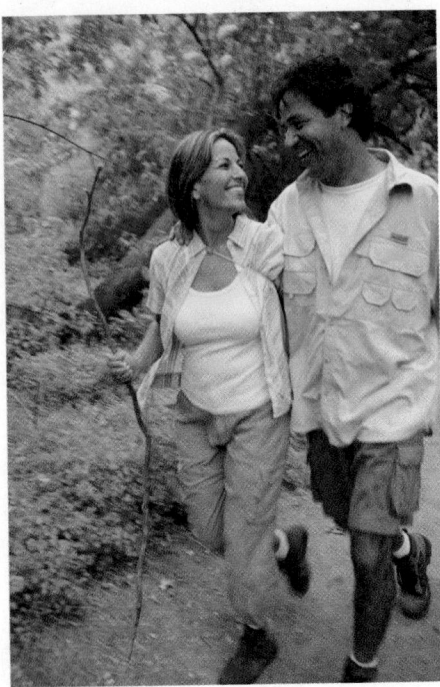

▲ Physical activity, such as walking, is an important component of our energy expenditure.

One BMI unit = 6 to 7 pounds

body mass index (BMI) Weight (in kilograms) divided by height (in meters) squared; a value of 25 and above indicates overweight and a value of 30 and above indicates obesity.

for each individual. For example, *athletes with large, lean body mass but low-fat content will have greater healthy weights than sedentary individuals.*

Overall, the individual, under a physician's guidance, should establish a "personal" healthy weight (or need for weight reduction) based on weight history, fat distribution patterns, family history of weight-related disease, and current health status. Indications that your weight is not healthy would include the following weight-related conditions:

- Hypertension
- Elevated LDL-cholesterol
- Family history of obesity, cardiovascular disease, or certain forms of cancer (e.g., uterus, colon)
- Pattern of fat distribution in the body
- Elevated blood glucose

This assessment points out how well the person is tolerating any existing excess weight. Thus, current height/weight standards are only a rough guide. On a more practical note, other questions can be pertinent: What is the least one has weighed as an adult for at least a year? What is the largest size clothing one would be happy with? What weight has one been able to maintain during previous diets without feeling constantly hungry? Furthermore, a healthy lifestyle may make a more important contribution to a person's health status than the number on the scale. Fit and overweight are not necessarily mutually exclusive (although not often seen together), and neither is thin synonymous with healthy if the person is not also physically active.

Body Mass Index (BMI)

For the past 50 years, weight-for-height tables issued by the Metropolitan Life Insurance Company have been the typical way healthy weight was established. These tables are organized by gender and frame size, predicting the weight range at a specific height that was associated with the greatest longevity. The latest table (issued in 1983) and methods for determining frame size can be found in Appendix G.

Currently, **body mass index (BMI)** is the preferred weight-for-height standard because it is the clinical measurement most closely related to body fat content (Fig. 7-7).

Body mass index is calculated as

$$\frac{\text{body weight (in kilograms)}}{\text{height}^2 \text{ (in meters)}}$$

An alternate method for calculating BMI is

$$\frac{\text{weight (pounds)} \times 703}{\text{height}^2 \text{ (inches)}}$$

Figure 7-8 lists the BMI for various heights and weights. A healthy weight for height is a BMI between 18.5 to 24.9. Health risks from excess weight may begin when the body mass index is 25 or more. What is your BMI? How much would your weight need to change to yield a BMI of 25? 30? These are general cutoff values for the presence of overweight and obesity, respectively. BMI offers another way to define obesity (Fig. 7-8).

| 30 to 39.9 | Obese | Increased health risk |
| 40 or greater | Severely obese | Major health risk (The number of North Americans falling into this category is increasing rapidly.) |

The concept of body mass index is convenient to use because the values apply to both men and women (i.e., gender neutral). However, any weight-for-height standard is a crude measure. Keep in mind, also, that a BMI of 25 to 29.9 is a marker of *overweight* (compared to a standard population) and not necessarily a marker of *overfat*. Many men (especially athletes) have a BMI greater than 25 because of extra muscle tissue. Also, very short adults (under 5 feet tall) may have high BMIs that may not reflect overweight or fatness. For this reason, BMI should be used only as a screening test for overweight or obesity. Even agreed upon weight standards for BMI are not for everyone. Adult BMIs should not be applied to children, still growing adolescents, frail older people, pregnant and lactating women, and highly muscular individuals. Pregnant women and children have unique BMI standards (see Chapters 14 and 15).

Still, overfat and overweight conditions generally appear together. The focus is on BMI in clinical settings mainly because this is easier to measure than total body fat.

Putting Healthy Weight into Perspective

Listening to the body for hunger cues, regularly eating a healthy diet, and remaining physically active (not to be overlooked) eventually helps one maintain an appropriate height/weight value. This concept will be further addressed in the upcoming discussion on treatment for obesity. Another school of thought is to let nature take its course with regard to body weight. Support for this proposal is that after weight is lost during dieting, people often regain their original weight plus more. The clearest idea regarding a healthy weight is that it is personal. Weight has to be considered in terms of health, not a mathematical calculation.

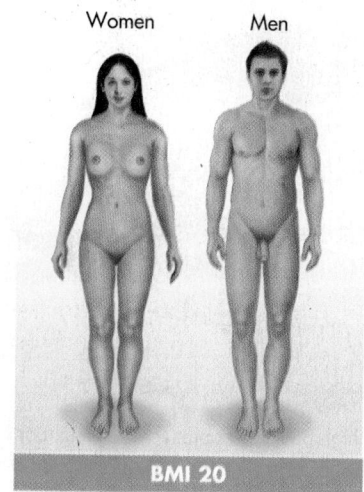

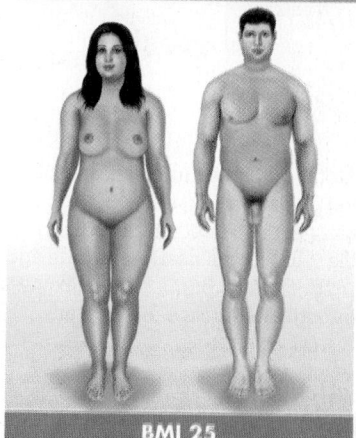

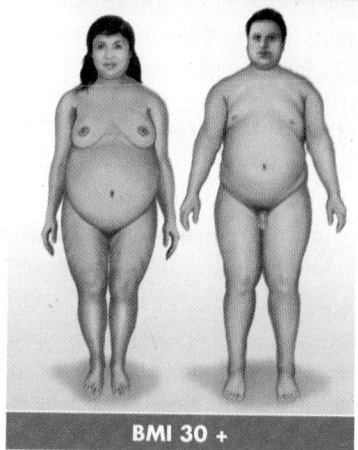

FIGURE 7-7 ▶ Estimates of body shapes at different BMI values.

Weight in pounds

Height	120	130	140	150	160	170	180	190	200	210	220	230	240	250
4'6"	29	31	34	36	39	41	43	46	48	51	53	56	58	60
4'8"	27	29	31	34	36	38	40	43	45	47	49	52	51	56
4'10"	25	27	29	31	34	36	38	40	42	44	46	48	50	52
5'0"	23	25	27	29	31	33	35	37	39	41	43	45	47	49
5'2"	22	24	26	27	29	31	33	35	37	38	40	42	44	46
5'4"	21	22	24	26	28	29	31	33	34	36	38	40	41	43
5'6"	19	21	23	24	26	27	29	31	32	34	36	37	39	40
5'8"	18	20	21	23	24	26	27	29	30	32	34	35	37	38
5'10"	17	19	20	22	23	24	26	27	29	30	32	33	35	36
6'0"	16	18	19	20	22	23	24	26	27	28	30	31	33	34
6'2"	15	17	18	19	21	22	23	24	26	27	28	30	31	32
6'4"	15	16	17	18	20	21	22	23	24	26	27	28	29	30
6'6"	14	15	16	17	19	20	21	22	23	24	25	27	28	29
6'8"	13	14	15	17	18	19	20	21	22	23	24	26	26	28

Height in feet and inches

☐ Healthy weight   ☐ Overweight   ☐ Obese

Developed by the National Center for Health Statistics in collaboration with the National Center for Chronic Disease Prevention and Health Promotion

FIGURE 7-8 ▶ Convenient height/weight table based on BMI. A healthy weight for height generally falls within a BMI range of 18.5 to 24.9 kilograms/meters².

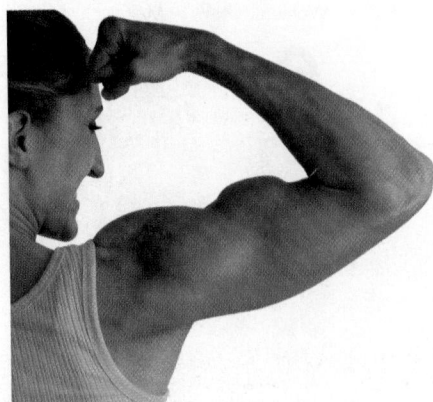

▲ A high BMI may not reflect overweight or fatness. Extra muscle tissue can result in a BMI greater than 25.

The total cost attributable to weight-related disease is about $147 billion annually in the United States. This is double what it was nearly a decade ago. Half of this cost is borne by the taxpayers through Medicare and Medicaid.

underwater weighing A method of estimating total body fat by weighing the individual on a standard scale and then weighing him or her again submerged in water. The difference between the two weights is used to estimate total body volume.

air displacement A method for estimating body composition that makes use of the volume of space taken up by a body inside a small chamber.

bioelectrical impedance The method to estimate total body fat that uses a low-energy electrical current. The more fat storage a person has, the more impedance (resistance) to electrical flow will be exhibited.

CONCEPT CHECK

Healthy body weight is generally determined in a clinical setting using a body mass index or another weight-for-height standard. The presence of existing weight-related diseases should be factored into the determination of healthy body weight. Total health history and lifestyle should be the major considerations when determining healthy weight.

7.4 Energy Imbalance

If calorie intake exceeds output over time, overweight (and often obesity) is a likely result. Often, health problems eventually follow (Table 7-1) (see Further Readings 1 and 12). As just discussed, BMI values can be used as a convenient clinical tool to estimate overweight (BMI ≥ 25), obesity (BMI ≥ 30), and severe obesity (BMI ≥ 40) in individuals greater than 20 years of age. Medical experts, however, recommend that an individual's diagnosis of obesity should not be based primarily on body weight but, rather, on the total amount of fat in the body, the location of body fat, and the presence or absence of weight-related medical problems.

Estimating Body Fat Content and Diagnosing Obesity

Body fat varies widely among individuals and can range from 2% to 70% of body weight. Desirable amounts of body fat are about 8% to 24% for men and 21% to 35% for women. Men with over 24% body fat and women with over about 35% body fat are considered obese. The higher range of body fat percentage for women is needed physiologically to maintain reproductive functions, including estrogen production.

To measure body fat content accurately using typical methods, both body weight and body volume of the person must be known. Body weight is easy to measure on a conventional scale. Of the typical methods used to estimate body volume, **underwater weighing** is the most accurate. This technique determines body volume using the difference between conventional body weight and body weight under water, along with the relative densities of fat tissue and lean tissue, and a specific mathematical formula. This procedure requires that an individual be totally submerged in a tank of water, with a trained technician directing the procedure (Fig. 7-9). **Air displacement** is another method of determining body volume. Body volume is quantified by measuring the space a person takes up inside a measurement chamber, such as the BodPod (Fig. 7-10). A less accurate method to measure body volume is to submerge a person in a tank and observe the level of the water before and after submersion. The volume of the displaced water is then calculated.

Once body volume is known, it can be used along with body weight in the following equation to calculate body density. Then using body density, body fat content finally can be determined.

$$\text{Body density} = \frac{\text{body weight}}{\text{body volume}}$$
$$\% \text{ body fat} = (495 \div \text{body density}) - 450$$

For example, assume that the individual in the underwater weighing tank in Figure 7-9 has a body density of 1.06 grams per centimeter^3. We can use the second formula to calculate that he has 17% body fat ([495 ÷ 1.06] − 450 = 17).

Skinfold thickness is also a common anthropometric method to estimate total body fat content, although there are some limits to its accuracy. Clinicians use calipers to measure the fat layer directly under the skin at multiple sites and then plug these values into a mathematical formula (Fig. 7-11).

The technique of **bioelectrical impedance** is also used to estimate body fat content. The instrument sends a painless, low-energy electrical current to and from the

TABLE 7-1 Health Problems Associated with Excess Body Fat

Health Problem	Partially Attributable To
Surgical risk	Increased anesthesia needs, as well as greater risk of wound infections (the latter is linked to a decrease in immune function)
Pulmonary disease and sleep disorders	Excess weight over lungs and pharynx
Type 2 diabetes	Enlarged adipose cells, which poorly bind insulin and poorly respond to the message insulin sends to the cell; less synthesis of factors that aid insulin action, and greater synthesis of factors by adipose cells that lessen insulin action
Hypertension	Increased miles of blood vessels found in the adipose tissue, increased blood volume, and increased resistance to blood flow related to hormones made by adipose cells
Cardiovascular disease (e.g., coronary heart disease and stroke)	Increases in LDL-cholesterol and triglyceride values, low HDL-cholesterol, decreased physical activity, and increased synthesis of blood clotting and inflamatory factors by enlarged adipose cells. A greater risk for heart failure is also seen, due in part to altered heart rhythm.
Bone and joint disorders (including gout)	Excess pressure put on knee, ankle, and hip joints
Gallstones	Increased cholesterol content of bile
Skin disorders	Trapping of moisture and microorganisms in tissue folds
Various cancers, such as in the kidney, gall-bladder, colon and rectum, uterus (women), and prostate gland (men)	Estrogen production by adipose cells; animal studies suggest excess calorie intake encourages tumor development
Shorter stature (in some forms of obesity)	Earlier onset of puberty
Pregnancy risks	More difficult delivery, increased number of birth defects, and increased needs for anesthesia
Reduced physical agility and increased risk of accidents and falls	Excess weight that impairs movement
Menstrual irregularities and infertility	Hormones produced by adipose cells, such as estrogen
Vision problems	Cataracts and other eye disorders are more often present
Premature death	A variety of risk factors for disease listed in this table
Infections	Reduced immune system activity
Liver damage and eventual failure	Excess fat accumulation in the liver
Erectile dysfunction in men	Low-grade inflammation caused by excess fat mass and reduced function of the cells lining the blood vessels associated with being overweight

The greater the degree of obesity, the more likely and the more serious these health problems generally become. They are much more likely to appear in people who show an upper-body fat distribution pattern and/or are greater than twice healthy body weight.

body via wires and electrode patches to estimate body fat. This estimation is based on the assumption that adipose tissue resists electrical flow more than lean tissue because it has a lower electrolyte and water content than lean tissue. More adipose tissue therefore means proportionately greater electrical resistance. Within a few seconds, bioelectrical impedance analyzers convert body electrical resistance into an approximate estimate of total body fat, as long as body hydration status is normal (Fig. 7-12). Body composition monitors, better known as body fat calculators, that use bioelectric impedence are now available for home use. These machines are similar in shape and use to bathroom scales but their main purpose is to measure body fat. A current passes easily through conductive foot pads and/or handheld electrodes. These in-home devices will hopefully encourage people to be less concerned with what they weigh than whether their weight comes from fat or muscle.

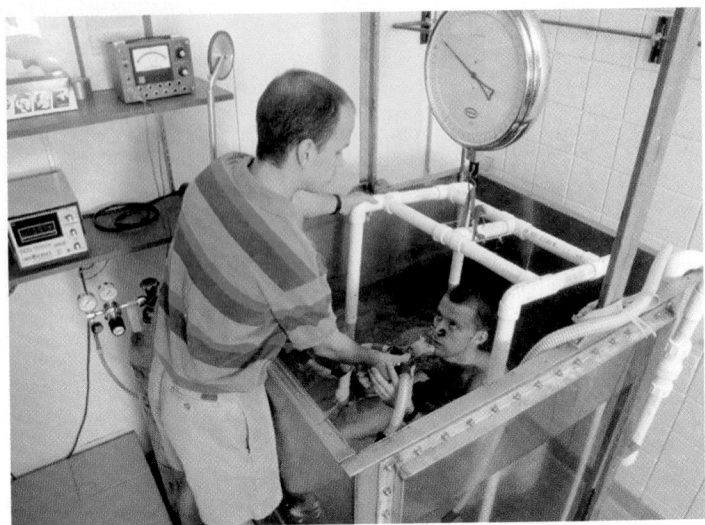

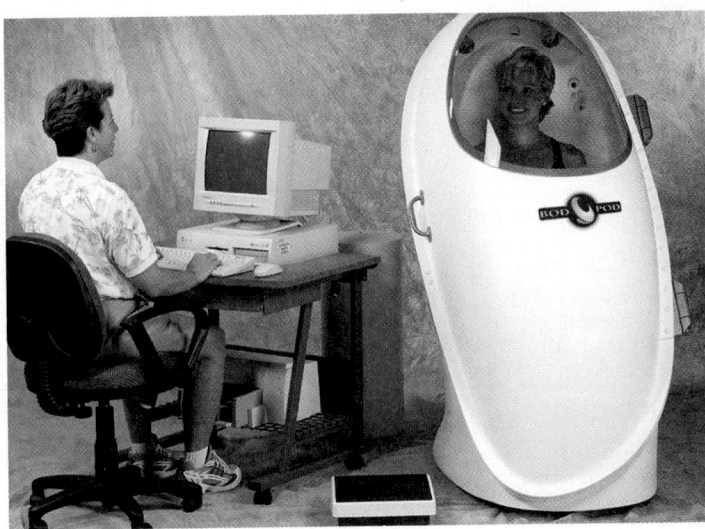

FIGURE 7-9 ▶ Underwater weighing. In this technique, the subject exhales as much air as possible and then holds his or her breath and bends over at the waist. Once the subject is totally submerged, the underwater weight is recorded. Using this value, body volume can be calculated.

FIGURE 7-10 ▶ BodPod. This device determines body volume based on the volume of displaced air, measured as a person sits in a sealed chamber for a few minutes.

FIGURE 7-11 ▶ Skinfold measurements. Using proper technique and calibrated equipment, skinfold measurements around the body can be used to predict body fat content in about 10 minutes. Measurements are made at several locations including the triceps (photo and drawing) skinfolds.

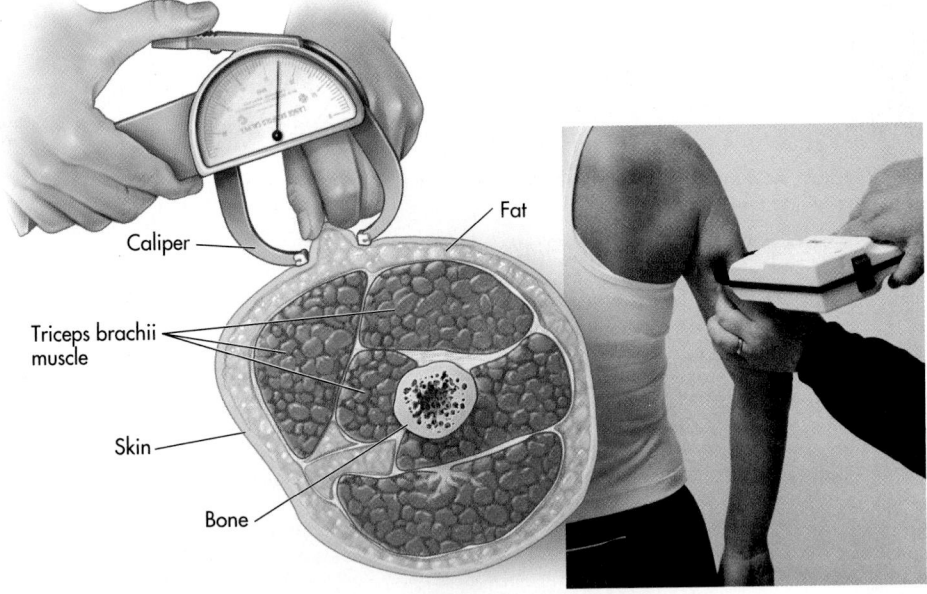

FIGURE 7-12 ▶ Bioelectrical impedance estimates total body fat in less than 5 minutes and is based on the principle that body fat resists the flow of electricity, since it is low in water and electrolytes. The degree of resistance to electrical flow is used to estimate body fatness.

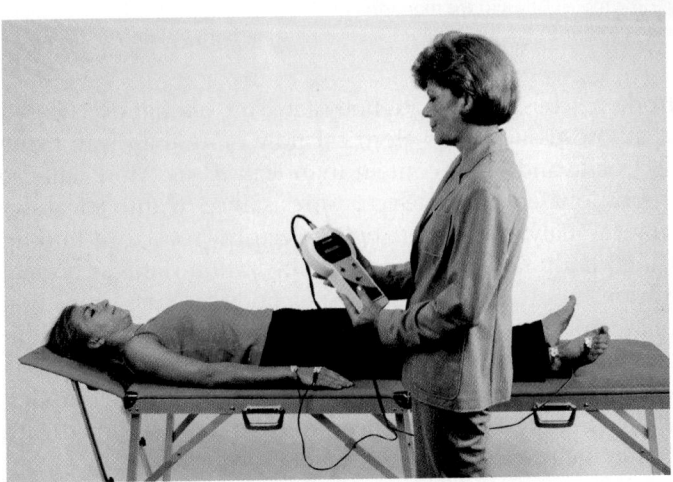

A more advanced determination of body fat content can be made using **dual energy X-ray absorptiometry (DEXA)**. DEXA is considered the most accurate way to determine body fat, but the equipment is expensive and not widely available for this use. This X-ray system allows the clinician to separate body weight into three separate components—fat, fat-free soft tissue, and bone mineral. The usual whole-body scan requires about 5 to 20 minutes and the dose of radiation is less than a chest X ray. An assessment of bone mineral density and the risk of osteoporosis also can be made using this method (Fig. 7-13).

Another method to assess body fat is to measure total-body electrical conductance (TOBEC) when placed in an electromagnetic field. Still another method, convenient and inexpensive, but not very accurate is **near-infrared reactance.** This method exposes the bicep muscle to a beam of near-infrared light and assesses the interactions of the light beam with fat and lean tissues in the upper arm after only 2 seconds.

In summary, although the DEXA is considered most accurate, the underwater weighing and air displacement methods of body fat estimation are also accurate because both body weight and body volume are measured. The adaptation of the bioelectrical impedence technology for in-home use is also a useful tool, providing valuable information about whether weight gain is coming from fat or muscle.

Using Body Fat Distribution to Further Evaluate Obesity

In addition to the amount of fat we store, the location of that body fat is an important predictor of health risks. Some people store fat in upper-body areas, whereas others store fat lower on the body. Excess fat in either location generally spells trouble, but each storage space also has its unique risks. **Upper-body obesity,** characterized by a large abdomen, is more often related to cardiovascular disease, hypertension, and type 2 diabetes. Whereas other adipose cells empty fat into general blood circulation, the fat released from abdominal adipose cells goes directly to the liver, by way of the portal vein. This process likely interferes with the liver's ability to use insulin and negatively affects lipoprotein metabolism by the liver. These abdominal adipose cells also make substances that increase insulin resistance, blood clotting, blood vessel constriction, and inflammation in the body. These changes can lead to long-term health problems.

High blood testosterone (primarily a male hormone) levels apparently encourage upper-body obesity, as does a diet with a high glycemic load, alcohol intake, and smoking. This characteristic male pattern of fat storage is also called android obesity and is commonly known as the apple shape (large abdomen [pot belly] and small buttocks and thighs). Upper-body obesity is assessed by measuring the waist at the widest point just above the hips when relaxed. A waist circumference more than 40 inches (102 centimeters) in men and more than 35 inches (88 centimeters) in women indicates upper-body obesity (Fig. 7-14). If BMI is also 25 or more, health risks are significantly increased.

Estrogen and progesterone (primarily female hormones) encourage lower-body fat storage and **lower-body (gynecoid or gynoid) obesity**—the typical female pattern. The small abdomen and much larger buttocks and thighs give a pearlike appearance. Fat deposited in the lower body is not mobilized as easily as the other type and often resists being shed. After menopause, blood estrogen falls, encouraging upper-body fat distribution.

dual energy X-ray absorptiometry (DEXA) A highly accurate method of measuring body composition and bone mass and density using multiple low-energy X rays.

upper-body obesity The type of obesity in which fat is stored primarily in the abdominal area; defined as a waist circumference more than 40 inches (102 centimeters) in men and more than 35 inches (89 centimeters) in women; closely associated with a high risk for cardiovascular disease, hypertension, and type 2 diabetes. Also known as android obesity.

lower-body obesity The type of obesity in which fat storage is primarily located in the buttocks and thigh area. Also known as gynoid or gynecoid obesity.

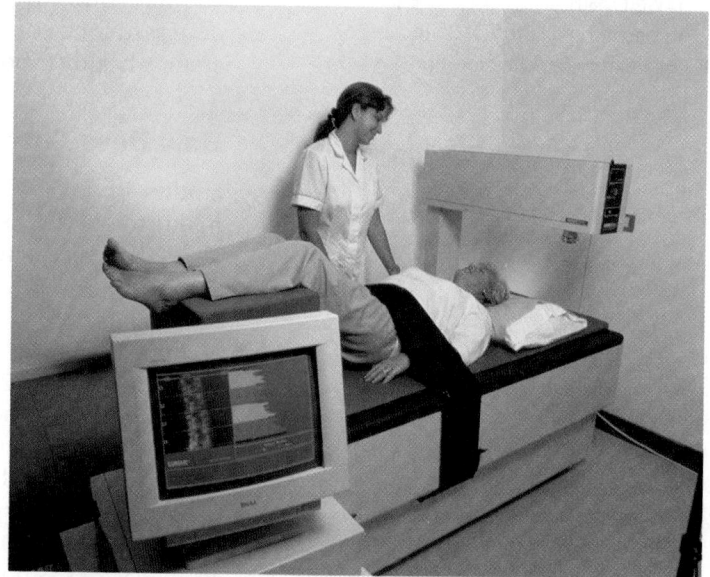

FIGURE 7-13 ▶ Dual energy X-ray absorptiometry (DEXA). This method measures body fat by passing small doses of radiation through the body. The radiation reacts differently with fat, lean tissue, or bone allowing these components to be quantified. The scanner arm moves from head to toe and in doing so can determine body fat as well as bone density. DEXA is currently considered the most accurate method for determining body fat (as long as the person can fit under the arm of the instrument). The radiation dose is minimal.

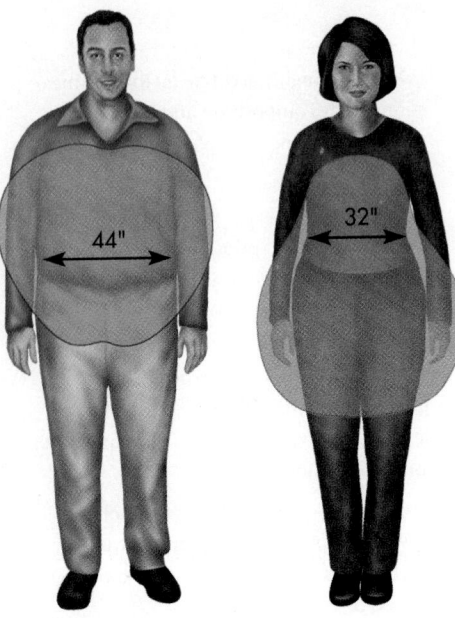

Upper-body fat
distribution
(android: apple shape)

Lower-body fat
distribution
(gynoid: pear shape)

FIGURE 7-14 ▶ Body fat stored primarily in the upper-body (android) form brings higher risks of ill health associated with obesity than does lower-body (gynoid) fat. The woman's waist circumference of 32 inches and the man's waist circumference of 44 inches indicate that the man has upper-body fat distribution but the woman does not, based on a cutoff of 35 inches for women and 40 inches for men.

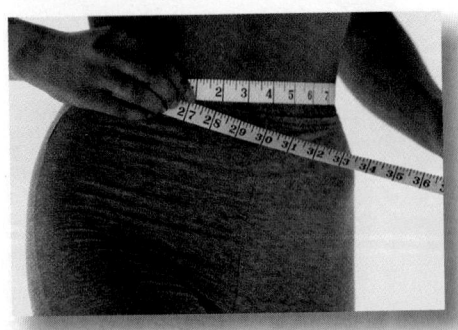

▲ Waist circumference is an important measure of weight-related health risk.

identical twins Two offspring that develop from a single ovum and sperm and, consequently, have the same genetic makeup.

CONCEPT CHECK

Overweight and obesity typically are associated with excessive body fat storage. The risk of health problems related to being overweight especially increases under the following conditions:

- A man's percentage of body fat exceeds 25%; a woman's exceeds about 35%.
- Excess fat is primarily stored in the upper-body region.
- Body mass index (BMI) is 30 or more (calculated as weight in kilograms divided by height squared in meters).

However, these are merely guidelines. A more individualized approach to assessment is warranted as long as a person is following a healthy lifestyle and has no existing health problems.

Body fat content can be estimated using a variety of methods such as underwater weighing, air displacement, skinfold thickness, bioelectrical impedance, and DEXA. Fat storage distribution further specifies an obese state as either upper-body or lower-body. Obesity leads to an increased risk for cardiovascular disease, some types of cancer, hypertension, type 2 diabetes, certain bone and joint disorders, and some digestive disorders. The risks for some of these diseases are greater with upper-body fat storage.

7.5 Why Some People Are Obese—Nature Versus Nurture

Both genetic (nature) and environmental (nurture) factors can increase the risk for obesity (Table 7-2). The eventual location of fat storage is strongly influenced by genetics. Consider the possibility that obesity is nurture allowing nature to express itself. Some obese people begin life with a slower basal metabolism; maintain an inactive lifestyle; and consume highly-refined, calorie-dense diets. These people in turn are nurtured into gaining weight, promoting their natural tendency toward obesity.

Still, genes do not fully control destiny. With increased physical activity and decreased food consumption, even those with a genetic tendency toward obesity can attain a healthier body weight.

How Does Nature Contribute to Obesity?

Studies in pairs of **identical twins** give us some insight into the contribution of nature to obesity. Even when identical twins are raised apart, they tend to show similar weight gain patterns, both in overall weight and body fat distribution. It appears that nurture—eating habits and nutrition, which varies between twins raised apart—has less to do with obesity than nature does. In fact, research suggests that genes account for up to 70% of weight differences between people. A child with no obese parent has only a 10% chance of becoming obese. When a child has one obese parent (common in our society), that risk advances up to 40%, and with two obese parents, it soars to 80%. Our genes help determine metabolic rate, fuel use, and differences in brain chemistry—all of which affect body weight.

We also inherit specific body types. Tall, thin people appear to have an inherently easier time maintaining healthy body weight. This is probably because basal metabolism increases as body surface increases, and therefore taller people use more calories than shorter people, even at rest.

Many of us probably have inherited a thrifty metabolism that enables us to store fat more readily than the typical human, so that we require fewer calories to get through the day. In earlier times, when food supplies were scarce, a thrifty metabolism would have been a built-in safeguard against starvation. Now, with a general abundance of food, people operating in this low gear require much physical activity and wise food choices to prevent obesity. If you think you are prone to weight gain, you likely have inherited a thrifty metabolism.

TABLE 7-2 What Encourages Excess Body Fat Stores and Obesity?

Factor	How Fat Storage is Affected
Age	Excess body fat is more common in adults and middle-age individuals.
Menopause	Increase in abdominal fat deposition is typical.
Gender	Females have more fat.
Positive energy balance	Over a long period promotes storage of fat.
Composition of diet	Excess calorie intake from fat, alcohol, and calorie dense (sugary, fat-rich) foods contributes to obesity.
Physical activity	Low physical activity ("couch potato") leads to positive energy balance and body fat storage.
Basal metabolism	A low BMR is linked to weight gain.
Thermic effect of food	Low for some obesity cases.
Increased hunger sensations	Some people have trouble resisting the abundant availability of food, which is likely linked to the activity of various brain chemicals.
Ratio of fat to lean tissue	A high ratio of fat mass to lean body mass is correlated with weight gain.
Fat uptake by adipose tissue	This is high in some obese individuals and remains high (perhaps even increases) with weight loss.
Variety of social and behavioral factors	Obesity is associated with socioeconomic status; familial conditions; network of friends; busy lifestyles that discourage balanced meals; binge eating; easy availability of inexpensive, "supersized" high-fat food; pattern of leisure activities; television time; smoking cessation; excessive alcohol intake; and number of meals eaten away from home.
Undetermined genetic characteristics	These affect components of energy balance, particularly energy expenditure, the deposition of the energy surplus as adipose tissue or as lean tissue, and the relative proportion of fat and carbohydrate used by the body.
Race	In some ethnic groups, higher body weight may be more socially acceptable.
Certain medications	Food intake increases.
Childbearing	Women may not lose all weight gained in pregnancy.
National region	Regional differences, such as high-fat diets and sedentary lifestyles in the Midwest and areas of the South, lead to geographically different rates of obesity.

Does the Body Have a Set Point for Weight?

The **set-point** theory of weight maintenance proposes that humans have a genetically predetermined body weight or body fat content, which the body closely regulates. Some research suggests that the **hypothalamus** region of the brain monitors the amount of body fat in humans and tries to keep that amount constant over time. The hypothalamus has two sites—the feeding center and the satiety center—that play a role in regulating hunger. The hormone **leptin** forms a communication link between adipose cells and the brain, which allows for some weight regulation.

Several physiological changes that occur during calorie reduction and weight loss also endorse the set-point theory (see Further Reading 2). For example, when calorie intake is reduced, the blood concentration of thyroid hormones falls, which slows basal metabolism. In addition, as weight is lost, the calorie cost of weight-bearing activity decreases, so that an activity that burned 100 kcal before weight loss may only burn 80 kcal after weight loss. Furthermore, with weight loss, the body becomes more efficient at storing fat by increasing the activity of the enzyme *lipoprotein lipase*, which takes fat into cells. All of these changes protect the body from losing weight.

If a person overeats, in the short run, basal metabolism tends to increase. This causes some resistance to weight gain. However, in the long run, resistance to weight

set point Often refers to the close regulation of body weight. It is not known what cells control this set point or how it functions in weight regulation. There is evidence, however, that mechanisms exist that help regulate weight.

hypothalamus A region at the base of the brain that contains cells that play a role in the regulation of hunger, respiration, body temperature, and other body functions.

leptin A harmone made by adipose tissue in proportion to total fat stores in the body that influences long-term regulation of fat mass. Leptin also influences reproductive functions, as well as other body processes, such as release of the hormone insulin.

▶ Studies in identical twins give us insight into the genetic contribution to obesity.

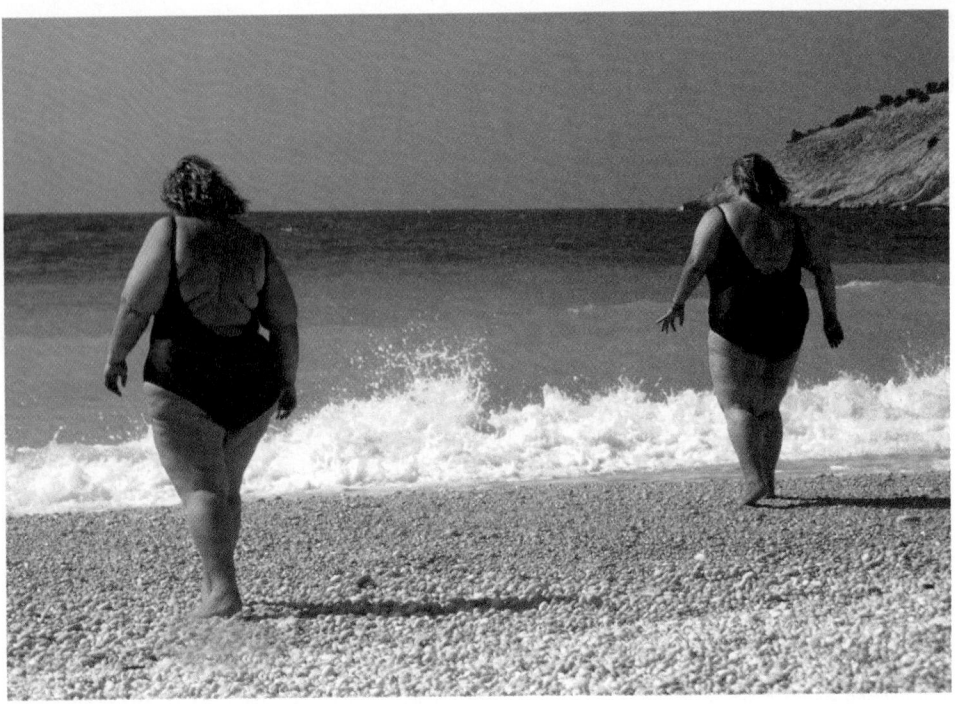

▼ Body weight is influenced by many factors related to both nature and nurture. We resemble our parents because of the genes we have inherited, as well as the lifestyle habits, including diet, that we have learned from them.

gain is much less than resistance to weight loss. When a person gains weight and stays at that weight for a while, the body tends to establish a new set point.

Opponents of the set-point theory argue that weight does not remain constant throughout adulthood—the average person gains weight slowly, at least until old age. Also, if an individual is placed in a different social, emotional, or physical environment, weight can be altered and maintained markedly higher or lower. These arguments suggest that humans, rather than having a set point determined by genetics or the number of adipose cells, settle into a particular stable weight based on their circumstances, often regarded as a "settling point."

The size-acceptance nondiet movement, "Health at Every Size," indirectly refers to a set point for weight by defining healthy weight as the natural weight the body adopts, given a healthy diet and meaningful levels of physical activity. Overall, the set point is weaker in preventing weight gain than in preventing weight loss. Even with a set point helping us, the odds are in favor of eventual weight gain unless we devote effort to a healthy lifestyle.

Does Nurture Have a Role?

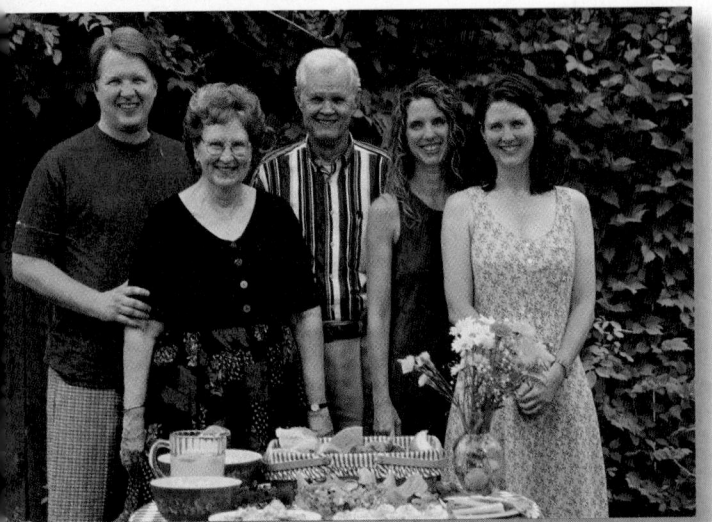

Some would argue that body weight similarities between family members stem more from learned behaviors rather than genetic similarities. Even couples, who have no genetic link, may behave similarly toward food and eventually assume similar degrees of leanness or fatness. Proponents of nurture pose that environmental factors, such as high-fat diets and inactivity, literally shape us. This seems likely when we consider that our gene pool has not changed much in the past 50 years, whereas according to the U.S. Centers for Disease Control and Prevention the ranks of obese people have grown in epidemic proportions over the last 25 years.

Adult obesity in women is often rooted in childhood obesity. In addition, relative inactivity and periods of stress or boredom, as well as excess weight gain during pregnancy, contribute to female obesity. (Chapter 14 notes that breastfeeding one's infant contributes to loss of some of the excess fat associated with pregnancy.) These patterns suggest both social and genetic links. Male obesity, however, is not strongly linked to childhood obesity and, instead, tends to appear after age 30. This powerful and prevalent pattern suggests a primary role of nurture in obesity, with less genetic influence.

Is poverty associated with obesity? Ironically, the answer is often yes. North Americans of lower socioeconomic status, especially females, are more likely to be obese than those in upper socioeconomic groups. Several social and behavioral factors promote fat storage. These factors include lower socioeconomic status, overweight friends and family, a cultural/ethnic group that prefers higher body weight, a lifestyle that discourages healthy meals and adequate exercise, easy availability of inexpensive high-calorie food, limited access to fresh fruits and vegetables, excessive television viewing, smoking cessation, lack of adequate sleep, emotional stress, and meals frequently eaten away from home.

7.6 Treatment of Overweight and Obesity

Treatment of overweight and obesity should be long-term, similar to that for any chronic disease. Treatments require long-term lifestyle changes, rather than a quick fix promoted by many popular (also called fad) diet books. We often view a "diet" as something one goes on temporarily, only to resume prior (typically poor) habits once satisfactory results have been achieved. This is a big reason that so many people regain lost weight. Instead, an emphasis on healthy, active living with acceptable dietary modifications will promote weight loss and later weight maintenance.

What to Look for in a Sound Weight-Loss Plan

A dieter can develop a plan of action by seeking advice from a health professional, such as a registered dietitian, or by using the interactive tools at www.ChooseMyPlate.gov. Either way, a sound weight-loss program (Fig. 7-15) should especially include these components:

1. Control of calorie intake. One recommendation is to decrease calorie intake by 100 kcal per day (and increase physical activity by 100 kcal per day). This should allow for slow and steady weight loss.
2. Increased physical activity.
3. Acknowledgment that maintenance of a healthy weight requires lifelong changes in habits, not a short-term weight-loss period.

A one-sided approach that focuses only on restricting calories is a difficult plan of action. Instead, adding physical activity and an appropriate psychological component

MAKING DECISIONS

Losing Body Fat

Rapid weight loss cannot consist primarily of fat loss because a high calorie deficit is needed to lose a large amount of adipose tissue. Adipose tissue, mostly fat, contains about 3500 kcal per pound. Weight loss, however, includes adipose tissue plus lean tissues that support it and represents approximately 3300 kcal per pound (about 7.2 kcal per gram). Therefore, to lose 1 pound of adipose tissue per week, calorie intake must be decreased by approximately 500 kcal per day, or physical activity must be increased by 500 kcal per day. Alternately, a combination of both strategies can be used. Diets that promise 10 to 15 pounds of weight loss per week cannot ensure that the weight loss is from adipose tissue stores alone. How many calories would need to be eliminated from the diet per day to lose 10 pounds per week? Is it possible to subtract enough calories from one's daily intake to lose that amount of adipose tissue? Lean tissue and water, rather than adipose tissue, account for the major part of the weight lost during these dramatic weight-loss programs.

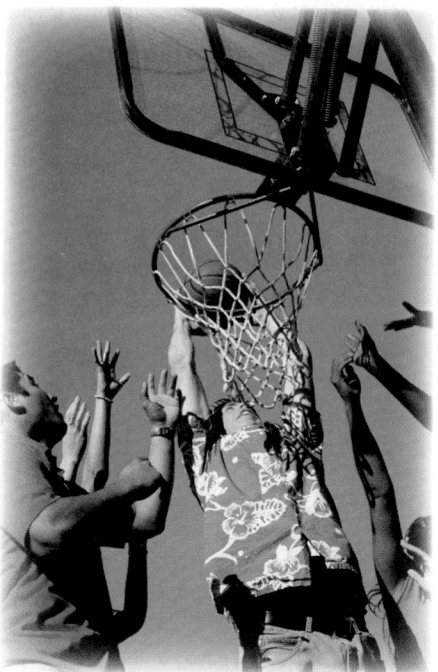

▲ Student life is often full of physical activity. This is not necessarily true for a person's later working life; hence, weight gain is a strong possibility.

▶ **Weight Status objectives from** *Healthy People 2020*

- Increase by 10% the proportion of adults who are at a healthy weight.
  - Target for 2020:   33.9%
  - Baseline in 2005–08: 30.8%
- Reduce by 10% the proportion of adults who are obese.
  - Target for 2020:   30.6%
  - Baseline in 2005–08: 34.0%
- Reduce by 10% the proportion of children and adolescents, 2 to 19 years, who are considered obese.
  - Target for 2020:   14.6%
  - Baseline in 2005–08: 16.2%
- Prevent inappropriate weight gain in youth and adults.

As you read brochures, articles, or research reports about specific diet plans, look beyond the weight loss promoted by the diet's advocate to see if the reported weight loss was maintained. If the weight-maintenance aspect was missing, then the program was not successful.

FIGURE 7-15 ▶ Characteristics of a sound weight-loss diet. Use this checklist to evaluate any new diet plan before putting it into practice.

The 2010 Dietary Guidelines for Americans provide the following recommendations regarding "Balancing Calories to Manage Weight" as part of healthy eating pattern and while staying within their calories need:

- Prevent and/or reduce overweight and obesity through improved eating and physical activity behaviors.

- Control total calorie intake to manage body weight. For people who are overweight or obese, this will mean consuming fewer calories from foods and beverages.

- Increase physical activity and reduce time spent in sedentary behaviors.

- Maintain appropriate calorie balance during each stage of life—childhood, adolescence, adulthood, pregnancy and breastfeeding, and older age.

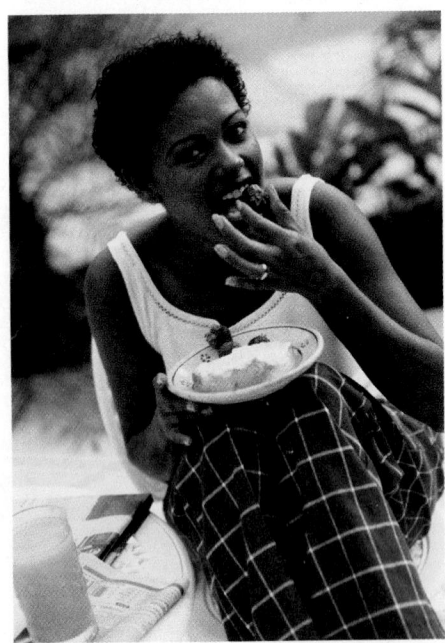

▲ Making a commitment to a healthier diet and lifestyle can be a challenge for many individuals. A sound weight-loss plan, however, does not require you to completely avoid certain favorite foods. Practical strategies include substituting lower-calorie choices, choosing high-calorie treats less often, and limiting portion sizes.

RATE OF LOSS

☐ Encourages slow and steady weight loss, rather than rapid weight loss, to promote lasting weight
☐ Sets goal of 1 pound of fat loss per week
☐ Includes a period of weight maintenance for a few months after 10% of body weight is lost
☐ Evaluates need for further dieting before more weight loss begins

FLEXIBILITY

☐ Supports participation in normal activities (e.g., parties, restaurants)
☐ Adapts to individual habits and tastes

INTAKE

☐ Meets nutrient needs (except for energy needs)
☐ Includes common foods, with no foods being promoted as magical or special
☐ Recommends a fortified ready-to-eat breakfast cereal or balanced multivitamin/mineral supplement, especially when intake is less than 1600 kcal per day
☐ Uses MyPlate as a pattern for food choices

BEHAVIOR MODIFICATION

☐ Focuses on maintenance of healthy lifestyle (and weight) for a lifetime
☐ Promotes reasonable changes that can be maintained
☐ Encourages social support
☐ Includes plans for relapse, so that one does not quit after a setback
☐ Promotes changes that control problem eating behaviors

OVERALL HEALTH

☐ Requires screening by a physician for people with existing health problems, those over 40 (men) to 50 (women) years of age who plan to increase physical activity substantially, and those who plan to lose weight rapidly
☐ Encourages regular physical activity, sufficient sleep, stress reduction, and other healthy changes in lifestyle
☐ Addresses underlying psychological weight issues, such as depression or marital stress

will contribute to success in weight loss and eventual weight maintenance (Fig. 7-16). From the 2010 Dietary Guidelines for Americans section on weight management, the key recommendations for those who need to lose weight is to aim for a slow, steady weight loss by decreasing calorie intake while maintaining an adequate nutrient intake and increasing physical activity.

Weight Loss in Perspective

These principles point to the importance of preventing obesity. This concept has wide support because conquering the disorder is so difficult. Public health strategies to address the current obesity problem must speak to all age groups. There is a particular need to focus on children and adolescents because patterns of excess weight and sedentary lifestyle developed during youth may form the basis for a lifetime

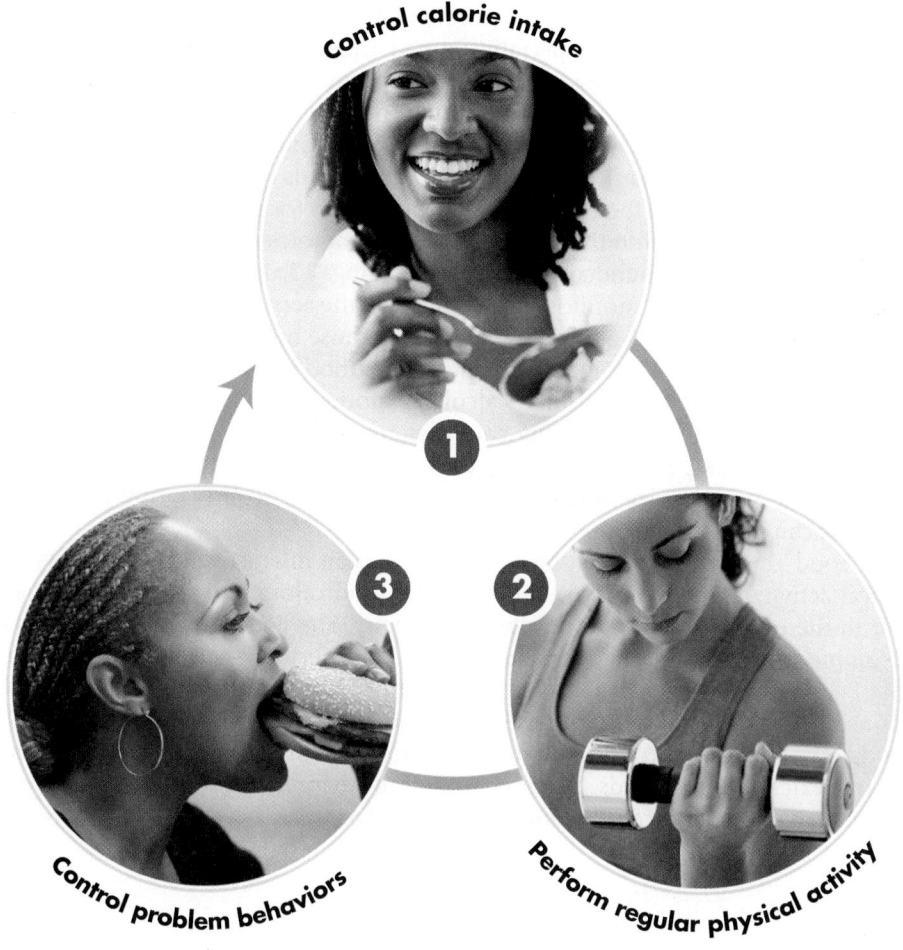

Control calorie intake

Control problem behaviors

Perform regular physical activity

FIGURE 7-16 ▶ Weight-loss triad. The key to weight loss and maintenance can be thought of as a triad, which consists of three parts: (1) controlling calorie intake, (2) performing regular physical activity, and (3) controlling problem behaviors. The three parts of the triad support each other in that without one part of the triad, weight loss and later maintenance become unlikely.

For more information on weight control, obesity, and nutrition, visit the Weight-Control Information Network (WIN) at http://win.niddk.nih.gov/index.htm or call 800-WIN-8098. Complete guidelines for weight management are available at www.nhlbi.nih.gov/guidelines/index .htm. Other websites include www .caloriecontrol.org, www.weight.com, www.obesity.org, and www.cyberdiet .com.

CONCEPT CHECK

Obesity is a chronic disease that necessitates lifelong treatment. Emphasis should be placed especially on preventing obesity, because overcoming this disorder is difficult. Appropriate weight-loss programs have the following characteristics in common: (1) They meet nutritional needs; (2) they can adjust to accommodate habits and tastes; (3) they emphasize readily obtainable foods; (4) they promote changing habits that discourage overeating; (5) they encourage regular physical activity; and (6) they help change obesity-promoting beliefs and rally healthy social support.

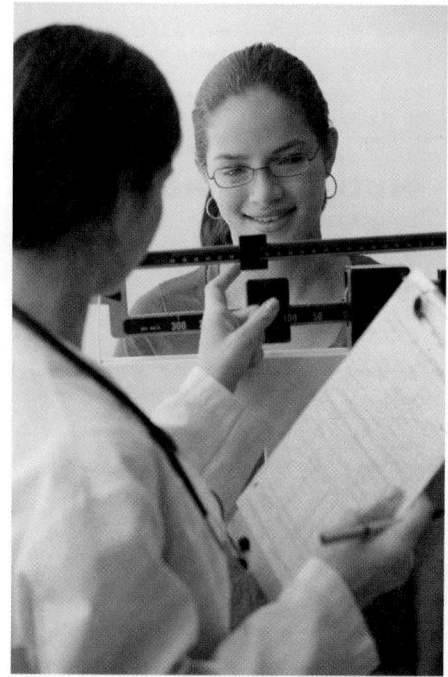

▲ Slow, steady weight loss is one of the characteristics of a sound weight-loss program.

For interactive dietary and physical activity tools, check out the Food Tracker and Food Planner at www.ChooseMyPlate.gov.

of weight-related illness and increased mortality. In the adult population, attention should be directed toward weight maintenance and increased physical activity.

7.7 Control of Calorie Intake—The Main Key to Weight Loss and Weight Maintenance

A goal of losing 1 pound or so of stored fat per week may require limiting calorie intake to 1200 kcal per day for women and 1500 kcal for men. The calorie allowance could also be higher for very active people. Keep in mind that, in our sedentary society, decreasing calorie intake is vital because it is difficult to burn much energy without ample physical activity. With regard to consuming fewer calories, some experts

NEWSWORTHY NUTRITION

Small changes result in large weight change over the years

Subjects in a large 20-year study of lifestyle factors and weight change gained an average of 20 pounds in 20 years. Less exercise led to weight gain but the kinds of foods people ate had a larger effect than changes in physical activity. Increased consumption of French fries alone led to an average weight gain of 3.4 pounds every 4 years. Greater intake of fruits, vegetables, whole grains, yogurt, and nuts resulted in weight loss or no gain. The result of this study show how small changes in eating, exercise, and other habits can result in large changes in body weight over the years.

Source: Mozaffarian D and others: Changes in diet and lifestyle and long-term weight gain in women and men. *New England Journal of Medicine* 364:2392 2011, (see Further Reading 8).

connect NUTRITION **Check out the Connect site www.mcgrawhillconnect.com to further explore long-term weight gain.**

suggest consuming less fat (especially saturated fat and *trans* fat), while others suggest consuming less carbohydrate, especially refined (high glycemic load) carbohydrate sources. Protein intakes in excess of what is typically needed by adults are also receiving attention. Using all these approaches simultaneously is fine. At this time, the low-fat, high-fiber approaches have been the most successful in long-term studies. A recent report (see Newsworthy Nutrition) confirms that the kinds of food we eat have a large effect on weight gain over the years. Finding what works for an individual is a process of trial and error. The notion that any type of diet promotes significantly greater calorie use by the body is unfounded (see Further Readings 13, 14, and 15).

One way for a dieter to monitor calorie intake at the start of a weight-loss program is by reading labels. Label reading is important, because many foods are more energy dense than people suppose (Fig. 7-17). Another method is to write down food intake for 24 hours (Appendix E) and then calculate calorie intake from the food table in the textbook supplement or by using your diet-analysis software. With knowledge of current calorie intake, future food choices can be adjusted as needed. People often underestimate portion size when recording food intake, so measuring cups and a food scale can help.

The Food Tracker at www.ChooseMyPlate.gov is an interactive online dietary and physical activity assessment tool that tracks the food calories you eat and compares them to the energy you expend in physical activity. The Food Planner is an interactive online tool for planning menus based on your personal ChooseMyPlate goals. Table 7-3 shows how to start reducing calorie intake. As you should realize, it is best to consider healthy eating a lifestyle change, rather than a weight-loss plan. Also, liquids deserve attention, because liquid calories do not stimulate satiety mechanisms to the same extent as solid foods. The corresponding advice from experts is to use beverages that have few or no calories and limit sugar-sweetened beverages.

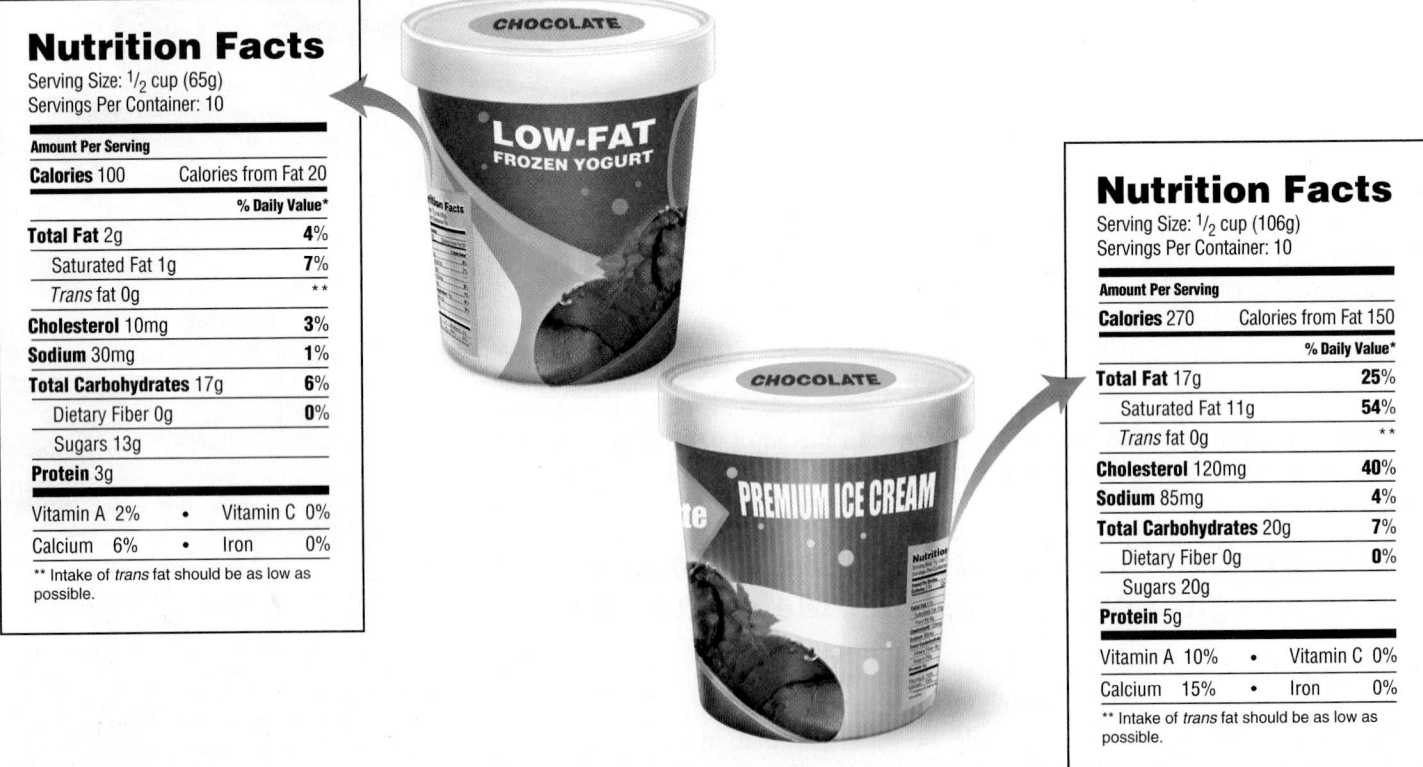

FIGURE 7-17 ▶ Reading labels helps you choose foods with fewer calories. Which of these frozen desserts is the best choice, per ½ cup serving, for a person on a weight-loss diet? The % Daily Values are based on a 2000 kcal diet. Read more about these dessert choices in What Would You Choose Recommendations.

TABLE 7-3 Lowering kcal: Point of Purchase and Consumption Decisions

Instead of	Try	Number of kcal Saved
3 oz well-marbled meat (prime rib)	3 oz lean meat (eye of round)	140
½ chicken breast, batter-fried	½ chicken breast, broiled with lemon	175
½ cup home-fried potatoes	1 medium baked potato	65
½ cup green bean-mushroom casserole	½ cup cooked green beans	50
½ cup potato salad	1 cup raw vegetable salad	140
½ cup pineapple chunks in heavy syrup	½ cup pineapple chunks canned in juice	25
2 tbsp bottled French dressing	2 tbsp low-calorie French dressing	150
⅛ 9-inch apple pie	1 baked apple, unsweetened	308
3 oatmeal-raisin cookies	1 oatmeal-raisin cookie	125
½ cup ice cream	½ cup ice milk	45
1 danish pastry	½ English muffin	150
1 cup sugar-coated corn flakes	1 cup plain corn flakes	60
1 cup whole milk	1 cup 1% low-fat milk	45
1 oz bag potato chips	1 cup plain popcorn	120
1/12 8-inch white layer cake with chocolate frosting	1/12 angel food cake, 10-inch tube	185
12-fluid-ounce cola	12-fluid-ounce diet cola	150

7.8 Regular Physical Activity—A Second Key to Weight Loss and Especially Important for Later Weight Maintenance

Regular physical activity is important for everyone, especially those trying to lose weight or maintain a lower body weight. Calorie burning is enhanced both during and after physical activity. Therefore, activity greatly complements a reduction in calorie intake for weight loss. Many of us rarely do more than sit, stand, and sleep. More calories are used during physical activity than at rest. Expending only 100 to 300 extra kcal per day above and beyond normal daily activity, while controlling calorie intake, can lead to a steady weight loss. Furthermore, physical activity has so many other benefits, including a boost for overall self-esteem. A Key Recommendation from the 2010 Dietary Guidelines is to increase physical activity and reduce time spent in sedentary behaviors. The Dietary Guidelines point to the 2008 Physical Activity Guidelines for Americans for specific recommendations. Weight management, as well as other health outcomes including diseases and risk factors for disease, was considered in developing the Physical Activity Guidelines. Although some adults will need a higher level of physical activity than others, it is recommended that adults should do the equivalent of 150 minutes of moderate-intensity aerobic activity each week to achieve and maintain a healthy body weight. Some may need more than the equivalent of 300 minutes per week of moderate-intensity activity.

Adding any of the activities in Table 7-4 to one's lifestyle can increase calorie use. Duration and regular performance, rather than intensity, are the keys to success with this approach to weight loss. One should search for activities that can be continued over time. In this regard, walking vigorously 3 miles per day can be as helpful as

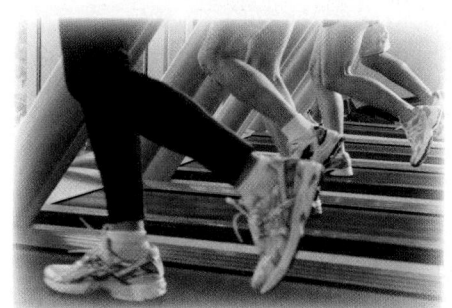

▲ Physical activity complements any diet plan.

TABLE 7-4 Approximate Calorie Costs of Various Activities and Specific Calorie Costs Projected for a 150-Pound (68-Kilogram) Person

Activity	kcal per kilogram per Hour	Total kcal per Hour	Activity	kcal per kilogram per Hour	Total kcal per Hour
Aerobics—heavy	8.0	544	Horseback riding	5.1	346
Aerobics—medium	5.0	340	Ice skating (10 mph)	5.8	394
Aerobics—light	3.0	204	Jogging—medium	9.0	612
Backpacking	9.0	612	Jogging—slow	7.0	476
Basketball—vigorous	10.0	680	Lying—at ease	1.3	89
Bowling	3.9	265	Racquetball—social	8.0	544
Calisthenics—heavy	8.0	544	Roller skating	5.1	346
Calisthenics—light	4.0	272	Running or jogging (10 mph)	13.2	897
Canoeing (2.5 mph)	3.3	224	Skiing downhill (10 mph)	8.8	598
Cleaning (female)	3.7	253	Sleeping	1.2	80
Cleaning (male)	3.5	236	Swimming (.25 mph)	4.4	299
Cooking	2.8	190	Tennis	6.1	414
Cycling (13 mph)	9.7	659	Volleyball	5.1	346
Cycling (5.5 mph)	3.0	204	Walking (3.75 mph)	4.4	299
Dressing/showering	1.6	106	Walking (2.5 mph)	3.0	204
Driving	1.7	117	Water skiing	7.0	476
Eating (sitting)	1.4	93	Weight lifting—heavy	9.0	612
Food shopping	3.6	245	Weight lifting—light	4.0	272
Football—touch	7.0	476	Window cleaning	3.5	240
Golf (using power cart)	3.6	244	Writing (sitting)	1.7	118

The values in Table 7-4 refer to total energy expenditure, including that needed to perform the physical activity, plus that needed for basal metabolism, the thermic effect of food, and thermogenesis. Use your diet-analysis software for your personal estimate.

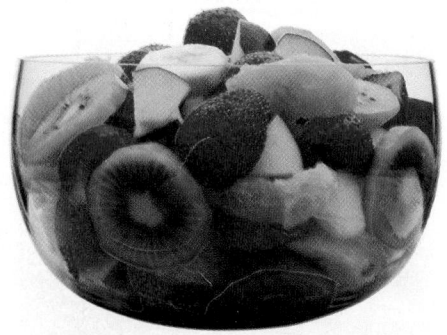

▲ Fruit is a great low-cal snack—high in nutrient density and low in calories.

aerobic dancing or jogging, if it is maintained. Moreover, activities of lighter intensity are less likely to lead to injuries. Some resistance exercises (weight training) also should be added to increase lean body mass and, in turn, fat use (see Chapter 10). As lean muscle mass increases, so will one's overall metabolic rate. An added benefit of including exercise in a weight-reduction program is maintenance of bone health.

Unfortunately, opportunities to expend calories in our daily lives are diminishing as technology systematically eliminates almost every reason to move our muscles. The easiest way to increase physical activity is to make it an enjoyable part of a daily routine. To start, one might pack a pair of athletic shoes and walk around the parking lot before coming home after school or work every day. Other ideas are avoiding elevators in favor of stairs and parking the car farther away from the shopping mall.

A pedometer is an inexpensive device that monitors activity as steps. A recommended goal for activity is to take at least 10,000 steps per day—typically we take half that many or less. A pedometer tracks this activity. Calorie counters, such as the Bodybugg, are new devices that track calorie expenditures throughout the day. The counters calculate calories by measuring heart rate, sweat rate, or heat loss and production. Like pedometers, calorie counters can motivate users to do more activity.

7.9 Behavior Modification—A Third Strategy for Weight Loss and Management

Controlling calorie intake also means modifying *problem* behaviors. Only the dieter can decide what behaviors are preventing calorie control. What events cause us to start (or stop) eating? What factors influence food choices?

The 2010 Dietary Guidelines identify the following behaviors as having the strongest evidence related to body weight:

- Focus on the total number of calories consumed.
- Monitor food intake.
- When eating out, choose smaller portions or lower-calorie options.
- Prepare, serve, and consume smaller portions of foods and beverages, especially those high in calories.
- Eat a nutrient-dense breakfast.
- Limit screen time.

Chain-breaking, stimulus control, cognitive restructuring, contingency management, and *self-monitoring* are behavior modification strategies used by psychologists that (Table 7-5) help place the problem in perspective and organize the intervention into manageable steps.

Chain-breaking separates behaviors that tend to occur together—for example, snacking on chips while watching television. Although these activities do not have to occur together, they often do. Dieters may need to break the chain reaction (see Rate Your Plate at the end of this chapter for more details).

Stimulus control puts us in charge of temptations. Options include pushing tempting food to the back of the refrigerator, removing fat-laden snacks from the kitchen counter, and avoiding the path by the vending machines. Provide a positive stimulus by keeping low-fat snacks available to satisfy hunger/appetite.

Cognitive restructuring changes our frame of mind. For example, after a hard day, avoid using alcohol or comfort foods as quick relief for stress. Instead, plan for healthful, relaxing activities for stress reduction. For example, take a walk around the neighborhood or have a satisfying talk with a friend.

Labeling some foods as "off limits" sets up an internal struggle to resist the urge to eat that food. This hopeless battle can keep us feeling deprived. We lose the fight. Managing food choices with the principle of moderation is best. If a favorite food becomes troublesome, place it off limits only temporarily, until it can be enjoyed in moderation.

Contingency management prepares one for situations that may trigger overeating (e.g., when snacks are served at a party) or hinder physical activity (e.g., rain).

A **self-monitoring** record can reveal patterns—such as unconscious overeating—that may explain problem eating habits. This record can encourage new habits that will counteract unwanted behaviors. Obesity experts note that this is the key behavioral tool to use in any weight-loss program (see Further Readings 4 and 6). See the margin for a list of free online tools available for self-monitoring.

Overall, it's important to address specific problems, such as snacking, compulsive eating, and mealtime overeating. Behavior Modification principles (review Table 7-5) are critical components of weight reduction and maintenance. Without them it is difficult to make lifelong lifestyle changes needed to meet weight-control goals.

Relapse Prevention Is Important

Preventing relapse is thought to be the hardest part of weight control—even harder than losing weight. A dieter needs to plan for lapses, not overreact, and take charge immediately. Change responses such as "I ate that cookie; I'm a failure" to "I ate that cookie, but I did well to stop after only one!" When dieters lapse from their diet plan, newly learned food habits should steer them back toward the plan. Without a strong behavioral program for **relapse prevention** in place, a lapse frequently turns into a relapse and a potential collapse. Once a pattern of poor food choices begins, dieters may feel

---

The motivation to lose weight and keep it off generally comes with a proverbial "flip of the switch," in which the desire to lose weight finally becomes more important than the desire to overeat.

chain-breaking Breaking the link between two or more behaviors that encourage overeating, such as snacking while watching television.

stimulus control Altering the environment to minimize the stimuli for eating—for example, removing foods from sight and storing them in kitchen cabinets.

cognitive restructuring Changing one's frame of mind regarding eating—for example, instead of using a difficult day as an excuse to overeat, substituting other pleasures for rewards, such as a relaxing walk with a friend.

contingency management Forming a plan of action to respond to a situation in which overeating is likely, such as when snacks are within arm's reach at a party.

self-monitoring Tracking foods eaten and conditions affecting eating; actions are usually recorded in a diary, along with location, time, and state of mind. This is a tool to help people understand more about their eating habits.

relapse prevention A series of strategies used to help prevent and cope with weight-control lapses, such as recognizing high-risk situations and deciding beforehand on appropriate responses.

Food and Activity Tracking
Here are some websites where you can record your food and physical activity online for free:

www.fitday.com
http://www.livestrong.com
www.mypyramidtracker.gov
http://nutritiondata.self.com
www.sparkpeople.com

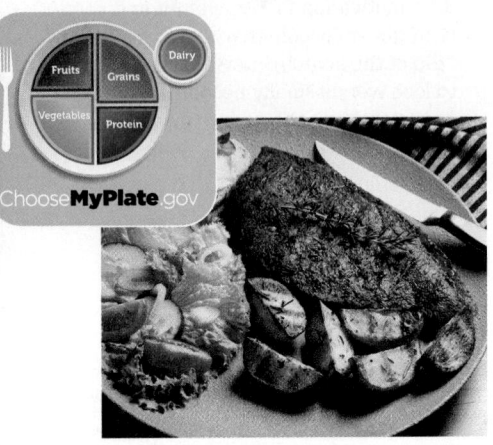

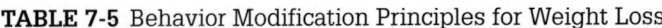

▲ Large portions of food, such as this steak, provide us with many opportunities to overeat. It takes much perseverance to eat sensibly. How do the portion sizes shown here compare to those recommended on MyPlate?

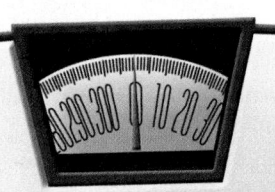

Successful weight losers and maintainers from the National Weight Control Registry:

- Eat a low-fat, high-carbohydrate diet (on average 25% of calorie intake as fat).
- Eat breakfast almost every day.
- Self-monitor by regularly weighing oneself and keeping a food journal.
- Exercise for about 1 hour per day.
- Eat at restaurants only once or twice per week.

Other recent studies support this approach, especially the last four characteristics.

TABLE 7-5 Behavior Modification Principles for Weight Loss

Shopping
1. Shop for food after eating—buy nutritious foods.
2. Shop from a list; limit purchases of irresistible "problem" foods. Shopping for fresh foods around the perimeter of the store first helps.
3. Avoid ready-to-eat foods.
4. Put off food shopping until absolutely necessary.

Plans
1. Plan to limit food intake as needed.
2. Substitute periods of physical activity for snacking.
3. Eat meals and snacks at scheduled times; don't skip meals.

Activities
1. Store food out of sight, preferably in the freezer, to discourage impulsive eating.
2. Eat all food in a "dining" area.
3. Keep serving dishes off the table, especially dishes of sauces and gravies.
4. Use smaller dishes and utensils.

Holidays and Parties
1. Drink fewer alcoholic beverages.
2. Plan eating behavior before parties.
3. Eat a low-calorie snack before parties.
4. Practice polite ways to decline food.
5. Don't get discouraged by an occasional setback.

Eating Behavior
1. Put fork down between mouthfuls.
2. Chew thoroughly before taking the next bite.
3. Leave some food on the plate.
4. Pause in the middle of the meal.
5. Do nothing else while eating (for example, reading, watching television).

Reward
1. Plan specific rewards for specific behavior (behavioral contracts).
2. Solicit help from family and friends and suggest how they can help you. Encourage family and friends to provide this help in the form of praise and material rewards.
3. Use self-monitoring records as basis for rewards.

Self-Monitoring
1. Note the time and place of eating.
2. List the type and amount of food eaten.
3. Record who is present and how you feel.
4. Use the diet diary to identify problem areas.

Cognitive Restructuring
1. Avoid setting unreasonable goals.
2. Think about progress, not shortcomings.
3. Avoid imperatives such as *always* and *never*.
4. Counter negative thoughts with positive restatements.

Portion Control
1. Make substitutions, such as a regular hamburger instead of a "quarter pounder" or cucumbers instead of croutons in salads.
2. Think small. Order the entrée and share it with another person. Order a cup of soup instead of a bowl or an appetizer in place of an entrée.
3. Use a doggie bag. Ask your server to put half the entrée in a doggie bag before bringing it to the table.

As we said at the start of this chapter, many of us need to become "defensive eaters." Know when to refuse food after satiety registers, and reduce portion sizes.

failure and stray farther from the plan. As the relapse lengthens, the diet plan collapses, and falls short of the weight-loss goal. Losing weight is difficult. Overall, maintenance of weight loss is fostered by the "3 *Ms*": motivation, movement, and monitoring.

Social Support Aids Behavioral Change

Healthy social support is helpful in weight control. Helping others understand how they can be supportive can make weight control easier. Family and friends can provide praise and encouragement. A registered dietitian or other weight-control professional can keep dieters accountable and help them learn from difficult situations. Long-term contact with a professional can be helpful for later weight maintenance. Groups of individuals attempting to lose weight or maintain losses can provide empathetic support.

Societal Efforts to Reduce Obesity

The incidence of obesity in the United States is now considered an epidemic. Improvement in the health of our nation requires an approach that includes many sectors. Although we ultimately make our own choices at an individual level, partnerships, programs, and policies that support healthy eating and active living must be coordinated. The 2010 Dietary Guidelines' Call to Action includes three guiding principles:

1. Ensure that all Americans have access to nutritious foods and opportunities for physical activity.
2. Facilitate individual behavior change through environmental strategies.
3. Set the stage for lifelong healthy eating, physical activity, and weight-management behaviors.

Public, private, and nonprofit organizations have begun to work together to address and reverse this public health crisis. For example, the U.S. Food and Drug Administration has brought together leaders from industry, government, academia, and the public health community to seek solutions to the obesity epidemic by making changes in foods eaten outside the home (restaurant and carry-out foods). These groups have collaborated and made recommendations to support the consumer's ability to manage calorie intake. Recommendations include "social marketing" programs that promote healthy eating and active living.

CRITICAL THINKING

With regard to readiness to lose weight, what would you say to a young woman who has just had a baby, needs to find a new job, and recently has gone back to school part-time?

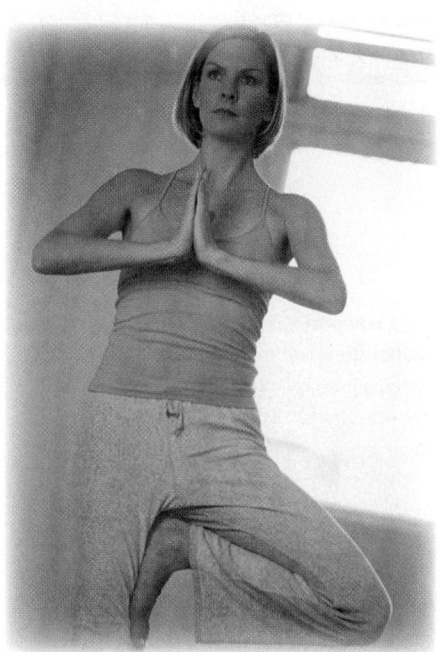

▲ Individuals who successfully maintain their weight loss employ a variety of strategies to cope with the stresses and challenges of changing problem behaviors.

CONCEPT CHECK

Increasing physical activity in daily life should be part of any weight-loss plan. Daily activity, such as walking and stair climbing, is recommended. Behavior Modification can improve conditions for losing weight. One key step is to break behavior chains that encourage overeating, such as snacking while watching television. Another tactic is to modify the environment to reduce temptation; for example, put foods into cupboards to keep them out of sight. In addition, rethinking attitudes about eating—for example, substituting pleasures other than food as a reward for coping with a stressful day—can be important for altering undesirable behavior. Advanced planning to prevent and deal with lapses is vital, as is rallying healthy social support. Finally, careful observation and recording of eating habits can reveal subtle cues that lead to overeating. Overall, weight loss and maintenance are fostered by controlling calorie intake, performing regular physical activity, and modifying "problem" behaviors.

7.10 Professional Help for Weight Loss

The first professional to see for advice about a weight-loss program is one's family physician. Doctors are best equipped to assess overall health and the appropriateness of weight loss. The physician may then recommend a registered dietitian for a specific weight-loss plan and answers to diet-related questions. Registered dietitians are uniquely qualified to help design a weight-loss plan because they understand both food composition and the psychological importance of food. Exercise physiologists can provide advice about programs to increase physical activity. The expense for such

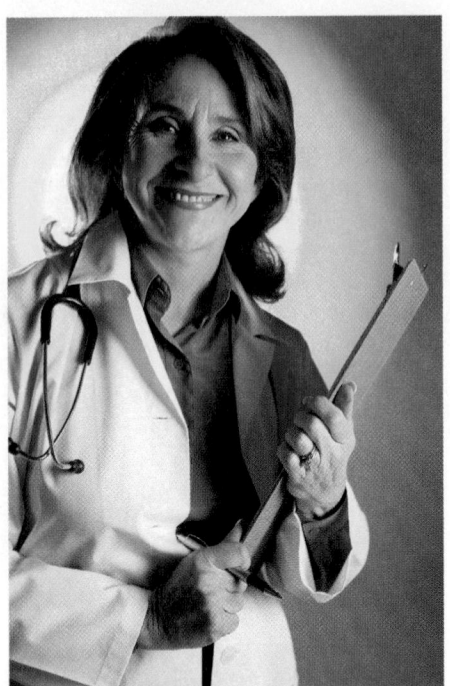

▲ All weight loss programs should begin with a visit to your family physician.

amphetamine A group of medications that induce stimulation of the central nervous system and have other effects in the body. Abuse is linked to physical and psychological dependence.

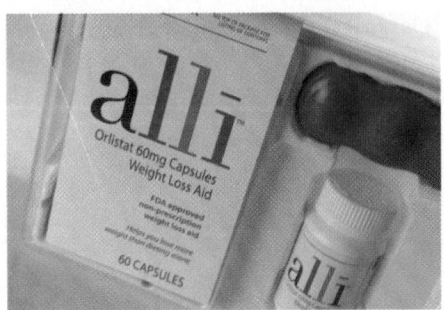

professional interventions is tax deductible in the United States in some cases (see a tax advisor) and often covered by health insurance plans if prescribed by a physician.

Many communities have a variety of weight-loss organizations. These include self-help groups, such as Take Off Pounds Sensibly and Weight Watchers. Other programs, such as Jenny Craig and Physicians' Weight Loss Center, are less desirable for the average dieter. Often, the employees are not registered dietitians or other appropriately trained health professionals. These programs also tend to be expensive because of their requirements for intense counseling or mandatory diet foods and supplements. In addition, the Federal Trade Commission has charged these and other commercial diet-program companies with misleading consumers through unsubstantiated weight-loss claims and deceptive testimonials.

North Americans are willing to try almost anything to shed unwanted pounds. Operation Waistline is a program designed by the U.S. Federal Trade Commission to terminate fraudulent claims being made by weight-loss charlatans with regard to diet products. The program hopes to put an end to the $6 billion spent annually in the United States on counterfeit products. The Enforma Natural Products Corporation had to pay $10 million in response to false claims for its "Fat Trapper" product.

Medications for Weight Loss

Candidates for medications for obesity include those with a BMI of 30 or more, or a BMI of 27 to 29.9 with weight-related health conditions, such as type 2 diabetes, cardiovascular disease, hypertension, or excess waist circumference; those with no contraindications to use the medication; and those ready to undertake lifestyle change. Drug therapy alone has not been found to be successful. Success with medications has been shown only in those who also modify their behavior, decrease calorie intake, and increase physical activity. In addition, if a person has not lost at least 4.4 pounds (2 kilograms) after 4 weeks, it is not likely that the person will benefit from further use of the medication.

Three main classes of medications have been used. An **amphetamine**-like medication (phenteramine [Fastin or Ionamin]) prolongs the activity of epinephrine and norepinephrine in the brain. This therapy is effective for some people in the short run but has not yet been proven effective in the long run. Most state medical boards limit use of this drug to 12 weeks unless the person is participating in a medical study using the product. The medication should not be used in pregnant or nursing women or those under 18 years of age.

The second class of medication approved by FDA for weight loss and the only weight-loss medication approved for long-term use is orlistat (Xenical). This medication reduces fat digestion by about 30% by inhibiting lipase enzyme action in the small intestine (Fig. 7-18). This cuts absorption of dietary fat by one-third for about 2 hours when taken along with a meal containing fat. This malabsorbed fat is deposited in the feces. *Fat intake has to be controlled*, however, because large amounts of fat in the feces cause numerous side effects, such as gas, bloating, and oily discharge. Interestingly, orlistat use can remind the person to follow a fat-controlled diet, as the symptoms resulting from consuming a high-fat meal are unpleasant and develop quickly. Orlistat is taken with each meal containing fat. The malabsorbed fat also carries fat-soluble vitamins into the feces, so the person taking orlistat must take a multivitamin and mineral supplement at bedtime. In this way, any micronutrients not absorbed during the day can be replaced; fat malabsorption from the dinner meal will not greatly influence micronutrient absorption in the late evening. A low-dose form of orlistat (alli™) is now available over the counter without a prescription.

Sibutramine (Meridia) is a third class of medication that was approved by FDA for weight loss and was available until October 2010. It enhances both norepinephrine and serotonin activity in the brain by reducing reuptake of these neurotransmitters by nerve cells. The neurotransmitters then remain active in the brain for

ZZZZZ

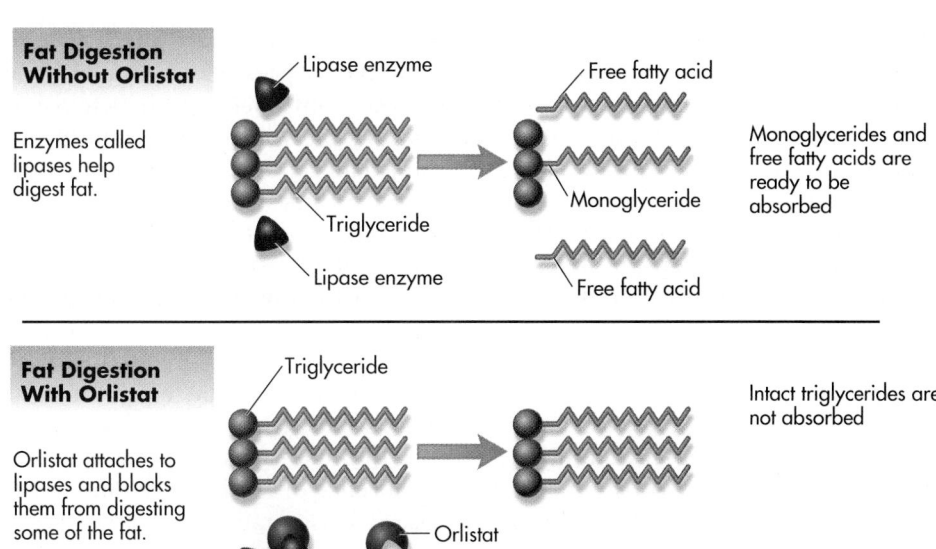

Fat Digestion Without Orlistat

Enzymes called lipases help digest fat.

Lipase enzyme

Triglyceride

Lipase enzyme

Free fatty acid

Monoglyceride

Free fatty acid

Monoglycerides and free fatty acids are ready to be absorbed

Fat Digestion With Orlistat

Orlistat attaches to lipases and blocks them from digesting some of the fat.

Triglyceride

Orlistat

Lipase enzyme

Intact triglycerides are not absorbed

FIGURE 7-18 ▶ Orlistat is a weight-loss drug that works in the digestive system to block digestion of about one-third of the fat in the food we eat. A low-dose form of this drug (alli™) is now available without a prescription.

a longer time and so prolong a sense of reduced hunger. The main effect is to moderately reduce appetite so that people eat less. Production of subutramine was voluntarily stopped at the request of FDA and based on increased risk of heart attacks and strokes observed in people taking sibutramine. Read more about this study in Newsworthy Nutrition.

Drug companies are working on many other types of medications and hopes that some of these will prove to be safe and effective for weight loss. In addition, physicians may prescribe medications not approved for weight loss but that have weight loss as a side effect. Certain antidepressants are an example. Such an application is termed *off-label*, because the product label does not include weight loss as an FDA-approved use. Over-the-counter medications and supplements are widely marketed as miracle cures for obesity, but in some cases, they do more harm than good (see Further Reading 11). Today more than ever, let the buyer beware concerning any purported weight-loss aid not prescribed by a physician.

Overall, in skilled hands, prescription medications can aid weight loss in some instances. However, they do not replace the need for reducing calorie intake, modifying "problem" behaviors, and increasing physical activity, both during and after therapy. Often, any weight loss during drug treatment can be attributed mostly to the individual's hard work at balancing calorie intake with calorie output.

Treatment of Severe Obesity

Severe (morbid) obesity, having a BMI greater than or equal to 40 or weighing at least 100 pounds over healthy body weight (or twice one's healthy body weight), requires professional treatment. Because of the serious health implications of severe obesity, drastic measures may be necessary. Such treatments are recommended only when traditional diets and medications fail. Drastic weight-loss procedures are not without side effects, both physical and psychological, making careful monitoring by a physician a necessity.

NEWSWORTHY NUTRITION | **Popular weight-loss drug withdrawn from the market**

In October 2010, the FDA withdrew the obesity drug sibutramine (Meridia) from the market based on the results of the Sibutramine Cardiovascular OUTcomes Trial. This study evaluated the cardiovascular safety of the drug in patients at high risk for cardiovascular events. Subjects receiving sibutramine long-term (~3.4 years) had 16% increased risk of nonfatal heart attacks and strokes. Based on these results and the small difference in weight loss among those taking the drug and those receiving a placebo, sibutramine should not be used in patients with preexisting cardiovascular disease. At the time of its withdrawal from the market in the United States and several other countries, about 100,000 people in the United States were taking Meridia.

Source: James WPT and others: Effect of sibutramine on cardiovascular outcomes in overweight and obese subjects. *New England Journal of Medicine* 363(10):905, 2010 (see Further Reading 5).

connect NUTRITION   **Check out the connect site** www.mcgrawhillconnect.com **to further explore long-term weight-loss medications.**

very-low-calorie diet (VLCD) Known also as *protein-sparing modified fast (PSMF)*, this diet allows a person 400 to 800 kcal per day, often in liquid form. Of this, 120 to 480 kcal is carbohydrate, and the rest is mostly high-quality protein.

bariatrics The medical specialty focusing on the treatment of obesity.

adjustable gastric banding A restrictive procedure in which the opening from the esophagus to the stomach is reduced by a hollow gastric band.

gastroplasty Gastric bypass surgery performed on the stomach to limit its volume to approximately 30 milliliters. Also referred to as stomach stapling.

Very-Low-Calorie Diets. If more traditional diet changes have failed, treating severe obesity with a **very-low-calorie diet (VLCD)** is possible, especially if the person has obesity-related diseases that are not well controlled (e.g., hypertension, type 2 diabetes). Some researchers believe that people with body weight greater than 30% above their healthy weight are appropriate candidates. VLCD programs are offered almost exclusively by medical centers or clinics since careful monitoring by a physician is crucial throughout this very restrictive form of weight loss. Major health risks include heart problems and gallstones. Optifast is one such commercial program. In general, the diet allows a person to consume only 400 to 800 kcal per day, often in liquid form. (These diets were previously known as protein-sparing modified fasts.) Of this amount, about 30 to 120 grams (120 to 480 kcal) is carbohydrate. The rest is high-quality protein, in the amount of about 70 to 100 grams per day (280 to 400 kcal). This low carbohydrate intake often causes ketosis, which may decrease hunger. However, the main reasons for weight loss are the minimal energy consumption and the absence of food choice. About 3 to 4 pounds can be lost per week; men tend to lose at a faster rate than women. When physical activity and resistance training augment this diet, a greater loss of adipose tissue occurs.

Weight regain remains a nagging problem, especially without a behavioral and physical activity component. If behavioral therapy and physical activity supplement a long-term support program, maintenance of the weight loss is more likely but still difficult. Any program under consideration should include a maintenance plan. Today, antiobesity medications also may be included in this phase of the program.

Bariatric Surgery. **Bariatrics** is the medical specialty focusing on the treatment of obesity. Bariatric surgery is only considered for people with severe obesity and includes operations aimed at promoting weight loss. Two types of bariatric operations are now common and effective (see Further Readings 7 and 10). Both procedures can be performed using an open (8- to 10-inch) incision in the middle of the abdomen or a laparoscopic approach in which several smaller (½- to 2-inch) incisions are used that allow cameras and instruments to enter the abdomen. **Adjustable gastric banding** (also known as the lap-band procedure) is a restrictive procedure in which the opening from the esophagus to the stomach is reduced by a hollow gastric band. This creates a small pouch and a narrow passage into the rest of the stomach and thus decreases the amount of food that can be eaten comfortably. The band can be inflated or deflated via an access port placed just under the skin. Studies have demonstrated that adjustable gastric banding is more effective long term than a very low-calorie diet (500 kcal) for people who are about 50 pounds overweight.

Gastric bypass (also called **gastroplasty** or stomach stapling) is another bariatric surgical procedure used for treating severe obesity. The most common and effective approach (the Roux-en-Y gastric bypass procedure) works by reducing the stomach capacity to about 30 milliliters (the volume of one egg or shot glass) and bypassing a short segment of the upper small intestine (Fig. 7-19). Weight loss is promoted mainly because overeating of solid foods is now less likely due to rapid satiety and discomfort or vomiting after overeating. About 75% of people with severe obesity eventually lose 50% or more of excess body weight with this method. In addition, the surgery's success at long-term maintenance often leads to dramatic health improvements, such as reduced blood pressure and elimination of type 2 diabetes. Risks of the surgery include bleeding, blood clots, hernias, and severe infections. In the long run, nutrient deficiencies can develop if the person is not adequately treated in the years following the surgery. Anemia and bone loss might then be the result. Risk of death from this demanding surgery can be as high as 2% (less risk with experienced surgeons).

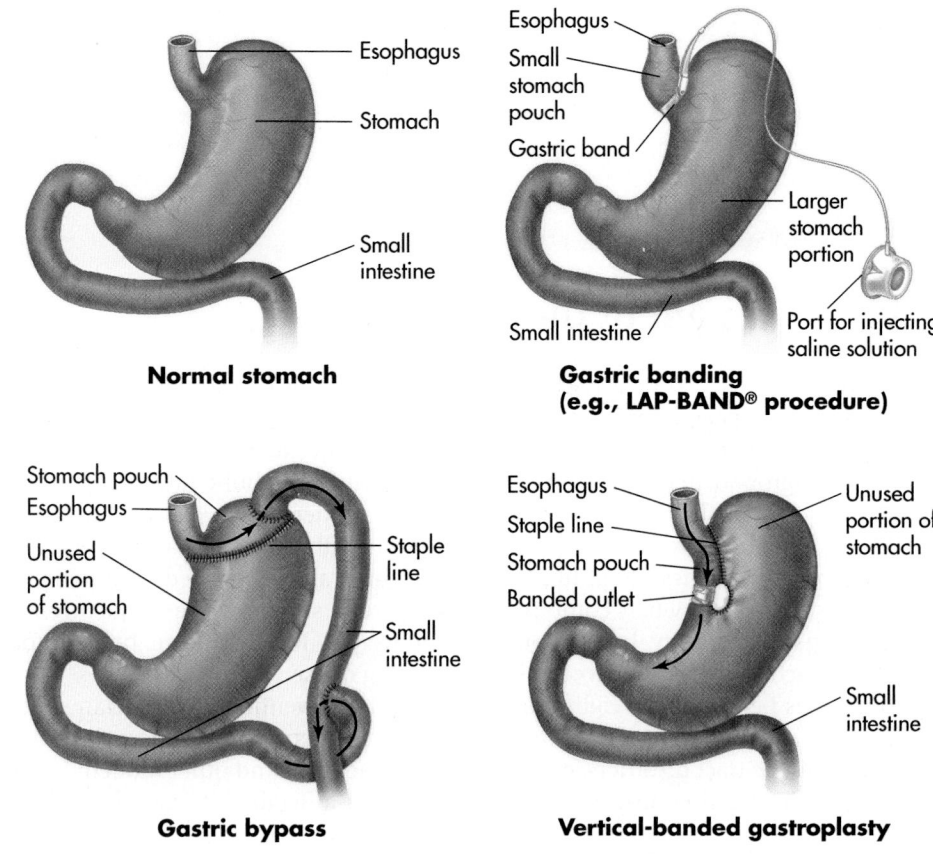

FIGURE 7-19 ▶ The most common forms of gastroplasty for treating severe obesity. The gastric bypass is the most effective method. In banded gastroplasty, the band prevents expansion of the outlet for the stomach pouch.

Patient selection criteria for bariatric surgery include:

- BMI should be greater than 40.
- BMI between 35 and 40 is considered when there are serious obesity-related health concerns.
- Obesity must be present for a minimum of 5 years, with several nonsurgical attempts to lose weight.
- There should be no history of alcoholism or major untreated psychiatric disorders.

The person also must consider that the surgery is costly and may not be covered by medical insurance. The average cost for gastric bypass produres is $18,000 to $35,000 and for adjustable gastric banding is $17,000 to $30,000. In addition, follow-up surgery is often needed after weight loss to correct stretched skin, previously filled with fat. Furthermore, the surgery necessitates major lifestyle changes, such as the need to plan frequent, small meals. Therefore, the dieter who has chosen this drastic approach to weight loss faces months of difficult adjustments.

MAKING DECISIONS

Lipectomy

Spot-reducing by using diet and physical activity is not possible. "Problem" local fat deposits can be reduced in size, however, using suction lipectomy. Lipectomy or liposuction means surgical removal of fat. A pencil-thin tube is inserted into an incision in the skin, and the fat tissue, such as that in the buttocks and thigh area, is suctioned. This procedure carries some risks, such as infection; lasting depressions in the skin; and blood clots, which can lead to kidney failure and sometimes death. The procedure is designed to help a person lose about 4 to 8 pounds per treatment. Cost is about $1800 per site; total costs range as high as $2600 to $9000.

CONCEPT CHECK

Severely obese people who have failed to lose weight with conservative weight-loss strategies may consider other options. Their doctors may recommend undergoing surgery such as reducing the volume of the stomach to approximately 30 milliliters or following a very-low-calorie diet plan containing 400 to 800 kcal per day. Careful monitoring by a physician is crucial in both cases.

7.11 Treatment of Underweight

underweight A body mass index below 18.5. The cutoff is less precise than for obesity because this condition has been less studied.

Underweight is defined by a BMI less than 18.5 and can be caused by a variety of factors, such as cancer, infectious disease (e.g., tuberculosis), digestive tract disorders (e.g., chronic inflammatory bowel disease), and excessive dieting or physical activity. Genetic background may also lead to a higher resting metabolic rate, a slight body frame, or both. Health problems associated with underweight include the loss of menstrual function, low bone mass, complications with pregnancy and surgery, and slow recovery after illness. Significant underweight is also associated with increased death rates, especially when combined with cigarette smoking. We frequently hear about the risks of obesity, but seldom of underweight. In our culture, being underweight is much more socially acceptable than being obese.

Sometimes being underweight requires medical intervention. A physician should be consulted first to rule out hormonal imbalances; depression; cancer; infectious disease; digestive tract disorders; excessive physical activity; and other hidden disease, such as a serious eating disorder (see Chapter 11 for a detailed discussion of eating disorders).

The causes of underweight are not altogether different from the causes of obesity. Internal and external satiety-signal irregularities, the rate of metabolism, hereditary tendencies, and psychological traits can all contribute to underweight.

In growing children, the high demand for calories to support physical activity and growth can cause underweight. During growth spurts in adolescence, active children may not take the time to consume enough calories to support their needs. Moreover, gaining weight can be a formidable task for an underweight person. An extra 500 kcal per day may be required to gain weight, even at a slow pace, in part because of the increased expenditure of energy in thermogenesis. In contrast to the weight loser, the weight gainer may need to increase portion sizes.

When underweight requires a specific intervention, one approach for treating adults is to gradually increase their consumption of calorie-dense foods, especially those high in vegetable fat. Italian cheeses, nuts, and granola can be good calorie sources with low saturated-fat content. Dried fruit and bananas are good fruit choices. If eaten at the end of a meal, they don't cause early satiety. The same advice applies to salads and soups. Underweight people should replace such foods as diet soft drinks with good calorie sources, such as fruit juices and smoothies.

Encouraging a regular meal and snack schedule also aids in weight gain and maintenance. Sometimes underweight people have experienced stress at work or have been too busy to eat. Making regular meals a priority may not only help them attain an appropriate weight but also help with digestive disorders, such as constipation, sometimes associated with irregular eating times.

Excessively physically active people can reduce activity. If their weight remains low, they can add muscle mass through a resistance training (weight-lifting) program, but they must also increase their calorie intake to support that physical activity. Otherwise, weight gain will be hindered.

If these efforts fail to help a person achieve a healthy weight, they should at least prevent the health problems associated with being underweight. After achieving that, they may have to accept their lean frames.

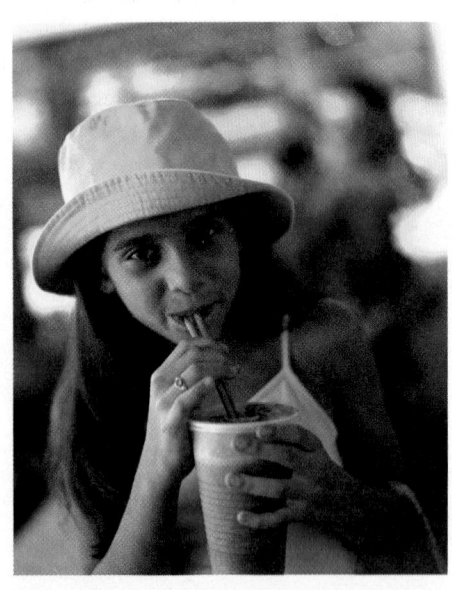

▲ Underweight people should increase their consumption of calorie-dense foods, such as smoothies, that are also loaded with nutrients.

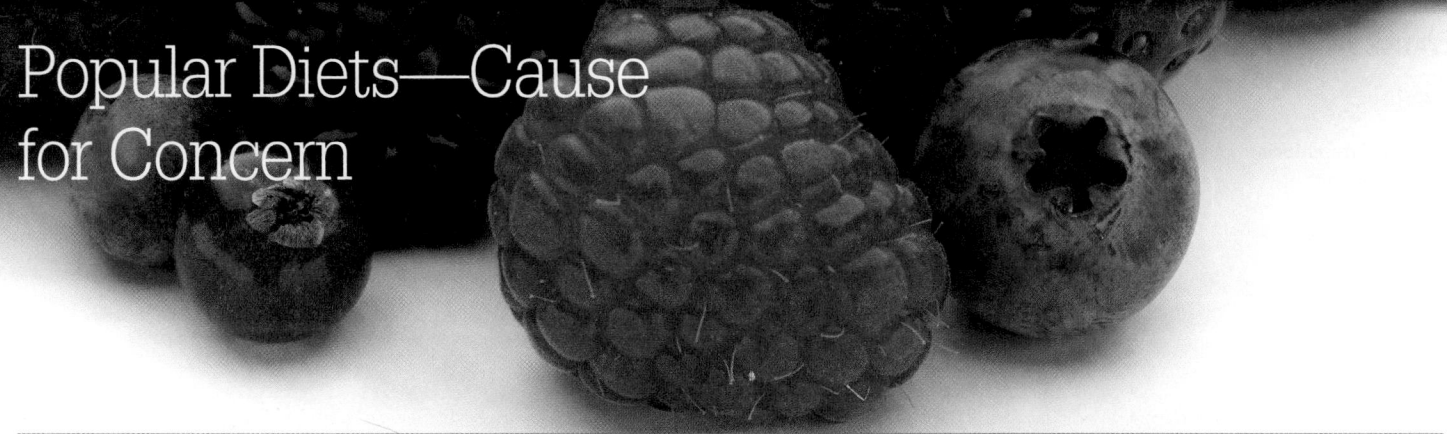

Popular Diets—Cause for Concern

Many overweight people try to help themselves by using the latest popular (also called fad) diet book. But, as you will see, most of these diets do not help, and some can actually harm those who follow them (Table 7-6). Research has shown that early dieting and other unhealthful weight control practices in adolescents lead to an increased risk of weight gain, overweight, and eating disorders.

Recently, weight-loss experts came together at the request of the USDA to evaluate weight-loss diets. They came to this conclusion: Forget these fads when it comes to dieting. Most of the popular diets are nutritionally inadequate and include certain foods that people would not normally choose to consume in large amounts. The experts stated that eating less of one's favorite foods and becoming more physically active can be much more effective when trying to implement a weight-loss diet. People need a plan they can live with in the long run so that weight control becomes permanent. The goal should be weight control over a lifetime, not immediate weight loss. Every popular diet leads to some immediate weight loss simply because daily in-take is monitored and monotonous food choices are typically part of the plan. A well-known example of the effectiveness of monotony contributing to weight loss is the experience of Jared Fogle. He ate primarily Subway sandwiches for 11 months and lost 245 pounds. He notes however that this is not a miracle diet—it takes a lot of hard work to lead to the success he experienced. There are also many other examples where diet monotony has led to weight loss. Overall, a traditional moderate diet coupled with regular physical activity is adequate for weight loss.

People on diets often fall within a healthy BMI of 18.5 to 25. Rather than worrying about weight loss, these individuals should be focusing on a healthy lifestyle that allows for weight maintenance. Incorporating necessary lifestyle changes and learning to accept one's particular body characteristics should be the overriding goals.

The dieting mania can be viewed as mostly a social problem, stemming from unrealistic weight expectations (especially for women) and lack of appreciation for the natural variety in body shape and weight. Not every woman can look like a fashion model, nor can every man look like a Greek god, but all of us can strive for good health and, if physically possible, an active lifestyle.

The size-acceptance nondiet movement, "Health at Every Size," has attempted to shift the paradigm away from the use of "popular" weight loss diets. The goals of the movement are all independent of body weight and include improvement of self-image, normalization of eating behavior, and increase in physical activity.

How to Recognize an Unreliable Diet

The criteria for evaluating weight-loss programs with regard to their safety and effectiveness were discussed previously (review Fig. 7-15). In contrast, unreliable diets typically share some common characteristics:

1. They promote quick weight loss. This is the primary temptation that the dieter falls for. As mentioned, this initial weight loss primarily results from water loss and lean muscle mass depletion.

2. They limit food selections and dictate specific rituals, such as eating only fruit for breakfast or cabbage soup every day.

3. They use testimonials from famous people and tie the diet to well-known cities, such as Beverly Hills and South Beach.

4. They bill themselves as cure-alls. These diets claim to work for everyone, whatever the type of obesity or the person's specific strengths and weaknesses.

5. They often recommend expensive supplements.

6. No attempts are made to change eating habits permanently. Dieters follow the diet until the desired weight is reached and then revert to old eating habits—they are told, for example, to eat rice for a month, lose weight, and then return to old habits.

7. They are generally critical of and skeptical about the scientific community. The lack of a quick fix from medical and dietetic professionals has led some of the public to seek advice from those who appear to have the answer.

8. They claim that there is no need to exercise.

Probably the cruelest characteristic of these diets is that they essentially guarantee failure for the dieter. The diets are not designed for permanent weight loss. Habits are not changed, and the food selection is so limited that the person cannot follow the diet in the long run. Although dieters assume they have lost fat, they have lost mostly muscle and other lean tissue mass. As soon as they begin

TABLE 7-6 Summary of Popular Diet Approaches to Weight Control

Approach	Examples*	Characteristics	Dietitian's Review
Moderate calorie restriction	• *Dieting for Dummies* (2003) • *Dieting with the Duchess* (2000) • *Dr. Phil's Ultimate Weight Solution* (2003, 2005) • *Flat Belly Diet* (2008) • *Jenny Craig* (1980s) • *Picture Perfect Weight Loss* (2003) • *Slim-fast* (1980s) • *Sonoma Diet* (2005) • *Volumetrics* (2000) • *Wedding Dress Diet* (2000) • *Weight Watchers* (1960s) • *You on a Diet* (2006)	• Generally 1200 to 1800 kcal per day • Moderate fat intake • Reasonable balance of macronutrients • Encourage exercise • May use behavioral approach	These diets are acceptable if a multivitamin and mineral supplement is used and permission of family physician is granted.
Carbohydrate focused	• *Carbohydrate Addicts Diet* (1993, 2001) • *Dr. Atkin's Diet Revolution* (1973, 2002) • *Dr. Gott's No Flour, No Sugar Diet* (2006) • *Eat, Drink & Weigh Less* (2006) • *G.I. (Glycemic Index) Diet* (2003) • *Healthy for Life* (2005) • *New Glucose Revolution* (2002) • Nutrisystem (2003) • *South Beach Diet* (especially initial phases) (2003) • *Sugar Busters Diet* (1998, 2003) • *Zone Diet* (1995)	• Restricted carbohydrate diets generally advise consumption of less than 100 grams of carbohydrate per day • Some plans focus on carbohydrate choices (e.g., choosing low rather than high glycemic index foods)	Selecting high-fiber, whole-grain sources of carbohydrates is an advisable practice for weight control and prevention of several chronic diseases. However, severe carbohydrate restriction may lead to ketosis, reduced exercise capacity (due to poor glycogen stores in the muscles), excessive animal fat intake, constipation, headaches, halitosis (bad breath), and muscle cramps. Severe carbohydrate restriction is not a nutritionally sound, long-term, weight-loss solution.
Low fat	• *20/30 Fat and Fiber Diet Plan* (2000) • *Complete Hip and Thigh Diet* (1989, 1999) • *Eat More, Weigh Less* (1993, 2001) • *Fit or Fat* (1977, 2005) • *Foods That Cause You to Lose Weight* (1992, 2003) • *McDougall Program* (1983, 1995) • *Pritikin Diet* (1984, 1995) • *Rice Diet Solution* (2005) • *T-Factor Diet* (1989, 2001) • *Okinawa Program* (2002)	• Generally less than 20% of calories from fat • Limited (or elimination of) animal protein sources; also limited plant oils, nuts, seeds	Low-fat diet plans are not necessarily to be avoided, but certain aspects may be unacceptable. Some potentially negative outcomes include flatulence, poor mineral absorption (from excess fiber intake), and a sense of deprivation (due to limited food choices).
Novelty diets	• *17-Day Diet* (2011) • *3-Hour Diet* (2005) • *Beverly Hills Diet* (1981, 1996) • *Cabbage-Soup Diet* (2004) • *Eat Right 4 Your Type* (1996) • *Fat Smash Diet* (2006) • *Fit for Life* (1987, 2001) • *Metabolic Typing Diet* (2002) • *New Hilton Head Metabolism Diet* (1983, 1996) • *Ultrametabolism* (2006) • *Weigh Down Diet* (2002)	• Promote certain nutrients, foods, or combinations of foods as having unique, magical, or previously undiscovered qualities	Novelty diets are usually not nutritionally balanced, thus malnutrition is a possible result. Also, failure to make long-term changes may lead to relapse, and unrealistic food choices lead to possible bingeing.

*Dates listed are original release date followed by most recent release date, if applicable.

eating normally again, much of the lost tissue is replaced. In a matter of weeks, most of the lost weight is back. The dieter appears to have failed, when actually the diet has failed. The gain and loss cycle is called weight cycling or "yo-yo" dieting. This whole scenario can add more blame and guilt, challenging the self-worth of the dieter. It can also come with some health costs, such as increased upper-body fat deposition. If someone needs help losing weight, professional help is advised. It is unfortunate that current trends suggest that people are spending more time and money on "quick fixes" rather than on such professional help.

Types of Popular Diets

Low- or Restricted-Carbohydrate Approaches

Low-carbohydrate diets have recently been the most popular diets. The low-carbohydrate intake leads to less glycogen synthesis, and therefore less water in the body (about 3 grams of water are stored per gram of glycogen). As discussed in Chapter 4, a very-low-carbohydrate intake also forces the liver to produce needed glucose. The source of carbons for this glucose is mostly proteins from tissues such as muscle resulting in loss of protein tissue, about 72% water. Essential ions, such as potassium are also lost in the urine. With the loss of glycogen stores, lean tissue and water, the dieter loses weight very rapidly. When a normal diet is resumed, the protein tissue is rebuilt and the weight is regained.

Although low-carbohydrate diets work in the short run primarily because they limit total food intake, recent results indicate that low-carbohydrate diets may be effective alternatives to low-fat diets. In a recent 2-year study published in the New England Journal of Medicine, moderately obese adults on a low-carbohydrate diet lost and kept off about 12 pounds, compared to 10 pounds for those following the traditional Mediterranean diet, and 7 pounds for those on a restricted-fat plan.

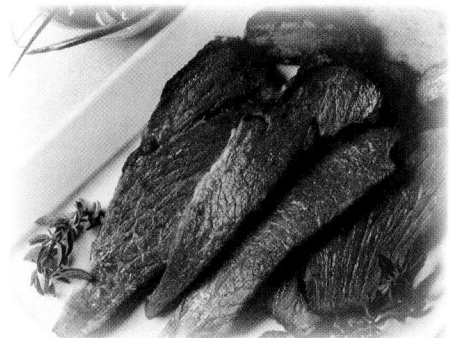

▲ In time, the very-low-carbohydrate, high-protein diets typically leave a person wanting more variety in meals, and so the diets are abandoned. Dropout rates are high on these diets.

The most popular diet using a low-carbohydrate approach is the Dr. Atkins' New Diet Revolution. More moderate approaches are found in the various Zone diets (40% of calorie intake as carbohydrate), Sugar Busters diet, and the South Beach diet (especially initial phases).

Carbohydrate-Focused Diets

Several recent diets, including Sugar Busters the Glucose Revolution, and Eat, Drink and Weigh Less, do not restrict carbohydrates, but rather emphasize the "good" carbohydrates in place of the "bad" or "harmful" ones. These diets recommend eating plenty of fruits, vegetables, whole grains, and cutting out simple sugars and processed grains. The carbohydrate-focused diets rely largely on low glycemic index and low glycemic load foods. In theory, these foods will cause a slow, steady rise in blood sugar, which will help control hunger.

Low-Fat Approaches

The very-low-fat diets contain approximately 5% to 10% of calories as fat and are very high in carbohydrates. The most notable are the Pritikin Diet and the Dr. Dean Ornish "Eat More, Weigh Less" diet plans. This approach is not harmful for healthy adults, but it is difficult to follow. People are quickly bored with this type of diet because they cannot eat many of their favorite foods. These dieters eat primarily grains, fruits, and vegetables, which most people cannot do for very long. Eventually, the person wants some foods higher in fat or protein. These diets are just too different from the typical North American diet for many adults to follow consistently, but may be acceptable for some people.

Novelty Diets

A variety of diets are built on gimmicks. Some novelty diets emphasize one food or food group and exclude almost all others. A rice diet was designed in the 1940s to lower blood pressure; now it has resurfaced as a weight-loss diet. The first phase consists of eating only rice and fruit. On the Beverly Hills Diet, you eat mostly fruit.

The rationale behind these diets is that you can eat only rice or fruit for just so long before becoming bored and, in theory, reducing your calorie intake. However,

chances are that you will abandon the diet entirely before losing much weight.

The most questionable of the novelty diets propose that "food gets stuck in your body." Fit for Life, the Beverly Hills Diet, and Eat Great, Lose Weight are examples. The supposition is that food gets stuck in the intestine, putrefies, and creates toxins, which invade the blood and cause disease. In response, recommendations are to not consume meat with potatoes or to consume fruits only after noon. These recommendations make no physiological sense.

Meal Replacements

Meal replacements come in many forms, including beverages or formulas, frozen or shelf-stable entrees, and meal or snack bars. Most meal replacements are fortified with vitamins and minerals and are appropriate to replace one or two regular meals or snacks per day. Although they are not a "magic bullet" for weight loss, they have been shown to help some people lose weight. Advantages of these convenient products are that they provide portion- and calorie-controlled foods that can serve as a visual education on appropriate portion sizes.

Quackery Is Characteristic of Many Popular Diets

Many popular diets fall under the category of quackery—people taking advantage of others. They usually involve a product or service that costs a considerable amount of money. Often, those offering the product or service don't realize that they are promoting quackery, because they were victims themselves. For example, they tried the product and by pure coincidence it worked for them, so they wish to sell it to all their friends and relatives.

Numerous other gimmicks for weight loss have come and gone and are likely to resurface. If in the future an important aid for weight loss is discovered, you can feel confident that major journals, such as the *Journal of the American Dietetic Association*, the *Journal of the American Medical Association*, or *The New England Journal of Medicine*, will report it. You don't need to rely on paperback books, infomercials, billboards, or newspaper advertisements for information about weight loss.

Case Study Choosing a Weight-Loss Program

Joe has a hectic schedule. During the day he works full-time at a warehouse distribution center filling orders. At night, three times a week, he attends class at the local community college in pursuit of computer certification. On weekends he likes to watch sports on TV, spend time with family and friends, and study. Joe has little time to think about what he eats—convenience rules. He stops for coffee and a pastry on his way to work, has a burger or pizza for lunch at a quick service restaurant, and for dinner picks up fried chicken or fish at the drive-through on his way to class. Unfortunately, over the past few years Joe's weight has been climbing. Watching a game on television a few nights ago, he saw an infomercial for a product that promises he can eat large portions of tasty foods but not gain weight. A famous actor supports the claim that this product allows one to eat at will and not gain weight. This claim is tempting to Joe.

Answer the following questions, and check your response in Appendix A.

1. Has Joe been experiencing positive or negative energy balance over the past few years?
2. What aspects of Joe's lifestyle (other than diet) are causing this effect on his energy balance? What changes could Joe make in his habits to promote weight loss or maintenance?
3. What changes could Joe make in his diet that would promote weight loss or maintenance?
4. Why should Joe be skeptical of the claims he heard about the weight-loss product in the infomercial?
5. What advice can you offer Joe for evaluation of weight-loss programs?

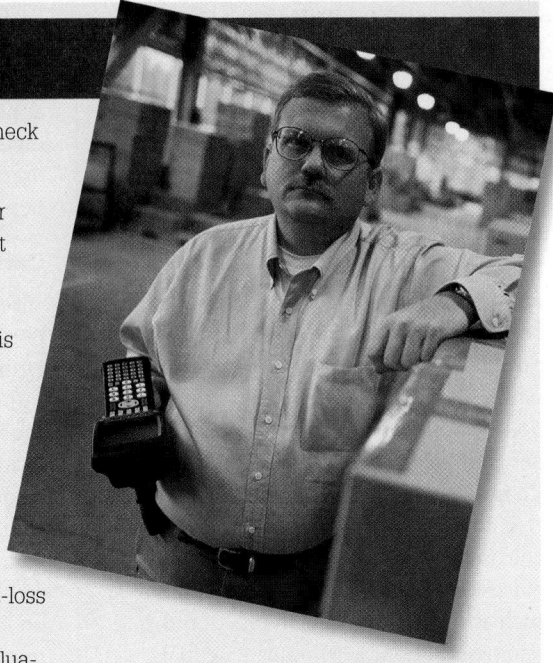

▲ What changes can Joe make in his daily routine and diet to stop his weight gain?

Summary (Numbers refer to numbered sections in the chapter.)

7.1 Energy balance considers energy intake and energy output. Negative energy balance occurs when energy output surpasses energy intake, resulting in weight loss. Positive energy balance occurs when calorie intake is greater than output, resulting in weight gain.

Basal metabolism, the thermic effect of food, physical activity, and thermogenesis account for total energy use by the body. Basal metabolism, which represents the minimum amount of calories required to keep the resting, awake body alive, is primarily affected by lean body mass, surface area, and thyroid hormone concentrations. Physical activity is energy use above that expended at rest. The thermic effect of food describes the increase in metabolism that facilitates digestion, absorption, and processing of the nutrients recently consumed. Thermogenesis is heat production caused by shivering when cold, fidgeting, and other stimuli. In a sedentary person, about 70% to 80% of energy use is accounted for by basal metabolism and the thermic effect of food.

7.2 Energy use by the body can be measured as heat given off by direct calorimetry or as oxygen used by indirect calorimetry. A person's Estimated Energy Requirement can be calculated based on the following factors: gender, height, weight, age, and amount physical activity.

7.3 A person of healthy weight shows good health and performs daily activities without weight-related problems. A body mass index (weight in kilograms ÷ height² in meters) of 18.5 to 25 is one measure of healthy weight. A healthy weight is best determined in conjunction with a thorough health evaluation by a physician. A body mass index of 25 to 29.9 represents overweight. Obesity is defined as a total body fat percentage over 25% (men) or 35% (women) or a body mass index of 30 or more.

7.4 If calorie intake exceeds output, an energy imbalance occurs that results in overweight. Fat distribution greatly determines health risks from obesity. Upper-body fat storage, as measured by a waist circumference greater than 40 inches (102 centimeters) for men or 35 inches (88 centimeters) for women typically results in higher risks of hypertension, cardiovascular disease, and type 2 diabetes than does lower-body fat storage.

7.5 Both genetic (nature) and environmental (nurture) factors can increase the risk of obesity. The set-point theory proposes that we have a genetically predetermined body weight or body fat content, which the body regulates.

7.6 A sound weight-loss program meets the dieter's nutritional needs by emphasizing a wide variety of low-calorie, bulky foods; adapts to the dieter's habits; consists of readily obtainable foods; strives to change poor eating habits; stresses regular physical activity; and stipulates the supervision by a physician if weight is to be lost rapidly or if the person is over the age of 40 (men) or 50 (women) and plans to perform substantially greater physical activity than usual.

7.7 A pound of adipose tissue contains about 3500 kcal. Loss or gain of a pound of adipose tissue—the fat itself plus lean support tissue—represents approximately 3300 kcal. Thus, if energy output exceeds calorie intake by about 500 kcal per day, a pound of adipose tissue can be lost per week.

7.8 Physical activity as part of a weight-loss program should be focused on duration rather than intensity. Ideally, vigorous activity for 60 minutes should be part of each day to prevent adult weight gain.

7.9 Behavior modification is a vital part of a weight-loss program because the dieter may have many habits that discourage weight maintenance. Specific behavior modification techniques, such as stimulus control and self-monitoring, can be used to help change problem behavior.

7.10 Medications to blunt appetite, such as phenteramine (Fastin), can aid weight-reduction strategies. Orlistat (Xenical) reduces fat absorption from a meal when taken with the meal. Weight-loss drugs are reserved for those who are obese or have weight-related problems, and they must be administered under close physician supervision.

The treatment of severe obesity may include surgery to reduce stomach volume to approximately 30 milliliters (1 ounce) or very-low-calorie diets containing 400 to 800 kcal per day. Both of these measures should be reserved for people who have failed at more conservative approaches to weight loss. They also require close medical supervision.

7.11 Underweight can be caused by a variety of factors, such as excessive physical activity and genetic background. Sometimes being underweight requires medical attention. A physician should be consulted first

to rule out underlying disease. The underweight person may need to increase portion sizes and learn to like calorie-dense foods. In addition, encouraging a regular meal and snack schedule aids in weight gain, as well as weight maintenance.

N&YH Many overweight people try popular diets that most often are not helpful and may actually be harmful. Unreliable diets typically share some common characteristics, including promoting quick weight loss, limiting food selections, using testimonials as proof, and requiring no exercise.

Check Your Knowledge (Answers to the following questions are below.)

1. Decreasing energy intake by about 500 kcal per day would mean a loss of 1 pound of body fat stores in _____ days.
   a. 2
   b. 7
   c. 10
   d. 14

2. Thermic effect of food represents the energy cost of
   a. chewing food.
   b. peristalsis
   c. basal metabolism.
   d. digesting, absorbing, and packaging nutrients.

3. A well-designed diet should
   a. increase physical activity.
   b. alter problem behaviors.
   c. reduce energy intake.
   d. All of the above.

4. All of the following factors are associated with a higher basal metabolic rate *except*
   a. stress.
   b. starvation.
   c. fever.
   d. pregnancy.

5. The intent of bariatric surgery is to
   a. limit stomach volume.
   b. speed transit time.
   c. surgically remove adipose tissue.
   d. prevent snacking.

6. Basal metabolism
   a. represents about 30% of total energy expenditure.
   b. is energy used to maintain heartbeat, respiration, and other basic functions and daily activities.
   c. represents about 60% to 70% of total calories used by the body during a day.
   d. includes energy to digest food.

7. Dr. Atkins' New Diet Revolution, The Zone, and the South Beach Diet are all examples of low- _____ diets.
   a. fat
   b. carbohydrate
   c. protein
   d. fiber

8. Probably the most important reason for obesity today in the United States is
   a. watching TV.
   b. snacking practices.
   c. inactivity.
   d. eating French fries.

9. The major goal for weight reduction in the treatment of obesity is the loss of
   a. weight.
   b. body fat.
   c. body water.
   d. body protein.

10. For most adults, the greatest portion of their energy expenditure is for
    a. physical activity.
    b. sleeping.
    c. basal metabolism.
    d. the thermic effect of food.

Answers: 1. b (LO 7.6), 2. d (LO 7.2), 3. d (LO 7.6), 4. b (LO 7.1), 5. a (LO 7.10), 6. c (LO 7.1), 7. b (LO 7.12), 8. c (LO 7.5), 9. b (LO 7.6), 10. c (LO 7.1)

Study Questions (Numbers refer to Learning Outcomes)

1. After reexamining the nature and nurture aspects of weight control, propose two hypotheses for the development of obesity. **(LO 7.5)**

2. Propose two hypotheses for the development of obesity, based on the four contributors to energy expenditure. **(LO 7.1)**

3. Define a healthy weight in a way that makes the most sense to you. **(LO 7.3)**

4. Describe a practical method to define obesity in a clinical setting. **(LO 7.3)**

5. What are the two most convincing pieces of evidence that both genetic and environmental factors play significant roles in the development of obesity? **(LO 7.5)**

6. List three health problems that obese people typically face and a reason that each problem arises. **(LO 7.4)**

7. What are three key characteristics of a sound weight-loss program? **(LO 7.6)**

8. Why is the claim for quick, effortless weight loss by any method always misleading? **(LO 7.6)**

9. Define the term *behavior modification*. Relate it to the terms *stimulus control*, *self-monitoring*, *chain-breaking*, *relapse prevention*, and *cognitive restructuring*. Give examples of each. **(LO 7.9)**

10. Why should obesity treatment be viewed as a lifelong commitment rather than a short episode of weight loss? **(LO 7.12)**

What Would You Choose Recommendations

Regular varieties of ice cream contain at least 10% milk fat by weight and are therefore a source of fat, saturated fat, and cholesterol. The milk fat gives the product the smooth, creamy texture for which ice cream is famous. You can see that the regular ice cream in the choices provided has 180 kcal, 10 grams of fat, 6 grams of saturated fat, and 65 mg of cholesterol. The sugar content is 19 grams—some of this comes from natural milk sugar (lactose), and some sugar is added for flavor.

Premium ice cream varieties, such as those you would find in an ice cream shop, may have up 300 kcal, 18 grams of fat, and 30 grams of sugar per ½-cup serving! That's equivalent to 4 teaspoons of butter and 7 teaspoons of sugar. Such decadent treats can be enjoyed in moderation, but are best reserved for special occasions.

Reduced-fat, low-fat, light, or fat-free varieties of ice cream have less than 10% milk fat. This can be accomplished by starting with lower-fat milk, using gelatin instead of eggs, using fat replacers incorporating more air into the product (e.g., "churned"), or any combination thereof. "Reduced fat" means the product has at least 25% less fat than the original product. "Low fat" sets the standard at 3 grams of fat or less per ½-cup serving. "Light" ice cream has at least 50% less fat than the original product. "Fat free" signifies 0.5 grams of fat or less per ½-cup serving. The brand shown here is "light"—it contains

lower fat and sugar than the regular ice cream. It has 110 kcal, 3 grams of fat, 2 grams of saturated fat, 10 mg cholesterol, and 14 grams of sugar per serving. For weight-management purposes, this saves you 70 kcals, 7 grams of fat, and 5 grams of sugar per serving compared to regular ice cream. Reducing the fat content of ice cream might also reduce the creamy texture, but for most reduced-fat, low-fat, and light products, the change is barely noticeable.

Frozen yogurt is not always a lower-calorie option than ice cream. It does not have to comply with the same 10% milk fat standard as ice cream does, so there may be a wide range of fat and sugar content. This brand of frozen yogurt has 180 kcal, 3 grams of fat, 1 gram of saturated fat, and 45 mg cholesterol—very similar to the regular ice cream. The product is marketed as "low fat"—and it does only contain 3 grams of fat per ½-cup serving—but there are still 22 grams of sugar. This is a great example of how low fat does not necessarily mean low calorie.

Serving size is the most important part of the Nutrition Facts panel when it comes to calorie control. No matter how low the calorie, fat, and sugar content are, if you consume multiple servings of any product, you are likely to take in too many calories.

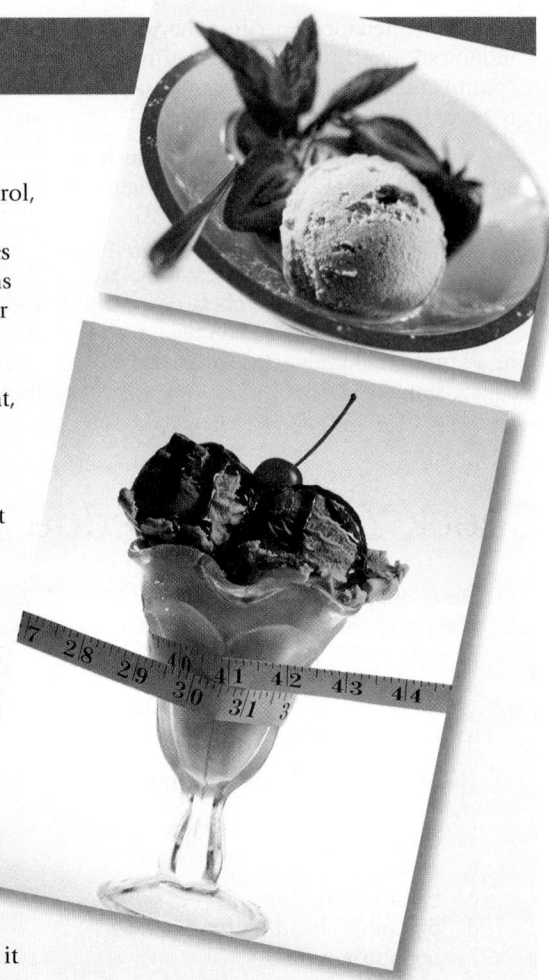

▲ One serving (one scoop) of ice cream with berries is a lower-calorie choice than several scoops with chocolate sauce and cherry.

NUTRITION FACTS		
Kroger Private Selection—Country Made Vanilla Ice Cream		
Serving: 1/2 cup		
Calories	180	Sodium 45 mg
Total Fat	10 g	Potassium 0 g
Saturated	6 g	Total Carbs 19 g
Polyunsaturated	0 g	Dietary Fiber 0 g
Monounsaturated	0 g	Sugars 19 g
Trans	0 g	Protein 6 g
Cholesterol	65 mg	
Vitamin A	8%	Calcium 10%
Vitamin C	2%	Iron 2%
*Percent Daily Values are based on a 2000 calorie diet. Your daily values may be higher or lower depending on your calories needs.		

NUTRITION FACTS		
Kroger Deluxe—Vanilla Bean Light Ice Cream		
Serving: 1/2 cup		
Calories	110	Sodium 50 mg
Total Fat	3 g	Potassium 0 g
Saturated	2 g	Total Carbs 17 g
Polyunsaturated	0 g	Dietary Fiber 0 g
Monounsaturated	0 g	Sugars 14 g
Trans	0 g	Protein 3 g
Cholesterol	10 mg	
Vitamin A	6%	Calcium 10%
Vitamin C	2%	Iron 0%
*Percent Daily Values are based on a 2000 calorie diet. Your daily values may be higher or lower depending on your calories needs.		

NUTRITION FACTS		
Haagen-Dazs—Yogurt Frozen Low Fat Vanilla		
Serving: 1/2 cup		
Calories	180	Sodium 45 mg
Total Fat	3 g	Potassium 0 g
Saturated	1 g	Total Carbs 30 g
Polyunsaturated	0 g	Dietary Fiber 0 g
Monounsaturated	0 g	Sugars 22 g
Trans	0 g	Protein 9 g
Cholesterol	45 mg	
Vitamin A	2%	Calcium 20%
Vitamin C	0%	Iron 0%
*Percent Daily Values are based on a 2000 calorie diet. Your daily values may be higher or lower depending on your calories needs.		

Further Readings

1. Adams KF and others: Overweight, obesity, and mortality in a large prospective cohort of persons 50 to 71 years old. *The New England Journal of Medicine* 355:763, 2006.

    Excess body weight during midlife was associated with an increased risk of death. Risk of death increased by 20% to 40% among overweight persons and by two to three times among obese persons.

2. Blackburn GL, Corliss J: *Break Through Your Set Point.* New York: Harper Collins, 2007.

    This book outlines strategies for "breaking through" weight-loss plateaus by working with the body's natural tendency to stay at a fixed weight. The key is slow, gradual weight loss, followed by a 6-month period of holding steady at your new weight.

3. Flegal KM and others: Prevalence and trends in obesity among U.S. adults, 1999–2008. *Journals of the American Medical Association* 303(3):235, 2010.

    In the United States adult obesity rates have increased significantly. In the late 1970s, 15% of adults were obese compared to 34% in 2008.

4. Hollis JF and others: Weight loss during the intensive intervention phase of the weight-loss maintenance trial. *American Journal of Preventive Medicine* 35:118, 2008.

    Overweight or obese participants lost an average of 12 pounds. Keeping a daily record of food and physical activity helped them succeed suggesting that the willingness to record your eating habits could lead to a healthier weight.

5. James WPT and others: Effect of sibutramine on cardiovascular outcomes in overweight and obese subjects. *New England Journal of Medicine* 363(10):905, 2010.

    Sibutramine (Meridia) was withdrawn from the market in October 2010 based primarily on results from the SCOUT study (Sibutramine Cardiovascular OUTcomes Trial). Among subjects who were receiving long-term sibutramine treatment (~3.4 years), those with preexisting cardiovascular conditions had an increased risk of nonfatal heart attacks and stroke. More than 90% of the 10,000 patients in the study had underlying cardiovascular disease and therefore should not have received sibutramine. It was concluded that sibutramine should not be used in patients with preexisting cardiovascular disease.

6. Kruger J and others: Dietary and physical activity behaviors among adults successful at weight-loss maintenance. *International Journal of Behavioral Nutrition and Physical Activity* 3:17, 2006.

    Strategies practiced more frequently by successful weight losers included weighing oneself, planning meals, tracking fat and calories, exercising 30 or more minutes daily, and adding physical activity to their daily routines.

7. Madan AT, Orth WD: Vitamin and trace mineral levels after laparoscopic gastric bypass. *Obesity Surgery* 16:603, 2006.

    Vitamin and mineral deficiencies are thought to be a common long-term outcome of bariatric surgery. In this study, of 100 patients who underwent laparoscopic Roux-en-Y gastric bypass, most vitamins and minerals were slightly lower at 1-year postoperative. Significant decreases were observed only for vitamin D and selenium.

8. Mozaffarian D and others: Changes in diet and lifestyle and long-term weight gain in women and men. *New England Journal of Medicine* 364:2392, 2011.

    Relationships between lifestyle factors and weight change were evaluated. Subjects gained an average of 3.35 pounds every 4 years, adding up to 20 pounds in 20 years. Those with the greatest increase in physical activity gained 1.76 fewer pounds. The kind of foods eaten had a larger effect than changes in physical activity. Weight gained was associated with greater intake of French fries, potato chips, potatoes, sugar-sweetened beverages, unprocessed red meats, and processed meats. Foods that resulted in weight loss or no gain were fruits, vegetables, whole grains, yogurt, and nuts. Results show how small changes in eating, exercise, and other habits can result in large changes in body weight over the years.

9. National Center for Chronic Disease Prevention and Health Promotion: *Obesity: Halting the Epidemic by Making Health Easier.* Center for Disease Control and Prevention, Department of Health and Human Services, 2009. www.cdc.gov/nccdphp/dnpa.

    In the United States, obesity rates did not increase significantly between 2003–2004 and 2005–2006. Increased awareness of obesity as a national health problem, innovative policy and environmental changes in communities, work sites, and schools, and increased exercise and reduced consumption of high-calorie and fatty foods have likely led to this leveling of rates.

10. O'Brien PE and others: Treatment of mild to moderate obesity with laparoscopic adjustable gastric banding or an intensive medical program: A randomized trial. *Annals of Internal Medicine* 144:625, 2006.

    Surgical patients lost weight more rapidly and also had greater improvement in the metabolic syndrome and quality of life.

11. Robb M, Robb N: Tiny pills, big promises. *Today's Diet & Nutrition* 4(4):58, 2008.

    Information is provided about the latest dietary aids/diet pills for weight loss. Diet pills rely on one of three strategies: suppressing appetite, boosting metabolism, or blocking absorption of fats or carbohydrates. Each strategy is reviewed.

12. See R and others: The association of differing measures of overweight and obesity with prevalent atherosclerosis: the Dallas Heart Study. *Journal of American College of Cardiologists* 50:752, 2007.

    A study of associations between different measures of obesity (body mass index, waist circumference, and waist-to-hip ratio) and atherosclerosis found that waist-to-hip ratio was more strongly associated with atherosclerosis than body mass index or waist circumference. These results indicate that apple-shaped people are at greater risk for obesity-related diseases and heart attack than pear-shaped ones.

13. Shai I and others: Weight loss with a low-carbohydrate, Mediterranean, or low-fat diet. *New England Journal of Medicine* 359:229, 2008.

    Moderately obese adults were assigned to either a low-fat Mediterranean or low-carbohydrate diet, and studied for 2 years. Participants on the low-carbohydrate diet lost and kept off about 12 pounds; those on the Mediterranean Diet, kept off a 10-pounds weight loss; and those on the restricted-fat plan kept off 7 pounds. The results indicate that Mediterranean and low-carbohydrate diets may be effective alternatives to low-fat diets.

14. Slavin J and others: How fiber affects weight regulation. *Food Technology*, p. 34, February 2008.

    Dietary fiber has intrinsic, hormonal, and intestinal effects that decrease food intake by promoting satiety. Effects include decreased gastric emptying and/or slowed energy and nutrient absorption.

15. Svetkey LP and others: Comparison of strategies for sustaining weight loss: The weight-loss maintenance randomized controlled trial. *Journal of the American Medical Association* 299:1139, 2008.

    Participants weighed an average of 213 pounds, followed the Dietary Approaches to Stop Hypertension (DASH) diet for 6 months, and were encouraged to do 180 minutes of moderate exercise a week. Average weight loss was 19 pounds. After 2 ½ years, dieters kept more weight off if they reported to a nutrition counselor every month.

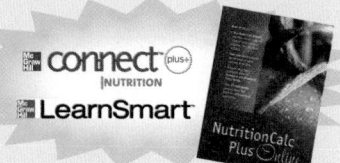

To get the most out of your study of nutrition, go to McGraw-Hill's online resources: Connect www.mcgrawhillconnect.com, where you will find NutritionCalc Plus, LearnSmart, and many other dynamic tools.

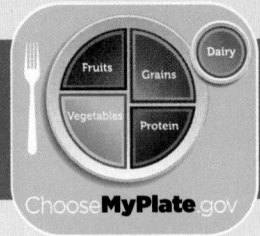

I. A Close Look at Your Weight Status

Determine the following two indices of your body status: body mass index and waist circumference.

Body Mass Index (BMI)

Record your weight in pounds: _____ pounds
Divide your weight in pounds by 2.2 to determine your weight in kilograms: _____ kilograms
Record your height in inches: _____ in
Divide your height in inches by 39.4 to determine your height in meters: _____ meters
Calculate your BMI using the following formula:
BMI = weight (kilograms)/height^2 (meters)
BMI = _____ kg/ _____ m^2 = _____

Waist Circumference

Use a tape measure to measure the circumference of your waist (at the umbilicus with stomach muscles relaxed). Circumference of waist (umbilicus) = _____ in

Interpretation

1. When BMI is greater than 25, health risks from obesity often begin. It is especially advisable to consider weight loss if your BMI exceeds 30. Does yours exceed 25 (or 30)?

   Yes _____ No _____

2. When a person has a BMI greater than 25 and a waist circumference of more than 40 inches (102 centimeters) in men or 35 inches (88 centimeters) in women, there is an increased risk of cardiovascular disease, hypertension, and type 2 diabetes. Does your waist circumference exceed the standard for your gender?

   Yes _____ No _____

3. Do you feel you need to pursue a program of weight loss?

   Yes _____ No _____

Application

From what you have learned in Chapter 7, what can you do to change your patterns of eating and physical activity to lose weight and help ensure maintenance of any loss?

_____

_____

_____

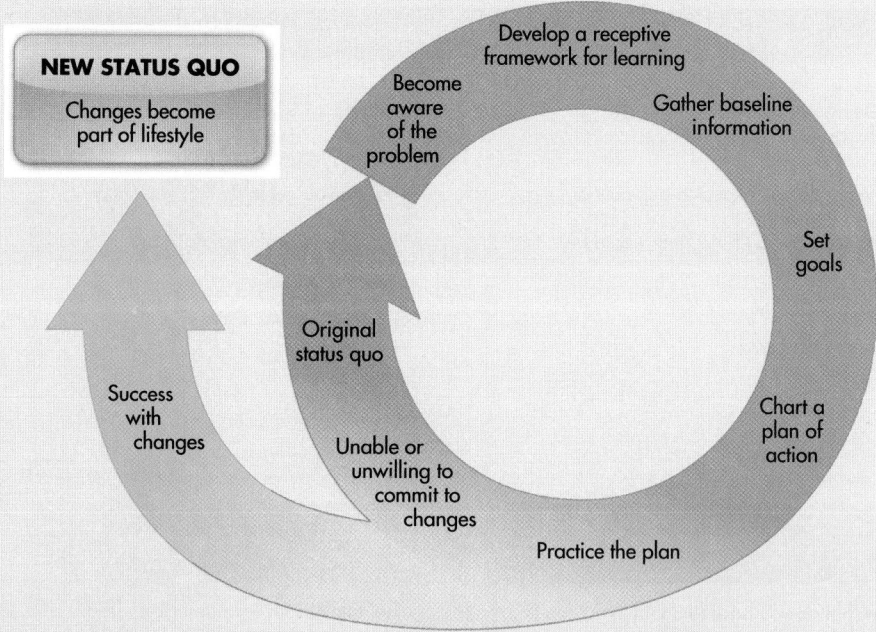

FIGURE 7-20 ▶ A model for behavior change. It starts with awareness of the problem and ends with the incorporation of new behaviors intended to address the problem.

II. An Action Plan to Change or Maintain Weight Status

Now that you have assessed your current weight status, do you feel that you would like to make some changes? Following is a step-by-step guide to behavioral change. This process can be useful even for those satisfied with their current weight, as it can be applied to changing exercise habits, self-esteem, and a variety of other behaviors (Fig. 7-20).

Becoming Aware of the Problem

By calculating your current weight status, you have already become aware of the problem, if one exists. From here, it is important to find out more information about the cause of the problem and whether it is worth working toward a change.

1. What are the factors that most influence your eating habits? Do you eat due to stress, boredom, or depression? Is volume of food your problem, or do you eat mainly the wrong foods for you? Take some time to assess the root causes of your eating habits.

2. Once you have more information about your specific eating practices, you must decide if it is worth changing these practices. A benefits and costs analysis can be a useful tool in evaluating whether it is worth your effort to make life changes. Use the following example as a guide for listing benefits and costs pertinent to your situation (Fig. 7-21).

Setting Goals

What can we accomplish, and how long will it take? Setting a realistic, achievable goal and allowing a reasonable amount of time to pursue it increase the likelihood of success.

1. Begin by determining the outcome you would like to achieve. If you are trying to change your eating behaviors to be more healthy, list your reasons for doing so (e.g., overall health, weight loss, self-esteem).

    Overall goal:

    _____

    _____

FIGURE 7-21 ▶ Benefits and costs analysis applied to increasing physical activity. This process helps put behavior change into the context of total lifestyle.

Benefits and Costs Analysis

1 Benefits of changing eating habits?

What do you expect to get, now or later, that you want?
What may you avoid that would be unpleasant?

feel better physically and psychologically
look better

2 Benefits of not changing eating habits?

What do you get to do that you enjoy doing?
What do you avoid having to do?

no need for planning
can eat without feeling guilty

3 Costs involved in changing eating habits?

What do you have to do that you don't want to do?
What do you have to stop doing that you would rather continue doing?

take time to plan meals and shop
must give up some food volume

4 Costs of not changing eating habits?

What unpleasant or undesirable effects are you likely to experience now or in the future?
What are you likely to lose?

creeping weight gain
low self-esteem and poor health

Reasons to pursue goal:

_____

_____

_____

2. Now list several steps that will be necessary to achieve your goal. Keep in mind, however, that it is generally best to change only a few specific behaviors at first—walking briskly for 60 minutes each day, reducing fat intake, using more whole-grain products, and not eating after 7 P.M. Attempting small and perhaps easier dietary changes first reduces the scope of the problem and increases the likelihood of success.

Steps toward achieving goal:

1. _____

2. _____

3. _____

If you are having trouble deciphering the steps needed to achieve your goal, health professionals are an excellent resource for aid in planning.

Measuring Commitment

Now that you have collected information and know what is required to reach your goal, you must ask yourself, "Can I do this?" Commitment is an essential component in the success of behavioral change. Be honest with yourself. Permanent change is not quick or easy. Once you have decided that you have the commitment required to see this through, continue on to the following sections.

Making It Official with a Contract

Drawing up a behavioral contract often adds incentive to follow through with a plan. The contract could list goal behaviors and objectives, milestones for measuring progress, and regular rewards for meeting the terms of the contract. After finishing a contract, you should sign it in the presence of some friends. This encourages commitment.

Initially, plans should reward positive behaviors, and then they should focus on positive results. Positive behaviors, such as regular physical activity, eventually lead to positive outcomes, such as increased stamina.

Figure 7-22 is a sample contract for increasing physical activity. Keep in mind that this sample contract is only a suggestion; you can add your ideas as well.

Psyching Yourself Up

Once your contract is in place, you need to psych yourself up. Discouragement from peers and your temptations to stray from your plan need to be anticipated. Psyching yourself up can enable you to progress toward your goals in spite of others' attitudes and

Name _Alan Young_

Goal

I agree to _ride my exercise bike_
(specify behavior)

under the following circumstances _for 30 minutes, 4 times per week in the evening_
(specify where, when, how much, etc.)

Substitute behavior and/or reinforcement schedule _I will reinforce myself if I've achieved my goal after a month with a weekend off campus with my roommate._

Environmental planning

In order to help me do this, I am going to (1) arrange my physical and social environment by _buying a new portable CD player_

and (2) control my internal environment (thoughts, images) by _coordinating riding the bike with the first T.V. watching I do in the evening_

Reinforcements

Reinforcements provided by me daily or weekly (if contract is kept):
I will buy myself a new piece of clothing for off campus trip

Reinforcements provided by others daily or weekly (if contract is kept):
at the end of a month if I've completed my goal my parents will buy me a fitness club membership for winter.

Social support

Behavior change is more likely to take place when other people support you. During the quarter/semester please meet with the other person at least three times to discuss your progress.

The name of my "significant helper" is: _Mr. and Mrs. Young_

This contract should include:

1. Baseline data (one week)
2. Well-defined goal
3. Simple method for charting progress (diary, counter, charts, etc.)
4. Reinforcements (immediate and long-term)
5. Evaluation method (summary of experiences, success, and/or new learnings about self).

FIGURE 7-22 ▶ Alan's behavior contract. Completing such a contract can help generate commitment to behavior change. What would your contract look like?

opinions. Almost everyone benefits from some assertiveness training when it comes to changing behaviors. The following are a few suggestions. Can you think of any others?

- No one's feelings should be hurt if you say, "No, thank you," firmly and repeatedly when others try to dissuade you from a plan. Tell them you have new diet behavior and your needs are important.

- You don't have to eat a lot to accommodate anyone—your mother, business clients, or the chef. For example, at a party with friends, you may feel you have to eat a lot to participate, but you don't. Another trap is ordering a lot just because someone else is paying for the meal.

- Learn ways to handle put-downs—inadvertent or conscious. An effective response can be to communicate feelings honestly, without hostility. Tell criticizers that they have annoyed or offended you, that you are working to change your habits and would really like understanding and support from them.

Practicing the Plan

Once you've set up a plan, the next step is to implement it. Start with a trial of at least 6 to 8 weeks. Thinking of a lifetime commitment can be overwhelming. Aim for a total duration of 6 months of new activities before giving up. We may have to persuade ourselves more than once of the value of continuing the program. The following are some suggestions to help keep a plan on track:

- *Focus on reducing but not necessarily extinguishing undesirable behaviors.* For example, it's usually unrealistic to say, "I'll never eat a certain food again." It's better to say, "I won't eat that *problem* food as often as before."

- *Monitor progress.* Note your progress in a diary and reward yourself according to your contract. While conquering some habits and seeing improvement, you may find yourself quite encouraged, even enthusiastic, about your plan of action. That can give you the impetus to move ahead with the program.

- *Control environments.* In the early phases of behavioral change, try to avoid problem situations, such as parties, coffee breaks, and favorite restaurants. Once new habits are firmly established, you can probably more successfully resist the temptations of these environments.

Reevaluating and Preventing Relapse

After practicing a program for several weeks to months, it is important to reassess the original plan. In addition, you may now be able to pinpoint other problem areas for which you need to plan appropriately.

1. Begin by taking a close and critical look at your original plan. Does it lead to the goals you set? Are there any new steps toward your goal that you feel capable of adding to your contract? Do you need new reinforcements? It may even be necessary to make a new contract. For permanent change, it is worth this time of reassessment.

2. In practicing your plan over the past weeks or months, you have likely experienced relapses. What triggered these relapses? To prevent a total retreat to your old habits, it is important to set up a plan for such relapses. You can do this by identifying high-risk situations, rehearsing a response, and remembering your goals.

You may have noticed a behavior chain in some of your relapses. That is, the relapse may stem from a series of interconnected habitual activities. The way to break the chain is to first identify the activities, pinpoint the weak links, break those links, and substitute other behaviors. Figure 7-23 illustrates a sample behavior chain and a substitute activities list. Consider compiling a list based on your behavior chains.

Epilogue

If you have used the activities in this section, you are well on your way to permanent behavioral change. Recall that this exercise can be used for a variety of desired changes, including quitting smoking, increasing physical activity, and improving study habits. It is by no means an easy process, but the results can be well worth the effort. Overall, the keys to success are motivation (keeping the problem in the forefront of your mind), having a plan of action, securing the resources and skills needed for success, and looking for help from family, friends, or a group.

SUBSTITUTE ACTIVITIES

Pleasant activities
1. _Singing / washing hair_
2. _Reading comics / biking_
3. _Sewing / calling a friend_

Necessary activities
1. _Ironing_
2. _Vacuuming_
3. _Straightening apartment_

Situations when used
1. _Wanted ice cream – delayed with bath_
2. _Wanted wheat thins – cleaned up apt._
3. _Wanted snack – went for walk_
4. _Wanted cookies – did dishes first_
5. _Saw leftovers – went for bike ride_
6. _Tempted by cookies – set timer_
7. _Wanted snack – read comics_

BEHAVIOR CHAIN

Identify the links in your eating response chain on the following diagram.
Draw a line through the chain where it was interrupted. Add the link you
substituted and the new chain of behavior this substitution started.

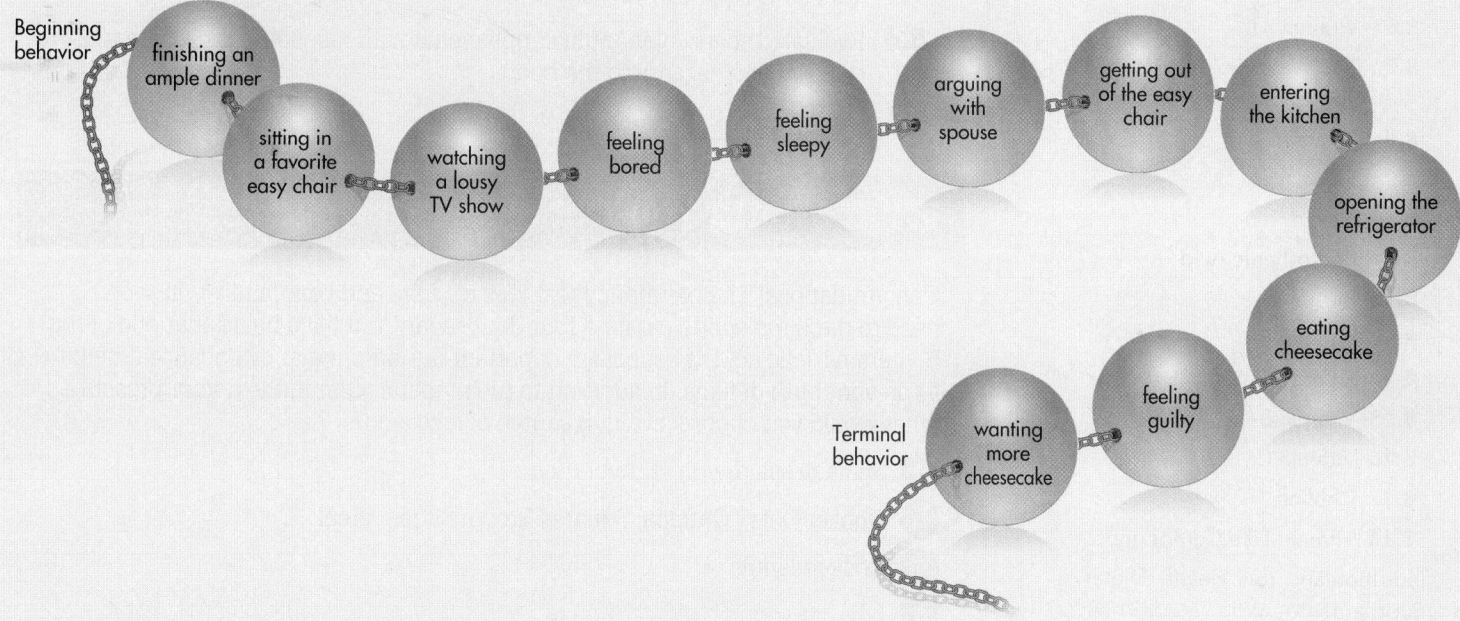

FIGURE 7-23 ▶ Identifying behavior chains. This is a good tool for understanding more about your habits and pinpointing ways
to change unwanted habits. The earlier in the chain you substitute a nonfood link, the easier it is to intervene. Four types of behaviors can be substituted in an ongoing behavior chain.

1. Fun activities (taking a walk, reading a book)
2. Necessary activities (cleaning a room, balancing your checkbook)
3. Incompatible activities (taking a shower)
4. Urge-delaying activities (setting a kitchen timer for 20 minutes before allowing yourself to eat)

Using activities to interrupt behavior patterns that lead to inappropriate eating (or inactivity) can be a powerful means of changing
habits.

Chapter 8 Vitamins

Student Learning Outcomes

Chapter 8 is designed to allow you to:

8.1 Define the term *vitamin* and list three characteristics of vitamins as a group.

8.2 Classify the vitamins according to whether they are fat soluble or water soluble.

8.3 List the major functions and deficiency symptoms for each vitamin.

8.4 List three important food sources for each vitamin.

8.5 Describe toxicity symptoms from excess consumption of certain vitamins.

8.6 Evaluate the use of vitamin supplements with respect to their potential benefits and hazards to the body.

What Would You Choose?

Congratulations! The pregnancy test was positive and your family will soon need to ditch the sports car for a four-door sedan! You have heard that one of the B vitamins, folic acid, is especially important during pregnancy because it helps to prevent birth defects. In addition to the prenatal vitamin the doctor prescribed, what would you choose as a rich source of folic acid?

a Spinach salad with strawberries

b Quaker Oats® Oatmeal Squares Brown Sugar cereal

c Cooked lentils

d Low-fat yogurt

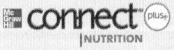 **Think about your choice as you read Chapter 8, then see our recommendations at the end of the chapter. To learn more about nutrient needs during pregnancy, check out the Connect site:** www.mcgrawhillconnect.com

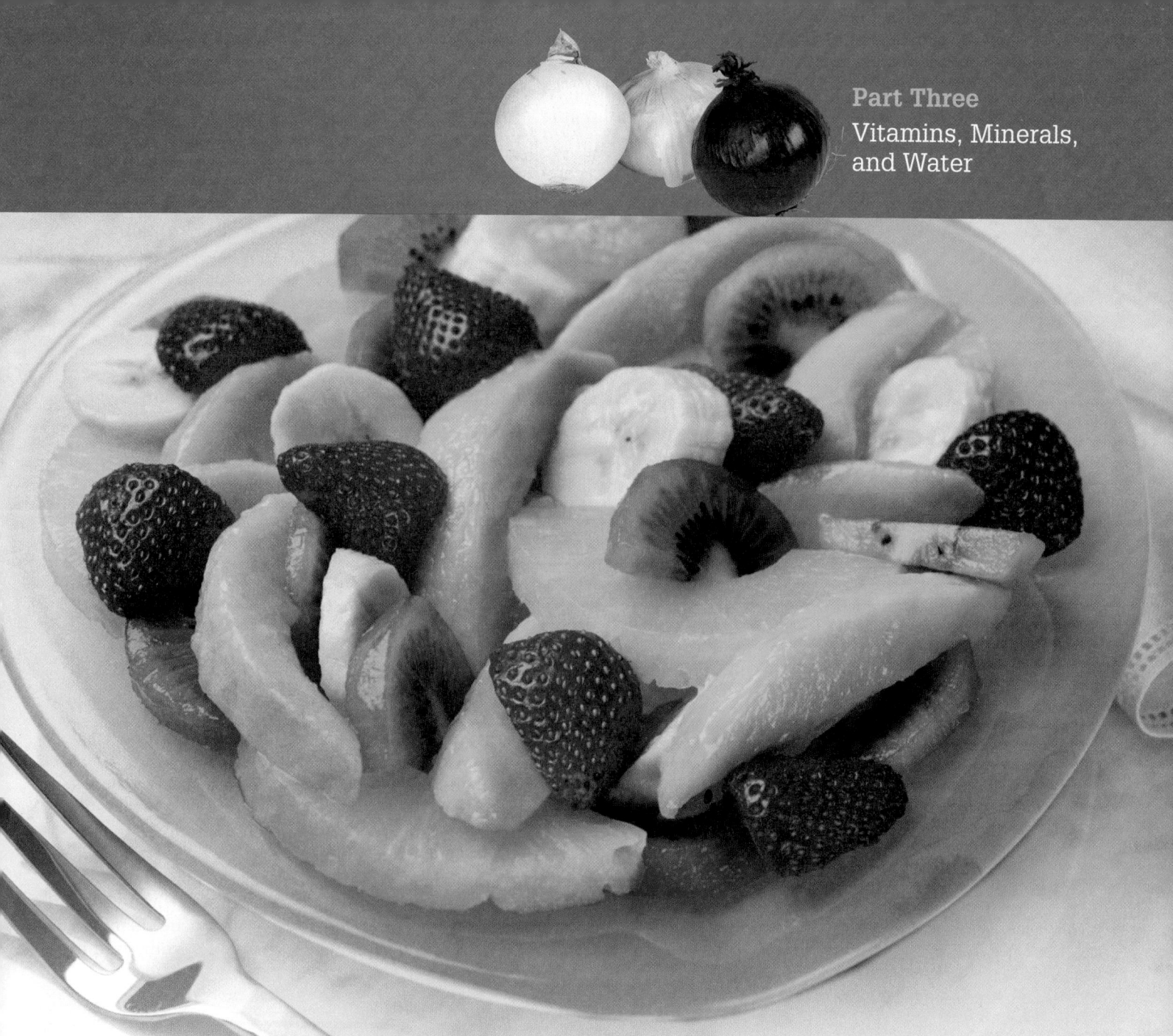

A lthough the vitamins are essential nutrients, the amount of vitamins we need to prevent deficiency is small. In general, humans require a total of about 1 ounce (28 grams) of vitamins for every 150 pounds (70 kilograms) of food consumed. Some people believe that consuming vitamins far in excess of their needs provides them with extra energy, protection from disease, and prolonged youth. They seem to think that if a little is good, then more must be better. More than half of the U.S. adult population have taken vitamin and/or mineral supplements on a regular basis, some at unsafe levels. In 2010, we spent $28.7 billion on dietary supplements. Sales for vitamin D at $550 million were up 30% over 2009. The health-related value of this practice is hotly debated.

Vitamins are found in plants and animals. Plants synthesize all the vitamins they need and, as the chapter comic suggests, are a healthy source of vitamins for animals. Animals vary in their ability to synthesize vitamins. For example, guinea pigs and humans are two of the few organisms unable to make their own supply of vitamin C.

Chapter 8 reviews some general properties of vitamins. These vital nutrients are divided into two groups: the fat-soluble vitamins and the water-soluble vitamins. The chapter focuses on the functions and sources of each vitamin and human needs for them. The current controversy over vitamin and mineral supplement use is also explored.

Refresh Your Memory

As you begin your study of vitamins in Chapter 8, you may want to review:

- Implications of the Dietary Supplement Health and Education Act (DSHEA) in Chapter 2
- The gastrointestinal system for the digestion and absorption of nutrients and the urinary system for vitamin D activation in Chapter 3
- The digestion and absorption of dietary lipids, the formation of lipoproteins, and the definition of antioxidants in Chapter 5
- Amino-acid metabolism, protein synthesis, and protein-calorie malnutrition in Chapter 6

8.1 Vitamins: Vital Dietary Components

By definition, **vitamins** are essential organic (carbon-containing) substances needed in small amounts in the diet for normal function, growth, and maintenance of the body. Although vitamins yield no energy to the body, they often participate in energy-yielding reactions. Vitamins A, D, E, and K are **fat soluble,** whereas the B vitamins and vitamin C are **water soluble.** In addition, the B vitamins and vitamin K function as parts of **coenzymes** (compounds that help enzymes function).

Vitamins are generally essential in human diets because they can't be synthesized in the human body or because their synthesis can be decreased by environmental factors. Notable exceptions to having a strict dietary need for a vitamin are vitamin A, which we can synthesize from certain pigments in plants; vitamin D, synthesized in

vitamin Compound needed in small amounts in the diet to help regulate and support chemical reactions and processes in the body.

fat-soluble vitamins Vitamins that dissolve in fat and such substances as ether and benzene but not readily in water. These vitamins are A, D, E, and K.

water-soluble vitamins Vitamins that dissolve in water. These vitamins are the B vitamins and vitamin C.

coenzyme A compound that combines with an inactive enzyme to form a catalytically active form. In this manner, coenzymes aid in enzyme function.

Increasing our intake of fruits and vegetables is one of the recurring Dietary Guidelines. Which vitamins are especially found in fruits and vegetables? What are some other health-related attributes of fruits and vegetables in general? Which chronic diseases are associated with a poor intake of fruits and vegetables? Should we take a daily vitamin supplement if we do not include fruits and vegetables in our diet? Chapter 8 provides some answers.

ZIGGY

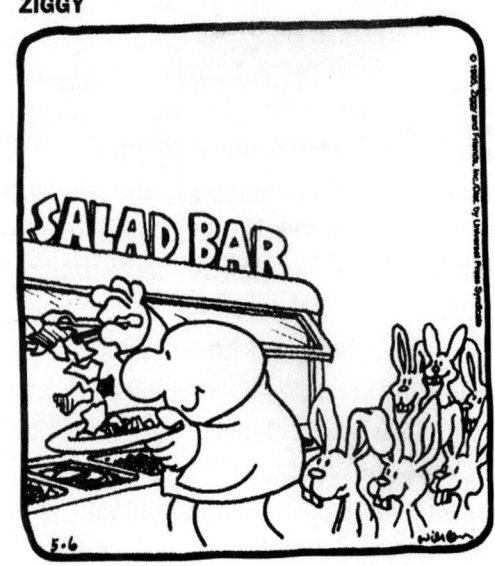

ZIGGY © ZIGGY AND FRIENDS, INC. Reprinted with permission of UNIVERSAL PRESS SYNDICATE. All rights reserved.

the body if the skin is exposed to adequate sunlight; niacin, synthesized from the amino acid tryptophan; and vitamin K and biotin, synthesized to some extent by bacteria in the intestinal tract.

To be classified as a vitamin, a compound must meet the following criteria to be an essential nutrient: (1) the body is unable to synthesize enough of the compound to maintain health; and (2) absence of the compound from the diet for a defined period produces deficiency symptoms that, if caught in time, are quickly cured when the substance is resupplied. A substance does not qualify as a vitamin merely because the body can't make it. Evidence must suggest that health declines when the substance is not consumed.

As scientists began to identify various vitamins, related deficiency diseases such as scurvy, beriberi, pellagra, and rickets were dramatically cured. For the most part, as the vitamins were discovered, they were named alphabetically: A, B, C, D, E, and so on. Later, many substances originally classified as vitamins were found not to be essential for humans and were dropped from the list. Other vitamins, thought at first to be only one chemical turned out to be several chemicals, so the alphabetical names had to be broken down by numbers (B-6, B-12, and so on).

In addition to their use in correcting deficiency diseases, a few vitamins have also proved useful in treating several nondeficiency diseases. These medical applications require administration of pharmacological amounts or **megadoses,** well above typical human needs for the vitamins. For example, megadoses of a form of niacin can be used as part of blood cholesterol–lowering treatment for certain individuals. This chapter will mention others as well. Still, any claimed benefits from use of vitamin supplements, especially intakes in excess of the Upper Level (if set), should be viewed critically because unproven claims are common.

Both plant and animal foods supply vitamins in the human diet. Vitamins isolated from foods or synthesized in the laboratory are the same chemical compounds and generally work equally well in the body. Contrary to claims in the health-food literature, "natural" vitamins isolated from foods are, for the most part, no more healthful than those synthesized in a laboratory, but there are exceptions. Vitamin E is much more potent in its natural form than in its synthetic form. In contrast, synthetic folic acid, the form of the vitamin added to ready-to-eat breakfast cereals and flour, is 1.7 times more potent than the natural vitamin form.

Have Scientists Found All the Vitamins?

You may wonder whether there are vitamins in foods that have yet to be discovered. After all, the first chemical formula of a vitamin (thiamin) was not determined until 1937, and the last structure was characterized in 1948 (vitamin B-12). Although some optimistic researchers hope to discover that one or more additional compounds (e.g., choline; see p. 330) are vitamins, most scientists are confident that all compounds that meet the criteria for classification as a vitamin have been discovered. Evidence supports this assumption. For example, people have lived well for years when receiving only intravenous administration of solutions that consist of protein, carbohydrate, fat, all the known vitamins, and the essential minerals. With appropriate medical monitoring, these people not only continue to live, but also build new body tissues, heal wounds, fight existing diseases, and even have babies.

Storage of Vitamins in the Body

Except for vitamin K, the fat-soluble vitamins are not readily excreted from the body. In contrast, excess amounts of the water-soluble vitamins are generally lost from the body rapidly, partly because the water in cells dissolves these vitamins and excretes them out of the body via the kidneys. Water-soluble vitamin B-6 and vitamin B-12 are exceptions; these are stored much more readily than the other water-soluble vitamins.

megadose Intake of a nutrient beyond estimates of needs to prevent a deficiency or what would be found in a balanced diet; 2 to 10 times human needs is a starting point for such a pharmacological dosage.

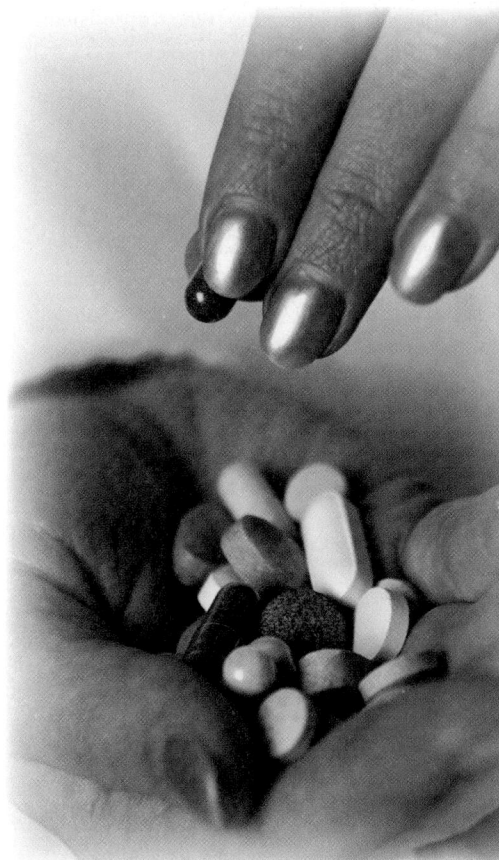

▲ Vitamins are not likely to be toxic unless taken in large amounts as supplements.

Because of the limited storage of many vitamins, they should be consumed in the diet daily, although an occasional lapse in the intake of even water-soluble vitamins generally causes no harm. Symptoms of a vitamin deficiency occur only when that vitamin is lacking in the diet and body stores are essentially exhausted. For example, an average person must consume no thiamin for 10 days or no vitamin C for 20 to 40 days before developing the first symptoms of deficiency of these vitamins.

Vitamin Toxicity

Fat-soluble vitamins are not readily excreted, so some can easily accumulate in the body and cause toxic effects. And, although a toxic effect from an excessive intake of any vitamin is theoretically possible, toxicity of the fat-soluble vitamin A is the most frequently observed. Vitamin E and the water-soluble vitamins niacin, vitamin B-6, and vitamin C can also cause toxic effects, but only when consumed in large amounts (15 to 100 times human needs or more). These five vitamins are unlikely to cause toxic effects unless taken in supplement (pill) form. Vitamin A even causes toxicity with long-term intake as little as two times human needs.

A "one-a-day" type of multivitamin and mineral supplement usually contains less than two times the Daily Values of the components, so daily use of these products is unlikely to cause toxic effects in men and nonpregnant women. But consuming many vitamin pills, especially highly potent sources of vitamin A, can cause problems. Today, concentrated vitamin A supplements are widely available in grocery, drug, and health-food stores and pose risks for toxicity when used inappropriately. See the later Nutrition and Your Health section to find out more about whether you should take a multivitamin and mineral supplement and, if so, how to do it safely.

Preservation of Vitamins in Foods

Substantial amounts of vitamins can be lost from the time a fruit or vegetable is picked until it is eaten. The water-soluble vitamins—particularly thiamin, vitamin C, and folate—can be destroyed with improper storage and excessive cooking. Heat, light, exposure to the air, cooking in water, and alkalinity are all factors that can destroy vitamins. The sooner a food is eaten after harvest, the less chance of nutrient loss. Food cooperatives, **community-supported agriculture (CSA)** and farmers' markets are great sources of freshly harvested fruits and vegetables.

In general, if the food is not eaten within a few days, freezing is the best preservation method to retain nutrients. Fruits and vegetables are often frozen immediately after harvesting, so frozen vegetables and fruits are often as nutrient-rich as freshly picked ones. As part of the freezing process, vegetables are quickly blanched in boiling water. This destroys the enzymes that would otherwise degrade the vitamins. Table 8-1 provides some tips to aid in preserving the vitamins in food.

See Nutrition and Your Health: Dietary Supplements—Who Needs Them? at the end of Chapter 8.

Community-supported agriculture (CSA) Farms that are supported by a community of growers and consumers who provide mutual support and share the risks and benefits of food production, usually including a system of weekly delivery or pick-up of vegetables and fruit, sometimes dairy products and meat.

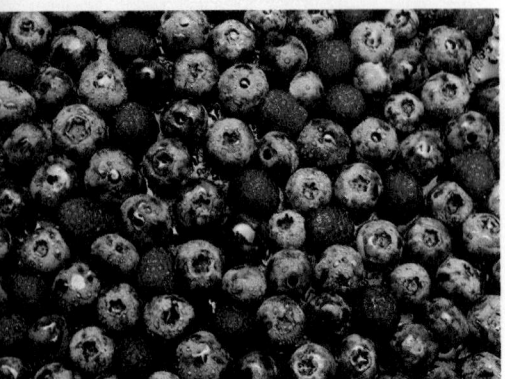

▲ Frozen fruits and vegetables are often as nutrient rich as freshly picked ones.

CONCEPT CHECK

In general, the fat-soluble vitamins—A, D, E, and K—are less readily excreted than the water-soluble B vitamins and vitamin C. Regular consumption of foods rich in both water-soluble and fat-soluble vitamins is important for health. However, the occasional inadequate consumption of any one vitamin is of little health concern, because even water-soluble vitamins persist in the body to some extent. For example, when a person ingests a vitamin-free diet, the first deficiency signs (due to lack of thiamin) will not appear for about 10 days. When taken in supplement form, the fat-soluble vitamin A poses the greatest risk of toxicity. For the most part, there is little risk of toxicity when vitamins are obtained from a variety of foods.

TABLE 8-1 Tips for Preserving the Vitamin Content of Foods

What to Do	Why
Keep fruits and vegetables cool.	Enzymes in food begin to degrade vitamins once the fruit or vegetable is picked. Chilling reduces this process. Refrigerate fresh produce (except for potatoes, tomatoes, onions, and bananas) until they are consumed.
Refrigerate foods in moisture-proof, air-tight containers.	Nutrients keep best at temperatures near freezing, at high humidity, and away from air.
Trim, peel, and cut fruits and vegetables minimally—just enough to remove rotten or inedible parts.	Oxygen breaks down vitamins faster when more surface is exposed. Outer leaves of lettuce and other greens have higher values of vitamins and minerals than the inner, tender leaves or stems. Potato skins and apple skins are higher in vitamins and minerals than the inner parts.
Microwave, steam, or use a pan or wok with very small amounts of fat and a tight-fitting lid to cook vegetables.	More nutrients are retained when there is less contact with water and shorter cooking time. Whenever possible, cook fruits or vegetables in their skins.
Minimize reheating food.	Prolonged reheating reduces vitamin content.
Do not add fats to vegetables during cooking if you plan to discard the liquid.	Fat-soluble vitamins will be lost in discarded fat. Add fats to vegetables after they are fully cooked and drained.
Do not add baking soda to vegetables to enhance the green color.	Alkalinity destroys much thiamin, and other vitamins.
Store canned foods in a cool place.	Canned foods vary in the amount of nutrients lost, largely because of differences in storage time and temperatures. To get maximal nutritive value from canned goods, serve any liquid packed with the food whenever possible.

▲ Rapid cooking of vegetables in minimal fluids aids in preserving vitamin content. Steaming is one effective method.

8.2 The Fat-Soluble Vitamins—A, D, E, and K

Let's look at what we know about the fat-soluble vitamins—vitamins A, D, E, and K.

Absorption of Fat-Soluble Vitamins

Vitamins A, D, E, and K are absorbed along with dietary fat, because they are fat-soluble. These vitamins then travel with dietary fats through the bloodstream to reach body cells. Special carriers in the bloodstream help distribute some of these vitamins. Fat-soluble vitamins are stored mostly in the liver and fatty tissues.

When fat absorption is efficient, about 40% to 90% of the fat-soluble vitamins are absorbed. Anything that interferes with normal digestion and absorption of fats, however, also interferes with fat-soluble vitamin absorption. For example, people with cystic fibrosis, a disease that often inhibits fat absorption, may develop deficiencies of fat-soluble vitamins. Some medications, such as the weight-loss drug orlistat (Xenical), that we discussed in Chapter 7, also interfere with fat absorption. Unabsorbed fat carries these vitamins to the large intestine, where they are excreted in the feces. People with such conditions are especially susceptible to vitamin K deficiency because body stores of vitamin K are lower than those of the other fat-soluble vitamins. Vitamin supplements, taken under a physician's guidance, are part of the treatment for preventing a vitamin deficiency associated with fat malabsorption. Finally, people who use mineral oil as a laxative at mealtimes risk fat-soluble vitamin deficiencies. The intestine does not absorb mineral oil, so fat-soluble vitamins are eliminated with the mineral oil in the feces.

8.3 Vitamin A

The amount of vitamin A you consume is important, as both deficiency and toxicity of this vitamin can cause severe problems. In addition, there is a narrow range of optimal intakes between these two states. Vitamin A is found in foods in a variety of forms. **Retinoids,** or preformed vitamin A, are only found in foods of animal origin, such as fish and organ meats. However, plants contain pigments called **carotenoids,** which can be turned into vitamin A in the body as needed. They can be termed **provitamin A.** Only three of the more than 600 carotenoids found in nature are known to serve as provitamin A in humans, but there may be more. Beta-carotene, the orange-yellow pigment in carrots, is the most potent form of provitamin A. The other known provitamin A carotenoids are lutein and zeaxanthin. Together, preformed vitamin A from animal sources and provitamin A carotenoids make up what is generally called vitamin A.

Functions of Vitamin A and Carotenoids

Vitamin A plays many important roles in the body. The best known and most clearly understood of its roles is in vision. Body changes that occur when vitamin A is lacking provide insight to this and other actions of this fat-soluble nutrient.

Vision. Vitamin A performs important functions in light-dark vision, and to a lesser extent, color vision. One form of vitamin A (retinal) allows certain cells in the eye to adjust from bright to dim light (such as after seeing the headlights of an oncoming car). Without sufficient dietary vitamin A, the cells in the eye cannot quickly readjust to dim light. This condition, known as **night blindness,** is an early sign of vitamin A deficiency.

If vitamin A deficiency progresses, the cells that line the cornea of the eye (the clear window of the eye) also lose their ability to produce **mucus.** The eye then becomes dry. Eventually, when dirt particles scratch the dry surface of the eye, bacteria infect it. The infection soon spreads to the entire surface of the eye and leads to blindness. This disease process is called **xerophthalmia,** which means *dry eye* (Fig. 8-1).

Vitamin A deficiency is second only to accidents as a worldwide cause of blindness. North Americans are at little risk because of generally good diets. However, people—especially children—in less-developed nations are susceptible to vitamin A deficiency. Poor vitamin A intakes, low fat intakes that do not allow for sufficient vitamin A absorption, and low stores of vitamin A lessen the ability of the children to meet high needs during rapid childhood growth. Hundreds of thousands of children in developing nations, especially Asia, become blind each year because of vitamin A deficiency and ultimately die from infections. In North America, the leading cause of blindness in adults is diabetes; in children, it is accidents. As covered in more detail in Chapter 12, worldwide attempts to reduce this problem have included giving large doses of vitamin A twice yearly and fortifying sugar, margarine, and monosodium glutamate with vitamin A. These food vehicles are used because they are commonly consumed by the populations of less-developed nations. This effort has proven effective in some countries.

Age-related **macular degeneration** is a leading cause of legal blindness among North American adults over the age of 65 (Fig. 8-2). The disease is associated with changes in the macular area of the eye, which provides the most detailed vision. Age, smoking, and genetics are risk factors. The macula contains the carotenoids lutein and zeaxanthin in high enough concentrations to impart a yellow color. In one study, the higher the total number of carotenoids (beta-carotene, lutein, and zeaxanthin) consumed in the diet, the lower was the risk for age-related macular degeneration. These carotenoids may also decrease the risk of cataracts in the eyes. Consumption of fruits and vegetables high in carotenoids, rather than the intake of these specific carotenoids in supplements, may reduce the risk for these eye disorders. Multivitamin and mineral supplements formulated for older adults (e.g., Centrum Silver™) are being marketed as a source of lutein.

retinoids Chemical forms of preformed vitamin A; one source is animal foods.

carotenoids Pigment materials in fruits and vegetables that range in color from yellow to orange to red; three of the various carotenoids yield vitamin A. Many are antioxidants.

provitamin/precursor A substance that can be made into a vitamin if the body needs it.

night blindness A vitamin A deficiency condition in which the retina (in the eye) cannot adjust to low amounts of light.

mucus A thick fluid secreted by many cells throughout the body. It contains a compound that has both carbohydrate and protein parts. It acts as a lubricant and means of protection for cells.

xerophthalmia Literally "dry eye." This is a cause of blindness that results from a vitamin A deficiency. A lack of mucus production by the eye, which leaves it at a greater risk of damage from surface dirt and bacteria.

macular degeneration A painless condition leading to disruption of the central part of the retina (in the eye) and, in turn, blurred vision.

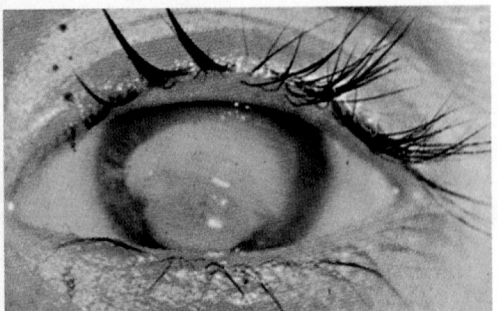

FIGURE 8-1 ▶ Vitamin A deficiency that eventually led to blindness. Note the severe effects on this eye. This problem is commonly seen today in southeast Asia.

Health of Other Cells. Vitamin A also maintains the health of cells that line internal and external surfaces of the lungs, intestines, stomach, vagina, urinary tract, and bladder, as well as those of the eyes and skin. These cells (called **epithelial cells**) serve as important barriers to bacterial infection. As just noted for the eye, some epithelial cells secrete mucus, a needed lubricant. Without vitamin A, mucus-forming cells deteriorate and no longer synthesize mucus. Vitamin A deficiency also causes insufficient mucus production in the intestines and lung cells, and poor health of cells in general. Vitamin A deficiency also reduces the activity of certain immune system cells. Together, these effects leave the vitamin A–deficient person at great risk for infections. For many years, vitamin A has been dubbed the "anti-infection" vitamin.

Growth, Development, and Reproduction. Vitamin A participates in the processes of growth, development, and reproduction in several ways. This role has been demonstrated in vitamin A deficient children experiencing growth retardation when vitamin A supplementation increased their growth. At the genetic level, vitamin A (as retinoic acid) binds to receptors on DNA to increase synthesis of a variety of proteins (review Fig. 6-1 regarding the role of DNA in protein synthesis). In doing so, vitamin A is said to be affecting **gene expression**. Some of these proteins are required for growth, such as bone growth. In laboratory animals, another consequence of vitamin A deficiency is an inability to reproduce.

Cardiovascular Disease Prevention. Carotenoids may play a role in preventing cardiovascular disease in persons at high risk, possibly linked to carotenoids' antioxidant capability. Until definitive studies are complete, many scientists recommend that we increase our intake of carotenoids and other nutrients and compounds by consuming at least 5 servings of fruits and vegetables per day as part of an effort to reduce the risk of cardiovascular disease (see Further Reading 13).

Cancer Prevention. Most forms of cancer arise from cells influenced by vitamin A. Coupled with its ability to aid immune system activity, vitamin A may be a valuable tool in the fight against cancer. This is especially true for skin, lung, bladder, and breast cancers. Still, because of the potential for toxicity, unsupervised use of megadose vitamin A supplements to reduce cancer risk is not advised.

Carotenoids by themselves also may help prevent cancer, acting again as antioxidants. Population studies show that regular consumption of foods rich in carotenoids decreases the risk of lung and oral cancers. Cancer of the **prostate gland** is one of the most common cancers among North American men. The dietary carotenoid found in tomatoes, (the red pigment lycopene) seems to protect against this type of cancer and may also decrease skin cancer risk.

In contrast to the potential benefits of carotenoids in food, recall from Chapter 1 that recent studies from the United States and Finland failed to show a reduction in lung cancer in male smokers and nonsmokers given supplements of the carotenoid beta-carotene for 5 or more years. In fact, beta-carotene use in male smokers increased the number of lung cancer cases compared with the control groups. No comparable studies have been done with women. Although further research continues, most researchers are now convinced that beta-carotene supplementation offers no protection against cancer. Thus, overwhelming advice is to rely on food sources of this or any other carotenoids.

Vitamin A Analogs for Acne. The acne medication tretinoin (Retin-A) is made of one **analog** form of vitamin A. It is used as a topical treatment (applied to the skin) for acne. It appears to work by irritating the skin, which leads to opening of pores and a generalized peeling of the skin layer. It also can block the deleterious effects that skin bacteria have on acne lesions. Similar vitamin A derivatives are also used in antiaging creams because they increase cell turnover and interrupt the path-

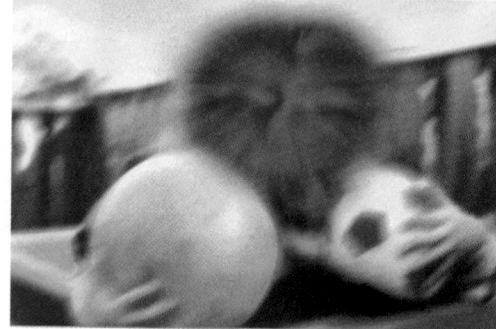

FIGURE 8-2 ▶ Age-related macular degeneration causing a blind spot in the center of the visual field. Increased dietary lutein and zeaxanthin are associated with decreased risk of macular degeneration. Further research is needed to better understand the relationship between macular degeneration and carotenoids.

epithelial cells The cells that line the outside of the body and the inside of all external passages within it, such as the GI tract.

gene expression Use of DNA information on a gene to produce a protein. This is a major determinant of cell development.

prostate gland A solid, chestnut-shaped organ surrounding the first part of the urinary tract in the male. The prostate gland secretes substances into the semen.

analog A chemical compound that differs slightly from another, usually natural, compound. Analogs generally contain extra or altered chemical groups and may have similar or opposite metabolic effects compared with the native compound. Also spelled *analogue*.

▼ Many vegetables are rich in provitamin A carotenoids.

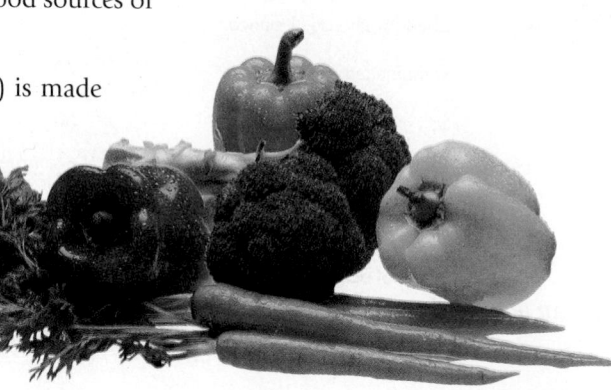

ways of UV skin damage. Another derivative of vitamin A, isotretinoin (Accutane), is an oral drug used to treat serious acne. It acts in part to regulate development of cells in the skin (the gene expression role discussed earlier). Taking high doses of vitamin A itself would not be safe. The use of isotretinoin (Accutane) is strictly monitored by the U.S. Food and Drug Administration (FDA) in order to prevent the use of the drug during pregnancy due to the high risk of birth defects. iPLEDGE is a mandatory distribution program required since March 2006 by the FDA. In order for women to receive this medication, they must have two negative pregnancy tests; sign a patient information/consent form; agree to use two effective forms of birth control; register, along with their doctors and pharmacists, with iPLEDGE by phone or on the Internet, and agree to follow all instructions in the iPLEDGE program.

Vitamin A Sources and Needs

Preformed vitamin A is found in liver, fish, fish oils, fortified milk and yogurt, and eggs (Fig. 8-3). Although liver is a rich food source of vitamin A and other nutrients that are stored in the liver. Focusing on liver to meet nutrient needs is not a good idea because it also provides a high concentration of cholesterol and other fats. Margarine is also fortified with vitamin A. The provitamin A carotenoids mentioned before are mainly found in dark green and yellow-orange vegetables and some fruits. Carrots, spinach and other greens, winter squash, sweet potatoes, broccoli, mangoes, cantaloupe, peaches, and apricots are examples of such sources. About 65% of the vitamin A in the typical North American diet comes from preformed vitamin A sources, whereas provitamin A dominates in the diet among poor people in other parts of the world.

Food Sources of Vitamin A

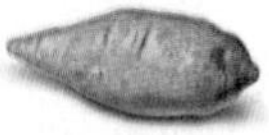

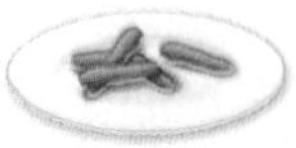

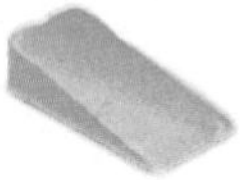

Food Item and Amount	Vitamin A (micrograms RAE*)	Adult Male RDA = 900 micrograms %RDA	Adult Female RDA = 700 micrograms %RDA
RDA	700-900 micrograms	100%	100%
Sweet potato, ½ cup	958	106%	137%
Spinach, ⅔ cup	494	55%	71%
Mango, 1	402	45%	57%
Baby carrots, 5	375	42%	54%
Acorn squash, ⅔ cup	244	27%	35%
Cooked kale, ½ cup	206	23%	29%
Nonfat milk, 1 cup	150	17%	21%
Broccoli, 1 cup	138	15%	20%
Apricot, 3	137	15%	20%
Cheddar cheese, 1 ounce	78	9%	11%
Romaine lettuce, 1 cup	72	8%	10%
Soft margarine, 1 tsp	50	6%	7%
Scallions, 1 tablespoon	32	4%	5%
Peach, 1	26	3%	4%

Daily Value = 1000 micrograms

Key:
- Grains
- Vegetables
- Fruits
- Dairy
- Protein
- Oils

ChooseMyPlate.gov

* Retinol activity equivalents.

FIGURE 8-3 ▶ Food sources of vitamin A compared to the RDA for adult males and females.

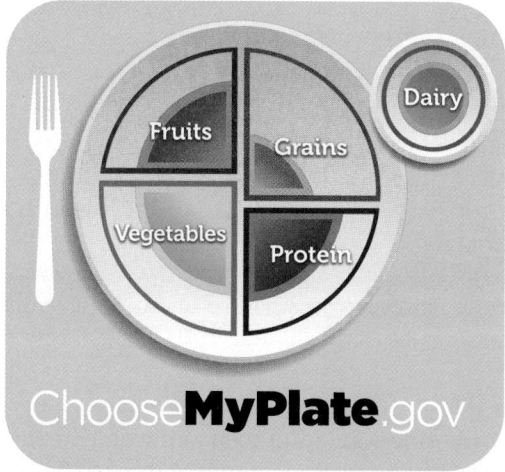

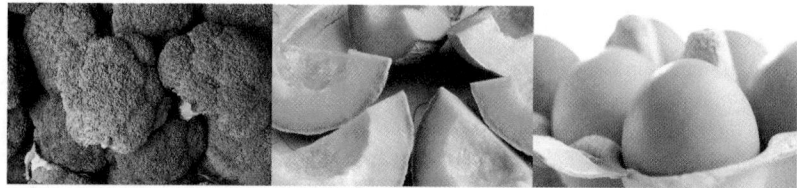

MyPlate:
Sources of Vitamin A

Grains	Vegetables	Fruits	Dairy	Protein
• Fortified break -fast cereals • Fortified meal replacement bars	• Carrots • Broccoli • Spinach • Squash • Sweet potatoes	• Peaches • Apricots • Cantaloupes • Mangoes • Papayas	• Fortified milk • Fortified yogurt • Cheese	• Liver • Eggs

FIGURE 8-4 ▶ Sources of vitamin A from MyPlate. The fill of the background color (none, 1/3, 2/3, or completely covered) within each group on the plate indicates the average nutrient density for vitamin A in that group. Overall, the vegetables group, fruits group, and certain choices in the protein group provide the richest sources. The grains group contains some foods that are nutrient-dense sources of vitamin A because they are fortified with the vitamin. With regard to physical activity, vitamin A plays no specific role *per se* in such endeavors.

Among common foods, those especially rich in vitamin A are carrots, spinach and other greens, sweet potatoes, winter squash, romaine lettuce, broccoli, apricots, and fat-free and low-fat milk. Many of the vegetables listed in Figs. 8-3 and 8-4 are good sources of beta-carotene and the other two provitamin A carotenoids. Marine oils are rich in vitamin A, and consumption of large amounts of such oils can lead to symptoms of vitamin A toxicity.

Beta-carotene accounts for some of the orange color of carrots. In vegetables such as broccoli, this yellow-orange color is masked by dark-green chlorophyll pigments. Still, green vegetables contain provitamin A. Green, leafy vegetables, such as spinach and kale, have a high concentration of lutein and zeaxanthin. Tomato juice and other tomato products, such as pizza sauce, contain significant amounts of lycopene.

The RDA for vitamin A is 700 to 900 micrograms of retinol activity equivalents (RAEs). These RAE units take into account the activity of both preformed vitamin A and the three carotenoids that also are known to yield vitamin A in humans. The total RAE value for a food is calculated by adding the concentration of preformed vitamin A to the amount of provitamin A carotenoids in the food that will be converted to vitamin A. The retinol equivalent (RE) is an older unit for vitamin A. This RE is similar to the RAE but assumed that there was a greater contribution to vitamin A needs from carotenoids than we assume today. Food composition tables and nutrient databases still contain some values based on this older RE standard. It will take some time to update these resources. The Daily Value used on food and supplement labels is 1000 micrograms (5000 IU).

▲ Provitamin A carotenoids are the safest way to meet vitamin A needs. A serving of these carrots would be an excellent addition to the vegetable section of MyPlate.

international unit (IU) A crude measure of vitamin activity, often based on the growth rate of animals in response to the vitamin. Today IUs have largely been replaced by more precise milligram or microgram measures.

fetus The developing human life form from 8 weeks after conception until birth.

MAKING DECISIONS

Expressing Vitamin A Content

In the past, most nutrient amounts in foods, including vitamin A, were formerly expressed in less precise **international units (IUs).** Some food and supplement labels still show the IU value for vitamin A. To compare the older IU standards to current RAE recommendations, assume that for any preformed vitamin A in a food or added to food, 3.3 IU = RAE. The same is true for any beta-carotene added to foods.

There is no easy way to convert IU units to RAE units for foods that naturally contain provitamin A carotenoids, such as carrots, spinach, and apricots. A general rule of thumb is to divide the IU units for foods containing carotenoids by 2, and then divide the result by 3.3 as just discussed.

Average intakes of vitamin A for North American adult men and women meet the RDA. Most adults in North America have liver reserves of vitamin A three to five times greater than needed to provide good health. Thus, the use of vitamin A supplements by most people is unnecessary. At present, there is no separate RDA for beta-carotene or any of the other provitamin A carotenoids.

Deficient vitamin A status in North America may be seen in preschool children who do not eat enough vegetables. The urban poor, older adults, and people with alcoholism or liver disease (which limits vitamin A storage) can also show diminished vitamin A status, especially with respect to stores. Finally, children and adults with severe fat-malabsorption may also experience vitamin A deficiency.

Upper Level for Vitamin A

The Upper Level for vitamin A intake is established at 3000 micrograms of preformed vitamin A (3000 RAE or 10,000 IU) per day for adult men and women. This is based on the increases in birth defects and liver toxicity that accompany intakes in excess of 3000 micrograms of vitamin A per day. Above the Upper Level, other possible side effects include an increased risk of hip fracture and poor pregnancy outcomes.

During the early months of pregnancy, a high intake of preformed vitamin A is especially dangerous because it may cause **fetal** malformations and spontaneous abortions. This is because vitamin A binds to DNA and so influences cell development. FDA recommends that women of childbearing age limit their overall intake of preformed vitamin A to a total of about 100% of the Daily Value (1000 micrograms RAE or 5000 IU). Therefore, it is important to limit consumption of rich food sources, such as liver. These precautions also apply to women who may possibly become pregnant. Vitamin A is stored in the body for long periods, so women who take large amounts during the months before pregnancy place their fetuses at risk.

The consumption of large amounts of vitamin A–yielding carotenoids does not cause toxic effects. A high carotenoid concentration in the blood can occur if someone consumes large amounts of carrots or takes pills containing beta-carotene (more than 30 milligrams daily) or if infants eat a great deal of squash. This can turn the skin yellow-orange. The palms of the hands and soles of the feet in particular become colored. This condition does not appear to cause harm and disappears when carotenoid intake decreases. Dietary carotenoids do not produce toxic effects because (1) their rate of conversion into vitamin A is relatively slow and regulated, and (2) the efficiency of carotenoid absorption from the small intestine decreases markedly as oral intake increases.

8.4 Vitamin D

Vitamin D is not just a vitamin. It is primarily considered a hormone. A cholesterol-like substance in the skin cells is converted to the prohormone vitamin D when exposed to ultraviolet B (UVB) rays from sunlight or tanning beds (Fig. 8-5). Liver and kidney cells then convert the prohormone to its active hormone form. The skin,

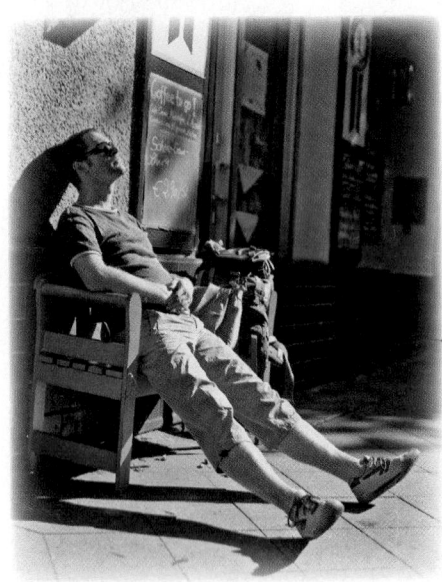

▲ Solar radiation on the skin provides about 80% to 100% of the vitamin D humans use. This is also the most reliable way to maintain vitamin D status. Dietary vitamin D is also effective, but less so.

8-4

liver, and kidney cells that participate in vitamin D synthesis are different from the bone and intestinal cells that are responsive to vitamin D. Having a site of synthesis different from the location of action is characteristic of hormones.

For many individuals, UVB exposure provides about 80% to 100% of our vitamin D needs. The amount of sun exposure needed by individuals to produce vitamin D depends on their skin color, age, time of day, season, and location. Experts recommend that people should expose their hands, face, and arms at least two to three times a week for 25% of the time it takes to turn one's skin pink (e.g., 5 to 10 minutes) to make enough vitamin D. Persons with dark skin would need additional exposure, about three to five times the amount just recommended (or maybe even more). The large amount of melanin pigment in dark-skinned people is a potent natural sunscreen.

Sun exposure is only effective for vitamin D synthesis between about 8:00 A.M. and 4:00 P.M. and without sunscreen over SPF 8. Although excessive exposure to the sun can increase the risk of skin cancer, the minimal amount of UVB exposure needed for vitamin D synthesis is encouraged. Still, this practice is not effective at all when there is little skin exposed to sun in the winter in northern climates. Although some people may have enough vitamin D stored in their adipose cells from summer months, most people in northern climates should find alternate vitamin D sources in the winter months. Overall, anyone who does not receive enough sunshine to synthesize an adequate amount of vitamin D must have a dietary source of the vitamin. About 80% of dietary vitamin D is absorbed.

FIGURE 8-5 ▶ The synthesis of vitamin D can take place in the body.

Functions of Vitamin D

The main function of the vitamin D hormone (1,25-dihydroxyvitamin D) is to help regulate calcium and bone metabolism. Working with other hormones, especially **parathyroid hormone (PTH),** the vitamin D hormone closely regulates blood calcium so that appropriate amounts of it will be supplied to all cells. This regulation involves two main processes: the vitamin D hormone helps regulate absorption of calcium and phosphorus from the intestine and the deposition of calcium in the bones.

More interestingly, the vitamin D hormone is also capable of ensuring normal development of some cells, such as skin, colon, prostate, ovary, and breast cells, in turn reducing cancer risk in these sites (see Further Readings 4 and 7). The vitamin D hormone controls the growth of the parathyroid gland; aids in the function of the immune system; and contributes to skin cell development, muscle and gum health, and blood pressure regulation.

The most obvious result of the vitamin D hormone action is increased calcium and phosphorus deposition in bones. Without adequate calcium and phosphorus deposition during bone synthesis, bones weaken and bow under pressure. A child with these symptoms has the disease **rickets.** Symptoms also include enlarged head, joints, and rib cage and a deformed pelvis (Fig. 8-6) (see Further Readings 6, 7, and 11).

Studies have shown rickets to be a problem in breastfed infants who receive little sun exposure. For the prevention of rickets, breastfed infants should be provided supplemental vitamin D (under a physician's guidance). Keep in mind that supplements need to be used very carefully to avoid vitamin D toxicity in the infant. Rickets in children is also associated with fat malabsorption, such as that occurring in children with cystic fibrosis.

Osteomalacia, which means *soft bones,* is an adult disease comparable to rickets. It results from inefficient calcium absorption in the intestine or poor conservation of calcium by the kidneys. Both of these calcium-related problems can be caused by vitamin D deficiency. Bones then lose their minerals and become porous and weak and break easily. This leads to fractures in the hip and other bones. The risk of vitamin D deficiency increases in older adults. Adults with limited sun exposure may also develop the disease as may many African-American individuals. Combinations of sun exposure, vitamin D intake, or both can prevent this problem. Older people are advised to get sun exposure during early morning and late afternoon to receive the benefit of vitamin D synthesis without also increasing skin cancer risk. Aging decreases production of vitamin D in the skin by about 70% by the time one reaches the age of 70. One study showed that treatment with 10 to 20 micrograms per day

parathyroid hormone (PTH) A hormone made by the parathyroid glands that increases synthesis of the vitamin D hormone and aids calcium release from bone and calcium conservation by the kidneys, among other functions.

rickets A disease characterized by poor mineralization of newly synthesized bones because of low calcium content. This deficiency disease arises in infants and children from insufficient amounts of the vitamin D hormone in the body.

osteomalacia Adult form of rickets. The weakening of the bones seen in this disease is caused by low calcium content. A reduction in the amount of the vitamin D hormone in the body is one cause.

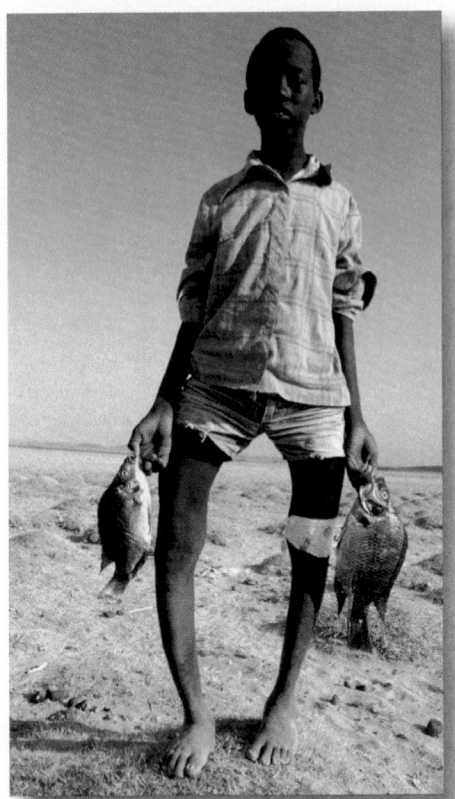

FIGURE 8-6 ▶ Vitamin D deficiency causes rickets, in which the bones and teeth do not develop normally.

Be careful not to confuse osteomalacia with osteoporosis, another type of bone disorder discussed in Chapter 9.

(400 to 800 IU per day) of vitamin D (in conjunction with adequate dietary calcium) greatly decreased fracture risk in older people in nursing homes. Follow-up studies support this role of vitamin D in reducing hip fracture risk (see Further Reading 16).

MAKING DECISIONS

New Benefits and Concerns about Vitamin D

Physicians are increasing the testing of blood levels of vitamin D. The jump in vitamin D testing stems from an abundance of emerging research linking vitamin D deficiency not only with osteoporosis and osteomalacia but also with some infectious diseases, cancers, autoimmune disorders, and cardiovascular disease. A recent study found that individuals with low vitamin D levels had a 60% greater risk of cardiac events such as heart attacks and stroke, and when both a vitamin D deficiency and high blood pressure were present, the risk for a serious cardiovascular event was doubled (see Further Readings 5 and 14). These results are of concern because vitamin D deficiency is becoming more common than previously believed in the United States, especially in people living at higher latitudes where vitamin D is less available from exposure to sunlight. Statistics indicate that 36% of Americans are vitamin D deficient and 40% of infants and toddlers have tested below the optimal blood threshold for vitamin D. A normal vitamin D test result is 30 nanograms/milliliter (ng/ml) or above, whereas under 20 ng/ml is considered deficient. Children are at risk of vitamin D insufficiency as a result of too little exposure to the sun stemming from concerns about skin cancer and increasing playtime indoors.

Vitamin D Sources and Needs

Few foods contain significant amounts of vitamin D. Rich sources are fatty fish (e.g., sardines and salmon), fortified milk and yogurt, and some ready-to-eat breakfast cereals (Fig. 8-7). In the United States and Canada, milk usually is fortified with 10 micrograms (400 IU) per quart. Although eggs, butter, liver, and a few brands of margarine contain some vitamin D, large servings must be eaten to obtain an adequate amount of the vitamin from these sources.

The Food and Nutrition Board established the first RDA for vitamin D in 2010. The RDA for healthy people ages 1 to 70 is 15 micrograms (600 IU) based on a daily intake that is sufficient to maintain bone health and normal calcium metabolism and on the basis of minimal sun exposure. The Daily Value used on food and supplement labels is 10 micrograms (400 IU). As mentioned, young, light-skinned people can synthesize all the vitamin D needed from casual sun exposure. For adults age 70 and over who have limited sun exposure, the RDA is set at 20 micrograms (800 IU) and can be obtained from a combination of vitamin D-fortified foods and a multivitamin and mineral supplement. Within the 2010 Dietary Guidelines for Americans, a key recommendation is to choose foods that provide more vitamin D, which is a nutrient of concern in American diets.

Upper Level for Vitamin D

The Upper Level for vitamin D is 100 micrograms per day (4000 IU per day) for children over age 9 and adults. Too much vitamin D taken regularly can create problems, especially in some infants and young children. For adults, intakes somewhat above the Upper Level appear to be safe. The Upper Level is based on the risk of too much vitamin D causing the overabsorption of calcium, which eventually leads to calcium deposits in the kidneys and other organs. These high intakes of vitamin D would also cause the typical symptoms of high blood calcium: weakness, loss of appetite, diarrhea, vomiting, mental confusion, and increased urine output. Calcium deposits in organs cause metabolic disturbances and cell death. However, vitamin D toxicity does not result from tanning in the sun too long because the body regulates the amount made in the skin.

Food Sources of Vitamin D

Food Item and Amount	Vitamin D (micrograms) Daily Value = 15 micrograms	Vitamin D (IU)	Adult Male and Female RDA = 15 micrograms %RDA
RDA	15	600	100%
Baked Salmon, 3 ounces	11.0	438	73%
Sardines, 1 ounce	3.4	136	23%
Canned tuna, 3 ounces	3.4	136	23%
1% milk, 1 cup	2.5	99	17%
Nonfat milk, 1 cup	2.5	98	17%
Soft margarine, 1 teaspoon	1.5	60	10%
Italian pork sausage, 3 ounces	1.1	44	7%
Soy milk, 1 cup	1.0	40	7%
Raisin Bran cereal, ¾ cup	1.0	38	7%
Baked bluefish, 3 ounces	0.9	34	6%
Special K cereal, ¾ cup	0.8	30	5%
Cooked egg yolk, 1	0.6	25	4%

Key:
- Grains
- Vegetables
- Fruits
- Dairy
- Protein
- Oils

ChooseMyPlate.gov

FIGURE 8-7 ▶ Food sources of vitamin D compared to the Adequate Intake for adults.

CONCEPT CHECK

Vitamin A is found in foods as preformed vitamin A and as provitamin A carotenoids. The most fully understood function of vitamin A is its importance in vision. Blindness caused by vitamin A deficiency is a major problem in many parts of the world. Vitamin A is also needed to maintain the health of many types of cells, support the immune system, and promote proper growth and development. Vitamin A and some carotenoids may be important in preventing cancer. However, because taking supplements of preformed vitamin A can be toxic, especially in pregnancy, the best recommendation is to focus primarily on eating plenty of provitamin A–rich foods, such as fruits and vegetables.

Vitamin D is a true vitamin only for people who fail to produce enough from sunlight, such as some older people and those with dark skin. Humans synthesize vitamin D from a cholesterol-like substance by the action of sunlight on their skin. The vitamin D is later acted on by the liver and kidneys to form the hormone 1,25-dihydroxyvitamin D. This hormone increases calcium absorption in the intestine and works with another hormone (parathyroid hormone) to maintain calcium in bones. Statistics indicating that 36% of Americans are vitamin D deficient have led to an increase in the recommended vitamin D intake and the first RDA for vitamin D. Rich food sources of vitamin D are fish oils and fortified milk. Megadose vitamin D intake can be toxic, especially in infancy and early childhood.

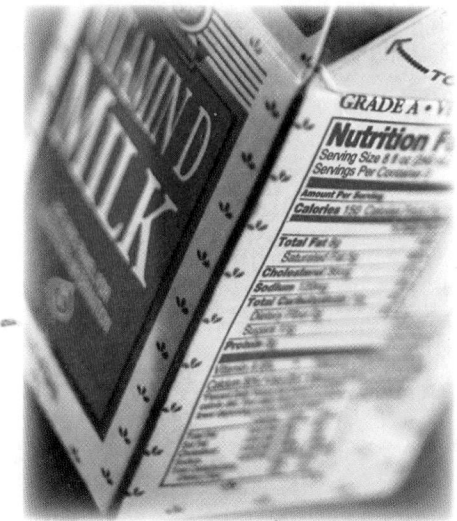

▲ Milk is usually fortified with vitamin D as well as vitamin A.

8.5 Vitamin E

In the past North Americans have spent more than $1 billion on vitamin E supplements each year. Sales of vitamin E supplements have declined in recent years, however, after studies raised concerns about higher deaths in those taking more than 800 IU of vitamin E per day. The following section attempts to sort out fact from fiction in the debate over this high-profile vitamin.

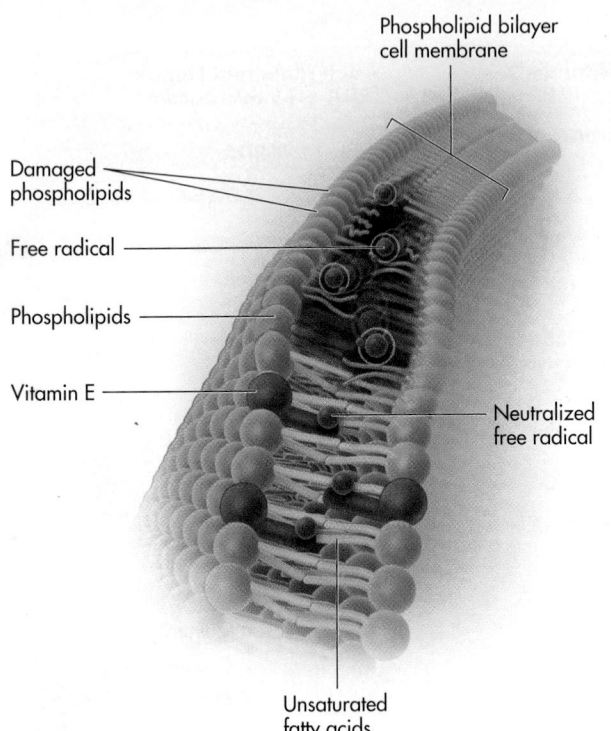

Phospholipid bilayer cell membrane

Damaged phospholipids

Free radical

Phospholipids

Vitamin E

Neutralized free radical

Unsaturated fatty acids

FIGURE 8-8 ▶ Fat-soluble vitamin E can donate an electron to stop free radical chain reactions. If not interrupted, these reactions cause extensive oxidative damage to cell membranes.

hemolysis Destruction of red blood cells. The red blood cell membrane breaks down, allowing cell contents to leak into the fluid portion of the blood.

Functions of Vitamin E

Acting as a fat-soluble antioxidant, vitamin E resides mostly in cell membranes. As discussed in Chapter 5, an antioxidant can form a barrier between a target molecule—an unsaturated fatty acid in a cell membrane, for example—and a compound seeking its electrons (Fig. 8-8). The antioxidant donates electrons or hydrogens to the electron-seeking compound. This protects other molecules or parts of a cell from having electrons stolen (such as from double bonds of unsaturated fatty acids).

Free radicals are highly reactive compounds containing an unpaired electron. Production of free-radicals is a normal result of cell metabolism and immune system function. For example, white blood cells generate free radicals as part of their action to stop infection. Some exposure to free radicals, then, is an important part of life. If vitamin E is not available to do its job, the electron-seeking free radicals can pull electrons from cell membranes, DNA, and other electron-dense cell components. This either alters the cell's DNA, which may increase the risk for cancer, or injures cell membranes, possibly causing the cell to die. Overall, the body needs antioxidants like vitamin E to carefully regulate exposure to free radicals and thereby prevent cellular damage.

Cells do not rely exclusively on vitamin E for protection from free radicals. Many other antioxidant systems exist in cells, some of which use minerals, such as copper, selenium, and manganese (see Chapter 9 for details). As discussed earlier in this chapter, carotenoids in fruits and vegetables also act as antioxidants. In addition, cells have mechanisms other than antioxidants to repair molecules (such as DNA) that have been damaged by free radicals.

Thus, vitamin E is just one component of the antioxidant system. There is evidence that vitamin E helps prevent or delay heart diseases and certain cancers. Consuming vitamin E as a dietary supplement, however, may not be the most effective way to produce these effects. Two large recent studies have shown no benefit from vitamin E supplements on the prevention of certain diseases in males (see Further Readings 8 and 12). In the Physician's Health Study II, neither vitamin E nor C had an effect on major cardiovascular events including heart attacks, stroke, or death. The major prostate cancer SELECT trial also found no benefit of vitamin E or selenium supplements on prostate cancer. These results suggest that pulling a nutrient out of the whole diet, may not produce the same effects. Furthermore, there is far stronger evidence to support the benefits of lifestyle changes such as improving diet (especially fruit, vegetable, and whole-grain bread and cereal intake), performing regular physical activity, not smoking, and maintaining a healthy body weight than there is for the postulated benefits of supplemental antioxidants, including vitamin E. Thus, as reviewed in Chapter 5, even if antioxidant supplements are eventually determined to be effective in preventing cardiovascular disease or cancer, they should be used only as an adjunct—not as an alternative—to a healthful lifestyle. In fact, the American Heart Association and a group of leading cardiologists stated that it is premature to recommend vitamin E supplements to the general population, based on current knowledge and the failure of major clinical trials to show any benefit (review Chapter 5). This conclusion is in agreement with the latest report on vitamin E by the Food and Nutrition Board of the National Academy of Sciences. In addition, FDA has denied the request of the supplement industry to make a health claim that vitamin E supplements reduce the risk of cardiovascular disease and cancer. Still, some experts recommend vitamin E supplements (50 IU to 400 IU per day), while at the same time noting that evidence supporting this recommendation is sketchy.

A deficiency of vitamin E causes cell membranes to break down. The double bonds in the unsaturated fatty acids in cell membranes are sensitive to attack by oxidizing compounds. Vitamin E neutralizes these compounds, so it protects cell membranes from damage. When oxidative damage causes the cell membranes of red blood cells to break down, it is called **hemolysis.**

Vitamin E Sources and Needs

Vitamin E is a family of four **tocopherols,** called alpha, beta, gamma, and delta. Alpha-tocopherol is the main form in the human body, whereas gamma-tocopherol is the main form in foods. Major sources of vitamin E include plant oils, the main components of products such as salad dressings and mayonnaise, ready-to-eat breakfast cereals, some fruits and vegetables (e.g., asparagus, tomatoes, and green leafy vegetables), eggs, and margarine. Also, whole grains, nuts (e.g., almonds), and seeds (e.g., sunflower seeds) are good sources of vitamin E (Fig. 8-9). Plant oils are made up of mainly unsaturated fatty acids, and the vitamin E in plant oils protects these unsaturated fats from oxidation. Animal fats and fish oils, on the other hand, have practically no vitamin E (Fig. 8-10). The actual vitamin E content of a food depends on how it was harvested, processed, stored, and cooked because vitamin E is susceptible to destruction by oxygen, metals, light, and especially repeated use in deep-fat frying.

The RDA of vitamin E for adults is 15 milligrams per day of alpha-tocopherol, the most active form of vitamin E. The 15-milligram allotment is equivalent to 22 IU of a natural source and 33 IU of a synthetic source. Typically, North American adults consume about two-thirds of the RDA for vitamin E from food sources. Daily intake of nuts and seeds, ready-to-eat breakfast cereals containing vitamin E, or use of a multivitamin and mineral supplement would close this gap between needs and actual intakes. A Daily Value of 30 IU is used to express the vitamin E content on food and supplement labels.

The chemical structure of vitamin E varies depending on its source. The dl form or isomer is found in synthetic vitamin E and the d isomer is found in natural sources of vitamin E. Within the older IU system, 1 IU equals about 0.45 milligrams vitamin E,

> **tocopherols** The chemical name for some forms of vitamin E. The alpha form is the most potent.

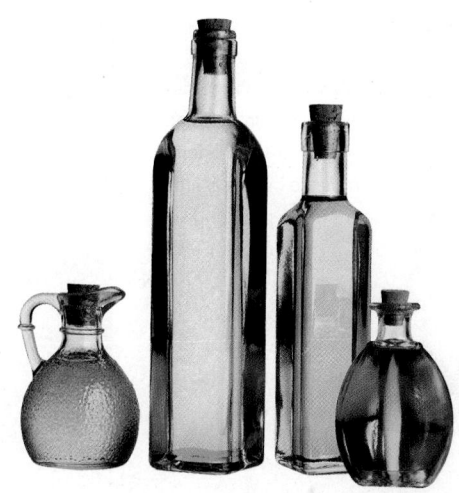

▲ Plant oils are rich sources of vitamin E.

Food Sources of Vitamin E

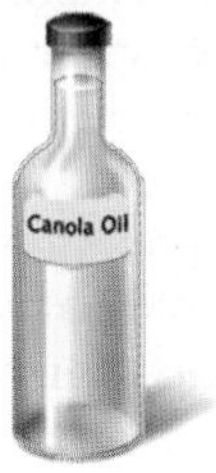

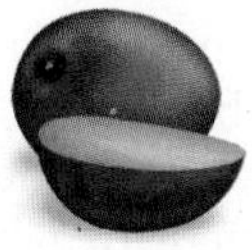

Food Item and Amount	Vitamin E (milligrams)	Vitamin E (IU)	Adult Male and Female RDA = 15 milligrams
	Daily Value = 30 IU		%RDA
RDA	15	22-33	100%
Fortified Bran cereal, ¾ cup	22.5	33.5	150%
Sunflower oil, 2 tablespoons	16.3	24.3	109%
Dry-roasted sunflower seeds, 1 ounce	14.3	21.2	95%
Dry-roasted almonds, 1 ounce	7.5	11.1	50%
Safflower oil, 1 tablespoon	5.9	8.7	39%
Canola oil, 2 tablespoons	5.7	8.5	38%
Wheat germ, ¼ cup	5.2	7.7	35%
Almonds, 1 ounce	4.5	6.8	30%
Oil-roasted sunflower seeds, 1 tablespoon	3.4	5.0	23%
Italian dressing, 2 tablespoons	3.1	4.5	21%
Mayonnaise, 1 tablespoon	3.0	4.5	20%
Avocado, 1	2.7	4.0	18%
Chunky peanut butter, 2 tablespoons	2.4	3.6	16%
Mango, 1	2.3	3.5	15%
Peanuts, 1 ounce	2.1	3.1	14%

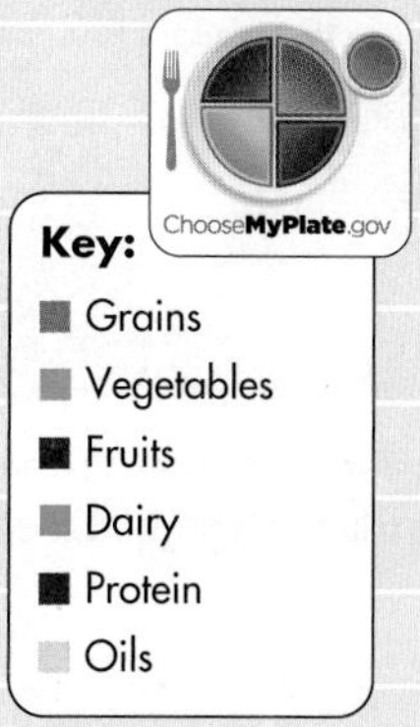

Key:
■ Grains
■ Vegetables
■ Fruits
■ Dairy
■ Protein
■ Oils

ChooseMyPlate.gov

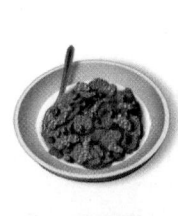

FIGURE 8-9 ▶ Food sources of vitamin E compared to the RDA for adults.

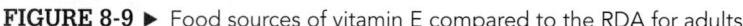

FIGURE 8-10 ▶ Sources of vitamin E from MyPlate. The fill of the background color (none, 1/3, 2/3, or completely covered) within each group on the plate indicates the average nutrient density for vitamin E in that group. Overall, plant oils are the richest source, followed by nuts and seeds in the protein group. With regard to physical activity, vitamin E has no primary role in the related energy metabolism *per se* but likely limits some oxidant damage during such endeavors.

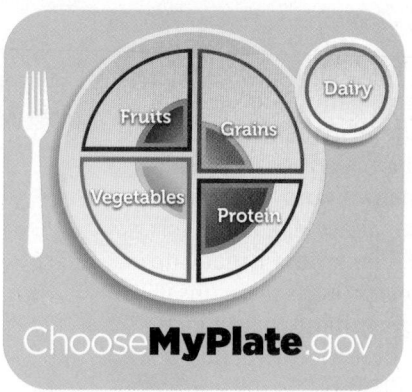

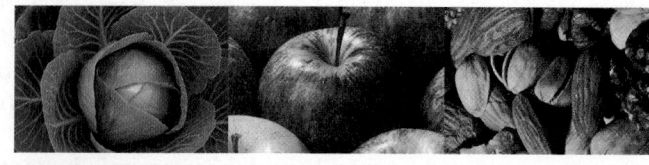

MyPlate: Sources of Vitamin E

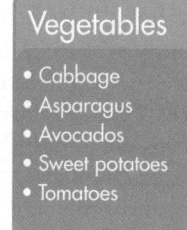
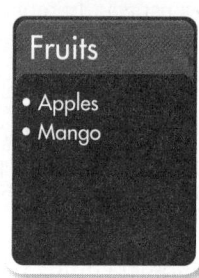
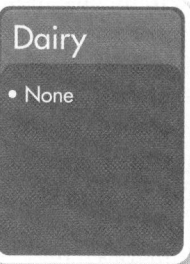
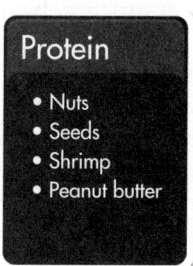

Grains
- Wheat germ (whole grains)
- Some fortified breakfast cereals

Vegetables
- Cabbage
- Asparagus
- Avocados
- Sweet potatoes
- Tomatoes

Fruits
- Apples
- Mango

Dairy
- None

Protein
- Nuts
- Seeds
- Shrimp
- Peanut butter

isomers Different chemical structures for compounds that share the same chemical formula.

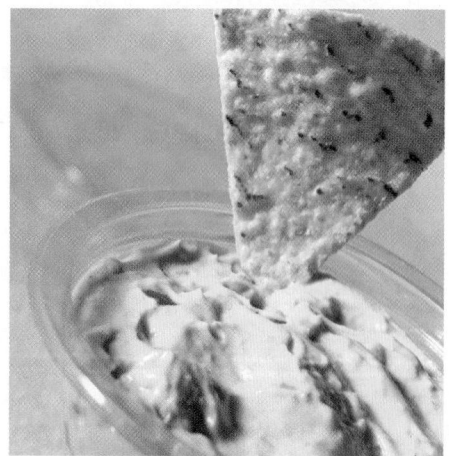

▲ The avocado in guacamole and the oil in the tortilla chip are good sources of vitamin E.

hemorrhage An escape of blood from blood vessels.

based on the synthetic form (dl **isomer**) of vitamin E found in most supplements. If vitamin E is from a natural source (d isomer), 1 IU equals 0.67 milligrams, because the natural form of vitamin E is more potent than the synthetic form.

The maximum dose the body can retain on a daily basis is thought to be 200 milligrams. This would represent 300 IU of the d isomer (200/0.67 = 300) to 450 IU of the dl isomer (200/0.45 = 450).

Cell damage by free radicals occurs over an extended period. Therefore, the beneficial effects of vitamin E and other antioxidants in counteracting this damage is most apparent when viewed over the long term. Research on a possible benefit of intakes of vitamin E in excess of the RDA for healthy adults is currently underway.

Several populations are especially susceptible to developing marginal vitamin E status. Preterm infants are born with low vitamin E stores, because this vitamin is transferred from mother to baby during late stages of pregnancy. Hemolysis (described on page 302) is of particular concern for preterm infants, due to red blood cell damage that occurs in the absence of adequate vitamin E. The rapid growth of preterm infants, coupled with the high oxygen needs of their immature lungs, greatly increases the stress on red blood cells. Special formulas and supplements designed for preterm infants can help compensate for their low vitamin E status. Smokers are another group at high risk for vitamin E deficiency, as smoking readily destroys vitamin E in the lungs. Still, one study showed that even using megadoses of vitamin E was ineffective in preventing this damage in smokers. Others at considerable risk of vitamin E deficiency include adults on very low-fat diets or those with fat malabsorption.

Upper Level for Vitamin E

The Upper Level for vitamin E for a healthy population is 1000 milligrams per day of supplemental alpha-tocopherol. The upper level has been established because excessive amounts of vitamin E can interfere with vitamin K's role in the clotting mechanism, leading to **hemorrhage**. Individuals who are vitamin K deficient or taking anticoagulants (e.g., Coumadin) or heavy doses of aspirin are especially at risk for hemorrhage from megadose vitamin E use. In international units, the Upper Level is 1500 IU for vitamin E isolated from natural sources (d isomer; 1000/0.67 = 1500) and 1100 IU for synthetic vitamin E (dl isomer; 1000/0.45/2 = 1100). The lower IU value for the synthetic form reflects the greater number of forms present in the synthetic product, only half or less of which contribute to vitamin E activity in cells, but are still absorbed. This Upper Level is set for a healthy population.

8.6 Vitamin K

A family of compounds known collectively as vitamin K is found in plants, plant oils, fish oils, and meats. While most vitamin K comes from our diet, another form is also synthesized by bacteria in the human intestine. This form supplies us with about 10% of the vitamin K we need.

Functions of Vitamin K

Vitamin K is vital for blood clotting, working along with various proteins and calcium. The *K* stems from the Danish spelling of **coagulation** because a Danish researcher first noted the relationship between vitamin K and blood clotting. Vitamin K is needed for the activation of several blood-clotting factors (Fig. 8-11). Vitamin K

coagulation Blood clotting; essentially a transition of blood from a liquid cell suspension into a solid, gel-like form.

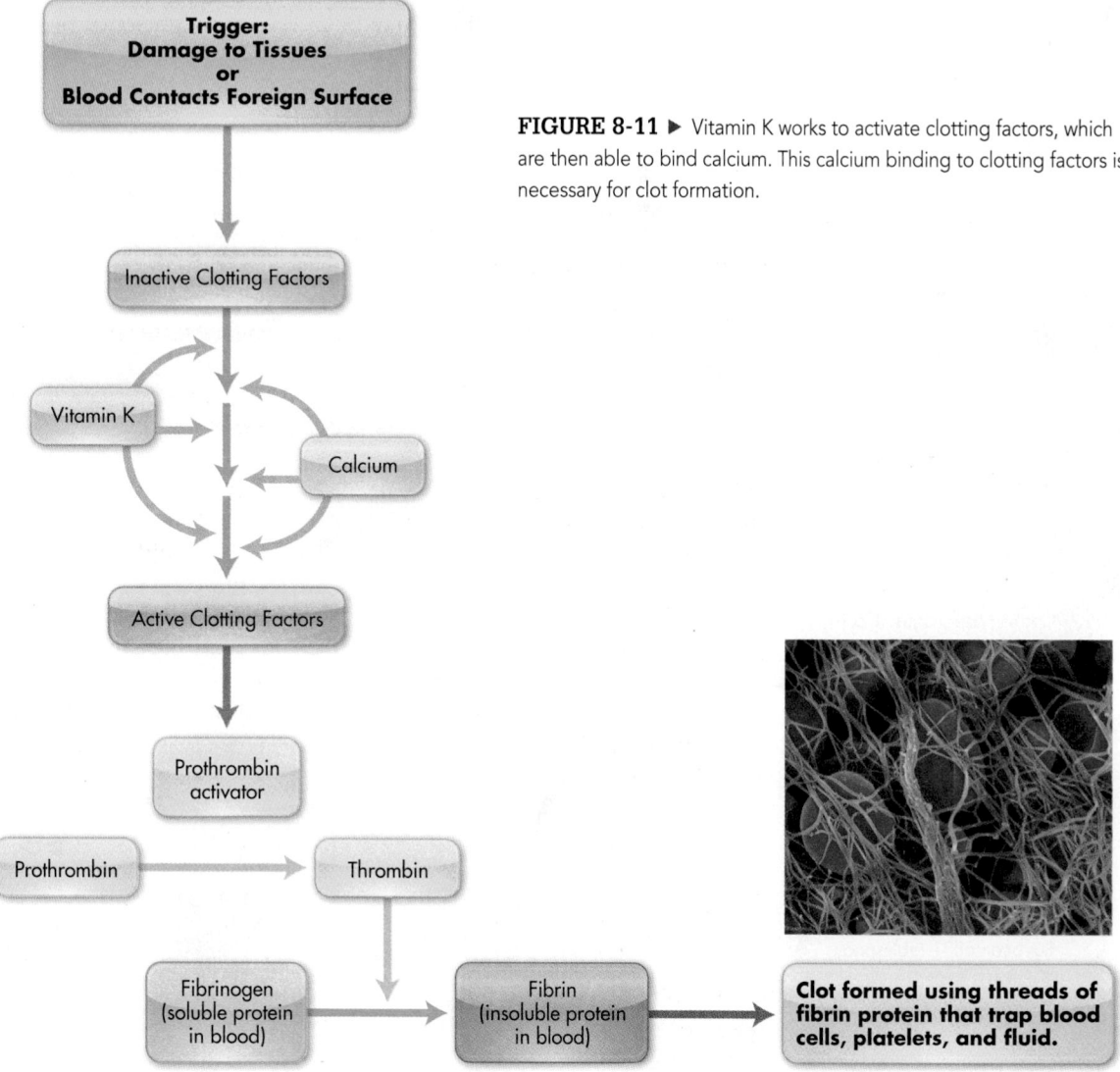

FIGURE 8-11 ▶ Vitamin K works to activate clotting factors, which are then able to bind calcium. This calcium binding to clotting factors is necessary for clot formation.

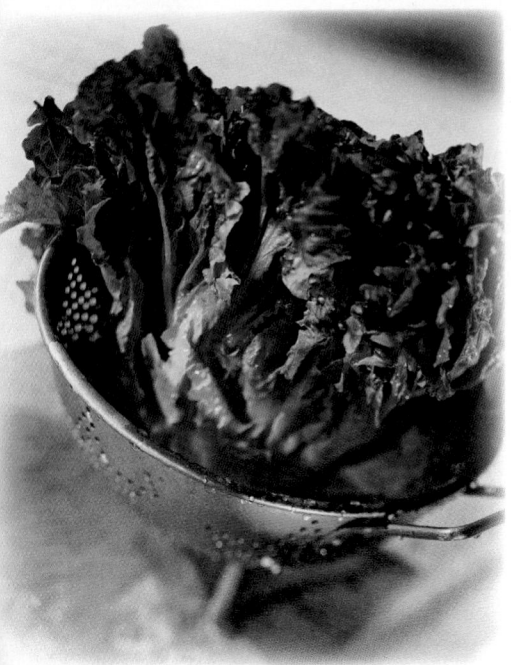

also activates proteins present in bone, muscle, and kidneys, to give calcium-binding ability to these organs. A poor vitamin K intake has been linked to an increase in hip fractures because of its effect on various proteins in bone (see Further Reading 16).

At birth, a newborn's intestinal tract lacks a sufficient amount of bacteria to produce enough vitamin K to allow for effective blood clotting. Therefore, vitamin K also is routinely given by injection shortly after birth to insure blood clotting if the infant is injured or needs surgery. In adults, deficiencies of vitamin K have occurred in the presence of severe, long-standing fat malabsorption or when a person takes long-term antibiotics that destroy many of the intestinal bacteria that produce vitamin K.

Vitamin K Sources and Needs

Major food sources of vitamin K are liver, green leafy vegetables (e.g., kale, turnip greens, dark-green lettuce, and spinach), broccoli, peas, and green beans (Fig. 8-12). Other sources are soybean and canola oils and certain fortified chocolate confections (these also contain extra calcium). Thus, another reason to consume a diet rich in green vegetables is to obtain sufficient vitamin K. Most vitamin K consumed in a day disappears from the body by the next day. Nevertheless, vitamin K is abundant in a balanced diet, and a deficiency is uncommon. Vitamin K is resistant to cooking losses.

The Adequate Intake for vitamin K is 90 and 120 micrograms per day for adult women and men, respectively. Most North Americans consume at least this much. A Daily Value of 80 micrograms is used to express vitamin K content on food and supplement labels. Older adults may be at risk of a deficiency because of low consumption of green vegetables.

▲ A salad containing dark greens (or other green vegetables) each day provides abundant vitamin K for a diet.

Food Sources of Vitamin K

Food Item and Amount	Vitamin K (micrograms)	Adult Male AI = 120 micrograms	Adult Female AI = 90 micrograms
		Daily Value = 80 micrograms	
		%AI	%AI
RDA	90-120	100%	100%
Cooked kale, ½ cup	530	442%	589%
Cooked turnip greens, 1 cup	520	433%	578%
Cooked spinach, 1 cup	480	400%	533%
Cooked Brussel sprouts, ½ cup	150	125%	167%
Raw spinach, 1 cup	144	120%	160%
Cooked asparagus, 1 cup	144	120%	160%
Cooked broccoli, ½ cup	110	92%	122%
Looseleaf lettuce, 1 cup	97	81%	108%
Cooked green beans, ½ cup	49	41%	54%
Raw cabbage, 1 cup	42	35%	47%
Sauerkraut, ½ cup	30	25%	33%
Green peas, ½ cup	26	22%	29%
Soybean oil, 1 tablespoon	25	21%	28%
Cooked cauliflower, 1 cup	20	17%	22%
Canola oil, 1 tablespoon	17	14%	19%

Key:
■ Grains
■ Vegetables
■ Fruits
■ Dairy
■ Protein
■ Oils

ChooseMyPlate.gov

FIGURE 8-12 ▶ Food sources of vitamin K compared to the Adequate Intake for adult males and females.
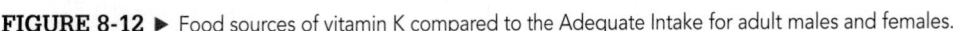

Oral vitamin K generally poses no risk of toxicity, so no Upper Level has been set. The main problem with megadose use is reduced effectiveness of oral medications used to reduce blood clotting (e.g., Coumadin). These medications are used to lessen blood clotting especially in those who have undergone recent cardiovascular surgery.

Table 8-2 reviews what we have covered so far regarding the fat-soluble vitamins.

TABLE 8-2 Summary of the Fat-Soluble Vitamins

Vitamin	Major Functions	RDA or Adequate Intake	Dietary Sources	Deficiency Symptoms	Toxicity Symptoms
Vitamin A (preformed vitamin A and provitamin A)	• Promote vision: night and color • Promote growth • Prevent drying of skin and eyes • Promote resistance to bacterial infection and overall immune system function	Females: 700 micrograms RAE Males: 900 micrograms RAE 2300–3000 IU if as preformed (vitamin A)	Preformed Vitamin A: • Liver • Fortified milk • Fortified breakfast cereals Provitamin A: • Sweet potatoes • Spinach • Greens • Carrots • Cantaloupe • Apricots • Broccoli	• Night blindness • Xerophthalmia • Poor growth • Dry skin	• Fetal malformations • Hair loss • Skin changes • Bone pain • Fractures Upper Level is 3000 micrograms of preformed vitamin A (10,000 IU) based on the risk of birth defects and liver toxicity
Vitamin D	• Increase absorption of calcium and phosphorus • Maintain optimal blood calcium and calcification of bone	15 micrograms (600 IU)	• Vitamin D fortified milk • Fortified breakfast cereals • Fish oils • Sardines • Salmon	• Rickets in children • Osteomalacia in adults	• Growth retardation • Kidney damage • Calcium deposits in soft tissue Upper Level is 100 micrograms (4000 IU) based on the risk of elevated blood calcium
Vitamin E	• Antioxidant prevents breakdown of vitamin A and unsaturated fatty acids	15 milligrams alpha-tocopherol 22 IU natural form, 33 IU (synthetic form)	• Plant oils • Products made from plant oils • Some greens • Some fruits • Nuts and seeds • Fortified breakfast cereals	• Hemolysis of red blood cells • Nerve degeneration	• Muscle weakness • Headaches • Nausea • Inhibition of vitamin K metabolism Upper Level is 1000 milligrams (1100 IU synthetic form, 1500 IU natural form) based on the risk of hemorrhage
Vitamin K	• Activation of blood-clotting factors • Activation of proteins involved in bone metabolism	Females: 90 micrograms Males: 120 micrograms	• Green vegetables • Liver • Some plant oils • Some calcium supplements	• Hemorrhage • Fractures	No Upper Level has been set

Abbreviations: RAE = retinol activity equivalents; IU = international units

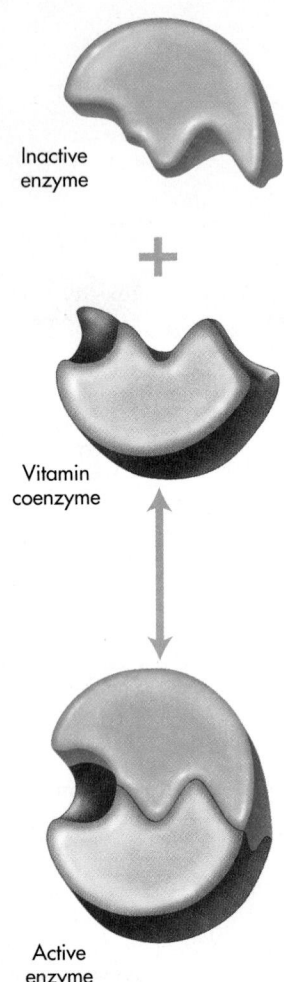

Inactive enzyme

+

Vitamin coenzyme

Active enzyme

FIGURE 8-13 ▶ Coenzymes, such as those formed from B vitamins, aid in the function of various enzymes. Without the coenzyme, the enzyme cannot function, and deficiency symptoms associated with the missing vitamin eventually appear. Health-food stores sell the coenzyme forms of some vitamins. These more expensive forms of vitamins are unnecessary. The body makes all the coenzymes it needs from vitamin precursors.

bioavailability The degree to which an ingested nutrient is absorbed and thus is available to the body.

CONCEPT CHECK

Vitamin E functions primarily as an antioxidant. It can donate electrons to electron-seeking free radical (oxidizing) compounds. By neutralizing these compounds, vitamin E helps prevent cell destruction, especially the destruction of red blood cell membranes. Vitamin E occurs in a wide variety of foods, but its richest sources are plant oils, foods rich in these oils, and nuts. Studies using dietary supplements of vitamin E have not shown beneficial effects on the risk of diseases including heart disease and cancer.

Vitamin K plays a key role in efficient blood clotting; it contributes to the activation of certain blood-clotting proteins. In addition, vitamin K contributes to the synthesis of the calcium-binding proteins in some organs, such as bones. About 10% of the vitamin K we absorb every day is synthesized by our intestinal bacteria; the rest comes from our diets. The amount in the diet alone generally meets our daily needs. Thus, except for newborns and possibly older adults, a deficiency of vitamin K is unlikely.

8.7 The Water-Soluble Vitamins and Choline

Regular consumption of good sources of the water-soluble vitamins is important. Most water-soluble vitamins are readily excreted from the body with any excess generally ending up in the urine or stool and very little being stored. They dissolve in water, so large amounts of these vitamins can be lost during food processing and preparation. Vitamin content is best preserved by light cooking methods, such as stir-frying, steaming, and microwaving (review Table 8-1).

The B vitamins are thiamin, riboflavin, niacin, pantothenic acid, biotin, vitamin B-6, folate, and vitamin B-12. Choline is a related nutrient, but currently is not classified as a vitamin. Vitamin C is also a water-soluble vitamin.

The B vitamins often occur together in the same foods, so a lack of one B vitamin may mean other B vitamins are also low in a diet. The B vitamins function as coenzymes, small molecules that interact with enzymes to enable the enzymes to function. In essence, the coenzymes contribute to enzyme activity (Fig. 8-13).

As coenzymes, the B vitamins play many key roles in metabolism. The metabolic pathways used by carbohydrates, fats, and amino acids all require input from B vitamins. Because of their role in energy metabolism, needs for many B vitamins increase somewhat as energy expenditure increases. Still, this is not a major concern because this increase in energy expenditure usually results in a corresponding increase in food intake, which contributes more B vitamins to a diet. Many B vitamins are interdependent because they participate in the same processes (Fig. 8-14). B vitamin deficiency symptoms typically occur in the brain and nervous system, skin, and GI tract. Cells in these tissues are metabolically active, and those in the skin and GI tract are also constantly being replaced.

After being ingested, the B vitamins are first broken down from their active coenzyme forms into free vitamins in the stomach and small intestine. The vitamins are then absorbed, primarily in the small intestine. Typically, about 50% to 90% of the B vitamins in the diet are absorbed, which means they have relatively high **bioavailability**. Once inside cells, the active coenzyme forms are resynthesized. There is no need to consume the coenzyme forms themselves. Some vitamins are sold in their coenzyme forms but these are broken down during digestion and we activate them when needed.

B Vitamin Intakes of North Americans

The nutritional health of most North Americans with regard to the B vitamins is generally good. Typical diets contain a good amount and variety of natural sources of

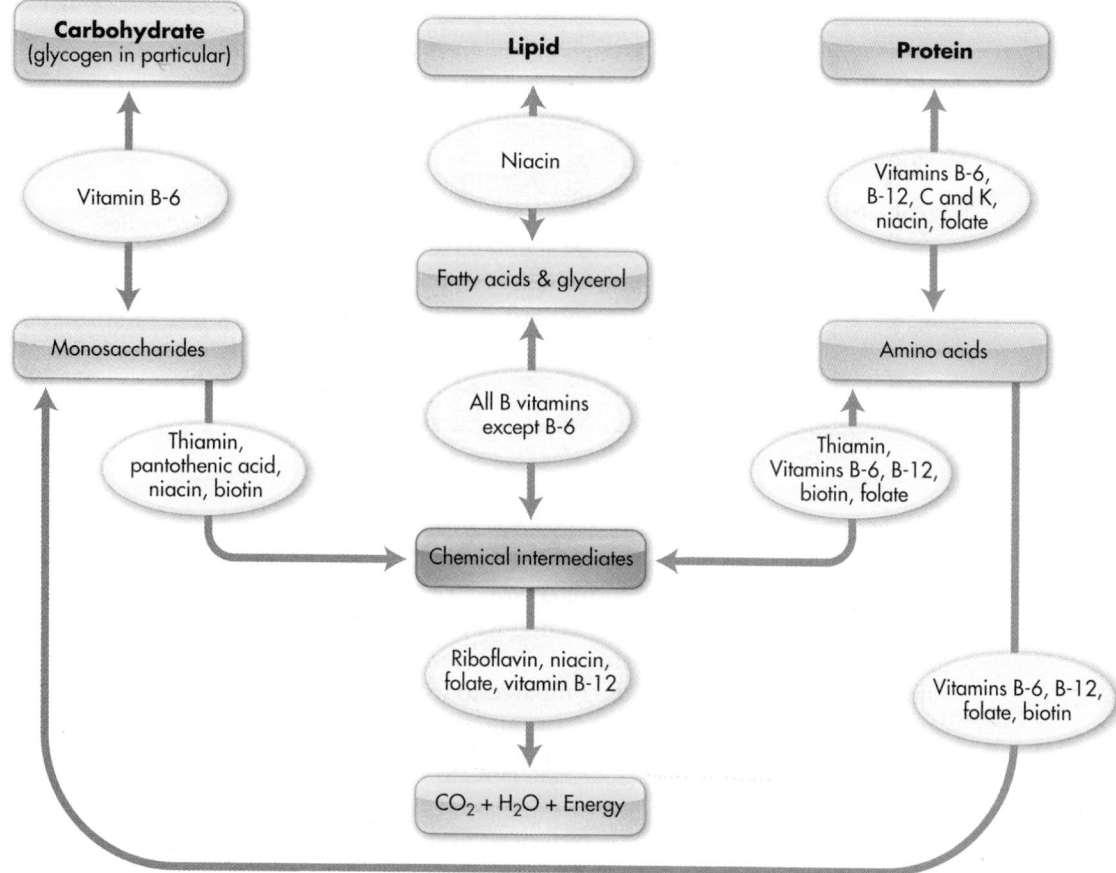

FIGURE 8-14 ▶ Examples of metabolic pathways for which water soluble vitamins are essential. The metabolism of energy-yielding nutrients requires vitamin input.

these vitamins. In addition, many common foods, such as ready-to-eat breakfast cereals, are fortified with one or more of the water-soluble vitamins. In some developing countries, however, deficiencies of the water-soluble vitamins are more common, and the resulting deficiency diseases pose significant public health problems. (A detailed discussion of nutritional deficiencies worldwide is presented in Chapter 12.)

Despite the generally good B vitamin status of North Americans, marginal deficiencies of the water-soluble vitamins may occur in some cases, especially in older people who eat little food and in people who follow poor dietary patterns. The long-term effects of such marginal deficiencies are unknown, but increased risk of cardiovascular disease, cancer, and cataracts of the eye is suspected. However, in the short run, such a marginal deficiency in most people likely leads only to fatigue or other bothersome and unspecific physical effects. With rare exceptions, healthy adults do not develop the more serious B vitamin deficiency diseases from dietary inadequacies alone. The main exceptions are people with alcoholism. The combination of extremely unbalanced diets and alcohol-induced alterations of vitamin absorption and metabolism creates significant risks for serious nutrient deficiencies among people with alcoholism (see Chapter 16).

Grains: One Important Source of B Vitamins The milling of grains leads to losses of vitamins and minerals. In the milling process, seeds are crushed and the germ, bran, and husk layers are discarded, leaving just the starch-containing endosperm in the refined grains. The starch is used to make flour, bread, and cereal products. Unfortunately, many nutrients are lost along with the discarded germ, bran, and husk materials. To counteract these losses, in the United States, bread and cereal products made from milled grains are enriched with four B vitamins (thiamin, riboflavin, niacin,

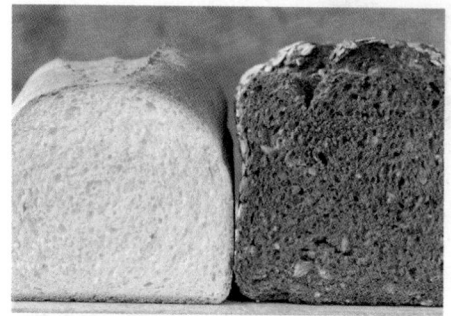

▲ The white bread on the left is made from refined flour that has been enriched with four B vitamins and iron to achieve the nutrient level in the whole-grain bread on the right.

FIGURE 8-15 ▶ Compare the relative nutrient contents of refined versus whole grains. Nutrients are expressed as a percentage of the nutrient contribution of the whole grain product.

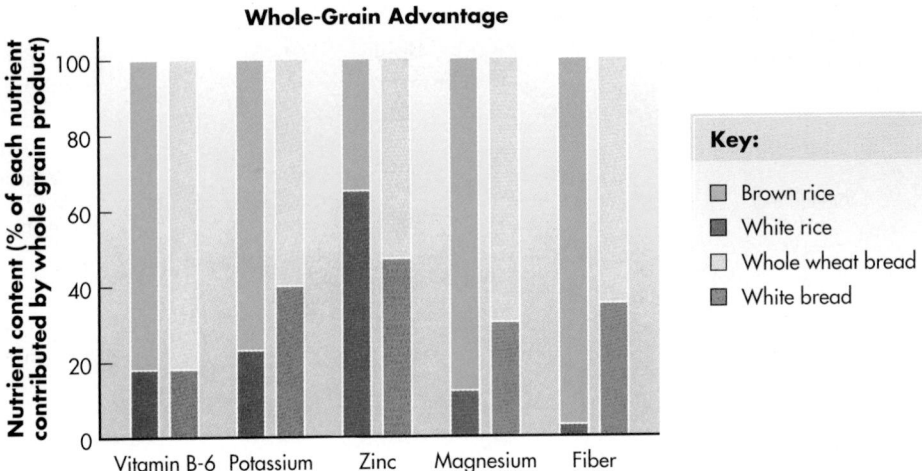

and folic acid) and with the mineral iron. This addition helps protect us from the common deficiency diseases associated with a dietary lack of these nutrients. Unfortunately, these products remain lower in vitamin E, vitamin B-6, potassium, magnesium, fiber, and other nutrients compared to whole-grain products (Fig. 8-15). This is one reason why nutrient experts advocate regular consumption of whole-grain products, such as whole-wheat bread and brown rice, rather than refined grain products.

8.8 Thiamin

beriberi The thiamin deficiency disorder characterized by muscle weakness, loss of appetite, nerve degeneration, and sometimes edema.

Thiamin (formerly called *vitamin B-1*) is used, among other purposes, to help release energy from carbohydrate. Its coenzyme form participates in reactions in which a carbon dioxide (CO_2) is lost from a larger molecule. This reaction is particularly important in the breakdown of carbohydrates and certain amino acids for energy needs (review Fig. 8-14).

The thiamin deficiency disease is called **beriberi,** a word that means "I can't, I can't" in the Sri Lanka language of Sinhalese. The symptoms include weakness, loss of appetite, irritability, nervous tingling throughout the body, poor arm and leg coordination, and deep muscle pain in the calves. A person with beriberi often develops an enlarged heart and sometimes severe edema.

Beriberi results when glucose, the primary fuel for brain and nerve cells, cannot be metabolized to release energy. The thiamin coenzyme participates in glucose metabolism, so problems with body functions associated with brain and nerve action are the first signs of a thiamin deficiency, some after only 10 days on a thiamin-free diet.

Beriberi is seen in areas where rice is a staple and polished (white) rice is consumed rather than brown (whole-grain) rice. In most parts of the world, brown rice has had its bran and germ layer removed to make white rice, a poor source of thiamin, unless it is enriched.

Thiamin Sources and Needs

Major sources of thiamin include pork products, whole grains (wheat germ), ready-to-eat breakfast cereals, enriched grains, green beans, milk, orange juice, organ meats, peanuts, dried beans, and seeds (Figs. 8-16 and 8-17).

The adult RDA for thiamin is 1.1 to 1.2 milligrams per day. The Daily Value of 1.5 milligrams is used to express the thiamin content on food and supplement labels. Average daily intakes for men exceed this by 50% or more, and women generally meet the RDA. Some groups, such as low-income and older people, may barely meet

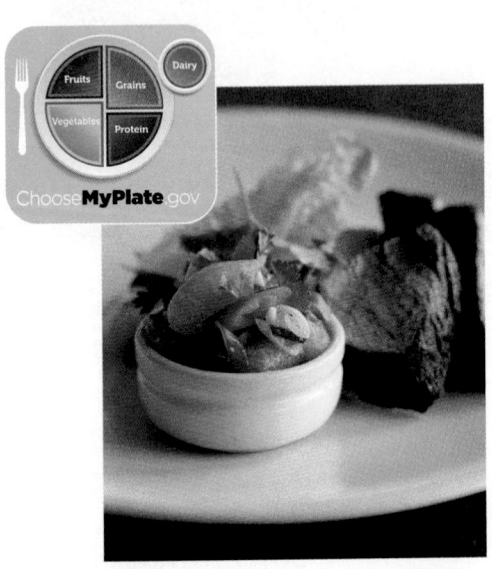

▲ The roasted pork filet and mandarin orange and chili pepper salad are good sources of thiamin from the protein, fruit, and vegetable sections of MyPlate. Which sections are missing?

Food Sources of Thiamin

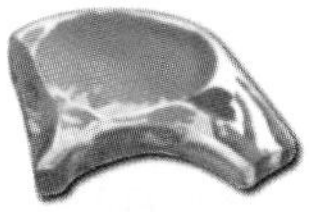

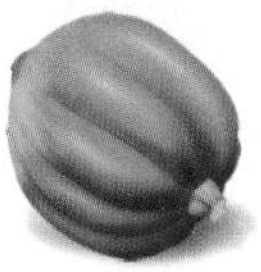

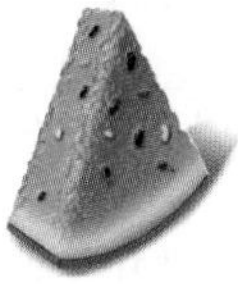

Food Item and Amount	Thiamin (milligrams)	Adult Male RDA = 1.2 milligrams		Adult Female RDA = 1.1 milligrams	
		Daily Value = 1.5 mg			
		%RDA		%RDA	
RDA	1.1-1.2	▬▬▬▬▬▬	100%	▬▬▬▬▬▬	100%
Canned lean ham, 3 ounces	0.9	▬▬▬▬▬	75%	▬▬▬▬▬	82%
Pork chops, 4 ounces	0.6	▬▬▬	50%	▬▬▬▬	55%
Wheat germ, ¼ cup	0.5	▬▬▬	42%	▬▬▬	45%
Canadian bacon, 2 ounces	0.5	▬▬▬	42%	▬▬▬	45%
Acorn squash, 1 cup	0.4	▬▬	33%	▬▬	36%
Soy milk, 1 cup	0.4	▬▬	33%	▬▬	36%
Flour tortilla, 1	0.4	▬▬	33%	▬▬	36%
Ham lunch meat, 2 pieces	0.3	▬▬	25%	▬▬	27%
Watermelon, 1 slice	0.2	▬	17%	▬	18%
Fresh orange juice, 1 cup	0.2	▬	17%	▬	18%
Cooked green peas, ½ cup	0.2	▬	17%	▬	18%
Baked beans, ½ cup	0.2	▬	17%	▬	18%
Navy beans, ½ cup	0.2	▬	17%	▬	18%
Corn, ½ cup	0.2	▬	17%	▬	18%

Key:
- Grains
- Vegetables
- Fruits
- Dairy
- Protein

FIGURE 8-16 ▶ Food sources of thiamin compared to the RDA for adult males and females.

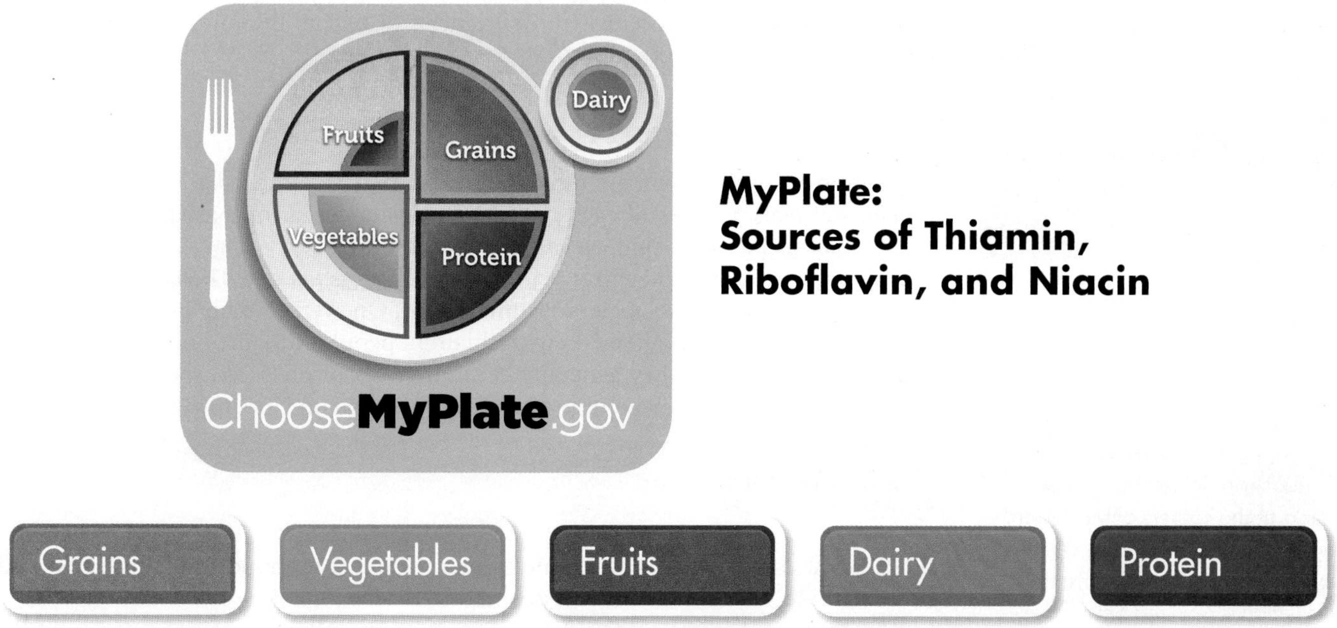

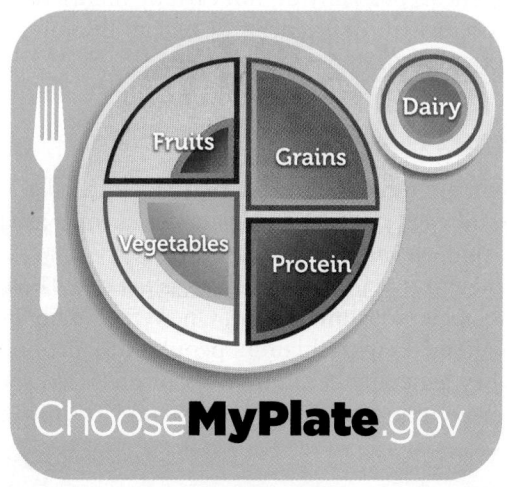

MyPlate: Sources of Thiamin, Riboflavin, and Niacin

Grains Vegetables Fruits Dairy Protein

FIGURE 8-17 ▶ Sources of thiamin, riboflavin, and niacin from MyPlate. The fill of the background color (none, 1/3, 2/3, or completely covered) within each group in the plate indicates the average nutrient density for these vitamins in that group. Overall, the protein group and the grains group contain many foods that are nutrient-dense sources of thiamin, riboflavin, and niacin. As well, foods from the dairy group are especially rich sources of riboflavin.

their needs for thiamin. A diet dominated by highly processed and unenriched foods, sugar, fat, and alcohol also creates a potential for thiamin deficiency. Oral thiamin supplements are typically nontoxic because excess thiamin is rapidly lost in the urine. Thus, no Upper Level has been set for thiamin.

MAKING DECISIONS

Thiamin and Alcohol

People with alcoholism are at the greatest risk for thiamin deficiency because absorption and use of thiamin are profoundly diminished and excretion is increased by consumption of alcohol. Furthermore, the low-quality diet that often accompanies severe alcoholism makes matters worse. There is limited thiamin storage in the body, so an alcoholic binge lasting 1 to 2 weeks may quickly deplete already diminished amounts of the vitamin and result in deficiency symptoms.

8.9 Riboflavin

The name *riboflavin* comes from its yellow color (*flavus* means yellow in Latin). Riboflavin was formerly referred to as *vitamin B-2*.

The coenzyme forms of riboflavin participate in many energy-yielding metabolic pathways. When cells generate energy using oxygen-requiring pathways, such as when fatty acids are broken down and burned for energy, the coenzymes of riboflavin are used (review Fig. 8-14). Some vitamin and mineral metabolism also requires riboflavin. In addition, because of its link to the activity of certain enzymes, riboflavin has an antioxidant role in the body.

The symptoms associated with riboflavin deficiency include inflammation of the mouth and tongue, dermatitis, cracking of tissue around the corners of the mouth (called *cheilosis*), various eye disorders, sensitivity to the sun, and confusion (Fig. 8-18). Such symptoms develop after approximately 2 months on a riboflavin-poor diet. In addition, riboflavin deficiencies probably do not exist by themselves. Instead, a riboflavin deficiency would occur with deficiencies of niacin, thiamin, and vitamin B-6 because these nutrients often occur in the same foods.

Riboflavin Sources and Needs

Major sources of riboflavin are milk and milk products, enriched grains, ready-to-eat breakfast cereals, meat, and eggs (Fig. 8-19). Vegetables such as asparagus, broccoli, and various greens (e.g., spinach) are also good sources.

The adult RDA of riboflavin is 1.1 to 1.3 milligrams per day. The Daily Value used on food and supplement labels is 1.7 milligrams. On average, daily intakes of riboflavin are slightly above the RDA. As with thiamin, people with alcoholism risk riboflavin deficiency because they generally eat nutrient-poor diets. No specific symptoms indicate that riboflavin taken in megadoses is toxic, so no Upper Level has been set.

8.10 Niacin

Niacin functions in the body as one of two related compounds: nicotinic acid and nicotinamide. Niacin was formerly referred to as *vitamin B-3*.

The coenzyme forms of niacin function in many cellular metabolic pathways. In general, when energy is being released from the energy nutrients and used by cells, a niacin coenzyme is used. Synthetic pathways in the cell—those that make new compounds—also often use a niacin coenzyme. This is especially true for fatty acid synthesis (review Fig. 8-14).

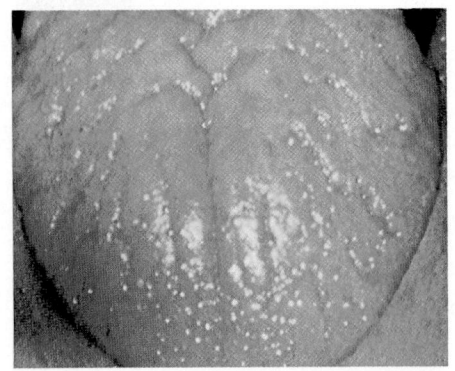
(a)

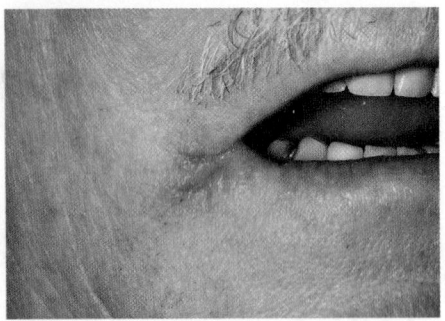
(b)

FIGURE 8-18 ▶ (a) Glossitis is a painful, inflamed tongue that can signal a deficiency of riboflavin, niacin, vitamin B-6, folate, or vitamin B-12. (b) Angular cheilitis, also called cheilosis or angular stomatitis, is another result of a riboflavin deficiency. It causes painful cracks at the corners of the mouth. Both glossitis and angular cheilitis can be caused by other medical conditions; thus, further evaluation is required before diagnosing a nutrient deficiency.

Food Sources of Riboflavin

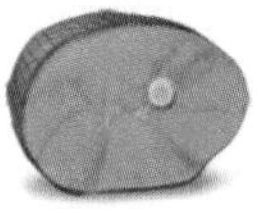

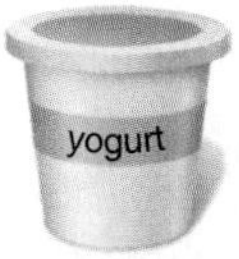

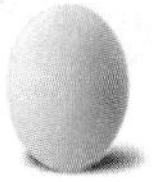

Food Item and Amount	Riboflavin (milligrams)	Adult Male RDA = 1.3 milligrams		Adult Female RDA = 1.1 milligrams	
		Daily Value = 1.7 milligrams			
		%RDA		%RDA	
RDA	1.1-1.3	▰▰▰▰	100%	▰▰▰▰	100%
Multigrain oat cereal, ¾ cup	1.3	▰▰▰▰	100%	▰▰▰▰ ≫	110%
Fried beef liver, 1 ounce	1.2	▰▰▰	92%	▰▰▰▰ ≫	109%
Steamed oysters, 10	1.1	▰▰▰	85%	▰▰▰▰	100%
Plain yogurt, 1 cup	0.5	▰	38%	▰	45%
Raw mushrooms, 5	0.5	▰	38%	▰	45%
Braunschweiger sausage,1	0.4	▰	31%	▰	36%
Cooked spinach, 1 cup	0.4	▰	31%	▰	36%
1% milk, 1 cup	0.4	▰	31%	▰	36%
Buttermilk, 1 cup	0.4	▰	31%	▰	36%
Boiled egg, 1	0.3	▰	23%	▰	27%
Sirloin steak, 3 ounces	0.3	▰	23%	▰	27%
Feta cheese, 1 ounce	0.2	▰	15%	▰	18%
Tortilla, 1	0.2	▰	15%	▰	18%
Lean ham, 3 ounces	0.2	▰	15%	▰	18%

Key:
- Grains
- Vegetables
- Fruits
- Dairy
- Protein

ChooseMyPlate.gov

FIGURE 8-19 ▶ Food sources of riboflavin compared to the RDA for adult males and females.

Almost every cellular metabolic pathway uses a niacin coenzyme, so a deficiency causes widespread changes in the body. The group of niacin deficiency symptoms is known as *pellagra*, which means rough or painful skin. The symptoms of the disease are **dementia,** diarrhea, and dermatitis (especially on areas of skin exposed to the sun) (Fig. 8-20). Later, death often results. Early symptoms include poor appetite, weight loss, and weakness.

dementia A general loss or decrease in mental function.

Pellagra is the only dietary deficiency disease ever to reach epidemic proportions in the United States. It became a major problem in the southeastern United States in the late 1800s and persisted until the late 1930s when standards of living and diets improved. Today, pellagra is rare in Western societies, but can be seen in the developing world.

High does of niacin, beyond what is available from food, are also prescribed as a treatment to increase HDL-cholesterol (good). Niacin can raise HDL-cholesterol by 15% to 35%, making niacin the most effective drug available for raising HDL-cholesterol.

MAKING DECISIONS

Niacin in Corn

Do you enjoy corn tortillas? Niacin in corn is bound by a protein that hampers its absorption. Soaking corn in an alkaline solution, such as lime water (water with calcium hydroxide), releases bound niacin and renders it more usable. Hispanic people in North America traditionally soak corn in lime water before making tortillas. This treatment is one reason this Hispanic population never experienced much pellagra.

FIGURE 8-20 ▶ The dermatitis of pellagra. (a) Dermatitis on both sides (bilateral) of the body is a typical symptom of pellagra. Sun exposure worsens the condition. (b) The rough skin around the neck is referred to as Casal's necklace.

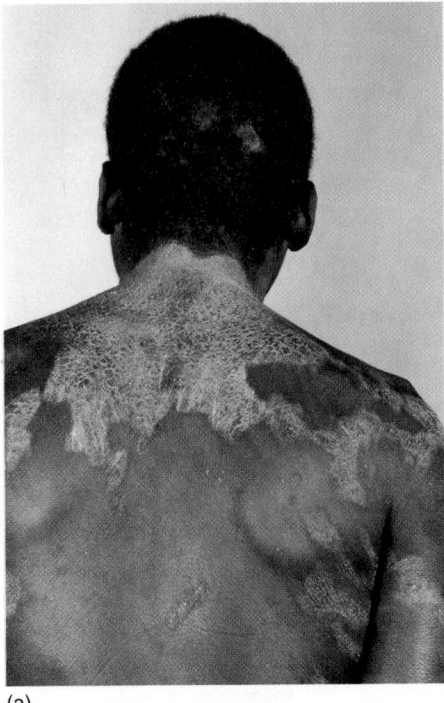 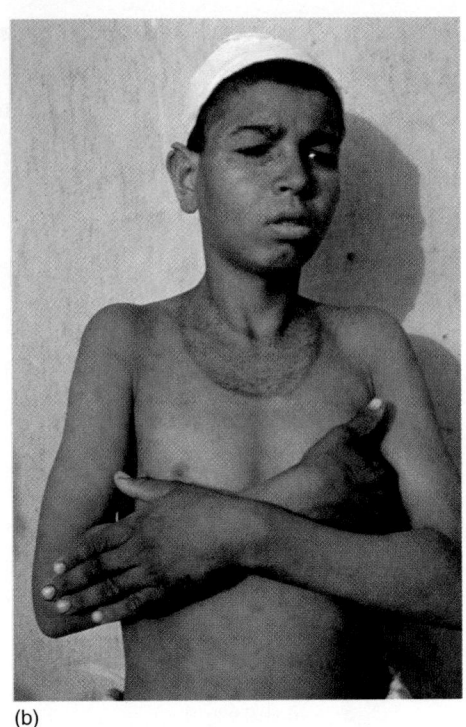

(a)   (b)

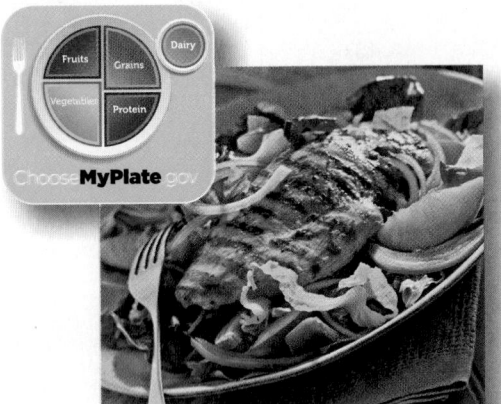

▲ Chicken is a good source of niacin. The tryptophan present can also be metabolized to niacin. How does this dish compare to ChooseMyPlate recommendations?

Niacin Sources and Needs

Major sources of niacin are poultry, ready-to-eat breakfast cereals, beef, wheat bran, tuna and other fish, asparagus, and peanuts (Fig. 8-21). Coffee and tea also contribute some niacin to the diet. Niacin is heat stable; little is lost in cooking.

Besides the preformed niacin found in protein foods, we can synthesize niacin from the amino acid tryptophan: 60 milligrams of tryptophan in a diet yield about 1 milligram of niacin. In this manner, we synthesize about 50% of the niacin we need.

The adult RDA of niacin is 14 to 16 milligrams per day. The RDA is expressed as niacin equivalents (NE) to account for niacin received intact from the diet, as well as that made from tryptophan. A Daily Value of 20 milligrams is used to express niacin content on food and supplement labels. Intakes of niacin by adults are about double the RDA, without considering the contribution from tryptophan. (Tables of food composition values also ignore this contribution.) People with alcoholism and those with rare disorders of tryptophan metabolism are generally the only groups to show a niacin deficiency.

Upper Level for Niacin

The Upper Level for niacin is 35 milligrams per day of the nicotinic acid form. Effects of high intakes include headache, itching, and increased blood flow to the skin, causing a general blood vessel dilation or flushing in various parts of the body, especially when intakes are above 100 milligrams per day. In the long run, GI tract and liver damage is possible, so any use of megadoses, including large doses recommended for treatment of cardiovascular disease, requires close physician scrutiny (review Chapter 5).

Food Sources of Niacin

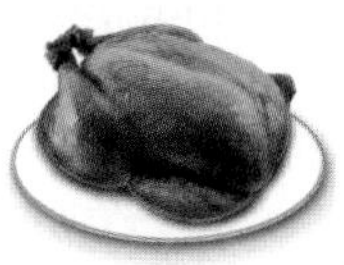

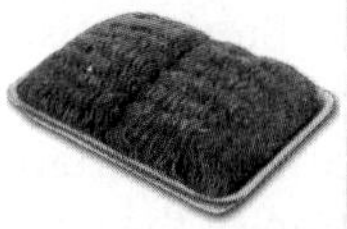

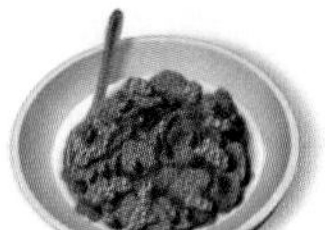

Food Item and Amount	Niacin (milligrams)	Adult Male RDA = 16 milligrams	Adult Female RDA = 14 milligrams
		Daily Value = 20 milligrams	
		%RDA	%RDA
RDA	14-16	100%	100%
Tuna, 3 ounces	11.3	71%	81%
Roasted chicken, 3 ounces	10.1	63%	72%
Peanuts, ½ cup	9.9	62%	71%
Baked salmon, 3 ounces	8.6	54%	61%
Turkey lunch meat, 3 ounces	5.4	34%	39%
Ground beef, 3 ounces	5.0	31%	36%
Raw mushrooms, 5	4.7	29%	34%
Lean steak, 4 ounces	4.5	28%	32%
Chunky peanut butter, 2 tablespoons	4.4	28%	31%
Fried beef liver, 1 ounce	4.1	26%	29%
Raisin Nut Bran cereal, ¾ cup	3.8	24%	27%
Tortilla, 1	2.6	16%	19%
Baked cod, 3 ounces	2.1	13%	15%
Potato, 1	2.1	13%	15%
Broiled halibut, 3 ounces	1.6	10%	11%

Key: ChooseMyPlate.gov
- Grains
- Vegetables
- Fruits
- Dairy
- Protein

FIGURE 8-21 ▶ Food sources of niacin compared to the RDA for adult males and females.

CONCEPT CHECK

The B vitamins thiamin, riboflavin, and niacin are important in the metabolism of carbohydrates, proteins, and fats. Energy metabolism in particular requires adequate amounts of the coenzyme forms of these three vitamins. Deficiency symptoms typically occur in the brain and nervous system, skin, and GI tract. Cells in these tissues are metabolically active, and those in the skin and GI tract are also constantly being replaced. Enriched grains and ready-to-eat breakfast cereals are adequate sources of all three vitamins. Additionally, pork is an excellent source of thiamin, milk is an excellent source of riboflavin, and protein foods in general—such as chicken—are excellent sources of niacin. Deficiencies of all three vitamins can occur with alcoholism; a thiamin deficiency is the most likely of the three.

8.11 Pantothenic Acid

Like the other B vitamins, pantothenic acid helps release energy from carbohydrates, fats, and protein. By forming its coenzyme (coenzyme A or CoA) pantothenic acid allows many energy-yielding metabolic reactions to occur (review Fig. 8-14). This coenzyme also activates fatty acids so they can yield energy. It is also used in the beginning steps of fatty acid synthesis. Pantothenic acid is so widespread in foods that a nutritional deficiency among healthy people who eat varied diets is unlikely.

Pantothenic Acid Sources and Needs

Rich sources of pantothenic acid are sunflower seeds, mushrooms, peanuts, and eggs. Other sources are meat, milk, and many vegetables (Fig. 8-22).

The Adequate Intake set for pantothenic acid is 5 milligrams per day for adults, and we generally consume that amount or more. A Daily Value of 10 milligrams is used to express pantothenic acid content on food and supplement labels. A deficiency of pantothenic acid might occur when alcoholism is accompanied by a nutrient-deficient diet. However, the symptoms would probably be hidden among deficiencies of thiamin, riboflavin, vitamin B-6, and folate, so the pantothenic acid deficiency might be unrecognizable. No toxicity is known for pantothenic acid, therefore no Upper Level has been set.

8.12 Biotin

In its coenzyme form, biotin aids in fat and carbohydrate metabolism. Biotin assists in the addition of carbon dioxide to other compounds. By doing so, it promotes the synthesis of glucose and fatty acids, while also helping to break down certain amino acids. Symptoms of biotin deficiency include a scaly inflammation of the skin, changes in the tongue and lips, decreased appetite, nausea, vomiting, a form of anemia, depression, muscle pain and weakness, and poor growth.

Biotin Sources and Needs

Cauliflower, egg yolks, peanuts, and cheese are good sources of biotin (Fig. 8-23). Intestinal bacteria synthesize and supply some biotin, making a biotin deficiency unlikely. However, scientists are not sure how much of the bacteria-synthesized biotin

FIGURE 8-22 ▶ Food sources of pantothenic acid compared to the Adequate Intake for adults.

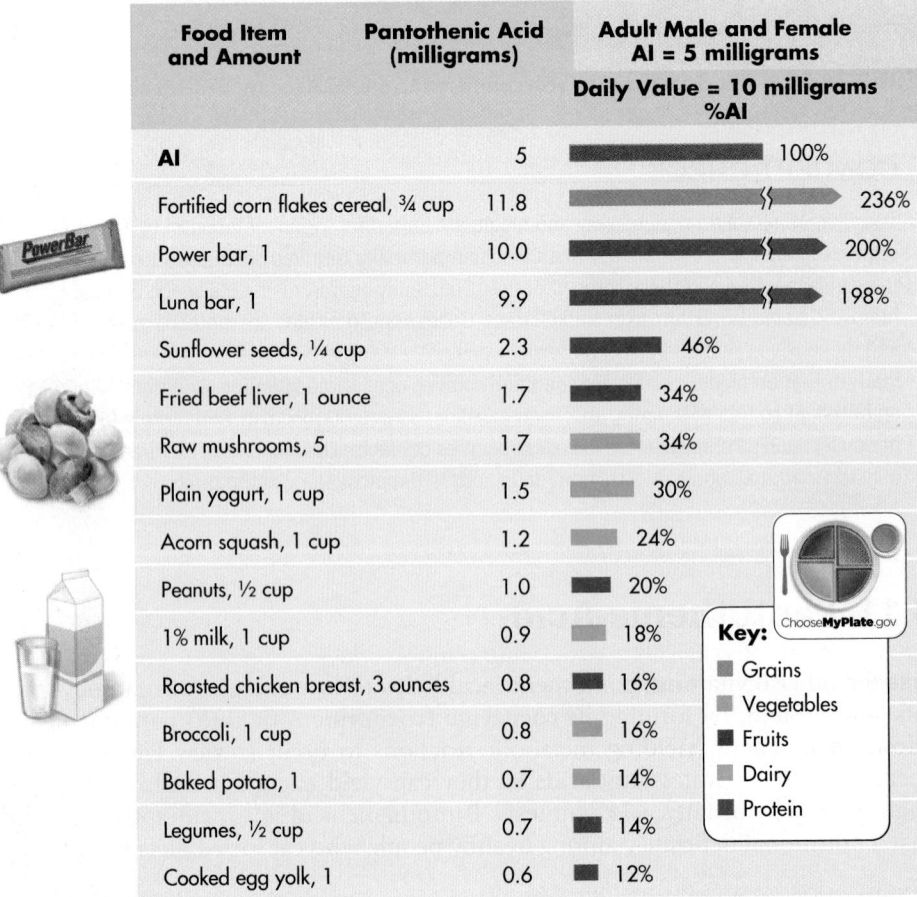

Food Sources of Pantothenic Acid

Food Item and Amount	Pantothenic Acid (milligrams)	Adult Male and Female AI = 5 milligrams Daily Value = 10 milligrams %AI
AI	5	100%
Fortified corn flakes cereal, ¾ cup	11.8	236%
Power bar, 1	10.0	200%
Luna bar, 1	9.9	198%
Sunflower seeds, ¼ cup	2.3	46%
Fried beef liver, 1 ounce	1.7	34%
Raw mushrooms, 5	1.7	34%
Plain yogurt, 1 cup	1.5	30%
Acorn squash, 1 cup	1.2	24%
Peanuts, ½ cup	1.0	20%
1% milk, 1 cup	0.9	18%
Roasted chicken breast, 3 ounces	0.8	16%
Broccoli, 1 cup	0.8	16%
Baked potato, 1	0.7	14%
Legumes, ½ cup	0.7	14%
Cooked egg yolk, 1	0.6	12%

Key:
- Grains
- Vegetables
- Fruits
- Dairy
- Protein

ChooseMyPlate.gov

Food Sources of Biotin

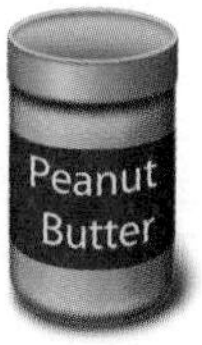

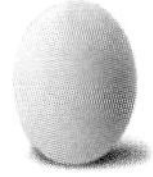

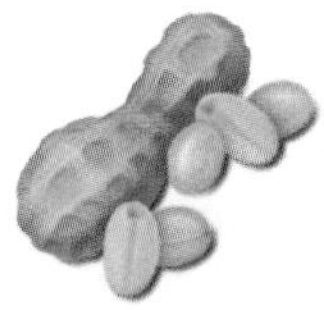

Food Item and Amount	Biotin (micrograms)	Adult Male and Female AI = 30 micrograms; Daily Value = 30 micrograms; %AI
AI	30.0	100%
Smooth peanut butter, 2 tablespoons	30.1	100%
Cooked lamb liver, 1 ounce	11.6	39%
Boiled egg, 1	9.3	31%
Cooked egg yolk, 1	8.1	27%
Yogurt, 1 cup	7.4	25%
Wheat germ, ¼ cup	7.2	24%
Roasted peanuts, 5	6.5	22%
Wheat bran, ¼ cup	6.4	21%
Nonfat milk, 1 cup	4.9	16%
Salmon, 3 ounces	4.3	14%
Egg noodles, 1 cup	4.0	13%
Swiss cheese, 2 ounces	2.2	7%
Cheddar cheese, 2 ounces	1.7	6%
Raw cauliflower, 1 cup	1.5	5%
American cheese, 2 ounces	1.4	5%

ChooseMyPlate.gov

Key:
- Grains
- Vegetables
- Fruits
- Dairy
- Protein

FIGURE 8-23 ▶ Food sources of biotin compared to the Adequate Intake for adults.

in our intestines is absorbed. If intestinal bacterial synthesis is not sufficient, as in people missing a large part of the small intestine or who take antibiotics for many months, special attention should be paid to meeting biotin needs. A protein called *avidin* in raw egg whites binds biotin and inhibits its absorption. Consuming many raw egg whites eventually leads to the deficiency disease. Cooking denatures avidin in eggs such that it cannot bind biotin.

The Adequate Intake set for biotin is 30 micrograms per day for adults. Our food supply is thought to provide 40 to 60 micrograms per person per day. A Daily Value of 30 micrograms is used to express biotin content on food and supplement labels and is 10 times our current estimate of needs. Biotin is relatively nontoxic. Large doses have been given over an extended period without harmful side effects to children who exhibit defects in biotin metabolism. Thus, no Upper Level for biotin has been set.

8.13 Vitamin B-6

Vitamin B-6 can exist in three chemical forms, all of which can be changed to the active vitamin B-6 coenzyme. Pyridoxine is the general vitamin name and form added to foods.

Functions of Vitamin B-6

The coenzymes of vitamin B-6 are needed for the activity of many enzymes involved in carbohydrate, protein, and fat metabolism. Vitamin B-6 is needed in many areas of metabolism, so a deficiency results in widespread symptoms, such as depression, vomiting, skin disorders, irritation of the nerves, and impaired immune response.

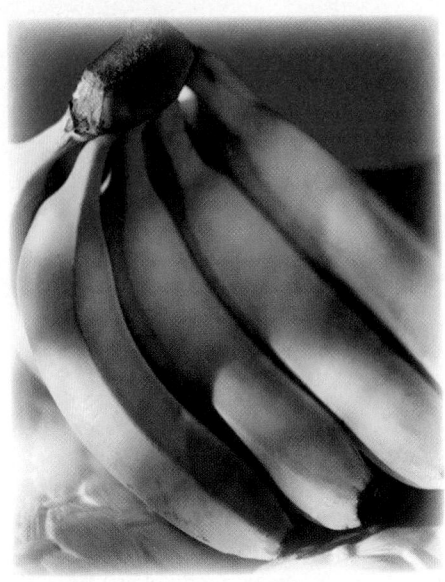

▲ Bananas are a plant source of vitamin B-6.

Vitamin B-6 plays a particularly important role in protein and amino acid metabolism (review Fig. 8-14). The coenzyme helps to remove the nitrogen group ($-NH_2$) from certain amino acids, making nitrogen available to another amino acid. These amino acid reactions allow a cell to synthesize nonessential (dispensable) amino acids. In a related function, vitamin B-6 plays a role in homocysteine metabolism.

Another important role of vitamin B-6 is the synthesis of many neurotransmitters. Recall from Chapter 3 that neurotransmitters allow nerve cells to communicate with each other and with other body cells. A vitamin B-6 deficiency can cause a decrease in these neurotransmitters and lead to symptoms, especially convulsions. This problem occurred in the 1950s when heat destroyed vitamin B-6 in formulas fed to infants.

The vitamin B-6 coenzyme is important for the synthesis of hemoglobin and its function as the oxygen-carrying part of the red blood cell. Vitamin B-6 is also necessary for the synthesis of white blood cells, which perform a major role in the immune system.

Vitamin B-6 Sources and Needs

Major sources of vitamin B-6 are animal products, ready-to-eat breakfast cereals, potatoes, and milk. Other sources are fruits and vegetables such as bananas, cantaloupes, broccoli, and spinach (Figs. 8-24 and 8-25). Overall, animal sources and fortified products are the most reliable because the vitamin B-6 they contain is more absorbable than that in plant foods.

The adult RDA of vitamin B-6 is 1.3 to 1.7 milligrams per day. A Daily Value of 2 milligrams is used to express vitamin B-6 content on food and supplement labels. Average daily consumption of vitamin B-6 for men and women is somewhat above the RDA.

FIGURE 8-24 ▶ Food sources of vitamin B-6 compared to the RDA for adults.

Food Sources of Vitamin B-6

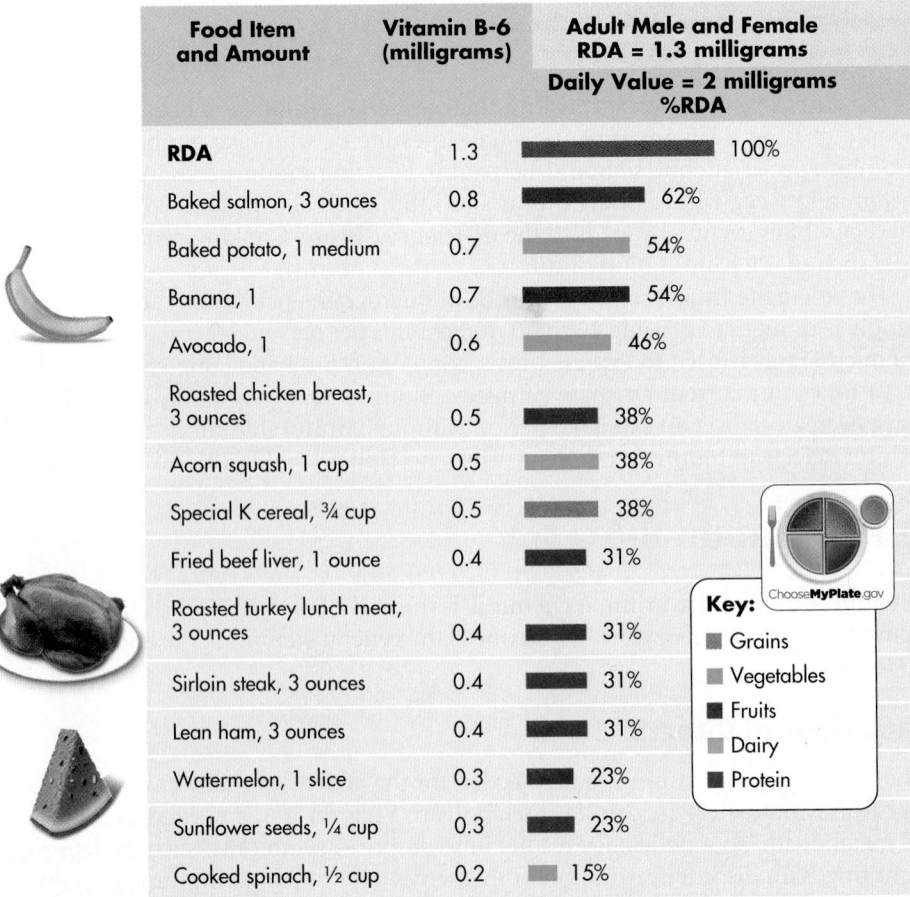

Food Item and Amount	Vitamin B-6 (milligrams)	Adult Male and Female RDA = 1.3 milligrams Daily Value = 2 milligrams %RDA
RDA	1.3	100%
Baked salmon, 3 ounces	0.8	62%
Baked potato, 1 medium	0.7	54%
Banana, 1	0.7	54%
Avocado, 1	0.6	46%
Roasted chicken breast, 3 ounces	0.5	38%
Acorn squash, 1 cup	0.5	38%
Special K cereal, ¾ cup	0.5	38%
Fried beef liver, 1 ounce	0.4	31%
Roasted turkey lunch meat, 3 ounces	0.4	31%
Sirloin steak, 3 ounces	0.4	31%
Lean ham, 3 ounces	0.4	31%
Watermelon, 1 slice	0.3	23%
Sunflower seeds, ¼ cup	0.3	23%
Cooked spinach, ½ cup	0.2	15%

Key:
- Grains
- Vegetables
- Fruits
- Dairy
- Protein

ChooseMyPlate.gov

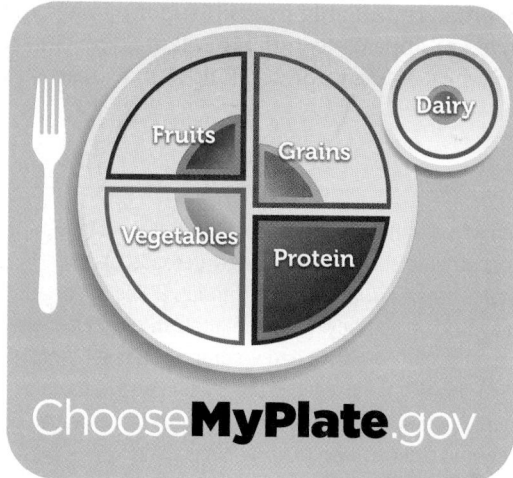

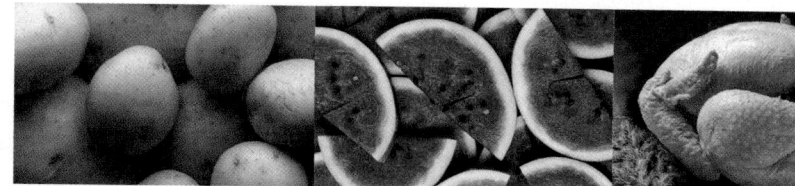

MyPlate:
Sources of Vitamin B-6

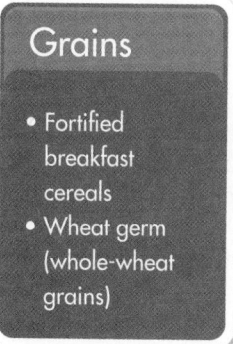

Grains
- Fortified breakfast cereals
- Wheat germ (whole-wheat grains)

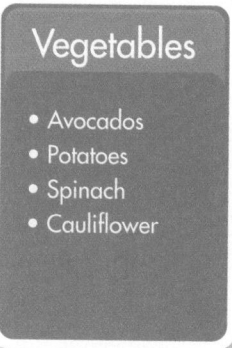

Vegetables
- Avocados
- Potatoes
- Spinach
- Cauliflower

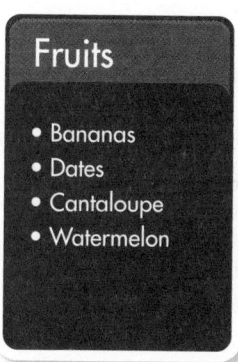

Fruits
- Bananas
- Dates
- Cantaloupe
- Watermelon

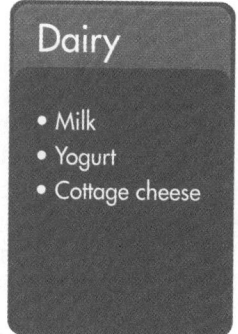

Dairy
- Milk
- Yogurt
- Cottage cheese

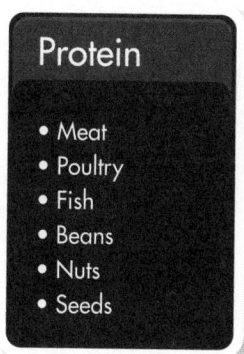

Protein
- Meat
- Poultry
- Fish
- Beans
- Nuts
- Seeds

FIGURE 8-25 ▶ Sources of vitamin B-6 from MyPlate. The fill of the background color (none, 1/3, 2/3, or completely covered) within each group in the plate indicates the average nutrient density for vitamin B-6 in that group. Overall, the protein group especially contains many foods that are nutrient-dense sources of vitamin B-6. With regard to physical activity, vitamin B-6 participates in the related energy metabolism during such endeavors.

Athletes may need slightly more vitamin B-6 than sedentary adults. The athlete's body processes a great deal of glycogen and ingested protein (in the form of amino acids) for fuel, and the metabolism of these compounds requires vitamin B-6. However, athletes are likely to consume plenty of protein-rich foods—enough to supply needed amounts of vitamin B-6.

People with alcoholism are susceptible to a vitamin B-6 deficiency because a metabolite formed in alcohol metabolism can displace the coenzyme form from enzymes, increasing its tendency to be destroyed. In addition, alcohol decreases the absorption of vitamin B-6 and the synthesis of its coenzyme form. Cirrhosis and hepatitis (both of which may accompany alcoholism) also disable liver tissue from metabolizing vitamin B-6, which decreases synthesis of its coenzyme form.

Nausea is experienced by 70% to 85% of women during the first trimester of pregnancy (see Chapter 14). Sometimes physicians recommend vitamin B-6 supplementation, typically 30 to 75 milligrams per day, to reduce nausea. A review of the research on treating nausea during pregnancy suggests that this therapy is both safe and likely to help reduce nausea. Even though vitamin B-6 supplements to treat nausea are available over-the-counter without a prescription, pregnant women should first discuss this treatment option with their physicians.

▲ This grilled salmon with red onion, potatoes, and lemon provides good sources of vitamin B-6 from the protein and vegetable sections of MyPlate. Which sections of MyPlate are missing?

Upper Level for Vitamin B-6

The Upper Level for vitamin B-6 is 100 milligrams per day, based on the risk of developing nerve damage. Studies have shown that intakes of 2 to 6 grams of vitamin B-6 per day for 2 or more months especially can lead to irreversible nerve damage. Symptoms of vitamin B-6 toxicity include walking difficulties and hand and foot numbness. Some nerve damage in individual sensory neurons is probably reversible, but damage to the ganglia (where many nerve fibers converge) appears to be permanent. With 500 milligram tablets of vitamin B-6 available in health-food stores, taking a toxic dose is easy.

CONCEPT CHECK

Pantothenic acid and biotin both participate in the metabolism of carbohydrate and fat. A deficiency of either vitamin is unlikely; pantothenic acid is found widely in foods, and our need for biotin is partially met by intestinal synthesis from bacteria. Vitamin B-6 is important for protein metabolism, neurotransmitter synthesis, homocysteine metabolism, and other key metabolic functions. Headache, a form of anemia, nausea, and vomiting can result from a vitamin B-6 deficiency. Increased risk of cardiovascular disease is also likely. Animal protein foods, ready-to-eat breakfast cereals, broccoli, spinach, and bananas are some food sources of vitamin B-6. Megadose supplements of vitamin B-6 can lead to nerve damage.

8.14 Folate

The term *folate* encompasses a variety of food forms of the vitamin. Folic acid is the synthetic chemical form added to foods and present in supplements. Folic acid is more readily absorbed (1.7 times greater) than natural forms of folate. The structure of natural food folate differs from folic acid by containing extra units of the amino acid, glutamic acid. These extra units must be removed before absorption, yielding free folic acid.

Functions of Folate

A key role of the folate coenzymes is to supply or accept single carbon compounds. In this role, the coenzymes help form DNA and also metabolize various amino acids and their derivatives, such as homocysteine.

One major result of a folate deficiency is decreased red blood cell synthesis. Without folate, the immature cells cannot divide because they cannot form new DNA. The cells grow progressively larger because they can still synthesize enough protein and other cell parts to make new cells. When the time comes for the cells to divide, however, the amount of DNA is insufficient to form two nuclei. The cells then remain in a large immature form, known as a **megaloblast** (Fig. 8-26).

The bone marrow of a folate-deficient person, therefore, produces mostly immature megaloblast cells, and very few mature red blood cells (called **erythrocytes**). With fewer mature red blood cells in the bloodstream, the blood's capacity to carry oxygen decreases, causing folate deficiency anemia called **megaloblastic anemia** (also called macrocytic anemia).

The changes in red blood cell formation occur after 7 to 16 weeks on a folate-free diet, depending on the person's folate stores. White blood cell formation is also affected, but to a lesser degree. In addition, cell division throughout the entire body is disrupted. Clinicians focus primarily on red blood cells because they are easy to collect and examine. Other symptoms of folate deficiency are inflammation of the tongue, diarrhea, poor growth, mental confusion, depression, and problems in nerve function.

About 10% of the North American population has a genetic defect in an important aspect of folate metabolism. They may need up to twice the RDA to compensate for the defect. Genetic testing for this defect is not routine in medical practice, but one day it may be.

A maternal deficiency of folate along with this genetic abnormality related to folate metabolism has been linked to development of **neural tube defects** in the fetus (Fig. 8-27). These defects include spina bifida (spinal cord or spinal fluid bulge

megaloblast A large, immature red blood cell that results from the particular cell's inability to divide normally.

erythrocytes Mature red blood cells. These have no nucleus and a life span of about 120 days; they contain hemoglobin, which transports oxygen and carbon dioxide.

megaloblastic anemia Anemia characterized by the presence of abnormally large red blood cells.

neural tube defect A defect in the formation of the neural tube occurring during early fetal development. This type of defect results in various nervous system disorders, such as spina bifida. Folate deficiency in the pregnant woman increases the risk that the fetus will develop this disorder.

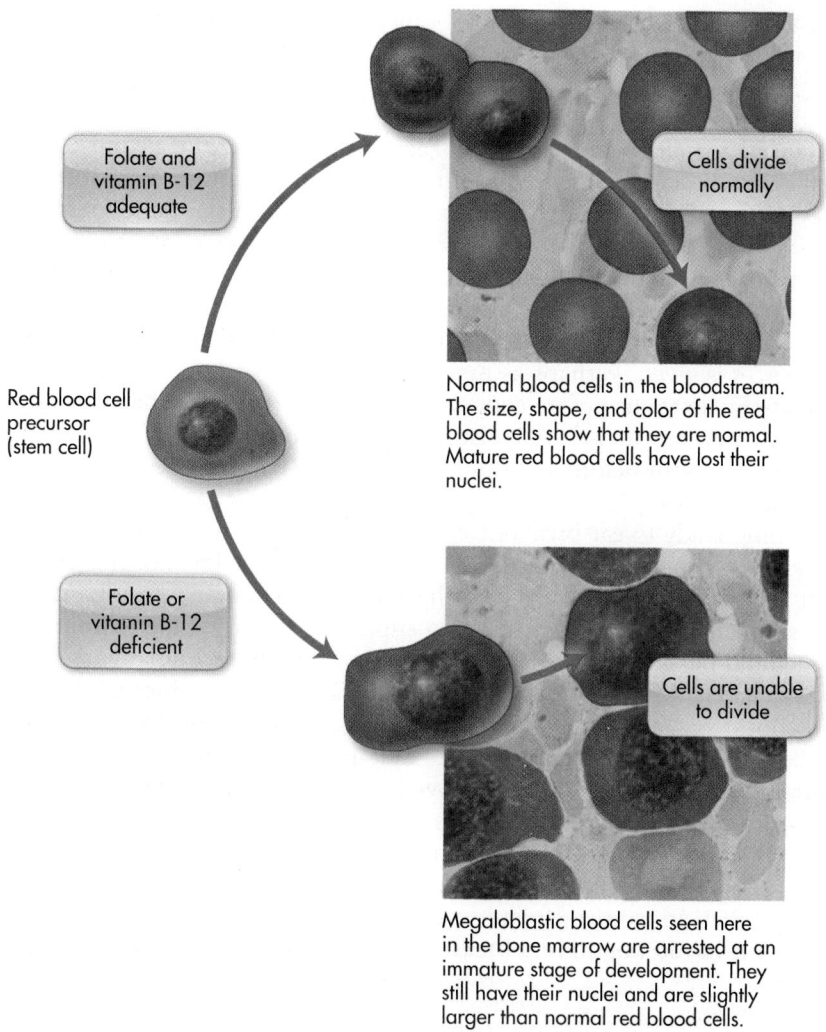

FIGURE 8-26 ▶ Megaloblastic anemia occurs when blood cells are unable to divide, leaving large, immature red blood cells. Either a folate or vitamin B-12 deficiency may cause this condition. Measurements of blood concentrations of both vitamins are taken to help determine the cause of the anemia.

Folate and vitamin B-12 adequate

Red blood cell precursor (stem cell)

Cells divide normally

Normal blood cells in the bloodstream. The size, shape, and color of the red blood cells show that they are normal. Mature red blood cells have lost their nuclei.

Folate or vitamin B-12 deficient

Cells are unable to divide

Megaloblastic blood cells seen here in the bone marrow are arrested at an immature stage of development. They still have their nuclei and are slightly larger than normal red blood cells.

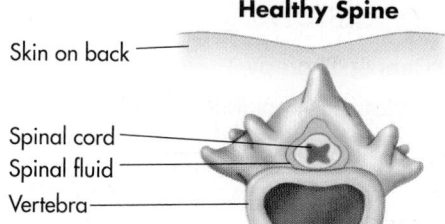

Healthy Spine

Skin on back
Spinal cord
Spinal fluid
Vertebra

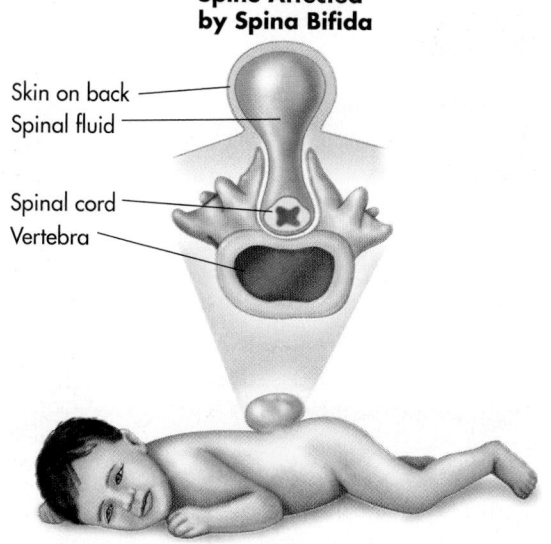

Spine Affected by Spina Bifida

Skin on back
Spinal fluid
Spinal cord
Vertebra

FIGURE 8-27 ▶ Neural tube defects result from a developmental failure affecting the spinal cord or brain in the embryo. Very early in fetal development, a ridge of neural-like tissue forms along the back of the embryo. As the fetus develops, this material develops into both the spinal cord and nerves at the lower end and into the brain at the upper end. At the same time, the bones that make up the back gradually surround the spinal cord on all sides. If any part of this sequence goes awry, many defects can appear. The worst case is total lack of a brain (anencephaly). Spina bifida, in which the back bones do not form a complete ring to protect the spinal cord, is much more common. Deficient folate status in the mother during the beginning of pregnancy, especially in combination with a genetic abnormality in folate metabolism, greatly increases the risk of neural tube defects.

NEWSWORTHY
NUTRITION

Folic acid added to cereal reduces number of neural tube defects

Fortification of cereal products with folic acid became mandatory in Canada and the United States in 1998. As a result of the fortification, the prevalence of neural tube defects decreased 46% in Canada from 1.58 per 1000 births before fortification to 0.86 per 1000 births after fortification. The reduction rate was greatest for spina bifida (a decrease of 53%). Declines have also been observed in the United States.

Source: DeWals P and others: Reduction in neural tube defects after folic acid fortification in Canada. *New England Journal of Medicine* 357:135, 2007 (see Further Reading 3).

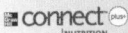

Check out the Connect site www.mcgrawhillconnect.com **to further explore vitamin-fortified foods.**

through the back) and anencephaly (absence of a brain). About 2000 infants are affected with neural tube defects annually in the United States. Victims of spina bifida exhibit paralysis, incontinence, learning disabilities, and other health problems. Children born with anencephaly die shortly after birth. Adequate folate nurture is crucial for all women of childbearing age because the neural tube closes within the first 28 days of pregnancy, a time when many women are not even aware that they are pregnant. Research that has been done with synthetic folic acid supplementation has resulted in a recommendation that ample folate, specifically 400 micrograms of synthetic folic acid per day, be consumed at least 6 weeks before conception. It appears that even those women with varied diets may not consume adequate synthetic folic acid to prevent neural tube defects unless specific attention to rich sources is given. Perhaps as many as 70% of these defects could be avoided by adequate folate status before conception. (Women who have had a child with a neural tube defect are advised to consume 4 milligrams per day of folic acid, beginning at least 1 month before any future pregnancy. This must be done under strict physician supervision.)

Consuming ready-to-eat breakfast cereals that contain 100% of the Daily Value for folate (this is the same as the RDA) is a good practice for meeting the goal for synthetic folic acid intake (see Newsworthy Nutrition in margin). A multivitamin and mineral supplement can also be used to supply adequate synthetic folic acid, but women should be careful to monitor the amount of any accompanying preformed vitamin A content (do not exceed 100% of the Daily Value). Since 1992, there has been an effort to get all women of childbearing age to take daily vitamins containing folic acid. A March of Dimes survey found that 40% of these women did so in 2007.

Research is underway on the link between folate and cancer protection. Folate aids in DNA synthesis, so it is hypothesized that even mild folate deficiency contributes to abnormal DNA integrity, which in turn affects certain cancer-protecting genes. Meeting the RDA for folate is thought to be one way to reduce cancer risk. A recent 7-year study found that, in women, folate supplements in combination with vitamin B-6 and vitamin B-12 did not prevent breast cancer or other invasive cancers (see Further Reading 15).

MAKING DECISIONS

Folate and Cancer Therapy

Some forms of cancer therapy provide a vivid example of the effects of a folate deficiency on DNA metabolism. A cancer drug, methotrexate, closely resembles a form of folate but cannot act in its place. Because of this resemblance, when methotrexate is taken in high doses, it hampers folate metabolism. In essence, methotrexate crowds out folate in the metabolic pathways. DNA synthesis and, consequently, cell division, then decrease. Cancer cells are among the most rapidly dividing cells in the body, so they are among those first affected. However, other rapidly dividing cells, such as intestinal cells and skin cells, are also affected. Not surprisingly, typical side effects of methotrexate therapy are diarrhea, vomiting, and hair loss. These are also typical symptoms of folate deficiency. Today when patients are given methotrexate, they need to follow a high-folate diet and/or take folic acid supplements because this reduces the toxic side effects of the drug. High supplemental doses generally have little or no influence on methotrexate's effectiveness as a cancer therapy.

Folate Sources and Needs

Green, leafy vegetables (*folate* is derived from the Latin word *folium*, which means *foliage* or *leaves*), organ meats, sprouts, other vegetables, dried beans, and orange juice are the richest sources of folate (Figs. 8-28 and 8-29). The vitamin C in orange juice also reduces folate destruction. Ready-to-eat breakfast cereals, milk, and bread also are important sources of folate for many adults.

Folate is susceptible to destruction by heat. Food processing and preparation destroy 50% to 90% of the folate in food. This underscores the importance of regularly eating fresh fruits and raw or lightly cooked vegetables. As mentioned, vegetables retain their nutrients best when cooked quickly in minimal water—steaming, stir-frying, or microwaving (review Table 8-1).

The RDA of folate for adults is 400 micrograms per day, as is the Daily Value used to express folate content on food and supplement labels. Folate recommendations for all but women of child-bearing age (these women should meet such recommendations with synthetic folic acid), are based on dietary folate equivalents (DFE). To compute folate intake in DFE units, one has to determine how much of a day's folate intake comes from food folate and how much comes from synthetic folic acid added to foods. When in doubt, assume all folate in a diet is in the food form, except that coming from ready-to-eat breakfast cereals and refined grain products. Also included in this second category is any folic acid in supplements. To calculate the DFE, multiply total synthetic folic acid intake by 1.7, and add that value to the food folate consumed. For example, if a person consumed 300 micrograms as food folate and 200 micrograms from a ready-to-eat breakfast cereal, total DFE would be 640 micrograms ($300 + [200 \times 1.7] = 640$). Compared to the RDA of 400 micrograms, this intake would be sufficient.

Prior to 1998, average daily folate intakes in the United States were approximately 320 micrograms for men and 220 micrograms for women. In 1998, the fortification of grain products with folate was mandated in the United States and Canada, with the aim of reducing birth defects of the spine. With this mandate, average intakes have increased by about 200 micrograms per day. Studies have shown this practice has decreased rates of neural tube defects in infants (see Further Reading 3).

Food Sources of Folate

Food Item and Amount	Folate (micrograms)	Adult Male and Female RDA = 400 micrograms Daily Value = 400 micrograms %RDA
RDA	400	100%
Asparagus, 1 cup	263	66%
Cooked spinach, 1 cup	262	66%
Cooked lentils, ½ cup	179	45%
Black-eyed peas, ½ cup	179	45%
Romaine lettuce, 1½ cups	114	29%
Great Grains cereal, ¾ cup	114	29%
Tortilla, 1	89	22%
Cooked turnips, ½ cup	85	21%
Cooked broccoli, 1 cup	78	20%
Sunflower seeds, ¼ cup	76	19%
Fresh orange juice, 1 cup	75	19%
Cooked beets, ½ cup	68	17%
Kidney beans, ½ cup	65	16%

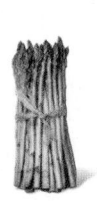
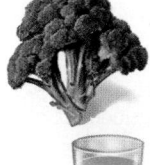
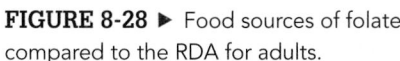

Key:
- Grains
- Vegetables
- Fruits
- Dairy
- Protein

CRITICAL THINKING

Suzanne and Ted are planning to start a family. They are especially concerned because Suzanne's sister gave birth last year to a baby with spina bifida. In preparation for her pregnancy, Suzanne takes a multivitamin supplement and eats fortified breakfast cereal most days. She also tries to include oranges, orange juice, broccoli, and spinach salads in her diet. What is spina bifida? How do Suzanne's diet and multivitamin supplement help prevent this serious disorder? Read more about this issue in What Would You Do Recommendations at the end of Chapter 8.

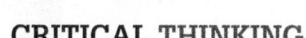

FIGURE 8-28 ▶ Food sources of folate compared to the RDA for adults.

FIGURE 8-29 ▶ Sources of folate from MyPlate. The fill of the background color (none, 1/3, 2/3, or completely covered) within each group in the plate indicates the average nutrient density for folate in that group. Overall, the vegetables group provides the richest sources, but the fruits group and the grains group contain some foods that are nutrient-dense sources of folate.

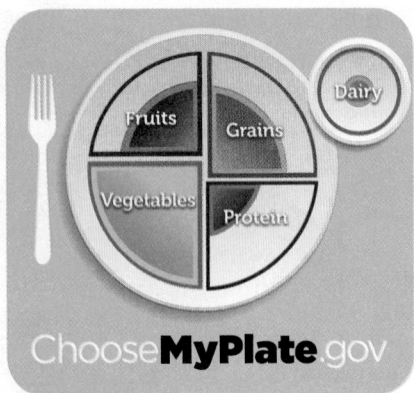

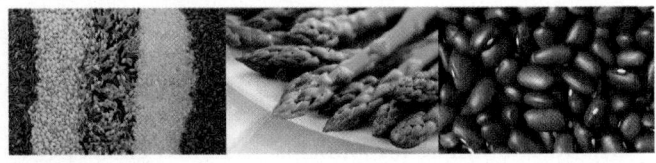

MyPlate:
Sources of Folate

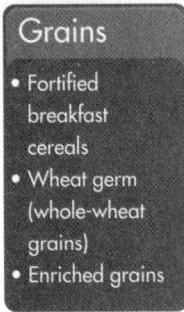

Grains
- Fortified breakfast cereals
- Wheat germ (whole-wheat grains)
- Enriched grains

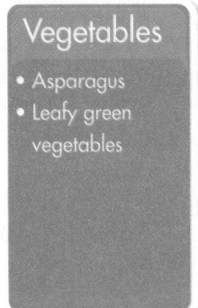

Vegetables
- Asparagus
- Leafy green vegetables

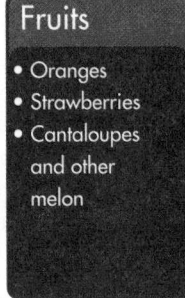

Fruits
- Oranges
- Strawberries
- Cantaloupes and other melon

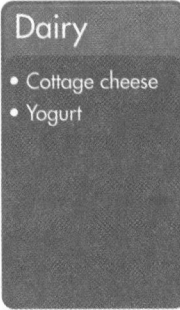

Dairy
- Cottage cheese
- Yogurt

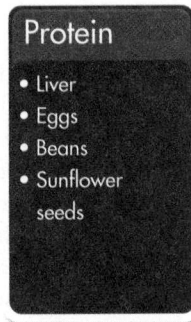

Protein
- Liver
- Eggs
- Beans
- Sunflower seeds

See Nutrition and Your Health: Dietary Supplements—Who Needs Them? at the end of Chapter 8.

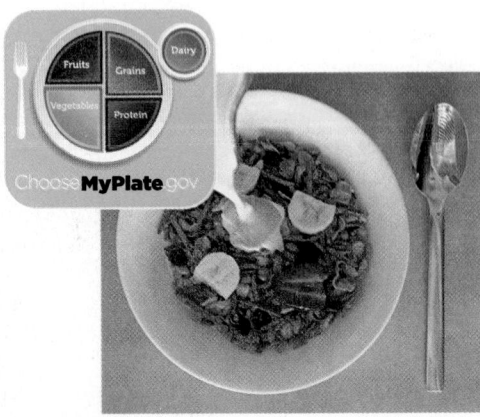

▲ Enriched grains and ready-to-eat breakfast cereals are good sources of synthetic folic acid. The cereal, fruit, and milk provide good sources of vitamins from the grains, fruit, and dairy sections of MyPlate.

Pregnant women need extra folate (a total of 600 micrograms DFE) to accommodate the increased rates of cell division and DNA synthesis in their own bodies and in the developing fetus. A healthy diet easily supplies this much. Although most vitamin supplements have no proven health benefits in most people (See the Nutrition and Your Health section at the end of this chapter), supplemental folic acid is effective at preventing birth defects. Prenatal care often includes a specially formulated multivitamin and mineral supplement enriched with synthetic folic acid to help compensate for the extra needs associated with pregnancy. Within the 2010 Dietary Guidelines for Americans, a key recommendation for women of childbearing age who may become pregnant and those in the first trimester of pregnancy is to consume 400 micrograms per day of synthetic folic acid daily (from fortified foods or supplements) in addition to food forms of folate from a varied diet.

Older people are also at risk for folate deficiency, possibly due to a combination of inadequate folate intake and decreased absorption. Perhaps these people fail to consume sufficient amounts of fruits and vegetables because of poverty or physical problems, such as poor dental health. In addition, folate deficiencies often occur with alcoholism, due mostly to poor intake and absorption. Symptoms of a folate-related anemia can alert a physician to the possibility of alcoholism.

MAKING DECISIONS

Dietary Folate Equivalents

The use of dietary folate equivalents (DFEs) instead of the actual amount of folate in a food has some important implications. Typically, many foods will be richer in folate than the Nutrition Facts label suggests because folate content is due primarily to synthetic folic acid added to the foods, such as in enriched grains and ready-to-eat breakfast cereals. This contributes substantially to the DFE calculation. Another implication is that food composition tables and diet-analysis software programs (such as that supplied with this book) also underestimate the true folate contribution of a diet compared to folate needs because these have not been updated to DFE units.

Upper Level for Folate

The Upper Level for folate is 1 milligram (1000 micrograms) per day but only refers to the synthetic source. This is because folate naturally present in foods has limited absorption. Large doses of folate can hide the signs of vitamin B-12 deficiency and therefore complicate its diagnosis. Specifically, regular consumption of large amounts of folate can prevent the appearance of an early warning sign of vitamin B-12 deficiency—enlarged red blood cell size. To prevent such masking of vitamin B-12 deficiency, the goal of the folate fortification of grains program is, to increase the folate status of women of childbearing age without causing excessive intake (over 1 milligram of synthetic folic acid per day) by other individuals. Also, because of risk of masking a vitamin B-12 deficiency, FDA limits supplements for nonpregnant adults and food fortification to 400 microgram amounts.

8.15 Vitamin B-12

Vitamin B-12 represents a family of compounds that contain the mineral cobalt. All vitamin B-12 compounds are synthesized by bacteria, fungi, and other lower organisms.

The body has a complex means of absorbing vitamin B-12. Vitamin B-12 in food enters the stomach and is digested from other materials, especially by stomach acid. The free vitamin B-12 in the stomach binds with a protein produced by the salivary glands in the mouth, and that protects vitamin B-12 from stomach acid. Vitamin B-12 is later freed from this protein in the small intestine. Finally, vitamin B-12 binds in the small intestine with a compound made in the stomach called **intrinsic factor.** The resulting intrinsic factor/vitamin B-12 complex travels to the last portion of the small intestine for absorption. After these digestion steps, approximately 50% of dietary vitamin B-12 is absorbed, depending on the body's need for it.

If a person has a defect in the digestion and absorption of vitamin B-12, the body may only be able to use 1% to 2% of dietary vitamin B-12. Monthly injections of vitamin B-12 or vitamin B-12 nasal gels are used to bypass the need for absorption or megadoses of a supplemental form (300 times the RDA) are needed to overcome the absorption defect by providing enough of the vitamin via simple diffusion across the intestinal tract.

About 95% of all cases of vitamin B-12 deficiencies in healthy people result from defective vitamin B-12 absorption, rather than from inadequate intakes. This is especially true for older people. As we age, our stomachs have a decreased ability to synthesize the intrinsic factor needed for vitamin B-12 absorption.

intrinsic factor A proteinlike compound produced by the stomach that enhances vitamin B-12 absorption.

Functions of Vitamin B-12

Vitamin B-12 participates in a variety of cellular processes. The most important function is in folate metabolism. Vitamin B-12 is required to convert folate coenzymes to the active forms needed for metabolic reactions, such as DNA synthesis. Without vitamin B-12, reactions that require certain active forms of folate do not take place in the cell. Thus, a vitamin B-12 deficiency can result in symptoms of a folate deficiency. Another vital function of vitamin B-12 is maintaining the myelin sheaths that insulate neurons from each other. People with vitamin B-12 deficiencies have destruction of segments of the myelin sheaths. This destruction eventually causes paralysis and, perhaps, death. Vitamin B-12 also participates in homocysteine metabolism and certain minor metabolic pathways.

In the past, the inability to absorb enough vitamin B-12 eventually led to death, mainly because it destroyed nerves. This phenomenon was

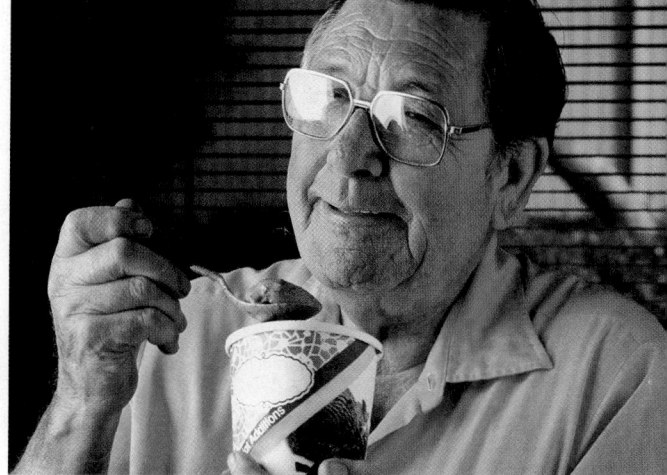

▼ As we age, our digestive system absorbs vitamin B-12 from food less efficiently.

pernicious anemia The anemia that results from a lack of vitamin B-12 absorption; it is pernicious because of associated nerve degeneration that can result in eventual paralysis and death.

called **pernicious anemia** (*pernicious* literally means "leading to death"). Clinically, the anemia looks much like a folate-deficiency anemia, characterized by the appearance of many large red blood cells in the bloodstream. However, the true cause of pernicious anemia is poor vitamin B-12 absorption rather than inadequate folate intakes.

Symptoms of pernicious anemia include weakness, sore tongue, back pain, apathy, and tingling in the extremities. We store significant amounts of vitamin B-12, so symptoms of nerve destruction generally do not develop until at least 3 years after the onset of the deficiency. Unfortunately, significant nerve destruction often occurs before the anemia is detected, and this destruction is irreversible. Pernicious anemia and its accompanying nerve destruction generally start after middle age, affecting up to 10% to 20% of older adults. The explanation for this age-associated pernicious anemia is twofold. First, aging is often associated with low production of stomach acid. Thus, vitamin B-12 is not properly cleaved from other food components during digestion. Second, aging may be accompanied by reduced output of intrinsic factor, resulting in decreased absorption of the vitamin (see Further Reading 2).

Infants who are breastfed by vegetarian or vegan mothers are at risk for vitamin B-12 deficiency accompanied by anemia and long-term nervous system problems, such as diminished brain growth, degeneration of the spinal cord, and poor intellectual development. The problems may have their origins during pregnancy, when the mother is deficient in vitamin B-12. Vegan diets supply little vitamin B-12 unless they include vitamin B-12–enriched food or supplements, so achieving an adequate vitamin B-12 intake is a key diet-planning goal for vegans (review Chapter 6).

Vitamin B-12 Sources and Needs

Major sources of vitamin B-12 include meat, milk, ready-to-eat breakfast cereals, poultry, seafood, and eggs (Fig. 8-30). Organ meats (especially liver, kidneys, and heart) are especially rich sources of vitamin B-12. Adults over age 50 are encouraged

FIGURE 8-30 ▶ Food sources of vitamin B-12 compared to the RDA for adults.

Food Sources of Vitamin B-12

Food Item and Amount	Vitamin B-12 (micrograms)	Adult Male and Female RDA = 2.4 micrograms Daily Value = 6 micrograms %RDA
RDA	2.4	100%
Baked clams, 1 ounce	15.7	654%
Boiled oysters, 2	14.4	600%
Lobster, 3 ounces	2.7	113%
Pot roast, 3 ounces	2.5	104%
Plain yogurt, 1 cup	1.4	58%
Corn Flakes cereal, ¾ cup	1.1	46%
Shrimp, 3 ounces	1.0	42%
1% milk, 1 cup	0.9	38%
Soy milk, 1 cup	0.8	33%
Boiled egg, 1	0.6	25%
Lean ham, 3 ounces	0.6	25%
Beef hot dog, 1	0.5	21%
Ham lunch meat, 2 ounces	0.4	17%

Key: ChooseMyPlate.gov
- Grains
- Vegetables
- Fruits
- Dairy
- Protein

to seek a synthetic vitamin B-12 source to aid absorption, which can be limited due to reduced intrinsic factor and stomach acid output seen in aging, as mentioned. Synthetic vitamin B-12 is not food bound, so it doesn't need stomach acid to release it from foods. Thus, it will be more readily absorbed than the food form. Ready-to-eat breakfast cereals and a multivitamin and mineral supplement are two possible synthetic sources.

The RDA of vitamin B-12 for adults is 2.4 micrograms per day. The Daily Value of 6 micrograms is used on food and supplement labels. On average, adults consume 2 times the RDA or more. This high intake provides the average meat-eating person with storage of vitamin B-12 in the liver for about 2 to 3 years.

It takes a person approximately 20 years of consuming a diet essentially free of vitamin B-12 to exhibit nerve destruction caused by a diet deficiency. Still, vegans, who eat no animal products, should find a reliable source of vitamin B-12, such as fortified soybean milk, ready-to-eat breakfast cereals, and a supplemental form of vitamin B-12 enriched yeast. Use of a multivitamin and mineral supplement containing vitamin B-12 is another option. As noted earlier, older persons are at significant risk for developing pernicious anemia due to the loss of vitamin B-12 absorption capacity. Within the 2010 Dietary Guidelines for Americans, a key recommendation for people over age 50 is to consume foods fortified with vitamin B-12, such as fortified cereals, or dietery supplements. Regular physical examinations should test for pernicious anemia in older adults. Vitamin B-12 supplements are essentially nontoxic, so no Upper Level has been set.

CONCEPT CHECK

Folate is needed for cell division because it influences DNA synthesis. A folate deficiency results in megaloblastic (macrocytic) anemia, as well as elevated blood homocysteine, inflammation of the tongue, diarrhea, and poor growth. Excess folate intake can mask a vitamin B-12 deficiency because these vitamins work together in metabolism. Folate is found in fruits and vegetables, beans, and organ meats. Emphasizing fresh and lightly cooked vegetables in the diet is important because much folate is lost during cooking. Women of childbearing age should meet needs by consuming a source of synthetic folic acid. Folate needs during pregnancy are especially high; a deficiency around the time of conception and in the first month of pregnancy may lead to neural tube defects in the fetus.

Vitamin B-12 is necessary for folate metabolism. Without dietary vitamin B-12, folate deficiency symptoms, such as macrocytic anemia, develop. In addition, vitamin B-12 is necessary for maintaining the nervous system. Paralysis can develop from a vitamin B-12 deficiency. Vitamin B-12 also participates in homocysteine metabolism. The absorption of vitamin B-12 requires a number of specific factors. If absorption is inhibited, the resulting deficiency can lead to pernicious anemia and its associated nerve destruction. Concentrated amounts of vitamin B-12 are found only in animal foods; meat-eaters generally have a 2- to 3-year supply stored in the liver. Vegans need to find an alternate source. Vitamin B-12 absorption may decline as we age. Monthly injections, nasal gels, or megadoses can make up for this.

People with HIV/AIDS also are at risk of vitamin B-12 deficiency, linked to long-standing malabsorption that they often experience. In a few studies, adequate vitamin B-12 status has been shown to lessen the decline in health experienced by those with HIV/AIDS.

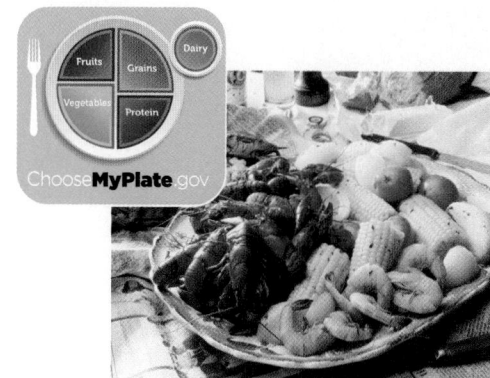

▲ Seafood, is a good source of vitamin B-12. Servings of seafood, corn, and potatoes can fill the protein and vegetables sections of MyPlate.

8.16 Vitamin C

Vitamin C (ascorbic acid) is found in all living tissues, and most animals (but not humans) synthesize it from the simple sugar glucose. Vitamin C is absorbed in the small intestine. About 70% to 90% of vitamin C is absorbed when a person eats between 30 and 180 milligrams of it per day. If someone ingests 1 gram (1000 milligrams) per day, absorption efficiency drops to about 50%. A common side effect of megadose vitamin C use is diarrhea. The unabsorbed vitamin C stays in the small intestine and attracts water, resulting in diarrhea (see the section on toxicity of vitamin C).

CRITICAL THINKING

Carlos just returned from a local mall and is excited because he saw an advertisement claiming that vitamin C will cure just about everything, from colds to heart disease. How would you explain vitamin C's main functions in the human body to Carlos?

Functions of Vitamin C

Collagen Synthesis The best understood function of vitamin C is its role in synthesizing the protein collagen. This protein is highly concentrated in connective tissue, bone, teeth, tendons, and blood vessels. It is important for wound healing. Vitamin C increases the cross-connections between amino acids in collagen, greatly strengthening the structural tissues it helps form.

On long sea voyages, captains often lost half or more of their crews to scurvy, the vitamin C deficiency disease. Its symptoms include weakness, slow wound healing, opening of previously healed wounds, bone pain, fractures, bleeding gums, diarrhea, and pinpoint hemorrhages around hair follicles on the back of the arms and legs. In 1740, the Englishman Dr. James Lind first showed that citrus fruits—two oranges and one lemon a day—could cure scurvy. Fifty years after Lind's discovery, rations for British sailors included limes to prevent scurvy (thus their nickname, limeys).

A vitamin C deficiency can cause widespread changes in tissue metabolism. Most symptoms of scurvy are linked to a decrease in collagen synthesis, such as in the skin. About 20 to 40 days with no vitamin C intake are required for the first symptoms of scurvy to appear (Fig. 8-31).

Antioxidant Activity Vitamin C has antioxidant properties. This may allow vitamin C to reduce the formation of cancer-causing nitrosamines in the stomach and also keep the folate coenzymes intact, preventing their destruction. Vitamin C may work as a free radical scavenger. Vitamin C also may aid in reactivating oxidized vitamin E so that it can be reused. The extent to which all this antioxidant activity happens in the body, however, is debatable and not proven as of now. Population studies suggest that vitamin C is effective in helping prevent certain cancers (of the esophagus, mouth, and stomach) and cataracts in the eye, probably because of its antioxidant properties.

Iron Absorption Vitamin C enhances iron absorption by keeping iron in its most absorbable form, especially as the mineral travels through the small intestine's alkaline environment. This is seen with a vitamin C intake of 75 milligrams or more at a meal. Increasing intake of vitamin C-rich foods is beneficial for those with poor iron stores. Within the 2010 Dietary Guidelines for Americans, a key recommendation for women of childbearing age who may become pregnant is to choose foods that supply heme iron, which is more readily absorbed by the body, additional iron sources, and enhancers of iron absorption, such as vitamin C-rich foods.

Immune Function Finally, vitamin C is vital for the function of the immune system, especially for the activity of certain immune cells. Thus, disease states that increase the need for immune function can increase the need for vitamin C, possibly above the RDA. Partly on the basis of this observation, Dr. Linus Pauling gained great notoriety by claiming that vitamin C could combat the common cold. He claimed that 1000 milligrams (1 gram) or more of vitamin C daily could reduce the number of colds for most people by nearly half. As a result of the popularity of his books and the respectability of his scientific credentials, millions of North Americans supplement their diets with vitamin C.

But does vitamin C reliably and effectively work against colds and other infections? Most medical and nutrition scientists disagree with Pauling's views of vitamin C. Numerous well-designed, double-blind studies have not shown megadoses of vitamin C to reliably prevent colds, though it seems to reduce the duration of symptoms by a day or so.

Vitamin C Sources and Needs

Major sources of vitamin C are citrus fruits, green peppers, cauliflower, broccoli, cabbage, strawberries, papayas, and romaine lettuce. Potatoes, ready-to-eat breakfast cereals, and fortified fruit drinks are also good sources of vitamin C (Figs. 8-32 and 8-33).

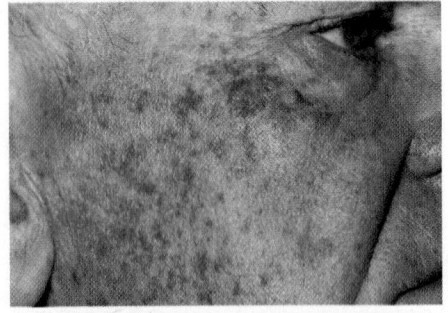
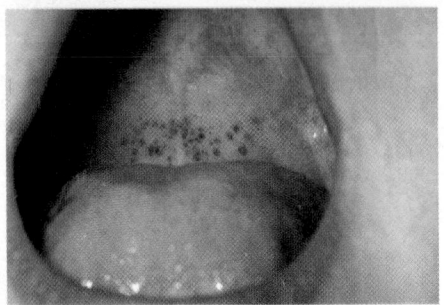

FIGURE 8-31 ▶ Pinpoint hemorrhages of the skin—an early symptom of scurvy. The spots on the skin are caused by slight bleeding. The person may experience poor wound healing. These are all signs of defective collagen synthesis.

Food Sources of Vitamin C

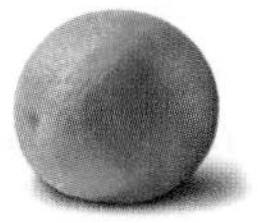

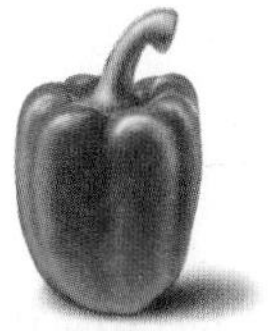

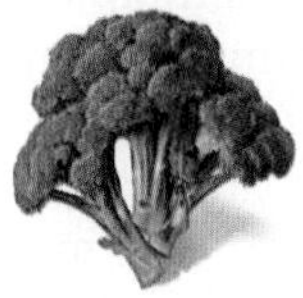

Food Item and Amount	Vitamin C (milligrams)	Adult Male RDA = 90 milligrams		Adult Female RDA = 75 milligrams	
		Daily Value = 60 milligrams			
		%RDA		%RDA	
RDA	75–90	▬▬▬▬▬ 100%		▬▬▬▬▬ 100%	
Orange, 1	98	▬▬▬▬▬≫ 109%		▬▬▬▬▬≫ 131%	
Cooked Brussels sprouts, 1 cup	97	▬▬▬▬▬≫ 108%		▬▬▬▬▬≫ 129%	
Strawberries, 1 cup	94	▬▬▬▬▬≫ 104%		▬▬▬▬▬≫ 125%	
Grapefruit juice, 1 cup	80	▬▬▬▬▬ 89%		▬▬▬▬▬≫ 107%	
Red peppers, ¼ cup	71	▬▬▬▬ 79%		▬▬▬▬▬ 95%	
Kiwi fruit, 1	57	▬▬▬ 63%		▬▬▬▬ 76%	
Green pepper rings, 5	45	▬▬▬ 50%		▬▬▬ 60%	
Tomato juice, 1 cup	45	▬▬▬ 50%		▬▬▬ 60%	
Cooked broccoli, ½ cup	33	▬▬ 37%		▬▬▬ 44%	
Kale, ½ cup	27	▬▬ 30%		▬▬ 36%	
Raw cauliflower, ½ cup	23	▬▬ 26%		▬▬ 31%	
Sweet potato, 1	17	▬ 19%		▬▬ 23%	
Baked potato, 1 medium	16	▬ 18%		▬ 21%	
Pineapple chunks, ½ cup	12	▬ 13%		▬ 16%	
Cooked spinach, ½ cup	9	▬ 10%		▬ 12%	

Key:
- ▮ Grains
- ▮ Vegetables
- ▮ Fruits
- ▮ Dairy
- ▮ Protein

FIGURE 8-32 ▶ Food sources of vitamin C compared to the RDA for adult males and females.

FIGURE 8-33 ▶ Sources of vitamin C from MyPlate. The fill of the background color (none, 1/3, 2/3, or completely covered) within each group on the plate indicates the average nutrient density for vitamin C in that group. Overall, the vegetables group and the fruits group contain many foods that are nutrient-dense sources of vitamin C. With regard to physical activity, vitamin C has no primary role in the related energy metabolism *per se*, but likely limits some oxidant damage during such endeavors.

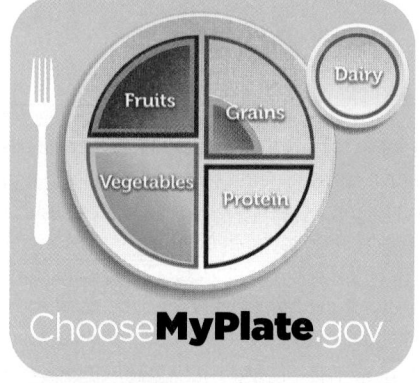

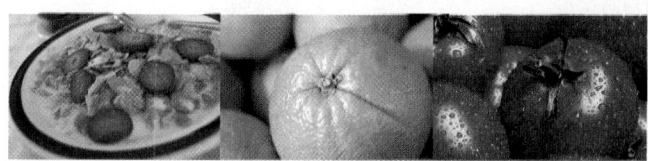

MyPlate: Sources of Vitamin C

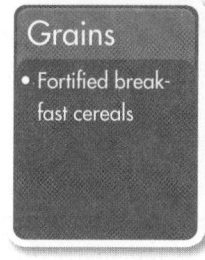
Grains
- Fortified breakfast cereals

Vegetables
- Tomatoes
- Potatoes
- Cauliflower
- Green vegetables

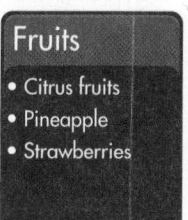
Fruits
- Citrus fruits
- Pineapple
- Strawberries

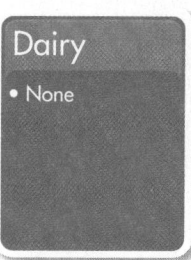
Dairy
- None

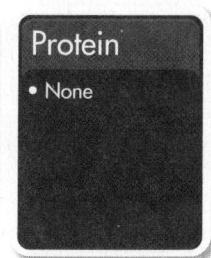
Protein
- None

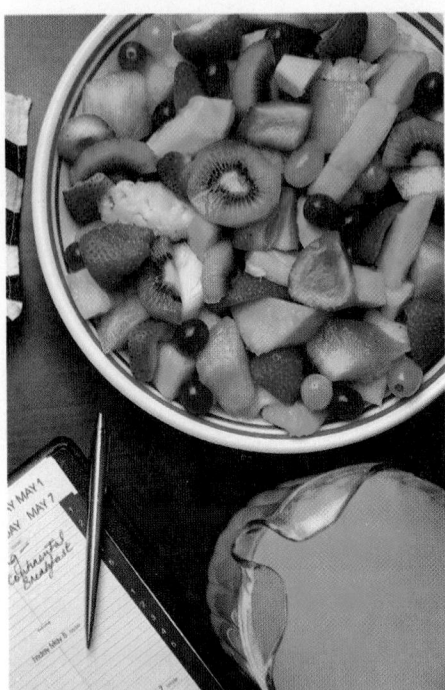

▲ In addition to orange juice, fruits such as strawberries and kiwis are excellent sources of vitamin C.

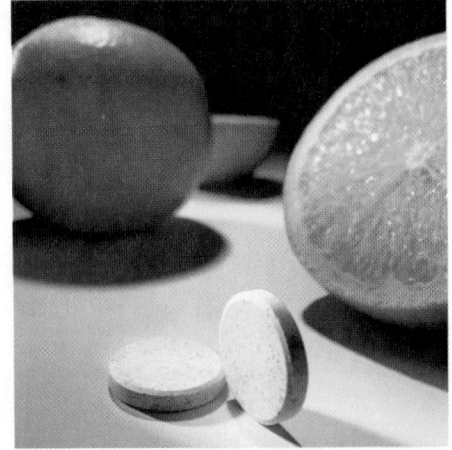

▲ Oranges are a rich source of vitamin C. The many phytochemicals they provide are an additional benefit and are not found in vitamin C supplements.

Meeting the servings for fruits and vegetables recommended by MyPyramid can easily provide enough vitamin C. Vitamin C is rapidly lost in processing and cooking as it is unstable in the presence of heat, iron, copper, or oxygen and is water soluble.

The adult RDA of vitamin C is 75 to 90 milligrams per day. The Daily Value of 60 milligrams is used to express vitamin C content on food and supplement labels. Cigarette smokers need to add an extra 35 milligrams per day to the RDA because of the great stress on their lungs from oxygen and toxic by-products of cigarette smoke. Nearly all North Americans likely meet their daily needs for vitamin C. We consume an average 70 to 100 milligrams per day. Respected nutrition experts who advocate increased use of vitamin C often recommend intakes of about 200 milligrams per day. Still, this amount can be obtained by sufficient fruit and vegetable intake. Today, vitamin C deficiency appears mostly in alcoholic people who eat nutrient-poor diets and in some older persons with inadequate food intakes.

Upper Level for Vitamin C

Most vitamin C consumed in large doses in supplements ends up in the feces or the urine. Only a small fraction of such large doses can be used. The kidneys start rapidly excreting excess vitamin C, beginning at intakes of about 100 milligrams per day. This means that if more than that is ingested, much is quickly excreted. At dosages of 500 milligrams per day, almost all of consumed vitamin C is excreted. The Upper Level for vitamin C is 2 grams per day. Regularly consuming more than that may cause stomach inflammation and diarrhea. Other suggested toxicity symptoms have been discounted in healthy people.

MAKING DECISIONS

High Doses of Vitamin C

If people want to experiment with large doses of vitamin C, they should alert their physician. High doses of vitamin C can change reactions to medical tests for blood in the feces and glucose in the urine (test for diabetes). Vitamin C can interact with the testing procedures because much of a high dose of vitamin C will not be absorbed and end up in the feces, or if absorbed, will be rapidly excreted in the urine. Physicians may misdiagnose conditions when large doses of vitamin C are consumed without their knowledge.

CONCEPT CHECK

Vitamin C is important in the synthesis of collagen, a major connective tissue protein. A vitamin C deficiency, known as scurvy, causes many changes in the skin and gums, such as small hemorrhages. This is mainly because of poor collagen synthesis. Vitamin C also modestly improves iron absorption, is involved in synthesizing certain hormones and neurotransmitters, and likely acts as a general body antioxidant. Citrus fruits, green peppers, cauliflower, broccoli, strawberries, and ready-to-eat breakfast cereals are good sources of vitamin C. As with folate, eating fresh or lightly cooked foods is important because vitamin C loses a lot of its potency in cooking. High doses of vitamin C can lead to diarrhea and foil various medical tests.

8.17 Choline

The dietary component choline is the latest addition to the list of essential nutrients. Choline is part of acetylcholine, a neurotransmitter associated with attention, learning and memory, muscle control, and many other functions. It is also part of phospholipids, such as **lecithin,** the major component of the cell membrane. Finally, choline participates in some aspects of homocysteine metabolism.

There has been only one published study examining the effect of inadequate dietary intake of choline in healthy humans. The study of male volunteers showed decreased choline stores and liver damage when humans were fed choline-deficient total parental (intravenous) nutrition solutions. Based on this human study and several laboratory animal studies, choline has been deemed essential, but is not yet classified as a vitamin.

lecithin A group of phospholipid compounds that are major components of cell membranes.

Choline Sources and Needs

Choline is widely distributed in foods (Fig. 8-34). Milk, liver, and peanuts are sources. Lecithins often are added to food during processing, so this is yet another source. There is so much choline available in ordinary foods that it is unlikely that a dietary deficiency exists naturally. Choline also can be synthesized from the nonessential (dispensable) amino-acid serine.

The Adequate Intake for choline for adults is 425 to 550 milligrams per day. We do not know if a dietary supply is needed at all life stages. Although Adequate Intakes are set for choline, it may be that the choline requirement can be met by body synthesis at some or all stages of life. We consume ample choline from food, at least 700 to 1000 milligrams per day.

Upper Level for Choline

The Upper Level for adults is 3.5 grams per day. This is based on development of a fishy body odor and low blood pressure at excessive intakes.

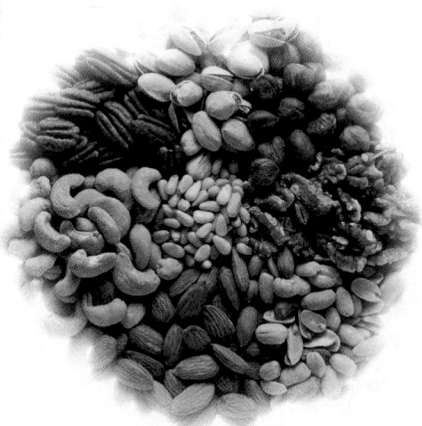

▲ Nuts, such as peanuts, are a good source of choline. Body cells also produce choline.

8.18 Vitamin-Like Compounds

A variety of vitamin-like compounds are found in the body. These include the following:

- Carnitine, needed to transport fatty acids into cell mitochondria
- Inositol, part of cell membranes

Food Sources of Choline

Food Item and Amount	Choline (milligrams)	Adult Male AI=550 milligrams %AI	Adult Female AI=425 milligrams %AI
AI	425-550	100%	100%
Egg, 1 each	126	23%	30%
Cod, 3 ounces	70	13%	16%
Chicken, 3 ounces	56	10%	13%
Fat-free milk, 1 cup	37	7%	9%
Beef, 3 ounces	36	7%	8%
Yogurt, 1 cup	31	6%	7%
Wheat germ, 2 tablespoons	21	4%	5%
Peanut butter, 2 tablespoons	20	4%	5%
Cottage cheese, ½ cup	20	4%	5%

Key:
- Grains
- Vegetables
- Fruits
- Dairy
- Protein

ChooseMyPlate.gov

FIGURE 8-34 ▶ Food sources of choline compared to the Adequate Intake for adult males and females.

- Taurine, part of bile acids
- Lipoic acid, which participates in carbohydrate metabolism and acts as an antioxidant

These vitamin-like compounds can be synthesized by cells using common building blocks, such as amino acids and glucose. Our diets are also a source. In disease states or periods of active growth, synthesis of vitamin-like compounds may not meet needs, so dietary intake can be crucial. The needs for vitamin-like compounds in certain groups of individuals, such as for preterm infants, are being investigated. Although promoted and sold by health-food stores, these vitamin-like compounds need not be included in the diet of the average healthy adult.

Table 8-3 summarizes much of what we know about the water-soluble vitamins. Now that you have studied the vitamins, review MyPlate and note how each food group can make an important vitamin contribution (Fig. 8-35).

Figure 8-36 summarizes much of what we have covered about the functions of the fat-soluble and water-soluble vitamins. Many vitamins work together for a common purpose.

TABLE 8-3 Summary of the Water-Soluble Vitamins and Choline

Vitamin	Major Functions	RDA or Adequate Intake	Dietary Sources*	Deficiency Symptoms	Toxicity Symptoms
Thiamin	• Coenzyme of carbohydrate metabolism • Nerve function	1.1–1.2 milligrams	• Sunflower seeds • Pork • Whole and enriched grains • Dried beans • Peas	*Beriberi* • Nervous tingling • Poor coordination • Edema • Heart changes • Weakness	None
Riboflavin†	• Coenzyme of carbohydrate metabolism	1.1–1.3 milligrams	• Milk • Mushrooms • Spinach • Liver • Enriched grains	• Inflammation of the mouth and tongue • Cracks at the corners of the mouth • Eye disorders	None
Niacin	• Coenzyme of energy metabolism • Coenzyme of fat synthesis • Coenzyme of fat breakdown	14–16 milligrams (niacin equivalents)	• Mushrooms • Bran • Tuna • Salmon • Chicken • Beef • Liver • Peanuts • Enriched grains	*Pellagra* • Diarrhea • Dermatitis • Dementia • Death	Upper Level is 35 milligrams from supplements, based on flushing of skin
Pantothenic acid	• Coenzyme of energy metabolism • Coenzyme of fat synthesis • Coenzyme of fat breakdown	5 milligrams	• Mushrooms • Liver • Broccoli • Eggs *Most foods have some*	• No natural deficiency disease or symptoms	None
Biotin	• Coenzyme of glucose production • Coenzyme of fat synthesis	30 micrograms	• Cheese • Egg yolks • Cauliflower • Peanut butter • Liver	• Dermatitis • Tongue soreness • Anemia • Depression	Unknown

Vitamin	Major Functions	RDA or Adequate Intake	Dietary Sources*	Deficiency Symptoms	Toxicity Symptoms
Vitamin B-6†	• Coenzyme of protein metabolism • Neurotransmitter synthesis • Hemogloblin synthesis *Many other functions*	1.3–1.7 milligrams	• Animal protein foods • Spinach • Broccoli • Bananas • Salmon • Sunflower seeds	• Headache • Anemia • Convulsions • Nausea • Vomiting • Flaky skin • Sore tongue	Upper Level is 100 milligrams, based on nerve destruction
Folate (folic acid)†	• Coenzyme involved in DNA synthesis *Many other functions*	400 micrograms (dietary folate equivalents)	• Green leafy vegetables • Orange juice • Organ meats • Sprouts • Sunflower seeds	• Megaloblastic anemia • Inflammation of tongue • Diarrhea • Poor growth • Depression	None likely Upper Level for adults set at 1000 micrograms for synthetic folic acid (exclusive of food folate), based on masking of B-12 deficiency
Vitamin B-12†	• Coenzyme of folate metabolism • Nerve function *Many other functions*	2.4 micrograms *Older adults and vegans should use fortified foods or supplements.*	• Animal foods (not natural in plants) • Organ meats • Oysters • Clams • Fortified, ready-to-eat breakfast cereals	• Macrocytic anemia • Poor nerve function	None
Vitamin C	• Connective tissue synthesis • Hormone synthesis • Neurotransmitter synthesis • Possible antioxidant activity	75–90 milligrams *Smokers should add 35 milligrams*	• Citrus fruits • Strawberries • Broccoli • Greens	• Scurvy • Poor wound healing • Pinpoint hemorrhages • Bleeding gums	Upper Level is 2 grams, based on development of diarrhea Can also alter some diagnostic tests
Choline†	• Neurotransmitter synthesis • Phospholipid synthesis	425–550 milligrams	Widely distributed in foods and synthesized by the body	No natural deficiency	Upper Level is 3.5 grams per day based on development of fishy body odor and reduced blood pressure

*Fortified ready-to-eat breakfast cereals are good sources for most of these vitamins and a common source of B vitamins for many of us.

†These nutrients also participate in homocysteine metabolism, which in turn may reduce the risk of developing cardiovascular disease.

FIGURE 8-35 ▶ Certain groups of MyPlate are especially rich sources of various vitamins and choline. This is true for those listed. Each may be also found in other groups on the plate but in lower amounts. Pantothenic acid is also present in moderate amounts in many groups.

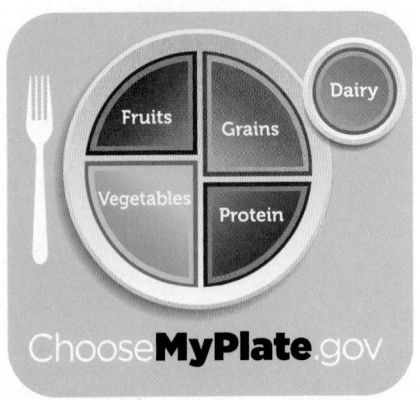

**MyPlate:
Sources of Vitamins
and Choline**

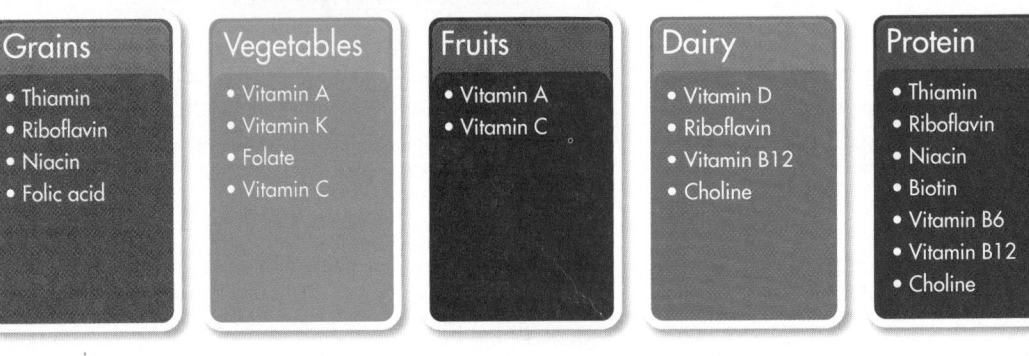

Grains
• Thiamin
• Riboflavin
• Niacin
• Folic acid

Vegetables
• Vitamin A
• Vitamin K
• Folate
• Vitamin C

Fruits
• Vitamin A
• Vitamin C

Dairy
• Vitamin D
• Riboflavin
• Vitamin B12
• Choline

Protein
• Thiamin
• Riboflavin
• Niacin
• Biotin
• Vitamin B6
• Vitamin B12
• Choline

FIGURE 8-36 ▶ Vitamins and related compounds (e.g., choline) work together to maintain health.

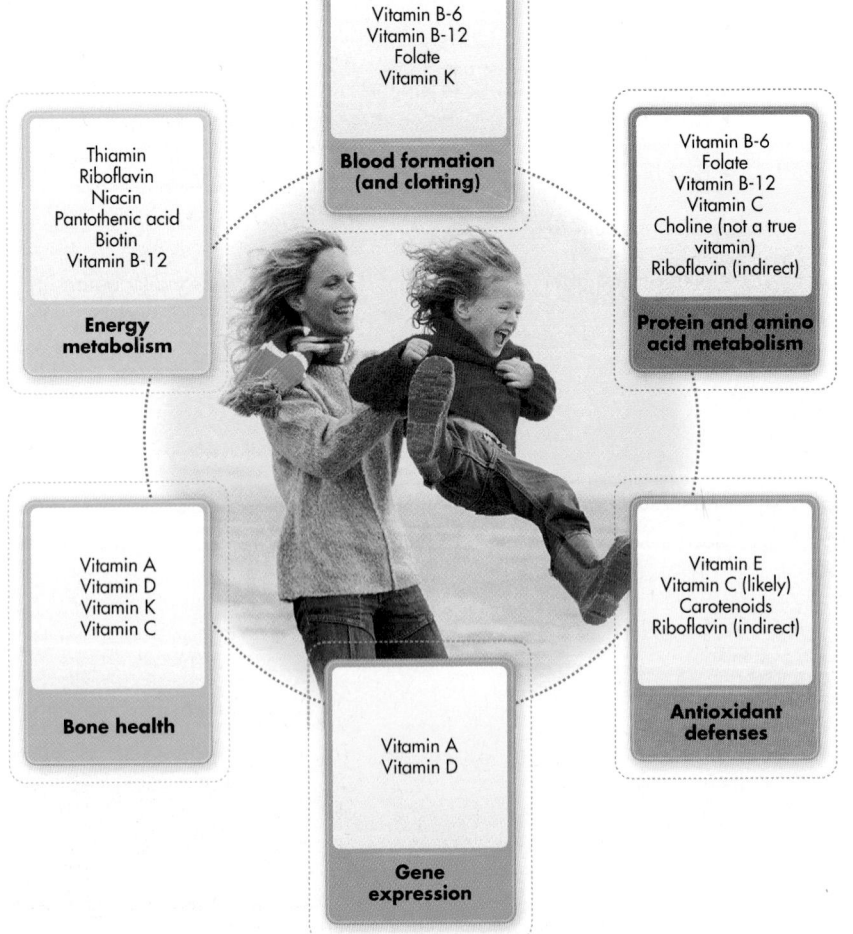

Vitamin B-6
Vitamin B-12
Folate
Vitamin K
**Blood formation
(and clotting)**

Thiamin
Riboflavin
Niacin
Pantothenic acid
Biotin
Vitamin B-12
**Energy
metabolism**

Vitamin B-6
Folate
Vitamin B-12
Vitamin C
Choline (not a true vitamin)
Riboflavin (indirect)
**Protein and amino
acid metabolism**

Vitamin A
Vitamin D
Vitamin K
Vitamin C
Bone health

Vitamin E
Vitamin C (likely)
Carotenoids
Riboflavin (indirect)
**Antioxidant
defenses**

Vitamin A
Vitamin D
**Gene
expression**

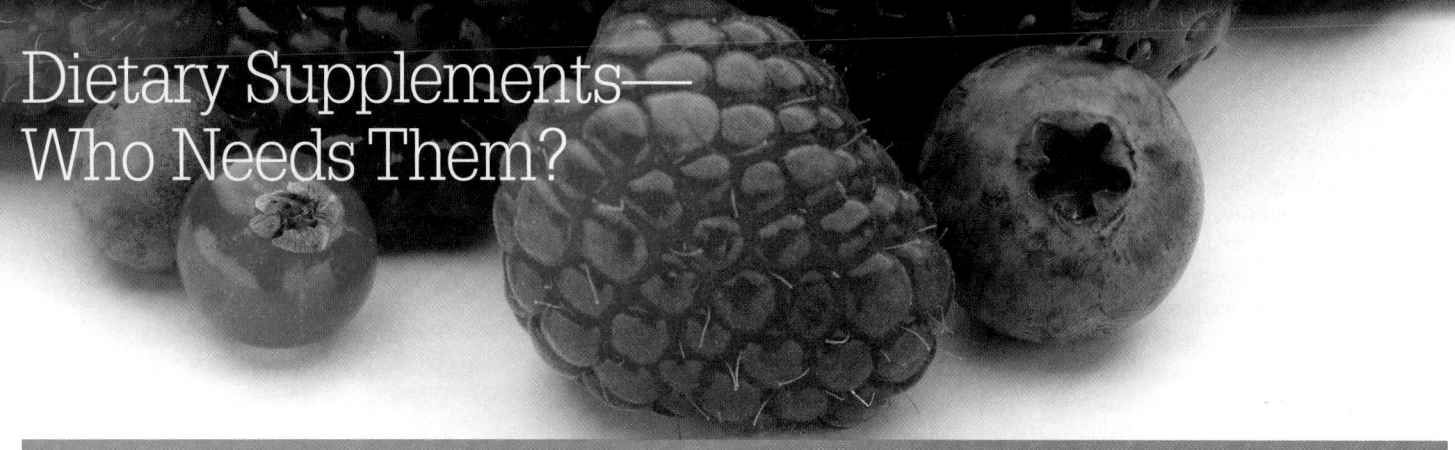

Dietary Supplements— Who Needs Them?

The term *multivitamin and mineral supplement* has been mentioned many times so far in this textbook. Often, these and other supplements are marketed as cures for anything and everything. This cure-all approach is promoted by the supplement industry and countless health-food stores, pharmacies, and supermarkets.

According to the Dietary Supplement Health and Education Act of 1994 (discussed in Chapter 1), a supplement in the United States is a product intended to supplement the diet that contains one or more of the following ingredients:

- A vitamin
- A mineral
- An herb or another botanical
- An amino acid
- A dietary substance to supplement the diet, which could be an extract or a combination of the first four ingredients in this list

The definition is broad and covers a wide variety of nutritional substances. The use of dietary supplements is a common practice among North Americans and generates about $28–29 billion annually for the industry in the United States (Fig. 8-37). Supplements can be sold without proof that they are safe and effective. Unless FDA has evidence that a supplement is inherently dangerous or marketed with an illegal claim, it will not regulate such products closely. (The vitamin folate is an exception.) FDA has limited resources to police supplement manufacturers and has to act against these manufacturers one at a time. Thus, we cannot rely on FDA to protect us from vitamin and mineral supplement overuse and misuse. We bear that responsibility ourselves, with the help of professional advice from a physician or registered dietitian.

The supplement makers can make broad claims about their products under the "structure or function" provision of the law. The products, however, cannot claim to prevent, treat, or cure a disease. Menopause in women and aging are not diseases *per se,* so products alleging to treat symptoms of these conditions can be marketed without FDA approval. For example, a product that claims to treat hot flashes arising during menopause can be sold without any evidence to prove that the product works, but a product that claims to decrease the risk of cardiovascular disease by reducing blood cholesterol must have results from scientific studies that justify the claim.

Why do people take supplements? Frequently given reasons include to:

- Reduce susceptibility to health problems (e.g., colds)
- Prevent heart attacks
- Prevent cancer
- Reduce stress
- Increase "energy"

FIGURE 8-37 ▶
The dietary supplement industry is a growing multibillion dollar business.

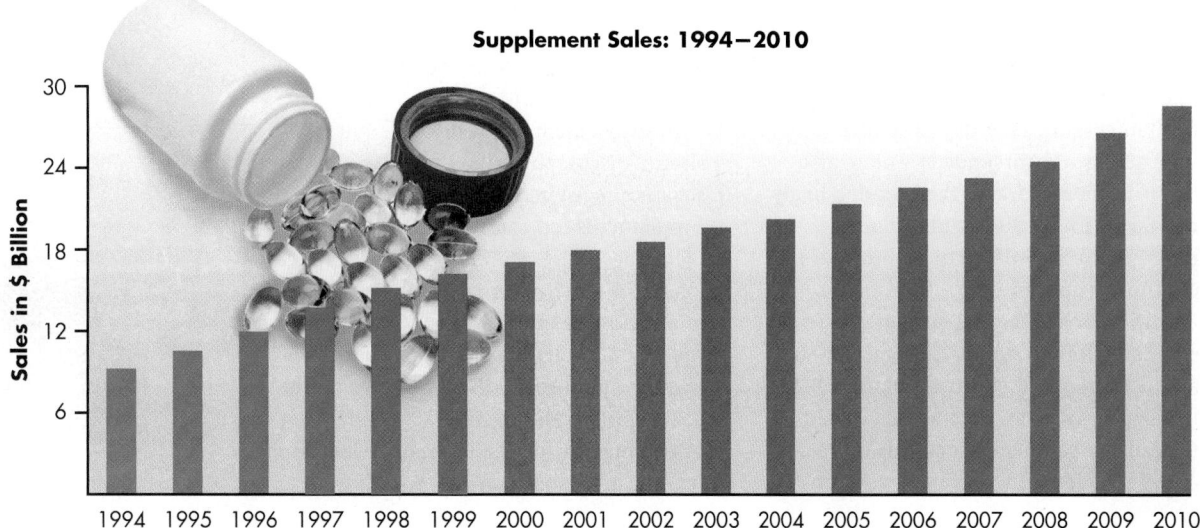

Supplement Sales: 1994—2010

Sales in $ Billion

30
24
18
12
6

1994 1995 1996 1997 1998 1999 2000 2001 2002 2003 2004 2005 2006 2007 2008 2009 2010

Should You Take a Supplement?

Opinions vary about the wisdom and safety of supplement use even among knowledgeable scientists. Typically, nutrition scientists have recommended that supplement use is needed only by a few groups (see Further Reading 9). The National Institutes of Health came to the same conclusion, noting there is insufficient evidence to support the recommendation of use of a multivitamin and mineral supplement by the general population. The experts found that only a few studies of vitamins and minerals demonstrate beneficial effects for the prevention of chronic disease, including increased bone mineral density and decreased fractures in postmenopausal women who use calcium and vitamin D supplements. (See the next section in this feature for more specific examples.) In contrast, several other studies provide disturbing evidence of risk, such as increased lung cancer risk with beta-carotene use among smokers. The NIH State-of-the-Science report (see Further Reading 10) concludes that the present evidence is insufficient to recommend either for or against the use of multivitamin/mineral supplements by Americans to prevent chronic disease.

The rationale for widespread use of a multivitamin and mineral supplement is primarily because many North Americans have been unwilling to change their food habits to include the recommended servings of fruits, vegetables, and whole grains. As for individual vitamins, there are specific cases in which supplements are advised. As discussed in Chapter 8, adequate folate status when a woman becomes pregnant helps reduce the risk of certain birth defects in her offspring (400 micrograms per day of synthetic folic acid is recommended). Folate also limits homocysteine in the blood, a likely risk factor for cardiovascular disease that can affect all of us. In addition, the committee appointed by the Food and Nutrition Board that set current nutrient standards for vitamin B-12 suggested that adults over age 50 consume vitamin B-12 in a synthetic form, such as that added to ready-to-eat breakfast cereals or present in supplements. Synthetic vitamin

B-12 is more easily absorbed than that found in food; this helps compensate for the fall in vitamin B-12 absorption often seen in one's older years.

Whether experts support use of a multivitamin and mineral supplement or not, they all emphasize that many of the health-promoting effects of foods cannot be found in a bottle. Recall the discussions of phytochemicals in Chapter 2 and the benefits of fiber in Chapter 4. Few or no phytochemicals and no fiber are present in supplements. Multivitamin and mineral supplements also contain little calcium to keep the pill size small, and the oxide forms of magnesium, zinc, and copper used in many supplements are not as well absorbed as forms found in foods.

Overall, supplement use cannot fix a poor diet in all respects. Uninformed megadose supplement use also can lead to harm—most cases of nutrient toxicity are a result of supplement use. Thus, we are advised to first take a good look at our dietary habits and then improve them, as outlined in Chapter 2 (Fig. 8-38). Then we should find out which nutrient gaps remain, and identify food sources that can help. Such a source could be ready-to-eat breakfast cereals to increase vitamin E, folic acid, and vitamin B-6 intake, and as well provide highly absorbable forms of vitamin B-12. Calcium-fortified orange juice could be used to increase calcium intake, or milk and yogurt to increase vitamin D and calcium intake. You need to be careful of highly fortified foods, however, as these products may provide the appropriate amount of nutrients in 1 serving, but the typical consumer may eat more than 1 serving. This can lead to an excessive intake of some nutrients, such as vitamin A, iron, and synthetic folic acid.

If supplement use is desired, you should discuss this practice with a physician or registered dietitian, as some supplements can interfere with certain medicines. For example, high intakes of vitamin K or vitamin E alter the action of anticlotting medications. Vitamin B-6 can offset the action of L-dopa (used in treating Parkinson's disease). Large doses of vitamin C can interfere with certain cancer therapy regimens, excessive zinc intake can inhibit copper absorption.

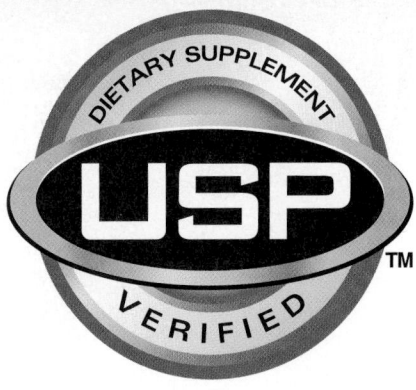

▲ The USP (United States Pharmacopeia) label indicates the product meets USP standards.

▶ Because research on a variety of nutrient supplements has revealed a lack of product quality, FDA now requires supplement makers to test the purity, strength, and composition of all their products. The USP (United States Pharmacopeia) designation, which has been extended to an increasing number of nutrient supplements, establishes professionally accepted standards for these products and can be used to evaluate supplements. The USP standards designate strength, quality, purity, packaging, labeling, speed of dissolution, and acceptable length of storage of ingredients for drugs.

Top Five Dietary Supplements in 2010:

1. Fish/Oil
2. Multivitamins
3. Vitamin D
4. Calcium
5. Coenzyme Q

Source: www.Consumerlab.com

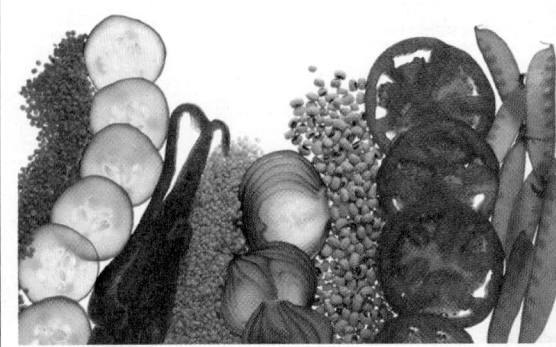

▲ Focus first on foods that meet nutrient needs.

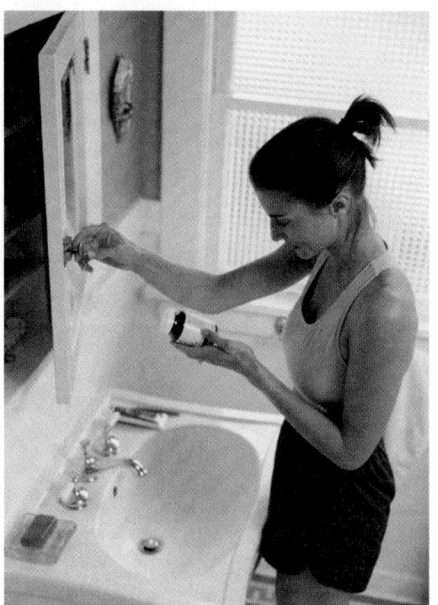

▲ Long-term intake of just three times the Daily Value for some fat-soluble vitamins—particularly preformed vitamin A—can cause toxic effects. Know what you are taking if you use supplements.

Healthy Diet Rich in Vitamins and Minerals

↓

Fortified Foods

↓

Possible Multivitamin and Mineral Supplement Use

↓

Individual Supplements in Some Cases

FIGURE 8-38 ▶ Supplement savvy—an approach to the use of nutrient supplementation. Emphasizing a healthy diet rich in vitamins and minerals is always the first option.

<u>CRITICAL THINKING</u>

Believing that supplements provide the nutrition her body needs, Janice regularly takes numerous supplements while paying relatively little attention to daily food choices. How would you explain to her that this practice may lead to health problems?

Large amounts of folate can mask signs and symptoms of a vitamin B-12 deficiency (review the section on toxicity of folate in this chapter). Remember, you *can* get too much of a good thing.

People Most Likely to Need Supplements

As you might guess, generally the people who take supplements in our society are already healthy. Various medical and health-related organizations suggest that the following vitamin and mineral supplements can be important for certain groups of healthy people:

- Women of childbearing age may need extra synthetic folic acid if their dietary patterns do not supply the recommended amount (400 micrograms).
- Women with excessive bleeding during menstruation may need extra iron.
- Women who are pregnant or breastfeeding may need extra iron, folate, and calcium.
- People with low calorie intakes (less than about 1200 kcal per day) may need a range of vitamins and minerals. This is true of some women and many older people.
- Strict vegans may need extra calcium, iron, zinc, and vitamin B-12.
- Newborns need a single dose of vitamin K, as directed by a physician.
- Some older infants may need fluoride supplements, as directed by a dentist.
- People with limited milk intake and sunlight exposure may need extra vitamin D. This includes breastfed infants and many African-American and older people.
- People with lactose maldigestion or lactose intolerance, and those with allergies to dairy products, may need extra calcium.
- Adults over age 50 may need a synthetic source of vitamin B-12.
- People on low-fat diets or diets low in plant oils and nuts may need some extra vitamin E.
- People who consume a large part of their diet as refined foods rather than as fruits, vegetables, or whole grains may need a range of vitamins and minerals.

Individuals with certain medical conditions (e.g., vitamin-resistant diseases or longstanding fat malabsorption) and those who use certain medications also may require supplementation with specific vitamins and minerals. Children who are "picky eaters" may require supplementation as well (see Chapter 15). Finally, smokers and alcohol abusers may benefit from supplementation, but cessation of these two activities is far more beneficial than any supplementation.

Which Supplement Should You Choose?

If you decide to take a multivitamin and mineral supplement, which one should you choose? As a start, choose a nationally recognized brand (from a supermarket or pharmacy) that contains about 100% of the Daily Values for the nutrients present. A multivitamin and mineral supplement should generally be taken with or just after meals to maximize absorption. Make sure also that intake from the total of this supplement, any other supplements used, and highly fortified foods (such as ready-to-eat breakfast cereals) provide no more than the Upper Level for each vitamin and mineral. (See the inside cover of this text book for Upper Levels.) This is especially important with regard to preformed vitamin A intake. Two exceptions are (1) both men and older women should make sure any product used is low in iron or iron-free to avoid possible iron overload (see Chapter 9 for details), and (2) somewhat exceeding the Upper Level for vitamin D is likely a safe practice for adults. One should read the labels carefully to be sure of what is being taken (Fig. 8-39).

Another consideration in choosing a supplement is avoiding superfluous ingredients, such as para-aminobenzoic acid (PABA), hesperidin complex, inositol, bee pollen, and lecithins. These are not needed in our diets. They are especially common in expensive supplements sold in health-food stores and by mail. In addition, use of l-tryptophan and high doses of beta-carotene or fish oils is discouraged.

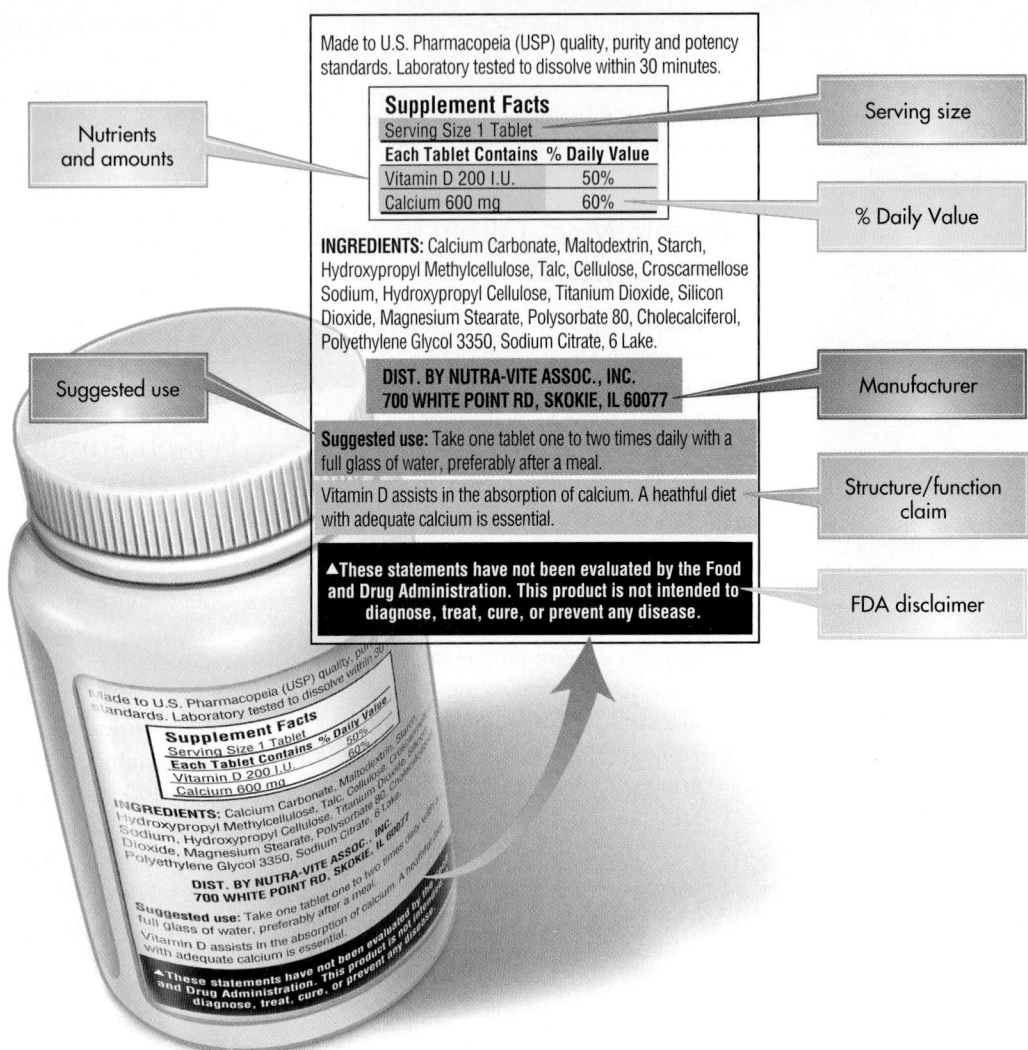

Nutrients and amounts

Suggested use

Serving size

% Daily Value

Manufacturer

Structure/function claim

FDA disclaimer

Made to U.S. Pharmacopeia (USP) quality, purity and potency standards. Laboratory tested to dissolve within 30 minutes.

Supplement Facts

Serving Size 1 Tablet

Each Tablet Contains	% Daily Value
Vitamin D 200 I.U.	50%
Calcium 600 mg	60%

INGREDIENTS: Calcium Carbonate, Maltodextrin, Starch, Hydroxypropyl Methylcellulose, Talc, Cellulose, Croscarmellose Sodium, Hydroxypropyl Cellulose, Titanium Dioxide, Silicon Dioxide, Magnesium Stearate, Polysorbate 80, Cholecalciferol, Polyethylene Glycol 3350, Sodium Citrate, 6 Lake.

DIST. BY NUTRA-VITE ASSOC., INC.
700 WHITE POINT RD, SKOKIE, IL 60077

Suggested use: Take one tablet one to two times daily with a full glass of water, preferably after a meal.

Vitamin D assists in the absorption of calcium. A heathful diet with adequate calcium is essential.

▲These statements have not been evaluated by the Food and Drug Administration. This product is not intended to diagnose, treat, cure, or prevent any disease.

FIGURE 8-39 ▶ Nutrient supplements display a nutrition label different from that of foods. This Supplement Facts label must list the ingredient(s), amount(s) per serving, serving size, suggested use, and % Daily Value if one has been established. This label also includes structure/function claims. Thus, it also must include the FDA warning that these claims have not been evaluated by the agency.

Six websites to help you evaluate ongoing claims and evaluate safety of supplements are:

www.acsh.org
www.quackwatch.com
www.ncahf.org
http://ods.od.nih.gov
www.eatright.org
www.usp.org/USPVerified/dietarySupplements/

These sites are maintained by groups or individuals committed to providing reasoned and authoritative nutrition and health advice to consumers. See Further Reading 1 for more advice on nutrient supplementation.

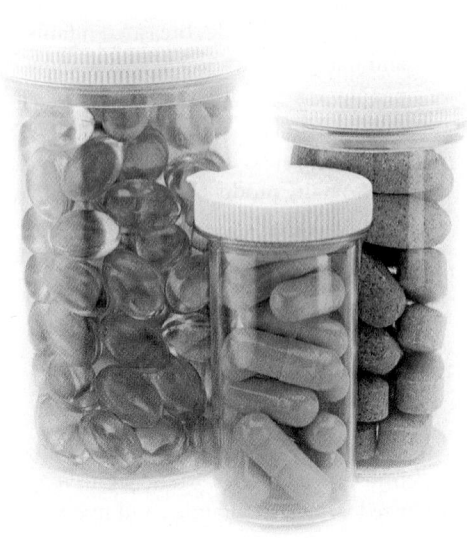

◀ The regular use of individual nutrient supplements could lead to health risks. These should be used with caution.

Case Study Choosing a Dietary Supplement

Amy works the "pre-dawn" shift as a baker at a popular bistro. Amy is also a full-time student, and the combination of taking a full course load at college and working early hours while her friends are sleeping has created a lot of stress for her. Amy's many commitments also make it important that she not become ill. Recently one of her coworkers suggested that she take *Nutramega* supplements to help prevent colds, flu, and other illnesses. The product's label suggests that *Nutramega* helps prevent such problems, especially those associated with the changing of seasons. The label recommends taking two to three tablets daily for health maintenance and two to three tablets every 3 hours at the first sign of feeling ill. Amy looks at the Supplement Facts label on the bottle and finds that each tablet contains (as percent of the Daily Value): 33% for vitamin A (three-quarters is preformed vitamin A), 700% for vitamin C, 200% for niacin, and 100% for vitamin B-6. A month's supply costs about $50.

Answer the following questions, and check your response in Appendix A.

1. Are there any health risks associated with taking the "maintenance" dose of two to three tablets per day? How does this dose compare with the Upper Tolerable Intake Levels for the four nutrients?

2. How many tablets would be taken per day if Amy was feeling ill?
   a. For vitamin A, use the % Daily Value to calculate the micrograms RAE that would be in this larger dose. How does this compare to the Upper Level for Vitamin A?
   b. Use the % Daily Value to calculate the milligrams of vitamin C in this larger dose. How does this compare to the Upper Level for vitamin C?
   c. Use the % Daily Value to calculate the milligrams of niacin in this larger dose. How does this compare to the Upper Level for niacin?
   d. Use the % Daily Value to calculate the micrograms of vitamin B-6 in this larger dose. How does this compare to the Upper Level for vitamin B-6?
   e. Does the recommended dosage of any of these nutrients pose any health risks?

3. Does the cost of this supplement seem reasonable? How does it compare to the

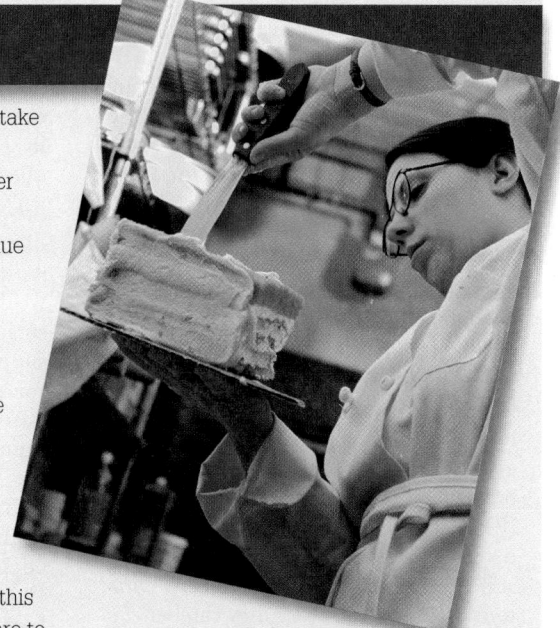

▲ Is a dietary supplement a safe way for Amy to prevent colds and the flu?

cost of a typical multivitamin supplement available at your local drug store?

4. Should Amy be concerned about meeting her nutrient needs? Does the type of stress she is under increase her nutrient needs?

5. After studying Chapter 8, what diet and supplement advice would you offer to Amy?

Summary (Numbers refer to numbered learning outcomes.)

8.1 Vitamins are carbon-containing compounds we generally need daily in small amounts from foods. They yield no energy directly, but many contribute to energy-yielding chemical reactions in the body and promote growth and development. Many vitamins act as coenzymes, which help enzymes function.

8.2 Vitamins A, D, E, and K are fat soluble, whereas the B vitamins, vitamin C and choline are water soluble.

8.3 Vitamin A is a family of compounds that includes several forms of preformed vitamin A. Three forms of carotenoids can also yield vitamin A; some also function as antioxidants. Vitamin A contributes to vision, immune function, and cell development. Vitamin D is both a hormone

and a vitamin. It can be synthesized in the human body using sunshine and a cholesterol-like substance in the skin. The active hormone form of vitamin D helps regulate blood calcium in part by increasing calcium absorption from the intestine. Infants and children who don't get enough vitamin D may develop rickets, and adults develop osteomalacia. Vitamin E functions primarily as an antioxidant. By donating electrons to electron-seeking, free-radical (oxidizing) compounds, it neutralizes them. This effect shields cell membranes and red blood cells from breakdown. Vitamin K helps blood clot and increases the calcium-binding potential of some organs. Vitamin K is poorly stored in the body, but our dietary intake alone is usually sufficient to meet needs. People who can't

absorb fat well or who are on antibiotics for long periods may need extra vitamin K. Thiamin, riboflavin, and niacin play key roles as coenzymes in energy-yielding reactions. They help metabolize carbohydrates, fats, and proteins. Alcoholism and a poor diet can create deficiencies of these three nutrients, which often show up as symptoms in the brain and nervous system, skin, and GI tract. Pantothenic acid, which participates in many aspects of cell metabolism. Biotin, which participates in glucose production, fatty acid synthesis, and DNA synthesis, can be synthesized by bacteria in the intestine. Vitamin B-6 performs a vital role in protein metabolism, especially in synthesizing nonessential amino acids. It also helps synthesize neurotransmitters and performs other metabolic roles, such as metabolism of homocysteine. Headaches, a form of anemia, nausea, and vomiting result from a B-6 deficiency. Folate plays an important role in DNA synthesis and homocysteine metabolism. Symptoms of a deficiency include generally poor cell division in various areas of the body, megaloblastic anemia, tongue inflammation, diarrhea, and poor growth. Pregnancy puts high demands for folate on the body; deficiency during the first month of pregnancy can result in neural tube defects in offspring. A deficiency can also occur in people with alcoholism. Vitamin B-12 is needed to metabolize folate and homocysteine, and maintain the insulation surrounding nerves. A deficiency results in anemia (because of its relationship to folate) and nerve degeneration. Older people often suffer from inefficient absorption of vitamin B-12, in which case they can benefit from monthly injections or megadoses of the vitamin. Vitamin C is mainly used to synthesize collagen, a major protein for building connective tissue. A vitamin C deficiency results in scurvy, evidenced by poor wound healing, pinpoint hemorrhages in the skin, and bleeding gums. Vitamin C also modestly enhances iron absorption, is likely a general antioxidant, and is needed for synthesizing some hormones and neurotransmitters. Deficiencies can occur in people with alcoholism and those whose diets lack sufficient fruits and vegetables. Smoking makes matters worse for people already at risk. Choline is used to form a neurotransmitter, and has other functions, including a role in homocysteine metabolism. Nutritional needs have recently been set. No natural deficiency of choline has been reported. The vitamin-like compounds carnitine, inositol, taurine, and lipoic acid, while participating in many important chemical reactions in the body, are not true vitamins because they can be synthesized in the body from readily available building blocks; they are also obtained from the diet.

8.4 Vitamin A is found in liver and fish oils; carotenoids are especially plentiful in dark green and orange vegetables. If we don't spend enough time in the sun, such foods as fish and fortified milk can supply vitamin D. Older people, African-Americans, and breastfed infants often need a supplemental source. Vitamin E is found in plant oils. Claims are made about the curative powers of vitamin E, but more information is needed before megadose vitamin E recommendations for healthy adults can be made with certainty. Some vitamin K absorbed each day comes from bacterial synthesis in the intestine, but most comes from foods, primarily green, leafy vegetables. Enriched grain products are common sources of thiamin, riboflavin, and niacin. Pantothenic acid is widely distributed among foods. Biotin comes from foods such as eggs, peanuts, and cheese. Regular consumption of animal protein foods and rich plant sources such as broccoli provide needed vitamin B-6. Food sources of folate are leafy vegetables, organ meats, and orange juice. Women of child-bearing age need to meet the RDA with synthetic folic acid. Great amounts of folate can be lost in prolonged cooking. Generally, a dietary deficiency is unlikely because vitamin B-12 is highly concentrated in animal foods, which constitute a major part of the North American diet. Vitamin B-12 does not occur naturally in plant foods. Vegans need a supplemental source, and adults over age 50 should consume a synthetic source, such as that in ready-to-eat breakfast cereals. Fresh fruits and vegetables, especially citrus fruits, are generally good sources. A great amount of vitamin C is lost in cooking, so a diet should emphasize fresh or lightly cooked vegetables. Choline is a dietary component available from a wide variety of foods and is synthesized in the body.

8.5 Vitamin A can be toxic, even when taken at just 3 times the RDA for preformed vitamin A (the Upper Level). High vitamin A intakes are especially dangerous during pregnancy. Vitamin D is potentially a toxic substance in infancy and early childhood. The Upper Level for vitamin E is set at about 50 times adult needs. Niacin has an Upper Level (2.5 times adult needs). Taking high doses of vitamin B-6 causes damage to the nervous system. The Upper Level is about 60 times adult needs. Excess folate in the diet can mask a vitamin B-12 deficiency, so an Upper Level has been set at 2½ times adult needs (refers to synthetic folic acid only). The Upper Level of vitamin C is set at about 20 times adult needs. The Upper Level of choline is set at about eight times adult needs.

N&YH Taking a multivitamin and mineral supplement to help meet nutrient needs is recommended by some experts, while other experts suggest that only some in the population need such supplementation. Taking many nutrient supplements can lead to nutrient-related toxicity, so any such use should be carefully considered. The clearest evidence is for a diet rich in fruits and vegetables and whole-grain breads and cereals, not reliance on supplements.

Check Your Knowledge (Answers to the following questions are below.)

1. Vitamins are classified as
   a. organic and inorganic.
   b. fat-soluble and water-soluble.
   c. essential and nonessential.
   d. elements and compounds.

2. Vitamin D is called the sunshine vitamin because
   a. it is available in orange juice.
   b. exposure to sunlight converts a precursor to vitamin D.
   c. it can be destroyed by exposure to sunlight.
   d. All of the above.

3. Vitamin E functions as
   a. a coenzyme.
   b. an antioxidant.
   c. a hormone.
   d. a peroxide.

4. A deficiency of vitamin A can lead to the disease called
   a. xerophthalmia.
   b. osteomalacia.
   c. scurvy.
   d. pellagra.

5. A high intake of vitamin E can
   a. inhibit vitamin K metabolism.
   b. lead to lead poisoning.
   c. inhibit copper absorption.
   d. cause baldness.

6. A vitamin synthesized by bacteria in the intestine is
   a. A.
   b. D.
   c. E.
   d. K.

7. Bowed legs, an enlarged and misshapen head, and enlarged knee joints in children are all symptoms of
   a. rickets.
   b. xerophthalmia.
   c. osteoporosis.
   d. vitamin D toxicity.

8. Thiamin, riboflavin, and niacin are called the "energy" vitamins because they
   a. can be broken down to provide energy.

   b. are coenzymes needed for release of energy from carbohydrates, fats, and proteins.
   c. are ingredients in energy drinks such as Powerade.
   d. are needed in large amounts by competitive athletes.

9. A deficient intake of _____ has been shown to increase the risk of having a baby with a neural tube defect such as spina bifida.
   a. vitamin A
   b. vitamin C
   c. vitamin E
   d. folic acid

10. Vitamin C is necessary for the production of
    a. stomach acid.
    b. collagen.
    c. hormones.
    d. clotting factors.

Answers: 1.b (LO 8.1), 2.b (LO 8.4), 3.b (LO 8.3), 4.a (LO 8.3), 5.a (LO 8.5), 6.d (LO 8.4), 7.a (LO 8.3), 8.b (LO 8.3), 9.d (LO 8.3), 10.b (LO 8.3)

Study Questions (Numbers refer to Learning Outcomes)

1. Why is the risk of toxicity greater with the fat-soluble vitamins A and D than with water-soluble vitamins in general? **(LO 8.2)**

2. How would you determine which fruits and vegetables displayed in the produce section of your supermarket are likely to provide plenty of carotenoids? **(LO 8.4)**

3. What is the primary function of the vitamin D hormone? Which groups of people likely need to supplement their diets with vitamin D, and on what do you base your answer? **(LO 8.3)**

4. Describe how vitamin E functions as an antioxidant. Use the term *free radical* **(LO 8.3)**

5. Describe how the RDA, Daily Value, and Upper Level for vitamin B-6 should be used in everyday life. How do the RDA and Daily Value for vitamin B-6 differ? **(LO 8.4)**

6. The need for certain vitamins increases as energy expenditure increases. Name two such vitamins and explain why this is the case. **(LO 8.3)**

7. Take one of the B vitamins that might be low in the North American diet and explain why a deficiency might occur. **(LO 8.3)**

8. Which vitamins are lost from cereal grains as a result of the "refining" process? Which vitamins must be replaced

by law in the subsequent enrichment process? **(LO 8.4)**

9. Why does FDA limit the amount of folate that may be included in supplements and fortified foods? **(LO 8.4)**

10. Is it necessary for North Americans to consume a great excess of vitamin C to avoid the possibility of a deficiency? Do vitamin C intakes well above the RDA have any negative consequences? **(LO 8.5)**

What Would You Choose Recommendations

Folate is especially important during pregnancy because it is required for DNA synthesis. During pregnancy, folate needs increase from 400 to 600 micrograms per day. Obstetricians typically prescribe prenatal vitamins that contain 800 micrograms of folic acid, but good food sources of folate have benefits besides the nutrient itself, such as phytochemicals and fiber.

Meats and other animal products are not particularly good sources of folate. Dairy foods do contribute some—your low-fat yogurt supplies about 27 micrograms of folate per 1-cup container. Other dairy products, such as skim milk, provide about 12 micrograms of folate. To find more folate, seek out plant sources.

Lentils and other dried beans are among the richest sources of folate. A 1/2-cup serving of cooked lentils provides about 179 micrograms of folate. Beans are also great sources of other nutrients that are typically low in American diets, such as fiber, potassium, magnesium. Plus, they are low in fat and cholesterol-free.

Spinach and other leafy green vegetables are excellent sources of folate. Two cups of fresh, chopped spinach provide 116 micrograms of folate. Half a cup of sliced strawberries adds an additional 20 micrograms, so this delicious spinach salad supplies almost 25% of the RDA for folate during pregnancy. Even with 1 tablespoon of low-fat vinaigrette, this salad is a very nutrient-dense source of folate (recall Chapter 2): 136 micrograms folate compared to only 50 kcal. Cooked spinach (as presented in Figure 8-28) is an even more concentrated source of folate because greens cook down to a smaller volume, so you are actually consuming more vegetables per cup.

Recall that grain products, such as the whole-wheat bread in your turkey sandwich, are fortified with folic acid. Fortified breakfast cereals are a fabulous source of synthetic folic acid. One cup of Oatmeal Squares cereal contains 400 micrograms (100% of the DV) of folic acid in one serving! Also, the synthetic folic acid incorporated into fortified foods is more bioavailable than natural sources of folate. During pregnancy—or any life stage—a fortified, whole-grain, ready-to-eat breakfast cereal is an excellent way to start the day.

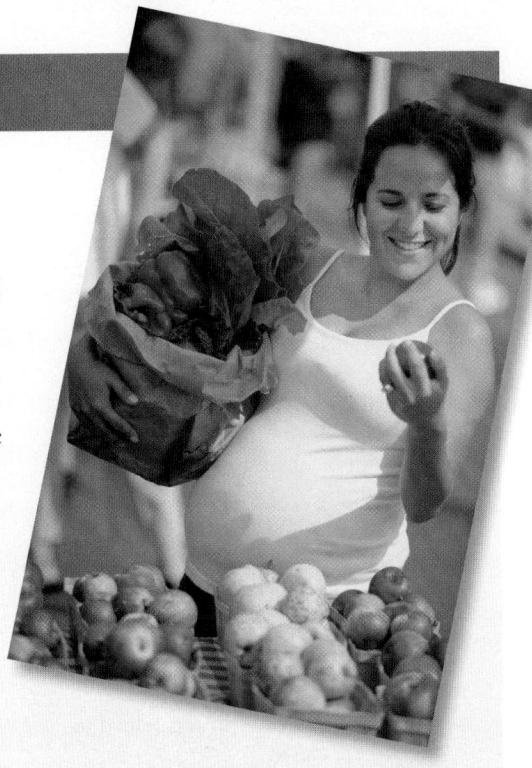

▲ Spinach and other leafy green vegetables are excellent sources of folate. Your next choice—should you decorate the nursery pink or blue?

Further Readings

1. ADA Reports: Position of the American Dietetic Association: Nutrient supplementation. *Journal of the American Dietetic Association* 109:2073, 2009.
   The best nutrition-based strategy for promoting optimal health and reducing the risk of chronic disease is to wisely choose a wide variety of foods. Additional nutrients and/or supplements can help some people meet their nutritional needs as set by science-based nutrition standards (e.g., the Dietary Reference Intakes).

2. Andres E and others: Food-cobalamin malabsorption in elderly patients: Clinical manifestations and treatments. *American Journal of Medicine* 118:1154, 2005.
   About 15% of older adults show defective vitamin B-12 absorption. This condition especially affects absorption of the vitamin B-12 found naturally in foods. Consumption of crystalline vitamin B-12 in contrast is not so affected and was found to be a useful form of therapy for the older adults in this study.

3. DeWals P and others: Reduction in neural tube defects after folic acid fortification in Canada. *New England Journal of Medicine* 357:135, 2007.
   Changes in the prevalence of neural tube defects were assessed in Canada before and after food fortification of cereal products with folic acid became mandatory in 1998. A 46% reduction in the prevalence of neural tube defects occurred during the full-fortification period, with a decrease from 1.58 per 1000 births before fortification to 0.86 per 1000 births after fortification. The reduction rate was greater for spina bifida (a decrease of 53%) than for anencephaly and encephalocele (decreases of 38% and 31%, respectively).

4. Garland CF and others: Vitamin D and prevention of breast cancer: Pooled analysis. *Journal of Steroid Biochemistry & Molecular Biology* 103:708, 2007.
   This review of all studies reported risk of breast cancer and assessed the dose-response association between serum 25(OH)D and risk of breast cancer. The conclusion of this review is that daily intake of 2000 IU of Vitamin D3, and, when possible, very moderate exposure to sunlight, could raise serum 25(OH)D to 52 ng/ml, a level associated with reduction by 50% in incidence of breast cancer, according to observational studies.

5. Giovannucci E and others: 25-Hydroxyvitamin D and risk of myocardial infarction in men: A prospective study. *Archives Internal Medicine* 168:1174, 2008.
   Vitamin D deficiency is thought to be involved in the development of atherosclerosis and coronary heart disease in humans. This study found men 40 to 75 years of age with vitamin D levels

below normal had a higher risk of heart attack even after controlling for factors known to be associated with coronary artery disease. Even men with intermediate vitamin D levels were at elevated risk of heart disease relative to those with sufficient vitamin D levels.

6. Gordon CM and others: Prevalence of vitamin D deficiency among healthy infants and toddlers. *Archives of Pediatric and Adolescent Medicine* 162:505, 2008.

    The prevalence of vitamin D deficiency was determined and 25-hydroxyvitamin D concentration was examined as a function of skin pigmentation, season, sun exposure, breastfeeding, and vitamin D supplementation. Suboptimal vitamin D status was common among otherwise healthy young children with 40% of infants and toddlers testing below average for vitamin D. One-third of the vitamin D deficient infant and toddlers exhibited demineralization a hallmark of the deleterious skeletal effects of this condition.

7. Holick MF: Vitamin D deficiency. *New England Journal of Medicine* 357:266, 2007.

    This is a review of numerous studies that have shown that vitamin D does more than just enhance bone health in children and adults. Studies show that vitamin D deficiency in adults has been linked to an increased risk for osteoporosis and osteomalacia but also certain cancers.

8. Lee I and others: Vitamin E in the primary prevention of cardiovascular disease and cancer: The women's health study: A randomized controlled trial. *Journal of the American Medical Association* 294:56, 2005.

    The data from this large trial indicated that 600 IU of natural-source vitamin E taken every other day provided no overall benefit for major cardiovascular events or cancer. These data do not support recommending vitamin E supplementation for cardiovascular disease or cancer prevention among healthy women, but more research is warranted, because a decrease in sudden cardiac death was seen in a subset of older women in this study.

9. Lichtenstein AH, Russell RM: Essential nutrients: Food or supplements? Where should the emphasis be? *Journal of the American Medical Association* 294:351, 2005.

    There is insufficient evidence to justify a shift in public health policy from one that emphasizes a food-based diet to fulfill nutrient requirements and promote optimal health to one that emphasizes dietary supplementation. Targeted nutrient supplementation is appropriate in some cases, however, as reviewed by these authors.

10. NIH State-of-the-Science Conference Statement on Multivitamin/Mineral Supplements and Chronic Disease Prevention. *NIH consensus State-of-the-Science Statements* 23(2):1, 2006.

    Use of multivitamins/minerals (MVMs) has grown rapidly over the past several decades. Due in part to the fortification of foods, there is still insufficient knowledge about the actual amount of total nutrients that Americans consume from diet and supplements. The cumulative effects of supplementation and fortification have raised safety concerns about exceeding upper levels. Most studies do not provide strong evidence for beneficial health-related effects of supplements taken singly, in pairs, or in combinations of three or more. Although there is encouraging evidence of increased bone mineral density and decreased fractures in postmenopausal women who use calcium and vitamin D supplements, several other studies provide disturbing evidence of risk, such as increased lung cancer risk with beta-carotene use among smokers. The present evidence is insufficient to recommend either for or against the use of MVMs by the American public to prevent chronic disease.

11. Nield LS and others: Rickets: Not a disease of the past. *American Family Physician* 74(4), 200:619, 2006.

    This review article emphasizes the current need to screen for rickets even in developed countries. Background and support is given for the recent recommendation by the American Academy of Pediatrics (AAP) to provide a daily vitamin D supplement for all solely breastfed babies beginning in the first 2 months of life. Until recently, vitamin D supplementation was not advised for breastfed infants. Multiple case reports of nutritional rickets in the United States have promoted the AAP recommendation.

12. Sesso HD and others: Vitamins E and C in the prevention of cardiovascular disease in men. The Physicians' Health Study II Randomized Controlled Trial. *Journal of American Medical Association* 300:2123, 2008.

    Men enrolled in the Physician's Health Study II were placed into four groups, which were given vitamin C and a placebo, vitamin E and a placebo, C and E together, and placebo only. Neither C nor E had an effect on major cardiovascular events, which include heart attacks, stroke, or death. The results suggest that when you pull a nutrient out of the whole diet, you do not see the same effects.

13. Voutilainen S and others: Carotenoids and cardiovascular health. *American Journal of Clinical Nutrition* 83:1265, 2006.

    This report reviews the role of carotenoids in the prevention of heart disease. Although fruit and vegetables are recognized as having protective effects against cardiovascular disease, the role of a single group of compounds such as carotenoids cannot be ascertained. Therefore, the consumption of carotenoids in supplemental forms cannot be recommended.

14. Wang TJ and others: Vitamin D deficiency and risk of cardiovascular disease. *Circulation* 117:503, 2008.

    This study was conducted over 5 years and examined the vitamin D levels in the blood of 1739 people with an average age of 59 years and no prior history of cardiovascular disease. Individuals with low vitamin D levels had a 60% greater risk of cardiac events such as heart attacks and stroke. For people with both a vitamin D deficiency and high blood pressure, the risk for a serious cardiovascular event was doubled. These results are of concern because vitamin D is becoming more common, especially in people living at higher latitudes where vitamin D is less available from exposure to sunlight.

15. Zhang SM and others: Effect of combined folic acid, vitamin B-6, and vitamin B-12 on cancer risk in women: A randomized trial. *Journal of the American Medical Association* 300(17):2012, 2008.

    Use of a combined supplement of folic acid, vitamin B-6, and vitamin B-12 had no significant effect on overall risk of total invasive cancer or breast cancer in a 7-year study of 5442 women. This was the longest-running trial of its kind and occurred at the time that background fortification of the food supply with folic acid had begun.

16. Yaegashi Y and others: Association of hip fracture incidence and intake of calcium, magnesium, vitamin D, and vitamin K. *European Journal of Epidemiology* 23(3):219, 2008.

    An association was found between the dietary intakes of magnesium, vitamin D, and vitamin K and the incidence of hip fractures and osteoporosis in Japanese men and women. The strongest inverse correlation was found between hip fracture incidence and vitamin K intake. It was concluded that vitamin K-2 consumption can aid recovery from hip fracture as well as have potenital osteoporosis benefits.

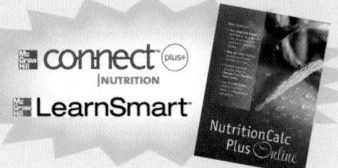

To get the most out of your study of nutrition, go to McGraw-Hill's online resources: Connect www.mcgrawhillconnect.com, where you will find NutritionCalc Plus, LearnSmart, and many other dynamic tools.

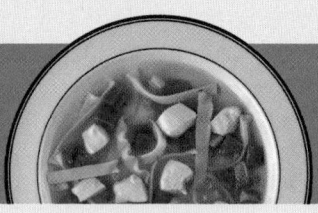
I. Spotting Fraudulent Claims on the Internet

Search for vitamins and vitamin-like substances sold over the Internet. Then write a report concerning any claims made on behalf of these products that you consider fraudulent or misleading. Are the websites selling vitamins, or are they a cover for selling something else? Compare the price of the vitamins from these sites with the price you would pay at the local supermarket or drugstore. Do any of these sites display any disclaimers or warnings about the products?

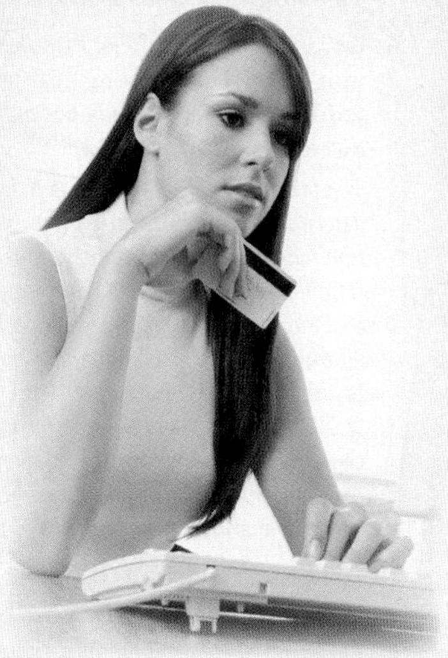

II. A Closer Look at Supplement Use

With the current popularity of vitamin and mineral supplements, it is more important than ever to understand how to evaluate a supplement. Study the label of a supplement you use or one readily available from a friend or the supermarket. Then answer the following questions.

1. What is the recommended dosage of this supplement?

_____

_____

2. Based on the recommended dosage, are there any individual vitamins for which the intake would be greater than 100% of the Daily Value? List these vitamins.

_____

_____

3. Are any suggested intakes above the Upper Level for the nutrient?

_____

_____

4. Are there any superfluous ingredients, such as herbs or flavors, in the supplement? You can often determine these by looking for ingredients that do not have a percent of Daily Value.

_____

_____

5. Does at least 50% of the vitamin A in the product come from beta-carotene or other provitamin A carotenoids (to reduce risk of preformed vitamin A toxicity)?

_____

_____

_____

6. Are there any warnings on the label as to populations who should not consume this product?

_____

_____

7. Are there any other signs that tip you off that this product may not be safe?

_____

_____

Chapter 9 Water and Minerals

Student Learning Outcomes

Chapter 9 is designed to allow you to:

9.1 List and briefly explain the functions of water in the body.

9.2 Discuss healthy water intake and output levels to maintain water balance.

9.3 List safety concerns about our water supply.

9.4 Classify the minerals as major or trace minerals.

9.5 List conditions of the body, dietary factors, and other pertinent relationships that influence the absorption, retention, and availability of specific minerals.

9.6 List key functions and at least two food sources of the major and trace minerals. Identify possible deficiency and toxicity symptoms associated with the major and trace minerals.

9.7 Explain the role of nutrition in maintaining a healthy blood pressure.

9.8 Describe the processes involving minerals that aid in maintaining bone health and preventing osteoporosis.

What Would You Choose?

Water is the best choice for everyday hydration—it quenches thirst without calories. There are currently many "water" choices available. Do you need water that contains vitamins and minerals? What's the difference between spring water and mineral water? Is bottled water safer to drink than tap water? As you peruse the convenience store shelves, which is the healthiest choice to take along to the student recreation center for your workout?

a 20-ounce reusable bottle filled with tap water

b 16.9-ounce bottle of Aquafina® Pure Water

c 16.9-ounce bottle of San Pellegrino Mineral Water

d 20-ounce bottle of vitaminwater®

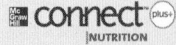 **Think about your choice as you read Chapter 9, then see our recommendations at the end of the chapter. To learn more about water choices, check out the Connect site:** www.mcgrawhillconnect.com

Part Three
Vitamins, Minerals, and Water

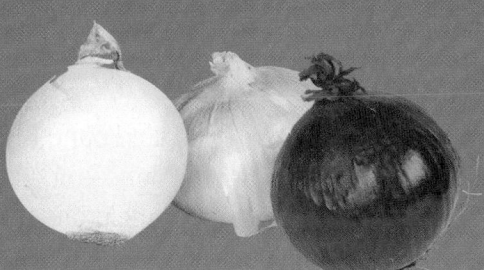

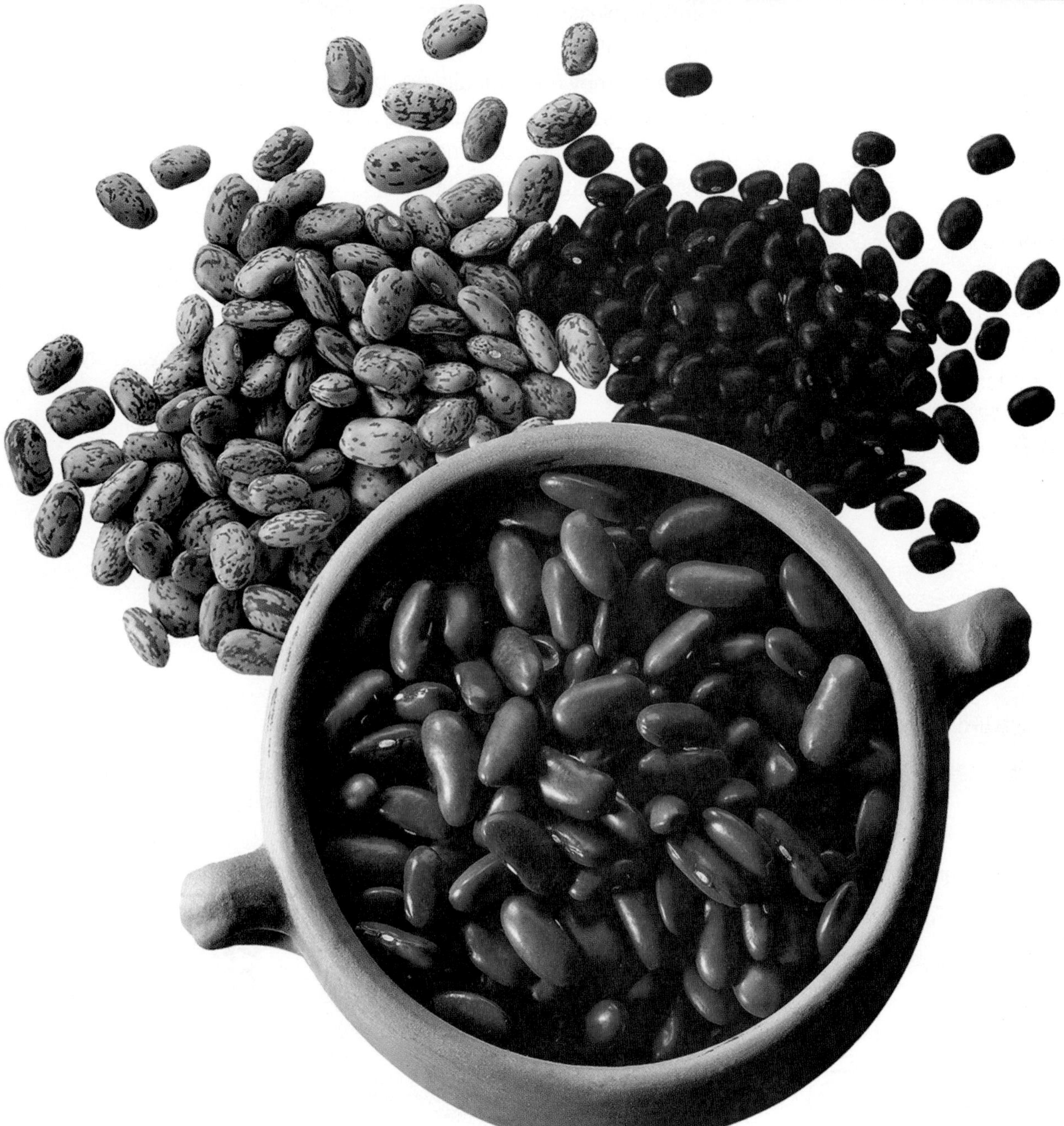

Water—the most versatile medium for a variety of chemical reactions—constitutes the major portion of the human body. Without water, biological processes necessary to life would cease in a matter of days. We must replenish water regularly, as the comic in the chapter suggests, because the body does not store it *per se*. We recognize this constant demand for water as thirst. Recent beverage guidelines recommend a water intake of approximately 50 fluid ounces (1.7 liters) per day, with other beverages total-ing about 48 fluid ounces (1.4 liters).

Many nutrients, including minerals, exist in the body dissolved in water. The functions of several minerals are related to the characteristics of water, so water and its roles in the body are explored first in Chapter 9.

Many minerals, like water, are vital to health. They are considered inor-ganic because they are typically not bonded to carbon atoms. Minerals are key participants in body metabolism, muscle movement, body growth, water balance, and other wide-ranging processes. We also know that some mineral deficiencies can cause severe health problems. For this reason, the study of minerals in Chapter 9 also is critical to understanding human nutrition.

 Refresh Your Memory

As you begin your study of water and minerals in Chapter 9, you may want to review:

- Cell structure and function, digestion and absorption of nutrients, cardiovas-cular function, immunity, and endocrine function in Chapter 3
- The functions of vitamin D and vitamin K related to calcium and bone health in Chapter 8
- The role of vitamin C in collagen synthesis in Chapter 8

9.1 Water

solvent A liquid substance in which other substances dissolve.

Life as we know it could not exist without water. Acting as a **solvent,** it dissolves many body compounds such as sodium chloride (table salt). Water is the perfect medium for body processes because it enables chemical reactions to occur. Water even participates directly in many of these reactions. It forms the greatest component

FRANK & ERNEST by Bob Thaves

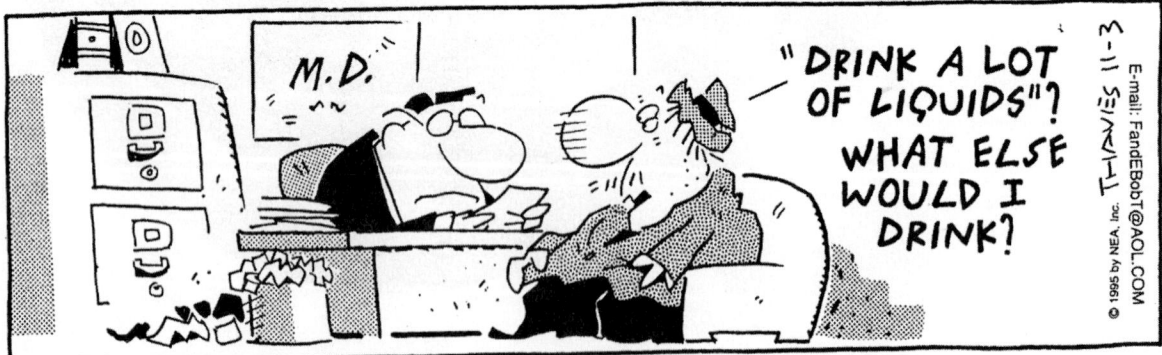

As suggested in the comic, replacing fluids—water as part of foods, beverages, and water itself—is an important daily task. Why is this so critical for maintaining health? And why are infants, athletes, and older adults particularly at risk for dehydration? In addition, how does water interact with some of the minerals used by the body? Chapter 9 provides some answers.

FRANK & ERNEST © Reprinted by permission of Newspaper Enterprise Association, Inc.

of the human body, making up 50% to 70% of the body's weight (about 10 gallons or 40 liters). Lean muscle tissue contains about 73% water. Adipose tissue is about 20% water. Thus, as fat content increases (and the percentage of lean tissue decreases) in the body, total body water content drifts downward toward 50%.

Depending on the amount of fat stores present, an adult can survive for about 8 weeks without eating food but only a few days without drinking water. This occurs not because water is more important than carbohydrate, fat, protein, vitamins, or minerals, but rather because we cannot conserve or store water as well as we can the other components of our diet.

Water in the Body—Intracellular and Extracellular Fluid

Water flows in and out of body cells through cell membranes. Water inside cells forms part of the **intracellular fluid.** When water is outside cells or in the bloodstream, it is part of the **extracellular fluid** (Fig. 9-1). Cell membranes are permeable to water, so water shifts freely in and out of cells. For example, if blood volume decreases, water can move into the bloodstream from the areas inside and around cells to increase blood volume. On the other hand, if blood volume increases, water can shift out of the bloodstream into cells and the surrounding areas, leading to edema (review Fig. 6-8 in Chapter 6).

The body controls the amount of water in the intracellular and extracellular compartments mainly by controlling *ion* movement and concentrations. Ions are minerals that have electrical charges and so are called **electrolytes.** Water is attracted to ions, such as sodium, potassium, chloride, phosphate, magnesium, and calcium. By controlling the movements of ions in and out of the cellular compartments, the body maintains the appropriate amount of water in each compartment using a process called **osmosis.** Overall, where ions go, water follows (Fig. 9-2).

intracellular fluid Fluid contained within a cell; it represents about two-thirds of body fluid.

extracellular fluid Fluid present outside the cells; represents about one-third of body fluid.

electrolytes Substances that separate into ions in water and, in turn, are able to conduct an electrical current. These include sodium, chloride, and potassium.

osmosis The passage of a solvent such as water through a semipermeable membrane from a less concentrated compartment to a more concentrated compartment.

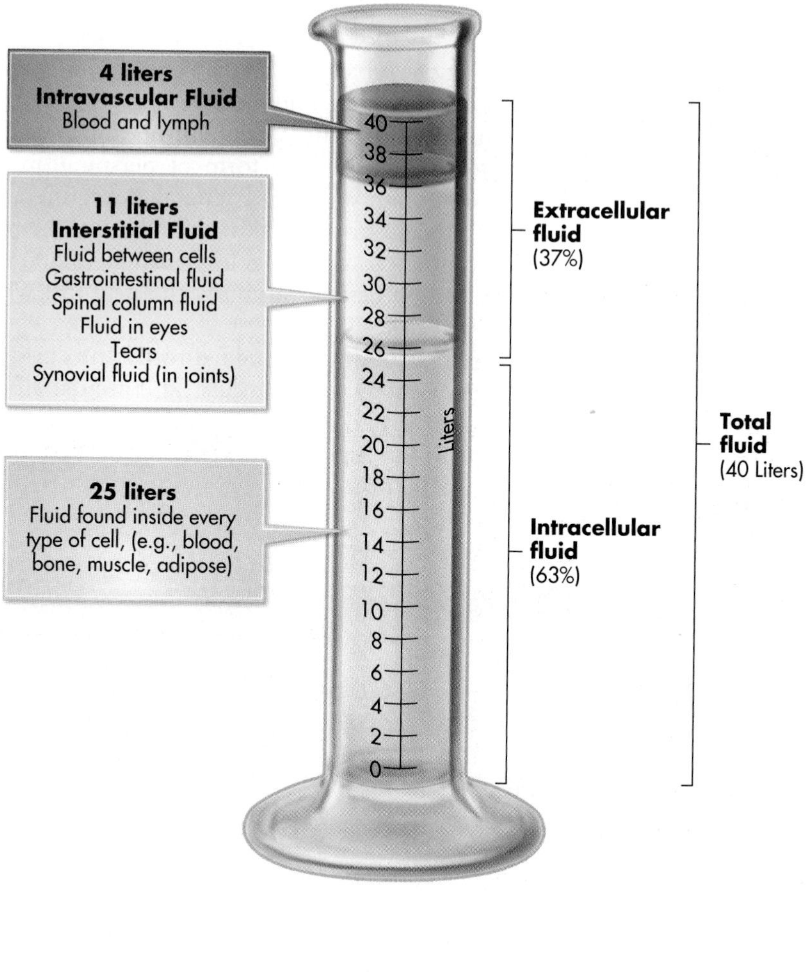

FIGURE 9-1 ▶ Fluid compartments in the body. Total fluid volume is about 10 gallons (40 liters).

FIGURE 9-2 ▶ Effects of various ion concentrations in a fluid on red blood cells. This shows the process of osmosis. Fluid is shifting in and out of the red blood cells in response to changing ion concentrations in the flasks.

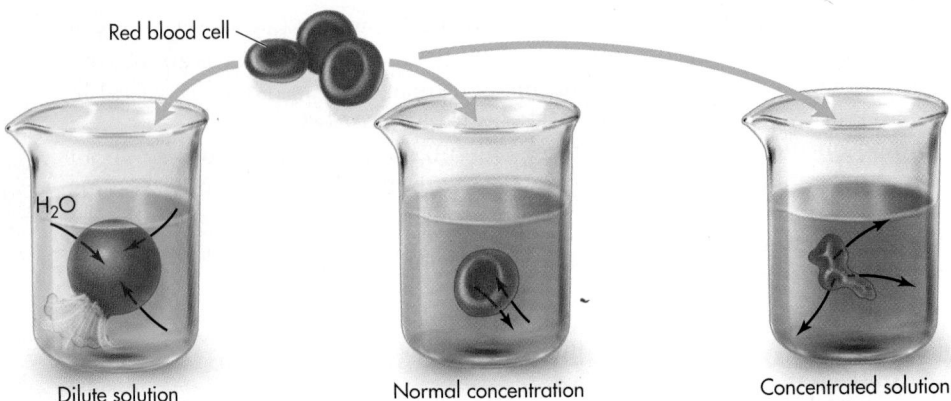

Red blood cell

H₂O

Dilute solution

Normal concentration

Concentrated solution

(a) A dilute solution with a low ion concentration results in swelling (*black arrows*) and subsequent rupture (*puff of red in the lower left part of the cell*) of a red blood cell placed into the solution.

(b) A normal concentration (a concentration of ions outside the cell equal to that inside the cell) results in a typically shaped red blood cell. Water moves into and out of the cell in equilibrium (*black arrows*), but there is no net water movement.

(c) A concentrated solution, with a high ion concentration, causes shrinkage of the red blood cell as water moves out of the cell and into the concentrated solution (*black arrows*).

Positive ions, such as sodium and potassium, end up pairing with negative ions, such as chloride and phosphate. Maintenance of intracellular water volume depends primarily on intracellular potassium and phosphate concentrations. Extracellular water volume depends primarily on the extracellular sodium and chloride concentrations.

Water Contributes to Body Temperature Regulation

Water temperature changes slowly because it has a great ability to hold heat. It takes much more energy to heat water than it does to heat fat. Water molecules are attracted to each other, and it takes much energy to separate them. Because water requires so much energy to change states—for example, from a liquid to a gas in the evaporation of perspiration—it forms an ideal medium for removing heat from the body.

When overheated, the body secretes fluids in the form of perspiration, which evaporates through skin pores. To evaporate water, heat energy is required. So, as perspiration evaporates, heat energy is taken from the skin, cooling it in the process. Each quart (liter) of perspiration evaporated represents approximately 600 kcal of energy lost from the skin and surrounding tissues. Similarly the heat lost when we have a fever increases one's need for calories.

About 60% of the chemical energy in food is turned directly into body heat; the other 40% is converted to forms of energy cells can use, and almost all of that energy eventually leaves the body in the form of heat. If this heat could not be dissipated, the body temperature would rise too high, preventing enzyme systems from functioning efficiently. Perspiration is the primary way to prevent this rise in body temperature.

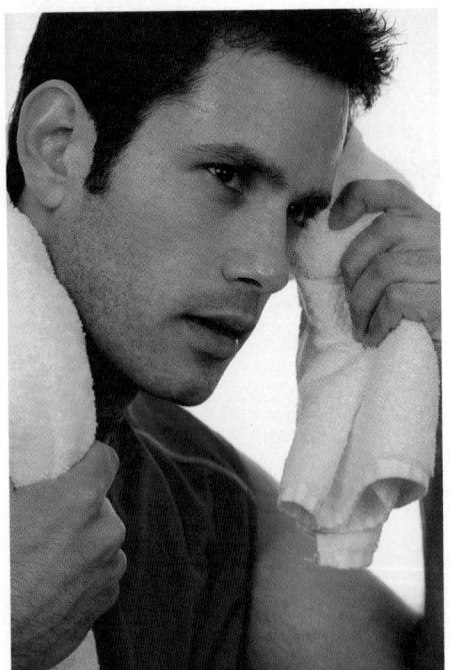

▲ The evaporation of sweat is an important part of temperature regulation.

MAKING DECISIONS

Importance of Perspiration

To cool efficiently, perspiration must be allowed to evaporate. If it simply rolls off the skin or soaks into clothing, perspiration doesn't cool the body as much. Evaporation of perspiration occurs quickly when humidity is low. This is why humans can cool off and therefore tolerate hot, dry climates far better than they do hot, humid climates. This is also why increasing air circulation with a fan cools the body during an exercise workout.

Water Helps Remove Waste Products

Water is an important vehicle for transporting substances throughout the body and for removing waste products from the body. Most unusable substances in the body can dissolve in water and exit the body through the urine.

Urea is a major body waste product. This by-product of protein metabolism contains nitrogen. The more protein we eat in excess of needs, the more nitrogen we remove from amino acids and excrete—in the form of urea—in the urine. Likewise, the more sodium we consume, the more sodium we excrete in the urine. Overall, the amount of urine a person needs to produce is determined primarily by excess protein and salt intake. By limiting excess protein and salt intakes, it is possible to limit urine output—a useful practice, for example, in space flights and in the treatment of some kidney diseases wherein the ability to produce urine is hampered.

A typical volume of urine produced per day is about 1 liter (1 quart) or more, depending mostly on the intake of fluid, protein, and sodium. A somewhat greater urine output than that is fine, but less—especially less than 500 milliliters (2 cups)—forces the kidneys to form concentrated urine. The simplest way to determine if water intake is adequate is to observe the color of one's urine. Whereas urine should be clear or pale yellow, concentrated urine is very dark yellow. The heavy ion content of concentrated urine in turn increases the risk of kidney stone formation in susceptible people (generally men). Kidney stones are formed from minerals and other substances that have precipitated out of the urine and accumulate in kidney tissues.

Other Functions of Water

Water helps form the lubricants found in knees and other joints of the body. It is the basis for saliva, bile, and **amniotic fluid.** Amniotic fluid acts as a shock absorber surrounding the growing fetus in the mother's womb. Ion concentrations vary in each fluid compartment to accommodate Specific needs, such as the ability to transfer nerve impulses.

How Much Water Do We Need per Day?

The Adequate Intake for total water intake per day is 2.7 liters (11 cups) for adult women and 3.7 liters (15 cups) for adult men. This is based primarily on our typical total water intakes from a combination of fluids and foods. For fluid alone this corresponds to about 2.2 liters (9 cups) for women and about 3 liters (13 cups) for men. (Keep in mind also that it does not indicate that water *per se* must be used to meet fluid needs.) At minimum, adults need 1 to 3 liters of fluid to replace daily water losses.

We consume water in various liquids, such as fruit juice, coffee, tea, soft drinks, and water itself. Note that coffee, tea, and soft drinks often contain caffeine, which increases urine output. However, the fluid consumed from these beverages is not completely lost in urine, so these fluids still help to meet water needs. Foods also supply water; many fruits and vegetables are more than 80% water (Fig. 9.3). Water as a by-product of metabolism provides approximately 250 to 350 milliliters (1 to 1½ cups) of additional water.

Much of the water needed is used to produce urine (500 to 1000 milliliters or more). The rest compensates for typical water losses through the lungs (250 to 350 milliliters), feces (100 to 200 milliliters), and skin (450 to 1900 milliliters) (Fig. 9.4). These are just estimates: altitude, caffeine intake, alcohol intake, and humidity can affect these individual losses.

When we consider the large amount of water used to lubricate the gastrointestinal (GI) tract, the loss of only 100 to 200 milliliters of water each day through the feces is remarkable. About 8000 milliliters of water enter the GI tract daily through secretions from the mouth, stomach, intestine, pancreas, and other organs, while the diet

urea Nitrogen-containing waste product of protein metabolism; major source of nitrogen in the urine.

Functions of water:
- Chemical processes
- Temperature regulation
- Removal of waste products
- Primary component of body fluids, such as in joints

amniotic fluid Fluid contained in a sac within the uterus. This fluid surrounds and protects the fetus during development.

FIGURE 9-3 ▶ Water content of foods by weight. In addition to the MyPlate food groups, pink is used for substances that do not fit easily into food groups (e.g., honey, candy, coffee, alcohol, and table salt).

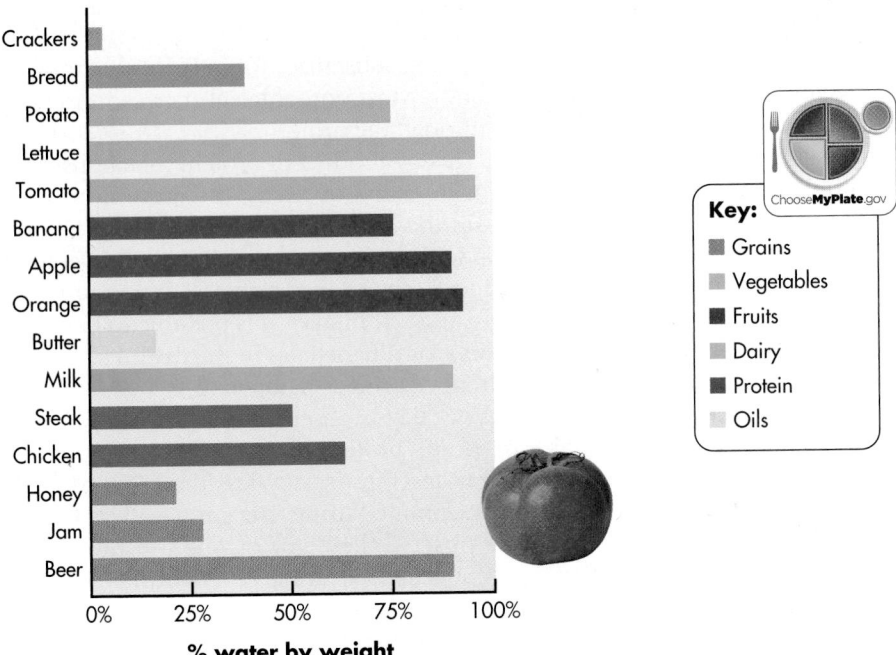

Key:
- Grains
- Vegetables
- Fruits
- Dairy
- Protein
- Oils

% water by weight

supplies an additional 30% to 50% or more. The small intestine reabsorbs most of this water, while the large intestine takes up a lesser—but still important—amount. The kidneys also greatly conserve water. They reabsorb about 97% of the water filtered from waste products.

MAKING DECISIONS

Hard Water or Soft Water?

Water can be classified by whether it is hard or soft. Hard water generally comes from underground wells and usually contains calcium, magnesium, and iron. The more minerals the water contains, the harder it is. Soft water has a low content of these minerals and is often produced by replacing other minerals with sodium.

▶ Regular intake of water and water-rich fluids are essential to replace daily fluid losses. One trend in North America is to carry bottles of water with us.

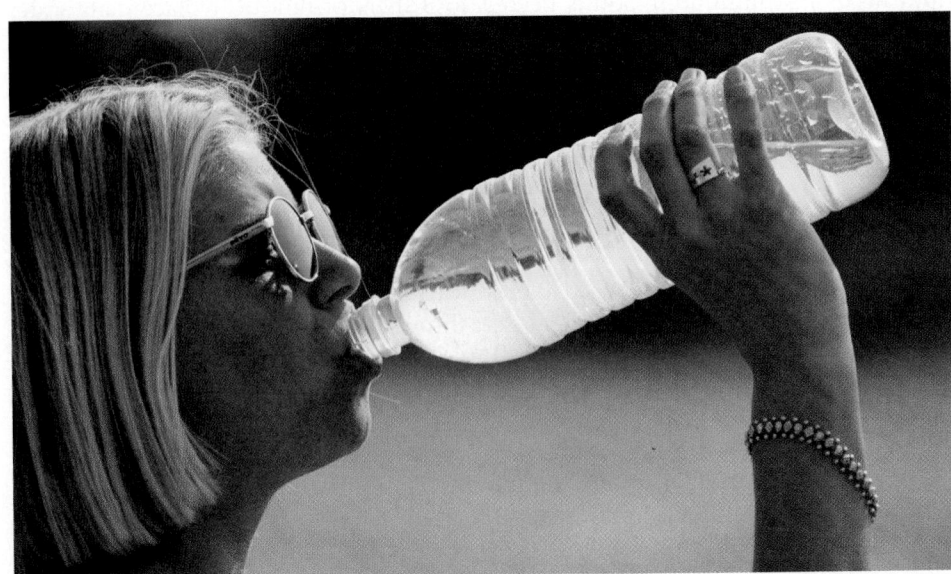

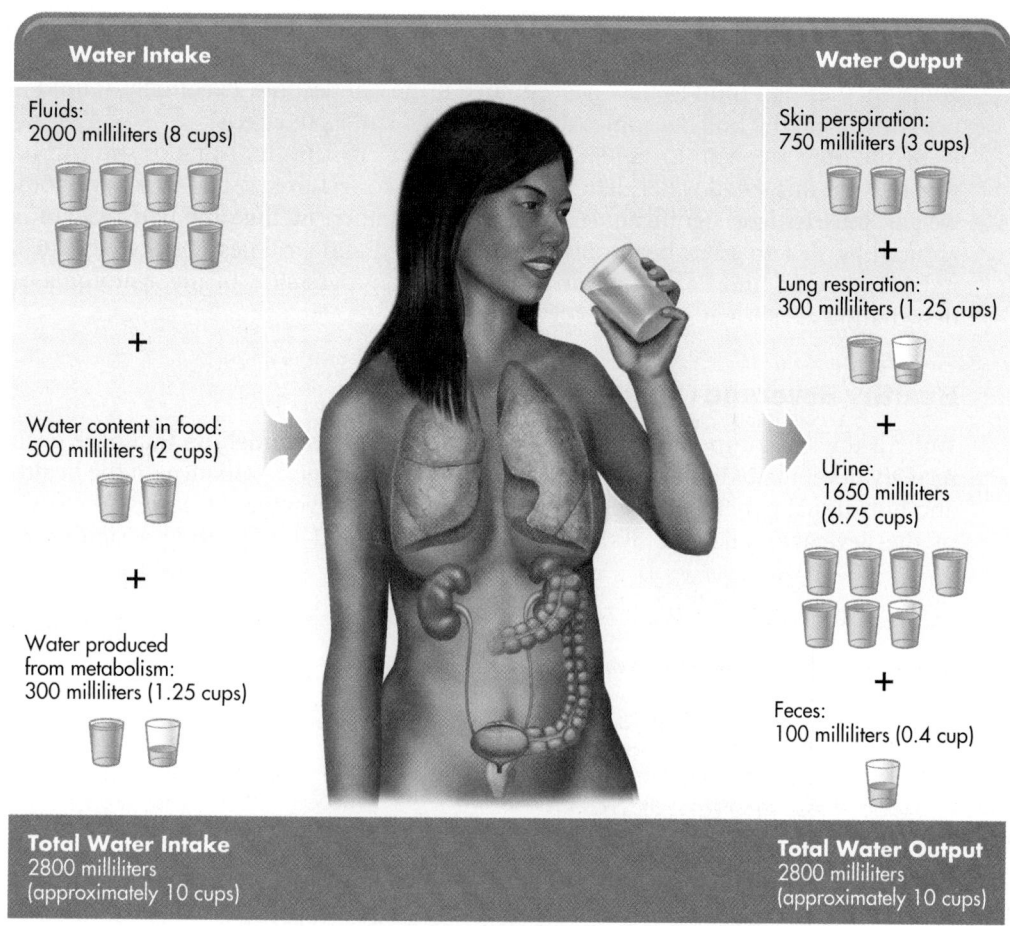

Water Intake

Fluids:
2000 milliliters (8 cups)

+

Water content in food:
500 milliliters (2 cups)

+

Water produced
from metabolism:
300 milliliters (1.25 cups)

Water Output

Skin perspiration:
750 milliliters (3 cups)

+

Lung respiration:
300 milliliters (1.25 cups)

+

Urine:
1650 milliliters
(6.75 cups)

+

Feces:
100 milliliters (0.4 cup)

Total Water Intake
2800 milliliters
(approximately 10 cups)

Total Water Output
2800 milliliters
(approximately 10 cups)

FIGURE 9-4 ▶ Estimate of water balance—intake versus output—in a woman. We primarily maintain body fluids at an optimum amount by adjusting water output to intake. As you can see for this woman, most water comes from the liquids we consume. Some comes from the moisture in more solid foods, and the remainder is manufactured during metabolism. Water output includes that lost via lungs, urine, skin, and feces.

Thirst

If you don't drink enough water, your body eventually lets you know by signaling thirst. Your brain is communicating the need to drink. This thirst mechanism can lag behind actual water loss, however, during prolonged exercise and illness, as well as in one's older years. For this reason, athletes should carefully monitor fluid status—they should weigh themselves before and after training sessions to determine their rate of water loss and, thus, their water needs. The current goal for athletes is to consume 2 to 3 cups of fluid for every pound lost (see Chapter 10 for details). Sick children—especially those with fever, vomiting, diarrhea, and increased perspiration—and older persons often need to be reminded to drink plenty of fluids (see Chapters 15 and 16 for details). As Chapter 15 discusses in further detail, infants can easily become dehydrated.

What If the Thirst Message Is Ignored?

Once the body registers a shortage of available water, it increases fluid conservation. Two hormones that participate in this process are **antidiuretic hormone** and **aldosterone.** The pituitary gland releases antidiuretic hormone to force the kidneys to conserve water. The kidneys respond by reducing urine flow. At the same time, as fluid volume decreases in the bloodstream, blood pressure falls. This eventually triggers the release of the hormone aldosterone, which signals the kidneys to retain more sodium and, in turn, more water.

Alcohol inhibits the action of antidiuretic hormone. One reason people feel so weak the day after heavy drinking is that they are dehydrated. Even though they may have consumed a lot of liquid in their drinks, they have lost even more liquid because alcohol has inhibited antidiuretic hormone.

antidiuretic hormone A hormone that is secreted by the pituitary gland and that acts on the kidneys to decrease water excretion.

aldosterone A hormone produced by the adrenal glands that acts on the kidneys to conserve sodium (and therefore water).

However, despite mechanisms that work to reduce water loss via the kidneys, fluid continues to be lost via the feces, skin, and lungs. Those losses must be replaced. In addition, there is a limit to how concentrated urine can become. Eventually, if fluid is not consumed, the body becomes dehydrated and suffers ill effects.

By the time a person loses 1% to 2% of body weight in fluids, he or she will be thirsty. Even this small water deficit can cause one to feel tired. At a 4% loss of body weight, muscles lose significant strength and endurance. By the time body weight is reduced by 10% to 12%, heat tolerance is decreased and weakness results. At a 20% reduction, coma and death may soon follow. The progression of the symptoms of dehydration are shown in Figure 9-5.

Healthy Beverage Consumption Guidelines

Water is the key component in the beverage consumption guidelines that have been recently developed (Table 9-1). These recommendations give guidance on the health and nutritional benefits as well as the risks of various beverage categories. The basis of the Beverage Guidance System is that fluids should not provide a significant

FIGURE 9-5 ▶ The effects of dehydration can range from thirst to death, depending on the extent of water weight lost.

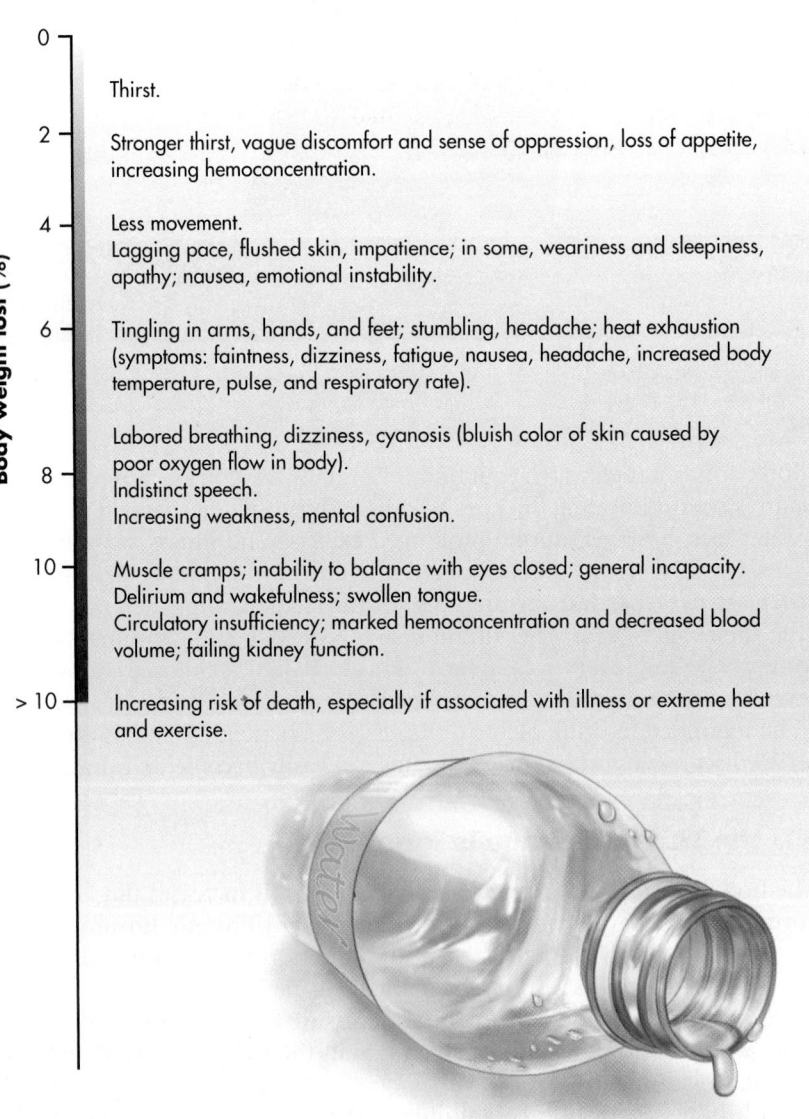

Body weight lost (%)

0 — Thirst.

2 — Stronger thirst, vague discomfort and sense of oppression, loss of appetite, increasing hemoconcentration.

4 — Less movement.
Lagging pace, flushed skin, impatience; in some, weariness and sleepiness, apathy; nausea, emotional instability.

6 — Tingling in arms, hands, and feet; stumbling, headache; heat exhaustion (symptoms: faintness, dizziness, fatigue, nausea, headache, increased body temperature, pulse, and respiratory rate).

Labored breathing, dizziness, cyanosis (bluish color of skin caused by poor oxygen flow in body).
Indistinct speech.
8 — Increasing weakness, mental confusion.

10 — Muscle cramps; inability to balance with eyes closed; general incapacity.
Delirium and wakefulness; swollen tongue.
Circulatory insufficiency; marked hemoconcentration and decreased blood volume; failing kidney function.

> 10 — Increasing risk of death, especially if associated with illness or extreme heat and exercise.

TABLE 9-1 The Beverage Guidance System

Level	Category*	Recommended Servings per day
1	Water	50 fluid ounces (1.7 liters)
2	Tea or coffee, unsweetened	0 to 40 fluid ounces (0 to 1.4 liters)
3	Low-fat and skim milk and soy beverages	0 to 16 fluid ounces (0 to 0.5 liter)
4	Non-calorically sweetened beverages (diet drinks)	0 to 32 fluid ounces (0 to 1 liter)
5	Calorie beverages with some nutrients (100% fruit juices, alcoholic beverages, whole milk, sports drinks)	0 to 8 fluid ounces (0 to 0.25 liter) 0 to 2 alcoholic drinks for men 0 to 8 fluid ounces (0 to 0.25 liter)
6	Calorically sweetened beverages (regular soft drinks)	0 to 1 alcoholic drinks for women,

*Categories established based on their possible health benefits or risks.

Adapted from Popkin and others: *Am J Clin Nutr* 83:529, 2006.

amount of the energy or nutrients in a healthy diet. More specifically, the system recommends that beverages provide less than 10% of total calories consumed for a 2200 kcal diet (see Further Reading 14).

Is There Such a Thing as Too Much Water?

Consuming too much water—whatever amount the kidneys are unable to excrete—can also lead to ill health, especially if concentrations of blood electrolytes, notably sodium, become too low. However, an excessive amount would have to approach many quarts (liters) each day. When excessive water intake overwhelms the kidneys' capacity to excrete fluid, blurred vision is one resulting symptom. Such water toxicity risks during athletic events are covered in Chapter 10.

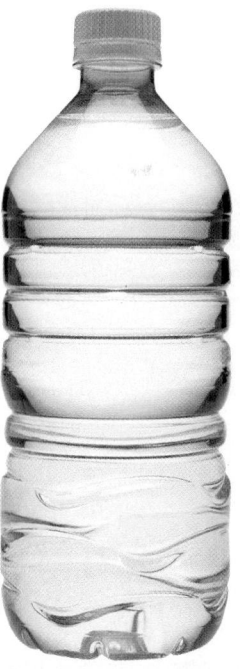

▲ Bottled water is a convenient but relatively expensive source of water. In most cases, tap water is just as healthy a choice to meet our water needs.

CONCEPT CHECK

The body can neither readily store nor conserve water, so we can survive only a few days without it. Water transports nutrients and waste products, serves as a medium for chemical reactions and as a lubricant, and aids in temperature regulation. Water accounts for 50% to 70% of body weight and distributes itself all over the body—among lean and other tissues (in both intracellular and extracellular fluids) and in urine and other body fluids. The Adequate Intake for total water intake is 2.7 liters (11 cups) for women and 3.7 liters (15 cups) for men per day. Thirst is the body's first sign of dehydration. If this thirst mechanism is faulty, as it may be during illness or vigorous exercise, hormonal mechanisms also help conserve water by reducing urine output. Excess fluid intake can be hazardous to a person's health. Overall, the United States enjoys a safe water supply. However, people with poor immune status should boil water used for drinking and cooking to avoid waterborne illness. Bottled water can also be used if desired.

Our Water Supply: Safety Issues

Many people choose bottled water over tap water because they doubt the safety of their public drinking water. Some concern over municipal water supplies is warranted. For example, contamination of the public water supply by the parasite *Cryptosporidium* is possible. This parasite is usually found in lakes and rivers; the typical chlorination procedures used to treat public water supplies do not kill *Cryptosporidium*.

This parasite poses little risk to healthy people—other than a case of diarrhea—but it can harm people who have AIDS or other diseases that compromise function of the immune system (such as some forms of cancer therapy or organ transplant therapy). High-risk people have been advised to boil for at least 1 minute any tap water they use for cooking or drinking to ensure that the parasite is destroyed. Alternatively, individuals can purchase a water filter that screens out *Cryptosporidium* (the National Sanitation Foundation at (800) 673-8010 can provide a list of manufacturers) or use bottled water certified to be free of the parasite (contact the supplier if in doubt). Generally, distilled water or that which has undergone reverse osmosis is parasite free.

Monitoring the Safety of Your Water

Under the Safe Water Drinking Act, all public drinking water supplies are monitored for contaminants such as bacteria, various chemicals, and toxic metals (such as lead and mercury). The local municipal water department must mail the results of these tests each year to its consumers. According to the Environmental Protection Agency (EPA), the U.S. water supply ranks among the safest in the world. However, this water does sometimes fail to meet the agency's standards for contaminants such as lead and nitrates. Generally, the public will be warned about the latter, because it is dangerous to use nitrate-rich water for mixing infant formulas (Chapter 15). Some studies indicate that in 1 year, about one in five Americans consumes water not up to standards, especially in rural areas. These people could consider using a home water filter or bottled water. The local water department can help a person evaluate whether health risks are worth the cost of home water filters or bottled water.

As a safeguard against contamination, chlorine and ammonia are added to kill bacteria. The addition of such chemicals has raised concern that drinking water may increase rectal and bladder cancer risk, though there is no conclusive proof of such risk. If chlorine in tap water does increase cancer risk, the risk is likely extremely small (perhaps two cases of cancer in 1 million people).

If you find the taste of chlorinated tap water unpleasant or are concerned about the possible cancer risk, you can remove the chlorine from tap water by boiling it or by letting a large container filled with water stand uncovered overnight. In both cases, the chlorine will evaporate, taking its characteristic flavor with it. Alternatively, you can install a filter on the household spigot from which you obtain your water. It should be designed to remove trihalomethanes, common chlorine by-products.

Options Regarding Your Water Source

Keep in mind that by most standards, bottled water ranges from moderately expensive to expensive. In many cases, you are paying for water not much different from the water you get from your tap. If you are concerned about the safety of your tap water, you can ask the municipal water department for its most recent test results, or you can have the water tested. A local testing laboratory or state health department can be of service, as can the EPA at (800) 426-4791, if local information is not available (for example, if you have a well). This testing can point out whether there are health risks associated with your water supply. Compared with the cost of bottled water, the testing fee will be insignificant. Letting cold water run for a minute or so before taking a drink or before using it in meal preparation is a good way to limit possible lead exposure, especially if the water has been off for more than two hours. In addition, do not use hot tap water for food preparation. For more information, see the website www.epa.gov/safewater.

9.2 Minerals—An Overview

cofactor A mineral or other substance that binds to a specific region on a protein, such as an enzyme, and is necessary for the protein's function.

The metabolic roles of minerals and the amounts of them in the body vary considerably (Fig. 9-6). Some minerals, such as copper and selenium, work as **cofactors,** enabling various proteins, such as enzymes, to function. Minerals also contribute

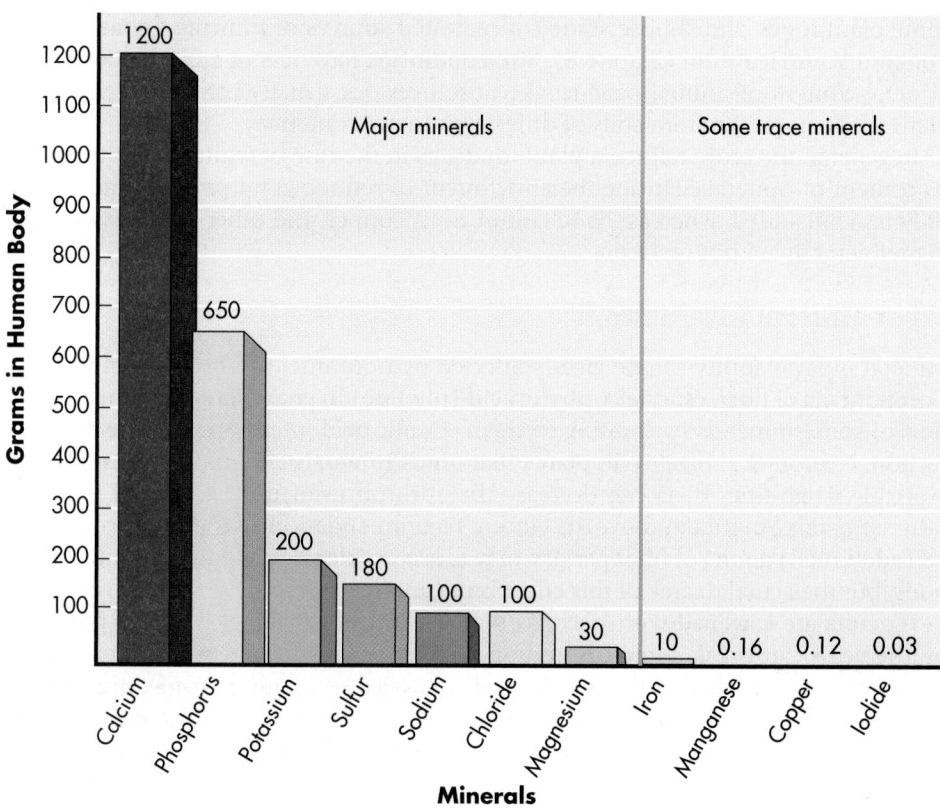

FIGURE 9-6 ▶ Approximate amounts of various minerals present in the average human body. Other trace minerals of nutritional importance not listed include chromium, fluoride, molybdenum, selenium, and zinc.

to many body compounds. For example, iron is a component of red blood cells. Sodium, potassium, and calcium aid in the transfer of nerve impulses throughout the body. Body growth and development also depend on certain minerals, such as calcium and phosphorus. Water balance requires sodium, potassium, calcium, and phosphorus. At all levels—cellular, tissue, organ, and whole body—minerals clearly play important roles in maintaining body functions.

Minerals are categorized based on the amount we need per day. Recall from Chapter 1 that if we require greater than 100 milligrams (1/50 of a teaspoon) of a mineral per day, it is considered a **major mineral;** otherwise, it is considered a **trace mineral.** For example, calcium and phosphorus are major minerals and iron and zinc are trace minerals.

The roles and nutritional significance of both the major and the trace minerals are discussed in this chapter. But before examining the properties of the individual minerals, let's consider some topics that apply to all these nutrients.

Mineral Bioavailability

Foods offer us a plentiful supply of many minerals, but the ability of our bodies to absorb and use them varies. The degree to which an ingested nutrient is absorbed from food sources and is available to the body is called **bioavailability.** The bioavailability of minerals depends on many factors. The mineral content listed in a food composition table for the amount of a mineral in a food is just a starting point for estimating the actual contribution the food will make to our mineral needs. Spinach, for example, contains plenty of calcium, but only about 5% of it can be absorbed because of the vegetable's high concentration of **oxalic acid (oxalate),** a calcium-binder. Usually, about 25% of dietary calcium is absorbed by adults.

The average North American diet derives minerals from both plant and animal sources. Overall, minerals from animal products are better absorbed than those from plants because binders such as fiber are not present to hinder absorption. The mineral content of plants greatly depends on mineral concentrations of the soil in which they are grown. Vegans must be aware of the potentially poor mineral content of

major mineral A mineral vital to health that is required in the diet in amounts greater than 100 milligrams per day.

trace mineral A mineral vital to health that is required in the diet in amounts less than 100 milligrams per day.

bioavailability The degree to which an ingested nutrient is absorbed and available to the body.

oxalic acid (oxalate) An organic acid found in spinach, rhubarb, and other leafy green vegetables that can depress the absorption of certain minerals present in the food, such as calcium.

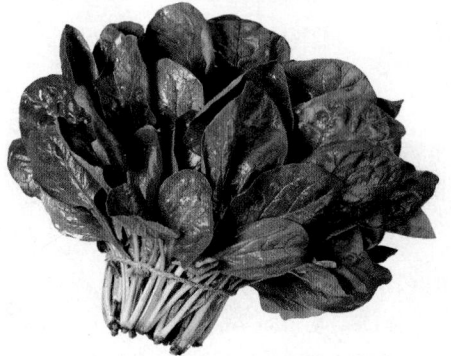

▲ Spinach is often touted as a rich source of calcium, but little of the calcium present is available to the body.

some plant foods and choose some concentrated sources of minerals (review Nutrition and Your Health in Chapter 6). Soil conditions have less of an influence on the mineral content of animal products because livestock usually consume a variety of plant products grown from soils of differing mineral contents.

In general, the more refined a plant food—as in the case of white flour—the lower its content of minerals. During the enrichment of refined grain products, iron is the only mineral added, whereas the selenium, zinc, copper, and other minerals lost during refinement are not replaced.

Fiber-Mineral Interactions

phytic acid (phytate) A constituent of plant fibers that binds positive ions to its multiple phosphate groups.

Mineral bioavailability can be greatly affected by nonmineral substances in the diet. Components of fiber, especially **phytic acid (phytate)** in grain fiber, can limit absorption of some minerals by binding to them. Oxalic acid, mentioned in the previous section, is another substance in plants that binds minerals and makes them less bioavailable. High-fiber diets can decrease the absorption of iron, zinc, and probably other minerals. An intake above the current recommendation of 25 (adult women) to 38 (adult men) grams of fiber per day may cause problems with mineral status of the body, but the actual degree of this effect is uncertain.

If grains are leavened with yeast, as they are in breadmaking, enzymes produced by the yeast can break some of the bonds between phytic acid and minerals. This increases mineral absorption. The zinc deficiencies found among some Middle Eastern populations are attributed partly to their consumption of unleavened breads, resulting in low bioavailability of dietary zinc. Zinc bioavailability is discussed in greater detail in a later section.

Mineral-Mineral Interactions

Many minerals, such as magnesium, calcium, iron, and copper, are of similar sizes and electrical charges. Having similar sizes and the same electrical charge causes these minerals to compete with each other for absorption, and therefore they affect each other's bioavailability. Simply stated, an excess of one mineral decreases the absorption and metabolism of other minerals. For example, a large intake of zinc decreases copper absorption. Because of this, people should avoid taking individual mineral supplements unless a dietary deficiency or medical condition specifically warrants it. Food sources, however, pose little risk for these mineral interactions, giving us another reason to emphasize foods in meeting nutrient needs.

Vitamin-Mineral Interactions

Several beneficial vitamin-mineral interactions occur during nutrient absorption and metabolism. When consumed in conjunction with vitamin C, absorption of certain forms of iron—such as that in plant products—improves. The active vitamin D hormone improves calcium absorption. Many vitamins require specific minerals to act as components in their structure and function. For example, the thiamin coenzyme requires magnesium or manganese to function efficiently.

Mineral Toxicities

An excessive mineral intake, especially of trace minerals, such as iron and copper, can have toxic results. For many trace minerals, the gap between just enough and too much is small. Taking minerals as supplements poses the biggest threat for mineral toxicity, whereas food sources are unlikely culprits. Mineral supplements exceeding current standards for mineral needs—especially those that supply more than 100% of the Daily Values on supplement labels—should be taken only under a physician's supervision. The Daily Values are for the most part higher than our current standards (e.g., RDA) for mineral needs. Without close monitoring, doses of minerals should not exceed any Upper Level set on a long-term basis.

▲ Mineral supplements pose a high risk for toxicity. Generally, mineral intake from a supplement should not exceed 100% of the Daily Value, unless otherwise specified by a physician.

The potential for toxicity is not the only reason to carefully consider the use of mineral supplements. Harmful interactions with other nutrients are possible. Also, contamination of mineral supplements—with lead, for example—is a possibility. Use of brands approved by the United States Pharmacopeia (USP) lessens this risk (review Nutrition and Your Health in Chapter 8). In summary, even with the best intentions, people may harm themselves using mineral supplements.

CONCEPT CHECK

Minerals are vital to the functioning of many body processes. Their bioavailability depends on many factors, including a mineral's interaction with fiber, vitamins, and other minerals. Animal products often yield better mineral absorption than do plants. Still, both animal and plant sources help us meet our mineral needs. Taking megadoses of an individual mineral supplement can greatly diminish the absorption and metabolism of other minerals. In addition, some minerals are potentially toxic in amounts not much in excess of body needs. These are two good reasons to carefully consider any use of mineral supplements exceeding the Daily Value on the label, particularly long-term use of supplements that lead to intakes in excess of the Upper Level set for any mineral.

9.3 Major Minerals

Up to now, some general characteristics of minerals and how some of them interact with water in the body have been covered. Now let us review the individual properties of the major minerals (also called macrominerals) in the context of the North American diet.

9.4 Sodium (Na)

Our primary dietary source of sodium is table salt, chemically known as sodium chloride, added during food processing. This mineral is an essential part of our diets and adds flavor to our foods, but there is concern that an overabundance of sodium in the diet may cause harm. Table salt is 40% sodium and 60% chloride. For example, dietary intake of 10 grams of salt translates into about 4 grams of sodium. A teaspoon of salt contains about 2 grams of sodium (2000 milligrams).

The human body absorbs almost all sodium that gets eaten. Once absorbed, sodium becomes the major positive ion outside of cells in extracellular fluid and a key factor for retaining body water. Fluid balance throughout the body depends partly on the variation in the sodium and other ion concentrations among the water-containing compartments in the body. Sodium ions also function in nerve impulse conduction and absorption of some nutrients (e.g., glucose).

A dietary deficiency of sodium is rare. However, a diet low in sodium—coupled with excessive perspiration, persistent vomiting, or diarrhea—has the ability to deplete the body of sodium. This state can lead to muscle cramps, nausea, vomiting, dizziness, and later, shock and coma. The likelihood of this happening, however, is low because the kidney responds early to low sodium status, eventually triggering the body to conserve sodium. This conservation of sodium by the body demonstrates how important small amounts of sodium are to body functions.

Only when perspiration leads to weight loss exceeding 2% to 3% of total body weight (or about 5 to 6 pounds) should sodium losses raise concern. Even then, merely salting foods is sufficient to restore body sodium for most people. Certain endurance athletes, however, may need to consume sports drinks during competition to replace sodium losses from perspiration in order to avoid depletion of sodium (see Chapter 10). Although perspiration tastes salty on the skin, sodium is not highly concentrated in perspiration. Rather, water evaporating from the skin leaves concentrated

For your information, the chemical symbols for the minerals discussed are given next to each mineral heading.

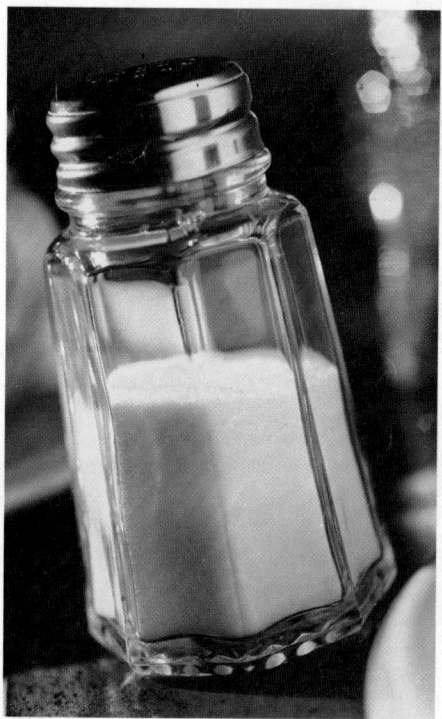

▲ Table salt is our primary source of the minerals sodium and chloride.

sodium behind. Perspiration contains about two-thirds the sodium concentration found in blood.

Sodium Sources and Needs

About 80% of the sodium we consume is added to foods during manufacturing and preparation at restaurants (Fig. 9-7). Sodium added in cooking provides about 10% of our intakes, and sodium naturally present in foods provides the rest, about another 10%. Almost all foods naturally contain a little sodium; the higher amount found in milk (about 120 milligrams per cup) is one exception.

The more processed and restaurant food one consumes, generally the higher one's sodium intake. Conversely, the more home cooking one does, the more sodium control that person has. The foods that contribute most of the sodium in the adult diet (white bread and rolls, hot dogs and lunch meats, cheese, soups, and foods with tomato sauce) do so partly because they are eaten so often. Other foods that generally are especially high in sodium include salted snack foods, French fries and potato chips, and sauces and gravies (Fig. 9-8).

If we ate only unprocessed foods and added no salt, we would consume about 500 milligrams of sodium per day. In comparison, the Adequate Intake for sodium for adults under age 51 is 1500 milligrams, a generous amount; this is reduced by 100 to 200 milligrams for older adults. (See the inside back cover for references to mineral needs for various age groups.) The 2010 Dietary Guidelines for Americans recommends that the general population consume less than 2300 milligrams (approximately 1 teaspoon of salt) of sodium per day. The Dietary Guidelines for individuals with hypertension, diabetes, or chronic kidney disease; blacks; and middle-aged and older adults are to aim to consume no more than 1500 milligrams of sodium per day. We really need only about 200 milligrams per day to maintain physiological functions. (Additional sodium above needs was added to establish the Adequate Intake to allow for a more varied diet where not all foods are low in sodium.)

If we compare 500 milligrams of sodium from unprocessed food with the amount typically eaten by adults (2300 to 4700 milligrams or more), it is clear that food processing and cooking contribute most of our dietary sodium. As discussed in Chapter 2, nutrition labels list a food's sodium content. When dietary sodium must be severely restricted, attention to food labels is of utmost importance. Under FDA food and supplement labeling rules, the Daily Value for sodium is 2400 milligrams (2.4 grams).

Most humans can adapt somewhat to various dietary salt intakes, though very high intakes can be toxic. For most people, today's sodium intake simply will be in tomorrow's urine output. However, approximately 10% to 15% of adults, such as African-Americans and people who have diabetes and/or are overweight, are especially *sodium sensitive*. For these people, high sodium intakes can increase blood pressure, whereas lower-sodium diets (about 2000 milligrams daily) often help correct the problem (see the Nutrition and Your Health section on minerals and hypertension at the end

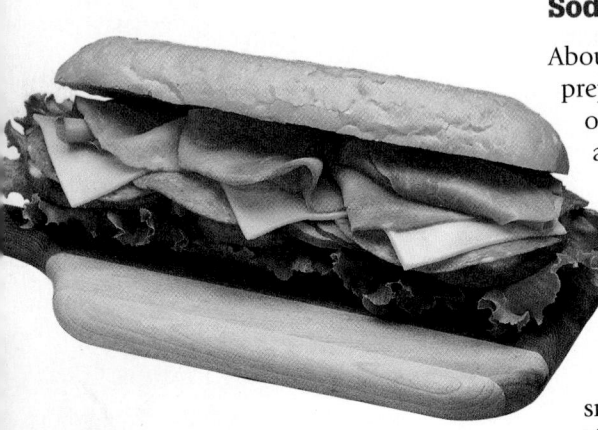

▲ Deli meats, such as ham, are high in sodium (salt).

FIGURE 9-7 ▶ Salt arrives in the American diet largely as a result of food processing.

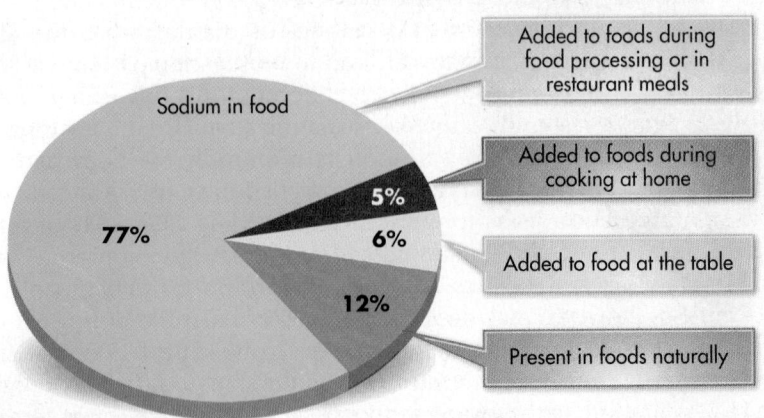

Sodium in food

- 77%
- 5% — Added to foods during food processing or in restaurant meals
- 6% — Added to foods during cooking at home
- 12% — Added to food at the table
- Present in foods naturally

Food Sources of Sodium

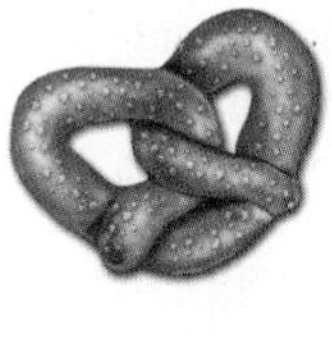

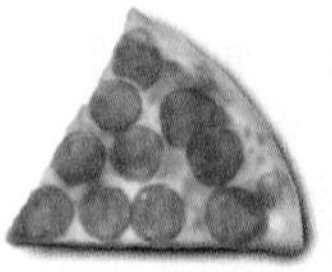

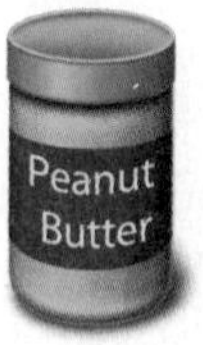

Food Item and Amount	Sodium Content (milligrams)	Adult Male and Female AI = 1500 milligrams Daily Value = 2400 milligrams %AI
AI*	1500	100%
Pepperoni pizza, 2 slices	2045	136%
Ham, sliced, 1 ounce	1215	81%
Chicken noodle soup, canned, 1 cup	1106	74%
V8 vegetable juice, 8 ounces	620	41%
Macaroni salad, ½ cup	561	37%
Hard pretzels, 1 ounce	486	32%
Hamburger with bun, 1 each	474	32%
Green beans, canned, ½ cup	390	26%
Saltine crackers, 6 each	234	16%
Cheddar cheese, 1 ounce	176	12%
Peanut butter, 2 tablespoons	156	10%
Nonfat milk, 1 cup	127	8%
Seven grain bread, 1 slice	126	8%
Animal crackers, 1 ounce	112	7%
Grape juice, 1 cup	10	1%

Key:
- Grains
- Vegetables
- Fruits
- Dairy
- Protein

ChooseMyPlate.gov

* For adults; see the DRI table in the back of this book for age-specific recommendations.

FIGURE 9-8 ▶ Food sources of sodium compared to the Adequate Intake.

of the chapter and the Newsworthy Nutrition in the margin). Still, keep in mind that other lifestyle factors, such as being overweight and inactive, are more likely to contribute to hypertension.

Scientific groups typically suggest that adults in general reduce sodium intake, mostly to limit the risk of developing hypertension later. It is also a good idea to have your blood pressure checked regularly. If you have hypertension, you should try to reduce your sodium intake as you follow a comprehensive plan to treat this disease. Reducing sodium intake also helps to maintain healthy calcium status, because urinary calcium loss is increased along with sodium when sodium intake is greater than about 2000 milligrams per day (see Further Reading 5).

It is not that hard to follow a low-sodium diet, but many typical food choices such as processed meats and salty snacks will have to be limited (see the first Rate Your Plate activity at the end of this chapter). At first, foods may also taste bland, but eventually you will perceive more flavor as the tongue becomes more sensitive to the salt content of foods. By slowly reducing dietary sodium and substituting lemon juice, herbs and spices, you can eventually become accustomed to a diet that contains minimal sodium but does not result in much of a flavor trade-off. Many new cookbooks offer excellent recipes for flavorful low-sodium foods.

Upper Level for Sodium

The Upper Level for sodium for adults is 2300 milligrams (2.3 grams). Intakes exceeding this amount are common but are not recommended because they typically

NEWSWORTHY NUTRITION

Lower sodium and higher potassium intakes reduce risk of cardiovascular disease

Increasing potassium intakes appears effective in lowering blood pressure and is most effective at reducing risk of cardiovascular disease when combined with lower intake of sodium. The sodium-to-potassium ratio in urine is a good predictor of cardiovascular disease.

Source: Cook NR and others: Joint effects of sodium and potassium intake on subsequent cardiovascular disease. *Archives of Internal Medicine* 169:32, 2009 (see Further Reading 3).

connect NUTRITION **Check out the Connect site** www.mcgrawhillconnect.com **to further explore the roles of sodium and potassium.**

increase blood pressure. About 95% of North American adults have sodium intakes that exceed the Upper Level.

CRITICAL THINKING

Mrs. Massa has recently seen and heard a lot about the amount of salt (sodium) in foods. She has been surprised by the number of articles that advise the public to decrease the amount of salt in their food. If sodium is such a bad thing, Mrs. Massa wonders, why do you need to have any at all? How would you respond to her question?

CONCEPT CHECK

Sodium is the major positive ion in the extracellular fluid. It is important for maintaining fluid balance and conducting nerve impulses. Sodium depletion is unlikely, because the typical North American's diet has abundant sources of sodium and most of it gets absorbed. Compared to dining out or buying commercially prepared foods, preparation of foods in the home allows greater control over sodium intake. The Adequate Intake for sodium for adults is 1500 milligrams per day. The average adult consumes 2300 to 4700 milligrams or more daily. About 10% to 15% of the population is especially sensitive to sodium, such as overweight individuals and African-Americans. In these people, hypertension can develop as a result of high-sodium diets, but many other lifestyle habits also contribute to hypertension. Nutrition experts suggest that for young adults, sodium intake should be about 1500 milligrams (1.5 grams) and not exceed 2300 milligrams (2.3 grams) on a regular basis. Sodium in the North American diet is provided predominantly through processed and restaurant foods.

9.5 Potassium (K)

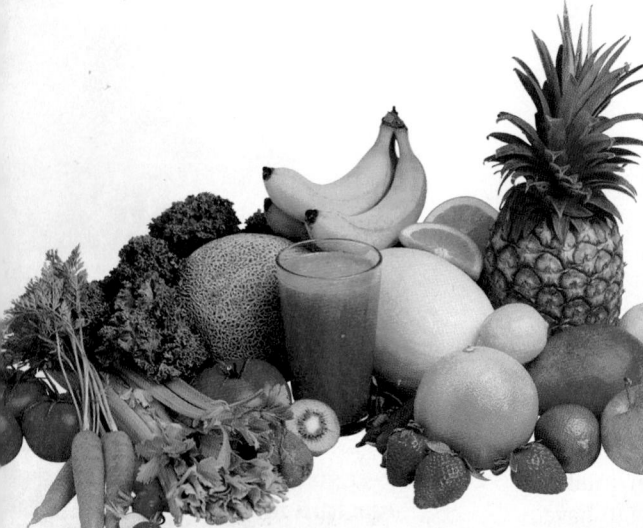

▲ Vegetables in general are a rich source of potassium, as are fruits.

diuretic A substance that increases the volume of urine.

Potassium performs many of the same functions as sodium, such as fluid balance and nerve impulse transmission. However, it operates inside, rather than outside cells. Intracellular fluids—those inside cells—contain 95% of the potassium in the body. Also, unlike sodium, increasing potassium intake is associated with lower rather than higher blood pressure values. We absorb about 90% of the potassium we eat.

Low blood potassium is a life-threatening problem. Symptoms often include a loss of appetite, muscle cramps, confusion, and constipation. Eventually, the heart beats irregularly, which decreases its capacity to pump blood.

Potassium Sources and Needs

Generally, unprocessed foods are rich sources of potassium. This includes fruits, vegetables, milk, whole grains, dried beans, and meats (Fig. 9-9). Major contributors of potassium to the adult diet include milk, potatoes, beef, coffee, tomatoes, and orange juice (Fig. 9-10).

The Adequate Intake for potassium for adults is 4700 milligrams (4.7 grams) per day. The Daily Value used to express potassium content on food and supplement labels is 3500 milligrams. On average, North Americans consume 2000 to 3000 milligrams per day. Thus, many of us need to increase our potassium intakes, preferably by increasing fruit and vegetable intake.

Diets are more likely to be lower in potassium than sodium because we generally do not add potassium to foods. Some **diuretics** used to treat high blood pressure also deplete the body's potassium. Thus, people who take potassium-wasting diuretics need to monitor their potassium intakes carefully. For these people, high-potassium foods are good additions to the diet, as are potassium chloride supplements if prescribed by a physician.

A chronically deficient food intake, as may be the case in alcoholism, can result in a severe potassium deficiency that requires medical attention. People with certain eating disorders, whose diets are poor and whose bodies can be depleted of nutrients because of vomiting, are also at risk for severe potassium deficiency (see Chapter 11).

Food Sources of Potassium

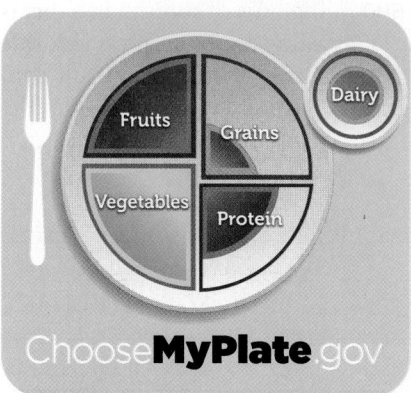

Food Item and Amount	Potassium (milligrams)	Adult Male and Female AI = 4700 milligrams
		Daily Value = 3500 milligrams %AI
AI*	4700	100%
Kidney beans, 1 cup	715	15%
Winter squash, ¾ cup	670	14%
Plain yogurt, 1 cup	570	12%
Orange juice, 1 cup	495	11%
Cantaloupe, 1 cup	495	11%
Lima beans, ½ cup	480	10%
Banana, 1 medium	470	10%
Zucchini, 1 cup	450	10%
Soybeans, ½ cup	440	9%
Artichoke, 1 medium	425	9%
Tomato juice, ¾ cup	400	9%
Pinto beans, ½ cup	400	9%
Baked potato, 1 small	385	8%
Buttermilk, 1 cup	370	8%
Sirloin steak, 3 ounces	345	7%

Key:
- Grains
- Vegetables
- Fruits
- Dairy
- Protein

ChooseMyPlate.gov

* For adults; see the DRI table in the back of this book for age-specific recommendations.

FIGURE 9-9 ▶ Food sources of potassium compared to the Adequate Intake.

ChooseMyPlate.gov

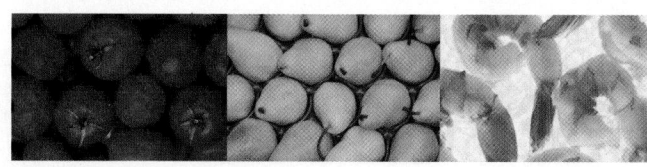

MyPlate: Sources of Potassium

FIGURE 9-10 ▶ Sources of potassium from MyPlate. The fill of the background color (none, 1/3, 2/3, or completely covered) within each group on the plate indicates the average nutrient density for potassium in that group. Overall, the vegetables group and the fruits group contain many foods that are nutrient-dense sources of potassium, with the dairy group and protein group following close behind.

Grains
- Whole-wheat bread
- Whole-grain products

Vegetables
- Avocados
- Spinach
- Squash
- Potatoes
- Tomatoes
- Lettuce
- Lima beans

Fruits
- Pears
- Prunes
- Peaches
- Cantaloupes
- Bananas

Dairy
- Milk
- Yogurt
- Cottage cheese
- Ricotta cheese

Protein
- Meat
- Chicken
- Fish
- Shrimp
- Beans

Other populations especially at risk for a severe potassium deficiency include people on very low-calorie diets and athletes who exercise heavily. As covered in Chapters 7 and 10, all of these people should compensate for potentially low body potassium by consuming potassium-rich foods.

If the kidneys function normally, typical food intakes will not lead to potassium toxicity. Thus, no Upper Level for potassium has been set. When the kidneys function poorly, potassium builds up in the blood. This inhibits heart function, causing slowed heartbeat. If untreated, this can be fatal, as the heart eventually stops beating. Consequently, in cases of reduced kidney function, close control of potassium intake becomes critical.

9.6 Chloride (Cl)

In our bodies, chloride—an ion form of chlorine—is an important negative ion for the extracellular fluid. Chlorine, on the other hand, is a poisonous gas. Chloride ions are a component of the acid produced in the stomach and are also used during immune responses as white blood cells attack foreign cells. In addition, nerve function relies on the presence of chloride. As is the case with sodium, most of the body's chloride is excreted by the kidneys; some is lost in perspiration. It is also thought to contribute to the blood pressure-raising ability of sodium chloride.

A chloride deficiency is unlikely because our dietary sodium chloride (salt) intake is so high. Frequent and lengthy bouts of vomiting—if coupled with a nutrient-poor diet—can, however, contribute to a deficiency because stomach secretions contain much chloride.

Chloride Sources and Needs

A few fruits and some vegetables are naturally good sources of chloride. Chlorinated water is also a source. However, the chloride we consume is mostly in the salt added to foods. Knowing a food's salt content allows for a close prediction of its chloride content; recall salt is 60% chloride.

The Adequate Intake for chloride for adults is 2300 milligrams per day. This is based on the 40:60 ratio of sodium to chloride in salt (1500 milligrams of sodium in a diet is accompanied by 2300 milligrams of chloride). The Daily Value used to express chloride content on food and supplement labels is 3400 milligrams. If the average adult consumes about 9 grams of salt daily, that yields 5.4 grams (5400 milligrams) of chloride.

Upper Level for Chloride

The Upper Level is 3600 milligrams. The average adult typically consumes an excess amount of this ion.

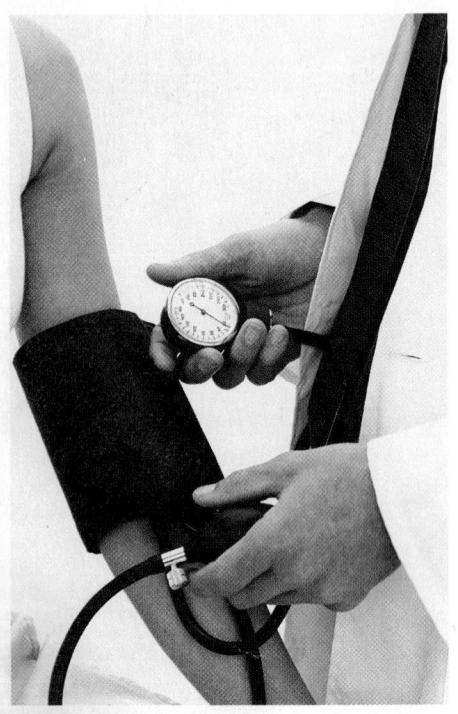

▲ Chloride is likely part of the blood pressure-raising property of sodium chloride (salt).

CONCEPT CHECK

The functions of potassium closely parallel those of sodium, but whereas sodium is found outside cells, potassium is the main positive ion found inside cells. Potassium is vital to fluid balance and nerve transmission. A potassium deficiency—caused by an inadequate intake of potassium, persistent vomiting, or use of some diuretics—can eventually lead to loss of appetite, muscle cramps, confusion, and heartbeat irregularities. Fruits and vegetables are generally rich sources of potassium. Potassium intake can be toxic if a person's kidneys do not function properly. Chloride is the major negative ion of extracellular fluid. Chloride also functions in digestion as part of stomach acid and in immune and nervous system responses. Deficiencies of chloride are highly unlikely because we eat so much sodium chloride (salt).

9.7 Calcium (Ca)

All cells need calcium, but more than 99% of the calcium in the body is used to strengthen bones and teeth. This calcium represents 40% of all the minerals present in the body and equals about 2.5 pounds (1200 grams). The calcium circulating in the bloodstream supplies the calcium needs of body cells. Growth and bone development require an adequate calcium intake.

Unlike sodium, potassium, and chloride, the amount of calcium in the body depends greatly on its absorption from the diet. Calcium requires an acidic environment in the GI tract to be absorbed efficiently. Absorption occurs primarily in the upper part of the small intestine. This area tends to be the most acidic portion of the small intestine because it receives the acidic stomach contents. Calcium absorption in the upper small intestine also depends on the active vitamin D hormone.

Adults absorb about 25% of the calcium in the foods eaten, but during times when the body needs extra calcium—such as in infancy and pregnancy—absorption increases to as high as 60%. Young people tend to absorb calcium better than do older people, especially those older than 70.

Many factors enhance calcium absorption, including:

- Blood levels of parathyroid hormone
- The presence of glucose and lactose in the diet
- The gradual flow (motility) of digestive contents through the intestine

On the other hand, several factors limit calcium absorption, such as:

- Large amounts of phytic acid in fiber from grains
- Great excess of phosphorus (and possibly magnesium) in the diet
- Polyphenols (tannins) in tea
- Vitamin D deficiency
- Diarrhea
- Old age

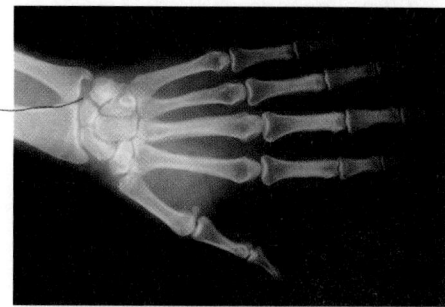

▲ Ninety-nine percent of calcium in the body is in bones.

We have excellent hormonal systems to control blood calcium, so a normal blood calcium value can be maintained despite an inadequate calcium intake. The bones, however, pay the price. Bones can be seen as a calcium bank to which calcium can be added or withdrawn. Bone loss caused by a net calcium loss from this bank proceeds slowly. Only after many years of calcium loss are clinical symptoms apparent. By not meeting calcium needs, some people—especially women—are most likely setting the stage for future bone fractures.

Functions of Calcium

Forming and maintaining bones are calcium's major roles in the body. This is discussed in detail in the second Nutrition and Your Health section on minerals and **osteoporosis** found at the end of this chapter. However, calcium is important in many other processes as well. Calcium is essential for blood clotting and for muscle contraction. If blood calcium falls below a critical point, muscles cannot relax after contraction; the body stiffens and shows involuntary twitching, called **tetany**. In nerve transmission, calcium assists in the release of neurotransmitters and permits the flow of ions in and out of nerve cells. Without sufficient calcium, nerve function fails, which can also cause tetany. Finally, calcium helps regulate cellular metabolism by influencing the activities of various enzymes and hormonal responses. It is the hormonal regulation of blood calcium that keeps all of these processes going, even if a person fails to consume enough calcium on a daily basis.

Other Possible Health Benefits of Calcium

Researchers have been examining links between calcium intake and risks for a variety of diseases including certain cancers, kidney stones, hypertension, high blood

osteoporosis Decreased bone mass related to the effects of aging, genetic background, and poor diet in both genders, and hormonal changes at menopause in women.

tetany A body condition marked by sharp contraction of muscles and failure to relax afterward; usually caused by abnormal calcium metabolism.

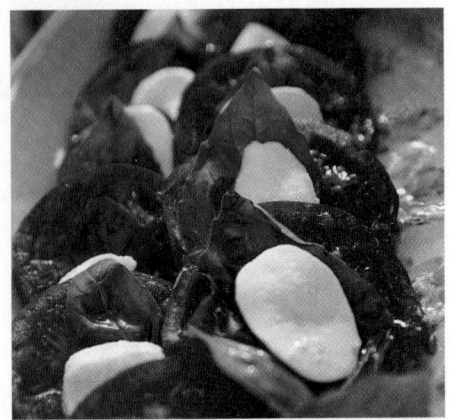

▲ To enhance intake of calcium and other nutrients, the 2010 Dietary Guidelines recommend an increased intake of fat-free or low-fat milk and milk products such as the mozzarella cheese on this tomato-basil salad.

cholesterol, and most recently, obesity. An adequate calcium intake can reduce the risk of colon cancer, especially in people who consume a high-fat diet (see Further Reading 13). A decreased risk of some forms of kidney stones and reduced lead absorption are other possible benefits when calcium is part of a meal. Calcium intakes of 800 to 1200 milligrams per day can also decrease blood pressure, compared with intakes of 400 milligrams per day or less. As covered in Chapter 5, calcium intakes of 1200 milligrams per day in combination with a low-fat, low-cholesterol diet can help people with elevated LDL cholesterol improve their blood lipid profiles. A link between a low calcium intake and overweight/obesity is also under study. Although the true benefit in this regard is not clear, studies suggest that an adequate calcium intake (compared to a very low intake [e.g., 400 milligrams per day]), coupled with a low calorie intake, may promote even more weight loss than the low calorie diet alone. Focusing on dairy sources of calcium is recommended because other components in dairy foods, such as some of the specific dairy proteins, contribute to this potential weight loss benefit. For women, an adequate calcium in-take might also reduce the risk of premenstrual syndrome and high blood pressure that can develop during pregnancy. Overall, the benefits of a diet providing adequate calcium extend beyond bone health.

Calcium Sources and Needs

Dairy products, such as milk and cheese, provide about 75% of the calcium in North American diets. The exception is cottage cheese, because most calcium is lost during production. Bread, rolls, crackers, and other foods made with milk products are secondary contributors. Other calcium sources are leafy greens (such as spinach), broccoli, sardines, and canned salmon (Fig. 9-11). It is important to remember that much of the calcium in some leafy green vegetables, notably spinach, is not absorbed because of the presence of oxalic acid. This effect is not as strong, however, in kale,

FIGURE 9-11 ▶ Food sources of calcium compared to the Adequate Intake.

Food Sources of Calcium

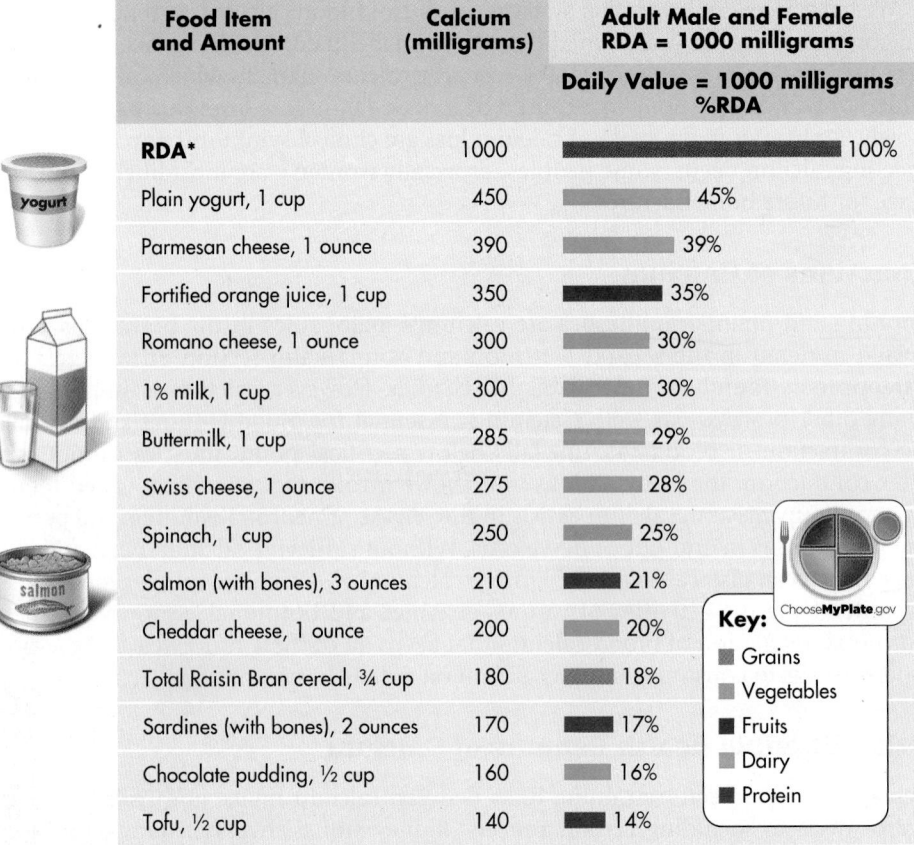

Food Item and Amount	Calcium (milligrams)	Adult Male and Female RDA = 1000 milligrams
		Daily Value = 1000 milligrams %RDA
RDA*	1000	100%
Plain yogurt, 1 cup	450	45%
Parmesan cheese, 1 ounce	390	39%
Fortified orange juice, 1 cup	350	35%
Romano cheese, 1 ounce	300	30%
1% milk, 1 cup	300	30%
Buttermilk, 1 cup	285	29%
Swiss cheese, 1 ounce	275	28%
Spinach, 1 cup	250	25%
Salmon (with bones), 3 ounces	210	21%
Cheddar cheese, 1 ounce	200	20%
Total Raisin Bran cereal, ¾ cup	180	18%
Sardines (with bones), 2 ounces	170	17%
Chocolate pudding, ½ cup	160	16%
Tofu, ½ cup	140	14%

Key:
■ Grains
■ Vegetables
■ Fruits
■ Dairy
■ Protein

*For adults; see the DRI table in the back of this book for age-specific recommendations.

collard, turnip, and mustard greens. Overall, fat-free milk is the most nutrient-dense (milligrams per kcal) source of calcium because of its high bioavailability and low calorie content, with some of the vegetables just noted following close behind (Fig. 9-12). The new calcium-fortified versions of orange juice and other beverages (e.g., soy milk), as well as calcium-fortified cottage cheese, breakfast cereals, breakfast bars, snacks, and certain chewable candies, also follow as close competitors. Another source of calcium is soybean curd (tofu) if it is made with calcium carbonate (check the label). Also, the bones in canned fish, such as salmon and sardines, supply calcium. High-calcium mineral waters appear to provide useful quantities of bioavailable calcium. Read more about these mineral waters in Further Reading 6 and in the What Would You Choose Recommendations at the end of this chapter.

Information about calcium is mandatory on food labels. The Daily Value used to express the calcium content on food and supplement labels is 1000 milligrams.

The Recommended Dietary Allowance for calcium for adults ranges from 1000 to 1200 milligrams per day for adults and is based on the amount of calcium needed each day to offset calcium losses in urine, feces, and other routes. The RDA for adolescents and teens is 1300 milligrams to allow for increases in bone mass during growth and development. In the United States, average calcium intakes are approximately 800 milligrams for women and 1000 milligrams for men. Thus, dietary intakes of calcium by many women, especially young women, are below the RDA, whereas intakes by most men are roughly equivalent to the RDA. It is also important for vegans to focus on eating good plant sources of calcium as well as on the total amount of calcium ingested.

To estimate your calcium intake, use the rule of 300s. Count 300 milligrams for the calcium provided by foods scattered throughout the diet. Add to that another 300 milligrams for every cup of milk or yogurt or 1.5 ounces of cheese. If you eat a lot of tofu, almonds, or sardines, or drink calcium-fortified beverages, use the second "Rate Your Plate" activity at the end of this chapter or your diet-analysis software to get a more accurate calculation of your calcium intake.

▲ Milk is a rich as well as convenient source of calcium.

Calcium Supplements

Calcium supplements can be used by people who do not like milk or who cannot incorporate enough calcium-containing foods into their diets. Calcium carbonate, the

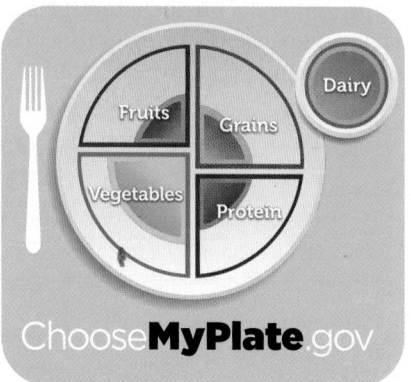

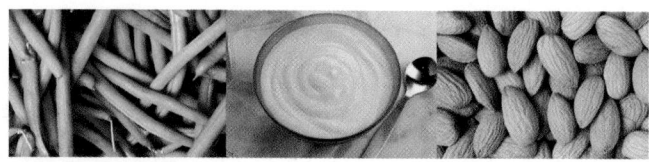

**MyPlate:
Sources of Calcium**

FIGURE 9-12 ▶ Sources of calcium from MyPlate. The height of the background color (none, 1/3, 2/3, or completely covered) within each group on the plate indicates the average nutrient density for calcium in that group. Overall, foods from the dairy group and many fortified foods are nutrient-dense and bioavailable sources of calcium. Additional calcium-fortified foods appear in stores each year and thus will add to the food sources listed for various groups.

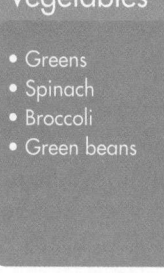

Grains

- Calcium-fortified snack foods
- Calcium-fortified flour tortillas
- Calcium-fortified breakfast cereals

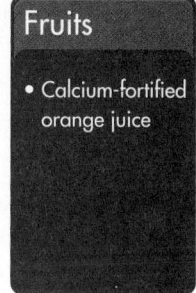

Vegetables

- Greens
- Spinach
- Broccoli
- Green beans

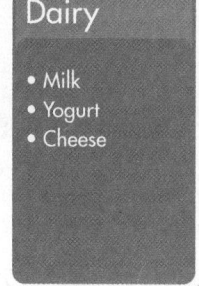

Fruits

- Calcium-fortified orange juice

Dairy

- Milk
- Yogurt
- Cheese

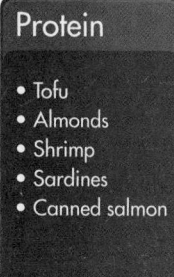

Protein

- Tofu
- Almonds
- Shrimp
- Sardines
- Canned salmon

MAKING DECISIONS

Choosing a Calcium Supplement

Here is how to determine the calcium content of typical supplements based on the form of calcium, as listed on the supplement label and the percentage of calcium per unit of weight.

- Calcium carbonate: 40%
- Calcium phosphate (tribasic): 38%
- Calcium citrate: 21%
- Calcium lactate: 13%
- Calcium gluconate: 9%

To calculate the amount of calcium in a supplement, multiply the weight of the capsule by the percentage listed above. For example, if 1 tablet of calcium citrate weighs 500 milligrams, it contains 105 milligrams of calcium.

500 milligrams × 0.21 = 105 milligrams

Some calcium supplements are poorly digested because they do not readily dissolve. To test for this, put a supplement in ¾ cup of cider vinegar. Stir every 5 minutes. It should dissolve within 30 minutes. You now see that the type of calcium supplement chosen can make a big difference in how much calcium is in each pill.

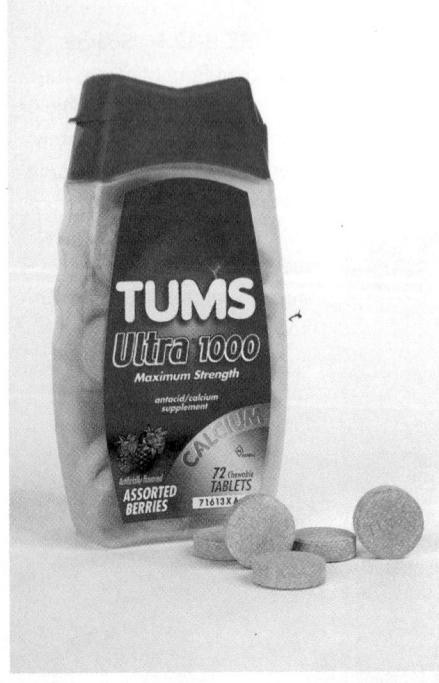

▲ Tums is an antacid that is also a good source of calcium carbonate.

form found in calcium-based antacid tablets, is the most common supplement used. People should take this supplement with or just after meals in doses of about 500 milligrams so that stomach acid produced during digestion can aid with absorption of this mineral. On the other hand, a supplement containing calcium citrate, which is acidic itself, can be taken without regard to meals. Studies have shown that supplements containing calcium citrate reduce bone loss and height loss in postmenopause women (see Further Reading 15).

With calcium supplements, interactions with other minerals are a valid concern. Perhaps most importantly, there is some evidence that calcium supplements may decrease zinc absorption. Therefore, calcium supplements should not be taken with meals rich in zinc. An effect of calcium supplementation on iron absorption is possible; however, this appears to be small over the long term. To be safe, people should notify their physician if using a calcium supplement on a regular basis.

Some calcium supplements also contain lead. FDA has no standards for lead content in food supplements, but does plan to regulate the lead content of supplements, including calcium, in the future. Until then, it is important to avoid supplements made from bonemeal, the worst offender when it comes to lead. Tablet or liquid calcium supplements with the USP seal of approval are less likely than others to contain high concentrations of contaminants.

No form of natural calcium, such as coral calcium, is superior to typical supplement forms. People making such claims of superiority have been prosecuted by the U.S. Federal Trade Commission for false advertising.

Upper Level for Calcium

The Upper Level for calcium intake is 2500 milligrams per day, based on the observation that greater intakes increase the risk for some forms of kidney stones. Excessive calcium intakes by some people also can cause high blood and urinary calcium concentrations, irritability, headache, kidney failure, soft tissue calcification, and decreased absorption of other minerals, as noted above.

So, which is better: calcium from food or supplements? Taking 1000 milligrams of calcium carbonate or calcium citrate daily in divided doses (about 500 milligrams per tablet) is probably safe in many instances. However, people often have difficulty adhering to a supplement regimen. If possible, modification of eating habits to include foods that are good sources of calcium is a better plan. In addition to this important mineral, foods that contain calcium also supply other vitamins, minerals, phytochemicals, and fats needed to support health. Plus, problems associated with excessive consumption of calcium are not likely when foods are one's sources of calcium.

CONCEPT CHECK

About 99% of calcium in the body is found in the bones. Aside from its critical role in bone, calcium also functions in blood clotting, muscle contraction, nerve-impulse transmission, and cell metabolism. Calcium requires a slightly acid pH and the vitamin D hormone for efficient absorption. Factors that reduce calcium absorption include a vitamin D deficiency, large amounts of fiber (especially excess wheat bran), and old age in general. Blood calcium is regulated primarily by hormones and does not closely reflect daily intake.

Dairy products are rich food sources of calcium. Other foods, such as calcium-fortified beverages, are rich sources as well. Supplemental forms, such as calcium carbonate, are well-absorbed by most people. However, overzealous supplementation can also result in the development of kidney stones and other health problems.

9.8 Phosphorus (P)

Although no disease is currently associated with an inadequate phosphorus intake, a deficiency may contribute to bone loss in older women. The body efficiently absorbs phosphorus, at about 70% of dietary intake. This high absorption, plus the wide availability of phosphorus in foods, makes this mineral less important than is calcium in diet planning. The active vitamin D hormone enhances phosphorus absorption, as it does for calcium. Blood phosphorus concentration is regulated primarily by kidney excretion and also by changes in the degree of absorption.

Phosphorus is a component of enzymes, other key compounds, DNA (genetic material), cell membranes, and bone. About 85% of the body's phosphorus is inside bone. The remaining phosphorus circulates freely in the bloodstream and functions inside cells.

Phosphorus Sources and Needs

Milk, cheese, meat, and bread provide most of the phosphorus in the adult diet. Breakfast cereals, bran, eggs, nuts, and fish are also good sources (Fig. 9-13). About 20% to 30% of dietary phosphorus comes from food additives, especially in baked goods, cheeses, processed meats, and many soft drinks with about 75 milligrams per 12-ounce ($\frac{1}{3}$-liter) serving of soft drinks. Next time you have a soft drink, look for a listing of phosphoric acid on the label.

The RDA for phosphorus for adults over age 18 is 700 milligrams daily, based on the amount needed to maintain normal blood concentrations of phosphorus. The Daily Value used to express phosphorus content on food and supplement labels is 1000 milligrams. Adults consume about 1000 to 1600 milligrams of phosphorus per day. Thus, deficiencies of phosphorus are unlikely in healthy adults, especially because it is so efficiently absorbed.

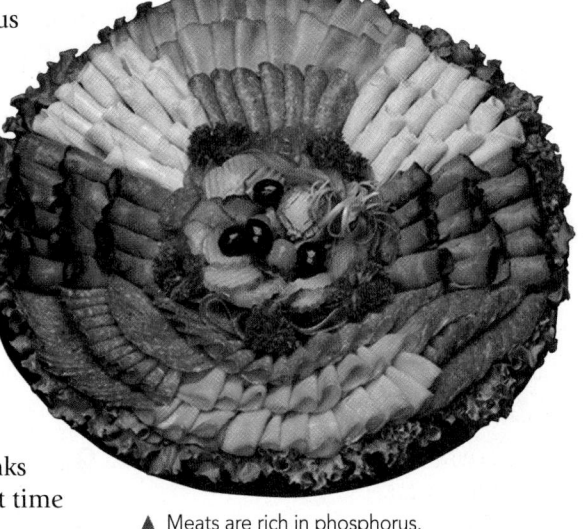

▲ Meats are rich in phosphorus.

Food Sources of Phosphorus

FIGURE 9-13 ▶ Food sources of phosphorus compared to the RDA.

Food Item and Amount	Phosphorus (milligrams)	Adult Male and Female RDA = 700 milligrams / Daily Value = 1000 milligrams %RDA
RDA*	700	100%
Plain yogurt, 1 cup	350	50%
Swiss cheese, 2 ounces	345	49%
Almonds, ½ cup	340	49%
Sunflower seeds, 1 ounce	330	47%
1% milk, 1 cup	235	34%
Cheddar cheese, 1.5 ounces	220	31%
Salmon, 3 ounces	220	31%
Raisin Bran cereal, 1 cup	215	31%
Sirloin steak, 3 ounces	210	30%
Egg, 2 hard boiled	200	29%
Chicken breast, 3 ounces	180	26%
Roasted turkey, 3 ounces	180	26%
Pot roast, 3 ounces	170	24%
Lean ham, 3 ounces	165	24%
American cheese, 1 slice	155	22%

Key:
- Grains
- Vegetables
- Fruits
- Dairy
- Protein

ChooseMyPlate.gov

*For adults; see the DRI table in the back of this book for age-specific recommendations.

Marginal phosphorus status can be found in preterm infants, vegans, people with alcoholism, older people on nutrient-poor diets, and people with long-term bouts of diarrhea.

Upper Level for Phosphorus

The Upper Level for phosphorus intake is 3 to 4 grams per day. Intakes greater than this impair kidney function. High intakes are especially a problem in people with certain kidney diseases. In addition, a chronically high phosphorus intake coupled with a low calcium intake can cause an imbalance in the calcium-to-phosphorus ratio in the diet, which can contribute to bone loss. This situation most likely arises when the Adequate Intake for calcium is not met, as can occur in adolescents and adults who regularly substitute soft drinks for milk or otherwise underconsume calcium.

9.9 Magnesium (Mg)

Magnesium is important for nerve and heart function and aids many enzyme reactions. It is found mostly in the plant pigment chlorophyll, where it functions in respiration. We normally absorb about 40% to 60% of the magnesium in our diets, but absorption efficiency can increase up to about 80% if intakes are low.

Bone contains 60% of the body's magnesium. The rest circulates in the blood and operates inside cells. Over 300 enzymes use magnesium, and many energy-yielding compounds in cells require magnesium to function properly, as does the hormone insulin.

In humans, a magnesium deficiency causes an irregular heartbeat, sometimes accompanied by weakness, muscle pain, disorientation, and seizures. Adequate magnesium intakes decrease cardiovascular disease risk by decreasing blood pressure by dilating arteries and preventing heart rhythm abnormalities. People with cardiovascular disease should closely monitor magnesium intake, especially because they are often on medications such as diuretics that reduce magnesium status. Keep in mind that a magnesium deficiency develops slowly because our bodies store it readily.

Magnesium Sources and Needs

Rich sources for magnesium are plant products, such as whole grains (like wheat bran), broccoli, potatoes, squash, beans, nuts, and seeds (Fig. 9-14). Animal products, such as milk and meats, and even chocolate supply some magnesium, although less than the foods in the magnesium plate (Fig. 9-15). Two other sources of magnesium are hard tap water, which contains a high mineral content, and coffee.

The adult RDA for magnesium is about 400 milligrams per day for men and about 310 milligrams per day for women. This is based on the amount needed to offset daily losses. The Daily Value used to express magnesium content on food and supplement labels is 400 milligrams. Adult men consume an average of 320 milligrams daily, whereas women consume closer to 220 milligrams daily. A study has shown that a diet high in magnesium-rich foods, especially whole grains, decreases the risk of type 2 diabetes in U.S. black women (see Further Reading 16). This suggests that many of us should improve our intakes of magnesium-rich foods, such as whole-grain breads and cereals.

The refined grain products that dominate the diets of many North Americans are poor sources of this mineral. If dietary means are not enough, a balanced multivitamin and mineral supplement containing approximately 100 milligrams of magnesium can help to close the gap between intake and needs. The typical form used in supplements (magnesium oxide) is not as well absorbed as the forms of magnesium found in foods but still contributes to meeting magnesium needs.

Poor magnesium status is found especially among users of certain diuretics. In addition, heavy perspiration for weeks in hot climates and bouts of long-standing

Diabetes and hypertension have both been linked with low levels of magnesium in the blood. However, the cause for low magnesium in people with these diseases is unclear. Research is underway to uncover the potential role of magnesium in treatment and/or prevention of these chronic diseases.

Food Sources of Magnesium

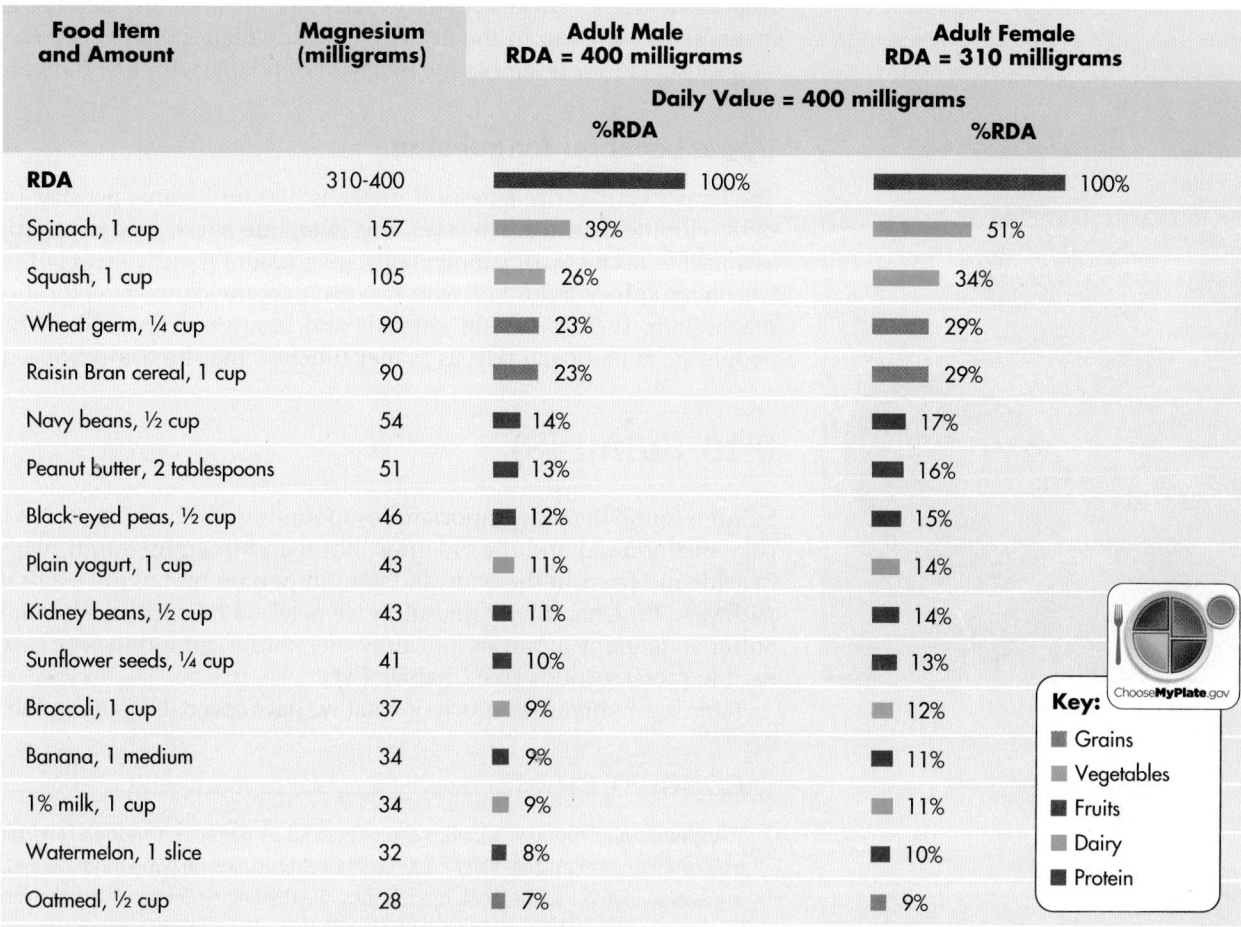

Food Item and Amount	Magnesium (milligrams)	Adult Male RDA = 400 milligrams		Adult Female RDA = 310 milligrams	
		Daily Value = 400 milligrams			
		%RDA		%RDA	
RDA	310-400		100%		100%
Spinach, 1 cup	157		39%		51%
Squash, 1 cup	105		26%		34%
Wheat germ, ¼ cup	90		23%		29%
Raisin Bran cereal, 1 cup	90		23%		29%
Navy beans, ½ cup	54		14%		17%
Peanut butter, 2 tablespoons	51		13%		16%
Black-eyed peas, ½ cup	46		12%		15%
Plain yogurt, 1 cup	43		11%		14%
Kidney beans, ½ cup	43		11%		14%
Sunflower seeds, ¼ cup	41		10%		13%
Broccoli, 1 cup	37		9%		12%
Banana, 1 medium	34		9%		11%
1% milk, 1 cup	34		9%		11%
Watermelon, 1 slice	32		8%		10%
Oatmeal, ½ cup	28		7%		9%
Whole-wheat bread, 1 slice	25		6%		8%

Key:
- ■ Grains
- ■ Vegetables
- ■ Fruits
- ■ Dairy
- ■ Protein

FIGURE 9-14 ▶ Food sources of magnesium compared to the RDA for adult males and females.

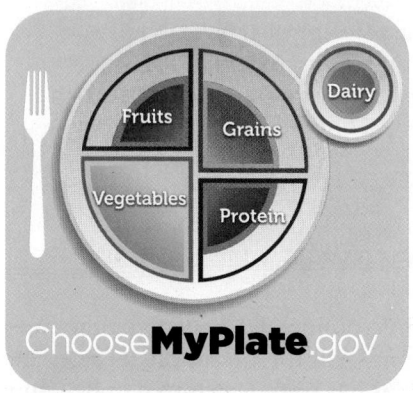

ChooseMyPlate.gov

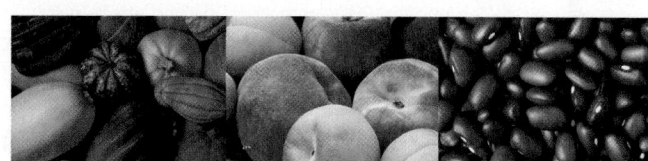

MyPlate: Sources of Magnesium

FIGURE 9-15 ▶ Sources of magnesium from MyPlate. The fill of the background color (none, 1/3, 2/3, or completely covered) within each group on the plate indicates the average nutrient density for magnesium in that group. Overall, the vegetables group provides the richest sources. Whole-grain choices in the grains group are also rich sources.

Grains
- Wheat bran
- Wheat germ
- Whole-grain products

Vegetables
- Avocados
- Spinach
- Greens
- Broccoli
- Lima beans
- Potatoes
- Squash

Fruits
- Figs
- Peaches
- Bananas
- Berries

Dairy
- Milk
- Yogurt

Protein
- Tofu
- Nuts
- Shrimp
- Kidney beans
- Sunflower seeds

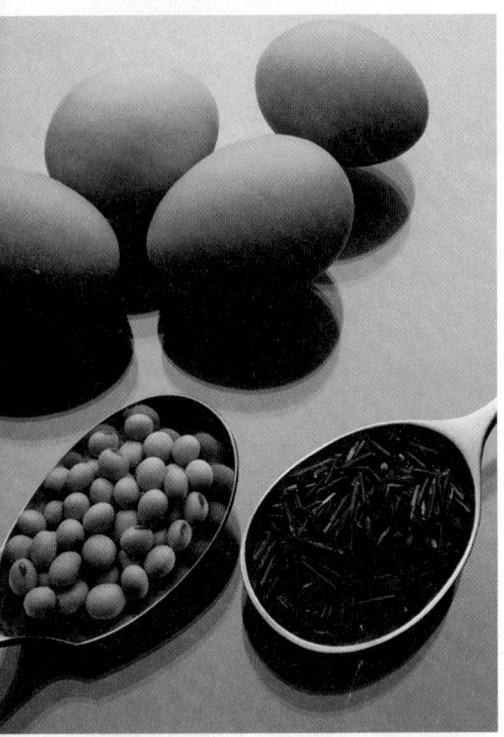

▲ Protein-rich foods supply sulfur in the diet.

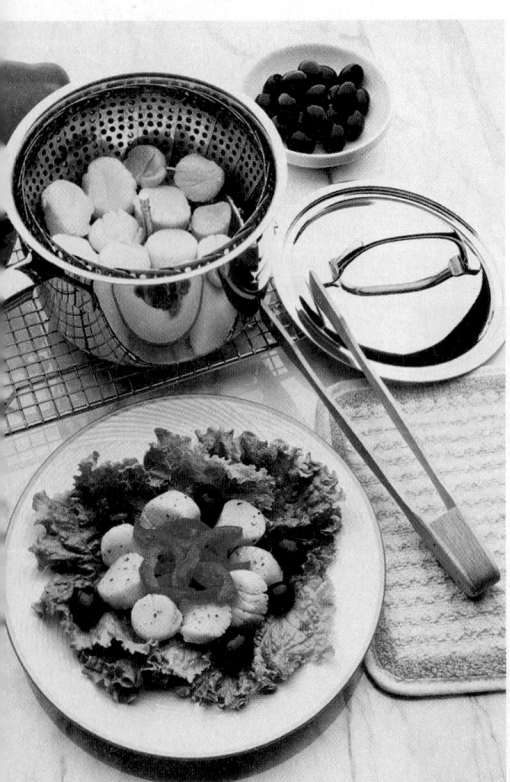

▲ Seafood, such as scallops, is a good source of many trace minerals.

diarrhea or vomiting cause significant magnesium loss. Alcoholism also increases the risk of a deficiency because dietary intake may be poor and because alcohol increases magnesium excretion in the urine. The disorientation and weakness associated with alcoholism closely resemble the behavior of people with low blood magnesium.

Upper Level for Magnesium

The Upper Level for magnesium intake is 350 milligrams per day, based on the risk of developing diarrhea. However, this guideline refers only to nonfood sources such as antacids, laxatives, or supplements. Magnesium toxicity especially occurs in people who have kidney failure or who overuse over-the-counter medications that contain magnesium, such as certain antacids and laxatives (e.g., milk of magnesia). Older people are at particular risk, as kidney function may be compromised.

9.10 Sulfur (S)

Sulfur is found in many important compounds in the body, such as some amino acids (like methionine) and the vitamins biotin and thiamin. Sulfur helps in the balance of acids and bases in the body and is an important part of the liver's drug-detoxifying pathways. Proteins supply the sulfur we need, so it is not an essential nutrient *per se.* Sulfur is naturally a part of a healthy diet. Sulfur compounds (e.g., sulfites) are also used to preserve foods (see Chapter 13).

Table 9-2 summarizes much of what we have covered regarding the major minerals.

CONCEPT CHECK

Phosphorus absorption is efficient and enhanced by the active vitamin D hormone. Urinary excretion mainly controls body content. Phosphorus aids enzyme function and is part of key metabolic compounds and cell membranes. No distinct deficiency symptoms caused by an inadequate phosphorus intake have been reported. Food sources for phosphorus include dairy products, baked goods, and meat. The RDA is met by most North Americans. An excess intake of phosphorus can compromise bone health, if sufficient calcium is not consumed, and can impair kidney function. Magnesium is required for nerve and heart function; it also aids activity for many enzymes. Food sources of magnesium are whole grains (wheat bran), vegetables, beef, coffee, beans, nuts, and seeds. People using certain diuretics and people with alcoholism are at greatest risk of developing a deficiency. Magnesium toxicity is most likely in people with kidney failure or people using certain forms of laxatives and antacids. Sulfur is a component of certain vitamins and amino acids. The protein we consume supplies sufficient sulfur for the body's needs.

9.11 Trace Minerals—An Overview

Information about trace minerals (also called microminerals) is perhaps the most rapidly expanding area of knowledge in nutrition. With the exceptions of iron and iodide, the importance of trace minerals to humans has been recognized only within the last 40 years. Although we need 100 milligrams or less of each trace mineral daily, they are as essential to good health as major minerals.

In some cases, discovering the importance of a trace mineral reads like a detective story, and the evidence is still unfolding. In 1961, researchers linked dwarfism among Middle Eastern villagers to a zinc deficiency. Other scientists recognized that a rare form of heart disease in an isolated area of China was linked to a selenium deficiency. In North America, some trace mineral deficiencies were first observed in the late 1960s and early 1970s when the minerals were not added to newly developed synthetic formulas used for intravenous feeding.

TABLE 9-2 Summary of the Major Minerals

Mineral	Major Functions	RDA, or Adequate Intake	Dietary Sources	Deficiency Symptoms	Toxicity Symptoms
Sodium	• Major positive ion of the extracellular fluid • Aids nerve impulse transmission • Water balance	*Age 19–50 years:* 1500 milligrams *Age 51–70 years:* 1300 milligrams *Age > 70 years* 1200 milligrams	• Table salt • Processed foods • Condiments • Sauces • Soups • Chips	• Muscle cramps	• Contributes to hypertension in susceptible individuals • Increases calcium loss in urine • Upper Level is 2300 milligrams
Potassium	• Major positive ion of intracellular fluid • Aids nerve impulse transmission • Water balance	4700 milligrams	• Spinach • Squash • Bananas • Orange juice • Milk • Meat • Legumes • Whole grains	• Irregular heart beat • Loss of appetite • Muscle cramps	• Slowing of the heartbeat, as seen in kidney failure
Chloride	• Major negative ion of extracellular fluid • Participates in acid production in stomach • Aids nerve impulse transmission • Water balance	2300 milligrams	• Table salt • Some vegetables • Processed foods	• Convulsions in infants	• Linked to hypertension in susceptible people when combined with sodium • Upper Level is 3600 milligrams
Calcium	• Bone and tooth structure • Blood clotting • Aids in nerve impulse transmission • Muscle contractions • Other cell functions	*Age 9–18 years:* 1300 milligrams *Age > 18 years:* 1000–1200 milligrams	• Dairy products • Canned fish • Leafy vegetables • Tofu • Fortified orange juice (and other fortified foods)	• Increased risk of osteoporosis	• May cause kidney stones and other problems in susceptible people • Upper Level is 2500 milligrams
Phosphorus	• Major ion of intracellular fluid • Bone and tooth strength • Part of various metabolic compounds • Acid/base balance	*Age 9–18 years:* 1250 milligrams *Age > 18 years:* 700 milligrams	• Dairy products • Processed foods • Fish • Soft drinks • Bakery products • Meats	• Possibility of poor bone maintenance	• Impairs bone health in people with kidney failure • Poor bone mineralization if calcium intakes are low • Upper Level is 3 to 4 grams
Magnesium	• Bone formation • Aids enzyme function • Aids nerve and heart function	*Men:* 400–420 milligrams *Women:* 310–320 milligrams	• Wheat bran • Green vegetables • Nuts • Chocolate • Legumes	• Weakness • Muscle pain • Poor heart function	• Causes diarrhea and weakness in people with kidney failure • Upper Level is 350 milligrams, but refers to nonfood sources (e.g., supplements) only
Sulfur	• Part of vitamins and amino acids • Aids in drug detoxification • Acid/base balance	None	• Protein foods	• None observed	• None likely

It is difficult to precisely define our trace mineral needs because we need only minute amounts. Highly sophisticated technology is required to measure such small amounts in both food and body tissues.

9.12 Iron (Fe)

Although the importance of dietary iron has been recognized for centuries, today, iron deficiency is still one of the most common nutrient deficiencies worldwide. Iron is the only nutrient for which young women have a greater RDA than do adult men. Iron is found in every living cell, adding up to about 5 grams (1 teaspoon) for the entire body.

Absorption and Distribution of Iron

Controlling absorption is important because our bodies cannot easily eliminate excess iron once it is absorbed. The body uses several mechanisms to regulate iron absorption. Overall, iron absorption depends on its form in the food, the body's need for it, and a variety of other factors. Healthy people absorb about 18% of that present in food, whereas people with iron deficiency absorb somewhat more.

The form of iron in foods especially influences how much is absorbed. About 40% of the total iron in animal flesh is in the form of **hemoglobin** (the same form as in red blood cells) and **myoglobin** (pigment found in muscle cells). This type of iron, called **heme iron,** is absorbed about two to three times more efficiently than the simple elemental iron, called **nonheme iron.** Nonheme iron is added to grain products during the enrichment process and is also present in animal flesh, as well as in eggs, milk, vegetables, grains, and other plant foods.

Consuming heme iron and nonheme iron together increases nonheme iron absorption. A protein factor in meats may also aid nonheme absorption. Overall, eating meat with vegetables and grain products enhances the absorption of all nonheme iron present.

Vitamin C in amounts of about 75 milligrams can also increase nonheme iron absorption. Drinking a glass of orange juice when taking an iron supplement, therefore, will enhance the iron absorbed from the supplement. Consuming more foods rich in vitamin C is particularly desirable if dietary iron is inadequate or if blood iron is low. Iron use in the body is also aided by copper, as explained in the later section on copper.

In contrast, several dietary factors interfere with our ability to absorb nonheme iron. Phytic acid and other factors in grain fibers and oxalic acid in vegetables can all bind this iron and reduce its absorption. Polyphenols (tannins) found in tea also reduce nonheme iron absorption. It is a good idea to moderate intake of tannins if one has iron deficiency and keep fiber intake within current recommendations. Taking zinc supplements will also interfere with nonheme iron because zinc will compete with iron for absorption.

Overall, the most important factor influencing nonheme iron absorption is the body's need for it. Iron needs are increased during pregnancy and growth. At high altitudes, the need for iron is also increased because the lower oxygen concentration of the air causes an increase in the hemoglobin concentration of blood. During an iron deficiency state, nonheme iron absorption can increase. When iron stores are inadequate, the main protein that carries iron in blood readily binds more iron from intestinal cells and shifts it into the bloodstream. When iron stores are adequate and the iron-binding protein in the blood is fully saturated with iron, iron stays bound in the intestinal cells and little will be absorbed.

By this mechanism, under normal circumstances, iron, especially the nonheme form, is absorbed as needed. If not needed, iron stored in intestinal cells will be excreted when intestinal cells are shed at the end of their 2- to 5-day life cycle. High doses of iron can still be toxic, but absorption is carefully regulated under typical dietary conditions in most people.

hemoglobin The iron-containing part of the red blood cell that carries oxygen to the cells and some carbon dioxide away from the cells. The heme iron portion is also responsible for the red color of blood.

myoglobin Iron-containing protein that binds oxygen in muscle tissue.

heme iron Iron provided from animal tissues in the form of hemoglobin and myoglobin. Approximately 40% of the iron in meat is heme iron; it is readily absorbed.

nonheme iron Iron provided from plant sources and animal tissues other than in the forms of hemoglobin and myoglobin. Nonheme iron is less efficiently absorbed than heme iron; absorption is closely dependent on body needs.

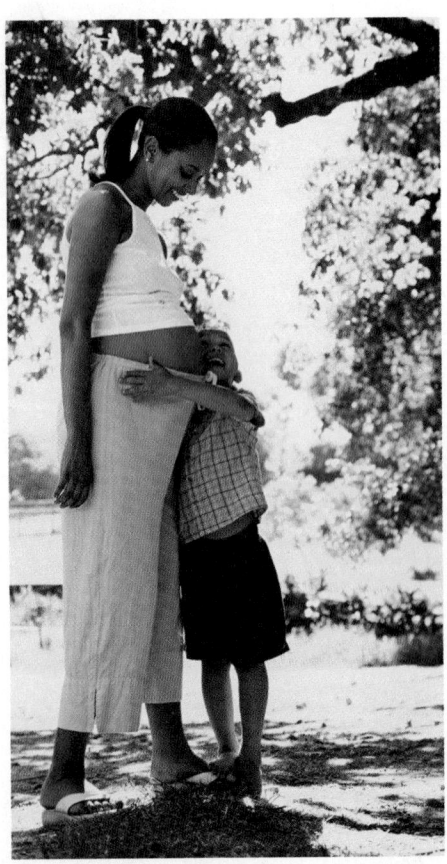

▲ Pregnancy greatly increases iron needs, as does growth in childhood.

Most iron in the body is contained in the hemoglobin molecules of the red blood cells. Some iron is stored in the bone marrow, and a small portion goes to other body cells, such as the liver, for storage. As iron is needed, it can be mobilized from these body stores. If dietary intake is chronically inadequate, these iron stores become depleted. Only then do signs of an iron deficiency appear.

Functions of Iron

Iron is part of the hemoglobin in red blood cells and myoglobin in muscle cells. Hemoglobin molecules in red blood cells transport oxygen (O_2) from the lungs to cells and assist in the return of some carbon dioxide (CO_2) from cells to the lungs for excretion. In addition, iron is used as part of many enzymes, some proteins, and compounds that cells use in energy production. Iron is also needed for brain and immune function and contributes to drug detoxification in the liver and to bone health.

If neither the diet nor body stores can supply the iron needed for hemoglobin synthesis, the number of red blood cells decreases in the bloodstream. The blood hemoglobin concentration also falls. Physicians use both the percentage of red blood cells (called the **hematocrit**) and the hemoglobin concentration in blood to assess iron status, along with the amount of iron and iron-containing proteins in the bloodstream. When hematocrit and hemoglobin fall, an iron deficiency is suspected. In severe deficiency, hemoglobin and hematocrit fall so low that the amount of oxygen carried in the bloodstream is decreased. Such a person has **anemia,** defined as a decreased oxygen-carrying capacity of the blood.

While there are many types of anemia, iron-deficiency anemia is the major type worldwide. About 30% of the world's population is anemic, and about half of those cases are caused by an iron deficiency. Probably about 10% of North Americans in high-risk categories have iron-deficiency anemia. This appears most often in infancy, the preschool years, and at puberty for both males and females. Growth, with accompanying expansion of blood volume and muscle mass, increases iron needs, making it difficult to consume enough iron. Women are also vulnerable during childbearing years from blood loss during menstruation. In addition, anemia is often found in pregnant women, as discussed in Chapter 14. Iron-deficiency anemia in adult men is usually caused by blood loss from ulcers, colon cancer, or hemorrhoids. Finally, athletes can develop iron-deficiency anemia, as discussed in Chapter 10.

Clinical symptoms of iron-deficiency anemia primarily include pale skin, fatigue upon exertion, poor temperature regulation, loss of appetite, and apathy. Insufficient iron for the synthesis of red blood cells and key cell compounds may cause the fatigue. Poor iron stores may also decrease learning ability, attention span, work performance, and immune status even before a person is anemic.

More North Americans have an iron deficiency without anemia than have iron-deficiency anemia. Their blood hemoglobin values are still normal, but they have no stores to draw from in times of pregnancy or illness, and basic functioning may be at decreased levels. These effects could range from having too little energy to perform everyday tasks in an efficient manner to difficulties staying alert in school or on the job.

To speed the cure of iron-deficiency anemia, a person needs to take iron supplements. A physician should determine the cause of the anemia, be it an inadequate diet or a bleeding ulcer, for example, so that the anemia does not recur. Changes in diet may prevent iron-deficiency anemia, but supplemental iron is the only reliable cure once it has developed.

Iron Sources and Needs

Because animal sources contain some heme iron, the most bioavailable form, they are our best iron sources. The major iron sources in the adult diet are ready-to-eat breakfast cereals, animal products, and bakery items, such as bread (Figs. 9-16 and 9-17). Most of the iron in bakery items has been added to refined flour in the

hematocrit The percentage of blood made up of red blood cells.

anemia Generally refers to a decreased oxygen-carrying capacity of the blood. This can be caused by many factors, such as iron deficiency or blood loss.

Food Sources of Iron

Food Item and Amount	Iron (milligrams)	Adult Male RDA = 8 milligrams %RDA	Adult Female RDA =18 milligrams %RDA
RDA		100%	100%
Oat bran cereal, 1 cup	15	188%	83%
Baked clams, 3 ounces	14	175%	78%
Spinach, 1 cup	6.4	80%	36%
Kidney beans, 1 cup	5.3	66%	29%
Pot roast, 4 ounces	3.9	49%	22%
Sirloin steak, 4 ounces	3.8	48%	21%
Parsley, 1 cup	3.7	46%	21%
Fried beef liver, 2 ounces	3.6	45%	20%
Shrimp, 3 ounces	2.7	34%	15%
Braunschweiger sausage, 1 piece	2.7	34%	15%
Flour tortilla, 1	2.4	30%	13%
Garbanzo beans, ½ cup	2.4	30%	13%
Navy beans, ½ cup	2.3	29%	13%
Baked potato, 1	1.7	21%	9%
Artichoke, 1	1.6	20%	9%

Daily Value = 18 milligrams

Key:
- Grains
- Vegetables
- Fruits
- Dairy
- Protein

FIGURE 9-16 ▶ Food sources of iron compared to the RDA for adult males and females.

FIGURE 9-17 ▶ Sources of iron from MyPlate. The fill of the background color (none, 1/3, 2/3, or completely covered) within each group on the plate indicates the average nutrient density for iron in that group. Overall, the protein group and the grains group contain many foods that are nutrient-dense sources of iron. Still, the iron content of a food containing mostly nonheme iron is only an approximate measure of the amount delivered to body cells, as body need greatly influences the absorption of nonheme iron.

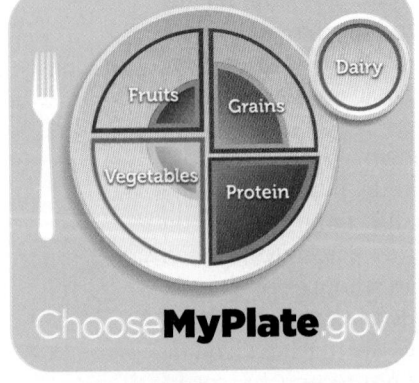

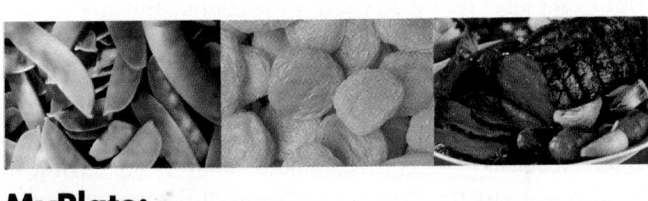

MyPlate: Sources of Iron

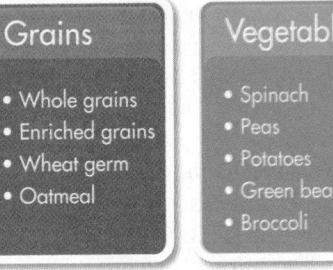
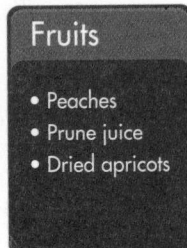
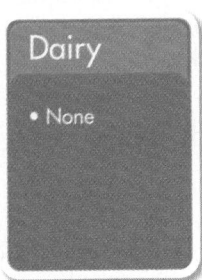
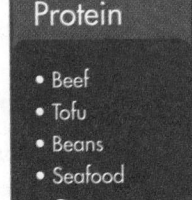

Grains
- Whole grains
- Enriched grains
- Wheat germ
- Oatmeal

Vegetables
- Spinach
- Peas
- Potatoes
- Green beans
- Broccoli

Fruits
- Peaches
- Prune juice
- Dried apricots

Dairy
- None

Protein
- Beef
- Tofu
- Beans
- Seafood
- Organ meats

enrichment process. Other iron sources are spinach, peas, and legumes, but the iron is less available from these foods than from animal products.

Milk is a poor source of iron. A common cause of iron-deficiency anemia in children is an overreliance on milk, coupled with an insufficient meat intake. Total vegetarians (vegans) are particularly susceptible to iron-deficiency anemia because of their lack of dietary heme iron.

The daily adult RDA for iron for men, and for women over 50 years, is 8 milligrams. For women ages 19 to 50 years the RDA is 18 milligrams. The higher RDA for young and middle-age women is primarily because of menstrual blood loss. The variation in menstrual blood loss, and hence, loss of iron, makes it difficult to set an RDA for iron for women. Women who menstruate more heavily and longer than average may need even more dietary iron than those who have lighter and shorter flows. The Daily Value used to express iron content on food and supplement labels is 18 milligrams.

Most women do not consume 18 milligrams of iron daily. The average daily intake is closer to 13 milligrams, while in men it is about 18 milligrams per day. Women can close this gap between average daily intakes and needs by seeking out iron-fortified foods, such as ready-to-eat breakfast cereals that contain at least 50% of the Daily Value. Use of a balanced multivitamin and mineral supplement containing up to 100% of the Daily Value for iron is another option. Consuming more than that much iron is not advised unless a physician suggests otherwise (e.g., compensating for heavy menstrual loss).

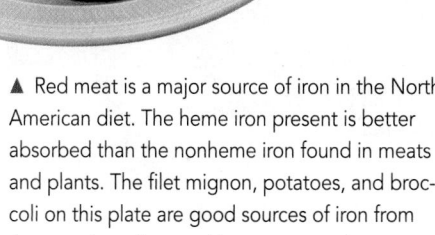

▲ Red meat is a major source of iron in the North American diet. The heme iron present is better absorbed than the nonheme iron found in meats and plants. The filet mignon, potatoes, and broccoli on this plate are good sources of iron from the protein and vegetable groups.

MAKING DECISIONS

Blood Donation

The adult human body contains about 21 cups (5 liters) of blood. Blood donations are generally 2 cups (500 milliliters). Thus, a blood donor gives about a tenth of his or her total supply with each donation. Healthy people generally can donate blood two to four times a year without harmful consequences. As a precaution, blood banks first screen potential donors' blood for the presence of anemia.

Upper Level for Iron

The Upper Level for iron is 45 milligrams per day. Higher amounts can lead to stomach irritation. Although iron overload is not as common as iron deficiency, it can be a serious result of misuse because iron can easily build up in the body and lead to toxic symptoms. Even a large single dose of 60 milligrams of iron can be life-threatening to a 1-year-old. Children are frequently victims of iron poisoning because iron pills and nutrient supplements containing iron are tempting when accessible on kitchen tables and even from cabinets.

FDA has ruled that all iron supplements must carry a warning about toxicity and that tablets with 30 milligrams of iron or more must be individually wrapped. Smaller doses of iron (but still greater than what is needed) over a long period can also cause problems. Repeated blood transfusions can also lead to iron toxicity.

Hemochromatosis. Iron toxicity can occur as a result of the genetic disease called hereditary **hemochromatosis**. The disease is associated with a substantial increase in iron absorption. Heme iron poses the greatest risk as body needs do not influence its absorption to a great extent. For people with this disease, iron in the body eventually builds up to dangerous amounts, especially in the blood and liver. Some iron is deposited in the muscles, pancreas, and heart. If not treated, the excess iron deposits contribute to severe organ damage, especially in the liver and heart.

Development of hereditary hemochromatosis requires that a person carry two defective copies of a particular gene. People with one defective gene and one normal

Chapter 8 noted that if men, in general, and older women take a multivitamin and mineral supplement, it should be low in iron or iron-free because of their increased risk for iron toxicity.

hemochromatosis A disorder of iron metabolism characterized by increased iron absorption and deposition in the liver and heart tissue. This eventually poisons the cells in those organs.

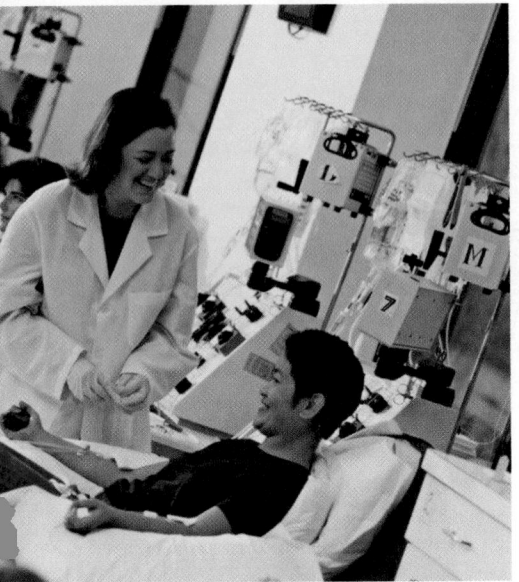

▲ Young adult women should avoid frequent blood donations because a significant amount of iron is lost in each donation. Blood donation, however, is an effective treatment for hemochromatosis.

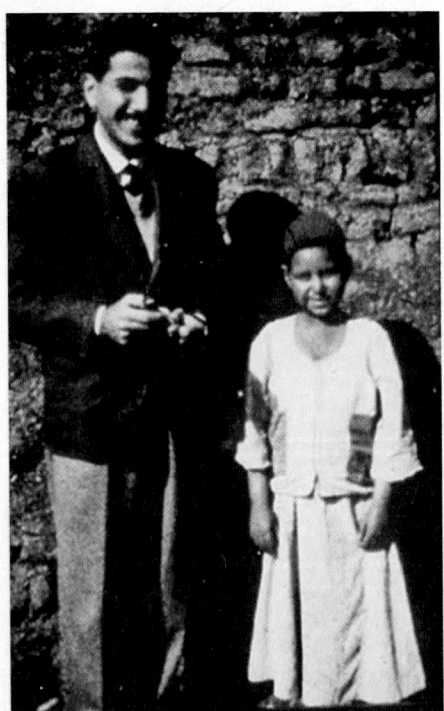

▲ Low intakes of zinc limit growth in people worldwide. On the right, an Egyptian farm boy, age 16 years old and 49 inches tall, with limited growth and sexual development associated with zinc deficiency.

gene, called carriers, may also absorb too much dietary iron but not to the same extent as those with two defective genes. About 5% to 10% of North Americans of Northern European descent are carriers of hemochromatosis. Approximately 1 in 250 North Americans has both hemochromatosis genes. These numbers are high considering that many physicians regard hemochromatosis as a rare disease and thus do not routinely test for it.

A reasonable approach is for you to ask to be screened for iron overload at your next visit to a physician (ask for a transferrin saturation test or a ferritin test to assess iron stores). Hemochromatosis can go undetected until a person is in their fifties or sixties, so some experts recommend screening for anyone over the age of 20. If the disease goes untreated, many organs will have become irreversibly damaged by one's middle years. If you show evidence of hemochromatosis, it would be wise to undergo therapy. This includes regular blood donations and avoidance of iron-rich foods and iron supplements (see the website www.americanhs.org).

Ideally, consent of a physician should precede any intake of iron from supplements, especially by men. When iron supplements are advised, there should be adequate follow-up so that supplementation does not exceed what is necessary. Probably the only factor keeping many people with hemochromatosis and carriers of one gene from experiencing serious effects of the disease is that they consume only a moderate amount of iron.

CONCEPT CHECK

Iron is absorbed depending mostly on its form and the body's need for it. Absorption is affected by iron needs but excess iron intake can override the system, leading to toxicity. Nonheme iron absorption increases somewhat in the presence of vitamin C and meat protein and decreases in the presence of large amounts of some components of grain fiber, such as phytic acid. Iron is used in synthesizing hemoglobin and myoglobin, in supporting immune function, and in energy metabolism. An iron deficiency can cause decreased red blood cell synthesis, which can lead to anemia. It is particularly important for women of childbearing age to consume adequate iron, primarily to replace that lost in menstrual blood. Sources include red meat, pork, liver, enriched grains and cereals, and oysters. Iron toxicity usually results from a genetic disorder called hemochromatosis. This disease causes overabsorption and accumulation of iron, which can result in severe liver and heart damage. Any use of iron supplements should be supervised by a physician because of the risk of toxicity.

9.13 Zinc (Zn)

Zinc deficiency was first recognized in humans in the early 1960s in Egypt and Iran. Zinc deficiencies were determined to cause growth retardation and poor sexual development in some groups of people, even though the zinc content of their diets was fairly high. The zinc bioavailability of the customary diet however, was decreased by the lack of animal protein and almost exclusive use of unleavened bread. Unleavened bread is very high in phytic acid and other factors that decrease zinc bioavailability.

In North America, zinc deficiencies were first observed in the early 1970s in hospitalized patients who were fed only intravenously via total parenteral nutrition containing individual amino acids as the protein source. Zinc deficiency symptoms quickly developed because amino-acid formulas are low in trace minerals compared to whole proteins.

Like iron, zinc absorption is influenced by the foods a person ingests. About 40% of dietary zinc is absorbed, especially when animal protein sources are used and when the body needs more zinc. Most people worldwide rely on cereal grains (low in zinc) for their sources of protein and calories. This makes consuming adequate zinc a problem. In addition, high-dose calcium supplementation with meals decreases zinc absorption. Finally, zinc competes with copper and iron for absorption, and vice versa, when supplemental sources are taken.

Functions of Zinc

Up to 200 or so enzymes, such as alcohol dehydrogenase, require zinc as a cofactor for optimal activity. Adequate zinc intake is necessary to support many bodily functions, such as:

- DNA synthesis and function
- Protein metabolism, wound healing, and growth
- Immune function (intakes in excess of the RDA do not provide any extra benefit to immune function)
- Development of sexual organs and bones
- Storage, release, and function of insulin
- Cell membrane structure and function
- Indirect antioxidant as a component of two forms of superoxide dismutase, an enzyme that aids in the prevention of oxidative damage to cells.

Other possible functions of zinc are slowing the progression of macular degeneration of the eye and reducing the risk for developing certain forms of cancer. One study has shown that megadose zinc supplements (80 milligrams per day of zinc oxide) reduces the progression of macular degeneration by 25% in people who had a moderate case of the disease. The zinc supplements worked even better when provided in combination with 400 IU of vitamin E, 500 milligrams of vitamin C, and 15 milligrams of beta-carotene. (Copper oxide [2 milligrams] was also included because zinc decreases copper absorption.) Experts suggest that adults who have evidence of moderate macular degeneration talk to their physicians and eyecare specialists about the possibility of following such a protocol.

Symptoms of adult zinc deficiency include an acnelike rash, diarrhea, lack of appetite, reduced sense of taste and smell, and hair loss. In children and adolescents with zinc deficiency, growth, sexual development, and learning ability may also be hampered.

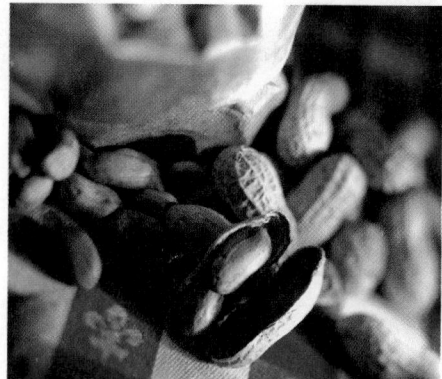

▲ Peanuts are a plant source of zinc.

Zinc Sources and Needs

In general, protein-rich diets are also rich in zinc. Animal foods supply almost half of an individual's zinc intake. Major sources of zinc are beef, fortified breakfast cereals, milk, poultry, and bread. As with iron, bioavailability is also important to consider for zinc. Animal foods are again our prime sources because zinc from animal sources is not bound by phytic acid. However, good plant sources of zinc—such as whole grains, peanuts, and legumes (beans)—should not be discounted. They can deliver substantial amounts of zinc to body cells (Figs. 9-18 and 9-19). Also, the form generally used in multivitamin and mineral supplements (zinc oxide) is not as well absorbed as zinc found naturally in foods, but still contributes to meeting zinc needs.

The adult RDA for zinc is 11 milligrams for men and 8 milligrams for women, based on the amount to cover daily losses of zinc. The Daily Value used to express zinc content on food and supplement labels is 15 milligrams. The average North American takes in 10 to 14 milligrams of zinc per day, with men consuming the higher values. There are no indications of moderate or severe zinc deficiencies in an otherwise healthy adult population. It is likely, however, that some North Americans—especially some women, poor children, vegans, older people, and people with alcoholism—have a marginal zinc status. These and other people who show deterioration in taste sensation, recurring infections, poor growth, or depressed wound healing should have zinc status checked. Unfortunately, it is difficult to detect early signs of a zinc deficiency (see Further Reading 9).

FIGURE 9-18 ▶ Sources of zinc from MyPlate. The fill of the background color (none, 1/3, 2/3, or completely covered) within each group on the plate indicates the average nutrient density for zinc in that group. Overall, the protein group and the grains group contain many foods that are nutrient-dense sources of zinc.

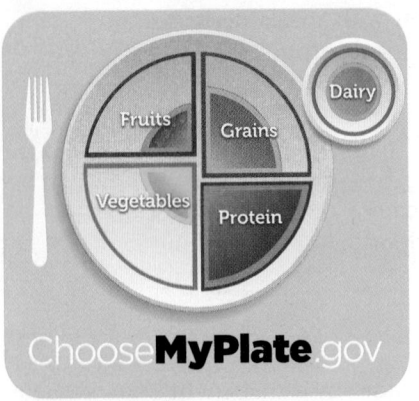

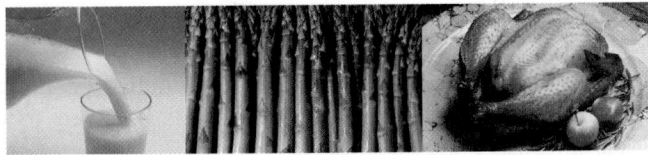

MyPlate: Sources of Zinc

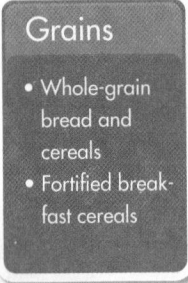

Grains
- Whole-grain bread and cereals
- Fortified breakfast cereals

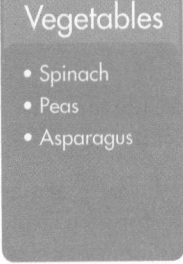

Vegetables
- Spinach
- Peas
- Asparagus

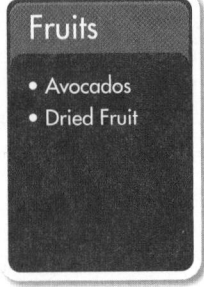

Fruits
- Avocados
- Dried Fruit

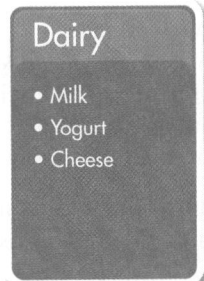

Dairy
- Milk
- Yogurt
- Cheese

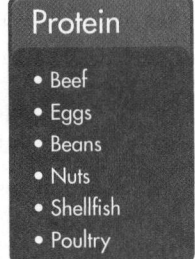

Protein
- Beef
- Eggs
- Beans
- Nuts
- Shellfish
- Poultry

Food Sources of Zinc

Food Item and Amount	Zinc (milligrams)	Adult Male RDA = 11 milligrams %RDA	Adult Female RDA = 8 milligrams %RDA
		Daily Value = 15 milligrams	
RDA		100%	100%
Steamed oysters, 3	24.9	226%	311%
Sirloin steak, 4 ounces	7.4	67%	93%
Pot roast, 3 ounces	4.6	42%	58%
Special K cereal, 1 cup	3.8	35%	48%
Wheat germ, ¼ cup	3.5	32%	44%
Lamb chops, 3 ounces	2.7	25%	34%
Peanuts, ½ cup	2.4	22%	30%
Black-eyed peas, 1 cup	2.2	20%	28%
Plain yogurt, 1 cup	2.2	20%	28%
Lean ham, 3 ounces	1.9	17%	24%
Swiss cheese, 1.5 ounces	1.7	15%	21%
Ricotta cheese, ½ cup	1.7	15%	21%
Sunflower seeds, 1 ounce	1.5	14%	19%
Cheddar cheese, 1.5 ounces	1.3	12%	16%
Enriched white rice, ½ cup	1.1	10%	14%

Key:
- Grains
- Vegetables
- Fruits
- Dairy
- Protein

FIGURE 9-19 ▶ Food sources of zinc compared to the RDA for adult males and females.

Upper Level for Zinc

The Upper Level for zinc is 40 milligrams per day based on the potential interference with copper metabolism. Excessive zinc intakes over time can lead to problems by interfering with copper metabolism. An increased risk for prostate cancer with high intakes of zinc is also under study. Overall, if a person uses megadose zinc supplements (e.g., to try to slow macular degeneration), he or she should be under close medical supervision and also take a supplement containing copper (2 milligrams per day). Zinc intakes over 100 milligrams per day also result in diarrhea, cramps, nausea, vomiting, and depressed immune system function, especially if intake exceeds 2 grams per day.

MAKING DECISIONS

Zinc and the Common Cold

Many companies are singing the praises of zinc as a cold remedy. Products such as Cold-EEZE are lozenges that contain zinc, and their claims are based largely on one study done with 100 participants. The 50 individuals in the experimental group took 13 milligrams of zinc via the lozenges every 2 hours for the duration of their symptoms. Cold symptoms subsided after 4 days in the experimental group and 7 days in the control group. Nausea was a common side effect of the zinc lozenges. Of 10 other follow-up studies, however, only half have shown beneficial results from zinc. This may be due to differences in the bioavailability of various forms of zinc. Experts also note that we also have no idea of how the zinc would treat a cold, if it did. Adults can determine if the benefits outweigh the taste. Zinc expert Dr. Ananda Prasad recommends discontinuing use of zinc lozenges after 3 to 4 days unless they are showing evidence of effectiveness. Any use of such amounts beyond a week or so is potentially dangerous.

9.14 Selenium (Se)

Selenium exists in many readily absorbed forms. Like zinc, selenium has an indirect antioxidant function. Selenium's best understood role is as part of the enzyme (glutathione peroxidase) that works to reduce damage to cell membranes from electron-seeking, free-radical (oxidizing) compounds. Selenium also contributes to thyroid hormone metabolism and other functions.

In Chapter 8 you saw that vitamin E helps prevent attacks on cell membranes by donating electrons to electron-seeking compounds. Thus, vitamin E and selenium work together toward the same goal. The potential for free-radical compounds to cause cancer was also discussed in Chapter 8. Although selenium could prove to have a role in prevention of cancers, such as prostate cancer, it is premature to recommend megadose selenium supplementation for this purpose. Animal studies in this area are conflicting; recent studies with humans using supplemental intakes of 200 micrograms per day have shown no benefit of selenium in cancer prevention (see Further Reading 11).

Selenium deficiency symptoms in humans include muscle pain and wasting and a certain form of heart damage. In some areas of China, people develop characteristic muscle and heart disorders associated with inadequate selenium intake. Other factors probably also contribute.

Selenium Sources and Needs

Fish, meats (especially organ meats), eggs, and shellfish are good animal sources of selenium (Fig. 9-20). Grains and seeds grown in soils containing selenium are good plant sources. Major selenium contributors to the adult diet are animal and grain products.

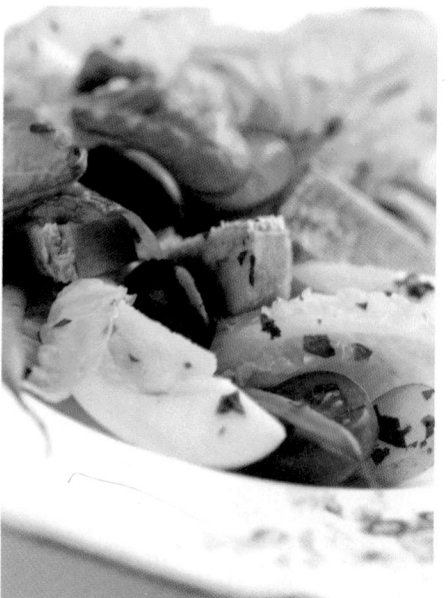

▲ The tuna and egg in this Salade Niçoise are excellent sources of selenium.

CRITICAL THINKING

Tammy read an article about antioxidants and their role in preventing free-radical damage to cells. When Tammy went to the drugstore to take a closer look at such supplements, she saw that selenium was one of the antioxidants in the supplements. Why does selenium deserve consideration as an antioxidant?

FIGURE 9-20 ▶ Food sources of selenium compared to the RDA.

Food Sources of Selenium

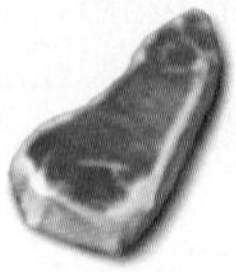

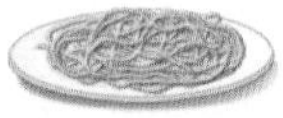

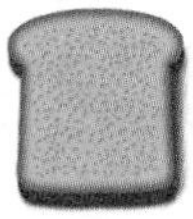

Food Item and Amount	Selenium (micrograms)	Adult Male and Female RDA = 55 micrograms
		Daily Value = 70 micrograms %RDA
RDA*	55	100%
Tuna, 3 ounces	68	124%
Sirloin steak, 5 ounces	47	85%
Lean ham, 3 ounces	42	76%
Clams, 3 ounces	41	75%
Salmon, 3 ounces	40	73%
Egg noodles, 1 cup	35	64%
Chicken breast, 3 ounces	20	36%
Special K cereal, 1 cup	17	31%
Oat bran cereal, 1 cup	14	25%
Whole-wheat bread, 1 slice	10	18%
Cooked oatmeal, 1 cup	10	18%
White bread, 1 slice	9	16%
Raisin bran cereal, 1 cup	4	7%

Key:
■ Grains
■ Vegetables
■ Fruits
■ Dairy
■ Protein

ChooseMyPlate.gov

*For adults; see DRI table in the back of this book for gender- and age-specific recommendations.

We eat a varied diet of foods supplied from many geographic areas, so it is unlikely that low soil selenium in a few locations will mean inadequate selenium in our diets.

The RDA for selenium is 55 micrograms per day for adults. This intake maximizes the activity of selenium-dependent enzymes. The Daily Value used to express selenium content on food and supplement labels is 70 micrograms. In general, adults meet the RDA, consuming on average 105 micrograms of selenium each day.

Upper Level for Selenium

The Upper Level for selenium is 400 micrograms per day for adults. This is based on overt signs of selenium toxicity, such as hair loss.

CONCEPT CHECK

Zinc functions as a cofactor for many enzymes (including those that act as antioxidants) and is important for growth, cell membrane structure and function, immune function, and sense of taste. Beef, seafood, and whole grains are good food sources. As in the case of iron, zinc absorption is regulated according to the body's needs for the mineral. If taken in excess amounts, zinc competes with copper for absorption. Selenium activates an enzyme that helps change electron-seeking, free-radical (oxidizing) compounds into less toxic compounds so these do not attack and break down cell membranes. By helping to dismantle the free-radical compounds, selenium works toward the same goal as vitamin E in providing antioxidant protection to the body. A selenium deficiency results in muscle and heart disorders. Animal products and grains are good selenium sources; however, the selenium content in plants depends on the selenium concentration in the soil. The misuse of both selenium and zinc supplements can readily lead to toxic results.

9.15 Iodide (I)

Iodine in foods is found in an ion form, called iodide. During World War I, a link was discovered between a deficiency of iodide and the production of a **goiter,** an enlarged thyroid gland. Men drafted from areas such as the Great Lakes Region of the United States had a much higher rate of goiter than did men from some other areas of the country. The soils in these areas have low iodide contents. In the 1920s, researchers in Ohio found that low doses of iodide given to children over a 4-year period could prevent goiter. That finding led to the addition of iodide to salt beginning in the 1920s.

Today, many nations such as Canada require iodide fortification of salt. In the United States, salt can be purchased either iodized or plain. Iodized salt is clearly marked on the label of a package of salt. Some areas of Europe, such as northern Italy, have low levels of iodide in soil, but have yet to adopt an iodide fortification program. People in these areas, especially women, still suffer from goiter, as do people in areas of Latin America, the Indian subcontinent, Southeast Asia, and Africa. About 2 billion people worldwide are at risk of iodide deficiency, and approximately 800 million of these people have suffered the widespread effects of the deficiency. Eradication of iodide deficiency is a goal of many health-related organizations worldwide.

Function of Iodide

The thyroid gland actively accumulates and traps iodide from the bloodstream to support thyroid hormone synthesis. Thyroid hormones are synthesized using iodide and the amino acid tyrosine. These hormones help regulate metabolic rate and promote growth and development throughout the body, including the brain.

If a person's iodide intake is insufficient, the thyroid gland enlarges as it attempts to take up more iodide from the bloodstream. This eventually leads to goiter. Simple goiter is a painless condition, but if uncorrected can lead to pressure on the trachea (windpipe), which may cause difficulty in breathing. Although iodide can prevent goiter formation, it does not significantly shrink a goiter once it has formed. Surgical removal may be required in severe cases.

If a woman has an iodide-deficient diet during the early months of her pregnancy, the fetus suffers iodide deficiency because the mother's body uses up the available iodide. The infant then may be born with short length and develop mental retardation. The stunted growth and mental retardation that results is known as **cretinism.** Cretinism appeared in North America before iodide fortification of table salt began. Today, cretinism still appears in Europe, Africa, Latin America, and Asia.

Iodide Sources and Needs

Saltwater fish, seafood, iodized salt, dairy products, and grain products contain various forms of iodide (Fig. 9-21). Sea salt found in health-food stores, however, is not a good source because the iodide is lost during processing.

The RDA for iodide for adults is 150 micrograms to support thyroid gland function. This is the same as the Daily Value used to express iodide content on food and supplement labels. A half teaspoon of iodide-fortified salt (about 2 grams) supplies that amount. Most adults consume more iodide than the RDA—an estimated 190 to 300 micrograms daily, not including that from use of iodized salt at the table. The iodide in our diets adds up because dairies and fast-food restaurants use it as a sterilizing agent, bakeries use it as a dough conditioner, food producers use it as part of food colorants, and it is added to salt. There is concern, however, that vegans may not consume enough unless iodized salt is used.

Upper Level for Iodide

The Upper Level for iodide is 1.1 milligrams per day. When high amounts of iodide are consumed, thyroid hormone synthesis is inhibited, as in a deficiency. This can

goiter An enlargement of the thyroid gland; this is often caused by insufficient iodide in the diet.

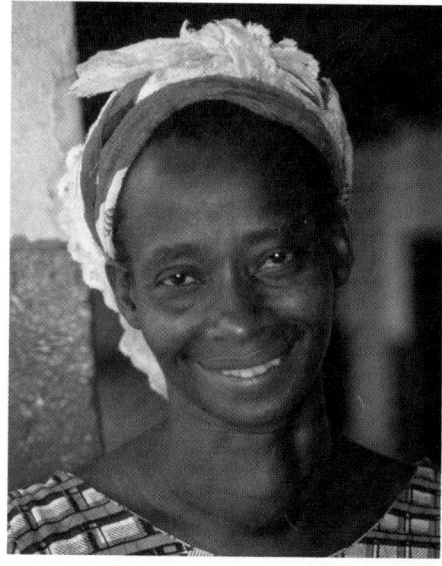

▲ This woman has an enlargement of the thyroid gland also known as a goiter caused by insufficient iodide in the diet.

cretinism The stunting of body growth and poor mental development in the offspring that results from inadequate maternal intake of iodide during pregnancy.

FIGURE 9-21 ▶ Food sources of Iodide compared to the RDA.

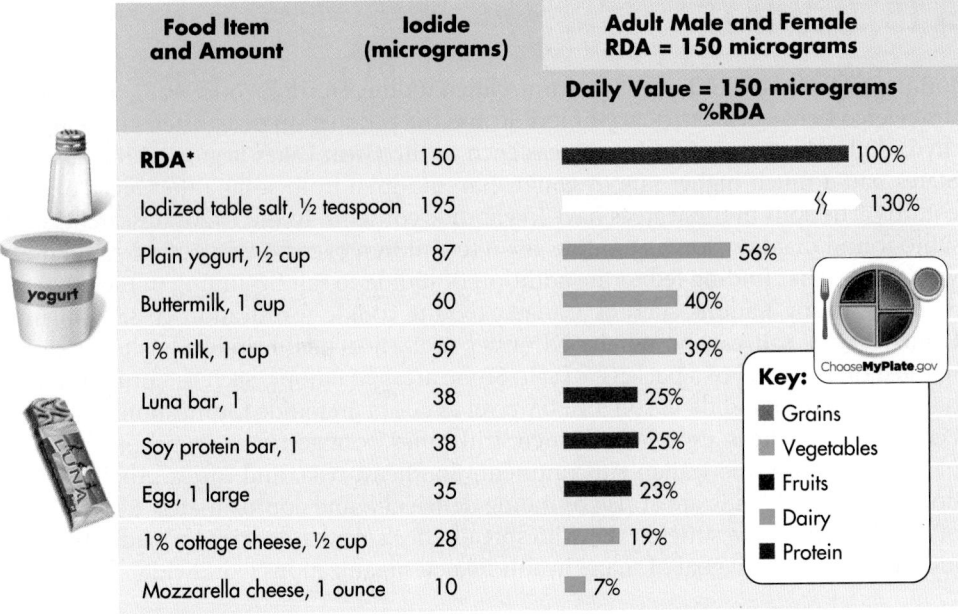

Food Item and Amount	Iodide (micrograms)	Adult Male and Female RDA = 150 micrograms Daily Value = 150 micrograms %RDA	
RDA*	150		100%
Iodized table salt, ½ teaspoon	195		130%
Plain yogurt, ½ cup	87		56%
Buttermilk, 1 cup	60		40%
1% milk, 1 cup	59		39%
Luna bar, 1	38		25%
Soy protein bar, 1	38		25%
Egg, 1 large	35		23%
1% cottage cheese, ½ cup	28		19%
Mozzarella cheese, 1 ounce	10		7%

Key:
- ■ Grains
- ■ Vegetables
- ■ Fruits
- ■ Dairy
- ■ Protein

ChooseMyPlate.gov

*For adults; see the DRI table in the back of this book for gender- and age-specific recommendations.

appear in people who eat a lot of seaweed, because some seaweeds contain as much as 1% iodide by weight. Total iodide intake then can add up to 60 to 130 times the RDA.

9.16 Copper (Cu)

Copper is involved in the metabolism of iron by functioning in the formation of hemoglobin and transport of iron. A copper-containing enzyme aids in the release of iron from storage. Copper is needed by enzymes that create cross-links in connective tissue proteins. Copper is also needed by other enzymes, such as those that defend the body against free-radical (oxidizing) compounds (e.g., a form of superoxide dismutase) and those that act in the brain and nervous system. Finally, copper performs in immune system function, blood clotting, and blood lipoprotein metabolism. About 12% to 75% of dietary copper is absorbed, with higher intakes associated with lower absorption. Absorption takes place primarily in the stomach and upper small intestine. Copper is excreted in the bile made by the liver and released by the gallbladder. Phytates, fiber, as well as zinc and iron supplements, may all interfere with copper absorption. Symptoms of copper deficiency include a form of anemia, low white blood cell count, bone loss, poor growth, and some forms of cardiovascular disease.

Copper Sources and Needs

Copper is found primarily in liver, seafood, cocoa, legumes, nuts, seeds, and whole-grain breads and cereals (Fig. 9-22).

The RDA for copper is 900 micrograms daily for adults, based on the amount needed for activity of copper-containing proteins and enzymes in the body. The Daily Value used to express copper content on food and supplement labels is 2 milligrams. The average adult intake is about 1 to 1.6 milligrams per day. Women generally consume the smaller amount. The form of copper typically found in multivitamin and mineral supplements (copper oxide) is not readily absorbed. It is best to rely on food sources to meet copper needs. The copper status of adults appears to be good, though we lack sensitive measures to determine copper status.

The groups most likely to develop copper deficiencies are preterm infants, infants recovering from semistarvation on a milk-dominated diet (a poor source of copper),

▲ Seafood is one source of copper in the diet

Food Sources of Copper

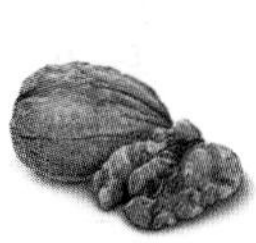

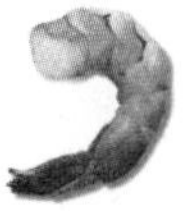

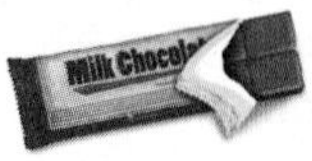

FIGURE 9-22 ▶ Food sources of copper compared to the RDA.

Food Item and Amount	Copper (milligrams)	Adult Male and Female RDA = 900 milligrams Daily Value = 2 milligrams %RDA
RDA*	900	100%
Fried beef liver, 3 ounces	3800	422%
Power bar, 1	700	78%
Walnuts, ½ cup	600	67%
Kidney beans, ½ cup	500	56%
Lobster, 3 ounces	400	44%
Molasses, 3 tablespoons	300	33%
Sunflower seeds, 2 tablespoons	300	33%
Shrimp, 3 ounces	300	33%
Raisin Bran cereal, 1 cup	300	33%
Great Grains cereal, 1 cup	300	33%
Black-eyed peas, ½ cup cooked	200	22%
Wheat germ, ¼ cup	200	22%
Milk chocolate, 1 ounce	110	12%
Whole-wheat bread, 1 slice	80	9%

ChooseMyPlate.gov

Key:
■ Grains
■ Vegetables
■ Fruits
■ Dairy
■ Protein
■ Discretionary calories

*For adults; see the DRI table in the back of this book for gender- and age-specific recommendations.

and people recovering from intestinal surgery (during which time copper absorption decreases). Recall that a copper deficiency can also result from overzealous supplementation of zinc, because zinc and copper compete with each other for absorption.

Upper Level for Copper

The Upper Limit for copper is 10 milligrams per day. High doses of copper can cause toxicity, including vomiting, at single doses of greater than 10 milligrams. Other effects, such as liver toxicity, are also possible with megadose uses.

9.17 Fluoride (F)

The fluoride ion (F⁻) is the form of this trace mineral essential for human health. Like chlorine, fluorine (F₂) is a poisonous gas. This link was found as dentists in the early 1900s noticed a lower rate of dental caries (cavities) in the southwestern United States. These areas contained high amounts of fluoride in the water. The amounts of fluoride were sometimes so high that small spots on the teeth, called **mottling**, appeared. Even though mottled teeth were quite discolored, they contained very few dental caries. After experiments showed that fluoride in the water did indeed decrease the rate of dental caries, controlled fluoridation of water in parts of the United States began in 1945.

Those who grew up drinking fluoridated water generally have 40% to 60% fewer dental caries than people who did not drink fluoridated water as children. Dentists can provide topical fluoride treatments, and schools can provide fluoride tablets, but it is much less expensive and more reliable to add fluoride to a community's drinking

mottling The discoloration or marking of the surface of teeth from fluorosis.

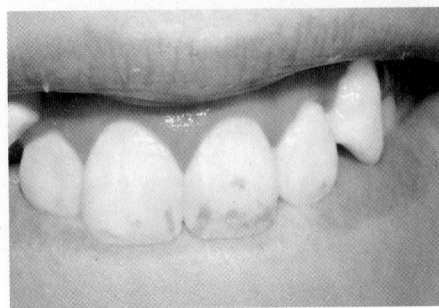

▲ Example of mottling in a tooth caused by overexposure to fluoride.

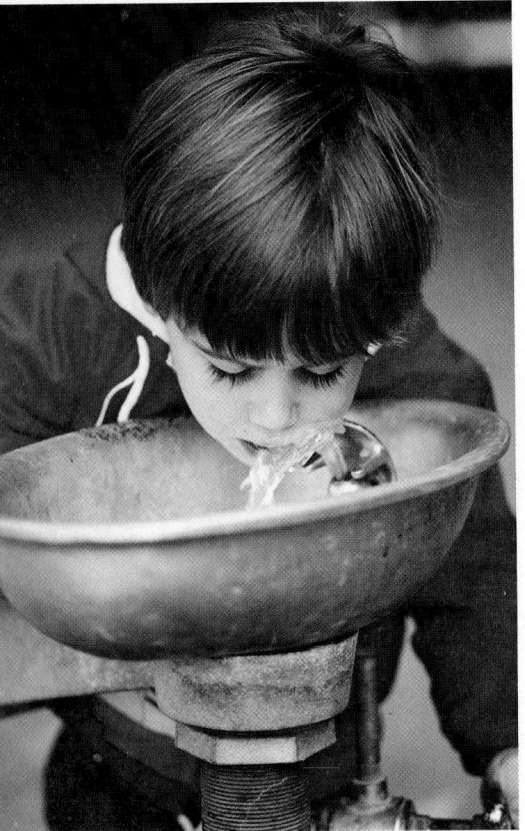

▲ Fluoridated water is responsible for much of the decrease in dental caries throughout North America.

water. State and private water sources do not always contain enough fluoride, however. When in doubt, contact your local water plant or have the water in your home analyzed for fluoride content. If it is less than 1 part fluoride per million parts of water (e.g., 1 milligram per kilogram or liter of water), talk to your dentist about the best means to obtain the fluoride.

Functions of Fluoride

Dietary fluoride consumed during childhood, when bones and teeth are developing, aids the synthesis of a form of tooth enamel that strongly resists acid. Therefore, teeth become resistant to dental caries. Fluoride also inhibits metabolism and growth of the bacteria that cause dental caries, and fluoride present in saliva directly inhibits tooth demineralization and enhances tooth remineralization.

Fluoride applied to the surface of the teeth by dentists or from toothpaste or rinses adds additional protection against dental caries. Thus, people of all ages benefit from the topical effects of fluoride, whether they consumed fluoridated water or fluoride supplements as children (see Further Reading 1).

Fluoride Sources and Needs

Tea, seafood, seaweed, and some natural water sources are the only good food sources of fluoride. Most of our fluoride intake comes from fluoride added to drinking water and toothpaste and from fluoride treatments performed by dentists. Fluoride is not added to bottled water. Therefore, if people such as children consume bottled water, they won't receive fluoride from such water intake.

The Adequate Intake for fluoride for adults is 3.1 to 3.8 milligrams per day. This range of intake provides the benefits of resistance to dental caries without causing ill effects. Typical fluoridated water contains about 1 milligram per liter, which works out to about 0.25 milligrams per cup.

Upper Level for Fluoride

The Upper Level for fluoride is set at 1.3 to 2.2 milligrams per day for young children, and 10 milligrams per day for children over 9 years of age and adults, based on skeletal and tooth damage seen with higher doses. If children swallow large amounts of fluoridated toothpaste as part of daily tooth care, tooth mottling may develop. Not swallowing toothpaste and limiting the amount used to "pea" size are the best ways to prevent this problem. In addition, children under 6 years should have toothbrushing supervised by an adult. Fluoride-related mottling only occurs during tooth development, so adults do not develop mottling from their fluoride exposure.

CONCEPT CHECK

Iodide is vital for the synthesis of thyroid hormones. A prolonged insufficient intake causes the thyroid gland to enlarge, resulting in a goiter. The use of iodized salt in North America has virtually eliminated this condition. Copper functions mainly in iron and free-radical metabolism, and in the cross-bonding of connective tissue. A deficiency can result in a type of anemia. Good food sources of copper are seafoods, legumes, nuts, dried fruits, and whole grains. Fluoride becomes incorporated into teeth during development and is present in salivary secretions. The presence of this trace mineral makes teeth resistant to acid and bacterial growth, in turn reducing development of dental caries. Fluoride also aids in remineralization of teeth once decay begins. Most of us receive adequate amounts of fluoride from that added to drinking water and toothpaste. An excessive fluoride intake during tooth development can lead to spotted (i.e., mottled) teeth and possibly bone damage.

9.18 Chromium (Cr)

The importance of chromium in human diets has been recognized only in the past 40 years. The most-studied function of chromium is the maintenance of glucose uptake into cells. Our current understanding is that chromium enters the cell and acts to enhance the transport of glucose across the cell membrane by aiding insulin function. Marginal to low chromium intakes may contribute to an increased risk for developing type 2 diabetes, but opinions are mixed on the true degree of this effect.

A chromium deficiency is characterized by impaired blood glucose control and elevated blood cholesterol and triglycerides. The mechanism by which chromium influences cholesterol metabolism is not known but may involve enzymes that control cholesterol synthesis. Chromium deficiency originally appeared in people maintained on intravenous total parenteral nutrition solutions not supplemented with chromium and in children with malnutrition. Sensitive measures of chromium status are not available, so marginal chromium deficiencies may go undetected.

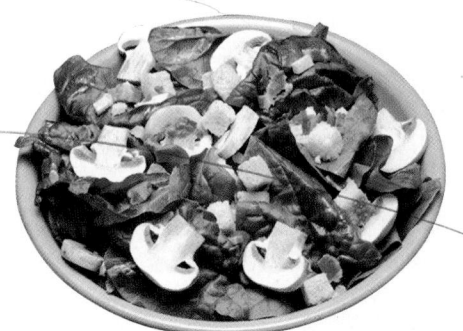

▲ The mushrooms in this spinach salad are a good source of chromium.

Chromium Sources and Needs

Specific data regarding the chromium content of various foods are limited, and most food composition tables do not include values for this trace mineral. Egg yolks, whole grains (bran), organ meats, other meats, mushrooms, nuts, and beer are good sources. Yeast is also a source. The amount of chromium in foods is closely tied to the local soil content of chromium. To provide yourself with a good chromium intake, regularly choose whole grains in place of mostly refined grains.

The Adequate Intake for chromium is 25 to 35 micrograms per day, based on the amount present in a balanced diet. The Daily Value used to express chromium content on food and supplement labels is about 4 times greater at 120 micrograms. Average adult intakes in North America are estimated at about 30 micrograms per day, but could be somewhat higher.

No Upper Level for chromium has been set because toxicity for that present in foods has not been observed. Chromium toxicity, however, has been reported in people exposed to industrial waste and in painters who use art supplies with a high chromium content. Liver damage and lung cancer can result. Use of any supplement should normally not exceed the Daily Value set unless supervised by a physician, because of the risk of toxicity.

Chromium supplements have been touted to help with exercise-induced increases in muscle mass and weight loss. Careful research, however, does not support this assertion.

9.19 Manganese (Mn)

The mineral manganese is easily confused with magnesium. Not only are their names similar, but they also often substitute for each other in metabolic processes. Manganese is needed by enzymes used in carbohydrate metabolism and by a form of superoxide dismutase used in free-radical metabolism. Manganese is also important in bone formation.

No human deficiency symptom is associated with a low manganese intake. Our need for manganese is low, and our diets tend to be adequate in this trace mineral.

Good food sources of manganese are nuts, rice, oats and other whole grains, beans, and leafy vegetables. The Adequate Intake for manganese is 1.8 to 2.3 milligrams to offset daily losses. Average intakes generally fall within this range. The Daily Value used to express manganese content on food and supplement labels is 2 milligrams.

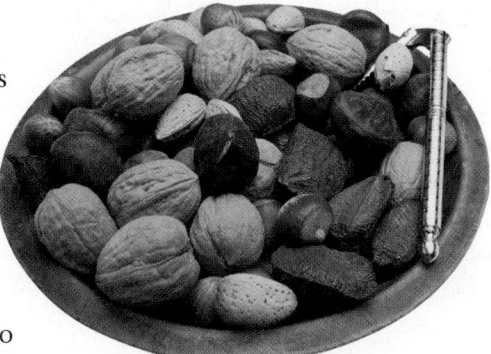

▲ Nuts are rich in manganese.

Upper Level for Manganese

Manganese is toxic at high doses. The Upper Level is 11 milligrams per day and is based on the development of nerve damage.

9.20 Molybdenum (Mo)

Several human enzymes use molybdenum. No molybdenum deficiency has been noted in people who consume normal diets, though deficiency symptoms have appeared in people maintained on intravenous total parenteral nutrition feedings. These symptoms include increased heart and respiration rates, night blindness, mental confusion, edema, and weakness.

Good food sources of molybdenum include milk and milk products, beans, whole grains, and nuts. The RDA for molybdenum is 45 micrograms to offset daily losses. The Daily Value used to express molybdenum content on food and supplement labels is 75 micrograms. Our daily intakes average 75 to 110 micrograms.

Upper Level for Molybdenum

The Upper Level for molybdenum is 2 milligrams per day. When consumed in high doses, molybdenum causes toxicity in laboratory animals, resulting in weight loss and decreased growth.

Table 9-3 summarizes what we have covered regarding the trace minerals, as does Figure 9-23. Figure 9-24 summarizes the various contributions of groups in MyPlate to mineral needs.

FIGURE 9-23 ▶ Water and minerals are involved in many processes in the body.

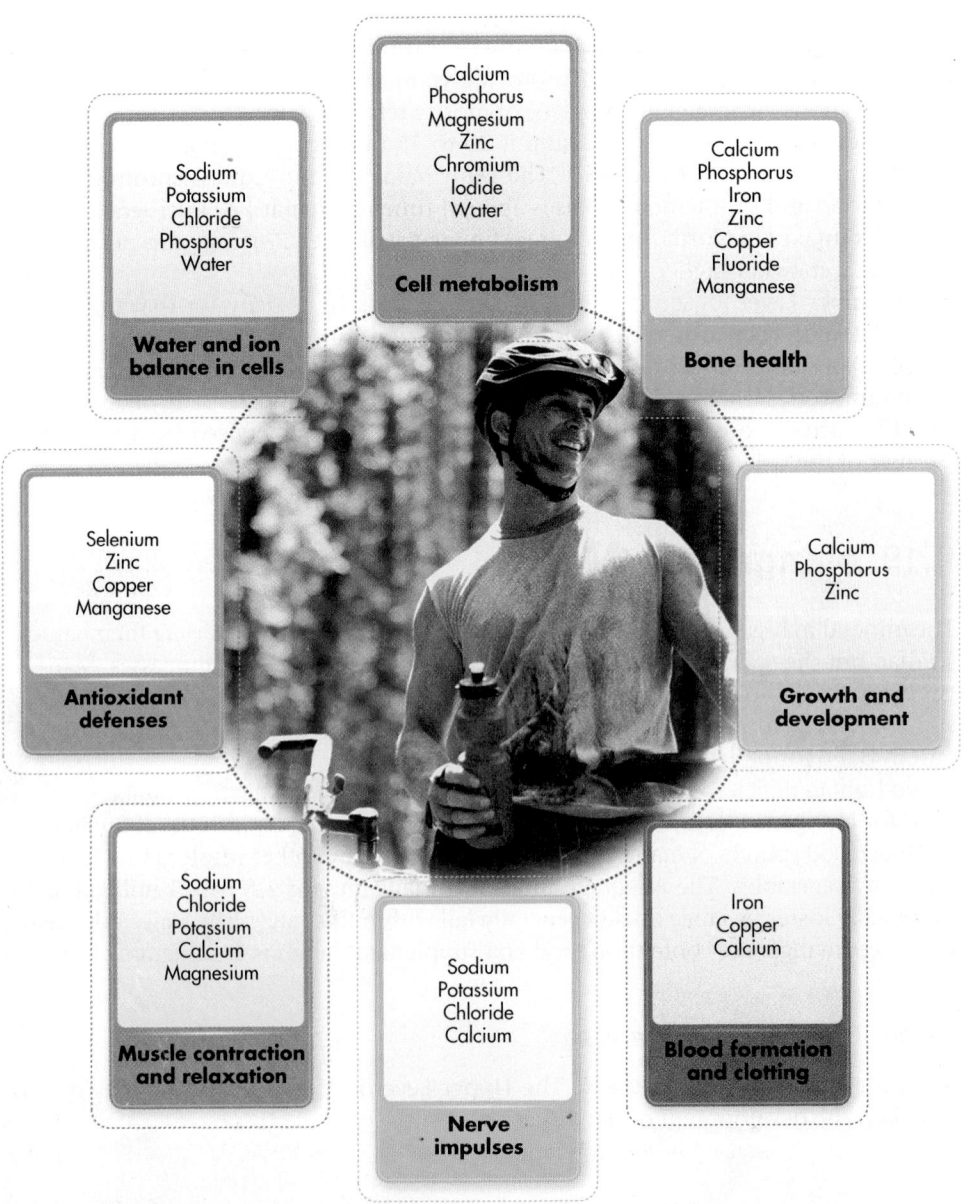

TABLE 9-3 A Summary of Key Trace Minerals

Mineral	Major Functions	RDA, or Adequate Intake	Dietary Sources	Deficiency Symptoms	Toxicity Symptoms
Iron	• Components of hemoglobin and other key compounds used in respiration • Immune function • Cognitive development	*Men:* 8 milligrams *Premenopausal Women:* 18 milligrams	• Meats • Seafood • Broccoli • Peas • Bran • Enriched breads	• Fatigue • Anemia • Low blood hemoglobin values	• Liver and heart damage (extreme cases) • GI upset • Upper Level is 45 milligrams
Zinc	• Required for nearly 200 enzymes • Growth • Immunity • Alcohol metabolism • Sexual development • Reproduction • Antioxidant protection	*Men:* 11 milligrams *Women:* 8 milligrams	• Seafood • Meats • Greens • Whole grains	• Skin rash • Diarrhea • Decreased appetite and sense of taste • Hair loss • Poor growth and development • Poor wound healing	• Reduced copper absorption • Diarrhea • Cramps • Depressed immune function • Upper Level is 40 milligrams
Selenium	• Part of an antioxidant system	55 micrograms	• Meats • Eggs • Fish • Seafood • Whole grains	• Muscle pain • Weakness • Form of heart disease	• Nausea • Vomiting • Hair loss • Weakness • Liver disease • Upper Level is 400 micrograms
Iodide	• Component of thyroid hormones	150 micrograms	• Iodized salt • White bread • Saltwater fish • Dairy products	• Goiter • Mental retardation • Poor growth in infancy when mother is iodide deficient during pregnancy	• Inhibition of thyroid gland function • Upper Level is 1.1 milligrams
Copper	• Aids in iron metabolism • Works with many antioxidant enzymes • Involved with enzymes of protein metabolism and hormone synthesis	900 micrograms	• Liver • Cocoa • Beans • Nuts • Whole grains • Dried fruits	• Anemia • Low white blood cell count • Poor growth	• Vomiting • Nervous system disorders • Upper Level is 8–10 milligrams
Fluoride	• Increases resistance of tooth enamel to dental caries	*Men:* 3.8 milligrams *Women:* 3.1 milligrams	• Fluoridated water • Toothpaste • Tea • Seaweed • Dental treatments	• Increased risk of dental caries	• Stomach upset • Mottling (staining) of teeth during development • Bone pain • Upper Level is 10 milligrams for adults
Chromium	• Enhances insulin action	25–35 micrograms	• Egg yolks • Whole grains • Pork • Nuts • Mushrooms • Beer	• High blood glucose after eating	Caused by industrial contamination, not dietary excesses, so no Upper Level has been set
Manganese	• Cofactor of some enzymes, such as those involved in carbohydrate metabolism • Works with some antioxidant systems	1.8–2.3 milligrams	• Nuts • Oats • Beans • Tea	None observed in humans	• Nervous system disorders • Upper Level is 11 milligrams
Molybdenum	• Aids in action of some enzymes	45 micrograms	• Beans • Grains • Nuts	None observed in healthy humans	• Poor growth in laboratory animals • Upper Level is 2 milligrams

FIGURE 9-24 ▶ Certain groups of MyPlate are especially rich sources of various minerals. This is true for the minerals listed. Each mineral may also be found in other groups, but in lower amounts. Other trace minerals are also present in moderate amounts in many groups. With regard to the grains group, whole-grain varieties are the richest sources of most trace minerals listed.

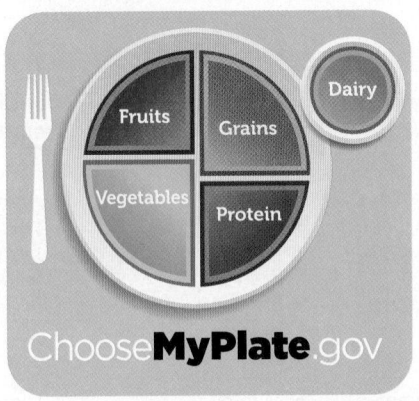

**MyPlate:
Sources of Minerals**

Grains
- Sodium chloride
- Calcium (fortified products)
- Phosphorus
- Magnesium
- Iron
- Zinc
- Copper
- Selenium
- Chromium

Vegetables
- Potassium
- Magnesium

Fruits
- Potassium
- Boron

Dairy
- Calcium
- Phosphorus
- Zinc

Protein
- Sodium chloride (processed foods)
- Potassium
- Phosphorus
- Magnesium
- Selenium
- Iron
- Zinc
- Copper

9.21 Other Trace Minerals

Although a variety of other trace minerals is found in humans, many of them have not yet been shown to be required. The list of minerals in this category includes boron, nickel, vanadium, arsenic, and silicon. Widespread deficiency symptoms in humans have never been noted, probably because typical diets provide adequate amounts of these minerals and they are needed by very few enzymes and metabolic systems. Their potential for toxicity should make one question any supplementation not supervised by a physician. These trace minerals may achieve more importance as more research is reported.

CONCEPT CHECK

Chromium contributes to insulin function. The amount of chromium found in food depends on chromium content of the soil on which it was grown. Meats, whole grains, and egg yolks are good sources. Manganese is a component of bone and is used by many enzymes, including those involved in glucose production. Our need for manganese is low, so deficiencies are rare. Nuts, rice, oats, and beans are good food sources. Molybdenum is another trace mineral required by a few enzymes. Good sources include milk, beans, whole grains, and nuts. Deficiencies have appeared only in people nourished by unsupplemented total parenteral nutrition. The needs for some other trace minerals—such as boron, nickel, arsenic, and vanadium—have not been fully established in humans. If required, these minerals are needed in such small amounts that our current diets are probably adequate sources of them.

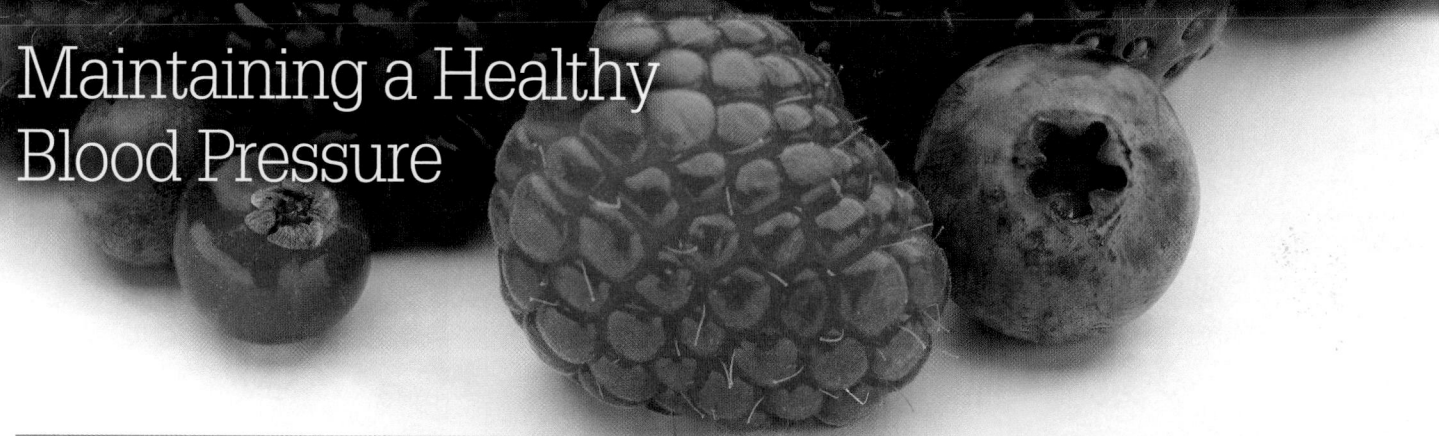

Maintaining a Healthy Blood Pressure

Among North Americans, an estimated 1 in 5 adults has hypertension. Over the age of 65, the number rises to 1 in every 2 adults. Only about half of cases are being treated. Blood pressure is expressed by two numbers. The higher number represents systolic blood pressure, the pressure in the arteries when the heart muscle is contracting and pumping blood into the arteries. Optimal systolic blood pressure is 120 millimeters of mercury (mm Hg) or less. The second value is diastolic blood pressure, the artery pressure when the heart is relaxed. Optimal diastolic blood pressure is 80 mm Hg or less. Elevations in both systolic and diastolic blood pressure are strong predictors of disease (Fig. 9-25).

Hypertension is defined as sustained systolic pressure exceeding 139 mm Hg or diastolic blood pressure exceeding 89 mm Hg. Most cases of hypertension (about 95% of cases) have no clear-cut cause. It is described as primary, or essential (i.e., essential hypertension). Kidney disease, sleep-disordered breathing (sleep apnea), and other causes often lead to the other 5% of cases, known as secondary hypertension. African-Americans are more likely than Caucasians to develop hypertension and to do so earlier in life.

Unless blood pressure is periodically measured, the development of hypertension is easily overlooked. Thus, it's described as a silent disorder, because it usually does not cause symptoms.

Why Control Blood Pressure?

Blood pressure needs to be controlled mainly to prevent cardiovascular disease, kidney disease, strokes and related declines in brain function, poor blood circulation in the legs, problems with vision, and sudden death. These conditions are much more likely to be found in individuals with hypertension than in people with normal blood pressure. Smoking and elevated blood lipoproteins make these diseases even more likely. Individuals with hypertension need to be diagnosed and treated as soon as possible, as the condition generally progresses to a more serious stage over time and even resists therapy if it persists for years.

Causes of Hypertension

A family history of hypertension is a risk factor, especially if both parents have (or had) the problem. In addition, blood pressure usually increases as a person ages. Some increase is caused by atherosclerosis. As plaque builds up in the arteries, the arteries become less flexible and cannot expand. When vessels remain rigid, blood pressure remains high. Eventually, the plaque begins to decrease the blood supply to the kidneys, decreasing their ability to control blood volume and, in turn, blood pressure.

An enzyme secreted by the kidneys and some hormonelike compounds are designed to maintain a healthy blood pressure. When blood pressure is elevated, the effect of these compounds can be reduced by anti-hypertension medications.

Overweight people have six times greater risk of having hypertension than lean people. Overall, obesity is considered the number one lifestyle factor related to hypertension.

This is especially the case in minority populations. Additional blood vessels

How High Is High?

If your systolic and diastolic pressures fall into different categories, your risk depends on the higher category

Hypertension (High)	
	SYSTOLIC 140 / DIASTOLIC 90
Pre-hypertension	
	120 / 80
Normal	

Numbers (in millimeters of mercury) apply to adults who aren't taking drugs to lower their blood pressure.

FIGURE 9-25 ▶ The cutoff for hypertension is 140/90 mm Hg, but the risk of heart attacks and stroke precedes the rise in blood pressure.

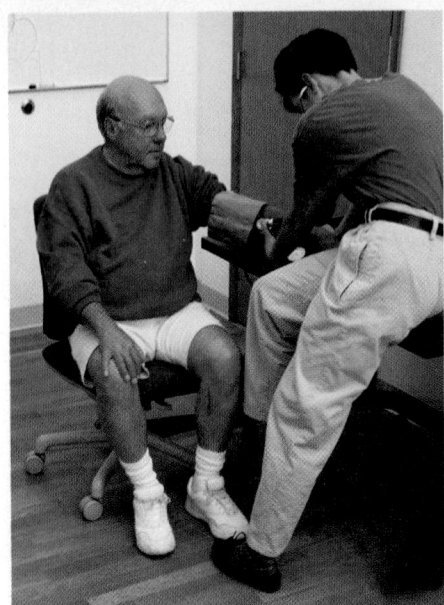

▲ Older adults are particularly at risk of hypertension.

develop to support excess tissue in overweight and obese individuals, and these extra miles of associated blood vessels increase work by the heart and also blood pressure. Hypertension is linked to obesity if elevated blood insulin levels result from insulin-resistant adipose cells. This increased insulin level increases sodium retention in the body and accelerates atherosclerosis. A weight loss of as little as 10 to 15 pounds often can help treat hypertension.

Inactivity is considered the number two lifestyle factor related to hypertension. If an obese person can engage in regular physical activity (at least 5 days per week for 30 to 60 minutes) and lose weight, blood pressure often returns to normal.

Third, excess alcohol intake is responsible for about 10% of all cases of hypertension, especially in middle-aged males and among African-Americans in general. When hypertension is caused by excessive alcohol intake, it is usually reversible. A sensible alcohol intake for people with hypertension is two or fewer drinks per day for men and one or no drinks per day for women and all older adults. Did you recognize that this is the same recommendation given in the 2010 Dietary Guidelines for Americans? Some studies suggest that such a minimal alcohol

intake may reduce the risk of ischemic stroke. These data, however, should not be used to encourage alcohol use.

In some people, particularly African-Americans and older overweight persons, blood pressure is especially sensitive to sodium. In these people, excess salt leads to fluid retention by the kidney and a corresponding increase in blood volume, which therefore increases blood pressure. It is not clear whether the sodium ion or the chloride ion is most responsible for the effect. Still, as reviewed in this chapter, if one reduces sodium intake, chloride intake naturally falls; the opposite is also true. For the most part, a recommendation to consume less sodium is equivalent to a call for less salt in the diet. Only some North Americans are very susceptible to increases in blood pressure from salt intake, so it is only the number four lifestyle factor related to hypertension. It is unfortunate that salt intake receives the major portion of public attention with regard to hypertension. Efforts to prevent hypertension should also focus on obesity, inactivity, and alcohol abuse.

Other Minerals and Blood Pressure

Minerals such as calcium, potassium, and magnesium also deserve attention when it comes to prevention and treatment of hypertension. Studies show that a diet rich in these minerals and low in salt can decrease blood pressure within days of beginning this type of diet, especially among African-Americans. The response is even similar to that seen with

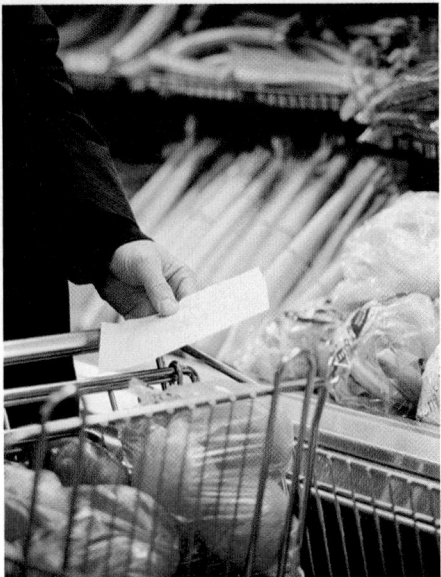

▲ Opting for the fruits, vegetables, and low-fat foods recommended by the DASH diet represents a sound approach to nutrition for most people regardless of hypertension risk.

commonly used medications. The diet is called the Dietary Approaches to Stop Hypertension (DASH) diet (Table 9-4). The diet, rich in calcium, phosphorus, and magnesium and low in salt, takes a standard MyPlate food plan and adds 1 to 2 extra vegetables and fruits servings and a serving of nuts, seeds, or legumes (beans) 4 to 5 days of the week. In DASH studies, participants also consumed no more than 3 grams of sodium and no more than one to two alcoholic drinks per day. A DASH 2 diet trial tested three daily sodium intakes (3300 milligrams, 2400 milligrams, and 1500 milligrams). People showed a steady decline in blood

TABLE 9-4 What Is the DASH Diet?
The DASH diet is characterized as low in fat and sodium and rich in fruits, vegetables, and low-fat dairy products. Here is the breakdown:

Per Day	Per Week
6–8 servings of grains and grain products	4–5 servings of nuts, seeds, or legumes
4–5 servings of fruit	5 servings of sweets and added sugars
4–5 servings of vegetables	
2–3 servings of low-fat or fat-free dairy products	
2 or less servings of meats, poultry, and fish	
2–3 servings of fats/oils	

pressure on the DASH diet as sodium intake declined. Over all, the DASH diet is seen as a total dietary approach to treating hypertension. It is not clear which of the many healthful practices of this diet are responsible for the fall in blood pressure (see Further Readings 2 and 4).

Other studies also show a reduction in stroke risk among people who consume a diet rich in fruits, vegetables, and vitamin C (recall that fruits and vegetables are rich vitamin C sources). Overall, a diet low in salt and rich in low-fat and fat-free dairy products, fruits, vegetables, whole grains, and some nuts can substantially reduce hypertension and stroke risk in many people, especially those with hypertension.

Medications to Treat Hypertension

Diuretic medications are one class of drugs used to treat hypertension. These "water pills" work to reduce blood volume (and therefore blood pressure) by increasing fluid output in the urine. Other medications act by slowing heart rate or by causing relaxation of blood vessels. A combination of two or more medications is commonly required to treat hypertension that does not respond to diet and lifestyle therapy. Read more about the importance of antihypertensive drugs compared to the reduction in salt intake in Further Reading 7.

Prevention of Hypertension

Many of the risk factors for hypertension and stroke are controllable, and appropriate lifestyle changes can reduce a person's risk (Fig. 9-26). Experts also recommend that those with hypertension lower blood pressure through diet and lifestyle changes before resorting to blood pressure medications.

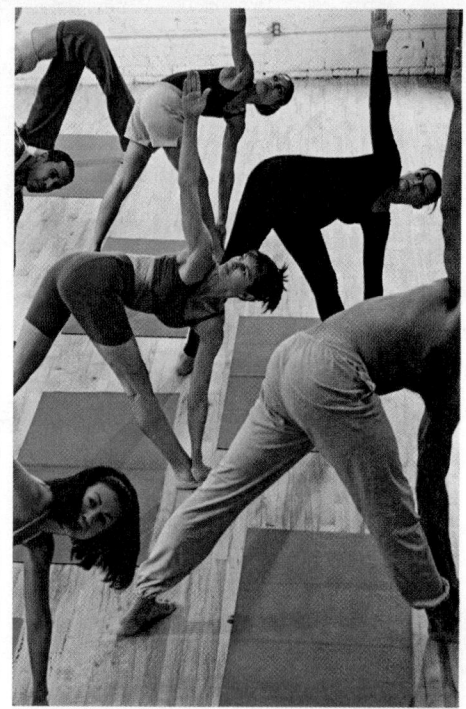

▲ Regular, moderate physical activity contributes to better blood pressure control.

FIGURE 9-26 ▶ What works? If your blood pressure is high, here's how much lifestyle changes should lower it.

Advice	Details	Drop in Systolic Blood Pressure
Lose excess weight	For every 20 pounds you lose	5 to 20 points
Follow a DASH diet	Eat a lower-fat diet rich in vegetables, fruits, and low-fat dairy foods	8 to 14 points
Exercise daily	Get 30 minutes a day of aerobic activity (such as brisk walking)	4 to 9 points
Limit sodium	Eat no more than 2400 mg per day (1500 mg per day is better)	2 to 8 points
Limit alcohol	Have no more than 2 drinks per day for men, 1 drink per day for women (1 drink = 12 oz. beer, 5 oz. wine, or 1.5 oz. 80-proof whiskey)	2 to 4 points

Source: *The Seventh Report of the Joint National Committee on Prevention, Detection, Evaluation, and Treatment of High Blood Pressure, May 2003* (www.nhibl.hih.gov/guidelines/hypertension).

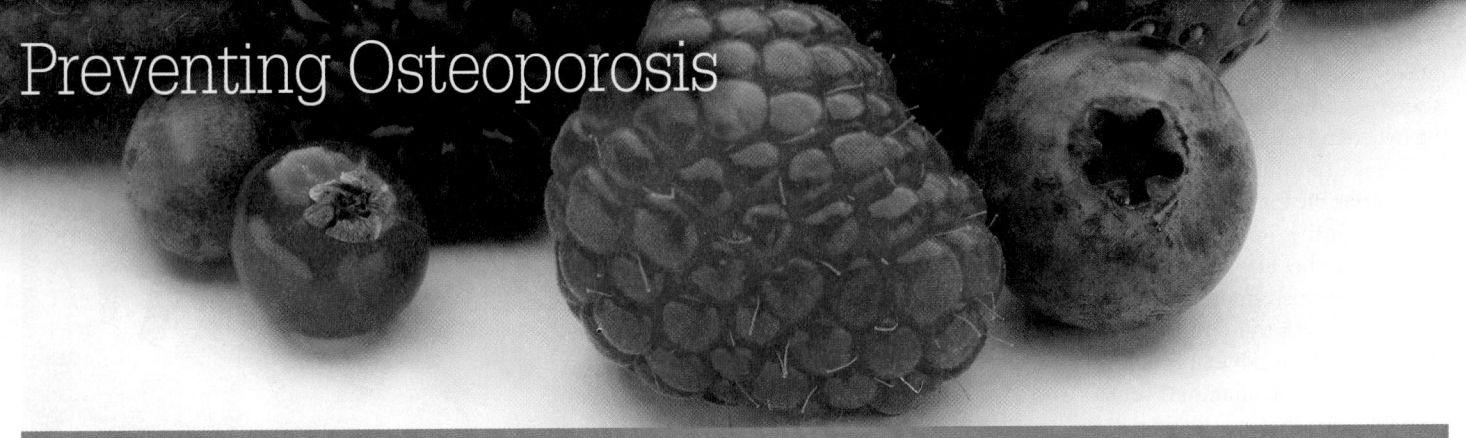

Preventing Osteoporosis

Widespread media attention has made it almost impossible for women to ignore osteoporosis. The crippling effect this disease has on older persons is now recognized as a major medical problem. Osteoporosis leads to approximately 1.5 million bone fractures per year in the United States, usually in the hip, spine, or wrist, leading to about $18 billion per year in health-care costs. Many older women in North America experience osteoporosis-related fractures in their lifetimes.

The slender, inactive woman who smokes is most susceptible to osteoporosis, but any person who lives long enough can suffer from the disease, including men. About 25% of women older than age 50 develop osteoporosis. Among people older than age 80, osteoporosis becomes the rule—not the exception. The spine fractures commonly found in women with osteoporosis cause considerable pain and deformity and decrease physical ability (Fig. 9-27); hip fractures are seen in both men and women with osteoporosis. Not only is this disease debilitating, it also can be fatal. Almost one-quarter of older persons who suffer hip fractures die within the first year from fracture-related complications.

Bone Structure and Strength

To better understand the role calcium plays in bone health and osteoporosis, it is important to understand how bone is constructed. Visual observation of the cross-sections of a bone reveals two primary bone structural types: **cortical bone** and **trabecular bone.** These interact within each bone to form an engineering marvel of strength (Fig. 9-28).

The entire outer surface of all bones is composed of cortical bone, also known as compact bone, which is very dense. The shafts of long bones, such as those of the arm, are almost entirely cortical bone. Trabecular bone, also known as spongy bone, is found in the ends of the long bones, inside the spinal vertebrae,

cortical bone Dense, compact bone that comprises the outer surface and shafts of bone; also called compact bone.

trabecular bone The spongy, inner matrix of bone, found primarily in the spine, pelvis, and ends of bones; also called spongy or cancellous bone.

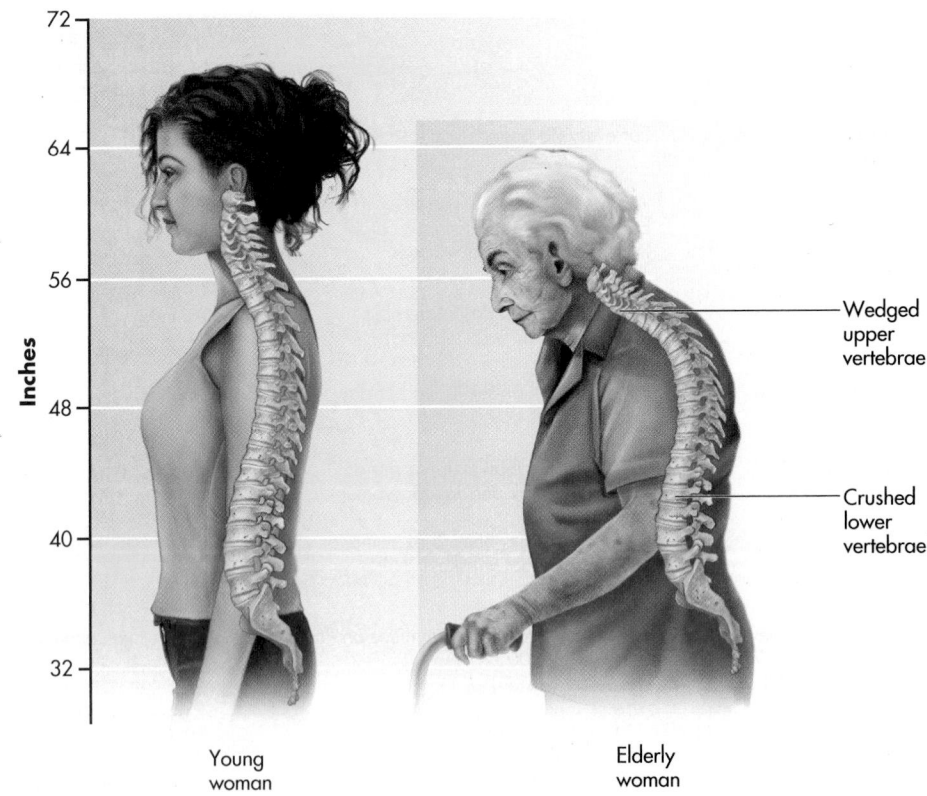

Young woman

Elderly woman

Wedged upper vertebrae

Crushed lower vertebrae

FIGURE 9-27 ▶ Normal and osteoporotic woman. Osteoporotic bones have less substance, so osteoporosis generally leads to loss of height, distorted body shape, fractures, and loss of teeth. Monitoring changes in adult height is one way to detect early evidence of osteoporosis.

and inside the flat bones of the pelvis. Trabecular bone is porous and forms an internal scaffolding-like network for a bone. It supports the outer cortical shell of the bone, especially in heavily stressed areas, such as joints. Like the beams of a building, the trabecular bone adds strength to the bone without the added weight of a more solid matrix. It is especially critical for the horizontal and vertical trabecular beams to extend continuously—without breaks. Any break in the trabecular beams weakens the support system of a bone and increases the risk for bone fracture. Once these beams are broken, there is no way to rebuild them. This is why it is so important to limit bone loss as people age.

Bone Mass Is Related to Age and Gender

Bone strength depends on a person's **bone mass** and **bone mineral density**. The more bone there is, and especially

the more densely packed bone crystals are in the bone, the stronger the bone structure. Rapid and continual bone growth and calcification occur throughout the adolescent years, ultimately resulting in what is called *peak bone mass*. In the adolescent growth spurt, bone mass is increasing at the rate of about 8.5% per year. Small increases in bone mass then continue between 20 and 30 years of age.

The ultimate amount of bone built by a person is clearly dependent on gender; race; familial patterns seen in the mother and father; and probably other genetically determined factors, such as the degree of calcium absorption. In addition, men have higher bone mass than women, and African-Americans have heavier skeletons than Caucasians. As a direct consequence, men and African-Americans in general have a somewhat lower risk of osteoporosis-related fractures than do other populations. Slender, small-framed Caucasian and Asian women show the

bone mass Total mineral substance (such as calcium or phosphorus) in a cross section of bone, generally expressed as grams per centimeter of length.

bone mineral density Total mineral content of bone at a specific bone site divided by the width of the bone at that site, generally expressed as grams per cubic centimeter.

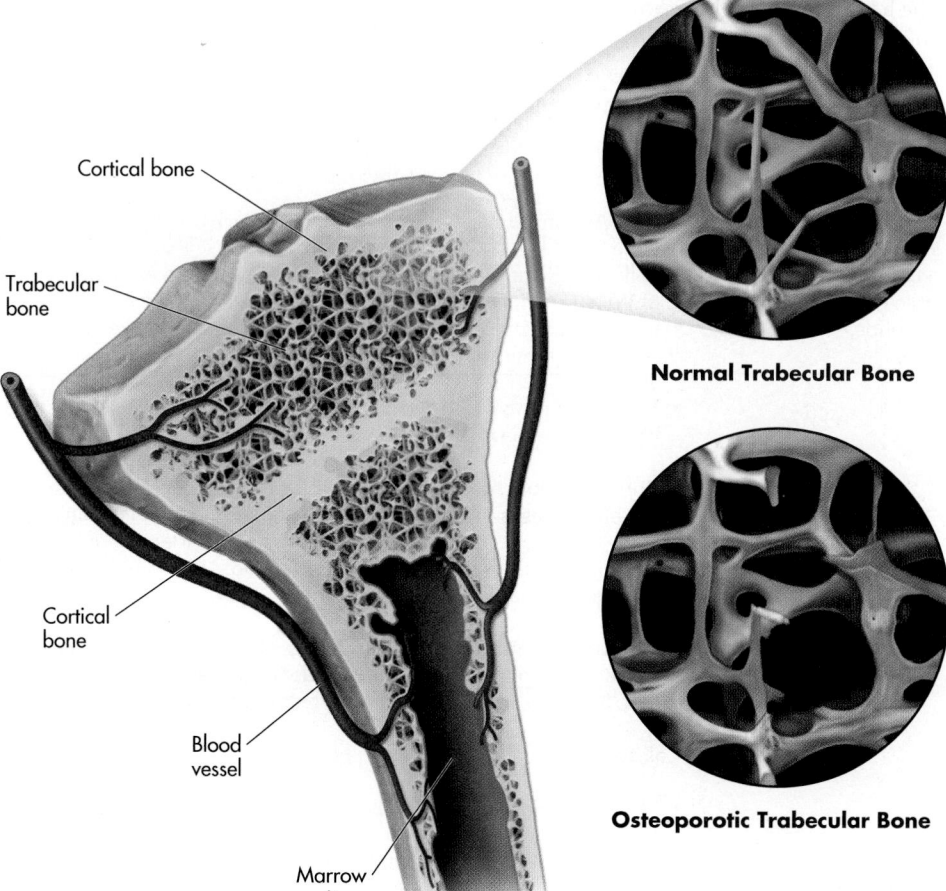

Cortical bone

Trabecular bone

Cortical bone

Blood vessel

Marrow cavity

Normal Trabecular Bone

Osteoporotic Trabecular Bone

FIGURE 9-28 ▶ Cortical and trabecular bone. Cortical bone forms the shafts of bones and their outer mineral covering. Trabecular bone supports the outer shell of cortical bone in various bones of the body, as in the illustration. Note how the osteoporotic bone has much less trabecular bone. This leads to a more fragile bone and is not reversible to any major extent with current therapies.

lowest bone mass values. Peak bone mass is also related to dietary intake of calcium and other nutrients, such as protein, phosphorus, vitamin A, vitamin D, vitamin K, magnesium, iron, zinc, and copper (Table 9-5). Recent studies also link a potassium-rich diet high in fruits and vegetables to osteoporosis prevention (see Further Reading 10). Thus, osteoporosis is not just a calcium story—many minerals and other nutrients play a part.

Bone mass varies among young adults; some have much denser bone than others, perhaps because they built more bone when they were young. Some people also may adapt more easily to lower-calcium diets. People who have developed more bone by early adulthood can sustain greater age-related bone loss with less risk of osteoporosis compared with those who reach adulthood with less bone. Thus, osteoporosis is considered to be a "pediatric disease" with geriatric (old age) consequences (Fig. 9-29).

For women, bone loss begins at age 30 and proceeds slowly and continuously to menopause (approximately age 50). It often speeds up at menopause with the decline in estrogen output and continues at a high rate of loss for the next 10 years. By age 65 to 70, the rate of bone loss falls to about the same rate as before menopause. In men, bone loss is slow and steady from around age 30. Overall, this bone loss in both males and females progresses without noticeable short-term symptoms.

Osteoporosis

Failure to maintain enough bone mass in the body is generally diagnosed as osteoporosis. Bone loss can also be caused by the vitamin D deficiency disease osteomalacia, the use of certain medications (such as cortisol and antiseizure drugs), and cancer.

All women age 65 and older should be screened for this disease. The most accurate screening involves a **dual energy X-ray absorptiometry (DEXA) bone scan** of the whole body. (Somewhat less accurate instruments measure bone mineral density at a single site, such as the heel.) Younger women with associated risk factors are advised to do the same at menopause, because the results of the screening would help them decide

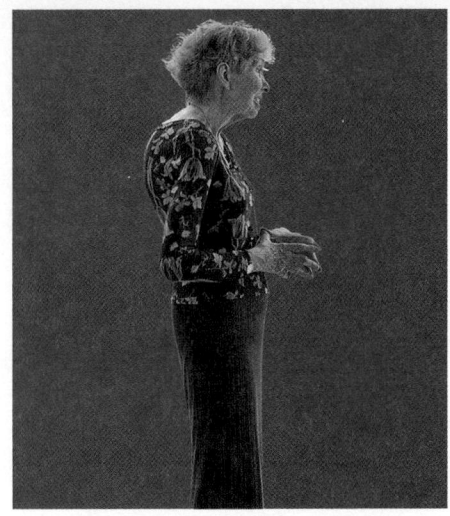

▲ Women with osteoporosis typically develop abnormal curvature of the upper spine. This results from fractures of the weakened vertebrae. This can lead to both physical and emotional pain.

Dual energy X-ray absorptiometry (DEXA) bone scan Method to measure bone density that uses small amounts of X-ray radiation. The ability of a bone to block the path of the radiation is used as a measure of bone density at that bone site.

TABLE 9-5 Diet and Lifestyle Factors Associated with Bone Status

Positive Diet and Lifestyle Factors	Call to Action
Adequate diet containing a sufficient amount of protein, calcium, phosphorus, magnesium, potassium, vitamin A, vitamin C, vitamin D, vitamin K, iron, zinc, copper, fluoride, and manganese and possibly boron.	• Follow MyPlate with special emphasis on adequate amounts of fruits, vegetables, and low-fat and fat-free dairy products. • Consider use of fortified foods (or supplements) to make up for specific nutrient shortfalls, such as vitamin D and calcium.
Healthy body weight	• Be aware that low body weight (slender figure) increases the risk for low bone mass.
Normal menses	• During childbearing years, seek medical advice if menses cease (such as in cases of anorexia nervosa or extreme athletic training). • Women at menopause and beyond should consider use of current medical therapies to reduce bone loss linked to the fall in estrogen output.
Weight-bearing physical activity	• Perform weight-bearing activity as this contributes to bone maintenance, whereas bed rest and a sedentary lifestyle lead to bone loss. Strength training is especially helpful for bone maintenance.
Negative Diet and Lifestyle Factors	**Call to Action**
Excessive intake of protein, phosphorus, sodium, caffeine, wheat bran, and alcohol	• Moderate intake of these dietary constituents is recommended. Problems primarily arise if adequate calcium is not consumed. • Excessive soft drink consumption is especially discouraged.
Smoking	• Smoking lowers estrogen output in women, so smoking cessation is advised.

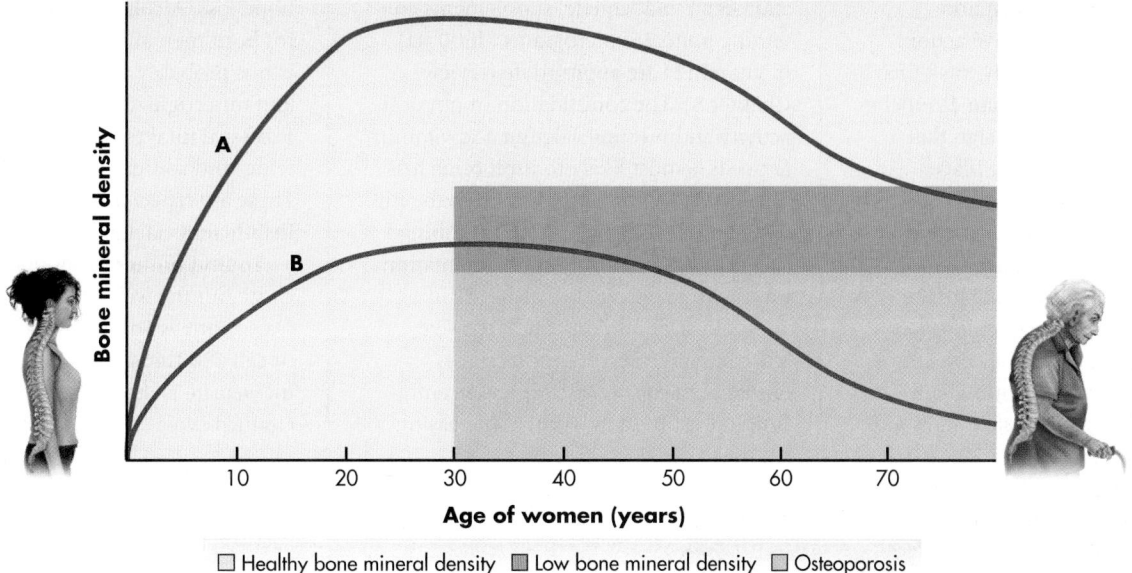

FIGURE 9-29 ▶ The relationship between peak bone mass and the ultimate risk of developing osteoporosis and related bone fractures
• **Woman A** had developed a high peak bone mass by age 30. Her bone loss was slow and steady between ages 30 and 50 and sped up somewhat after age 50 because of the effects of menopause. At age 75, the woman had a healthy bone mineral density value and did not show evidence of osteoporosis.
• **Woman B** with low peak bone mass experienced the same rate of bone loss as woman A. By age 50, she already had low mineral density and by age 70 kyphosis and spinal fractures had occurred.
Given the low calcium intakes that are common among young women today, line B is a sobering reality. Following a diet and lifestyle pattern that contributes to maximal bone mineral density can help women follow line A and significantly reduce their risk of developing osteoporosis.

whether medical therapy for bone loss is an appropriate plan for menopause.

For the DEXA test, a person will lie down on his or her back on a padded table while a movable imaging arm moves over the length of the body. The procedure usually takes about 20 to 30 minutes. The ability of a bone to block the path of radiation is used as a measure of bone mineral density at that bone site. A low dose of radiation is used for the DEXA—about one-tenth of the exposure from a chest X ray.

From the DEXA measurement of bone density, a T score is generated, which compares the observed bone density to that of a person at peak bone strength (e.g., age 30). Such a T score is interpreted as follows:

0 to −1	Normal
−1 to −2.4	Low bone mineral density
−2.5 or lower	Osteoporosis

Preventing Osteoporosis

Once osteoporosis is present, there is no way to repair the bone damage. This makes prevention important. Strategies for prevention of osteoporosis vary based on age and individual risk factors.

For young women, osteoporosis prevention involves three main elements. First, young women should focus on meeting calcium, vitamin D, protein, and other nutrient needs. Second, because the hormones of regular menstruation contribute to bone maintenance in young women, any sign of menstrual irregularities is reason to see a physician. Some non-menstruating female athletes and other women with irregular menstrual cycles (e.g., women with anorexia nervosa) already exhibit low bone mineral density. Third, an active lifestyle that includes weight-bearing physical activity is also important. The increased muscle mass that stems from weight-bearing physical activity is associated with greater bone mineral density, as muscle keeps tension on bone. However, physical activity cannot prevent the bone loss associated with irregular menstruation. Even though female athletes may do plenty of weight-bearing physical activity, they should

be closely monitored by a physician if they have irregular menstrual cycles.

Once they have reached menopause, women should discuss approved osteoporosis-related therapies with a physician. The most common medications are **bisphosphonates.** These lessen bone breakdown. Estrogen replacement previously was the most common therapy for bone protection, but it has been shown to increase the risks in some women for cardiovascular disease and strokes, as well as cancers of the breast and ovaries. Estrogen replacement is now reserved for short-term use to control menopausal symptoms in most cases.

bisphosphonates Compounds primarily composed of carbon and phosphorus that bind to bone mineral and in turn reduce bone breakdown. Examples are alendronate (Fosamax), risedronate (Actonel), and ibandronate (Boniva).

As age advances, both men and women need to take preventive action. First, adults need to accurately track their height. A decrease of more than 1½ inches from young adult height is a sign that significant bone loss is taking place.

Older adults especially need to stay physically active—including some weight-bearing and resistance activities—and they should meet the Adequate Intake for calcium set for their particular age. Regular sun exposure and the consumption of food sources of vitamin D are also important. If sun exposure and food sources are inadequate, supplements containing up to 25 micrograms (1000 IU) of vitamin D are appropriate (review Chapter 8). The combination of physical activity and meeting calcium and vitamin D needs is most likely to limit bone loss in some areas of the body, such as the hip. Read more about the effect of combined calcium and vitamin D supplementation on hip bone density in Further Reading 8.

At any age, smoking and excessive alcohol intake decrease bone mass. Smoking lowers the estrogen concentration in the blood in women, increasing bone loss. Alcohol is toxic to bone cells for both men and women, and alcoholism is probably a major undiagnosed and unrecognized cause of osteoporosis. Excessive intakes of phosphorus, caffeine, and sodium are also discouraged. These are especially problematic when insufficient calcium is consumed.

To find out more about osteoporosis, check out the website of the National Osteoporosis Foundation (www.nof.org) or call (800)464-6700. Another helpful website is that of the National Dairy Council (www.nationaldairycouncil.org).

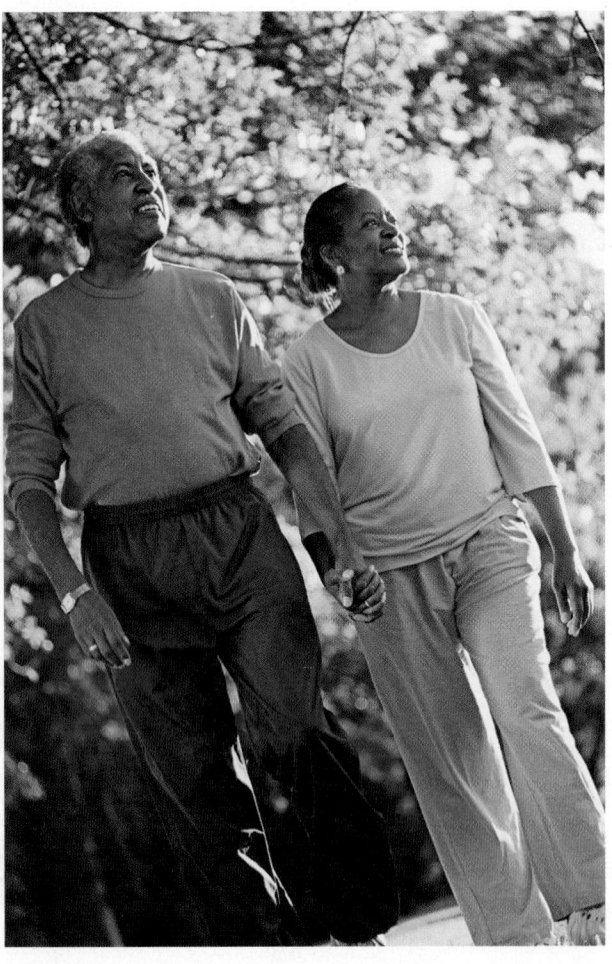

◀ Regular, moderate, weight-bearing physical activity contributes to bone health in both men and women. Note that men can also develop osteoporosis as they age.

Case Study Giving Up Milk

Ashley, a 19-year-old sophomore in college, recently gave up drinking milk. She thought this would help her stay slim by avoiding the calories in milk. Ashley's mother is concerned about her diet change. One of her primary concerns is the future risk of osteoporosis. Ashley also started smoking, and her only physical activity is practice for Women's Glee Club.

Ashley's typical diet consists of oatmeal made with water, a banana and a cup of fruit juice for breakfast. At midmorning, she buys a snack cake or candy bar from the vending machine. At lunch, she has pasta with vegetables, bread with olive oil, a side salad, 1 ounce of mixed nuts, and a soft drink. For dinner, she has a chicken or hamburger sandwich along with mixed vegetables and another soft drink. As an evening snack, she has some cookies and hot tea.

Answer the following questions about Ashley's situation and check your responses in Appendix A.

1. What nutrients are low in Ashley's typical diet that put her at risk of osteoporosis in the future?
2. Which of Ashley's lifestyle factors contribute to this increased risk of osteoporosis?
3. Is there any evidence that consumption of milk or other dairy products leads to weight gain?
4. What changes to her current diet could reduce the risk of osteoporosis and also help Ashley maintain her weight?
5. What lifestyle changes (other than the dietary changes) could Ashley make to decrease her risk of osteoporosis and maintain a healthy weight?

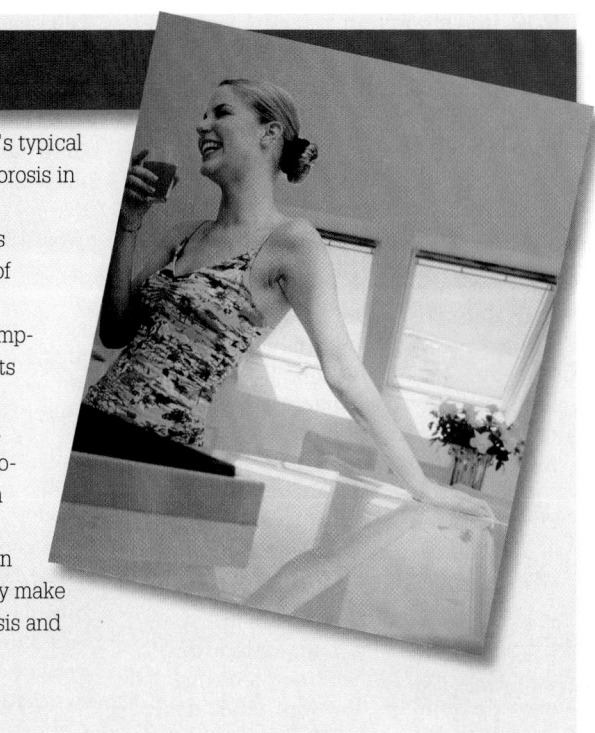

Summary (Numbers refer to numbered sections in the chapter.)

9.1 Water constitutes 50% to 70% of the human body. Its unique chemical properties enable it to dissolve substances as well as serve as a medium for chemical reactions, temperature regulation, and lubrication. Water also helps regulate the acid-base balance in the body.

For adults, daily water needs are estimated at 9 cups (women) to 13 cups (men) per day; fluid intake contributes to meeting this need.

Overall, the United States enjoys a safe water supply. However, people with poor immune status should boil water used for drinking and cooking to avoid waterborne illness. Bottled water can be used, but reliance on it to meet fluid needs is costly to the environment and our personal budgets.

9.2 Minerals are categorized based on the amount we need per day. If we require greater than 100 milligrams of a mineral per day, it is considered a major mineral; otherwise it is considered a trace mineral.

9.3 Many minerals are vital for sustaining life. For humans, animal products are the most bioavailable sources of most minerals. Supplements of minerals exceeding 100%

of the Daily Values listed on the label should be taken only under a physician's supervision. Toxicity and nutrient interactions are especially likely if the Upper Level (when set) is exceeded on a long-term basis.

9.4 Sodium, the major positive ion found outside cells, is vital in fluid balance and nerve impulse transmission. The North American diet provides abundant sodium through processed foods and table salt. About 10% to 15% of the adult population, such as overweight people, is especially sodium-sensitive and at risk for developing hypertension from consuming excessive sodium.

9.5 Potassium, the major positive ion found inside cells, has a similar function to sodium. Milk, fruits, and vegetables are good sources.

9.6 Chloride is the major negative ion found outside cells. It is important in digestion as part of stomach acid and in immune and nerve functions. Table salt supplies most of the chloride in our diets.

9.7 Calcium forms a part of bone structure and plays a role in blood clotting,

muscle contraction, nerve transmission, and cell metabolism. Calcium absorption is enhanced by stomach acid and the active vitamin D hormone. Dairy products are important calcium sources. Women are particularly at risk for not meeting calcium needs.

9.8 Phosphorus aids enzyme function and forms part of key metabolic compounds, cell membranes, and bone. It is efficiently absorbed, and deficiencies are rare, although there is concern about possible poor intake by some older women. Good food sources are dairy products, bakery products, and meats.

9.9 Magnesium is a mineral found mostly in plant food sources. It is important for nerve and heart function and as an activator for many enzymes. Whole-grain breads and cereals (bran portion), vegetables, nuts, seeds, milk, and meats are good food sources.

9.10 Sulfur is incorporated into certain vitamins and amino acids.

9.11 Trace minerals are essential to good health even though we only need 100 milligrams or less of each daily.

9.12 Iron absorption depends mainly on the form of iron present and the body's need for it. Heme iron from animal sources is better absorbed than the nonheme iron obtained primarily from plant sources. Consuming vitamin C or meat simultaneously with nonheme iron increases absorption. Iron operates mainly in synthesizing hemoglobin and myoglobin and in the action of the immune system. Women are at great risk for developing iron deficiency, which decreases blood hemoglobin and hematocrit. When this condition is severe, iron-deficiency anemia develops. This decreases the amount of oxygen carried in the blood. Iron toxicity usually results from a genetic disorder called hemochromatosis. This disease causes overabsorption and accumulation of iron, which can result in severe liver and heart damage.

9.13 Zinc aids in the action of up to 200 enzymes important for growth, development, cell membrane structure and function, immune function, antioxidant protection, wound healing, and taste. A zinc deficiency results in poor growth, loss of appetite, reduced sense of taste and smell, hair loss, and a persistent rash. Zinc is best absorbed from animal sources. The richest sources of zinc are oysters, shrimp, crab, and beef. Good plant sources are whole grains, peanuts, and beans.

9.14 An important role of selenium is decreasing the action of free-radical (oxidizing) compounds. In this way, selenium acts along with vitamin E in providing antioxidant protection. Muscle pain, muscle wasting, and a form of heart damage may result from a selenium deficiency. Meats, eggs, fish, and shellfish are good animal sources of selenium. Good plant sources include grains and seeds.

9.15 Iodide forms part of the thyroid hormones. A lack of dietary iodide results in the development of an enlarged thyroid gland or goiter. Iodized salt is a major food source.

9.16 Copper is important for iron metabolism, cross-linking of connective tissue, and other functions, such as enzymes that provide antioxidant protection. A copper deficiency can result in a form of anemia. Copper is found mainly in liver, seafood, cocoa, legumes, and whole grains.

9.17 Fluoride as part of regular dietary intake or toothpaste use makes teeth resistant to dental caries. Most North Americans receive the bulk of their fluoride from fluoridated water and toothpaste.

9.18–9.21 Chromium aids in the action of the hormone insulin. Egg yolks, meats, and whole grains are good sources of chromium. Manganese and molybdenum are used by various enzymes. One enzyme that uses manganese provides antioxidant protection. Clear deficiencies in otherwise healthy people are rarely seen for any of these three nutrients. Human needs for other trace minerals are so low that deficiencies are uncommon

N&YH Controlling weight and alcohol intake; exercising regularly; decreasing salt intake; and ensuring adequate potassium, magnesium, and calcium in the diet all can play a part in controlling high blood pressure.

Women are particularly at risk for developing osteoporosis as they age. Numerous lifestyle and medical options can help reduce this risk, including an adequate intake of calcium and many other minerals.

Check Your Knowledge (Answers to the following questions are below.)

1. Dietary heme iron is derived from
   a. elemental iron in food.
   b. animal flesh.
   c. breakfast cereal.
   d. vegetables.

2. Chloride is
   a. a component of hydrochloric acid.
   b. an intracellular fluid ion.
   c. a positively charged ion.
   d. converted to chlorine in the intestinal tract.

3. Minerals involved in fluid balance are
   a. calcium and magnesium.
   b. copper and iron.
   c. calcium and phosphorus.
   d. sodium and potassium.

4. In a situation where there is an insufficient intake of dietary iodide, the thyroid-stimulating hormone promotes the enlargement of the thyroid gland. This condition is called
   a. Graves' disease.
   b. goiter.
   c. hyperparathyroidism.
   d. cretinism.

5. Ninety-nine percent of the calcium in the body is found in
   a. intracellular fluid.
   b. bones and teeth.
   c. nerve cells.
   d. the liver.

6. At the end of long bones, inside the spinal vertebrae, and inside the flat bones of the pelvis, is a spongy type of bone known as _____ bone.
   a. osteoclastic
   b. osteoblastic
   c. trabecular
   d. compact

7. Which compartment contains the greatest amount of body fluid?
   a. intracellular
   b. extracellular
   c. They contain the same amount.

8. The primary function of sodium is to maintain
   a. bone mineral content.
   b. hemoglobin concentration.
   c. immune function.
   d. fluid distribution.

9. Hypertension is defined as a blood pressure greater than
   a. 110/60.
   b. 120/65.
   c. 140/90.
   d. 190/80.

10. Which of the following individuals are most likely to develop osteoporosis?
    a. premenopausal women athletes
    b. women taking estrogen replacement therapy
    c. slender, inactive women who smoke
    d. women who eat a lot of high-fat dairy products

Answer Key: 1. b (LO 9.6), 2. a (LO 9.6), 3. d (LO 9.6), 4. b (LO 9.6), 5. b (LO 9.6), 6. c (LO 9.8), 7. a (LO 9.1), 8. d (LO 9.6), 9. c (LO 9.7), 10. c (LO 9.8)

Study Questions (Numbers refer to Learning Outcomes)

1. Approximately how much water do you need each day to stay healthy? Identify at least two situations that increase the need for water. Then list three sources of water in the average person's diet. (LO 9.2)

2. What is the relationship between sodium and water balance, and how is that relationship monitored as well as maintained in the body? (LO 9.6)

3. Identify four factors that influence the bioavailability of minerals from food. (LO 9.5)

4. What are two similarities and differences between sodium and potassium? Sodium and chloride? (LO 9.6)

5. In terms of total amounts in the body, calcium and phosphorus are the first and second most abundant minerals, respectively. What function do these minerals have in common? (LO 9.6)

6. What are the best food sources for zinc and copper? (LO 9.6)

7. Describe the symptoms of iron-deficiency anemia and explain possible reasons they occur. (LO 9.6)

8. Which trace minerals are lost from cereal grains when they are refined? Are any of these nutrients replaced by enrichment? (LO 9.6)

9. Describe the chief functions of fluoride, copper, and chromium in the body. (LO 9.6)

10. What are the practical consequences of the Daily Values on food and supplement labels exceeding the RDA or Adequate Intake for many trace minerals? (LO 9.6)

What Would You Choose Recommendations

Bottled water has become very popular. In 2009, each American consumed almost 28 gallons of bottled water, adding up to about 8.5 billion gallons for the nation. The public perception that bottled water is safer and healthier than tap water has stimulated the current bottle-toting habit. The truth is that bottled and tap water are both regulated: bottled water by the FDA and tap water by the Environmental Protection Agency (EPA). The FDA requirements for bottled water mimic those of the EPA for water quality, but neither has to be contaminant-free.

"Pure" is an advertising term and means nothing about the quality of the water. Recent controversy over misleading advertising by major companies such as Pepsico and Coca-Cola that use public source water in their respective products, Aquafina and Dasani, has led to the printing of "Public Source Water" or "PSW" on labels (see Further Reading 12).

Mineral water must contain consistent levels of natural elements from an underground source; no minerals may be added to the water. The precise mineral content varies by source, but some common minerals found in water include calcium, magnesium, potassium, sodium, sulfur, iron, fluoride, zinc, and some ultratrace minerals. The minerals impart some taste to the water but are typically a minor contributor to overall mineral intake.

There is no legal definition for "vitamin water." Manufacturers of vitamin water (i.e., soft-drink companies) usually use filtered or distilled water and add sweeteners (e.g., high-fructose corn syrup) and citric acid as flavoring agents, plus several vitamins (mostly vitamin C and an assortment of B vitamins). In 2010, the Coca-Cola Bottling Company was sued by the Center for Science in the Public Interest for false marketing of its popular vitaminwater® brand as "nutritious." These products are marketed as healthy because they contain added vitamins, but most of them also supply a surprising amount of sugar. Recall that the American Heart Association recommends that men and women get no more than 150 or 100 kcal per day, respectively, from added sugars. A 20-ounce bottle of vitaminwater® has 33 grams of sugar, providing 132 kcal from added sugar. This is about half the sugar in a regular soft drink, but you can see how this can add up to excess. Furthermore, most North

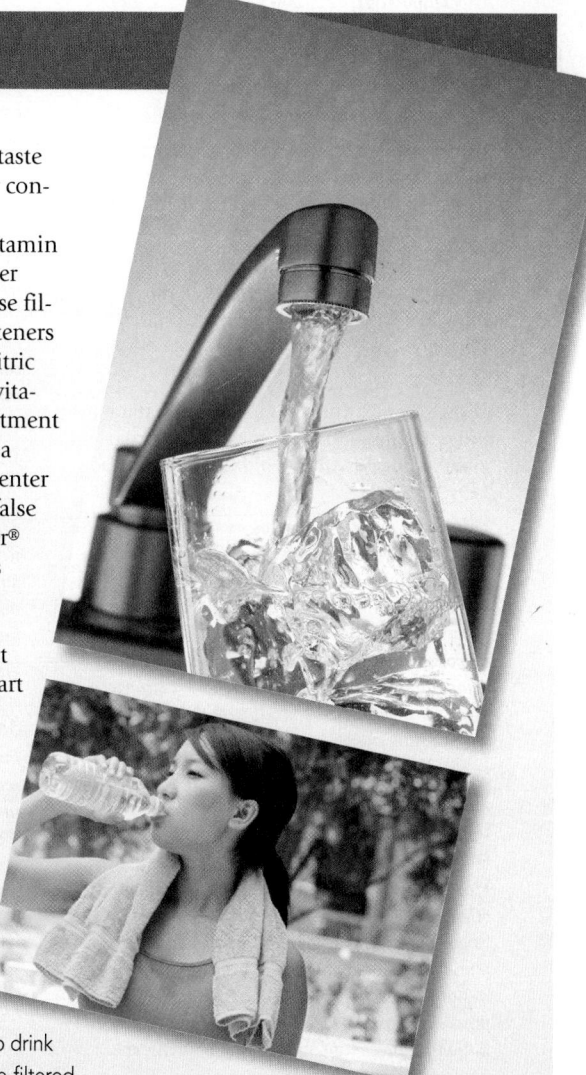

▲ While following the recommendations to drink more water, hydrate with tap water or home-filtered water in a reusable container.

Americans consume adequate amounts of vitamin C and the B vitamins without the aid of these beverages.

Consumers should also be aware of the FDA definitions for other types of bottled water.

- Artesian water must come from a confined aquifer.
- Springwater must flow naturally to the surface.

- Purified water is produced through an approved process such as distillation or reverse osmosis.

Relying on bottled water is an expensive habit, personally and environmentally. If you use bottled water to meet your recommended fluid needs, you will spend close

to $1500 per year compared with about 50 cents for the same volume of tap water. On a larger scale, it is estimated that close to 90% of water bottles end up in the trash, clogging our landfills or being shipped to other countries for recycling. It is well known that America has some of the cleanest, safest tap water in the world.

Further Readings

1. ADA Reports: Position of the American Dietetic Association: The impact of fluoride on health. *Journal of the American Dietetic Association* 105:1620, 2005.

   The American Dietetic Association reaffirms that fluoride is an important element for all mineralized tissues in the body. Appropriate fluoride intake is beneficial to bone and tooth health.

2. Appel LJ and others: Dietary approaches to prevent and treat hypertension: A scientific statement from the American Heart Association. *Hypertension* 47:296, 2006.

   Latest advice from the American Heart Association on diet and hypertension. Key preventive factors are to avoid overweight and inactivity and to moderate alcohol and salt intake.

3. Cook NR and others: Joint effects of sodium and potassium intake on subsequent cardiovascular disease. *Archives of Internal Medicine* 169: 32, 2009.

   This study suggests that potassium is effective in lowering blood pressure. Furthermore, the combination of a higher intake of potassium and a lower intake of sodium seems to be more effective than either on its own in reducing the risk of cardiovascular disease. The sodium-to-potassium ratio in subjects' urine was a stronger predictor of cardiovascular disease than sodium or potassium alone.

4. Elliott P and others: Dietary phosphorus and blood pressure: International study of macro- and micro-nutrients and blood pressure. *Hypertension* 51:669, 2008.

   Little attention has been given to the possible effects of phosphorus intake on blood pressure. The results of this study indicate that increased phosphorus intake, as well as calcium and magnesium intake, have the potential to lower blood pressure. This may be an important recommendation for prevention and control of prehypertension and hypertension.

5. Havas S and others: The urgent need to reduce sodium consumption. *Journal of the American Medical Association* 298:1439, 2007.

   In the United States, 77% of sodium comes from processed and restaurant foods, with many processed foods containing 1000 mg or more per serving. There is a general consensus that sodium levels should be reduced substantially in processed and restaurant foods. Policy developments and possible solutions to address this problem are presented in this article.

6. Heaney RP: Absorbability and utility of calcium in mineral waters. *American Journal of Clinical Nutrition* 84(2):371, 2006.

   Published absorbability and utility of high-calcium mineral waters are summarized and integrated in this article. The absorbability of all the high-calcium mineral waters was equal to or slightly better than milk calcium. The utility of calcium as measured by increased urinary calcium, decreased serum parathyroid hormone, decreased bone resorption biomarkers, and protection of bone mass indicated that a significant quantity of calcium was absorbed. High-calcium mineral waters, therefore, appear to provide useful quantities of bioavailable calcium.

7. Hollenberg NK: The influence of dietary sodium on blood pressure. *Journal of the American College of Nutrition* 25:240S, 2006.

   Evidence relating salt intake to blood pressure is reviewed. The merit of mandating a reduction in salt intake is discussed. The author indicates that the evidence supporting such a policy is inconsistent and small. The importance of antihypertensive drugs is emphasized.

8. Jackson RD and others: Calcium plus vitamin D supplementation and the risk of fractures. *New England Journal of Medicine* 354 (7):669, 2006.

   Postmenopausal women, 50 to 79 years of age, who were enrolled in a Women's Health Initiative (WHI) clinical trial were assigned to receive 1000 mg of elemental calcium as calcium carbonate with 400 IU of vitamin D_3 daily or a placebo. The occurrence of fractures and bone density was determined for 7 years. Calcium with vitamin D supplementation resulted in a small but significant increase in hip bone density, but did not significantly reduce hip fracture and increased the risk of kidney stones.

9. King JC: Zinc: An essential but elusive nutrient. *American Journal of Clinical Nutrition* 94:679S, 2011.

   Zinc is essential for many biochemical functions. When zinc is insufficient in the diet, body stores give up zinc immediately to conserve the nutrient. There is probably a small zinc reserve in all cells in addition to the zinc in blood. Zinc concentrations in blood decline quickly with severe deficiencies and more slowly with marginal depletion. Blood zinc concentrations also decrease with conditions such as infection, trauma, stress, and steroid use due to redistribution of zinc from blood to tissues. This redistribution confuses the interpretation of low blood zinc concentrations and determining whether this redistribution is the cause of low blood zinc rather than poor nutrition.

10. Lanham-New SA. The balance of bone health: Tipping the scales in favor of potassium-rich, bicarbonate-rich foods. *Journal of Nutrition* 137:1725, 2008.

    About 10 million Americans have osteoporosis. This review article summarizes the current evidence linking potassium-rich, bicarbonate-rich foods (e.g., fruits and vegetables) to osteoporosis prevention.

11. Lippman SM and others: Effect of selenium and vitamin E on risk of prostate cancer and other cancers: The selenium and vitamin E cancer prevention trial (SELECT). *Journal of the American Medical Association* 301:39, 2009.

The results of this study showed no benefit to taking a supplement of selenium or vitamin E alone or in combination for the prevention of prostate cancer, colon cancer, lung cancer, all cancers, and cardiovascular disease and for overall survival.

12. Palmer S: Busting bottled water. *Today's Dietitian* 9(12):60, 2007.

    This article highlights several reasons why consumers have been wrong in assuming that bottled water is always better than tap water. The ecological, environmental, and economic problems with relying on bottled water for our fluids needs. The laws regulating bottled and tap water are also compared, suggesting that bottled water is generally not safer and healthier than tap water. The author recommends that we drink more water, but do it from the tap.

13. Park Y and others: Dairy food, calcium, and risk of cancer in the NIH-AARP diet and health study. *Archives of Internal Medicine* 169:391, 2009.

The 7-year study of 493,000 older men and women provides evidence that diets rich in calcium may lower risk of total cancer and cancers of the digestive system, especially colorectal cancer. Benefits were mostly associated with foods high in calcium, rather than calcium supplements. Getting more than the recommended 1200 milligrams of calcium for older people did not result in greater cancer protection.

14. Popkin BM and others: A new proposed guidance system for beverage consumption in the United States. *American Journal of Clinical Nutrition* 83:529, 2006.

    Drinking water is recommended as the preferred beverage to fulfill water needs, with tea, coffee, and low-fat and skim milk also ranked high. The Beverage Guidance Panel suggests that beverages with no or few calories should be consumed more often than calorie-containing beverages. An intake of 98 fluid ounces is recommended daily for a person consuming 2200 calories.

15. Reid IR and others: Randomized controlled trial of calcium in healthy older women.

American Journal of Medicine 119(9):777, 2006.

In this study of postmenopausal women receiving 1 g/day as calcium citrate over 5 years, height loss was reduced by calcium but constipation was more common. The authors conclude that calcium results in a sustained reduction in bone loss and turnover, but its effect on fracture is uncertain.

16. Van Dam RM and others: Dietary calcium and magnesium, major food sources, and risk of type 2 diabetes in U.S. black women. *Diabetes Care* 29:2238, 2006.

Magnesium and calcium intakes have been inversely associated with risk of type 2 diabetes in predominantly white populations. The results of this study of 41,186 participants of the Black Women's Health Study indicated that a diet high in magnesium-rich foods, particularly whole grains, is associated with a significantly lower risk of type 2 diabetes in U.S. black women.

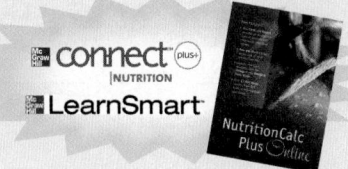

To get the most out of your study of nutrition, go to McGraw-Hill's online resources: Connect www.mcgrawhillconnect.com, where you will find NutritionCalc Plus, LearnSmart, and many other dynamic tools.

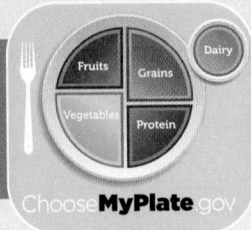

RATE YOUR PLATE

I. How High Is Your Sodium Intake?

Complete this questionnarie to evaluate your sodium habits with respect to typically rich sources.

How Often Do You...	Rarely	Occasionally	Often	Regularly (Daily)
1. Eat cured or processed meats, such as ham, bacon, sausage, frankfurters, and other luncheon meats?	☐	☐	☐	☐
2. Choose canned or frozen vegetables with sauce?	☐	☐	☐	☐
3. Use commercially prepared meals, main dishes, or canned or dehydrated soups?	☐	☐	☐	☐
4. Eat cheese, especially processed cheese?	☐	☐	☐	☐
5. Eat salted nuts, popcorn, pretzels, corn chips, or potato chips?	☐	☐	☐	☐
6. Add salt to cooking water for vegetables, rice, or pasta?	☐	☐	☐	☐
7. Add salt, seasoning mixes, salad dressings, or condiments—such as soy sauce, steak sauce, catsup, and mustard—to foods during preparation or at the table?	☐	☐	☐	☐
8. Salt your food before tasting it?	☐	☐	☐	☐
9. Ignore labels for sodium content when buying foods?	☐	☐	☐	☐
10. When dining out, choose obviously salty sauces or foods?	☐	☐	☐	☐

The more checks you put in the "often" or "regularly" columns, the higher your dietary sodium intake is. However, not all the habits in the table contribute the same amount of sodium. For example, many natural cheeses such as cheddar are relatively moderate in sodium, whereas processed cheeses and cottage cheese are much higher. To moderate sodium intake, choose lower-sodium foods from each food group more often and balance high-sodium food choices with low-sodium ones.

Adapted from *USDA Home and Garden Bulletin* No. 232–6, April 1986.

II. Working for Denser Bones

Osteoporosis and related low bone mass affect many adults in North America, especially older women. One-third of all women experience fractures because of this disease, amounting to about 2 million bone fractures per year.

Osteoporosis is a disease you can do something about. Some risk factors can't be changed, but others, such as a poor calcium intake, can. Is this true for you? To find out, complete this tool for estimating your current calcium intake. For all the following foods, write the number of servings you eat in a day. Total the number of servings in each category and then multiply the total number of servings by the amount of calcium for each category. Finally, add the total amount for each food category to estimate your calcium intake for that day.

Does your intake meet your RDA set for calcium?

Food	Serving Size	Number of Servings	Calcium (mg)	Total Calcium (mg)
Plain low-fat yogurt	1 cup	_____		
Fat-free dry milk powder	1/2 cup	_____		
Total servings		_____	× 400	= _____ mg
Canned sardines (with bones)	3 ounces	_____		
Fruit-flavored yogurt	1 cup	_____		
Milk: fat-free, reduced-fat, whole, chocolate, buttermilk	1 cup	_____		
Calcium-fortified soy milk (e.g., Silk)	1 cup	_____		
Parmesan cheese (grated)	1/4 cup	_____		
Swiss cheese	1 ounce	_____		
Total servings		_____	× 300	= _____ mg
Cheese (all other hard cheese)	1 ounce	_____		
Pancakes	3	_____		
Total servings		_____	× 200	= _____ mg
Canned pink salmon	3 ounces	_____		
Tofu (processed with calcium)	4 ounces	_____		
Total servings		_____	× 150	= _____ mg
Collards or turnip greens, cooked	1/2 cup	_____		
Ice cream or ice milk	1/2 cup	_____		
Almonds	1 ounce	_____		
Total servings		_____	× 75	= _____ mg
Chard, cooked	1/2 cup	_____		
Cottage cheese	1/2 cup	_____		
Corn tortilla	1 medium	_____		
Orange	1 medium	_____		
Total servings		_____	× 50	= _____ mg
Kidney, lima, or navy beans, cooked	1/2 cup	_____		
Broccoli	1/2 cup	_____		
Carrot, raw	1 medium	_____		
Dates or raisins	1/4 cup	_____		
Egg	1 large	_____		
Whole-wheat bread	1 slice	_____		
Peanut butter	2 tablespoons	_____		
Total servings		_____	× 25	= _____ mg
Calcium-fortified orange juice	6 ounces	_____		
Calcium-fortified snack bars	1 each	_____		
Calcium-fortified breakfast bars	1/2 bar	_____		
Total servings		_____	× 200	= _____ mg
Calcium-fortified chocolate candies	1 each	_____		
Calcium supplements*	1 each	_____	× 500	= _____ mg
Total servings		_____	Total calcium intake	= _____ mg

Other calcium sources to consider include many breakfast cereals (100 to 250 mg per cup) and some vitamin/mineral supplements (200 to 500 mg or more per tablet).

*Amount varies, so check the label for the amount in a specific product and then adjust the calculation as needed.

Reprinted with permission from *Topics in Clinical Nutrition*, "Putting Calcium into Perspective for Your Clients," G. Wardlaw and N. Weese, 11:1, p. 29. © 1995 Aspen Publishers, Inc.

Chapter 10 Nutrition: Fitness and Sports

Student Learning Outcomes

Chapter 10 is designed to allow you to:

10.1 List five positive health-related outcomes of a physically active lifestyle.

10.2 Design a fitness regimen.

10.3 Describe when and how glycogen, blood glucose, fat, and protein are used to meet energy needs during different types of physical activity.

10.4 Differentiate between anaerobic and aerobic use of glucose, and identify advantages and disadvantages of each.

10.5 Show how muscles and related organs adapt to an increase in physical activity.

10.6 Outline how to estimate an athlete's calorie needs and discuss the general principles for meeting overall nutrient requirements in the training diet.

10.7 Examine the problems associated with rapid weight loss by dehydration and outline the importance of water and/or sports drinks during exercise.

10.8 Understand how athletes can optimize performance by consuming foods and fluids before, during, and after exercise.

10.9 List several ergogenic aids and describe their effects, if any, on an athlete's performance.

What Would You Choose?

You are gearing up to run your first half-marathon in a few weeks. When your race packet arrived in the mail, it included your T-shirt, race number, and a bunch of free samples and coupons for sports nutrition products. From your long training runs, you know that you tend to lose your speed and motivation around mile nine. What would you choose to take along during the race to help you make it to the finish line?

a Clif Shot Turbo energy gel with 100 milligrams caffeine, 22 grams of carbohydrate, and electrolytes

b PowerBar ProteinPlus energy bar with 23 grams of protein

c Powerade sports drink with electrolytes, vitamins, and 14 grams of carbohydrate

d Essential Amino Energy drink with branched-chain amino acids

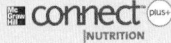 **Think about your choice as you read Chapter 10, then see our recommendations at the end of the chapter. To learn more about store-bought and homemade sports nutrition products, check out the Connect site:**
www.mcgrawhillconnect.com

Part Four

Nutrition: Beyond the Nutrients

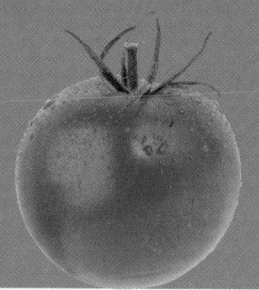

Athletes invest a lot of time and effort in training. Most athletes don't want to miss out on any advantage, whether real or perceived, that might give them the winning edge. Athletes often seek ways to enhance their diets to improve performance, so they make easy targets for purveyors of nutrition misinformation.

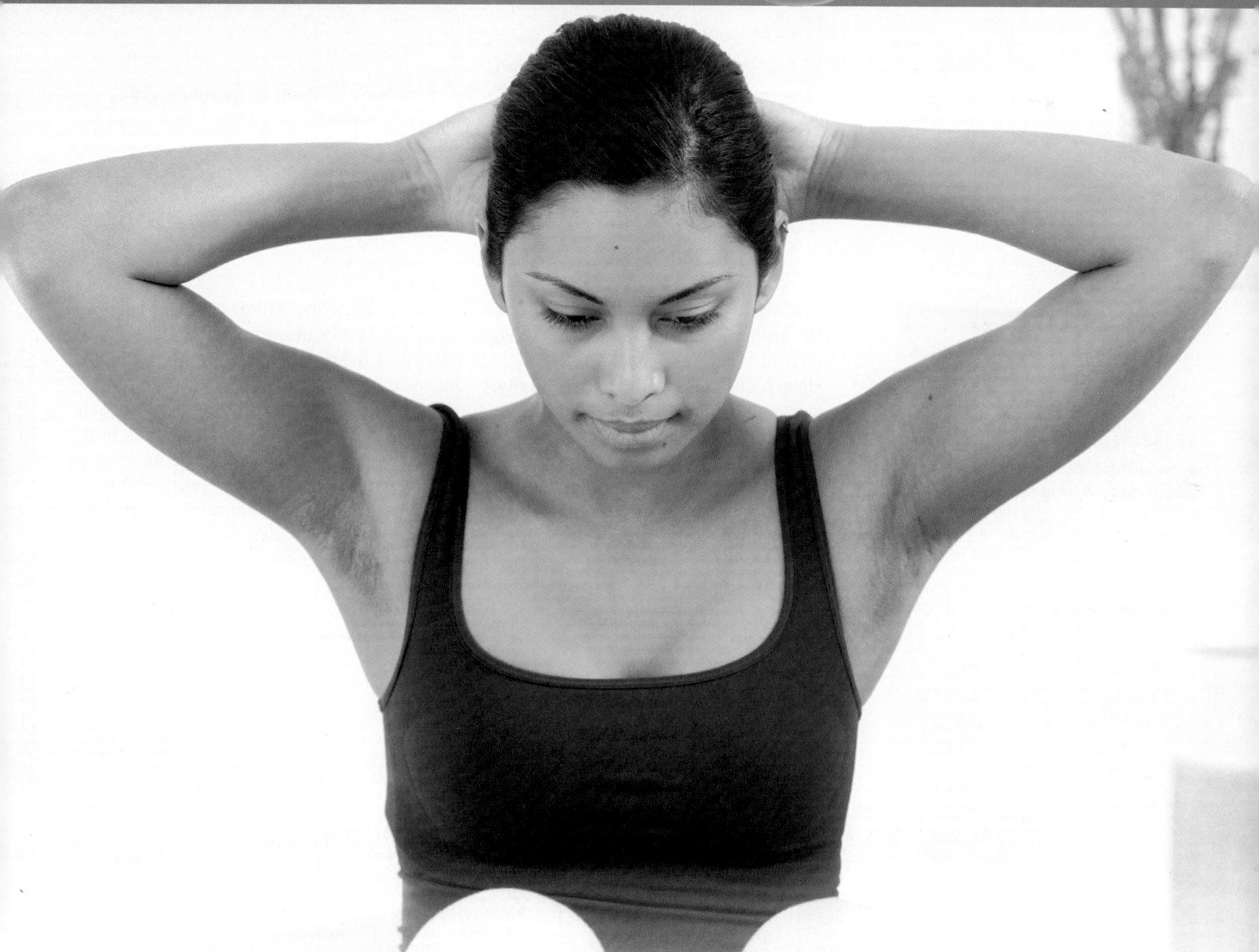

Although good eating habits can't substitute for physical training and genetic endowment, proper food and beverage choices are crucial for top-notch performance, contributing to endurance and helping to speed the repair of injured tissues.

Although experts might disagree on how much carbohydrate, protein, and fat we should consume, there is no argument over the health benefits of regular physical activity. It is even beneficial for overweight people who remain at that excess weight. As the comic in this chapter suggests, it takes a strong commitment to reap the benefits.

In Chapter 10, you will discover how physical fitness benefits the entire body and how nutrition relates to fitness and sports performance.

Refresh Your Memory

As you begin your study of nutrition for fitness and sports in Chapter 10, you may want to review:

- The current trend of consuming "energy bars" in Chapter 1
- Components of the cell in Chapter 3
- Concept of glycemic load in Chapter 4
- Various food sources of carbohydrates, proteins, and lipids in Chapters 4–7
- Food sources of calcium and iron in Chapter 9

10.1 The Close Relationship Between Nutrition and Fitness

Healthy people 2020 objectives focus on reducing the proportion of adults who engage in no leisure time physical activity and increasing the proportion of adults who meet the 2008 Physical Activity Guidelines for aerobic and muscle-strengthening physical activity.

Without a doubt, physical fitness has many health benefits. Physical fitness refers to the ability to perform moderate to vigorous activity without undue fatigue. The benefits of regular physical activity include enhanced heart function, less injury, better sleep habits, and improvement in body composition. Physical activity also can reduce stress and positively affect blood pressure, blood cholesterol, blood glucose regulation, and immune function. In addition, physical activity aids in weight control, both by raising resting energy expenditure for a short time after exercise and by increasing overall energy expenditure. In fact, as physical fitness improves, so does your ability to mobilize fat as a source of energy. See Figure 10-1 and Further Readings 8 and 11 for a further look at these and other benefits of a physically active lifestyle.

Unfortunately, as noted in Chapter 7, many North American adults lead sedentary lives. Most adults do not regularly practice moderate to vigorous physical activity and about half of all adults quit an exercise program within 3 months of initiation.

To help yourself stay with an exercise program, experts recommend the following:

- Start slowly.
- Vary your activities; make it fun.

Sherman's Lagoon by J.P. Toomey

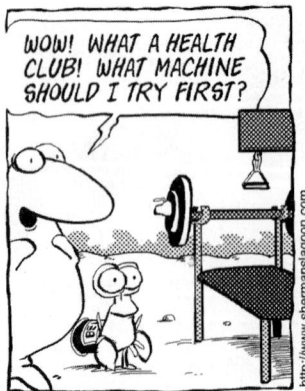
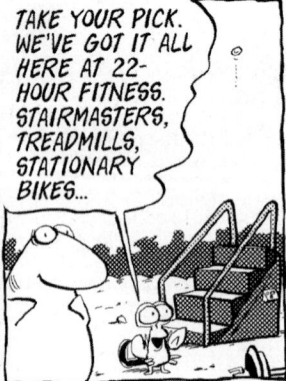
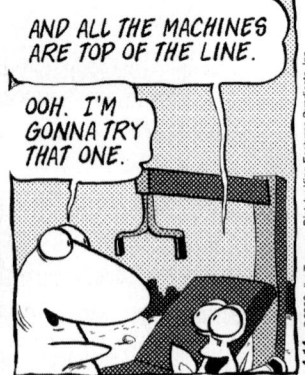
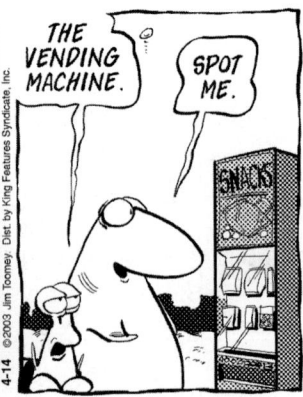

Why is regular physical activity—including some strength-building activities—generally advocated for all of us? What benefits accrue from this practice? How do strength-training and endurance athletes need to tailor their diets to support their vigorous physical activities? Chapter 10 provides some answers.

© Jim Toomey. Reprinted with special permission of King Features Syndicate.

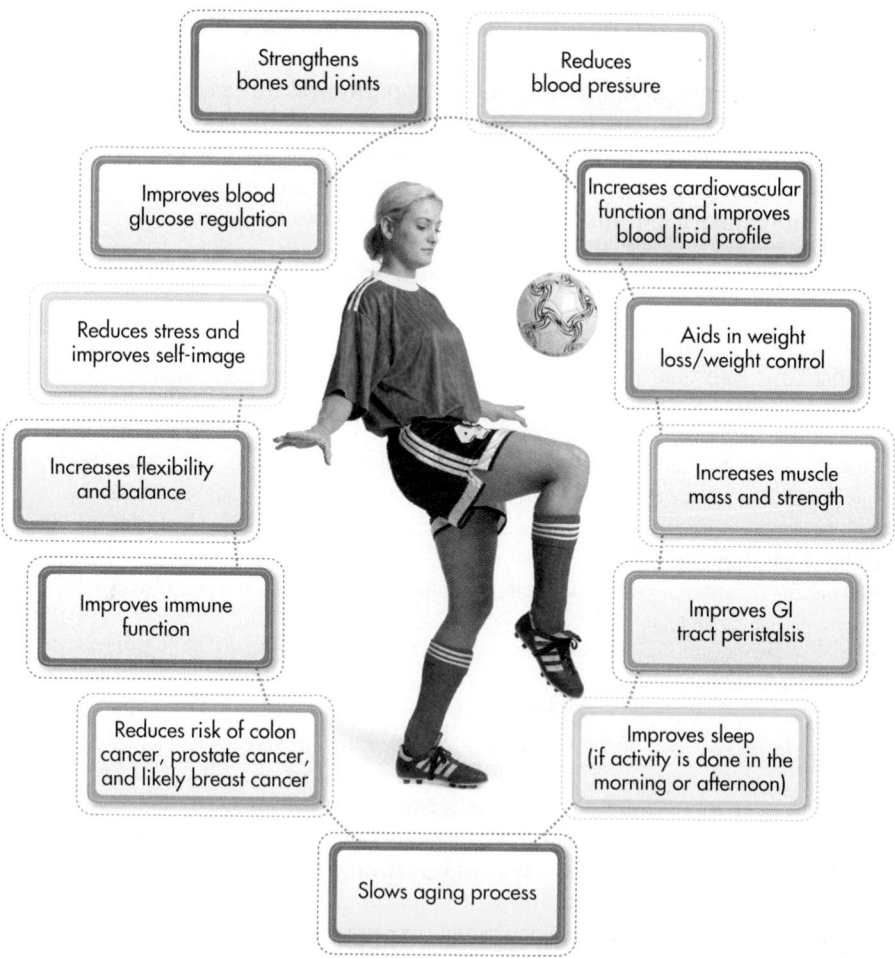

FIGURE 10-1 ▶ The benefits of regular, moderate physical activity and exercise.

- Include friends and family members.
- Set specific, attainable goals and monitor progress.
- Set aside a specific time each day for exercise; build it into your routine, but make it convenient.
- Reward yourself for being successful in keeping up with your goals.
- Don't worry about occasional setbacks; focus on the long-term benefits to your health.

The 2008 Physical Activity Guidelines for Americans recommend that all adults should avoid inactivity. Some physical activity is better than none, and adults who participate in any amount of physical activity gain some health benefits. The Physical Activity Guidelines set specific time goals for adults (review Chapter 2):

- For substantial health benefits, adults should do at least 150 minutes (2 hours and 30 minutes) a week of **moderate-intensity,** or 75 minutes (1 hour and 15 minutes) a week of **vigorous-intensity aerobic physical activity**, or an equivalent combination of moderate- and vigorous-intensity aerobic activity. Aerobic activity should be performed in episodes of at least 10 minutes, and preferably, it should be spread throughout the week.
- For additional and more extensive health benefits, adults should increase their aerobic physical activity to 300 minutes (5 hours) a week of moderate-intensity, or 150 minutes a week of vigorous-intensity aerobic physical activity, or an equivalent combination of moderate- and vigorous-intensity activity. Additional health benefits are gained by engaging in physical activity beyond this amount.
- Adults should also include **muscle-strengthening activities** that involve all major muscle groups on 2 or more days a week.

moderate-intensity aerobic physical activity Aerobic activity that increases a person's heart rate and breathing to some extent (5–6 on RPE scale). Examples include brisk walking, dancing, swimming, or bicycling on level terrain.

vigorous-intensity aerobic physical activity Aerobic activity that greatly increases a person's heart rate and breathing (7–8 on RPE scale). Examples include jogging, singles tennis, swimming continuous laps, or bicycling uphill.

muscle-strengthening activity Physical activity, including exercise, that increases skeletal muscle strength, power, endurance, and mass. Examples include strength training, resistance training, and muscle strength and endurance exercises.

These recommendations are consistent with guidance from the American College of Sports Medicine (see Further Reading 3).

The Physical Activity Guidelines aim to develop physical fitness and reduce risk of chronic diseases. Performing at least 150 minutes per week of moderate-intensity or 75 minutes per week of vigorous-intensity aerobic physical activity can assist efforts at preventing weight gain during adulthood. Weight loss and maintenance of weight loss require more than 150 minutes of physical activity per week.

▶ To earn yourself a place in the *Guinness Book of World Records* for the Physical Fitness Challenge, you'll need to complete:

2 miles swimming,

12 miles running,

12 miles hiking with a 25-pound backpack,

1250 push-ups,

1250 leg lifts,

1250 jumping jacks,

110 miles cycling,

20 miles rowing,

20 miles cross-training on elliptical equipment,

3250 abdominal crunches, and

300,000 pounds lifting through various upper-body repetitions.

Oh, and by the way, this will all need to be accomplished (on videotape and with at least three official witnesses) within 18 hours, 25 minutes, and 40 seconds!

MAKING DECISIONS

Planning Your Exercise

Consider applying the dietary principles of variety, balance, and moderation to your exercise plan:

- Variety: Enjoy many different activities to exercise different muscles.
- Balance: Different activities have different benefits, so balance your exercise pattern. For overall fitness, you need exercises that build cardiovascular endurance, muscular strength, and flexibility.
- Moderation: Exercise to keep fit without overdoing it. You don't need a heavy workout every day to achieve fitness.

CONCEPT CHECK

Regular physical activity is a vital part of a healthy lifestyle, ideally consisting of a total of at least 150 minutes of moderate-intensity or 75 minutes of vigorous-intensity aerobic physical activity per week. In addition, muscle-strengthening activities should be included at least twice per week. Physically active people benefit from lower risks of cardiovascular disease, type 2 diabetes, obesity, and other common chronic diseases.

10.2 Guidelines for Achieving and Maintaining Physical Fitness

For healthy people, a gradual increase to a goal of regular physical activity is recommended. Men 40 years of age or older and women 50 years of age or older who have been inactive for many years, or who have an existing health problem, should discuss their fitness goals with their physician before increasing activity. Health problems that require medical evaluation before beginning an exercise program are obesity, cardiovascular disease (or family history of it), hypertension, diabetes (or family history), shortness of breath after mild exertion, and arthritis.

During the first phase of a fitness program to promote health, you should begin to incorporate short periods of physical activity into your daily routine. This includes walking, taking the stairs instead of the elevator, house cleaning, gardening, and other activities that cause you to "huff and puff" a bit. The goal is a total of 30 minutes of this moderate type of physical activity on most (and preferably all) days. If necessary, this can be broken up into increments lasting at least 10 minutes. Experts suggest starting with short intervals, building up to a total of 30 minutes of activity incorporated into each day's tasks. If there is not much time for activity, you can even go for more intensity in the activities over shorter periods to get the same benefits. Clearly, many of the activities just recommended are not very vigorous.

Once you can perform physical activity for 30 minutes per day, turn your attention to more specific goals, such as increasing muscle mass and strength, to reap even more benefits. Guidelines for designing a fitness program are listed in Table 10-1.

Aerobic, strength, and stretching activities are included, as well as considerations for duration, frequency, intensity, and progression.

Begin by warming up with 5 to 10 minutes of low-intensity exercises, such as walking, slow jogging, or any slow version of the anticipated activity. This warms up your muscles so that muscle filaments more easily slide over one another to increase range of motion and decrease the risk of injury.

Aerobic Workout

Daily aerobic activity is recommended. As you learned in Chapter 3, "aerobic" means "with oxygen." Aerobic exercises use large muscle groups in a rhythmic fashion. They are usually of low or moderate intensity and long duration (i.e., 30 minutes of brisk walking). Health benefits from regular physical activity are especially seen when you can achieve a moderate level of intensity of exercise.

There are a few ways to determine the intensity of exercise. A popular and simple method is to use a percentage of your age-predicted maximum heart rate (Fig. 10-2). To find maximum heart rate, subtract your age from 220. Multiplying maximum heart rate by 0.60 and 0.90 will result in a range of heart rates, sometimes called the *target zone*. For a 20-year-old person beginning an exercise program, maximum heart rate equals 200 beats per minute ($220 - 20 = 200$). Then, (200×0.6) and (200×0.9) yields a target zone of 120 to 180 beats per minute. Measuring heart rate (pulse) is easy: Stop and count your pulse for 10 seconds and then multiply that number by 6 to determine your heart rate for one minute. Some exercise equipment and high-tech watches contain heart rate monitors.

At the initiation of an exercise program, aim for the lower end of the target zone. As you progress and become more physically fit, you can work up to a higher heart rate. As with many of the prediction formulas, calculation of maximum heart rate is just an estimate. Medications, such as those for hypertension and other health conditions, may impact heart rate. If you have health concerns, a physician can help to personalize your target zone.

▲ What is the best exercise? One you want to continue to do.

TABLE 10-1 Designing a Fitness Program

Type of Activity	Aerobic (uses large muscle groups in rhythmic fashion)	Strength (resistance activity)	Stretching (uses major muscle groups; most beneficial when muscles are warm, such as during cooldown.)
Examples	Brisk walking, running, cycling, swimming, basketball, tennis, soccer	Weight lifting, pilates, push-ups, pull-ups	Yoga
Duration (time spent in exercise session)	20 to 60 minutes	8 to 12 repetitions of 8 to 10 different exercises	4 repetitions of 10 to 30 seconds per muscle group
Frequency (times activity is performed)	5 days per week	2 to 3 days per week	2 to 3 days per week and during warm-up and cooldown
Intensity (level of exertion)	55% to 90% maximum heart rate or RPE of 4 or above (see Figure 10-3)	Enough to condition major muscle groups of the upper and lower body	5 to 10 minutes during warm-up and cooldown
Progression (increase in frequency, intensity, and duration over time)	**Initiation phase:** 3 to 6 weeks **Improvement phase:** 5 to 6 months **Maintenance phase:** plateau in gains in fitness		Start with smaller muscle groups (e.g., arms) and work toward large muscle groups (e.g., legs and abdomen)

FIGURE 10-2 ▶ Heart rate training chart. This chart shows the number of heart beats per minute that corresponds to various exercise intensities.

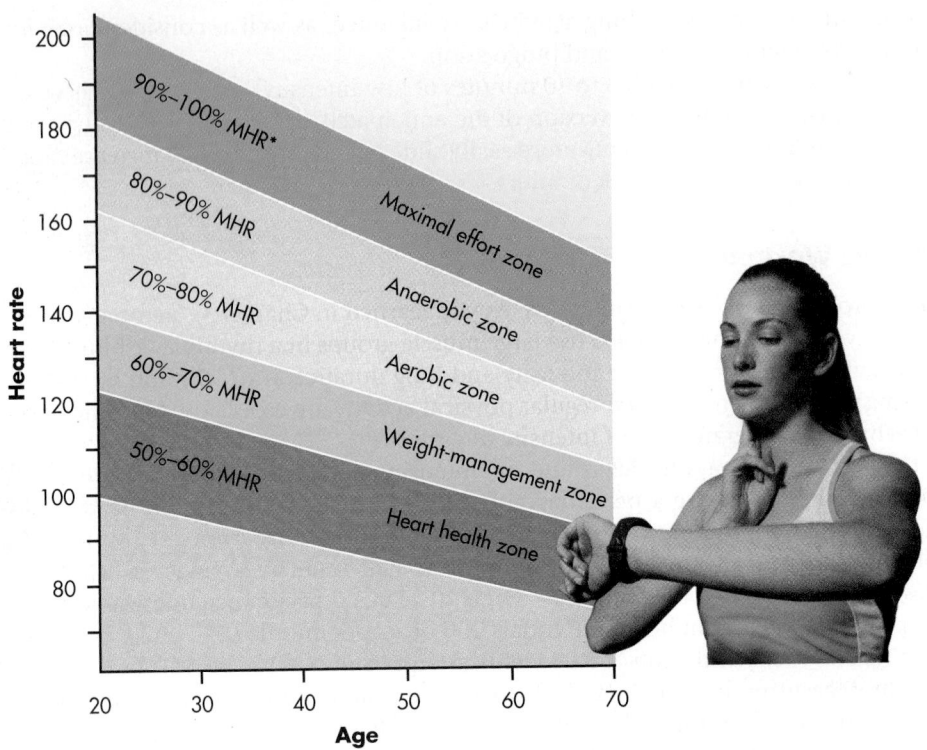

*MHR (maximum heart rate) = 220 - Age in years

Another way of determining the intensity of exercise is the Rating of Perceived Exertion scale (RPE). One version includes a range of 1 to 10, with each number corresponding to a subjective feeling of exertion. For example, the number 0 is "nothing at all" (sitting at a table) and the number 10 is considered close to maximal effort or "very, very strong" (all-out sprint) (Fig. 10-3).

When using the RPE scale, the goal is to aim for the number 4, which corresponds to the beginning of "somewhat strong." This is the point at which you begin to see significant fitness results. You should be working hard, but still be able to talk to an exercise partner (sometimes called the "talk test").

During cooldown, follow a reverse pattern of the warm-up: 5 to 10 minutes of low-intensity activity and add 5 to 10 minutes of stretching. The same exercises performed during warm-up are appropriate. The cooldown is essential to the prevention of injury and soreness.

10.3 Energy Sources for Exercising Muscles

Like other cells, muscle cells cannot directly use the energy released from breaking down glucose or triglycerides. Muscle cells need a specific form of energy for contraction. Body cells must first convert food energy (i.e., calories) to **adenosine triphosphate (ATP)**.

The chemical bonds between phosphates in ATP and related molecules are high-energy bonds. Using the energy obtained from foodstuffs, cells make ATP from its breakdown product **adenosine diphosphate (ADP)** and a phosphate group (abbreviated P_i).

$$ADP + Energy \ from \ food + P_i \rightarrow ATP$$

Conversely, to release energy from ATP, cells partially break the compound down into ADP and P_i. The released energy is used for many cell functions.

$$ATP \rightarrow Energy \ to \ do \ work + ADP + P_i$$

Structure of ATP

High-energy bonds

adenosine triphosphate (ATP) The main energy currency for cells. ATP energy is used to promote ion pumping, enzyme activity, and muscular contraction.

adenosine diphosphate (ADP) A breakdown product of ATP. ADP is synthesized into ATP using energy from foodstuffs and a phosphate group (abbreviated P_i).

RPE Scale*

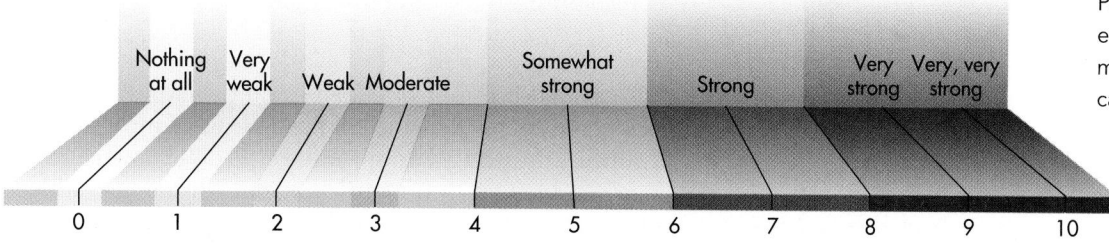

Nothing at all — Very weak — Weak — Moderate — Somewhat strong — Strong — Very strong — Very, very strong

0   1   2   3   4   5   6   7   8   9   10

* Rating of Perceived Exertion (RPE) beyond 10 is considered maximal.

FIGURE 10-3 ▶ Rating of Perceived Exertion scale. When exercising, aim for 4 for light/moderate activity or up to 8 for cardiorespiratory fitness.

Essentially, ATP is the immediate source of energy for body functions (Table 10-2). The primary goal in the use of any fuel, whether carbohydrate, fat, or protein, is to make ATP. A resting muscle cell contains only a small amount of ATP that can be used immediately. This amount of ATP could keep the muscle working maximally for only about 2 to 4 seconds if no resupply of ATP were possible. Fortunately, another type of high-energy compound—**phosphocreatine (PCr)**—is also present in muscle cells and can be quickly broken down to release enough energy to make more ATP. This supports the working muscle cells until metabolism of carbohydrate and fat for fuel begins in earnest. Overall, cells must constantly and repeatedly use and then re-form ATP, using a variety of energy sources.

Phosphocreatine Is the First Line of Defense for Resupplying ATP in Muscles

As soon as ATP stored in muscle cells begins to be used, another source of energy just mentioned, PCr, is used to produce ATP. An enzyme in the muscle cell is activated to split PCr into phosphate and **creatine.** This releases energy that can be used to re-form ATP from its breakdown products. If no other source of energy for ATP resupply were available, PCr could probably maintain maximal muscle contractions

phosphocreatine (PCr) A high-energy compound that can be used to re-form ATP. It is used primarily during bursts of activity, such as lifting and jumping.

creatine An organic (i.e., carbon-containing) molecule in muscle cells that serves as a part of a high-energy compound (termed creatine phosphate or phosphocreatine) capable of synthesizing ATP from ADP.

TABLE 10-2 Energy Sources Used by Resting and Working Muscle Cells

Energy Source*	When in Use	Activity
ATP	At all times	All types
Phosphocreatine (PCr)	All exercise initially; short bursts of exercise thereafter	Shotput, high jump, bench press
Carbohydrate (anaerobic)	High-intensity exercise, especially lasting 30 seconds to 2 minutes	200-yard (about 200 meters) sprint
Carbohydrate (aerobic)	Exercise lasting 2 minutes to 3 hours or more; the higher the intensity (for example, running a 6-minute mile), the greater the use	Basketball, swimming, jogging, power walking, soccer, tennis
Fat (aerobic)	Exercise lasting more than a few minutes; greater amounts are used at lower exercise intensities	Long-distance running, long-distance cycling; much of the fuel used in a 30-minute brisk walk is fat
Protein (aerobic)	Low amount during all exercise; slightly more in endurance exercise, especially when carbohydrate fuel is depleted	Long-distance running

*At any given time, more than one source is used. The relative amount of use differs during various activities.

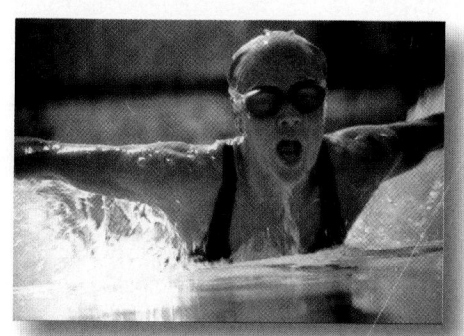

▲ Bursts of muscle activity use a variety of energy sources, including PCr and ATP.

See the Nutrition and Your Health Section: Ergogenic Aids and Athletic Performance at the end of Chapter 10.

aerobic Requiring oxygen.

anaerobic Not requiring oxygen.

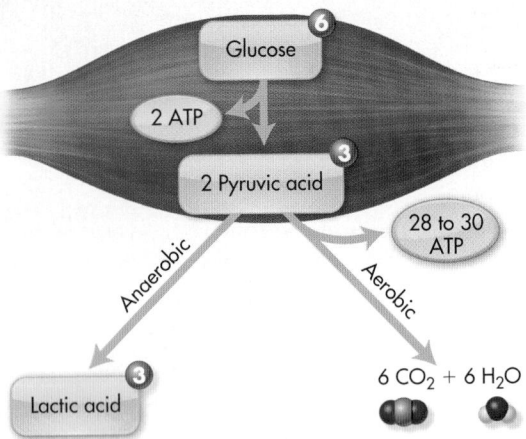

FIGURE 10-4 ▶ ATP yield from aerobic versus anaerobic glucose use. Encircled numbers indicate the number of carbons in each molecule.

pyruvic acid A three-carbon compound formed during glucose metabolism; also called *pyruvate*.

lactic acid A three-carbon acid formed during anaerobic cell metabolism; a partial breakdown product of glucose; also called *lactate*.

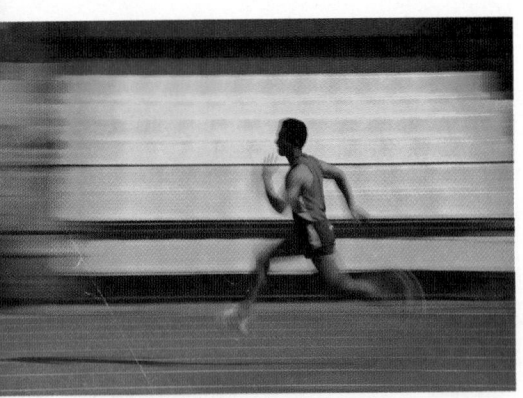

▲ Sprinting relies primarily on anaerobic glucose breakdown.

for about 10 seconds. Other sources of ATP resupply kick in, however, so PCr ends up as a source of energy for events lasting about 1 minute or less.

$$PCr + ADP \rightarrow ATP + Cr$$

The main advantage of PCr is that it can be activated instantly and can replenish ATP at rates fast enough to meet the energy demands of the fastest and most powerful actions, including jumping, lifting, throwing, and sprinting. The disadvantage of PCr is that not much of it is made and stored in the muscles. Strength-training athletes have begun to use creatine supplements in an effort to increase PCr in muscles.

Carbohydrate Fuel for Muscles

Carbohydrates are an important fuel for muscles. The most useful form of carbohydrate fuel is the simple sugar glucose, available to all cells from the bloodstream. As you will recall from Chapter 4, glucose is stored as glycogen in the liver and muscle cells. Blood glucose is maintained by the breakdown of liver glycogen. Breakdown of glycogen stored in a specific muscle also helps meet the carbohydrate demand of that muscle, but the actual amount of glycogen stored in muscle is limited (about 350 grams for all the muscles in the body, which would yield about 1400 kcal).

Depending on whether oxygen is available to exercising muscles, use of glucose to make ATP can be either **anaerobic** or **aerobic**.

Anaerobic Glucose Breakdown Yields Energy Fast. When oxygen supply in the muscle is limited (anaerobic conditions), glucose is broken down into a three-carbon compound called **pyruvic acid**. The pyruvic acid accumulates in the muscle and is then converted to **lactic acid**. Only about 5% of the total amount of ATP that could be formed from complete breakdown of glucose, is released through this anaerobic process (glucose → → lactic acid).

The advantage of anaerobic glucose breakdown is that it is the fastest way to resupply ATP, other than PCr breakdown. It therefore provides most of the energy needed for events that require a quick burst of energy, ranging from about 30 seconds to 2 minutes. Examples of activities that primarily rely on anaerobic glucose breakdown include sprinting 400 meters or swimming 100 meters.

The two major disadvantages of the anaerobic process are that (1) the high rate of ATP production cannot be sustained for long periods, and (2) the rapid accumulation of lactic acid greatly increases the acidity of the muscle. Acidity inhibits the activities of key enzymes in the muscle cells, slowing anaerobic ATP production and causing short-term fatigue. The acidity also leads to a net potassium loss from muscle cells, providing another cause of fatigue. We learn by trial-and-error a pace that will control muscle lactic acid concentrations during these anaerobic events.

For the most part, lactic acid builds up in active muscle cells until it is released into the bloodstream. The liver (and the kidneys, to some extent) takes up the lactic acid and resynthesizes it into glucose. Glucose can then reenter the bloodstream, where it is available for cell uptake and breakdown.

Aerobic Glucose Breakdown Is a Sustained Energy Source. If plenty of oxygen is available in the muscle (aerobic conditions), such as when the exercise is of low to moderate intensity, the bulk of the three-carbon pyruvic acid is shuttled to the mitochondria of the cell, where it is fully metabolized into carbon dioxide (CO_2) and water (H_2O) (Fig. 10-5). This aerobic breakdown of glucose yields approximately 95% of the ATP made from complete glucose metabolism (glucose → → CO_2 + H_2O).

Aerobic glucose breakdown supplies more ATP than does the anaerobic process, but it releases the energy more slowly. This slower rate of aerobic energy supply can be sustained for hours. One reason is that the products are carbon dioxide and water, not lactic acid. Aerobic glucose breakdown makes a major energy contribution to activities that last anywhere from 2 minutes to 3 hours or more. Examples of such activities include jogging or distance swimming (review Table 10-2).

Many researchers have studied the ability of various types of carbohydrate feeding regimens to maximize glucose supply to muscles during prolonged exercise. Overall, the techniques have succeeded. Consuming about 30 to 60 grams of carbohydrate per hour during strenuous endurance exercise that lasts 1 hour or more, such as cycling, can aid in maintaining adequate blood glucose, resulting in a delay of fatigue by 30 to 60 minutes. This attention to carbohydrate intake also helps one tolerate vigorous training on a daily basis.

As blood glucose declines during exercise, so does mental function. Cyclists refer to this diminished mental ability as "bonking." The fall in blood glucose is related to depletion of liver glycogen, not muscle glycogen, because liver glycogen is used to maintain blood glucose. See the later section, "Sports Drinks," to learn more about carbohydrate replacement during exercise.

CRITICAL THINKING

Marty started going to the gym about 8 weeks ago. At first, he noticed that he began "huffing and puffing" about 7 minutes into his aerobic workout. Now, however, he can work out for about 25 minutes without tiring. What is a possible explanation for this ability to work out longer?

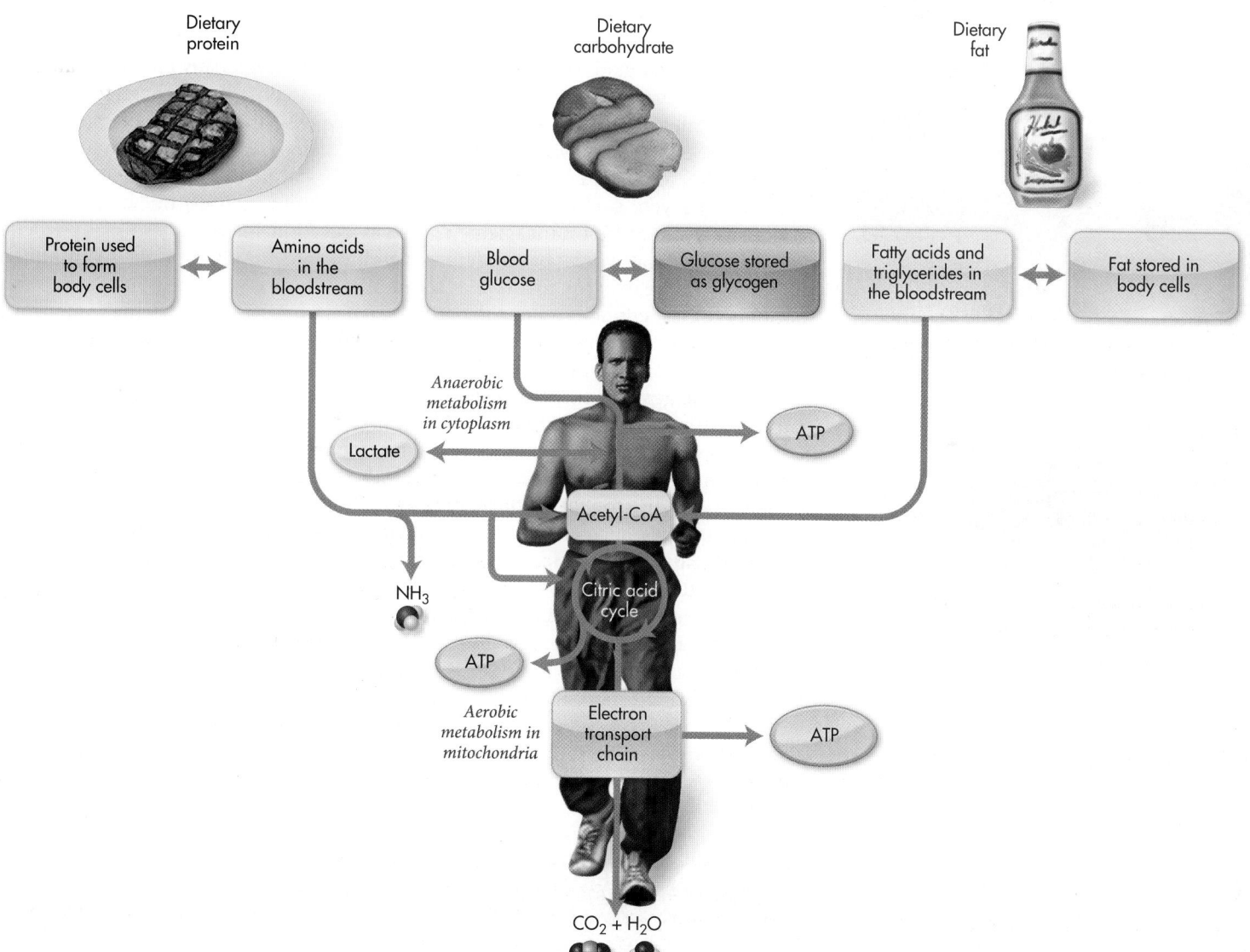

FIGURE 10-5 ▶ Simplified view of ATP formation from carbohydrate, fat, and protein. Along with phosphocreatine (PCr), all three macronutrients may be used for ATP synthesis, but glucose and fatty acids are primary sources. Glucose may be broken down anaerobically or may undergo complete aerobic metabolism. The products of fatty acid breakdown are channeled into aerobic metabolism. Although limited, products of amino-acid breakdown are channeled into the aerobic pathway as well. Recall also from Chapters 8 and 9 that many vitamins and minerals participate in these metabolic pathways.

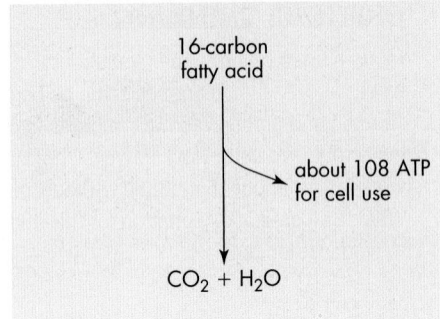

▲ ATP yield from aerobic fatty acid utilization.

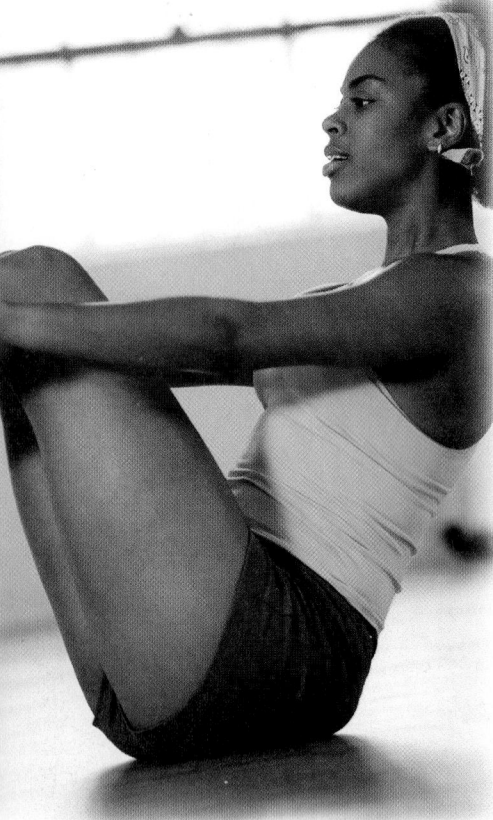

▲ Fatty acids can come from all over the body, not necessarily from fat stored near the active muscles. *This is why spot reducing does not work.* Exercise can tone the muscles near adipose tissue but does not preferentially use those stores.

Carbohydrate intake during exercise is not as important in shorter events (e.g., 30 minutes or so) because the muscles do not take up much blood glucose during short-term exercise, relying instead primarily on their glycogen stores for fuel.

Fat: The Main Fuel for Prolonged Low-Intensity Activity

When fat stores in body tissues begin to be broken down for energy, each triglyceride first yields three fatty acids and a glycerol. The majority of the stored energy is found in the fatty acids. During physical activity, fatty acids are released from various adipose tissue depots into the bloodstream and travel to the muscles, where they are taken into each cell and broken down aerobically to carbon dioxide and water. Some of the fat stored in muscles also is used, especially as activity increases from a low to a moderate pace (see Further Reading 2).

The rate at which muscles use fatty acids partly depends on the concentration of fatty acids in the bloodstream. In other words, the more fatty acids released from adipose tissue stores into the bloodstream, the more fat will be used by the muscles. Some cyclists and other endurance athletes have attempted to raise their blood concentrations of fatty acids by consuming caffeinated beverages. This practice can actually increase fatty acid release from the adipose tissue depots and is therefore helpful to certain athletes, but it is illegal under NCAA rules if the amount of caffeine in the body exceeds the equivalent of 6 to 8 cups of coffee (see the Nutrition and Your Health section at the end of this chapter).

Fat is not a very useful muscle fuel for intense, brief exercise, but it becomes a progressively more important energy source as duration increases, especially when exercise remains at a low or moderate (aerobic) rate for more than 20 minutes (Fig. 10-6). The reason for this is that some of the steps involved in fat breakdown cannot occur fast enough to meet the ATP demands of short-duration, high-intensity exercise. If fat were the only available fuel, we would be unable to exercise beyond a fast walk or jog.

The advantage of fat fuel is that it provides stores of energy in a relatively concentrated form, and we generally have a lot of it stored. For a given weight of fuel, fat supplies more than twice as much energy as carbohydrate does. For lengthy activities at a moderate pace (for example, hiking) or even sitting at a desk for 8 hours a day, fat supplies about 70% to 90% of the energy required. Carbohydrate use is much less. As intensity increases, such as in a 3-hour marathon run at a competitive pace, muscles use about a 50:50 ratio of fat to carbohydrate. In comparison, for short events, such as a 100-meter sprint or even a 1500-meter race, the contribution of fat to resupply ATP is minimal. To summarize, remember that the only fast-paced (anaerobic) fuel we eat is carbohydrate; slow and steady (aerobic) activity uses fat in addition to carbohydrate.

MAKING DECISIONS

Training Effect

As people start exercising regularly four or five times per week, they experience a "training effect." Initially, these individuals might be able to exercise for 20 minutes before tiring. Months later, exercise can be extended to an hour before they feel tired. During the months of training, muscle cells have produced more mitochondria and thus can burn more fat. Training also increases the number of capillaries in muscles, which increases oxygen supply to the muscles. As a result, lactic acid production from anaerobic glucose metabolism decreases. Lactic acid contributes to short-term muscle fatigue, so the less lactic acid produced, the longer the exercise can be sustained. Other contributors to the training effect include increased aerobic efficiency of the heart and muscles and elevations in muscle triglyceride content, with an enhanced ability of muscles to use triglycerides for energy needs.

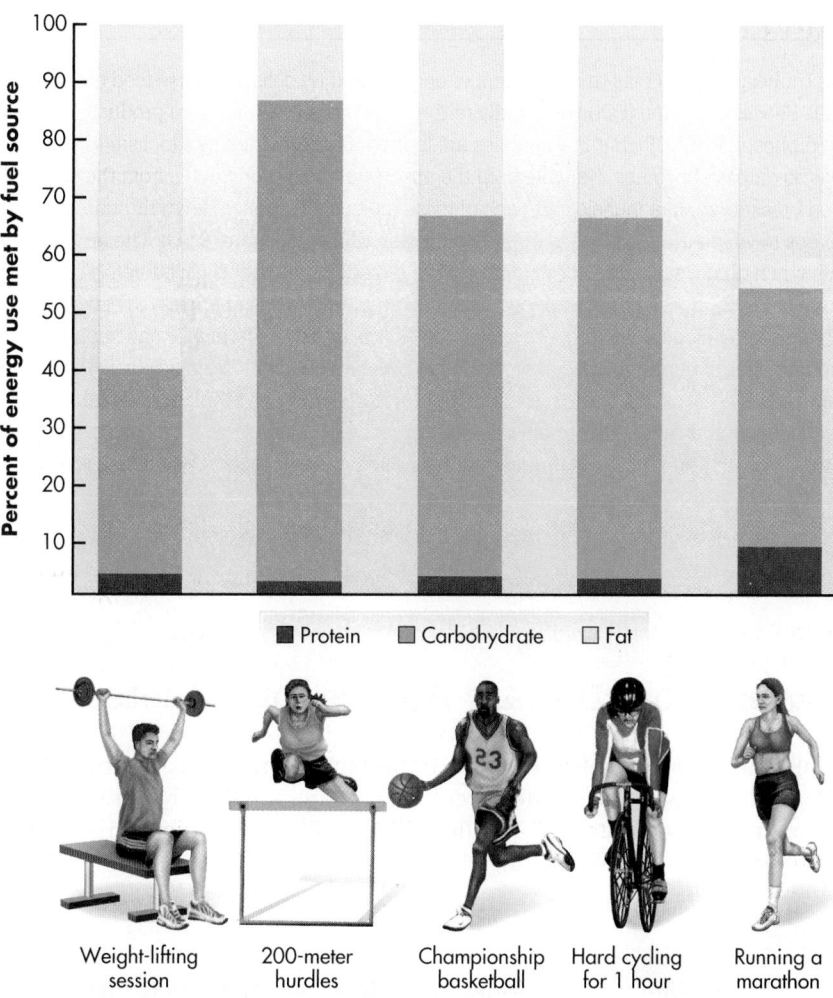

Weight-lifting session — 200-meter hurdles — Championship basketball — Hard cycling for 1 hour — Running a marathon

■ Protein ■ Carbohydrate □ Fat

Percent of energy use met by fuel source

FIGURE 10-6 ▶ Rough estimates of fuel use during various forms of physical activity. With regard to the weight-lifting session, carbohydrate use could be somewhat greater and fat use somewhat less if the session is intense and fast-paced (e.g., circuit training). Fat use generally is higher because much of the time spent weight lifting is for rest periods and equipment-related activities.

Protein: A Minor Fuel Source, Primarily for Endurance Exercise

Although amino acids derived from protein can be used to fuel muscles, their contribution is relatively small, compared with that of carbohydrate and fat. As a rough guide, only about 5% of the body's general energy needs, as well as the typical energy needs of exercising muscles, is supplied by the metabolism of amino acids.

During endurance exercise, proteins can contribute importantly to energy needs, perhaps as much as 10% to 15%, especially as glycogen stores in the muscle are exhausted. Most of the energy supplied from protein comes from metabolism of the branched-chain amino acids—leucine, isoleucine, and valine. A normal diet provides ample branched-chain amino acids to supply this amount of fuel, so protein or amino-acid supplements are not needed. Contrary to what many athletes believe, protein is used for fuel less in resistance types of exercise (e.g., weight lifting) than in endurance exercise (e.g., running) (review Fig. 10-6). The primary muscle fuels for weight lifting are phosphocreatine (PCr) and carbohydrate for the brief bursts of activity, with fat providing energy during the resting stages, and with little use of protein overall. Despite this, high-protein products such as Pro-Complex, Amino Fuel 2000, High Voltage Protein Drink, and Instant Egg Protein are marketed specifically to weight lifters and bodybuilders in nearly every health-food and fitness store. Consuming high-carbohydrate, moderate-protein foods immediately after a weight-training workout enhances the muscle-building effect of the activity, most likely by increasing the concentrations of insulin and growth hormone released into the blood and contributing to protein synthesis. Still, it is impossible to increase muscle mass simply by eating protein. Overloading muscle through strength training or other physical activity is needed.

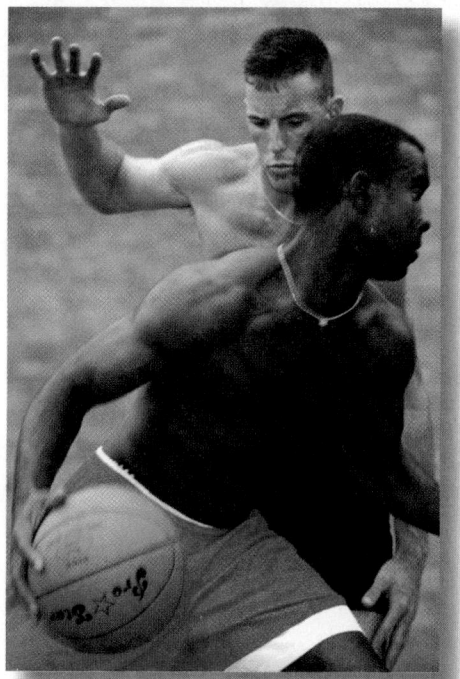

▲ The calories needed to perform come from carbohydrate, fat, and protein. The relative mix depends on the pace.

CONCEPT CHECK

Adenosine triphosphate (ATP) is the main form of energy used by cells. Cells use food energy to form ATP. Phosphocreatine (PCr) can rapidly re-form ATP from its breakdown product adenosine diphosphate (ADP), but PCr supplies are limited. Carbohydrate metabolism to form ATP begins as glucose becomes available from the absorption of carbohydrates from the diet or glycogen breakdown. In a muscle cell, each glucose molecule is broken down through a series of steps to yield either lactic acid or carbon dioxide (CO_2) plus water (H_2O). The process that occurs when glucose is broken down into carbon dioxide and water is called *aerobic* because oxygen is used. The conversion of glucose to lactic acid is called *anaerobic* because no oxygen is used. The anaerobic process allows the cell to quickly re-form ATP and supports the demand for energy during intense exercise. Fat is a key aerobic fuel for muscle cells, especially at low exercise outputs. At rest and during light activity, muscles burn primarily fat for energy needs. In comparison, little protein generally is used to fuel muscles. At most, protein supplies 10% to 15% of energy needs during endurance activities, especially when glycogen stores are depleted.

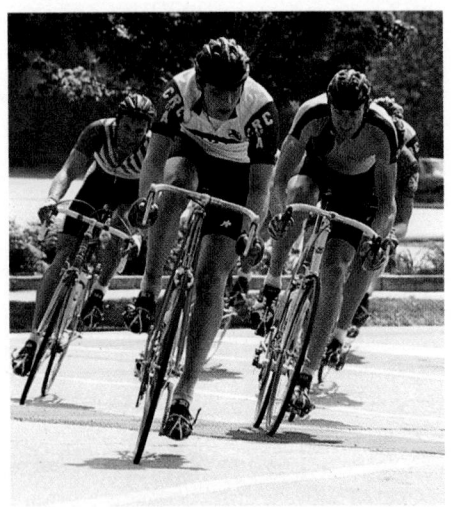

▲ Intense athletic training may require thousands of additional calories. This increased food intake should easily provide ample protein and other nutrients to support activity.

Review Table 7-4 in Chapter 7, which listed the energy costs of typical forms of physical activity.

10.4 Power Food: Dietary Advice for Athletes

Athletic training and genetic makeup are two important determinants of athletic performance. A good diet won't substitute for either factor, but diet can help to enhance and maximize an athlete's potential. On the other hand, a poor diet can seriously reduce performance (see Further Readings 12 and 15).

Calorie Needs

Athletes need varying amounts of calories, depending on each athlete's body size, body composition, and the type of training or competition being considered. A small person may need only 1700 kcal daily to sustain normal daily activities without losing body weight; a large, muscular man may need 4000 kcal. Review Chapter 7 or visit www.ChooseMyPlate.gov to calculate Estimated Energy Requirements (EERs) at various activity levels. These rough estimates can be viewed as starting points that need to be individualized by trial and error for each athlete.

An estimate of the calories required to sustain moderate activity is 5 to 8 kcal per minute. The calories required for sports training or competition then have to be added to those used to carry on normal activities. For example, an hour of bowling requires few calories in addition to that required to sustain normal daily living. At the other extreme, a 12-hour endurance bicycle race over mountains can require an additional 4000 kcal per day. Therefore, some athletes may need as much as 7000 kcal or more daily to maintain body weight while training, whereas others may need 1700 kcal or less. If an athlete experiences daily fatigue, the first consideration should be whether he or she is consuming enough food. Up to six meals per day may be needed, including one before each workout.

How can we know if an athlete is getting enough calories? Estimating daily intake from a food diary kept by the athlete is one way. Another step is to estimate the athlete's body fat percentage via skinfold measurements, bioelectrical impedance, or underwater weighing (review Chapter 7). Body fat should be the typical amount found for athletes in the specific sport practiced. This corresponds to 5% to 18% for most male athletes and 17% to 28% for most female athletes. The next step is to monitor body weight changes on a daily or weekly basis. If body weight starts to fall, calories should be increased; if weight rises and it is because of increases in body fat, the athlete should eat less.

MAKING DECISIONS

Making Weight

Wrestlers, boxers, judoists, jockeys, and oarsmen often try to lose weight before a competition, so that they can be certified to compete in a lower weight class. This helps them gain a mechanical advantage over an opponent of smaller stature. They usually lose this weight before stepping on the scale for weight certification. Athletes can lose up to 22 pounds (10 kilograms) of body weight as water in 1 day by sitting in a sauna, exercising in a plastic sweat suit, or taking diuretic drugs, which speed water loss from the kidneys. Losing as little as 2% of body weight by dehydration, however, can adversely affect endurance and performance, especially in hot weather. A pattern of repeated weight loss or gain of more than 5% of body weight by dehydration carries risk of kidney malfunction and heat-related illness. Death is also a possibility.

To prevent future deaths from such weight loss in athletes, the National Collegiate Athletic Association and many states have authorized physicians or athletic trainers to set safe weight and body fat content minimums (e.g., 7% or more of total body weight for male athletes and 12% or more for females) in weight-class sports. Under new guidelines, athletes are assigned to weight classes at the beginning of the season and are not allowed to "cut weight" to gain a competitive advantage. Weight gain in the days after a competition (reflecting regain of body water) can now be no greater than 2 pounds. If athletes, such as wrestlers, wish to compete in a lower-bodyweight class and have enough extra fat stores, they should begin a gradual, sustained reduction in calorie intake long before the competitive season starts.

If the body composition test shows that an athlete has too much body fat, the athlete should lower food intake by about 200 to 500 kcal per day, while maintaining a regular exercise program, until the desirable fat percentage is achieved. Reducing fat intake is the best nutrient-related approach. On the other hand, if an athlete needs to gain weight, increasing food intake by 500 to 700 kcal per day will eventually lead to the needed weight gain. A mix of carbohydrate, fat, and protein is advised, coupled with exercise to make sure this gain is mostly in the form of lean tissue and not fat stores.

Carbohydrate Needs

Anyone who exercises vigorously, especially for more than 1 hour per day on a regular basis, needs to consume a diet that includes moderate to high amounts of carbohydrates. The diet should provide a variety of foods, such as those portrayed by MyPlate. Numerous servings of grains, starchy vegetables, and fruits provide enough carbohydrate to maintain adequate liver and muscle glycogen stores, especially for replacing glycogen losses from workouts on the previous day. Relatively low-carbohydrate/ high-protein diets, such as the Zone Diet, are not recommended. Recall that Chapter 7 discussed the Zone Diet. The carbohydrate content of this diet is only 40% of calories, rather than the 60% or more typically recommended for athletes.

Carbohydrate intake should be at least 5 grams per kilogram body weight. People engaged in aerobic training and endurance activities (60 minutes or more per day) may need as much as 7 grams per kilogram body weight. When exercise duration approaches several hours per day, the carbohydrate recommendation increases to up to 10 grams per kilogram of body weight. In other words, triathletes and marathoners should consider eating close to 500 to 600 grams of carbohydrates daily, and even more if necessary, to (1) prevent chronic fatigue and (2) load the muscles and liver with glycogen. Attention to carbohydrate intake is especially important when performing multiple training bouts in a day, such as swim practices, or heavy training on successive days, as in cross-country running. Depletion of carbohydrate ranks just behind depletion of fluid and electrolytes as a major cause of fatigue. Table 10-3 shows sample menus, based on MyPlate's Daily Food Plan recommendations, for

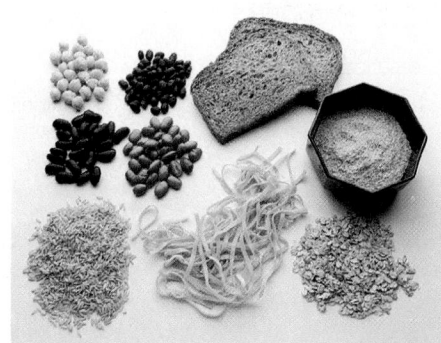

▲ High-carbohydrate foods should form the basis of the diet for athletes.

TABLE 10-3 Sample Daily Menus Based on MyPlate's Daily Food Plan* Recommendations That Provide Various Total Calorie Intakes

1500 kcal	2000 kcal	3000 kcal	4000 kcal	5000 kcal
Breakfast Fat-free milk, 1 cup Cheerios, 1/2 cup Bagel, 1/2 Cherry jam, 2 tsp Margarine, 1 tsp	**Breakfast** Fat-free milk, 1 cup Cheerios, 1 cup Bagel, 1/2 Cherry jam, 1 tbsp Margarine, 1 tsp	**Breakfast** Fat-free milk, 1 cup Cheerios, 2 cups Bagel, 1 Cherry jam, 2 tsp Margarine, 1 tsp Bran muffins, 2	**Breakfast** Fat-free milk, 1 cup Cheerios, 2 cups Orange, 1 Bran muffins, 2	**Breakfast** Fat-reduced milk, 1 cup Cheerios, 2 cups Bran muffins, 2 Orange, 1
			Snack Chopped dates, 3/4 cup	**Snack** Low-fat yogurt, 1 cup Chopped dates, 1 cup

Lunch
Chicken breast (roasted),
  2 oz
Figs, 1
Fat-free milk, 1/2 cup
Banana, 1
	Lunch
	Chicken breast (roasted),
	  2 oz
	Wheat bread, 2 slices
	Mayonnaise, 1 tsp
	Raisins, 1/4 cup
	Cranberry juice,
	  1 1/2 cups
	Banana, 1
		Lunch
		Chicken breast (roasted),
		  2 oz
		Wheat bread, 2 slices
		Provolone cheese, 1 oz
		Mayonnaise, 1 tsp
		Raisins, 1/3 cup
		Cranberry juice,
		  1 1/2 cups
		Low-fat fruit yogurt, 1 cup
			Lunch
			Romaine lettuce, 1 cup
			Garbanzo beans, 1 cup
			Grated carrots, 1/2 cup
			French dressing, 2 tbsp
			Macaroni and cheese,
			  3 cups
			Apple juice, 1 cup
				Lunch
				Chicken enchilada, 1
				Romaine lettuce, 1 cup
				Garbanzo beans, 1 cup
				Shredded carrots, 3/4 cup
				Chopped celery, 1/2 cup
				Seasoned croutons, 1 oz
				French dressing, 2 tbsp
				Wheat bread, 2 slices
				Margarine, 1 tbsp
				Apple juice, 1 cup

Snack Oatmeal-raisin cookie, 1 Low-fat fruit yogurt, 1 cup	**Snack** Oatmeal-raisin cookies, 3 Low-fat fruit yogurt, 1 cup	**Snack** Banana, 1 Oatmeal-raisin cookies, 3	**Snack** Wheat bread, 2 slices Margarine, 1 tsp Jam, 2 tbsp	**Snack** Banana, 1 Bagel, 1 Cream cheese, 1 tbsp

Dinner
Spaghetti w/meatballs,
  1 cup
Romaine lettuce, 1 cup
Italian dressing, 2 tsp
Green beans, 1/2 cup
Cranberry juice, 1 1/2 cups
	Dinner
	Broiled beef sirloin, 3 oz
	Romaine lettuce, 1 cup
	Italian dressing, 2 tsp
	Green beans, 1 cup
	Fat-free milk, 1/2 cup
		Dinner
		Broiled beef sirloin, 3 oz
		Romaine lettuce, 1 cup
		Garbanzo beans, 1 cup
		Italian dressing, 2 tsp
		Spinach pasta noodles,
		  1 1/2 cups
		Margarine, 1 tsp
		Green beans, 1 cup
		Fat-free milk, 1/2 cup
			Dinner
			Skinless turkey breast, 2 oz
			Mashed potatoes, 2 cups
			Peas and onions, 1 cup
			Banana, 1
			Fat-free milk, 1 cup
				Dinner
				Beef sirloin, 5 oz
				Mashed potatoes, 2 cups
				Spinach pasta noodles,
				  1 1/2 cups
				Grated parmesan cheese,
				  2 tbsp
				Green beans, 1 cup
				Oatmeal-raisin cookies, 3
				Fat-reduced milk, 1 cup

			Snack Pasta, 1 cup cooked Margarine, 2 tsp Parmesan cheese, 2 tbsp Cranberry juice, 1 cup	**Snack** Air-popped popcorn, 4 cups Raisins, 1/3 cup Cranberry juice, 2 cups
18% protein (68 grams) 64% carbohydrate (240 grams) 19% fat (32 grams)	17% protein (85 grams) 63% carbohydrate (315 grams) 20% fat (44 grams)	17% protein (128 grams) 62% carbohydrate (465 grams) 21% fat (70 grams)	14% protein (140 grams) 61% carbohydrate (610 grams) 26% fat (116 grams)	14% protein (175 grams) 63% carbohydrate (813 grams) 24% fat (136 grams)

* Daily Food Plans are available online for diets supplying 1000 to 3200 kcal/day (see www.ChooseMyPlate.gov). Additional servings from each food group have been added to supply increased calories while maintaining healthy proportions of protein, carbohydrate and fat.

diets providing food energy ranging from 1500 to 5000 kcal per day. In addition, the Exchange System described in Appendix D is a very useful tool for planning all types of diets, including high-carbohydrate diets for athletes.

As noted, athletes should obtain at least 60% of their total energy needs from carbohydrate (rather than the 50% typical of most North American diets), especially if exercise duration is expected to exceed 2 hours and total caloric intake is about 3000 kcal per day or less. Diets providing 4000 to 5000 kcal per day can be as low as 50% carbohydrate, as these will still provide sufficient carbohydrate (e.g., 500 to 600 grams or so per day).

One does not have to give up any specific food when planning a high-carbohydrate diet. The focus is to include more high-carbohydrate foods while moderating concentrated fat sources. Sports nutritionists emphasize the difference between a high-carbohydrate meal and a high-carbohydrate/high-fat meal. Before endurance events, such as marathons or triathlons, some athletes seek to increase their carbohydrate reserves by eating foods such as potato chips, French fries, banana cream pie, and pastries. Although such foods provide carbohydrate, they also contain a lot of fat. Better high-carbohydrate food choices include pasta, rice, potatoes, bread, fruit and fruit juices, and many breakfast cereals (check the label for carbohydrate content) (Table 10-4). Sports drinks appropriate for carbohydrate loading, such as GatorLode and UltraFuel, can also help. Consuming a moderate rather than a high amount of fiber during the final day of training is a good precaution to reduce the chances of bloating and intestinal gas during the next day's event.

Carbohydrate Loading

For athletes who compete in continuous, intense aerobic events lasting more than 60 to 90 minutes (or in shorter events taking place more than once within a 24-hour period), a **carbohydrate-loading** regimen can help to maximize the amount of energy stored in the form of muscle glycogen for the event. (However, this amount of activity applies to few athletes.) In one possible regimen, during the week prior to the event, the athlete gradually reduces the intensity and duration of exercise ("tapering") while simultaneously increasing the percentage of total calories supplied by carbohydrate.

For example, consider the carbohydrate-loading schedule of a 25-year-old man preparing for a marathon. His typical calorie needs are about 3500 kcal per day. Six days before competition, he completes a final hard workout of 60 minutes. On that day, carbohydrates contribute 45% to 50% of his total calorie intake. As he goes through the rest of the week, the duration of his workouts decreases to 40 minutes, and then to about 20 minutes by the end of the week. Meanwhile, he increases the amount of carbohydrate in his diet to reach 70% to 80% of total calorie intake as the week continues. Total calorie intake should decrease as exercise time decreases throughout the week. On the final day before competition, he rests while maintaining the high-carbohydrate intake.

Carbohydrate Loading Regimen

Days Before Competition	6	5	4	3	2	1
Exercise time (minutes)	60	40	40	20	20	Rest
Carbohydrate (grams)	450	450	450	600	600	600

This carbohydrate-loading technique usually increases muscle glycogen stores by 50% to 85% over typical conditions (that is, when dietary carbohydrate constitutes only about 50% of total calorie intake).

A potential disadvantage of carbohydrate loading is that additional water (about 3 grams) is incorporated into the muscles along with each gram of glycogen. Although the additional water aids in maintaining hydration, for some individuals this additional water weight and related muscle stiffness detract from their sports performance, making carbohydrate loading inappropriate. Athletes considering a carbohydrate-loading regimen should try it during training (and well before an important competition) to experience its effects on performance. They can then determine whether it is worth the effort. Also, consuming carbohydrates during a competition provides about the same advantage as carbohydrate loading prior to the event. Expert advice is shifting away from carbohydrate loading and more toward this second method, coupled with a daily diet high in carbohydrate. In addition, remember the importance of the "training effect" discussed in " Making Decisions: Training Effect " on page 415.

page 415

CRITICAL THINKING

Joe is a wrestler who qualified for the 125-pound weight classification in the annual state high school competition. After a few matches, Joe began to feel dizzy and faint. He was disqualified because he was unable to continue the match. Later, the coach found out that Joe had spent 2 hours in the sauna before weighing in, which had made him dehydrated. What are the consequences of dehydration? What can you suggest as a safer alternative for weight loss?

carbohydrate loading A process in which a high carbohydrate intake is consumed for 6 days before an athletic event while tapering exercise duration in an attempt to increase muscle glycogen stores.

▶ **Carbohydrate Loading May Be Beneficial for These activities**

Marathons

Long-distance swimming

Cross-country skiing

30-kilometer runs

Triathlons

Tournament-play basketball

Soccer

Cycling time trials

Long-distance canoe racing

Carbohydrate Loading Is Not Beneficial for These Activities

American football games

10-kilometer or shorter runs

Walking and hiking

Most swimming events

Single basketball games

Weight lifting

Most track and field events

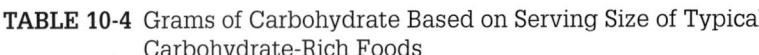

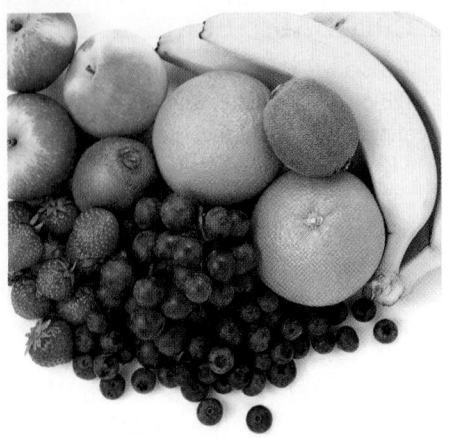

▲ Fruits provide a good source of carbohydrate, especially starch and natural sugars, for athletes.

TABLE 10-4 Grams of Carbohydrate Based on Serving Size of Typical Carbohydrate-Rich Foods

Starches—15 grams Carbohydrate per Serving (80 kcal)

One Serving

dry breakfast cereal*, 1/2–3/4 cup	baked potato, 1/4 large
cooked breakfast cereal, 1/2 cup	bagel, 1/4 (4 ounces)
cooked grits, 1/2 cup	English muffin, 1/2
cooked rice, 1/3 cup	bread, 1 slice
cooked pasta, 1/3 cup	pretzels, 3/4 ounces
baked beans, 1/3 cup	saltine crackers, 6
cooked corn, 1/2 cup	pancake, 4 inches in diameter, 1
cooked dry beans, 1/2 cup	taco shells, 2 (add 45 kcal)

Vegetables—5 grams Carbohydrate per Serving (25 kcal)

One Serving
cooked vegetables, 1/2 cup
raw vegetables, 1 cup
vegetable juice, 1/2 cup
Examples: carrots, green beans, broccoli, cauliflower, onions, spinach, tomatoes, vegetable juice

Fruits—15 grams Carbohydrate per Serving (60 kcal)

One Serving

canned fruit or berries, 1/2 cup	grapes (small), 17
fruit juice, 1/2 cup	grapefruit, 1/2
figs (dried), 1 1/2	dates, 3
apple or orange, 1 small	peach, 1
apricots (dried), 8	watermelon cubes, 1 1/4 cups
banana, 1 small	

Milk—12 grams Carbohydrate per Serving

One Serving	soymilk, 1 cup
milk, 1 cup	
plain low-fat yogurt, 2/3 cup	

Sweets—15 grams Carbohydrate per Serving (variable calories)

One Serving	
cake, 2-inch square	ice cream, 1/2 cup
cookies, 2 small	sherbet, 1/2 cup

*The carbohydrate content of dry cereal varies widely. Check the labels of the ones you choose and adjust the serving size accordingly.

Modified from *Choose Your Foods: Exchange Lists for Diabetes* by the American Diabetes Association and American Dietetic Association, 2008, Chicago, American Dietetic Association.

Fat Needs

A diet containing up to 35% of calories from fat is generally recommended for athletes. Rich sources of monounsaturated fat, such as canola oil, should be emphasized, and saturated fat and *trans* fat intake should be limited.

Protein Needs

For athletes, the American College of Sports Medicine, American Dietetic Association, and Dietitians of Canada recommend protein intake within the range of 0.8 to 1.7 grams of protein per kilogram of body weight. The International Society of Sports Nutrition recommends up to 2.0 grams of protein per-kilogram (see Further Reading 7). This advice is considerably higher than the RDA of 0.8 grams per kilogram body weight for nonathletes recommended by the Food and Nutrition Board for all adults, including athletes. Estimates of protein needs vary by the type of physical activity (Table 10-5).

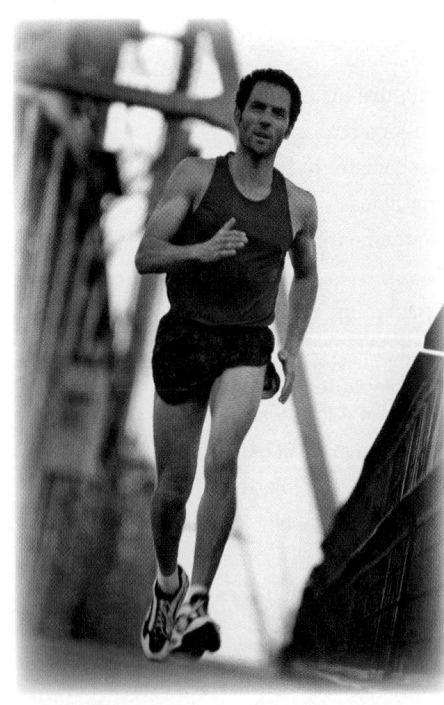

▲ Carbohydrate loading is appropriate only for endurance activities such as a long-distance race.

TABLE 10-5 Estimated Protein Needs of Athletes Based on Kilograms Body Weight[1]

Activity Level	Males	Females	Amount for a 70-kilogram (154-pound) Man
Sedentary adults[2]	0.8 g/kg	0.8 g/kg	56 g/d
Recreational endurance athletes[3]	0.8–1.0 g/kg	0.8–0.9 g/kg	56–70 g/d
Moderate-intensity endurance athletes[4]	1.2 g/kg	1.0–1.1 g/kg	84 g/d
Elite endurance athletes	1.6 g/kg	1.3–1.4 g/kg	112 g/d
Football, power sports	1.4–1.7 g/kg	1.1–1.5 g/kg	98–119 g/d
Resistance athletes (early training)	1.5–1.7 g/kg	1.2–1.5 g/kg	105–119 g/d
Resistance athletes (steady state)	1.0–1.2 g/kg	0.8–1.1 g/kg	70–84 g/d

Source: Adapted from Burke L, Deakin V: *Clinical Sports Nutrition*, 4th ed., McGraw-Hill, Australia, 2009.

[1]Calculate kilograms by dividing pounds by 2.2.

[2]RDA, as recommended by the Food and Nutrition Board.

[3]Exercising four to five times per week for 30 minutes.

[4]Exercising four to five times per week for 45–60 minutes.

For athletes beginning a strength-training program, some experts recommend up to 2.0 grams of protein per kilogram of body weight. That is more than twice the RDA for protein. To date, the value of such an excessive protein intake during the initial phases of strength training has not been supported by sufficient research. In addition, protein intakes above this amount result in an increased use of amino acids for energy needs; no further increase in muscle protein synthesis is seen. Recall from earlier in this chapter that phosphocreatine and carbohydrate (not extra protein) primarily fuel the body during strength-training activities. The extra protein, theoretically, is required for the synthesis of new muscle tissue brought on by the loading effect of strength training. Once the desired muscle mass is achieved, protein intake need not exceed 1.2 grams per kilogram of body weight.

Table 10-5 summarizes recommended ranges of protein intakes for various types of activity. Any athlete not specifically on a low-calorie regimen can easily meet these protein recommendations by eating a variety of foods (review Table 10-3). To illustrate, a 123-pound (53-kilogram) woman performing moderate-intensity endurance activity can consume 58 grams of protein (53 × 1.1) during a single day by including 3 ounces of chicken (one chicken breast), 3 ounces of beef (a small, lean hamburger), and two glasses of milk in her diet. Similarly, a 180-pound (77-kilogram) man who aims to gain muscle mass through strength training needs to consume only 6 ounces of chicken (a large chicken breast), ½ cup of cooked beans, a 6-ounce can of tuna, and three glasses of milk to achieve an intake of 130 grams of protein (77 × 1.7) in a day. And, for both athletes, these calculations do not even include the protein present in grains or vegetables they will also eat. As you can see, by meeting their calorie needs, many athletes consume much more protein than is required. Despite marketing claims, protein supplements are an expensive and unnecessary part of a fitness plan.

Consuming excessive amounts of protein has drawbacks. As noted in Chapter 6, it increases calcium loss somewhat in the urine. It also leads to increased urine production, possibly compromising body hydration. It also may lead to kidney stones in people with a history of this or other kidney problems. Finally, enough carbohydrate fuel may not be consumed on such a diet, leading to fatigue. Athletes who either feel they must significantly limit their calorie intake or are vegetarians should specifically determine how much protein they eat. They should make sure to follow a diet that provides at least 1.2 grams of protein per kilogram of body weight per day, the upper recommendation for most athletes.

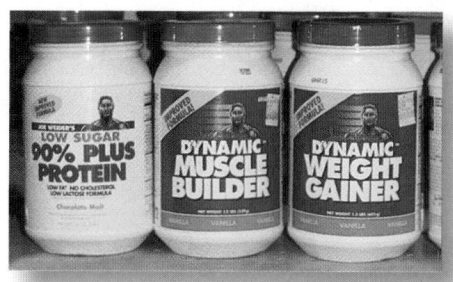

▲ High-protein products, often marketed to athletes, are unnecessary. The same holds true for high-protein bars, a trend in marketing products to athletes.

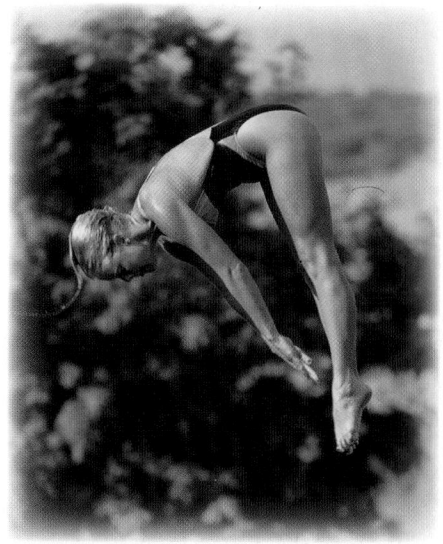

▲ Weight-restricted athletes especially should make sure they are consuming enough protein as well as other essential nutrients.

Vitamin and Mineral Needs

Vitamin and mineral needs are the same or slightly higher for athletes, compared with those of sedentary adults. Athletes usually have high calorie intakes, so they tend to consume plenty of vitamins and minerals. An exception is athletes consuming low-calorie diets (about 1200 kcal or less), such as seen with some female athletes participating in events in which maintaining a low body weight is crucial. These diets may not meet B-vitamin and other micronutrient needs. Vegetarian athletes are also a concern. In these cases, consuming fortified foods, such as ready-to-eat breakfast cereals or a balanced multivitamin and mineral supplement is recommended.

Athletes' needs for antioxidants such as vitamin E and vitamin C may be somewhat greater because of the potential protection these nutrients provide; this effect could be especially important in the face of high oxygen use by muscles. The use of large doses of vitamin E and vitamin C, however, requires more study and is not currently an accepted part of the dietary guidance for athletes. Experts suggest consuming a diet containing foods rich in antioxidants, such as fruits, vegetables, whole-grain breads and cereals, and vegetable oils. In addition, there is evidence that antioxidant systems in the body increase in activity as exercise training progresses. There is also speculation that the "oxidative stress" produced during exercise might have benefits, such as for muscle adaptation to exercise, and so trying to block this process may not be advantageous (see Further Reading 9).

Iron Deficiency Impairs Performance. Iron is involved in red blood cell production, oxygen transport, and energy production, so a deficiency of this mineral can noticeably detract from optimal athletic performance. The potential causes for iron deficiency in athletes vary (see Further Reading 1). As in the general population, female athletes are most susceptible to low iron status due to monthly menstrual losses. Special diets followed by athletes, such as low-calorie and vegetarian (especially vegan) diets are likely to be low in iron. Distance runners should pay special attention to iron intake, because their intense workouts may lead to gastrointestinal bleeding. Another concern is *sports anemia*—which occurs because exercise causes blood plasma volume to expand, particularly at the start of a training regimen before the synthesis of red blood cells increases. This results in dilution of the blood. In this case, even if iron stores are adequate, blood iron tests may appear low.

Sports anemia is not detrimental to performance, but it is hard to differentiate between sports anemia and true anemia. If iron status is low and not replenished, iron-deficiency anemia and markedly impaired endurance performance can eventually result. Although true anemia (a depressed blood hemoglobin level) is not that common among athletes, it is a good idea for athletes (especially adult women), to have their iron status checked at the beginning of a training season and at least once during midseason to monitor dietary iron intake.

Any blood test indicating low iron status—sports anemia or not—is cause for follow-up. For some, the use of iron supplements may be advisable. However, indiscriminate use of iron supplements is not advised because toxic effects are possible. It is important that physicians investigate the cause of the deficiency because iron deficiency can be caused by blood loss. If caught early, some serious medical conditions such as this can be treated or prevented.

Some studies have suggested that iron deficiency without anemia may also have a negative effect on physical activity and performance. Also, once depleted, iron stores can take months to replenish. For this reason, athletes must be especially careful to meet iron needs.

Calcium Intake Is Important, Especially in Women. Athletes, especially women trying to lose weight by restricting their intake of dairy products, can have marginal or low dietary intakes of calcium. This practice compromises optimal bone health. Of still greater concern are women athletes who have stopped menstruating because their arduous training and low body fat content interferes with the normal secretion of reproductive hormones. Disturbing reports show that female athletes who do not menstruate regularly have spinal bones far less dense than those of both nonathletes

Recall from Chapter 8 that nutrients in dietary supplements should not exceed any Upper Levels set over the long term. As well, men should be cautious about any use of supplements containing iron.

"Blood doping" is the injection of red blood cells, naturally containing iron, to enhance aerobic capacity. This is an illegal practice under Olympic guidelines.

See the Nutrition and Your Health: Ergogenic Aids and Athletic Performance at the end of Chapter 10.

and female athletes who menstruate regularly. This places them at increased risk for bone fractures during training and competition and osteoporosis in later life. The negative impacts of low dietary calcium intake and irregular menses in female athletes outweigh the benefits of weight-bearing exercise on bone density. Increasing energy intake to restore body weight and body fat stores is important to correct hormonal imbalances and prevent further bone loss. This topic is discussed further in Chapter 11, with respect to the female athlete triad, and in Chapter 9, where osteoporosis was reviewed in detail (also see Further Readings 5 and 11).

Research has clearly documented the importance of regular menstruation to maintain bone mineral density. Studies show that a woman runner who does not menstruate regularly may also have a higher risk for the development of a **stress fracture.** Thus, female athletes whose menstrual cycles become irregular should consult a physician to determine the cause. Decreasing the amount of training or increasing energy intake and body weight often restores regular menstrual cycles. If irregular menstrual cycles persist, severe bone loss (much of which is not reversible) and osteoporosis can result. Extra calcium in the diet does not necessarily compensate for these damaging effects of menstrual irregularities, but inadequate dietary calcium can make matters worse.

stress fracture A fracture that occurs from repeated jarring of a bone. Common sites include bones of the foot.

10.5 A Focus on Fluid Needs

Fluid needs for an average adult are about 9 cups per day for women and 13 cups per day for men. Athletes generally need even more water to regulate internal temperature and keep cool. Heat production in contracting muscles can rise 15 to 20 times above that of resting muscles. Unless this heat is quickly dissipated, heat exhaustion, heat cramps, and potentially fatal heatstroke may ensue.

Fluid intake during exercise, when possible, should be adequate to minimize body weight loss; following this practice is a good idea even when sweating can go unnoticed, such as when swimming or during the winter. Fluid and electrolyte needs vary widely, based on differences in body mass, environmental conditions, level of training, event duration, and even genetics. Because fluid needs are highly individualized and dynamic, it is not appropriate to make general recommendations for fluid replacement (see Further Reading 14). Rather, an athlete should aim to replace the total amount of fluid lost during exercise. This can be accomplished by knowing the body's hourly sweat rate, which can be calculated from the weight lost during exercise per hour plus the fluid consumed during exercise per hour.

The American College of Sports Medicine recommends losing no more than 2% of body weight during exercise, especially in hot weather. Athletes should first calculate 2% of their body weight and then by trial and error determine how much fluid they must take in to avoid excessive losses. Monitoring pre- and post-workout body weight is the most straightforward method of determining fluid losses. Much of this fluid replacement will have to take place after exercise because it is difficult to consume enough fluid during exercise to prevent weight loss. If weight change can't be monitored, urine color is another measure of hydration status. Urine color should be no more yellow than lemonade.

Thirst is a late sign of dehydration. An athlete who drinks only when thirsty may take 48 hours to replenish fluid losses. After several days of training, an athlete relying on thirst can build up a fluid debt that will impair performance. The following fluid-replacement approach can meet athletes' fluid needs in most cases:

- Freely drink beverages (e.g., water, diluted fruit juice, sports drinks) during the 24-hour period before an event, even if not particularly thirsty.
- Drink 5 to 7 milliliters per kilogram of body weight (about 1.5 to 2 cups for a 150-pound male) of water or sports drink at least 4 hours before exercise. This allows time for both adequate hydration and excretion of excess fluid.
- During events lasting more than 30 minutes, athletes should consume fluid to prevent dehydration (i.e., losses of >2% body weight). Research in marathon runners suggests about 1 ½ to 3 ½ cups (400 to 800 milliliters) per hour to prevent

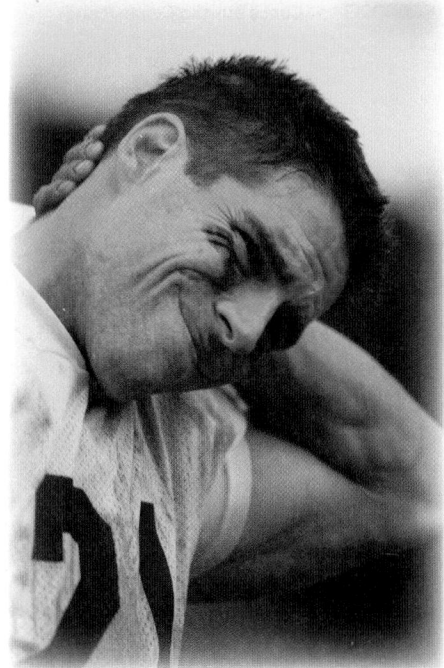

▲ Dehydration, which can lead to illness and death, is a problem that must be avoided during physical activity in hot, humid environments.

NEWSWORTHY
NUTRITION

Sports drinks and energy drinks are not interchangeable

The value of electrolyte- and carbohydrate-containing *sports* drinks (e.g., Gatorade) is well documented for replenishing fluids during physical activity lasting more than 1 hour. However, an assortment of *energy* drinks are now marketed alongside sports drinks to young people, especially male athletes. Experts caution athletes against using energy drinks, such as the top-selling Red Bull, Rockstar, Monster, and Throttle, to meet fluid needs during exercise. The sugar content is too high, and a multitude of additives, including caffeine, taurine, ginseng, guarana, and others, have limited if any documented benefits for athletes. In fact, binge consumption of energy drinks with stimulants has led to illness and at least four deaths. Combining energy drinks with alcohol can mask the symptoms of intoxication and result in hazardous behavior and accidents. Experts recommend limiting use of energy beverages to 1 serving (500 milliliters) per day, avoiding combinations with alcohol, and, for people with cardiac problems, consulting a physician before use. Athletes should use a sports drink rather than an energy drink for the purpose of rehydration during physical activity.

Source: Higgins JP and others: Energy beverages: Content and safety. *Mayo Clinic Proceedings* 85:1033, 2010.

■ connect
| NUTRITION

Check out the Connect site
www.mcgrawhillconnect.com
to further explore sports and energy drinks.

heat exhaustion The first stage of heat-related illness that occurs because of depletion of blood volume from fluid loss by the body. This increases body temperature and can lead to headache, dizziness, muscle weakness, and visual disturbances, among other effects.

heat cramps A frequent complication of heat exhaustion. They usually occur in people who have experienced large sweat losses from exercising for several hours in a hot climate and have consumed a large volume of water. The cramps occur in skeletal muscles and consist of contractions for 1 to 3 minutes at a time.

dehydration. Football players wearing equipment for two-a-day practices during the heat of August may need even more than 800 milliliters per hour to prevent dehydration. The best plan is to determine individual rate of fluid losses during training and plan accordingly. In many cases, athletes, especially children and teenagers, need to be reminded to consume fluids during exercise. Colder drinks also enhance body cooling.

- Within 4 to 6 hours after exercise, about 2 to 3 cups of fluid should be consumed for every pound lost. It is important that weight be restored before the next exercise period. Skipping fluids before or during events will almost certainly impair performance.

The popularity of caffeine-containing energy drinks has surged in recent years. Some studies show that caffeine improves athletic performance during endurance events (e.g., cycling) or sports that require a high level of mental alertness (e.g., archery). However, excessive caffeine consumption can lead to shakiness, nervousness, anxiety, nausea, and insomnia. In addition, the diuretic effect of caffeine may not support optimal hydration, particularly for athletes who are not accustomed to caffeine. Compare the caffeine and kilocalorie contents of several top-selling energy drinks (Table 10-6).

As environmental temperature rises above 95°F (35°C), virtually all body heat is lost through the evaporation of sweat from the skin. Sweat rates during prolonged exercise range from 3 to 8 cups (750 to 2000 milliliters) per hour.

Wearing football equipment in hot weather can lead to a loss of 2% of body weight in 30 minutes. Marathon runners have been shown to lose 6% to 10% of body weight during a race. Dehydration reduces endurance, strength, and overall performance. As humidity rises, especially above 75%, evaporation slows and sweating becomes an inefficient way to cool the body. The result is rapid fatigue, increased work for the heart, and difficulty with prolonged exertion. Heat-related injuries—heat exhaustion, heat cramps, and heatstroke—can be as dangerous as extreme cold.

Heat exhaustion occurs when heat stress causes loss of body fluid and then depletion of blood volume. Common symptoms of heat exhaustion include profuse sweating, headache, dizziness, nausea, vomiting, muscle weakness, visual disturbances,

TABLE 10-6 Caffeine, Kilocalorie, and Sugar Content of Popular Energy Drinks

Beverage	Container Size (fl oz)	Caffeine (mg)	Energy (kcal)	Sugars (g)
5-Hour Energy	1.93	80+*	4	0
Amp	16	142	220	58
Full Throttle	16	197	220	58
Monster	16	160	200	54
Red Bull	8.4	80	110	27
Red Bull Sugarfree	8.4	80	10	0
Red Rain Energy Shot	2	80+*	0	0
Rockstar	16	160	280	62
Slap Energy Frost	16	200	220	52
SoBe Energize	20	160	88	23

*Caffeine content is not specified by the manufacturer but rather as part of a total amount of "energy blend." The labels state these products have approximately the same amount of caffeine as a strong cup of coffee (typical range: 80–175 milligrams). An independent lab analysis of 5-Hour Energy determined caffeine content was 207 milligrams.

and flushing of the skin. A person with heat exhaustion should be taken to a cool environment immediately, and excess clothing should be removed. The body should be sponged with tap water. Fluid replacement, as tolerated, then should suffice to correct the condition.

Heat cramps are a frequent complication of heat exhaustion, but they may appear without other symptoms of dehydration. Cramps usually occur in individuals who have exercised for several hours in a hot climate, experienced significant sweating, and have consumed a large volume of water without replacing sodium losses. It is important not to confuse heat cramps with other forms of muscle cramps, such as those caused by GI tract upset. Heat cramps occur in skeletal muscles, including those of the abdomen and extremities. They consist of a contraction lasting 1 to 3 minutes at a time. The cramp moves down the muscle and is associated with excruciating pain. To prevent heat cramps, exercise moderately at first; aim to have adequate salt intake before engaging in long, strenuous activity in the heat; and avoid dehydration.

Heatstroke can occur when the internal body temperature reaches 104°F or more. Related symptoms include nausea, confusion, irritability, poor coordination, seizures, and coma. Exertional heatstroke results from high blood flow to exercising muscles, which overloads the body's cooling capacity. Sweating generally ceases, and the body temperature may become dangerously high. If left untreated, circulatory collapse, nervous system damage, and death are likely. The death rate from heatstroke is high, approximately 10%, making heatstroke the number 3 killer of athletes in the United States. Since 1995, at least 40 football players have died as a result of heatstroke.

Many individuals faint during heatstroke, and their skin becomes hot and dry. Cooling the skin with ice packs or cold water is the usual recommended immediate treatment until medical help can be summoned. To decrease the risk of developing heatstroke, athletes should watch for rapid body-weight changes (2% or more of body weight), replace lost fluids, and avoid exercising under extremely hot, humid conditions.

Sports Drinks

A question that often arises is whether to drink water or a sports-type carbohydrate-electrolyte drink (e.g., All Sport, Exceed Energy Drink, Gatorade, PowerAde, and Amino Force) during competition (Fig. 10-7). For sports that require less than 60 minutes of exertion or when total weight loss is less than 5 to 6 pounds, the primary concern is replacing the water lost in sweat, because losses of carbohydrate stores and electrolytes (sodium, chloride, potassium, and other minerals) are not usually very great. Although electrolytes are lost in sweat, the quantities lost in exercise of brief to moderate duration can be easily replaced later by consuming normal foods, such as orange juice, potatoes, and tomato juice. Keep in mind that sweat is about 99% water and only 1% electrolytes and other substances.

When exercise extends beyond 60 minutes, electrolyte (especially sodium) and carbohydrate replacement becomes increasingly important. Use of sports drinks during long bouts of exercise—especially in hot weather—offers several advantages.

Water by itself, as you have learned, increases blood volume to allow for efficient cooling and transport of fuels and waste products to and from cells. The addition of carbohydrate to a sports drink supplies glucose to muscles as they become depleted of glycogen, and thus can enhance performance when administered during endurance activities (see the later section on carbohydrate replacement). Carbohydrate also adds flavor, which encourages athletes to drink. Finally, the electrolytes in sports drinks help to maintain blood volume, enhance the absorption of water and carbohydrate from the intestine, and stimulate thirst. For these reasons, some experts prefer sports drinks over water for all athletes.

Overall, the decision to use a sports drink hinges primarily on the duration of the activity. As the projected duration of continuous activity approaches 60 minutes or longer, the advantages of the use of a sports drink over plain water clearly emerge. However, athletes should first experiment with sports drinks during practice, instead of trying them for the first time during competition.

heatstroke Heatstroke can occur when internal body temperature reaches 104°F. Sweating generally ceases if left untreated, and blood circulation is greatly reduced. Nervous system damage may ensue, and death is likely. Often the skin of individuals who suffer heatstroke is hot and dry.

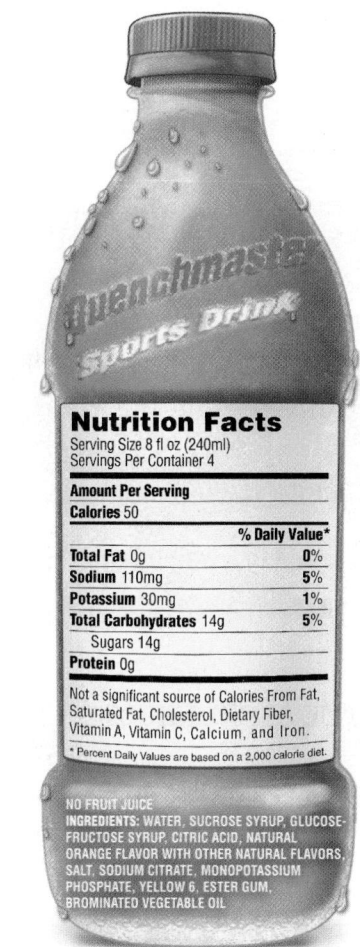

FIGURE 10-7 ▶ Sports drinks for fluid and electrolyte replacement typically contain a form of simple carbohydrate plus sodium and potassium. The various sugars in this product total 14 grams per 1 cup (240 milliliters) serving. In percentage terms based on weight, the sugar content is about 6% ([14 grams sugar per serving ÷ 240 grams per serving] × 100 = 5.8%). Sports drinks typically contain about 6% to 8% sugar. This provides ample glucose and other monosaccharides to fuel working muscles, and it is well tolerated. Drinks with a sugar content above 10%, such as soft drinks or fruit juices, may cause stomach distress and are not recommended.

General Guide for Approximate Pre-event Carbohydrate Intake

Hours Before	Grams per kilogram Body Weight	For a 70-kilogram Person
1	1	70
2	2	140
3	3	210
4	4	280

It is also possible for some athletes to drink too much water and thereby develop water intoxication (hyponatremia). Endurance athletes (especially poorly trained individuals) may compete at relatively low exercise intensities for prolonged periods and therefore may not sweat as much as one might predict. Thus, water losses are not high. Drinking less fluid, choosing a sports drink containing sodium (usually in the form of sodium chloride), and not gaining weight during the activity can help prevent this problem. (A drop in blood sodium can occur in both hot and cold weather.)

10.6 Specialized Dietary Advice for Before, During, and After Endurance Exercise

Pre-event Meals Optimize Performance

A light meal supplying up to 1000 kcal should be eaten about 2 to 4 hours before an endurance event to top off muscle and liver glycogen stores, prevent hunger during the event, and provide extra fluid. The longer the period before an event, the larger the meal can be, because there will be more time available for digestion. A pre-event meal should consist primarily of carbohydrate (about 200 grams), contain little fat or fiber, and include a moderate amount of protein (Table 10-7). A meal eaten 1 hour or so before an event should be blended or liquid to promote rapid stomach emptying. Examples are low-fat smoothies, juices, and sports drinks.

Good food choices for a pre-event meal include spaghetti, muffins, bagels, pancakes with fresh fruit topping, oatmeal with fruit, baked potato topped with a small amount of sour cream, toasted bread with jam, bananas, and low-sugar breakfast cereals with reduced-fat or fat-free milk. Liquid meal-replacement formulas, such as Carnation Instant Breakfast, also can be used. Foods especially rich in fiber should be eaten the previous day to help empty the colon before an event, but they should not be eaten the night before or on the morning of the event. Avoid fatty or fried foods, such as sausage, bacon, sauces, and gravies. Some foods (e.g., dairy products) may cause

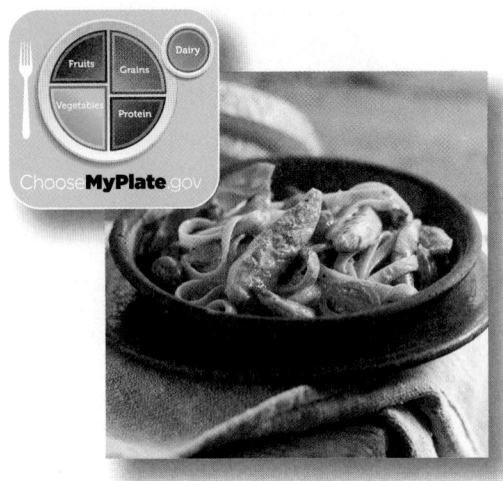

CRITICAL THINKING

Pre-event meals may require a higher proportion of grains than suggested by MyPlate to boost carbohydrate content. Choose starchy vegetables and grain-based snacks to help top off glycogen stores. How does this pasta meal compare to MyPlate?

TABLE 10-7 Convenient Pre-event Meals

Breakfast	
Cheerios, ¾ cup Reduced-fat milk, 1 cup Blueberry muffin, 1 Orange juice, 4 ounces	450 kcal 92 grams (82%) carbohydrate
or	
Low-fat fruit yogurt, 1 cup Plain bagel, ½ Apple juice, 4 ounces Peanut butter (for bagel), 1 tbsp	482 kcal 84 grams (68%) carbohydrate
Lunch or Dinner	
Broiled pork chop, 3 ounces White rice, 1½ cups Steamed zucchini, 1 cup Chocolate milk, 1 cup Jello, ½ cup	839 kcal 120 grams (57%) carbohydrate
or	
Spaghetti noodles, 2 cups Spaghetti sauce, 1 cup Reduced-fat milk, 1½ cups Green beans, 1 cup	761 kcal 129 grams (66%) carbohydrate

With regard to the timing of pre-activity meals, a general guide is to allow 4 hours for a big meal (about 1200 kcal), 3 hours for a moderate meal (about 800 to 900 kcal), 2 hours for a light meal (about 400 to 600 kcal), and an hour or less for a snack (about 300 kcal).

gastrointestinal upset. Athletes should experiment with the size, timing, and composition of pre-event meals during training to determine what will be tolerated.

Replenishing Fuel During Endurance Exercise

We've already established the importance of consuming adequate fluids during endurance exercise. For sporting events longer than 60 minutes, consumption of carbohydrate during activity can also improve athletic performance. This is because prolonged exercise depletes muscle glycogen stores and low levels of blood glucose lead to fatigue, both physical and mental. When the supply of carbohydrate calories runs low, athletes often complain of "hitting the wall," the point at which maintaining a competitive pace seems impossible. One way to overcome this obstacle is to maintain normal blood glucose concentrations by carbohydrate feedings.

A general guideline for endurance events is to consume 30 to 60 grams of carbohydrate per hour. Some experts suggest that consuming protein with carbohydrate during exercise provides added benefit. In particular, branched-chain amino acids, which can be used for fuel, are thought to delay fatigue. This is an area of ongoing research, but there is not enough evidence at this time to support a recommendation for ingesting protein during exercise. Compared to carbohydrates, fat is more slowly digested, absorbed, and metabolized. Thus, although it serves as fuel during prolonged aerobic activity, consumption of fat during activity is not likely to improve athletic performance.

Sports drinks are a good source of carbohydrate calories during endurance events. They supply the necessary fluid, electrolytes, and carbohydrate to keep an athlete performing at his or her best. As an alternative to sports drinks, some athletes use carbohydrate gels (e.g., PowerGel and Clif Shot) and energy bars (e.g., PowerBar). Check the label on these products to gauge the amount of gel or bar that provides 30 to 60 grams of carbohydrate per hour. Whereas sports drinks contain about 14 grams of carbohydrate per 8-oz serving, gels contain about 25 grams of carbohydrate per serving, and depending on the type, popular energy bars range from 2 to 45 grams of carbohydrate per serving (Table 10-8). The wide range of carbohydrate content in energy bars is due to a variety of marketing trends in the sports supplement industry. Overall, choosing a bar with about 40 grams of carbohydrate and no more than 10 grams of protein, 4 grams of fat, and 5 grams of fiber is recommended. The bars may also be fortified with up to 100% of the Daily Values of certain vitamins and minerals. These bars can be seen as a convenient, although somewhat expensive, source of nutrients. Caution should be exercised to avoid toxicities from such fortified products.

If solid sources of carbohydrate are one's preference, Teddy Grahams, Gummy Bears, and jellybeans can also yield a quick source of glucose at a much lower cost. However, any carbohydrate-containing food, including energy bars and gels, must be accompanied by fluid to ensure adequate hydration.

MAKING DECISIONS

Energy Bars

As discussed, food manufacturers have begun to promote meal replacement bars (also called "energy" bars) to all kind of athletes. These bars typically contain about 180 to 250 kcal, with a macronutrient distribution typical of common diets. However, some bars replace much of the carbohydrate with protein. The bars are fortified with vitamins and minerals in amounts ranging from about 25% to 100% of typical human needs. Some people find these bars provide a convenient way to consume a meal (or snack) on the run, while also focusing on certain nutrients they may underconsume, such as the B-vitamin folate or the mineral calcium. These bars generally cost $1 to $2. The energy and nutrient contents of popular energy bars are shown in Table 10-8. Critics suggest these products are essentially the nutritional equivalent of a cup of low-fat yogurt and piece of fruit.

It cannot be emphasized enough that any nutrition strategies should be tested during practice and trial runs before being used in a meet or key event. An athlete should never try a new food or beverage on the day of competition. Some food items and beverages may not be well tolerated, and the day of competition is not the time to find out.

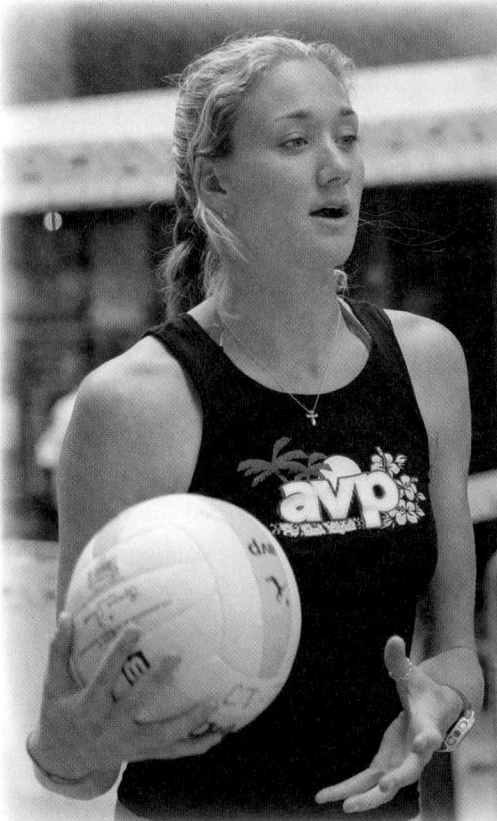

▲ Elite athletes such as Olympic beach volleyball gold medal winner Kerri Walsh are well aware that modifying their diet and training regimen to match the specific needs of their sport is key to optimum performance. Replenishing carbohydrate and fluids is especially important when training.

TABLE 10-8 Energy and Macronutrient Content of Popular Energy Bars, Gels, and Chews

Energy Bars	Serving (oz)	Energy (kcal)	Carbohydrates (g)	Fiber (g)	Protein (g)	Fat (g)
Balance Bar (peanut butter)	1.76	200	21	1	14	7
Clif Bar (chocolate chip)	2.4	240	44	5	10	4.5
Clif Builder's (peanut butter)	2.4	270	30	4	20	8
Clif Kid Z-Bar (honey graham)	1.27	130	26	3	3	2
EAS Myoplex (chocolate peanut butter)	2.65	290	35	1	25	9
Genisoy Bar (cookies & cream)	2.2	230	33	1	14	4.5
Kashi GoLean Bar (malted chocolate chip)	1.94	190	31	5	12	4.5
LARABAR (peanut butter cookie)	1.7	220	23	4	7	12
LUNA Bar (nutz over chocolate)	1.69	180	25	4	9	6
MET-Rx Big 100 Bar (super cookie crunch)	3.52	410	41	3	32	14
Met-Rx Protein Plus (chocolate fudge deluxe)	3.0	310	32	2	32	9
Power Crunch Bar (peanut butter crème)	1.4	200	10	1	13	12
PowerBar Harvest (toffee chocolate chip)	2.29	250	42	5	10	5
PowerBar Performance (peanut butter)	2.3	240	44	1	9	4
PowerBar Pria (French vanilla crisp)	0.98	110	17	1	5	3
PowerBar ProteinPlus (chocolate crisp)	2.75	290	37	2	23	6
PowerBar TripleThreat	1.94	230	31	3	10	9
Premier Nutrition Titan (cookie & cream)	2.8	320	27	<1	26	8
Promax Energy Bar (German chocolate cake)	2.7	280	37	2	20	6
Pure Protein (chocolate deluxe)	1.76	180	17	2	20	4.5
Snickers Marathon Protein Bar (caramel nut rush)	2.82	290	40	10	20	10
Tiger's Milk (peanut butter and honey)	1.23	140	19	<1	5	5
Zone Perfect (chocolate mint)	1.76	210	24	3	14	7
Energy Gels & Chews						
Carb BOOM! Energy Gel (strawberry kiwi)	1.4	110	27	0	0	0
Clif Shot (vanilla)	1.1	100	24	0	0	0
Clif Shot Blocks (cran-razz)	1.0	100	24	0	0	0
GU Energy Gel (lemon sublime)	1.1	100	25	0	0	0
Hammer Gel (raspberry)	1.2	90	21	0	0	0
Honey Stinger Energy Gel (orange blossom)	1.8	160	39	1	1	0
Jelly Belly Sport Beans (berry)	1.0	100	24	0	0	0
PowerBar Energy Bites (chocolate)	3.0	340	58	2	11	7
PowerBar Gel (strawberry banana)	1.44	110	27	0	0	0

Overall, choosing energy bars is preferable to choosing candy bars and packaged cakes. When used in sports situations, energy bars can be handy. Better yet, however, is to eat a variety of wholesome foods; these offer more health-protective compounds. This is also a less expensive choice, especially for day-to-day snacking. An additional concern is that micronutrient toxicity might occur if numerous bars are eaten in a day, as many are highly fortified. Vitamin A and iron are two nutrients of special concern in this regard.

Carbohydrate Intake During Recovery from Prolonged Exercise

An athlete's need for nutrition during recovery from exercise depends on the type of workout completed and the timing of the next workout. For example, multiple events in the same day will require rapid restoration of glycogen stores. However, if an athlete will be able to rest for 1 or 2 days before the next exercise session, immediate consumption of a postworkout meal is not as crucial.

To rapidly restore glycogen stores, carbohydrate-rich foods providing 1 to 1.5 grams of carbohydrate per kilogram body weight should be consumed within 30 minutes after extended (endurance) exercise (Table 10-9). Immediately after exercise is when glycogen synthesis is greatest, because the muscles are insulin-sensitive at this point. This process should then be repeated every 2 hours for the next 4 to 6 hours. Athletes training hard can consume a sugar candy, sugared soft drink, fruit or fruit juice, or a sports-type carbohydrate supplement right after training as they attempt to reload their muscles with glycogen.

Later, enriched bread, mashed potatoes, and short-grain white rice can contribute to additional carbohydrate consumption. These high-glycemic-load carbohydrates especially contribute to glycogen synthesis. Recall that Table 4-4 shows the glycemic load for various foods. Adding an appropriate amount of protein (3 grams of carbohydrate: 1 gram of protein) during recovery can be especially helpful for meeting overall calorie and nutrient needs. For a 154-pound (70-kilogram) athlete, this corresponds to about 70 grams of carbohydrate and 25 grams of protein in each 2-hour interval (Table 10-9 contains sample meals of this composition). In summary, the following are key factors for achieving the most rapid replenishment of muscle glycogen after exercise: (1) availability of adequate carbohydrate, (2) ingestion of carbohydrate as soon as possible after completion of exercise, and (3) selection of high-glycemic-load carbohydrates.

Fluid and electrolyte (i.e., sodium and potassium) intake is also an essential component of an athlete's recovery diet. This helps replenish body fluids as quickly as possible. This is especially important if two workouts a day are performed or if the environment is hot and humid. If food and fluid intake is sufficient to restore weight loss, it generally will also supply enough electrolytes to meet needs during recovery from endurance activities.

TABLE 10-9 Sample Postexercise Meals for Rapid Muscle Glycogen Replacement

Option 1
1 regular bagel
2 tbsp peanut butter, smooth
8 fl oz fat-free milk
1 medium banana
562 kcal, 77 grams carbohydrate, 23 grams protein, 18 grams fat

Option 2 (blend until smooth)
1 packet Carnation Instant Breakfast
8 oz fat-free milk
1 medium banana
1 tbsp peanut butter
438 kcal, 70 grams carbohydrate, 17 grams protein, 10 grams fat

Option 3
1.5 cans GatorPro (11 fl oz per can)
559 kcal, 89 grams carbohydrate, 26 grams protein, 11 grams fat

For more information on sports nutrition, visit the Gatorade Sports Science Institute webpage (www.gssiweb.com). For more information on sports medicine, visit https://physsportsmed.org. This homepage of *The Physician and Sportsmedicine* journal details current issues in sports medicine, including injury prevention, nutrition, and exercise. Also helpful are the webpages of the American College of Sports Medicine (www.acsm.org), Centers for Disease Control and Prevention Division of Nutrition, Physical Activity and Obesity (www.cdc.gov/nccdphp/dnpao), and the American Council on Exercise (www.acefitness.org).

CONCEPT CHECK

All athletes would do well to plan a diet that conforms to MyPlate recommendations. High-carbohydrate foods should be emphasized, and these should dominate in pre-event meals. Protein intake above 1.7 grams per kilogram of body weight is not supported by scientific evidence. Most athletes easily consume enough protein from typical food choices. If nutrient supplements are used, dosages generally should not exceed the Upper Level set for each nutrient. Fluid should be consumed as liberally as possible before, during, and after an event. Carbohydrate and electrolytes in the fluid are especially helpful to help delay fatigue and maintain electrolyte balance when exercise duration exceeds 60 minutes.

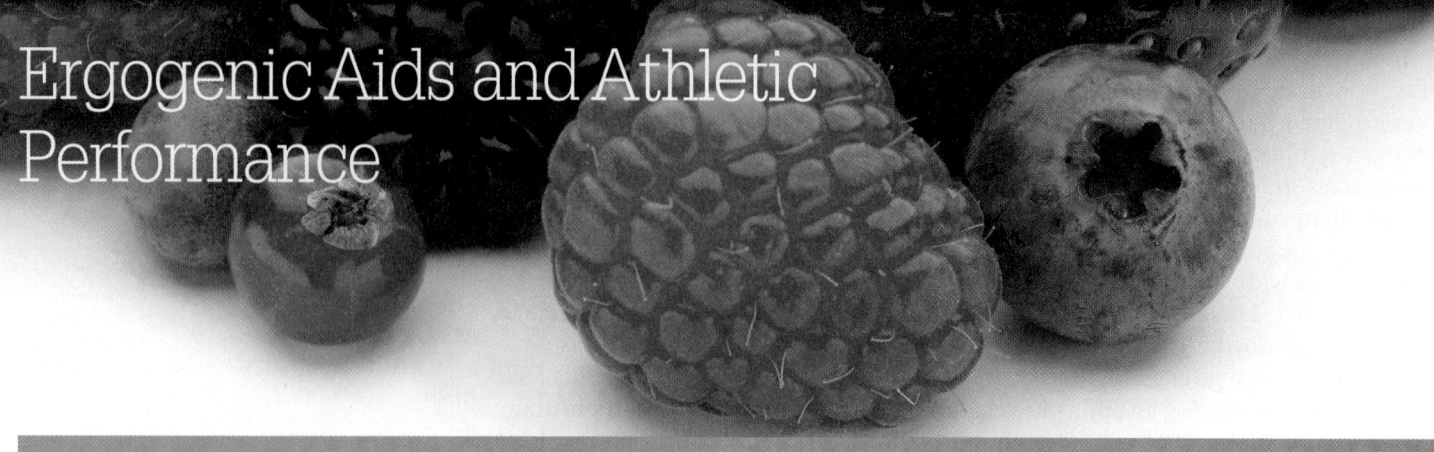

Ergogenic Aids and Athletic Performance

Ergogenic Aids to Enhance Athletic Performance

Extreme diet manipulation to improve athletic performance is not a recent innovation. As long as 30 years ago, American football players were encouraged on hot practice days to "toughen up" for competition by liberally consuming salt tablets before and during practice and by not drinking water. Now it is widely recognized that this practice can be fatal. Today's athletes are as likely as their predecessors to experiment with any substance that promises a competitive advantage. In 2010, consumers spent more than $22.7 billion on sports nutrition and weight loss supplements. Artichoke hearts, bee pollen, dried adrenal glands from cattle, seaweed, freeze-dried liver flakes, gelatin, and ginseng are just some of the ineffective substances used by athletes in hopes of gaining an **ergogenic** (work-producing) edge.

Based on what is known at this time, today's athletes can benefit from scientific evidence documenting the ergogenic properties of a few dietary substances. These ergogenic aids include sufficient water and electrolytes, lots of carbohydrates, and a balanced and varied diet consistent with MyPlate. Protein and amino acid supplements are not among those aids because athletes can easily meet protein needs from foods, as Table 10-3 demonstrated. The use of nutrient supplements should

> **ergogenic** Work-producing. An ergogenic aid is a mechanical, nutritional, psychological, pharmacological, or physiological substance or treatment intended to directly improve exercise performance.

be designed to meet a specific dietary shortcoming, such as an inadequate iron intake. These and other aids, which often have dubious benefits and may pose health risks, must be given close scrutiny before use. The risk-benefit ratio of any ergogenic aid merits careful evaluation (see Further Readings 6 and 13).

As summarized in Table 10-10, no scientific evidence supports the effectiveness of many substances touted as performance-enhancing aids. Many are useless; some are dangerous. Athletes should be skeptical of any substance until its ergogenic effect is scientifically validated. FDA has a limited ability to regulate these dietary supplements (review Chapter 1), and the manufacturing processes for dietary supplements are not as tightly regulated by FDA as they are for prescription drugs. Some supplements may contain substances that will cause athletes to "test positive" for various banned substances. This was demonstrated in the 2002 Winter Olympics. Studies also have called into question the quality control associated with the manufacturing of dietary supplements. Many do not contain the substance and/or the amount listed on the label.

These results add yet another worry for the athlete. Not only must he or she determine whether there is evidence that a dietary supplement is safe and effective, but must also question if the dietary supplement contains what it is supposed to contain.

Even substances whose ergogenic effects have been supported by systematic scientific studies should be used with caution, as the testing conditions may not match those of the intended use. Caution should be exercised when it comes to using the appropriate dose of supplements or using multiple types of supplements concurrently.

Finally, rather than waiting for a magic bullet to enhance performance, athletes are advised to concentrate their efforts on improving their training routines and sport techniques, while consuming well-balanced diets as described in this chapter.

MAKING DECISIONS

NCAA and Supplements

The NCAA's Committee on Competitive Safeguards and Medical Aspects of Sports has developed lists of permissible and nonpermissible supplements for athletic departments to dispense. The NCAA advises students to discuss their use of *any* dietary supplement with their coaches to avoid unknowingly ingesting banned substances. Following are a few key examples:

Permissible	Nonpermissible
Vitamins and minerals	Amino acids
"Energy" bars (if no more than 30% protein)	Creatine
Sports drinks	Glycerol
Meal replacement drinks such as Ensure Plus or Boost	HMB
	L-carnitine
	Protein powders

For a complete explanation of NCAA's rules regarding dietary supplements, see www.ncaa.org.

TABLE 10-10 An Evaluation of Popular Ergogenic Aids

Substance/Practice	Rationale	Reality
Useful in Some Circumstances		
Creatine	Increase phosphocreatine (PCr) in muscles to keep ATP concentration high	Use of 20 grams per day for 5 to 6 days and then a maintenance dose of 2 grams per day may improve performance in those who undertake repeated bursts of activity, such as in sprinting and weight lifting. Vegetarian athletes benefit the most because their diets are low in or devoid of creatine. Some of the muscle weight gain noted with use results from water contained in muscles. Endurance athletes do not benefit from use. Little is known about the safety of long-term creatine use. Continual use of high doses has led to kidney damage in a few cases. Cost: $25 to $65 per month.
Sodium Bicarbonate (baking soda)	Counter lactic acid buildup	Partially effective in some circumstances (when lactic acid is rapidly produced), such as wrestling, but induces nausea and diarrhea. The dose used is 300 milligrams/kilogram, given 1 to 3 hours before exercise. Cost: nil.
Caffeine	Increase use of fatty acids to fuel muscles, promote mental alertness	Drinking two to three 5-ounce cups of coffee (equivalent to 3 to 9 milligrams of caffeine per kilogram of body weight) about 1 hour before events lasting about 5 minutes or longer is useful for some athletes; benefits are less apparent in those who have ample stores of glycogen, are highly trained, or habitually consume caffeine; intake of more than about 600 milligrams (six to eight cups of coffee) elicits a urine concentration illegal under NCAA rules (greater than 15 micrograms per milliliter). Possible side effects include shakiness, nervousness, nausea, anxiety, and insomnia. Cost: $0.08 per 300 milligrams.
Possibly Useful, Still Under Study		
Beta-hydroxy-beta methylbutyric acid (HMB)	Decrease protein catabolism, causing a net growth-promoting effect	Some research suggests that supplementation with this substance may increase muscle mass by 0.5 to 1 kilogram beyond unsupplemented diets when taken during initial phases of weight training. Still, safety and effectiveness of-long term HMB use in humans is unknown. Cost: $100 per month.
Glutamine (an amino acid)	Enhance immune function, preserve lean body mass	Some preliminary studies show decreased occurrence of upper respiratory tract infections in athletes with use. It also may promote muscle growth, but long-term studies are lacking. Protein foods are a rich source of glutamine. Cost: $10 to $20 per month for 1 to 2 grams per day.
Branched-chain amino acids (BCAA) (leucine, isoleucine, valine)	Increase gains in muscle mass during resistance training Important energy source, especially when carbohydrate stores are depleted	Several studies point to positive effects of BCAA on increases in muscle mass when taken before or after resistance training. This effect is most dramatic among untrained athletes who are just beginning a resistance-training program. Protein-rich foods (especially dairy proteins) are also rich in BCAA. Cost: $20 per month. For endurance athletes, supplementation of BCAA (10 to 30 grams per day) during exercise can increase BCAA in the blood when it has been depleted due to exercise, although there is no consistent evidence of improved endurance performance. Carbohydrate feeding, by delaying use of BCAA as fuel, may negate the need for BCAA supplementation in endurance activities.
Dangerous or Illegal Substances/Practices		
Anabolic steroids (and related substances, such as androstenedione and tetrahydrogestrinone)	Increase muscle mass and strength	Although effective for increasing protein synthesis, anabolic steroids are illegal in the United States unless prescribed by a physician. They have numerous potential side effects, such as premature closure of growth plates in bones (thus possibly limiting the adult height of a teenage athlete), bloody cysts in the liver, increased risk of cardiovascular disease, increased blood pressure, and reproductive dysfunction. Possible psychological consequences include increased aggressiveness, drug dependence (addiction), withdrawal symptoms (such as depression), sleep disturbances, and mood swings (known as "roid rage"). Use of needles for injectable forms adds further health risk. Banned by the International Olympic Committee.

TABLE 10-10 *(continued)*

Substance/Practice	Rationale	Reality
Growth hormone	Increase muscle mass	At critical ages, may increase height; may also cause uncontrolled growth of the heart and other internal organs and even death; potentially dangerous; requires careful monitoring by a physician. Use of needles for injections adds further health risk. Banned by the International Olympic Committee.
Blood doping	To enhance aerobic capacity by injecting red blood cells harvested previously from the athlete, or alternately the athlete may use the hormone erythropoietin (Epogen) to increase red blood cell number	May offer aerobic benefit; very serious health consequences are possible, including thickening of the blood, which puts extra strain on the heart; is an illegal practice under Olympic guidelines.
Gamma hydroxybutyric acid (GHB)	Promoted as a steroid alternative for bodybuilding	FDA has never approved it for sale as a medical product; is illegal to produce or sell GHB in the United States. GHB-related symptoms include vomiting, dizziness, tremors, and seizures. Many victims have required hospitalization, and some have died. Clandestine laboratories produced virtually all of the chemical accounting for GHB abuse. FDA is working with the U.S. Attorney's office to arrest, indict, and convict individuals responsible for the illegal operations.

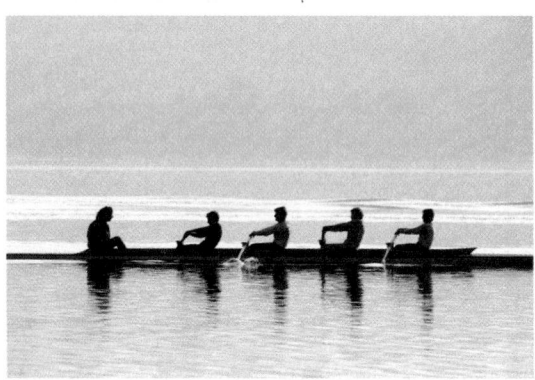

◀ Attention to carbohydrate and fluid needs—along with meeting overall nutrient needs—is the most important ergogenic aid.

Case Study Planning a Training Diet

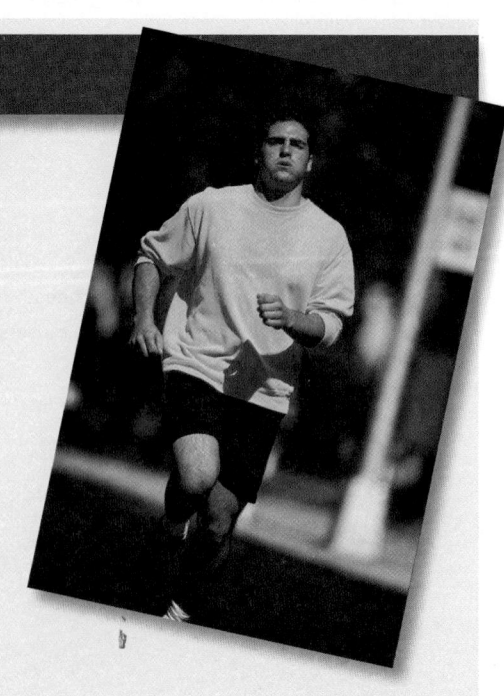

Michael is training for a 10K run coming up in 3 weeks. He has read a lot about sports nutrition and especially about the importance of eating a high-carbohydrate diet while in training. He also has been struggling to keep his weight in a range that he feels contributes to better speed and endurance. Consequently he is also trying to eat as little fat as possible. Unfortunately, over the past week his workouts in the afternoon have not met his expectations. His run times are slower, and he shows signs of fatigue after just 20 minutes into his training program.

His breakfast yesterday was a large bagel, a small amount of cream cheese, and orange juice. For lunch, he had a small salad with fat-free dressing, a large plate of pasta with marinara sauce and broccoli, and a diet soft drink. For dinner, he had a small broiled chicken breast, a cup of rice, some carrots, and iced tea. Later, he snacked on fat-free pretzels.

Answer the following questions, and check your responses in Appendix A.

1. Is the high-carbohydrate diet a good idea during Michael's training?
2. Are there any important components missing in Michael's diet? Are missing components contributing to his fatigue?
3. Describe some changes that should be made in Michael's diet including some specific foods that should be emphasized.
4. How should fluid needs be met during workouts?
5. Should Michael focus on fueling his body before, during, or after workouts?

Summary (Numbers refer to numbered sections in the chapter.)

10.1 A gradual increase in regular physical activity is recommended for all healthy persons. Benefits include improvements in cardiovascular health, gastrointestinal function, blood glucose regulation, and sleep; reduced risk of certain cancers; and enhanced muscle and bone strength.

10.2 The Physical Activity Guidelines for Americans advise adults to do at least 150 minutes of moderate-intensity or 75 minutes of vigorous-intensity aerobic physical activity per week. In addition, adults should perform muscle-strengthening activities at least twice per week. Workouts should allow time for warm-up exercises to increase blood flow and warm the muscles, and then end with cooldown exercises, including stretching.

10.3 Human metabolic pathways extract chemical energy from carbohydrate, fat, and protein to yield ATP, the compound that provides energy for body functions. Phosphocreatine is another high-energy compound that can be used to resupply ATP during short, intense activities. The mix of macronutrients used for fuel depends on the intensity and duration of activity: short-term, intense exercises primarily use carbohydrate for fuel, whereas low- or moderate-intensity endurance exercises use more fat for fuel. Protein makes a minor contribution as a fuel source.

10.4 To support physical activity, athletes require 5 to 8 kcal per minute of activity above energy needs for a sedentary person. Monitoring weight changes over time is a good way to assess the adequacy of energy intake. Athletes should obtain energy from a varied diet that includes sources of carbohydrates (6 to 10 grams of carbohydrate per kilogram of body weight; usually 60% of total energy), protein (0.8 to 2.0 grams of protein per kilogram, depending on the type of training), and fat (up to 35% of energy, focusing on vegetable oils instead of solid fats). The increased overall food intake of athletes typically furnishes adequate vitamins and minerals. Some micronutrients concern are iron and calcium, especially for women.

10.5 Athletes should consume enough fluid to both minimize loss of body weight and ultimately restore pre-exercise weight. Sports drinks help replace fluid, electrolytes, and carbohydrates lost during workouts that last beyond 60 minutes.

10.6 In the 24 hours before an event, athletes should drink fluids freely and consume plenty of carbohydrates. During endurance events, athletes should consume enough fluid and electrolytes to prevent losses of more than 2% of body weight, as determined by individuals during training. Sports drinks and energy gels are two options for fueling during events. In the recovery period, endurance athletes should consume high-glycemic-load carbohydrates and some protein soon after a workout to begin restoration of muscle glycogen stores. To replace fluid losses, athletes should drink 2 to 3 cups of fluid for every pound lost.

N&YH Athletes can benefit from ergogenic properties of sufficient water and electrolytes, lots of carbohydrates, and a balanced and varied diet consistent with the Dietary Guidelines and MyPlate. Under some circumstances, creatine, sodium bicarbonate, and caffeine are useful for enhancing athletic performance. Protein and amino-acid supplements are not beneficial because athletes meet protein needs from foods.

Check Your Knowledge (Answers to the following questions are below.)

1. An energy-rich compound, phosphocreatine (PCr), is found in _____ tissue.
   a. adipose
   b. muscle
   c. liver
   d. kidney

2. A fitness program should include
   a. aerobic exercises 5 days per week.
   b. strength-training exercises 2 to 3 days per week.
   c. stretching exercises 2 to 3 days per week.
   d. All of the above.

3. During muscle-building regimes, athletes should consume _____ grams of protein per kilogram body weight.
   a. 0.5 to 0.7
   b. 0.8
   c. 1.5 to 1.7
   d. 2 to 2.5

4. Which of these foods is the best choice for carbohydrate loading before endurance events?
   a. potato chips
   b. French fries
   c. All-Bran (high-fiber) cereal
   d. rice

5. As the body adapts to regular exercise, the "training effect" results in
   a. decreased blood flow to muscles.
   b. increased lactic acid production.
   c. decreased muscle triglyceride content.
   d. decreased resting heart rate.

6. A physically active lifestyle leads to
   a. increased bone strength.
   b. decreased risk of colon cancer.
   c. reduced stress.
   d. All of the above.

7. How many cups of fluid are required to replace each pound of weight lost during an athletic event or workout?
   a. 0.5 to 0.75
   b. 1 to 1.5
   c. 2 to 3
   d. 4 to 5

8. The benefit of a "sports" drink is to provide
   a. water to hydrate.
   b. electrolytes to enhance water absorption in the intestine and maintain blood volume.
   c. carbohydrate for energy.
   d. All of the above.

9. Compared to anaerobic glucose metabolism, aerobic glucose metabolism produces more
   a. lactic acid.
   b. ATP.
   c. phosphocreatine.
   d. fatty acids.

10. Caffeine is used as an ergogenic aid by some athletes because it is thought to
    a. increase use of fatty acids.
    b. decrease the buildup of lactic acid.
    c. serve as an energy source.
    d. increase muscle mass and strength.

Answers: 1. b (LO 10.3), 2. d (LO 10.2), 3. c (LO 10.6), 4. d (LO 10.8), 5. d (LO 10.5), 6. d (LO 10.1), 7. c (LO 10.7), 8. d (LO 10.7), 9. b (LO 10.4), 10. a (LO 10.9)

Study Questions (Numbers refer to Learning Outcomes)

1. How does greater physical fitness contribute to better overall health? Explain the process. **(LO 10.1)**

2. You have set a goal to increase muscle mass and decrease body fat. Plan a weekly fitness regime, specifying activity types, frequency, intensity, duration, and progression. **(LO 10.2)**

3. How are carbohydrates, fat, and protein used to supply energy during a 100-meter sprint? During a weight-lifting session? During a 3-mile walk? **(LO 10.3)**

4. What is the difference between anaerobic and aerobic exercise? Explain why aerobic metabolism is increased by a regular exercise routine. **(LO 10.4)**

5. Is fat from adipose tissue used as an energy source during exercise? If so, when? **(LO 10.5)**

6. What are some typical measures used to assess whether an athlete's calorie intake is adequate? **(LO 10.6)**

7. List five specific nutrients that athletes need and the appropriate food sources from which these nutrients can be obtained. **(LO 10.6)**

8. You plan to participate in half-marathon. Plan your menu for the day, being sure to include appropriate levels of macro-nutrients and fluids before, during, and after the athletic event. **(LO 10.8)**

9. What advice would you give your neighbor, planning to run a 5-kilometer (km) race, concerning fluid intake before and during the event? **(LO 10.7)**

10. One of your friends, a competitive athlete, asks your opinion about an amino-acid supplement sold in a local sporting-goods store. She has read that such supplements can help improve athletic performance. What would you tell her about the general effectiveness of such products? **(LO 10.9)**

What Would You Choose Recommendations

In this chapter, you have learned that it's important to replenish carbohydrates, fluids, and electrolytes for optimal performance during endurance events, like this half-marathon. General guidelines are to consume ½ to 1 ½ cups of fluid every 15 minutes and 30 to 60 grams of carbohydrate per hour. Choosing a sports nutrition product is something you should do during training. With a few weeks to go, you have time to experiment with a product that can help you avoid "hitting the wall" at mile nine.

The PowerBar ProteinPlus energy bar provides 300 kcal, 6 grams of fat, 39 grams of carbohydrate, and 23 grams of protein. This might be a tasty and convenient meal replacement during your busy weeks of training. Alternatively, it could serve as a recovery meal to help replenish your muscle glycogen stores after the race. However, during the race, its high fat and protein content would slow digestion, possibly leading to abdominal cramps. Furthermore, this product would not contribute to fluid replenishment.

The Essential Amino Energy drink provides 2 grams of carbohydrate and 5 grams of essential amino acids in free form, including branched-chain amino acids. The drink may help meet fluid needs, but the carbohydrate content is not sufficient to maintain blood glucose during the race. It is true that BCAAs are utilized for fuel during endurance activities and that they can enhance muscle building during weight

training, but there is no consistent evidence that supplying BCAAs during endurance exercise enhances performance.

A sports drink, such as Powerade, is superior to water for events lasting more than 60 minutes. The added carbohydrates help to supply energy to the brain and muscles. The added flavor encourages consumption. The electrolytes replace those lost in sweating, increase fluid absorption, and stimulate thirst. A 32-ounce bottle of Powerade (4 servings) contains a total of 200 kcal and 56 grams of carbohydrate in 4 cups of fluid. One bottle of Powerade per hour while you compete would meet your fluid and carbohydrate needs, but may be inconvenient to tote while running.

The energy gel is small enough to take along during the race—and the chocolate cherry flavor sounds delicious! The label says it has 110 kcal, 1.5 grams of fat, 22 grams of carbohydrate, 12 grams of sugar, and 100 milligrams of caffeine. A Clif Shot during the race could help replenish blood glucose and electrolytes, but it definitely won't meet your fluid requirements while racing. However, there will be water available at numerous stops along the course.

Some energy gels are caffeine-free, but this one contains as much caffeine as a strong cup of coffee. Research shows that caffeine can increase the ability of muscles to use fatty acids for energy and increase mental alertness among people who are not habitual caffeine consumers. On the other hand, negative effects of excessive

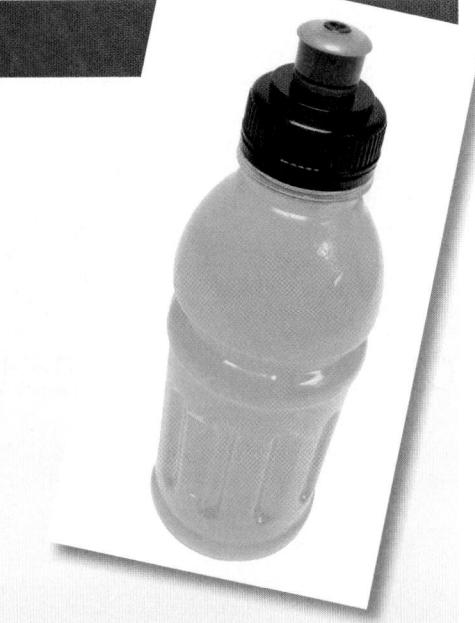

▲ Sports drinks replenish carbohydrates and electrolytes lost during prolonged exercise.

caffeine include dehydration, heart palpitations, and gastrointestinal discomfort, so moderation is necessary.

In summary, both the Powerade and the Clif Shot would replenish carbohydrates and electrolytes. The Powerade would also fulfill your fluid needs, whereas you'd need to grab water along the course if you choose the energy gel. The energy gel has the advantage of being light and portable, plus the caffeine may have an ergogenic effect. Give both the Powerade and the Clif Shot energy gel a trial run during your training sessions and see which one helps you most around mile nine.

Further Readings

1. Adamidou J, Bell-Wilson J: Iron deficiency anemia and exercise. *IDEA Fitness Journal* May:82, 2006.

    This article reviews why athletes may have increased iron requirements. The best food sources to prevent iron depletion and sports anemia are also suggested.

2. DeJonge L, Smith MR: Macronutrients and exercise. *Obesity Management* February:11, 2008.

    Body stores of carbohydrate and fat are used preferentially as fuel for exercising muscles, whereas protein is conserved. Exercise not only leads to increased fat oxidation during exercise, but also in the post-exercise period. Furthermore, the body's ability to burn fat is improved by training.

3. Garber CE and others: American College of Sports Medicine Position Stand: Quantity and quality of exercise for developing and maintaining cardiorespiratory, musculo-skeletal, and neuromotor fitness in apparently healthy adults: Guidance for prescribing exercise. *Medicine and Science in Sports and Exercise* 43:1334, 2011.

    These exercise guidelines from the American College of Sports Medicine generally agree with advice conveyed by the 2008 Physical Activity Guidelines for Americans. The benefits of and recommendations for endurance, strength, and flexibility exercises are reviewed. Sedentary behavior is discouraged.

4. Gleeson M: Can nutrition limit exercise-induced immunodepression? *Nutrition Reviews* March:119, 2006.

    Intense or prolonged exercise can lead to immunodepression, resulting in increased incidence of infections among athletes. These effects are due to the activity of stress hormones on immune cells. Optimal nutrition, including adequate habitual dietary intake of protein, essential fatty acids, zinc, iron, and antioxidants supports immune function. Consuming carbohydrate and staying hydrated are important strategies to prevent the stress response that leads to immune dysfunction.

5. Harber VJ: Energy balance and reproductive function in active women. *Canadian Journal of Applied Physiology* 29:48, 2004.

    It is important for female athletes engaged in rigorous training programs to meet their calorie needs. If not, the resulting negative calorie balance will likely lead to a variety of menstrual cycle disturbances that can lead to other health problems.

6. Jenkinson DM, Harbert AJ. Supplements and sports. *American Family Physician* 78:1039, 2008.

    Use of dietary supplements among athletes is widespread and supplement users are often uninformed about the risks and benefits of supplementation. Some supplements, including anabolic steroids and ephedrine, have dangerous effects. Most supplements do not demonstrate consistent benefits for athletic performance. A few substances, including creatine, caffeine, and sodium bicarbonate, are useful under certain circumstances.

7. Kreider RB and others: ISSN exercise and sport nutrition review: Research and recommendations. *Journal of the International Society of Sports Nutrition* 7:7, 2010.

    This detailed and comprehensive review covers fluid and nutrient needs for optimal athletic performance, timing of food intake, and up-to-date research on an array of dietary supplements. Of note, ISSN recommends up to 2.0 grams of protein per kilogram of body weight for some athletes involved in intense training— more than twice the recommendations of the Food and Nutrition Board.

8. Laaksonen DE and others: Physical activity in the prevention of type 2 diabetes: The Finnish Diabetes Prevention Study. *Diabetes* 54:158, 2005.

    Regular physical activity can substantially reduce the risk of developing type 2 diabetes in high risk individuals. People who increased their activity from moderate to vigorous amounts reduced their risk of developing type 2 diabetes by 65% compared to people who remained inactive.

9. Margaritis I, Rousseau AS: Does physical exercise modify antioxidant requirements? *Nutrition Research Reviews* 21:3, 2008.

    Exercise induces oxidative stress, leading to the hypothesis that exercise may increase antioxidant nutrient requirements among athletes. To date, however, research does not support use of antioxidant supplements to enhance athletic performance. In fact, some studies show detrimental effects of supplementation on endpoints such as muscle recovery and even all-cause mortality. Except in cases of pre-existing nutrient deficiencies, consuming a well-balanced diet is the best advice for optimizing athletic performance.

10. Maughan RJ, Shirreffs SM: Development of individual hydration strategies for athletes. *International Journal of Sport and Nutrition and Exercise Metabolism* 18:457, 2008.

    Both dehydration and hyperhydration are detrimental to athletic performance and can be lethal. Despite the popular devaluation of thirst as an indicator of dehydration, recent research demonstrates that adherence to physiologic cues for consumption of fluid and electrolytes supports optimal athletic performance even when

    100% body weight is not maintained. For optimal performance, hydration strategies should account for carbohydrate and electrolyte replacements in addition to fluid intake.

11. Nichols DL and others: Bone density and young athletic women. An update. *Sports Medicine* 37:1001, 2007.

    Athletes have 5–30% higher bone density than their non-athletic counterparts. In combination with prolonged negative energy balance, however, high levels of physical activity may lead to the female athlete triad, in which low dietary intake and weight loss lead to amenorrhea and subsequent bone loss. Although current research does not point to augmented requirements for female athletes, meeting DRIs for protein, calcium, and vitamin D intake is an important dietary goal to support optimal bone development.

12. Rodriguez NR and others: Position of the American Dietetic Association, Dietitians of Canada, and the American College of Sports Medicine: Nutrition and athletic performance. *Journal of the American Dietetic Association* 109:509, 2009.

    This position statement summarizes recommendations for nutrient and fluid intake before, during, and after exercise to optimize athletic performance. Guidance for special population groups, such as vegetarian athletes,is provided. Dietary supplements and ergogenic acids are discouraged because food intake usually provides adequate micronutrients and supplements may be contaminated with banned and/or dangerous ingredients.

13. Rosenbloom C, Rosbruck M. Popular dietary supplements used in sports. *Nutrition Today* 43:60, 2008.

    The authors review four dietary supplements that are popular as ergogenic and weight loss aids creatine, caffeine, epigallocatechin (EGCG), and nitric oxide and its metabolite, L-arginine.

14. Sawka MN and others: American College of Sports Medicine Position Stand: Exercise and fluid replacement. *Medicine and Science in Sports and Exercise* 39:377, 2007.

    This review summarizes the water intake recommendations for healthy humans, emphasizing that hydration is well maintained as long as food and fluid are readily available. The review concludes that exercise and heat can greatly increase water needs, and that the individual variability between athletes can be significant.

15. Williams MH: Nutrition for health, fitness, & sport. 9th ed. Boston: McGraw-Hill, 2009.

    Excellent textbook for reviewing nutrient needs of athletes, as well as learning more about ergogenic aids; also provides a detailed look at metabolism in exercise.

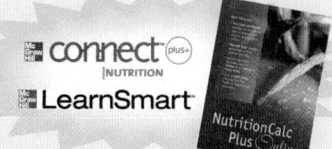

To get the most out of your study of nutrition, go to McGraw-Hill's online resources: Connect www.mcgrawhillconnect.com, **where you will find NutritionCalc Plus, LearnSmart, and many other dynamic tools.**

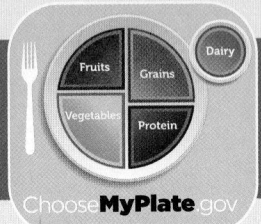

RATE YOUR PLATE

I. Evaluating Protein Intake—A Case Study

Mark is a college student who has been lifting weights at the student recreation center. The trainer at the center recommended a protein drink to help Mark build muscle mass. Answer the following questions about Mark's current food intake and determine whether a protein drink is needed to supplement Mark's diet.

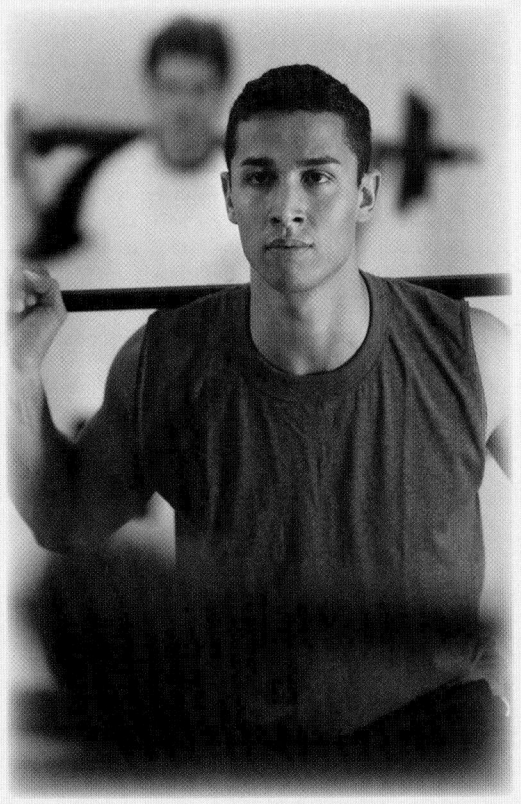

1. The following is a tally of yesterday's intake.

Breakfast	Frosted Mini-Wheats cereal, 2 oz 1% milk, 1½ cups Orange juice, chilled, 6 oz Glazed yeast doughnut, 1 Brewed coffee, 1 cup
Lunch	Double hamburger with condiments, 1 French fries, 30 Cola, 12 oz Medium apple, 1
Dinner	Frozen lasagna w/meat, 2 pieces 1% milk, 1 cup Looseleaf lettuce, chopped, 1 cup Creamy Italian salad dressing, 2 tsp Medium tomato, ½ Whole carrot, raw, 1
Evening snack	Vanilla ice milk, 1 cup Hot fudge chocolate topping, 2 tsp Soft chocolate chip cookies, 2

Evaluate Mark's diet using NutritionCalc Plus—is he meeting the minimum recommendations of MyPlate's Daily Food Plan for his calorie needs?

_____

2. Mark's weight has been stable at 70 kilograms (154 pounds). Determine his protein needs based on the RDA (0.8 grams per kilogram).
    a. Mark's estimated protein RDA: _____
    b. What are the maximum recommendations for protein intake for strength-training athletes (see p. 423)? _____
    c. Calculate the maximum protein recommendation for Mark. _____

    _____

3. An analysis of the total calorie and protein content of Mark's current diet is 3470 kcal, 125 grams of protein (14% of total calories supplied by protein). This diet is representative of the food choices and amounts of food that Mark chooses on a regular basis.
    a. What is the difference between Mark's estimated protein needs as an athlete (from number 2) and the amount of protein that his current diet provides? _____
    b. Is his current protein intake inadequate, adequate, or excessive? _____

4. Mark takes his trainer's advice and goes to the supermarket to purchase a protein drink to add to his diet. Four products are available; they contain the following label information.

	Amino Fuel	Joe Weider's Sugar-Free 90% Plus Protein	Joe Weider's Dynamic Muscle Builder	Victory Super Mega Mass 2000
Serving size	3 tbsp	3 tbsp	3 tbsp	¼ scoop
Kcal	104	110	103	104
Protein (grams)	15	24	10	5

The trainer recommends adding the supplement to Mark's diet two times a day. Mark chooses the Muscle Builder protein drink.

a. How much protein would be added to Mark's diet daily from two servings of the supplement alone (prior to mixing it with a beverage)?

b. Mark mixes the powder with the milk he already consumes at breakfast and dinner. How much protein total would Mark now consume in 1 day? (Add the protein amount from the nutrition analysis to the value from question 4a.)

c. What is the difference between Mark's estimated protein needs as an athlete and this total intake?

5. What is your conclusion—does Mark need the protein supplement?

(from above): 145 grams −119 grams = 26 grams protein.

4c. Difference between Mark's estimated maximum protein needs for muscle mass gain and total protein consumption with protein supplement

4b. Mark's total protein consumption: 125 grams + 20 grams = 145 grams protein.

4a. Two servings of protein supplement alone = 20 grams of protein.

3b. Mark's current protein intake exceeds maximum protein needs.

3a. Difference between Mark's estimated maximum protein needs for muscle mass gain and the amount of protein provided by his current diet:
125−119 = 6 grams protein.

2c. Applied to Mark: 1.7 × 70 = 119 grams.

2b. Maximum recommendation for protein intake for athletes = 1.7 grams per kilogram.

2a. Mark's estimated protein RDA: 70 kilograms × 0.8 grams per kilogram = 56 grams.

Answers to Calculations

II. How Physically Fit Are You?

The fitness assessments presented here are easy to do and require little equipment. Also included are charts to compare your results to those typical of your peers.

Cardiovascular Fitness: One-Mile Walk

Measure a mile on a running track (usually four laps) or on a little-trafficked neighborhood street (use a car's odometer to get the right distance). With a stopwatch or watch with a second hand, walk the mile as fast as you can. Note the time it took.

Strength: Push-ups

Men: Get up on your toes and hands. Keep your back straight, with hands flat on the floor directly below your shoulders. Women: Same position, but you can support your body on your knees if necessary.

Lower your body, bending your elbows, until your chin grazes the floor. Push back up until your arms are straight. Continue until you can't do any more push-ups (you can rest when in the up position).

Strength: Curl-ups

Lie on the floor on your back with your knees bent, feet flat. Your hands should rest on your thighs. Now squeeze your stomach muscles, push your back flat, and raise your upper body high enough for your hands to touch the tops of your knees. Don't pull with your neck or head, and keep your lower back on the floor. Count how many curl-ups you can do in one minute.

Flexibility: Sit-and-Reach

Place a yardstick on the floor and apply a two-foot piece of tape on the floor perpendicular to the yardstick, crossing at the 15-inch mark. Sit on the floor with your legs extended and the soles of your feet touching the tape at the 15-inch mark, the zero-inch facing you. Your feet should be about 12 inches apart. Put one hand on the other, exhale, and very slowly reach forward as far as you can along the yardstick, lowering your head between your arms. Don't bounce! Note the farthest inch mark you reach. Don't hurt yourself by reaching farther than your body wants to. Relax, and then repeat two more times.

Now check your results. Want to improve? You know the answer:

- Do aerobic exercise that makes you breathe hard for at least half an hour on most or all days of the week.
- Lift weights that challenge you two to three times per week.
- Stretch after activity at least a couple of times per week.
- Walk more.

Cardiovascular: One-mile walk (time, in minutes)

| | Under 40 Years | | Over 40 Years | |
	Men	Women	Men	Women
Excellent	13:00 or less	13:30 or less	14:00 or less	14:30 or less
Good	13:01–15:30	13:31–16:00	14:01–16:30	14:31–17:00
Average	15:31–18:00	16:01–18:30	16:31–19:00	17:01–19:30
Below average	18:01–19:30	18:31–20:00	19:01–21:30	19:31–22:00
Poor	19:31 or more	20:01 or more	21:31 or more	22:01 or more

Source: Cooper Institute.

Strength: Push-ups (number completed without rest)

	Men						
Age	17–19	20–29	30–39	40–49	50–59	60–65
Excellent	>56	>47	>41	>34	>31	>30
Good	47–56	39–47	34–41	28–34	25–31	24–30
Above average	35–46	30–39	25–33	21–28	18–24	17–23
Average	19–34	17–29	13–24	11–20	9–17	6–16
Below average	11–18	10–16	8–12	6–10	5–8	3–5
Poor	4–10	4–9	2–7	1–5	1–4	1–2
Very poor	<4	<4	<2	0	0	0

	Women						
Age	17–19	20–29	30–39	40–49	50–59	60–65
Excellent	>35	>36	>37	>31	>25	>23
Good	27–35	30–36	30–37	25–31	21–25	19–23
Above average	21–27	23–29	22–30	18–24	15–20	13–18
Average	11–20	12–22	10–21	8–17	7–14	5–12
Below average	6–10	7–11	5–9	4–7	3–6	2–4
Poor	2–5	2–6	1–4	1–3	1–2	1
Very poor	0–1	0–1	0	0	0	0

Source: Golding LA, YMCA of the USA: *YMCA Fitness Testing and Assessment Manual*, 4th ed, 2000. www.topendsports.com.

Strength: Curl-ups (number completed in 60 seconds)

	Men					
Age	**18–25**	**26–35**	**36–45**	**46–55**	**56–65**	**65+**
Excellent	>49	>45	>41	>35	>31	>28
Good	44–49	40–45	35–41	29–35	25–31	22–28
Above average	39–43	35–39	30–34	25–28	21–24	19–21
Average	35–38	31–34	27–29	22–24	17–20	15–18
Below average	31–34	29–30	23–26	18–21	13–16	11–14
Poor	25–30	22–28	17–22	13–17	9–12	7–10
Very poor	<25	<22	<17	<13	<9	<7

	Women					
Age	**18–25**	**26–35**	**36–45**	**46–55**	**56–65**	**65+**
Excellent	>43	>39	>33	>27	>24	>23
Good	37–43	33–39	27–33	22–27	18–24	17–23
Above average	33–36	29–32	23–26	18–21	13–17	14–16
Average	29–32	25–28	19–22	14–17	10–12	11–13
Below average	25–28	21–24	15–18	10–13	7–9	5–10
Poor	18–24	13–20	7–14	5–9	3–6	2–4
Very poor	<18	<13	<7	<5	<3	<2

Source: Golding LA, YMCA of the USA: *YMCA Fitness Testing and Assessment Manual*, 4th ed, 2000.

Flexibility: Sit-and-reach (in centimeters)

	Men	Women
Super	>+27	>+30
Excellent	+17 to +27	+21 to +30
Good	+6 to +16	+11 to +20
Average	0 to +5	+1 to +10
Fair	−8 to −1	−7 to 0
Poor	−19 to −9	−14 to −8
Very poor	<−20	<−15

Source: Golding LA, YMCA of the USA: *YMCA Fitness Testing and Assessment Manual*, 4th ed, 2000.

These charts are typical charts used by health and fitness experts. For a more thorough assessment of fitness or for development of an exercise plan appropriate for your fitness level, consult a certified personal trainer or other fitness professional.

Chapter 11 Eating Disorders:
Anorexia Nervosa, Bulimia Nervosa, and Other Conditions

Chapter Outline

Student Learning Outcomes

Chapter 11 is designed to allow you to:

11.1 Contrast healthy attitudes toward uses of food with behavior patterns that could lead to unhealthy uses of food.

11.2 Outline the causes of, effects of, typical persons affected by, and treatment for anorexia nervosa.

11.3 Outline the causes of, effects of, typical persons affected by, and treatment for bulimia nervosa.

11.4 Describe still other forms of eating disorders: binge-eating disorder, night eating syndrome, and the female athlete triad.

11.5 Relate the presence of eating disorders to current social trends.

11.6 Describe methods to reduce the development of eating disorders, including the use of warning signs to identify early cases.

What Would You Choose?

Your college roommate has been acting strangely lately, and you are starting to suspect she has an eating disorder. Over the first few months at college, she gained the "freshman fifteen." She got kind of depressed about it when her jeans started to fit too snugly and declared she was going on a diet. Her weight has not really changed much since then, but her eating behaviors have. She stopped joining your group of friends for meals in the dining hall, opting instead to eat by herself in your dorm room. She has been spending at least 2 hours a day in the campus recreation center, sometimes going in the morning and evening. A few days ago, you thought you heard her throwing up in the restroom, but when she came out of the stall, she said she was fine. What would you choose to help your roommate?

a Tell her she has bulimia and needs to get some treatment.

b Give her some weight-management advice that you learned in Chapter 7.

c Express your concern and ask her if you can go with her to the student health center to talk to someone about it

d Ignore her behavior; she is just trying to draw attention to herself, and this phase will pass in a few weeks.

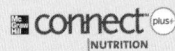 **connect** plus+ NUTRITION **Think about your choice as you read Chapter 11, then see our recommendations at the end of the chapter. To learn more about warning signs of eating disorders, check out the Connect site:** www.mcgrawhillconnect.com

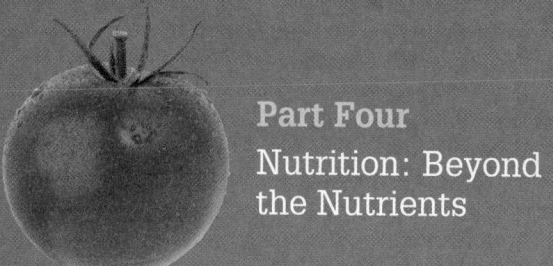

Part Four
Nutrition: Beyond
the Nutrients

Many of us occasionally eat until we're stuffed and uncomfortable, such as at Thanksgiving dinner. Faced with savory and tempting foods, we find that we can't easily stop eating. Usually we forgive ourselves, vowing not to overeat the next time. Nevertheless, many of us have problems controlling our food intake and body weight. The combination of too many instances of simple overeating, and too little physical activity eventually leads to progressive weight gain.

The obesity epidemic tends to upstage all other nutrition-related problems. However, the eating disorders discussed here are just as serious, if not more, than obesity, and can develop into life-threatening conditions if left untreated. What's most alarming about these disorders—anorexia nervosa, bulimia nervosa, binge-eating disorder, and the female athlete triad—is the increasing number of cases reported each year.

Some people are more susceptible to these eating disorders than other people are—for genetic, psychological, and physical reasons. Successful treatment of eating disorders, therefore, is complex and must go beyond nutritional therapy. Keep in mind that eating disorders are not restricted to any socioeconomic class or ethnicity. They can also strike, as suggested in the comic in this chapter, at any age in both females and males. Let's examine the causes and treatments of these conditions in detail, because eating disorders touch many of our lives.

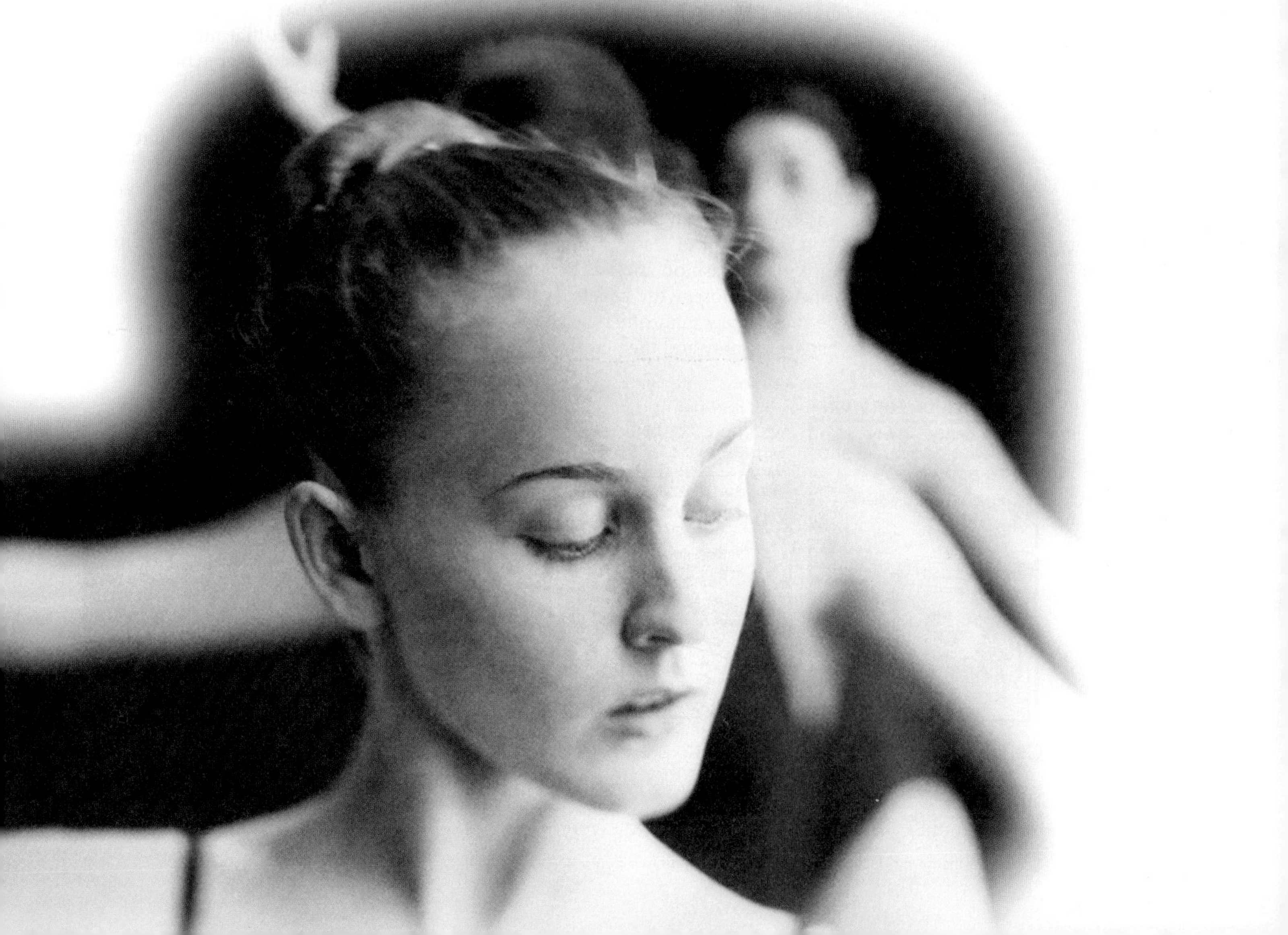

Refresh Your Memory

As you begin your study of eating disorders, such as anorexia nervosa and bulimia nervosa, in Chapter 11, you may want to review:

- The effects of neurotransmitters on food intake in Chapter 1
- The role of genetic risk in disease susceptibility in Chapter 3
- Calculation of BMI in Chapter 7
- The effects and treatment of osteoporosis in Chapter 9
- The effects and treatment of iron-deficiency anemia in Chapter 9

11.1 From Ordered to Disordered Eating Habits

Eating—a completely instinctive behavior for animals—serves an extraordinary number of psychological, social, and cultural purposes for humans. Eating practices may take on religious meanings; signify bonds within families and ethnic groups; and provide a means to express hostility, affection, prestige, or class values. Within the family, supplying, preparing, and distributing food may be a means of expressing love, hatred, or even power.

We are bombarded daily with images of our society's portrayal of the "ideal" body. Dieting is promoted to achieve this ideal body—eternally young and admired. Television programs, billboard and Internet advertisements, magazine pictures, movies, and newspapers suggest that an ultraslim body will bring happiness, love, and ultimately, success. This fantasy notion is contradictory to the fact that much of society is becoming fatter, even obese. In response to this social pressure, some of us take an extreme approach—the pathological pursuit of weight control or weight loss.

Early in life, we develop images of "acceptable" and "unacceptable" body types. Of the attributes that constitute attractiveness, many people view body weight as the most important, partly because we can control our weight somewhat. Fatness is the most dreaded deviation from our cultural ideals of body image, the one most derided and shunned, even among schoolchildren.

It is difficult to resist comparing ourselves to the "ideal" body. Not everyone can look like a fashion model. People who are overly impressed by media messages, especially those with genetic, psychological, and environmental influences, may be more likely than others to develop eating disorders in an effort to close the gap between reality and the perceived ideal.

FOR BETTER OR FOR WORSE

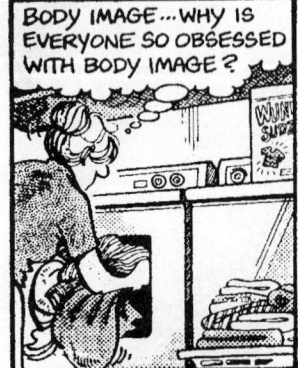
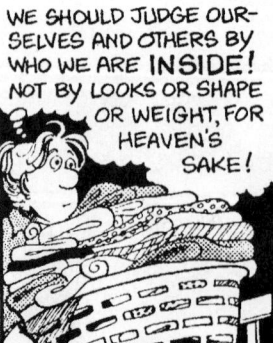
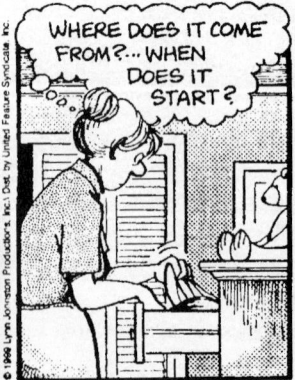
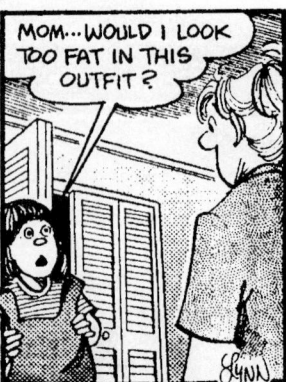

Concern with body image often starts early in life. Why do you think this is so? What societal trends have fostered this concern? Are some people more vulnerable, based on genetics and environment? Chapter 11 provides some answers.

© Lynn Johnston Productions, Inc. Distributed by United Features Syndicate, Inc.

Given the multiple functions associated with normal eating and constant exposure to our culture's ideal body image, it is not surprising that some people progress from typical responses to hunger and satiety cues to obsessive weight-loss behaviors, and then to a full-blown eating disorder.

Food: More than Just a Source of Nutrients

From birth, we link food with personal and emotional experiences. As infants, we associate milk with security and warmth so the breast or bottle becomes a source of comfort as well as food. As noted in Chapter 1, even when older, most people continue to derive comfort and great pleasure from food. This is both a biological and a psychological phenomenon. Food can be a symbol of comfort, but eating can also stimulate the release of certain neurotransmitters (e.g., serotonin) and *natural opioids* (including **endorphins**), which produce a sense of calm and euphoria in the human body. Thus, in times of great stress, some people turn to food for a druglike, calming effect.

Food is also used as a reward or a bribe. Haven't you heard or spoken something similar to the following comments?

You can have your dessert if you eat five more bites of your vegetables.
You can't play until you clean your plate.
I'll eat the broccoli if you let me watch TV.
If you love me, you'll eat your dinner.

On the surface, using food as a reward or bribe seems harmless enough. Eventually, however, this practice encourages both caregivers and children to use food to achieve goals other than satisfying hunger and nutrient needs. Food may then become much more than a source of nutrients. Regularly using food as a bargaining chip can contribute to abnormal eating patterns. Carried to the extreme, these patterns can lead to **disordered eating.**

Disordered eating can be defined as mild and short-term changes in eating patterns that occur in response to a stressful event, an illness, or even a desire to modify the diet for a variety of health and personal appearance reasons (see Further Reading 14). The problem may be no more than a bad habit, a style of eating adapted from friends or family members, or an aspect of preparing for athletic competition. While disordered eating can lead to weight loss or weight gain, as well as certain nutritional problems, it rarely requires in-depth professional attention. If, however, disordered eating becomes sustained, distressing, or starts to interfere with everyday activities and is linked to physiological changes, it may require professional intervention.

Overview of Anorexia Nervosa and Bulimia Nervosa

Given the common practice of dieting in North America, it can sometimes be difficult to tell where disordered eating stops and an **eating disorder** begins. Indeed, many eating disorders start with a simple diet. Eating disorders then go on to involve physiological changes associated with food restriction, binge eating, purging, and fluctuations in weight. They also involve a number of emotional and cognitive changes that affect the way a person perceives and experiences his or her body, such as feelings of distress or extreme concern about body shape or weight. Eating disorders are not due to a failure of will or behavior; rather, they are real, treatable medical illnesses in which certain maladaptive patterns of eating take on a life of their own.

The main types of eating disorders are **anorexia nervosa** and **bulimia nervosa.** Another type, **binge-eating disorder**, is not yet approved as a formal psychiatric diagnoses, but this will likely change with the update of the American Psychiatric Association's *Diagnostic and Statistical Manual of Mental Disorders,* expected in 2013. The various classifications of eating disorders are all rooted in an overvaluation of body shape or body weight as a source of self-identity. Although it is convenient to label patients with a particular diagnosis, the various types of eating disorders have more similarities than distinctions, particularly in the psychological processes that underlie them. Furthermore, people who cope with eating disorders tend to migrate from one type to another.

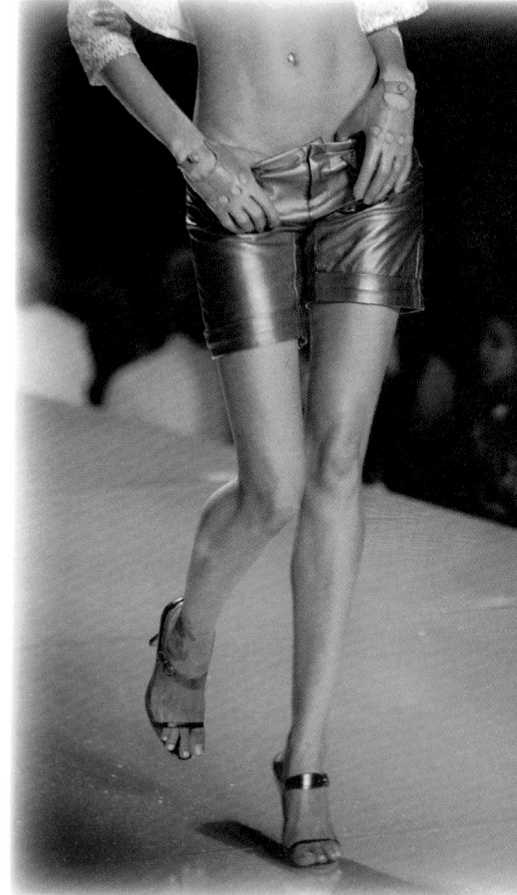

▲ Maintaining an anorexic body type is an all too common goal in today's culture. The media and the fashion world bombard us with body images that are unrealistic for most people.

endorphins Natural body tranquilizers that may be involved in the feeding response and function in pain reduction.

disordered eating Mild and short-term changes in eating patterns that occur in relation to a stressful event, an illness, or a desire to modify one's diet for a variety of health and personal appearance reasons.

eating disorder Severe alterations in eating patterns linked to physiological changes. The alterations are associated with food restriction, binge eating, purging, and fluctuations in weight. They also involve a number of emotional and cognitive changes that affect the way a person perceives and experiences his or her body.

anorexia nervosa An eating disorder involving a psychological loss or denial of appetite, followed by self-starvation; related in part to a distorted body image and to various social pressures commonly associated with puberty.

bulimia nervosa An eating disorder in which large quantities of food are eaten at one time (binge eating) and then purged from the body by vomiting, or misuse of laxatives, diuretics, or enemas. Alternate means to counteract the binge behavior are fasting and excessive exercise.

binge-eating disorder An eating disorder characterized by recurrent binge eating that is not followed by purging and has lasted at least 6 months. Binge episodes are characterized by loss of control over eating and can be triggered by frustration, anger, depression, anxiety, permission to eat forbidden foods, and excessive hunger.

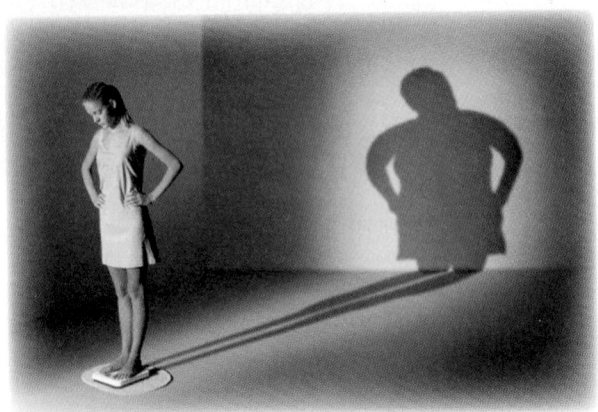

▲ Self-image is an important part of adolescence. For people with eating disorders, the difference between the real and desired body images may be too difficult to accept. See the website www.4women.gov/body-image.

Progression from Ordered to Disordered Eating

Attention to hunger and satiety signals; limitation of calorie intake to restore weight to a healthful level

↓

Some disordered eating habits begin as weight loss is attempted, such as very restricted eating

↓

Clinically evident eating disorder recognized

Early detection is important

According to the National Eating Disorders Association, as many as 10 million people in the United States have an eating disorder. Eating disorders typically develop during adolescence or young adulthood, but increasingly, the onset occurs during childhood (an alarming trend; see Further Reading 2). Eating disorders frequently co-occur with other psychological disorders, such as depression, substance abuse, and anxiety disorders. *People who suffer from eating disorders, especially anorexia nervosa and bulimia nervosa, can experience a wide range of health complications, including heart conditions and kidney failure, which may even lead to death.* Recognition of eating disorders as important and treatable diseases, therefore, is critical.

Common to both eating disorders, *nervosa* refers to an attitude of disgust with one's body. The term *anorexia* implies a loss of appetite; however, a denial of one's appetite more accurately describes the behavior of people with anorexia nervosa. Anorexia nervosa is characterized by extreme weight loss; a distorted body image; and an irrational, almost morbid, fear of obesity and weight gain. Anorexic patients irrationally believe they are fat, even though others constantly comment on their thin physique. Some anorexics realize they are thin but continue to be haunted by certain areas of their bodies that they believe to be fat (such as thighs, buttocks, and stomach).

Bulimia nervosa (*bulimia* means "great [ox] hunger") is characterized by episodes of binge eating followed by attempts to purge the calories by vomiting or misusing laxatives, diuretics, or enemas. People with this disorder may be difficult to identify because they keep their binge-purge behaviors secret, and their symptoms are not obvious. Four percent or more of adolescent and college-age women suffer from bulimia nervosa. And, as with anorexia nervosa, about 10% of the cases occur in men.

Specific criteria are used by clinicians to diagnose eating disorders (e.g., *Diagnostic and Statistical Manual of Mental Disorders* of the American Psychiatric Association). Some characteristics are listed in Table 11-1. It is possible that people exhibit some symptoms of eating disorders but not enough to enable a medical worker to diagnose one of the two recognized diseases. Also, as suggested in the diagnostic criteria, some people show characteristics of both anorexia nervosa and bulimia nervosa because the diseases overlap considerably. About half of the women diagnosed as having anorexia nervosa eventually develop bulimic symptoms. As shown in Table 11-1, bulimic characteristics also can be seen in anorexia nervosa, which blurs the distinction. Still, appreciating the differences between the disorders helps us to understand the various approaches to prevention and treatment.

Certainly, women outnumber men when it comes to eating disorders—by at least 5 to 1. Currently, up to 5% of women in North America develop some form of anorexia nervosa or bulimia nervosa during their lifetimes. By rough estimate, approximately 0.5% (1 in 200) of women in North America eventually develop anorexia nervosa. Approximately 2% to 3% of women will develop bulimia nervosa. An estimated 95% of all cases of eating disorders occur among young women (ages 12 to 25). This high number may be due to the tendency of females to blame themselves for weight gain typical of their age group.

Men only account for 10% to 15% of all cases of eating disorders, partly because the image conveyed for men is big and muscular (see Making Decisions on page 463). Among men, exercise status and sexual orientation are factors that particularly influence development of eating disorders. Male athletes are more prone than nonathletes to develop eating disorders, especially those who participate in sports that require weight classes, such as boxers, wrestlers, and jockeys (see Further Readings 3 and 10). The rate of eating disorders among athletes lies between 10% and 20%. Other activities that may foster eating disorders in men include swimming, dancing and modeling. The prevalence of eating disorders in gay men is two to three times that of heterosexual men (see Further Reading 5).

ppl @ risk → Until recently, most researchers have reported that eating disorders primarily affect middle- and upper-class Caucasian women. Now, studies show greater similarities in the rates of body dissatisfaction and disordered eating behaviors across ethnic and cultural groups. Perhaps minorities with eating disorders have been less likely to seek

TABLE 11-1 Typical Characteristics of Anorexic and Bulimic Persons

Anorexia Nervosa	Bulimia Nervosa
• Rigid dieting causing dramatic weight loss, generally to less than 85% of what would be expected for one's age (or BMI of 17.5 or less) • False body perception—thinking "I'm too fat," even when extremely underweight; relentless pursuit of control • Rituals involving food, excessive exercise, and other aspects of life • Maintenance of rigid control in lifestyle; security found in control and order • Feeling of panic after a small weight gain; intense fear of gaining weight • Feelings of purity, power, and superiority through maintenance of strict discipline and self-denial • Preoccupation with food, its preparation, and observing another person eat • Helplessness in the presence of food • Lack of menstrual periods (after what should be the age of puberty) for at least 3 months • Possible presence of bingeing and purging practices	• Secretive binge eating; generally not overeating in front of others • Eating when depressed or under stress • Bingeing on a large amount of food, followed by fasting, laxative or diuretic abuse, self-induced vomiting, or excessive exercise (at least twice a week for 3 months) • Feelings of shame, embarrassment, deceit, and depression; low self-esteem and guilt (especially after a binge) • Fluctuating weight (±10 pounds or 5 kilograms) resulting from alternate bingeing and fasting • Loss of control; fear of not being able to stop eating • Perfectionism; "people pleaser"; food as the only comfort/escape in an otherwise carefully controlled and regulated life • Erosion of teeth, swollen glands • Purchase of syrup of ipecac, a compound sold in pharmacies that induces vomiting

Those who exhibit only one or a few of these characteristics may be at risk but probably do not have either disorder. They should, however, reflect on their eating habits and related concerns and take appropriate action, such as seeking a careful evaluation by a physician.

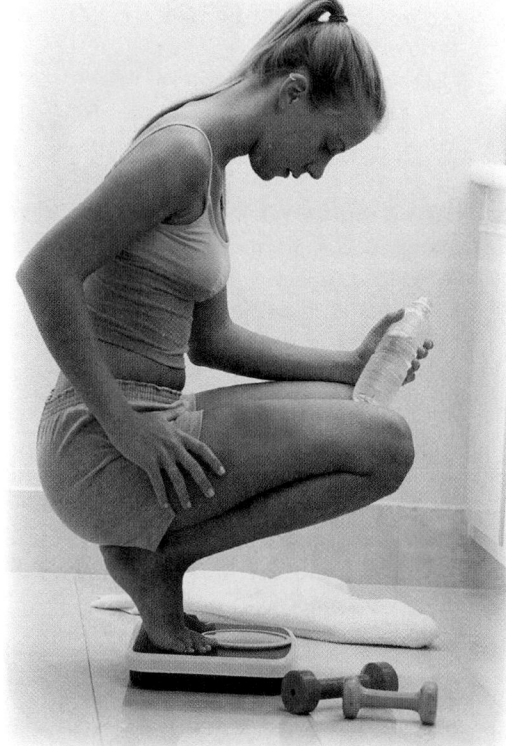

▲ Anorexia nervosa is characterized by a feeling of panic after only a small weight gain; bulimia nervosa is characterized by frequent weight fluctuations from alternate bingeing and fasting.

help in the past due to fear of shame or stigma, lack of resources, or language barriers. It seems more likely, however, that health care workers are less likely to diagnose non-Caucasians as having eating disorders. Previously, it seemed that non-Caucasian cultures were more accepting of larger body shapes, but mainstream pressures for thinness now seem to cut across racial differences. Our overall cultural change may be associated with increased vulnerability to eating disorders.

There are no simple causes of eating disorders, and there are no simple treatments. Stress may have an especially strong role in the development of eating disorders. An underlying commonality seems to be the lack of appropriate coping mechanisms as individuals begin to reach adolescence and young adulthood, coupled with dysfunctional family relationships.

The influence of genetics on the development of eating disorders is an area of active research. In general, twin studies have shown that identical twins have a higher likelihood of sharing eating disorders than do fraternal twins. This indicates that genetics is a strong risk factor in development of such disorders, because identical twins share the same DNA. One study found genetic background to describe 56% of the overall risk of developing anorexia nervosa. A variety of genes could be implicated in the development of eating disorders, including those that code for the expression of hormones and neurotransmitters involved in weight regulation and eating behaviors (review Chapter 1), as well as genes that lead to depression or individual responses to stress. In addition to the genetic code itself, researchers are also studying **epigenetics**, the interaction between genes and environmental influences as it relates to the development of eating disorders see Further Reading 4. Some studies suggest that maternal stress or hormone levels during pregnancy can predict the future development of an eating disorder in the offspring. Identifying genes that cause eating disorders eventually could

Our passion for thinness may have its roots in the Victorian era of the nineteenth century, which specialized in denying "unpleasant" physical realities, such as appetite and sexual desire. Flappers of the 1920s cemented the twentieth century trend for thinness. Since 1922, the BMI values of Miss America winners have steadily decreased; during the last three decades, most winners had a BMI in the "underweight" range (less than 18.5).

epigenetics The study of changes in gene function that are independent of DNA sequence. For example, malnutrition during pregnancy may modify gene expression in the fetus and affect long-term body weight regulation in the offspring.

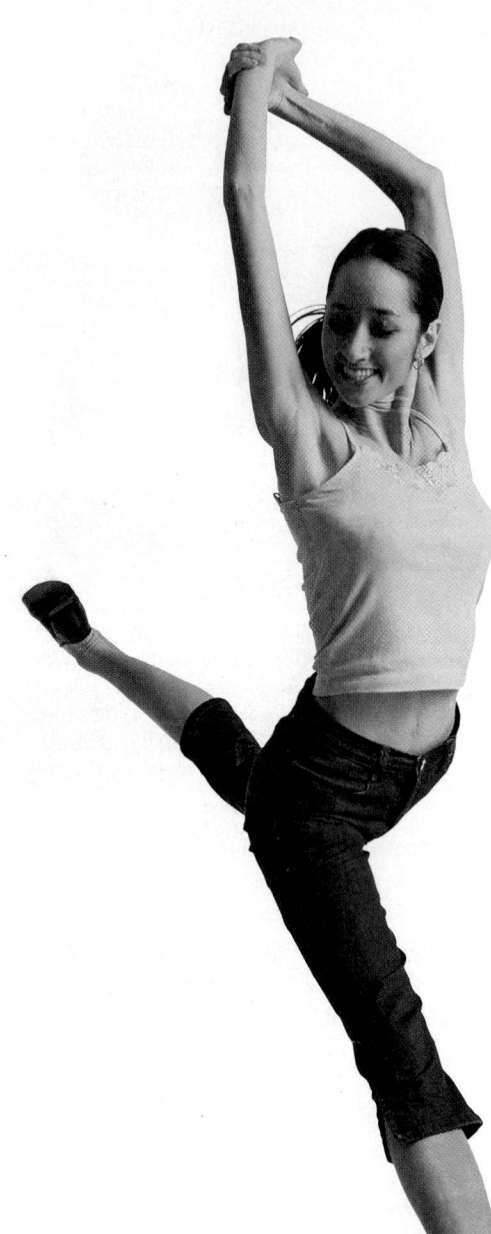

▲ Eating disorders are commonly seen in people who must maintain low body weight, such as ballet dancers (see Further Reading 16).

help in tailoring prevention and treatment efforts for at-risk individuals. However, the psychiatric counseling that is part of current therapy will still be of value.

Do you know someone who is at risk of these eating disorders? If so, suggest that the person seek a professional evaluation because, the sooner treatment begins, the better the chances for recovery. However, do not try to diagnose eating disorders in your friends or family members. Only a professional can exclude other possible diseases and correctly evaluate the diagnostic criteria required to make a diagnosis of anorexia nervosa or bulimia nervosa. Once an eating disorder is diagnosed, immediate treatment is advisable. As a friend, the best you can do is to encourage an affected person to seek professional help. Such help is commonly available at student health centers and student guidance/counseling facilities on college campuses.

11.2 A Closer Look at Anorexia Nervosa

Anorexia nervosa evolves from a dangerous mental state to an often life-threatening physical condition. As first described in the early medical literature in 1689, people suffering from this disorder think they are fat and intensely fear obesity and weight gain. They lose much more weight than is healthful. Although food is entwined in this disease, it stems more from psychological conflict.

About 3% of people with anorexia nervosa eventually die from the disease—from suicide, heart ailments, and infections. About one quarter of those with anorexia nervosa recover within 6 years, whereas the rest simply exist with the disease or go on to develop another form of eating disorder. The longer someone suffers from this eating disorder, the poorer the chances for complete recovery. A young patient with a brief episode and a cooperative family has a better outlook than an older patient with a long history of disordered eating and dysfunctional family relationships. Overall, prompt and vigorous treatment and close long-term follow-up improve the chances for success.

Anorexia nervosa may begin as a simple attempt to lose weight. A comment from a well-meaning friend, relative, or coach suggesting that the person seems to be gaining weight or is too fat may be all that is needed. The stress of having to maintain a certain weight to look attractive or competent on a job can also lead to disordered eating. Physical changes associated with puberty, the stress of leaving childhood, or the loss of a friend are examples of triggers for extreme dieting. Leaving home for college or starting a job can reinforce the desire to appear more "socially acceptable." Still, looking "good" does not necessarily help people deal with anger, depression, low self-esteem, or past experiences with sexual abuse. If these issues are behind the disorder and are not resolved as weight is lost, the individual may intensify efforts to lose weight "to look even better," rather than work through unresolved psychological concerns.

During adolescence, a period of turbulent sexual and social tensions, teenagers seek—and are often expected—to establish separate and independent lives. While declaring independence, they seek acceptance and support from peers and parents and react intensely to how they think others perceive them. At the same time, their bodies are changing, and much of the change is beyond their control. In response to the adolescent's or teenager's lack of control and coping mechanisms, dieting may start and then lead to a failure to gain appropriate weight-for-height. This may not be readily identified as a problem because the child has not actually lost any weight. Stunting (failure to grow in height) may also occur if inadequate calories are ingested during a period of growth. If anorexia develops before puberty, sexual maturation and menstruation also may be delayed.

Teens with chronic illnesses, such as type 1 diabetes or asthma, are at even greater risk for disordered eating. Any evidence of poor weight gain/maintenance or excessive exercise among these individuals needs to be investigated as a possible sign of disordered eating.

Extreme dieting is the most important predictor of an eating disorder. (Adolescents expressing concern about their weight should be advised to focus on exercise, which does not appear to impart a risk for subsequent problems.) Once dieting begins, a person developing anorexia nervosa does not stop. The result is a long period of rigidly self-enforced semistarvation, practiced almost with a vengeance, in a relentless pursuit of control. Anorexia nervosa may eventually lead to bingeing on large amounts of food in a short time, then purging. Purging occurs primarily through vomiting, but laxatives, diuretics, and enemas are also used. Thus, a person with anorexia nervosa may exist in a state of semistarvation or may alternate periods of starvation with periods of bingeing and purging.

Profile of the Typical Person with Anorexia Nervosa

A person with anorexia nervosa refuses to eat enough food to maintain an acceptable weight. This refusal is a hallmark of the disease, whether or not other practices, such as binge-purge cycles, appear. The most typical anorexic person is a Caucasian female from the middle or upper socioeconomic class. Perhaps her mother also has distorted views of desirable body shape and acceptable food habits. The girl is often described by parents and teachers as responsible, meticulous, and obedient.

She is competitive and often obsessive. Her parents set high standards for her. At home, she may not allow clutter in her bedroom. Physicians note that, after a physical examination, she may fold her examination gown very carefully and clean up the examination room before leaving. Even though such behavior may seem odd, only a skilled professional can tell the difference between anorexia nervosa and other adolescent complaints, such as delayed puberty, fatigue, and depression.

A common thread underlying many—but not all—cases of anorexia nervosa is conflict within the family structure, typically with an overbearing mother and an emotionally absent father. When family expectations are always too high—including those regarding body weight—frustration results and leads to fighting. Overinvolvement, rigidity, over-protection, and denial are typical daily transactions of such families.

Issues of control are central to the development of anorexia nervosa. Often, the eating disorder allows an anorexic person to exercise control over an otherwise powerless existence. Losing weight may be the first independent success the person has had. People with anorexia evaluate their self-worth almost entirely in terms of self-control. Some sexually abused children develop anorexia nervosa, believing that if they control their appetite for food, sexual relations, and human contact, they will feel in control and competent and will eliminate shameful feelings. Moreover, food restriction, which arrests development and shuts down sexual impulses, may be a strategy to prevent future victimization and guilt feelings. Often anorexic persons feel hopeless about human relationships and socially isolated because of their dysfunctional families. They focus on food, eating, and weight instead of human relationships.

Early Warning Signs

A person developing anorexia nervosa exhibits important warning signs. At first, dieting becomes the life focus. The person may think, "The only thing I am good at is dieting. I can't do anything else." This innocent beginning often leads to very abnormal self-perceptions and eating habits, such as cutting a pea in half before eating it. Other habits include hiding and storing food or spreading food around a plate to make it look as if much has been eaten. An anorexic person may cook a large meal and watch others eat it while refusing to eat anything. Anorexic persons may also exercise compulsively to the point that it is obsessive. Exercise can interfere with life activities or occur at unusual times or settings—for example, doing squats while brushing teeth.

As the disorder progresses, the range of foods may narrow and be rigidly divided into safe and unsafe ones, with the list of safe foods becoming progressively shorter. For people developing anorexia nervosa, these practices say "I am in control." These people may be hungry, but they deny it, driven by the belief that good things will happen by just becoming thin enough. It becomes a question of willpower.

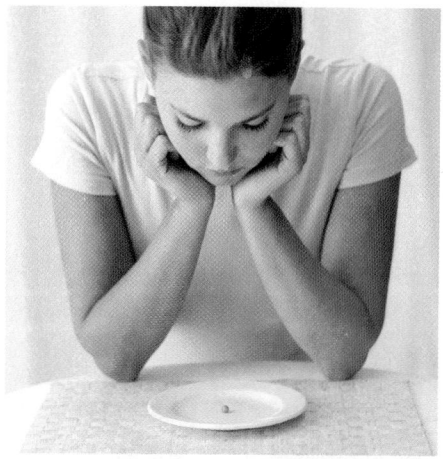

▲ Extreme dietary rules severely limit nutritional intake among people with anorexia nervosa.

Links exist between disordered eating behaviors and substance abuse, particularly alcohol abuse. Some people may use food restriction or purging to offset the calories consumed during drinking binges. Popularly called "drunkorexia," this practice can lead to severe nutrient deficiencies and dehydration.

Anorexia Nervosa

By severely limiting calorie intake for long periods, adolescent girls and young adult women greatly compromise their nutritional status, impair their reproductive systems, and restrict growth. The harm produced by milder, shorter periods of diet restriction is not clear. Evidence, however, suggests that even moderate diet restriction, if continued, contributes to the risks for various forms of anemia, future pregnancy complications and delivery of low-birth-weight infants, and permanently reduced bone mass.

[handwritten: animal products: ready to eat cereal, potato & milk]

[handwritten: B6: Spinach, broccoli, banana, sunflower seed]

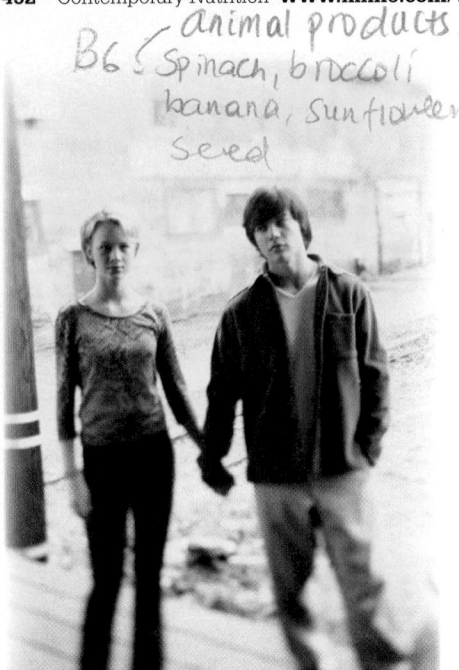

▲ Anorexia nervosa occurs much more frequently in young women than in young men.

[handwritten: Thiamin: pork, sunflower, milk, whole & enriched grains, orange juice, organ meat, dried beans, & peanuts breakfast cereal]

Parents may not consider a teenager mature enough to make decisions. If the teen disagrees and the situation is very tense, she may turn to purging or starving as a way to show her power: "You may try to control my life, but I can do anything I want with my body."

In the words of one young woman, "I couldn't get angry, because it would be like destroying someone else, like my mother. It felt like she would hate me forever. I got angry through anorexia nervosa. It was my last hope. It's my own body and this was my last-ditch effort."

lanugo Downlike hair that appears after a person has lost much body fat through semistarvation. The hair stands erect and traps air, acting as insulation for the body to compensate for the relative lack of body fat, which usually functions as insulation.

People with anorexia become irritable and hostile and begin to withdraw from family and friends. School performance generally crumbles. They refuse to eat out with family and friends, thinking, "I won't be able to have the foods I want to eat," or "I won't be able to throw up afterward."

Anorexic persons see themselves as rational and others as irrational. They also tend to be excessively critical of themselves and others. Nothing is good enough. Because it cannot be perfect, life appears meaningless and hopeless. A sense of joylessness pervades everything.

As stress increases in the person's life, sleep disturbances and depression are common. Many of the psychological and physical problems associated with anorexia nervosa arise from insufficient calorie intake, as well as deficiencies of nutrients, such as thiamin and vitamin B-6. For a female, the combination of problems—coupled with lower and lower body weight and fat stores—causes menstrual periods to cease. This may be the first sign of the disease that a parent notices and represents an additional hallmark of the disease.

Ultimately, an anorexic person eats very little food; 300 to 600 kcal daily is not unusual. In place of food, the person may consume up to 20 cans of diet soft drinks and chew many pieces of sugarless gum each day.

Physical Effects of Anorexia Nervosa

Rooted in the emotional state of the victim, anorexia nervosa produces profound physical effects. The anorexic person often appears to be skin and bones. Body weight less than 85% of that expected is one clinical indicator of anorexia nervosa. This percentage can be calculated using the Metropolitan Life Insurance Company tables (see Appendix G), but body build and weight history should also be used when estimating an appropriate weight. BMI is a more reliable indicator of the degree of malnourishment; generally, a BMI of 17.5 or less indicates a severe case (review Chapter 7 for more on BMI). For children under age 18, growth charts should be used to assess weight status (see Chapter 15). *[handwritten: Bd weigh in kg / height² in meter or wei, hei]*

The state of semistarvation disturbs many body systems as it forces the body to conserve energy stores as much as possible (Fig. 11-1). This attempt to conserve energy stores is the cause of most of the physical effects. Thus, many complications can be reversed by returning to a healthy weight, provided the duration of the insult has not been too long. The following are predictable effects caused by hormonal responses to and deficient nutrient intakes from semistarvation:

- Lowered body temperature and cold intolerance from loss of insulating fat layer.
- Slowed metabolic rate from decreased synthesis of thyroid hormones.
- Decreased heart rate as metabolism slows, leading to premature fatigue, fainting, and an overwhelming need for sleep. Other changes in heart function may occur as well, including loss of heart tissue and irregular heart rhythm.
- Iron-deficiency anemia, which leads to further weakness.
- Rough, dry, scaly, and cold skin, which may show multiple bruises because of the loss of the protective fat layer normally present under the skin.
- Low white blood cell count, which increases the risk of infection—one cause of death in people with anorexia nervosa.
- Abnormal feeling of fullness or bloating, which can last for several hours after eating.
- Loss of hair.
- Appearance of **lanugo**—downy hairs on the body that trap air to partially counteract heat loss that occurs with loss of fat tissue.
- Constipation due to deterioration of the gastrointestinal tract and abuse of laxatives.

- Low blood potassium, worsened by potassium losses during vomiting and use of some types of diuretics. This increases the risk of heart rhythm disturbances, another leading cause of death in anorexic people.
- Loss of menstrual periods because of low body weight, low body fat content, and the stress of the disease. Accompanying hormonal changes contribute to bone loss.
- Changes in neurotransmitter function in the brain, which lead to depression
- Osteopenia (i.e., low bone mass, evident in 90% of adult women with anorexia nervosa) and osteoporosis (evident in at least one site in 40% of adult women with anorexia nervosa). Bone loss is due to decreased body weight and lean mass, several related hormonal changes, and prolonged use of some antidepressant medications.
- Eventual loss of teeth caused by acid erosion of tooth enamel if frequent vomiting occurs. Until vomiting ceases, one way to reduce this effect on teeth is to rinse the mouth with water right away and brush the teeth as soon as possible. Loss of teeth (along with low bone mass) can be lasting signs of the disease, even if the other physical and mental problems are resolved.
- Muscle tears and stress fractures in athletes because of decreased bone and muscle mass.

A person with this disorder is psychologically and physically ill and needs help.

CONCEPT CHECK

Anorexia nervosa is an eating disorder characterized by semistarvation. It is found primarily—but not exclusively—in adolescent girls, starting at or around puberty. People with anorexia dwindle essentially to skin and bones yet still believe they are fat. Semistarvation produces hormonal changes and nutrient deficiencies, which lower body temperature; slow the heart rate; decrease immune response; stop menstrual periods; and contribute to hair, muscle, and bone loss. It is a serious disease, which often produces lifelong consequences and may be fatal.

CRITICAL THINKING

Jennifer is an attractive 13-year-old. However, she's very compulsive. Everything has to be perfect—her hair, her clothes, even her room. Her body is beginning to mature, so she's obsessed with having perfect physical features as well. Her parents are worried about her behavior. Given her behavioral traits, what symptoms of an eating disorder should they watch for? What should Jennifer's parents do if they suspect an eating disorder?

Erika Goodman, former dancer with the Joffrey Ballet, became crippled from osteoporosis resulting from years of restricting food intake to maintain a low body weight. Her food restriction led to irregular or absent menstrual periods for many years. She died in 2004 at the age of 59 after falling in her Manhattan apartment.

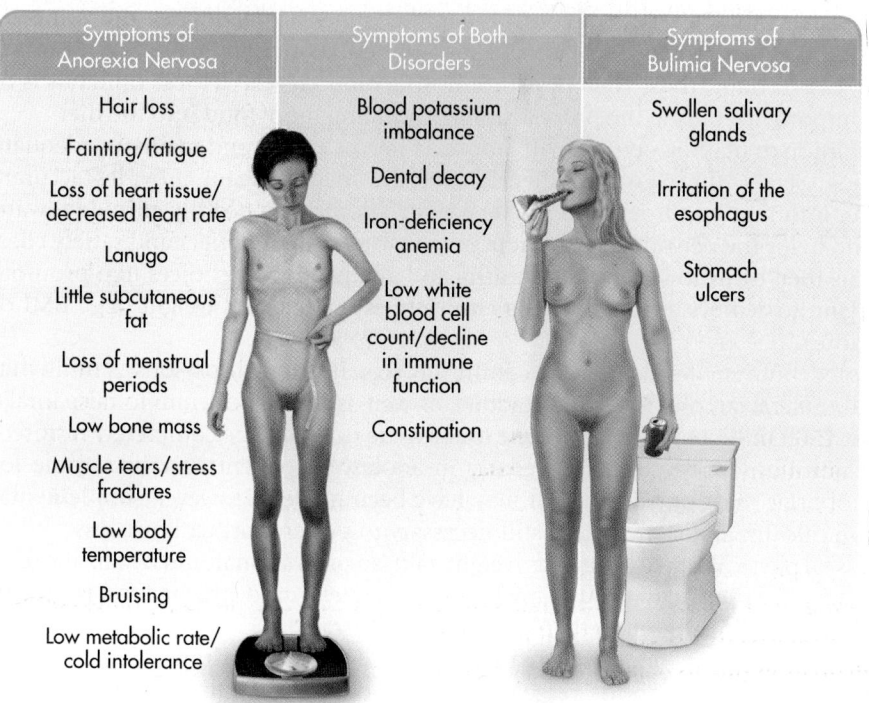

Symptoms of Anorexia Nervosa	Symptoms of Both Disorders	Symptoms of Bulimia Nervosa
Hair loss	Blood potassium imbalance	Swollen salivary glands
Fainting/fatigue	Dental decay	Irritation of the esophagus
Loss of heart tissue/ decreased heart rate	Iron-deficiency anemia	Stomach ulcers
Lanugo	Low white blood cell count/decline in immune function	
Little subcutaneous fat		
Loss of menstrual periods	Constipation	
Low bone mass		
Muscle tears/stress fractures		
Low body temperature		
Bruising		
Low metabolic rate/ cold intolerance		

FIGURE 11-1 ▶ Signs and symptoms of eating disorders. A vast array of physical effects are associated with anorexia nervosa and bulimia nervosa. This figure contains many but is not an exhaustive list of all potential consequences. These physical effects can also serve as warning signs that a problem exists. Professional evaluation is then indicated.

Singer Karen Carpenter's death from complications of anorexia nervosa in 1983 increased awareness of the serious nature of this disease. Currently, the average time for recovery from anorexia nervosa is 7 years; many insurance companies cover only a fraction of the estimated $150,000 cost of treatment.

A young woman in a self-help group for those with anorexia nervosa explained her feelings to the other group members: "I have lost a specialness that I thought it gave me. I was different from everyone else. Now I know that I'm somebody who's overcome it, which not everybody does."

A disturbing trend is the attempt to promote eating disorders as a way of life. Some anorexic individuals have personified their illness into a role model named "Ana," who tells them what to eat and mocks them when they don't lose weight. Ana websites reject the serious health risks of anorexia behaviors and instead dispense unsafe "thinspiration" to vulnerable individuals (see Further Reading 12).

Treatment of Anorexia Nervosa

People with anorexia often sink into shells of isolation and fear. They deny that a problem exists. Frequently, their friends and family members meet with them to confront the problem in a loving way. This is called an *intervention*. They present evidence of the problem and encourage immediate treatment. Treatment then requires a multidisciplinary team of experienced physicians, registered dietitians, psychologists, and other health professionals working together. An ideal setting is an eating disorders clinic in a medical center. Outpatient therapy generally begins first. This may be extended to 3 to 5 days per week. Day hospitalization (6 to 12 hours) is another option, as is total hospitalization. Hospitalization is necessary once a person falls below 75% of expected weight, experiences acute medical problems, and/or exhibits severe psychological problems or suicidal risk. Still, even in the most skilled hands at the finest facilities, efforts may fail. This tells us that the prevention of anorexia nervosa is of utmost importance.

Once a medical team has gained the cooperation and trust of an anorexic person, the team attempts to work together to restore a sense of balance, purpose, and future possibilities. As previously stated, anorexia nervosa is usually rooted in psychological conflict. However, the anorexic person who has been barely existing in a state of semi-starvation cannot focus on much besides food. Dreams and even morbid thoughts about food will interfere with therapy until sufficient weight is regained.

Nutrition Therapy. The first goal of nutrition therapy is to gain the person's cooperation and trust, with the ultimate objective of increasing oral food intake. Ideally, weight gain must be enough to raise the metabolic rate to normal and reverse as many physical signs of the disease as possible. Food intake is designed first to minimize or stop any further weight loss. Then, the focus shifts to restoring appropriate food habits. After this, the expectation can be switched to slowly gaining weight. A gain of 2 to 3 pounds per week is appropriate. Tube and/or intravenous (IV) feeding is used only if immediate renourishment is required, as this can frighten the person and cause him or her to distrust medical staff.

Persons with anorexia nervosa need considerable reassurance during the refeeding process because of uncomfortable and unfamiliar effects—such as bloating, increase in body heat, and increase in body fat. This is a frightening process because these changes can symbolize a loss of control. Rapid changes in electrolytes and minerals in the blood associated with refeeding, especially potassium, phosphorus, and magnesium, can be dangerous. Therefore, monitoring blood levels of these minerals is of critical importance during the process of incorporating more food into the diet.

In addition to helping persons with anorexia nervosa reach and maintain adequate nutritional status, the registered dietitian on the medical team provides accurate nutrition information throughout the treatment, promotes a healthy attitude toward food, and helps the person learn to eat in response to natural hunger and satiety cues. The focus then turns to identifying healthy and adequate food choices that promote weight gain to achieve and maintain a clinically estimated goal weight (e.g., BMI of 20 or more).

As noted, nutrient deficiencies are commonly seen in anorexic persons. A multivitamin and mineral supplement will be added, as well as enough calcium to raise intake to about 1500 milligrams per day. Bone loss will be not likely be completely restored, even if nutrition is adequate. Particularly in adolescent patients, a critical time for accrual of bone mass or gains height may have been missed. However, supplementation with calcium and vitamin D is still necessary to prevent further bone loss.

Excessive physical activity prevents weight gain, so professionals must help anorexic persons regulate their activity. At many treatment centers, moderate bed rest is used in the early stages of treatment to help promote weight gain.

Experienced professional help is the key (see Further Readings 1 and 11). An anorexic person may be on the verge of suicide and starvation. In addition, anorexic people are often very clever and resistant to therapy. They may try to hide weight loss by wearing many layers of clothes, putting coins in their pockets or underwear, and drinking numerous glasses of water before stepping on the scale.

Psychological and Related Therapy. Once the physical problems of anorexia nervosa are addressed, the treatment focus shifts to the underlying emotional problems that led to excessive dieting and other symptoms of the disorder. To heal, these anorexic persons must reject the sense of accomplishment they have associated with an emaciated body and begin to accept themselves at a healthy body weight. If therapists can discover reasons for the disorder, they can develop strategies for restoring normal weight and eating habits that involve resolving psychological conflicts. Education about the medical consequences of semistarvation is also helpful. A key aspect of psychological treatment is showing affected individuals how to regain control of other facets of their lives and cope with difficult situations. As eating evolves into a normal routine, they can turn to previously neglected activities.

Therapists may use **cognitive behavior therapy,** which involves helping the person confront and change irrational beliefs about body image, eating, relationships, and weight. Underlying issues that may be the cause for the disease, such as sexual abuse, also must be identified and addressed by the therapist.

Family therapy often is important in treating anorexia nervosa, especially for younger persons who still live with their families. It focuses on the role of the illness among family members, the reactions of individual family members and ways in which their subconscious behavior might contribute to the abnormal eating patterns. Frequently, a therapist finds family struggles at the heart of the problem. As the disorder resolves, patients must relate to family members in new ways to gain the attention that was needed and previously tied to the disease. For example, the family may need to help the young person ease into adulthood and accept its responsibilities as well as its advantages. Self-help groups for anorexic (and bulimic) people, as well as their families and friends, represent nonthreatening first steps into treatment.

Food is the drug of choice in the treatment of anorexic patients. Generally, medications are not effective in management of the primary symptoms of anorexia nervosa. Fluoxetine (Prozac®) and related medications may stabilize recovery once 85% of expected body weight has been attained. These medications work by prolonging serotonin activity in the brain, which in turn regulates mood and feelings of satiety. A variety of other pharmacologic agents, such as olanzapine (Zyprexa®), may have some role in treating mood changes, anxiety, or psychotic symptoms associated with anorexia nervosa, but they have limited value unless weight gain is also achieved.

With professional help, many people with anorexia nervosa can lead normal lives. Although they may not be totally cured, anorexic individuals do not have to depend on unusual eating habits to cope with daily problems. They recover a sense of normalcy in their lives. Longer follow-up—sometimes several years—is associated with better outcomes. No universal approach exists, because each case is unique. Establishing a strong relationship with either a therapist or another supportive person is an especially important key to recovery. Once anorexic persons feel understood and accepted by another person, they can begin to build a sense of self and exercise some autonomy. As they learn alternative coping mechanisms, they can relinquish their dysfunctional relationships with food and instead develop healthy personal relationships.

cognitive behavior therapy Psychological therapy in which the person's assumptions about dieting, body weight, and related issues are confronted. New ways of thinking are explored and then practiced by the person. In this way, an individual can learn new ways to control disordered eating behaviors and related life stress.

CONCEPT CHECK

To relieve the semistarved condition of most anorexic persons, the initial treatment focuses on moderately increased food intake and slow weight gain. Once this is accomplished, psychotherapy can begin to uncover the causes of the disease and help the individual develop the skills needed to return to a healthy life. Family therapy can be an important tool in treatment, whereas medications have a limited role.

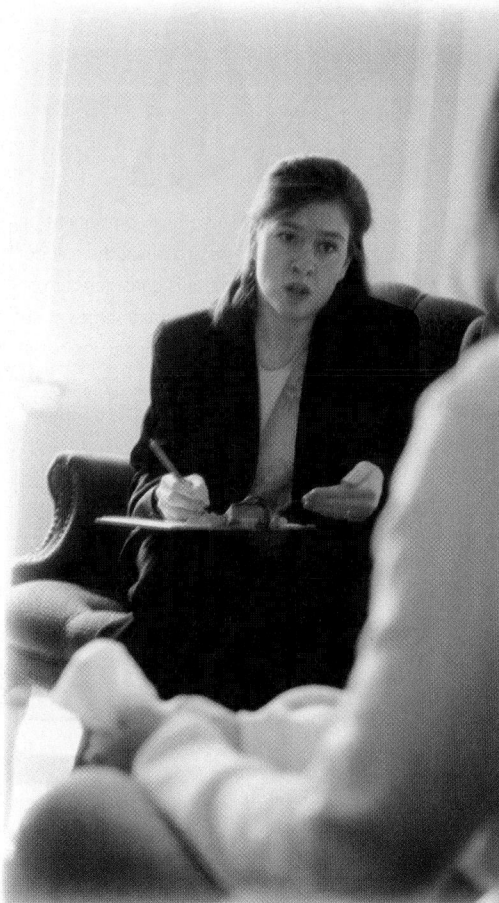
▲ Early treatment for an eating disorder, such as anorexia nervosa, improves chances of success.

Bingeing and purging (via vomiting) was evident in pre-Christian Roman times, but was practiced in a group setting. The eating disorder bulimia nervosa is generally practiced in private. It was first described in the medical literature in 1979.

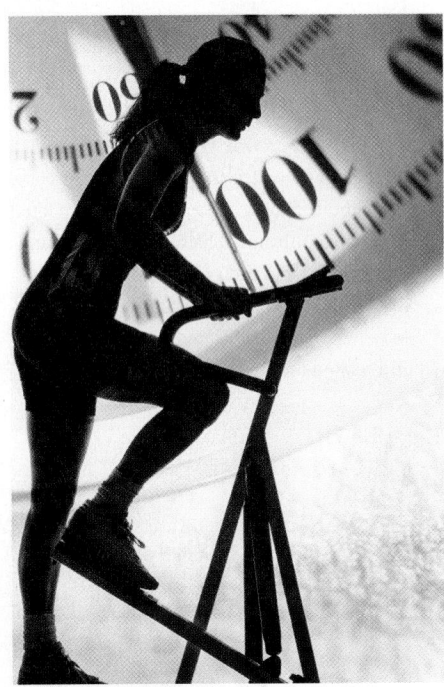

▲ Excessive exercise can be one component of bulimia if it is used as a way to offset the calorie intake from a binge. Exercise is considered excessive when it is done at inappropriate times or settings or when a person does it despite injury or other medical complications.

11.3 A Closer Look at Bulimia Nervosa

Bulimia nervosa involves episodes of binge eating followed by various means to purge the food. It is most common among young adults of college age, although some high school students are also at risk. Susceptible people often have genetic factors and lifestyle patterns that predispose them to becoming overweight, and many try frequent weight-reduction diets as teenagers. Like people with anorexia nervosa, those with bulimia nervosa are usually female and successful. Unlike anorexic individuals, however, they are usually at or slightly above a normal weight. Females with bulimia nervosa are also more likely to be sexually active than those with anorexia nervosa.

The person with bulimia nervosa may think of food constantly. But unlike the anorexic person, who turns away from food when faced with problems, the bulimic person turns toward food in critical situations. Also, unlike those with anorexia nervosa, people with bulimia nervosa recognize their behavior as abnormal. These people often have low self-esteem and are depressed. Approximately half of the people with bulimia nervosa have major depression. Lingering effects of child abuse may be one reason for these feelings. Many bulimic persons report that they have been sexually abused. They appear competent to outsiders, while they actually feel out of control, ashamed, and frustrated.

Bulimic people tend to be impulsive, which may be expressed in behaviors such as stealing, increased sexual activity, drug and alcohol abuse, self-mutilation, or attempted suicide. Some experts have suggested that part of the problem may actually arise from an inability to control responses to impulse and desire. Some studies have demonstrated that bulimic people tend to come from disengaged families—ones that are loosely organized. In these families, roles for family members are not clearly defined, rules are disregarded, and a great deal of conflict exists. (In contrast, anorexic people tend to have families so actively engaged that roles may be too well defined.)

Typical Behavior in Bulimia Nervosa

It is likely that many people with bulimic behavior are never diagnosed; the diagnostic criteria specify that a person must binge and purge at least twice a week for 3 months. People with bulimia nervosa lead secret lives, hiding their abnormal eating habits. Moreover, it is impossible to recognize the disorder simply by appearance. Most diagnoses of bulimia nervosa rely on self-reports, so estimates of the number of cases are probably low. The disorder, especially in its milder forms, may be much more widespread than commonly thought.

For intake to qualify as a binge, an atypically large amount of food must be consumed in a short time and the person must exhibit a lack of control over his or her behavior. Among sufferers of bulimia nervosa, bingeing often alternates with attempts to rigidly restrict food intake. Elaborate food rules are common, such as avoiding all sweets. Thus, eating just one cookie or donut may cause individuals with this disorder to feel as though they have broken a rule. At that point, in the mind of a bulimic person, the objectionable food must be eliminated. Usually this leads to further overeating, partly because it is easier to regurgitate a large amount of food than a small amount.

Binge-purge cycles may be practiced daily, weekly, or across longer intervals. A specific time often is set aside. Most binge eating occurs at night, when other people are less likely to interrupt, and usually lasts from ½ to 2 hours. A binge can be triggered by a combination of stress, boredom, loneliness, and depression. It often follows a period of strict dieting and thus can be linked to intense hunger. The binge is not at all like normal eating; once begun, it seems to propel itself. The person not only loses control, but generally doesn't even taste or enjoy food during a binge. This separates the practice from overeating.

Most commonly, bulimic people consume cakes, cookies, ice cream, and other high-carbohydrate convenience foods during binges because these foods can be purged relatively easily and comfortably by vomiting. In a single binge, foods supplying 3000 kcal or more may be eaten. Purging follows in hopes that no weight will be gained. However, even when vomiting follows the binge, 33% to 75% of the calories taken in are still absorbed, inevitably causing some weight gain. When laxatives or enemas are used, about 90% of the calories are absorbed, as laxatives act in the large intestine, beyond the point of most nutrient absorption. The belief that purging soon after bingeing will prevent excessive calorie absorption and weight gain is a misconception.

At the onset of bulimia nervosa, sufferers often induce vomiting by placing their fingers deep into the mouth. They may bite down on these fingers inadvertently, resulting in bite marks and scars around the knuckles, a characteristic sign of this disorder. Once the disease is established, however, a person may be able to vomit simply by contracting the abdominal muscles. Vomiting may also occur spontaneously.

Another way bulimic persons attempt to compensate for a binge and control their weight is by engaging in excessive exercise to expend a large amount of calories. In this practice, referred to as "debting," bulimic individuals try to estimate the amount of calories eaten during a binge, and then exercise to counteract the excess.

People with bulimia nervosa are not proud of their behavior. After a binge, they usually feel guilty and depressed. Over time, they experience low self-esteem, feel hopeless about their situation, and are caught in a vicious cycle of obsession (Fig. 11-2). Compulsive lying, shoplifting to obtain food, and drug abuse can further intensify these feelings. Bulimic people discovered in the act of bingeing by a friend or family member may order the intruder to "get out" and "go away." Sufferers gradually distance themselves from others, spending more time preoccupied by and engaging in bingeing and purging.

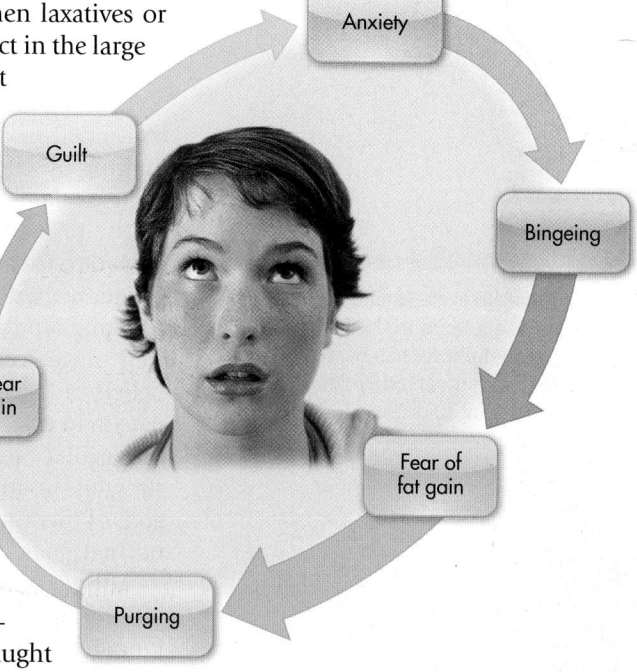

FIGURE 11-2 ▶ Bulimia nervosa's vicious cycle of obsession.

Health Problems Stemming from Bulimia Nervosa

The vomiting that many bulimic sufferers induce is a physically destructive method of purging. Indeed, the majority of health problems associated with bulimia nervosa, as noted here, arise from vomiting:

- Repeated exposure of teeth to stomach acid causes demineralization, making the teeth painful and sensitive to heat, cold, and acids. Eventually, the teeth may decay severely, erode away from fillings, and finally fall out. Dental professionals are sometimes the first health professionals to notice signs of bulimia nervosa. As noted, it is important to rinse the mouth with water after any vomiting episode, especially before brushing the teeth.
- Blood potassium can drop significantly with regular vomiting or the use of certain diuretics. This can disturb the heart's rhythm and even produce sudden death.
- Salivary glands may swell as a result of infection and irritation from persistent vomiting.
- Stomach ulcers and bleeding and tears in the esophagus develop in some cases.
- Constipation may result from frequent laxative use.
- Ipecac syrup, sometimes used to induce vomiting, is toxic to the heart, liver, and kidneys. It has caused accidental poisoning when taken repeatedly.

Overall, bulimia nervosa is a potentially debilitating disorder that can lead to death, usually from suicide, low blood potassium, or overwhelming infections.

Treatment of Bulimia Nervosa

Therapy for bulimia nervosa, as for anorexia nervosa, requires a team of experienced clinicians (see Further Reading 1). Bulimic individuals are less likely than those with anorexia to enter treatment in a state of semistarvation. However, if a bulimic person has lost significant weight, this must be treated before psychological treatment begins.

People with type 1 diabetes may intentionally skip doses of insulin to induce weight loss. This practice, so called "diabulimia," can have dangerous consequences, such as eye damage, kidney damage, diabetic coma, or death (see Further Reading 6).

Although clinicians have yet to agree on the best therapy for bulimia nervosa, they generally agree that treatment should last at least 16 weeks. Hospitalization may be indicated in cases of extreme laxative abuse, regular vomiting, substance abuse, and depression, especially if physical harm is evident.

The first goal of treatment for bulimia nervosa is to decrease the amount of food consumed in a binge session to decrease the risk of esophageal tears from related purging by vomiting. A decrease in the frequency of this type of purging will also decrease damage to the teeth.

The primary aim of psychotherapy is to improve a persons' self-acceptance and help one to be less concerned about body weight. Cognitive behavior therapy is generally used (see Further Reading 11). Psychotherapy helps correct the all-or-none thinking typical of bulimic persons: "If I eat one cookie, I'm a failure and might as well binge." The premise of this psychotherapy is that, if abnormal attitudes and beliefs can be altered, normal eating will follow. In addition, the therapist guides the person in establishing food habits that will minimize bingeing: avoiding fasting, eating regular meals, and using alternative methods—other than eating—to cope with stressful situations. Group therapy is often useful to foster strong social support. One goal of therapy is to help bulimic persons accept some depression and self-doubt as normal.

Although pharmacological agents should not be used as the sole treatment for bulimia nervosa, studies indicate that some medications may be beneficial in conjunction with other therapies. Fluoxetine (Prozac®) is the only antidepressant that has been approved by FDA for use in the treatment of bulimia nervosa, but physicians also may prescribe other similar forms of antidepressants, other classes of psychiatric medications, or certain antiseizure medications, (e.g., topiramate [Topamax®]).

Nutritional counseling has two main goals: correcting misconceptions about food and re-establishing regular eating habits. Bulimic persons are given information about bulimia nervosa and its consequences. Avoiding binge foods and not constantly stepping on a scale may be recommended early in treatment. The primary goal, however, is to develop a normal eating pattern. To achieve this goal, some specialists encourage these individuals to develop daily meal plans and keep a food diary in which they record food intake, internal sensations of hunger, environmental factors that precipitate binges, and thoughts and feelings that accompany binge-purge cycles. Keeping a food diary not only is an accurate way to monitor food intake but also may help identify situations that seem to trigger binge episodes. With the help of a therapist, bulimic persons can develop alternative coping strategies.

In general, the focus is not on stopping bingeing and purging *per se* but on developing regular eating habits. Once this is achieved, the binge-purge cycle should start to break down. Individuals are discouraged from following strict rules about healthy food choices, because this mimics the typical obsessive attitudes associated with bulimia nervosa. Rather, encouraging a mature perspective on nutrient intake—that is, regular consumption of moderate amounts of a variety of foods balanced among the food groups—helps one overcome this disorder.

Setting time limits for the completion of meals and snacks is important for people with eating disorders. Many bulimic persons eat quickly, reflecting their difficulties with satiety. Suggesting that the person put his or her utensil down after each bite is a behavioral technique that a therapist might try during recovery for bulimia. (In comparison, many anorexic persons eat in an excessively slow manner—for example, taking 1 hour to eat a muffin cut into tiny, bite-size pieces.)

People with bulimia nervosa must recognize that they have a serious disorder that can have grave medical complications if not treated. Relapse is likely, so therapy should be long term. Those with bulimia nervosa need professional help because they can be very depressed and are at a high risk for suicide. About 50% of people with bulimia nervosa recover completely from the disorder. Others continue to struggle with it to varying degrees for the rest of their lives. Such a difficult course of treatment underscores the need for prevention.

The binge-purge cycle can create an initial state of euphoria in the person. Giving up this euphoria has been equated to giving up an addiction. Still, it is important to do so.

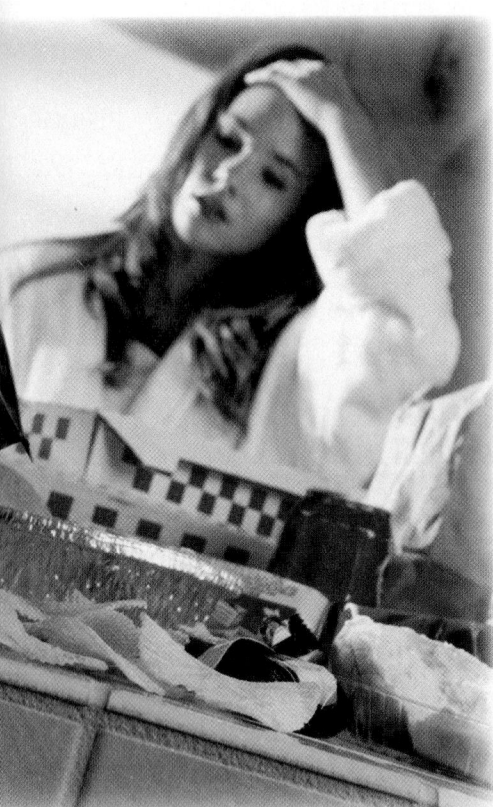

▲ Developing regular eating habits helps a person with bulimia nervosa to stop the binge-purge cycle.

CONCEPT CHECK

Bulimia nervosa is characterized by episodes of binge eating followed by purging, usually by vomiting. Vomiting is very destructive to the body, often causing severe dental decay, stomach ulcers, irritation of the esophagus, and blood potassium imbalances. Treatment using nutrition counseling and psychotherapy attempts to restore normal eating habits, to help the person correct distorted beliefs about diet and lifestyle, and to find tools to cope with the stresses of life. Medications, such as fluoxetine (Prozac®), can aid recovery when added to this regimen.

11.4 Other Disordered Eating Patterns

In recent years, other patterns of disordered eating have been recognized (see Further Readings 6, 8, 9, and 10). Several of these patterns fall under the diagnosic category, *eating disorder not otherwise specified* (EDNOS). EDNOS is described in the American Psychiatric Association diagnostic manual as a "category [of] disorders of eating that do not meet the criteria for any specific eating disorder."

The EDNOS category is frequently used for people who have some, but not all, of the characteristics of anorexia nervosa or bulimia nervosa. Each EDNOS has distinctive qualities. For example, a person may experience episodes of bingeing and purging, but not frequently enough to meet the diagnosis of bulimia nervosa. A person may also engage in bingeing episodes without the use of inappropriate compensatory behaviors; this is referred to as binge-eating disorder. Another disordered eating pattern under study is night eating syndrome. **Night eating syndrome** is characterized by eating a lot of food in the late evening and nocturnal awakening with ingestion of food. Finally, the **female athlete triad** is a condition characterized by disordered eating, lack of menstrual periods, and osteoporosis. These conditions have been recognized as requiring professional treatment and are discussed in the following sections.

Binge-Eating Disorder

The typical characteristics for binge-eating disorder are listed in Table 11-2. Generally, it can be defined as binge-eating episodes not accompanied by purging (as typifies bulimia nervosa) at least two times per week for at least 6 months. First officially described in 1994, today health care professionals recognize binge-eating disorder as a growing, complex, and potentially serious problem. It is likely that binge-eating disorder will move from the EDNOS category and be recognized as a district eating disorder in the *DSM-V*, expected in 2013.

Approximately 30% of subjects in organized weight-control programs have binge-eating disorder, whereas among the general U.S. population, about 4 million have this disorder. However, many more people in the general population are likely to have less severe forms of the disorder that do not meet all the criteria that describe the problem. The number of cases of binge-eating disorder is far greater than that of either anorexia nervosa or bulimia nervosa. This disorder is also more common among the severely obese and those with a long history of frequent restrictive dieting, although obesity is not a criterion for having binge-eating disorder.

Development and Characteristics of Binge-Eating Disorder. Individuals with binge-eating disorder (about 40% of whom are males) often perceive themselves as hungry more often than normal. They usually started dieting at a young age, began bingeing during adolescence or in their early twenties, and did not succeed in commercial weight-control programs. Almost half of those with severe binge-eating disorder exhibit clinical depression. Some people also may have a genetic predisposition for this disorder.

Up to 25% of college-age women exhibit some degree of binge eating. Such behavior may have a negative impact on physical appearance, health, social life, and academics.

night eating syndrome Eating a lot of food in the late evening and nocturnal awakenings with ingestion of food.

female athlete triad A condition characterized by disordered eating, lack of menstrual periods (amenorrhea), and osteoporosis.

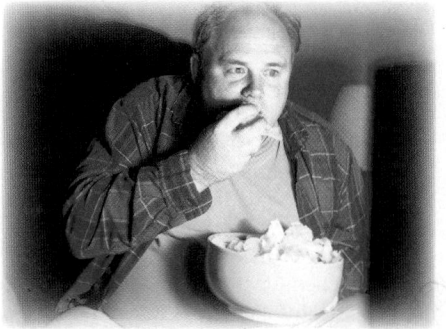
▲ Binge-eating disorder is seen in both men and women.

TABLE 11-2 Some Characteristics of Binge-Eating Disorder

A. Recurrent episodes of binge eating, which is characterized by:
   (1) Eating, in a discrete period (e.g., within any 2-hour period), an amount of food definitely larger than most people would eat during a similar period in similar circumstances
   (2) A sense of lack of control during the episodes (e.g., a feeling that one can't stop eating or control what or how much one is eating)

B. During most binge episodes, at least three of the following occur:
   (1) Eating much more rapidly than usual
   (2) Eating until feeling uncomfortably full
   (3) Eating large amounts of food when not feeling physically hungry
   (4) Eating alone because of being embarrassed by how much one is eating
   (5) Feeling disgusted with oneself, depressed, or guilty after overeating

C. Marked distress regarding binge eating

D. The binge eating occurs, on average, at least 2 days a week for 6 months.

E. The behavior does not occur only during the course of bulimia nervosa or anorexia nervosa.

Based on information from the *Diagnostic and Statistical Manual of Mental Disorders,* Fourth Edition (DSM-IV-TR). Washington DC: American Psychiatric Association, 2000.

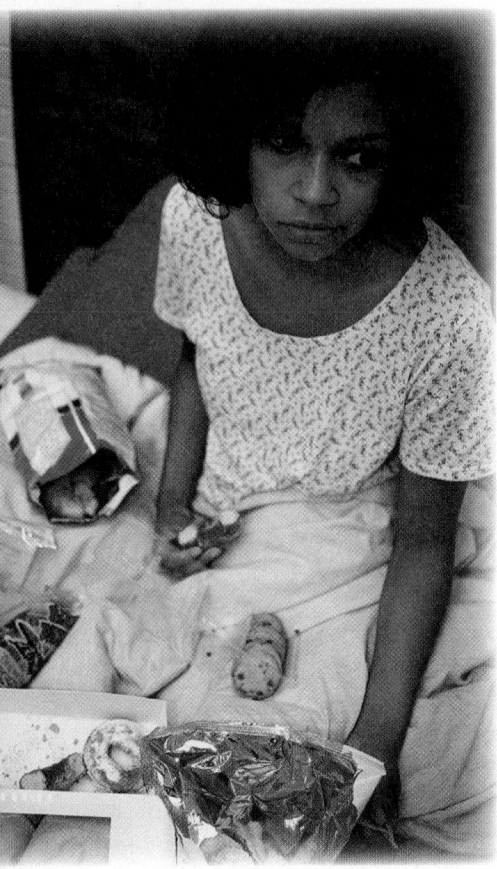

▲ Professional help is advised for people with a binge-eating disorder.

As noted in Chapter 2, spreading one's dietary intake into numerous, small meals (grazing) over a day provides some health advantages if overall calorie intake remains appropriate.

People with binge-eating disorder may come from families with alcoholism or may have suffered sexual abuse. Members of such dysfunctional families often do not know how to deal effectively with emotions. They cope by turning to substances. Family members learn to cover up dysfunctional patterns for the alcoholic person and to nurture him or her at the expense of each other and their own needs.

Typical binge eaters isolate themselves and eat large quantities of a favorite food. Stressful events and feelings of depression or anxiety can trigger this behavior. Giving themselves permission to eat a forbidden food can also precipitate a binge. Other triggers include loneliness, anxiety, self-pity, depression, anger, rage, alienation, and frustration (see Further Reading 15). They sometimes binge on whatever is easy to eat in large amounts—noodles, rice, bread, leftovers. Characteristically, however, binge eaters consume foods that carry the social stigma of "junk" or "bad" foods—ice cream, cookies, sweets, potato chips, and similar snack foods.

In general, people engage in binge eating to induce a sense of well-being and perhaps even numbness, usually in an attempt to avoid feeling and dealing with emotional pain and anxiety. They eat without regard to biological need and often in a recurrent, ritualized fashion. Some people with this disorder eat food continually over an extended period, called *grazing;* others cycle episodes of bingeing with normal eating. For example, someone with a stressful or frustrating job might come home every night and graze until bedtime. Another person might eat normally most of the time but find comfort in consuming large quantities of food when an emotional setback occurs.

Although people with anorexia nervosa and bulimia nervosa exhibit persistent preoccupation with body shape, weight, and thinness, binge eaters do not necessarily share these concerns. Thus, neither purging nor prolonged food restriction is characteristic of binge-eating disorder. Some physicians classify binge-eating disorder as an addiction to food, involving psychological dependence. The person becomes attached to the behavior and has a drive to continue it, senses only limited control over it, and needs to persist at it despite negative consequences. Food is used to reduce stress, produce feelings of power and well-being, avoid feelings of intimacy with others, and avoid life problems. Obesity and binge eating are not necessarily linked. Not all obese people are binge eaters, and, although obesity may result from trying to numb emotional pain with food, it is not necessarily an outcome of binge eating.

Binge-eating disorder is most likely to develop in people who never learned to express and deal appropriately with their feelings. Rather than face their frustration, anger, and pain, they turn to food. The frustration will continue because they never confront the basic problem. Binge eating makes them feel they cannot control the behavior pattern and therefore cannot control their lives. Worse, the binge eating usually increases feelings of guilt, embarrassment, and shame.

Often, people who practice binge eating have been shaped by families who do not address and express feelings in healthful ways. The parents nurture and comfort their children with food rather than engage in healthy exchanges of self-disclosure of feelings and potential solutions. Members of such families learn to eat in response to emotional needs and pain instead of hunger. Those who regularly practice binge eating may grow up nurturing others instead of themselves, avoiding their own feelings and taking little time for themselves. Not knowing how to satisfy their personal and emotional needs in more healthful ways, people in these families turn to food.

For some people, frequent dieting beginning in childhood or adolescence is a precursor to binge-eating disorder. During periods when little food is eaten, they get very hungry and obsessive about food. When allowed to eat more food, they feel driven to eat in a compulsive, uncontrolled way. The pattern of strict dieting alternating with binge eating may continue over time.

Help for the Person with Binge-Eating Disorder. Those with binge-eating disorder must learn to eat in response to hunger—a biological signal—rather than in response to emotional needs or external factors (such as the time of day or the simple presence of food). Counselors often direct binge eaters to record their perceptions of physical hunger throughout the day and at the beginning and end of every meal. These people must learn to respond to a prescribed amount of fullness at each meal. They should initially avoid weight-loss diets because feelings of food deprivation can lead to more disruptive emotions and a greater sense of unmet needs. Diets are likely to encourage more intense problems, such as extreme hunger. Many people with binge-eating disorder may experience difficulty in identifying personal emotional needs and expressing emotions. This problem is a common predisposing factor in binge eating, so communication issues should be addressed during treatment. Binge eaters often must be helped to recognize their buried emotions in anxiety-producing situations, and then encouraged to share them with their therapist or therapy group. Learning simple but appropriate phrases to say to oneself can help stop bingeing when the desire is strong.

Self-help groups, such as Overeaters Anonymous, aim to help recovery from binge-eating disorder. Their treatment philosophy, which parallels that of Alcoholics Anonymous, attempts to create an environment of encouragement and accountability to overcome this eating disorder. Dietary advice typically ranges from avoiding restraint in eating in general to limiting binge foods. Some experts feel that learning to eat all foods—but in moderation—is an effective goal for binge eaters. This practice can prevent the feelings of desperation and deprivation that come from limiting particular foods. Antidepressants, such as fluoxetine (Prozac®), and other types of medications (e.g., topiramate [Topamax®]) also have been found to help reduce binge eating in these individuals by decreasing depression. Overall, people who have this disorder are usually unsuccessful in controlling it on their own. Professional help is advised.

Night Eating Syndrome

Night eating syndrome is characterized by evening hyperphagia (eating more than one-third of total daily calories after the evening meal) and nighttime awakening accompanied by the ingestion of food. Although night eating syndrome was first observed among obese patients, it also occurs among nonobese persons. It has been estimated to occur in 1.5% of the general population and in 8.9% of persons treated in obesity clinics (see Further Reading 8).

Signs and Symptoms of Night Eating Syndrome

- Not feeling hungry in the morning and delaying the first meal until several hours after waking
- Overeating in the evening with more than one-third of daily food intake after dinner

NEWSWORTHY NUTRITION

Strong connection between eating disorders and binge drinking

A survey of 480 college-age women at high risk for eating disorders found a positive correlation between binge drinking (consuming four or more drinks in one sitting) and disordered eating behaviors. At baseline, 67% of the women in the study engaged in binge drinking at least once per month, and 30% did so frequently (three or more times per month). Additional research also supports this interplay between substance abuse and disordered eating behavior—purging, skipping meals, or fasting to compensate for calories consumed during drinking episodes—particularly among women. These studies exemplify how disordered eating behaviors and abuse of substances such as alcohol are used as inappropriate coping mechanisms. The stress of college and the influence of peers in this age group demand university-based intervention programs to educate students on the dangers of both eating disorders and substance abuse and to help students develop effective coping mechanisms.

Sources: Khaylis A and others: Binge drinking in women at risk for developing eating disorders. *International Journal of Eating Disorders* 42:409, 2009.

Kelly-Weeder S: Binge drinking and disordered eating in college students. *Journal of the American Academy of Nurse Practitioners* 23:33, 2011.

connect Check out the Connect site www.mcgrawhillconnect.com to further explore eating disorders and binge drinking.

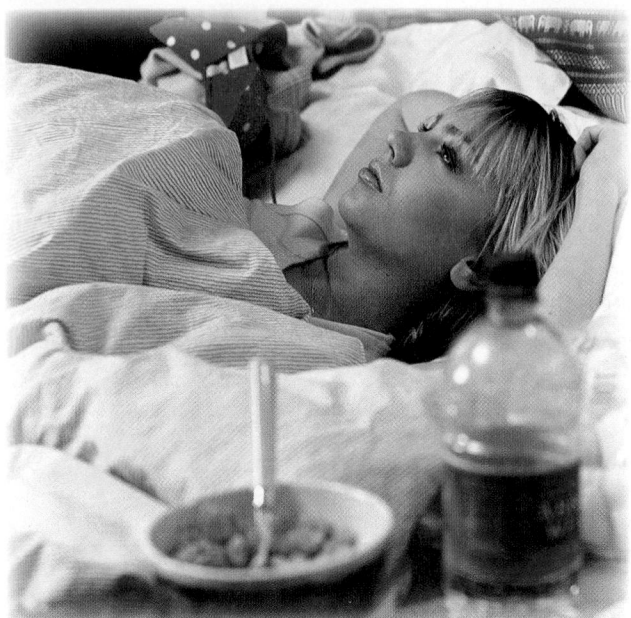

▲ Night eating syndrome is characterized by waking at least once during the night and needing to eat to be able to fall asleep again.

It is often difficult to get female athletes to accept necessary treatment plans. They frequently have a single-minded approach to their sport, while ignoring future health consequences.

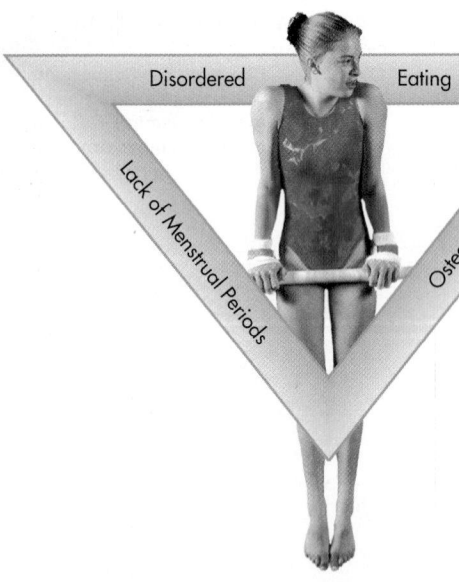

FIGURE 11-3 ▶ The female athlete triad occurs when the athlete has disordered eating, lack of menstrual periods, and osteoporosis. Stress fractures and chronic fatigue also occur. This triad often is seen in appearance-related sports, such as gymnastics. Long-term health is at risk; thus, prevention and early treatment are crucial.

- Difficulty falling asleep and a need to eat something to help fall asleep faster
- Waking at least once during the night with a need to eat to be able to fall asleep again
- Eating produces feelings of guilt and shame
- Feeling depressed, especially at night

Research shows that the cause of night eating syndrome may be an abnormal food cycle in the body, resulting in a delayed intake of food during the day. The circadian rhythm (your body's 24-hour clock) of food intake appears to be disturbed in night eating syndrome. Studies have also shown that night eating syndrome is prevalent among outpatients with psychiatric conditions and that the symptoms, including nocturnal ingestion and evening hyperphagia, are significantly improved with use of the antidepressant setraline (Zoloft®).

Female Athlete Triad

Women participating in appearance-based and endurance sports are at risk of developing an eating disorder. One study of college-age female athletes found that 15% of swimmers, 62% of gymnasts, and 32% of varsity athletes exhibited disordered eating patterns. Estimates of eating disorders for college women not involved in competitive sports are much lower.

In addition to disordered eating, college women athletes tend to experience irregular menstruation more frequently than other college women. Disordered eating, particularly food restriction, and stress can precipitate this, causing women to have less dense and weaker bones than normal because of lower estrogen concentrations in the blood. Some of these young women have bone mass values equivalent to those of 50- to 60-year-olds, increasing their risk for bone and stress fractures during sports as well as general activities. Much of the bone loss is irreversible.

The American College of Sports Medicine (ACSM) has named this syndrome "female athlete triad" because it consists of three parts: disordered eating, lack of menstrual periods, and osteoporosis (Fig. 11-3). The ACSM has issued a plea to teachers, coaches, health professionals, and parents to educate female athletes about the triad and its health consequences.

Many coaches/trainers and even some health professionals wrongly believe that loss of menstrual periods is a normal consequence of a high level of physical activity. However, loss of menstrual periods in female athletes stems from a dramatic decrease in female reproductive hormones, particularly estrogen. Loss of estrogen has other negative consequences on the body, such as fragile bones, as mentioned. Correcting the hormonal imbalance and menstrual irregularities by increasing caloric intake should stabilize bone mass. During therapy, a physician may prescribe a multivitamin and mineral supplement as well as calcium supplements as needed to maintain an intake of 1200 to 1500 milligrams.

Those exhibiting symptoms of the female athlete triad should seek treatment from a multidisciplinary team of health professionals. Involving the coach or trainer in therapy is usually a key factor in the success of the treatment plan. Suggestions for treatment are as follows:

- Reduce preoccupation with food, weight, and body fat.
- Gradually increase meals and snacks to an appropriate amount.
- Achieve an appropriate weight-for-height.
- Establish regular menstrual periods.
- Decrease training time and/or intensity by 10% to 20%.

The tragic case of Christy Henrich illustrates why anyone at risk for the female athlete triad should seek professional help. As a young teenager, Christy weighed 95 pounds and was 4 feet 11 inches tall. She showed promise as a gymnast but was told that she was too fat to excel in gymnastics. Christy continued her training but often starved herself, some days consuming just an apple and frequently purging by vomiting. Her success in gymnastics continued, but at age 22 her weight had fallen to 52 pounds, and she died from the effects of long-term semistarvation.

MAKING DECISIONS

Muscle Dysmorphia: The Pursuit of "Bigness"

Muscle dysmorphia has gained attention as a psychological condition with many similarities to eating disorders. First identified among male bodybuilders in the 1990s, muscle dysmorphia was initially termed "reverse anorexia." Men (and some women) with this disorder perceive themselves as *too thin*, rather than too fat, and are preoccupied with strict weight-lifting and diet regimens to achieve a high level of muscularity. Among high school and college-aged men, in particular, body dissatisfaction may lead to disordered eating and exercise practices. In muscle dysmorphia, numerous hours are devoted to working out at the gym; planning and eating low-carbohydrate, high-protein meals; and keeping meticulous records of exercise, body measurements, and food intake. The dietary practices (e.g., high-volume eating, protein intakes of up to 5 grams per kilogram) and use of unproven ergogenic aids or anabolic steroids can result in physical impairment. Such exercise and eating routines also interfere with social, occupational, and recreational activities. People with muscle dysmorphia may avoid social contact, eating in restaurants, and being seen without clothes because of distress over appearing too thin. Considering its many similarities with anorexia nervosa and a tendency for people with muscle dysmorphia to cross over to other forms of eating disorders over time, some experts support recognition of muscle dysmorphia as an eating disorder.

11.5 Prevention of Eating Disorders

A key to developing and maintaining healthful eating behavior is to realize that some concern about diet, health, and weight is normal. It is also normal to experience variation in what we eat, how we feel, and even how much we weigh. For example, it is normal to experience some minimal weight change (up to 2 to 3 pounds) throughout the day and even more over the course of a week. A large weight fluctuation or ongoing weight gain or weight loss is more likely to indicate that a problem is present. If you notice a large change in your eating habits, how you feel, or your body weight, it is a good idea to consult your personal physician. Treating physical and emotional problems early helps lead you to peace of mind and good health.

With a view on society as a whole, many people begin to form opinions about food, nutrition, health, weight, and body image prior to or during puberty. Parents, friends, and professionals working with young adults should consider the following advice for preventing eating disorders:

- Discourage restrictive dieting and meal skipping. Fasting is also discouraged (except for religious occasions).
- Provide information about normal changes that occur during puberty.
- Correct misconceptions about nutrition, healthy body weight, and approaches to weight loss.
- Carefully phrase any weight-related recommendations and comments.
- Don't overemphasize numbers on a scale. Instead, primarily promote healthful eating.
- Encourage normal expression of disruptive emotions.
- Encourage children to eat only when they're hungry.
- Teach the basics of proper nutrition and regular physical activity in school and at home.
- Provide adolescents with an appropriate, but not unlimited, degree of independence, choice, responsibility, and self-accountability for their actions.

A female high school athlete recently admitted her 3-year struggle with anorexia nervosa and bulimia nervosa. Even after her athletic performance declined and she suffered a sports-related injury, which sidelined her for a year and required surgery, she continued to think that controlling her weight and eating behaviors would make her the best—academically and physically. This example demonstrates several important points about eating disorders: certain groups of people are at greater risk for developing eating disorders; these people are often high achievers and are careful about concealing their eating disorder; and eating disorders such as the female athlete triad, bulimia nervosa, and anorexia nervosa frequently overlap.

CRITICAL THINKING

Tom, a high school teacher, is concerned about eating disorders. He wants to try to prevent young adults from falling into the discouraging traps of anorexia nervosa and bulimia nervosa. What are some of the topics and issues he should discuss with students in his health classes?

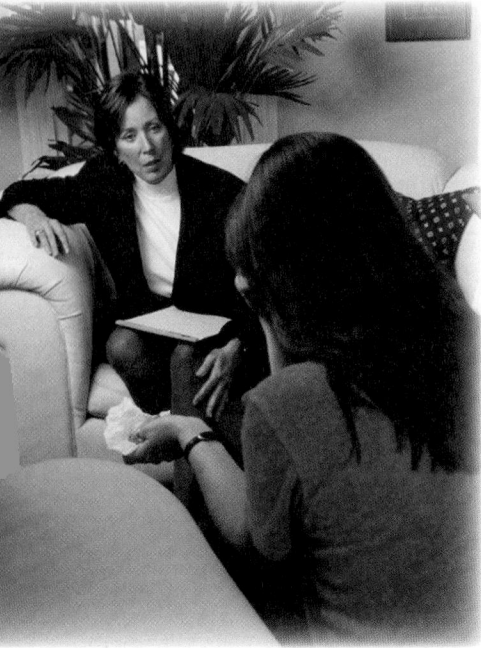

▲ Bulimia nervosa affects many college students. Counselors are aware of this and are available to help.

For further information on eating disorders, contact:

Academy for Eating Disorders, 111 Deer Lake Road, Suite 100, Deerfield, IL 60015 847-498-4274; www.aedweb.org

The National Eating Disorders Association, 603 Stewart St., Suite 803, Seattle, WA 98101; 206-382-3587 or 800-931-EDAP; www.nationaleatingdisorders.org

The National Institute of Mental Health has published a concise review of eating disorders (www.nimh.nih.gov/publicat/ eatingdisorders.cfm).

- Increase self-acceptance and appreciation of the power and pleasure emerging from one's body.
- Enhance tolerance for diversity in body weight and shape.
- Build respectful environments and supportive relationships.
- Encourage coaches to be sensitive to weight and body-image issues among athletes.
- Emphasize that thinness is not necessarily associated with better athletic performance.

Our society as a whole can benefit from a fresh focus on nutritious food practices and a healthful outlook toward food and body weight. Not only is treatment of eating disorders far more difficult than prevention, these disorders also have devastating effects on the entire family. For this reason, caregivers and health care professionals must emphasize the importance of an overall healthful diet that focuses on moderation, as opposed to restriction and perfection. Restricted diets are especially detrimental to children because they do not supply enough calories to sustain growth. In response, nutritional counseling can assure caregivers that including some sweets and fast-food in a child's diet is acceptable (see Chapter 15 for more details).

Overall, the challenge facing many North Americans is achieving a healthy body weight without excessive dieting. This means adopting and maintaining sensible eating habits, a physically active lifestyle, and realistic and positive attitudes and emotions while practicing creative ways to handle stress. Eating disorders develop in part from certain cultural values; changing these values might reduce the pressures predisposing some people to various types of disordered eating behavior. Some feminists, for example, assert that true liberation means being free to find one's natural weight. Women who combine careers and motherhood are saying that they have more important things to worry about; some fashion leaders are tolerating more curves; exercise programs are encouraging regular brisk walking, rather than high-intensity activities such as jogging. Finally, writers, therapists, and registered dietitians are working to help women accept their bodies, as noted in the "size acceptance" approach discussed in Chapter 7.

MAKING DECISIONS

Polycystic Ovary Syndrome and Eating Disorders

Polycystic ovary syndrome (PCOS) is a complex hormonal disorder and is the leading cause of infertility. PCOS is characterized by hormonal imbalances in women with high levels of male hormones such as testosterone secreted by the ovaries. The hormonal imbalance causes tiny cysts to surround the ovaries like a strand of pearls. The signs and symptoms of PCOS include difficulty losing weight, intense cravings for carbohydrates, and irregular or absent periods. Most of these have a direct effect on body image and self-esteem, so a relationship between PCOS and eating disorders is suspected. The overlap in symptoms means it is important that persons with these characteristics be screened for both PCOS and eating disorders before recommendations for treatment are made (see Further Reading 7).

CONCEPT CHECK

Food bingeing (without purging) and grazing are two characteristic behaviors of binge-eating disorder. Treatment addresses the deeper emotional issues that undermine healthy eating practices, while shifting the person's focus away from food deprivation and restrictive diets and toward more normal eating behaviors. Night eating syndrome involves overeating in the evening and a need to eat to be able to fall asleep. The female athlete triad consists of disordered eating, amenorrhea, and osteoporosis, and most commonly affects those in appearance-related and endurance sports. Parents, coaches, teachers, and health professionals need to be involved in efforts to prevent and treat this problem.

Eating Disorder Reflections

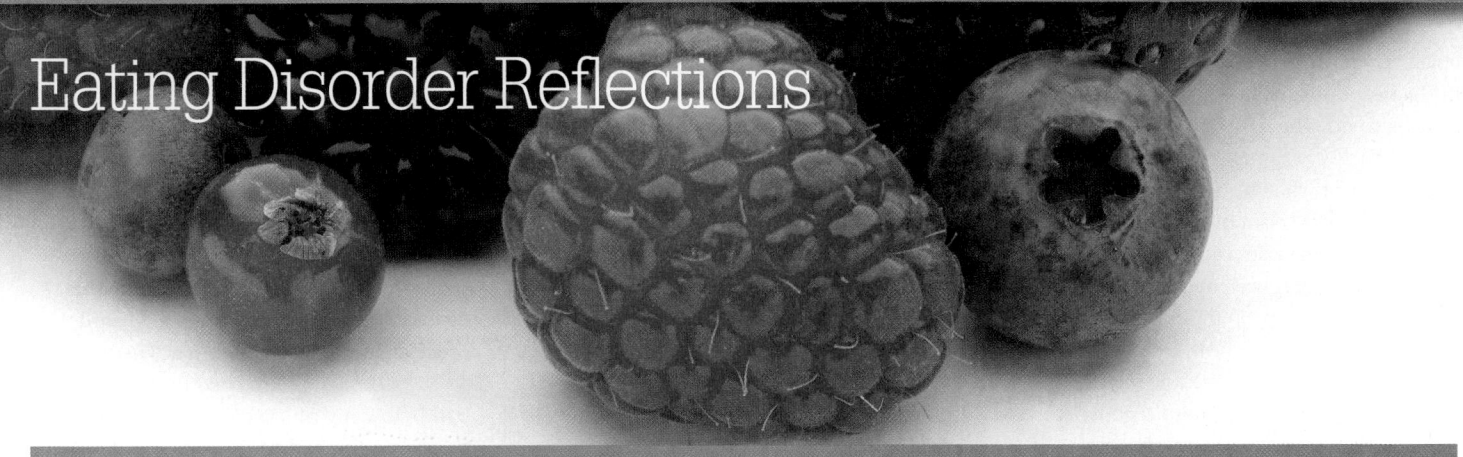

Thoughts of an Anorexic Woman

It was the spring of my freshman year of high school, and I had just turned 15. I wanted to get a leading role in the upcoming high school musical *West Side Story*. I thought I should lose some weight to look more attractive to the student director Shawn, so I decided to give up "junk" food. The next day my friend Sandra looked at my lunch, spread out neatly on a napkin before me, and squawked, "Dill pickles?! Who brings dill pickles for lunch in a zip-lock baggie?" The other girls at the table fell into a fit of hysterics. "Casting for *West Side Story* is coming up,"

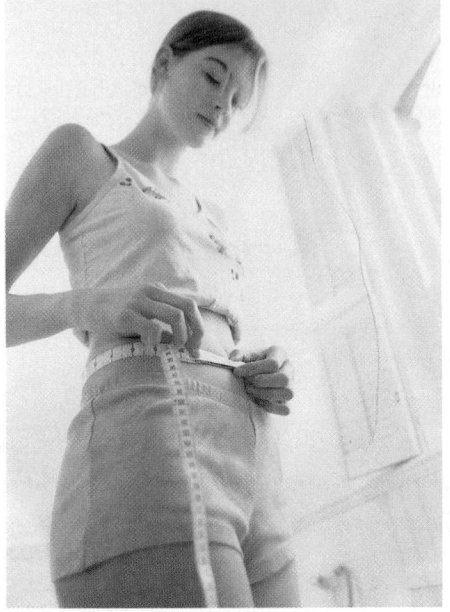

▲ A history of anorexia nervosa can harm physical as well as mental health.

I said, "and I gave up 'junk' food to try to lose a few pounds." One of my friends thought it would be funny to give me an M&M—just to smell. Ha, ha. I put it in a little Tupperware container and kept it for days in my backpack as a reminder. Every once in a while, I did smell it.

For the next few weeks there were times when I would find myself cracking open the refrigerator door and just staring down what I knew to be a deliciously crunchy, crisp, and cold Kit Kat bar in the dairy bin. I didn't eat it though. At the mall with my friends (since at 15, that's about all my parents allowed me to do), Bridgette and Nora wanted to stop and get a cinnamon bun. They chided me, but I didn't budge. The cinnamon bun smelled so good. But as I sat opposite them in the food court and watched them over-dramatize its ooey-gooey goodness, I felt a sense of pride that I could make a decision and stick with it. I could see that they were jealous of my willpower.

When Easter came around, I took a look at the contents of the Easter basket my mom insisted on preparing and turned up my nose at it. I had proven to myself that I could resist temptation . . . why stop now?

I was eventually offered only a minor part in the musical, but I wasn't that disappointed. I was looking so much better as the pounds kept coming off. Every morning, just after going to the bathroom and before getting any breakfast, I would pop onto the scale in my mom's bathroom. One hundred and fifteen pounds and still going. At 5 feet 7 inches, that wasn't too bad.

Also at this time, I started running, and my friend Laura became my running partner. She was getting in shape for the next season of field hockey. After school, we met in the locker room, changed out of our school clothes, and out we went. I had never been much of an athlete—I thought that being part of a team, whether in sports or academics, diluted the excellence I could achieve on my own. Running, however, could just be me and the road—no mediocrity there.

Cheese and butter had made it to the "no" list by the time I was 16 and down to 105 pounds. Fat-free was my mantra. For my 16th birthday, my friends threw a little surprise party for me. Nora, knowing I would put up a fight, made me a cake. "It's your birthday! You can have a piece of cake!" I politely said no, that I would cut it for everyone else, but I really didn't want any. They pestered me and Nora started to feel offended, so finally I took a few bites so she wouldn't burst into tears. It had been so long since I'd had so much sugar. I felt bloated and sick. I ate nothing for the rest of the day, and only 6 saltines, 1 apple, and 2 stalks of celery the next day. Those foods were on the "yes" list. Salads also were okay, but only lettuce with salt and vinegar. I told my parents that the dissections in biology class had given me a distaste for meat, but really, I just didn't want all those calories. For a while, I craved food day and night, but I was getting better and better at holding my ground.

By my senior year, I was skipping lunches altogether, opting instead to hang out in the library and read over my AP Bio text. "Where were you at lunch today?" Bridgette would ask later. "Oh, I had some reading to do. The AP exam is going to be tough." At 100 pounds, I was getting closer to finding out what "tough" really meant.

Even though Laura moved out of state, I didn't give up on exercising. Now, the stair stepper in the gym was my favorite. I'd take my biology notes, prop them up in front of me, and step-step-step until I had burned 400 kcal. I felt so efficient knowing that I could multi-task. Sometimes I'd go twice a day. As senior year wore on, though, it got harder and harder to get up in the morning and put on my tennis shoes. And then one morning, in the shower, I just collapsed under the stream of hot water.

I ended up in this hospital bed with an IV tube in my arm. At 92 pounds, my body was starving. As it turns out, if you don't give your body any fuel, you start to cannibalize yourself, in a sense. My body had been so hungry, my muscles had been wasting away, and the episode in the shower was due to a problem with my heart. It's a problem I have created . . . not my parents or my distant group of friends . . . just me. My mom was there, next to me, caressing the arm with the IV tube, putting her whole life on hold because of me. Isn't this what I'd wanted—to be in control of my own destiny?

Where do I go from here?

Thoughts of a Bulimic Woman

From Hall L, Cohn L: *Bulimia—A Guide to Recovery*. Gurze Books: Carlsbad, CA, 1992.

I am wide awake and immediately out of bed. I think back to the night before, when I made a new list of what I wanted to get done and how I wanted to be. My husband is not far behind me on his way into the bathroom to get ready for work. Maybe I can sneak onto the scale to see what I weigh this morning before he notices me. I am already in my private world. I feel overjoyed when the scale says that I stayed the same weight as I was the night before, and I can feel that slightly hungry feeling. Maybe it will stop today; maybe

today everything will change. What were the projects I was going to get done?

We eat the same breakfast, except that I take no butter on my toast, no cream in my coffee, and never take seconds (until Doug gets out the door). Today I am going to be really good, and that means eating certain predetermined portions of food and not taking one more bite than I think I am allowed. I am very careful to see that I don't take more than Doug. I judge myself by his body. I can feel the tension building. I wish Doug would hurry up and leave so I can get going!

As soon as he shuts the door, I try to get involved with one of the myriad responsibilities on my list. I hate them all! I just want to crawl into a hole. I don't want to do anything. I'd rather eat. I am alone; I am nervous; I am no good; I always do everything wrong anyway; I am not in control; I can't make it through the day, I know it. It has been the same for so long. I remember the starchy cereal I ate for breakfast. I am into the bathroom and onto the scale. It measures the same, but I don't want to stay the same! I want to be thinner! I look into the mirror. I think my thighs are ugly and deformed looking. I see a lumpy, clumsy, pear-shaped wimp. There is always something wrong with what I see. I feel frustrated, trapped in this body, and I don't know what to do about it.

I float to the refrigerator knowing exactly what is there. I begin with last night's brownies. I always begin with the sweets. At first I try to make it look like nothing is missing, but my appetite is huge and I resolve to make another batch of brownies. I know there is half of a bag of cookies in the bathroom, thrown out the night before, and I polish them off immediately. I take some milk so my vomiting will be smoother. I like the full feeling I get after downing a big glass. I get out six pieces of bread and toast one side of each in the broiler, turn them over and load

them with pats of butter, and put them under the broiler again until they are bubbling. I take all six pieces on a plate to the television and go back for a bowl of cereal and a banana to have along with them. Before the last piece of toast is finished, I am already preparing the next batch of six more pieces. Maybe another brownie or five, and a couple of large bowls full of ice cream, yogurt, or cottage cheese.

My stomach is stretched into a huge ball below my rib cage. I know I'll have to go into the bathroom soon, but I want to postpone it. I am in never-never land. I am waiting, feeling the pressure, pacing the floor in and out of the rooms. Time is passing. Time is passing. It is getting to be time. I wander aimlessly through each of the rooms again, tidying, making the whole house neat and put back together. I finally make the turn into the bathroom. I brace my feet, pull my hair back and stick my finger down my throat, stroking twice, and get up a huge pile of food. Three times, four times, and another pile of food. I can see everything come back. I am so glad to see those brownies because they are so fattening. The rhythm of the emptying is broken and my head is beginning to hurt. I stand up feeling dizzy, empty, and weak. The whole episode has taken about an hour.

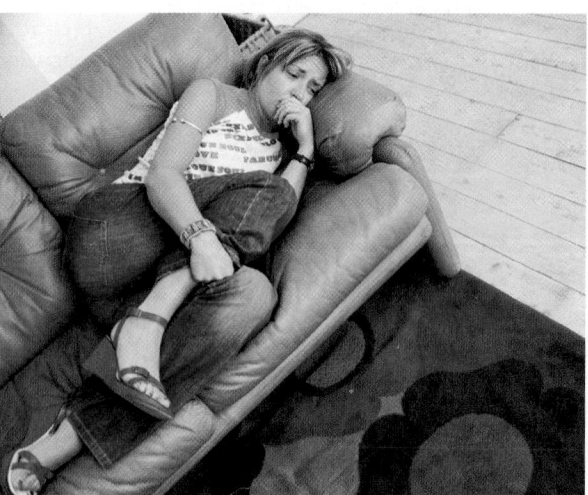

▲ Bulimic episodes add to the despair felt in this disorder.

Case Study Eating Disorders—Steps to Recovery

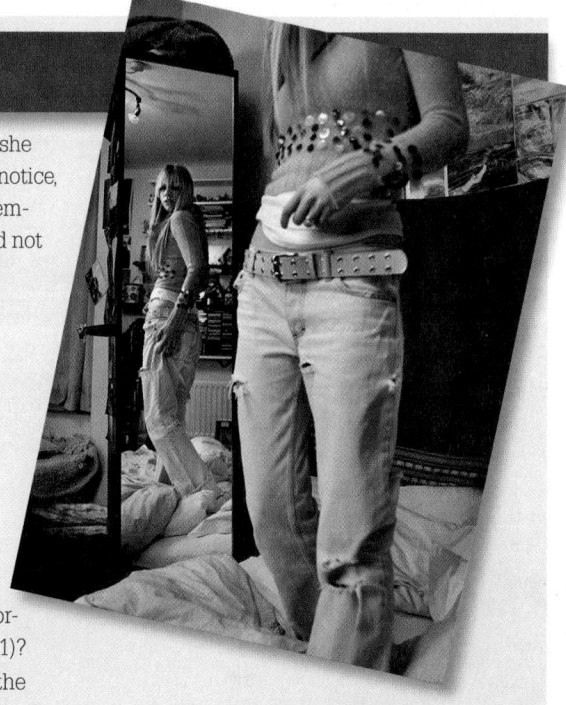

At age 16, Sarah suddenly became self-conscious about her body when her peers teased her about being overweight. She began exercising to an aerobics video for an hour each day and found that she had success in losing weight; this was the beginning of her obsession to be thin. Next, Sarah turned to eating less food to lose even more weight and began eliminating certain foods from her diet, such as candy and meat. She increased her water and vegetable intake and chewed sugarless gum to curb her appetite. Once she began dieting, it was impossible for her to stop. She enjoyed having a high degree of self-control over her body. Still, she was literally obsessed with food, even staring at others while they were eating a meal. She occasionally cooked large meals and then refused to eat all but a few bites. By the time Sarah was 19 years old and 5 feet 6 inches tall, her weight had dropped from 150 pounds to 85 pounds in 20 months. Her family was concerned about her weight status, demanding that she go to a physician for an evaluation. Sarah was not happy about this idea but believed that her family would stop pestering her if she went. Sarah did not think she had a problem; she thought she was still grotesquely overweight. She did notice, however, that she was intolerant of cold temperatures and was concerned that she had not menstruated in a year.

Answer the following questions, and check your responses in Appendix A.

1. Sarah appears to have an eating disorder. Which eating disorder best describes her behavior?
2. List the behaviors that Sarah developed between age 16 and 19 years that are signs of the development of this eating disorder.
3. What physical symptoms of this disorder does Sarah have (review Fig. 11-1)?
4. What types of therapy do you think the physician will suggest for Sarah?
5. Do you think Sarah has developed any vitamin or mineral deficiencies? Which ones would be most likely? How could these deficiencies be best treated?
6. Where could she go for the therapy she needs?
7. What type of professionals would most likely provide therapy for Sarah's condition?
8. What is the likelihood that she will fully recover from her condition?

Summary (Numbers refer to numbered sections in the chapter.)

11.1 Healthy eating, which incorporates the principals of balance, variety, and moderation, provides fuel for the body and a source of pleasure. Disordered eating encompasses mild and short-term changes in eating patterns that occur as a result of life stress, illness, or a desire to change body weight. When carried to the extreme, disordered eating may progress to an eating disorder, in which severe changes in eating patterns have lasting and detrimental effects.

11.2 Anorexia nervosa is most common among high-achieving, perfectionist girls from families marked by conflict, high expectations, rigidity, and denial. The disorder usually starts with dieting in early puberty and proceeds to the near-total refusal to eat. Early warning signs include intense concern about weight gain and dieting, as well as abnormal food habits, such as cooking food that they won't allow themselves to eat.

Anorexia nervosa may be defined as a denial of appetite. Anorexic persons become irritable, hostile, overly critical, and joyless; they tend to withdraw from family and friends. Eventually, anorexia nervosa can lead to numerous physical effects, including a profound decrease in body weight and body fat, a fall in body temperature and heart rate, iron-deficiency anemia, a low white blood cell count, hair loss, constipation, low blood potassium, and the loss of menstrual periods. Those with anorexia nervosa are in a state of physical illness. Treatment of anorexia nervosa includes increasing food intake to support gradual weight gain. Psychological counseling attempts to help establish regular food habits and to find means of coping with the life stresses that led to the disorder. Hospitalization may be necessary, as well as use of certain medications.

11.3 Bulimia nervosa is characterized by secretive bingeing on large amounts of food within a short time span, and then purging by vomiting or misusing laxatives, diuretics, or enemas. Alternately, fasting and excessive exercise may be used. Both men and women are at risk. Vomiting as a means of purging is especially destructive to the body; it can cause severe tooth decay, stomach ulcers, irritation of the esophagus, low blood potassium, and other problems. Bulimia nervosa poses a serious health problem and is associated with significant risk of suicide. Treatment of bulimia nervosa includes psychological as well as nutritional counseling. During treatment, bulimic persons learn to accept themselves and to cope with problems in ways that do not involve food. Regular eating patterns are developed as these bulimic persons begin to plan meals in an informed, healthful manner. Certain medications can be a helpful addition to the regimen.

11.4 Besides anorexia nervosa and bulimia nervosa, there are several categories of eating disorders not otherwise specified (EDNOS). Binge-eating disorder, more widespread than either anorexia nervosa or bulimia nervosa, is most common among people with a history of frequent, unsuccessful dieting. Binge eaters typically either practice bingeing (without purging) or grazing (i.e., eating continually over extended periods). Emotional disturbances are often at the root of this disordered form of eating. Night eating syndrome is overeating in the evening with more than one-third of daily food intake after dinner, difficulty falling asleep and a need to eat something to help fall asleep faster, and waking at least once during the night and a need to eat to be able to fall asleep again. The female athlete triad consists of disordered eating, loss of menstrual periods, and osteoporosis. It is particularly common in appearance-related and endurance sports. If not corrected, this disorder eventually leads to decreased athletic performance and general health problems.

11.5 Prevention of eating disorders is crucial because treatments are expensive and lengthy and are not 100% effective. Encouraging healthy attitudes about eating and exercise from a young age will aid in preventing the development of eating disorders. Those who work closely with children and young adults should encourage acceptance of diversity in body sizes and carefully phrase comments about body weight. Helping children to develop healthy ways to cope with emotions is also important.

Check Your Knowledge (Answers to the following questions are below.)

1. Anorexia nervosa generally is a disease of
   a. children.
   b. middle-aged women.
   c. young boys.
   d. teenage women.

2. Anorexia nervosa can be defined as
   a. compulsive eating.
   b. hyperactivity.
   c. psychological denial of appetite.
   d. purging.

3. A long-term health consequence of anorexia nervosa could be
   a. fractures resulting from bone loss.
   b. atherosclerotic heart disease.
   c. esophageal ulcers.
   d. cancer.

4. Bulimia is most frequently diagnosed by a
   a. dietitian.
   b. physician.
   c. dentist.
   d. physical therapist.

5. The *major* health risk from frequent vomiting due to bulimia nervosa is
   a. a drop in blood potassium.
   b. constipation.
   c. weight gain.
   d. a swelling of salivary glands.

6. Initial treatment of bulimia nervosa includes all of the following *except*
   a. psychotherapy to improve body image.
   b. emphasis on regular eating habits.
   c. nutritional counseling.
   d. refeeding via tube feedings.
   e. Both a and c.

7. Binge-eating disorder can be characterized as
   a. bingeing accompanied by purging.
   b. secretive eating.
   c. eating to avoid feeling and dealing with emotional pain.
   d. the early phase of bulimia nervosa.

8. Binge-eating disorder is different from anorexia nervosa, and particularly bulimia nervosa, because it doesn't involve
   a. females.
   b. a persistent concern with body shape, weight, and thinness.
   c. purging, such as regular vomiting.

   d. health risks.
   e. Both b and c.

9. Night eating syndrome is characterized by
   a. eating dinner but no breakfast or lunch.
   b. the need to eat to fall asleep.
   c. waking at night to purge by vomiting.
   d. consuming all of the daily calories at night.

10. Female athlete triad consists of
    a. anorexia nervosa, lack of family support, and overtraining.
    b. disordered eating, overtraining, and lack of menstrual periods.
    c. osteoporosis, lack of menstrual periods, and disordered eating.
    d. osteoporosis, lack of sleep, and disordered eating.

Answers: 1. d (LO 11.2), 2. c (LO 11.2), 3. a (LO 11.2), 4. c (LO 11.3), 5. a (LO 11.3), 6. d (LO 11.3), 7. c (LO 11.4), 8. e (LO 11.4), 9. b (LO 11.4), 10. c (LO 11.4)

Study Questions (Numbers refer to Learning Outcomes)

1. What are the typical characteristics of a person with anorexia nervosa? What may influence a person to begin rigid, self-imposed dietary patterns? (LO 11.2)

2. List the detrimental physical and psychological side effects of bulimia nervosa. Describe important goals of the psychological and nutrition therapy used to treat bulimic patients. (LO 11.3)

3. What is the current thinking concerning medication use for anorexia nervosa and bulimia nervosa? (LOs 11.2 and 11.3)

4. Explain the role of excessive exercise in eating disorders. (LO 11.1)

5. How might parents significantly contribute to the development of an eating disorder? Suggest an attitude that a parent or an adult friend of yours displayed that may not have been conducive to developing a normal relationship to food. (LO 11.5)

6. Based on your knowledge of good nutrition and sound dietary habits, answer the following questions:
   a. How can repeated bingeing and purging lead to significant nutrient deficiencies?

b. How can significant nutrient deficiencies contribute to major health problems in later life?

c. A friend asks you, the nutrition expert, if it is okay to "cleanse" the body by eating only grapefruit for a week. What is your response? **(LO 11.1)**

7. How, in your opinion, has society contributed to the development of various forms of disordered eating? Provide an example. **(LO 11.5)**

8. List the three symptoms that constitute the female athlete triad. What is the major health risk associated with loss of menstrual periods in the female athlete? **(LO 11.4)**

9. How does binge-eating disorder differ from bulimia nervosa? Describe the factors that contribute to the development and treatment of binge-eating disorder. **(LO 11.4)**

10. Provide two recommendations to reduce the problem of eating disorders in our society. **(LO 11.6)**

What Would You Choose Recommendations

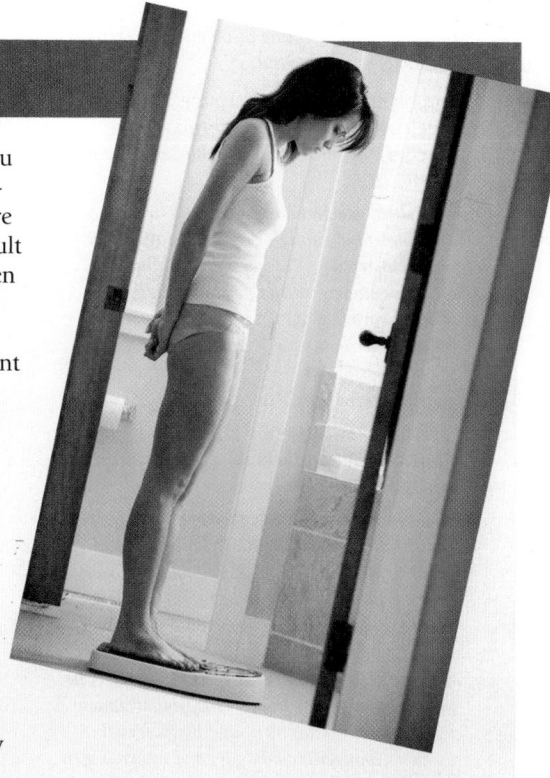

It can be uncomfortable to confront a friend about an unhealthy behavior. You may worry about compromising your friendship. The eating and excessive exercise behaviors you have witnessed may be short-term disordered eating and may pass in a few weeks. On the other hand, they might just be the tip of the iceberg. Ignoring her behavior will not make it go away. As you have learned in this chapter, eating disorders can have very serious consequences, and the earlier they are treated, the better the outcome. If you feel unable to address your concerns one on one with your roommate, you can seek help from a resident assistant in your dorm, a school counselor, or a nurse in the student health center. You will not be betraying your friendship; you will be showing how much you care about her by taking action.

Diagnosing an eating disorder is a complex task. People with eating disorders may deny the problem, hide their behaviors, and be irrational and uncooperative with those who try to help them. Do not try to diagnose your friend, but do try to keep the lines of communication open. Tell her what you have observed and ask her how you can help. She may open up to you and be glad she is not alone in her struggle. Then again, she may get angry and withdraw from you. Try to share what you know about eating disorders without lecturing or admonishing her. Also, be aware that your friend is going through a difficult emotional struggle that has probably been years in the making. Do not assume you know what she is going through.

Discussing healthy weight-management techniques with your roommate is not likely to help her if she has fallen prey to an eating disorder. She is already critical of her appearance and weight; your advice, although well intended and backed by the nutrition knowledge you have picked up in this course, may be construed as judgmental. Eating disorders are not about food. Rather, they involve issues of self-concept and control. It is important to be supportive but not critical. Taking the focus off food and body weight is important. Do not try to force her to eat or slow down on her exercise. If you can help get your roommate to seek professional treatment, psychiatric counseling will help to address her unhealthy relationship with food; eventually, nutrition counseling will help her to establish better eating habits.

Get prepared before you confront your roommate. Find out what information and resources are available on campus so you can share them with her. Recognize that you are not going to cure her disorder—she needs professional help. You can be supportive and patient as she deals with her inner turmoil. Listen and offer to go with her to seek care. Someday, you may be a health professional who is able to diagnose and counsel victims of eating disorders. For now, leave it to a qualified professional.

Further Readings

1. ADA Reports: Position of the American Dietetic Association: Nutrition intervention in the treatment of anorexia nervosa, bulimia nervosa, and other eating disorders. *Journal of the American Dietetic Association* 106:2073, 2006.

    Eating disorders are complex and serious illnesses that span a continuum from extreme dieting to diagnosed conditions. For effective treatment the expert interaction between professionals in many disciplines, including dietetics, is required.

2. American Academy of Pediatrics: Clinical Report—Identification and management of eating disorders in children and adolescents. *Pediatrics* 126:1240, 2010.

    Physicians should screen children and adolescents annually by looking for evidence of disordered eating, delayed development, and especially by monitoring weight and height. In children, eating disorders may appear not as weight loss, but as failure to grow appropriately. Early detection and treatment of eating disorders are especially important for younger patients because problems with growth, brain development, and bone mineralization can be irreversible.

3. Bonci CM: National Athletic Trainers' Association position statement: Preventing, detecting, and managing disordered eating in athletes. *Journal of Athletic Training* 43:80, 2008.

Disordered eating is common among athletes, particularly in sports with weight classifications or those in which appearance is related to success. As training intensity increases nutrient needs, nutrient deficiencies impair athletic performance. Athletic trainers, coaches, and others who regularly interact with athletes should be trained to promote healthful dietary behaviors, recognize signs of eating disorders, and exercise sensitivity to weight issues.

4. Campbell IC and others: Eating disorders, gene-environment interactions and epigenetics. *Neuroscience and Behavioral Reviews* 35:784, 2011.

The role of genetics and epigenetics in the development of eating disorders is a relatively new field of study. Environmental influences, including undernutrition, overnutrition, and stress at various stages of the life cycle, may impact a person's genetic predisposition for eating disorders.

5. Feldman MB, Meyer IH: Eating disorders in diverse lesbian, gay, and bisexual populations. *International Journal of Eating Disorders* 40:218, 2007.

This study assessed prevalence of eating disorders in a diverse community sample. Rates of eating disorders are higher among gay and bisexual men compared to heterosexual men. Whereas many heterosexual men are motivated to attain a large, muscular physique, gay and bisexual men tend to desire a slender build. The prevalence of eating disorders is similar among lesbians, bisexual women, and heterosexual women. Younger lesbian, gay, and bisexual men and women were more susceptible to disordered eating practices than older study participants.

6. Goebel-Fabbri AE: Eating disorders in type 1 diabetes: Clinical significance and treatment recommendations. *Current Diabetes Reports* 9:133, 2009.

Type 1 diabetes increases risk for eating disorders. Dietary restrictions and fear of hypoglycemia may precipitate binge eating. Some individuals may restrict insulin therapy as a means of purging calories without regard to the detrimental outcomes of impaired glucose control. Girls and women with diabetes should be screened for the presence of eating disorders.

7. Grassi A: Are polycystic ovary syndrome & eating disorders related? *Today's Dietitian* p. 32, October 2006.

Polycystic ovary syndrome (PCOS) is a complex hormonal disorder and is the leading cause of infertility. The symptoms of PCOS have a direct effect on body image and self-esteem and may lead to the development of eating disorders.

8. Lundgren JD and others: Prevalence of the night eating syndrome in a psychiatric population. *American Journal of Psychiatry* 163 (1):156, 2006.

Night eating syndrome is characterized by evening hyperphagia and waking during the night to consume food. The results of this study show that night eating syndrome is a common disorder among psychiatric outpatients and is associated with substance use and obesity.

9. Mathieu J: What is orthorexia? *Journal of the American Dietetic Association* 105:1510, 2005.

"Orthorexia," although not currently classified as an eating disorder, describes an emerging condition in which healthful eating becomes an obsession. A need for perfection or purity lies at the heart of orthorexia. Healthful or not, strict dietary practices become a problem when they interfere with a person's ability to take part in society. Such extreme dietary perfectionism may be related to obsessive-compulsive disorder.

10. McFarand MB and Kaminski PL: Men muscles, and mood: The relationship between self-concept, dysphoria, and body image disturbances. *Eating Behaviors* 10:68, 2009.

Just as women are under societal pressure to maintain unnatural thinness. men are unduly influenced by the extremely lean and muscular male body ideal portrayed by the media. This study of college-age men found that body dissatisfaction is predicted by low self-concept and increased levels of interpersonal sensitivity, depression, and anxiety. The study also noted associations between muscle dysmorphia and disordered eating.

11. Murphy R and others: Cognitive behavioral therapy for eating disorders. *Psychiatric Clinics of North America* 33:611, 2010.

The success of cognitive behavioral therapy (CBT) for patients with bulimia nervosa has spawned interest in applying CBT to anorexia nervosa and other eating disorders. This is based on the conclusion that all eating disorders, regardless of classification, stem from placing too much value on body shape and weight. This type of therapy aims to identify and modify the pathological thought patterns, such as strict dieting rules, that support an eating disorder.

12. Norris ML and others: Ana and the Internet: A review of pro-anorexia websites. *International Journal of Eating Disorders* 39:443, 2006.

Searching for "anorexia" using common search engines results in hundreds of links, many of which are "pro-anorexia." These websites provide information that is supportive of anorexia nervosa but is largely controversial and dangerous. Key characteristics of pro-anorexia websites include control, success, and perfection. It is important that health care providers and caregivers be aware of these websites and their content.

13. Ringham R and others: Eating disorder symptomatology among ballet dancers. *International Journal of Eating Disorders* 39:503, 2006.

Ballet dancers are at high risk of developing eating disorders. In this study, 29 female ballet dancers were compared to women with anorexia nervosa, bulimia nervosa, and not eating pathology. The results showed that the eating patterns of dancers were more similar to eating-disordered individuals than to control individuals. The majority of the dancers (83%) met lifetime criteria for eating disorders.

14. Robinson-O'Brien R and others: Adolescent and young adult vegetarianism: Better dietary intake and weight outcomes but increased risk of disordered eating behaviors. *Journal of the American Dietetic Association* 109:648, 2009.

This study of more than 2500 young men and women contributes to the body of evidence demonstrating that appropriately planned vegetarian and vegan lifestyles can be healthfully practiced by people of all ages. However, some young adults may use these socially acceptable eating patterns as a means of unhealthful dietary restriction for extreme weight loss. A history of vegetarian dietary practices is associated with disordered eating practices. If weight loss is the primary motive for choosing a vegetarian lifestyle, parents should be on alert for warning signs of eating disorders.

15. Stuppy P: Eating disorders in women at midlife. *Today's Dietitian* p. 12, January 2006.

Several emotional changes that occur in middle age, such as death of a spouse, divorce, the "empty nest" syndrome, and caring for aging parents, may precipitate eating disorders. Women, who already experience a high level of dissatisfaction with their bodies, may use dietary restriction or bingeing behaviors as coping mechanisms. Registered dietitians can help clients by facilitating recognition of the emotional underpinnings of clients' eating problems and by appropriately referring clients to mental health professionals, when needed.

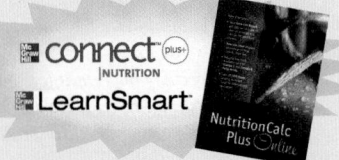

To get the most out of your study of nutrition, go to McGraw-Hill's online resources: Connect www.mcgrawhillconnect.com, where you will find NutritionCalc Plus, LearnSmart, and many other dynamic tools.

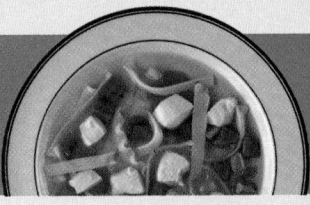

I. Assessing Risk of Developing an Eating Disorder

British investigators have developed a five-question screening tool called the **SCOFF** Questionnaire for recognizing eating disorders:[†]

1. Do you make yourself **S**ick because you feel full?
2. Do you lose **C**ontrol over how much you eat?
3. Have you lost more than **O**ne stone (about 13 pounds) recently?
4. Do you believe yourself to be **F**at when others say you are thin?
5. Does **F**ood dominate your life?

Two or more positive responses suggest an eating disorder.

1. After completing this questionnaire, do you feel that you might have an eating disorder or the potential to develop one?

   _____

   _____

2. Do you think any of your friends might have an eating disorder?

   _____

   _____

3. What counseling and education resources exist in your area or on your campus to help with a potential eating disorder?

   _____

   _____

4. If a friend has an eating disorder, what do you think is the best way to assist him or her in getting help?

   _____

   _____

[†]Morgan JF and others: The SCOFF Questionnaire, *British Medical Journal* 319:1467, 1999.

II. Helping Prevent Eating Disorders

You have been asked to speak to a junior high school class about eating disorders. What are four major points that you would make to help prevent disordered eating in this population?

1. _____
2. _____
3. _____
4. _____

Here are points you may consider:

1. Extreme thinness is oversold in the media. Extremely low weight (i.e., BMI of less than 17.5) is generally not healthy.
2. Self-induced vomiting is dangerous. Damage to the teeth, stomach, and esophagus often results.
3. Loss of menstrual periods is a sign of illness. It is important to see a physician about this. Bone deterioration is a common result.
4. The treatment of eating disorders in early phases aids success. These diseases are difficult to treat once firmly established.

Chapter 12 Undernutrition Throughout the World

Student Learning Outcomes

Chapter 12 is designed to allow you to:

12.1 Define and characterize the terms *hunger, malnutrition,* and *undernutrition.*

12.2 Examine undernutrition in the United States and highlight several programs established to combat this problem.

12.3 Examine undernutrition in the developing world and evaluate the major obstacles that hinder a solution.

12.4 Outline some possible solutions to under-nutrition in the developing world.

12.5 Evaluate the consequences of undernutrition during critical periods in a person's life.

What Would You Choose?

"You'd better clean your plate! There are starving children in Africa who would love to eat that dinner!"

Mom was right—we often overlook the fact that we live in a rich nation with access to plentiful food and clean water, whereas something as simple as clean drinking water is merely a dream in many developing nations. In fact, the problems of hunger and food insecurity exist in your own community. It is probably not feasible (or sanitary) to send your rejected green beans overseas, but there are some simple steps you can take at home to support agencies seeking to provide clean water and nutritious food for people in need. What would you choose to help put an end to world hunger?

a Organize a group of friends to prepare and hand out peanut butter and jelly sandwiches to homeless people downtown.

b Donate $10 per month to an international aid organization that supplies food to starving children in Africa.

c Participate in a 5K run/walk event that raises funds and awareness to combat world hunger.

d Buy locally grown fruits and vegetables at your community's farmers' market.

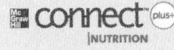 **connect** NUTRITION **Think about your choice as you read Chapter 12, then see our recommendations at the end of the chapter. To learn more about combating hunger, check out the Connect site:** www.mcgrawhillconnect.com

Part Four
Nutrition: Beyond the Nutrients

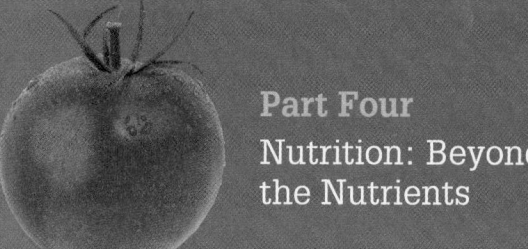

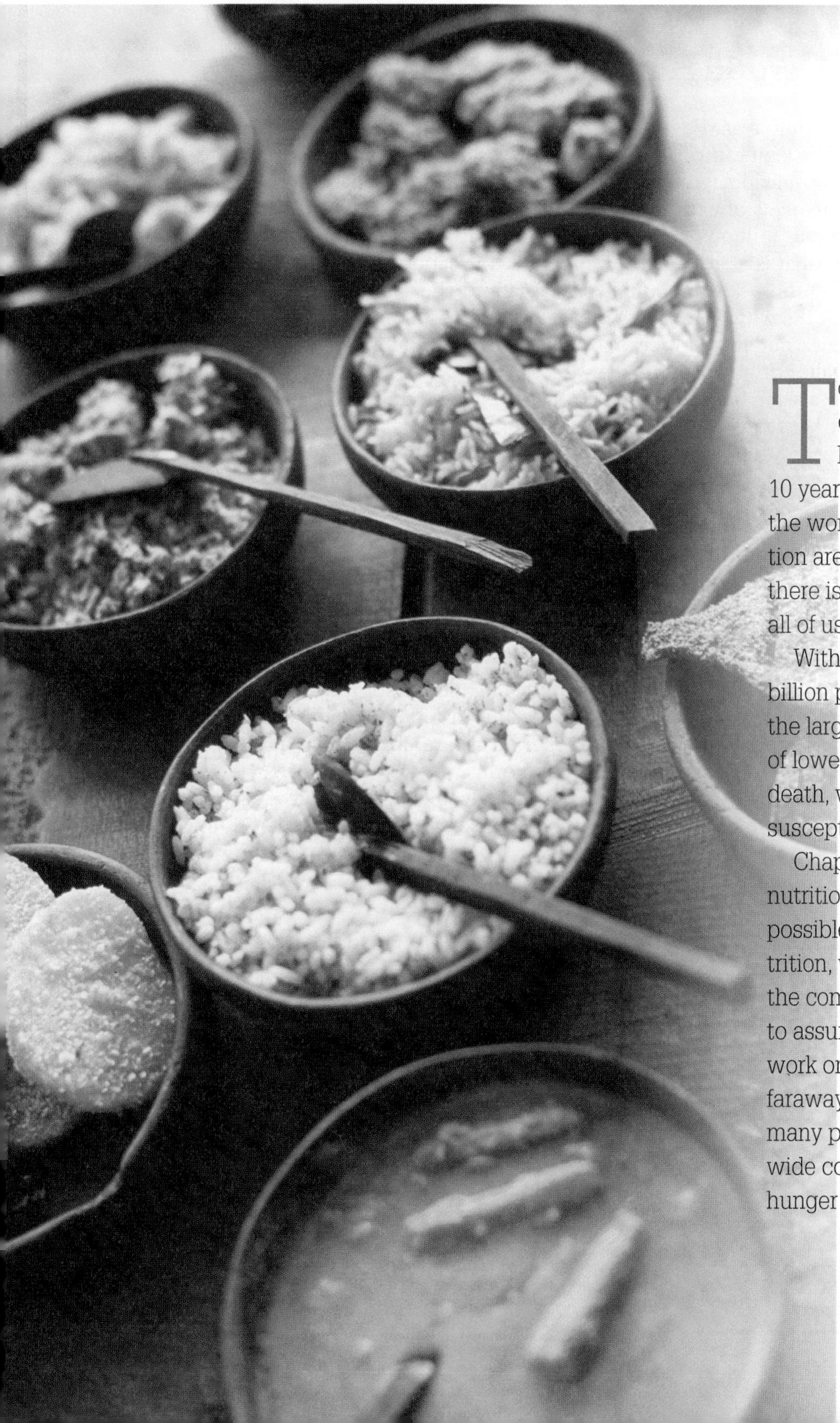

Today, nearly one in six people worldwide is chronically undernourished— too hungry to lead a productive, active life. Over the past 10 years, this problem has worsened. Throughout the world, the problems of poverty and undernutrition are widespread and growing—even though there is enough food available to sufficiently feed all of us.

Within the developing world, approximately 1 billion people are malnourished, with Asia having the largest number. Malnutrition is the main cause of lowered resistance to disease, infection, and death, with children under 5 years being the most susceptible.

Chapter 12 examines the problem of undernutrition, the conditions that create it, and some possible solutions. If we are to eradicate undernutrition, we all have to understand the problem. As the comic in the chapter suggests, we must begin to assume responsibility today, not tomorrow, to work on solutions to hunger close to home and in faraway nations. It is important to recognize that many political, economic, and social factors worldwide contribute directly and indirectly to the hunger problem.

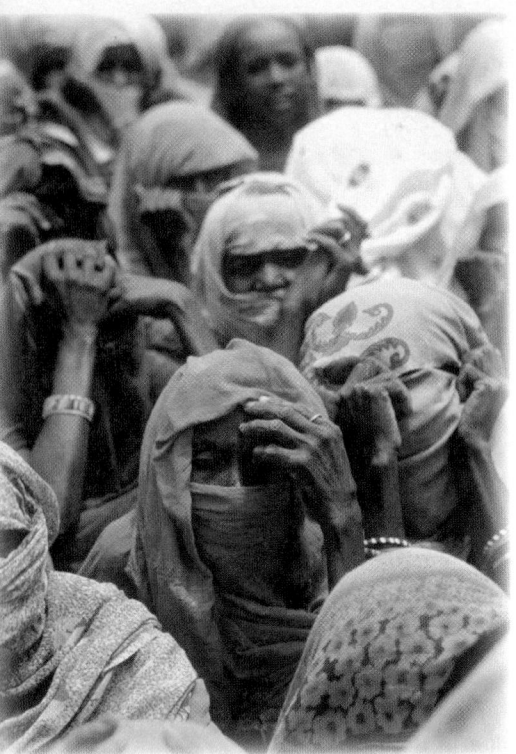

▲ Malnutrition is associated with or exacerbated by overpopulation in some developing countries.

food insecure Condition in which the quality, variety, and/or desirability of the diet is reduced and there is difficulty at times providing enough food for everyone in the household.

hunger The primarily physiological (internal) drive to find and eat food.

 Refresh Your Memory

As you begin your study of world hunger in Chapter 12, you may want to review:

- The health effects of protein-calorie malnutrition in Chapter 6
- The role of vitamin A and rich food sources in Chapter 8
- The roles and rich food sources of iron, zinc, and iodide in Chapter 9

12.1 World Hunger: A Crisis on the Rise

Uncertainty regarding the source of one's next meal remains a daily experience for close to 1 billion people around the world. This situation is troubling considering that worldwide agriculture produces more than enough food to meet the energy requirements of each of the nearly 7 billion persons. Even with this abundance, in 2008, 963 million people were unable to access enough food to lead active, healthy lives—that is, they were **food insecure.** The serious problems of food insecurity and malnutrition exist in virtually every nation. They are most common in the developing world, with Asia having the largest number, along with sub-Saharan Africa, Latin America, and the Caribbean. Nearly all people suffering from food insecurity, hunger, or malnutrition are poor.

Let's begin our look at the problem of world hunger and malnutrition by defining some key terms.

Hunger

The physiological state that results when not enough food is eaten to meet energy needs is **hunger.** It also describes an uneasiness, a discomfort, a weakness, or a pain caused by lack of food. The medical and social costs of the undernutrition that can result from hunger are high—preterm births, mental disabilities, inadequate growth and development in childhood, poor school performance, decreased work output in adulthood, and chronic disease. Although malnutrition does occur in North America, it is not due to extreme poverty over a large section of the population. Instead, there are usually specific causes such as an eating disorder, alcoholism, problems in nursing home settings, or homelessness. There is also some degree of moderate malnutrition in some of the poorer segments of North American society (i.e., those earning less than the current poverty level). Fortunately, there are resources such as food banks and food stamps, though sometimes there are bureaucratic obstacles to getting these

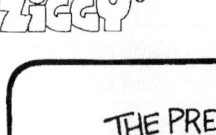

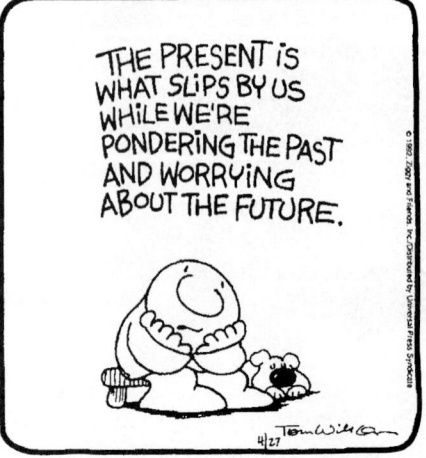

THE PRESENT IS WHAT SLIPS BY US WHILE WE'RE PONDERING THE PAST AND WORRYING ABOUT THE FUTURE.

Millions of people worldwide die each year from health problems related to undernutrition. Rising food prices, war, and environmental catastrophe combine with the global threat of AIDS as important causes. Why must we act today to stem this tide of undernutrition? Why is Ziggy's concern an important one? Chapter 12 provides some answers.

ZIGGY © ZIGGY AND FRIENDS, INC. Reprinted with permission of UNIVERSAL PRESS SYNDICATE. All rights reserved.

resources to the people who need them. In addition, there is the problem known as **food insecurity,** which describes a state of anxiety about running out of food or running out of money to buy more food. In 2009, 14.7% of households in the United States reported that they experienced food insecurity. Food insecurity is also a problem in Canada with 8% living in food-insecure households in 2008.

Around the world, poverty is a primary cause of malnutrition. In the United States, at least 13 million children, 18% of all children under the age of 18, are in families living below the federal poverty level, defined as a family of four having an income less than $22,350 a year in 2011 (more information available at http://aspe.hhs.gov/poverty/11poverty.shtml). Research, however, estimates that families need an income of about twice that level to cover basic expenses. Using this income standard, 39% of children live in low-income families. Living in poverty impairs a child's ability to learn and contributes to behavioral problems and poor health. The risks of poverty are greatest for young children. Fortunately, the United States does have food assistance programs for low-income families, and therefore most children in the United States are shielded from hunger.

Malnutrition and Micronutrient Deficiences

A condition of impaired development or function caused by either a long-term deficiency or excess in calorie and/or nutrient intake is **malnutrition.** When food supplies are low and the population is large, **undernutrition** is common, leading to nutritional deficiency diseases, such as goiter (from an iodide deficiency) and xerophthalmia (eye problems caused by poor vitamin A intake). However, when the food supply is ample or overabundant, incorrect food choices coupled with an excessive intake can lead to overnutrition and its related chronic diseases, such as type 2 diabetes.

Undernutrition is the most common form of malnutrition among the poor in both developing and developed countries. Undernutrition is also the primary cause of specific nutrient deficiencies that can result in muscle wasting, blindness, scurvy, pellagra, beriberi, anemia, rickets, goiter, and a host of other problems (Table 12-1).

The most critical micronutrients missing from diets worldwide (see Fig. 12-1) are iron, vitamin A, iodide, zinc, and various B vitamins (e.g., folate), as well as selenium and vitamin C (see Further Readings 7 and 11). About 1 billion people, mostly in the developing world, are affected by iron deficiency. The same is true for zinc deficiencies. With poor iron status, cognitive development will likely be impaired, particularly if prolonged deficiency occurs during early infancy. An estimated 50 million people worldwide also suffer brain damage from preventable maternal iodide deficiency. Although severe vitamin A deficiency, which causes blindness, is on the decline, up to 500,000 preschool-age children are still blinded by it each year. UNICEF reports that the lives of 1 million to 3 million children could be saved annually in the developing world if vitamin A supplements were provided a few times each year. The annual cost per child would be about 6 cents.

Of the 6.4 billion people in the world, about 2 billion may experience episodes of food shortages and be affected by some form of micronutrient malnutrition. Death and disease from infections, particularly those causing acute and prolonged diarrhea or respiratory disease, increase dramatically when the infections occur during a state of chronic undernutrition. Chronic undernutrition leaves many people in the developing world in a continual state of depressed immune function, in turn greatly increasing the risk of death, especially in childhood.

Protein-calorie malnutrition (PCM) is a form of undernutrition caused by an extremely deficient intake of calories or protein generally accompanied by an illness. The dramatic results of PCM—kwashiorkor and marasmus—were described in Chapter 6. This chapter focuses on the more subtle effects of a chronic lack of food.

Famine

The extreme form of chronic hunger is **famine.** Periods of famine are characterized by large-scale loss of life, social disruption, and economic chaos that slows food production. As a result of these extreme events, the affected community experiences

food insecurity A condition of anxiety regarding running out of either food or money to buy more food.

malnutrition Failing health that results from longstanding dietary practices that do not coincide with nutritional needs.

undernutrition Failing health that results from a longstanding dietary intake that is not enough to meet nutritional needs.

famine An extreme shortage of food, which leads to massive starvation in a population; often associated with crop failures, war, and political unrest.

The Irish potato famine of 1840 to 1850 caused an estimated 2 million deaths and resulted in nearly as many people emigrating to other countries, such as the United States and Canada. More than 3 million people may have perished in the great famine of 1943 in Bengal, India. China suffered a famine from 1959 to 1961—estimates of mortality range from 16 million to 64 million. In 1974, another 1.5 million starved in the country of Bangladesh.

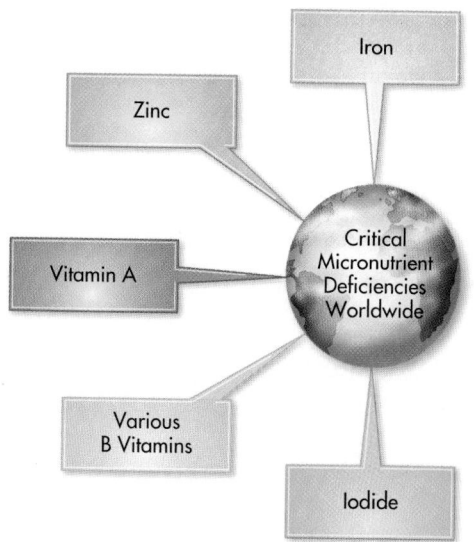

FIGURE 12-1 ▶ Critical micronutrient deficiencies worldwide.

TABLE 12-1 Nutrient-Deficiency Diseases That Commonly Accompany Undernutrition

Disease and Key Nutrient Involved*	Typical Effects	Foods Rich in Deficient Nutrient	Target Populations for Intervention
Xerophthalmia Vitamin A	Blindness from chronic eye infections, restricted growth, dryness and keratinization of epithelial tissues	Fortified milk, sweet potatoes, spinach, greens, carrots, cantaloupe, apricots	Asia, Africa
Rickets Vitamin D	Poorly calcified bones, bowed legs, other bone deformities	Fortified milk, fish oils, sun exposure	Asia, Africa, and parts of the world where religious dress codes prevent women and children from receiving adequate sun exposure; older adults in developed nations
Beriberi Thiamin	Nerve degeneration, altered muscle coordination, cardiovascular problems	Sunflower seeds, pork, whole and enriched grains, dried beans	Victims of famine in Africa
Ariboflavinosis Riboflavin	Inflammation of tongue, mouth, face and oral cavity, nervous system disorders	Milk, mushrooms, spinach, liver, enriched grains	Victims of famine in Africa
Pellagra Niacin	Diarrhea, dermatitis, dementia	Mushrooms, bran, tuna, chicken, beef, peanuts, whole and enriched grains	Victims of famine in Africa, survivors of war-torn Eastern Europe
Megaloblastic anemia Folate	Enlarged red blood cells, fatigue, weakness	Green leafy vegetables, legumes, oranges, liver	Asia, Africa
Scurvy Vitamin C	Delayed wound healing, internal bleeding, abnormal formation of bones and teeth	Citrus fruits, strawberries, broccoli	Victims of famine in Africa
Iron-deficiency anemia Iron	Reduced work output, retarded growth, increased health risk in pregnancy	Meats, seafood, broccoli, peas, bran, whole-grain and enriched breads	Worldwide
Goiter Iodide	Enlarged thyroid gland in teenagers and adults, possible mental retardation, cretinism	Iodized salt, saltwater fish	South America, Eastern Europe, Africa

*Although the nutrients are listed separately to illustrate the important role of each one, often two or more nutrition-deficiency diseases are found in an undernourished person in the developing world.

a downward spiral characterized by human distress; sales of land, livestock, and other farm assets; migration; division and impoverishment of the poorest families; crime; and the weakening of customary moral codes, as seen in Sudan and Rwanda. In the midst of all this, undernutrition rates soar; infectious diseases, such as cholera, spread; and many people die.

Special efforts are needed to eradicate the fundamental causes of famine. Causes vary by region and decade, but the most common is crop failure. The most obvious reasons for crop failure are extreme weather conditions such as floods or drought, war, and civil strife. War deserves a special focus and will be specifically addressed in a separate section on war and political/civil unrest.

General Effects of Semistarvation

In the initial stages, the results of undernutrition from semistarvation are often so mild that physical symptoms are absent and blood tests do not usually detect the slight metabolic changes. Even in the absence of clinical symptoms, however, undernourishment may affect reproductive capacity, resistance to and recovery from disease, and physical activity and work output, and lead to fatigue and behavior problems. Recall from Chapter 2 that, as tissues continue to be depleted of nutrients, blood tests eventually detect biochemical changes, such as a drop in blood hemoglobin concentration. Physical symptoms, such as body weakness, appear with further depletion. Finally, the full-blown symptoms of the predominating deficiency are recognizable, such as when blindness accompanies a vitamin A deficiency.

When a few people in a population develop a severe deficiency, this may represent only the "tip of the iceberg." Typically, a much greater number have milder degrees of undernutrition. These deficiencies should not, therefore, be dismissed as trivial, especially in the developing world. It is becoming clear that combined deficiencies of specific vitamins and the minerals iron and zinc can seriously reduce work performance, even when they do not cause obvious physical symptoms. This resulting state of ill health, in turn, diminishes the ability of individuals, communities, and even whole countries to perform at peak levels of physical and mental capacity (Fig. 12-2).

Added to their lack of nourishment, the inhabitants of poorer countries must also contend with recurrent infections, poor sanitation, extreme weather conditions, and regular exposure to infectious diseases. They require greater amounts of certain nutrients—especially iron—to combat rampant parasite and other infections. Deficiencies of both iron and zinc can lead to reduced immune function and thereby increase the risk of diseases, such as diarrhea and pneumonia.

The effects of hunger are widespread:

- Reduced energy and strength
- Diminished concentration
- Impaired ability to learn
- Lowered productivity
- Worsening of chronic health conditions
- Increased susceptibility to infectious diseases
- Deterioration of mood
- Slowed recovery from illness and injury

Historical Research on Undernutrition

In the 1940s a group of researchers led by Dr. Ansel Keys examined the general effects of undernutrition on adults. Previously healthy men were fed a diet averaging about 1800 kcal daily for 6 months. During this time, the men lost an average of 24% of their body weight. After about 3 months, the participants complained of fatigue, muscle soreness, irritability, intolerance to cold, and hunger pains. They exhibited a lack of ambition, self-discipline, and concentration, and were often moody, apathetic, and depressed. Their heart rate and muscle tone decreased, and they developed edema. When the men were permitted to eat normally again, feelings of recurrent hunger and fatigue persisted even after 12 weeks of rehabilitation. Full recovery required about 8 months. This study helps us understand the general state of undernourished adults worldwide.

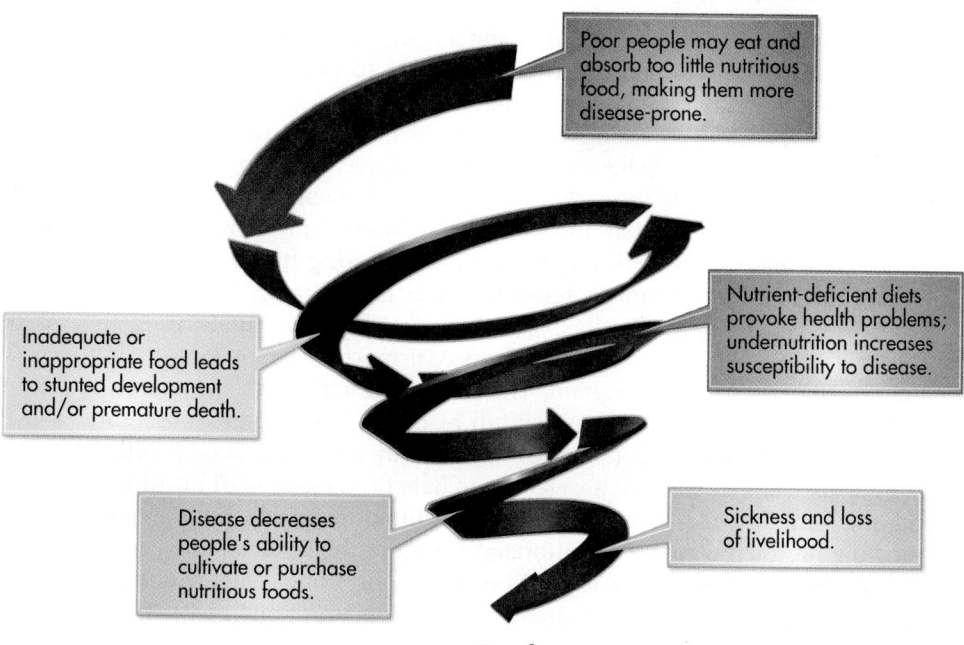

Death

FIGURE 12-2 ▶ The downward spiral of poverty and illness can ultimately end in death (based on World Food Program graphic).

CONCEPT CHECK

Hunger provokes uneasiness and pain when insufficient food is eaten to meet calorie needs. Food insecurity is anxiety about running out of food or money to buy more food. Chronic hunger leads to undernutrition, which can cause growth failure in children and physical weakness in adults. Risk of infection increases, and nutrient-deficiency diseases result. The primary cause of undernutrition is poverty. The critical periods for undernutrition occur during pregnancy, infancy, childhood, and old age. Chronic undernutrition decreases work performance, motivation, and immune function. The adverse effects in pregnancy and infancy are dramatic, as evidenced by mortality rates much higher than those of healthy populations. Irreversible developmental damage in surviving children is also common.

12.2 Undernutrition in the United States

About 50 million (14.7%) people in the United States live at or below the poverty level, estimated at about $22,350 annually for a family of four. Of those 50 million, 17 million (34%) are children. The percentage of the population living in food-insecure households in Canada is lower than in the United States (see Further Reading 14).

Ten percent of Caucasians, 24% of African-Americans, and 20.6% of Hispanics live in poverty. Many Native Americans are also poor, as are 18% of Asian Americans. (Many Native Americans in Canada also live in poverty.)

The poor often face difficult choices: whether to buy groceries for the family or pay this month's rent; whether to have dental work done or pay the current utility bill; whether to replace clothes the children have outgrown or pay for transportation to apply for a job. Food is one of the few flexible items in a poor person's budget. Whereas housing and utility costs, medical care, and transportation fares are non-negotiable, a person can always eat less. The short-term consequences of eating less may be less dramatic than getting evicted, but the long-term cumulative effects are significant.

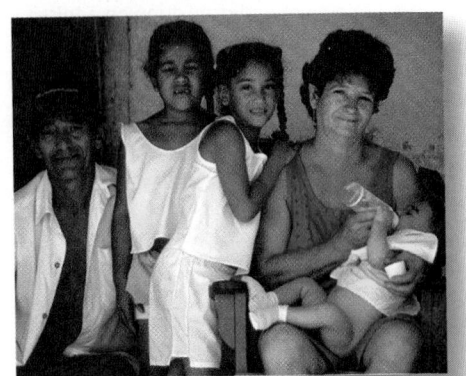

▲ Food insecurity is part of the North American landscape. A "safety net" of programs exists, but it is "porous."

Helping the Hungry in the United States

Until the twentieth century, individuals and a wide variety of charitable, often church-related organizations, provided most of the help to poor, undernourished people in the United States. Early programs rarely distributed direct cash payments to poor people because these were thought to reduce recipients' motivation to improve their circumstances or change behaviors, such as excessive drinking, that contributed to their poverty. Beginning in the early 1900s, the involvement of local, county, and state governments in providing assistance to the poor has steadily increased.

After observing extensive hunger and poverty during his presidential campaign in the 1960s, John F. Kennedy revitalized the Food Stamp Program, which had begun two decades earlier, and expanded commodity distribution programs. As of October 1, 2008, Supplemental Nutrition Assistance Program (SNAP) is the new name for the Food Stamp Program. The new name reflects the program's focus on nutrition and putting healthy food within reach for low-income households. SNAP helps low-income people and families buy food they need for good health. The program allows recipients to use an Electronic Benefit Transfer (EBT) card to purchase food and garden seeds—but not tobacco, cleaning items, alcoholic beverages, and nonedible products—at stores authorized to accept them. In recent years, each participating household received about $190 per month, on average. About 39 million people in the United States participate in this program (Table 12-2). The American Recovery and Reinvestment Act of 2009 increased benefits for SNAP participants. The increase for a participating household of four was $80 in monthly benefits.

The U.S. Congress established the School Breakfast Program in 1965 as politicians became aware of the number of hungry children coming to school. School breakfast and lunch programs still enable low-income students—11.7 million for breakfast

TABLE 12-2 Some Current Federally Subsidized Programs That Supply Food for People in the United States

Program	Eligibility	Description
Supplemental Nutrition Assistance Program (formerly Food Stamp Program)*	Low-income families	Electronic Benefit Transfer (debit) cards are given to purchase food at grocery stores; the amount is based on size of household and income.
The Emergency Food Assistance Program (TEFAP)*	Low-income families	Provides nutrition assistance to needy Americans through distribution of USDA food commodities.
Commodity Supplemental Food Program	Certain low-income populations, such as pregnant women, children until the age of 6 years, and seniors	USDA surplus foods are distributed by county agencies; not found in all states; may be based on nutritional risk.
Special Supplemental Nutrition Program for Women, Infants, and Children (WIC)*	Low-income pregnant/lactating women, infants, and children less than 5 years old at nutritional risk	Coupons are given to purchase milk, cheese, fruit juice, cereal, infant formula, and other specific food items at grocery stores; includes nutrition education component. Includes new Farmers' Market Nutrition Program (FMNP).
National School Lunch Program*	Low-income children of school age	Free or reduced-price lunch is distributed by the school; meal follows USDA pattern based on MyPyramid; cost for the child depends on family income. For students who do not participate in the lunch program, special milk program may be available.
School Breakfast Program	Low-income children of school age	Free or reduced-price breakfast is distributed by the school; meal follows USDA pattern; cost for the child depends on family income.
Child and Adult Care Food Program	Child enrolled in organized child-care program and seniors in adult-care programs; income guidelines are the same as those for the School Lunch Program	Reimbursement is given for meals supplied to children at the site; meals must follow USDA guidelines based on MyPlate.
Congregate Meals for the Elderly	Age 60 or over (no income guidelines)	Free noon meal is furnished at a site; meal follows specific pattern based on one-third of nutrient needs.
Home-Delivered Meals	Age 60 or over, homebound	Noon meal is delivered at no cost or for a donation at least 5 days a week. Sometimes additional meals for later consumption are delivered at the same time; often referred to as "Meals on Wheels."
Summer Food Service Program	Residence in a low-income neighborhood or participation in a program	Free, nutritious meals and snacks are given to children in a low-income area at a central site, such as a school or a community center during long school vacations.
Food Distribution Program on Indian Reservations*	Low-income American Indian and non-Indian households on reservations; members of federally recognized tribes	Alternative to Supplemental Nutrition Assistance Program, distribution of monthly food packages; includes nutrition education component.
Fresh Fruit and Vegetable Program	Low-income elementary schools	Provides free fresh fruits and vegetables to increase their consumption and to combat childhood obesity.

* Benefits increased through the American Recovery and Reinvestment Act of 2009.

and 31.7 million for lunch in 2010—to receive meals free or at reduced cost if certain income guidelines are met (under $29,055 to $41,348, respectively, for annual income of a family of four). In the same year, the U.S. Congress funded group noon-time (called *congregate*) meals and home-delivered meals for all citizens over 60 years of age, regardless of income (donations are requested, however). Both remain active programs, serving about 1 million meals each day, but they still do not reach all who need help. In addition, in 1972, the Special Supplemental Nutrition Program for Women, Infants, and Children (WIC) was authorized. This program provides food

CRITICAL THINKING

While studying early childhood development, Nakia was surprised to learn that some children in the United States are undernourished. What evidence might Nakia observe in children that would suggest undernourishment?

vouchers and nutrition education to low-income pregnant and lactating women and their young children. It serves about 9.2 million people. Read more about child and adolescent nutrition assistance programs in Further Reading 4.

Between 1969 and 1971, some already large federal food programs were expanded and others were created. For example, the Food Stamp Program served only 2 million people in 1968, but by 1971 it was serving 11 million. The National School Lunch Program, which served only 2 million poor children before 1970, was serving 8 million children by 1971. Soon after, the School Breakfast Program, a pilot program for children living in impoverished areas, became available nationally.

Sometimes, severe undernutrition due to involuntary hunger does occur in the United States. More often, though, Americans experience periodic episodes of hunger and food insecurity. Unemployment, medical and housing expenses, and even occasional holiday shopping can cause a household to be hungry or food insecure.

Government food assistance programs are like a "safety net"—they are strong, yet porous. The Recovery Act that was signed by President Obama in February 2009 was an unprecedented effort to increase benefits and services offered by the federal food and nutrition programs (Table 12-2). The enhancement of these programs has helped those workers and families hardest hit by the economic crisis. Privately funded programs have stepped in to add to state and federal efforts to combat hunger and related food insecurity in the United States. There are more than 150,000 charitable food providers (such as food banks and food pantries) helping to cope with this problem. They serve about 23 million Americans. Many low-income U.S. households rely on food pantries, and one survey found that slightly more than two of every three people requesting such emergency food assistance are members of families—children and their parents.

MAKING DECISIONS

Food Insecurity and Overweight?

Undernutrition in North America is a much more subtle problem than in developing countries. To the untrained eye, undernourished children may just seem skinny, when, in fact, their growth is being stunted by insufficient nutrients. More likely, though, children from food-insecure households are prone to be overweight. This may be the result of considerable reliance on convenience foods that provide mostly fat and sugar. Also, food-insecure families may buy candies and snack foods as treats when expensive toys and clothing aren't affordable.

The availability of cooking facilities affects nutrient intake among the poor. Without cooking facilities, people may buy expensive convenience foods that require no preparation. These are typically highly processed snack foods, which provide calories but are often lacking in nutrients.

Socioeconomic Factors Related to Undernutrition

In the United States, persistent hunger and food insecurity are largely associated with two interrelated conditions: poverty and homelessness. Thus, the economic, social, and political changes that lead to an increase in the number of poor or homeless people also tend to intensify the problem of undernutrition.

Poverty. Underemployment leads to poverty. This relationship has increased significantly with the economic recession that began late in 2007. The recent economic crisis is the worst in decades and has caused unemployment to soar. Between December 2007 and September 2009, 7.6 million jobs were lost. These job losses occurred across all major private-sector industries, including manufacturing, retail trade, leisure and hospitality, financial, transportation, and warehousing. In June 2011, the number of unemployed persons was 14.1 million, resulting in an unemployment rate of 9.2%. The impact of the increase in unemployment has been enhanced because, during the economic downturn, many states have cut their welfare assistance. This combination of events has resulted in more people living in poverty and in need of food assistance, at risk of homelessness, and without sufficient healthcare.

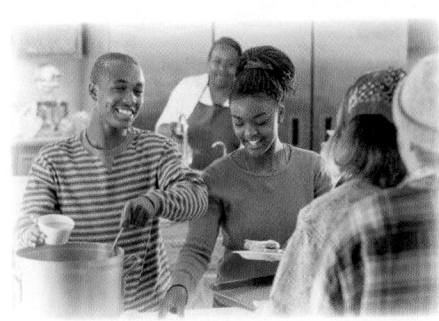

▲ Food pantries and soup kitchens are important sources of nutrients for a growing number of people in the United States. Consider volunteering some of your time to a local program.

Access to Healthy Food. Access to affordable and nutritious foods is also a challenge to many (see Further Reading 6). In 2011, 23.5 million Americans, including 6.5 million children, lived in low-income areas lacking stores likely to sell affordable healthy foods such as fresh fruits and vegetables. These impoverished areas with little access to healthy foods have been named "food deserts." The USDA defines a food desert as an area where 33% or 500 people, whichever is less, live more than a mile from a grocery store in an urban area, or more than 10 miles away in a rural area. In 2011, several national retail stores, including Wal-Mart, Walgreens, and SuperValu, as well as some regional companies, agreed to bring more nutritious and fresh food to underserved communities by opening or expanding more than 1500 stores. These changes were aimed to serve about 9.5 million people and to create tens of thousands of jobs.

Homelessness. The growing shortage of affordable rental housing and a simultaneous increase in poverty are the two trends largely responsible for the rise in homelessness over the past 25 years. The more recent foreclosure and economic crises have added to this situation and created a significant increase in homelessness and the number of families at risk of homelessness across the country. In 2009, data from major cities indicated increases of homelessness by as much as 20% since the foreclosure crisis began in 2007. A study done by the National Law Center on Homelessness and Poverty estimates that 3.5 million people, including 1.35 million children are likely to experience homelessness in a given year. Families with children are one of the fastest growing homeless groups, especially in rural areas, and make up about 23% of the homeless population. Single mothers in their late 20s with approximately two children are the most common heads of homeless families. Poor people must make difficult choices when limited resources cover only some necessities such as housing, food, childcare, health care, and education. Because housing absorbs a high percentage of income, it is often given up. Currently the largest gap on record exists between the number of affordable housing units and the number of people needing them. The homelessness created by this gap impacts the health and well-being of all individuals. Homeless children are most vulnerable and are twice as likely to experience hunger compared to children with a home.

Possible Solutions to Poverty and Hunger in the United States

Government-funded food assistance programs have helped to alleviate some problems of undernutrition in the United States. The question is, *Can government programs provide a permanent solution to poverty and undernutrition . . . and should they?* (see Further Reading 2).

It is documented that an increasing number of people who are experiencing poverty are accessing the Supplemental Nutrition Assistance Program (SNAP; formerly called the Food Stamp Program) benefits as well as other federal programs. As a result of the American Recovery and Reinvestment Act of 2009 (www.recovery.gov), more federal funds have been infused into assistance programs. There is no guarantee, however, that benefits from these programs will suitably meet the needs of the poor. In addition, there is a growing sentiment that state and federal support programs and policies are ineffective and inappropriate. These concerns are especially expressed by those who are falling deeper into poverty and those who are at increased risk of poverty and homelessness.

Obtaining food to survive is a tremendous challenge, especially when homeless people are forced to live outside. Surveys on hunger and homelessness in U.S. cities indicate that indoor food programs are not adequate to meet the need in some cities. A national survey by the Interagency Council on Homelessness also revealed that 40% of homeless people did not have anything to eat on one or more days during the month previous to the survey.

Although many people assume that food pantries and soup kitchens are abundant and accessible for every needy person there are many obstacles to these resources. Food pantries are often ineffective because they can give only one box of food to

food desert An area where 33% or 500 people, whichever is less, live more than a mile from a grocery store in an urban area or more than 10 miles away in a rural area.

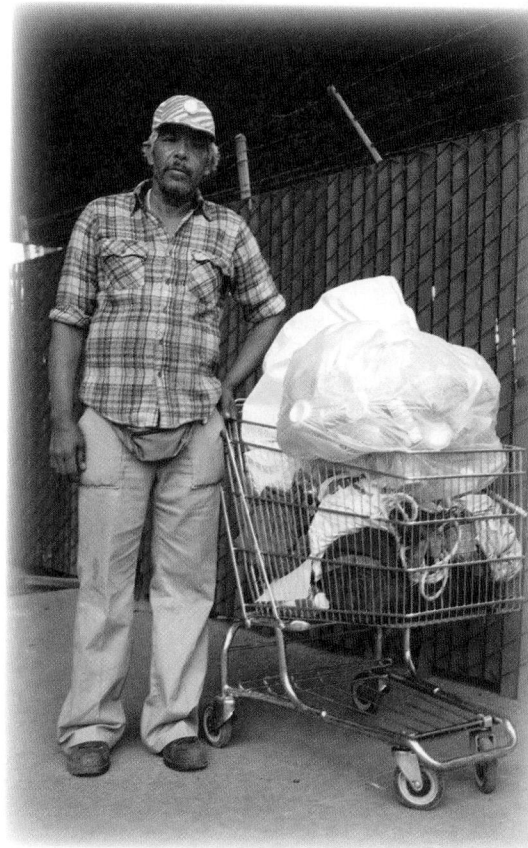

▲ Homelessness can be the result of many problems, including poverty.

families per month, which does not meet their needs. Furthermore, homeless people lack the cooking facilities necessary to prepare the food. Food availability through soup kitchens is also limited in many cities. An additional challenge is that cities have recently begun to use ordinances and policies to discourage or prohibit the sharing of food with poor or homeless persons by individuals and groups. These laws are troubling, considering that most cities do not have adequate food resources to meet the need of their poor and homeless. Advocacy groups raise questions about individual rights and freedoms and have challenged these practices in court cases. Advocates and food providers appear eager to work with cities and other government agencies to help address the problems of hunger and homelessness by improving access to federal food benefits and other food resources.

Despite even the highest motivation, the outlook is bleak for many people who attempt to gain independence from assistance programs. Teen pregnancy may have cut short the education or vocational training of one or both parents, thwarting efforts to earn adequate income. Often, the expense of reliable and safe child care far exceeds the meager income from a minimum-wage job. Illness of either the parents or children may prevent the adults from holding steady employment. Poor communication skills, inability to relocate, and a lack of economic reserves also complicate financial independence. Regardless of how wasteful government assistance appears to some people, it will probably always be necessary to some extent.

Many consider an increase in individual responsibility as a critical goal. Government programs cannot easily fix poverty and the resulting hunger that stem from irresponsible individual behavior. Government programs can, however, help reduce or prevent the poverty that results largely from lack of education or opportunity.

Long-term undernutrition—especially among children—has both individual and societal consequences, so everyone in the United States is affected by this problem, either directly or indirectly. As government programs are redesigned, it is likely that some will suffer. The hope is that these new approaches will lead to long-term progress and the eventual relief of poverty and hunger.

Two objectives of *Healthy People 2020* are to eliminate very low food security among children from 1.3% of households in 2008 to 0.2% in 2020 and to reduce hunger by reducing household food insecurity from 14.6% of households in 2008 to 6% in 2020.

CONCEPT CHECK

In response to reports of widespread poverty and hunger during the 1960s, the U.S. Congress established several food assistance programs and substantially increased funding for already existing programs. Largely as a result of these federal programs, undernutrition had decreased substantially by the mid-1970s. The presence of poverty, homelessness, and undernutrition is influenced by economic, cultural, and individual factors, as well as government policies. The serious questions about the long-term effectiveness of many government assistance programs are causing major changes in their program design. All citizens can help reduce the problem of undernutrition.

12.3 Undernutrition in the Developing World

Undernutrition in the developing world is also tied to poverty, and any true solution must address this problem. However, these countries have a multitude of problems so complex and interrelated that they cannot be treated separately. Programs that have proved immensely helpful in the United States (and throughout the rest of North America) are only a starting point in this context. The following major obstacles challenge those seeking a solution:

- Extreme imbalances in the food/population ratio in different regions of a country
- War and political/civil unrest, especially in Africa

- The rapid depletion of natural resources, such as farmland, fish, and water
- The disease AIDS, especially in sub-Saharan Africa and Asia
- High external (foreign) debt, much of which is owed to developed nations
- Poor **infrastructure,** especially poor housing, sanitation and storage facilities, education, communications, and transportation systems

Each problem deserves individual consideration (Fig. 12-3).

infrastructure The basic framework of a system of organization. For a society, this includes roads, bridges, telephones, and other basic technologies.

Food/Population Ratio

The world has 6.85 billion inhabitants. Population growth exceeds economic growth in much of the developing world, and as a result, poverty is increasing. This disrupts the balance in the food/population ratio, tipping it toward food shortages. If we want to ensure a decent life for a widening segment of humanity, many experts suggest that the growth in the earth's most vulnerable populations should slow. If not, by 2050 the world may have 1 to 3 billion more people than it does today—most of them in countries where the average person earns less than $2 per day. In developing countries, nearly 29% of people live on less than $1 per day. Unless a catastrophe occurs, more than 9 of 10 infants in the next generation will be born in the poorest parts of the world.

More than three-quarters of people in the world live in developing countries, and more than half live in Asia. A United Nations report on worldwide hunger revealed that almost two-thirds of the world's undernourished live in Asia and the Pacific Rim. The world's food supplies also are not distributed equally among consumers. Gross disparities exist between developed and developing countries, among the rich and the poor within countries, and even within families (males may be fed before females).

Still, economists estimate that world food production will continue to increase more rapidly than the world population in the near future, allowing the food/population ratio to increase through the year 2020. This will come at a high cost, however, in terms of the water, fertilizer, and pesticides needed to allow for this production. Overall, in the short run, the primary problem appears not to be food production *but* distribution and use, especially in poverty-stricken areas of developing nations.

Eventually, though, food production will begin to lag behind population growth. Most good farmland in the world is already in use, and because of poor farming practices or competing land-use demands, the number of farmable acres worldwide decreases annually. For many reasons, sustainable world food output—an amount that doesn't deplete the earth's resources—is now running well behind food consumption. This discrepancy suggests that food production in less-developed countries will barely keep up with population growth and will soon lag behind.

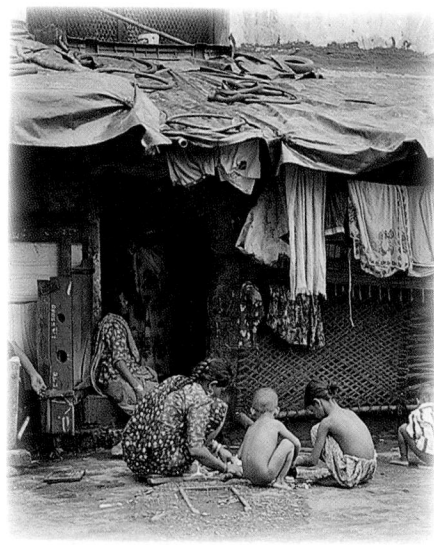

▲ Poverty aggravates the problem of hunger in the developing world

FIGURE 12-3 ▶ Many factors contribute to undernutrition in the developing world. Any solutions to the problem must take these factors into consideration.

AIDS

War and political/civil unrest

Rapid depletion of natural resources, such as farmland, fish, and water

Hunger in the Developing World

Extreme imbalances in the food/population ratio

Poor infrastructure

High external (foreign) debt

Birth control programs, an obvious brake on population expansion, have been effective in developed countries but relatively ineffective in many developing countries that could really benefit from them. Among women, family planning and contraceptive use worldwide has increased to 63% today, up from 10% in 1969. If the United Nations, voluntary organizations, and governments had not started promoting family planning and contraceptive use, the population today might be as high as 7 or 8 billion. However, women (and men) in many developing countries are still lacking adequate access to contraceptives. The United Nations estimates that at least 200 million women want to use safe and effective family planning methods, but they lack access to information and services or the support of their husbands and communities. Organizations such as Population Services International are trying to keep distribution costs low and make the products available to as many people as possible by subsidizing condoms and oral contraceptives to areas such as Bangladesh.

human immunodeficiency virus (HIV) The virus that leads to acquired immune deficiency syndrome (AIDS).

acquired immune deficiency syndrome (AIDS) A disorder in which a virus (human immunodeficiency virus [HIV]) infects specific types of immune system cells. This leaves the person with reduced immune function and, in turn, defenseless against numerous infectious agents; typically contributes to the person's death.

MAKING DECISIONS

Benefits of Breastfeeding

Promoting breastfeeding also contributes to the goal of birth control. Although it is not a completely reliable method of contraception, exclusively breastfeeding an infant lessens ovulation, thereby lowering the likelihood of fertilization, for an average of 6 months. (Women who do not breastfeed generally begin to ovulate within a month or so after giving birth.) When childbirths are more widely spaced, not only do fewer total births occur, but the mother has a longer chance to recover from pregnancy, and the infant receives feeding priority for a longer time. One possible exception to the healthful nature of breastfeeding occurs, however, when mothers are infected with the **human immunodeficiency virus (HIV).** The risk of transferring the virus through human milk is about 10%. Depending on the circumstances, this may outweigh the benefits of breastfeeding.

Experience with family planning programs in developing countries and historical changes in birth rates in many developed countries suggest an important conclusion. Generally, only when people have enough to eat and are financially secure do they feel confident that having fewer children will still result in enough surviving sons and/or daughters to provide for their care in later years. Increasing per capita income and improving education, especially for women in developing nations, are considered to be the most likely long-term solutions to excessive population growth. In the last few years, this effort has led to a decline in family size in Brazil, Egypt, India, and Mexico. A major concern is whether there are enough resources worldwide to raise per capita income and provide enough education to slow population growth.

CONCEPT CHECK

World food production is sufficient to meet the calorie needs of the world's population. Despite these adequate food resources, undernutrition continues to exist because of poverty, politics, and unequal food distribution. In addition, projected population growth may soon overwhelm food production. Most scientists and world leaders recommend limiting population growth, especially in developing countries where birth rates are high.

▲ Lasting gains have come slowly in the world's battle against undernutrition.

The conflicts in the Darfur region of Sudan have led to high rates of death and undernutrition among people displaced by war.

War and Political/Civil Unrest

The Millennium Summit of the United Nations in September 2000 resulted in the Millennium Declaration that included the resolution to "spare no effort to free our peoples from the scourge of war." Against that background stands the reality that worldwide military spending is reported to be over $2.1 trillion in annual expenditure and has been rising in recent years since 2001. The entire budget of the United Nations is only a fraction of the world's military expenditure at approximately 1.5%. In the twentieth century, deadly weapons of war took an enormous toll on civilians living in poor, politically vulnerable, war-torn nations. Less than one-half of 1% of the world's yearly production of goods and services is devoted to economic development assistance, whereas approximately 6% goes to military expenditures.

Aside from the economic impact of military spending, civil disruptions and wars are setting back the progress of the poor and contributing to massive undernutrition. Many regions of Africa have been involved in numerous civil wars and conflicts in recent years. These include conflicts in the countries directly involved in the Democratic Republic of Congo, the Sierra Leone crisis, and the war in Ethiopia/Eritrea. These conflicts have resulted in millions of deaths as well as over 9 million refugees and internally displaced people. While war has raged, health, education, and public services have declined for African people, and poverty has increased in Sub-Saharan Africa. War-related famine affects at least 20 million people in southern and northeastern Africa. The border war between Ethiopia and neighboring Eritrea has had a tremendous negative impact on food resources. A World Bank official stated that the food shortage in Ethiopia is a problem that will persist until political changes are made. Approximately 12.4 million people in Ethiopia, Eritrea, Djibouti, Kenya, Somalia, and Zimbabwe are at risk for food shortages. Other conflicts continue between Congo (formerly Zaire) and the Republic of Congo, as well as in Angola and Sudan, where millions have been put at risk of starvation (see Further Reading 12). In the capitol of war-torn Iraq, Baghdad, child malnutrition has increased dramatically. Disruptions in infrastructure from bombing and looting limit the safety of water, and as a result, health officials have observed a 250% increase in cases of diarrhea. Furthermore, health facilities needed to cope with undernutrition and dehydration have been damaged and looted throughout Baghdad and the surrounding area. Overall, most people in war-torn areas are without sufficient shelter, clothing, food, or means of obtaining them. Worldwide, this entire problem is projected to worsen over the next 15 years.

Even when food is available, political divisions may impede its distribution to the point that undernutrition will plague many people for years. Especially during emergencies, programs designed to help the poor have been undermined by unstable administration, corruption, and political influence. During such political chaos, relief agencies are often caught between warring factions and those they are trying to help. This has been the case in Sudan where non-governmental relief organizations, such as the Children's Hunger Relief Fund, have been expelled in recent years. This has caused continued deterioration in the Darfur region, and hundreds of thousands of refugees are left without the help they depended on from relief organizations.

During the 1960s and 1970s, the problem of undernutrition in developing countries was perceived as a technical one: how to produce enough food for the growing world population. The problem is now seen as largely political: how to achieve cooperation among and within nations, so that gains in food production and infrastructure are not wiped out by war. The best answer lies in a combination of approaches—finding technical solutions to help with the problems of chronic hunger and poverty and resolving political crises that have pushed developing nations into a state of acute hunger and chaos.

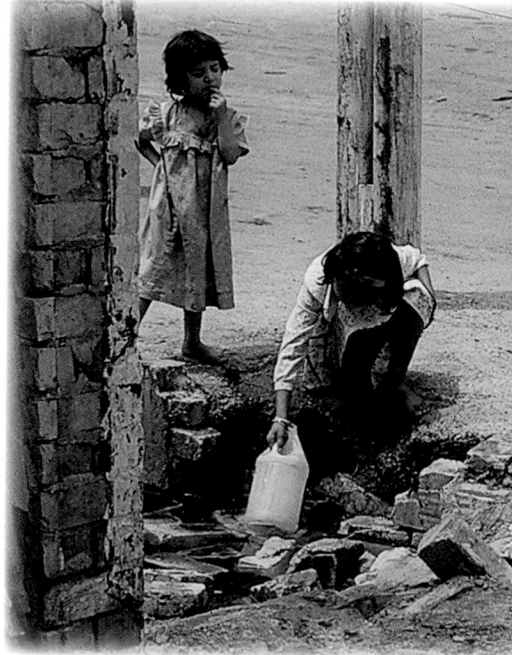

▲ Homes and infrastructure are often damaged during times of war and political unrest.

Rapid Depletion of Natural Resources

As we quickly deplete the earth's resources, population control grows increasingly critical. Agriculture production is approaching its limits in many areas worldwide. Environmentally unsustainable farming methods are undermining food production, especially in developing countries.

The **green revolution** was a phenomenon that began in the 1960s when crop yields rose dramatically in some countries, such as the Philippines, India, and Mexico (countries in Africa did not benefit because climates were not compatible with the

green revolution This refers to increases in crop yields that accompanied the introduction of new agricultural technologies in less-developed countries, beginning in the 1960s. The key technologies were high-yielding, disease-resistant strains of rice, wheat, and corn; greater use of fertilizer and water; and improved cultivation practices.

crops used). The increased use of fertilizers, irrigation, and the development of superior crops through careful plant breeding made this boost in agricultural production possible. Many of the technologies associated with the green revolution have now achieved their potential. Rice yields, for example, have not increased significantly since the release of superior varieties in 1966. (The green revolution was intended as a stopgap measure until world leaders could control population growth.)

Future gains in productivity may be much harder to accomplish because of the existence of less productive farmland. Until the introduction of another superior strain of rice or other grain, developing countries will not benefit greatly from recent, more modest breakthroughs in biotechnology (see the section on use of biotechnology).

Areas of the world that remain uncultivated or ungrazed are mostly too rocky, steep, infertile, dry, wet, or inaccessible to sustain farming. Nearly all irrigation water available worldwide is being used, and groundwater supplies are becoming depleted at rapid rates in many regions. An eventual water shortage is projected to increase war and civil unrest in arid areas of the world, such as Northern Africa and the Middle East. China, which has more than 20% of the world's irrigated land, is also plagued with a growing scarcity of fresh water. In the future, billions of people will face ongoing water shortages.

The prospects of obtaining substantially more food from the oceans are also poor. In recent years, the amount of fish caught worldwide has leveled off. Fish was once considered the poor person's protein, but this is not likely to continue because farming of fish does not come close to compensating for the degree of reduction in wild fish populations.

Clearly, we can exploit the earth's resources only so far—the world population probably cannot continue to expand as it does today without the potential for serious famine and death. The Food and Agriculture Organization (FAO) of the United Nations works on this principle: "The fight to ensure that all people have enough nutritious food to eat is worthy of our greatest efforts, but it must be fought with the full recognition that it cannot be won unless agricultural, fishery, and forestry production returns to the earth as much as—or more than—it takes." Thus, if food production is to keep up with the expanding population, immediate action is needed to protect the earth's already deteriorated environment from further destruction (see Further Reading 10).

Inadequate Shelter and Sanitation

When people die from undernutrition in developing countries, other factors, such as inadequate shelter and sanitation, almost always contribute. Poor sanitation along with undernutrition particularly raises the risk of infection. Inadequate and deteriorating shelters threaten the lives of more than 500 million people. Many of the 15 million annual deaths of children—half of them under 5 years old—in developing countries could be prevented by improving the standards of environmental hygiene. Urban populations of some developing countries are growing at an annual rate of 5% to 7%. Such a skewed population distribution will result in more poverty. The urban explosion is the result of both high birth rates and continuing migration of people to the cities from rural areas. People go to the cities to find employment and resources the countryside can no longer provide. Worldwide, 38% of people lived in urban areas in 1975. The figure is now about 50% and is expected to reach 70% by 2050. Nine of the world's 10 largest cities will be in poor countries 20 years from now. The World Bank reports that 16 of the 20 most polluted cities in the world are in China.

In developing countries, the poor make up most of the urban population, and their needs for housing and community services often go beyond available governmental resources. Most of these urban poor live in overcrowded, self-made shelters, which lack a safe and adequate water supply and are only partially served by public

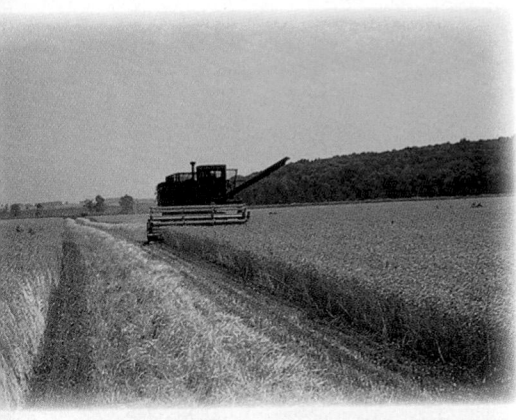

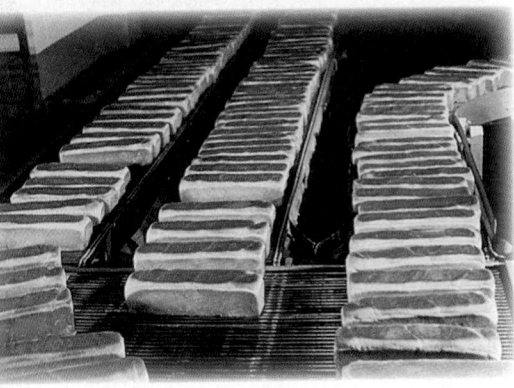

▲ Rich agricultural resources in North America, seen in the wheat fields above, results in a bounty of food to enjoy, such as these loaves of fresh bread.

In Brazil, migrants displaced by multinational land developers have flooded from the north and northeast into Rio de Janeiro and São Paulo, attracted by the prospect of jobs. There they have built shantytowns next to apartment towers and affluent suburbs, but the jobs do not materialize, and urban poverty replaces rural impoverishment.

utilities. The shantytowns and ghettos of the developing world are often worse than the rural areas the people left behind. The urban poor need cash to purchase food, so they often subsist on diets even more meager than the homegrown rural fare. Making matters worse, haphazard shelters often lack facilities to protect food from spoilage or damage by insects and rodents. This inability to protect food supplies in some developing countries leads to the loss of as much as 40% of all perishable foods.

The shift from rural to urban life takes its greatest toll on infants and children. Infants are often weaned early from the breast to infant formula, partly because the mother must find employment and partly because she may be influenced by advertisements depicting images of sophisticated, formula-feeding women. Unfortunately, because infant formulas are relatively expensive, poor parents may try to conserve the formula by either overdiluting the mixture or using too little to meet the infant's needs. The water supply may not be safe, so the prepared formula is also likely to be contaminated with bacteria. Human milk, in contrast, is much more hygienic, readily available, and nutritious. It also provides infants with immunity to some ailments. Promoting breastfeeding is important when it is safe for the infant (review the earlier discussion of AIDS, HIV, and breastfeeding).

Overall, the single most effective health advantage for people, wherever they live, is a safe and convenient water supply. Inadequate sanitation and the consumption of contaminated water cause 75% of all diseases and more than one-third of deaths in developing countries. The World Health Organization (WHO) estimates that 1.1 billion people, about one-sixth of all people, have an unsafe and inadequate water supply. In addition, up to 90% of the diseases seen in developing countries may be attributed to contaminated water.

Poor sanitation, another example of inadequate infrastructure in the developing world, creates a critical public health problem. Human feces, rotting garbage, and associated insect and rodent infestations are potent sources of disease organisms commonly seen in urban areas of the developing world. Two of the most dangerous substances encountered in routine daily living are human urine and feces. The inability to dispose of the massive numbers of dead people (and dead animals) resulting from civil wars causes additional sanitation problems. In some developing countries, diarrheal diseases account for as many as one-third of all deaths in children under 5 years of age. WHO estimates that even with improvements in housing, 2 billion people in the world still lack proper sanitation facilities. Read more about the sanitation crisis in Further Reading 16.

High External Debt

Since the 1970s many developing countries have become trapped in a cycle of borrowing repeatedly from foreign countries and international banks. Servicing these external debts has brought several countries to the verge of economic collapse. About $6 billion is owed to the United States. The external debt of Latin America represents 45% of the region's gross regional output of goods and services.

Many African nations also carry large debt burdens. This problem is made worse by drops in prices for the raw commodities they export, higher prices for imported oil, and embezzlement of funds by high-ranking officials. To make up the difference between export income and import expenses, countries have been forced to borrow millions of dollars from international banks. Although the African debts are much smaller in absolute terms than those of Brazil, Argentina, and Mexico, for example, the burden is greater when national incomes and export earnings are considered. Nearly half the money African nations earn from exports goes to paying off the continent's multibillion-dollar debt. Much of the rest goes to fund imports of machinery, concrete, trucks, and consumer goods from developed countries. This leaves little for domestic programs, necessitating cutbacks that translate into fewer resources to counter already widespread undernutrition.

Blood loss caused by intestinal and blood-borne parasite infections is another common cause of anemia among poor populations, especially when people do not wear shoes. Parasites, such as hookworms, can easily penetrate the soles of the feet and legs and enter the bloodstream. Although hookworm disease has been largely eradicated through improved sanitation in the United States and other industrialized nations, it continues to plague more than one-eighth of the world's population, mostly in tropical regions.

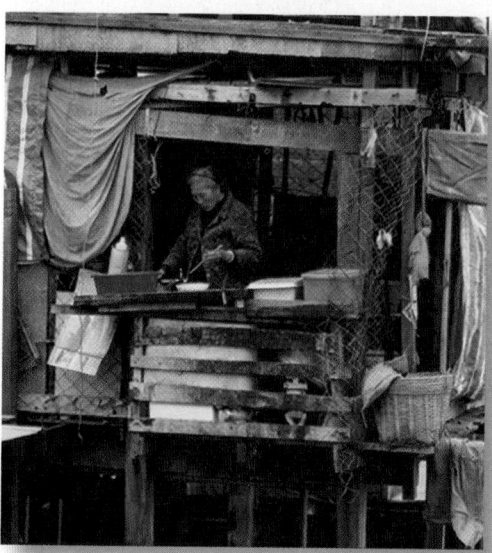

▲ Inadequate sanitation facilities and the consumption of contaminated water cause the majority of all diseases. About 1 billion people in developing countries often lack access to a safe water supply.

CONCEPT CHECK

War and civil strife, along with a decline in the world's natural resources, contribute to the difficulty of ending undernutrition in many developing countries. In addition, substandard housing conditions, impure water, and inadequate sanitation worldwide increase the risk for infection and disease. Infection then combines with undernutrition to compromise further the health of impoverished people. Finally, many developing countries are burdened by extremely high external debts, which severely limit their ability to implement programs to reduce undernutrition.

NEWSWORTHY
NUTRITION

Should HIV-positive women choose breastfeeding for their infants?

Exclusive breastfeeding is recommended for infants of HIV-positive women during the first months of life if available replacement feeding methods are not acceptable, feasible, affordable, sustainable, or safe for their circumstances. This study of South African HIV-positive women found that exclusive breastfeeding was successful when the women had a strong belief in the benefits of breastfeeding and a supportive home environment and when they could recall key messages on mother-to-child transmission risks and mixed feeding and could resist pressure from the family to introduce other fluids.

Source: Doherty T and others: A longitudinal qualitative study of infant-feeding decision making and practices among HIV-positive women in South Africa. *Journal of Nutrition* 136:2421, 2006 (see Further Reading 8).

connect NUTRITION   **Check out the Connect site** www.mcgrawhillconnect.com **to further explore HIV and breastfeeding.**

The Impact of AIDS Worldwide

About 33 million people around the world are infected with the human immunodeficiency virus (HIV) or have gone on to develop acquired immune deficiency syndrome (AIDS) from the infection. The male to female ratio is about 1:1 but is now increasing faster in women than in men in several countries. Although the annual number of AIDS deaths has declined worldwide since 2005, 1.8 million adults and children died with AIDS in 2009.

An individual can be infected with HIV through contact with bodily fluids including blood, semen, vaginal secretions, and human milk. Thus the virus can be transmitted through sexual contact; through blood-to-blood contact; as well as from a mother to an infant during pregnancy, delivery, or breastfeeding. The virus has a very limited ability to exist outside the body. Read more about HIV and breastfeeding in Newsworthy Nutrition and Further Readings 5 and 8.

Once infected with HIV, the individual is said to be HIV-positive. If untreated, the viral disease progresses over the next few years, and the individual develops symptoms of opportunistic infections such as diarrhea, lung disease, weight loss, and a form of cancer. Once the individual has developed these symptoms, they are said to have AIDS. Without treatment, an individual will likely die from AIDS within 4 to 5 years.

Global efforts are having some effect in that the HIV epidemic worldwide is stabilizing and the rate of new HIV infections has decreased in several countries (see Further Reading 13). From 2001 to 2009 the annual number of new HIV infections decreased from 3.1 to 2.6 million. In Africa, particularly sub-Saharan countries, HIV is rampant throughout the entire population, both in men and women. This region contains over 34% of the world's HIV-positive people (Fig. 12-4). In most areas of sub-Saharan Africa, AIDS is reducing life expectancy by one-half, especially if the person also has tuberculosis. In many countries, AIDS is also creating orphans, with an estimated 12 million in Africa alone.

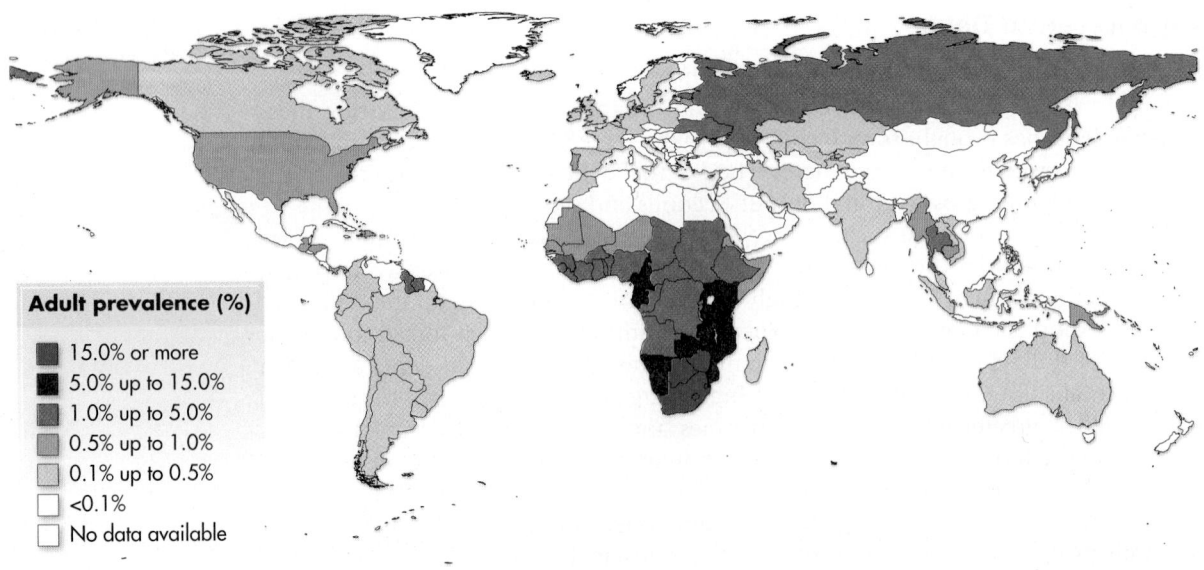

Adult prevalence (%)
- 15.0% or more
- 5.0% up to 15.0%
- 1.0% up to 5.0%
- 0.5% up to 1.0%
- 0.1% up to 0.5%
- <0.1%
- No data available

FIGURE 12-4 ▶ A global view of 33 million people living with HIV infection in 2009.

Source: Report on the Global HIV/AIDS Epidemic 2010: Executive Summary, 2010.

The largest regional increase in HIV prevalence has been in Eastern Europe and Central Asia. The number of people living with HIV in these areas has tripled since 2000.

North America also has an AIDS problem. In the United States, it is estimated that about 1 million people are infected with HIV, with 1 in 5 (21%) unaware of their infections. (Reports show 1 in every 100 persons in New York City is infected with HIV.) About 580,000 people in the United States have died from the disease since it surfaced in the early 1980s, and each year about 56,300 new cases are reported. HIV affects a greater percentage of minority populations in the United States.

The face of AIDS is quickly becoming the face of a child. In 2009, 2.5 million children under 15 years were living with HIV/AIDS globally. Most of those children, almost 9 in 10, live in sub-Saharan Africa. Fortunately there has been an estimated 19% decrease in AIDS-related deaths among children worldwide from 2004 to 2009.

Although no vaccine is available to prevent AIDS, the latest antiviral drugs can significantly slow the progression of the disease. However, there are many barriers to the use of these drugs in the developing world. For example, the newest therapies require a person to take at least three different drugs in the form of about 14 pills each day. A few missed doses can significantly reduce the effectiveness of the drugs and result in faster disease progression. Another barrier is economic: a typical drug regimen can cost approximately $14,000 per year, not including unforeseen hospital stays. Certain drug companies and governments are working to lower the cost of AIDS drugs for developing nations. Still, in most cases, the drugs will remain out of reach to those who need them. It has been suggested that developed nations should step in and cover most or all of the costs. The United Nations is spearheading an effort to raise the $8 to $10 billion needed to fight the disease.

MAKING DECISIONS

Nutrition and AIDS

Can eating a balanced diet prevent AIDS? The answer, unfortunately, is no. Healthy eating does not cure the disease, but it can help to lessen the impact of infections associated with AIDS. Poor nutritional status, such as a low status of vitamin A and vitamin E, contributes to a quicker onset of symptoms such as body wasting and fever, and a more rapid demise. This explains why daily use of a balanced vitamin and mineral supplement was shown to slow health declines in such people in one study. Overall, maintenance of nutritional status should be an integral part of the treatment for AIDS.

The devastating effects of AIDS on our civilization have been rapid when measured by earth's scale of time. One study warns us that 57 countries risk major HIV outbreaks. Reported HIV cases are increasing rapidly in Africa, the Indian subcontinent, Southeast Asia, China, the Caribbean, Russia, and much of Eastern Europe. The main goal for addressing the problem of AIDS in the developing world is prevention of new cases through education regarding safer sex and the importance of clean needles, and other behavior-linked approaches. Providing AIDS drugs to pregnant women is also important. If a woman begins taking AIDS drugs such as zidovudine (AZT) by the fourteenth week of pregnancy, the risk of transferring the virus to her offspring is greatly reduced. Providing the drug immediately before birth also helps (see Further Reading 9).

Behind the mind-boggling statistics on AIDS are less obvious costs to businesses, families, schools and universities, and society in general. For example, worker productivity will plummet because AIDS victims produce less and demand more, especially in the latter stages of the disease. Business productivity drops even further when relatives take time away from work and school to care for family members afflicted with AIDS. Furthermore, AIDS demands a considerable amount of family income. Hard-pressed families, who have to devote much of their income to doctors and medicines, have little left for living expenses. Other family members must struggle to keep up with daily duties because they must care for orphans left behind in the disease's wake. To learn more about AIDS, check out the website www.unaids.org.

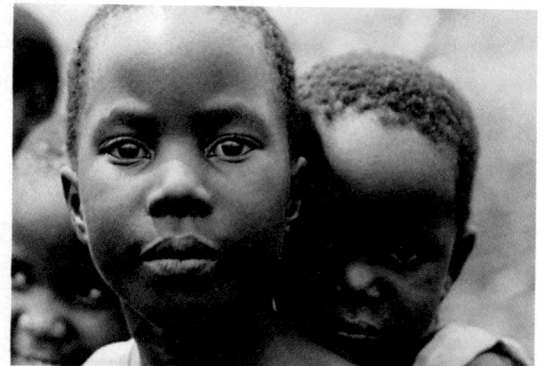

▲ A particularly sad consequence of AIDS in Africa is the number of AIDS orphans, children whose parents have both died of AIDS. The United Nations reports that about 15 million AIDS orphans have become responsible for the care of their siblings and other family members.

CONCEPT CHECK

About 40 million people around the world are infected with the human immunodeficiency virus (HIV) or have gone on to develop acquired immunodeficiency syndrome (AIDS) from the infection. The virus can be transmitted through sexual contact; through blood-to-blood contact; or from a mother to a baby during pregnancy, delivery, and breastfeeding. Without treatment, an individual once infected will likely die from AIDS within 4 to 5 years. The main hope for addressing the problem of AIDS in the developing world is prevention of new cases.

Reducing Undernutrition in the Developing World

As you have probably guessed, greatly reducing undernutrition in the developing world will be complicated and will take considerable time to accomplish (Fig. 12-5). It is a common practice for the more affluent nations to supply famine areas with direct food aid. However, direct food aid is not a long-term solution. Although it reduces the number of deaths from famine, it can also reduce incentives for local production by driving down prices. In addition, the affected countries may have little or no means of transporting the food to those who need it most, and the donated foods may not be culturally acceptable.

In the short run, there is no choice—aid must be given because people are starving (see Further Reading 3). Still, improving the infrastructure for poor people, especially rural people, needs to be the long-term focus. This future-minded approach is

FIGURE 12-5 ▶ Possible solutions to the puzzle of hunger in the developing world. Putting all the pieces together employs the action steps that contribute to meeting the overall goal.

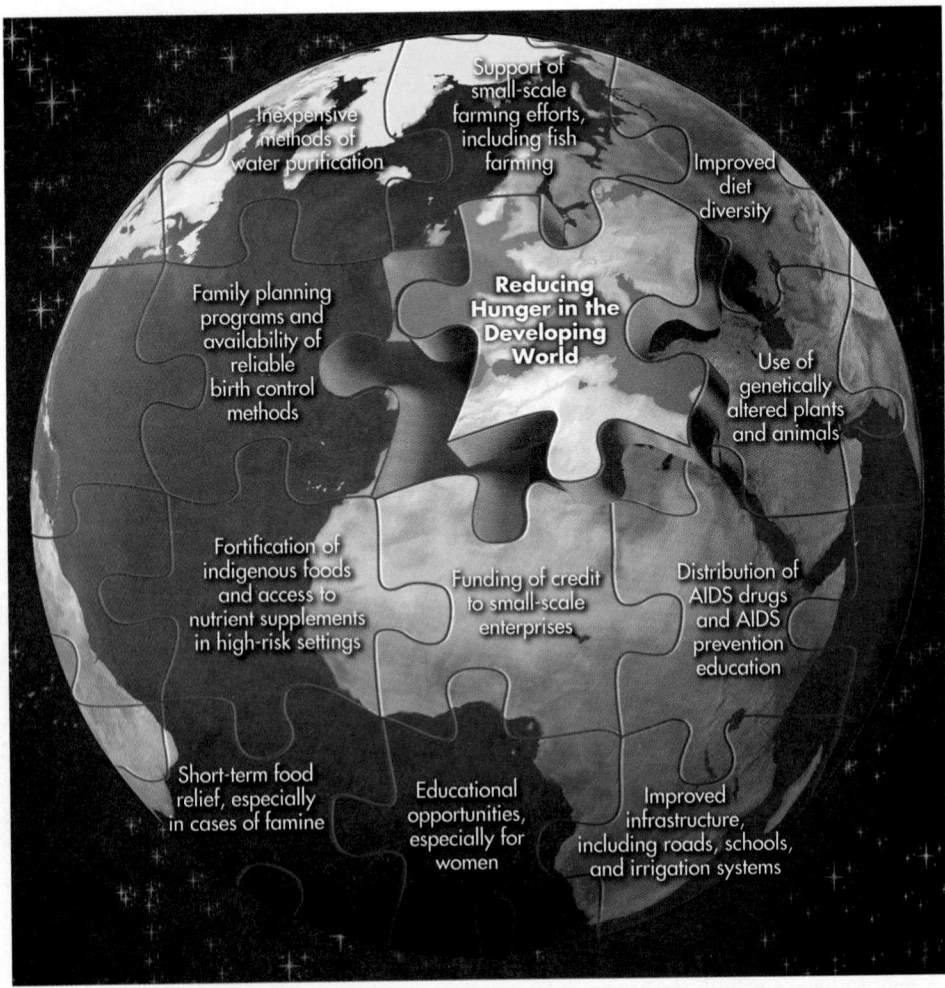

necessary because the most significant factor affecting the undernutrition of people in impoverished areas of the world is their reliance on outside sources for basic needs. Their dependence makes them constantly vulnerable.

Three basic approaches to counteract micronutrient deficiencies are suggested by the World Bank: increase diversity of the food supply; fortify specific foods with nutrients; and provide nutrient supplementation for individuals when necessary.

Development Tailored to Local Conditions Is Important. Recall that, in the past 40 years, world food supplies have grown faster than the population. Thus, the increase in undernutrition during this period has been caused by an increase in the number of people cut off from their share of this supply. Millions of farmers are losing access to resources they need to be self-reliant. There is a growing realization that unless economic opportunities can be created as part of a plan for sustainable development, rural people who own no land will flock to the overcrowded cities. In response, careful, small-scale regional development is one option.

For the most part, the solution lies in helping people meet their own needs and directing them to resources and employment opportunities, rather than giving them resources. Experience has shown that the provision of credit—along with training, food storage facilities, and marketing support—allows rural people to actively participate in their development, which will benefit their families and communities.

One U.S. program, the Peace Corps, has helped improve conditions in developing nations by providing education, distributing food and medical supplies, and building structures for local use. The aim of the Peace Corps is to help create independent, self-sustaining economies around the world.

Impoverished women are a special concern. In addition to working longer hours than men, they grow most of the food for family consumption and make up three-fourths of the labor force in the informal sector of the economy and an increasing proportion in the formal sector. Economic opportunities for women and education regarding family planning must be augmented. Of the 3 billion people in the world living on less than $2 a day, 70% are women. Moreover, among the developing world's 900 million illiterate people, women outnumber men 2 to 1. Thus, an important means of propelling nations out of poverty is to end the cycle of female neglect.

Suitable technologies for processing, preserving, marketing, and distributing nutritious local staples also need to be encouraged, so that small farmers can flourish. Education on how to use these foods to create healthful diets, such as preparing vitamin A-rich vegetables, adds further benefit. Supplementing indigenous foods with nutrients that are in short supply, such as iron, various B vitamins, zinc, and iodide, also deserves consideration. One program involves adding iron to sugar in various parts of the world. The next section examines the role of biotechnology in improving nutrient quality and other plant and animal characteristics, another possible positive step in lessening undernutrition. In addition, advances in water purification need to be employed.

Promoting extensive land ownership may also be one part of the solution. Increasing the availability of food is one of its many advantages. If food resources are concentrated among a minority of people, as often happens with unequal land ownership, food is not likely to be equally distributed unless efficient transportation systems are in place. Inequitable distribution then proves to be a difficult problem to resolve.

Raising the economic status of impoverished people by employing them is as important as expanding the food supply. If an increase in food supply is achieved without an accompanying rise in employment, there may be no long-term change in the number of undernourished people. Although food prices may fall with increased mechanization, use of fertilizers, and other modern technologies, it needs to be realized that these advances can also displace people from jobs, a result that worsens rather than helps the population.

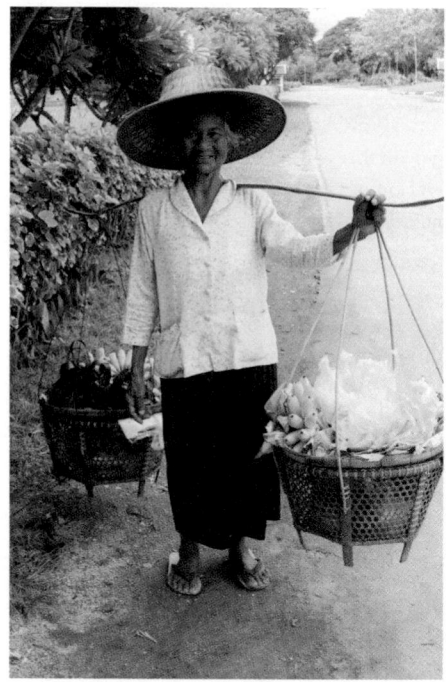

▲ Food security is fostered by communities raising and distributing locally grown food.

CRITICAL THINKING

Stan has read about various relief efforts to help undernourished people in developing countries, especially the emergency food aid programs for famine-ravaged areas. Many of these efforts appear to be only temporary, and he wonders what long-range approaches might help alleviate the problem of undernutrition. What suggestions would you give Stan about possible long-term solutions for undernutrition in developing countries?

sustainable development Economic growth that will simultaneously reduce poverty, protect the environment, and preserve natural capital.

gender and development (GAD) approach Understanding the roles and responsibilities of both men and women in the process of sustainable development.

MAKING DECISIONS

Sustainable Development and the Gender and Development (GAD) Approach

Sustainable development is economic growth that will reduce poverty while at the same time protect the environment and preserve natural capital. In its 2005 World Summit Outcome Document, the United Nations cites economic development, social development, and environmental protection as the "reinforcing pillars" of sustainable development. During the past 20 years, an understanding of the roles and responsibilities of both women and men in the community and the relationship of men and women to each other have been important components of sustainable development. The **gender and development (GAD) approach** works toward improving the status of women through the active participation of both men and women. By increasing women's access to education, information and communication technologies, economic resources, and governance, the GAD approach reduces poverty, promotes development, achieves gender equality, protects women's human rights, and eliminates violence against women.

12.4 The Role of Sustainable Agriculture and Biotechnology in Worldwide Food Availability

Sustainable Agriculture

Over the years, changes in agricultural practices have had many positive results on the availability of food around the world. Along with the positive effects on farming, however, there have been significant negative impacts. Most significant among these are depletion of topsoil, contamination of groundwater, the decline of family farms, neglect of living and working conditions for farm laborers, increasing costs of production, and the lack of integration of economic and social conditions in rural communities.

During the past two decades, the role of the agriculture industry in promoting practices that contribute to environmental and social problems has been debated. As a result, interest in alternative farming practices has grown and a movement toward **sustainable agriculture** has emerged. Sustainable agriculture describes farming systems that can indefinitely maintain their productivity and usefulness to society. Sustainable agriculture depends on the integration of several goals including environmental health, economic profitability, and social and economic equity. It addresses many environmental and social concerns, and offers innovative and economically viable opportunities for many in the food system including growers, laborers, consumers, and policymakers. Today sustainable agriculture is gaining support and acceptance from conventional farmers in many countries.

sustainable agriculture Agricultural system that provides a secure living for farm families; maintains the natural environment and resources; supports the rural community; and offers respect and fair treatment to all involved, from farm workers to consumers to the animals raised for food.

Sustainable agriculture involves maintaining or enhancing the land and natural resources for use long into the future. In addition, the social responsibilities of human resources, including working and living conditions of laborers, the needs of rural communities, and consumer health and safety, must be considered both in the present and the future. The potential of sustainability is best understood when the consequences of farming practices on both human communities and the environment are considered.

Farmers around the globe can succeed in their transition to sustainable agriculture by taking small realistic steps based on their personal goals and family economics. Reaching the goal of worldwide sustainable agriculture will require participation by all stakeholders including farmers, laborers, retailers, consumers, researchers, and policymakers.

The ability of humans to manipulate nature has enabled us to improve the production and yield of many important foods. Traditional **biotechnology** is almost as old as agriculture. The first farmer to improve stock by selectively breeding the best bull with the best cows was implementing biotechnology in a simple sense. The first baker to use yeast to make bread rise took advantage of biotechnology.

By the 1930s, biotechnology made possible the selective breeding of better plant hybrids. As a result, corn production in the United States quickly doubled. Through similar methods, agricultural wheat was crossed with wild grasses to confer more desirable properties, such as greater yield, increased resistance to mildew and bacterial diseases, and tolerance to salt or adverse climatic conditions.

Another type of biotechnology uses hormones rather than breeding. In the last decade, Canadian salmon have been treated with a hormone that allows them to mature three times faster than normal—without changing the fish in any other way. In general terms, biotechnology can be understood as the use of living things—plants, animals, bacteria—to manufacture products.

Biotechnology

The new biotechnology used in agriculture includes several methods that directly modify products. It differs from traditional methods because it more directly changes some of the genetic material (DNA) of organisms to improve characteristics. Crossbreeding plants or animals is no longer the only tool. Development of the new process, called **genetic engineering,** began in the 1970s. The field now features a wide range of cell and subcell techniques for the synthesis and placement of genetic material in organisms (Fig. 12-6).

This process of **recombinant DNA technology** allows access to a wider gene pool, and it permits faster and more accurate production of new and more useful microbial, plant, and animal species. Conventional breeding is inefficient and has inconsistent results; biotechnology uses genetic material more precisely. Scientists select the traits they want and genetically engineer or introduce the gene that produces the desired trait into plants or animals (now called a **genetically modified organism [GMO]** or **transgenic**). Genetic engineering has not replaced conventional breeding practices; both work together.

Biotechnology has been used to enhance crops in three main categories. The primary category is the addition of a unique characteristic called an *input trait* to a crop. These enhanced input traits include herbicide tolerance, insect and virus protection, and tolerance to environmental stressors such as drought. Other categories are

biotechnology A collection of processes that involves the use of biological systems for altering and, ideally, improving the characteristics of plants, animals, and other forms of life.

genetic engineering Manipulation of the genetic makeup of any organism with recombinant DNA technology.

recombinant DNA technology A test tube technology that rearranges DNA sequences in an organism by cutting the DNA, adding or deleting a DNA sequence, and rejoining DNA molecules with a series of enzymes.

genetically modified organism (GMO) Any organism created by genetic engineering.

transgenic Organism that contains genes originally present in another organism.

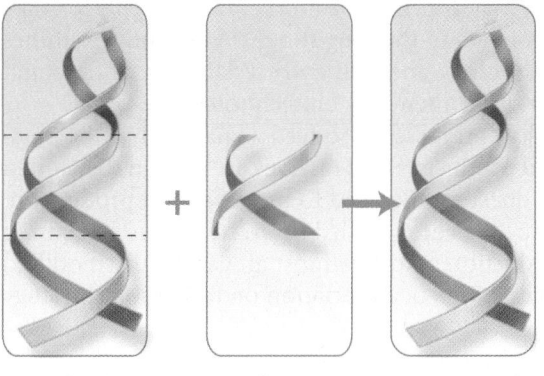

DNA of the host plant, corn.

Gene from bacteria (Bt gene) that produces a protein toxic to the European corn borer.

Bt gene inserted into DNA of corn plant. Now the corn plant is genetically modified. It makes the Bt toxin and, so, is resistant to the European corn borer.

FIGURE 12-6 ▶ Biotechnology involves various techniques for transferring foreign DNA into an organism. In this diagram, a sample of DNA is cleaved out of a larger DNA fragment and inserted into the DNA of a host cell. Thus, the host cell contains new genetic information, with the potential of providing the cell with new capabilities. For corn, this could mean resistance to the European corn borer. The corn plant is now referred to as a genetically modified organism (GMO). In another application, bacteria can be engineered to produce the human form of the hormone insulin.

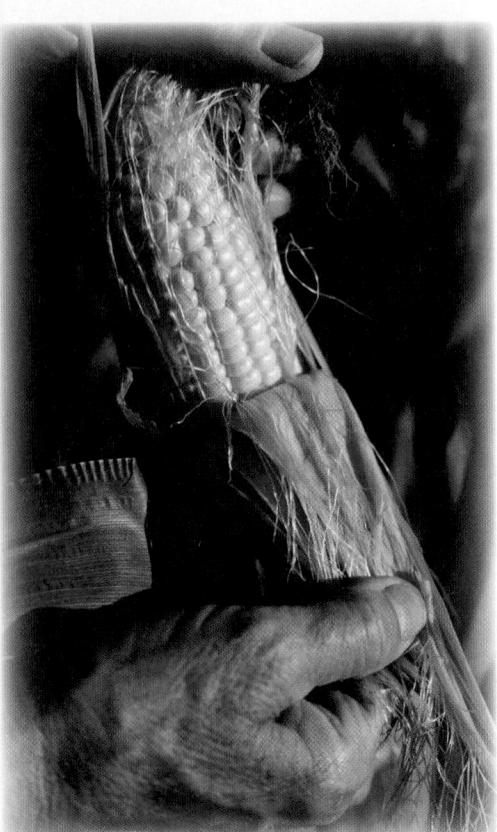

▲ Both traditional plant breeding and biotechnology have produced high-yielding and disease-resistant plant varieties, including new varieties of corn.

value-added output traits, such as plant oils with increased levels of omega-3 fatty acids, and crops that produce pharmaceuticals. Scientists have engineered plants that grow with the use of less pesticides and new forms of potatoes that can be stored longer without preservatives. In addition, biotechnology allows scientists to create fruits and grains with greater amounts of nutrients such as beta-carotene (e.g., "golden rice") and vitamins E and C. Biotechnology is being used cautiously and conservatively, so benefits of the new biotechnology will strike us as only subtly different. The ultimate benefits, however, could be important if foods eaten by people in the developing world can be so enhanced.

Few consumers in the United States realize that at least 72% of corn and 94% of soybeans produced in the United States have been genetically engineered to either resist certain insects, thereby reducing pesticide use, and/or survive when sprayed with herbicides that kill surrounding weeds. Papaya plants have been genetically engineered for viral resistance.

Genetic modification of corn has received a lot of media attention. Corn can be genetically altered by inserting a gene from the bacterium *Bacillus thuringiensis*, usually referred to as the Bt gene, into the corn DNA (Fig. 12-6). The gene allows the corn plant to make a protein lethal to certain caterpillars that destroy the plant. The Bt protein in the corn, however, is present in the plant in low concentrations and has no effect on humans—it is digested along with the other proteins in corn. For many years organic farmers have used the Bt bacteria as a dust on plants to destroy pests. (Dusting crops, however, does not change the DNA of the plant.)

FDA is confident that approved varieties of genetically engineered foods are safe to consume. Food manufacturers, therefore, are not required to disclose the genetically modified ingredient content on food labels. FDA does not believe labeling of GMO products is needed because they pose no health risk.

Public response to use of GMO biotechnology, however, has been mixed. Even the scientific community has conflicting opinions about this technology, with supporters as convinced about the benefits as opponents are of the risks. The biggest debate in the United States surrounds the potential environmental hazards of introducing genes from one species to another. Some challengers even question the reduction in pesticide use that accompanies the cultivation of genetically modified crops. Although the use of genetically modified crops may reduce the need for environmentally harmful activities, such as spraying crops with pesticides, critics point out that seeds produced with additional insecticide potentially will lead to rapid insect resistance because the insecticides are continuously emitted. Use of traditional pesticides involves prudent application, in part to avoid insect resistance. In addition, accidental release of genetically modified animals, such as fish, may go on to harm wild varieties.

Although the risks of biotechnology may appear to be momentarily negligible, they may be cumulative and therefore of concern in the long run. FDA carefully examines all products developed using this technology and will enforce labeling of potential allergens that may be newly present in food altered by biotechnology.

The public has long been opposed to processes perceived as harmful to the environment, such as producing unnatural products. Food reserves are high in the United States, Canada, and Europe, so some question the need to increase food production. Skepticism surrounds unnatural products, as exemplified by Western Europe's ban of hormones used in beef and milk production, and of almost all genetically modified foods. Read the position of the American Dietetic Association on food biotechnology in Further Reading 1.

Role of the New Biotechnology in the Developing World

Twenty-nine countries planted 366 million acres of crops enhanced through biotechnology in 2010. These crops included improved varieties of soybeans, corn, cotton, canola, papaya, and squash. The United States maintained the largest growth of biotech crops with nearly 165 million acres of soybeans, corn, and cotton. Brazil was second with 62 million acres. Developing countries also saw an increase, growing 48% of the biotech crops in 2010. Columbia, Honduras, and Iran were the second leading producers of biotechnology crops with acreage of 13.2 million. These countries aimed to increase crop production in rural areas to improve incomes and supply growing urban populations.

Whether applications of genetic engineering will help to significantly reduce undernutrition in the developing world remains to be seen. Unless price cuts accompany the increased production, only landowners and suppliers of biotechnology will enjoy the benefits. Small farmers may benefit if they can afford to purchase the genetically modified seeds. This point deserves emphasis: The person who cannot afford to buy enough food today will still face that same predicament in the future.

As with most innovations, the more successful farmers—often those with larger farms—will adopt the new biotechnology first. Because of this, the present trend toward fewer and larger farms will continue in the developing world, a movement that undermines the solution to one of the most pressing undernutrition issues there. Furthermore, biotechnology does not promise dramatic increases in the production of most grains and cassava, the primary food resources in developing parts of the world.

With the introduction of drought- and pest-resistant, as well as self-fertilizing crops, agricultural biotechnology may help to lessen world hunger. Perhaps the most promising potential of genetically modified foods today lies within the realm of plant breeding for micronutrients. Developing countries will then have a tool to treat and prevent selected nutrient deficiencies among their populations if they have access to farming resources to augment the micronutrient composition of crops. In addition, greater yields for indigenous plants, such as tomatoes that tolerate high soil salinity, are another hopeful outcome. Biotechnology will likely be a useful tool against the complex scourge of world undernutrition. Improved crops produced by this technology, together with political and other efforts, can contribute to success in the battle against worldwide undernutrition.

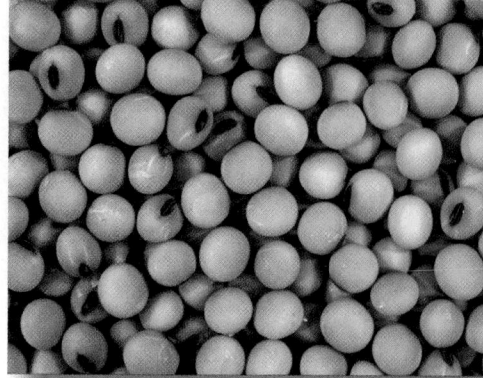

▲ Soybeans are a common GMO food in the marketplace. Over 90% of the soybeans grown in the United States are genetically modified.

Some Concluding Thoughts

The economic loss from undernutrition is staggering, and the amount of human pain and suffering is incalculable. With all the international relief efforts and assistance from governments and private organizations combined, we are still failing in our battle against undernutrition. Read more about the progress toward the goal of halving global hunger by 2015 in Further Reading 15.

Ultimately, the depletion of world resources, the massive debt incurred by poorer countries, the threat of danger to more prosperous countries nearby, and the toll taken in human lives affect the world economy and well-being. The resulting instability can go on to affect the developing world, as has been apparent in recent years. Life is not necessarily fair, but the aim of civilization should be to make it more so. The world has both enough food and the technical expertise to end hunger. What is lacking is the concerted political will to do so.

CONCEPT CHECK

Overall, one important strategy to reducing undernutrition in the developing world lies in providing sufficient employment, so that people can purchase the food their families need. Providing access to land and other food production resources will also counteract undernutrition. Development programs must be sensitive to regional conditions to ensure that the new technologies introduced do not intensify existing problems for the poorest people.

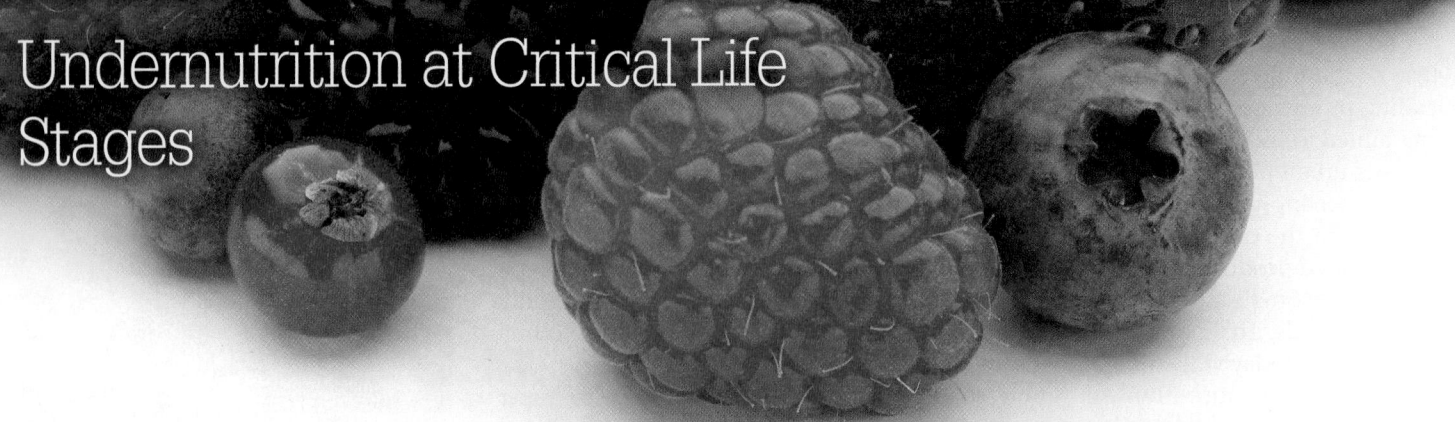

Undernutrition at Critical Life Stages

Critical Life Stages When Undernutrition Is Particularly Devastating

Prolonged undernutrition is detrimental to many aspects of human health (Fig. 12-7). It is particularly damaging during some periods of growth and old age. The United Nations Children's Fund developed a conceptual framework of malnutrition in 1990 (Fig. 12-8). According to this framework, the immediate causes of malnutrition (inadequate dietary intake and unsatisfactory health) affect individuals. The underlying causes relate to families and include inadequate access to food, inadequate care for women and children, and insufficient health services. Basic causes relate to human and economic resources and have their effect on communities and nations.

Pregnancy

Undernutrition poses the greatest health risk during pregnancy. About 500,000 women worldwide die each year from complications of pregnancy and childbirth. A pregnant woman needs extra nutrients to meet both her own needs and those of her developing offspring. Nourishing the fetus may deplete maternal stores of nutrients. Maternal iron deficiency anemia is one possible consequence (Chapter 14).

In Africa, women in their lifetimes give birth, on average, to more than six live babies. Coupled with chronic undernutrition, these high birth rates result in a 1 in 20 in chance that a woman will die from pregnancy-related causes. In contrast, North American women only face a risk of 1 death in about 8000 births from pregnancy-related causes. Pregnancy-related death is the social indicator showing the largest disparity between the developing and industrialized worlds. Smaller differences exist for literacy, life expectancy, and infant mortality.

Fetal and Infant Stages

The fetus faces major health risks from undernutrition during gestation. To support growth and development of the brain and other body tissues, a growing fetus requires a rich supply of protein, vitamins, and minerals. When these needs are not met, the infant is often born before 37 weeks of gestation, well before the ideal 40 weeks of gestation. The consequences of this pre-term birth include reduced lung function and a weakened immune system. These conditions not only compromise health but also increase the likelihood of premature death. Long-term problems in growth and development can result if the infant survives. In extreme cases, low-birth-weight infants (about 5.5 pounds [2.5 kilograms] or less) face 5 to 10 times the normal risk of dying before the age of 1 year, primarily because of reduced lung development. When low birth weight is accompanied by other physical abnormalities, medical intervention can cost $200,000 or more. These costs can be met only in developed countries.

Worldwide, more than 30 million infants are born each year with low birth weight. About 8% of infants born in the United States and 6% in Canada have low birth weights. In the United States, low birth weight accounts for more than half of all infant deaths and 75% of deaths of infants younger than 1 month old. Whereas undernutrition is a major contributor to low birth weight in developing countries, the primary cause for this problem in industrialized countries is cigarette smoking. Pregnancy during the teenage years, while a girl's body is still growing, contributes to low birth weight in developing and industrialized countries alike.

The percentage of infants born with low birth weight in the United States has been increasing steadily during the past 20 years. One reason is that more twins, triplets, and higher-order multiple births are being born because of improvements in medicine and fertility procedures. Rates of low birth weight also vary by race. About 13% of infants born to African-American women have low birth weights. Among Hispanics in the United States, infants of Mexican origin have the lowest rate of low birth weight (6%), while infants of Puerto Rican heritage have the highest (9%). Among Asian subgroups, low-birth-weight rates range from 5% for infants of Chinese heritage to nearly 9% for Filipino infants.

Childhood

Early childhood, when growth is rapid, is another period when undernutrition is extremely risky. The central nervous system— including the brain—continues to be vulnerable because of rapid growth through early childhood. After the

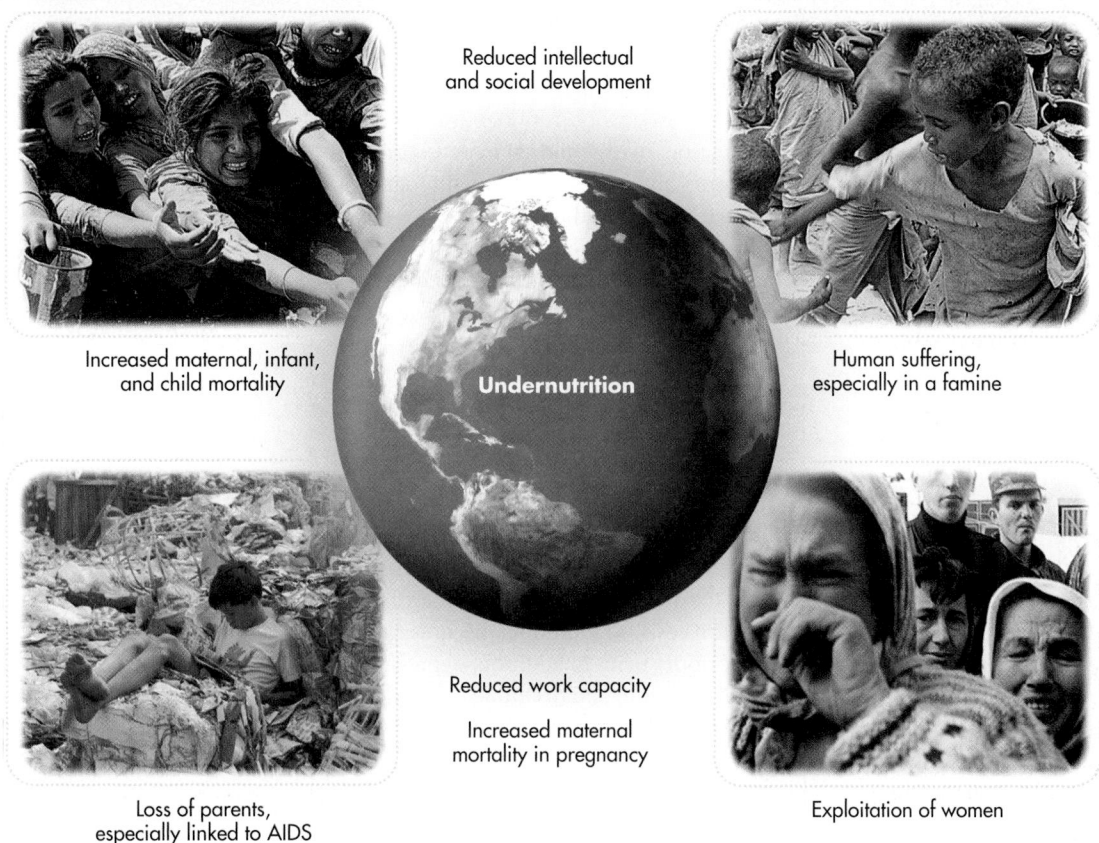

Reduced intellectual
and social development

Increased maternal, infant,
and child mortality

Undernutrition

Human suffering,
especially in a famine

Reduced work capacity

Increased maternal
mortality in pregnancy

Loss of parents,
especially linked to AIDS

Exploitation of women

FIGURE 12-7 ▶ Undernutrition results from and affects many aspects of human health and humanity.

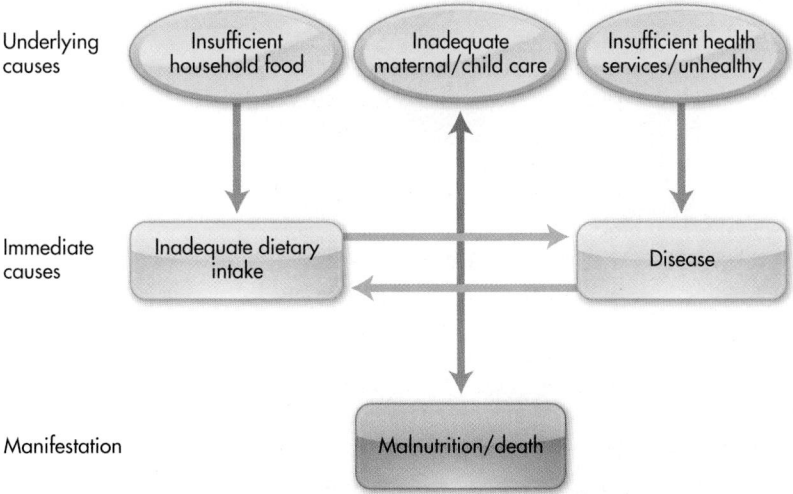

Underlying
causes

Insufficient
household food

Inadequate
maternal/child care

Insufficient health
services/unhealthy

Immediate
causes

Inadequate dietary
intake

Disease

Manifestation

Malnutrition/death

FIGURE 12-8 ▶ The UNICEF conceptual framework of the causes of malnutrition takes into account food, health, and caring practices. The causes are separated into three causes: immediate, underlying, and basic (not shown). Basic causes include human, economic, and organizational resources. The framework is used as a guide in health policy decision making.

preschool years, brain growth and development slow dramatically until maturity. Nutritional deprivation, especially in early infancy, can lead to permanent brain impairment. Without an effective intervention, it is projected that ongoing undernutrition could leave more than 1 billion children with mental impairment by 2020.

In general, poor children are at the greatest risk for nutritional deprivation and subsequent illness. Stunted growth is an obvious effect, seen in about one-third of children under 5 years of age worldwide. In addition, iron-deficiency anemia is much more common among low-income children than children from less deprived families. This deficiency can lead to fatigue upon exertion, reduced stamina, stunted growth, impaired motor development, and learning problems. Undernutrition in childhood can also weaken resistance to infection because immune function decreases when nutrients such as protein, vitamin A, and zinc are low in a diet. Clearly, undernutrition and illness have a cyclical relationship. Not only does undernutrition lead to illness, but illness, particularly diarrhea and infectious diseases, worsens undernutrition. For this reason, many children in developing countries are dying from the combination of malnutrition and infection. Conversely, when missing nutrients such as vitamin A and zinc are restored to children's diets, improvements in health can be obvious.

Later Years

Older adults, especially older women living alone in poverty, are also at risk for undernutrition. Older adults in general require nutrient-dense foods, in amounts dependent on their state of health and degree of physical activity. Many of them have fixed incomes and incur significant medical costs, so food often becomes a low-priority item. In addition, depression, social isolation, and declining physical and mental health can compound the problem of undernutrition in older adults.

▶ Compared to other children, homeless children suffer higher rates of many medical problems, some of which include:

- Upper respiratory tract infections
- Scabies and lice
- Tooth decay
- Ear and skin infections
- Diaper rash
- Eye infections
- Developmental delays
- Trauma-related injuries

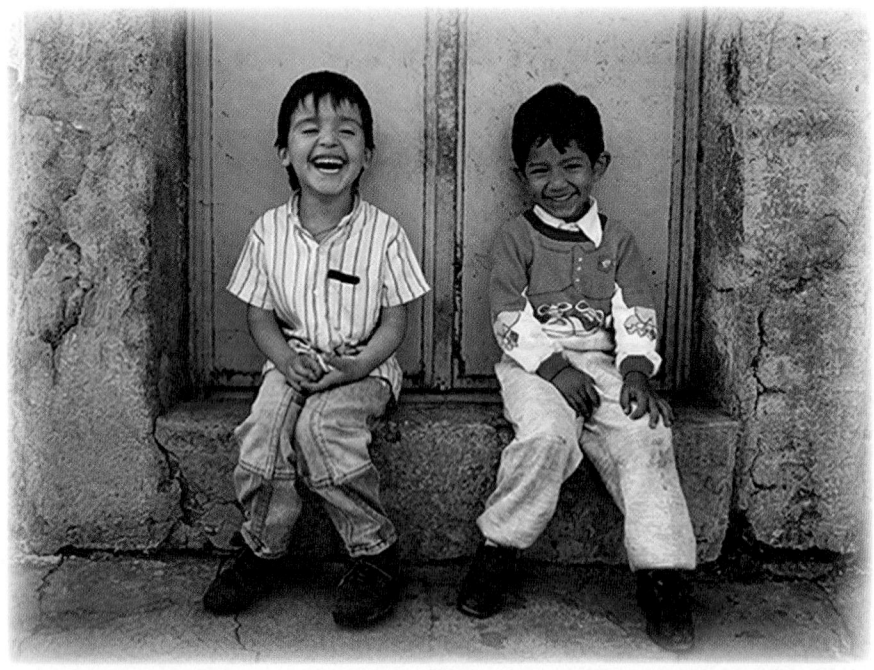

◀ Minimal intakes of protein and zinc limit the growth of children worldwide. About 30% of children in developing countries show evidence of poor growth rates.

Case Study Undernutrition During Childhood

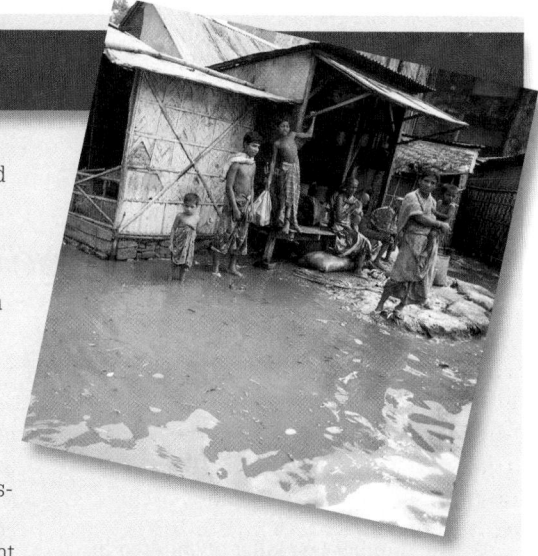

Jamal traveled to the Philippines with his church group last summer. During their stay, they helped build shelters for people in a village where, a few weeks before, a storm had destroyed several houses. Jamal noticed that many of the children were very short, much shorter than the children in his neighborhood in the United States. His group worked in a remote, low-elevation area where the storm and subsequent flooding had caused the most damage. On several occasions he noticed young mothers crouched on curbs or in doorways, holding their children. These children rarely moved—they appeared pale and listless. In contrast to the children Jamal's group had met at a church in the capital city, most of the children in this village were not active and lively. One evening a nurse from the local clinic came to speak to Jamal's group. She said that many children in this area do not get enough to eat and that health problems were rampant. She considered the recent storm a blessing in disguise, hoping

it would spur the Philippine government to send supplies to the village, particularly food and medicines. Jamal is shocked by such a degree of suffering. He wonders why children in the Philippines can be starving to death while many children in his hometown in the United States are overweight.

Answer the following questions, and check your responses in Appendix A.

1. Should Jamal have been surprised by widespread disease and general listlessness in the Philippine children?
2. Which nutrients are likely to be deficient in the diets of these children?
3. Which nutrient deficiencies contribute to poor growth or "stunting" of growth?
4. Which nutrient deficiencies may be causing diarrhea and illness?
5. Are these children likely to be consuming adequate calories? What effect does consumption of inadequate calories have on growth?
6. Why might the recent storm be a blessing for this small village?
7. List some reasons why the children in Jamal's neighborhood at home are more likely to be overweight

Summary (Numbers refer to numbered sections in the chapter.)

12.1 Poverty is commonly linked to chronic or periodic undernutrition. Malnutrition can occur when the food supply is either scarce or abundant. The resulting deficiency conditions and degenerative diseases contribute to poor health.

Undernutrition is the most common form of malnutrition in developing countries. It results from inadequate intake, absorption, or use of nutrients or food energy. Many deficiency conditions consequently appear, and infectious diseases thrive because the immune system cannot function properly.

Undernutrition diminishes both physical and mental capabilities. In poor countries, this is worsened by recurrent infections, unsanitary conditions, extreme weather, inadequate shelter, and exposure to diseases.

12.2 In North America, famine is not seen but food insecurity and undernutrition

remain problems. Soup kitchens, food stamps, the school lunch and breakfast programs, and the Special Supplemental Nutrition Program for Women, Infants, and Children (WIC) have focused on improving the nutritional health of poor and at-risk people. When adequately funded, these programs have proved effective in reducing undernutrition. The need to reduce out-of-wedlock pregnancies remains a national priority because single parents and their children are much more likely to live in poverty.

12.3 Multiple factors contribute to the problem of undernutrition in the developing world. In densely populated countries, food resources, as well as the means for distributing food, may be inadequate. Farming methods often encourage erosion, which deprives the soil of valuable nutrients and thereby hampers future efforts to grow food. Limited water availability

hinders food production. Naturally occurring devastation from droughts, excessive rainfall, fire, crop infestation, and human causes—such as urbanization, war and civil unrest, debt, poor sanitation, and AIDS—all contribute to the major problem of undernutrition.

12.4 Proposed solutions to world undernutrition must consider multiple interacting factors, many thoroughly embedded in cultural traditions. Family planning efforts, for example, may not succeed until life expectancy increases. Through education, efforts should be made to upgrade farming methods, improve crops, limit pregnancies, encourage breastfeeding when it is safe to do so, and improve sanitation and hygiene.

Direct food aid is only a short-term solution. In what may appear to be a step backward, many experts recommend more sustainable subsistence-level farming. Small-scale industrial development is another way to create meaningful employment and purchasing power for vast numbers of the rural poor. Various biotechnology applications may also prove beneficial.

N&YH The greatest risk of undernutrition occurs during critical periods of growth and development: gestation, infancy, and childhood. Low birth weight is a leading cause of infant deaths worldwide. Many developmental problems are caused by nutritional deprivation during critical periods of brain growth. People in their later years are also at great risk.

Check Your Knowledge (Answers to the following questions are below.)

1. There are an estimated _____ chronically undernourished people in the world.
   a. 14 million
   b. 800 million to 1.1 billion
   c. 3 billion
   d. 6 billion

2. The number one killer of children in developing countries is
   a. xerophthalmia.
   b. iron deficiency anemia.
   c. iodide deficiency.
   d. diarrhea.

3. The human organism is particularly susceptible to the effects of undernutrition during
   a. pregnancy.
   b. infancy.
   c. childhood.
   d. All of the above.

4. A barrier to solving undernutrition in the developing world is NOT
   a. external debt.
   b. poor infrastructure.
   c. a lack of manpower.
   d. expanding population

5. Many of the child deaths each year in developing countries could be prevented if

   a. technology was improved.
   b. doctors were more specialized.
   c. mothers would learn more about nutrition.
   d. sanitation and hygiene were improved.

6. The food stamp program, recently renamed the Supplemental Nutrition Assistance Program, allows
   a. low-income families to buy surplus food at government stores with government-issued Electronic Benefit Transfer cards.
   b. low-income people to purchase food, cleaning supplies, alcoholic beverages, and anything else sold in supermarkets with Electronic Benefit Transfer cards.
   c. low-income people to turn in government-issued Electronic Benefit Transfer cards for cash to buy food.
   d. low-income people to purchase food and seeds with government-issued Electronic Benefit Transfer cards.

7. A long-term solution to world hunger is
   a. the green revolution.
   b. cash crops.

   c. jobs and self-sufficiency.
   d. government/private aid.

8. Bt corn has been genetically modified to make
   a. the bacterium *Bacillus thuringiensis*.
   b. a protein toxic to caterpillars that can destroy the corn plant.
   c. a sugar that makes the corn sweeter.
   d. a fat that makes corn oil healthier.

9. Genetically modified soybeans make up _____% of the soybeans grown in the United States.
   a. 50
   b. 75
   c. 80
   d. 90

10. FDA requires the statement "contains genetically modified ingredients" on the label of all foods containing genetically modified ingredients.
    a. True   b. False

Answer key: 1. b (LO 12.1), 2. d (LO 12.3), 3. d (LO 12.5), 4. c (LO 12.3), 5. d (LO 12.3), 6. d (LO 12.2), 7. c (LO 12.4), 8. b (LO 12.4), 9. d (LO 12.4), 10. b (LO 12.4)

Study Questions (Numbers refer to Learning Outcomes)

1. Describe the difference between malnutrition and undernutrition. (LO 12.1)

2. Describe in a short paragraph any evidence of undernutrition that you saw while you were growing up, such as on television. What are/were the likely roots of these problems? (LO 12.1)

3. What do you believe are the major factors contributing to undernutrition in wealthy nations, such as the United States? What are some solutions to this problem? (LO 12.2)

4. What three points would you make to a group of seventh grade girls concerning the economic perils of teen pregnancy and parenting? (LO 12.2)

5. What federal programs are available to address the problem of under nutrition in the United States? (LO 12.2)

6. Outline how war and civil unrest in developing countries have worsened problems of chronic hunger over the past few years. (LO 12.3)

7. How important is population control in addressing the problem of world hunger

now and in the future? Support your answer with three main points. (LO 12.3)

8. Why is solving the problem of undernutrition a key factor in the ability of developing countries to reach their full potential? (LO 12.3)

9. Name three nutrients often lacking in the diets of undernourished people. What effects can be expected with each deficiency? (LO 12.1)

10. Describe how sustainable agriculture and biotechnology can improve food availability worldwide. (LO 12.4)

What Would You Choose Recommendations

The correct response for the question posed at the beginning of this chapter is *all of the above*! Do what comes naturally to you—whether it is donating your spare change or volunteering your spare time—to move thought into action against world hunger. Indeed, the need is great—both globally and locally—and opportunities to get involved abound.

As you learned in this chapter, there are basically two ways to address the problem of hunger: direct food aid or empowering others to help themselves. Direct aid (e.g., donating money each month) is a short-term solution—one that necessarily fills an immediate gap between resources and requirements. However, in the long run, solving the problem of world hunger will take bottom-up changes that enable struggling communities to provide their own food and clean water.

It may be easier and more comfortable to visualize the hunger problem in a faraway place, such as in a developing country. In reality, however, poverty and hunger lurk in your own community. You can help local efforts by donating nonperishable items to local food pantries, volunteering at Summer Food Service Programs for school-age children, or simply by shopping for locally grown foods direct from farmers in your neighborhood.

In your quest to get involved, look for organizations whose focus is to help set up sustainable solutions in communities—empowering local citizens to grow their own food, maintain their own clean water supplies, or build their own local economies.

Action Against Hunger: www.actionagainsthunger.org
Alliance to End Hunger: www.alliancetoendhunger.org
Blood:Water Mission: www.bloodwatermission.com
Bread for the World: www.bread.org
The Hunger Project: www.thp.org
The International Food Policy Research Institute: www.ifpri.org

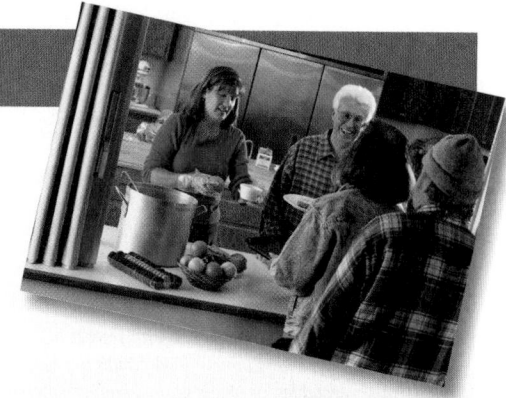

▲ Volunteer your time at a local food pantry or soup kitchen. Check out www.serve.gov/endhunger.asp to find a volunteer opportunity near you.

MAZON: A Jewish Response to Hunger: http://mazon.org
Stop Hunger Now: www.stophungernow.org

There are many creative ideas for raising funds and awareness to end world hunger. Check out the Rate Your Plate section at the end of Chapter 12 for more ideas, and put your own talents and passions to work for a good cause!

Further Readings

1. ADA Reports: Position of the American Dietetic Association: Agricultural and food bio-technology. *Journal of the American Dietetic Association* 106:285, 2006.

   It is the position of the American Dietetic Association that agricultural and food biotechnology techniques can enhance the quality, safety, nutritional value, and variety of food available for human consumption and increase the efficiency of food production, food processing, food distribution, and environmental and waste management.

2. ADA Reports: Position of the American Dietetic Association: Food insecurity in the United States. *Journal of the American Dietetic Association* 110:1368, 2010.

   It is the position of the American Dietetic Association that systematic and sustained action is needed to achieve food and nutrition security for all in the United States. Interventions are needed, including adequate funding for and increased use of food and nutrition assistance programs, inclusion of food and nutrition education in such programs, and innovative programs to promote and support individual and household economic self-sufficiency.

3. ADA Reports: Position of the American Dietetic Association: Addressing world hunger, malnutrition and food security. *Journal of the American Dietetic Association* 103:1046, 2003.

   It is the position of the American Dietetic Association that access to adequate amounts of safe, nutritious, and culturally appropriate foods is a fundamental human right. Still, hunger continues to be a worldwide problem of staggering proportions. In response, it is important to encourage programs and practices that combat hunger and malnutrition, increase food security, promote self-sufficiency, and are environmentally and economically sustainable.

4. ADA Reports: Position of the American Dietetic Association: Child and adolescent nutrition assistance programs. *Journal of the American Dietetic Association* 110:791, 2010.

   Children and adolescents should have access to an adequate supply of healthful and safe foods that promote optimal physical, social, and cognitive growth and development. Nutrition assistance programs, such as food assistance and meal service programs and nutrition initiatives, play a vital role in meeting this critical need.

5. Coutsoudis A: Infant feeding dilemmas created by HIV: South African experiences. *Journal of Nutrition* 135:956, 2005.

   This paper discusses the dilemma surrounding the risks and benefits of breastfeeding by an HIV-infected mother. The impact of the South African Safer Breastfeeding Programme, implemented to reduce some of the risk factors associated with HIV transmission, is reported.

6. Dammann KW, Smith C: Race, homelessness, and other environmental factors associated with the food-purchasing behavior of low-income women. *Journal of the American Dietetic Association* 110:1351, 2010.

The hunger-obesity paradox has increased interest in the quality of low-income households' food purchases. This study of low-income, urban women's food purchases showed that rates of "less healthy" food group purchases were higher compared to "healthy" food group purchases. Racial differences were found with respect to purchasing healthy protein food groups but not fruits, vegetables, or whole grains. Homelessness reduced the likelihood of purchasing most food groups, regardless of nutrient density. These findings indicate that we must strategize to help low-income, urban women make best use of food resources within their local food system.

7. Darton-Hill I and others: Micronutrient deficiencies and gender: Social and economic costs. *American Journal of Clinical Nutrition* 81:1198S, 2005.

Micronutrient deficiencies, such as for vitamin A, iodine, iron, and zinc, in developing countries, lead to health problems, especially in females. Addressing these micronutrient deficiencies is important in order to improve economic status at the personal, community, and national level in developing countries.

8. Doherty T and others: A longitudinal qualitative study of infant-feeding decision making and practices among HIV-positive women in South Africa. *Journal of Nutrition* 136:2421, 2006.

HIV-positive women face challenges regarding infant-feeding decisions. This study examined these challenges and found that successful breastfeeding resulted from a supportive home environment, a strong belief in the benefits of breastfeeding, and the ability to resist pressure to introduce other fluids.

9. Dworkin SL, Ehrhardt AA: Going beyond "ABC" to include "GEM": Critical reflections on progress in the HIV/AIDS epidemic. *American Journal of Public Health* 97:13, 2007.

This article discusses the feminization of HIV/AIDS and the limitations of the "ABC" (abstinence, be faithful, condom use) strategy.

Strategies focused on gender relation, economics, and migration (GEM) are suggested as more appropriate prevention measures.

10. Food and Agriculture Organization of the United Nations: *The state of food insecurity in the world 2008: High food prices and food security-threats and opportunities.* FAO, Rome, Italy, 2008

This report of the FAO food security meeting in Rome, Italy in June 2008, emphasizes that in 2008 alone, millions more became food-insecure, demanding urgent action and substantial investments. The worldwide concern about threats to global food security, largely triggered by soaring food prices, is discussed. Representatives of 180 countries plus the European Union met to express their conviction "that the international community needs to take urgent and coordinated action to combat the negative impacts of soaring food prices on the world's most vulnerable countries and populations."

11. Gibson RS: Zinc: The missing link in combating micronutrient malnutrition in developing countries. *Proceedings of the Nutrition Society* 65:51, 2006.

Although zinc deficiency is included as a major risk factor in the global burden of disease, zinc is still not included in the United Nations micronutrient priority list. Certain countries are at risk of zinc deficiency and should be targeted for zinc interventions. Zinc intervention strategies are discussed in this article.

12. Grandesso F and others: Mortality and malnutrition among populations living in South Darfur, Sudan. *Journal of the American Medical Association* 293:1490, 2005.

The conflicts in the Darfur region of Sudan have led to high rates of death and undernutrition among people displaced by war. This article describes what has been seen numerous times in the last 50 years—undernutrition and related death is a typical casualty of war.

13. Joint United Nations Programme on HIV/AIDS (UNAIDS) and World Health Organization. UNAIDS Report on the Global AIDS Epidemic 2010.

This UNAIDS report contains the 2010 global estimates on the scale of the AIDS pandemic. It

is reported that approximately 33 million people were living with HIV in 2009. The world has halted and begun to reverse the spread of HIV. Since 1999, the number of new infections has fallen by 19%.

14. Nord M, Hopwood H: A comparison of household food security in Canada and the United States. *Economic Research Report* 67, December 2008. www.ers.usda.gov/publications/err67/.

Differences in the prevalence of household food insecurity between Canada and the United States are described in this report. The percentage of the population living in food-insecure households was lower in Canada (7.0%) than in the United States (12.6%). The difference between the percentage of children living in food-insecure households in Canada vs. the United States was greater (8.3% vs. 17.9%) than that for adults (6.6% vs. 10.8%).

15. Shetty P: Achieving the goal of halving global hunger by 2015. *Proceedings of the Nutrition Society* 65:7, 2006.

This article reviews the goal of the FAO World Food Summit (WFS) and the United Nations Millennium Development Goals (MDG) to halve the numbers of the global population suffering from hunger by the year 2015. To date, the efforts have fallen short of the pace needed to achieve this goal. Developing countries are facing new challenges of hunger co-existing with new epidemics of diet-related diseases.

16. United Nations: *Tackling a global crisis: International year of sanitation 2008.* UN-Water, 2008. www.unwater.org.

The International Year of Sanitation in 2008 focused global attention on the need for improved health and hygiene. It is estimated that around the world, 2.6 billion people do not have a clean and safe place to perform their bodily functions because they lack access to a basic necessity, a toilet. This report helps to expose the scandal of human indignity, unnecessary child death, and lost economic opportunities associated with the sanitation crisis and provides a call to action for organizations to redouble their efforts and bring this silent crisis to an end.

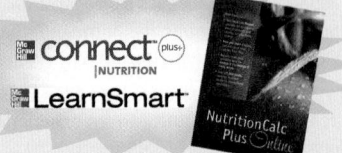

To get the most out of your study of nutrition, go to McGraw-Hill's online resources: Connect www.mcgrawhillconnect.com, where you will find NutritionCalc Plus, LearnSmart, and many other dynamic tools.

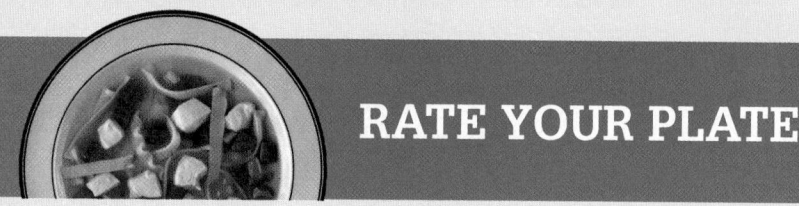

I. Fighting World Undernutrition on a Personal Level

If you want to do something about world and domestic undernutrition, consider the following activities. It is a noble act to try to make a difference, even if you make only one small step. As with any change in behavior, do not try to do too many things at once. Try one or two activities that represent your commitment to solving this problem.

1. Volunteer at a local soup kitchen or homeless shelter for a time (1 month, for example). What insights did you gain?

2. Coordinate the efforts of a campus organization to donate money to an antihunger agency such as the following:

Bread for the World
50 F Street NW, Suite 500
Washington, DC 20001
www.bread.org/

Catholic Relief Services
228 W. Lexington St
Baltimore, MD 21201
www.crs.org

Oxfam America
226 Causeway St., 5th Floor
Boston, MA 02114
www.oxfamamerica.org/

Feeding America
35 E. Wacker Dr., #2000
Chicago, IL 60601
http://feedingamerica.org

CARE USA
151 Ellis Street, NE
Atlanta, GA 30303
www.care.org/

EarthSave International
PO Box 96
New York, NY 10108
www.earthsave.org/

Save the Children Foundation
54 Wilton Rd.
Westport, CT 06880
www.savethechildren.org/

3. Make a contribution of nonperishable foods to the ongoing offering at a place of worship near you. If such an offering does not exist, start one.

4. Get on a food recovery program's mailing list, read its newsletters for information on upcoming fund-raisers and other activities, and become involved.

5. Utilize your love of good food and healthy cooking skills to organize a local meal for the hungry or a benefit dinner to raise money for local food banks. Resources to set up projects may be available from mission organizations. For example, with Blood: Water Mission's Lemon: Aid project, students or families can use something as simple as the sale of a refreshing drink to fund potable drinking water in rural communities in Africa.

6. Participate in food drives organized by local grocery stores by contributing food or services. Food-drive organizers may need volunteers to transport the donations to a food pantry. Pay attention to events around World Food Day, October 16.

7. Point, click, and fight hunger. Internet users can find information on hunger at several sites, including the following:

- Someone somewhere dies of hunger every 3.6 seconds. You can help stop the clock: go to www.thehungersite.com and click on Donate Free Food to send a meal to a needy someone. This site is affiliated with the UN World Food Program, which tracks the number of clicks and then sends a bill to one of its corporate or nonprofit sponsors.

- The Food and Agriculture Organization of the United Nations has worked to alleviate poverty and hunger by promoting agricultural development, improved nutrition, and the pursuit of food security. This website will keep you up-to-date on recent issues and provides an extensive list of publications related to food security. www.fao.org

- America's Second Harvest, the largest domestic hunger-relief organization, shows you how to help online and has information about the latest updates. www.secondharvest.org

- Bread for the World is a nationwide Christian citizens' movement seeking justice for the world's hungry people by lobbying our nation's decision makers. www.bread.org

- CARE is one of the world's largest private international relief and development organizations, with the goal of saving lives, building opportunities, and bringing hope to people in need. www.care.org

- Turn your personal fitness goals into a campaign to raise funds and awareness for projects that provide food and clean water to communities around the world. Water Walks (see www.bloodwatermission.com) or Crop Walks (see www.churchworld service.org) are great ways to walk a mile in someone else's shoes.

II. Joining the Battle Against Undernutrition

Imagine that you recently spent your summer vacation in a developing country and saw evidence of undernutrition and hunger. Then imagine that you are now asking a large corporation to support your efforts to ease hunger and suffering in this area. Develop a two-paragraph statement outlining why addressing hunger issues in this area is important. Include how the corporation could assist you.

Chapter 13 Safety of Our Food Supply

Chapter Outline

Student Learning Outcomes

Chapter 13 is designed to allow you to:

13.1 List some of the types and common sources of viruses, bacteria, fungi, and parasites that can make their way into food.

13.2 Compare and contrast food-preservation methods.

13.3 Understand the foodborne illnesses caused by bacteria, viruses, and parasites.

13.4 Describe the main reasons for using chemical additives in foods, the general classes of additives, and the functions of each class.

13.5 Identify sources of toxic environmental contaminants in food and the consequences of their ingestion.

13.6 Understand the reasons behind pesticide use, the possible long-term health complications, and the safety limits set for their use.

13.7 Understand the effects of conventional and sustainable agriculture on our food choices.

13.8 Describe the procedures that can be used to limit the risk of foodborne illness.

What Would You Choose?

By now, you have learned the importance of including more fruits and vegetables in your diet. You are choosing fresh or frozen produce more often than canned to cut back on sodium and other preservatives. You are steaming or stir-frying your vegetables to retain nutrients and avoid adding too much fat during preparation. In the grocery store, you have seen the growing selection of organic products including produce. Do they have health benefits that make them worth the extra cost? If cost was not a concern, what type of fruits and vegetables would you choose from the following list to satisfy your desire for increased nutritional value, decreased exposure to preservatives, lower risk for foodborne illness, and decreased exposure to pesticides?

a Canned low-sodium

b Organically grown

c Frozen

d Fresh

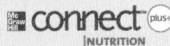 **Think about your choice as you read Chapter 13, then see our recommendations at the end of the chapter. To learn more about organic foods, check out the Connect site:** www.mcgrawhillconnect.com

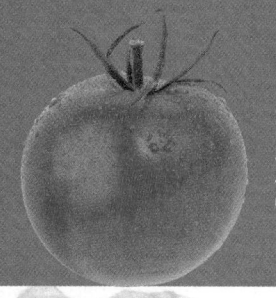

Over 100 years ago, in 1906, increasing public pressure forced the passage of the first Food and Drug Act in the United States and generally improved food preparation standards. Today, warnings about the safety of food and water appear everywhere. Attention has turned to more contemporary concerns, such as microbial and chemical contamination. Whereas we are told to eat more fruits, vegetables, fish, and poultry and to drink more water, we are also warned that these may contain dangerous substances. We still must ask, "How safe is our food and water?"

Scientists and health authorities agree that North Americans enjoy a relatively safe food supply, especially if foods are stored and prepared properly. Over the past 100 or so years, tremendous progress has been made to allow for this. Nonetheless, microorganisms and certain chemicals in foods still can pose a health risk. Thus, the nutritional and health benefits of food must be balanced against any food-related hazards. Chapter 13 focuses on these hazards—how real they are and how you can minimize their effect on your life. As the comic in the chapter suggests, you bear some responsibility for this—government agencies and industry can only do so much. Recall from Chapter 2 that the 2010 Dietary Guidelines for Americans encourage us to prepare and store foods safely.

pasteurizing The process of heating food products to kill pathogenic microorganisms and reduce the total number of bacteria.

virus The smallest known type of infectious agent, many of which cause disease in humans. A virus is essentially a piece of genetic material surrounded by a coat of protein. They do not metabolize, grow, or move by themselves. They reproduce only with the aid of a living cellular host.

bacteria Single-cell microorganisms; some produce poisonous substances, which cause illness in humans. Bacteria can be carried by water, animals, and people. They survive on skin, clothes, and hair and thrive in foods at room temperature. Some can live without oxygen and survive by means of spore formation.

spores Dormant reproductive cells capable of turning into adult organisms without the help of another cell. Various bacteria and fungi form spores.

fungi Simple parasitic life forms, including molds, mildews, yeasts, and mushrooms. They live on dead or decaying organic matter. Fungi can grow as single cells, like yeast, or as a multicellular colony, as seen with molds.

parasite An organism that lives in or on another organism and derives nourishment from it.

foodborne illness Sickness caused by the ingestion of food containing harmful substances.

Refresh Your Memory

As you begin your study of food safety in Chapter 13, you may want to review:

- Alternative sweeteners in Chapter 4
- The disease phenylketonuria (PKU) in Chapter 4
- Fat substitutes in Chapter 5
- Food biotechnology in Chapter 12

13.1 Food Safety: Setting the Stage

During the early stages of urbanization in North America, contaminated water and food—notably, milk—were responsible for many large outbreaks of typhoid fever, septic sore throat, scarlet fever, diphtheria, and other devastating human diseases. These experiences led to the development of processes for purifying water, treating sewage, and **pasteurizing** milk. Since that time, safe water and milk have become universally available, with only occasional problems from either.

The greatest health risk from food today is contamination by **viruses** and **bacteria** and, to a lesser extent, by various forms of **fungi** and **parasites.** These microorganisms can all cause **foodborne illness.** In a recent outbreak in the United States, 199 persons in 26 states were infected with *Escherichia coli* (*E. coli*) bacteria O157:H7 from fresh spinach. Of these ill persons, 102 were hospitalized, 31 developed kidney failure, and 22 were children under 5 years. Three deaths were associated with the outbreak. A deadlier outbreak of Escherichia coli O104:H4 occurred in Germany during the summer of 2011, resulting in over 3000 infections, hundreds of cases of kidney failure, and a death toll of at least 36. Read more about this outbreak that was linked to sprouts in Table 13.1.

Although microbial contamination is the cause of most incidents of foodborne illness, North Americans seem more concerned about health risks from chemicals in foods. In the long run, this concern has some merit. On a day-to-day basis, however, food additives cause only about 4% of all cases of foodborne illness in North America. Microbial contamination of food is by far the more important issue for our day-to-day health, so it will be discussed first. Chapter 13 will then cover chemical food safety hazards, including the use and safety of food additives, and discuss the risks of pesticides in foods.

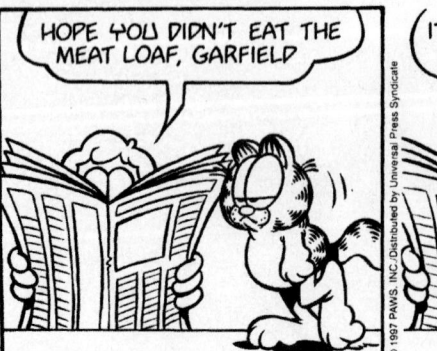
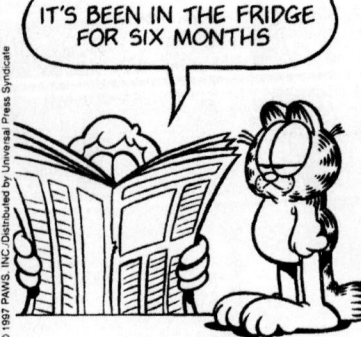
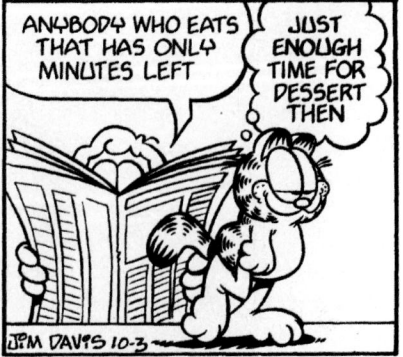

Which foods pose the greatest risk for foodborne illness? Is any food safe after being stored in the refrigerator for 6 months? Are food additives and pesticides an even greater day-to-day concern? Chapter 13 provides some answers.

GARFIELD © Paws, Inc. Reprinted with permission of Universal Press Syndicate. All rights reserved.

Effects of Foodborne Illness

According to the U.S. Centers for Disease Control and Prevention, foodborne illness causes 48 million illnesses, 128,000 hospitalizations, and 3000 deaths in the United States each year. Some people are particularly susceptible to foodborne illness, including the following:

- Infants and children
- Older adults
- Those with liver disease, diabetes, HIV infection (and AIDS), or cancer
- Postsurgical patients
- Pregnant women
- People taking immunosuppressant agents (e.g., transplant patients)

Some bouts of foodborne illness, especially when coupled with ongoing health problems, are lengthy and lead to food allergies, seizures, blood poisoning (from **toxins** or microorganisms in the bloodstream), or other illnesses. Foodborne illnesses often result from the unsafe handling of food at home, so we each bear some responsibility for preventing them (see Further Readings 2 and 10). You can't usually tell so by taste, smell, or sight that a particular food contains harmful microorganisms; therefore, you might not even be aware that food has caused your distress. In fact, your last case of diarrhea may have been caused by foodborne illness (Table 13-1). In response to the significant public health burden of foodborne illness that is largely preventable, the FDA Food Safety Modernization Act was signed into law by President Obama on January 4, 2011. This new law strengthens the food safety system, enabling FDA to better protect public health. It allows FDA to focus on prevention of food safety problems before they occur. The law also provides new tools for inspection and compliance and for holding imported foods to the same standards as domestic foods. The law also directs FDA to build a national food safety system that is integrated and in partnership with state and local authorities. Although government agencies are at work on problems regarding food safety, this does not substitute for individual safety efforts (Table 13-2).

toxins Poisonous compounds produced by an organism that can cause disease.

Read more about the Food Safety Modernization Act at www.fda.gov./Food/FoodSafety/FSMA/default.htm.

Why Is Foodborne Illness So Common?

Foodborne illness is carried or transmitted to people by food. Most foodborne illnesses are transmitted through food in which microorganisms are able to grow rapidly. These foods are generally moist, rich in protein, and have a neutral or slightly acidic pH. Unfortunately, this describes many of the foods we eat every day, such as meats, eggs, and dairy products.

Our food industry tries whenever possible to increase the shelf life of food products; however, a longer shelf life allows more time for bacteria in foods to multiply. Some bacteria even grow at refrigeration temperatures. Partially cooked—and some fully cooked—products pose a particular risk because refrigerated storage may only slow, not prevent, bacterial growth. The risk of contracting foodborne illness also is high because of consumer trends. First, there is greater consumer interest in eating raw or undercooked animal products. In addition, more people receive medication that suppresses their ability to combat foodborne infectious agents. Another factor is the continuing increase in the number of older adults in the population.

The risk of illness from foodborne microorganisms increases as more of our foods are prepared in kitchens outside the home. Supermarkets have become an alternative to cooking at home by offering a variety of prepared foods from specialty meat shops, salad bars, and bakeries. With the increasing number of two-income families, more people are looking for convenient, easy-to-prepare, nutritious foods. Supermarkets offer entrées that can be served immediately or reheated. The foods are usually prepared in central kitchens or processing plants and shipped to individual stores.

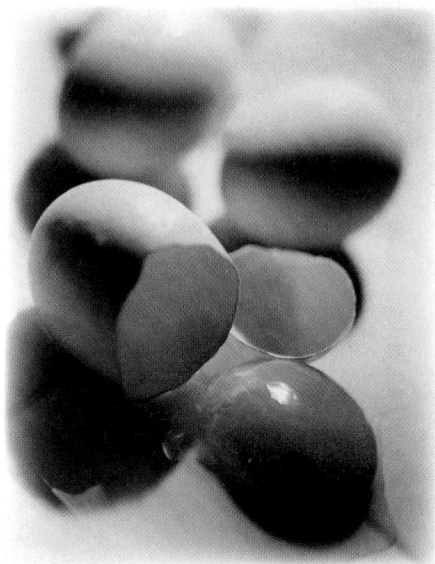

▲ Some restaurants that serve requested undercooked food are now warning patrons (on the menu) of the health risks of ordering such foods, particularly with undercooked eggs and meats.

TABLE 13-1 Some Examples of Cases of Foodborne Illness. We generally have a safe food supply, but there are occasional instances of foodborne illnesses, such as those listed.

Viruses

- *Norovirus:* Over 380 passengers and crew members of the largest cruise ship, Royal Caribbean's Freedom of the Seas, were sickened by *Norovirus.* The ship was sanitized, but one week later a second outbreak of the gastrointestinal illness afflicted 97 passengers and 11 crew members.

- *Hepatitus A:* Over 500 adults in the United States contracted hepatitis A after eating raw green onions in a Mexican restaurant. These were contaminated during growth in Mexico and not properly washed by food service workers.

Bacteria

- *Salmonella:* In 2008–2009, two outbreaks of salmonella cost their industries millions of dollars. The first outbreak was traced to imported jalapeno and serrano peppers from one Mexican farm. Illnesses led to 282 hospitalizations and 2 deaths. The second outbreak, traced to peanut butter from a processing plant in Georgia may have caused at least eight deaths.

- *Shigella:* More than 600 people on a cruise ship developed shigellosis and one person died.

- *Listeria:* Forty-eight deaths were associated with foodborne illness caused by *Listeria* organisms in soft, Mexican-style cheeses. A listeriosis outbreak associated with undercooked hot dogs and cold cuts resulted in more than 82 illnesses and 17 deaths in 19 states.

- *E. coli:* The world's deadliest outbreak of *Escherichia coli* occurred during the summer of 2011 with 3332 persons infected, more than 600 in intensive care, and a death toll of 36. The outbreak occurred mainly in Germany and involved the rare *E.coli* O104:H4 strain. Several hundred also contracted its potentially fatal kidney complication. The *E.coli* infection was caused by tainted vegetable sprouts from a small, rather traditional organic sprout farm. The sprout seeds were mostly imported from overseas and the *E.coli* bacteria were antibiotic

resistant. In the United States, the largest *E. coli* 0157:H7 outbreak on record infected more than 1000 people in upstate New York at a county fair. The bacterium was found in infected well water. It killed a 79-year-old man and a 4-year-old girl, and it caused 10 other children to undergo kidney dialysis. Six adults and a 2-year-old child were killed after an *E. coli* outbreak from contaminated drinking water in Canada. The bacteria entered the water supply from animal manure after flooding from a heavy storm. In an outbreak of 199 persons infected with *E. coli* from fresh spinach, *E. coli* 0157:H7 was isolated from 13 packages of fresh spinach in 10 states.

- *C. botulinum:* A man in Arkansas developed botulism after eating stew that was cooked and then kept at room temperature for 3 days. He spent—42 days on mechanical ventilation.

- *Vibrio:* Since 1992, 17 people in Florida have died of *Vibrio vulnificus* infections after eating raw oysters.

- *B. cereus:* A teenage boy and his father experienced abdominal pain, vomiting, and diarrhea within 30 minutes of eating 4-day-old homemade pesto that had been reheated and left out a number of times and was apparently contaminated with *Bacillus cereus.* The boy died of liver failure.

Parasites

- *Cryptosporidium:* A group attending a banquet developed diarrhea 3 to 9 days after eating green onions. Stool specimens were positive

for *Cryptosporidium.* Restaurant workers reported they did not consistently wash green onions before using them.

Risks from Seafood

- *Ciguatera:* An outbreak of ciguatera fish poisoning involved 17 crew members of a cargo ship that caught, cooked, and ate a barra-cuda in the Bahamas. All became ill with nausea, vomiting, abdominal

cramps, and diarrhea within hours of eating the fish. Within 2 days, all suffered from muscle pain and weakness; dizziness; and numb or itchy feet, hands, and mouth.

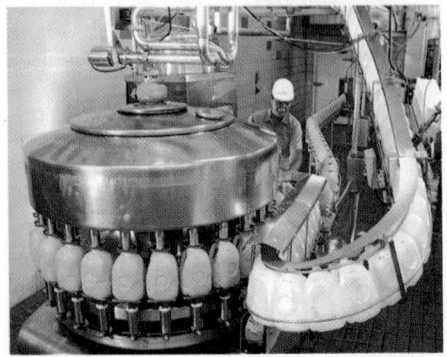

▲ Food contaminated in a central plant can go on to produce illness in people across the nation. In the case of juices, pasteurization is an effective method of reducing the risk of foodborne illness.

This centralization of food production by the food-processing and restaurant industry enhances the risk of foodborne illness. If a food product is contaminated in a central processing plant, consumers over a wide area can suffer foodborne illness. For example, a malfunction in an ice cream plant in Minnesota resulted in 224,000 suspected cases of *Salmonella* bacterial infections, which were linked to use of contaminated ice cream mix. At least 4 people died and 700 became ill in Washington and surrounding western states after eating at a chain of fast-food restaurants. The source of the problem was undercooked hamburger contaminated with the bacterium *E. coli* 0157:H7. Restaurants are inspected by health departments only about every 6 months so we must rely on each restaurant to practice good food safety.

Greater consumption of ready-to-eat foods imported from foreign countries is still another cause of increased foodborne illness in North America. In the past, food imports were mostly raw products processed here under strict sanitation standards. Now, however, we import more ready-to-eat processed foods—such as berries from Guatemala and shellfish from Asia—some of which are contaminated. U.S. authorities are re-examining inspection procedures for these imports.

TABLE 13-2 Agencies Responsible for Monitoring the Food Supply in the United States

Agency Name	Responsibilities	Methods	How to Contact
United States Department of Agriculture (USDA)	• Enforces wholesomeness and quality standards for grains and produce (while in the field), meat, poultry, milk, eggs, and egg products	• Inspection • Grading • "Safe Handling Label"	www.fsis.usda.gov
Bureau of Alcohol, Tobacco, Firearms and Explosives (ATF)	• Enforces laws on alcoholic beverages	• Inspection	www.atf.gov
Environmental Protection Agency (EPA)	• Regulates pesticides • Establishes water quality standards	• Approval required for all U.S. pesticides • Sets pesticide residue limits in food	www.epa.gov
Food and Drug Administration (FDA)	• Ensures safety and wholesomeness of all foods in interstate commerce (except meat, poultry, and processed egg products) • Regulates seafood • Controls product labels	• Inspection • Food sample studies • Sets standards for specific foods	www.fda.gov or call 1-800-FDA-4010
Centers for Disease Control and Prevention (CDC)	• Promotes food safety	• Responds to emergencies concerning foodborne illness • Surveys and studies environmental health problems • Directs/enforces quarantines • National programs for prevention and control of foodborne and other diseases	www.cdc.gov
National Marine Fisheries Service or NOAA Fisheries	• Domestic and international conservation and management of living marine resources	• Voluntary seafood inspection program • Can use mark to show federal inspection	www.nmfs.noaa.gov
State and local governments	• Milk safety • Monitors food industry within their borders	• Inspection of food-related establishments	Government pages of telephone book

Government agencies responsible for monitoring food safety in Canada and the specific laws followed are listed in Appendix C.

The use of antibiotics in animal feeds is also increasing the severity of cases of foodborne illness. This antibiotic use encourages bacteria such as *E.coli* O157:H7 and O104:H4 to develop antibiotic-resistant strains, those that can grow even if exposed to typical antibiotic medicines. This issue is receiving considerable attention by scientists in the field.

Finally, more cases of foodborne disease are reported now because scientists are more aware of the roles of various players in the process. Every decade the list of microorganisms suspected of causing foodborne illness lengthens. In addition, physicians are more likely to suspect foodborne contaminants as a cause of illness. Furthermore, we now know that food, besides serving as a good growth medium for some microorganisms, transmits many others as well. Seafood is receiving greater scrutiny and surveillance by FDA as a cause of foodborne illness. For more information about food safety, contact FDA's Center for Food Safety and Applied Nutrition information line at 1-888-SAFEFOOD or log on to www.FoodSafety.gov (see Further Reading 5).

One tool in the battle against foodborne illness is HACCP, or Hazard Analysis Critical Control Point. By applying the principles of HACCP, food handlers critically analyze how they approach food preparation and what conditions may exist that might allow pathogenic microorganisms to enter and thrive in the food system. Once specific hazards and critical control points (potential problems) are identified, preventive measures can be used to reduce specific sources of contamination.

13.2 Food Preservation—Past, Present, and Future

For centuries, salt, sugar, smoke, fermentation, and drying have been used to preserve food. Ancient Romans used sulfites to disinfect wine containers and preserve wine. In the age of exploration, European adventurers traveling to the New World preserved their meat by salting it. Most preserving methods work on the principle of decreasing water content. Bacteria need abundant stores of water to grow; yeasts and molds can grow with less water, but some is still necessary. Adding sugar or salt binds water and so decreases the water available to these microbes. The process of drying evaporates off free water.

Decreasing the water content of some high-moisture foods, however, would cause them to lose essential characteristics. To preserve such foods—cucumber pickles, sauerkraut, milk (yogurt), and wine—fermentation has been a traditional alternative. Selected bacteria or yeast are used to ferment or pickle foods. The fermenting bacteria or yeast make acids and alcohol, which minimize the growth of other bacteria and yeast.

Today we can add pasteurization, sterilization, refrigeration, freezing, food **irradiation**, canning, and chemical preservation to the list of food preservation techniques. An additional method of food preservation—**aseptic processing**—simultaneously sterilizes the food and package separately before the food enters the package. Liquid foods, such as fruit juices, are especially easy to process in this manner. With aseptic packaging, boxes of sterile milk and juices can remain on supermarket shelves, free of microbial growth, for many years.

Food irradiation uses minimal doses of radiation to control pathogens such as *E. coli* O157:H7 and *Salmonella*. The radiation energy used does not make the food radioactive. The energy essentially passes through the food, as in microwave cooking, and no radioactive residues are left behind. However, the energy is strong enough to break chemical bonds, destroy cell walls and cell membranes, break down DNA, and link proteins together. Irradiation thereby controls growth of insects, bacteria, fungi, and parasites in foods.

FDA approved the use of irradiation for raw red meat to reduce risk of *E. coli* and other infectious microorganisms. Other additions to the approved list are shell eggs and seeds. Prior to this, the only animal products so treated were pork and chicken. Irradiation also extends the shelf life of spices, dry vegetable seasonings, meats, and fresh fruits and vegetables.

Irradiated food, except for dried seasonings, must be labeled with the international food irradiation symbol, the Radura, and a statement that the product has been treated by irradiation. Foods treated in this way are safe in the opinion of FDA and many other health authorities, including the American Academy of Pediatrics. Although the demand for irradiated foods is still low in the United States, other countries, including Canada, Japan, Italy, and Mexico, all use food irradiation technology widely. Certain consumer groups continually try to block its use in the United States, claiming that irradiation diminishes the nutritional value of food and that it can lead to the formation of harmful compounds, such as carcinogens. Future research should be able to sort out this controversy, but in any case the risk is very low. Keep in mind that, even when foods, especially meats, have been irradiated, it is still important to follow basic food-safety procedures, as later contamination during food preparation is possible.

13.3 Foodborne Illness Caused by Microorganisms

Most cases of foodborne illness are caused by specific viruses, bacteria, and other fungi. Prions—proteins involved in maintaining nerve cell function—can also turn infectious and lead to diseases such as mad cow disease. Bacteria specifically cause health problems either directly by invading the intestinal wall and producing an *infection* via a toxin contained in the organism, or indirectly by producing a toxin

irradiation A process in which **radiation** energy is applied to foods, creating compounds (free radicals) within the food that destroy cell membranes, break down DNA, link proteins together, limit enzyme activity, and alter a variety of other proteins and cell functions of microorganisms that can lead to food spoilage. This process does not make the food radioactive.

radiation Literally, energy that is emitted from a center in all directions. Various forms of radiation energy include X-rays and ultraviolet rays from the sun.

aseptic processing A method by which food and container are separately and simultaneously sterilized; it allows manufacturers to produce boxes of milk that can be stored at room temperature.

▲ This is the Radura, the international label denoting prior irradiation of the food product.

secreted into the food, which later harms us (called an *intoxication*). The main way to distinguish an infectious route from an intoxication is time: If symptoms appear in 4 hours or less, it is an intoxication.

Bacteria

Bacteria are single-cell organisms found in the food we eat, the water we drink, and the air we breathe. Many types of bacteria cause foodborne illness, including *Bacillus*, *Campylobacter*, *Clostridium*, *Escherichia*, *Listeria*, *Vibrio*, *Salmonella*, and *Staphylococcus* (Table 13-3). Bacteria are everywhere: each teaspoon of soil contains about 2 billion bacteria. Luckily, only a small number of all bacteria pose a threat. Some foodborne bacteria cause infections, whereas others cause intoxications. *Salmonella*, for example, causes an infection because the bacteria cause the illness. *Clostridium botulinum*, *Staphylococcus aureus*, and *Bacillus cereus* produce toxins and therefore cause illness from intoxication. In addition, while most strains of *E. coli* are harmless, *E. coli* O157:H7 and O104:H4 produce a toxin that can cause severe illness, including severe bloody diarrhea and hemolytic uremic syndrome (HUS). Bacterial foodborne illnesses typically cause gastrointestinal symptoms such as vomiting, diarrhea, and abdominal cramps. *Salmonella*, *Listeria*, *E. coli* O157:H7 and O104:H4, and *Campylobacter* are the bacterial foodborne illnesses of particular interest because they are the ones most often associated with death. *E. coli* O157:H7 and O104:H4 has caused deaths when HUS has developed. Of the 1600 cases of Listeriosis in the United States each year, 255 cases are fatal. Listeriosis is of particular concern for pregnant women because they are about 20 times more likely to get this infection than other healthy adults, and Listeriosis can cause spontaneous abortion or stillbirth because the *Listeria* bacteria can cross the placenta and infect the fetus.

To proliferate, bacteria require nutrients, water, and warmth. Most grow best in **danger zone** temperatures of 40° to 140°F (4° to 60°C) (Fig. 13-1). Pathogenic bacteria

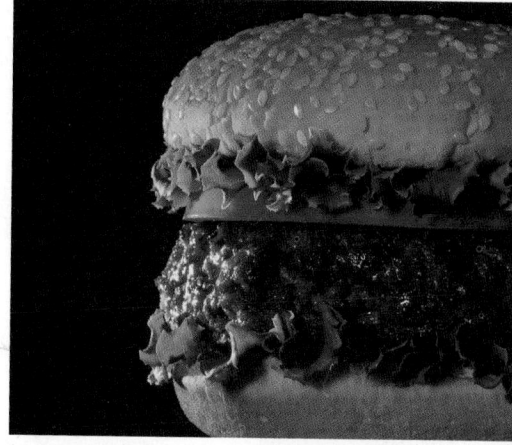

▲ Ground meats are a typical source of foodborne infection because bacteria on the surface of whole meats are distributed throughout the meat during grinding.

FIGURE 13-1 ▶ Effects of temperature on microbes that cause foodborne illness.

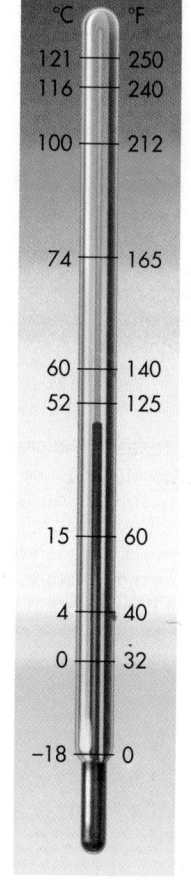
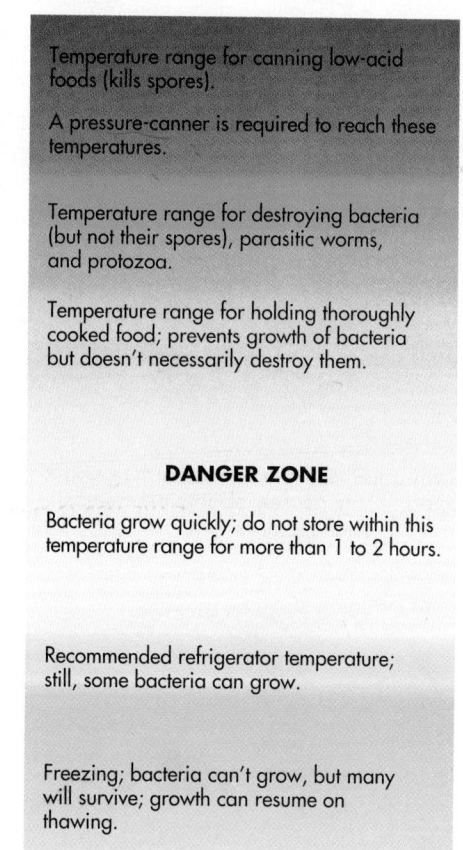

°C	°F	
121	250	Temperature range for canning low-acid foods (kills spores).
116	240	
100	212	A pressure-canner is required to reach these temperatures.
74	165	Temperature range for destroying bacteria (but not their spores), parasitic worms, and protozoa.
		Temperature range for holding thoroughly cooked food; prevents growth of bacteria but doesn't necessarily destroy them.
60	140	
52	125	**DANGER ZONE**
15	60	Bacteria grow quickly; do not store within this temperature range for more than 1 to 2 hours.
4	40	Recommended refrigerator temperature; still, some bacteria can grow.
0	32	
–18	0	Freezing; bacteria can't grow, but many will survive; growth can resume on thawing.

$$C = (F - 32) \times 5/9$$

$$F = \frac{9}{5} \times (C°) + 32$$

TABLE 13-3 Bacterial Causes of Foodborne Illness

Bacteria	Typical Food Sources	Symptoms	Additional Information
Salmonella species	Raw and undercooked meats, poultry, eggs, and fish; produce, especially raw sprouts; peanut butter; unpasteurized milk (see Further Reading 4.)	Onset: 12–72 hours; nausea, fever, headache, abdominal cramps, diarrhea, and vomiting; can be fatal in infants, the elderly, and those with impaired immune systems; lasts 4–7 days	Estimated 1 million infections/year; bacteria live in the intestines of animals and humans; food is contaminated by infected water and feces; about 2000 strains of *Salmonella* bacteria can cause disease, but 3 strains account for almost 50% of cases; *Salmonella enteritidis* infects the ovaries of healthy hens and contaminates eggs; almost 20% of cases are from eating undercooked eggs or egg-containing dishes; reptiles, such as turtles, also spread the disease
Campylobacter jejuni	Raw and undercooked meat and poultry (more than half of raw poultry in the United States is contaminated), unpasteurized milk, contaminated water	Onset: 2–5 days; muscle pain, abdominal cramping, diarrhea (sometimes bloody), fever; lasts 2–7 days	Estimated 845,000 infections/year; produces a toxin that destroys intestinal mucosal surfaces; can cause Guillain-Barré syndrome, a rare neurological disorder that causes paralysis
Escherichia coli (O157:H7 O104:H4 and other strains)	Undercooked ground beef; produce—lettuce, spinach, sprouts; unpasteurized juice and milk	Onset: 1–8 days; bloody diarrhea, abdominal cramps; in children under age 5 and the elderly, hemolytic uremic syndrome (HUS) is a serious complication; red blood cells are destroyed and kidneys fail; can be fatal; lasts 5–10 days	Leading cause of bloody diarrhea in the United States; estimated 73,000 cases/year; lives in the intestine of healthy cattle; cattle and cattle manure are chief sources; illness caused by a powerful toxin made by the bacteria; petting zoos, lakes, and swimming pools can contain pathogenic *E. coli*
Shigella species	Fecal/oral transmission; water supplies, produce, and other foods contaminated by infected food handlers with poor hygiene	Onset: 1–3 days; abdominal cramps, fever, diarrhea (often bloody); lasts 5–7 days	Estimated 448,000 cases/year; humans and primates are the only sources; common in day-care centers and custodial institutions from poor hygiene; traveler's diarrhea often caused by *Shigella dysenteriae*
Staphylococcus aureus	Ham, poultry, egg salads, cream-filled pastries, custards, whipped cream	Onset: 1–6 hours; diarrhea, vomiting, nausea, abdominal cramps; lasts 1–3 days	Bacteria on skin and nasal passages of up to 25% of people; can be passed to foods; multiplies rapidly when contaminated foods are held for extended time at room temperature; illness caused by a heat-resistant toxin that cannot be destroyed by cooking

TABLE 13-3 (continued)

Bacteria	Typical Food Sources	Symptoms	Additional Information
Clostridium perfringens	Beef, poultry, gravy, Mexican food	Onset: 8–24 hours; abdominal pain and diarrhea, usually mild; can be more serious in elderly or ill persons; lasts 1 day or less	Estimated 966,000 cases/year; anaerobic bacteria widespread in soil and water; multiplies rapidly in prepared foods, such as meats, casseroles, and gravies, held for extended time at room temperature
Listeria monocytogenes	Unpasteurized milk and soft cheeses, raw meats, uncooked vegetables, ready-to-eat deli meats and hotdogs, refrigerated smoked fish (see Further Reading 6.)	Onset: 9–48 hours for early symptoms, 14–42 days for severe symptoms; fever, muscle aches, headache, vomiting; can spread to nervous system, resulting in stiff neck, confusion, loss of balance, or convulsion; can cause premature birth and stillbirth	Estimated 1600 cases with 260 fatalities/year; widespread in soil and water and can be carried in healthy animals; grows at refrigeration temperatures; about one-third of cases occur during pregnancy; high-risk persons should avoid uncooked deli meats, soft cheeses (e.g., feta, Brie, and Camembert), blue-veined cheeses, Mexican-style cheeses (e.g., queso blanco made from unpasteurized milk), refrigerated meat spreads or pates, uncooked refrigerated smoked fish
Clostridium botulinum	Incorrectly home-canned vegetables, meats, and fish; incorrectly canned commercial foods; herb-infused oils; bottled garlic; potatoes baked in foil and held at room temperature; honey	Onset: 18–36 hours but can be 6 hours to 10 days; neurological symptoms—double and blurred vision, drooping eyelids, slurred speech, difficulty swallowing, muscle weakness, and paralysis of face, arms, respiratory muscles, trunk, and legs; can be fatal; lasts days to weeks	Estimated 100 cases/year; caused by a neurotoxin; *C. botulinum* grows only in the absence of air in non-acidic foods; incorrect home canning causes most botulism, but in 2007 commercially canned chili sauce caused an outbreak; honey can contain botulism spores and should not be given to infants younger than 1 year of age
Vibrio	*V. parahemolyticus:* raw and undercooked shellfish, especially oysters	Onset: 24 hours; watery diarrhea, nausea, vomiting, fever, chills; lasts 3 days	Found in coastal waters; more infections in summer; number of infections hard to determine because it is difficult to isolate in the lab
	V. vulnificus: raw and undercooked shellfish, especially oysters	Onset: 1–2 days; vomiting, diarrhea, abdominal pain; in more severe cases, bloodstream infection with fever, chills, decreased blood pressure, blistering skin lesions; lasts 3 or more days	Estimated 95 cases/year; found in coastal waters; more infections in summer; those with impaired immune systems and liver disease at higher risk of infection; fatality rate of 50% with bloodstream infection
	V. cholerae: contaminated water and food, human carriers	Onset: 2–3 days; severe, dehydrating diarrhea, vomiting; dehydration, cardiovascular collapse, and death can occur	Occurs mainly in countries without adequate water purification and sewage treatment
Yersinia enterocolitica	Raw or undercooked pork, particularly pork intestines (chitterlings); tofu; water; unpasteurized milk	Onset: 4–7 days; fever, abdominal pain, diarrhea (often bloody); lasts 1–3 weeks or longer	Yersinosis most common in children under age 5 years; relatively rare; bacteria live mainly in pigs but can be found in other animals

typically do not multiply when food is held at temperatures above 140°F (60°C) or stored at safe refrigeration temperatures, 32° to 40°F (0° to 4.4°C). One important exception is *Listeria* bacteria, which can multiply at refrigeration temperatures. Also note that high temperatures can kill toxin-producing bacteria, but any toxin produced in the food will not be inactivated by high temperatures. Most pathogenic bacteria also require oxygen for growth, but *Clostridium botulinum* and *Clostridium perfringens* grow only in anaerobic (oxygen-free) environments, such as those found in tightly sealed cans and jars. Food acidity can affect bacterial growth, too. Although most bacteria do not grow well in acidic environments, some, such as disease-causing *E. coli*, can grow in acidic foods, such as fruit juice.

Viruses

Viruses, like bacteria, are widely dispersed in nature. Unlike bacteria, however, viruses can reproduce only after invading body cells, such as those that line the intestines. Experts speculate that about 70% of foodborne illness cases go un-diagnosed because they result from viral causes, and there is no easy way to test for these pathogens. Table 13-4 describes the two most common viral causes of foodborne illness and describes typical food sources and symptoms of the illnesses they cause. Norovirus is the number one pathogen contributing to domestically acquired foodborne illnessses. It causes an illness commonly misdiagnosed as the "stomach flu." Norovirus infection has a sudden onset and usually a short duration of only one to two days. Noroviruses have become a problem on cruise ships. They are hardy and survive freezing, relatively high temperatures, and chlorination up to 10 ppm. A website coordinating the U.S. efforts on food safety is the www.FoodSafety.gov site mentioned earlier. Another useful website is www.homefoodsafety.org.

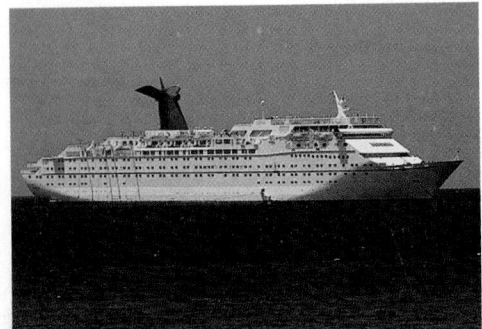

▲ Norovirus epidemics commonly occur on cruise ships. Noroviruses were originally called "Norwalk viruses" from Norwalk, Ohio, where they were first known to cause an epidemic of gastroenteritis.

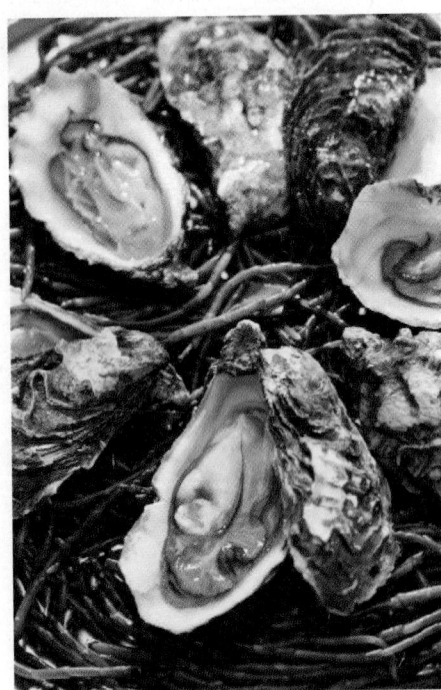

▲ Raw shellfish, especially bivalves (e.g., oysters and clams), present a particular risk related to foodborne viral disease. These animals filter feed, a process that concentrates viruses, bacteria, and toxins present in the water as it is filtered for food. Adequate cooking of shellfish will kill viruses and bacteria, but toxins may not be affected. It's important to buy shellfish from reliable sources who have harvested these foods from safe areas.

TABLE 13-4 Viral Causes of Foodborne Illness

Viruses	Typical Food Sources	Symptoms	Additional Information
Norovirus (Norwalk and Norwalk-like viruses), human rotavirus	Foods prepared by infected food handlers; shellfish from contaminated waters; vegetables and fruits contaminated during growing, harvesting, and processing (see Further Reading 13.)	Onset: 1–2 days; "stomach flu"—severe diarrhea, nausea, vomiting, stomach cramping, low-grade fever, chills, muscle aches; lasts 1–2 days or longer	Estimated over 5 million cases per year and 150 deaths. Viruses found in stool and vomit of infected persons; food handlers can contaminate foods or work surfaces; noroviruses are very infectious—as few as 10–100 particles can lead to infection; workers with norovirus symptoms should not work until 2 or 3 days after they feel better.
Hepatitis A virus	Foods prepared by infected food handlers, especially uncooked foods or those handled after cooking, such as sandwiches, pastries, and salads; shellfish from contaminated waters; vegetables and fruits contaminated during growing, harvesting, and processing	Onset: 15–50 days; anorexia, diarrhea, fever, jaundice, dark urine, fatigue; may cause liver damage and death; lasts several weeks up to 6 months	Infected food handlers contaminate food and transmit the disease to dozens of persons; children and young adults are more susceptible; a vaccine is available, decreasing the number of infections dramatically; immunoglobulin given within 1 week to those exposed to hepatitis A virus can also decrease infection.

CONCEPT CHECK

Viruses and bacteria pose the greatest risk for foodborne illness. In the past, the addition of sugar and salt to foods, as well as smoking and drying, were used to prevent the growth of microorganisms. Commercial processes, such as pasteurization and irradiation, offer protection from foodborne illness. Treat all raw animal products, cooked food, and raw fruits and vegetables as potential sources of foodborne illness.

Parasites

Parasites live in or on another organism, known as the host, from which they absorb nutrients. Humans may serve as a host to parasites. These tiny ravagers rob millions of people around the globe of their health and, in some cases, their lives. Those hardest hit live in tropical countries where poor sanitation fosters the growth of parasites.

The more than 80 foodborne parasites known to affect humans include mainly **protozoa** (one-celled animals), such as *Cryptosporidium* and *Cyclospora,* and **helminths,** such as tapeworms and the roundworm *Trichinella spiralis.* Table 13-5 describes common parasites and typical food sources and symptoms of the illnesses they cause. Parasitic infections spread via person-to-person contact and contaminated food, water, and soil.

13.4 Food Additives

By the time you see a food on the market shelf, it usually contains substances added to make it more palatable or increase its nutrient content or shelf life. Manufacturers also add some substances to foods to make them easier to process. Other substances may have accidentally found their way into the foods you buy. All of these extraneous substances are known as **additives,** and, although some may be beneficial, others, such as sulfites, may be harmful for some people. All purposefully added substances must be evaluated by FDA.

Why Are Food Additives Used?

Most additives are used to limit food spoilage. Common food additives serve the general function of **preservatives,** including acidic or alkaline agents, antioxidants, antimicrobial agents, curing and pickling agents, and **sequestrants.** Table 13-6 helps you to understand exactly why these are used and to learn more about the specific substances used. Food additives, such as potassium sorbate, are used to maintain the safety and acceptability of foods by retarding the growth of microbes implicated in foodborne illness.

Additives are also used to combat some enzymes that lead to undesirable changes in color and flavor in foods but don't cause anything as serious as foodborne illness. This second type of food spoilage occurs when enzymes in a food react to oxygen—for example, when apple and peach slices darken or turn rust color as they are exposed to air. Antioxidants are a type of preservative that slow the action of oxygen-requiring enzymes on food surfaces. These preservatives are not necessarily novel chemicals. They include vitamins E and C and a variety of sulfites.

Without the use of some food additives, it would be impossible to produce massive quantities of foods and safely distribute them nationwide or worldwide, as is now done. Despite consumer concerns about the safety of food additives, many have been extensively studied and proven safe when FDA guidelines for their use are followed.

protozoa One-celled animals that are more complex than bacteria. Disease-causing protozoa can be spread through food and water.

helminth Parasitic worm that can contaminate food, water, feces, animals, and other substances.

additives Substances added to foods, such as preservatives.

preservatives Compounds that extend the shelf life of foods by inhibiting microbial growth or minimizing the destructive effect of oxygen and metals.

sequestrants Compounds that bind free metal ions. By so doing, they reduce the ability of ions to cause rancidity in foods containing fat.

TABLE 13-5 Parasitic Causes of Foodborne Illness

Parasite	Typical Food Sources	Symptoms	Additional Information
Trichinella spiralis	Pork, wild game	Onset: weeks to months; GI symptoms followed by muscle weakness, fluid retention in the face, fever, flulike symptoms	The number of trichinosis infections has decreased greatly because pigs are now less likely to harbor this parasite; cooking pork to 160°F (72°C) will kill *trichinella*, as will freezing it for 3 days at −4°F (−20°C).
Anisakis	Raw or undercooked fish	Onset: 12 hours or less; violent stomach pain, nausea, vomiting	Caused by eating the larvae of roundworms; the infection is more common where raw fish is routinely consumed.
Tapeworms	Raw beef, pork, and fish	Abdominal discomfort, diarrhea	
Toxoplasma gondii	Raw or undercooked meat, unwashed fruits and vegetables	Onset: 5–20 days; most people are asymptomatic; those with symptoms have fever, headache, sore muscles, diarrhea; can be fatal to the fetus of pregnant women	Parasite is spread to humans from animals, including cats, the main reservoir of the disease; humans acquire the disease from ingesting contaminated meat or from fecal contamination from handling cat litter.
Cyclospora cayetanensis	Water, contaminated food	Onset: 1 week; watery diarrhea, vomiting, muscle aches, fatigue, anorexia, weight loss; lasts 10–12 weeks	Most common in tropical and subtropical areas, but since 1990 about a dozen outbreaks, affecting 3600 people, have occurred in the United States and Canada.
Cryptosporidium	Water, contaminated food	Onset: 2–10 days; watery diarrhea, abdominal pain, fever, nausea, vomiting, weight loss; those with impaired immune systems become more ill; lasts 1–2 weeks in otherwise healthy persons	Outbreaks occur worldwide; the largest U.S. outbreak was in 1993 in Milwaukee, with more than 443,000 persons affected; also can be spread in water parks and community swimming pools.

TABLE 13-6 Types of Food Additives—Sources and Related Health Concerns

Food Additive Class	Attributes	Health Risks
Acidic or alkaline agents, such as citric acid, calcium lactate, and sodium hydroxide	Acids impart a tart taste to soft drinks, sherbets, and cheese spreads; inhibit mold growth; lessen discoloration and rancidity. They also reduce the risk of botulism in naturally low-acid vegetables, such as canned green beans. Alkaline agents neutralize acids produced during fermentation, and so improve flavor.	No known health risks when used properly.
Alternative low-calorie sweeteners, such as saccharin, sucralose, ascesulfame potassium, aspartame, neotame, and tagatose	Sweeten foods without adding more than a few calories	Moderate use of these alternative sweeteners is considered safe (except for use of aspartame by people with the disease PKU).
Anticaking agents, such as calcium silicate, magnesium stearate, and silicon dioxide	Absorb moisture to keep table salt, baking powder, or powdered sugar and powdered food products free-flowing and prevent caking and lumping	No known health risks when used properly.
Antimicrobial agents, such as salt, sodium benzoate, sorbic acid, and calcium propionate	Inhibit mold and fungal growth	Salt increases the risk of developing hypertension, especially in some individuals. No known health risks from other agents when used properly.
Antioxidants, such as BHA (butylated hydroxyanisole), BHT (butylated hydroxytoluene), alpha-tocopherol (vitamin E), ascorbic acid (vitamin C), and sulfites	Delay food discolorations from oxygen exposure; Reduce rancidity from the breakdown of fats; Maintain the color of luncheon meats; Prevent the formation of cancer-causing nitrosamines	Sulfites can cause an allergic reaction in about 1 in every 100 people. Symptoms include difficulty breathing, wheezing, hives, diarrhea, abdominal pain, cramps, and dizziness. Salad bars, dried fruit, and wine are typical sources of sulfites.
Color additives, such as tartrazine	Make foods more appealing	Tartrazine (FD&C yellow number 5) can cause allergic symptoms such as hives and nasal discharge in some people, especially those allergic to aspirin. FDA requires manufacturers to list all forms of synthetic colors on the labels of foods that contain them.
Curing and pickling agents, such as salt, nitrates, and nitrites	Nitrates and nitrites act as preservatives, especially to prevent the growth of *Clostridium botulinium*; often used in conjunction with salt	Salt increases the risk of developing hypertension, especially in some individuals. Nitrate and nitrite consumption from both cured foods and that found naturally in some vegetables has been associated with synthesis of nitrosamines. (An adequate

Sugar, salt, corn syrup, and citric acid constitute 98% of all additives (by weight) used in food processing.

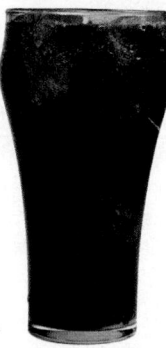

▲ Soft drinks are typical sources of alternative sweeteners for many of us. Moderate use of these products generally poses no health risk in most people.

You might wonder why, if nitrates and nitrites form chemical substances that can cause cancer, they aren't banned by the Delaney Clause. In the United States, USDA regulates the use of chemicals in meats. The laws that govern USDA regulation of foods are separate from those that govern FDA regulation. Because of this, the Delaney Clause does not apply to USDA actions. USDA sees no clear threat to public safety from the regulated use of nitrates and nitrites in meats, so no action has been taken.

TABLE 13-6 *(continued)*

Food Additive Class	Attributes	Health Risks
		vitamin C intake may reduce this synthesis.) Some nitrosamines are cancer-causing agents, particularly for the stomach, esophagus, and colon, but the risk is low. The National Cancer Institute advises consuming these foods in moderation.
Emulsifiers, such as monoglycerides and lecithins	Suspend fat in water to improve uniformity, smoothness, and body of foods, such as baked goods, ice cream, and mayonnaise	No known health risks when used properly.
Fat replacements, such as Paselli SA2, Dur-Low, Oatrim, Sta-Slim 143, Stellar, and Olean	Limit calorie content of foods by reducing some of the fat content	Generally no known health risks when used properly.
Flavor and flavoring agents (such as natural and artificial flavors), sugar, and corn syrup	Impart more or improve flavor of foods	Sugar and corn syrup can increase risk for dental caries. Generally no known health risks for flavoring agents when used properly.
Flavor enhancers, such as monosodium glutamate (MSG) and salt	Help bring out the natural flavor of foods, such as meats	Some people (especially infants) are sensitive to the glutamate portion of MSG and after exposure experience flushing, chest pain, facial pressure, dizziness, sweating, rapid heart rate, nausea, vomiting, increase in blood pressure, and headache. Those so affected should look for the word glutamate on food labels, as well as isolated protein, yeast extract, bullion, and soup stock. Salt increases the risk of developing hypertension, especially in some people.
Humectants, such as glycerol, propylene glycol, and sorbitol	Retain more moisture, texture, and fresh flavor in foods such as candies, shredded coconut, and marshmallows	No known health risk when used properly.
Leavening agents, such as yeast, baking powder, and baking soda	Introduce carbon dioxide into food products	No known health risk when used properly.
Maturing and bleaching agents, such as bromates, peroxides, and ammonium chloride	Shorten the time needed for maturation of flour to become usable for baking products	No known health risk when used properly.
Nutrient supplements, such as vitamin A, vitamin D, and potassium iodide	Enhance the nutrient content of foods such as margarine, milk, and ready-to-eat breakfast cereals	No known health risk if intake from such supplemental sources combined with other natural food sources of a nutrient does not exceed the Upper Level set for a particular nutrient (iron may be one exception; review Chapter 9).

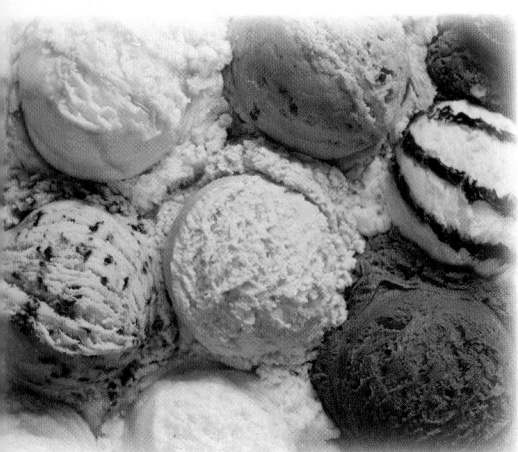

▲ Emulsifiers improve the texture of foods such as ice cream, baked goods, and cookies.

CRITICAL THINKING

Recognizing that Joseph is taking a nutrition class, his roommate asks him, "What is more risky: the bacteria that can be present in food or the additives listed on the label of my favorite snack cake?" How should Joseph respond? On what information should he base his conclusions?

TABLE 13-6 *(continued)*

Food Additive Class	Attributes	Health Risks
Stabilizers and thickeners, such as pectins, gums, gelatins, and agars	Impart a smooth texture and uniform color and flavor to candies, ice cream and other frozen desserts, chocolate milk, and beverages containing alternative sweeteners. Prevent evaporation and deterioration of flavorings used in cakes, puddings, and gelatin mixes	No known health risk when used properly.
Sequestrants, such as EDTA and citric acid	Bind free ions, helping preserve food quality by reducing ability of ions to cause rancidity in products containing fat	No known health risk when used properly.

[handwritten: marbling – is fat]

[handwritten: product of decomposed fatty acid that have unpleasant flavor/odor]

Intentional Versus Incidental Food Additives

Food additives are classified into two types: **intentional food additives** (directly added to foods) and **incidental food additives** (indirectly added as contaminants). Both types of agents are regulated by FDA in the United States. Currently, more than 2800 different substances are intentionally added to foods. As many as 10,000 other substances enter foods as contaminants. This includes substances that may reasonably be expected to enter food through surface contact with processing equipment or packaging materials.

The GRAS List

In 1958, all food additives used in the United States and considered safe at that time were put on a **generally recognized as safe (GRAS)** list. The U.S. Congress established the GRAS list because it believed manufacturers did not need to prove the safety of substances that had been used for a long time and were already generally recognized as safe. Since that time, FDA has been responsible for proving that a substance does not belong on the GRAS list. Substances may be added to the GRAS list if data and information about the use of the substance are known and accepted widely by qualified experts, and establish that the substance is safe under the conditions of its intended use.

Since 1958, some substances on the list have been reviewed. A few, such as cyclamates, failed the review process and were removed from the list. The additive red dye #3 was removed because it is linked to cancer. Many chemicals on the GRAS list have not yet been rigorously tested, primarily because of expense. These chemicals have received a low priority for testing, mostly because they have long histories of use without evidence of toxicity or because their chemical characteristics do not suggest they are potential health hazards.

Are Synthetic Chemicals Always Harmful?

Nothing about a natural product makes it inherently safer than a synthetic product. Many synthetic products are laboratory copies of chemicals that also occur in nature (see the discussion in Chapter 12 on biotechnology for some examples). Moreover, although human endeavors contribute some toxins to foods, such as synthetic pesticides and industrial chemicals, nature's poisons are often even more potent and

intentional food additives Additives knowingly (directly) incorporated into food products by manufacturers.

incidental food additives Additives that appear in food products indirectly, from environmental contamination of food ingredients or during the manufacturing process.

generally recognized as safe (GRAS) A list of food additives that in 1958 were considered safe for consumption. Manufacturers were allowed to continue to use these additives, without special clearance, when needed for food products. FDA bears responsibility for proving they are not safe, but can remove unsafe products from the list.

Some important definitions:

toxicology	Scientific study of harmful substances
safety	Relative certainty that a substance won't cause injury
hazard	Chance that injury will result from use of a substance
toxicity	Capacity of a substance to produce injury or illness at some dosage

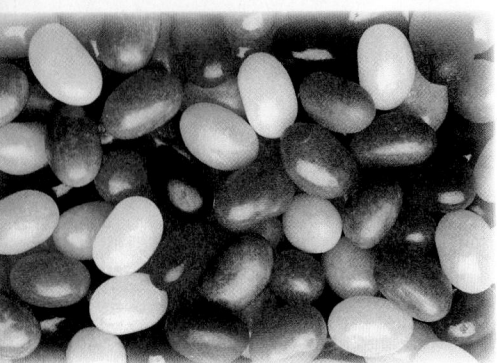

▲ Color additives make some foods more desirable.

The 100-fold margin of safety is 25 times less than that for vitamin A, when you compare the RDA for healthy women (700 micrograms) to a potentially harmful dose of vitamin A for pregnant women (3000 micrograms).

Delaney Clause A clause to the 1958 Food Additives Amendment of the Pure Food and Drug Act in the United States that prevents the intentional (direct) addition to foods of a compound shown to cause cancer in laboratory animals or humans.

widespread. Some cancer researchers suggest that we ingest at least 10,000 times more (by weight) natural toxins produced by plants than we do synthetic pesticide residues. (Plants produce these toxins to protect themselves from predators and disease-causing organisms.) This comparison does not make synthetic chemicals any less toxic, but it does put them in a more accurate perspective.

Consider vitamin E, often added to food to prevent rancidity of fats. This chemical is safe when used within certain limits. However, high doses have been associated with health problems, such as interfering with vitamin K activity in the body (review Chapter 8). Thus, even well-known chemicals we are comfortable using can be toxic in some circumstances and at some concentrations.

Tests of Food Additives for Safety

Food additives are tested by FDA for safety on at least two animal species, usually rats and mice. Scientists determine the highest dose of the additive that produces *no observable effects* in the animals. These doses are proportionately much higher than humans are ever exposed to. The maximum dosage that produced no observable effects is then divided by at least 100 to establish a margin of safety for human use. This 100-fold margin is used because it is assumed that we are at least 10 times more sensitive to food additives than are laboratory animals and that any one person might be 10 times more sensitive than another. This broad margin essentially ensures that the food additive in question will cause no harmful health effects in humans. In fact, many synthetic chemicals are probably less dangerous at these low doses than some of the natural compounds in common foods such as apples or celery.

One important exception applies to the schema for testing intentional food additives: If an additive is shown to cause cancer, even though only in high doses, no margin of safety is allowed. The food additive cannot be used, because it would violate the **Delaney Clause** in the 1958 Food Additives Amendment. This clause prohibits intentionally adding to foods a compound introduced after 1958 and that causes cancer at any level of exposure. Evidence for cancer could come from either laboratory animal or human studies. Few exceptions to this clause are allowed; exceptions are discussed regarding curing and pickling agents in Table 13-6.

Incidental food additives are another matter. FDA cannot ban various industrial chemicals, pesticide residues, and mold toxins from foods, even though some of these contaminants can cause cancer. These products are not purposely added to foods. FDA sets an acceptable level for these substances. An incidental substance found in a food cannot contribute to more than one cancer case during the lifetimes of 1 million people. If a higher risk exists, the amount of the compound in a food must be reduced until the guideline is met.

In general, if you consume a variety of foods in moderation, the chances of food additives jeopardizing your health are minimal. Pay attention to your body. If you suspect an intolerance or a sensitivity, consult your physician for further evaluation. Remember that in the short run, you are more likely to suffer either from foodborne illness due to poor food-handling practices that allow viral and bacterial contamination in food, or from the consumption of raw animal foods, than from consuming additives. Excess calories, saturated fat, cholesterol, *trans* fat, salt, and other potential "problem" nutrients in our diets pose the greatest long-term health risk.

Approval for a New Food Additive

Before a new food additive can be added to foods, FDA must approve its use. Besides rigorously testing an additive to establish its safety margins, manufacturers must give FDA information that (1) identifies the new additive, (2) gives its chemical composition, (3) states how it is manufactured, and (4) specifies laboratory methods used to measure its presence in the food supply at the amount of intended use.

Manufacturers must also offer proof that the additive will accomplish its intended purpose in a food, that it is safe, and that it is to be used in no higher amount than needed. Additives cannot be used to hide defective food ingredients, such as rancid oils; to deceive customers; or replace good manufacturing practices. A manufacturer must establish that the ingredient is necessary for producing a specific food product.

MAKING DECISIONS

Processed or Whole Foods?

If you are bewildered or concerned about all the additives in your diet, you can easily avoid most of them by consuming unprocessed whole foods. However, no evidence shows that this will necessarily make you healthier, nor can you avoid all additives, because some are used even on whole foods, such as with pesticides. It amounts to a personal decision. Do you have confidence that FDA and food manufacturers are adequately protecting your health and welfare, or do you want to take more personal control by minimizing your intake of compounds not naturally found in foods?

CONCEPT CHECK

Food additives are used to reduce spoilage from microbial growth, oxygen, metals, and other compounds. Additives are also used to adjust acidity, improve flavor and color, leaven, provide nutritional fortification, thicken, and emulsify food components. Additives are classified as intentional (direct; purposely added to foods), and incidental (indirect; present in foods from environmental contamination or various manufacturing practices). The amount of an additive allowed in a food is limited to one-one-hundredth of the highest amount that has no observable effect when fed to animals. The Delaney Clause allows FDA to limit intentional addition of cancer-causing compounds to food in the United States under its jurisdiction. Also set by law in the United States are the permissible amounts of carcinogens that incidentally enter foods.

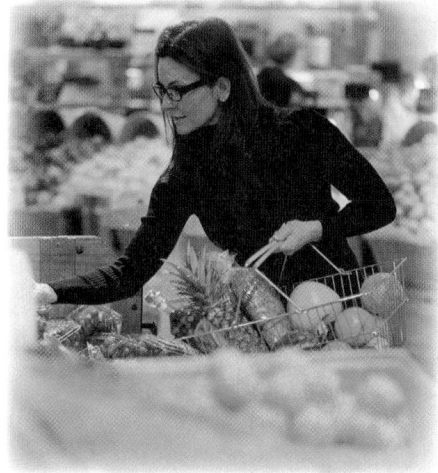

▲ Depending on whether you choose fresh versus processed foods, a diet can be either essentially free of or contain food additives. For most of us, this specific concern regarding food choice is not worth worrying about.

13.5 Substances That Occur Naturally in Foods and Can Cause Illness

Foods contain a variety of naturally occurring substances that can cause illness. Here are some of the more important examples:

- *Safrole*—found in sassafras, mace, and nutmeg; causes cancer when consumed in high doses
- *Solanine*—found in potato shoots and green spots on potato skins; inhibits the action of neurotransmitters
- *Mushroom toxins*—found in some species of mushrooms such as aminita; can cause stomach upset, dizziness, hallucinations, and other neurological symptoms. The more lethal varieties can cause liver and kidney failure, coma, and even death. FDA regulates commercially grown and harvested mushrooms. These are cultivated in concrete buildings or caves. However, there are no systematic controls on individual gatherers harvesting wild species, except in Illinois and Michigan.
- *Avidin*—found in raw egg whites (cooking destroys avidin); binds the vitamin biotin in a way that prevents its absorption, so a biotin deficiency may ultimately develop over the long term
- *Thiaminase*—found in raw fish, clams, and mussels; destroys the vitamin thiamin
- *Tetrodotoxin*—found in puffer fish; causes respiratory paralysis
- *Oxalic acid*—found in spinach, strawberries, sesame seeds, and other foods; binds calcium and iron in the foods, and so limits absorption of these nutrients
- *Herbal teas* containing senna or comfrey—can cause diarrhea and liver damage

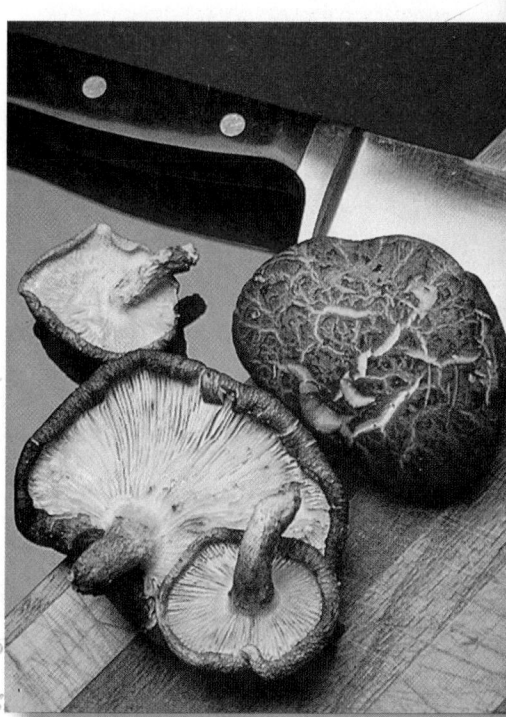

▲ When hunting wild mushrooms, know what you are looking for. Many varieties contain deadly toxins.

People have coexisted for centuries with these naturally occurring substances and have learned to avoid some of them and limit intake of others. They pose little health risk. Farmers know potatoes must be stored in the dark, so that solanine won't be synthesized. Furthermore, we've developed cooking and food-preparation methods to limit the potency of other substances, such as thiaminase. Spices are used in such small amounts that health risks don't result. Nevertheless, it's important to understand that some potentially harmful chemicals in foods occur naturally.

Is Caffeine a Cause for Concern?

Why all the controversy over a cup of coffee? Researchers have spent a great deal of time on the study of caffeine, the substance of greatest concern in the favorite beverage of many of us. So why do caffeine recommendations change from year to year?

Caffeine is a stimulant found as a natural or added ingredient in many beverages and chocolate. On average, we consume 75% of our caffeine intake as coffee, 15% as tea, 10% as soft drinks, and 2% as chocolate (Table 13-7). (For teenagers and young adults this ratio is often relatively higher for soft drinks and lower for coffee.)

Caffeine is not often consumed by itself. With the popularity of trendy coffee shops that serve everything from mocha java to flavored lattes, it is difficult to separate caffeine intake from cream, sugar, alternative sweeteners, and flavorings. So what is the conscientious coffee drinker to think? Let's explore the myths and facts of caffeine intake.

Caffeine does not accumulate in the body and is normally excreted within several hours following consumption. Caffeine can cause anxiety, increased heart rate, insomnia, increased urination (possibly resulting in dehydration), diarrhea, and gastrointestinal upset in high doses. In addition, those already suffering from ulcers may experience irritation due to increased acid production; those who have anxiety

TABLE 13-7 Caffeine Content of Common Sources

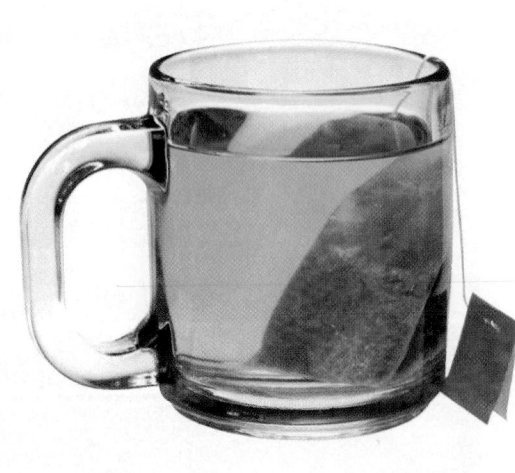

Item	Milligrams of Caffeine	
	Typical	Range*
Coffee (8 fl oz)		
Brewed, drip method	85	65–120
Brewed, percolator	75	60–85
Decaffeinated, brewed	3	2–4
Espresso (1 fl oz serving)	40	30–50
Teas (8 fl oz)		
Brewed, Black tea	40	20–90
Brewed, Green tea	20	8–30
Iced	25	9–50
Instant	28	24–31
Some soft drinks (8 fl oz)	24	20–40
"Energy drinks" such as Red Bull (8.3 fl oz)	80	0–80
Cocoa beverage (8 fl oz)	6	3–32
Chocolate milk beverage (8 fl oz)	5	2–7
Milk chocolate (1 oz)	6	1–15
Dark chocolate, semi-sweet (1 oz)	20	5–35
Baker's chocolate (1 oz)	26	26
Chocolate-flavored syrup (1 fl oz)	4	4

*For the coffee and tea products, the range varies due to brewing method, plant variety, brand of product, and so on.

Source: International Food Information Council. *Caffeine and women's health,* August 2002.

or panic attacks may find that caffeine worsens their symptoms; and those prone to heartburn may find that caffeine worsens this symptom because it relaxes sphincter muscles in the esophagus. Some people need little caffeine to feel such effects, and the dosage for children is likely even lower than that for adults.

Withdrawal symptoms are also real. Former coffee drinkers may experience headache, nausea, and depression for a short time after discontinuing use. These symptoms can be expected to peak at 20 to 48 hours following the last intake of caffeine. Symptoms hold true even for those trying to quit as little as one cup of coffee per day. Slow tapering of use over a few days is recommended to avoid these problems.

Are there more serious consequences of consuming caffeine regularly? It has been hypothesized that caffeine consumption can lead to certain types of cancer, such as pancreatic and bladder cancers. The association of caffeine with cancer has not been supported in recent literature. In fact, regular coffee consumption has been linked to a decreased risk of colon cancer.

Negative press has dwindled with regard to a link between cardiovascular disease and moderate coffee consumption. Heavy use does increase blood pressure for a short period of time. Coffee consumption also has been linked to increased LDL-cholesterol and triglycerides in the blood. This association was found to be caused by cafestol and kahweol, two oils in ground coffee. However, filtered and instant coffees do not contain the harmful oils. It is prudent, though, to limit the amount of coffee in general, especially from French coffee presses and from espresso as these beverages are not filtered.

Women are thought to be at higher risk for a variety of deleterious effects with caffeine consumption, including miscarriages, osteoporosis, and birth defects in their offspring. It is true that heavy caffeine use mildly increases the amount of calcium excreted in urine. For this reason, it is important that heavy coffee drinkers check their diets for adequate calcium sources. Some studies do show a higher likelihood for miscarriages in women consuming more than 500 milligrams of caffeine per day (about five 8-ounce cups of coffee). FDA warns women to consume caffeine in moderation (no more than the equivalent of one to two 8-ounce cups of coffee per day).

In contrast to these possibly harmful effects of caffeine consumption, many people are convinced of the benefits of a "cup of joe." Though some women testify to the idea that caffeine improves premenstrual symptoms, no study proves this theory. Some weight-loss drugs previously contained caffeine, under the assumption that it made the drugs more effective. FDA has since banned this use as it was found to be ineffective. Some newer research findings suggest caffeine may reduce the risk of developing headaches, cirrhosis of the liver, some forms of kidney stones, gallbladder stones, some nerve-related diseases, and furthermore, that it aids in blood glucose regulation. You may have heard that caffeine can improve physical performance. This has been shown in highly trained athletes; recall that use of large amounts of caffeine is banned by the NCAA (review Chapter 10). For those below professional status, though, no benefit has been shown. Also keep in mind that coffee will not "sober up" a person who is drunk.

Though the debate over caffeine will likely continue as long as North Americans drink coffee, research does not support many of the concepts previously thought of as fact. These studies are reinforcing the idea of moderation—the equivalent of about two to three 8-ounce cups of coffee per day. A prudent dose of caffeine is 200 to 300 milligrams per day. Review Table 13-7 concerning the caffeine content of typical sources.

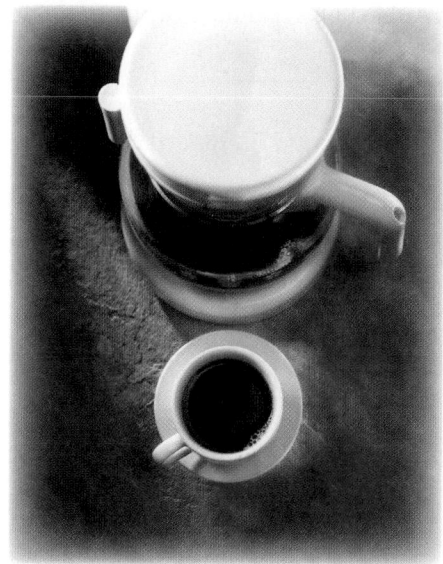

▲ Coffee is a common source of caffeine for many adults.

13.6 Environmental Contaminants in Food

A variety of environmental contaminants can be found in foods. Aside from pesticide residues, other potential contaminants that deserve attention are listed in Table 13-8. To reduce exposure to environmental toxins present in our foods that cause disease, find out which foods pose a risk. In addition, emphasize variety and moderation in food selection. Tips provided in Tables 13-8 and 13-9 also apply to reducing exposure to environmental contaminants.

Genetic alteration of foods such as corn and soybeans has created concern, especially in Europe. FDA considers genetically altered products safe if approval for human use has been granted (see Chapter 12 for details).

TABLE 13-8 Potential Environmental and Other Contaminants in Our Food Supply

Chemical Substance	Sources	Toxic Effects	Preventive Measures
Acrylamide	Fried foods rich in carbohydrate cooked at high temperatures for extended periods, such as French fries and potato chips	Potential neurotoxin and carcinogen. Known carcinogen for laboratory animals; however, studies have not clearly proven the relationship between acrylamide ingestion and the development of cancer in humans.	Limit intake of deep-fat fried foods rich in carbohydrate.
Cadmium	Plants in general if much cadmium is in the soil Clams, shellfish, tobacco smoke Occupational exposure in some cases	Kidney disease Liver disease Prostate cancer (debatable) Bone deformities Lung disease (when inhaled)	Consume a wide variety of foods, including seafood sources.
Dioxin	Trash-burning incinerators Bottom-feeding fish from the Great Lakes Animal fats from animals exposed to such contamination via water or soil	Abnormal reproduction and fetal/infant development Immune suppression Cancer (to date only clearly shown in laboratory animals)	Pay attention to warnings of dioxin risks from local fish; if risk exists, limit intake as suggested on the fishing license. Consume a variety of fish from local waters rather than mostly one specific species.
Lead	Lead-based paint chips and related dust in older homes Occupational exposure (e.g., radiator repair) Lead caps on wine bottles Fruit juices and pickled vegetables stored in galvanized or tin containers or leaded glass Some types of solder used in joining copper pipes (mostly in older homes) Mexican pottery dishes Koo Soo herbal remedies Leaded glass containers (see Further Reading 8.)	Anemia Kidney disease Nervous system damage (tiredness and changes in behavior are symptoms) Reduced learning capacity in childhood (even from mild lead exposure)	Avoid paint chips and related dust in older homes; regular cleaning of these homes is also important (see **www.hud.gov/offices/lead**). Meet iron and calcium needs to reduce lead absorption. Wipe the inside and outside neck of wine bottles before use if the bottle has a lead cap. Store fruit juices and pickled vegetables in glass or plastic or waxed paper containers. Let water run 1 minute or so if off for more than 2 hours, and use only cold water for cooking; do not soften drinking water. Do not store alcoholic beverages in leaded glass containers.
Mercury	Swordfish, shark, king mackerel, and tilefish. Fresh and canned albacore tuna also is a possible source. (In contrast, the more typical light chunk tuna is very low in mercury.)	Reduced fetal/child development and birth defects; toxic to nervous system	Consume these sources no more than once per week, no more than two times per week for albacore tuna. Pregnant women should avoid these species of fish, but some albacore tuna consumption is fine. Two to three fish meals per week is appropriate for pregnant (and nursing) women if different types of fish are eaten.
Polychlorinated biphenyls (PCBs)	Fish from the Great Lakes and Hudson River Valley (e.g., coho salmon) Farmed salmon are a possible source, but less so	Cancer (to date only clearly shown in laboratory animals), as well as a potential for liver, immune, and reproductive disorders	Pay attention to warnings of PCB contamination from local fish; if risk exists, limit intake as suggested on the fishing license or on state advisories. Vary the type of fish eaten during a specific week.
Urethane	Alcoholic beverages such as sherry, bourbon, sake, and fruit brandies	Cancer (to date only clearly shown in laboratory animals)	Avoid generous amounts of typical sources.

CONCEPT CHECK

A general program to minimize exposure to environmental contaminants includes knowing which foods pose greater risks and consuming a wide variety of foods in moderation.

Pesticides in Food

Pesticides used in food production produce both beneficial and unwanted effects (see Further Reading 3). Most health authorities believe that the benefits outweigh the risks. Pesticides help ensure a safe and adequate food supply and help make foods available at reasonable cost. However, there is sentiment nationwide that pesticides pose avoidable health risks. Consumers have come to assume that synthetic is dangerous and organic is safe. Some researchers believe this sentiment is grounded in fear and fueled by unbalanced reports. Other researchers say concern about pesticides is valid and overdue.

Most concern about pesticide residues in food appropriately focuses on chronic rather than acute toxicity because the amounts of residue present, if any, are extremely small. These low concentrations found in foods are not known to produce adverse effects in the short term, although harm has been caused by the high amounts that occasionally result from accidents or misuse. For humans, pesticides pose a danger mainly in their cumulative effects, so their threats to health are difficult to determine. However, growing evidence, including the problems of the contamination of underground water supplies and destruction of wildlife habitats, indicates that North Americans would probably be better off if we could reduce our use of pesticides. Both the U.S. federal government and many farmers are working toward that end. Chapter 12 discussed the lastest use of biotechnology to reduce pesticide use.

What Is a Pesticide?

Federal law defines a pesticide as any substance or mixture of substances intended to prevent, destroy, repel, or mitigate any pest. The built-in toxic properties of pesticides lead to the possibility that other, nontarget organisms, including humans, might also be harmed. The term *pesticide* tends to be used as a generic reference to many types of products, including insecticides, herbicides, fungicides, and rodenticides. A pesticide product may be chemical or bacterial, natural or synthetic. For agriculture, EPA allows about 10,000 pesticides to be used, containing some 300 active ingredients. About 1.2 billion pounds of pesticides are used each year in the United States, much of which is applied to agricultural crops.

Once a pesticide is applied, it can turn up in a number of unintended and unwanted places. It may be carried in the air and dust by wind currents, remain in soil attached to soil particles, be taken up by organisms in the soil, decompose to other compounds, be taken up by plant roots, enter groundwater, or invade aquatic habitats. Each is a route to the food chain; some are more direct than others.

Why Use Pesticides?

In the United States, pests destroy nearly $20 billion of food crops yearly, despite extensive pesticide use. The primary reason for using pesticides is economic—the use of agricultural chemicals increases production and lowers the cost of food, at least in the short run. Many farmers believe that it would be impossible to stay in business without pesticides, which help protect farmers from ruinous losses.

Consumer demands also have changed over the years. At one time, we wouldn't have thought twice about buying an apple with a worm hole; we took it home, cut out

One of the problems with pesticides is that they create new pests because they destroy the predators (spiders, wasps, and beetles) that naturally keep most plantfeeding insect populations in check. The brown plant hopper, which has plagued Indonesian rice fields, was not a serious problem before heavy pesticide use began to kill its predators in the early 1970s. In the United States, such major pests as spider mites and the cotton bollworm were merely nuisances until pesticides decimated their predators.

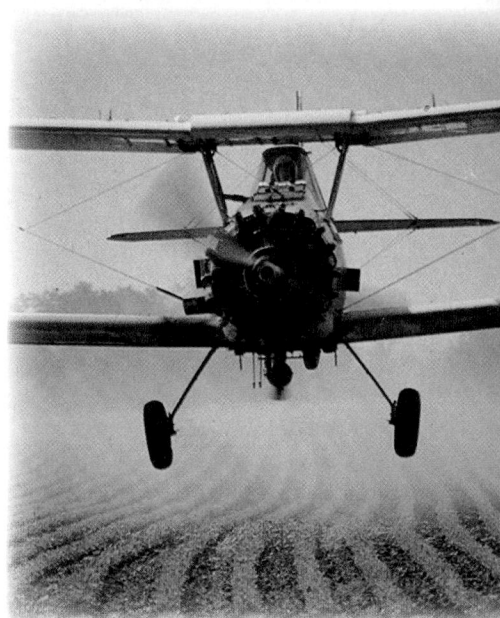

▲ Pesticide use poses a risk-versus-benefit question. Each side has points that deserve to be considered. Rural communities, where exposure is more direct, experience the greatest short-term risk.

the wormy part, and ate the apple. Today, consumers find worm holes less acceptable, so farmers rely more on pesticides to produce cosmetically attractive fruits and vegetables. On the practical side, pesticides can protect against the rotting and decay of fresh fruits and vegetables. This is helpful because our food distribution system doesn't usually permit consumer purchase within hours of harvest. Also, food grown without pesticides can contain naturally occurring organisms that produce carcinogens at concentrations far above current standards for pesticide residues. For example, fungicides help prevent the carcinogen aflatoxin (caused by growth of a fungus) from forming on some crops. Thus, although some pesticides may do little more than improve the appearance of food products, others help keep foods fresher and safer to eat.

Regulation of Pesticides EPA

The responsibility for ensuring that residues of pesticides in foods are below amounts that pose a danger to health is shared by FDA, EPA, and the Food Safety and Inspection Service of USDA in the United States. Table 13-2 listed the roles of various food protection agencies. FDA is responsible for enforcing pesticide tolerances in all foods except meat, poultry, and certain egg products, which are monitored by USDA. A newly proposed pesticide is exhaustively tested, perhaps over 10 years or more, before it is approved for use. EPA must decide that the pesticide causes no unreasonable adverse effects on people and the environment and that benefits of use outweigh the risks of using it. However, there is concern about older chemicals registered before 1970, when less stringent testing conditions were permitted. EPA is now asking chemical companies to retest the old compounds using more rigorous tests. Unfortunately, inadequate funding at EPA has hampered the review of older pesticides. The slow pace of this retesting has angered the critics of pesticide use. When weighing whether to approve or cancel a pesticide, EPA considers how much more it would cost the farmer to use an alternative pesticide or process and whether cancellation would decrease productivity. After determining the dollar cost to the farmer, EPA then looks at costs to processors and consumers. Once a pesticide is approved for use, it must follow the margin of safety provisions required of food additives (see previous section, "Tests of Food Additives for Safety").

How Safe Are Pesticides?

Dangers from exposure to pesticides through food depend on how potent the chemical toxin is, how concentrated it is in the food, how much and how frequently it's eaten, and the consumer's resistance or susceptibility to the substance. Accumulating information links pesticide use to increased cancer rates in farm communities. For rural counties in the United States, the incidence of lymph, genital, brain, and digestive tract cancers increases with higher-than-average pesticide use. Respiratory cancer cases increase with greater insecticide use. In tests using laboratory animals, scientists have found that some of the chemicals present in pesticide residues cause birth defects, sterility, tumors, organ damage, and injury to the central nervous system. Some pesticides persist in the environment for years.

Still, some researchers argue that the cancer risk from pesticide residues is hundreds of times less than the risk from eating such common foods as peanut butter, brown mustard, and basil. Plants manufacture toxic substances to defend themselves against insects, birds, and grazing animals (including humans). When plants are stressed or damaged, they produce even more of these toxins. Because of this, many foods contain naturally occurring chemicals considered toxic, and some are even carcinogenic. Other scientists argue that if natural carcinogens are already in the food supply, then we should reduce the number of added carcinogens whenever possible. In other words, we should do what we can to decrease our overall exposure.

Tests of the Amounts of Pesticides in Foods

FDA tests thousands of raw products each year for pesticide residues. (A pesticide is considered illegal in this case if it is not approved for use on the crop in question or

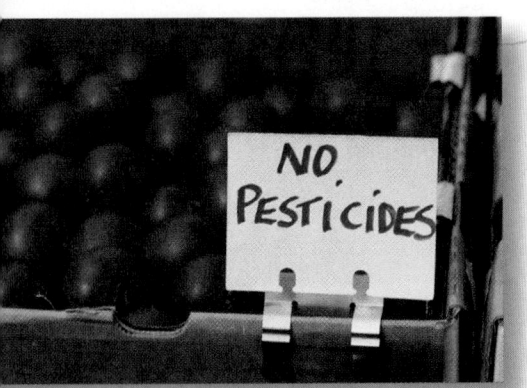

▲ Fruits and vegetables grown without use of pesticides are available and may bear an "organic" label (see Table 2-10 for rules regarding the use of the term "organic" on food labels). These products generally are more expensive than those grown using pesticides. Consumers need to decide if the potential benefits of the products are worth the extra cost.

if the amount used exceeds the allowed tolerance.) The latest FDA studies show no residues in about 60% of samples. Less than 1% of domestic and about 3% of import samples have residues continually over tolerance. These findings continue to support previous FDA studies over the past 10 years that pesticide residues in food are generally well below EPA tolerances, and they confirm the safety of the food supply relative to pesticide residues.

Personal Action

We often take risks in our lives, but we prefer to have a choice in the matter after weighing the pros and cons. With regard to pesticides in food, however, someone else is deciding what is acceptable and what is not. Our only choice is whether to buy or avoid pesticide-containing foods. In reality, it's almost impossible to avoid pesticides entirely, because even organic produce often contains traces of pesticides, probably as the result of cross-contamination from nearby farms.

Short-term studies of the effects of pesticides on laboratory animals cannot precisely pinpoint long-term cancer risks in humans. It should be clearly understood, however, that the presence of minute traces of an environmental chemical in a food does not mean that any adverse effect will result from eating that food.

FDA and other scientific organizations believe that the hazards are comparatively low and in the short run are less dangerous than the hazards of foodborne illness created in our kitchens. We cannot avoid pesticide risks entirely, but we can limit exposure by following some simple advice (Table 13-9).

We can also encourage farmers to use fewer pesticides to reduce exposure to our foods and water supplies, but we'll have to settle for produce that isn't perfect in appearance or that has been grown with the aid of biotechnology (again, see Chapter 12 for details). Are you concerned enough about pesticides on food to change your shopping habits or take more political action?

13.7 Food Production Choices

Agriculture, the production of food and livestock, has supplied humans with food for millennia. At one time, nearly everyone was involved in food production. Only about 1 in 3 people around the globe and far fewer in the United States (less than 1%), is now involved in farming. Today, numerous advances in agricultural sciences are affecting our food supply; of particular note are organic food production and sustainable agriculture.

TABLE 13-9 What You Can Do to Reduce Exposure to Pesticides

FDA's sampling and testing show that pesticide residues in foods do not pose a health hazard. Nevertheless, if you want to reduce dietary exposure to pesticides, follow this advice from the Environmental Protection Agency:

- Consume a wide variety of foods, especially regarding fruits, vegetables, and fish.
- Thoroughly rinse and scrub (with a brush if possible) fruits and vegetables. Peel them, if appropriate—although some nutrients will be peeled away.
- Remove the outer leaves of leafy vegetables, such as lettuce and cabbage.
- Residues of some pesticides in animal feed concentrate in the animals' fat, so trim fat from meat, poultry, and fish; remove skin (which contains most of the fat) from poultry and fish; and discard fats and oils in broths and pan drippings.
- When fishing, throw back the big fish—the little ones have had less time to take up and concentrate pesticides and other harmful residues. In addition, pay attention to any warnings by local authorities (and on the fishing license) about the high risk for contamination in specific waters or species of fish.
- Avoid lawns, gardens, and flower beds that have recently been treated with pesticides and herbicides.

Adapted from Food and Drug Administration: Safety first: Protecting America's food supply, *FDA Consumer*, p. 26, November 1988.

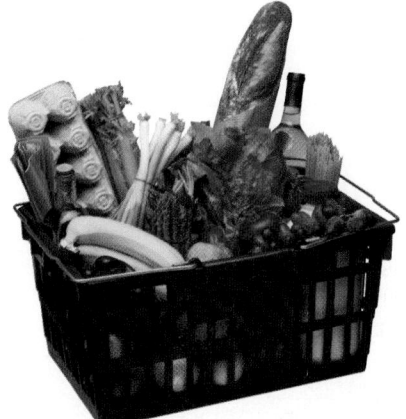

▲ FDA's yearly evaluation of a "market basket" of typical foods shows that pesticide content is minimal in most foods.

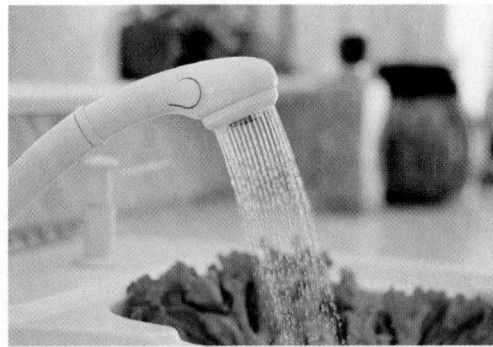

▲ Wash fresh fruits and vegetables under running water to remove bacteria and soil. Special antibacterial washing products are not necessary.

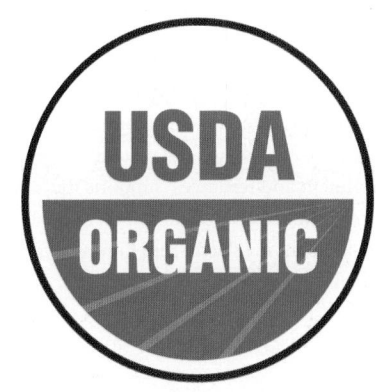

▲ The USDA organic seal identifies organic foods grown on USDA-certified organic farms.

▲ Organic fruits and vegetables experienced the highest growth in food sales at 11.8% over 2009 sales and representing over 11% of all fruit and vegetable sales.

biological pest management Control of agricultural pests by using natural predators, parasites, or pathogens. For example, ladybugs can be used to control an aphid infestation.

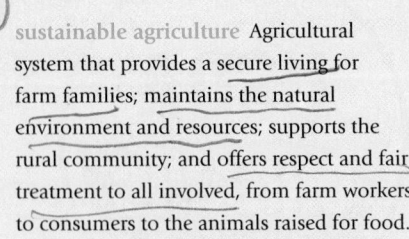

sustainable agriculture Agricultural system that provides a secure living for farm families; maintains the natural environment and resources; supports the rural community; and offers respect and fair treatment to all involved, from farm workers to consumers to the animals raised for food.

Organic Foods

Organic foods are increasingly available in supermarkets, specialty stores, farmers' markets, and restaurants (see Further Readings 11 and 14). Consumers can select organic fruits, vegetables, grains, dairy products, meats, eggs, and many processed foods, including sauces and condiments, breakfast cereals, cookies, and snack chips. Interest in personal and environmental health has contributed to the increasing availability and sales of organic foods. According to the Organic Trade Association, U.S. sales of organic foods reached $26.7 billion by the end of 2010. This was a 7.7% increase over 2009 sales, despite tough economic times. Despite this rapid growth, only 4% of foods sold are organic. Organic foods, because they often cost more to grow and produce, are typically more expensive than comparable conventional foods.

The term **organic** refers to the way agricultural products are produced. Organic production relies on farming practices such as **biological pest management**, composting, manure applications, and crop rotation to maintain healthy soil, water, crops, and animals. Synthetic pesticides, fertilizers, and hormones; antibiotics; sewage sludge (used as fertilizer); genetic engineering; and irradiation are not permitted in the production of organic foods. Additionally, organic meat, poultry, eggs, and dairy products must come from animals allowed to graze outdoors and are fed only organic feed.

The Organic Foods Production Act of 1990 established standards for the production of foods that bear the USDA organic seal. Foods labeled and marketed as organic must be grown on farms that are certified by the USDA as following all of the rules established in the 1990 act. Foods made from multiple ingredients (e.g., breakfast cereal) labeled as organic must have at least 95% of their ingredients (by weight) meet organic standards. The term "made with organic" can be used if at least 70% of the ingredients are organic. Small organic producers and farmers with sales less than $5000 per year are exempt from the certification regulation. Some farmers use organic production methods but choose not to be USDA certified. Their foods cannot be labeled as organic, but many of these farmers market and sell to those seeking organic foods.

The organic food market received a boost in 2009 when USDA offered $50 million in new funding to encourage greater production of organic food in the United States. The Organic Trade Association (www.ota.com/index.html) believes that this funding will further encourage farmers to use organic practices and help increase the U.S. production of organic food to meet growing consumer demand. With tough economic times, consumers have used various strategies in continuing to buy organic products. Because most stores now offer organic products, consumers have the opportunity to shop around. Increased availability and use of coupons, the proliferation of private label and store brands, and better value products offered by major organic brands all have contributed to increased sales.

Organic Foods and Health Consumers may choose to eat organic foods to reduce their pesticide intake, to protect the environment, and to improve the nutritional quality of their diets. Those who consume organic produce do ingest lesser amounts of pesticides (only 1 in 4 organically grown fruits and vegetables contains pesticides and in lower amounts than conventional produce), but it's still not known whether or how this affects the health of most consumers. However, organic foods may be a wise choice for young children because pesticide residues may pose a greater risk to them. Consumers also may opt for organic foods to encourage environmentally friendly **sustainable agriculture** practices.

Most studies do not show that organic foods have higher amounts of vitamins and minerals (see Further Reading 5). However, researchers have found that, in some cases, organic fruits and vegetables contain more vitamin C and antioxidants that help protect cells against damage. At this point, it's not possible to recommend organic foods over conventional foods based on nutrient content—both can meet nutritional needs. A healthy dose of common sense also is important—an "organic" label does not change a less healthy food into a more healthy food. Organic potato chips have the same calorie and fat content as conventional potato chips.

One concern raised about organic foods is that food safety may be jeopardized because animal manures used for fertilizers might cause more pathogen contamination of food. The recent outbreaks of foodborne illness linked to organically grown sprouts in Europe confirm that an organic label does not guarantee good health. However, research does not show that certified organic food has higher contamination with bacterial pathogens. Consumers should wash or scrub all produce—organic as well as conventional—under running water.

The term "natural" is not regulated. Products labeled as "natural" are generally those derived from natural ingredients, such as a plant source, which retain their natural properties in the finished product. Meat or poultry labeled "natural" must be minimally processed, and contain no artificial flavoring, coloring, chemical preservative, or other artificial or synthetic ingredient. No one is really checking these products, and there is some debate over what constitutes "minimally processed." Although all organic products fit this definition of natural, not all natural products are necessarily organic.

Sustainable Agriculture

Conventional agriculture focuses on maximizing production through the use of large acreages, powerful machines, chemicals to control pests, and petroleum-based fertilizers to boost growth. In contrast, sustainable agriculture is an integrated system of plant and animal production that will, over the long-term, satisfy human food needs, enhance environmental quality, efficiently use nonrenewable resources, sustain the economic viability of farm operations, and enhance the quality of life for farmers and society as a whole. A culture of sustainability has emerged, including a clear trend for sustainable food choices manufactured in an environmentally responsible way. The food industry has responded with a move toward "green" initiatives that should be sustainable for the long-term. A new demographic term, LOHAS (Lifestyle of Health and Sustainability), describes a growing demographic group focused on sustainable living. An increasing number of today's college students are joining this market segment and developing behaviors associated with social responsibility. These consumers are driving changes in many areas, including the food industry. Slow Food Nation is an example of a non-profit group dedicated to creating a framework for a deeper environmental connection to our food and aiming to inspire and empower Americans to build a food system that is sustainable, healthy, and delicious.

Locally Grown Foods

With people everywhere more interested in the origins of their food, more grocery store shelves are devoted to "locally grown" products. Consumers are demanding increased transparency with the food supply, and local food helps answer questions about where food comes from and how it was grown. Retailers are using the "locally grown" label to respond to consumer desires for fresh, safe products that also support small, local farmers and help the environment. Local products provide fresher options, do not have the added costs of long transportation, and thus, use less fossil fuel. Foodservice establishments are giving greater emphasis to local producers, focusing on where food was grown and how it was handled.

Farmers' markets are the most obvious way that consumers have access to locally grown, farm-fresh produce. Farmers' markets are also an integral part of the urban/farm linkage and continue to gain popularity. In 2010 there were 6132 farmers' markets operating throughout the United States, which was a 16% increase from 2009.

The interest in "local" foods has become such a phenomenon that the term "locavore" was the 2007 Word of the Year in the New Oxford American Dictionary. **Locavore** is defined as someone who eats food grown or produced locally or within a certain radius such as 50, 100, or 150 miles. The locavore movement has gained prominence due to food-safety concerns by consumers and the search for local, sustainable foods. It encourages consumers to buy from farmers' markets or even to produce their own food, with the argument that fresh, local products are more nutritious and taste better.

CRITICAL THINKING

Stephanie, a college sophomore, is adamant about eating only organic foods. She frequently states that conventionally grown and processed foods are unhealthy, full of harmful chemicals, and almost nutrient-free. Knowing that you are studying nutrition, Stephanie discusses her beliefs with you and asks for your opinion. What are some ways you might respond to her?

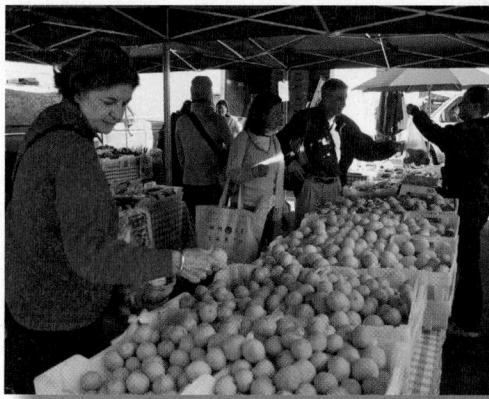

▲ The locavore movement is based on the assumption that local products are more nutritious and taste better and encourages consumers to buy from farmers' markets or even to produce their own food.

locavore Someone who eats food grown or produced locally or within a certain radius such as 50, 100, or 500 miles.

NEWSWORTHY NUTRITION

German organic sprouts cause deadly *E. coli* outbreak

The world's deadliest outbreak of *Escherichia coli* occurred during the summer of 2011. The outbreak occurred mainly in Germany and involved a rare enterohemorrhagic strain of *E. coli* known as O104:H4. In June 2011, 3332 persons had been infected, more than 600 were in intensive care, and the death toll from the outbreak had reached 36. Several hundred also contracted its potentially fatal kidney complication, known as hemolytic uremic syndrome. The European Centre for Disease Prevention and Control concluded that the *E. coli* infection was caused by tainted vegetable sprouts from a small, rather traditional organic sprout farm. The sprout seeds were mostly imported from overseas and the *E. coli* bacteria were antibiotic resistant. Experts say these types of outbreaks are becoming more common due to large-scale industrial farming and the widespread use of antibiotics.

Source: Dempsey J, Neuman W: Deadly *E. coli* outbreak linked to German sprouts. *New York Times*, June 5, 2011.

connect NUTRITION **Check out the Connect site**
www.mcgrawhillconnect.com
to further explore *E. coli*.

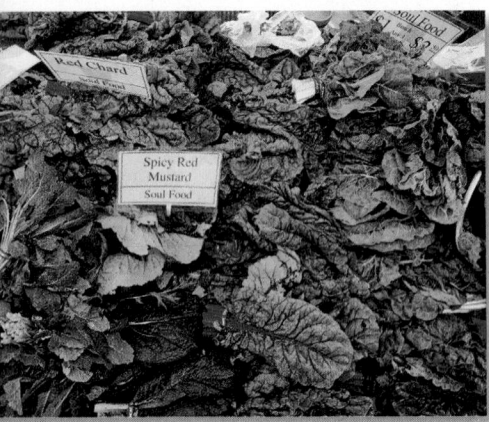

▲ Farmers participating in community supported agriculture (CSA) offer a share of foods from each growing season, to individuals, families or companies who support the CSA financially and/or by working for the CSA.

There is no evidence, however, that locally grown products are safer. Although many small producers have good food-safety practices, they often lack the expensive food-safety audits more common among big producers. Food-safety auditors determine such things as whether or not there is evidence of insects on produce and whether or not producers have enough bathrooms for workers. In addition, undetected foodborne illness outbreaks are more likely with "local" products delivered in small quantities and sold in a small area. Local products are not necessarily pesticide-free and may not be cheaper, given that smaller growers lack the economic advantages of bigger growers. Read about the outbreak of foodborne illness linked to a local organic farm in Newsworthy Nutrition.

Unlike organic products, there are no regulations specifying the meaning of "locally grown." Whole Foods Market, Inc. is the biggest retailer of natural and organic food and probably the best-known for buying and selling locally grown produce. Whole Foods considers local to be anything produced within seven hours of one of its stores, with most local producers within 200 miles of a store. Wal-Mart, the world's largest retailer, has also become a large buyer of locally grown fruits and vegetables and considers anything local if it is grown in the same state as it is sold. Searchable databases and mapping resources such as MarketMaker (http://national.marketmaker.uiuc.edu/) are now available to connect growers with buyers, restaurants with distributors, and consumers with local farmers' markets. These tools make it easier for people to find and sell locally grown foods.

Community Supported Agriculture

Consumers are not only taking comfort in knowing where their food comes from, but are also starting to have interest in community connections with local/regional farmers. Stemming from the interest in locally grown food, there is growing national support for local food collaboratives and community supported agriculture. Community Supported Agriculture programs (CSA) involve a partnership between local food producers and local consumers. During each growing season, CSA farmers offer a share of foods to individuals, families, or companies who have pledged support to the CSA either financially and/or by working for the CSA.

Another example of a farm-community partnership is the National Farm to School Program (www.farmtoschool.org/), a nonprofit effort to connect farmers with nearby school cafeterias. Between 1997 and 2011, this program grew from only six local programs to 2352 programs in 48 states resulting in 9756 schools incorporating the local bounty into their menus. Administrators of the program have found that if kids can meet the farmer who actually grew the food, they are much more likely to eat it.

Preventing Foodborne Illness

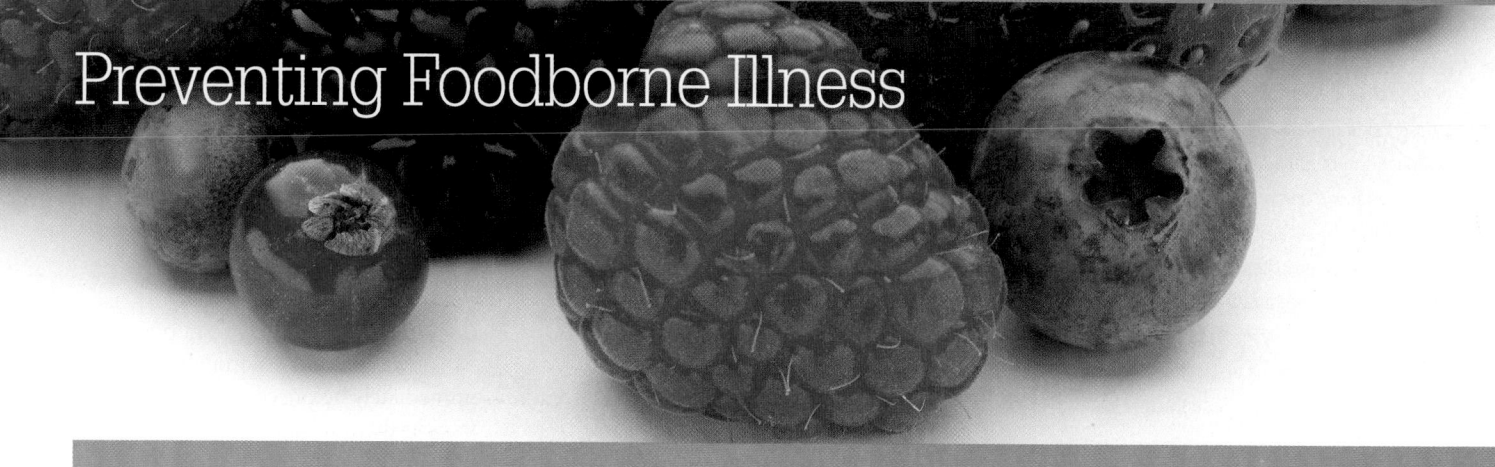

General Rules for Preventing Foodborne Illness

You can greatly reduce the risk of foodborne illness by following some important rules (see Further Reading 7). It's a long list, because many risky habits need to be addressed.

Purchasing Food

- When shopping, select frozen foods and perishable foods, such as meat, poultry, or fish, last. Always have these products put in separate plastic bags, so that drippings don't contaminate other foods in the shopping cart. Don't let groceries sit in a warm car; this allows bacteria to grow. Get the perishable foods such as meat and egg and dairy products home and promptly refrigerate or freeze them.
- Don't buy or use food from damaged containers that leak, bulge, or are severely dented or from jars that are cracked or have loose or bulging lids. Don't taste or use food that has a foul odor or spurts liquid when the can is opened; the deadly *Clostridium botulinum* toxin may be present.
- Purchase only pasteurized milk and cheese (check the label). This is especially important for pregnant women because highly toxic bacteria and viruses that can harm the fetus thrive in unpasteurized milk.
- Purchase only the amount of produce needed for a week's time. The longer you keep fruits and vegetables, the more time is available for bacteria to grow.
- When purchasing precut produce or salads, avoid those that look slimy,

brownish, or dry; these are signs of improper holding temperatures.
- Observe sell-by and expiration dates on food labels.

Preparing Food

- Thoroughly wash your hands for 20 seconds with hot, soapy water before and after handling food. This practice is especially important when handling raw meat, fish, poultry, and eggs, after using the bathroom, after playing with pets, or after changing diapers (see Further Reading 2).
- Make sure counters, cutting boards, dishes, and other equipment are thoroughly sanitized and rinsed before use. Be especially careful to use hot, soapy water to wash surfaces and equipment that have come in contact with raw meat, fish, poultry, and eggs as soon as possible to remove *Salmonella* bacteria that may be present. Otherwise, bacteria on the surfaces will infect the next foods that come in contact with the surface, a process called cross-contamination. In addition, replace sponges and wash kitchen towels frequently. (Microwaving sponges for 30 to 60 seconds also helps rid them of live bacteria.)
- If possible, cut foods to be eaten raw on a clean cutting board reserved for that purpose. Then clean this cutting board using hot, soapy water. If the same board must be used for both meat and other foods, cut any potentially contaminated items, such as meat, last. After cutting the meat, wash the cutting board thoroughly.

FDA recommends cutting boards with unmarred surfaces made of easy-

to-clean, non-porous materials, such as plastic, marble, or glass. If you prefer a wooden board, make sure it is made of a nonabsorbent hardwood, such as oak or maple, and has no obvious seams or cracks. Then reserve it for a specific purpose; for example, set it aside for cutting raw meat and poultry. Keep a separate wooden cutting board for chopping produce and slicing bread to prevent these products from picking up bacteria from raw meat. Many foods are served raw, so any bacteria clinging to them are not destroyed.

Furthermore, FDA recommends that all cutting boards be replaced when they become streaked with hard-to-clean grooves or cuts, which may harbor bacteria. In addition, cutting boards should be sanitized once a week in a dilute bleach solution. Flood the board with the solution, let it sit a few minutes, then rinse thoroughly.

- When thawing foods, do so in the refrigerator, under cold potable running water, or in a microwave oven. Also, cook foods immediately after thawing under cold water or in the microwave. Never let frozen foods thaw unrefrigerated all day or night. Also, marinate food in the refrigerator.
- Avoid coughing or sneezing over foods, even when you're healthy. Cover cuts on hands with a sterile bandage. This helps stop *Staphylococcus* from entering food.
- Carefully wash fresh fruit and vegetables under running water to remove dirt and bacteria clinging to the surface, using a vegetable brush if the skin is to

▶ The World Health Organization's Golden Rules for Safe Food Preparation

1. Choose foods processed for safety.
2. Cook food thoroughly.
3. Eat cooked foods immediately.
4. Store cooked foods carefully.
5. Reheat cooked foods thoroughly.
6. Avoid contact between raw and cooked foods.
7. Wash hands repeatedly.
8. Keep all kitchen surfaces meticulously clean.
9. Protect foods from insects, rodents, and other animals.
10. Use pure water.

The USDA simplified these rules into four actions as a part of their Fight BAC! Program (check out www.fightbac.org):

1. Clean. Wash hands and surfaces often.
2. Separate. Don't cross-contaminate.
3. Cook. Cook to proper temperatures.
4. Chill. Refrigerate promptly.

The 2010 Dietary Guidelines for Americans also stress the importance of these four actions.

be eaten. People have become ill from *Salmonella* introduced from melons used in making a fruit salad and from oranges used for fresh-squeezed orange juice. The bacteria were on the outside of the melons and oranges (see Further Reading 10).

- Completely remove moldy portions of food or don't eat the food. *When in doubt, throw the food out.* Mold growth is prevented by properly storing food at cold temperatures and using the food promptly.

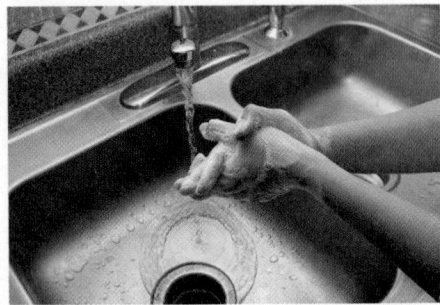

▲ Washing hands thoroughly (for at least 20 to 30 seconds) with hot water and soap should be the first step in food preparation. The 4 "F's" of food contamination are fingers, foods, feces, and flies. Handwashing especially combats the finger and fecal routes.

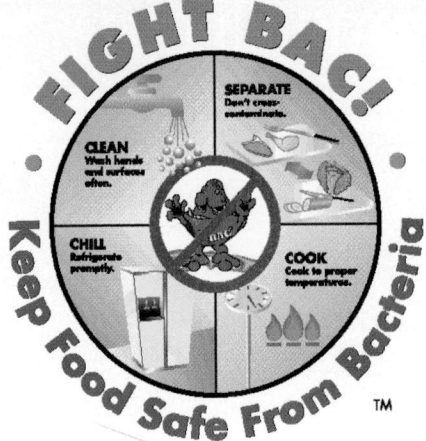

▲ Food safety logo of USDA.

- Use refrigerated ground meat and patties in 1 to 2 days and frozen meat and patties within 3 to 4 months. The 6-month interval mentioned in the comic at the beginning of this chapter is too long a time to be safe.

Cooking Food

- Cook food thoroughly using a bimetallic thermometer to check for doneness, especially for fresh beef and fish (145°F [63°C]), pork (160°F [71°C]), and poultry (165°F [74°C]) (Fig. 13-2). Eggs should be cooked until the yolk and white are hard. Alfalfa sprouts and other types of sprouts should be cooked until they are steaming. Cooking is by far the most reliable way to destroy foodborne viruses and bacteria, such as Norovirus and toxic strains of *E. coli*. Freezing only halts viral and bacterial growth. FDA does not recommend that eggs be prepared sunny-side-up.

As noted, many restaurants now include an advisory on menus stating that an increased risk of foodborne illness is associated with eating undercooked eggs. As long as restaurants provide this warning on their menus, however, they are allowed to cook eggs to any temperature requested by the consumer. FDA warns us not to consume homemade ice cream, eggnog, and mayonnaise if made with unpasteurized, raw eggs because of the risk of *Salmonella* foodborne illness. It is safer to use eggs or egg products that have been pasteurized, which kills *Salmonella* bacteria. Overall, a good general precaution is to eat no raw animal products.

USDA answers questions about the safe use of animal products (800-535-4555, 10 A.M. to 4 P.M. weekdays, Eastern time).

Seafood also poses a risk of foodborne illness, especially oysters. Properly cooked seafood should flake easily and/ or be opaque or dull and firm. If it's translucent or shiny, it's not done.

- Cook stuffing separately from poultry (or wash poultry thoroughly, stuff immediately before cooking, and then transfer the stuffing to a clean bowl immediately after cooking). Make sure the stuffing reaches 165°F (74°C). *Salmonella* is the major concern with poultry.

- Once a food is cooked, consume it right away, or cool it to 40°F (4°C) within 2 hours. If it is not to be eaten immediately, in hot weather (80°F and above) make sure this cooling is done within 1 hour. Do this by separating the food into as many shallow pans as needed to provide a large surface area for cooling. Be careful not to recontaminate cooked food by contact with raw meat or juices from hands, cutting boards, dirty utensils, or in other ways.

- Serve meat, poultry, and fish on a clean plate—never the same plate used to hold the raw product. For example, when grilling hamburgers, don't put cooked items on the same plate used to carry the raw product out to the grill.

- For outdoor cooking, cook food completely at the picnic site, with no partial cooking in advance.

Storing and Reheating Cooked Food

- Keep foods out of the "danger zone" (Fig. 13-1) by keeping hot foods hot and cold foods cold. Hold food below 40°F (4°C) or above 140°F (60°C). Foodborne microorganisms thrive in more moderate temperatures (60°F to 110°F [16°C to 43°C]). Some microorganisms can even grow in the refrigerator. Again, don't leave cooked or refrigerated foods, such as meats and salads, at room temperature for more than 2 hours (or 1 hour in hot weather) because that gives microorganisms an opportunity to grow. Store dry food at 60°F to 70°F (16°C to 21°C).

- Reheat leftovers to 165°F (74°C); reheat gravy to a rolling boil to kill *Clostridium*

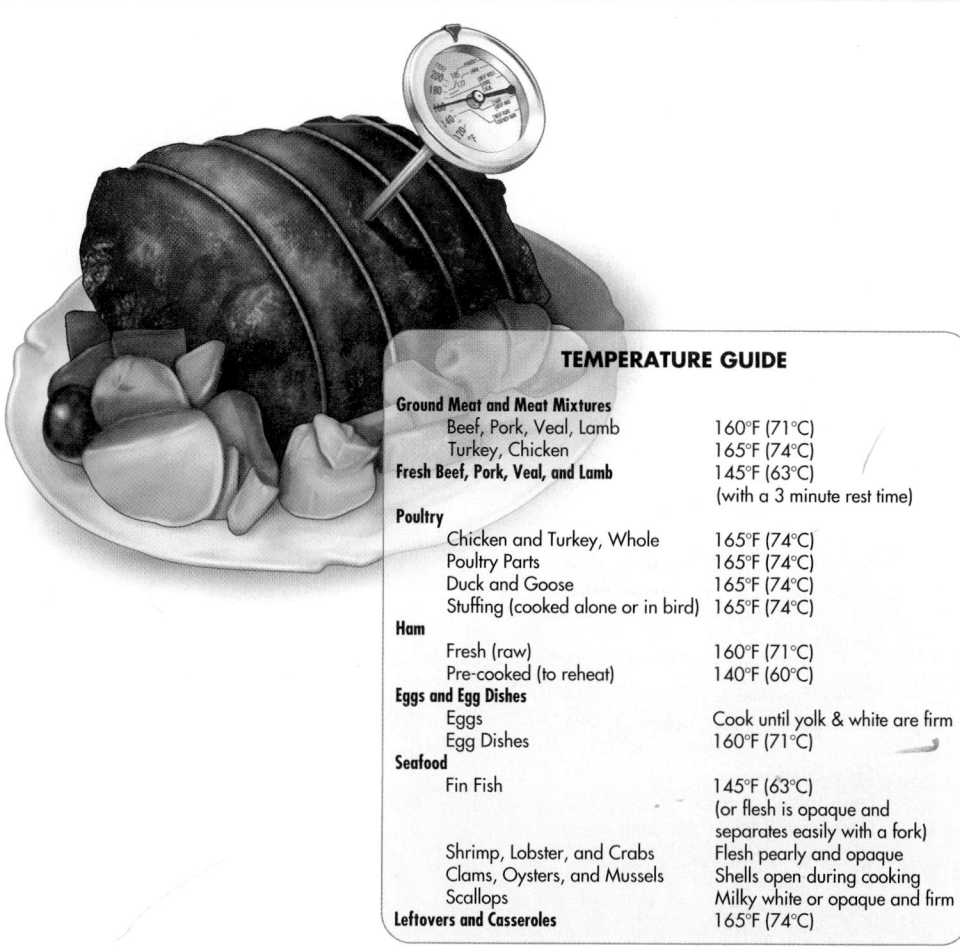

TEMPERATURE GUIDE

Ground Meat and Meat Mixtures	
Beef, Pork, Veal, Lamb	160°F (71°C)
Turkey, Chicken	165°F (74°C)
Fresh Beef, Pork, Veal, and Lamb	145°F (63°C)
	(with a 3 minute rest time)
Poultry	
Chicken and Turkey, Whole	165°F (74°C)
Poultry Parts	165°F (74°C)
Duck and Goose	165°F (74°C)
Stuffing (cooked alone or in bird)	165°F (74°C)
Ham	
Fresh (raw)	160°F (71°C)
Pre-cooked (to reheat)	140°F (60°C)
Eggs and Egg Dishes	
Eggs	Cook until yolk & white are firm
Egg Dishes	160°F (71°C)
Seafood	
Fin Fish	145°F (63°C)
	(or flesh is opaque and separates easily with a fork)
Shrimp, Lobster, and Crabs	Flesh pearly and opaque
Clams, Oysters, and Mussels	Shells open during cooking
Scallops	Milky white or opaque and firm
Leftovers and Casseroles	165°F (74°C)

▲ Sushi, like all raw fish or meat dishes, is a high-risk food. For maximum protection from foodborne illness, animal foods should be cooked thoroughly before eating.

FIGURE 13-2 ▶ Minimum internal temperatures when cooking or reheating foods.

Source: "Safe Cooking Temperatures as Measured with a Food Thermometer." (FDA, 2011)

perfringens bacteria, which may be present. Merely reheating to a good eating temperature isn't sufficient to kill harmful bacteria.

- Store peeled or cut-up produce, such as melon balls, in the refrigerator.
- Make sure the refrigerator stays below 40°F (4°C). Either use a refrigerator thermometer or keep it as cold as possible without freezing milk and lettuce.
- Keep leftovers in the refrigerator only for the recommended length of time (Fig. 13-3).

Cross-contamination is not only a threat during food preparation; it can also become a problem during food storage. Make sure all foods, including leftovers, are contained and covered in the refrigerator to prevent drippings from uncooked and potentially hazardous foods from tainting other foods. It is a good idea to store foods likely to pose risk of foodborne illness on lower shelves of the refrigerator, beneath other foods to be eaten raw.

MAKING DECISIONS

Raw Fish

Raw fish dishes, such as sushi, can be safe for most people to eat if they are made with very fresh fish that has been commercially frozen and then thawed. The freezing is important to eliminate potential health risks from parasites. FDA recommends that the fish be frozen to an internal temperature of −10°F for 7 days. If you choose to eat uncooked fish, purchase the fish from reputable establishments that have high standards for quality and sanitation. If you are at high risk for foodborne illness, it is wise to avoid raw fish products.

This product was prepared from inspected and passed meat and/or poultry. Some food products may contain bacteria that could cause illness if the product is mishandled or cooked improperly. For your protection, follow these handling instructions.

Keep refrigerated or frozen.

Thaw in refrigerator or microwave.

Keep raw meat and poultry separate from other foods.

Wash working surfaces (including cutting boards), utensils, and hands after touching raw meat or poultry.

Cook thoroughly.

Keep hot foods hot. Refrigerate leftovers immediately or discard.

► Safe Handling Instructions for Eggs

To prevent illness from bacteria: keep eggs refrigerated, cook eggs until yolks are firm, and cook foods containing eggs thoroughly.

► To reduce the risk of bacteria surviving during microwave cooking,

- Cover food with glass or ceramic when possible to decrease evaporation and heat the surface.

- Stir and rotate food at least once or twice for even cooking. Then, allow microwaved food to stand, covered, after heating is completed to help cook the exterior and equalize the temperature throughout.

- Use the oven temperature probe or a meat thermometer to check that food is done. Insert it at several spots.

- If thawing meat in the microwave, use the oven's defrost setting. Ice crystals in frozen foods are not heated well by the microwave oven and can create cold spots, which later cook more slowly.

► Regularly cleaning surfaces and equipment with a dilute bleach solution (1:10) is helpful in reducing the risk of cross-contamination of foods.

When in doubt, throw it out!

Food	Refrigerator Storage Time (days)
Meats	
Cooked ground beef/turkey	3–4
Deli meat	2–3
Cooked pork	3–4
Cooked poultry	3–4
Cooked beef, bison, lamb	3–4
Seafood	
Raw (e.g. sushi/sashimi)	Must consume on day of purchase
Cooked	2
Other Entrees	
Pizza	1–2
Pasta/rice	1–2
Casserole	3–4
Soups and Chili	
Chili with meat	2–3
Chili without meat	3–4
Soup/stew	3–4
Side Dishes	
Fresh salad	1–2
Fresh vegetables	1–2
Pasta or potato salad	2–3
Deviled egg	2–3
Hard boiled egg	7
Potato (any style)	3–4
Cooked vegetables	3–4
Dessert	
Cream pie	2–3
Fruit pie	2–3
Pastries	7
Cake	7
Cheesecake	7

FIGURE 13-3 ► Length of time to keep leftovers in the refrigerator.

CONCEPT CHECK

Thoroughly cook all meat and poultry to reduce the risk of foodborne illness from *E. coli*, and *Salmonella*. In addition, always separate raw meats and poultry products from cooked foods. To prevent foodborne intoxication from *Staphylococcus* organisms, cover cuts on hands and avoid sneezing on foods. To avoid intoxication from *Clostridium perfringens*, rapidly cool leftover foods and thoroughly reheat them. To avoid intoxication from *Clostridium botulinum*, carefully examine canned foods. Overall, don't allow cooked food to stand for more than 1 to 2 hours at room temperature. For other causes of foodborne illness, precautions already mentioned generally apply as well. In addition, thoroughly cook fish and other seafood; consume only pasteurized dairy products; wash all fruits and vegetables; and thoroughly wash your hands with soap and water before and after preparing food and after using the bathroom.

Case Study Preventing Foodborne Illness at Gatherings

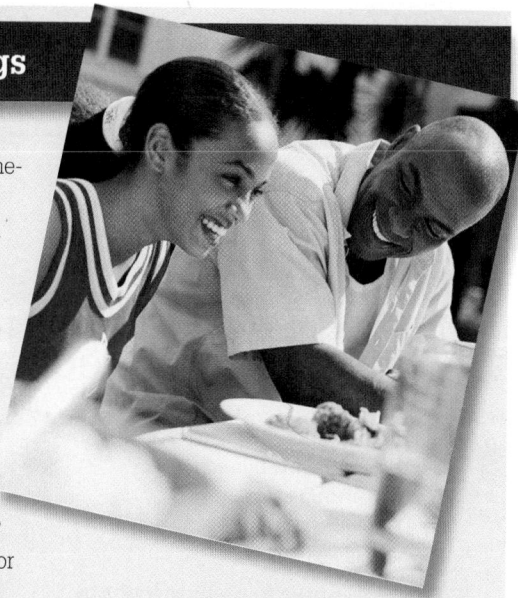

Nicole attended a gathering of her co-workers on a warm Saturday in July. The theme of the party was international dining. Nicole and her husband were asked to bring an Argentinian dish, potato and beef empanadas. They followed the recipe and cooking time carefully, removing the dish from the oven at 1 P.M. and keeping it warm by wrapping the pan in a towel. They traveled in their car to the party and set the dish out on the buffet table at 3 P.M. Dinner was to be served at 4 P.M. However, the guests were enjoying themselves so much lounging around the host's pool and drinking ginger beer (also on the menu) that no one began to eat until 6 P.M. Nicole made sure she sampled the empanadas that she and her husband made, while her husband did not. She also had some salad, garlic bread, and a sweet dessert made with coconut.

The couple returned home at 11 P.M. and went to bed. At about 2 A.M., Nicole knew something was wrong. She had severe abdominal pain and had to make a dash to the bathroom. She spent most of the next 3 hours in the bathroom with severe diarrhea. By dawn, the diarrhea subsided and she started to feel better. After a few cups of tea and a light breakfast, she was feeling like herself by noon.

Answer the following questions, and check your responses in Appendix A.

1. Based on her symptoms, what type of foodborne illness did Nicole contract?
2. Why is the beef the most likely vehicle for this type of foodborne illness?
3. Why is consuming food at large gatherings risky?
4. What precautions for avoiding foodborne illness were ignored by Nicole and the rest of the people at the party?
5. How could this scenario be rewritten to substantially reduce the risk of foodborne illness?

Summary (Numbers refer to numbered sections in the chapter.)

13.1, 13.3 Viruses, bacteria, and other microorganisms in food pose the greatest risk for foodborne illness. Major causes of foodborne illness are Norovirus and the bacteria *Campylobacter jejuni*, *Salmonella*, *Staphylococcus aureus*, and *Clostridium perfringens*. In addition, such bacteria as *Clostridium botulinum*, *Listeria monocytogenes*, and *Escherichia coli* have been found to cause illness.

13.2 In the past, salt, sugar, smoke, fermentation, and drying were used to protect against foodborne illness. Today, careful cooking, pasteurization, keeping hot foods hot and cold foods cold, and thorough handwashing provide additional insurance.

13.4 Food additives are used primarily to extend shelf life by preventing microbial growth and the destruction of food components by oxygen, metals, and other substances. Food additives are classified as those intentionally added to foods and those that incidentally appear in foods. An intentional additive is limited to no more

than one-one-hundredth of the greatest amount that causes no observed symptoms in animals. Under its jurisdiction in the United States, the Delaney Clause allows FDA to ban the use of any intentional food additive that causes cancer.

Antioxidants, such as BHA, BHT, vitamins E and C, and sulfites, prevent oxygen and enzyme destruction of food products. Emulsifiers suspend fat in water, improving the uniformity, smoothness, and body of foods such as ice cream. Common preservatives include salt, sodium benzoate, and sorbic acid, which prevent bacterial growth. Sequestrants bind metals and thus prevent spoilage of food from metal contamination. Various natural products such as natural flavors, sugar, and corn syrup, as well as artificial flavors and sweeteners, such as aspartame, improve the flavor of food.

13.5 Toxic substances occur naturally in a variety of foods, such as green potatoes, raw fish, mushrooms, and raw egg whites. Cooking foods limits their toxic effects in

some cases; others are best to avoid altogether, such as toxic mushroom species and the green parts of potatoes.

13.6 A variety of environmental contaminants and pesticide residues can be found in foods. It is helpful to know which foods pose the greatest risks and act accordingly to reduce exposure, such as washing fruits and vegetables before use.

13.7 Conventional agriculture focuses on maximizing production through the use of large farms, machines, and chemicals. A more recent culture of sustainability demands food choices produced in an environmentally responsible way. U.S. sales of organic foods have grown dramatically in recent years, despite tough economic times. Consumers are more interested in the origins of their food, resulting in grocery stores providing more "locally grown" products. Although there is no evidence that locally grown products are safer, local products provide fresher options and do not have the added transportation costs. Consumers also have an interest in connecting with local/regional farmers, resulting in growing national support for community-supported agriculture.

N&YH To protect against viruses and bacteria, cook susceptible foods thoroughly. In addition, cover cuts on the hands, do not sneeze or cough on foods, avoid contact between raw meat or poultry products

and other food products, rapidly cool and thoroughly reheat leftovers, and use pasteurized dairy products. Overall, be careful when foods are in the "danger zone" (40°F to 140°F).

Cross-contamination commonly causes foodborne illness. It occurs particularly when bacteria on raw animal products

contact foods that can support bacterial growth. Because of the risk of cross-contamination, no perishable food should be kept in the "danger zone" for more than 1 to 2 hours (depending on the environmental temperature), especially if it may have come in contact with raw animal products.

Check Your Knowledge (Answers to the following questions are below.)

1. Nitrite prevents the growth of *Canned Food*
   a. *Clostridium botulinum.*
   b. *Escherichia coli.*
   c. *Staphylococcus aureus.*
   d. yeasts.

2. Substances used to preserve foods by lowering the pH are
   a. smoke and irradiation.
   b. baking powder and soda.
   c. salt and sugar.
   d. vinegar and citric acid.

3. Food additives widely used for many years without apparent ill effects are on the _____ list.
   a. FDA
   b. GRAS
   c. USDA
   d. Delaney

4. The foodborne illness organism often associated with small cuts and boils is
   a. *Listeria.*
   b. *Staphylococcus.*
   c. *C. botulinum.*
   d. *Salmonella.*

5. Salmonella bacteria are usually spread via
   a. raw meats, poultry, and eggs.
   b. pickled vegetables.
   c. home-canned vegetables.
   d. raw vegetables.

6. It is unwise to thaw meats or poultry *- warm*
   a. in a microwave oven.
   b. in the refrigerator.
   c. under cool running water.
   d. at room temperature.

7. Milk that can remain on supermarket shelves, free of microbial growth, for many years has been processed by which of the following methods?
   a. use of humectants
   b. using antibiotics in animal feed
   c. use of sequestrants
   d. aseptic processing

8. Those at greatest risk for food-borne illness include
   a. pregnant women.
   b. infants and children.
   c. immunosuppressed individuals.
   d. All of the above.

9. Pasteurization involves the
   a. exposure of food to high temperatures for short periods to destroy harmful microorganisms.
   b. exposure of food to heat to inactivate enzymes that cause undesirable effects in foods during storage.
   c. fortification of foods with vitamins A and D.
   d. use of irradiation to destroy certain pathogens in foods.

10. Food can be kept for long periods by adding salt or sugar because these substances
    a. make the food too acidic for spoilage to occur.
    b. bind to water, thereby making it unavailable to the microorganisms.
    c. effectively kill microorganisms.
    d. dissolve the cell walls in plant foods.

Answers: 1. a (LO 13.4), 2. d (LO 13.2), 3. b (LO 13.4), 4. b (LO 13.1), 5. a (LO 13.1), 6. d (LO 13.8), 7. d (LO 13.2), 8. d (LO 13.3), 9. a (LO 13.2), 10. b (LO 13.4)

Study Questions (Numbers refer to Learning Outcomes)

1. What three trends in food purchasing and production have led to a greater number of cases of foodborne illness? **(LO 13.1)**

2. Which types of foods are most likely to be involved in foodborne illness? Why are they targets for contamination? **(LO 13.2)**

3. Identify three major classes of microorganisms responsible for foodborne illness. **(LO 13.3)**

4. Define the term *food additive,* and give examples of four intentional food

additives. What are their specific functions in foods? What is their relationship to the GRAS list? **(LO 13.4)**

5. Describe the federal process that governs the use of food additives, including the Delaney Clause. **(LO 13.4)**

6. Put into perspective the benefits and risks of using additives in food. Point out an easy way to reduce the consumption of food additives. Do you think this is worth the effort in terms of maintaining health? Why or why not? **(LO 13.4)**

7. Name some substances that occur naturally in foods but may cause illness **(LO 13.5)**.

8. Describe four recommendations for reducing the risk of toxicity from environmental contaminants. **(LO 13.6)**

9. Why is thoroughly cooking food an important practice for reducing the risk of foodborne illness? **(LO 13.8)**

10. List four techniques other than thorough cooking that are important in preventing foodborne illness. **(LO 13.8)**

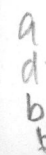
a
d
b
a
d

What Would You Choose Recommendations

Some organic fruits and vegetables do have higher levels of vitamin C, iron, phosphorus, magnesium, and phytochemicals. Exposure to environmental stressors may cause plants to produce more phytochemicals that have a positive impact on human health. However, current research is insufficient to recommend organic over conventional produce on the basis of nutrient content. Canned and frozen fruits and vegetables have greater nutrient content compared to fresh or organic products that are purchased several days or weeks after harvest.

Products labeled organic must comply with standards regarding use of fertilizers, pesticides, hormones, antibiotics, genetic engineering, and irradiation. Organic food producers may use natural preservatives. Most preservatives are used to prevent food spoilage and are not linked to negative health effects. Buying fresh or frozen produce and preparing meals at home are the best ways to avoid excessive preservative intake.

Organic produce is no less likely to be contaminated with microorganisms than conventionally grown foods. Although manure is used as organic fertilizer, statistics show similar levels of foodborne pathogens from either type of food. It is still important to follow food-safety advice, such as washing all fresh produce before eating it.

Exposure to pesticides makes organically grown produce stand apart. Because of

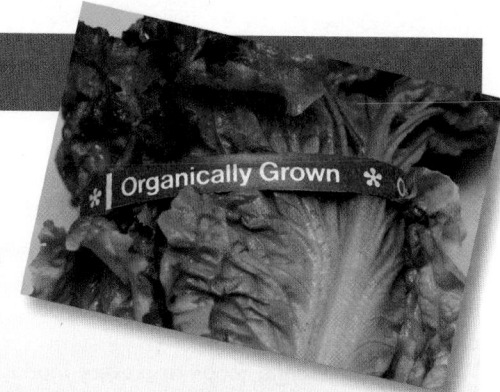

▲ Exposure to pesticides is lower from organic foods.

strict production standards we can expect a dramatically lower intake of pesticides from organic produce compared to conventionally grown produce. The health benefits of lower pesticide intake is greatest for children.

Further Readings

1. ADA Reports: Position of the American Dietetic Association: Food and water safety. *Journal of the American Dietetic Association* 109:1449, 2009.

   The public has a right to a safe food and water supply. The ADA supports collaboration among food and nutrition professionals, academics, representatives of the agriculture and food industries, and appropriate government agencies to ensure the safety of the food and water supply.

2. Anderson JB and others: A camera's view of consumer food-handling behaviors. *Journal of the American Dietetic Association* 104:186, 2004.

   Improper food handling was common in households studied. Implementing Fight BAC! recommendations would improve food handling practices.

3. Calvert GM: Health effects of pesticides. *American Family Physician* 69:1613, 2004.

   Clear cases of disease from high pesticide exposure are seen. Effects of low dose, chronic exposure have been hard to quantify, but most adults have detectable pesticide levels in their blood.

4. Consumers Union: Dirty birds: Even "premium" chickens harbor dangerous bacteria. *Consumer Reports* p. 20, January 2007.

   An analysis of fresh, whole chickens bought in the United States revealed that 83% contained two leading causes of foodborne disease.

5. Dangour AD and others: Nutritional quality of organic foods: A systematic review. *American Journal of Clinical Nutrition* 90:680, 2009.

   This systematic review found there is inadequate evidence of a nutritional benefit to consuming organic foods over conventionally produced foods. Organic and conventional food production methods had minimal impact on the nutrient content and therefore minimal health benefit.

6. Food Safety and Inspection Service: A century of progress in food safety. *Be Food Safe* Fall:12, 2006.

   This article summarizes the 100-year history of federal inspection of meat and poultry.

7. Gerner-Smidt P and others: Invasive listeriosis in Denmark 1994–2003: A review of 299 cases with special emphasis on risk factors for mortality. *Clinical Microbiological Infections* 11:618, 2005.

   Listeria infections lead to death primarily in older people and those with underlying cases of cancer.

8. McCabe-Sellers BJ, Beattie SF: Food safety: emerging trends in foodborne illness surveillance and prevention. *Journal of the American Dietetic Association* 104:1708, 2004.

   Recommendations are given to reduce risk of foodborne illness, with proper personal hygiene being a major focus.

9. Schardt D: Get the lead out—What you don't know can hurt you. *Nutrition Action Healthletter* p. 1, March 2005.

   Hypertension, renal disease, impaired brain function, and cataracts have been linked to lead exposure.

10. Sivapalasingam S and others: Fresh produce: A growing cause of outbreaks of foodborne illness in the United States. *Journal of Food Protection* 67:2342, 2004.

    Caution should be used with fresh produce, just as one would with raw meat and dairy products.

11. Spano M: Organics in overdrive—the explosion of natural food products. *Today's Dietitian* 9:66, October 2007.

    Increased availability of organic products and fear of hormones and antibiotics, has led to a dramatic growth in organic food sales.

12. U.S. Food and Drug Administration: *Food Code.* U.S. Department of Health and Human Services, Public Health Service, Food and Drug Administration: College Park, MD, 2009.

    The FDA Food Code is the model for local, state, tribal, and federal regulators to develop or update their food safety rules consistent with national policy.

13. Widdowson MA and others: Norovirus and foodborne disease, United States, 1991–2000. *Emerging Infectious Diseases* 11:95, 2005.

    The Norovirus leads to more causes of foodborne illness than any other agent.

14. Yeager D: Got organic? *Today's Dietitian* 10:60, October 2008.

    The USDA regulates the organic industry and the National Organic Program certifies that food is produced using organic practices.

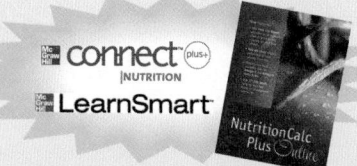

To get the most out of your study of nutrition, go to McGraw-Hill's online resources: Connect www.mcgrawhillconnect.com, **where you will find NutritionCalc Plus, LearnSmart, and many other dynamic tools.**

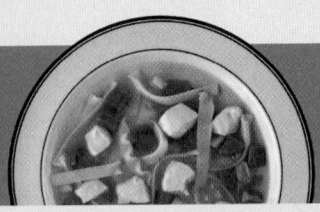
I. Can You Spot the Improper Food-Safety Practices?

In this chapter you learned that (1) foodborne illness strikes up to 76 million U.S. citizens each year and (2) about 5000 deaths each year in the United States are caused by foodborne organisms.

Carefully preparing foods to prevent foodborne illness can minimize its occurrence for most of us. Read the following excerpt and find the food-safety violations that could lead to illness.

A Local Health Department Inspector Gives the Following Account of His Visit to a Local Diner

As I walked through the kitchen of the Morningside Diner, I noticed that all food handlers washed their hands thoroughly with hot, soapy water before handling the food, especially after handling raw meat, fish, poultry, or eggs. Before preparing raw foods, they also thoroughly washed the cutting boards, dishes, and other equipment. As they used their cutting boards after cutting foods, they wiped them with a damp rag and used them again to cut more food.

When preparing fresh fruits and vegetables, they washed them but were careful to leave a little dirt on for fear of washing important nutrients from the outside. The cooks generally cooked meats to an internal temperature of 180°F (82°C). However, to preserve the flavor, pork was cooked to an internal temperature of 140°F (60°C). Some cooked foods to be served later were cooled to below 41°F (5°C) within 2 hours, and foods like beef stew were cooled in shallow pans.

The diner served canned foods, even when the cans were dented. When leftovers were reheated, they were raised to an internal temperature of 130°F (55°C) and served immediately. Food handlers took great care to remove moldy portions of food. The cooks prepared stuffing separately from the poultry. The temperature of refrigerators was approximately 45°F (7°C).

1. List the violations of food-safety practices that could contribute to foodborne illness.

   _____
   _____
   _____
   _____
   _____

2. If you were writing a report describing ways to correct these practices, what would you say?

   _____
   _____
   _____
   _____
   _____
   _____

3. List the food-safety practices that follow the general rules for preventing foodborne illness.

   _____
   _____
   _____
   _____
   _____

II. Take a Closer Look at Food Additives

Evaluate a food label of a convenience food item (e.g., frozen entree, ready-to-eat baked good) either in the supermarket or one you have available.

1. Write out the list of ingredients.

_____
_____
_____
_____

2. Identify the ingredients that you think may be food additives.

_____
_____
_____
_____
_____

3. Based on the information available in this chapter, what are the functions of these food additives?

_____
_____
_____
_____

4. How might this food product differ without these ingredients?

_____
_____
_____
_____

III. Take a Closer Look at Organic Foods

Visit one or more supermarkets to see what organic foods are available. Note your findings below.

	Available	Not Available
Meat		
Poultry		
Milk		
Eggs		
Cheese		
Lettuce		
Apples		
Bananas		
Broccoli		
Other produce		
Breakfast cereal		
Snack chips		
Crackers		
Bread		
Pasta		
Beer		

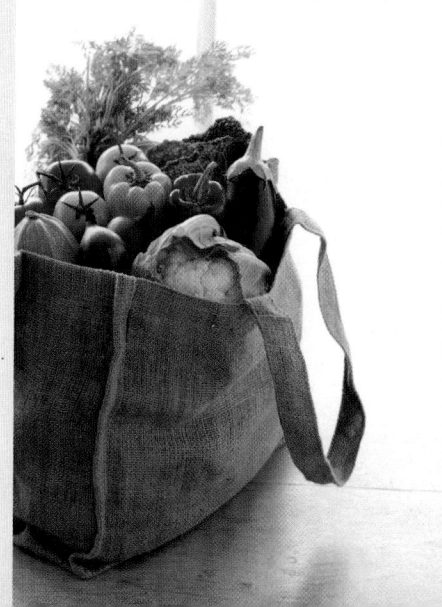

Do you currently purchase organic foods? Why or why not?

Chapter 14 Pregnancy and Breastfeeding

Student Learning Outcomes

Chapter 14 is designed to allow you to:

14.1 List major physiological changes that occur in the body during pregnancy and how nutrient needs are altered.

14.2 List factors that predict a successful pregnancy outcome and some that do not.

14.3 Specify the optimal weight gain during pregnancy for a healthy adult woman.

14.4 Design an adequate, balanced meal plan for a pregnant or breastfeeding woman based on the Dietary Guidelines and MyPlate.

14.5 Identify the nutrients that may need to be supplemented during pregnancy and explain the reason for each.

14.6 Explain the typical discomforts of pregnancy that can be minimized by dietary changes.

14.7 Describe the physiological processes involved in breastfeeding, as well as some advantages of breastfeeding for both the infant and mother.

What Would You Choose?

As a pregnant vegetarian, which of the following meals would you choose as the best source of iron?

a Spinach salad with hard boiled eggs and a whole-wheat roll

b Lean hamburger with cheese, lettuce, and tomato and roasted red potatoes

c Bean and cheese soft taco and stewed tomatoes

d Kellogg's Smart Start cereal, fat-free milk, and orange juice

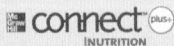 **Think about your choice as you read Chapter 14, then see our recommendations at the end of the chapter. To learn more about pregnancy and vegetarian diets, check out the Connect site:** www.mcgrawhillconnect.com

Part Five

Nutrition: A Focus on Life Stages

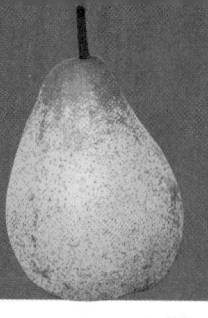

Pregnancy can be a special time. Exhilaration and amazement accompany parents' tremendous responsibility of helping a child develop and grow. Parents-to-be often feel an overriding desire to produce a healthy baby, which can arouse new interest in nutrition and health information. They usually want to do everything possible to maximize their chances of having a robust, lively newborn.

Despite these intentions, the infant mortality rate in North America is higher than that seen in many other industrialized nations. In Canada, about 6.1 of every 1000 infants per year die before their first birthday, while in the United States, it is 6.9. These are alarming statistics for two countries that have such a high per capita expenditure for health care compared to many other countries in the world. Comparatively, the rate of infant mortality in Sweden is roughly 3 of every 1000 infants. In addition, in the United States, about 20% of pregnant women receive inadequate prenatal care in the early months of pregnancy. Expectant teenagers are at the highest risk for this.

Producing a healthy baby is not just a matter of luck. True, some aspects of fetal and newborn health are beyond our control. Still, as the comic in this chapter suggests, conscious decisions about social, health, environmental, and nutritional factors during pregnancy significantly affect the baby's future. Choosing to breastfeed the infant adds further benefits. Let's examine how eating well during pregnancy and breastfeeding can help a baby to have a healthy start in life.

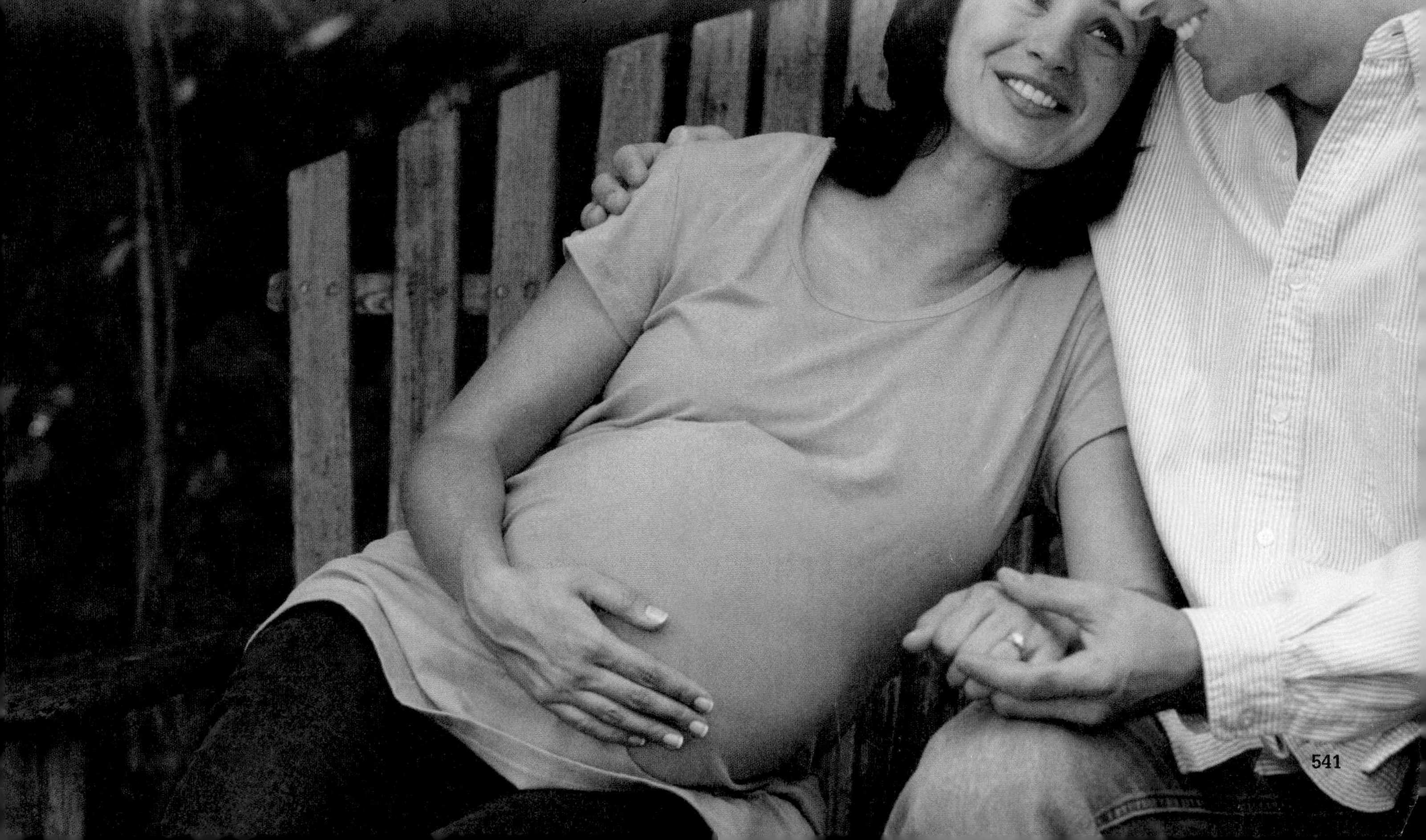

Refresh Your Memory

As you begin your study of nutrition in pregnancy and breastfeeding in Chapter 14, you may want to review:

- Typical fortification in meal replacement bars in Chapter 1 and ready-to-eat breakfast cereals in Chapter 2
- Causes and effects of ketosis in Chapter 4
- Components of the macronutrient classes—carbohydrates, proteins, and lipids—in Chapters 4 to 6, especially omega-3 fatty acids
- Calculation of body mass index in Chapter 7
- Food sources of folate in Chapter 8 and calcium, iron, and zinc in Chapter 9

14.1 Planning for Pregnancy

In an effort to reduce the occurrence of neural tube defects, *Healthy People 2020* includes a goal of increasing by 10% the proportion of women of child-bearing potential who consume at least 400 micrograms of folic acid per day. Currently, about 24% of women of child-bearing potential consume adequate folic acid from fortified foods or dietary supplements.

Controlling or correcting existing health conditions and modifying potentially harmful habits before conception can improve the chances for a successful pregnancy. About 50% of all pregnancies are unplanned. Even when planned, women often do not suspect they are pregnant during the first few weeks after conception. They may not seek medical attention until after the first 2 to 3 months of pregnancy. Still, even without fanfare, the child-to-be grows and develops daily. For that reason, the health and nutrition habits of a woman who is trying to become pregnant—or who has the ability to become pregnant—are particularly important. Although some aspects of fetal and newborn health are beyond the parents' control, a woman's conscious decisions about social, health, environmental, and nutritional factors affect her infant's health and future.

The time to address ongoing health concerns is before conception. Poor control of existing diabetes, hypertension, phenylketonuria, and HIV-positive status or AIDS may lead to serious complications in pregnancy, including birth defects and fetal death. In addition, women should aim to achieve a healthy weight prior to becoming pregnant. Prepregnancy weight and nutrient stores affect the woman's ability to become pregnant. Many underweight women experience amenorrhea, which may reduce their ability to ovulate. The chances of ovulating and becoming pregnant improve when body fat increases to a healthy level.

Infants born to women who began pregnancy substantially above or below a healthy weight are more likely to experience problems than women who began

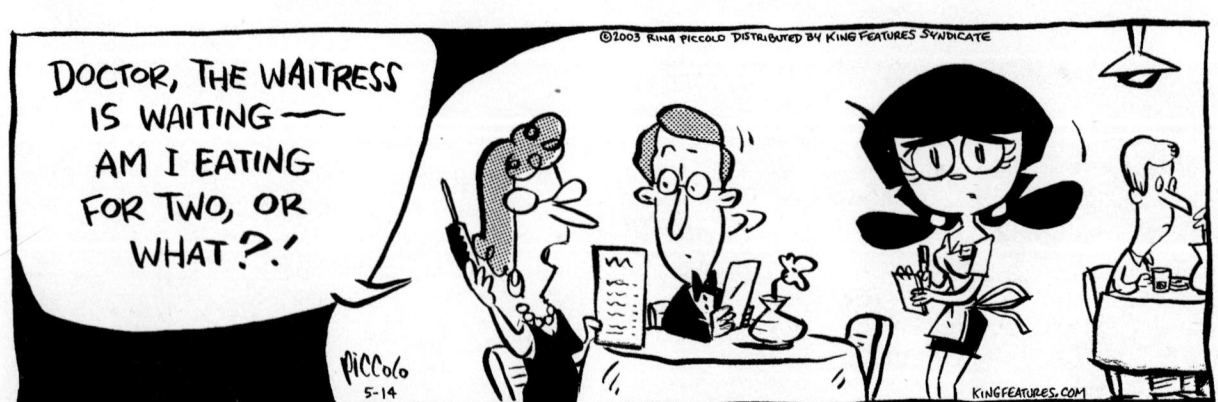

Which diet and lifestyle habits contribute to a successful pregnancy? Which are likely to be harmful?

Why should a woman begin to prepare for pregnancy months before conception of her new baby?

When pregnant, does the mother need to "eat for two?" Chapter 14 provides some answers.

© Rina Piccolo. Reprinted with special permission of King Features Syndicate.

pregnancy at a normal weight. For instance, babies born to obese women are at increased risk of having birth defects, death in the first few weeks after birth, and obesity in childhood. Many obese pregnant women experience high blood pressure, gestational diabetes, and difficult deliveries. At the other extreme, women who begin pregnancy underweight (BMI < 18.5) are more likely to have infants who are low birth weight and preterm than women at a normal weight. These differences may be because underweight women tend to have lighter placentas and lower nutrient stores, especially iron, than heavier women, which can affect fetal growth negatively. An underweight woman can improve her nutrient stores and pregnancy outcome by gaining weight before pregnancy or gaining extra weight during pregnancy.

Figure 14-1 depicts how and when toxic agents can harm the developing fetus. To prepare for a healthy pregnancy, the mother should undoubtedly eliminate tobacco, alcohol, and illicit drugs (e.g., marijuana and cocaine). Certain medicines, such as aspirin and related NSAIDs (e.g., ibuprofen [Advil]), as well as typical medicines to treat the common cold and many herbal therapies, have the potential to damage the fetus. Lower doses and/or safer alternatives should be used when planning for pregnancy. Health hazards in the mother's environment, including job-related hazards and exposure to x-rays, should be minimized. Caffeine intake also should be limited.

Much research suggests that an adequate vitamin and mineral intake at least 8 weeks before conception and then during pregnancy can improve outcomes of pregnancy. In particular, meeting folate needs (400 micrograms of synthetic folic acid per day) helps to prevent birth defects such as neural tube defects (review Fig. 8-27 in Chapter 8) and decrease the risk of preterm delivery. Recall from Chapter 8 that adequate folate status before and during pregnancy reduces the risk of neural tube defects by about 70%. Low intakes of calcium and iron or excessive intakes of vitamin A also are cause for concern during pregnancy. Careful dietary choices, often with the help of a balanced multivitamin and mineral supplement, will contribute to a healthy pregnancy for both mother and infant.

Folate—organ meat, sprout, dried beans, orange juice, Green leafy veg.

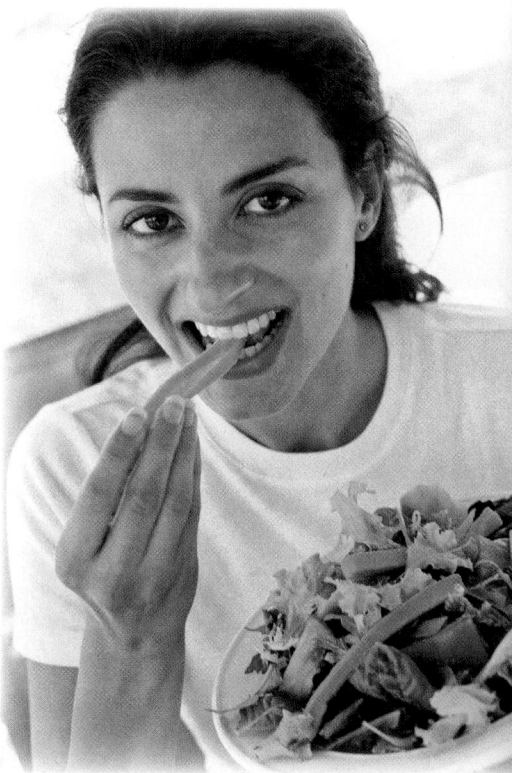

▲ The time to begin thinking about prenatal nutrition is before becoming pregnant. This includes making sure folic acid intake is adequate (400 micrograms of synthetic folic acid per day) and that any supplemental intake of preformed vitamin A does not exceed 100% of the Daily Value (1000 micrograms RAE or 5000 IU).

MAKING DECISIONS

Folate Supplements

Women who have previously given birth to an infant with a neural tube defect such as spina bifida should consult their physician about the need for folate supplementation; an intake of 4 milligrams of synthetic folic acid per day at least one month prior to conception is recommended for these women, but must be taken under a physician's supervision.

14.2 Prenatal Growth and Development

For 8 weeks after conception, a human **embryo** develops from a fertilized **ovum** into a **fetus.** For about another 32 weeks, the fetus continues to develop. When its body finally matures, the infant is born. Until birth, the mother nourishes it via a **placenta,** an organ that forms in her uterus to accommodate the growth and development of the fetus (Fig. 14-2). The role of the placenta is to exchange nutrients, oxygen and other gases, and waste products between the mother and the fetus. This occurs through a network of capillaries that bring the fetal blood close to the maternal blood supply, but the two blood supplies do not mix.

Early Growth—The First Trimester Is a Very Critical Time

In the formation of the human organism, egg and sperm unite to produce the **zygote** (Fig. 14-1). From this point, the reproductive process occurs very rapidly:

- Within 30 hours—zygote divides in half to form 2 cells.
- Within 4 days—cell number climbs to 128 cells.

embryo In humans, the developing offspring in utero from about the beginning of the third week to the end of the eighth week after conception.

ovum The egg cell from which a fetus eventually develops if the egg is fertilized by a sperm cell.

fetus The developing life form from about the beginning of the ninth week after conception until birth.

placenta An organ that forms in the uterus in pregnant women. Through this organ, oxygen and nutrients from the mother's blood are transferred to the fetus, and fetal wastes are removed. The placenta also releases hormones that maintain the state of pregnancy.

zygote The fertilized ovum; the cell resulting from the union of an egg cell (ovum) and sperm until it divides.

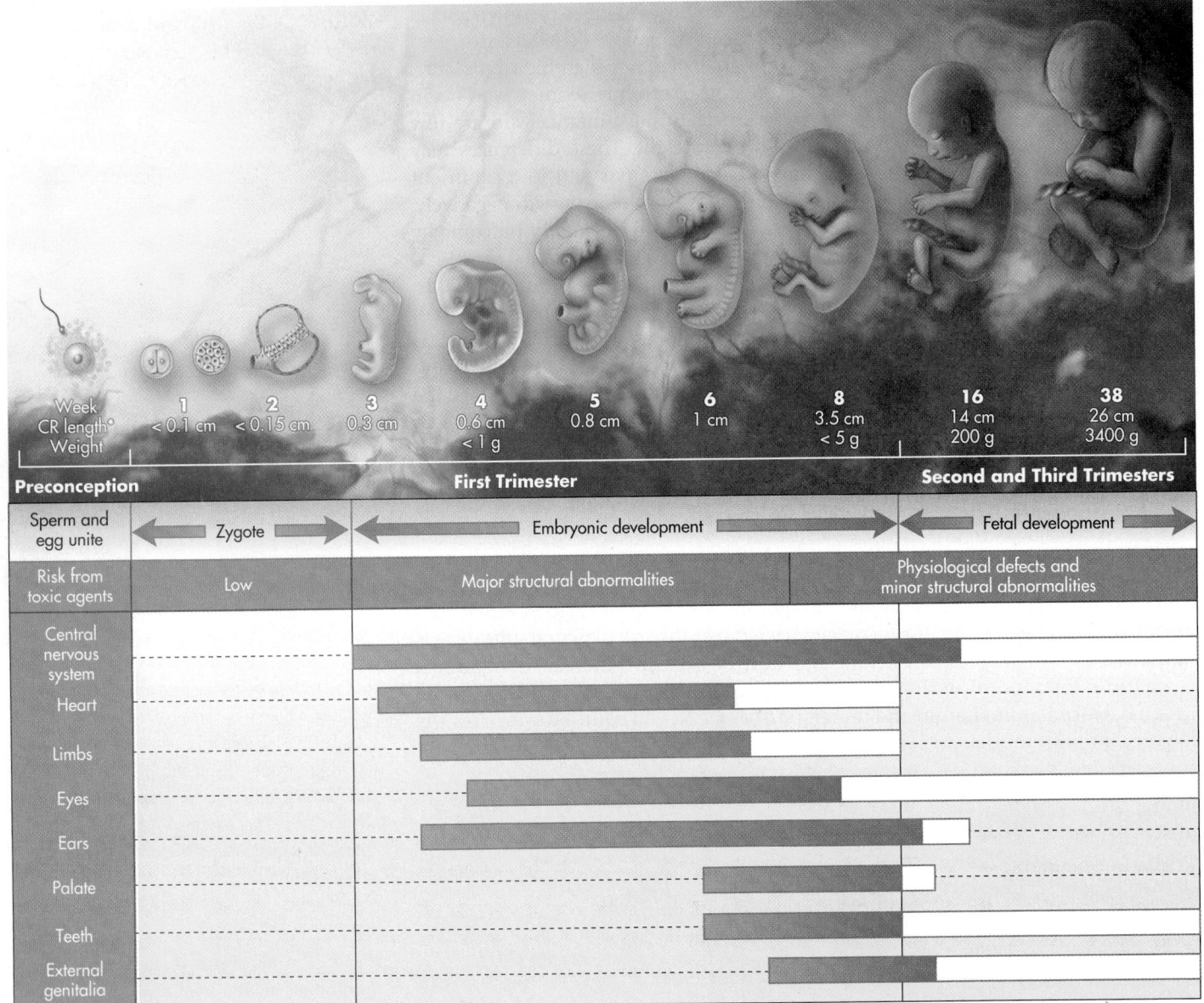

| Week
CR length*
Weight | | 1
< 0.1 cm | 2
< 0.15 cm | 3
0.3 cm | 4
0.6 cm
< 1 g | 5
0.8 cm | 6
1 cm | 8
3.5 cm
< 5 g | 16
14 cm
200 g | 38
26 cm
3400 g |

| Preconception | First Trimester | | Second and Third Trimesters |

Sperm and egg unite	Zygote	Embryonic development	Fetal development
Risk from toxic agents	Low	Major structural abnormalities	Physiological defects and minor structural abnormalities
Central nervous system			
Heart			
Limbs			
Eyes			
Ears			
Palate			
Teeth			
External genitalia			

FIGURE 14-1 ▶ Harmful effects of toxic agents during pregnancy. Vulnerable periods of fetal development are indicated with purple bars. The purple shading indicates the time of greatest risk to the organ. The most serious damage to the fetus from exposure to toxins is likely to occur during the first 8 weeks after conception, two-thirds of the way through the first trimester. As the white bars in the chart show, however, damage to vital parts of the body—including the eyes, brain, and genitals—can also occur during the later months of pregnancy.

trimesters Three 13- to 14-week periods into which the normal pregnancy (the length of a normal pregnancy is about 40 weeks, measured from the first day of the woman's last menstrual period) is divided somewhat arbitrarily for purposes of discussion and analysis. Development of the offspring, however, is continuous throughout pregnancy, with no specific physiological markers demarcating the transition from one trimester to the next.

- At 14 days—the group of cells is called an embryo.
- Within 35 days—heart is beating, embryo is 1/30 of an inch (8 millimeters) long, eyes and limb buds are clearly visible.
- At 8 weeks—the embryo is known as a fetus.
- At 13 weeks (end of first trimester)—most organs are formed, and the fetus can move.

For purposes of discussion, the duration of pregnancy—normally, 38 to 42 weeks—is commonly divided into three periods, called **trimesters.** Growth begins in the first trimester with a rapid increase in cell number. This type of growth dominates embryonic and early fetal development. The newly formed cells then begin to grow larger. Further growth is a mix of increases in cell number and cell size. By the end of 13 weeks—the first trimester—most organs are formed and the fetus can move (see Fig. 14-1).

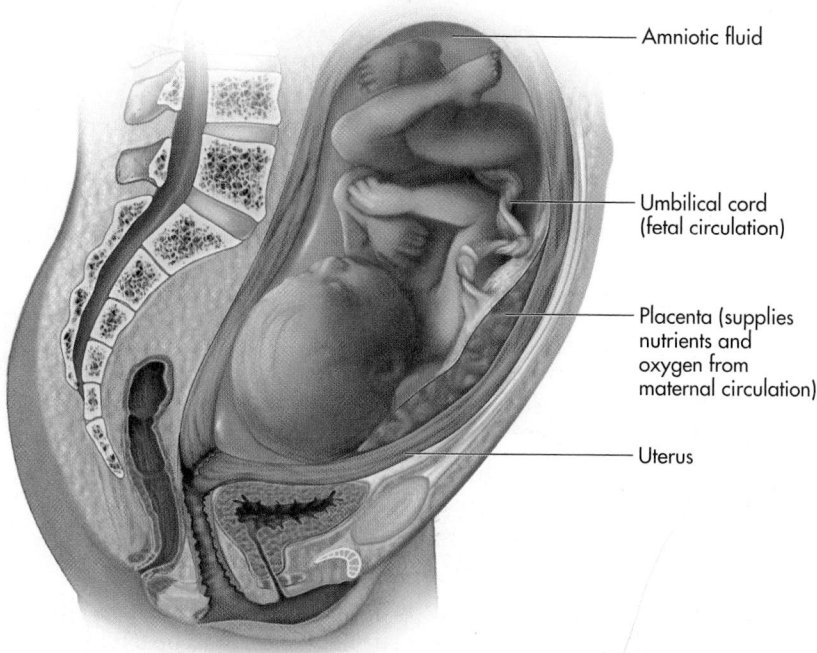

Amniotic fluid

Umbilical cord
(fetal circulation)

Placenta (supplies
nutrients and
oxygen from
maternal circulation)

Uterus

FIGURE 14-2 ▶ The fetus in relationship to the placenta. The placenta is the organ through which nourishment flows to the fetus.

As the embryo or fetus develops, nutritional deficiencies and other insults have the potential to impose damage or risk to organ systems. For example, adverse reactions to medications, high intakes of vitamin A, exposure to radiation, or trauma can alter or arrest the current phase of fetal development, and the effects may last a lifetime (review Fig. 14-1). The most critical time for these potential problems is during the first trimester. Most **spontaneous abortions**—premature terminations of pregnancy that occur naturally—happen at this time. About one-half or more pregnancies end in this way, often so early that a woman does not even realize she was pregnant. (An additional 15% to 20% are lost before normal delivery.) Early spontaneous abortions usually result from a genetic defect or fatal error in fetal development. Smoking, alcohol abuse, use of aspirin and NSAIDs, and illicit drug use raise the risk for spontaneous abortion.

A woman should avoid substances that may harm the developing fetus, especially during the first trimester. This holds true, as well, for the time when a woman is trying to become pregnant. As previously mentioned, she is unlikely to be aware of her pregnancy for at least a few weeks. In addition, the fetus develops so rapidly during the first trimester that, if an essential nutrient is not available, the fetus may be affected even before evidence of the nutrient deficiency appears in the mother.

For this reason, the *quality*—rather than the *quantity*—of the woman's nutritional intake is most important during the first trimester. In other words, women should consume the same amount of calories, but the foods chosen should be more nutrient dense. Although some women lose their appetite and feel nauseated during the first trimester, they should be careful to meet nutrient needs as much as possible.

Although a mother's decisions, practices, and precautions during pregnancy contribute to the health of her fetus, she cannot guarantee her fetus good health because some genetic and environmental factors are beyond her control. She and others involved in the pregnancy should not hold an unrealistic illusion of total control.

spontaneous abortion Cessation of pregnancy and expulsion of the embryo or nonviable fetus prior to 20 weeks gestation. This is the result of natural causes, such as a genetic defect or developmental problem; also called *miscarriage*.

Second Trimester

By the beginning of the second trimester, a fetus weighs about 1 ounce. Arms, hands, fingers, legs, feet, and toes are fully formed. The fetus has ears and begins to form tooth sockets in its jawbone. Organs continue to grow and mature, and, with a stethoscope or Doppler instrument, physicians can detect the fetal heartbeat. Most bones

▶ A healthy 1-week-old baby. At birth, a baby usually weighs about 7.5 pounds and is 20 inches long.

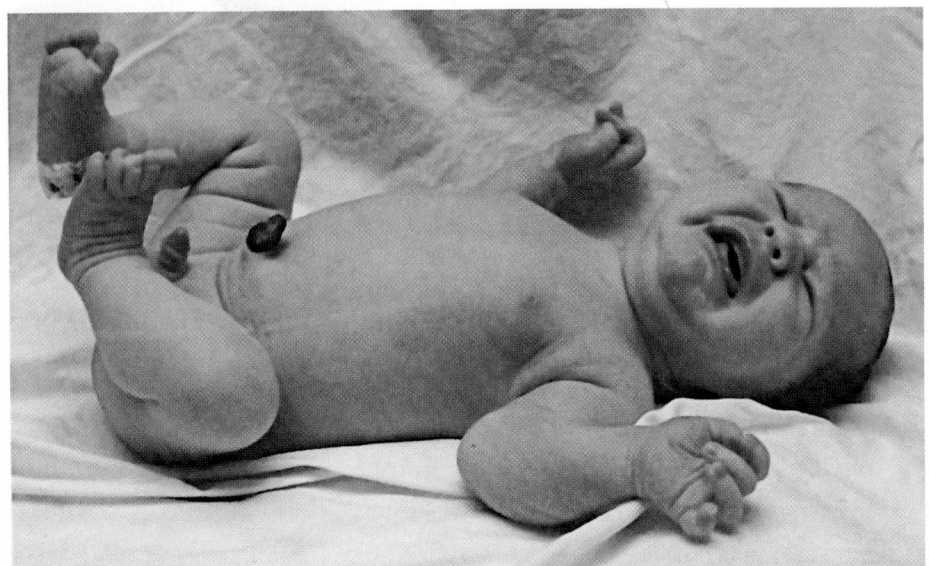

lactation The period of milk secretion following pregnancy; typically called *breastfeeding.*

gestation The period of intrauterine development of offspring, from conception to birth; in humans, gestation lasts for about 40 weeks after the woman's previous menstrual period.

A goal of *Healthy People 2020* is to reduce low birth weight by 5% and preterm births by 10%. Currently about 8% of live births are of low birth weight and about 13% are preterm.

are distinctly evident through the body. Eventually, the fetus begins to look more like an infant. It may suck its thumb and kick strongly enough to be felt by the mother. As was shown in Figure 14-1, the fetus can still be affected by exposure to toxins, but not to the degree seen in the first trimester.

During the second trimester, the mother's breast weight increases by approximately 30% due to the development of milk-producing cells and the deposition of 2 to 4 pounds of fat for **lactation.** This stored fat serves as a reservoir for the extra calories needed to produce breast milk.

Third Trimester

By the beginning of the third trimester, a fetus weighs about 2 to 3 pounds. The third trimester is a crucial time for fetal growth. The fetus will double in length and will increase its weight by three to four times. The fetus takes higher priority than the mother with regard to iron and will deplete the stores of the mother. If the mother is not meeting her iron needs, she can be severely depleted after delivery. An infant born after about 26 weeks of **gestation** has a good chance of survival if cared for in a nursery for high-risk newborns. However, the infant will not contain the stores of minerals (mainly iron and calcium) and fat normally accumulated during the last month of gestation. This and other medical problems, such as a poor ability to suck and swallow, complicate nutritional care for preterm infants.

By full term, the fetus usually weighs about 7 to 9 pounds (3 to 4 kilograms) and is about 20 inches (50 centimeters) long. A soft spot on the top of the head indicates where the skull bones (fontanels) are growing together. The bones finally close by the time the baby is about 12 to 18 months of age.

14.3 Success in Pregnancy

The goal of pregnancy is to achieve optimal health for both the baby and the mother. For the mother, a successful pregnancy is one in which her physical and emotional health is protected so that she can return to her prepregnancy health status. For the infant, two widely accepted criteria are (1) a gestation period longer than 37 weeks and (2) a birth weight greater than 5.5 pounds (2.5 kilograms). Sufficient lung development, likely to have occurred by 37 weeks of gestation, is critical to the survival of a newborn. The longer the gestation, the greater the ultimate birth weight and maturation state, leading to fewer medical problems and better quality of life for the infant. Overall, a successful pregnancy is the outcome of a complex interplay between genes, various lifestyle practices, and the environment.

Infant Birthweight

Low-birth-weight (LBW) infants are those weighing less than 5.5 pounds (2.5 kilograms) at birth. Most commonly, LBW is associated with **preterm** birth. Medical costs during the first year of life for LBW infants are higher than those for normal-weight infants. In fact, hospital-related costs of caring for LBW newborns total more than $4 billion per year in the United States. Full-term and preterm infants who weigh less than the expected weight for their duration of gestation, the result of insufficient growth, are described as **small for gestational age (SGA).** Thus, a full-term infant weighing less than 5.5 pounds at birth is SGA but not preterm, whereas a preterm infant born at 30 weeks' gestation is probably LBW without being SGA. Infants who are SGA are more likely than normal-weight infants to have medical complications, including problems with blood glucose control, temperature regulation, growth, and development in the early weeks after birth.

Prenatal Care and Counseling

Adequate prenatal care is a primary determinant of success in pregnancy. Ideally, women should receive examinations and counseling before becoming pregnant and continue regular prenatal care throughout pregnancy. If prenatal care is inadequate, delayed, or absent, untreated maternal nutritional deficiencies can deprive a developing fetus of needed nutrients. In addition, untreated health conditions, such as anemia, AIDS, hypertension, or diabetes, must be carefully addressed to minimize complications of pregnancy. Treating ongoing infections will also decrease risks of fetal damage. Without prenatal care, a woman is three times more likely to deliver an LBW baby—one who will be 40 times more likely to die during the first 4 weeks of life than a normal-birth-weight infant. According to the Physicians Committee for Responsible Medicine, early and consistent prenatal care could reduce the number of LBW births by 12,600 per year in the United States. Although the ideal time to start prenatal care is before conception, about 20% of women in the United States receive *no* prenatal care throughout the first trimester—a critical time to positively influence the outcome of pregnancy.

Food habits cannot be predicted from income, education, or lifestyle. Although some women already have good dietary habits, most can benefit from nutritional advice. All should be reminded of habits that may harm the growing fetus, such as severe dieting or fasting. By focusing on appropriate prenatal care, nutrient intake, and health habits, parents give their fetus—and later, their infant—the best chance of thriving. Overall, the chances of producing a healthy baby are maximized with education, an adequate diet, and early and consistent prenatal medical care.

Effects of Maternal Age

The age of the mother is another factor that determines pregnancy outcome. The ideal age for pregnancy is between 20 and 35 years of age. Outside that age range—at either extreme—complications are more likely to arise. The rates of teen pregnancy have declined since 1990; still, approximately 400,000 babies are born to teen mothers each year—the highest of any industrialized country. Teen pregnancy increases risk for negative outcomes for both mother and child (Table 14-1) and costs taxpayers an estimated $9.1 billion each year. A portion of these burdens stems from a disadvantaged background, but teenage pregnancy cuts across socioeconomic classes and the effects are evident even after controlling for background factors. Pregnant teens frequently exhibit a variety of risk factors that can complicate pregnancy and pose risk to the fetus. For instance, teenagers are more likely than adult women to be underweight at the start of pregnancy and to gain too little weight during pregnancy. In addition, their bodies lack the physical maturity needed to carry a fetus safely. Even with prenatal care—and 7% of teenage mothers receive none at all—10% of children born to teenage mothers are of low birth weight and 15% are preterm.

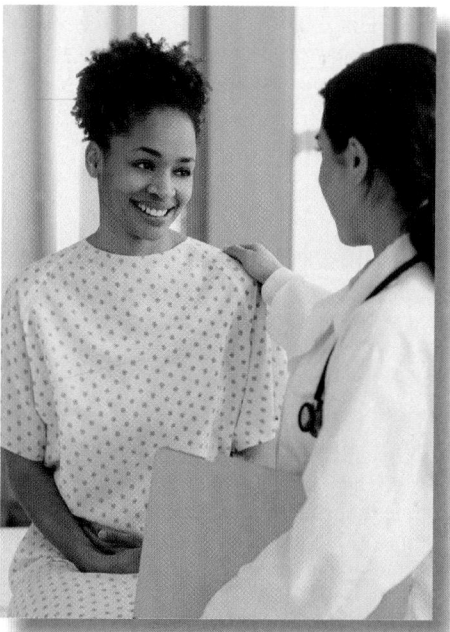

▲ To ensure optimal health and rapid treatment of medical conditions that develop during pregnancy, a pregnant woman should consult with her health-care provider on a regular basis. Ideally, this consultation should begin before she becomes pregnant.

low birth weight (LBW) Referring to any infant weighing less than 2.5 kilograms (5.5 pounds) at birth; most commonly results from preterm birth.

preterm An infant born before 37 weeks of gestation; also referred to as *premature*.

small for gestational age (SGA) Referring to infants who weigh less than the expected weight for their length of gestation. This corresponds to less than 2.5 kilograms (5.5 pounds) in a full-term newborn. A preterm infant who is also SGA will most likely develop some medical complications.

TABLE 14-1 The Burdens of Teenage Pregnancy

For Mother	For Child
↑ Depression and other mental health problems	↓ Birth weight
↑ Use of illicit drugs and alcohol	↑ Preterm birth
↑ Poverty and reliance on public assistance	↑ Infant mortality
↓ Graduation rates from high school and college	↑ Hospital admissions during childhood
↑ Single parenthood	↓ Academic performance
	↓ Nutritional status
	↑ Rates of imprisonment during adulthood

At the other end of the spectrum, advanced maternal age poses special risks for pregnancy. The risks of LBW and preterm delivery increase modestly, but progressively, with maternal age beyond 35 years. Given close monitoring, however, a woman older than 35 years has an excellent chance of producing a healthy infant.

Closely Spaced and Multiple Births

Siblings born in succession to a mother with less than a year between birth and subsequent conception are more likely to be born with low birth weights than are those farther apart in age. The risks of low birth weight, preterm birth, or small size for gestational age are 30% to 40% higher for infants conceived less than 6 months following a birth compared to those conceived 18 to 23 months following a birth. These poor outcomes are probably linked to a lack of enough time to rebuild nutrient stores depleted by the pregnancy. Similarly, multiple births (i.e., twins) increase the risk for preterm birth.

Smoking, Medication Use, and Drug Abuse

Smoking, use of some medications, and illicit drug use during pregnancy all lead to harmful effects. Smoking is linked to preterm birth and appears to increase the risk of birth defects, sudden infant death, and childhood cancer. Problem drugs include aspirin (especially when used heavily), hormone ointments, nose drops and related "cold" medications, rectal suppositories, weight-control pills, antidepressants, and medications prescribed for previous illnesses. Illicit drug use is particularly harmful during pregnancy. Many chemicals in recreational drugs cross the placenta and affect the fetus, whose detoxification systems are immature. During organ development, such insults can cause malformations. Marijuana, the most common illegal drug used during the reproductive years, can result in reduced blood flow to the uterus and placenta, leading to poor fetal growth. Low birth weight and higher risk of preterm delivery often are seen in infants whose mothers used marijuana during pregnancy. Use of psychoactive drugs, such as cocaine and methamphetamines, restricts fetal growth and brain development, the effects of which may plague the child for a lifetime.

Food Safety

Any foodborne illness during any stage of life is a concern. One type of foodborne illness that poses particular danger for pregnant women is caused by the bacterium *Listeria monocytogenes* (review Chapter 13). Infection with this microorganism typically causes mild flulike symptoms, such as fever, headache, and vomiting, about 7 to 30 days after exposure. However, pregnant women, newborn infants, and people with depressed immune function may suffer more severe symptoms, including spontaneous abortion and serious blood infections. In these high-risk people, 25% of infections may be fatal. Unpasteurized milk, soft cheeses made from raw milk (e.g., brie, Camembert, feta, and blue cheeses), and raw cabbage can be sources of *Listeria* organisms, so it is especially important that pregnant women (and other people at high risk for infection) avoid these products. Experts advise consuming only pasteurized milk products and cooking meat, poultry, and seafood thoroughly to kill this and other foodborne organisms. It is unsafe in pregnancy to eat any raw meats or other raw animal products, uncooked hot dogs, or

Women with acquired immune deficiency syndrome (AIDS) may pass the virus that causes this disease to the fetus during pregnancy or delivery. About one in three infected newborns will develop AIDS symptoms and die within just a few years. Studies show that these odds of mother-infant transmission can be cut significantly if the woman begins taking highly active antiretroviral therapy (HAART) and receiving routine obstetrical care. Before HAART was available, up to 45% of babies born to mothers with the AIDS virus were infected. Now, transmission is less than 2%. Thus, screening pregnant women for AIDS and providing HAART to those with AIDS are advocated by many experts.

The USDA warns pregnant women to thoroughly cook (e.g., microwave) all ready-to-eat meats, including hot dogs and cold cuts, until they are steaming to reduce risk of *Listeria* infections.

undercooked poultry. These food safety recommendations are included in the Dietary Guidelines for Americans discussed later in the chapter (Table 14-3 on page 554).

Nutritional Status

Is attention to good nutrition worth the effort? Yes; evidence shows that the effort is justified (see Further Readings 3, 5, and 19). Extra nutrients and calories are used for fetal growth, as well as for the changes the mother's body undergoes to accommodate the fetus. Her uterus and breasts grow, the placenta develops, her total blood volume increases, the heart and kidneys work harder, and stores of body fat increase.

Although it is difficult to predict to what degree poor nutrition will affect each pregnancy, a daily diet containing only 1000 kcal has been shown to greatly restrict fetal growth and development. Increased maternal and infant death rates seen in famine-stricken areas of Africa provide further evidence.

Genetic background can explain little of the observed differences in birth weight between developed and developing countries. Both environmental factors and nutritional factors are important. The worse the nutritional condition of the mother at the beginning of pregnancy, the more valuable a healthy prenatal diet and/or use of prenatal supplements are in improving the course and outcome of her pregnancy.

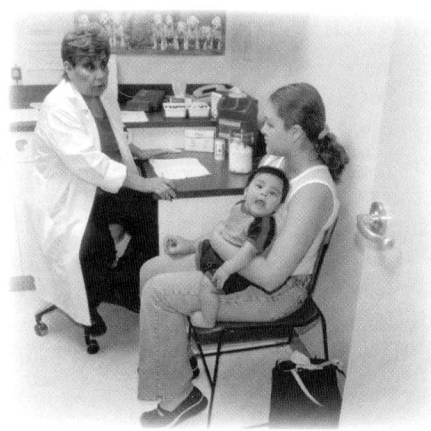

▲ In the United States, low-income pregnant women and their infants (and children) benefit from the nutritional and medical attention provided by the WIC program.

Nutrition Assistance for Low-Income Families

A low socioeconomic status is also associated with problems in pregnancy. Typical characteristics of low socioeconomic status include poverty, inadequate health care, poor health practices, lack of education, and unmarried status. In the United States, about 4 of every 10 births are to unwed mothers, and about 25% of unwed mothers and children live in poverty.

Several U.S. government programs provide high-quality health care and foods to reduce infant mortality. These are designed to alleviate the negative impact of poverty, insufficient education, and inadequate nutrient intake on pregnancy outcome. An example of such a program is the Special Supplemental Nutrition Program for Women, Infants, and Children (WIC). This program offers health assessments and vouchers for foods that supply high-quality protein, calcium, iron, and vitamins A and C to pregnant women, infants, and children (up to age 5 years) from low-income populations. The WIC program is available in all areas of the United States and has a staff trained to help women have healthy babies. More than 9 million women, infants, and young children are benefiting from this program, but many eligible pregnant women are not participating.

CONCEPT CHECK

To help ensure the optimal health of both the mother and her offspring, adequate nutrition is vital both before and during pregnancy. In particular, meeting folate needs from a synthetic source starting at least 3 months before pregnancy begins, is effective at preventing a variety of fetal malformations. The first trimester is a critical period when inadequate nutrient intake or alcohol and drug use can result in birth defects.

Infants born after 37 weeks of gestation who weigh more than 5.5 pounds (2.5 kilograms) have the fewest medical problems at birth. To reduce infant and maternal medical problems or death, the expectant mother, family, and medical care providers should take the steps necessary to allow the mother to carry the baby in her uterus for the entire 40 weeks. Good nutrition and health practices aid in this goal.

14.4 Increased Nutrient Needs to Support Pregnancy

Pregnancy is a time of increased nutrient needs. It is important to recognize the need for individual assessment and counseling of mothers-to-be, as the nutritional and health status of each woman is different. Still, there are some general principles true for most women with regard to increased nutrient needs.

CRITICAL THINKING

Alexandra wants to have a baby. She has read that it is very important for the woman to be healthy during the pregnancy. However, Jane, her sister, tells her that the time to begin to assess her nutritional and health status is before she becomes pregnant. What additional information should Jane have given Alexandra?

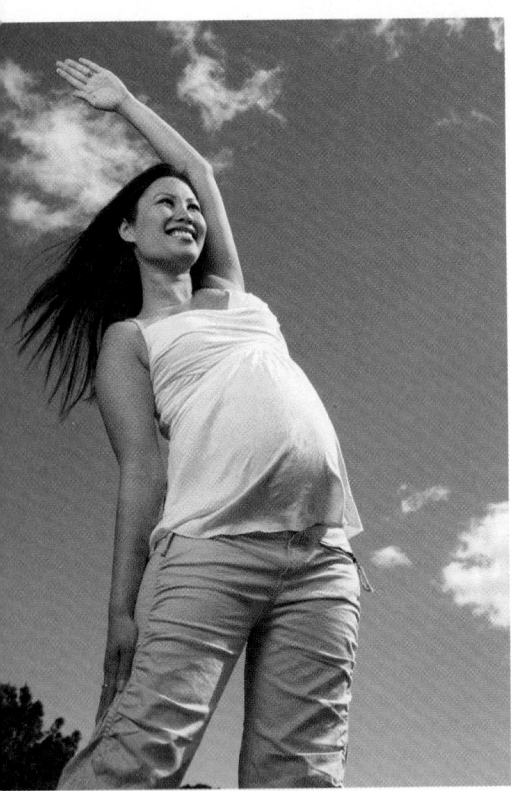

▲ The 2008 Physical Activity Guidelines for Americans recommend that healthy women should get at least 150 minutes of moderate-intensity aerobic activity each week during pregnancy.

Increased Calorie Needs

To support the growth and development of the fetus, pregnant women need to increase their calorie intake. Calorie needs during the first trimester are essentially the same as for nonpregnant women. However, during the second and third trimesters, it is necessary for a pregnant woman to consume approximately 350 to 450 kcal more per day than her prepregnancy needs (the upper end of the range is needed in the third trimester).

Rather than seeing this as an opportunity to fill up on sugary desserts or fat-filled snacks, these extra calories should be in the form of nutrient-dense foods. For example, throughout the day, about six whole-wheat crackers, 1 ounce of cheese, and ½ cup of fat-free milk would supply the extra calories (and also some calcium). Although she "eats for two," the pregnant woman must not double her normal calorie intake. The "eating for two" concept refers more appropriately to increased needs for several vitamins and minerals. Micronutrient needs are increased by up to 50% during pregnancy, whereas calorie needs during the second and third trimesters represent only about a 20% increase.

If a woman is active during her pregnancy, she may need to increase her calorie intake by even more than the estimated 350 to 450 kcal per day. Her greater body weight requires more calories for activity. Many women find that they are inactive during the later months, partly because of their increased size, so an extra 350 to 450 kcal in their daily diets is usually enough.

MAKING DECISIONS

Staying Active During Pregnancy

While pregnancy is not the time to begin an intense fitness regimen, women can generally take part in most low- or moderate-intensity activities during pregnancy. Walking, cycling, swimming, or light aerobics for at least 150 minutes per week is generally advised. Such exercise may prevent pregnancy complications and promote an easier delivery. Some research indicates that regular physical activity during pregnancy lowers a woman's risk of developing gestational diabetes by 50% and preeclampsia by 40%. Women who were highly active prior to pregnancy can maintain their activities as long as they remain healthy and discuss with their health care providers. A few types of activities can potentially harm the fetus and should be avoided, especially those with inherent risk of falls and abdominal trauma. Examples of exercises to avoid, especially during the second and third trimesters, include downhill skiing, weightlifting, soccer, basketball, horseback riding, certain calisthenics (e.g., deep knee bends), any contact sports (e.g., hockey), and SCUBA diving.

Women with high-risk pregnancies, such as those experiencing preterm labor contractions, may need to restrict their physical activity. To ensure optimal health for both herself and her infant, a pregnant woman should first consult her physician about physical activity and possible limitations (see Further Reading 13).

Adequate Weight Gain

Key recommendations for weight management during pregnancy and lactation are included in the Dietary Guidelines for Americans (see Table 14-3 on page 554). Healthy prepregnancy weight and appropriate weight gain during pregnancy are excellent predictors of pregnancy outcome (see Further Readings 8, 10, and 11). Her diet should allow for approximately 2 to 4 pounds (0.9 to 1.8 kilograms) of weight gain during the first trimester and then a subsequent weight gain of 0.8 to 1 pound (0.4 to 0.5 kilogram) weekly during the second and third trimesters (Fig. 14-3). A healthy goal for total weight gain for a woman of normal weight (based on BMI; Table 14-2) averages about 25 to 35 pounds (11.5 to 16 kilograms). Pregnant adolescents and women of various racial and ethnic groups are advised to meet these weight gain goals until further research determines any special recommendations. Women of normal prepregnancy BMI carrying twins should aim to gain within the range of 37 to

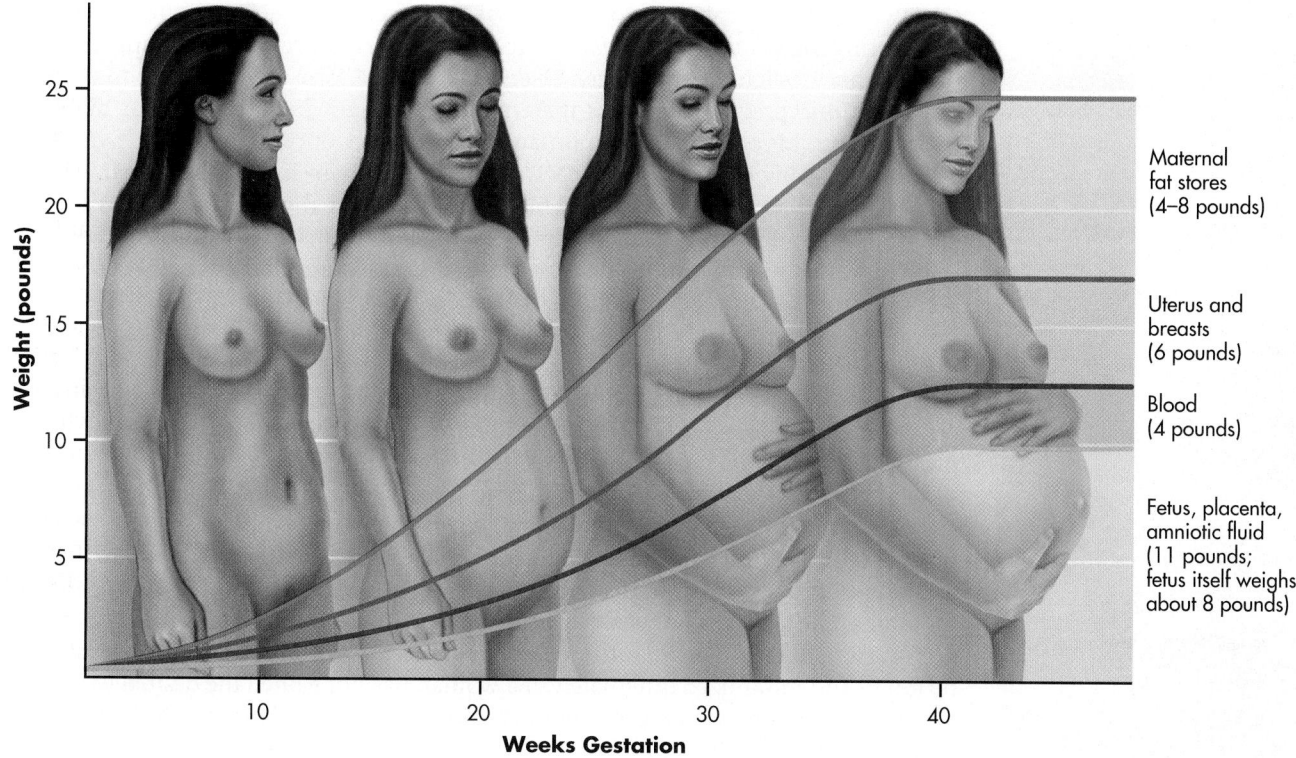

FIGURE 14-3 ▶ The components of weight gain in pregnancy. A weight gain of 25 to 35 pounds is recommended for most women. The various components total about 25 pounds.

54 pounds, whereas overweight or obese women should gain less (31 to 50 pounds or 25 to 42 pounds, respectively).

For women who begin pregnancy with a low BMI, the goal increases to 28 to 40 pounds (12.5 to 18 kilograms). The goal decreases to 15 to 25 pounds (7 to 11.5 kilograms) for overweight women. Target weight gain for obese women is 11 to 20 pounds (5 to 9 kilograms). Figure 14-3 shows why the typical recommendation begins at 25 pounds.

A weight gain of between 25 and 35 pounds for a woman starting pregnancy at normal weight has repeatedly been shown to yield optimal health for both mother and fetus if gestation lasts at least 38 weeks. The weight gain should yield a birth weight of 7.5 pounds (3.5 kilograms). Although some extra weight gain during pregnancy is

TABLE 14-2 Recommended Weight Gain in Pregnancy Based on Prepregnancy Body Mass Index (BMI)

Prepregnancy BMI Category	Total Weight Gain*	
	(pounds)	(kilograms)
Low (BMI less than 18.5)	28 to 40	12.5 to 18
Normal (BMI 18.5 to 24.9)	25 to 35	11.5 to 16
High (BMI 25.0 to 29.9)	15 to 25	7 to 11.5
Obese (BMI greater than 30.0)	11 to 20	5 to 9

*The listed values are for pregnancies with one fetus. For women of normal BMI carrying twins, the range is 37 to 54 pounds (17 to 24.5 kilograms), or less for heavier women.

Reprinted in part with permission from *Weight Gain During Pregnancy: Reexamining the Guidelines*, Copyright 2009 by the Institute of Medicine and National Research Council of the National Academies. Courtesy of the National Academies Press, Washington, DC.

During pregnancy, women in North America are more likely to gain excess weight and make poor food choices than to eat too little.

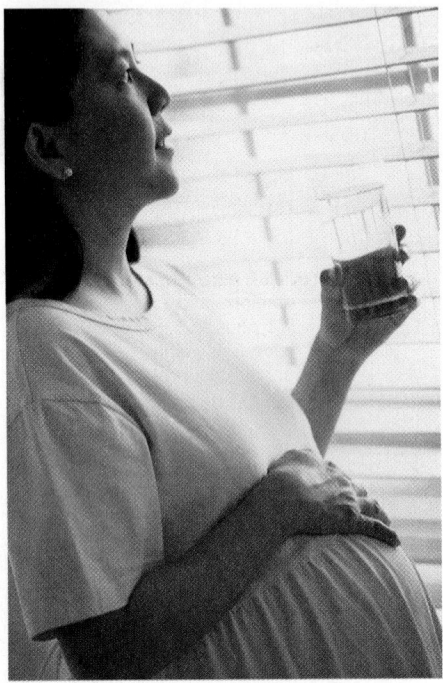

▲ During pregnancy, the Adequate Intake for total water increases 0.3 liters (1¼ cups) above prepregnancy needs to 3.0 liters (about 12½ cups) per day. For breastfeeding, consume 3.8 liters (16 cups) daily.

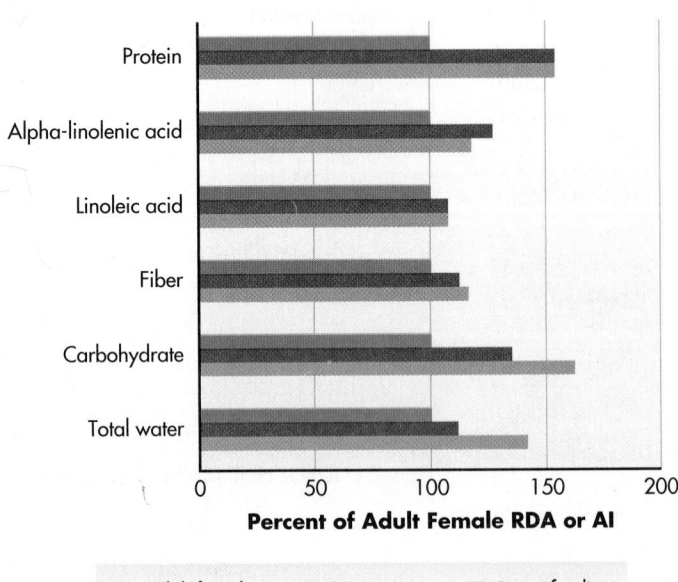

Adult female   Pregnancy   Breastfeeding

FIGURE 14-4 ▶ Relative macronutrient and water requirements for pregnancy and breastfeeding. Note that there is no RDA or AI for total fat.

usually not harmful (about 5 to 10 pounds), it can set the stage for a pattern of weight gain during the child-bearing years if the mother does not return to her approximate prepregnancy weight after delivery. Overweight and obesity do contribute to complications during pregnancy. Excess maternal body weight increases risk for diabetes, hypertension, blood clots, and spontaneous abortions during pregnancy. Even after childbirth, lasting effects of excess gestational weight gain include high BMI, central body fat distribution, and elevated blood pressure. For the baby, there is a greater chance of birth defects and macrosomia, in which the fetus grows larger than average in utero. Larger infants contribute to a greater need for surgical delivery (i.e., Cesarean sections) among overweight and obese mothers.

Weight gain during pregnancy should generally follow the pattern in Figure 14-3. Monitoring weekly records of a pregnant woman's weight gain helps assess how much to adjust her food intake. Weight gain is a key issue in prenatal care and a concern of many mothers-to-be. Remember that inadequate weight gain can cause many problems.

If a woman deviates from the desirable pattern, she should make the appropriate adjustment. For example, if a woman begins to gain too much weight during her pregnancy, she should not lose weight to get back on track. Even if a woman gains 35 pounds in the first 7 months of pregnancy, she must still gain more during the last 2 months. She should, however, slow the increase in weight to parallel the rise on the prenatal weight gain chart. In other words, the sources of the unnecessary calories should be found and minimized. Alternately, if a woman has not gained the desired weight by a given point in pregnancy, she shouldn't gain the needed weight rapidly. Instead, she should slowly gain a little more weight than the typical pattern to meet the goal by the end of the pregnancy. A registered dietitian can help make any needed adjustments.

Increased Protein and Carbohydrate Needs

The RDA for protein increases by an additional 25 grams per day during pregnancy. A cup of milk alone contains 8 grams. Many nonpregnant women already consume protein in excess of their needs and therefore do not need to increase protein intake any further. However, all women should check to make sure they are eating enough protein as well as enough calories, so this protein is not used to meet energy needs.

The RDA for carbohydrate increases to 175 grams daily, primarily to prevent ketosis. Ketone bodies, a by-product of metabolism of fat for energy, are thought to be poorly used by the fetal brain, implying possible slowing of fetal brain development. Carbohydrate intakes of most women, pregnant or not, already exceed the RDA (Fig. 14-4).

A Word About Lipids

Fat intake should increase proportionally with calorie intake during pregnancy to maintain around 20% to 30% of total calories from fat. Pregnancy is not a time for a low-fat diet, as lipids are a source of extra calories and essential fatty acids needed during pregnancy. Recommendations for the types of lipids during pregnancy are generally the same as for nonpregnant adults. To reduce risk for cardiovascular disease, the American Heart Association recommends no more than 7% of total calories from saturated fat and no more than 1% from *trans* fat. Consumption of dietary cholesterol is not required, but keeping cholesterol intake at a maximum of 300 milligrams per day is also a good goal for maintenance of maternal cardiovascular health.

During pregnancy, it is particularly important to make sure to consume adequate essential fatty acids—linoleic acid (omega-6) and alpha-linolenic acid (omega-3). As you learned in Chapter 5, essential fatty acids cannot be synthesized in the body and must be consumed in the diet. For the developing fetus, essential fatty acids are required for growth, brain development, and eye development. Recommendations are slightly increased by pregnancy: 13 grams per day of omega-6 fatty acids and 1.4 grams per day of omega-3 fatty acids. These needs can be met by consuming 2 to 4 tablespoons per day of plant oils. Consumption of fish at least two times per week is also helpful in meeting needs for essential fatty acids in the diet (see Further Reading 15). (See the "Nutrition and Your Health" section at the end of this chapter for a discussion of mercury in fish.)

Increased Vitamin Needs

Vitamin needs generally increase from prepregnancy RDAs/Adequate Intakes by up to 30% for most of the B vitamins and even greater for vitamin B-6 (45%) and folate (50%) (Fig 14-5). Vitamin A needs only increase by 10%, so a specific focus on this vitamin is not needed. And remember, excess amounts of vitamin A are harmful to the developing fetus.

The extra amount of vitamin B-6 and other B vitamins (except folate) needed in the diet is easily met via wise food choices, such as a serving of a typical ready-to-eat breakfast cereal and some animal protein sources. Folate needs, however, often merit specific diet planning and possible vitamin supplementation. The synthesis of DNA, and therefore cell division, requires folate, so this nutrient is especially crucial during pregnancy. Ultimately, both fetal and maternal growth depend on an ample supply of folate. Red blood cell formation, which requires folate, increases during pregnancy. Serious folate-related anemia therefore can result if folate intake is inadequate. The RDA for folate increases during pregnancy to 600 micrograms DFE per day (review Chapter 8 for calculation of DFE). This is a critical goal in the nutritional care of a pregnant woman. Increasing folate intakes to meet 600 micrograms DFE per day for a pregnant woman can be achieved through dietary sources, a supplemental source of folic acid, or a combination of both. Choosing a diet rich in synthetic folic acid, such as from ready-to-eat breakfast cereals or meal replacement bars (look for approximately 50% to 100% of the Daily Value), is especially helpful in meeting folate needs. Recall from Chapter 8 that synthetic folic acid is much more easily absorbed than the various forms of folate found naturally in foods (see Further Readings 14 and 17).

Increased Mineral Needs

Mineral needs generally increase during pregnancy, especially the requirements for iodide and iron (Fig. 14-6). Zinc needs also increase. (Calcium needs do not increase but still may deserve special attention because many women have deficient intakes.)

Pregnant women need the extra iodide (total of 220 micrograms per day) for prevention of goiter. Typical iodide intakes are enough if the woman uses iodized salt. Animal proteins or a fortified ready-to-eat breakfast cereal in the diet can easily provide enough extra zinc. The extra iron (total of 27 milligrams per day) is needed to synthesize the greater amount of hemoglobin needed during pregnancy and to provide iron stores for the fetus. Women often need a supplemental source of iron, especially if they do not consume iron-fortified foods, such as highly fortified breakfast cereals containing close to 100% of the Daily Value for iron (18 milligrams). Iron supplements decrease appetite and can cause nausea and constipation, so if used, these should be taken between meals or just before going to bed. Milk, coffee, or tea should not be consumed with an iron supplement because these beverages have substances that interfere with iron absorption. Eating foods rich in vitamin C along with nonheme iron-containing foods and iron supplements helps increase iron absorption from those sources. Pregnant women who are not anemic may wait until the second trimester, when pregnancy-related nausea generally lessens, to start iron supplementation if needed.

The consequences of iron-deficiency anemia—especially during the first trimester—can be severe. Negative outcomes include preterm delivery, LBW infants, and increased risk for fetal death in the first weeks after birth.

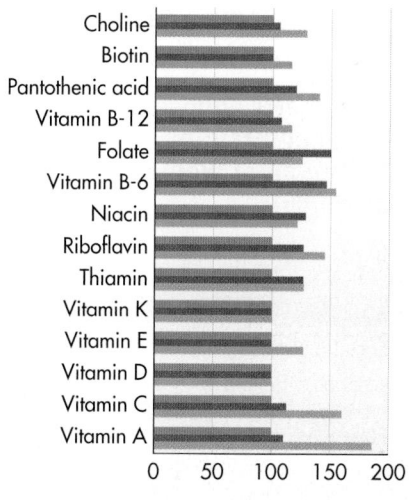

Percent of Adult Female RDA or AI

- Adult female
- Pregnancy
- Breastfeeding

FIGURE 14-5 ▶ Relative vitamin requirements for pregnancy and breastfeeding.

The Dietary Guidelines for Americans recommend that women who may become pregnant eat foods high in iron and consume adequate amounts of the synthetic form of folate (see Table 14-3).

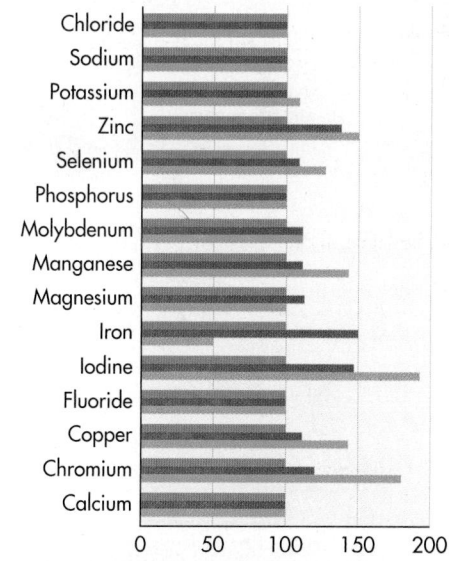

Percent of Adult Female RDA or AI

- Adult female
- Pregnancy
- Breastfeeding

FIGURE 14-6 ▶ Relative mineral requirements for pregnancy and breastfeeding.

NEWSWORTHY NUTRITION

Experts advocate higher vitamin D for pregnant women

Emerging evidence indicates that low maternal levels of vitamin D during pregnancy affect multiple health parameters in their children. Aside from its well-known role in bone health and prevention of rickets, poor vitamin D status is implicated in serious complications of pregnancy, including higher rates of gestational diabetes, pregnancy-induced hypertension, and a fourfold increased rate of Cesarean section. Vitamin D's role in immune regulation is underscored by higher rates of respiratory infections and mother-to-child transmission of HIV. Because of the ability of vitamin D to modulate gene expression, vitamin D status is critically important during early fetal development through infancy. Diseases that develop later in childhood or adulthood, such as type 1 diabetes, multiple sclerosis, asthma, schizophrenia, and certain types of cancer, are associated with low vitamin D status during gestation. The RDA for pregnant women is 15 micrograms (600 IU) of vitamin D daily, but many experts advocate increasing this recommendation to 25 micrograms (1000 IU) or more.

Source: Dror DK, Allen LH. Vitamin D inadequacy in pregnancy: Biology, outcomes, and interventions. *Nutrition Reviews* 68: 464, 2010.

Check out the Connect site www.mcgrawhillconnect.com **to further explore vitamin D and pregnancy.**

TABLE 14-3 Targeted Recommendations for Women from the Latest Dietary Guidelines for Americans

Balancing Calories to Manage Weight

Women capable of becoming pregnant
- Achieve and maintain a healthy weight before becoming pregnant.

Women who are pregnant
- Gain weight within the 2009 Institute of Medicine gestational weight-gain guidelines (review Table 14-2).

Foods and Food Components to Reduce

Women capable of becoming pregnant and women who are pregnant
- During pregnancy or when conception is possible, avoid alcohol. No safe level of alcohol consumption during pregnancy has been established.

Women who are pregnant
- Only eat foods with seafood, meat, poultry, or eggs that have been cooked to recommended safe minimum internal temperatures.
- Do not consume unpasteurized (raw) juice or milk or foods made from unpasteurized milk, like some soft cheeses (e.g., feta, queso blanco, queso fresco, Brie, Camembert, blue-veined cheeses, and Panela).
- Reheat deli and luncheon meats and hot dogs to steaming hot to kill *Listeria* and do not eat raw sprouts).

Women who are breastfeeding
- Wait at least 4 hours after drinking alcohol before breastfeeding.
- Alcohol should not be consumed at all until consistent latch on and breastfeeding patterns are established.

Foods and Nutrients to Increase

Women capable of becoming pregnant
- Choose foods that supply heme iron, which is more readily absorbed by the body, additional iron sources, and enhancers of iron absorption such as vitamin C–rich foods.
- Consume 400 micrograms per day of synthetic folic acid (from fortified foods and/or supplements) in addition to food forms of folate from a varied diet.

Women who are pregnant
- Take an iron supplement, as recommended by an obstetrician or other health care provider.
- Consume 600 micrograms of dietary folate equivalents daily from all food sources.

Women who are pregnant or breastfeeding
- Consume 8 to 12 ounces of seafood per week from a variety of seafood types.
- Due to their methyl mercury content, limit white (albacore) tuna to 6 ounces per week and do not eat the following four types of fish: tilefish, shark, swordfish, and king mackerel.

Use of Prenatal Vitamin and Mineral Supplements

Special supplements formulated for pregnancy are prescribed routinely for pregnant women by most physicians. Some are sold over the counter, while others are dispensed by prescription because of the high synthetic folic acid content (1000 micrograms), which could pose problems for others, such as older people (see Chapter 16). These supplements are high in iron (27 milligrams per pill). There is no evidence that use of such supplements causes significant health problems in pregnancy, aside perhaps from the combined amounts of supplementary and dietary vitamin A (see Nutrition and Your Health at the end of this chapter).

Instances when prenatal supplements may especially contribute to a successful pregnancy are with poor women, teenagers, those with a generally deficient diet, women carrying multiple fetuses, those that smoke or use alcohol or illegal drugs, and vegans. In other cases, healthy diets can provide the needed nutrients. When choosing a multivitamin, rely on brands that display the USP symbol on their label, signifying that the supplement meets the content, quality, purity, and safety standards of the

U.S. Pharmacopoeia. Also, avoid megadoses of any nutrient. In particular, toxicity of vitamin A is linked with birth defects. Skip supplements containing herbs, enzymes, and amino acids. Many of these ingredients have not been evaluated for safety during pregnancy or breastfeeding and may be toxic to the fetus. Furthermore, discard supplements that are past the expiration date, as some ingredients lose potency over time.

14.5 Food Plan for Pregnant Women

One dietary approach to support a successful pregnancy is based on MyPlate. For an active 24-year-old woman, about 2200 kcal is recommended during the first trimester (the same as recommended for such a woman when not pregnant). The plan should include:

- 3 cups of calcium-rich foods from the dairy group or use of calcium-fortified foods to make up for any gap between calcium intake and need
- 6 ounce-equivalents from the protein group
- 3 cups from the vegetables group
- 2 cups from the fruits group
- 7 ounce-equivalents from the grains group
- 6 teaspoons of vegetable oil

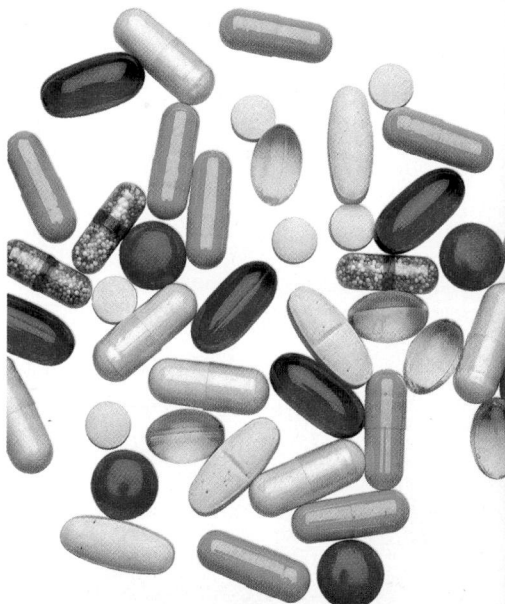

▲ Pregnancy, in particular, is not a time to self-prescribe vitamin and mineral supplements. For example, although vitamin A is a routine component of prenatal vitamins, intakes over three times the RDA for vitamin A have been shown to have toxic effects on the fetus.

MAKING DECISIONS

Cravings During Pregnancy

It is a common myth that women instinctively know what to eat during pregnancy. Cravings of the last two trimesters are often related to hormonal changes in the mother, or family traditions. Such "instinct" cannot be trusted, however, based on observations that some women crave nonfood items (called **pica**) such as laundry starch, chalk, cigarette ashes, and soil (clay). This practice can be extremely harmful to the mother and the fetus. Overall, though women may have a natural instinct to consume the right foods in pregnancy, humans are so far removed from living by instinct that relying on our cravings to meet nutrient needs is risky. Nutrition advice by experts is more reliable.

pica The practice of eating nonfood items, such as dirt, laundry starch, or clay.

At www.ChooseMyPlate.gov, moms-to-be can find individualized dietary information by clicking on the link for Daily Food Plans for Moms. Based on age, height, physical activity, and prepregnancy weight, calorie and food group recommendations are generated for each trimester.

Specifically, choices from the dairy group should include low-fat or fat-free versions of milk, yogurt, and cheese. These foods supply extra protein, calcium, and carbohydrate, as well as other nutrients. Choices from the protein group should include both animal and vegetable sources. Besides protein, these foods help provide the extra iron and zinc needed. The vegetables and fruits group choices provide a variety of vitamins and minerals. One cup from this combination should be a good vitamin C source, and 1 cup should be a green vegetable or other rich source of folate. Choices from the grains group should focus on whole-grain and enriched foods. One ounce of a whole-grain, ready-to-eat breakfast cereal significantly contributes to meeting many vitamin and mineral needs. Finally, inclusion of plant oils in the diet contributes essential fatty acids. Calories from solid fats and added sugars should be limited to 270 kcal per day.

In the second and third trimesters, about 2600 kcal is recommended for this woman. The plan should now include:

- 3 cups of calcium-rich foods from the dairy group or use of calcium-fortified foods
- 6 ½ ounce-equivalents from the protein group
- 3 ½ cups from the vegetables group
- 2 cups from the fruits group
- 9-ounce equivalents from the grains group
- 8 teaspoons of vegetable oil

Solid fats and added sugars should contribute no more than 360 kcal per day. Table 14-4 illustrates one daily menu based on the 2600 kcal plan for pregnancy for women in the second or third trimesters. This menu meets the extra nutrient needs associated with pregnancy. Women who need to consume more than this—and some do for various reasons—should incorporate additional fruits, vegetables, and whole-grain breads and cereals, not poor nutrient sources such as desserts and sugared soft drinks.

Pregnant Vegetarians

pl dairy egg   *pl & dairy*

Women who are either lactoovovegetarians or lactovegetarians generally do not face special difficulties in meeting their nutritional needs during pregnancy. Like

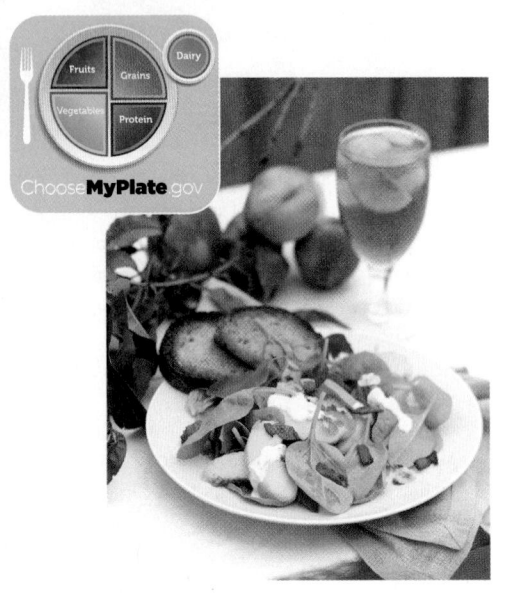

Choose **MyPlate** gov

CRITICAL THINKING

How does this lunch of spinach and fruit salad and whole-wheat toast compare to MyPlate? Is iced tea a good beverage choice? Why or why not?

TABLE 14-4 Sample 2600 kcal Daily Menu That Meets the Nutritional Needs of Most Pregnant and Breastfeeding Women

	Vitamin B-6	Folate	Iron	Zinc	Calcium
Breakfast					
1 cup Kellogg's Smart Start cereal	✓	✓	✓	✓	✓
1 cup orange juice		✓			
1 cup fat-free milk	✓				✓
Snack					
2 tbsp peanut butter	✓	✓	✓	✓	
2 stalks of celery		✓			
1 slice whole-wheat toast		✓	✓	✓	
1 cup plain low-fat yogurt	✓				✓
½ cup strawberries		✓			
Lunch					
2 cups spinach and fruit salad with 2 tbsp oil and vinegar dressing		✓			✓
2 slices whole-wheat toast		✓	✓	✓	✓
1 ½ ounces provolone cheese	✓				✓
Snack					
5 whole-wheat crackers		✓	✓	✓	
1 cup grape juice					
Dinner					
3 ounces lean hamburger, broiled (with condiments)	✓		✓	✓	
½ cup baked beans	✓	✓	✓	✓	
1 hamburger bun		✓	✓		
½ sliced tomato					
1 cup cooked broccoli		✓			✓
1 tsp soft margarine					
Iced tea					
Snack					
Granola bar (2 ounces)		✓	✓	✓	
½ banana	✓				
Foods or beverages containing solid fats or added sugars can be included (up to 360 kcal per day) to support adequate weight gain.					

*Amount of solid fats and added sugars will vary based on the actual food choices made within each MyPlate group.

This diet meets nutrient needs for pregnancy and breastfeeding. Lack of a check (✓) indicates a poor source of the nutrient. The vitamin- and mineral-fortified breakfast cereal used in this example makes an important contribution to meeting nutrient needs. Fluids can be added as desired. Total intake of fluids, such as water, should be 10 cups per day for pregnant women or about 13 cups per day for breastfeeding women.

nonvegetarian women, they should be concerned primarily with meeting vitamin B-6, iron, folate, and zinc needs.

On the other hand, for a vegan, careful diet planning during preconception and pregnancy is crucial to ensure sufficient protein, vitamin D (particularly in the absence of sufficient sun exposure), vitamin B-6, iron, calcium, zinc, and especially a supplemental source of vitamin B-12. The basic vegan diet listed in Chapter 6 should be modified to include more grains, beans, nuts, and seeds to supply the necessary extra amounts of some of these nutrients. As mentioned, use of a prenatal multivitamin and mineral supplement also is generally advocated to help fill micronutrient gaps. However, although these are high in iron, this is not true for calcium (200 milligrams per pill). If iron and calcium supplements are used, they should not be taken together, to avoid possible competition for absorption.

CONCEPT CHECK

Calorie needs increase by an average of about 350 to 450 kcal per day during the second and third trimesters of pregnancy, respectively. Weight gain should be slow and steady up to a total of 25 to 35 pounds for a woman of normal weight (i.e., prepregnancy BMI of 18.5 to 24.9). Protein and certain vitamin and mineral needs increase during pregnancy. Most important to consider are vitamin B-6, folate, iron, iodide, and zinc. A pregnant woman's diet should be varied and generally comply with MyPlate standards. A prenatal multivitamin and mineral supplement is commonly prescribed but may not be necessary, depending on one's diet and health status. Taking too many supplements—especially vitamin A—can be hazardous to the fetus.

14.6 Physiological Changes of Concern During Pregnancy

During pregnancy, the fetus's needs for oxygen and nutrients, as well as excretion of waste products increase the burden on the mother's lungs, heart, and kidneys. Although a mother's digestive and metabolic systems work efficiently, some discomfort accompanies the changes her body undergoes to accommodate the fetus.

Heartburn, Constipation, and Hemorrhoids

Hormones (such as progesterone) produced by the placenta relax muscles in the uterus and the gastrointestinal tract. This often causes heartburn as stomach acid refluxes into the esophagus (review Chapter 3). When this occurs, the woman should avoid lying down after eating, eat less fat so that foods pass more quickly from the stomach into the small intestine, and avoid spicy foods she cannot tolerate. She should also consume most liquids between meals to decrease the volume of food in the stomach after meals, and thus relieve some of the pressure that encourages reflux. Women with more severe cases may need antacids or related medications.

Constipation often results as the intestinal muscles relax during pregnancy. It is especially likely to develop late in pregnancy, as the fetus competes with the GI tract for space in the abdominal cavity. To offset these discomforts, a woman should perform regular exercise and consume more fluid, fiber, and dried fruits, such as prunes (dried plums). The Adequate Intake for fiber in pregnancy is 28 grams, slightly more than for the nonpregnant woman. Fluid needs are 10 cups per day. These practices can help prevent constipation and a problem that frequently accompanies it, hemorrhoids. Straining during elimination can lead to hemorrhoids, which are more likely to occur during pregnancy because of other body changes. A re-evaluation of the need for and dose of iron supplementation also should be considered, as high iron intakes are linked to constipation.

Edema

Placental hormones cause various body tissues to retain fluid during pregnancy. Blood volume also greatly expands during pregnancy. The extra fluid normally causes some swelling (edema). There is no reason to restrict salt severely or use diuretics to limit mild edema. However, the edema may limit physical activity late in pregnancy and occasionally requires a woman to elevate her feet or wear compression stockings to control the symptoms. Overall, edema generally spells trouble only if hypertension and the appearance of extra protein in the urine accompany it (see a following section, "Pregnancy-Induced Hypertension").

Morning Sickness

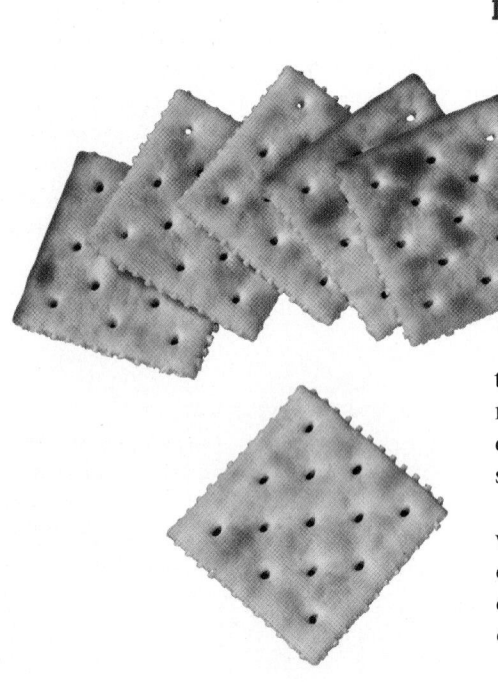

About 70% to 85% of pregnant women experience nausea during the early stages of pregnancy. This nausea may be related to the increased sense of smell induced by pregnancy-related hormones circulating in the bloodstream. Although commonly called "morning sickness," pregnancy-related nausea may occur at any time and persist all day. It is often the first signal to a woman that she is pregnant. To help control mild nausea, pregnant women can try the following: avoiding nauseating foods, such as fried or greasy foods; cooking with good ventilation to dissipate nauseating smells; eating saltine crackers or dry cereal before getting out of bed; avoiding large fluid intakes early in the morning; and eating smaller, more frequent meals. The iron in prenatal supplements triggers nausea in some women, so changing the type of supplement used or postponing use until the second trimester may provide relief in some cases. If a woman thinks her prenatal supplement is related to morning sickness, she should discuss switching to another supplement with her physician.

Overall, if a food sounds good to a pregnant woman with morning sickness, whether it is broccoli, soda crackers, or lemonade, she should eat it and eat when she can, while also striving to follow her prenatal diet. The American College of Obstetricians and Gynecologists recommends the following for the prevention and treatment of nausea and vomiting of pregnancy:

▲ A few saltine crackers upon waking or between meals can help lessen pregnancy-related nausea.

- History of use of a balanced multivitamin and mineral supplement at the time of conception
- Use of megadoses of vitamin B-6 (10–25 milligrams taken three to four times a day), especially coupled with the antihistamine doxylamine (10 milligrams) with each dose
- Ginger may also be helpful (350 milligrams taken three times per day)

Usually, nausea stops after the first trimester; however, in about 10% to 20% of cases, it can continue throughout the entire pregnancy. In cases of serious nausea, the preceding practices offer little relief. Excessive vomiting can cause dangerous dehydration and must be avoided. When vomiting persists (about 0.5% to 2% of pregnancies), medical attention is needed.

Anemia

physiological anemia The normal increase in blood volume in pregnancy that dilutes the concentration of red blood cells, resulting in anemia; also called *hemodilution*.

To supply fetal needs, the mother's blood volume expands to approximately 150% of normal. The number of red blood cells, however, increases by only 20% to 30%, and this occurs more gradually. As a result, a pregnant woman has a lower ratio of red blood cells to total blood volume in her system. This hemodilution is known as **physiological anemia.** It is a normal response to pregnancy, rather than the result of inadequate nutrient intake. If during pregnancy, however, iron stores and/or dietary iron intake are not sufficient to meet needs, any resulting iron-deficiency anemia requires medical attention. The Dietary Guidelines for Americans recommend that women who may become pregnant eat foods high in iron (Table 14-3).

Gestational Diabetes

Hormones synthesized by the placenta decrease the efficiency of insulin. This leads to a mild increase in blood glucose, which helps supply calories to the fetus. If the rise in blood glucose becomes excessive, this leads to **gestational diabetes,** often beginning in weeks 20 to 28, particularly in women who have a family history of diabetes or who are obese. Other risk factors include maternal age over 35 and gestational diabetes in a prior pregnancy. In North America, gestational diabetes develops in about 4% of pregnancies; however, it increases to 7% in the Caucasian population. Today, pregnant women with risk factors for type 2 diabetes (e.g., obesity, family history) should be screened for undiagnosed type 2 diabetes at the first prenatal visit. Pregnant women without type 2 diabetes should be screened for diabetes at 24 to 28 weeks by checking for elevated blood glucose concentration 1 to 2 hours after consuming 75 grams of glucose (see Further Reading 16). If gestational diabetes is detected, a special diet that distributes low glycemic load carbohydrates throughout the day needs to be implemented. Sometimes insulin injections or oral medications are also needed. Regular physical activity also helps control blood glucose.

The primary risk of uncontrolled diabetes during pregnancy is that the fetus can grow quite large. This is a result of the oversupply of glucose from maternal circulation coupled with an increased production of insulin by the fetus, which allows fetal tissues to take up an increased amount of building materials for growth. The mother may require a Cesarean section if the size of the fetus is not compatible with a vaginal delivery. Another threat is that the infant may have low blood glucose at birth, because of the tendency to produce extra insulin that began during gestation. Other concerns are the potential for early delivery and increased risk of birth trauma and malformations. Although gestational diabetes often disappears after the infant's birth, it increases the mother's risk of developing diabetes later in life, especially if she fails to maintain a healthy body weight. Studies show that infants of mothers with gestational diabetes may also have higher risks of developing obesity and type 2 diabetes as they grow to adulthood. For all these reasons, proper control of gestational diabetes (and any diabetes present in the mother before pregnancy) is extremely important.

Pregnancy-Induced Hypertension

Pregnancy-induced hypertension is a high-risk disorder that occurs in about 3% to 5% of pregnancies. In its mild forms, it is also known as *preeclampsia* and, in severe forms, as *eclampsia*. Early symptoms include a rise in blood pressure, excess protein in the urine, edema, changes in blood clotting, and nervous system disorders. Very severe effects, including convulsions, can occur in the second and third trimesters. If not controlled, eclampsia eventually damages the liver and kidneys, and mother and fetus may die. The populations most at risk for this disorder are women under age 17 or over age 35, overweight or obese women, and those who have had multiple-birth pregnancies. A family history of pregnancy-induced hypertension in the mother's or father's side of the family, diabetes, African-American race, and a woman's first pregnancy also raise risk.

Pregnancy-induced hypertension resolves once the pregnancy ends, making delivery the most reliable treatment for the mother. However, because the problem often begins before the fetus is ready to be born, physicians in many cases must use treatments to prevent the worsening of the disorder. Bed rest and magnesium sulfate are the most effective treatment methods, although their effectiveness varies. Magnesium likely acts to relax blood vessels, and so leads to a fall in blood pressure. There is good evidence of the role of adequate calcium intake in reducing incidence of pregnancy-induced hypertension. However, results of a recent trial showed that vitamin C and E supplementation during pregnancy is not effective in preventing the disorder. Several other treatments, such as various antiseizure and antihypertensive medications, fish oils, selenium, and vitamin D are under study (see Further Reading 6).

gestational diabetes A high blood glucose concentration that develops during pregnancy and returns to normal after birth; one cause is the placental production of hormones that antagonize the regulation of blood glucose by insulin.

pregnancy-induced hypertension A serious disorder that can include high blood pressure, kidney failure, convulsions, and even death of the mother and fetus. Although its exact cause is not known, an adequate diet (especially adequate calcium intake) and prenatal care may prevent this disorder or limit its severity. Mild cases are known as *preeclampsia*; more severe cases are called *eclampsia* (formerly called *toxemia*).

CRITICAL THINKING

Sandy, 4 months pregnant, has been having heartburn after meals, constipation, and difficult bowel movements. As a student of nutrition, you understand the digestive system and the role of nutrition in health. What remedies might you suggest to Sandy to relieve her problems?

CONCEPT CHECK

Heartburn, constipation, hemorrhoids, nausea and vomiting, edema, anemia, and gestational diabetes are possible discomforts and complications of pregnancy. Changes in food habits can often ease these problems. Pregnancy-induced hypertension, with high blood pressure and kidney failure, can lead to severe complications or even death of the mother and fetus if not treated.

14.7 Breastfeeding

Breastfeeding the new infant further fosters his or her health, and so complements the attention given to diet during pregnancy. The American Dietetic Association and the American Academy of Pediatrics (AAP) recommend breastfeeding exclusively for the first 6 months, with the continued combination of breastfeeding and infant foods until 1 year (see Further Readings 2 and 4). The World Health Organization goes beyond that to recommend breastfeeding (with appropriate solid food introduction; see Chapter 15) for at least 2 years. Still, surveys show that only about 70% of North American mothers now begin to breastfeed their infants in the hospital, and at 4 and 6 months only 33% and 20%, respectively, are still breastfeeding their infants. The number falls to 18% at 1 year of age. These statistics refer to Caucasian women; minority women are even less likely to be breastfeeding at these time intervals.

Women who choose to breastfeed usually find it an enjoyable, special time in their lives that strengthens the bond with their new infant. Although bottle feeding with an infant formula is also safe for infants, as discussed in Chapter 15, it does not equal the benefits derived from human milk in all aspects. If a woman doesn't breastfeed her child, breast weight returns to normal soon after birth.

Planning to Breastfeed

Almost all women are physically capable of breastfeeding their children (see later section "Medical Conditions Precluding Breastfeeding" for exceptions). In most cases, problems encountered in breastfeeding are due to a lack of appropriate information. Anatomical problems in breasts, such as inverted nipples, can be corrected during pregnancy. Breast size generally increases during pregnancy and is no indication of success in breastfeeding. Most women notice a dramatic increase in the size and weight of their breasts by the third or fourth day of breastfeeding. If these changes do not occur, a woman needs to speak with her physician or a lactation consultant.

Breastfed infants must be followed closely over the first days of life to ensure that feeding and weight gain are proceeding normally. Monitoring is especially important with a mother's first child, because the mother will be inexperienced with the technique of breastfeeding. Mothers and healthy infants are commonly discharged from the hospital 1 to 2 days after delivery, whereas 20 years ago they stayed in the hospital for 3 or 4 days or longer. One result of such rapid discharge is a decreased period of infant monitoring by health care professionals. Incidents have been reported of infants developing dehydration and, in turn, blood clots soon after hospital discharge when breastfeeding did not proceed smoothly. Careful monitoring in this first week by a physician or lactation consultant is advised.

First-time mothers who plan to breastfeed should learn as much as they can about the process early in their pregnancy. Interested women should learn the proper technique, what obstacles to anticipate, and how to respond to them. Overall, breastfeeding is a learned skill, and mothers need knowledge to breastfeed, especially with the first child.

Many of the benefits of breastfeeding can be found in Table 14-5 and at **www.womenshealth.gov/Breastfeeding/index.cfm**, sponsored by the U.S. Surgeon General.

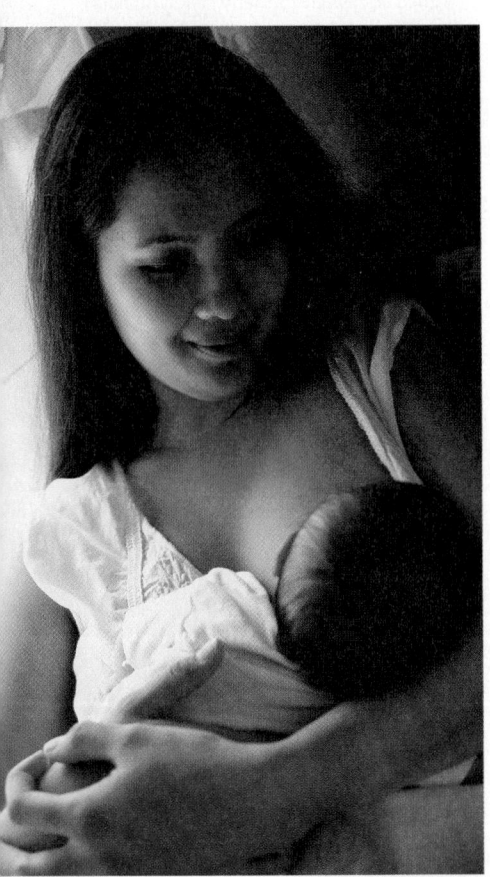

▲ Breastfeeding is the preferred way to feed a young infant.

*H*ealthy People 2020 has set a goal of 82% of women breastfeeding their infants at time of hospital discharge, 60% breastfeeding for 6 months, and 34% still breastfeeding at 1 year.

Production of Human Milk

During pregnancy, cells in the breast form milk-producing cells called **lobules** (Fig. 14-7). Hormones from the placenta stimulate these changes in the breast. After birth, the mother produces more **prolactin** hormone to maintain the changes in the breast and therefore the ability to produce milk. During pregnancy, breast weight increases by about 1 to 2 pounds.

The hormone prolactin also stimulates the synthesis of milk. Infant suckling stimulates prolactin release from the pituitary gland. Milk synthesis then occurs as an infant nurses. The more the infant suckles, the more milk is produced. Because of this, even twins (and triplets) can be breastfed adequately.

Most protein found in human milk is synthesized by breast tissue. Some proteins also enter the milk directly from the mother's bloodstream. These proteins include immune factors (e.g., antibodies) and enzymes. Fats in human milk come from both the mother's diet and those synthesized by breast tissue. The sugar galactose is synthesized in the breast, whereas glucose enters from the mother's bloodstream. Together, these sugars form lactose, the main carbohydrate in human milk.

Let-Down Reflex

An important brain-breast connection—commonly called the **let-down reflex**—is necessary for breastfeeding. The brain releases the hormone **oxytocin** to allow the breast tissues to let down (release) the milk from storage sites (Fig. 14-8). It then travels to the nipple area. A tingling sensation signals the let-down reflex shortly before milk flow begins. If the let-down reflex doesn't operate, little milk is available to the infant. The infant then gets frustrated, and this can frustrate the mother.

The let-down reflex is easily inhibited by nervous tension, a lack of confidence, and fatigue. Mothers should be especially aware of the link between tension and a weak let-down reflex. They need to find a relaxed environment where they can breastfeed.

lobules Saclike structures in the breast that store milk.

prolactin A hormone secreted by the pituitary gland that stimulates the synthesis of milk in the breast.

let-down reflex A reflex stimulated by infant suckling that causes the release (ejection) of milk from milk ducts in the mother's breasts; also called *milk ejection reflex.*

oxytocin A hormone secreted by the pituitary gland. It causes contraction of the muscle-like cells surrounding the ducts of the breasts and the smooth muscle of the uterus.

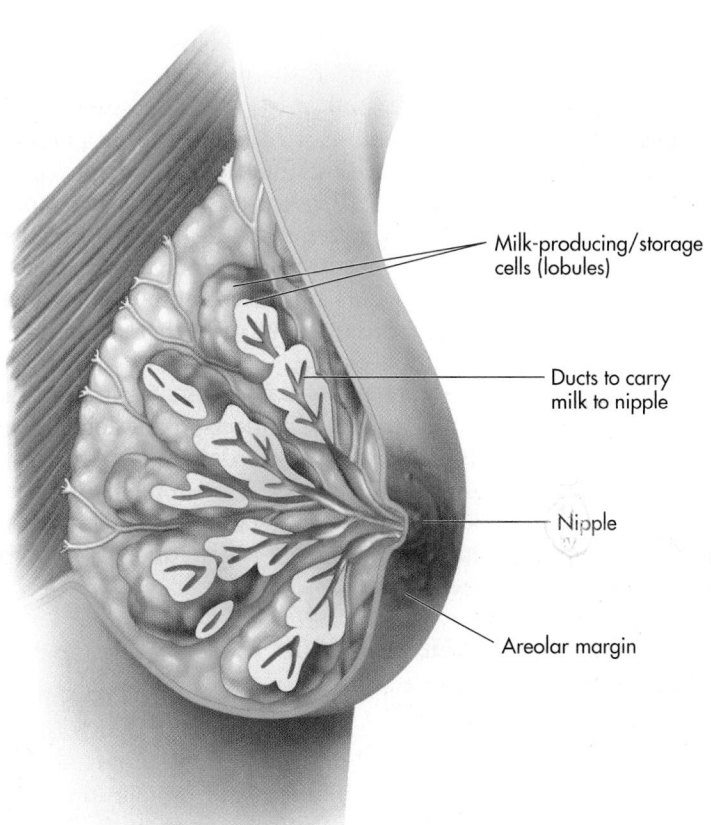

FIGURE 14-7 ▶ The anatomy of the breast. Many types of cells form a coordinated network to produce and secrete human milk.

Milk-producing/storage cells (lobules)

Ducts to carry milk to nipple

Nipple

Areolar margin

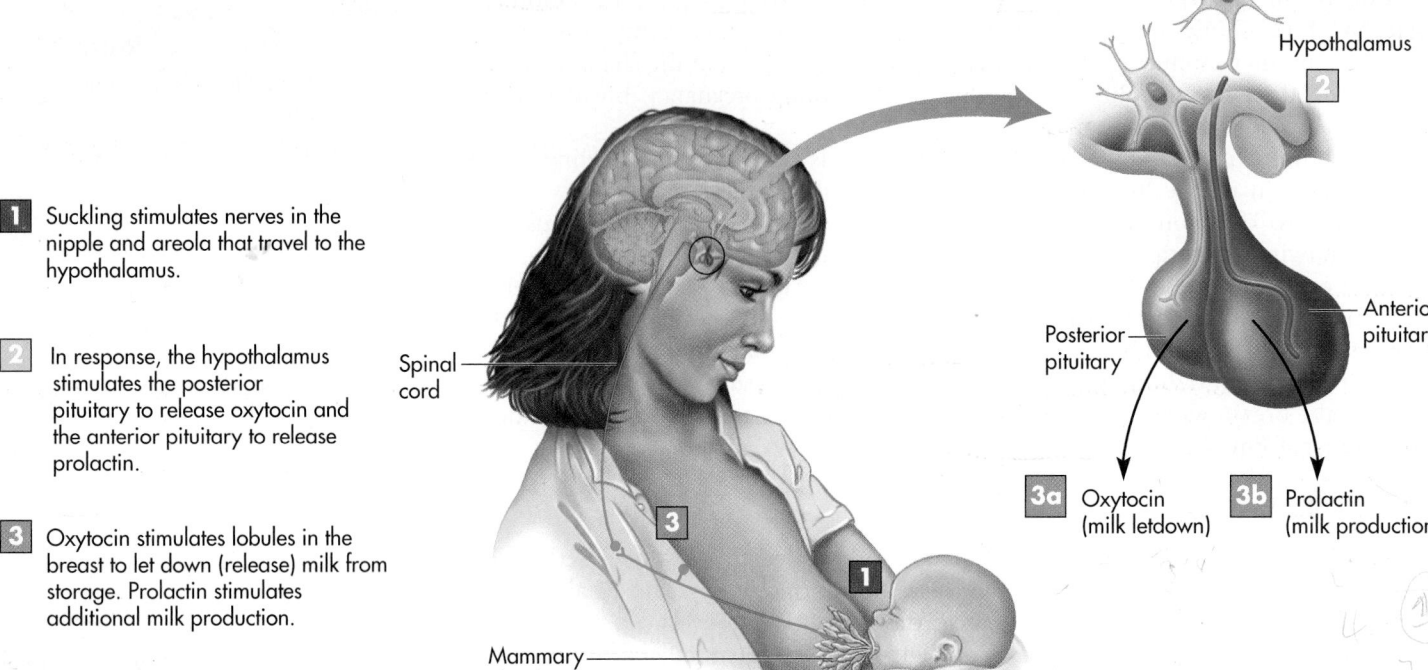

1 Suckling stimulates nerves in the nipple and areola that travel to the hypothalamus.

2 In response, the hypothalamus stimulates the posterior pituitary to release oxytocin and the anterior pituitary to release prolactin.

3 Oxytocin stimulates lobules in the breast to let down (release) milk from storage. Prolactin stimulates additional milk production.

FIGURE 14-8 ▶ Let-down reflex. Suckling sets into motion the sequence of events that lead to milk let-down, the flow of milk into ducts of the breast.

Disposable diapers can absorb so much urine that it is difficult to judge when they are wet. A strip of paper towel laid inside a disposable diaper makes a good wetness indicator. Alternatively, cloth diapers may be used for a day or two to assess whether nursing is supplying sufficient milk.

After a few weeks, the let-down reflex becomes automatic. The mother's response can be triggered just by thinking about her infant or seeing or hearing another one cry. At first, however, the process can be a bit bewildering. A mother cannot measure the amount of milk the infant takes in, so she may fear that she is not adequately nourishing the infant.

As a general rule, a well-nourished breastfed infant should (1) have three to five wet diapers per day by 3 to 5 days of age and four to six wet diapers per day thereafter, (2) show a normal weight gain, and (3) pass at least one or two stools per day that look like lumpy mustard. In addition, softening of the breast during the feeding helps indicate that enough milk is being consumed. Parents who sense their infant is not consuming enough milk should consult a physician immediately because dehydration can develop rapidly. Losing more than 7% of birth weight is an indicator of a feeding problem that requires intervention.

It generally takes 2 to 3 weeks to fully establish the feeding routine: Infant and mother both feel comfortable, the milk supply meets infant demand, and initial nipple soreness disappears. Establishing the breastfeeding routine requires patience, but the rewards are great. The adjustments are easier if supplemental formula feedings are not introduced until breastfeeding is well established, after at least 3 to 4 weeks. Then it is fine if a supplemental bottle or two of infant formula per day is needed, but supplemental feedings will decrease milk production.

Nutritional Qualities of Human Milk

Human milk is different in composition from cow's milk. Unless altered, cow's milk should never be used in infant feeding until the infant is at least 12 months old. Cow's milk is too high in minerals and protein and does not contain enough carbohydrate to meet infant needs. In addition, the major protein in cow's milk is harder for an infant to digest than the major proteins in human milk. The proteins in cow's milk also may spur allergies in the infant. Finally, certain compounds in human milk presently under study show other possible benefits for the infant.

Colostrum. At the end of pregnancy, the first fluid made by the human breast is **colostrum.** This thick, yellowish fluid may leak from the breast during late pregnancy and is produced in earnest for a few days to a week after birth. Colostrum contains antibodies and immune system cells, some of which pass unaltered through the infant's immature GI tract into the bloodstream. The first few months of life are the only time when we can readily absorb whole proteins across the GI tract. These immune factors and cells protect the infant from some GI tract diseases and other infectious disorders, compensating for the infant's immature immune system during the first few months of life.

One component of colostrum, the *Lactobacillus bifidus* **factor,** encourages the growth of *Lactobacillus bifidus* bacteria. These bacteria limit the growth of potentially toxic bacteria in the intestine. Overall, breastfeeding promotes the intestinal health of the breastfed infant in this way.

Mature Milk. Human milk composition gradually changes until it achieves the normal composition of mature milk several days after delivery. Human milk looks very different from cow's milk. (Table 15-1 in Chapter 15 provides a direct comparison.) Human milk is thin and almost watery in appearance and often has a slightly bluish tinge. Its nutritional qualities, however, are impressive.

Human milk's proteins form a soft, light curd in the infant's stomach and are easy to digest. Some human milk proteins bind iron, reducing the growth of iron-requiring bacteria, some of which can cause diarrhea. Still other proteins offer the important immune protection already noted.

The lipids in human breast milk are high in linoleic acid and cholesterol, needed for brain development. Breast milk also contains long-chain omega-3 fatty acids, such as docosahexaenoic acid (DHA). This polyunsaturated fatty acid is used for the synthesis of tissues in the brain and the rest of the central nervous system and in the retina of the eye.

The fat composition of human milk changes during each feeding. The consistency of milk released initially (fore milk) resembles that of skim milk. It later has a greater fat proportion, similar to whole milk. Finally, the milk released after 10 to 20 minutes (hind milk) is essentially like cream. Babies need to nurse long enough (e.g., a total of 20 or more minutes) to get the calories in the rich hind milk to be satisfied between feedings and to grow well. The overall calorie content of human milk is about the same as that of infant formulas (67 kcal per 100 milliliters).

Human milk composition also allows for adequate fluid status of the infant, provided the baby is exclusively breastfed. A question commonly asked is whether the infant needs additional water if stressed by hot weather, diarrhea, vomiting, or fever. The AAP recommends against supplemental water or juice during the first 6 months of life. The practice may unnecessarily introduce pathogens or allergens. Excessive water can lead to brain disorders, low blood sodium, and other problems. Thus, supplemental water and juice should be given only with a physician's guidance before 6 months of age.

Food Plan for Women Who Breastfeed

Nutrient needs for a breastfeeding mother change to some extent from those of the pregnant woman in the second and third trimester (see the inside cover of this book). There is a decrease in folate and iron needs and an increase in the needs for calories, vitamins A, E, and C, riboflavin, copper, chromium, iodide, manganese, selenium, and zinc. Still, these increased needs of the breastfeeding mother will be met by the general diet plan proposed for a woman in the latter stages of pregnancy. Recall that each day of this diet plan includes at least:

- 3 cups of calcium-rich foods such as from the dairy group or use of calcium-fortified foods to make up for any gap between calcium intake and need
- 6 ½ ounce-equivalents from the protein group
- 3 ½ cups from the vegetables group

colostrum The first fluid secreted by the breast during late pregnancy and the first few days after birth. This thick fluid is rich in immune factors and protein.

Lactobacillus bifidus **factor** A protective factor secreted in the colostrum that encourages growth of beneficial bacteria in the newborn's intestines.

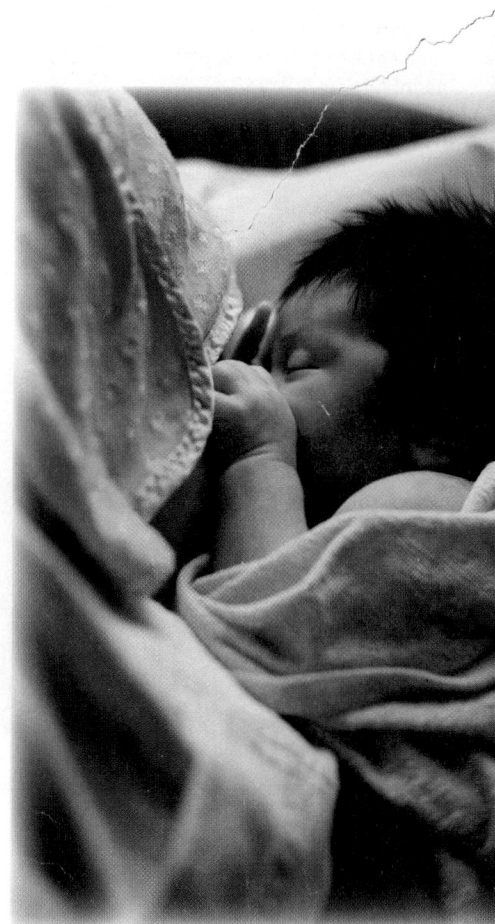

▲ Breastfeeding promotes the intestinal health of the breastfed infant.

Most substances that the mother ingests are secreted into her milk. For this reason, she should limit intake of or avoid all alcohol and caffeine and check all medications with a pediatrician. Some mothers believe that certain foods, such as garlic and chocolate, flavor the breast milk and upset the infant. If a woman notices a connection between a food she eats and the infant's later fussiness, she could consider avoiding that food. However, she might experiment again with it later, as infants become fussy for other reasons. Some researchers, on the other hand, feel that the passage of flavors from the mother's diet into her milk affords an opportunity for the infant to learn about the flavor of the foods of its family long before solids are introduced. These researchers suspect that bottle-fed infants are missing significant sensory experiences that, until recent times in human history, were common to all infants.

- 2 cups from the fruits group
- 9 ounce-equivalents from the grains group
- 8 teaspoons of vegetable oil

Foods containing solid fats and added sugars (up to about 360 kcal) can then be added to allow for weight maintenance or gradual weight loss, whichever is needed.

Table 14-4 provided a menu for such a plan. Substituting a soyburger (veggie burger) for the hamburger in that menu would make this a practical guide for a lacto-vegetarian woman as well.

As in pregnancy, a serving of a highly fortified ready-to-eat breakfast cereal (or use of a balanced multivitamin and mineral supplement) is advised to help meet extra nutrient needs. And, as mentioned for pregnant women, breastfeeding mothers should consume fish at least twice a week (or 1 gram per day of omega-3 fatty acids from a fish oil supplement) because the omega-3 fatty acids present in fish are secreted into breast milk and are likely to be important for development of the infant's nervous system.

Milk production requires approximately 800 kcal every day. The Estimated Energy Requirement during lactation is an extra 400 to 500 kcal daily above prepregnancy recommendations. The difference between that needed for milk production and the recommended intake—about 300 kcal—should allow a gradual loss of the extra body fat accumulated during pregnancy, especially if breastfeeding is continued for 6 months or more and the woman performs some physical activity. This shows just one of the natural benefits of following pregnancy with at least several months of breastfeeding.

After giving birth, women are often eager to shed the excess "baby fat." Breastfeeding, however, is no time for crash diets. A gradual weight loss of 1 to 4 pounds per month by the nursing mother is appropriate. At significantly greater rates of weight loss—when calories are restricted to less than about 1500 kcal per day—milk output decreases. A reasonable approach for a breastfeeding mother is to eat a balanced diet that supplies at least 1800 kcal per day; has moderate fat content; and includes a variety of dairy products, fruits, vegetables, and whole grains.

To promote the best possible feeding experience for the infant, there are several other dietary factors to consider. Hydration is especially important during breastfeeding; the woman should drink fluids every time her infant nurses. Drinking about 13 cups of fluids per day encourages ample milk production. Poor health habits, such as smoking cigarettes or drinking more than two alcoholic drinks a day, can decrease milk output. (Even less alcohol can have a deleterious effect on milk output in some women.) To avoid exposure to harmful levels of mercury, precautions concerning fish likely to contain mercury should extend past pregnancy for the breastfeeding mother. There is no evidence that maternal diet restrictions (e.g., peanuts, eggs, fish) during pregnancy or breastfeeding prevent food allergies in their infants. The AAP recommends exclusive breastfeeding and delaying introduction of solid foods until 4 to 6 months of age as the best approaches for preventing **atopic diseases** (see Further Reading 9).

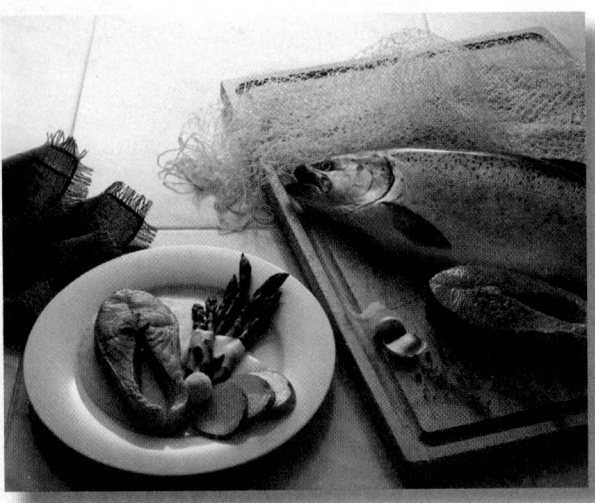

▲ Eating fish at least twice a week will help breastfeeding women ensure that their infants receive important omega-3 fatty acids. It is important, however, to avoid those fish likely to be contaminated with mercury (swordfish, shark, king mackerel, and tile fish).

atopic disease Condition resulting from an inappropriate immune response, such as asthma, allergic rhinitis, food allergies, or eczema.

CONCEPT CHECK

Recognition of the importance of breastfeeding has contributed to its greater popularity. Almost all women have the ability to breastfeed. The hormone prolactin stimulates breast tissue to synthesize milk. Infant suckling triggers a let-down reflex, which releases the milk. The more an infant nurses, the more milk is synthesized. Some components of human milk come directly from the mother's bloodstream. The nutrient composition of human milk is different from that of cow's milk and changes as the infant matures. The first fluid produced, colostrum, is rich in immune factors. The mother's diet during breastfeeding is generally similar to that for pregnancy, except for necessary additional fluids.

Breastfeeding Today

As noted, the vast majority of women are capable of breastfeeding and their infants benefit from it (see Table 14-5 and Further Reading 18). Nonetheless, some circumstances may make breastfeeding impractical or undesirable for a woman. Mothers who don't want to breastfeed their infants should not feel pressured to do so. Breastfeeding provides advantages, but none so great that a woman who decides to bottle feed should feel she is compromising her infant's well being.

Advantages of Breastfeeding. Human milk is tailored to meet infant nutrient needs for the first 4 to 6 months of life. However, there are some cases when infant dietary supplements, used under a pediatrician's guidance, are recommended:

- The AAP recommends all infants, including exclusively breastfed infants, be given 400 IU of vitamin D per day, beginning shortly after birth and continuing until the infant consumes that much from food (e.g., at least 2 cups (0.5 liters) of infant formula per day). Some sun exposure also helps in meeting vitamin D needs.
- Iron supplements are generally necessary for infants who were preterm, LBW, have blood disorders, or who were born with low iron stores.
- The AAP does not advise fluoride supplements before 6 months of age. After 6 months, the pediatrician or dentist may recommend supplemental fluoride if the infant's intake of fluoridated water, food sources, and use of toothpaste is insufficient.
- Vitamin B-12 supplements are recommended for the breastfed infant whose mother is a complete vegetarian (vegan).

Fewer Infections. Due in part to the antibodies in human milk, breastfeeding reduces the infant's overall risk of developing infections (see Further Reading 7). Breastfed

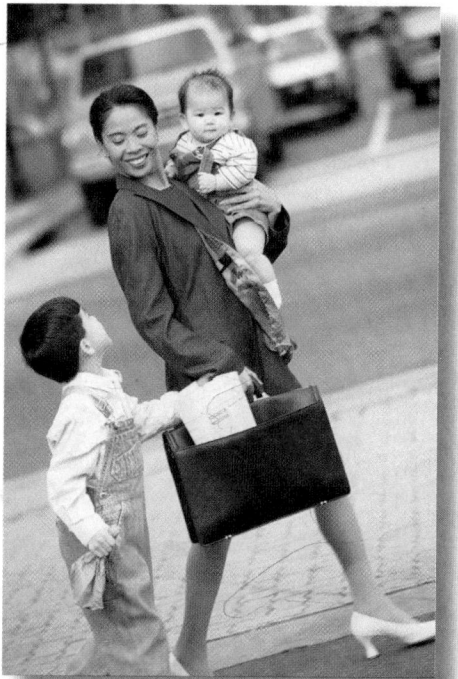

▲ Mothers who return to work outside the home can continue to breastfeed with the aid of a breastpump. In 2010, President Obama signed an amendment to the Fair Labor Standards Act that requires most U.S. employers to allow break time and a private setting for breastfeeding mothers to express milk.

TABLE 14-5 Advantages of Breastfeeding

For Infant
• Bacteriologically safe
• Always fresh and ready to go
• Provides antibodies and substances that contribute to maturation of the immune system
• Contributes to maturation of gastrointestinal tract via *Lactobacillus bifidus* factor; decreases incidence of diarrhea and respiratory disease
• Reduces risk of food allergies and intolerances, as well as some other allergies
• Establishes habit of eating in moderation, linked to 20% lower risk of obesity later in life
• Contributes to proper development of jaws and teeth for better speech development
• Decreases ear infections
• May enhance nervous system development (by providing DHA) and eventual learning ability
• May reduce the risk of chronic diseases (e.g., hypertension and diabetes)

For Mother
• Contributes to earlier recovery from pregnancy due to the action of hormones that promote a quicker return of the uterus to its prepregnancy state
• Decreases the risk of ovarian and premenopausal breast cancer
• Potential for quicker return to prepregnancy weight
• Potential for delayed ovulation, thus reducing chances of pregnancy in the short term

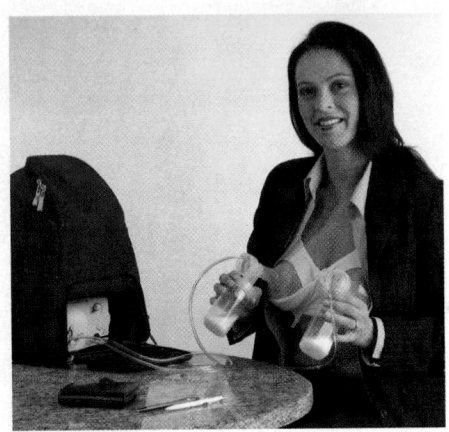

▲ Breast milk can be expressed by the mother using a manual, battery-operated, or electric (shown) breast pump. The expressed milk can be stored for times when the mother is not available to breastfeed the infant.

Useful breastfeeding resources on the Web:

www.lalecheleague.org

www.breastfeeding.com

www.breastfeeding.org

nal.usda.gov/wicworks

www.cdc.gov/breastfeeding

www.usbreastfeeding.org

www.breastfeedinginc.ca

Nipple piercings should have no impact on a woman's ability to breastfeed, but the jewelry should be removed before each feeding. Repeated removal and reinsertion of the jewelry may be inconvenient and irritating, so it may be best to leave the jewelry out for the entire period of breastfeeding. Breast tattoos will not impair breastfeeding, either. However, getting a new nipple piercing or breast tattoo while breastfeeding is not advised due to the pain of healing and possibility of infection. Past breast augmentation or reduction surgeries may impair a woman's ability to breastfeed if milk-producing tissue was damaged during the surgery.

infants also have fewer ear infections (otitis media) because they do not sleep with a bottle in their mouths. Experts strongly discourage allowing any infants to sleep with a bottle in their mouths; milk can pool in the mouth, throat, and inner ear, creating a growth medium for bacteria. By reducing these common infections parents can decrease discomfort for the infant, avoid related trips to the doctor, and prevent possible hearing loss. Tooth decay from nighttime bottles is another likely consequence of sleeping with a bottle in the mouth (see Chapter 15).

Fewer Allergies and Intolerances. Breastfeeding also reduces the chances of some allergies, especially in allergy-prone infants (see Chapter 15). The key time to attain this benefit from breastfeeding is during the first 4 to 6 months of an infant's life. A longer commitment is best, but breastfeeding for even a few weeks is beneficial. Infants are also better able to tolerate human milk than formulas. Formulas sometimes must be switched several times until caregivers find the best one for the infant.

Convenience and Cost. Breastfeeding frees the mother from the time and expense involved in buying and preparing formula and washing bottles. Human milk is ready to go and sterile. This allows the mother to spend more time with her baby.

Possible Barriers to Breastfeeding. Widespread misinformation, the mother's need to return to a job, and social reticence serve as barriers to breastfeeding.

Misinformation. The major barriers to breastfeeding are misinformation, such as the idea that one's breasts are too small, and the lack of role models. One positive note has been the widespread increase in the availability of lactation consultants over the past several years. First-time mothers who are interested in breastfeeding can find invaluable support from lactation consultants or by talking to women who have experienced it successfully. In almost every community, a group called La Leche League offers classes in breastfeeding and advises women who have problems with it (800-LALECHE or www.lalecheleague.org). Online resources are listed in the margin.

Return to an Outside Job. Working outside the home can complicate plans to breastfeed. One possibility after a month or two of breastfeeding is for the mother to express and save her own milk. She can use a breast pump or manually express milk into a sterile plastic bottle or nursing bag (used in a disposable bottle system). Saving human milk requires careful sanitation and rapid chilling. It can be stored in the refrigerator for 3 to 5 days or be frozen for 3 to 6 months. Thawed milk should be used within 24 hours. There is a knack to learning how to express milk, but the freedom can be worth it, because it allows others to feed the infant the mother's milk. A schedule of expressing milk and using supplemental formula feedings is most successful if begun after 1 to 2 months of exclusive breastfeeding. After 1 month or so, the baby is well adapted to breastfeeding and probably feels enough emotional security and other benefits from nursing to drink both ways.

Some women can juggle both a job and breastfeeding, but others find it too cumbersome and decide to formula-feed. A compromise—balancing some breastfeedings, perhaps early morning and night, with infant formula feedings during the day—is possible. However, too many supplemental infant formula feedings decrease milk production.

Social Concerns. Another barrier for some women is embarrassment about nursing a child in public. Historically, our society has stressed modesty and has discouraged public displays of breasts—even for as good a cause as nourishing babies. In the United States, no state or territory has a law prohibiting breastfeeding. However, indecent exposure (including the exposure of women's breasts) has long been a common law or statutory offense. Now, 45 states, the District of Columbia, and the Virgin Islands have specific laws that protect a woman's right to breastfeed in any location. Women who feel reluctant should be reassured that they do have social support and that breastfeeding can be done discreetly with little breast exposure.

Medical Conditions Precluding Breastfeeding. Breastfeeding may be ruled out by certain medical conditions in either the infant or mother. For example, breastfeeding is contraindicated for infants with galactosemia, an inherited disorder in which the body cannot break down galactose. Recall from Chapter 4 that lactose, the main carbohydrate in human breast milk, is made of glucose and galactose. When galactose is not properly broken down, its by-products can damage body organs.

Certain medications, which pass into the milk and adversely affect the nursing infant, are best avoided while breastfeeding. In addition, a woman in North America or other developed region of the world who has a serious chronic disease (such as tuberculosis, AIDS, or HIV-positive status) or who is being treated with chemotherapy medications should not breastfeed.

Environmental Contaminants in Human Milk. There is some legitimate concern over the levels of various environmental contaminants in human milk. However, the benefits of human milk are well established and the risks from environmental contaminants are still largely theoretical. Thus, it is probably best to continue with what has been shown to work until sufficiently strong research data contradict it. A few measures a woman could take to counteract some known contaminants are to (1) consume a variety of foods within each food group; (2) avoid freshwater fish from polluted waters; (3) carefully wash and peel fruits and vegetables; and (4) remove the fatty edges of meat, as pesticides concentrate in fat. In addition, a woman should not try to lose weight rapidly while nursing (more than ¾ to 1 pound per week) because contaminants stored in her fat tissue might then enter her bloodstream and affect her milk. If a woman questions whether her milk is safe, especially if she has lived in an area known to have a high concentration of toxic wastes or environmental pollutants, she should consult her local health department.

Phenylketonuria (PKU), a disorder of phenylalanine metabolism described in Chapter 6, was once thought to be a contraindication for breastfeeding. However, with complementary use of specialized phenylalanine-free formulas, infants with PKU can now enjoy the health and emotional benefits of breastfeeding.

MAKING DECISIONS

Breast Milk for Preterm Infants

There is no universal answer to whether a woman can breastfeed a preterm infant. In some cases, human milk is the most desirable form of nourishment, depending on infant weight and length of gestation. If so, it must usually be expressed from the breast and fed through a tube until the infant's sucking and swallowing reflex develops. This type of feeding demands great maternal dedication. Fortification of the milk with such nutrients as calcium, phosphorus, sodium, and protein is often necessary to meet the needs of a rapidly growing preterm infant. In other cases, special feeding problems may prevent the use of human milk or necessitate supplementing it with specialized formula. Sometimes total parenteral nutrition (intravenous feeding) is the only option. Working as a team, the pediatrician, neonatal nurses, and registered dietitian must guide the parents in this decision.

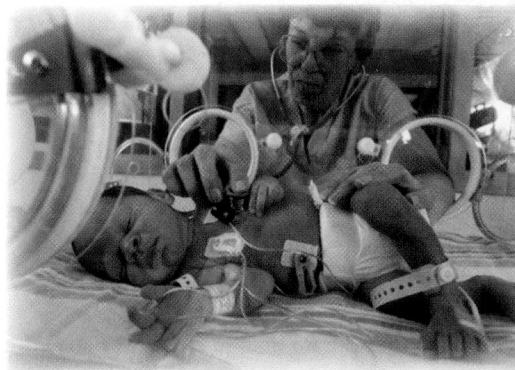

▲ If human milk is used to feed the preterm infant, fortification of the milk with certain nutrients is often needed.

CONCEPT CHECK

Human milk supplies most of an infant's nutritional needs for the first 6 months, although supplementation with vitamin D, iron, and fluoride may be needed. Breastfeeding is often more convenient than formula feeding. Compared with formula-fed infants, breastfed infants have fewer intestinal, respiratory, and ear infections and are less susceptible to some allergies and food intolerances. Despite the advantages of breastfeeding, misinformation, job responsibilities, and social reticence may dissuade a mother from breastfeeding. A combination of breastfeeding and formula feeding is possible when a mother is regularly away from the infant and is not able to express and store her milk for later use. Breastfeeding is not desirable if a mother has certain diseases or must take medication potentially harmful to the infant. The preterm infant, depending on its condition, may benefit from consuming human milk.

Preventing Birth Defects

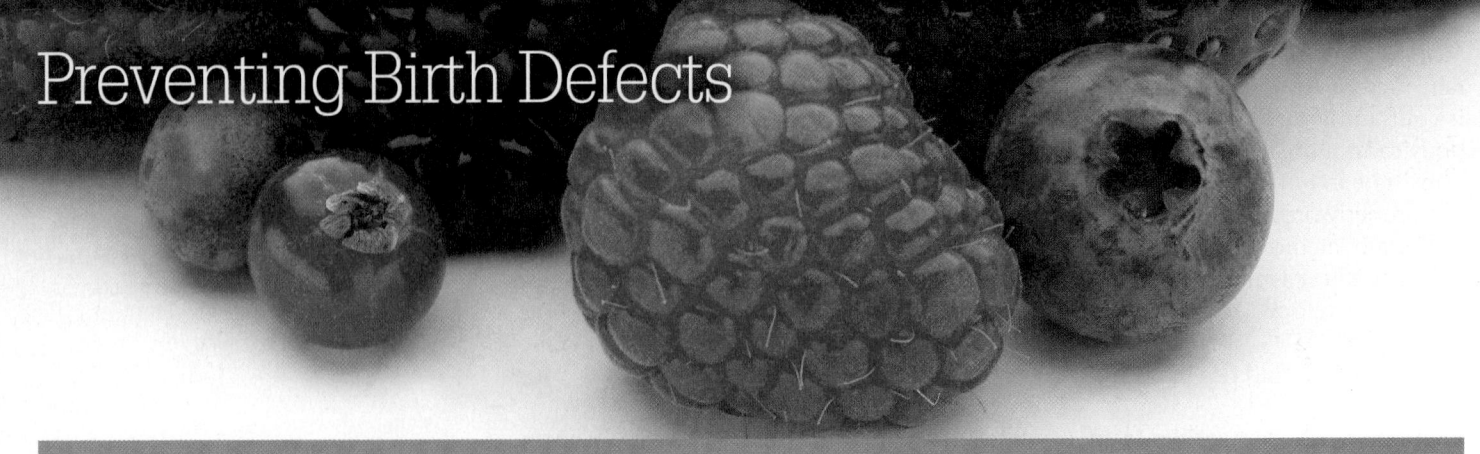

Eating well for a healthy pregnancy not only supplies materials for fetal growth and development, but also helps to direct the amazing process of building a new life. Considering the complexity of the human body and its more than 20,000 genes, it's not surprising that abnormalities of structure, function, or metabolism are sometimes present at birth. Birth defects impact one of every 33 babies born in the United States. In some cases, they are so severe that a baby cannot survive or thrive. Birth defects are the presumed cause of many spontaneous abortions and are at the root of about 20% of infant deaths before one year of age. However, with medical intervention, many babies with birth defects can go on to live healthy and productive lives.

A wide range of physical or mental disabilities result from birth defects. Heart defects are present in approximately 1 of every 100 to 200 newborn babies, accounting for a large proportion of infant deaths. Cleft lip and/or cleft palate are malformations of the lip or roof of the mouth and occur in approximately 1 in 700 to 1000 births. Neural tube defects are malformations of the brain or spinal cord that occur in early stages of pregnancy, during embryonic development. Examples include spina bifida, in which all or part of the spinal cord is exposed, and anencephaly, in which some or all of the brain is missing. Babies born with spina bifida can survive to adulthood, but in many cases, have extreme disabilities. Babies born with anencephaly die soon after birth. Neural tube defects occur in 1 in 1000 births. Down syndrome, a condition in which an extra chromosome

leads to mental retardation and other physical alterations, occurs in about 1 in 800 births. Other common birth defects include musculoskeletal defects, gastrointestinal defects, and metabolic disorders.

What causes a birth defect? About 15%–25% of birth defects are known to be genetic (i.e., inherited or spontaneous mutations of the genetic code). Another 10% are due to environmental influences (e.g., exposure to **teratogens**). The specific cause of the remaining 65%–75% of birth defects is unknown. Although the etiology of birth defects is multifactorial and many elements are beyond human control, good nutrition practices are an important way a mother-to-be can have a positive influence on the outcome of her pregnancy.

Folic Acid

During the 1980s, researchers in the United Kingdom noticed a relationship between poor dietary habits and a high rate of neural tube defects among children of impoverished women. Subsequent intervention studies demonstrated that administration of a multivitamin supplement during the periconceptional period—the months before conception and during early pregnancy—reduced the recurrence of these birth defects. The specific link between dietary folic acid and neural tube defects was tested and confirmed in several follow-up studies. As you learned in Chapter 8, folate plays a leading role in the synthesis of DNA and the metabolism of amino acids. The rapid cell growth of pregnancy increases needs for folate during pregnancy to 600 micrograms DFE per day. Some women, for genetic reasons,

may have an even higher requirement. Adequate folic acid in the periconceptional period decreases the risk of neural tube defects by about 70% and has also been associated with decreased risk of cleft lip/palate, heart defects, and Down syndrome.

In 1998, the FDA mandated fortification of grain products to provide 140 micrograms of folic acid per 100 grams of grain consumed. In Canada, the level of fortification is 150 micrograms of folate per 100 grams of grain consumed. In general, this increases the average consumption of dietary folic acid by 100 micrograms per day.

A well-planned diet can meet the RDA for folic acid, but the U.S. Public Health Service and the March of Dimes recommend that all women of childbearing age take a daily multivitamin and mineral supplement that contains 400 micrograms of folic acid. A physician may recommend prenatal vitamins or a higher dose of folic acid for some women, particularly those who have had a prior pregnancy complicated by a neural tube defect. The Dietary Guidelines for Americans recommend that women who may become pregnant and those in the first few months of pregnancy consume an adequate amount of the synthetic form of folate, folic acid (Table 14-3).

teratogen A substance that may cause or increase the risk of a birth defect. Exposure to a teratogen does not always lead to a birth defect; its effects on the fetus depend on the dose, timing, and duration of exposure.

Iodide

The relationship between folic acid and neural tube defects is a dramatic example of how a nutrient deficiency can negatively impact pregnancy outcome, but it is not the only nutrient of concern. Low iodide status during the first trimester of pregnancy—a critical period of brain development—may lead to cretinism (see Further Reading 20). This is a congenital form of hypothyroidism that leads to diminished physical and mental development if left untreated. When the defect is identified early (by newborn screening tests), cretinism can be prevented by treatment with thyroid hormones. With use of iodized salt, however, iodide deficiencies are rare.

Antioxidants

A case can be made for antioxidants in the prevention of birth defects as well. Free radicals are constantly generated within the body as a result of normal metabolic processes. An abundance of free radicals results in damage of cells and their DNA, which can lead to gene mutations or tissue malformations. Some research points to free radicals as a source of damage during embryo development and organogenesis. Antioxidant systems within the body act to minimize the damage caused by free radicals, and researchers hypothesize that dietary sources of antioxidants may aid in the prevention of birth defects. At this time, there is insufficient evidence to support supplementation of individual nutrients that participate in antioxidant systems—vitamin E, vitamin C, selenium, zinc, and copper—for the prevention of birth defects. However, use of a balanced multivitamin and mineral supplement while consuming a diet rich in whole grains, legumes, and a variety of fruits and vegetables will provide enough of these nutrients to meet current recommendations.

Vitamin A

Whereas the needs for most vitamins and minerals increase by about 30% during pregnancy, the requirement for vitamin A increases by only 10%. Studies have shown the teratogenic potential of vitamin A in doses as low as approximately 3000 micrograms RAE per day. This is just over three times the RDA of 770 micrograms RAE/per day for pregnant adult women.

Fetal abnormalities resulting from vitamin A toxicity primarily include facial and cardiac defects, but a wide range of defects have been reported. It is rare that food sources of vitamin A would lead to toxicity. Recall from Chapter 8 that preformed vitamin A is found in liver, fish, fish oils, fortified milk and yogurt, and eggs. Carotenoids, found in fruits and vegetables, are precursors of vitamin A that are converted to vitamin A in the small intestine. However, the efficiency of absorption of carotenoids decreases as intake increases. Vitamin A excesses typically arise from high-dose dietary supplements rather than food sources. Typical North American diets supply adequate vitamin A from foods, so supplemental use is not generally necessary. During pregnancy, supplemental preformed vitamin A should not exceed 3000 micrograms RAE per day (15,000 IU per day). Most multivitamins and prenatal vitamins supply less than 1500 micrograms RAE per day. A balanced diet and prudent use of dietary supplements are actions that can sidestep potential problems with vitamin A toxicity.

Caffeine

Caffeine has been scrutinized for its safety during pregnancy, especially for any link with rate of birth defects. Caffeine decreases the mother's absorption of iron and may reduce blood flow through the placenta. In addition, the fetus is unable to detoxify caffeine. Research shows that as caffeine intake increases, so does the risk of miscarriage or delivering an LBW infant. Heavy caffeine use during pregnancy may also lead to caffeine withdrawal symptoms in the newborn. These risks are reported with caffeine intakes in excess of 500 milligrams, or the equivalent of about 5 cups of coffee per day. Moderate use of caffeine (up to the equivalent of 3 cups of coffee per day), however, is not associated with risk for birth defects. Based on current evidence, drinking no more than three cups of coffee and no more than four cups of caffeinated soft

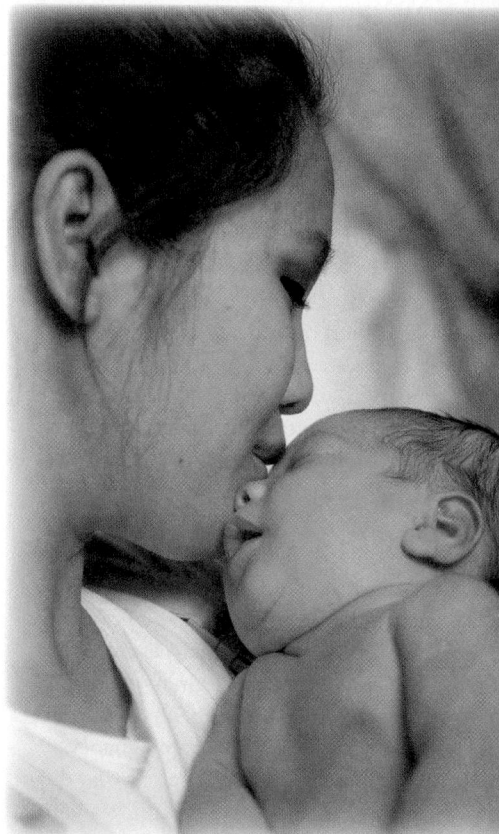

▲ Delivering a healthy baby is more than just luck. Many nutrition- and health-related practices need to be considered.

drinks per day during pregnancy (or when pregnancy is possible) is advocated. Paying attention to caffeine intake from tea, over-the-counter medicines containing caffeine, and chocolate is also important.

Aspartame

Phenylalanine, a component of the artificial sweetener aspartame (NutraSweet® and Equal®), causes concern for some pregnant women. High amounts of phenylalanine in maternal blood disrupt fetal brain development if the mother has a disease known as *phenylketonuria* (see next section). If the mother does not have this condition, however, it is unlikely that the baby will be affected by moderate aspartame use.

For most adults, diet soft drinks are the primary source of artificial sweeteners. Of greater concern than the safety of sweeteners during pregnancy is the quality of foods and beverages consumed. A high intake of diet soft drinks may crowd out healthier beverages, such as water and low-fat milk.

Obesity and Chronic Health Conditions

Even before becoming pregnant, women of childbearing age should have regular medical checkups to keep an eye on any health conditions that already exist or to identify any developing health problems. In some cases, the condition itself increases risk for birth defects. Obesity, high blood pressure, and uncontrolled diabetes are common health problems known to increase the risk for birth defects, including neural tube defects. In other cases, medications used to control illnesses may pose a risk to the developing fetus. Other health issues, such as seizure disorders and metabolic disorders, could also affect fetal development. A preconception visit with a health professional can help to sort out and make plans to minimize such risks. Once a woman has become pregnant, early and regular prenatal care can aid in the success of a pregnancy.

Women with diabetes are two to three times more likely to give birth to a baby with birth defects compared to women with normal glucose metabolism. Examples of birth defects common in this group include malformations of the spine, legs, and blood vessels of the heart. Some experts speculate that the mechanism by which diabetes increases birth defects is via excessive free radicals, which lead to oxidative damage of DNA during early gestation. Careful control of blood glucose drastically lowers risk for women with diabetes. Optimal blood glucose control can be achieved through a combination of dietary modifications and medications. Given that diabetes is on the rise among women of childbearing age, this elevated rate of birth defects has become an area of heightened awareness.

Another health condition for which maternal nutritional control is of utmost importance is PKU. Recall from Chapter 6 that PKU is an error of metabolism in which the liver lacks the ability to process phenylalanine, leading to an accumulation of this amino acid and its metabolites in body tissues. Babies born to women who have phenylketonuria that is not controlled by diet are at heightened risk for brain defects, such as microcephaly and mental retardation (see Further Reading 1).

Alcohol

Conclusive evidence shows that repeated consumption of four or more alcoholic drinks at one sitting harms the fetus (see Further Reading 12). Such binge drinking is especially perilous during the first 12 weeks of pregnancy, as this is when critical early developmental events take place in utero. Although scientists don't know whether pregnant women must totally eliminate alcohol use to avoid risk of damage to the fetus, women are advised not to drink any alcohol during pregnancy or when there is a chance pregnancy might occur—until a safe level can be established. The embryo (and, at later stages, the fetus), has no means of detoxifying alcohol.

Women with chronic alcoholism produce children with a variety of physical and intellectual problems collectively called **fetal alcohol spectrum disorders (FASDs)**. The most severe of these disorders is **fetal alcohol syndrome (FAS)**. A diagnosis of FAS is based mainly on poor fetal and infant growth, physical deformities (especially of facial features), and mental retardation (Fig. 14-9). Irritability, hyperactivity, short attention span, and limited hand-eye coordination are other symptoms of FAS. Defects in vision, hearing, and mental processing may also develop over time. Other FASDs consist of some but not all of the defects of FAS. **Alcohol-related neurodevelopmental disorders (ARNDs)** include behavior and learning problems resulting from exposure to alcohol in utero. **Alcohol-related birth defects (ARBDs)** typically include malformations of the heart, kidneys, bones, and/or ears.

Exactly how alcohol causes these defects is not known. One line of research suggests that alcohol, or products produced by the metabolism of alcohol (e.g., acetaldehyde), cause faulty movement of cells in the brain during early stages of nerve cell development or block the action of certain brain neurotransmitters. In addition, inadequate nutrient intake, reduced nutrient and oxygen transfer across the placenta, cigarette smoking commonly associated with alcohol intake, drug use, and possibly other factors contribute to the overall result.

The Dietary Guidelines for Americans recommend that alcoholic beverages

not be consumed by pregnant women (Table 14-3). For more information about fetal alcohol syndrome, visit the website www.cdc.gov/ncbddd/fasd/.

Environmental Contaminants

There is little evidence to link birth defects with the amounts of pesticides, herbicides, or other contaminants in foods or public water supplies in North America. However, evaluating such a link can be methodologically difficult and many would argue that regulations concerning contaminants in the food and water supply are too permissive. Thus, it seems prudent to take measures to decrease intake of pesticides and herbicides wherever possible. For fruits and vegetables, peeling, removing outer leaves, and/or thoroughly rinsing and scrubbing with a brush under running water will remove the majority of contaminants. In animal products, pesticides and other contaminants are most likely to accumulate in fatty tissues. Therefore, removing skin, discarding drippings, and trimming visible fat will decrease exposure from meat, poultry, and fish.

For fish, mercury is of particular concern because it can harm the nervous system of the fetus. Thus, FDA warns pregnant women to avoid swordfish, shark, king mackerel, and tile fish because of possible high mercury contamination. Largemouth bass are also implicated. In general, intake of other fish and shellfish

▶ A goal of *Healthy People 2020* is 98.3% abstinence from alcohol, cigarettes, and illicit drugs by pregnant women, a 10% improvement over current statistics.

fetal alcohol spectrum disorders (FASDs) A group of irreversible physical and mental abnormalities in the infant that result from the mother's consuming alcohol during pregnancy.

fetal alcohol syndrome (FAS) Severe form of FASD that involves abnormal facial features and problems with development of the nervous system and overall growth as a result of maternal alcohol consumption during pregnancy.

should not exceed 12 ounces per week. Canned albacore tuna is a potential mercury source, so it should not be consumed in amounts exceeding 6 ounces per week. As a rule of thumb, consuming a variety of foods minimizes risk of exposure to contaminants from the food supply.

Summing Up

Although many risk factors for birth defects are beyond our control, a woman of childbearing potential can make some wise nutrition choices to improve her chances of having a healthy baby without birth defects. A varied and balanced diet, such as the food plan for pregnant women described in this chapter, along with a daily multivitamin and mineral supplement with 400 micrograms of folic acid will ensure adequate nutrient status. It is estimated that daily use of a multivitamin and mineral supplement containing folic acid will decrease the rate of all birth defects by 50%. Discuss use of any other

dietary supplements with a physician to be sure that the fetus will not be exposed to toxic levels of vitamin A or other dangerous ingredients. Early and consistent prenatal care can help control obesity and any chronic health conditions that may complicate a pregnancy. Also, avoiding alcohol during pregnancy will eliminate any risk for fetal alcohol spectrum disorders.

Although it seems that advice for a healthy pregnancy is always directed at the mother, fathers-to-be are not off the hook. Health is a family affair, so encouraging healthy eating habits and avoiding smoking and alcohol are important for fathers, too. Less research has been done in the area, but the genetics of the baby are certainly an outcome of both parents. Indeed, inadequate supplies of zinc, folate, and vitamin C affect the quality of sperm, which may impair fertility. Considering that spermatogenesis takes approximately 70 days, the periconceptional period is a time for good nutrition and careful lifestyle practices for the father as well.

▶ In North America, maternal death as a result of childbirth is uncommon—only about 11 deaths in every 100,000 live births. The infant mortality rate, however, is much higher: for each 100,000 live births, about 600 to 700 infants die within the first year. The infant death rate among African-Americans is more than double the rates among Whites and Hispanics in the United States.

▶ Pregnant women should recognize that many cough syrups contain alcohol. Cases have been reported of infants with FASDs born to mothers who consumed generous amounts of such cough syrups but no other alcoholic beverages.

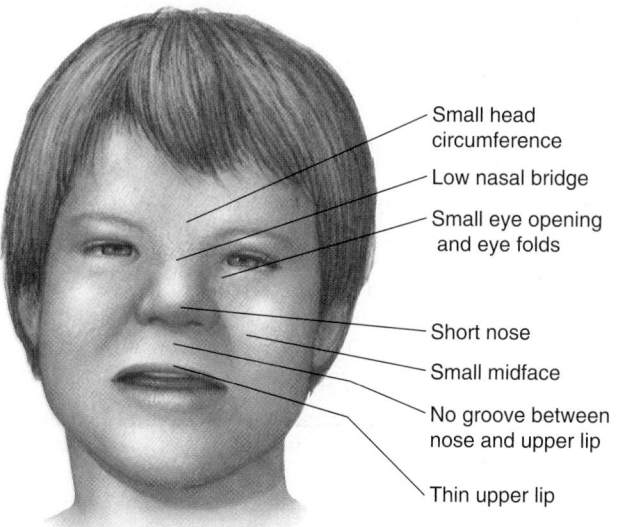

Small head circumference

Low nasal bridge

Small eye opening and eye folds

Short nose

Small midface

No groove between nose and upper lip

Thin upper lip

FIGURE 14-9 ▶ Fetal alcohol syndrome. The facial features shown are typical of affected children. Additional abnormalities in the brain and other internal organs accompany fetal alcohol syndrome but are not immediately apparent from simply looking at the child. Milder forms of alcohol-induced changes from a lower alcohol exposure to the fetus are known as alcohol-related neurodevelopmental disorders (ARNDs) and alcohol-related birth defects (ARBDs).

Case Study Preparing for Pregnancy

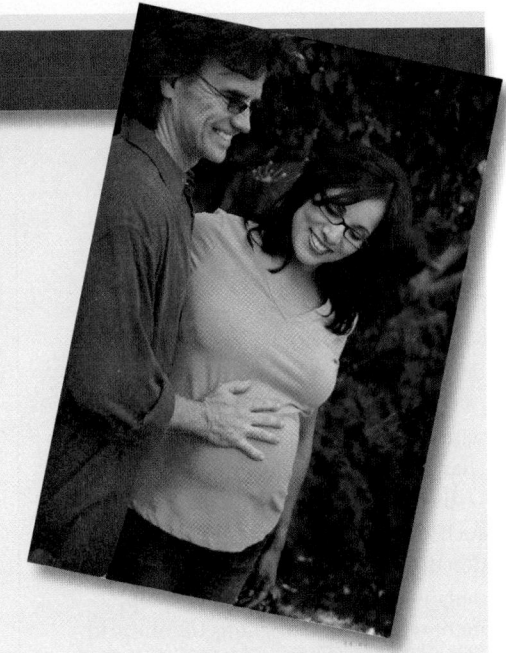

Lily and her husband have decided that they are ready to prepare for Lily's first pregnancy. She is 25 years old, weighs 135 pounds, and is 67 inches tall. Lily has been reading everything she can find on pregnancy because she knows that her prepregnancy health is important to the success of her pregnancy.

She knows she should avoid alcohol, especially because alcohol is potentially toxic to the growing fetus in the first weeks of pregnancy, and she could become pregnant and not know about it right away. Lily is not a smoker, does not take any medications, and limits her coffee intake to 4 cups a day and soft drink intake to 3 colas per day. Based on her reading, she has decided to breastfeed her infant and has already inquired about childbirth classes. She has modified her diet to include some extra protein, along with more fruits and vegetables. She has also started taking an over-the-counter vitamin and mineral supplement. Lily has always kept in good shape, and

she is admittedly worried about gaining too much weight during pregnancy. Recently, she started a running program 5 days a week, and she plans to continue running throughout her pregnancy.

Answer the following questions, and check your responses in Appendix A.

1. What recommendations do you have regarding Lily's use of dietary supplements?
2. What is Lily doing to prevent neural tube defects? What else could she do?
3. What recommendations would you make regarding Lily's caffeine consumption?
4. Lily is wise to pay attention to her protein intake to prepare for pregnancy and breastfeeding. Should she include fish as a source of protein in her diet? Why or why not?
5. Constipation is a common complaint during pregnancy. What suggestions do

you have to help Lily avoid this health concern?
6. What information would you share with Lily about appropriate weight gain during pregnancy?

Summary (Numbers refer to numbered sections in the chapter.)

14.1 The best time to prepare for pregnancy is before conception even occurs. Achieving a healthy body weight, avoiding toxic agents, correcting nutritional deficiencies, and controlling existing medical conditions will set the stage for a successful pregnancy.

14.2 Pregnancy is arbitrarily divided into three trimesters of 13 to 14 weeks each. The first trimester is characterized by a rapid increase in cell number as the zygote grows to be an embryo, then a fetus. During the first trimester, the growing organism is most susceptible to damage from exposure to toxic agents or nutrient deficiencies. By the start of the second trimester, the organs and limbs have formed and will continue to grow and develop. The third trimester is marked by rapid fetal growth and storage of nutrients in preparation for life outside the womb.

14.3 A successful pregnancy results in optimal health for both the infant and

the mother. Pregnancy success is defined as (1) gestation longer than 37 weeks and (2) birth weight greater than 5.5 pounds (2.5 kilograms). Factors that predict pregnancy success include early and regular prenatal care, maternal age within the range of 20 to 35 years, and adequate nutrition. Factors that contribute to poor pregnancy outcome include inadequate prenatal care, obesity, underweight, teenage pregnancy, smoking, alcohol consumption, use of certain prescription medications and all illicit drugs, inadequate nutrition, heavy caffeine use, and various infections, such as listeriosis.

14.4 For women with a healthy prepregnancy BMI (18.5 to 24.9), total weight gain should be within the range of 25 to 35 pounds. Underweight women and those carrying multiple fetuses should gain more; overweight and obese women should gain less. During the first trimester, although she need not increase diet

quantity, the woman should focus on diet quality to meet increased requirements for protein, carbohydrate, essential fatty acids, fiber, water, and many vitamins and minerals. A woman typically needs an additional 350 to 450 kcal per day during the second and third trimesters.

14.5 Following a plan based on the Dietary Guidelines for Americans as exemplified by MyPlate is recommended for pregnant and breastfeeding women. The mother-to-be should especially emphasize good sources of vitamin B-6, folate, iron, zinc, and calcium. Vegetarian diets are safe during pregnancy, but vegan mothers should specifically seek out good sources of vitamin B-12 and vitamin D. Prenatal multivitamin and mineral supplements are useful for meeting increased nutrient requirements during pregnancy.

14.6 Pregnancy-induced hypertension, gestational diabetes, heartburn, constipation, nausea, vomiting, edema, and anemia are all possible discomforts and complications of pregnancy. Nutrition therapy can help minimize some of these problems.

14.7 Almost all women are able to breastfeed their infants. The nutritional composition of human milk is different from that of unaltered cow's milk and is much more desirable for the infant.

For the infant, the advantages of breastfeeding over formula feeding are numerous, including fewer intestinal, respiratory, and ear infections and fewer allergies and food intolerances. Benefits for the mother include reduced risk of certain cancers, earlier recovery from pregnancy, and faster return to prepregnancy weight. For mothers who choose not to breastfeed or in medical situations that contraindicate breastfeeding (e.g., galactosemia), infants can be adequately nourished with formula.

N&YH There are several steps pregnant women can take to help prevent birth defects. Achieve a healthy body weight before pregnancy and strive to gain weight within the ranges recommended by the Institute of Medicine. Adequate intakes of folic acid, iodide, and antioxidant nutrients are essential for prevention of many types of birth defects. Excesses of vitamin A and caffeine should be avoided. There is no safe level of alcohol intake known during pregnancy. Dietary control of diseases (e.g., diabetes and PKU) will also protect the fetus.

Check Your Knowledge (Answers to the following multiple choice questions are below.)

1. The fetus is most susceptible to damage from nutrient deficiencies; teratogens; and use of certain medications, alcohol, and illicit drugs during
   a. the first trimester.
   b. the second trimester.
   c. the third trimester.
   d. labor and delivery.

2. An infant born at 38 weeks' gestation weighing 5.0 pounds can be described as
   a. preterm.   c. SGA.
   b. LBW.   d. LBW and SGA.

3. If a woman is 5'2" and weighs 150 pounds before becoming pregnant, how much weight should she gain during pregnancy?
   a. 28 to 40 pounds (12.5 to 18 kilograms)
   b. 25 to 35 pounds (11.5 to 16 kilograms)
   c. 15 to 25 pounds (7 to 11.5 kilograms)
   d. As little as possible

4. Increased carbohydrate needs during pregnancy are set to
   a. prevent ketosis.
   b. alleviate nausea.
   c. prevent pregnancy-induced hypertension.
   d. supply adequate folate.

5. Which of the following is best paired with an iron supplement during pregnancy?
   a. skim milk
   b. orange juice
   c. coffee
   d. tea

6. A food plan for a woman in the third trimester of pregnancy differs from her prepregnancy diet in that
   a. fluid needs are higher.
   b. additional solid fats and added sugars are allowed.
   c. there are more servings from the grains group.
   d. All of the above.

7. Consuming one cup of coffee per day is associated with
   a. spontaneous abortions.
   b. LBW.
   c. birth defects.
   d. None of the above.

8. Which of the following may help to alleviate nausea during pregnancy?

   a. postponing meals until the afternoon
   b. drinking large amounts of water
   c. postponing use of iron supplements until the second trimester
   d. All of the above.

9. Which of the following conditions medically prevents a woman from breastfeeding her infant?
   a. breasts are too small
   b. infant has galactosemia
   c. inverted nipples
   d. None of the above.

10. Physiologically, milk production requires _____ kcals per day.
   a. 300
   b. 500
   c. 800
   d. 1000

Answer Key: 1. a (LO 14.2), 2. d (LO 14.2), 3. c (LO 14.3), 4. a (LO 14.1), 5. b (LO 14.5), 6. d (LO 14.4), 7. d (LO 14.2), 8. c (LO 14.6), 9. b (LO 14.7), 10. c (LO 14.4)

Study Questions (Numbers refer to Learning Outcomes)

1. Provide three key pieces of advice for parents seeking to maximize their chances of having a healthy infant. Why did you identify those specific factors? (LO 14.2)

2. Outline current weight-gain recommendations for pregnancy. What is the basis for these recommendations? (LO 14.3)

3. Identify four key nutrients for which intake should be significantly increased during pregnancy. (LO 14.1)

4. Describe a diet based on the Dietary Guidelines as exemplified by MyPlate that meets the increased nutrient needs of pregnancy. (LO 14.4)

5. Why does teenage pregnancy receive so much attention these days? At what age do you think pregnancy is ideal? Why? (LO 14.2)

6. Give three reasons a woman should give serious consideration to breastfeeding her infant. (LO 14.7)

7. Describe the physiological mechanisms that stimulate milk production and release. How can knowing about these help mothers breastfeed successfully? **(LO 14.7)**

8. Describe two nutrients that may require supplementation during pregnancy and give reasons for each. **(LO 14.5)**

9. How should the basic food plan suitable for pregnancy be modified during breastfeeding? **(LO 14.4)**

10. What nutrition advice would you give to a friend who suffers from morning sickness? **(LO 14.6)**

What Would You Choose Recommendations

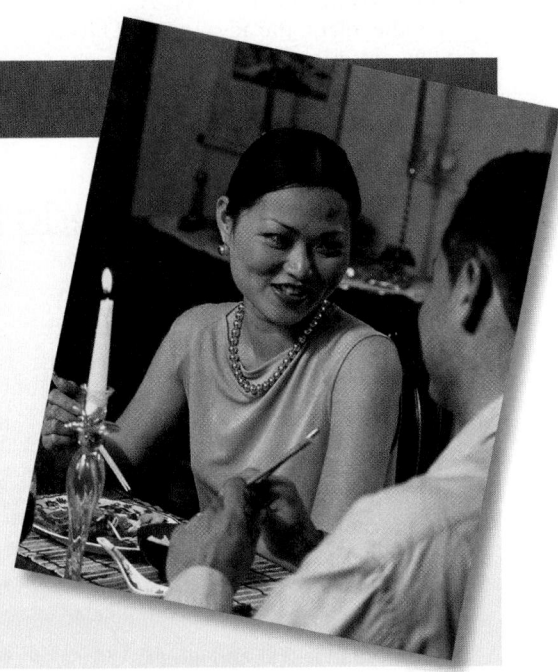

The spinach salad meal with hard-boiled egg and whole-wheat roll provides only about 2 grams of iron. It is a healthy, nutrient-dense choice that provides some protein, but does not make a significant contribution to meeting iron needs.

A hamburger is a source of iron—this meal would provide about 4.5 milligrams of iron—but it would not be a choice for a person who follows a vegetarian diet.

The bean and cheese taco option provides just as much iron (4.5 milligrams) as the hamburger meal and would be appropriate for a vegetarian.

Even though the nonheme iron in beans is not as well absorbed as the heme iron in beef, the 20 milligrams of vitamin C in the stewed tomatoes will enhance iron absorption.

All of these meals, however, pale in comparison to the iron contribution of the fortified, ready-to-eat breakfast cereal. One cup of Kellogg's Smart Start cereal provides 18 milligrams of iron, and the 72 milligrams of vitamin C in 1 cup of orange juice will enhance iron absorption. In one easy meal, any pregnant woman could obtain more than half of the 27-milligram RDA for iron during pregnancy.

Further Readings

1. AAP Committee on Genetics: Policy Statement: Maternal phenylketonuria. *Pediatrics* 122:445, 2008.

   Uncontrolled maternal phenylketonuria (PKU) leads to exposure of the fetus to elevated phenylalanine levels in the blood, which can lead to birth defects, poor physical growth, and altered brain development. All girls and women with PKU should be educated and counseled throughout life about controlling phenylalanine levels to minimize risks during pregnancy.

2. AAP Section on Breastfeeding: American Academy of Pediatrics Policy Statement: Breastfeeding and the use of human milk. *Pediatrics* 115:496, 2005.

   AAP firmly supports breastfeeding as the ideal nutrition for infants. A few contraindications to breastfeeding are discussed, such as HIV infection and galactosemia. Exclusive breastfeeding is recommended for the first 6 months of life. Breastfeeding should continue with age-appropriate introduction of complementary solid foods until 1 year of age or longer. Guidelines are provided for infant nutrient supplementation.

3. ADA Reports: Position of the American Dietetic Association: Nutrition and lifestyle for a healthy pregnancy outcome. *Journal of the American Dietetic Association* 108:553, 2008.

   The key components of a healthy lifestyle during pregnancy include appropriate weight gain; consumption of a variety of foods; appropriate and timely vitamin and mineral intake; avoidance of alcohol, tobacco, and other harmful substances; and safe food handling. Supplementation is appropriate for some nutrients.

4. James DC and others: Position of the American Dietetic Association: Promoting and supporting breastfeeding. *Journal of the American Dietetic Association* 109:1926, 2009.

   The American Dietetic Association strongly supports the breastfeeding of infants. This article discusses the benefits of breastfeeding for the mother and infant, as well as dietary considerations that need to be addressed, such as avoiding consumption of species of fish known to contain high amounts of mercury.

5. Barger MK. Maternal nutrition and perinatal outcomes. *Journal of Midwifery and Women's Health* 55:502, 2010.

   This review details the roles and requirements of various nutrients during pregnancy with an emphasis on the developmental origins of disease hypothesis. Nutritional status influences infant growth, length of gestation, and several pregnancy complications, such as gestational diabetes and preeclampsia.

6. Bodnar LM and others: Periconceptional multivitamin use reduces the risk of preeclampsia. *American Journal of Epidemiology* 164:470, 2006.

   In the Pregnancy Exposures and Preeclampsia Prevention Study, women who regularly consumed a multivitamin during the periconceptional period had a 45% lower risk of developing preeclampsia during their first pregnancy than those who did not consume multivitamins. Women with BMI less than 25 benefited most from multivitamin use.

7. Field CJ: The immunological components of human milk and their effect on immune development in infants. *Journal of Nutrition* 135:1, 2005.

   Human milk contains many factors that improve immune function in the infant. This article reviews a number of these complex factors.

8. Fraser A and others: Associations of gestational weight gain with maternal body mass index, waist circumference, and blood pressure measured 16 years after pregnancy: The Avon Longitudinal Study of Parents and Children (ALSPAC). *American Journal of Clinical Nutrition* 93:1285, 2011.

    Researchers examined long-term health effects of prepregnancy weight and gestational weight gain. Mothers with high prepregnancy BMI and gestational weight gain above recommended ranges had higher BMI, waist circumference, and blood pressure measurements 16 years after pregnancy. Of interest, even among women with normal prepregnancy weight, high rates of weight gain during midpregnancy were associated with higher blood pressure later in life. The results confirm that adherence to the 2009 IOM guidelines for prepregnancy weight and weight gain during pregnancy optimizes long-term maternal health.

9. Greer FR and others: Effects of early nutritional interventions on the development of atopic disease in infants and children: The role of maternal dietary restriction, breastfeeding, timing of introduction of complementary foods, and hydrolyzed formulas. *Pediatrics* 121:183, 2008.

    The American Academy of Pediatrics revised previous recommendations for prevention of atopic disease. Current evidence does not support a role of maternal dietary restrictions in prevention of atopic disease in children. The best course of action for at-risk infants is to breastfeed exclusively and delay introduction of solid foods until 4 to 6 months of age. Delaying introduction of complementary feedings beyond 6 months is not advantageous.

10. Han Z and others: Maternal underweight and the risk of preterm birth and low birth weight: A systematic review and meta-analysis. *International Journal of Epidemiology* 40:65, 2011.

    Despite the increasing prevalence of overweight and obesity among women of childbearing age, maternal underweight is related to higher risk of preterm birth and low birth weight.

11. Institute of Medicine and National Research Council: *Weight gain during pregnancy: Reexamining the guidelines.* Washington, DC: The National Academies Press, 2009.

    Excess maternal weight affects the health of both the fetus (size at birth, gestational age, and impact on childhood obesity) and the mother (postpartum weight retention and requirement for surgical delivery). The revised guidelines for weight gain during pregnancy recommended relatively narrow ranges based on mother's prepregnancy BMI, which was found to be an important predictor of pregnancy outcome. New guidelines for obese mothers now advise a weight gain of only 11 to 20 pounds (5 to 9 kilograms). Provisional recommendations are given for women carrying multiple fetuses.

12. Jones KL: The effects of alcohol on fetal development. *Birth Defects Research (Part C)* 93:3, 2011.

    This comprehensive review traces research on fetal alcohol spectrum disorders and describes its many physiological and neurological defects with color photos. Several maternal risk factors can increase risk for FASD, including maternal age >30 years, low socioeconomic status, previous children with FASD, genetics, and malnutrition.

13. Kelly, AKW: Practical exercise advice during pregnancy. *The Physician and Sports Medicine* 33(6):24, 2005.

    It is safe for pregnant women to exercise if they are experiencing uncomplicated pregnancies. Most non-weight-bearing exercises (e.g., swimming) and walking are safe for pregnant women. Women should begin with 15 minutes of exercise three times a week and progress as tolerated.

14. Lucas RM and others: Future health implications of prenatal and early-life vitamin D status. *Nutrition Reviews* 66:710, 2008.

    In addition to its role in bone health, preventive effects of vitamin D on autoimmune disorders, diabetes, cancer, cardiovascular disease, osteoporosis, and psychiatric illness are mediated by the vitamin's involvement in gene expression. Maternal vitamin D supplementation could lead to widespread improvements in public health.

15. Makrides M: Outcomes for mothers and their babies: Do n-3 long-chain polyunsaturated fatty acids and seafoods make a difference? *Journal of the American Dietetic Association* 108: 1622, 2008

    Omega-3 fatty acids are important for brain and eye development of the fetus and infant. These fats have been implicated in prevention of preeclampsia, preterm birth, LBW, and SGA, but current evidence does not support supplementation for these purposes. Despite the importance of n-3 fatty acids for fetal development, many women have inadequate intakes of these fats. Available data indicate that pregnant and lactating women should aim to consume at least 200 milligrams per day of omega-3 fatty acids from dietary sources, including oily fish, eggs, and lean red meats.

16. Rubin RC: Change is good—evidence to support lowering the diagnostic threshold for GDM. *Today's Dietitian* 13:10, 2011.

    Gestational diabetes may lead to macrosomia, birth injuries, and postnatal hypoglycemia for infants. For mothers, GDM increases risk of type 2 diabetes later in life. The American Diabetes Association updated its guidelines on diagnosis and treatment of GDM: high-risk women should be screened for undiagnosed type 2 diabetes at their first prenatal visit; all women should undergo a standardized 75-gram oral glucose tolerance test to screen for GDM between 24 and 28 weeks of gestation; after birth, mothers with GDM should be monitored for development of type 2 diabetes.

17. Tamura T, Picciano MF: Folate and human reproduction. *American Journal of Clinical Nutrition* 83:993, 2006.

    Folic acid supplementation for the prevention of megaloblastic anemia and neural tube defects represents a major public health advancement. Folate status may also be linked to placental abruption, preeclampsia, spontaneous abortion, stillbirth, low birth weight, and risk for birth defects other than neural tube defects.

18. Taylor JS and others: A systematic review of the literature associating breastfeeding with type 2 diabetes and gestational diabetes. *Journal of the American College of Nutrition* 24:320, 2005.

    Breastfed infants have lower rates of obesity, type 1 diabetes, and type 2 diabetes in adulthood compared to formula-fed infants. In addition, mothers who breastfeed have improved glucose tolerance and lower risk for postpartum diabetes compared to nonlactating mothers.

19. Ward EM: Prime the body for pregnancy— preconception care and nutrition for moms-to-be. *Today's Dietitian* 10:26, 2008.

    Women of childbearing potential should take steps to ensure a healthy pregnancy before becoming pregnant. The article provides practical guidelines for intakes of key nutrients (e.g., folic acid and iron), supplement use, weight management, physical activity, and caffeine and alcohol consumption.

20. Zimmerman MB: Iodine deficiency in pregnancy and the effects of maternal iodine supplementation on the offspring: A review. *American Journal of Clinical Nutrition* 89(suppl):668S, 2009.

    Iodine deficiency leads to cretinism or more subtle deficits in brain function. Recently, the World Health Organization augmented recommendations for iodine deficiency during pregnancy from 200 to 250 micrograms per day. Annual supplementation with 400 milligrams of iodine in the form of iodized oil or daily supplementation with potassium iodide are effective strategies for reducing maternal iodine deficiency and associated birth defects.

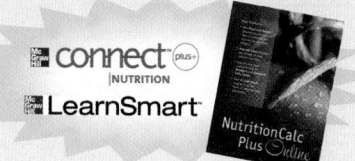

To get the most out of your study of nutrition, go to McGraw-Hill's online resources: Connect www.mcgrawhillconnect.com, where you will find NutritionCalc Plus, LearnSmart, and many other dynamic tools.

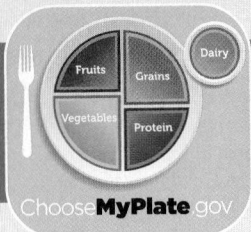

RATE YOUR PLATE

I. Targeting Nutrients Necessary for Pregnant Women

This chapter mentioned that pregnant women may have difficulty meeting their increased needs for folate, vitamin B-6, iron, and zinc. List six foods rich in each of these nutrients next to the appropriate heading. Refer to Chapters 8 and 9 if necessary.

Nutrient	Foods	Nutrient	Foods
Folate	_____	Iron	_____
	_____		_____
	_____		_____
	_____		_____
	_____		_____
	_____		_____
Vitamin B-6	_____	Zinc	_____
	_____		_____
	_____		_____
	_____		_____
	_____		_____
	_____		_____

1. Foods rich in more than one of these nutrients would be especially valuable for pregnant women. Write on the line any foods you listed that are good sources of more than one of these critical nutrients.

   _____

2. The needs for folate, vitamin B-6, iron, and zinc increase during pregnancy. For which of these nutrients can pregnant women usually obtain adequate intakes from dietary sources?

   _____

3. Which of these nutrients are commonly taken in supplement form during pregnancy?

   _____

   _____

4. Why might it be hard for pregnant women to meet their increased needs for these nutrients from food alone?

   _____

   _____

II. Putting Your Knowledge About Nutrition and Pregnancy to Work

A college friend, Angie, tells you that she is newly pregnant. You are aware that she usually likes to eat the following foods for her meals:

Breakfast

Skips this meal, or eats a granola bar
Coffee

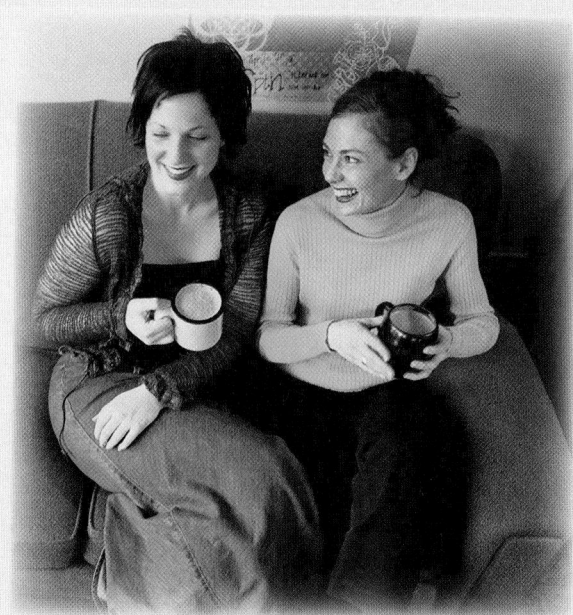

Lunch

Sweetened yogurt, 1 cup
Small bagel with cream cheese
Occasional piece of fruit
Regular caffeinated soda, 12 ounces

Snack

Chocolate candy bar

Dinner

2 slices of pizza, macaroni and cheese, or 2 eggs with 2 slices of toast
Seldom eats a salad or vegetable
Regular caffeinated soda, 12 ounces

Snacks

Pretzels or chips, 1 ounce
Regular caffeinated soda, 12 ounces

1. Using NutritionCalc Plus software, evaluate Angie's diet for protein, carbohydrate, folate, vitamin B-6, iron, and zinc. How does her intake compare with the recommended amounts for pregnancy?

   _____

   _____

   _____

2. Now redesign her diet and make sure that her intake meets pregnancy needs for protein, carbohydrate, folate, vitamin B-6, and zinc. (Hint: Fortified foods, such as breakfast cereal, are generally nutrient-rich foods, which can more easily help meet one's needs.) Increase the iron content as well, but it still may be below the RDA for pregnancy.

   _____

   _____

   _____

Chapter 15 Nutrition from Infancy Through Adolescence

Student Learning Outcomes

Chapter 15 is designed to allow you to:

15.1 Describe the extent to which nutrition affects infant and child growth and physiological development.

15.2 Identify diet guidelines to meet the basic nutritional needs for normal growth and development for an infant and discuss some do's and don'ts associated with infant feeding.

15.3 List several challenges parents might face in dealing with childhood eating habits.

15.4 List the nutrients often found to be lacking in the diets of infants, toddlers, preschoolers, and teenagers and make recommendations to remedy the problems.

15.5 Describe the long-term effects of childhood obesity and suggest ways to prevent or treat the problem.

15.6 Identify common food allergens and suggest several practices that may reduce the risk of developing a food allergy.

What Would You Choose?

Your brother and his wife have asked you to watch your 18-month-old niece, Lila, while they enjoy a weekend getaway at the lake to celebrate their anniversary. Before they drop her off, you make a trip to the grocery store to pick up some kid-friendly foods. Lila does not have any food allergies, but your brother warned you that she has gotten into some picky eating behaviors. Which of the following snack foods would you choose for your little houseguest?

a Reduced-fat popcorn

b Raw baby carrots with ranch dressing

c Fat-free light yogurt

d Whole-grain crackers with sliced cheddar cheese

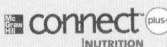 **Think about your choice as you read Chapter 15, then see our recommendations at the end of the chapter. To learn more about appropriate feeding practices for infants and preschoolers, check out the Connect site:** www.mcgrawhillconnect.com

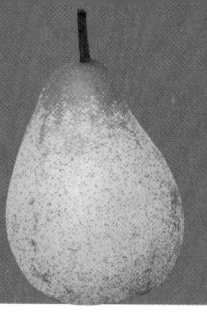

Part Five
Nutrition: A Focus
on Life Stages

From infancy through adolescence, rapid growth dictates calorie, protein, vitamin, and mineral requirements. The growth rate of infants is the highest of any life stage, so nutrient needs per pound of body weight are highest. As a child gets older, the rate of growth slows and nutrient needs per pound of body weight decrease proportionately. As the chapter comic suggests, this can lead to picky eating behaviors, which can be a source of frustration for parents and other caregivers. Nonetheless, these early years of life are an important time to establish healthful eating and exercise habits.

Influences on eating behaviors shift over time. During infancy and early childhood, the family mostly controls food intake, informs food preferences, and models eating behaviors. For school-age children and adolescents, peer and media influences take on more importance. Education designed to change the nutrition habits of children should start early and involve the family. Whenever possible, families should share meals together. Family mealtimes help children establish healthy eating habits; aid in prevention of childhood obesity; and, as children grow older, teach communication skills and improve self-esteem. Chapter 15 examines the specific nutrition issues facing each of these life stages and demonstrates how food choices should be tailored to adapt to changing needs of growing children.

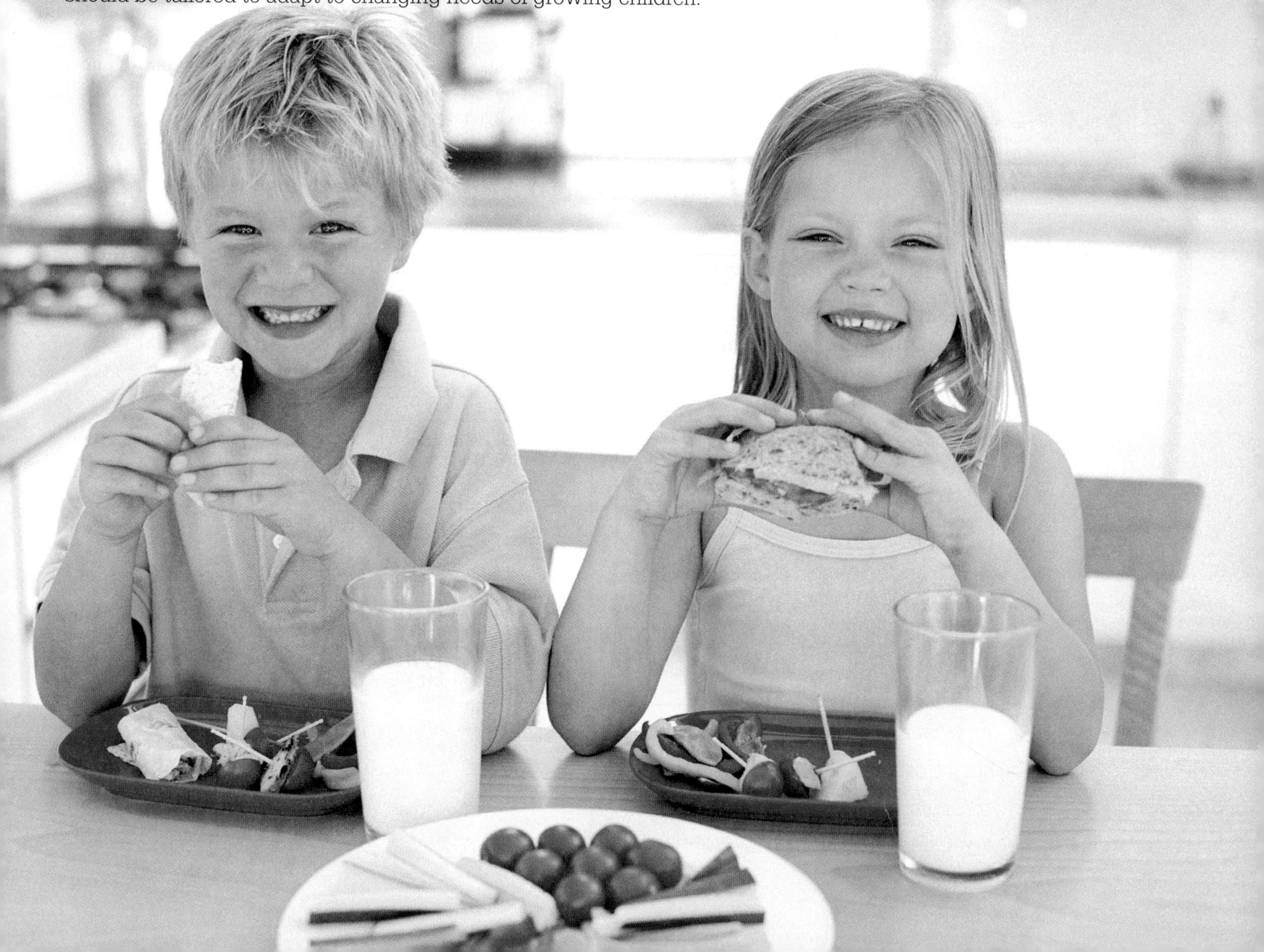

Refresh Your Memory

As you begin your study of nutrition from infancy through adolescence in Chapter 15, you may want to review:

- MyPlate and the 2010 Dietary Guidelines in Chapter 2
- The immune system in Chapter 3
- Diagnosis and treatment of type 2 diabetes in Chapter 4
- Common sources of saturated fat, cholesterol, and *trans* fat in Chapter 5
- Vegetarianism in Chapter 6

15.1 Nutrition and Child Health— an Introduction

Current statistics describing nutrition and overall health among children and adolescents in North America have shown both positive and negative trends. On a positive note, more children are receiving vaccinations than ever before and fewer teenagers are giving birth. In contrast to this good news, the number of children and teenagers with obesity and type 2 diabetes is rising, and physical activity in general is on the decline as more time is spent sitting in front of computer screens and television sets. Low calcium intakes are also receiving much attention, as soft drinks and energy drinks have replaced much of the milk that children and teenagers previously consumed on a daily basis. Fruits, vegetables, and whole grains are also often in short supply in their diets. In this chapter, we will look at these trends and their effects on nutrition and overall health of this age group.

15.2 Infant Growth and Nutrition Needs

During infancy, attitudes toward foods and the eating process begin to take shape. If parents and other caregivers practice good nutrition and are flexible, they can lead an infant into lifelong healthful food habits. A family environment that encourages healthy eating will provide the nutrients needed to optimize physical growth and development. However, these advantages don't guarantee that a child will thrive.

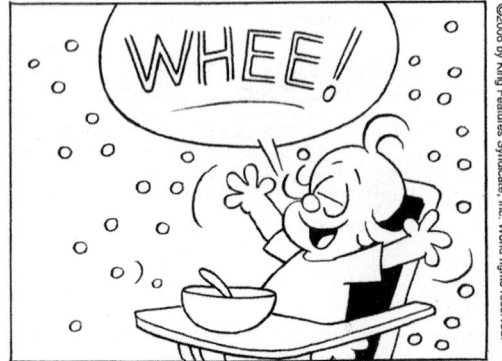
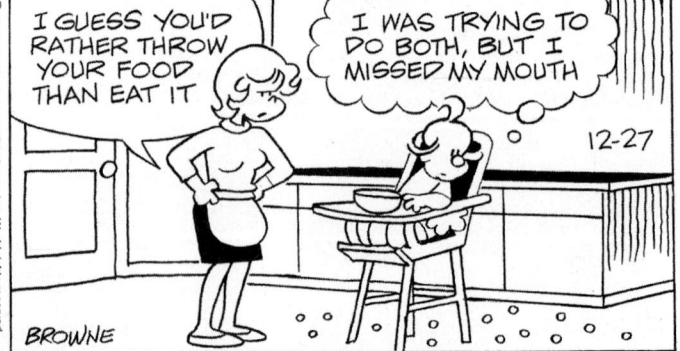

At what age should an infant be fed solid foods? Which foods are most appropriate for those early stages of solid food introduction? Which foods should not be fed to infants? Why? Chapter 15 provides some answers.

MARVIN © Reprinted with special permission of King Features Syndicate, Inc.

Children also need specific attention focused on them; they need to grow in a stimulating environment, and they need a sense of security. For example, children hospitalized for growth failure gain weight more quickly when more caring stimulation, such as holding and rocking the infant, accompanies needed nutrients.

The Growing Infant

All babies seem to do is eat and sleep. There's a good reason for this. An infant's birth weight doubles in the first 4 to 6 months and triples within the first year. Never again is growth so rapid. Such rapid growth requires a lot of nourishment and sleep. After the first year, growth is slower; it takes 5 more years to double the weight seen at 1 year. An infant also increases in length in the first year by 50% and then continues to gain height through the teen years. These gains are not necessarily continuous—spurts of growth alternate with plateaus. Height is essentially maximized by age 19, although increases of several inches may occur in the early twenties, especially for boys (Fig. 15-1). Head size in proportion to total height shrinks from one-fourth to one-eighth during the climb from infancy to adulthood.

The human body needs a lot more food to support growth and development than it does to merely maintain its size once growth ceases. When nutrients are missing at critical phases of this process, growth and development may slow or even stop.

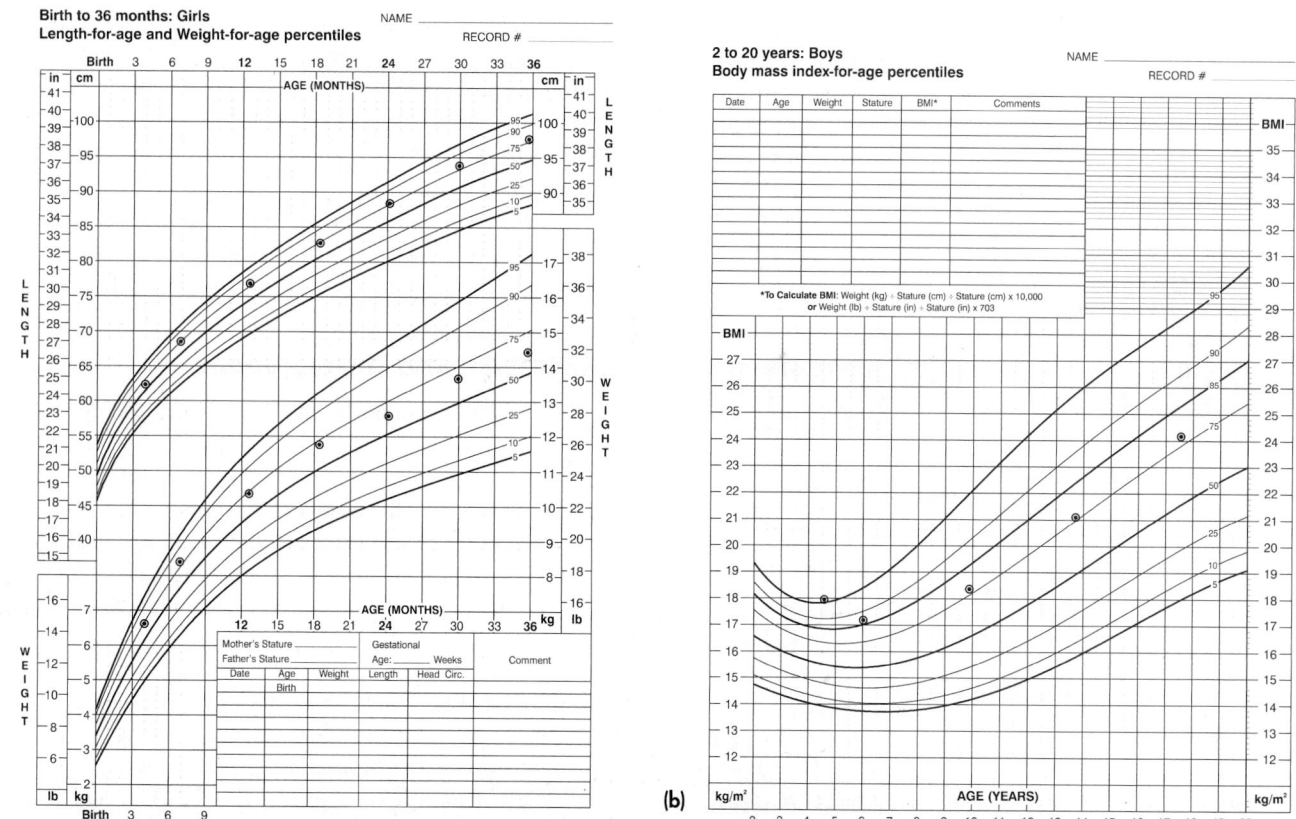

FIGURE 15-1 ▶ Growth charts for assessment of children in the growing years. The growth of a youngster is plotted to show how the charts are used in health care settings. (a) Growth charts used to assess length (height) and weight in young girls. A certain length (height) and weight correspond to a percentile value (i.e., a ranking of the person among 100 peers). This chart shows that at 36 months of age, the girl was at the 75th percentile for length and the 62nd percentile for weight. (b) Growth charts used to assess weight-for-height relationships in boys ages 2 to 20 years. Today, growth charts for older children and adolescents typically use BMI for evaluation purposes. At 6 years of age, the boy was at the 85th percentile for BMI.

Source: Developed by the National Center for Health Statistics in collaboration with the National Center for Chronic Disease Prevention and Health Promotion (2000). www.cdc.gov/growthcharts. *Revised November 21, 2000.*

undernutrition Failing health that results from a long-standing dietary intake that is not enough to meet nutritional needs.

percentile Classification of a measurement of a unit into divisions of 100 units.

In countries of the developing world, about one-third of the children under 5 years of age are short and underweight for their ages. Poor nutrition—called **undernutrition**—is at the heart of the problem. This occurs to a lesser extent in North America. The undernourished children are smaller versions of nutritionally fit children. In poorer countries, when breastfeeding ceases, children are often fed a high-carbohydrate, low-protein diet. This diet supports some growth but does not allow children to attain their full genetic potential. To grow, children must consume adequate amounts of calories, protein, calcium, iron, zinc, and other nutrients.

Effect of Undernutrition on Growth

As with the fetus in utero, the long-term effects of nutritional problems in infancy and childhood depend on the severity, timing, and duration of the nutritional insult to cell processes.

The single best indicator of a child's nutritional status is growth, particularly weight gain in the short run and length (height) in the long run. Mild zinc deficiencies in North American children have been linked to poor growth. Improving the diets of these children then leads to improved growth. Overall, eating a poor diet during a critical stage of infancy or childhood hampers the cell division that occurs at that stage. Consuming an adequate diet later usually won't compensate for lost growth, however, as the hormonal and other conditions needed for growth will not likely be present. In addition, growth ceases in girls and boys when the skeleton reaches its final size. This happens as growth plates at the ends of the bones fuse, which begins around 14 years of age in girls and 15 years of age in boys. The final stages of this process end at about 19 years of age in girls and 20 years of age in boys. Furthermore, muscles can increase in diameter later in life but their linear growth is limited by the length of the bone.

For these reasons, a 15-year-old Central American girl who is 4 feet 8 inches tall cannot attain the adult height of a typical North American girl simply by eating better. Girls experience their peak rate of growth right before the onset of menses. Once the time for growth ceases (in women, this is about 5 years after they start menstruating), a sufficient nutrient intake helps maintain health and weight but cannot make up for lost growth.

Assessment of Infant Growth and Development

Health professionals assess a child's increases in height and weight by comparing them with typical growth patterns recorded on charts (review Fig. 15-1). The charts contain **percentile** divisions, which represent the typical measurements for 90% to 96% of children. A percentile represents the rank of the person among 100 peers matched for age and gender. If a young boy, for example, is at the 90th percentile of height-for-age, he is shorter than 10% and taller than 89% of children his age. A child at the 50th percentile is considered average. Fifty of 100 children will be taller than this child; 49 will be shorter.

Individual growth charts are available for both males and females from the National Center for Health Statistics (as shown in Fig. 15-1). For ages ranging from birth to 36 months, options for growth charts include weight-for-age, length-for-age, weight-for-length, and head circumference-for-age. For males and females who are 2 to 20 years old, growth charts are available to determine weight-for-age and height-for-age; however, the preferred growth chart for children and adolescents is body mass index (BMI)-for-age. For adults, BMI has fixed cutoff points (for example, a BMI of 25 for an adult is considered overweight). As Figure 15-1 shows, this is not true for children, as BMI reference ranges are both gender- and age-specific.

In 2006, the World Health Organization released a new set of growth standards for children from birth through five years of age to replace the NCHS charts currently in use. The WHO growth charts provide a way to assess the same parameters listed (e.g., height or length, weight, BMI, and head circumference) but they are based on data collected from children from various regions of the world raised under conditions for optimal growth and development: breastfed as infants, followed recommended infant and child feeding practices set forth by WHO, had adequate health care, and mothers did not use tobacco during or after pregnancy. In contrast, the NCHS growth charts are based on data from primarily Caucasian children who were mostly formula-fed during infancy. The new WHO growth standards stress that breastfeeding is the biological norm for infant nutrition. The CDC advises clinicians to use WHO growth charts to monitor growth in infants and children from birth to 2 years, then use NCHS growth charts for children from 2 to 19 years.

Infants and children should have their growth assessed during regular health checkups. It takes 1 to 3 years for the genetic potential (in terms of percentile ranking on growth charts) of infant growth to be established. By 3 years of age, a child's measurements, such as length (height) for age, should generally track along the established percentile. If the child's growth does not keep up with his or her length for age percentile, the physician needs to investigate whether a medical or nutritional problem is impeding the predicted growth. Inappropriate weight gain—too little or too much—should also be investigated.

Infants born preterm may catch up in growth in 2 to 3 years. This requires that the child move up in the percentiles. If this occurs—especially in length for age—it is usually no cause for alarm. On the other hand, moving up in the percentiles for weight for height can be disturbing if the child approaches the 80th to 90th percentiles. A child between the 85th and 95th percentile for BMI is considered overweight. At or above the 95th percentile, the child is considered obese. At the 95th percentile, the diagnosis of obesity can also be established if the physical exam of the child indicates he or she is truly overfat. This is generally the case at this percentile.

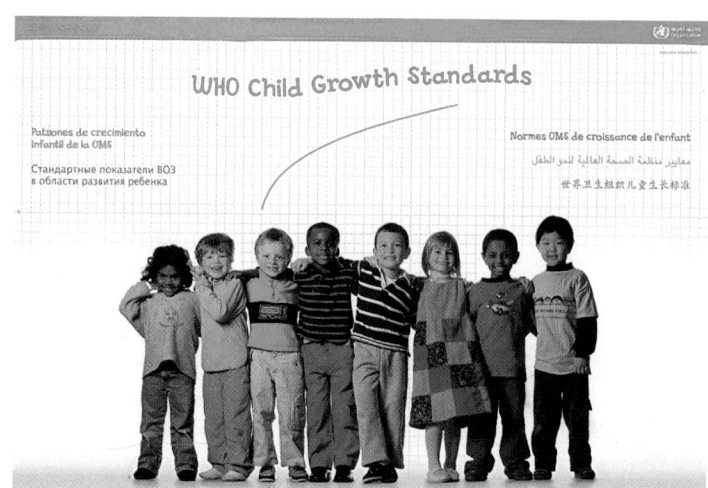

▲ The new WHO Growth Standards for Children differ from previous standards in part because they reflect data gathered from children from around the world who were raised in conditions for optimal growth and development. Go to www.who.int/childgrowth/en/ for more information on the WHO Child Growth Standards.

Children under 2 to 3 years of age are measured lying on their backs with knees unflexed, so the term *length* is used rather than *height*.

MAKING DECISIONS

Head Circumference and Brain Development

The brain grows faster in infancy than at any other time of life. To accommodate this growth, an infant's head circumference must be very large in proportion to the rest of the body. The rapid growth stops at about 18 months of age. In early physical checkups, a health professional usually measures the head circumference as one means of assessing growth, especially brain growth. How nutritional status affects brain development and intelligence quotient (IQ) is difficult to measure because scientists have not determined how to separate the effects of nature from those of nurture. However, several studies have determined that breastfed babies have higher IQs than do babies who were fed with infant formula. At the same time, studies from Central America suggest that IQ after age 5 years relates more closely to the amount of schooling a child receives than to nutritional intake during early childhood.

Adipose Tissue Growth

Since 1970, researchers have speculated that overfeeding during infancy may increase the number of adipose tissue cells. Today, we know that the number of adipose cells can also increase as adulthood obesity develops. Still, if calorie intake is limited during infancy to keep down the number of adipose cells, the growth of other organ systems may also be severely restricted. Special concern revolves around body growth and development, especially brain and nervous system development. In addition, most overweight infants become normal-weight preschoolers without excessive diet restrictions. For these reasons, it is unwise to greatly restrict diet, and especially fat intake in infants. After the first 12 months, fat intake can range from 30% to 40% of total kcal for ages 1 to 3 years, and 25% to 35% of calorie intake for older children (and teenagers).

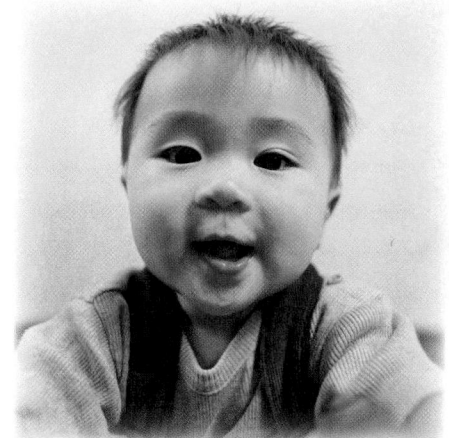

▲ Brain growth is faster in infancy than in any other stage of life. Therefore an infant's head needs to be larger in comparison to the body to allow for such growth.

Failure to Thrive

Occasionally, an infant doesn't grow much in the first few months. Physical problems that may contribute to restricted growth range from poor oral cavity development, infections, and heart irregularities to constant diarrhea associated with intestinal problems. However, more than half the infants who fail to thrive have no apparent disease. Sometimes the cause is poor infant-parent interaction. This stems from misinformation, lack of a parent role model, too little concern about the child's welfare, or even from exerting too much control over feedings (e.g., maternal anxiety, force feeding). Poverty or food insecurity may also be at the root of infant or child undernutrition. In general, the problems arise from the parents' inexperience, rather than intentional negligence. Consequences of failure to thrive include poor physical growth, impaired mental development, and behavioral problems. When health professionals encounter an infant failing to thrive, the true causes need to be identified and then treated.

CONCEPT CHECK

Growth occurs rapidly during infancy: Birth weight doubles in about 4 to 6 months and triples within the first year. Undernutrition in childhood can irreversibly inhibit growth and maturation, so that an individual never attains his or her full genetic potential for height. Infant and child growth is assessed by tracking body weight, length (height), and head circumference over time. Body mass index (BMI) is generally used to assess weight-for-height after 2 years of age. It is not desirable for infants to become overweight, although no evidence strongly indicates that overweight infants become overweight adults. Severe calorie restriction is not recommended for infants because it may slow the growth of organ systems. When infants do not grow properly, their failure to thrive may stem from physical disorders or inadequate care, including inappropriate feeding practices.

Infant Nutritional Needs

Infants' nutritional needs vary as they grow. Initially, human milk or infant formula (usually made from heat-treated cow's milk) supplies needed nutrients. Solid foods are not needed until around 6 months. Even after solid foods are added, the basis of an infant's diet for the first year is still human milk or infant formula. Because of the critical importance of adequate nutrition in infancy and the difficulties encountered in feeding some infants, there is more discussion in this chapter on this developmental period than on the later periods of childhood.

Calories. During infancy, energy needs per pound of body weight are the highest of any life stage. For example, a 6-month-old infant requires two to four times more kcal per pound of body weight than an adult:

Healthy 6-month-old infant
700 kcal/15 pounds = 47 kcal/pound

Healthy 20-year-old woman
2200 kcal / 135 pounds = 16 kcal/pound

Infants need a concentrated source of calories to meet these high demands. Exclusive feeding of either human milk or infant formula is ideal for the first 6 months of life; both are high in fat and supply about 640 kcal/quart (670 kcal/liter; Table 15-1). After 6 months of age, human milk or infant formula, supplemented by developmentally appropriate solid foods, can provide more calories, nutrients, and variety for the developing infant.

The infant's high calorie needs are primarily driven by rapid growth and high metabolic rate. The high metabolic rate is caused in part by the ratio of the infant's body surface area to its weight. More body surface area allows more heat loss from the skin; the body must use extra calories to replace that heat.

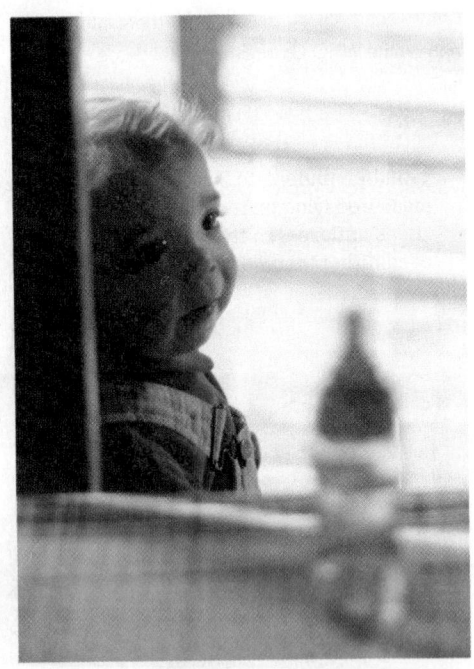

▲ Children older than 2 years are less likely to experience failure to thrive because they can often get food for themselves. Younger children, for the most part, are limited to what caregivers provide.

Age	EER* Equation
0 to 3 months	(89 kcal × weight**) + 75
4 to 6 months	(89 kcal × weight) - 44
7 to 12 months	(89 kcal × weight) – 78
13 to 35 months	(89 kcal × weight) – 80

*EER = Estimated Energy Requirements
**Weight is in kilograms.

TABLE 15-1 Composition of Human and Cow's Milk and Infant Formulas per liter. At 3 Months of Age, Infants Typically Consume 0.75 to 1 liter of Human Milk or Formula per Day.

	Energy (kcal)	Protein (grams)	Fat (grams)	Carbohydrate (grams)	Minerals* (grams)
Milk					
Human milk	670**	11	45	70	2
Cow's milk, whole†	670	36	36	49	7
Cow's milk, fat-free†	360	36	1	51	7
Casein/Whey-Based Formulas					
Similac	680	14	36	71	3
Enfamil	670	15	37	69	3
Good Start	670	16	34	73	3
Soybean Protein-Based Formulas					
ProSobee	670	20	35	67	4
Isomil	680	16	36	68	4
Transition Formulas/Beverages‡					
Similac Toddler's Best	670	25	33	75	3
Enfamil Next Step	670	17	33	74	3
Carnation Follow-Up	670	17	27	88	3

*Calcium, phosphorus, and other minerals.

**Rough estimate; ranges from 650–700 kcal per liter.

†Not appropriate for infant feeding, based primarily on high protein and mineral content.

‡For use after 6 months of age or later (see label).

Carbohydrate. Carbohydrate needs in infancy are 60 grams per day at 0 to 6 months and 95 grams per day at 7 to 12 months. These needs are based on the typical intakes of human milk by breastfed infants and their eventual use of solid foods. Both carbohydrate goals are satisfied by usual intakes of infants on a proper diet.

Protein. Daily protein needs in infancy are about 9 grams per day for younger infants and about 14 grams per day for older infants. These needs also are based on the typical intakes of human milk by breastfed infants for 0 to 6 months, and then on the needs for growth for older infants. About half of total protein intake should come from essential (indispensable) amino acids. As with carbohydrate, protein needs are easily satisfied by either human milk or infant formula. Protein intake should not greatly exceed this standard. Excess nitrogen and minerals supplied by high-protein diets would exceed the ability of an infant's kidneys to excrete the waste products of protein metabolism, thus putting much stress on overall kidney function.

In North America, infant protein deficiency is unlikely, except in cases of mistakes in formula preparation, such as when an infant's formula is excessively diluted with water. Protein deficiency may also be induced by elimination diets used to detect food **allergies** (hypersensitivities). As foods are eliminated from the diet, infants may not be offered enough protein to compensate for the high-protein sources no longer present (see the "Nutrition and Your Health" section later in this chapter).

Fat. Infants need about 30 grams of fat per day. Essential fatty acids should make up about 15% of total fat intake (about 5 grams per day). Both recommendations are again based on the typical intakes of human milk by breastfed infants and the eventual intake of solid foods. Fats are an important part of the infant's diet because they are vital to the development of the nervous system. As a concentrated source of calories, fat also helps resolve the potential problem of the infant's high calorie needs and small stomach capacity. Again, restriction of fat intake is not advised for infants or children under age 2 (Fig. 15-2).

Looking at Table 15-1, it is easy to see why fat-free milk products are not recommended for infants—these do not supply adequate fat and calories to meet needs. Fat-free milk (and reduced fat and whole milk as well) also would provide too much protein and minerals if it were used to meet calorie needs.

See Nutrition and Your Health: Food Allergies and Intolerances at the end of this chapter.

allergy A hypersensitive immune response that occurs when immune bodies produced by us react with a protein we sense as foreign (an antigen).

FIGURE 15-2 ▶ The labels on infant foods, like those on adult foods, contain a Nutrition Facts panel. However, the information provided on infant food labels differs from that on adult food labels, especially with respect to total fat, saturated fat, and cholesterol content (see Fig. 2-16 for a comparison). Some cereal brands are fortified with various other micronutrients.

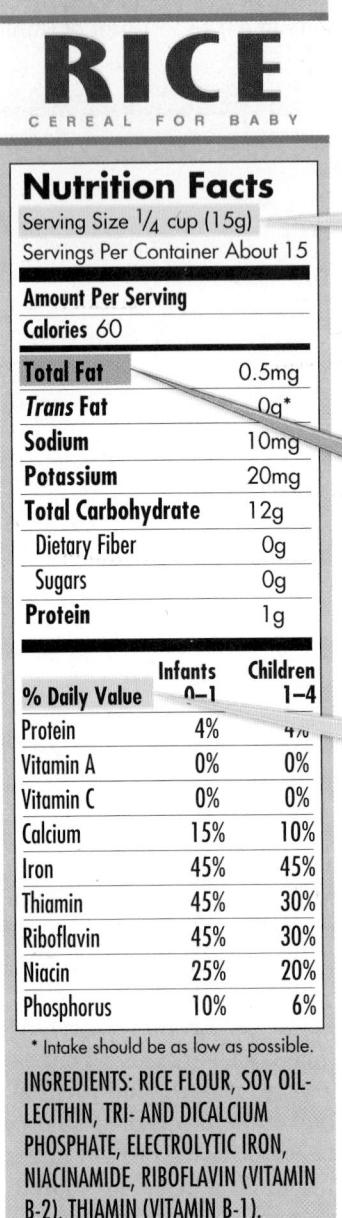

Serving Size
Serving sizes for infant foods are based on the average amount eaten at one time by a child under 2 years.

Total Fat
Shows the amount of total fat in a serving of the food. Unlike adult food labels, labels on infant foods do not list calories from fat, saturated fat, or cholesterol, since infants and toddlers under 2 years need fat. Parents should not attempt to limit their infant's fat intake.

Daily Values
Food labels for infants and children under 4 years list the Daily Value percentages for protein, vitamins, and minerals. Unlike adult food labels, Daily Values for fat, cholesterol, sodium, potassium, carbohydrate, and fiber are not listed.

Arachidonic acid (AA) and docosahexaenoic acid (DHA) are two long-chain fatty acids that have important roles in infant development. The nervous system, especially the brain and eyes, depend on these fatty acids for proper development. During the last trimester, DHA and AA provided by the mother accumulate in the brain and retinas of the eyes in the fetus. Breastfed infants are able to continue to acquire these fatty acids from human milk, especially if their mothers are regularly eating fish. Until recently, no infant formulas sold in the United States included AA or DHA, but many brands are now available with both AA and DHA. These are particularly useful for feeding preterm infants.

Vitamins of Special Interest. As noted in Chapter 8, vitamin K is routinely given by injection to all infants at birth. Formula-fed infants receive the rest of the vitamins they need from the formula. For bone health, immune function, and chronic disease prevention, the American Academy of pediatrics recommends that all infants and children consume 400 IU vitamin D per day starting soon after birth. For all breastfed infants and formula-fed infants who consume less than 1 quart of formula per day, supplemental vitamin D is necessary until they are weaned to infant formula and are consuming at least

500 milliliters of it per day (see Further Reading 14). Breastfed infants whose mothers are total vegetarians (vegans) should also receive vitamin B-12 in supplement form.

Minerals of Special Interest. Infants are born with some internal stores of iron. However, by the time birth weight doubles (4 to 6 months of age), iron stores are generally depleted if not otherwise part of the diet. If the mother was iron deficient during the pregnancy, these iron stores will be exhausted even sooner. As you will recall from Chapter 9, iron-deficiency anemia can lead to poor mental development in infants. Several studies indicate that iron deficiency anemia during infancy, even if corrected, has a lasting impact in terms of impaired cognition, motor development, and behavioral problems later in life. To maintain a desirable iron status, the American Academy of Pediatrics recommends that formula-fed infants should be given an iron-fortified formula from birth. Low-iron infant formulas are sometimes prescribed to treat infants with various GI tract problems, but otherwise their use is discouraged. In contrast, breastfed infants at about 4 to 6 months of age need solid foods to supply extra iron. This need for iron is a major consideration in the decision to introduce solid foods. Liquid iron supplements may be needed until food intake provides sufficient iron. Supplements are also indicated for preterm or LBW infants, those with blood disorders, or those born with inadequate stores of iron (i.e., due to maternal iron deficiency during pregnancy) (see Further Reading 2).

Breast milk is a poor source of fluoride—and formula manufacturers use fluoride-free water in formula preparation, so intake of this mineral during the first 6 months of life is low. However, fluoride supplementation is not advised before 6 months of age. After 6 months, the pediatrician or dentist may recommend fluoride supplements to aid in tooth development if fluoride supplied by tap water, foods, and toothpaste is inadequate.

Infants also need adequate amounts of zinc and iodide to support growth. However, when human milk and infant formula are provided in quantities to meet calorie needs, sufficient zinc and iodide are generally supplied.

Water. An infant needs about 3 cups (700 to 800 milliliters) of water per day. Infants typically consume enough human milk or formula to supply this amount. Even in hot weather, the American Academy of Pediatrics does not recommend supplemental water or juice during the first 6 months. Excess water can cause hyponatremia in infants.

Infants are easily dehydrated, a condition that has serious effects if not remedied. Early signs of dehydration in infants include:

- More than 6 hours without a wet diaper
- Dark yellow or strong-smelling urine
- Unusual lethargy
- Dry mouth and lips
- Absence of tears when crying

Special fluid-replacement formulas containing electrolytes such as sodium and potassium are available in supermarkets and pharmacies to treat mild to moderate dehydration. A physician should guide any use of these products. As dehydration becomes more severe, the infant's eyes and/or the soft spot on the head may appear sunken, hands and feet may be cold and splotchy, and he or she may be excessively tired and

The American Dental Association does not recommend fluoridated bottled water for use by infants because it creates risk for enamel fluorosis during early tooth development.

MAKING DECISIONS

Extra Fluid for Infants

In some stores, bottled water products marketed specifically for infants may be placed alongside infant formulas and electrolyte-replacement solutions. This placement may give parents and caregivers the mistaken impression that bottled water products are an appropriate feeding supplement or substitute for fluid replacement for infants; they are not and should not be used for such purposes. It is important to remember that excessive fluid can also be harmful, especially to the brain.

fussy. Such severe dehydration can result in rapid loss of kidney function and warrants medical intervention. Hospitalization and intravenous fluid treatment may be necessary for extreme cases or when the infant is unable to keep anything in the stomach.

Overall, it is best to rely exclusively on breast milk or infant formula to meet infant fluid needs up to 6 months of age unless a physician suggests otherwise. In sum, extremes in fluid intake—either too little or too much—can lead to health problems.

CONCEPT CHECK

Most nutrient needs in the first 6 months are met by human milk or infant formula. All infants and children should receive 400 IU of vitamin D, which necessitates supplementation for breastfed and some formula-fed infants. Some infants, especially after 4 months of age, with low iron stores may require iron supplements. Formula-fed infants and breastfed infants may need fluoride supplements after 6 months of age. Infants usually receive enough water from the human milk or infant formula they drink.

Formula Feeding for Infants

Breastfeeding was covered in detail in Chapter 14. Let's now focus on formula feeding. You'll recall that a major advantage of breastfeeding is the provision of immune protection to the infant. Although it lacks the full spectrum of benefits of breastfeeding, formula feeding is a safe alternative for infants in areas of the world with clean water supplies.

Formula Composition. Infants cannot tolerate cow's milk as such because of its high protein and mineral content. Cow's milk is perfect for the greater growth needs of calves, but not for human infants. Thus, cow's milk must be altered by formula manufacturers to be safe for infant feeding. Altered forms of cow's milk, known as infant formulas, must conform to strict federal guidelines for nutrient composition and quality. Formulas generally contain lactose and/or sucrose for carbohydrate, heat-treated proteins from cow's milk, and vegetable oils for fat (review Table 15-1). Soy protein–based formulas are available for infants who can't tolerate lactose or the types of proteins found in cow's milk. If the soybean-based formula is not tolerated, the next step is to try a predigested formula in which the proteins have been broken down into small polypeptides and amino acids. A variety of other specialized formulas also are available for specific medical conditions. In any case, it is important to use an iron-fortified formula unless a physician recommends otherwise.

Some transition formulas/beverages have been introduced for older infants and toddlers (review Table 15-1). Some of these products are intended for use after 6 months of age if the infant is consuming solid foods, whereas others are intended for use only by toddlers. These transition products are lower in fat than human milk or standard infant formulas; their iron content is higher than that of cow's milk; and their overall mineral content is generally more like that of human milk than cow's milk. According to the manufacturers, the advantages of these transition formulas/beverages over standard formulas for older infants and toddlers include reduced cost and better flavor. Parents should consult their physician with regard to the use of these products.

Formula Preparation. Some infant formulas come in ready-to-feed form. These are poured into a clean bottle and fed immediately. Room-temperature formula is acceptable for many infants. Otherwise, to warm a bottle of formula, a caregiver can run hot water over it or place it briefly in a pan of simmering water. Infant formulas should not be heated in a microwave oven because hot spots may develop, which can burn the infant's mouth and esophagus.

Powdered and concentrated fluid formula preparations are also commonly used. All utensils used to prepare formula should be washed and thoroughly rinsed.

Parents should consult a physician when choosing an appropriate infant formula. Not all formula-like products are designed for infant use. A 5-month-old girl was admitted to a hospital in Arkansas with symptoms of heart failure, rickets, inflamed blood vessels, and possible nerve damage after being fed Soy Moo (a soy beverage sold in health stores) since 3 days of age. The symptoms suggest severe vitamin deficiencies.

Bisphenol A (BPA) is a chemical used in the manufacture of many plastics, including some baby bottles. Human exposure to BPA, mainly through leaching of the chemical from packaging into foods and beverages, is widespread. Concern about exposure stems from animal studies that link BPA with reproductive and developmental defects. However, the consensus among regulatory agencies in the United States and Canada is that current levels of BPA exposure are not harmful, even for infants. For parents who wish to limit exposure, BPA-free baby bottles are available.

Powdered or concentrated formulas should be combined with clean, cold water, exactly following the directions on the formula label. The formula is then warmed, if desired, and fed immediately to the infant. Hot water from the faucet should not be used to make formula, since it poses a risk for high lead content (see Chapter 13). Cold water poses much less risk. For infants up to 6 months of age, pediatricians commonly recommend boiling (and then cooling) the water to be used in formula preparation and sterilizing bottles and utensils by immersion in boiling water.

Refrigerating prepared formula for 1 day is safe. However, formula left over from a feeding should be discarded because it will be contaminated by bacteria and enzymes from the infant's saliva. If well water is used, it should be boiled before making formula for at least the infant's first 3 months of life, and it should be analyzed for excessive concentration of naturally occurring nitrates, which can lead to a severe form of anemia. If nitrates are high in municipal water systems, consumers will be warned (such as in a local newspaper) not to use the water for making infant formula until the concentration falls to a safe amount. The American Dental Association does not recommend that formula be mixed with bottled nursery water, available alongside infant formula in most supermarkets, to limit risk of tooth discoloration from high fluoride levels.

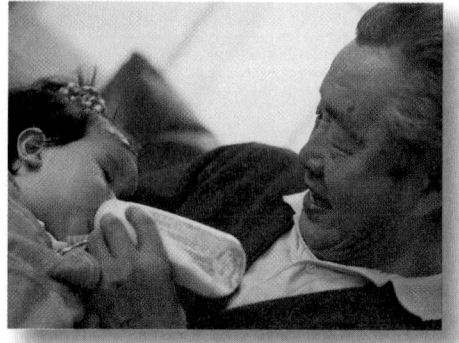

▲ Careful attention during feeding allows the caregiver to notice the infant's signal as to when the feeding should cease.

Feeding Technique

Infants swallow a lot of air as they ingest either formula or human milk, so it's important to burp an infant after either 10 minutes of feeding or 1 to 2 ounces (30 to 60 milliliters) has been consumed from a bottle and again at the end of feeding. Spitting up a bit of milk is normal at this time.

When the infant begins acting full, bottle feeding should be stopped, even if some milk is left in the bottle. Common cues that signal that an infant has had enough include turning the head away, being inattentive, falling asleep, and becoming playful. Generally, the infant's appetite is a better guide than standardized recommendations concerning feeding amounts. Breastfeeding infants usually have had enough to eat after about 20 minutes. Although it's difficult to tell how much milk breastfed infants are getting, they also give signs when full. By carefully observing bottle-feeding or breastfeeding infants and responding to their cues appropriately, caregivers not only can be assured that the infants' calorie needs are being met but also can foster a climate of trust and responsiveness.

Once fed, an infant should not be placed on its stomach. Placing the infant on its back is recommended by the American Academy of Pediatrics. The reason that an infant should not be placed on its stomach is because this sleeping position has been linked to sudden infant death syndrome (SIDS). The Back to Sleep campaign, started in 1994 in the United States, has reduced SIDS by 40%.

The Back to Sleep campaign, however, has led to a problem known as flattened head syndrome (clinically known as positional plagiocephaly). Infant skulls are soft and therefore can change in shape. Flattened head syndrome can occur if an excessive amount of an infant's day is spent on his or her back or against a highchair/car seat. In response to this concern, the American Academy of Pediatrics has recommended periodic repositioning of an infant's head while asleep and allowing for supervised time on his or her stomach while awake. In addition, some infants may need to wear specially fitted helmets to correct the shape of their heads.

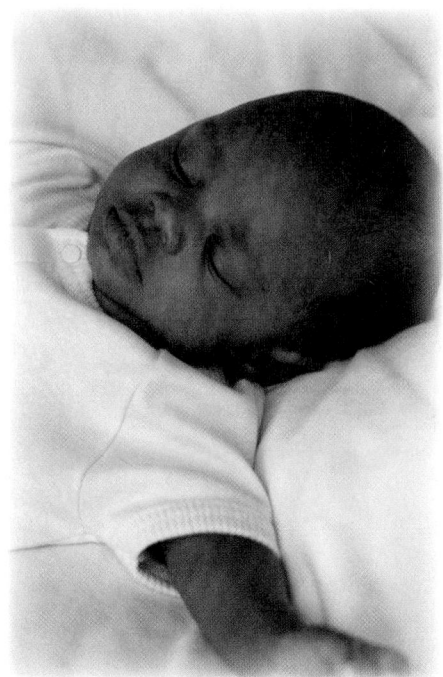

▲ The Back to Sleep campaign aims to reduce risk of sudden infant death syndrome.

Expanding the Infant's Mealtime Choices

By about 6 months of age, the infant is ready to start eating "table food." Initially, table foods add to—rather than replace—formula or human milk. In the first attempts to introduce solid foods, just getting the food into the infant's mouth may prove to be a challenge. By the end of the first year, though, the infant should be eating a variety of protein sources, vegetables, fruits, and grains so that the diet begins to resemble a balanced pattern, setting the stage for lifelong preferences and dietary habits (Table 15-2).

TABLE 15-2 Sample Daily Menu for a 1-Year-Old Child*

Breakfast	**Snack**
1 to 2 tbsp applesauce	½ ounce cheddar cheese
¼ cup Cheerios	4 wheat crackers
½ cup whole milk	½ cup whole milk

Snack	**Dinner**
½ hard-cooked egg	1 ounce hamburger (crumbled)
½ slice wheat toast with ½ tsp margarine	1 to 2 tbsp mashed potatoes with ½ tsp margarine
½ cup orange juice	1 to 2 tbsp cooked carrots (cut in strips, not coins)
	½ cup whole milk

Lunch	**Snack**
1 ounce roasted chicken, minced	½ banana
1 to 2 tbsp rice with ½ tsp margarine	2 oatmeal cookies (no raisins)
1 to 2 tbsp cooked peas	½ cup whole milk
½ cup whole milk	

Nutritional Analysis	
Total energy (kcal)	1100
% energy from	
Carbohydrate	40%
Protein	19%
Fat	41%

*This diet is just a start. A 1-year-old may need more or less food. In those cases, serving sizes should be adjusted. The milk can be fed by cup; some can be put into a bottle if the child has not been fully weaned from the bottle. The juice should be fed in a cup.

Throughout the process of expanding the infant's mealtime choices, it is essential to allow the infant to control the situation—the caregiver must proceed slowly and respond to the infant's cues that he or she is hungry or has had enough to eat.

Recognizing the Infant's Readiness for Solid Foods. How does the caregiver know it is time to introduce solid foods? Infant size can serve as a rough indicator of readiness—reaching a weight of at least 13 pounds (6 kilograms) is a preliminary sign of readiness for solid foods. Another physiological cue is frequency of feeding, such as consuming more than 32 ounces (1 liter) of formula daily or breastfeeding more than 8 to 10 times within 24 hours. Underlying these noticeable signals are several important developmental factors:

1. *Nutritional need.* Before the infant is 6 months old, nutritional needs can generally be met with human milk and/or formula. After 6 months of age, however, many infants need the additional calories supplied by solid foods. In terms of individual nutrients, iron stores are exhausted by about 6 months of age. Either solid foods or iron supplements are then needed to supply iron if the child is breastfed or fed a low-iron or iron-free formula. (As previously mentioned, a vitamin D supplement should also be provided.)

2. *Physiological capabilities.* As the infant ages, the ability to digest and metabolize a wider range of food components improves. Before about 3 months of age, an infant's digestive tract cannot readily digest starch. Also, kidney function is limited until about 4 to 6 weeks of age. Until then, waste products from excessive amounts of dietary protein or minerals are difficult to excrete.

3. *Physical ability.* Three physical markers indicate that a child is ready for solid foods: (1) the disappearance of the extrusion reflex (thrusting the tongue forward and pushing food out of the mouth), (2) head and neck control, and (3) the ability to sit up with support. These usually occur around 4 to 6 months of age, but they vary with each infant.

4. *Allergy prevention.* An infant's intestinal tract is "leaky"—whole proteins can readily be absorbed from birth until 4 to 5 months of age. If the infant is exposed too early to some types of proteins—particularly those in cow's milk

and egg whites—the infant may be predisposed to future allergies and other health problems, such as diabetes. For this reason, it is best to minimize the number of different types of proteins in an infant's diet, especially during the first 3 months (see the "Nutrition and Your Health" section on food allergies at the end of this chapter for details).

With these considerations in mind—nutritional need, physiological and physical readiness, and allergy prevention—the American Academy of Pediatrics recommends that solid foods not be introduced until about 6 months of age and that infants receive no unaltered cow's milk before 1 year.

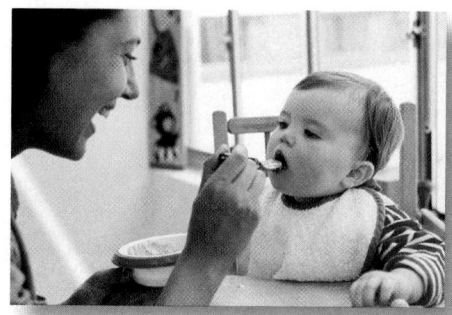

▲ Iron-fortified rice cereal is recommended as the first solid food to be fed to infants.

MAKING DECISIONS

Introducing Solid Foods

Parents may believe that the early addition of solid foods will help an infant sleep through the night. Actually, this achievement is a developmental milestone, and the amount of food consumed by the infant is of little relevance to the achievement of a good night's sleep. Before 4 to 6 months of age, infants are not physically mature enough to consume much solid food. Only occasionally does a rapidly growing infant need solid foods to meet calorie and nutrient needs before 6 months of age.

Foods to Match Needs and Developmental Abilities During the First Year. If solid foods are introduced before 6 months of age, the primary goal of the food should be to meet iron needs. Therefore, the first solid foods should be iron-fortified cereals. Some pediatricians may recommend lean ground (strained) meats for more absorbable forms of iron. Rice is the best cereal to begin with because it is least likely to cause allergies.

When starting solid foods, it is important to start with a teaspoon serving size of a single-ingredient food item, such as rice cereal, and increase the serving size gradually. Once the new food has been fed for about a week without ill effects, another food can be added to the infant's diet. At first, this can be another type of cereal or perhaps a cooked and strained (or mashed) vegetable, meat, fruit, or egg yolk.

Waiting about 7 days between the introduction of each new food is important because it can take that long for evidence of an allergy or intolerance to develop. Also, it is important to avoid introducing mixed foods until each component of the combination dish has been given separately without an adverse reaction. Signs of food allergies include diarrhea, vomiting, a rash, or wheezing. If one or more of these signs appears, the suspected problem food should be avoided for several weeks and then reintroduced in a small quantity. If the problem continues, a physician should be consulted. Fortunately, many babies outgrow food allergies later in childhood.

Until recently, parents and caregivers were advised to avoid feeding children a wide range of highly allergenic foods, including egg whites, chocolate, peanuts, tree nuts, fish, and other seafood. Now, the American Academy of Pediatrics acknowledges that there is no evidence that delaying introduction of solid foods—including these highly allergenic foods—beyond 6 months of age is of any benefit for prevention of food allergies and other atopic diseases. (See Nutrition and Your Health at the end of this chapter.)

Many strained foods for infant feeding are available at the supermarket. Single-food items are more desirable than mixed dinners and desserts, which are less nutrient-dense. Most brands have no added salt, but some fruit desserts contain a lot of added sugar.

As an alternative, plain, unseasoned cooked foods—vegetables, fruits, and meats—can be ground up in an inexpensive plastic baby food grinder/mill. Another option is to puree a larger amount of food in a blender, freeze it in ice-cube portions, store in plastic bags, and defrost and warm as needed. Careful attention to cleanliness is necessary. Seasonings that may please the rest of the family should not be added to infant foods made at home. The infant doesn't notice the difference if salt, sugar, or

▶ **Typical Solid Food Progression, Starting at 6 Months***

Week 1	Rice cereal
Week 2	Add strained carrots
Week 3	Add applesauce
Week 4	Add oat cereal
Week 5	Add cooked egg yolk
Week 6	Add strained chicken
Week 7	Add strained peas
Week 8	Add plums

*Extending the rice cereal step for a month or so is advised if solid food introduction begins at 4 months of age. Also, if at any point signs of allergy or intolerance develop, substitute another similar food item.

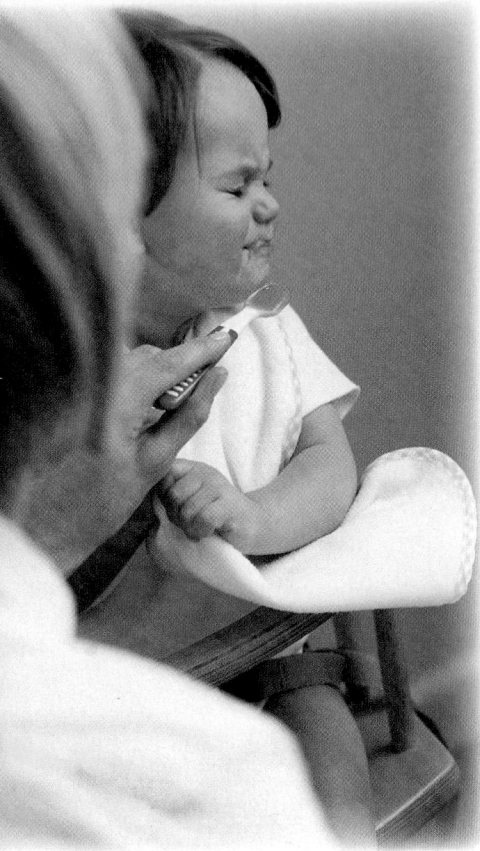

▲ Repeated exposure fosters acceptance of new tastes and textures.

early childhood caries Tooth decay that results from formula or juice (and even human milk) bathing the teeth as the child sleeps with a bottle in his or her mouth. The upper teeth are mostly affected as the lower teeth are protected by the tongue; formerly called *nursing bottle syndrome* and *baby bottle tooth decay*.

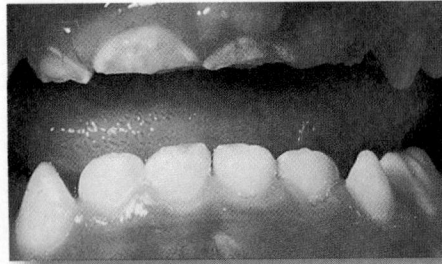

▲ Early childhood caries. An extreme example of tooth decay probably resulting from frequently putting the child to bed with a bottle. The upper teeth have decayed almost all the way to the gum line.

spices are omitted. It is best to introduce infants to a variety of foods, so that by the end of the first year, the infant is consuming many foods—human milk or formula, meats, fruits, vegetables, and grains.

Self-feeding skills require coordination and can develop only if the infant is allowed to practice and experiment. By 6 to 7 months of age, the infant has learned to handle finger foods and transfer objects from one hand to the other with some dexterity. At about this time, teeth also begin to appear. Dry toast, sliced in strips, offers hours of enjoyment. By age 7 to 8 months, infants can push food around on a plate, play with a drinking cup, hold a bottle, and self-feed a cracker or a piece of toast. Through mastery of these manipulations, infants develop confidence and self-esteem. It is important that parents be patient and support these early feeding attempts, even though they appear inefficient.

At 9 to 10 months of age, the infant's desire to explore, experience, and play with foods may hinder feeding. Food is used as a means to explore the environment, and therefore feeding time is often very messy—a bowl of macaroni may end up in the child's hair. Presenting a new food on several consecutive days can aid in an infant's acceptance of that food. Caregivers need to relax and take this phase of infant development in stride. Sloppy, friendly mealtimes make for good memories. By the end of the first year, finger-feeding becomes more efficient and chewing is easier as more teeth erupt. Still, experimentation and unpredictability are to be expected.

To ease the efforts in feeding solid foods, consider the following tips:

- Use a baby-sized spoon; a small spoon with a long handle is best.
- Hold the infant comfortably on the lap, as for breastfeeding or bottle feeding, but a little more upright to ease swallowing. When in this position, the infant expects food.
- Put a small dab of food on the spoon tip and gently place it on the infant's tongue.
- Convey a calm and casual approach to the infant, who needs time to get used to food.
- Expect the infant to take only two or three bites of the first meals.

Weaning from the Breast or Bottle

Around the age of 6 months, juices can be offered in a sippy cup with a wide, flat bottom. Drinking from a cup rather than from a bottle helps prevent **early childhood caries.** If an infant drinks continuously from a bottle, the carbohydrate-rich fluid bathes the teeth, providing an ideal growth medium for bacteria adhering to the teeth. These bacteria then make acids, which dissolve tooth enamel. To avoid dental caries, infants should not be put to bed with a bottle or placed in an infant seat with a bottle propped up.

By about 10 months of age, infants are learning to self-feed and likewise to drink independently from a cup. As children drink from a cup more frequently, fewer bottle feedings and/or breastfeedings are necessary. The added mobility of crawling and walking should naturally lead to gradual weaning from the bottle or breast. Even so, getting a baby out of the bedtime-bottle habit can be difficult. Determined caregivers can either wince through a few nights of their baby's crying or slowly wean the baby away from the bottle with either a pacifier or water (for a week or so).

Dietary Guidelines for Infant Feeding

It can be difficult for new parents to make sense of nutrition goals for infants in the face of changing dietary recommendations from health authorities, cultural preferences, and outdated advice from friends and family. In response to various controversies surrounding infant feeding, the American Academy of Pediatrics has issued a number of statements concerning infant diets. The following guidelines are based on these statements:

- *Build to a variety of foods.* For the first months of life, human milk (or infant formula) is all an infant needs. (Vitamin D supplementation is an exception.)

When the infant is ready, start adding new foods, one at a time. During the first year, the goal is to teach an infant to enjoy a variety of nutritious foods. A lifetime of healthy eating habits begins with this important first step.

- *Pay attention to your infant's appetite to avoid overfeeding or underfeeding.* Feed infants when they are hungry. Never force an infant to finish an unwanted serving of food. Watch for signs that indicate hunger or fullness. This will reinforce the infant's natural capability to self-regulate food intake.
- *Infants need fat.* Although fat contributes to many adult health problems, it's an essential source of calories for growing infants. Fat also helps the nervous system develop.
- *Choose fruits, vegetables, and grains, but don't overdo high-fiber foods.* During the second half of the first year, infants are fed a variety of fruits and vegetables. However, studies show that by 1 year of age, vegetable choices are dominated by white potatoes. Continuing to offer choices of green and yellow vegetables during infancy and the toddler years will enhance intake of important vitamins, minerals, and phytochemicals. In terms of fiber, although many adults benefit from high-fiber diets, they are not good for infants. They are bulky, filling, and often low in calories. The natural amounts of fiber and nutrients in fruits, vegetables, and grains are appropriate as part of a healthy infant diet.
- *Infants need sugars in moderation.* Sugars are an additional source of calories for active, rapidly growing infants. Foods such as human milk, fruits, and 100% juices are natural sources of sugars and other nutrients as well. Foods that contain artificial sweeteners should be avoided; they don't provide the calories growing infants need. On the other hand, excessive intake of sugars, particularly from fruit-flavored drinks and soft drinks, contribute to the epidemic of childhood obesity.
- *Infants need sodium in moderation.* Sodium is a necessary mineral found naturally in almost all foods. As part of a healthy diet, infants need sodium for their bodies to work properly. However, average intakes of sodium among infants and toddlers are above the AI. Caregivers should delay introduction of cow's milk (a source of sodium for infants) until 1 year of age and refrain from offering heavily-seasoned and processed foods.
- *Choose foods containing iron, zinc, and calcium.* Infants need good sources of iron, zinc, and calcium for optimum growth in the first 2 years. These minerals are important for healthy blood, optimal growth, and strong bones. Many infant and toddler foods (e.g., cereal, crackers, and biter biscuits) are fortified with these minerals.

In essence, there is no evidence that restrictive diets during infancy have positive effects, whereas their hazards are well documented.

What Not to Feed an Infant

Following are several foods and practices to avoid when feeding an infant:

- *Honey.* This product may contain spores of *Clostridium botulinum*. The spores can eventually develop into bacteria in the stomach and lead to a foodborne illness known as *botulism*. This can be fatal, especially in children under 1 year old (see Chapter 13).
- *Excessive infant formula or human milk.* After 6 to 8 months, solid foods should play a greater role in satisfying an infant's increasing appetite. The main reason to switch is that solid foods contain considerably more bioavailable iron than do human milk and low-iron formulas. About 24 to 32 ounces (¾ to 1 liters) of human milk or formula daily is ideal after 6 months, with food supplying the rest of the infant's calorie needs.
- *Foods that tend to cause choking.* These foods include hot dogs (unless finely cut into sticks, not coin shapes), candy, whole nuts, grapes, coarsely cut meats, raw carrots, popcorn, and peanut butter. Caregivers should not allow younger children to gobble snack foods during playtime and should supervise all meals.

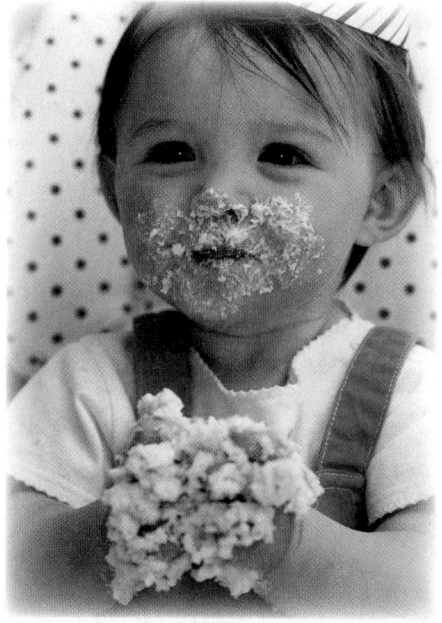

▲ Early feeding attempts should be encouraged, even though they're messy.

▶ **A Summary of Infant Feeding Recommendations**

Breastfed Infants

- Breastfeed for 6 months or longer, if possible. Then introduce infant formula if and when breastfeeding declines or ceases. (Breast milk can also be pumped and placed in a bottle for later use.)
- Provide a vitamin D supplement (400 IU per day).
- Investigate the need for vitamin B-12, fluoride, and iron supplementation to prevent deficiencies.

Formula-Fed Infants

- Use infant formula for the first year of life, preferably an iron-fortified type.
- Provide a vitamin D supplement if formula intake provides less than 400 IU per day.
- Investigate the need for a fluoride supplement if the water supply is not fluoridated.

All Infants

- Add iron-fortified cereal at about 6 months of age.
- Provide a variety of basic, soft foods after 6 months of age, advancing to a varied diet.

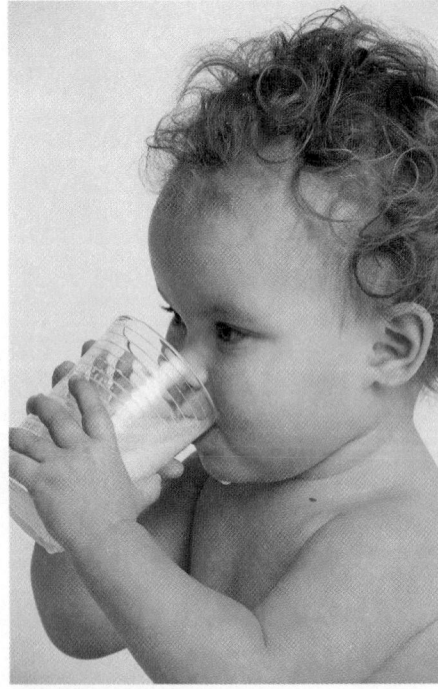

▲ Infants should begin drinking from a cup by 1 year of age. Cups with lids help to prevent spills, but allow a toddler to practice without a lid as his dexterity and coordination improve.

- *Cow's milk, especially low-fat or fat-free cow's milk.* The American Academy of Pediatrics strongly urges parents not to give children under age 2 fat-reduced, 1%, or fat-free milk. Before age 2, the amount of this milk needed to meet calorie needs would supply too many minerals and in turn could overwhelm the kidneys' ability to excrete the excess. The lower fat intake might also harm nervous system development. Beyond 2 years, children can drink fat-reduced, 1%, or fat-free milk, because by this age they are consuming enough solid foods to supply calorie and fat needs.
- *Feeding excessive fruit juice.* The fructose and sorbitol contained in some fruit juices, especially apple and pear juices, can lead to diarrhea because they are slowly absorbed. Also, if fruit juice or related drink products are replacing formula or milk in the diet, the infant may not be receiving adequate calories, calcium, or other nutrients essential for proper growth. Studies have shown a link between excessive amounts of fruit juice and failure to thrive, GI tract complications, obesity, short stature, and poor dental health. Thus, these substances should be used sparingly. Limit fruit juice to 4 to 6 ounces per day for infants from 6 months to 6 years of age.

Inappropriate Infant Feeding Practices

Parents and other caregivers should be aware of a variety of potential health problems related to infant nutrition, so that corrective action can be taken quickly. In some cases, such problems stem from inappropriate feeding practices and inadequate nutrient intakes, including the following:

- Diet providing insufficient iron
- Absence from the diet of an entire MyPlate food group as solid foods are introduced and become the main source of nutrients
- Use of cow's milk before 1 year of age
- Introduction of potential allergy-causing foods, such as egg whites and nuts, prior to 6 months of age
- Drinking raw (unpasteurized) milk, which may be contaminated with bacteria or viruses
- Drinking goat's milk, which is low in folate, iron, vitamin C, and vitamin D
- Failure to begin drinking from a cup by 1 year of age
- Continuing to feed from a bottle past 18 months of age
- Intake of supplemental vitamins or minerals above 100% of the appropriate RDA or other nutrient standard
- Drinking more than 6 ounces of fruit juice per day after 6 months of age, especially as a substitute for infant formula or human milk. (Recall that fruit juice is not to be fed at all before 6 months of age.)

The website of the American Academy of Pediatrics (www.aap.org) can also provide useful information on these and other nutrition-related problems in infancy.

CONCEPT CHECK

Infant formulas generally contain lactose or sucrose, heat-treated proteins from cow's milk, and vegetable oil. Formulas may or may not be fortified with iron. Sanitation is important in preparing and storing formula. Solid foods should not be added to an infant's diet until the child is both ready for and needs solid food, usually at about 6 months of age. The first solid foods can be iron-fortified infant cereals, with gradual additions of other foods—one at a time. Some foods to avoid giving to infants in the first year are honey, cow's milk (particularly fat-reduced, 1%, or fat-free milk), foods that may cause the child to choke, and excessive amounts of fruit juice or related products (e.g., fruit drinks).

15.3 Preschool Children: Nutrition Concerns

The rapid growth rate that characterizes infancy tapers off quickly during the subsequent few years. The average annual weight gain is only 4.5 to 6.6 pounds (2 to 3 kilograms), and the average annual height gain is only 3 to 4 inches (7.5 to 10 centimeters) between the ages of 2 and 5. As a toddler's growth rate tapers off, eating behavior changes. For example, the decreased growth rate leads to a decreased appetite, often called "picky eating," compared with infants.

Because of a reduced appetite, planning a diet that meets the nutrient needs of a preschool child poses a special challenge to caregivers. The USDA's MyPlate, in combination with Team Nutrition, available at www.teamnutrition.usda.gov, offers resources for planning nutritious, age-appropriate meals and snacks. Additional nutrition guidance, starting with pregnancy and extending through the preschool years, is available from the *Start Healthy, Stay Healthy* Resource Center at www.gerber.com. Choosing nutrient-dense foods is particularly important with children who eat relatively little. This is a good time to emphasize some whole grains, fruits, and vegetables without increasing fat and simple sugar intake. A whole-grain ready-to-eat breakfast cereal with limited fat and sugar is an excellent choice. There is no need to decrease fat or simple sugar intake severely, but fatty and sweet food choices should not overwhelm more nutritious ones.

Excessive sodium intake is a concern for preschool children as well (see Further Reading 11). Caregivers can lower sodium intake by limiting salt added during cooking and at the table; cutting back on use of processed foods (e.g., luncheon meats, hot dogs); rinsing canned beans and vegetables before cooking; and encouraging consumption of fruits, vegetables, and whole grains in place of prepackaged snacks. The preschool years are the best time for a child to start a healthful pattern of living and eating, focusing on regular physical activity and nutritious foods. Parents and other caregivers are role models: If they eat a variety of foods, the children will eat a variety of foods. One possible policy is the one-bite rule: Within reason, children should take at least one bite or taste of the foods presented to them. For snacks, parents should select several possibilities of acceptable choices and allow children to choose one; responsibility for food choice by the child ideally should start early.

How to Help a Child Choose Nutritious Foods

One way adults can encourage young children to eat nutritious, well-balanced meals is to serve new foods and repeat exposure to them. The dinner hour is a good time for children to experience new foods and to develop food preferences. Preschool children especially tend to be wary of new foods. One reason is that they have more taste buds, and their taste buds are more sensitive than those of adults. In addition, they have a general distrust of unfamiliar foods. If adults can be patient and persevere, children will build good food habits. It may take 8 to 10 exposures to a new food before a child finds it acceptable. Above all, the dinner table should not become a battleground, and using one food as a bribe to eat another—for example, a piece of pie for peas—is strongly discouraged.

Certain food characteristics, such as crisp textures and mild flavors, are appealing to children. Familiarity also plays an important role in food acceptance. In contrast, young children are especially wary of hot-temperature foods and tend to reject them.

Preschoolers eventually develop skill with spoons and forks and can even use dull knives. However, it's still a good idea to serve some finger foods. A goal should be to make mealtime a happy, social time to share and enjoy healthful foods (see Further Readings 1 and 9).

Childhood Feeding Problems

Tensions between parents, or between parents and children, especially during mealtime, often contribute to eating problems. Getting to the root of family problems and

▶ **Quick Guide to Child Nutrition Needs**

Carbohydrates

- 130 grams per day to supply energy for the central nervous system and prevent ketosis

Protein

- 13–19 grams per day (ages 1–3)
- 34–52 grams per day (older children)

Fat

- at least 5 grams per day of essential fatty acids
- eventually aim for 20% to 35% of total calorie intake by age 19

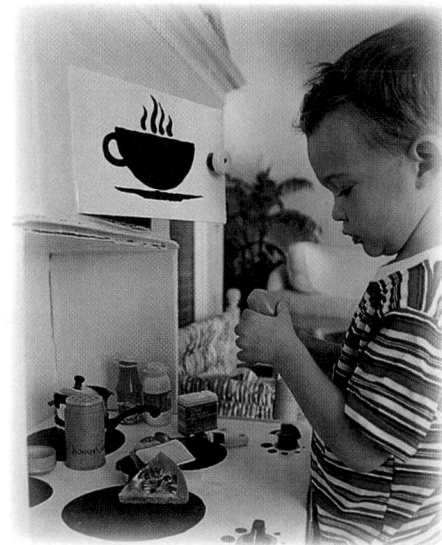

▲ Interest in food starts early in life.

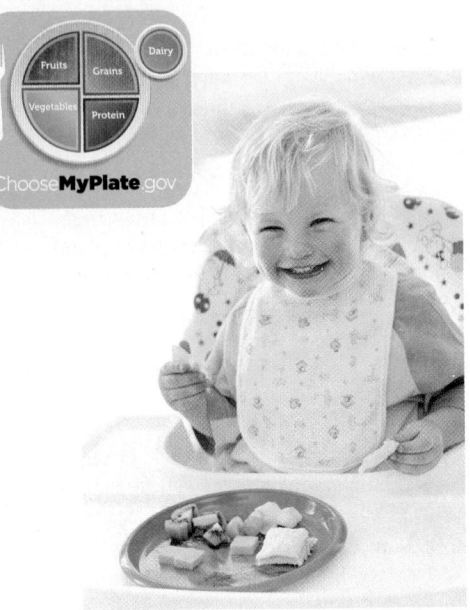

▲ How does this toddler's lunch of a peanut butter sandwich, cubed cheese, kiwi, and grapes compare to MyPlate?

creating a more harmonious family atmosphere are important steps toward resolving many childhood feeding problems. In addition, many parents must be educated as to what to expect of a preschool child and what food-related goals to set. Let's consider some typical complaints and concerns of parents, the causes of the problems, and suggestions for correcting them.

"My Child Won't Eat as Much or as Regularly as He Did as an Infant." This behavior is typical of preschoolers, because their growth rate slows after infancy; thus, they don't need as much food. Parents often need reminding that a 3-year-old can't be expected to eat as voraciously as an infant or to eat adult-size portions. MyPlate is a useful easy-to-understand tool for children, too. The proportions apply to all ages even though the portions will be smaller. Table 15-3 shows a general food plan that conforms to MyPlate proportions and is appropriate for preschool and school-age children. Until about 5 years of age, portion sizes in the vegetables group, fruits group, and protein group should be about 1 tablespoon per year of life, and can be increased as needed. The same advice does not apply to the grains or dairy groups, but consuming too much milk can leave the diet short on iron. Luckily, normal-weight children have a built-in feeding mechanism, which adjusts hunger to regulate food intake at each stage of growth. If a child is developing and growing normally and the caregiver is providing a variety of healthful foods, all can be confident of the child's well-being.

A pattern of picky eating is usually just another expression of independence for children, who have a strong desire to establish a self-determined routine. Caregivers should avoid nagging, forcing, and bribing children to encourage eating. Indirectly, these tactics reinforce picky-eating behaviors due to the added attention given to them. Overall, parents should focus on offering a variety of healthy choices, allowing the child to exert some autonomy over the specific type of food and the amount eaten. A child's sudden loss of appetite, however, may be reason for concern, as a poor appetite may be a sign of underlying illness.

Parents should also be reminded that food likes and dislikes change rapidly in childhood and are influenced by food temperature, appearance, texture, and taste. Sometimes children object to having foods mixed, as in stews and casseroles, even if they normally like the ingredients separately.

In addition, parents should recognize that this is an important age for children to explore the world around them. Even good eaters are sometimes more interested in

TABLE 15-3 Food Plans for Children Based on MyPlate Daily Food Plans

Food Group	Serving Size	Approximate Number of Servings [1]				
		Age 2 [2]	Age 5 [3]	Age 8 [3]	Age 12 [3,4]	Age 16 [3,4]
Grains	ounce	3	5	5	6–7	6–10
Vegetables	cup	1	1.5	2	2.5–3	2.5–3.5
Fruits	cup	1	1.5	1.5	2	2–2.5
Dairy	cup	2	2.5	3	3	3
Protein	ounce	2	4	5	5.5–6	5.5–7
Oils	teaspoon	3	4	5	6	6–8
Solid fats and added sugars	kcal	up to 140	up to 120	up to 120	up to 260–270	up to 260–400

[1]Log on to www.chooseMyPlate.gov for other ages and other physical activity levels.

[2]Based on less than 30 minutes of physical activity.

[3]Based on 30–60 minutes of physical activity.

[4]The lower amounts refer to girls.

exploring than eating. There's room for occasional indulgences, a skipped meal or two, or once in a while "less than ideal" choices. It's eating and lifestyle habits over the course of a month (and lifetime) that matter. Children master their eating when adults set a good example, provide opportunities to learn, give support for exploration, and limit inappropriate behavior.

"My Child Is Always Snacking, Yet She Never Finishes Her Meal." Children have small stomachs. Offering them six or so small meals succeeds better than limiting them to three meals each day. Sticking to three meals a day offers no special nutritional advantages; it's just a social custom. Snacking is fine, as long as good dental habits are practiced. When we eat isn't nearly as important as what we eat. If nutritious snacks are readily available, these are good to offer at midmorning or midafternoon when the child becomes hungry. Fruits and vegetables (fresh, frozen, or canned) and whole-grain breads and crackers are good snack choices. It is important that these snack choices be planned ahead in order to have healthy choices available. Working parents should make sure their children are provided with nutritious snacks to tide them over until dinnertime.

When a child refuses to eat, it's best not to overreact. Doing so may give the child the idea that not eating is a means of getting attention or manipulating a scene. Most children don't starve themselves to any point approaching physical harm. When children refuse to eat, have them sit at the table for a while; if they still aren't interested in eating, remove the food and wait until the next scheduled meal or snack.

"My Child Never Eats Vegetables." Children generally eat enough fruit but not an adequate amount of vegetables. Again, the one-bite policy can be used, including vegetable servings. It takes time for a child to become enthusiastic about a new food; however, with continual exposure and a positive role model, chances are the child may even grow to like it.

Children cannot and should not be forced to eat. They need to develop independence and identities separate from their parents. As stated earlier, children have to choose for themselves—a practice that should be encouraged. No one food is an essential part of a diet. Hunger is still the best means for getting a child to eat. It may be effective to feed children vegetables at the start of a meal, when they are hungriest. Offer new foods with familiar ones. A platter of raw or lightly cooked carrots, broccoli, green and red peppers, cabbage, and mushrooms eaten as a snack with friends may be accepted. A 4- or 5-year-old child can safely eat raw vegetables without fear of choking. Recall that children often are more sensitive than adults to strong flavors and odors. Nutritious dips, such as Ranch dressing, "sell" vegetables to many children. Vegetables may acquire more appeal when children help prepare them. And, as with any food, it is important to remember that children are entitled to their own likes and dislikes, too.

Do Children Need a Multivitamin and Mineral Supplement?

Major scientific groups, such as the American Dietetic Association and the American Society for Clinical Nutrition, believe that multivitamin and mineral supplements are generally unnecessary for healthy children; it's better to emphasize good foods. In fact, consuming fortified foods as well as supplements may lead to intakes above the UL for some nutrients, such as vitamin A and zinc. Children's supplements that are made to look like candy may result in accidental overdose, such as for iron. Fortified ready-to-eat breakfast cereals with milk are especially helpful in closing any gap between current micronutrient intake and needs, such as for vitamin E, folate, and vitamin D. Two micronutrients of particular concern are iron and zinc. These may be lacking in children's diets because they consume such small portions of rich sources, such as animal protein foods. In addition, since the 2010 Dietary Guidelines for Americans suggest that all Americans ages 2 years and older follow a diet low in saturated fat and cholesterol, rich sources of iron and zinc may be lacking in their diets. To compensate,

Food jags, common among preschoolers, are no cause for alarm. A child may switch from one specific food focus to another with equal intensity (older infants may also act this way). If the caregiver continues to offer choices, the child will soon begin to eat a wider variety of foods again, and the specific food focus will disappear as suddenly as it appeared.

Choking is a very preventable hazard for young children. Some suggestions for caregivers include:

- Set a good example at the table by taking small bites and chewing foods thoroughly.

- Have children sit at the table, take their time, and focus on their food during meals and snacks.

- Avoid giving children any foods that are round, firm, sticky, or cut into large chunks. Some examples of foods to avoid are nuts, grapes, raisins, popcorn, peanut butter, and hard pieces of raw fruits or vegetables.

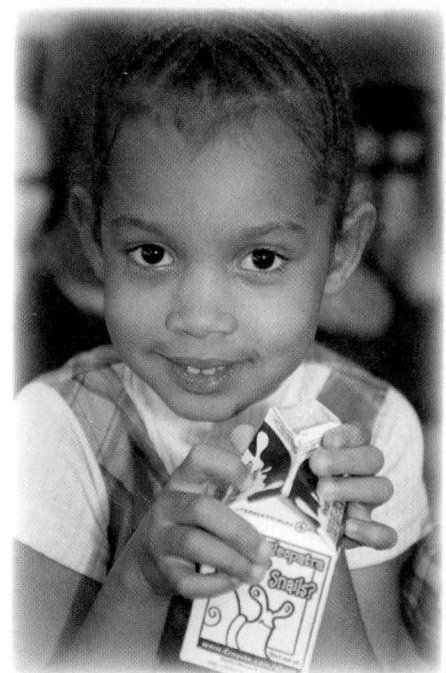

▲ Milk is a nutrient-dense source of protein, calcium, zinc, and other nutrients to support growth. It is especially challenging to meet calcium needs in childhood without regular dairy product consumption (see Chapter 9 for alternative sources of calcium).

parents can search for a whole-grain breakfast cereal that the child likes that also has about 50% of the Daily Value for iron and 25% of the Daily Value for zinc. (This will supply sufficient amounts of both nutrients because the Daily Values are based on the higher needs of adults.) If that's not possible, especially for a child who is ill, has a very erratic food preference pattern or appetite, or is on a weight-loss diet, the American Academy of Pediatrics states that the child may benefit from a children's multivitamin and mineral supplement not exceeding 100% of Daily Values on the label, especially if these conditions persist. Still, as mentioned many times in this textbook, such a practice does not substitute for an otherwise healthy diet—children included.

If current childhood feeding practices are to become more healthful, the focus should be on whole-grain breads and cereals, fruits, vegetables, and low-fat milk and milk products. Children do not need to be severely restricted but, rather, should modify food habits with small changes. Some easy diet changes to begin with are bagels instead of doughnuts, fat-free frozen yogurt instead of ice cream, fat-reduced or 1% milk instead of whole milk, dried fruit instead of candy for snacks, and air-popped popcorn instead of chips.

Nutritional Problems in Preschool Children

Three nutrition-related problems found in preschool children are iron-deficiency anemia, constipation, and dental caries. Proper diet can help correct or relieve these conditions. Vegetarian diets can also pose problems. Autism and lead poisoning are additional conditions that can be affected by nutritional status.

Iron-Deficiency Anemia. The best way to prevent iron-deficiency anemia in children is to provide foods that are adequate sources of iron. Iron-fortified breakfast cereals and a few ounces of lean meat are convenient means of increasing iron in a child's diet. The high proportion of heme iron in many animal foods allows the iron to be more readily absorbed than is iron from plant foods. Consuming a vitamin C source along with the less readily absorbed iron in plants and supplements aids absorption.

Childhood iron-deficiency anemia is most likely to appear in children between the ages of 6 and 24 months. It can lead to decreases in both stamina and learning ability because the oxygen supply to cells decreases. Another effect is lowered resistance to disease. Fortunately, childhood anemia is not common today in North America, probably because of children's use of iron-fortified breakfast cereals. Also deserving of credit in the United States is the Special Supplemental Nutrition Program for Women, Infants, and Children (WIC), sponsored by the U.S. federal government. This program emphasizes the importance of iron-fortified formulas and cereals and distributes these foods—along with nutrition education—to low-income parents of infants and preschool children considered to be at nutritional risk.

Constipation. Constipation may be associated with a more serious disease, yet some young children experience constipation unrelated to any medical condition. When presented with a constipated child, a physician first has to rule out a medical cause, such as intestinal blockage. And, although the most common GI tract symptom that reflects intolerance to cow's milk is diarrhea, chronic constipation may also result. Treatment for constipation generally consists of first evacuating the bowels, generally with an enema. The promotion of regular bowel habits then follows, with laxative use as directed by the physician. Several months to years of supportive intervention may be required for effective treatment.

The primary dietary interventions to alleviate constipation include eating more fiber and drinking more fluids. In the initial stages of treatment, providing certain fruit juices (e.g., prune, grape, and apple) and substituting soy milk for cow's milk may relieve constipation. In the long run, however, whole fruits (e.g., plums, peaches, and apricots) are better choices than juices because whole fruits are less concentrated sources of calories. Other foods to emphasize for fiber include vegetables,

For children who follow a totally vegetarian diet, attention should also focus on protein and vitamin B-12 intake.

Chapter 4 noted that it's unlikely that the use of sugar is the cause of hyperactivity or antisocial behavior in most children.

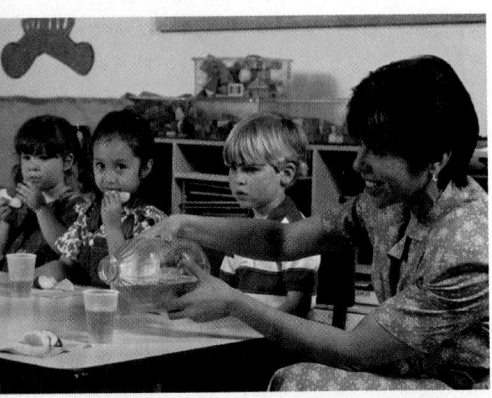

▲ Excessive fruit drink and fruit juice use is another potential problem in preschool (and later adolescent) years. The American Academy of Pediatrics recommends no more than 4 to 6 ounces per day for children 1 to 6 years (and 8 to 12 ounces per day for ages 7 to 18 years). Sweetened soft drinks should also be limited.

whole-grain breads and cereals, and beans. The daily fiber goals for children set by the Food and Nutrition Board vary by age (see margin). Few children meet these goals. Accompanying fluid recommendations are 4 cups (900 milliliters) per day for toddlers and about 5 cups (1200 milliliters) per day for older children.

Dental Caries. A proper diet goes a long way in reducing the risk for dental caries in young children. The following tips can help reduce dental problems in children:

- Begin oral hygiene when teeth start to appear.
- Seek early pediatric dental care.
- Drink fluoridated water.
- Use small amounts of fluoridated toothpaste twice daily.
- Snack in moderation.
- Have a dentist apply tooth sealants if needed.
- Avoid sticky, high-sugar snacks, especially between meals.
- If toddlers or preschoolers are chewing gum, sugarless gum is the best choice, as this has been shown to reduce the incidence of dental caries.

Vegetarianism in Childhood. Vegetarian diets can pose several risks for young children. These include the possibility of developing iron-deficiency anemia, a deficiency of vitamin B-12, and rickets from a vitamin D deficiency. During the first few years of life, children also may not consume enough calories when following a bulky vegetarian diet. These known pitfalls are easily avoided by informed diet planning (see Nutrition and Your Health: Vegetarian and Plant-Based Diets in Chapter 6). Diets for children who eat totally vegetarian fare should focus on protein, vitamin B-12, iron, and zinc content, with additional emphasis on vitamin D (or regular sun exposure) and calcium. Some of these dietary inadequacies can be compensated for by increasing oils, nuts, seeds, ready-to-eat breakfast cereals, and fortified soy milk in the diet.

Autism. Autism spectrum disorder (ASD) is characterized by a range of problems with social interaction, verbal and nonverbal communication, and/or unusual, repetitive, or limited activities and interests. These disorders usually are diagnosed in early childhood and affect an estimated 1 in every 150 children, with higher prevalence in boys than girls. The causes for ASD are not well understood, but there is a definite genetic component.

ASD can both affect and be affected by nutritional status (see Further Reading 6). In addition to developmental and behavioral abnormalities, many children with ASD also experience GI disorders, such as constipation, diarrhea, or reflux disease. Such disorders may impair nutrient intake or absorption. Some autistic children may have feeding problems related to developmental impairments. Also, picky eating behaviors may affect nutrient intake. Thus, careful attention to nutrient-dense food choices is warranted.

There are many nutrient-based theories concerning the causes and treatment of ASD. Nutritional interventions, such as dietary restrictions or nutrient supplements, are commonly employed by families affected by ASD. A widely used nutritional intervention is the gluten-free, casein-free (GFCF) diet, which eliminates all wheat, barley, rye, and milk products (see Further Reading 8). Proponents of this treatment propose that sensitivities to certain food proteins may have effects on neurotransmitter synthesis, thereby altering nervous system function. Clinical evidence supporting the effectiveness of the GFCF diet is limited, but promising. If the GFCF diet is used, families should enlist the aid of a registered dietitian to ensure dietary adequacy, particularly for protein, calcium, vitamin D, folic acid, and some B vitamins.

Other popular therapies for ASD include supplementation with probiotics, vitamin B-6 (0.6 mg/kg/d), magnesium (6.0 mg/kg/d), and omega-3 fatty acids (not exceeding 800 mg/d). Although sparse, research on these therapies is encouraging. There is evidence of altered absorption or metabolism of nutrients among children

▶ **Food and Nutrition Board Fiber Recommendations for Children**

Young Children

1–3 years	19 grams/day
4–8 years	25 grams/day

Boys

9–13 years	31 grams/day
14–18 years	38 grams/day

Girls

9–13 years	26 grams/day
14–18 years	26 grams/day

Despite a popularly held belief, scientific evidence does not support a causal relationship between mercury in vaccines and autism. Although small risks are inherent with routine vaccinations, the risks of infectious diseases are far worse.

with autism, so even with adequate nutrient intake, availability of some nutrients for metabolic processes may be low. Even though these supplements carry a low risk of adverse effects, caution is warranted to avoid overdoses. Because of the rising incidence of ASD and the lack of curative treatments, nutritional interventions for ASD will continue to be an active area of research.

Lead Poisoning. Humans may be exposed to lead from drinking contaminated water, consuming or inhaling lead dust (e.g., from cracked and peeling lead paint), contaminated dietary supplements (e.g., calcium supplements derived from bone meal), or foods stored or prepared in lead-containing vessels. In 2008, nearly 30,000 children were diagnosed with lead poisoning in the United States. Young children are particularly susceptible to the damaging effects of lead poisoning, which include long-term intellectual and behavioral impairments as well as increased risk for several chronic diseases in adulthood. Although it does not address the source of exposure, proper nutrition can reduce the risks of lead poisoning for children. Consuming regular meals, moderating fat intake, and ensuring adequate iron and calcium status are dietary practices known to reduce lead absorption. Adequate zinc, thiamin, and vitamin E intakes also reduce the harmful effects of absorbed lead. For lowest lead levels, only cold water should be used for drinking and preparation of formula or food. Letting cold water run from the tap for 2 to 3 minutes after a long period of inactivity (e.g., overnight) will limit the amount of lead that has accumulated in tap water. If the public water supply contains a high concentration of lead, bottled water is a safer alternative, particularly for formula preparation. Overall, a balanced meal plan that offers a variety of whole grains, lean meats, and low-fat dairy products is especially useful for protecting children from lead poisoning.

Objectives of *Healthy People 2020* include reducing mean blood lead level by 10% and eliminating elevated blood lead levels in children.

CONCEPT CHECK

The rapid growth rate of an infant's first year slows during the toddler and preschool years (ages 1 to 5). As a child's appetite decreases, adults need to serve nutrient-dense foods and allow the child to decide how much to eat. Sudden shifts in food preferences are to be expected. Snacking is fine if attention is given to the selection of healthful foods and good dental hygiene. Although a children's multivitamin and mineral supplement is usually not needed—a plan following MyPlate's Daily Food Plan that includes a serving of fortified ready-to-eat breakfast cereal should meet nutrient needs—use of such a supplement is a reasonable practice. Children need plenty of iron-rich food to prevent iron-deficiency anemia, as well as zinc for growth. Adequate mineral status also reduces risk of lead poisoning. Adequate fiber and fluid help prevent constipation. Diets for children who eat totally vegetarian fare should focus on meeting needs for protein, vitamin D, vitamin B-12, calcium, iron, and zinc. Potentially useful nutritional treatments for autism include the gluten-free, casein-free diet and supplementation with vitamin B-6, magnesium, probiotics, and essential fatty acids; research in this area is ongoing.

▲ How does this boy's dinner of broiled fish, broccoli, green beans, carrots, and zucchini compare to MyPlate?

15.4 School-Age Children: Nutrition Concerns

The diets of many school-age students can stand general improvement, particularly with regard to fruit, vegetable, whole-grain, and dairy choices. Drinking minimal amounts of sugared soft drinks is also advised. One survey of U.S. schoolchildren revealed that on the day of the survey, 40% of the children ate no vegetables, except for potatoes or tomato sauce, and 20% ate no fruits. Less than 20% of school-age girls consume adequate calcium. In general, the nutritional concerns and goals applicable to school-age children are the same as those discussed in relation to preschoolers. However, with the added pressures of peers, health messages from the media, and an increasing desire for independence, these goals may be harder to achieve as children grow older. MyPlate's daily food plans, which are tailored to age, gender, height, weight, and activity level, continue to be a good basis for diet planning, with an emphasis on moderating fat and sugar intake and ensuring adequate iron, zinc, and calcium intake (Fig. 15-3). Now let's look at several nutritional issues of particular concern during the school-age years.

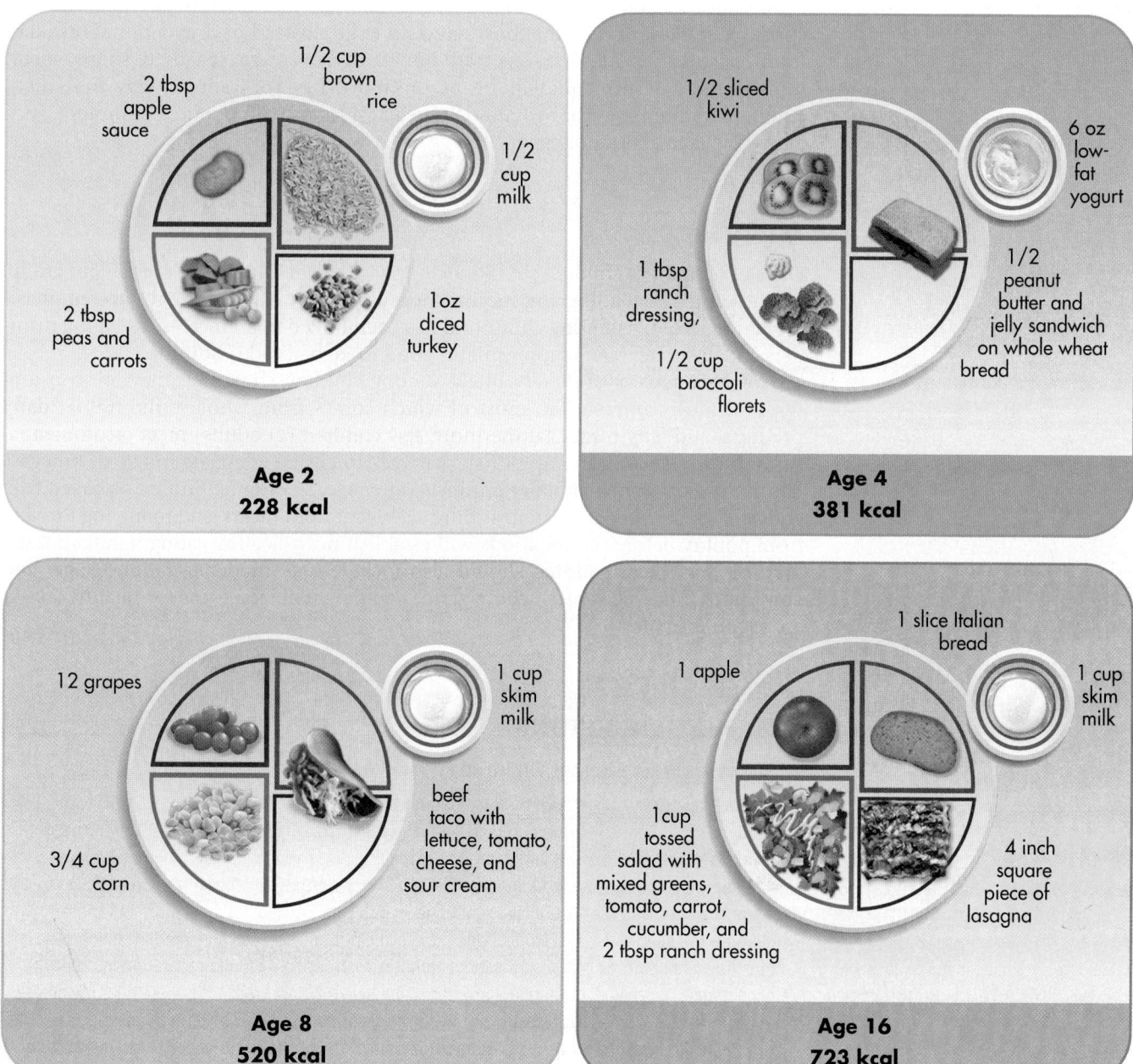

FIGURE 15-3 ▶ Using MyPlate to build a healthy meal for children. MyPlate is useful tool for all Americans, ages 2 and older. MyPlate proportions apply to children as well as adults, but portion sizes and food choices may vary by age.

NEWSWORTHY
NUTRITION

Healthy eating behaviors start at home

Parenting style and frequency of family meals are two important predictors of healthy eating behaviors among children, according to a recent review of family correlates of pediatric obesity. Of four basic parenting styles, authoritative parenting, which is demanding yet responsive to children, promotes healthy eating and physical activity and is associated with low rates of pediatric obesity. Eating family meals is also associated with healthy eating and lower BMI in children. When parents and children enjoy meals together, children are supervised and engaged while parents have the opportunity to communicate and model healthy behaviors. Thus, children eat more fruits and vegetables, leading to better nutrient intake, and are less likely to have disordered eating behaviors. Family meals and an authoritative parenting style promote health at the table and beyond.

Source: Berge JM: A review of family correlates of child and adolescent obesity: What has the 21st century taught us so far? *International Journal of Adolescent Medicine and Health* 21:457, 2009.

■ connect
NUTRITION
Check out the Connect site
www.mcgrawhillconnect.com
to further explore healthy eating behaviors.

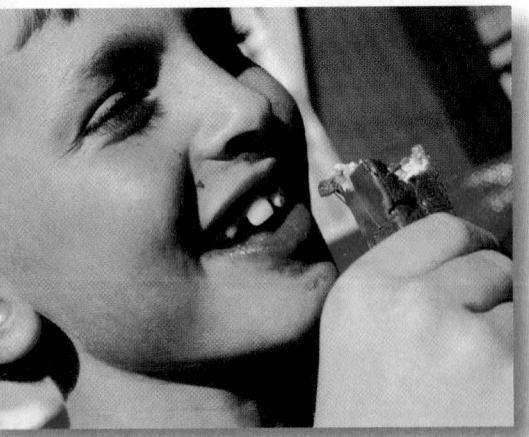

▲ Sweets should be consumed in moderation in childhood, but do not have to be avoided altogether.

CRITICAL THINKING

Tim refuses to eat breakfast before school. He doesn't like cereal, toast, or any of the other usual breakfast foods. What can Tim's parents do to ensure that he eats nutritious foods before leaving for school?

Breakfast

Once children enter school, their eating patterns become more scheduled, and the consumption of regular meals—especially breakfast—becomes an important focus. A fortified ready-to-eat breakfast cereal is typically the greatest source of iron, vitamin A, and folic acid for children ages 2 to 18. Although there is controversy over the true benefit of breakfast for cognitive ability, children who eat breakfast are more likely to meet their daily needs for vitamins and minerals compared to children not eating breakfast. To influence morning test performance, it appears that breakfast must be eaten within a few hours of a test; the subsequent rise in blood glucose is thought to enhance performance.

Breakfast menus need not be limited to traditional fare. A little imagination can spark the interest of even the most reluctant child. Instead of conventional breakfast foods, parents can offer leftovers from dinner, such as pizza, spaghetti, soups, yogurt topped with trail mix, chili with beans, or sandwiches. For lasting energy and satiety, combine traditional carbohydrate-rich breakfast foods with a source of protein, such as low-fat cheese, nuts, or eggs.

Fat Intake

Diets of school-age children should include a variety of foods from each major group, not necessarily excluding any specific food because of its fat content. Overemphasis on fat-reduced diets during childhood has been linked to an increase in eating disorders and encourages an inappropriate "good food, bad food" attitude.

However, surveys of dietary intake among children show that they are consuming too much saturated fat, most of which comes from whole milk, full-fat dairy products, and fatty meats. Furthermore, few children (or adults) meet recommendations to include two servings of fish per week to ensure adequate intake of omega-3 fats. Emphasizing low-fat dairy products (after age 2), offering broiled or baked fish, choosing leaner cuts of meat, trimming visible fat from meats, and removing the skin from poultry before serving foods will establish heart-healthy eating habits to last a lifetime. Snacks for children should also include only moderate fat and sugar and emphasize fruit, vegetables, whole grain, and dairy choices. Ideas for healthy snacks are found in Table 15-4.

MAKING DECISIONS

Nutrition Education for Children

Children spend the majority of their waking hours in school, so it is a great place to learn about positive, healthy eating habits (see Further Reading 3). A strong emphasis on nutrition in schools can help children understand why healthy diet habits will make them feel more energetic, look better, and work more efficiently. Federally-funded programs such as USDA's Team Nutrition and the CDC's National Bone Health Campaign are a good start, but more changes are needed. School foodservice outlets, including cafeterias and vending machines, must present healthier options for school children. Instruction on food preparation in home economics classes and after-school programs will help children learn to prepare healthy meals and snacks. Increased participation in physical education classes and recreational sports is more likely to improve academic performance than detract from it. However, positive nutrition influences must extend beyond the classroom to change persistent trends toward obesity and chronic diseases. Caregivers and other adult role models need to create safe opportunities for children to be active and must practice what they preach when it comes to healthy habits.

TABLE 15-4 Twenty Healthy Snack Ideas for School-Age Children

	Iron	Zinc	Calcium	Vitamin C	Fiber
Almonds (1 oz)			✓		✓
Applesauce (1/2 cup)				✓	✓
Bean and cheese burrito (1)	✓	✓	✓		✓
Cheese (1 oz) and whole-wheat crackers (6)	✓	✓	✓		✓
Dried cranberries (1/4 cup)				✓	✓
Frozen fruit pieces (1 cup)				✓	✓
Fruit salad (1 cup)				✓	✓
Fruit smoothie (1 cup)				✓	✓
Hard-boiled egg	✓	✓			
Hummus (2 tbsp) with bell pepper rings (1 cup)				✓	✓
Low-fat microwave popcorn (3 tbsp unpopped)					✓
Mini-pizzas on whole-grain English muffins (2)	✓	✓	✓	✓	✓
Peanut butter (2 tbsp) and apple slices (1 cup)		✓		✓	✓
Quick breads, such as banana bread, 1 slice	✓				✓
String cheese (1 stick)			✓		
Trail mix (1/4 cup)	✓	✓		✓	✓
Tuna salad (1/2 cup) in whole-wheat pita pocket	✓	✓			✓
Whole-grain cereal (1 cup)	✓	✓			✓
Whole-wheat pasta salad with veggies (1 cup)	✓	✓		✓	✓
Yogurt (8 oz) with granola (2 tbsp)		✓	✓		✓

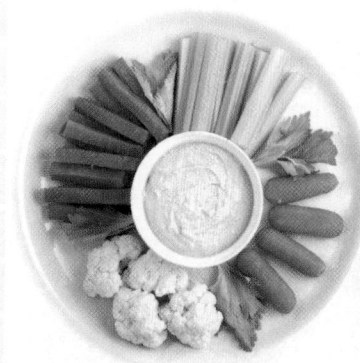

Type 2 Diabetes

Type 2 diabetes is generally thought to be an adult condition. As reviewed in the Nutrition and Your Health section, Diabetes—When Blood Glucose Regulation Fails in Chapter 4, it frequently occurs in overweight people older than 40. However, physicians have noted an alarming increase in the frequency of the disease among children (and teenagers). This is primarily due to the rise in obesity in this age group, coupled with minimal physical activity. Up to 85% of children with the disease are overweight at diagnosis. Experts are calling for screening for diabetes in at-risk children every 2 years, starting at age 10 or at the onset of puberty. Besides obesity and a sedentary lifestyle, other risk factors include having a first- or second-degree relative with the disease or belonging to a nonwhite population. Appropriate diet and lifestyle intervention should be implemented, along with the use of diabetes medications when necessary. A regular intake of low-glycemic-load fruits, vegetables, and whole-grain breads and cereals is especially recommended.

Early Signs of Cardiovascular Disease

Also paralleling the increase in childhood obesity, early signs of cardiovascular disease have become increasingly prevalent among children and adolescents. One out of five youths between the ages of 12 and 19 years has abnormal blood lipids. Therefore, lifestyle modifications to delay the progression of the disease are important throughout the lifespan. The American Academy of Pediatrics now recommends that at-risk children first undergo cholesterol screening sometime between the ages of 2 and 10, followed by repeated cholesterol screening every 3 to 5 years (see Further Reading 7). Children are considered "at risk" if they are overweight, have high blood pressure, smoke, or have diabetes; if they have a family history of cardiovascular disease; or if family history is unknown. For children whose cholesterol is elevated, lifestyle approaches, such as weight management through dietary modification and increased physical activity, are the first line of therapy. Following a meal plan that is based on the Dietary Guidelines and conforms to MyPlate's Daily Food Plan would be appropriate for prevention of cardiovascular disease. Some high-risk children may be candidates for cholesterol-lowering medications.

Overweight and Obesity

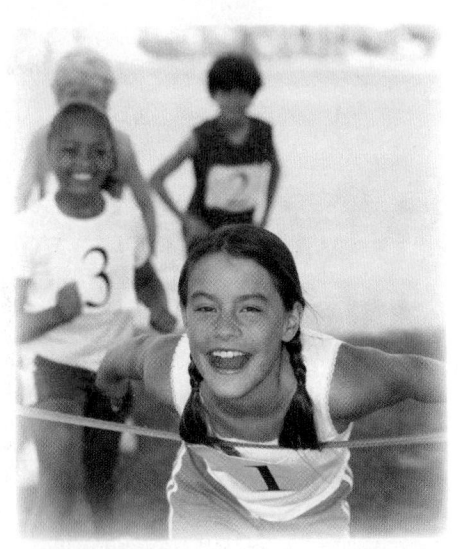

▲ Regular physical activity is an important part of prevention and treatment of weight problems in childhood. The goal is about 60 minutes of such activity each day. Many children do not meet this goal.

In the United States, more than 30% of school-age children are overweight or obese. The number of cases is increasing, especially in minority populations. In the short run, ridicule, embarrassment, possibly depression, and short stature linked to early puberty are the main consequences of such obesity. In the long run, significant health problems associated with obesity, such as cardiovascular disease, type 2 diabetes, and hypertension, usually will appear in adulthood or earlier. Childhood obesity is a serious health threat because about 40% of obese children (and about 80% of obese adolescents) become obese adults. Significant weight gain generally begins between ages 5 and 7, during puberty, or during the teenage years.

Research points to many potential causes of childhood obesity. Recall the nature versus nurture discussion in Chapter 7. Some infants are born with lower metabolic rates; they use calories more efficiently and in turn can more easily produce fat stores. Studies also suggest, though, that this genetic link accounts for only one-third of individual differences in body weight.

Researchers believe that, although diet is an important factor, inactivity is also a contributor to the increase in childhood obesity (see Further Readings 4 and 5). Studies show that as children age, physical activity steadily declines. By age 15, only one-third of children are getting the recommended 60 minutes of exercise per day. It doesn't help that physical education classes are now elective in many high schools. Today's generation of children now glues itself to the TV for an average of 24 hours per week; many children spend another 10 hours or so playing computer and video games. The American Academy of Pediatrics recommends a limit of 14 hours of TV and video time per week for children over age 2 (no television is recommended for children younger than 2 years). In addition, excessive snacking, overreliance on fast-food restaurants, parental neglect, the media in general, lack of safe areas to play, and the abundant availability of high-calorie food choices contribute to childhood obesity. Soft drinks and other sugared beverages are especially implicated.

The initial approach in treating an obese child is to assess how much physical activity he or she engages in. If a child spends much free time in sedentary activities (such as watching television or playing video games), more physical activities should be encouraged. The Physical Activity Guidelines for Americans recommend 60 minutes or more of moderate to intense physical activity per day for children and adolescents. Learning to engage in and enjoy regular physical activity will help children not only to attain a healthy body weight but also to keep a similar body weight later in life. An increase in physical activity won't just happen; parents and other caregivers need to plan for it. Getting the family together for a brisk walk after dinner encourages healthy habits for all involved. Age-appropriate activities for elementary school-age children include walking, dancing, jumping rope, and participation in organized sports that focus on fun rather than intense competition. For middle school-age children, more complex organized sports (e.g., football and basketball) are of interest and some weight training with small weights can also be beneficial.

Moderation in calorie intake is important, especially the limitation of high-calorie foods, such as sugared soft drinks and whole milk. The focus should be on more vitamin- and mineral-dense foods and healthy snacks. An emphasis on appropriate portion sizes may help youth learn to curb excessive food intake. Making small changes such as substituting low-fat for whole milk, or canned fruit in its own juice instead of heavy syrup, can moderately cut calories without sacrificing taste or disrupting normal eating patterns. To specifically address the increased burden of overweight and obesity among minority populations, health professionals must become versed in varied cultural food preferences.

Resorting to a weight-loss diet is usually not necessary—it is best to emphasize changing habits that allow for weight maintenance. Children have an advantage over adults in dealing with obesity; their bodies can use stored energy for growth. Thus, if weight gain can be moderated, increases in height and resulting lean body tissue may reduce the percentage of body weight accounted for as stored fat, yielding a more healthful weight-to-height ratio. This is one reason it is desirable to treat obesity in childhood. Further growth can contribute to success. If weight loss is necessary in younger children, it should be gradual, about ½ to 1 pound per week. In some cases, the child should be watched closely to ensure that the rate of growth continues to be normal. The child's calorie intake should not be so low that gains in height diminish. In some cases, medications may be prescribed under a physician's care (e.g., orlistat [Xenical]). For the 3% of American children who are morbidly obese, bariatric surgery may be an option for weight management (see Further Readings 12 and 13).

CONCEPT CHECK

The school-age child is advised to use MyPlate as a guide for eating and especially moderate choices high in fat and simple sugars. Breakfast is an important meal to refuel the body for a new school day and to help ensure fulfilling nutrient needs for the day. Attention to regular physical activity and healthy diet should help prevent/treat childhood obesity and build a desirable lifestyle pattern for later life.

15.5 Teenage Years: Nutrition Concerns

Most girls begin a rapid growth spurt between the ages of 10 and 13, and most boys experience rapid growth between the ages of 12 and 15. Nearly every organ in the body grows during these periods. Most noticeable are increases in height and weight and the development of secondary sexual characteristics. Girls usually begin menstruating (reach **menarche**) during this growth spurt, and they grow very little beyond 2 years after menarche. Early-maturing girls may begin their growth spurt as early as age 7 to 8, whereas early-maturing boys may begin growing by age 9 to 10.

During this adolescent growth spurt, girls gain about 10 inches (25 centimeters) in height, and boys gain about 12 inches (30 centimeters). Girls also tend to accumulate both lean and fat tissue, whereas boys tend to gain mostly lean tissue. This growth spurt provides about 50% of ultimate adult weight and about 15% of ultimate adult height (review Fig. 15-1).

As the growth spurt begins, teenagers begin to eat more. If teens choose nutritious food, they can take advantage of their increased hunger and easily satisfy their nutrient

To get kids involved in exercise, new physical education classes have been introduced into schools. These classes provide lifelong fitness lessons in such activities as rock climbing, in-line skating, and recreational jogging. These classes help promote activity because they take the focus away from teams and competition, which often discourage and embarrass kids who lack athletic talent.

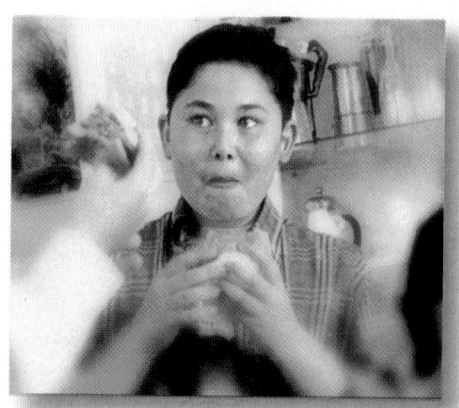

▲ Supersized portions of foods such as hamburgers and sugared soft drinks served to children are contributing to the obesity and type 2 diabetes epidemics they are experiencing.

menarche The onset of menstruation. Menarche usually occurs around age 13, 2 or 3 years after the first signs of puberty start to appear.

Drinking soft drinks in place of milk causes many teenagers to have inadequate calcium intake. Over the last 20 years, soft drinks have been replacing milk as the preferred beverage of adolescents. Only half of school-age boys and 20% of girls meet recommendations for calcium intake. This trend has been linked to decreased bone mass and increased bone fractures in this age group.

A strictly vegetarian diet must be monitored for adequate energy, protein, iron, vitamin B-12, calcium, and vitamin D (the latter if sun exposure is not sufficient). These nutrients become particularly important in teenagers, as their diets are often already compromised.

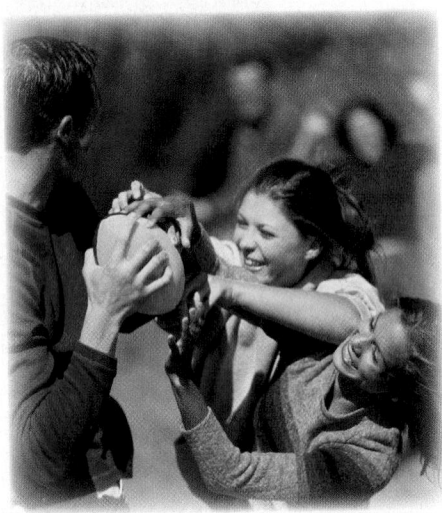

▲ An active lifestyle coupled with a healthy diet should be part of the teen years. Both habits contribute to bone development and bone strength.

Alcoholism is a significant health problem that may have its roots in the teen years. Smoking—another habit that compromises health—also often begins in teen years. Some of the impetus for smoking is the desire to control body weight—but this is not an advisable method.

needs. As discussed for younger age groups, MyPlate can serve as a guide for meeting these nutrient needs (Table 15-3). Following such a plan will meet carbohydrate needs (130 grams per day) and protein needs (52 grams per day for males and 46 grams per day for females).

Nutritional Problems and Concerns of Teens

Anorexia nervosa and bulimia nervosa are nutritional concerns of the teen years, as covered in detail in Chapter 11. Other nutritional problems are more common during the teen years. A survey of high school students showed that only a little over 25% had eaten five servings of fruits and vegetables on the previous day, and they are consuming approximately 25% more sodium than recommended. Another concern is that many teenage girls stop drinking milk, so they may not consume enough calcium to allow for maximal mineralization of bones through their early twenties. Inadequate calcium intake during the teenage years sets the stage for development of osteoporosis later in life.

Inadequate Calcium Intake. Many teenagers are not meeting their needs for calcium. The RDA for calcium for both males and females between ages 9 and 18 years is 1300 milligrams per day, compared with only 1000 milligrams per day for younger children. Three servings per day from the dairy group are recommended for all teenagers and young adults to meet calcium needs. Figure 2-1 in Chapter 2 shows the stark contrast between milk and typical soft drinks with respect to calcium and other nutrients. If dairy products are not consumed, alternative calcium sources need to be included.

Iron Deficiency. A further concern is iron deficiency. Iron-deficiency anemia sometimes appears in girls after they start menstruating (menarche) and in boys during their growth spurt. About 10% of teenagers have low iron stores or related anemia. Teens who strive to forge an identity by adopting dietary patterns unfamiliar to their families—vegetarianism, for example—may not know enough about the alternative diet pattern to keep from developing health problems, such as iron-deficiency anemia. It's important that teenagers choose good food sources of iron, such as lean meats, whole grains, and enriched cereals. Teenage girls, particularly those with heavy menstrual flows, need to eat good sources of iron (or regularly consume an iron supplement). Iron-deficiency anemia is a highly undesirable condition for a teen. It can produce increased fatigue and decreased ability to concentrate and learn. School and physical performance may suffer.

MAKING DECISIONS

Nutrition and Acne

Acne is a common teen concern—about 80% of teens experience it. Although it's popularly believed that eating nuts, chocolate, and pizza can make acne worse, scientific studies have failed to show a strong link between these dietary factors and acne. Based on the results of observational research, two dietary practices currently under study for possible roles in the development of acne include high glycemic load and consumption of cow's milk or whey protein-based product (e.g., body building supplements). However, sufficient evidence is not currently available to support any drastic dietary changes to control acne. A balanced diet and adequate fluid intake combined with sensible hygiene practices remain the best practices to promote skin health.

Acne medications, such as Accutane, contain analogs of vitamin A (e.g., 13-*cis* retinoic acid). Although these treatments can be effective, close supervision by a physician is crucial, as vitamin A analogs can be toxic. Vitamin A itself is no help in treating acne, and excess amounts of vitamin A or related analogs taken during pregnancy can cause birth defects. Thus, girls taking these vitamin A medications should not become pregnant.

Helping Teens Eat More Nutritious Foods

Teenagers face a variety of challenges. They pursue their independence, experience identity crises, seek peer acceptance, and worry about physical appearance. These factors affect food choice. Advertisers take advantage of this by pushing a vast array of products—candy, gum, soft drinks, and snacks—at the teenage market. Potato chips and French fries make up more than one-third of the vegetable servings consumed by teens. Additionally, many schools offer French fries on a regular basis, and soft drink machines can be found in school hallways and cafeterias, in turn competing with the school lunch. The increased consumption of fast-foods, sugary beverages, and snack foods crowds out nutrient-dense foods, thus limiting intake of calcium, iron, zinc, fat-soluble vitamins, and folate.

Teens often do not think about the long-term benefits of good health. They have a hard time relating today's actions to tomorrow's health outcomes. Many teenagers tend to think they can change habits later; there's no hurry.

Still, healthful teen food habits do not require giving up favorite foods. Small portions of fatty foods can complement larger portions of fat-free and reduced-fat dairy products, lean meats, vegetable proteins, fruits, vegetables, and whole-grain products. An example of this type of meal is a plain hamburger with a garden salad (minimize the amount of regular dressing or use a low-fat variety), small order of French fries or chili, and a medium diet soft drink or reduced-fat or fat-free milk.

Are Teenage Snacking Practices Harmful?

Teens often obtain one-fourth to one-third of all their calories and major nutrients from snacks. Unfortunately, studies have found just what you might expect—that teens snack mostly on potato and corn chips, cookies, candies, and ice cream. Key reasons for snacking include an opportunity to get out and socialize with friends, accessibility, hunger, and celebration of a special event. Teenagers can obtain many nutrients from snacking. Even fast-food restaurants offer some good food choices. By choosing wisely and eating in moderation, teens can eat at fast-food restaurants occasionally and still consume a very healthful diet. Snacks and fast-food restaurants themselves are not the problem; poor food choices in terms of type and quantity are.

Lack of exercise and poor dietary habits formed during teenage years often continue into adulthood and may increase risk of chronic diseases, such as cardiovascular disease, osteoporosis, and some types of cancer. Getting this message across to teenagers is an important and challenging task for parents and educators.

Obesity is a growing problem among teenagers, and about 30% of obese teenagers have the metabolic syndrome (Syndrome X) discussed in Chapters 4 and 5. If a teen attains ultimate adult height and is still obese, a weight-loss regimen may be necessary. This is especially appropriate after the adolescent growth spurt. Weight loss should be gradual, perhaps 1 pound per week, and generally follow the advice in Chapter 7. Weight loss medications may also be prescribed.

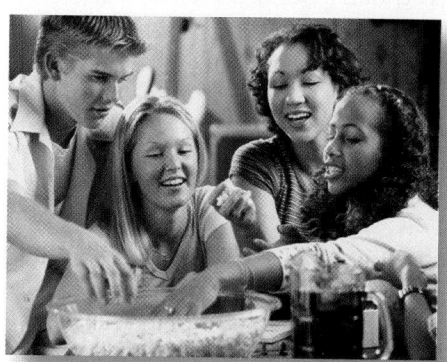

▲ The teenage years are noted for snacking. With reasonable food choices, teenagers can have healthful diets.

CONCEPT CHECK

A second period of rapid growth occurs during the teen years. Girls generally start this growth spurt earlier than boys. MyPlate's Daily Food Plan can direct meal planning. Common nutritional problems in these years arise from poor food choices and include inadequate calcium intake in girls and iron-deficiency anemia. Changes occur so rapidly during these years, and in so many areas—psychological, social, and physical—it may be difficult to stress the relevance of nutrition to teenagers. Moderation in fat and sugar intake are important goals to consider when choosing snacks.

Food Allergies and Intolerances

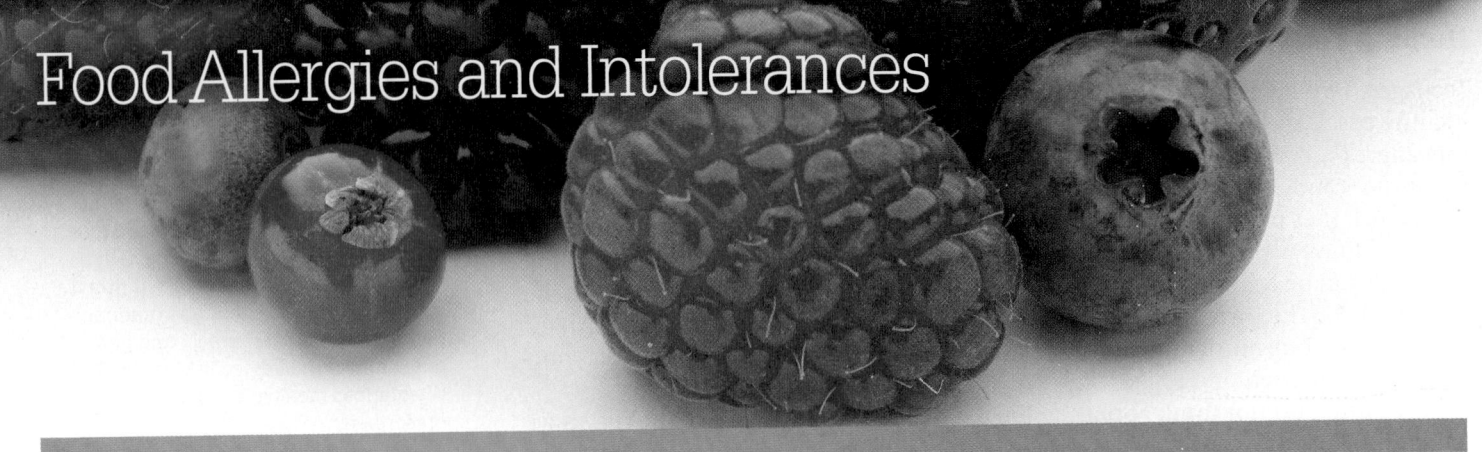

Food allergies are on the rise. Between 1997 and 2007, food allergies among children increased by 18%. What used to be a rare medical incident is now the cause for 30,000 emergency room visits and 150 to 200 deaths per year. Food allergies cost Americans more than $500 million per year. Today, food allergies affect about 8% (5.9 million) of children in the United States, one-third of whom suffer from multiple food allergies (see Further Reading 10).

Adverse reactions to foods—indicated by sneezing, coughing, nausea, vomiting, diarrhea, hives, and other rashes—are broadly classed as food allergies (also called hypersensitivities) or **food intolerances.** Whereas allergies involve an immune response to a foreign protein (**allergen**), intolerances are caused by an individual's inability to digest a certain food component or by the direct effect of a food component or contaminant on the body. Let's examine each process, first allergies and then intolerances.

FOOD ALLERGIES: SYMPTOMS AND MECHANISM

Allergic reactions to foods are common (Fig. 15-4) and occur more frequently in females than males. Food allergies occur most often during infancy and young adulthood. Three types of reactions may occur after the ingestion of problem foods by susceptible people:

- *Classic*–itching, reddening skin, asthma, swelling, choking, and a runny nose
- *GI tract*–nausea, vomiting, diarrhea, intestinal gas, bloating, pain, constipation, and indigestion

- *General*–headache, skin reactions, tension and fatigue, tremors, and psychological problems

Any reaction milder than these is a **food sensitivity.**

Allergic reactions vary not only in the body system affected, but also in their duration, ranging from seconds to a few days. A generalized, all-systems reaction is called **anaphylactic shock.** This severe allergic response results in low blood pres-

food intolerance An adverse reaction to food that does not involve an allergic reaction.

allergen A foreign protein, or antigen, that induces excess production of certain immune system antibodies; subsequent exposure to the same protein leads to allergic symptoms. Whereas all allergens are antigens, not all antigens are allergens.

food sensitivity A mild reaction to a substance in a food that might be expressed as slight itching or redness of the skin.

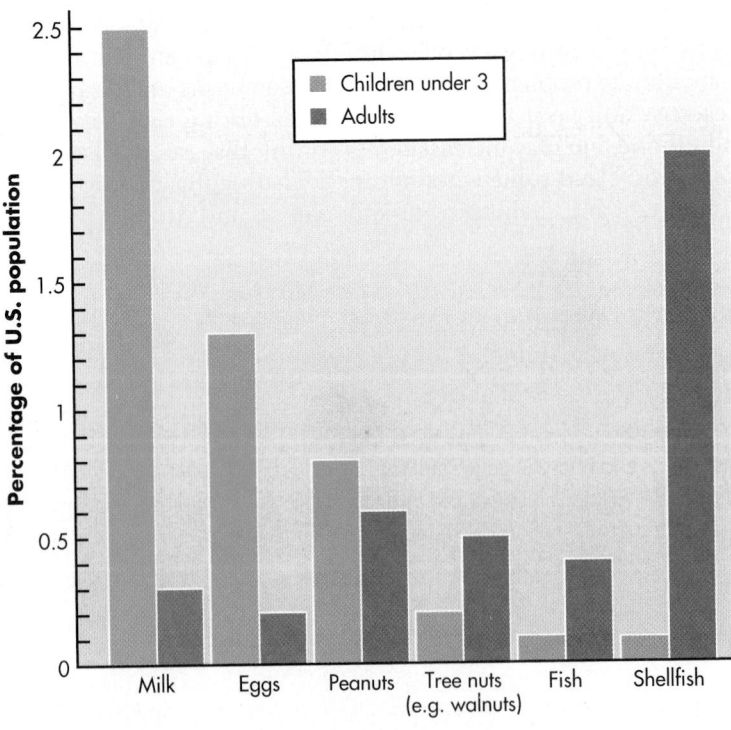

FIGURE 15-4 ▶ Types of allergies and percentage of U.S. population with those allergies.

Source: Journal of Allergy and Clinical Immunology (study done by Mount Sinai School of Medicine).

sure and distress of the respiratory system and GI tract. It can be fatal. A person who is extremely sensitive to a food may not be able to touch the food or even be in the same room where it is being cooked without reacting to it. Although any food can trigger anaphylactic shock, the most common culprits are peanuts (a legume, not a nut), tree nuts (e.g., walnuts, pecans, etc.), shellfish, milk (look for an ingredient called casein on the label), eggs (look for the ingredient albumin on the label), soybeans, wheat, and fish. Other foods frequently identified with adverse reactions include meat and meat products, fruits, and cheese. For a small number of people, avoiding foods such as peanuts or shellfish is a matter of life and death.

Basically, allergies are an inappropriate response of the immune system. When immune cells identify a harmful foreign protein (**antigen**), they destroy it and produce antibodies to it, so that the next response to the harmful substance will be swift and effective. Almost all food allergies are caused by proteins in foods that act as antigens (also called **allergens**). In these cases, the immune system mistakes the food protein for a harmful substance and mounts an immune response, leading to symptoms such as hives, runny nose, and GI disturbances.

No one is sure why the immune system sometimes overreacts to harmless proteins. The early introduction (e.g., before 4 to 6 months of age) of solid foods to infants may trigger food allergies. The reasoning is that the infant's GI tract is immature and "leaky," allowing some undigested proteins to be absorbed into the bloodstream. This is beneficial for breastfed infants, who can absorb immune proteins from breast milk. However, if some food proteins are introduced before the GI tract has matured, these antigens may enter the bloodstream and stimulate an immune response.

The hygiene hypothesis offers another interesting explanation: in our "germophobic" society, with the protection of antibiotics, hand sanitizers, and antimicrobial soaps and cleaners, our immune systems aren't vigorously challenged by antigens. As a result, the immune system may become sensitized to innocuous substances, such as food proteins. Recent research supports the hygiene hypothesis. Children who

grow up on farms or who have pets, and are thereby exposed to many antigens, have fewer allergies and asthma than children who grow up in more sterile environments.

Recently, researchers have proposed a link between low levels of vitamin D and food allergies. The rise in incidence of food allergies has paralleled an increase in vitamin D deficiency. The relationship between vitamin D and food allergies may be mediated by the vitamin's role in immune function.

Whatever the explanation, one thing is clear: food allergies are an important concern for many parents and others who work with children.

Testing for a Food Allergy

The diagnosis of a food allergy can often be a difficult task (Table 15-5). It requires the participation of a skilled physician. The first step in determining whether a food allergy is present is to record a detailed history of symptoms, including the time from ingestion to onset of symptoms, duration of symptoms, most recent reaction, food suspected of causing a reaction, and quantity and nature of food needed to produce a reaction. A family history of allergic diseases can also help, as allergic reactions tend to run in families. A physical examination may reveal evidence of an allergy, such as skin diseases and asthma. Various diagnostic tests can rule out other conditions. The diagnostic first step is to eliminate from the diet—for 1 to 2 weeks—all tested compounds that appear to cause allergic symptoms, plus all other foods suspected of causing an allergy based on the person's food history. The person generally starts out eating foods to which almost no one reacts, such as rice, vegetables, noncitrus fruits, and fresh meats and poultry. If symptoms are still present, the person can more severely restrict the diet or even use special formula diets that are hypoallergenic.

Once a diet is found that causes no symptoms, called an **elimination diet,** foods can be added back one at a time. This type of food challenge is an option only when the culprit foods are known to pose no risk of anaphylactic shock in the person. Doses of ½ to 1 teaspoon (2.5 to 5 milliliters) are given at first. The amount is increased until the dose approximates usual intake. Any reintroduced food that

anaphylactic shock A severe allergic response that results in lowered blood pressure and respiratory and gastrointestinal distress. This can be fatal.

antigen Any substance that induces a state of sensitivity and/or resistance to microorganisms or toxic substances after a lag period; substance that stimulates a specific aspect of the immune system.

▶ People with a history of serious allergic reactions and those who have asthma should carry a self-administered form of epinephrine, such as EpiPen, to subside an episode of anaphylactic shock, should it occur.

▶ The American Academy of Allergy, Asthma, and Immunology has a 24-hour toll-free hot line (800-822-2762) to answer questions about food allergies and to help direct people to specialists. Free information on food allergies is available by contacting The Food Allergy & Anaphylaxis Network. The telephone number is (800-929-4040); the website is **www.foodallergy.org**.

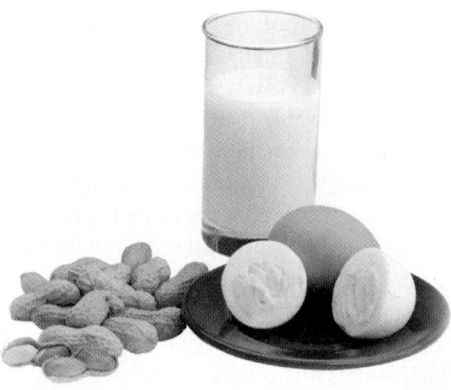

▲ Eggs, milk, and peanuts are three of the foods that pose the greatest risk for food allergies in childhood.

TABLE 15-5 Assessment Strategies for Food Allergies

History	Include description of symptoms, time between food ingestion and onset of symptoms, duration of symptoms, most recent allergic episode, quantity of food required to produce reaction, suspected foods, and allergic diseases in other family members.
Physical examination	Look for signs of an allergic reaction (rash, itching, intestinal bloating, etc.).
Elimination diet	Establish a diet lacking the suspected offending foods and stay on it for 1 to 2 weeks or until symptoms clear.
Food challenge	Add back small amounts of excluded foods, one at a time, as long as anaphylactic shock is not a possible consequence.
Blood test	Determine presence of antibodies in blood that bind to food antigens tested.
Skin test	Place a sample of the suspected allergen under the skin and watch for an inflammatory reaction.

causes significant symptoms to appear is identified as an allergen for the person.

Laboratory tests can also aid in diagnosis of food allergies. Skin testing involves pricking the skin with a small amount of purified food extract and observing any allergic response (e.g., a red eruption at the prick site). These types of tests are easy and safe, even for infants, but they may not clearly diagnose a food allergy. A positive skin-prick test merely indicates that a person has been sensitized to a food; it can't definitively identify if that food is the cause for the symptoms in question. Newer types of blood testing, however, have more diagnostic value. Blood tests estimate the blood concentration of antibodies that bind certain foodborne antigens.

Living with Food Allergies

Once potential allergens are identified, dietary modifications must be made. In some cases, small amounts of the offending food can be consumed without an observable reaction. Also, some food allergens are destroyed by heating, so cooking may eliminate the allergic response. This is effective primarily for allergies to fruits or vegetables, not for the more common allergies to milk, peanuts, or seafood. For most cases, though, complete avoidance of allergy-causing food ingredients is the safest course of action. This makes careful reading of food labels essential. As of 2006, the Food Allergen Labeling and Consumer Protection Act now requires manufacturers to clearly identify the presence of major food allergens (milk, eggs, fish, shellfish, peanuts, tree nuts, wheat, and soy) on food product labels.

A major challenge when treating a person with a food allergy is to make sure that what remains in the diet can still provide essential nutrients. The small food intake of children permits less leeway in removing offending foods that may contain numerous nutrients. A registered dietitian can help guide the diet-planning process to ensure that the remaining food choices still meet nutrient needs or to guide supplement use, if that is necessary.

About 80% of young children with food allergies outgrow them before 3 years. Parents should be made aware of this and not assume the allergy will be long-lived. Food allergies diagnosed after 3 years of age are often more long-lived, but not always. In these cases, about 33% of people outgrow their food allergies within 3 years. For others, the condition may be prolonged; some food allergies can last a lifetime, such as those for peanuts, tree nuts, and shellfish. Periodic reintroduction of offending foods can be tried every 6 to 12 months or so to see whether the allergic reaction has decreased. If no symptoms appear, tolerance to the food has developed.

Several strategies are under study to ease the dietary restrictions imposed by food allergies. One possibility includes treatment with antibodies that will increase the threshold at which an allergic response occurs. For a person with an allergy to peanuts, for example, this would alleviate some anxiety about severe reactions to trace amounts of peanuts found in foods. Similarly, immunotherapy, which exposes allergic individuals to very small, but progressively larger amounts of food allergens, may help some people build up a tolerance to certain food components. Vaccines are another area of research. Also, scientists are working on genetically engineered foods that do not contain common allergens.

Preventing Food Allergies

With the rising number of cases of food allergies, many new parents wonder when and how to introduce new foods during infancy and early childhood. It is evident that introducing foods other than human milk or infant formula before 4 months of age is associated with higher risk of allergic diseases. Most experts, including the American Academy of Pediatrics and the American College of Allergy, Asthma, and Immunology, advise waiting to introduce solid foods until 4 to 6 months of age for lowest risk of food allergies. Delaying introduction of solid foods beyond 6 months of age is not advised.

Any food can contain a potential allergen, but certain foods have been found to have high allergenic potential: peanuts, tree nuts, eggs, cow's milk, fish, and seafood. The American Academy of Pediatrics and the National Institute of Allergy and Infectious Disease no longer advise delaying introduction of highly allergenic foods beyond 6 months of age, even for infants with a family history of food allergies.

Until recently, allergy-prone women were advised to avoid highly allergenic foods during pregnancy and breastfeeding. Allergens can cross the placenta during

elimination diet A restrictive diet that systematically tests foods that may cause an allergic response by first eliminating them for 1 to 2 weeks and then adding them back, one at a time.

pregnancy and are secreted in breast milk. However, research does not demonstrate a benefit of maternal dietary restrictions in preventing food allergies in infants.

The best course of action is to breast-feed the infant exclusively for 6 months and continue to breastfeed through 12 months with appropriate introduction of solid foods to meet the infant's nutritional needs. Human milk contains factors that play a role in the maturation of the small intestine. Formula-fed infants, especially those on cow's milk–based formulas, have a greater risk for developing food allergies. There is evidence that hydrolyzed infant formulas (in which the large proteins have been broken down into smaller peptides) may be useful in allergy prevention for infants at risk of developing food allergies. However, hydrolyzed formulas are about three times as costly as iron-fortified cow's milk–based formulas.

Food Intolerances

Food intolerances are adverse reactions to foods that do not involve allergic mechanisms. Generally, larger amounts of an offending food are required to produce the symptoms of an intolerance than to trigger allergic symptoms. Common causes of food intolerances include:

- Constituents of certain foods (e.g., red wine, tomatoes, pineapples) that have a druglike activity, causing physiological effects such as changes in blood pressure
- Certain synthetic compounds added to foods, such as sulfites, food-coloring agents, and monosodium glutamate (MSG)
- Food contaminants, including antibiotics and other chemicals used in the production of livestock and crops, as well as insect parts not removed during processing
- Toxic contaminants, which may be ingested with improperly handled and prepared foods containing *Clostridium botulinum*, *Salmonella* bacteria, or other foodborne microorganisms (see Chapter 13)
- Deficiencies in digestive enzymes, such as lactase (review Chapter 4)

Almost everyone is sensitive to one or more of these causes of food intolerance, many of which produce GI tract symptoms.

Sulfites, added to foods and beverages as antioxidants, cause flushing, spasms of the airway, and a loss of blood pressure in susceptible people. Wine, dehydrated potatoes, dried fruits, gravy, soup mixes, and restaurant salad greens commonly contain sulfites. A reaction to MSG may include an increase in blood pressure, numbness, sweating, vomiting, headache, and facial pressure. MSG is commonly found in restaurant food and many processed foods (e.g., soups). A reaction to tartrazine, a food-coloring additive, includes spasm of the airway, itching, and reddening skin. Tyramine, a derivative of the amino acid tyrosine, is commonly found in "aged" foods, such as cheeses and red wines. This natural food constituent can cause high blood pressure in people taking monoamine oxidase (MAO) inhibitor medications, which may be prescribed for clinical depression.

The basic treatment for food intolerances is to avoid specific offending components. However, total elimination often is not required because people generally are not as sensitive to compounds causing food intolerances as they are to allergens.

Case Study Undernutrition During Infancy

Damon is a 7-month-old boy who has been taken into a clinic for a routine checkup. On examination, he was found to be moderately underweight relative to his age and body length. His physician scheduled a follow-up appointment in 3 months. At the 10-month visit, Damon appeared sluggish and was now even more underweight for his age and length.

A registered dietitian interviewed Damon's 16-year-old mother to collect information on Damon's dietary intake. His intake over the previous 24 hours consisted of two bottles of infant formula, three 8-ounce bottles of Kool-Aid, and a hot dog. However, the mother was still in school, and at night she often left Damon with the neighbor, so that she could go out with friends for a few hours. Thus, she was not aware of all that he ate.

Answer the following questions, and check your responses in Appendix A.

1. Damon's mother did not specify what type of formula he takes. What questions would you ask about his formula?
2. What potential dangers await Damon if his growth continues to lag behind?
3. What foods should Damon's caregivers offer that are appropriate for his age and nutritional needs?
4. What problems might arise from consumption of sugary drinks from a bottle?
5. Does Damon need any vitamin or mineral supplements?

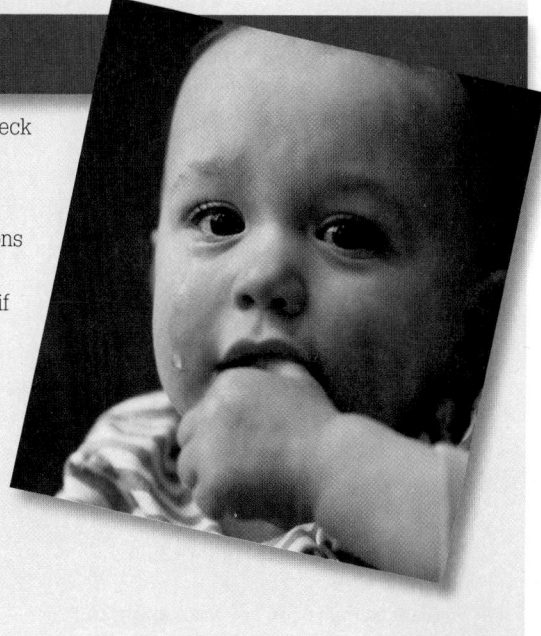

Summary (Numbers refer to numbered sections in the chapter.)

15.1 Alarming trends in child nutrition include an increase in childhood overweight and obesity, cardiovascular disease, and type 2 diabetes. A general lack of physical activity and failure to follow a healthy dietary pattern, such as that suggested by MyPlate's Daily Food Plan, are to blame.

15.2 Growth is rapid during infancy; birth weight doubles in 4 to 6 months, and length increases by 50% in the first year. An adequate diet, especially in terms of calories, protein, and zinc, is essential to support normal growth. Growth charts aid nutritional assessment of infants and children by tracking changes in body weight, height (or length), head circumference, and body mass index over time.

Nutrient needs in the first 6 months can be met by human milk or iron-fortified infant formula. Supplementation with vitamin D, iron, and fluoride may be appropriate for some infants.

Most infants do not need solid foods before 6 months of age. Introduction of solid foods should be based on an infant's nutritional needs, physical and physiological abilities, and developmental readiness. Solid foods should be introduced one at a time, starting with iron-fortified infant cereals or ground meats (sources of iron). Some foods to avoid giving infants in the first year include honey, cow's milk (especially fat-reduced varieties), foods with added salt or sugar, and foods that may cause choking.

15.3 A slower growth rate results in decreased appetite among preschool children. Other common nutrition-related concerns include iron-deficiency, constipation, and dental caries. With smaller portion sizes and picky eating behaviors, it is crucial to offer several small meals and snacks with a variety of nutrient-dense foods. Follow the example set forth by MyPlate, but use smaller portions (e.g., 1 tablespoon of food per year of life). For autism spectrum disorders, several nutritional interventions, including the gluten-free, casein-free diet and some dietary supplements, are under study.

15.4 Among school-age children, excessive energy and fat intakes have led to an alarming increase in overweight, obesity, type 2 diabetes, and cardiovascular disease. Parents can provide healthful food choices and encourage at least 60 minutes of physical activity per day. When controlled early through diet and exercise interventions, the problem of obesity may correct itself as the child continues to grow in height.

15.5 During the adolescent growth spurt, both boys and girls have increased needs for iron and calcium. Inadequate calcium intake by teenage girls is a major concern because it can set the stage for the development of osteoporosis later in life. Teenagers generally should moderate their intake of high-fat and sugar-rich foods—especially snacks and fast-food, which they often consume in abundance—and perform regular physical activity.

N&YH The most common food allergies are associated with peanuts, tree nuts, shellfish, milk, eggs, soybeans, wheat, and fish. Food allergies occur most often during infancy and young adulthood.

Check Your Knowledge (Answers to the following questions are below.)

1. Inadequate intake of which of the following results in poor growth?
   a. calories
   b. iron
   c. zinc
   d. All of the above.

2. An 11-month-old girl who weighs 19 pounds needs approximately _____ kcal per day.
   a. 690   c. 845
   b. 810   d. 930

3. Introduction of cow's milk should be delayed until 12 months of age because it
   a. contains too much fat.
   b. supplies too much lactose.
   c. contains too much protein.
   d. All of the above.

4. You are trying to introduce an apple and blueberry puree to a seven-month-old infant, but she rejects it. You should
   a. assume she doesn't like apples and blueberries.
   b. offer the food again on another day.
   c. force a spoonful into her mouth.
   d. None of the above.

5. Milk is a nutrient-dense source of all of the following except
   a. protein.   c. calcium.
   b. iron.   d. zinc.

6. A gluten-free, casein-free diet may be used to treat
   a. rickets.   c. lead poisoning.
   b. anemia.   d. autism.

7. To ensure adequate vitamin and mineral intake for a picky eater,
   a. provide a fortified breakfast cereal.
   b. promise dessert as a reward for eating meats and vegetables.
   c. use a multivitamin and mineral supplement.
   d. None of the above.

8. For treatment of overweight, school-age children should
   a. eat fewer meals.
   b. follow a low-carbohydrate eating plan.

   c. exercise for 60 minutes per day or more.
   d. avoid dairy products.

9. The prevailing dietary habits of North American teenagers contribute to all of the following except
   a. acne.
   b. high blood pressure.
   c. low bone mass.
   d. type 2 diabetes.

10. Your niece breaks out in hives and feels nauseous after eating a salad containing mango. She probably has a food
    a. sensitivity.   c. intolerance.
    b. allergy.   d. All of the above.

Answer key: 1. d (LO 15.1), 2. a (LO 15.2), 3. c (LO 15.2), 4. b (LO 15.2), 5. b (LO 15.4), 6. d (LO 15.3), 7. a (LO 15.3), 8. c (LO 15.5), 9. a (LO 15.4), 10. b (LO 15.6)

Study Questions (Numbers refer to Learning Outcomes)

1. List two factors that limit "catch-up" growth when a nutrient-deficient diet has been consumed throughout childhood. **(LO 15.1)**

2. Outline three key factors that help determine when to introduce solid foods into an infant's diet. **(LO 15.2)**

3. A 3-month-old infant is taken to a clinic with failure to thrive. What are two possible explanations? **(LO 15.2)**

4. List three reasons why preschoolers are noted for "picky" eating. For each, describe an appropriate parent response. **(LO 15.3)**

5. What three factors are likely to contribute to obesity in a typical 10-year-old child? **(LO 15.5)**

6. Compare the guidelines for infant feeding summarized in Chapter 15 with the 2010 Dietary Guidelines for Americans for children over age 2 and adults discussed in Chapter 2. Which guidelines are similar? Do any contradict each other? If so, why? **(LO 15.2)**

7. Describe three pros and cons of snacking. What is the basic advice for healthful snacking from childhood through the teenage years? **(LO 15.3)**

8. Which two nutrients are of particular concern in planning diets for teenagers? Why does each deserve to be singled out? **(LO 15.4)**

9. List three nutrients of concern for a teenage vegetarian. **(LO 15.4)**

10. Recommend two steps that a woman with a family history of food allergies can take to reduce risk of food allergies in her infant. **(LO 15.6)**

What Would You Choose Recommendations

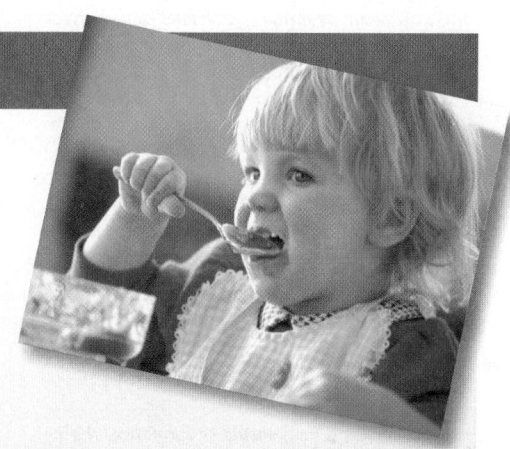

At 18 months of age, Lila's diet should include small portions of a variety of foods from each MyPlate food group. She should have several teeth by now, but her chewing ability is still limited. As a young child, Lila has high nutrient needs and yet has a small stomach capacity, so snacking makes an important contribution to meeting overall nutrient needs.

Reduced-fat popcorn is a healthy, low-fat snack for older children and adults. Feeding children bulky foods with low energy density, however, can lead to fullness without meeting nutritional needs. Furthermore, popcorn is a choking hazard.

Although baby carrots with ranch dressing would be a good source of beta-carotene and healthy vegetable oils, toddlers are not expert chewers just yet, and large pieces of hard, crunchy foods present a choking hazard. Slicing the carrots into long, thin strips would be a better idea.

Fat-free, light yogurt is a good source of calcium and vitamin D for building healthy bones and certainly does not present choking risk. However, infants and toddlers need the fat and sugar in dairy products to supply calories for their growing bodies. Whole-milk yogurt, such as YoBaby, would be a better choice.

Whole-grain crackers with sliced cheddar cheese would be an excellent snacking option for Lila. This snack provides a healthy balance of carbohydrates, protein, and fat. Using whole-grain crackers, rather than those made with refined flour, will boost the vitamin and mineral content (review Chapter 4).

Toddlers are known for picky eating behaviors. Lila's slower pace of growth may reduce her appetite and she may be more interested in exploring the world around her than sitting down for a meal. Make sure Lila sits down to eat and supervise her while she is eating. Finally, be a good role model. If she sees you eat the healthy snacks you have offered, she will be more likely to accept them.

Further Readings

1. ADA Reports: Position of the American Dietetic Association: Nutrition guidance for healthy children ages 2 to 11 years. *Journal of the American Dietetic Association* 108:1716, 2008.

   MyPyramid combined with the Dietary Guidelines for Americans provide an appropriate blueprint for feeding children. Diets of many children are not following this advice and in turn are contributing to the nutritional problems common in childhood and later adulthood.

2. Baker RD and others: Clinical report— Diagnosis and prevention of iron deficiency and iron-deficiency anemia in infants and young children (0–3 years of age). *Pediatrics* 126:1040, 2010.

   Healthy, full-term infants are born with sufficient iron stores to last through 4 months of age. After 4 months, exclusively and partially breastfed infants need additional iron from liquid iron supplements until consumption of solid foods provides a daily iron intake of 1 milligram per kilogram of body weight. For formula-fed infants, use of iron-fortified infant formula through 12 months of age will meet iron needs. Between 6 and 12 months of age, iron intake should be 11 milligrams per day from iron-rich foods or liquid iron supplements. Preterm infants require 2 milligrams of iron per kilogram for the first 12 months, provided as liquid supplements by 1 month of age until food and/or formula intake provides sufficient iron. Between 1 and 3 years of age, iron intake should be 7 milligrams per day from iron-rich foods, augmented by vitamin C-rich foods, and/ or use of a liquid iron supplement.

3. Briggs M and others: Position of the American Dietetic Association, School Nutrition Association, and Society for Nutrition Education: Comprehensive school nutrition services. Journal of the American Dietetic Association 110:1738, 2010.

   More than 31 million children participate in the National School Lunch Program. In addition, school-based nutrition education programs (e.g., garden-based education and farm-to-school programs), increased availability of healthy food choices on school campuses, school-home-community partnerships, and school-based health services for children in need can foster healthy behaviors.

4. Council on Communications and Media: Children, adolescents, obesity, and the media. Pediatrics 128:201, 2011.

   Exposure to media is associated with increases in obesity among children and adolescents. This relationship may be mediated by a sedentary lifestyle, the influence of food advertising, unhealthful snacking practices, or poor sleep habits. The American Academy of Pediatrics urges health care providers to curb media exposure by counseling children and their parents, lobbying government, and initiating public health campaigns.

5. Council on Sports Medicine and Fitness and Council on School Health. Active healthy living: Prevention of childhood obesity through increased physical activity. Pediatrics 117:1834, 2006.

   Physical activity should be encouraged during and after school and as part of home life. Benefits of regular physical activity among children and adolescents include physical changes (e.g., improved insulin sensitivity, lowered blood pressure) and psychological improvements (e.g., increased self-esteem, less depression).

6. Curtis LT and others: Nutritional and environmental approaches to preventing and treating autism and attention-deficit hyperactivity disorder (ADHD): A review. Journal of Alternative and Complementary Medicine 14:79, 2008.

   This article reviews hypothesized environmental and nutritional links to autism and attention-deficit hyperactivity disorder. Evidence does not support a relationship between autism and environmental exposure to mercury. Nutritional interventions of scientific merit in the treatment of autism include avoidance of food allergens and correcting deficiencies of some B vitamins, magnesium, iron, zinc, and omega-3 fatty acids. For treatment of ADHD, some studies show a benefit of eliminating refined sugars and food additives such as coloring agents and preservatives.

7. Daniels SR and others: Lipid screening and cardiovascular health in childhood. Pediatrics 122:198, 2008.

   In light of evidence of cardiovascular disease among youth, the American Academy of Pediatrics urges children with risk factors for cardiovascular disease to undergo regular lipid screening starting by age 10. Treatments for dyslipidemia in children include dietary modifications, physical activity, and lipid-lowering medications.

8. Elder JH: The gluten-free, casein-free diet in autism: An overview with clinical implications. Nutrition in Clinical Practice 23:583, 2008.

   The gluten-free, casein-free (GFCF) diet is a popular but intense treatment for children with autism spectrum disorders. Some researchers hypothesize that intestinal absorption in autistic children is altered (i.e., "leaky gut syndrome"), such that food sensitivities to wheat and dairy proteins develop, leading to inflammation and other effects on the central nervous system. The GFCF diet may be useful for alleviating symptoms in some children with autism, but proper dietary planning is essential to prevent nutrient deficiencies.

9. Gidding SS and others: Dietary recommendations for children and adolescents: A guide for practitioners. Pediatrics 117:544, 2006.

   The American Heart Association recognizes that the dietary patterns of children and adolescents put them at risk for cardiovascular diseases in adulthood and even during childhood. Age-appropriate recommendations are provided for total energy intake, dietary fats, added sugars, sodium, and physical activity.

10. Gupta RS and others: The prevalence, severity, and distribution of childhood food allergy in the United States. Pediatrics 128:e9, 2011.

    Based on data collected from more than 38,000 children, the prevalence of food allergies is now estimated at 8% of children in the United States. About 40% of these children experience severe food allergies, and about one-third have multiple food allergies. Racial and income disparities are discussed.

11. Monsen ER: New findings from the Feeding Infants and Toddlers Study. Journal of the American Dietetic Association 106:S5, 2006.

    The Gerber-sponsored Feeding Infants and Toddlers Study (FITS) examined usual intakes of nutrients from foods and supplements, as well as other dietary practices, with an emphasis on dietary habits of Hispanic infants and children. Infants and toddlers do not consume enough fruits, vegetables, or fiber, and that intakes of total kilocalories, dietary fats, and sodium are on the rise.

12. Rao G: Childhood obesity: Highlights of AMA expert committee recommendations. American Family Physician 78:56, 2008.

    Weight management should be addressed yearly at medical checkups with all children. For those children who are overweight or obese (based on BMI for age), additional screening of blood lipids, glucose, and liver and kidney function is warranted. The four-stage approach for treatment of childhood obesity includes reducing consumption of sweetened beverages and fast foods; limiting time spent watching TV, playing video games, and sitting at the computer; participating in 60 minutes or more of physical activity each day; and encouraging family meals.

13. Spruijt-Metz D: Etiology, treatment, and prevention of obesity in childhood and adolescence: A decade in review. Journal of Research on Adolescence 21:129, 2011.

    This comprehensive review of pediatric obesity provides demographic data on obesity and associated health problems in children and adolescents, and discusses etiological factors contributing to the condition (e.g., genetics and environment), physical and mental health consequences, and strategies for prevention and treatment.

14. Wagner CL and others: Prevention of rickets and vitamin D deficiency in infants, children, and adolescents. Pediatrics 122(5):1142, 2008.

    Rickets and vitamin D deficiency are of concern for infants as well as older children and adolescents in the United States and are attributable to inadequate vitamin D intake and decreased exposure to sunlight. The American Academy of Pediatrics recommends that all infants and children, including adolescents, have a minimum daily intake of 400 IU of vitamin D beginning soon after birth.

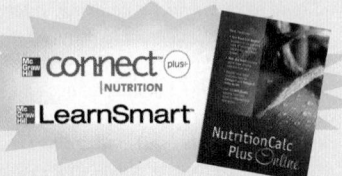

To get the most out of your study of nutrition, go to McGraw-Hill's online resources: Connect www.mcgrawhillconnect.com, where you will find NutritionCalc Plus, LearnSmart, and many other dynamic tools.

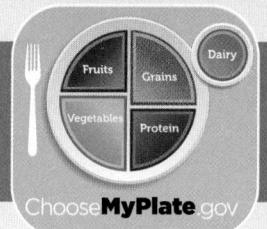

I. Getting Young Bill to Eat

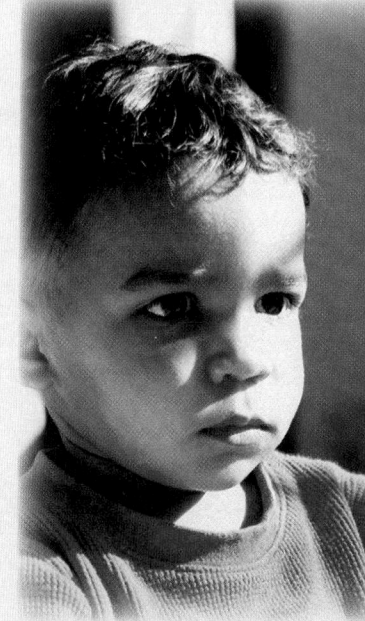

Bill is 3 years old, and his mother is worried about his eating habits. He refuses to eat vegetables, meat, and dinner in general. Some days he eats very little food. He wants to eat snacks most of the time. Mealtime is a battle because Bill says he isn't hungry, and his mother wants him to eat a sit-down lunch and dinner to make sure he gets all the nutrients he needs and to eat everything served on his plate. He drinks five or six glasses of whole milk per day because that is the one food he likes.

When his mother prepares dinner, she makes plenty of vegetables, boiling them until they are soft, hoping this will appeal to Bill. Bill's dad waits to eat his vegetables last, regularly telling the family that he eats them only because he has to. He also regularly complains about how dinner has been prepared. Bill saves his vegetables until last and usually gags when his mother orders him to eat them. Bill has been known to sit at the dinner table for an hour until the war of wills ends. Bill's mother serves casseroles and stews regularly because they are convenient. Bill likes to eat breakfast cereal, fruit, and cheese and regularly requests these foods for snacks. However, his mother tries to deny his requests, so that he will have an appetite for dinner. Bill's mother comes to you and asks you what she should do to get Bill to eat.

Analysis

1. List four mistakes Bill's parents are making that contribute to Bill's poor eating habits.

_____

_____

_____

_____

2. List four strategies they might try to promote good eating habits in Bill.

_____

_____

_____

_____

II. Evaluating a Teen Lunch

The following are two typical teen lunches and nutritional information for each:

Meal 1	Meal 2		
2 pieces cheese pizza	1 large hamburger sandwich with condiments		
1 milk chocolate candy bar	30 French fries		
20 fluid ounces cola	20 fluid ounces cola		
	Meal 1	Meal 2	Nutrient Needs for Teens
Energy (kcal)	990	1000	Males: 3000 Females: 2200
Protein	32	20	Males: 59 Females: 44
Vitamin C (milligrams)	5	18	Both genders: 45 to 75
Vitamin A (micrograms RAE)	300	10	Males: 900 Females: 700
Iron (milligrams)	3	4	Males: 11 Females: 15
Calcium (milligrams)	545	100	Both genders: 1300

1. Keeping in mind that meals should meet about one-third of nutrient needs, what are the shortcomings and excesses of these meals (i.e., given the nutritional information, compare these meals with one-third the RDA for protein, vitamin C, vitamin A, iron, and calcium)?

_____

_____

_____

2. How would you change these meals to improve balance and to meet the nutrient needs above? (Hint: Use NutritionCalc Plus.)

_____

_____

_____

3. Reflect on your food choices as a teenager. Do you think your meal choices were balanced and varied? Why or why not? What could you have done to improve your nutritional habits at that time?

_____

_____

_____

III. Public Health Efforts to Combat Childhood Obesity

Major public health initiatives aim to counter the rapid rise in childhood obesity and related health conditions. Whether school-based, community-driven, or targeted at families, the overarching goals are to promote healthy eating habits and increased physical activity.

1. Find out what is going on in your area to combat childhood obesity. As a starting point, here are a few examples:

   - *We Can!™* (Ways to Enhance Children's Activity and Nutrition): http://wecan.nhlbi.nih.gov
   - **HealthCorps:** www.healthcorps.net
   - **Action for Healthy Kids:** www.actionforhealthykids.org
   - **The President's Council on Fitness, Sports, and Nutrition:** www.fitness.gov

   _____

   _____

   _____

   _____

Imagine that you have been appointed to develop a public health campaign to decrease childhood obesity in your community.

2. What are the specific needs in your community (e.g., lack of safe space for physical activity, overabundance of fast-food outlets)?

   _____

   _____

   _____

   _____

3. Who will be your target audience? Why?

   _____

   _____

   _____

   _____

4. What activities will you undertake to reach your target audience? What will set your program apart from other efforts in your community?

   _____

   _____

   _____

   _____

5. How will you define the success of your program? List two or more measurable objectives for your campaign.

   _____

   _____

   _____

   _____

Chapter 16 Nutrition During Adulthood

Student Learning Outcomes

Chapter 16 is designed to allow you to:

16.1 Discuss demographic trends among adults in North America and how they impact health care.

16.2 List several hypotheses about the causes of aging.

16.3 Describe how physiological changes that occur during adulthood affect nutritional needs.

16.4 Compare the dietary intake of adults with current recommendations.

16.5 Make recommendations for lifestyle changes in the prevention and treatment of nutritional problems in older adults.

16.6 Identify nutrition-related health issues of the adult years and describe the prevention and treatment options.

16.7 Compare benefits of moderate alcohol use to risks of alcohol abuse.

16.8 List several nutritional programs available to help meet nutritional needs of older adults.

What Would You Choose?

In your family, there is a history of colon cancer. Your grandmother died from complications of colon cancer, and your father has already had some polyps removed from his colon. Even though you have not experienced any digestive abnormalities that would indicate a problem, your desire to learn about the role of lifestyle choices in disease prevention is part of what prompted you to take this nutrition course. What would you choose as the best nutrition strategy for cancer prevention?

a Take a variety of phytochemical supplements.

b Buy a juicer to make antioxidant-rich fruit and vegetable concoctions.

c Focus on filling half your plate at mealtimes with fruits and vegetables.

d Don't worry about making changes now, because colon cancer occurs in older adults.

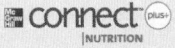 **connect** |NUTRITION **Think about your choice as you read Chapter 16, then see our recommendations at the end of the chapter. To learn more about links between nutrition and cancer, check out the Connect site:** www.mcgrawhillconnect.com

Part Five
Nutrition: A Focus on Life Stages

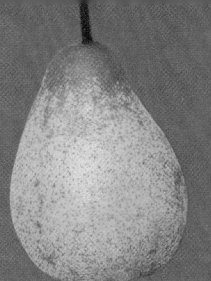

Eating is one of our great pleasures. Guided by common sense and moderation, eating well is also a means to good health. Most of us want a long, productive life, free of illness. Yet, as the comic in this chapter suggests, aging is inevitable. Unfortunately, many people from early middle age onward suffer from obesity, cardiovascular disease, hypertension and strokes, type 2 diabetes, osteoporosis, and other chronic diseases. We can slow the development of—and in some cases even prevent—these diseases by following a dietary pattern such as that exemplified by MyPlate. The effect of such a diet is most profitable if we begin early and continue throughout adulthood. We serve ourselves best—as individuals and as a nation—by striving to maintain vitality even in the later decades of life. This concept was first explored in Chapter 1 and is discussed again in this chapter, in light of the nutrition needs of adults.

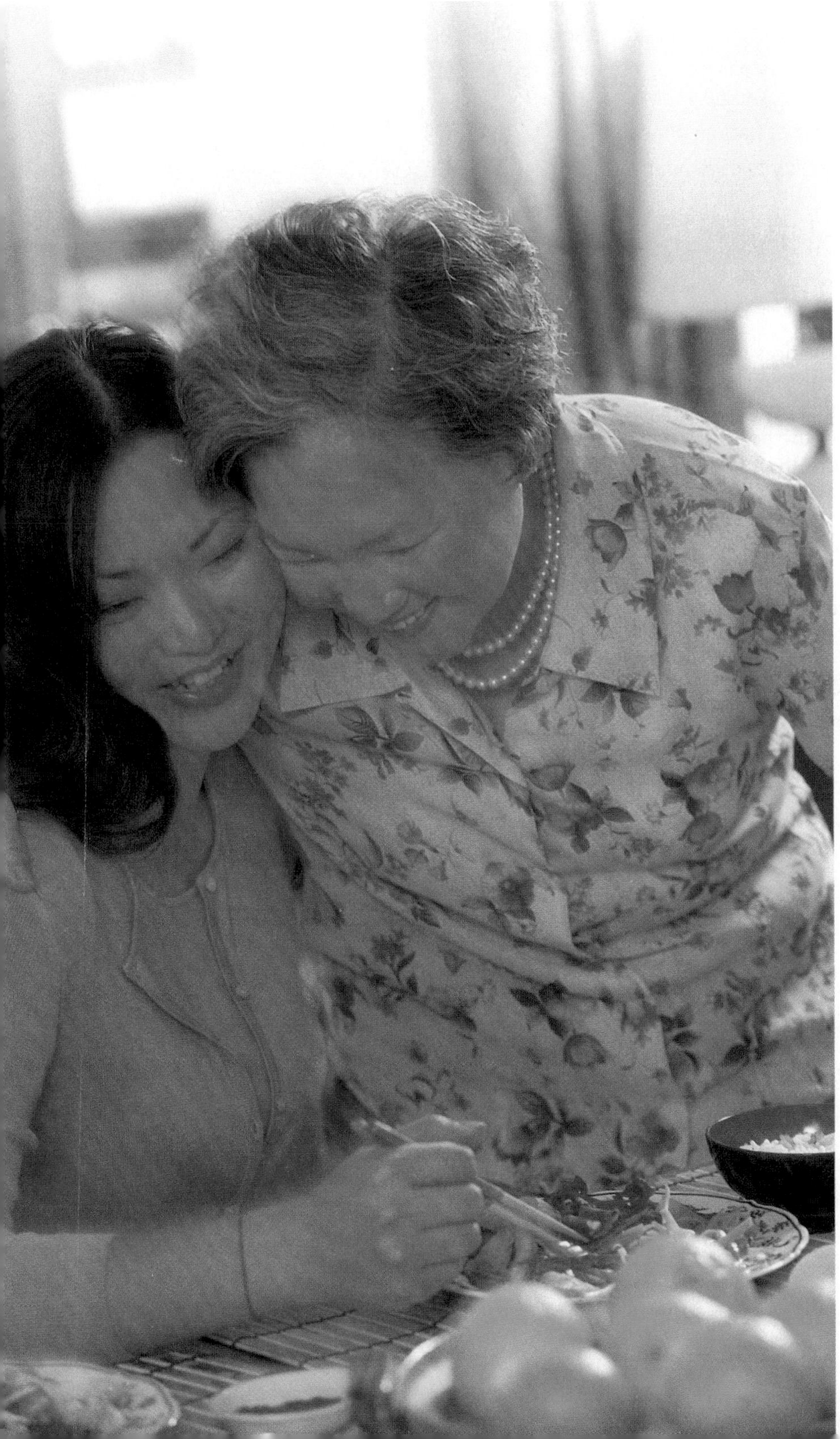

Keep in mind that present day-to-day health practices can significantly influence health during later life. Although genetics does play a role, as discussed in Chapter 3, many of the health problems that occur with age are not inevitable; they result from diet-related disease processes that influence physical health. Much can be learned from healthy older people whose attention to a healthy diet and physical activity—along with a little luck—keeps them active and vibrant well beyond typical retirement years. Successful aging is the goal. Age quickly or slowly—it is partly your choice.

Refresh Your Memory

As you begin your study of adult nutrition issues in Chapter 16, you may want to review:

- Implications of the 1994 Dietary Supplement Health and Education Act in Chapter 1
- The effect of genetics on health in Chapter 3
- The various body systems covered in Chapter 3
- The sources of fiber and sugar in Chapter 4
- Definition of healthy body weight in Chapter 7
- The dietary sources of vitamin D, the various B vitamins, and calcium in Chapters 8 and 9
- Recommendations for salt intake in Chapter 9
- The benefits of regular physical activity in Chapter 10

16.1 The Graying of North America

Due to advances in health care and sanitation, the demographics of developed countries are shifting so that as a population, we are getting older. In North America, the group constituting those aged 85+ years is the fastest growing segment. Between 1997 and 2050, the population aged 85+ years in the United States is expected to increase from 3.4 million to 19 million. Even more amazing, 1 million or more people in the United States could be over 100 years old in 2050.

This "graying" of North America poses some problems. Although people older than age 65 account for just 13% of the U.S. population, they account for more than 25% of all prescription medications used, 40% of acute hospital stays, and 50% of the federal health budget. Hip fractures alone cost the nation about $12 billion per year. Of older persons, 65% or more have nutrition-related problems, such as cardiovascular disease, type 2 diabetes, hypertension, and osteoporosis.

Postponing these chronic diseases for as long as possible will help control health care costs. Health and independence contribute quality—not just quantity—to life as

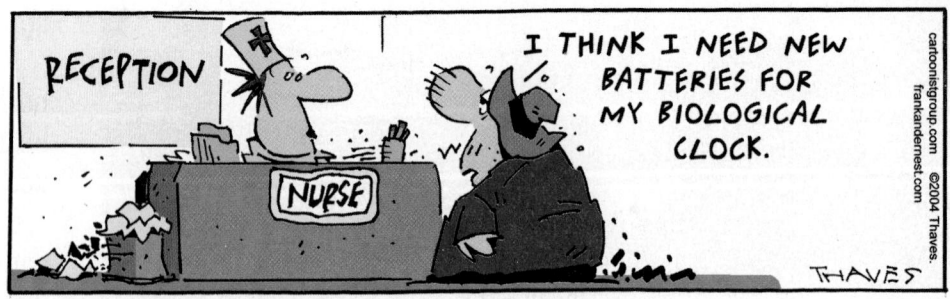

Is a decline in health inevitable as we age? Which diet and lifestyle interventions have been shown to slow (or reverse) the aging process? Which nutrition problems are typically seen in older adults? How should one compensate for these? Chapter 16 provides some answers.

"Frank and Ernest" used with the permission of the Thaves and the Cartoonist Group. All rights reserved. 2/28/1997

age advances and lessen the load on an already overburdened healthcare system. Keep in mind that aging is not a disease. Furthermore, diseases that commonly accompany old age—osteoporosis and atherosclerosis, for example—are not an inevitable part of aging. Many can be prevented or managed. Some people do die of old age, not as a direct result of disease.

16.2 Physiological Changes During Adulthood

Adulthood, the longest stage of the life cycle, begins when an adolescent completes his or her physical growth. Unlike earlier stages of the life cycle, nutrients are used primarily to maintain the body rather than support physical growth. (Pregnancy is the only time during adulthood when substantial amounts of nutrients are used for growth.) As adults get older, nutrient needs change. For example, vitamin D needs increase for older adults. Based on the needs for various nutrients, the Food and Nutrition Board divided the adult years into four stages: ages 19 to 30, 31 to 50, 51 to 70, and beyond 70 years of age. The intervals encompassing ages 19 through 50 are often referred to as young adulthood, 51 to 70 as middle adulthood, and beyond 70 years of age as older adulthood.

Adulthood is characterized by body maintenance and gradual physical and physiological transitions, often referred to as aging. **Aging** can be defined as the time-dependent physical and physiological changes in body structure and function that occur normally and progressively throughout adulthood as humans mature and become older. One view of aging describes it as a process of slow cell death, beginning soon after fertilization. When we are young, aging is not apparent because the major metabolic activities are geared toward growth and maturation. We produce plenty of active cells to meet physiological needs. During late adolescence and adulthood, the body's major task is to maintain cells. From the beginning of adulthood until age 30 or so, body systems are at their peak efficiency rate. Stature, stamina, strength, endurance, efficiency, and health are at their lifetime highs. Rates of cell synthesis and breakdown are balanced in most tissues. Inevitably, though, cells age and die. After about age 30, the rate of cell breakdown slowly begins to exceed the rate of cell renewal, leading to a gradual decline in organ size and efficiency. Eventually, the body can't adjust to meet all physiological demands, and body functioning begins to decrease (Fig. 16-1). Still, body systems and organs usually retain enough **reserve capacity** to handle normal, everyday demands throughout one's entire lifetime.

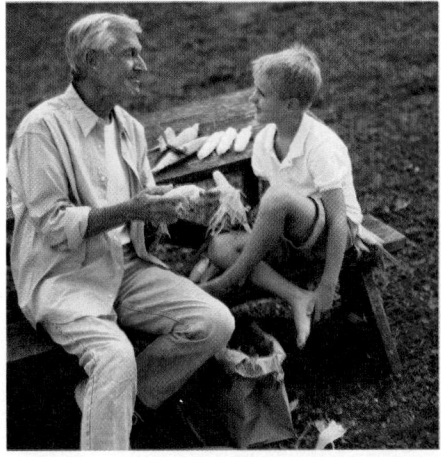

▲ The "baby boom" turned 65 in 2011, and now the health concerns of an aging population will demand increasing attention.

aging Time-dependent physical and physiological changes in body structure and function that occur normally and progressively throughout adulthood as humans mature and become older.

reserve capacity The extent to which an organ can preserve essentially normal function despite decreasing cell number or cell activity.

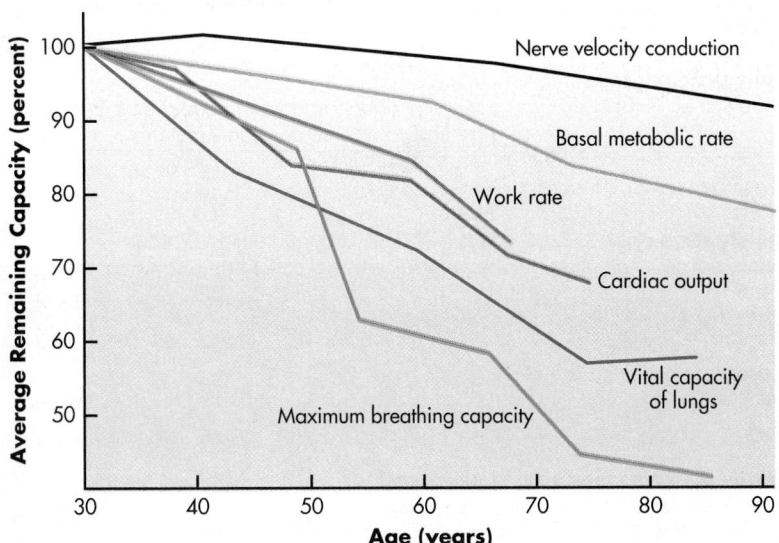

FIGURE 16-1 ▶ Declines in physiological function seen with aging. The decline in many body functions is especially evident in sedentary people.

Problems caused by diminished capacity typically don't arise unless severe demands are placed on the aging body. For example, alcohol intake can overtax an aging liver. The stress of shoveling a snow-covered sidewalk can exceed the capacity of the heart and lungs. Coping with an illness also can push an older body beyond its capacity.

The causes of aging remain a mystery. Most likely, the physiological changes of aging are the sum of automatic cellular changes, lifestyle practices, and environmental influences, as listed in Table 16-1. Even with the most supportive environment and healthy lifestyle, cell structure and function still decline over time. The eventual death of deteriorating cells is actually beneficial because it likely prevents diseases such as cancer. Unfortunately, there are negative consequences to this natural cell progression because, as more and more cells in an organ die, organ function decreases. For example, **kidney nephrons** are continually lost as we age. In some people, this loss exhausts the kidneys' reserve capacity and ultimately leads to kidney failure. Most people, however, maintain sufficient kidney function throughout life.

The diseases and degenerative processes commonly observed in older people have long been assumed to be unavoidable consequences of aging. Certainly, some of the declines we blame on aging may be inevitable, such as gradual reductions in tissue

kidney nephrons The units of kidney cells that filter wastes from the bloodstream and deposit them into the urine.

glycosylation The process by which glucose attaches to (glycates) other compounds, such as proteins.

TABLE 16-1 Current Hypotheses About the Causes of Aging

Errors occur in copying the genetic blueprint (DNA).
Once sufficient errors in DNA copying accumulate, a cell can no longer synthesize the major proteins needed to function, and it therefore dies.

Connective tissue stiffens.
Parallel protein strands, found mostly in connective tissue, cross-link to each other. This decreases flexibility in key body components.

Electron-seeking compounds damage cell parts.
Electron-seeking free radicals can break down cell membranes and proteins. One way to prevent some damage from these compounds is to consume adequate amounts of vitamins E and C, selenium, and carotenoids.

Hormone function changes.
The blood concentration of many hormones, such as testosterone in men, falls during the aging process. Replacement of these and other hormones is possible, but the resulting risks and benefits are largely unknown.

Glycosylation of proteins.
Blood glucose, when chronically elevated, attaches to (glycates) various blood and body proteins. This decreases protein function and can encourage immune system attack on such altered proteins.

The immune system loses some efficiency.
The immune system is most efficient during childhood and young adulthood, but with advancing age, it is less able to recognize and counteract foreign substances, such as viruses, that enter the body. Nutrient deficiencies, particularly of protein, vitamin E, vitamin B-6, and zinc, also hamper immune function.

Autoimmunity develops.
Autoimmune reactions occur when white blood cells and other immune system components begin to attack body tissues in addition to foreign proteins. Many diseases, including some forms of arthritis, involve this autoimmune response.

Death is programmed into the cell.
Each human cell can divide only about 50 times. Once this number of divisions occurs, the cell automatically succumbs.

Excess calorie intake speeds body breakdown.
Experimentally, underfed animals, such as spiders, mice, and rats, live longer. Usual calorie intake must be reduced by about 30% to see this effect. This approach is the only proven way to substantially slow the aging process (see Further Readings 8 and 11).

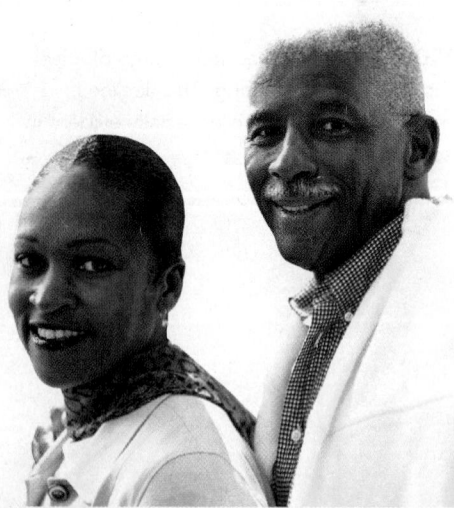

▲ Adopting diet and lifestyle practices that minimize a decline in body function is an investment in your future health. Visit www.nia.nih.gov for a free fact sheet on healthy aging.

and organ cell numbers, graying hair, and reduced lung capacity. However, many of the so-called usual or degenerative age-related changes can, in fact, be minimized, prevented, and/or reversed by healthy lifestyles (e.g., eating nutritious diets, exercising regularly, getting enough sleep) and avoiding adverse environmental factors (e.g., excessive exposure to sunlight and cigarette smoke). These discoveries have led researchers to introduce the concepts of "usual aging" and "successful aging."

Usual and Successful Aging

Body cells age, no matter what health practices we follow. However, to a considerable extent, you can choose how quickly you age throughout your adult years. *Usual aging* refers to those changes commonly thought to be a typical or expected part of aging, such as increasing body fatness, decreasing lean body mass, rising blood pressure, declining bone mass, and increasingly poor health. Researchers point out that many of these changes really represent an acceleration of the aging process induced by unhealthy lifestyle choices, adverse environmental exposures, and/or chronic disease. For instance, blood pressure does not tend to rise with age among people whose diets are traditionally low in sodium. Also, lean body mass is maintained much better in older people who exercise than in those who don't.

Successful aging, on the other hand, describes physical and physiological function declines that occur only because one grows older, not because lifestyle choices, environmental exposures, and chronic disease have aggravated or sped up the rate of aging. Those who are successful agers experience age-related declines at a slower rate and the onset of chronic disease symptoms at a later age than usual agers. Striving to have the greatest number of healthy years and the fewest years of illness is often referred to as **compression of morbidity**. In other words, a person tries to delay the onset of disabilities caused by chronic disease and to compress significant sickness related to aging into the last few years–or months–of life.

Factors Affecting the Rate of Aging

Life span refers to the maximum number of years a human can live. As far as we know, this hasn't changed in recorded time. The longest human life documented to date is 122 years for a woman and 114 years for a man. **Life expectancy,** alternatively, is the time an average person born in a specific year, such as 2009, can expect to live. Life expectancy in North America is about 75 years for men and about 80 years for women, with a span of "healthy years" of about 64. Furthermore, a person who survives to age 80 can expect to live an additional 7 to 10 years.

The rate at which one ages is individual; it is determined by heredity, lifestyle, and environment. With the exception of heredity, most of the factors that influence the rate of aging are directly linked to choices that are under our control.

Heredity

Heredity defines who you are biochemically and, to some extent, it defines how long you will live (longevity). Living to an old age tends to run in some families. If your parents and grandparents lived a long time, you are likely to have the potential to live to an old age, too. One of the most obvious genetic characteristics influencing longevity is gender. In the case of humans, as well as most other species, females tend to live longer than males.

Another genetic characteristic that can influence longevity is metabolic efficiency. Individuals with a "thrifty metabolism" require fewer calories for metabolic processes and are able to store body fat more easily than those with faster metabolic rates. Throughout history, it was the individuals with thrifty metabolism who tended to live the longest because they efficiently stored fat during times of plenty and thus had the energy stores needed to survive frequent periods of food scarcity. In today's

Keep in mind that extending life without delaying onset of chronic disease prolongs suffering in many cases. In addition, the greater number of disabled years is costly to all North Americans. For these reasons, prolonging life without compressing the number of disabled years is called the "failure of success."

compression of morbidity Delay of the onset of disabilities caused by chronic disease.

life span The potential oldest age a person can reach.

life expectancy The average length of life for a given group of people born in a specific year (such as this year).

Besides having other long-lived family members, people who live to 100 years generally:

- Do not smoke and do not drink heavily
- Gain little weight in adulthood
- Eat many fruits and vegetables
- Perform daily physical activity
- Challenge their minds
- Have a positive outlook
- Maintain close friendships
- Are (or were) married (especially true for men)
- Have a healthy rate of HDL cholesterol production

environment of labor-saving devices and abundant, energy-dense foods, however, a thrifty metabolism may actually reduce longevity. Accumulation of excessive body fat increases the risk of developing health problems that reduce life expectancy (e.g., heart disease, hypertension, and certain cancers).

As you know, heredity is largely unchangeable. However, heredity is not necessarily destiny—individuals can exert some control over the expression of their genetic potential. Lifestyle and environment both can modify the expression of genetic potential.

Lifestyle

Lifestyle is one's pattern of living—it includes food choices, exercise patterns, and substance use (e.g., alcohol, drugs, and tobacco). Lifestyle choices can have a major impact on health and longevity, as well as on the expression of genetic potential. If individuals have a family history of premature heart disease, they can adjust their diet, exercise, and tobacco use patterns to slow the progression of the disease, get needed medical care, and possibly extend their lifetime. The converse is true, too. That is, lifestyle choices (e.g., high-fat diet and couch potato mentality) can increase susceptibility to diseases that hasten the rate of aging, ultimately shortening life expectancy, even if a person's genetic potential is for a very long life.

Worldwide, the highest average life expectancy is in Okinawa, a stretch of islands off the coast of Japan: 86 years for women and 78 years for men. Researchers suggest that these statistics are rooted in the traditional diet and lifestyle of inhabitants of Okinawa. The Okinawan diet is based on rice, fish, vegetable protein sources, fruits, vegetables, tea, herbs for seasonings, and small amounts of meat. Alcohol and salt intake is minimal. The low energy density translates into a generally low calorie intake, and BMI averages 21 kg/m². A desire to mimic their weight management success, compression of morbidity, and longevity has given rise to several popular books and websites that promote Okinawan dietary practices.

Followers of the traditional Mediterranean Diet also enjoy some of the lowest recorded rates of chronic disease in the world (See Chapter 2, p. 63). As introduced in Chapter 5, the Mediterranean Diet features the following:

- Olive oil, a source of heart-healthy monounsaturated fat, as the main dietary fat
- Abundant daily intake of fruits, vegetables (especially leafy greens), whole grains, beans, nuts, and seeds
- An emphasis on minimally processed and, wherever possible, seasonally fresh and locally grown foods
- Daily intake of small amounts of cheese and yogurt
- Weekly intake of low to moderate amounts of fish
- Limited use of eggs and red meat
- Regular exercise
- Moderate drinking of wine at mealtime

Common themes among these life-prolonging dietary practices are their focus on unprocessed, fiber-rich foods, healthy sources of fat (e.g., vegetable oils and fish), and lean sources of protein. Besides diet, populations who enjoy extended quality and quantity of life include physical activity as a major part of their daily routines. Compare these lifestyle choices with those of typical North Americans.

Environment

Some aspects of the environment that exert a powerful influence on the rate of aging are income, education level, health care, shelter, and psychosocial factors. For instance, being able to purchase nutritious foods, quality health care, and safe housing helps decrease the rate of aging. Having the education needed to earn a sufficient income, as well as the knowledge required to select a nutritious diet and make

CRITICAL THINKING

The "fountain of youth" remains a mystery. Many people believe a source exists that can stop the aging process, allowing youth to remain. However, Neil, a history student, asserts that the fountain of youth is not a place or a particular thing but, rather, a combination of diet and lifestyle. How can he justify this claim?

wise lifestyle choices, also can slow the aging process. In addition, the willingness to seek health care promptly when it is needed, the capacity to follow the instructions of a health-care provider, and the desire to accept the responsibility for one's own health can slow the rate of aging. Likewise, shelter that protects individuals from physical danger, climatic extremes, and solar radiation helps slow the aging process. Allowing people to make at least some decisions for themselves and control their own activities (autonomy) and providing psychosocial support (informational and emotional resources) promote successful aging and psychological well-being. In contrast, aging is likely to accelerate if any or all of the converse (i.e., insufficient income, low education level, lack of health care, inadequate shelter, and/or lack of autonomy and psychosocial support) are true.

CONCEPT CHECK

Although lifespan has not changed, life expectancy has increased dramatically over the past century. This means an increasing proportion of the North American population is over 65 years of age and will live for decades longer. Avoiding continually rising health care costs and maximizing satisfaction with life require postponing and minimizing chronic illness. Aging begins early in life and is influenced by heredity, lifestyle, and environment. A healthy diet and regular physical activity can play a pivotal role in slowing the aging process.

16.3 Nutrient Needs During Adulthood

The challenge of the adult years is to maintain the body, preserve its function, and avoid chronic disease—that is, to age successfully. A healthy diet can help achieve this goal. One blueprint for a healthy diet comes from the 2010 Dietary Guidelines for Americans, discussed in Chapter 2. The advice from those guidelines can be summarized into three main goals:

1. Balance calories with physical activity to manage weight.
2. Consume more of certain foods and nutrients, such as fruits, vegetables, whole grains, fat-free and low-fat dairy products, and seafood.
3. Consume fewer foods with sodium, saturated fats, *trans* fats, cholesterol, added sugars, and refined grains.

Overall, good nutrition benefits adults in many ways. Meeting nutrient needs delays the onset of certain diseases; improves the management of some existing diseases; speeds recovery from many illnesses; increases mental, physical, and social well-being; and often decreases the need for and length of hospitalization (see Further Readings 1 and 9). As you know, American adults are fairly well nourished, although some dietary excesses and inadequacies do exist. For instance, common dietary excesses are calories, fat, sodium, and, for some, alcohol. The diets of adult women tend to fall short of the recommended amounts of vitamins D and E, folate, magnesium, calcium, zinc, and fiber. The diets of adult men tend to be low in the same nutrients, except vitamin D, which does not become problematic until age 50. The iron intake of most women during their childbearing years (19 to 50) is insufficient to meet their needs; however, due to a reduced iron need after **menopause,** older women do get enough iron (see Further Reading 3).

menopause Cessation of menses in women, usually beginning at about age 50.

People age 65 and up, particularly those in long-term care facilities and hospitals, are the single largest group at risk of malnutrition. They may become underweight and show signs of numerous micronutrient deficiencies (e.g., vitamins B-6 and B-12 and folate). Friends, relatives, and health care professionals should monitor nutrient intake in all older people, including those who live in long-term care facilities. Family

FIGURE 16-2 ▶ A nutrition checklist for older adults.

Reprinted with permission by the Nutrition Screening Initiative, a project of the American Academy of Family Physicians, the American Dietetic Association, and the National Council on Aging, Inc., and funded in part by a grant from Ross Products Division, Abbott Laboratories.

A Nutrition Test for Older Adults

Here's a nutrition check for anyone over age 65. Circle the number of points for each statement that applies. Then compute the total and check it against the nutritional score.

Points	
2	1. The person has a chronic illness or current condition that has changed the kind or amount of food eaten.
3	2. The person eats fewer than two full meals per day.
2	3. The person eats few fruits, vegetables, or milk products.
2	4. The person drinks three or more servings of beer, liquor, or wine almost every day.
2	5. The person has tooth or mouth problems that make eating difficult.
4	6. The person does not have enough money for food.
1	7. The person eats alone most of the time.
1	8. The person takes three or more different prescription or over-the-counter drugs each day.
2	9. The person has unintentionally lost or gained 10 pounds within the last 6 months.
2	10. The person cannot always shop, cook, or feed himself or herself.
Total	

Nutritional score:

0–2: Good. Recheck in 6 months.

3–5: Marginal. A local agency on aging has information about nutrition programs for the elderly. The National Association of Area Agencies on Aging can assist in finding help; call (800) 677-1116. Recheck in 6 months.

6 or more: High risk. A doctor should review this test and suggest how to improve nutritional health.

members can play a valuable role in making sure nutrient needs are met by looking for weight maintenance and regular, healthful meal patterns. To pinpoint those over age 65 at risk of nutrient deficiencies, the American Academy of Family Physicians, the American Dietetic Association, and the National Council on Aging developed the Nutrition Screening Initiative checklist (Fig. 16-2). Older Americans, family members, and health care providers can use the checklist to identify those at nutritional risk *before* health deteriorates significantly. If problems arise in consuming a healthful diet, registered dietitians can offer professional and personalized advice.

Defining Nutrient Needs

The DRIs for adults are divided by gender into four age groups to reflect how nutrient needs change as adults grow older. These changes in nutrient needs take into consideration aging-related physiological alterations in body composition, metabolism, and organ function.

Calories. After age 30 or so, total calorie needs of physically inactive adults fall steadily throughout adulthood. This is caused by a gradual decline in basal metabolism. To a considerable extent, adults can exert control over this reduction in calorie need by

ostomy Surgically created short circuit in intestinal flow where the end point usually opens from the abdominal cavity rather than the anus—for example, a colostomy. Short circuiting the intestinal flow means more water is lost in fecal matter than would be if the intestinal tract were intact.

exercising. Exercise can halt, slow, and even reverse reductions in lean body mass and subsequent declines in calorie need. Also, keeping calorie needs high makes it easier to meet one's nutrient needs and avoid becoming overweight.

Protein. The protein intake of adults of all ages in North America tends to exceed current recommended levels. However, some recent studies indicate that consuming protein in amounts slightly higher than the RDA may help preserve muscle and bone mass (see Further Reading 5). Adults who have limited food budgets, have difficulty chewing meat, or are lactose intolerant may not get enough protein. Recall from Chapter 6 that any protein consumed in excess of that needed for the maintenance of body tissue will be broken down and used as energy or stored as fat. The waste products of metabolism of protein must be removed by the kidneys; excessive protein intake may accelerate kidney function decline.

Fat. The fat intake of adults of all ages is often at or above the recommendations. It's a good idea for almost all adults to reduce their fat intake because of the strong link between high-fat diets and obesity, heart disease, and certain cancers. In addition, reducing fat intake "frees up" some calories that can be better "spent" on complex carbohydrates (see Further Reading 12).

Carbohydrates. The total carbohydrate intake of adults of all ages in North America is often lower than recommended. In addition, many adults need to shift the carbohydrate composition of their diets to emphasize complex carbohydrates while minimizing intake of sugary, simple carbohydrates. A diet rich in complex carbohydrates helps us achieve nutrient needs and stay within calorie bounds because many highly sweetened foods are low in nutrients and high in calories. Substituting foods rich in complex carbohydrates for sweets also makes it easier for the body to control blood glucose levels—a function that becomes less efficient as the increases in body fatness and inactivity associated with usual aging occur. Declines in carbohydrate metabolism are so common that more than 25% of those age 65 years or older have diabetes. A diet rich in fiber helps adults reduce their risk of colon cancer and heart disease, lower their blood cholesterol levels, and avoid constipation. The typical American adult gets slightly more than half the recommended amount of dietary fiber.

Water. Many adults, especially those in the later years, fail to consume adequate quantities of water. In fact, many are in a constant state of mild dehydration and at risk of electrolyte imbalances. Low fluid intakes in older adults may be caused by a fading sensitivity to thirst sensations, chronic diseases, and/or conscious reductions in fluid intake in order to reduce the frequency of urination. Some also may have increased fluid output because they are taking certain medications (i.e., diuretics and laxatives), have an **ostomy,** and/or experience an age-related decline in the kidneys' ability to concentrate urine. Dehydration is very dangerous and, among other symptoms, can cause disorientation and mental confusion, constipation, impacted fecal matter, and death.

Minerals and Vitamins. Adequate intake of all vitamins and minerals is important throughout the adult years (Figs. 16-3 and 16-4). The micronutrients that need special attention because they tend to be present in less than optimal amounts in the diets of many adults are calcium, vitamin D, iron, zinc, magnesium, folate, and vitamins B-6, B-12, and E. Adults with impaired absorption or who are unable to consume a nutritious diet may benefit from mineral or vitamin supplements matched with their needs. In fact, many nutrition experts recommend a daily balanced multivitamin and mineral supplement for older adults, especially for those 70 years of age and older. Supplements or fortified foods can be especially helpful when it comes to meeting vitamin D and vitamin B-12 needs.

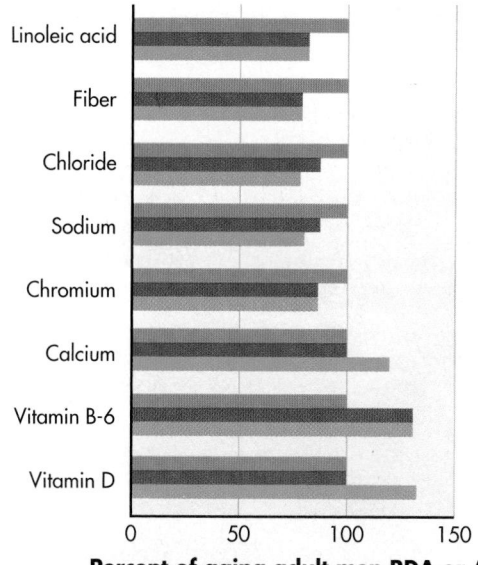

Percent of aging adult men RDA or AI

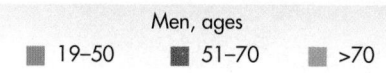

FIGURE 16-3 ▶ Relative nutrient requirements for aging adult men. Only nutrients that vary by age are shown.

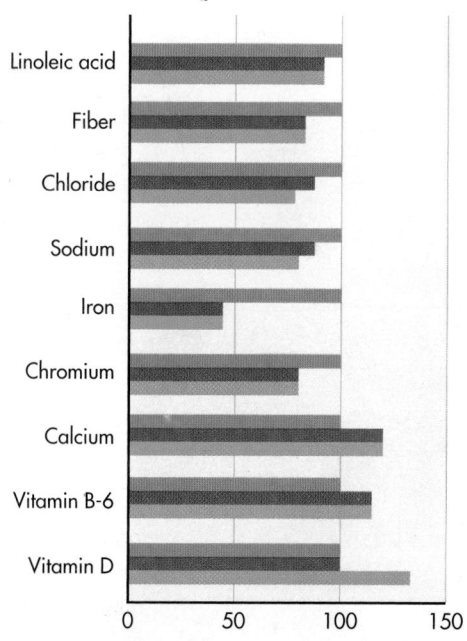

Percent of aging adult women RDA or AI

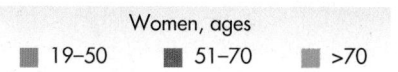

FIGURE 16-4 ▶ Relative nutrient requirements for aging adult women. Only nutrients that vary by age are shown.

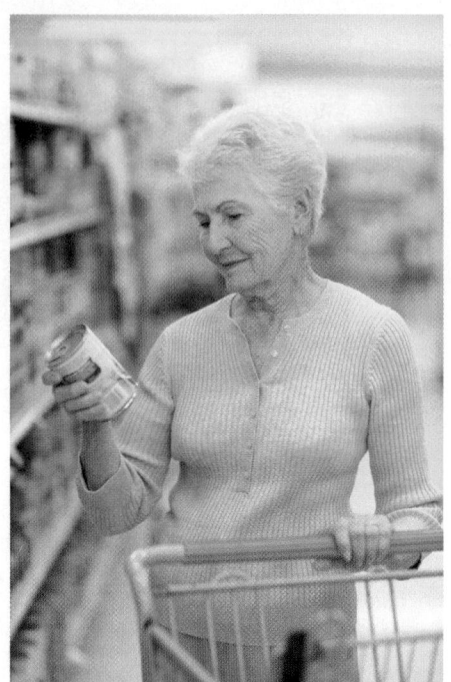

▲ Sodium needs for older adults are 1200 to 1300 milligrams per day. Older adults routinely consume at least this much sodium. Potassium needs are 4700 milligrams per day. Many older adults do not meet this goal.

Calcium and Vitamin D These bone-building nutrients tend to be low in the diets of all adults. They become particularly problematic after age 50. Inadequate intake of these nutrients, coupled with their reduced absorption, the reduced synthesis of vitamin D in the skin, and the kidneys' decreased ability to put vitamin D in its active form, greatly contributes to the development of osteoporosis. Getting enough of these nutrients is a challenge for many older adults because food sources of vitamin D are limited in the North American diet, and the major sources—fatty fish and fortified milk—are not widely consumed by older adults. Plus, with increasing age, lactase production frequently decreases. As you know, one of the richest and most absorbable sources of these nutrients, milk, contains lactose. To get the vitamin D and calcium needed, many with lactose intolerance can consume small amounts of milk at mealtime with no ill effects. Calcium-fortified foods, cheese, yogurt, fish eaten with bones (e.g., canned sardines or salmon), and dark green leafy vegetables can help those with lactose intolerance meet calcium needs—but these foods often do not provide vitamin D. Just 10 to 15 minutes per day of sunlight can make a large difference in vitamin D status.

Iron Iron deficiency anemia, the most common type of malnutrition during the adult years, is found most frequently in women in their reproductive years because their diets do not provide enough iron to compensate for the iron lost monthly during menstruation. Other common causes of iron deficiency in adults of all ages include digestive tract injuries that cause bleeding (i.e., bleeding ulcers or hemorrhoids) and the use of medicines, such as aspirin, that cause blood loss. Impaired iron absorption due to age-related declines in stomach acid production may contribute to iron deficiency in older adults.

Zinc In addition to less than optimal dietary zinc intake during adulthood, zinc absorption declines as stomach acid production diminishes with age. Poor zinc status may contribute to the taste sensation losses, mental lethargy, and delayed wound healing many elderly adults experience.

Magnesium This mineral tends to be low in adults' diets. Inadequate magnesium intakes may contribute to the bone loss muscular weakness, and mental confusion seen in some elderly adults. It also can lead to sudden death from poor heart rhythm and is linked to cardiovascular disease, osteoporosis, and diabetes. The best source of magnesium is the diet; supplements can cause loose stools and diarrhea.

Folate and Vitamins B-6 and B-12 Sufficient folate, because of its role in prevention of neural tube defects, is very important to women during the childbearing years. In later years, folate and vitamins B-6 and B-12 are especially important because they are required to clear homocysteine from the bloodstream. Introduced in Chapter 5, elevated blood concentrations of homocysteine are associated with the increased risk of cardiovascular disease, stroke, bone fracture, and neurological decline seen in some elderly people. Vitamin B-12 is a particular problem for the older population because a deficiency may exist even when intake appears to be adequate. As people age, the stomach slows its production of acid and intrinsic factor, which leads to poor absorption of vitamin B-12 and eventually pernicious anemia. Adults age 51 years and older need to meet vitamin B-12 needs with supplements or foods fortified with synthetic vitamin B-12.

Vitamin E The dietary intake of most of the population falls short of recommendations for vitamin E. Low vitamin E intake means the body has a reduced supply of antioxidants, which may increase the degree of cell damage caused by free radicals, promote the progression of chronic diseases and cataracts, and speed aging. In addition, low vitamin E levels can lead to declines in physical abilities.

Carotenoids. Dietary intakes of certain carotenoids have been shown to have a variety of important anti-aging and health protective effects. Specifically, lutein and zeaxanthin have been linked with the prevention of cataracts and age-related macular degeneration. Diets high in fruit and vegetables, the major sources of carotenoids and other beneficial phytochemicals, are consistently shown to be protective of a wide variety of age-related conditions.

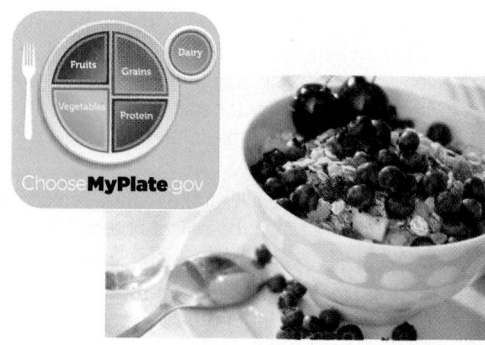

▲ How does this breakfast of whole-grain cereal, fruit, and milk compare to MyPlate?

Are Adults Following Current Dietary Recommendations?

In general, adults in North America are trying to follow many of the diet recommendations described in this chapter. Since the mid-1950s, they have consumed less saturated fat as more people substitute fat-free and low-fat milk for cream and whole milk. However, they eat more cheese, usually a concentrated form of saturated fat. Since 1963, they have eaten less butter, fewer eggs, less animal fat, and more vegetable oils and fish. These changes generally follow recommendations to reduce the intake of saturated fat and cholesterol in favor of unsaturated fat choices. Animal breeders are raising much leaner cattle and hogs than those produced in 1950, which also helps reduce saturated fat intake.

Other aspects of the average adult diet are less promising. The latest nutrition survey of eating habits in the United States shows that the major contributors of calories to the adult diet are white bread, beef, doughnuts, cakes and cookies, soft drinks, milk, chicken, cheese, alcoholic beverages, salad dressing, mayonnaise, potatoes, and sugars/syrups/jams. If the trend in diets were truly toward decreasing sugar and saturated fat intake, and increasing fiber intake, many of these foods would not appear at the top of the list.

CONCEPT CHECK

The 2010 Dietary Guidelines for Americans direct people to maintain healthy weight; choose more vegetables, fruits, legumes (beans), whole-grain products, fat-free and low-fat dairy products, and seafood; and choose fewer foods with sodium, saturated fats, *trans* fats, added sugars, and refined grains. Micronutrients of concern for an aging population include calcium, iron, zinc, magnesium, folate, carotenoids, and vitamins D, B-6, B-12, and E.

16.4 Factors Related to Food Intake and Nutrient Needs

Diet is one of the main factors directly involved in the development of several health conditions during adulthood. The effects of diet and nutrients on many of these conditions, including atherosclerosis, cancer, constipation, diabetes, diverticular disease, heartburn, hypertension, obesity, and osteoporosis, were discussed in earlier chapters. Still other health problems, including arthritis, Alzheimer's disease, and depression, are not directly diet-related, but nutrition is implicated in their prevention and/or treatment.

An important concept to remember is that an aging body loses resilience—it becomes less able to handle stressors and restore balance (homeostasis). For example, compared to a healthy 30-year-old adult, it takes twice as long for the kidneys of an 80-year-old to remove wastes and restore blood levels to normal after eating excess protein. Similarly, the breakdown of alcohol, drugs, and even nutrient supplements is

Researchers believe that maintaining lean muscle mass may be the most important strategy for successful aging. This is because maintaining lean muscle mass:

- Maintains basal metabolic rate, which helps decrease the risk of obesity

- Keeps body fat low, which helps control blood cholesterol levels and helps avoid the onset of type 2 diabetes

- Maintains body water, which decreases the risk of dehydration and improves body temperature regulation

sarcopenia In general, loss of muscle tissue. Among older adults this loss of lean mass greatly increases their risk of illness and death.

sarcopenic obesity Loss of muscle mass accompanied by gains in fat mass.

slowed. Consequently, blood levels of these substances rise higher and have a stronger and longer effect in older adults than in younger people. Taking steps to avoid stressing the body's capabilities (e.g., avoiding excessive protein intake or megadose dietary supplements) can help preserve optimal physiological function in older adults.

Like those of other age groups, the food choices and nutritional adequacy of adults' diets depend on the interplay of physiological, psychosocial, and economic factors. Alterations in any one of these factors can result in deteriorations in the quality of dietary intake, nutritional status, and health.

Physiological Factors

The implications of many of the physiological changes that occur during adulthood on dietary intake and nutrient needs are summarized in Table 16-2. Some of the changes listed (e.g., tooth loss, loss in taste and smell perceptions) can influence dietary intake. Other changes (e.g., loss of lean body tissue) can alter nutrient and/or calorie needs. Still other changes (e.g., reduced stomach acidity, diminished kidney function) can cause changes in nutrient utilization. Chronic diseases and the need for medications are additional physiological changes many adults experience that can influence food intake and nutrient needs. The following section details the interactions of several of these factors on nutritional status during adulthood.

Body Composition. The primary changes in body composition that occur as the adult years progress are diminished lean body mass, increased fat stores, and decreased body water. The loss of lean body mass is termed **sarcopenia.** Some muscle cells shrink and others are lost as muscles age; some muscles lose their elasticity as they accumulate fat and collagen. Loss of muscle mass leads to a decrease in basal metabolism, muscle strength, and energy needs. Less muscle mass also leads to lower physical activity, which makes the prognosis for maintaining muscle even worse. Clearly, it is best to avoid this downward spiral.

Lifestyle greatly determines the rate of muscle mass deterioration. As you might predict, an active lifestyle helps maintain muscle mass, whereas an inactive one encourages its loss. In fact, much of what we associate with old age is due to a lifetime of physical inactivity. Ideally, an active lifestyle should be maintained throughout life and include both aerobic and strength training (see Making Decisions). Physical activity increases muscle strength and mobility, improves balance and decreases the risk of falling, eases daily tasks that require some strength, improves sleep, slows bone loss, and increases joint movement, thus reducing injuries. It also has a positive impact on a person's mental outlook. Strength training (resistance) helps reverse some of the decline in daily function associated with the muscle loss typically seen in older adulthood.

As lean tissue declines with age, body fat often increases, a condition called **sarcopenic obesity** (see Further Reading 13). Much of this increase in body fat results from overeating and limited physical activity, although even athletic men and lean women typically gain some degree of midsection fat after age 50. A small fat gain in adulthood may not compromise health, but large gains are problematic. Recall that obesity can raise blood pressure and blood glucose and make walking and performing daily tasks more difficult.

Decreases in body weight are common in adults age 70 and older. Weight loss is a problem for older people in particular because it increases the risk of nutrition-related illness and death. It may indicate illness, reduced tolerance to medication, or withdrawal from life. The effects of current medication, as well as changes in taste and smell, may inhibit appetite, too. In addition, many older people live alone, a circumstance associated with depressed appetite.

Skeletal System. Recall from Chapter 9 that bone loss in women occurs primarily after menopause. Bone loss in men is slow and steady from middle age throughout later life. Many older people may suffer from undiagnosed osteomalacia, a condition

TABLE 16-2 Typical Physiological Changes of Aging and Recommended Diet and Lifestyle Responses

Physiological Changes	Recommended Responses
Appetite (↓)	• Monitor weight and strive to eat enough to maintain healthy weight. • Use meal replacement products, such as Boost® and Ensure Plus®.
Sense of taste and smell (↓)	• Vary the diet. • Experiment with herbs and spices.
Chewing ability (↓)	• Work with a dentist to maximize chewing ability. • Modify food consistency as necessary. • Eat calorie-rich snacks.
Sense of thirst (↓)	• Consume plenty of fluid each day. • Stay alert for evidence of dehydration (e.g., minimal output or dark-colored urine).
Stomach acidity (↓)	• Consume iron-rich foods with a source of vitamin C. • Choose foods fortified with vitamin B-12 or use a supplemental source of vitamin B-12.
Bowel function (↓)	• Consume enough fiber daily, choosing primarily fruits, vegetables, and whole-grain breads and cereals. • Meet fluid needs.
Lactase production (↓)	• Limit milk serving size at each use. • Substitute yogurt or cheese for milk. • Use reduced-lactose or lactose-free products. • Seek nondairy calcium sources.
Iron status (↓)	• Include some lean meat and iron-fortified foods in the diet. • Ask physician to monitor blood iron status.
Liver function (↓)	• Consume alcohol in moderation, if at all. • Avoid consuming excess vitamin A.
Insulin function (↓)	• Maintain healthy body weight. • Perform regular physical activity.
Kidney function (↓)	• If necessary, work with physician and registered dietitian to modify protein and other nutrients in diet.
Immune function (↓)	• Meet nutrient needs, especially protein, vitamin E, vitamin B-6, and zinc. • Perform regular physical activity.
Lung function (↓)	• Avoid tobacco products. • Perform regular physical activity.
Vision (↓)	• Regularly consume sources of carotenoids, vitamin C, vitamin E, and zinc (e.g., fruits, vegetables and whole-grain breads and cereals). • Moderate total fat intake. • Wear sunglasses in sunny conditions. • Avoid tobacco products. • Perform regular physical activity (to lessen insulin resistance). • In the case of diagnosed moderate macular degeneration, talk with a physician about following a protocol of zinc, copper, vitamin E, vitamin C, and beta-carotene supplementation.
Lean tissue (↓)	• Meet nutrient needs, especially protein and vitamin D. • Perform regular physical activity, including strength training.
Cardiovascular function (↓)	• Use diet modifications or physician-prescribed medications to keep blood lipids and blood pressure within desirable ranges. • Stay physically active. • Achieve and maintain a healthy body weight.
Bone mass (↓)	• Meet nutrient needs, especially calcium and vitamin D (regular sun exposure helps meet needs for vitamin D). • Perform regular physical activity, especially weight-bearing exercise. • Women should consider use of approved osteoporosis medications at menopause. • Remain at a healthy weight (especially avoid unneeded weight loss).
Mental function (↓)	• Meet nutrient needs (e.g., vitamin E, vitamin C, vitamin B-6, folate, and vitamin B-12) and consume seafood twice a week. • Strive for lifelong learning. • Perform regular physical activity. • Obtain adequate sleep.
Fat stores (↓)	• Avoid overeating. • Perform regular physical activity.

Registered dietitians, physicians, and pharmacists can help with any needed adjustments arising from these and other drug-related problems.

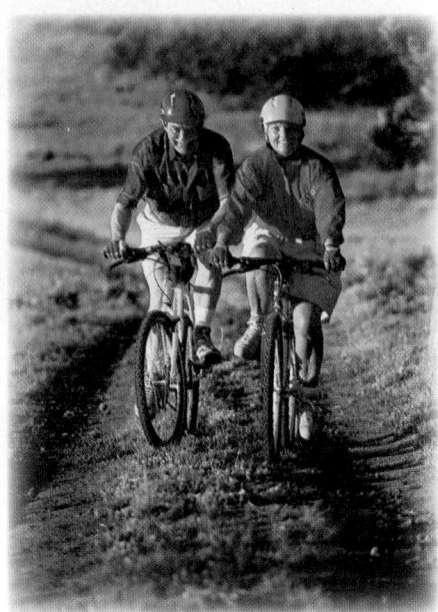

▲ Older people benefit from aerobic and strength-training (resistance) exercises. Download a free copy of *Exercise & Physical Activity: Your Everyday Guide* from the National Institute on Aging at www.nia.nih.gov.

The 2008 Physical Activity Guidelines for Americans provide the following guidelines specifically for older adults:

- When older adults cannot do 150 minutes of moderate-intensity aerobic activity a week because of chronic conditions, they should be as physically active as their abilities and conditions allow.

- Older adults should do exercises that maintain or improve balance if they are at risk of falling.

- Older adults should determine their level of effort for physical activity relative to their level of fitness.

- Older adults with chronic diseases should understand whether and how their conditions affect their ability to do regular physical activity safely.

mainly caused by insufficient vitamin D. Osteoporosis can limit the ability of older people to move about, shop, prepare food, and live normally. Consuming adequate vitamin D, calcium, and protein; not smoking; drinking alcohol moderately or not at all; and engaging in weight-bearing exercises can help preserve bone mass. Medications also can help lessen bone loss.

MAKING DECISIONS

Exercise Guidelines for Older Adults

Aerobic Exercise: All adults should engage in moderate-intensity aerobic exercise for at least 150 minutes per week, or vigorous intensity aerobic exercise for 75 minutes per week, or an equivalent combination of the two. This amount of aerobic activity aids in prevention of chronic diseases. Longer duration of daily exercise may be required for weight loss or weight maintenance. Weight bearing exercises are particularly helpful for preservation of bone mass.

Strength Training: To maintain lean tissue and basal metabolic rate, strength training should include eight to ten different exercises (each with two sets of eight to fifteen repetitions), performed two to three times per week. Exercises that involve the large muscle groups (e.g., arms, back, and legs) and exercises that enhance grip strength should be emphasized. Start slowly, concentrate on breathing, rest between sets, avoid locking joints in the arms and legs, and stop an exercise if it becomes painful.

Flexibility Exercises: To prevent injuries, stretching exercises for each major muscle group should accompany aerobic or strength exercises at least 2 days per week.

Balance Exercises: For those over age 65 who are at risk for falling, exercises that improve balance (e.g., yoga, tai chi) are recommended in addition to aerobic, strength, and flexibility exercises.

All older adults should avoid inactivity. Having an exercise plan, developed with a health professional to accommodate individual health risks and needs, will enhance success for older adults. Men older than age 40; women older than age 50; those with heart conditions, diabetes, or joint problems; and anyone who has been sedentary should consult a physician before beginning an exercise program.

Learn more at www.acsm.org and see Further Reading 4.

Digestive System. The production of HCl, intrinsic factor, and lactase declines with advancing age and, as a result, impairs the absorption of several nutrients. Constipation is the main intestinal problem for older people. To prevent constipation, older people should meet fiber needs, drink enough fluids, and exercise. Fiber medications are generally unnecessary but may be useful when total energy consumption does not allow for enough fiber intake. Because some medications can cause constipation, a physician should be consulted to determine if a laxative or stool softener is needed.

In addition to changes in the GI tract, the functions of the accessory organs decline as we age. For instance, the liver functions less efficiently. A history of significant alcohol consumption or liver disease will cause the liver to function even less efficiently. As liver efficiency declines, its ability to detoxify many substances, including medications, alcohol, and vitamin and mineral supplements, drops. The possibility for vitamin toxicity increases.

The gallbladder also functions less efficiently in later years. Gallstones can block the flow of bile out of the gallbladder into the small intestine, thereby interfering with fat digestion. Obesity is a major risk factor for gallbladder disease, especially in older women. A low-fat diet or surgery to remove the gallbladder may be necessary.

Although pancreatic function may decline with age, this organ has a large reserve capacity. One sign of a failing pancreas is high blood glucose, although this can occur as the result of several conditions. The pancreas may be secreting less insulin, or cells may be resisting insulin action (as is commonly seen in obese people with upper-body fat storage). Where appropriate, improved nutrient intake, regular physical activity, and loss of excess body weight can improve insulin action and blood glucose regulation.

Nervous System. A gradual loss of nerve cells that transmit signals may decrease taste and smell perceptions and impair neuromuscular coordination, reasoning, and memory. Both hearing and vision decline with age. Hearing impairment is greatest in those who have been exposed constantly to loud noises, such as urban traffic, aircraft noise, and music. Because they cannot hear well, older people may avoid social contacts, which increases their risk of poor dietary intake.

Declining eyesight, frequently caused by retina degeneration and cataracts, can affect a person's abilities to grocery shop, locate desired foods, read labels for nutritional content, and prepare foods at home. Vision losses also may cause people to curtail social contacts, reduce physical activity, and not practice daily personal health and grooming routines. Macular degeneration, one form of failing eyesight in old age, is quite common, affecting about 9.1 million adults in the United States. A major risk factor is cigarette smoking. Diets rich in carotenoids help reduce the risk of macular degeneration. The risk of developing cataracts is decreased by consuming a diet rich in fruits and vegetables.

Neuromuscular coordination losses may make it difficult to shop for and prepare food. Physical tasks as simple as opening food packages can become so difficult that individuals restrict dietary intake to foods that require little preparation and depend on others to provide food that is ready to eat. Eating may become difficult, too. Loss of coordination makes it a challenge to grasp cup handles and manipulate eating utensils. As a result, older adults may avoid foods that can be easily spilled (e.g., soups and juices) or that need to be cut (e.g., meats, large vegetable pieces) and restrict food intake to easy-to-eat finger foods. Some may even withdraw from social interaction and eat alone, which can lead to inadequate nutrient intake.

Immune System. With age, the immune system often operates less efficiently. Consuming adequate protein, vitamins (especially folate and vitamins A, D, and E), iron, and zinc helps maximize immune system function. Recurrent sicknesses and poor wound healing are warning signs that a deficient diet (especially of protein and zinc) may be hindering the function of the immune system. On the other hand, overnutrition appears to be equally harmful to the immune system. For example, obesity and excessive fat, iron, and zinc intakes can suppress immune function.

Endocrine System. As adulthood progresses, the rate of hormone synthesis and release can slow. A decrease in insulin release or sensitivity to insulin, for instance, means that it takes longer for blood glucose levels to return to normal after a meal. Maintaining a healthy weight, exercising regularly, eating a diet low in fat and high in fiber, and avoiding foods with a high glycemic index can enhance the body's ability to use insulin and restore elevated blood glucose levels to normal after a meal.

Chronic Disease. The prevalence of obesity, heart disease, osteoporosis, cancer, hypertension, and diabetes rises with age. More than eight out of every ten elderly people have one of these chronic and potentially debilitating diseases. Half of all elderly people have at least two chronic conditions. Chronic diseases may have a strong impact on dietary intake. For instance, excessive fatness, heart disease, and osteoporosis may impair physical mobility to the extent that victims are unable to shop for and prepare food. Chronic disease also can influence nutrient and calorie needs. Cancer, for example, boosts both nutrient and calorie needs. Hypertension may indicate a need to lower sodium intake. Nutrient utilization can be affected by chronic disease, too. For instance, diabetes alters the body's ability to utilize glucose. In addition, the effects of heart disease on the kidneys may impair their ability to reabsorb glucose, amino acids, and vitamin C.

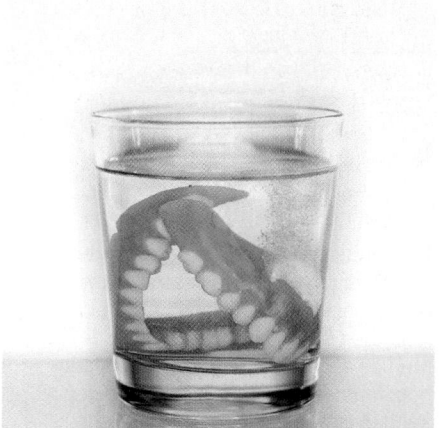

▲ Poor dental health contributes to decreased food intake and digestive problems. Serving softer, easier to chew foods and allowing extra time for chewing and swallowing improves food intake.

MAKING DECISIONS

Nutrition Interventions for Arthritis

There are over 100 forms of arthritis, a disease that causes the degeneration and roughening of the cartilage that covers and cushions the joints. Such changes in the joints cause them to ache and become inflamed and painful to move. Osteoarthritis, which increases in prevalence with advancing age, is the leading cause of disability among older persons. Rheumatoid arthritis, which is not as common, is more prevalent in younger adults.

Although precise causes or cures are unknown, many unproven "remedies" have been publicized. Unusual diets, food restrictions, and nutrient supplements are some of the more popular treatments. However, no special diet, food, or nutrient has been proven to reliably prevent, relieve, or cure arthritis in humans. As far as supplements go, glucosamine and/or chondroitin have been most extensively studied in relation to arthritis. Many but not all studies demonstrate these supplements can relieve pain, slow the progression of joint degeneration, or rebuild cartilage. Maintaining a healthy weight, which reduces stress on painful arthritic joints, is the only diet-related treatment known to offer some relief. MyPlate can be used as a guide in making healthy food choices for weight management.

CRITICAL THINKING

Jamila went to her local pharmacy yesterday to look for a product to help her stay awake while studying. On the shelves she found a dietary supplement claiming to be a Chinese herbal remedy for sleepiness and fatigue. She thought that because a pharmacy carried the product, it should be safe and work as indicated on the label.

Is she correct in these assumptions? Are there specific risks associated with taking such herbal remedies?

Numerous reports have documented significant health risks associated with the use of some herbal and alternative remedies, sometimes resulting in death. Studies especially implicate germander, pokeroot, sassafras, mandrake, pennyroyal, comfrey, chaparral, yohimbe, lobelia, jin bu huan, kava kava, products containing stephanie and magnolia, senna, hai gen fen, paraguay tea, kombucha tea, tung shueh (Chinese black balls), and willow bark.

Medications. Older adults are major consumers of medications (prescription and over-the-counter) and nutrient supplements. Half of all people over age 65 take several medicines each day. The rate of supplement use increases throughout adulthood, such that by age 50, approximately half of all adults are using supplements daily. Physiological declines that occur during aging (e.g., reduced body water, reduced liver and kidney function) cause the effects of medications and nutrient supplements to be exaggerated and persist longer in older adults.

Medications can improve health and quality of life, but some also adversely affect nutritional status, particularly of those who are older and/or take many different medications. For instance, some medications depress taste and smell acuity or cause anorexia or nausea that can blunt interest in eating and lead to reduced dietary intake. Some medications alter nutrient needs. Aspirin, for example, increases the likelihood of stomach bleeding, so long-term use may elevate the need for iron, as well as other nutrients. Antibiotics may deplete the body of vitamin K. Some medications may impair nutrient utilization—diuretics and laxatives may cause excessive excretion of water and minerals. Even vitamin and mineral supplements may have unanticipated effects on nutritional status. Iron supplements taken in large doses can interfere with the functioning of zinc and copper. Folate supplements can mask vitamin B-12 deficiencies.

People who must take medications should eat nutrient-dense foods and avoid any specific food or supplement that interferes with the function of their medications. For example, vitamin K can reduce the action of oral anticoagulants, aged cheese can interfere with certain drugs used to treat hypertension and depression, and grapefruit can interfere with medications such as tranquilizers and those that lower cholesterol levels. A physician or pharmacist should be consulted about any restrictions on food and/or supplements.

Alternative Medicine and Aging

At least half of adults report using some kind of dietary or herbal supplement. Recall from Chapter 2 that these products are not evaluated by FDA for effectiveness or safety since they are governed by the 1994 Dietary Supplement Health and Education Act (DSHEA). Purity and quantity of the product in the bottle are also suspect. Table 16-3 reviews some popular herbal remedies used by older adults. Note from the table that these products can pose health risks in certain people. In addition, they may be expensive ($100 per month or more in some cases) and are not covered by health insurance plans. Use of many herbal products has declined because of expense and questionable benefits. Instead, consumers are opting to spend their money on tried-and-true products, such as multivitamins, vitamin D, omega-3 fatty acids, fiber, and probiotics.

A rational approach to the use of herbal products is to use only one product at a time, keep a diary of symptoms, and check with one's physician first before discontinuing a prescribed medication. In addition, FDA advises anyone who experiences adverse side effects from an herbal remedy to contact a physician. Physicians are then encouraged to report such adverse events to FDA, state and local health departments, and consumer protection agencies.

For additional information about herbal remedies, access the following websites. These are regularly updated and cover the herbals listed in Table 16-3, as well as many others.

National Institutes of Health National Center for Complementary and Alternative Medicine (NCCAM)
www.nccam.nih.gov/
American Botanical Council
http://abc.herbalgram.org/
Complementary and Alternative Medicine Program at Stanford (CAMPS)
http://camps.stanford.edu/
National Institutes of Health Office of Dietary Supplements
http://ods.od.nih.gov/
Natural Medicines Comprehensive Database
www.naturaldatabase.com

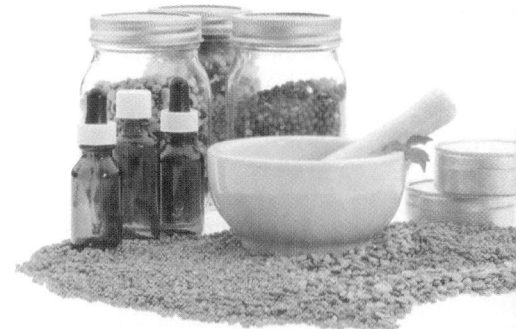

▲ Some herbal products are effective for treating specific medical problems. Follow label instructions carefully. Note potential side effects listed, as well as who should not use the product. The best advice is to only use these substances under strict supervision of a physician.

TABLE 16-3 A Close Look at Some Popular Herbal Remedies

Product	Purported Effects	Side Effects	Who Should Especially Seek Physician Guidance Before Use
Black cohosh	• Mild reduction of postmenopausal symptoms (shown to be effective in some but not all women; use should not go beyond 6 months in general)	• Nausea • Liver damage	• Women who have had breast cancer • Pregnant women • Anyone taking estrogen, hypertension medications, or blood-thinning medications*
Cranberry	• Prevention or treatment of urinary tract infections (some evidence of efficacy)	• Use of concentrated tablets may increase risk of kidney stones	• People susceptible to kidney stones • Anyone taking antidepressants or prescription painkillers
Echinacea	• Stimulation of the immune system • Prevention or treatment of colds or other infections (mild effect at best)	• Nausea • Skin irritation • Allergic reactions • Minor GI tract upset • Increased urination	• Anyone with an autoimmune disease • Pre- or postsurgical patients • Anyone with allergies to daisies
Garlic	• Antibiotic properties • Slight reduction of blood cholesterol or blood pressure in some, but not all, studies	• GI tract upset (e.g., heartburn, flatulence) • Unpleasant odor	• Pre- or postsurgical patients • Perinatal women • People with a history of gallstones • Anyone taking blood-thinning medications or AIDS medications
Ginkgo biloba	• Increased circulation • Improvement of memory (especially for people with Alzheimer's disease; low evidence of efficacy)	• Mild headache • GI tract upset • Allergic reactions • Irritability • Reduced blood clotting • Seizures (if contaminated with toxic ginkgo seeds)	• People with bleeding disorders • Pre- or postsurgical patients • Anyone with allergies to the plant • Concurrent use of feverfew, garlic, ginseng, dong quai, or red clover • Anyone taking diabetes medications, blood-thinning medications, vitamin E supplements, antidepressants, or diuretics

TABLE 16-3 *(continued)*

Product	Purported Effects	Side Effects	Who Should Especially Seek Physician Guidance Before Use
Ginseng	• Increased energy • Stress relief • Decreased weakness and fatigue (efficacy largely unknown)	• Hypertension • Asthma attacks • Irregular heartbeat • Insomnia • Headache • Nervousness • GI tract upset • Reduced blood clotting • Menstrual irregularities and breast tenderness	• Anyone who takes a prescription drug should consult a physician before using • Women on hormone replacement therapy • Women who have had breast cancer • Anyone with chronic GI tract disease • Anyone with uncontrolled hypertension • Anyone taking blood-thinning medications, diabetes medications, antidepressants, or heart failure medications
St. John's wort	• Alleviation of depression (mild effect at best)	• Mild GI tract upset • Rash • Tiredness • Restlessness • Increased sensitivity to sunlight	• Anyone who takes a prescription drug • People with UV sensitivity, including that induced by medications or other treatments** • People with bipolar disorder • Anyone recovering from a graft or organ transplant • Anyone taking ritalin, caffeine, HIV medications, heart failure medications, cholesterol-lowering medications, blood-thinning medications, chemotherapy, oral contraceptives, antidepressants, antipsychotic medications, or asthma medications
Valerian	• Alleviation of restlessness and other sleeping disorders that stem from nervous conditions • Reduction of anxiety (some evidence of efficacy)	• Impaired attention • Headache • Morning grogginess • Irregular heartbeat • GI tract upset • Disagreeable odor • Withdrawal delerium	• Anyone taking central nervous system depressants*** • Anyone who drinks alcohol • People about to operate heavy machinery or drive

Pregnant or breastfeeding women, children under 2 years of age, anyone over the age of 65 years, and anyone with a chronic disease should never take supplements unless under the guidance of a physician. A concern has been raised with regard to patients who abruptly end alternative medicines at the start of hospital treatments or deny that they are involved in alternative therapy. Interactions between alternative therapies and pharmaceutical drugs can be drastic and include complications such as delirium, clotting abnormalities, and rapid heartbeat, resulting in the need for intensive care. Full disclosure of all prescription and nonprescription treatments aids in prevention of such complications. Experts recommend that, if time permits, patients stop taking herbal products for about a week before a scheduled surgery or otherwise take all original supplement containers to the hospital, so that the anesthesiologist can evaluate what was taken.

*Coumadin, aspirin, Heparin, Lovenox, or Fragmin

**Sulfa medications, anti-inflammatory medications, or acid-reflux medications

***Valium, halcion, seconal

Psychosocial Factors

Worries about possible embarrassment caused by deteriorating physical capabilities may cause older adults to withdraw from social interaction and eat alone rather than with others. Those who eat alone, regardless of the reason, seldom eat as much or as nutritiously as they should. Both young and old people who eat without companionship tend to feel unmotivated to shop for or prepare foods. Many become apathetic toward life, which over time causes health and nutritional status to decline. As you'll see later in the chapter, several nutrition assistance programs can help older people obtain the food and social support needed for good health.

Depression A positive outlook on life and intact support networks help make food and eating interesting and satisfying. In contrast, social isolation, grief, chronic pain and infirmity, or a change in lifestyle can lead to depression, loss of appetite, lack of interest in food, and disability. Major depression affects 5% to 8% of adults in the United States. This statistic increases to about 18% among Americans ages 65 or older. Left untreated, depression can lead to a continual decline in appetite, which results in weakness, poor nutrition, mental confusion, and increased feelings of isolation and loneliness (Fig. 16-5). In contrast, some people cope by overeating, which can lead

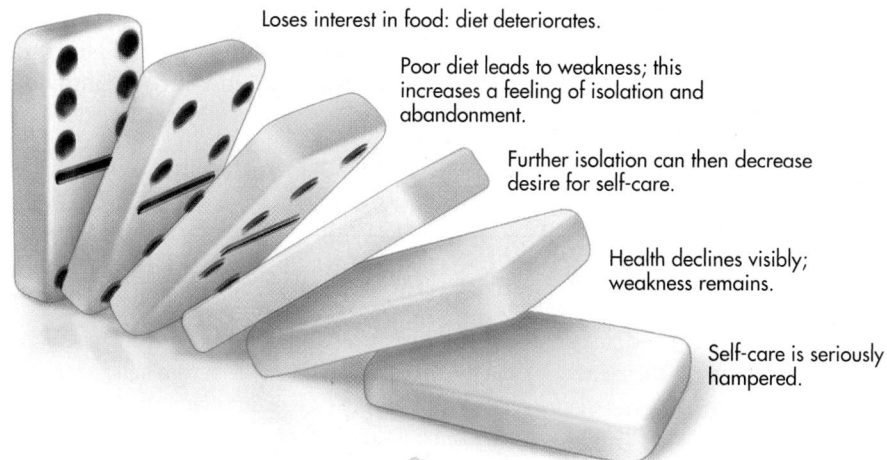

Social isolation; perhaps spouse has died.

Loses interest in food: diet deteriorates.

Poor diet leads to weakness; this increases a feeling of isolation and abandonment.

Further isolation can then decrease desire for self-care.

Health declines visibly; weakness remains.

Self-care is seriously hampered.

FIGURE 16-5 ▶ The decline of health often seen in older adults. A small change leads to a chain of events or "domino effect" that results in poor health. Early intervention can prevent declines in physical health related to psychosocial factors.

to obesity and its associated problems. Depression may signal an underlying illness and can also impair recovery from other illnesses or injuries. As many as 15% of cases end in suicide. For these reasons, early detection of depression is important in older adults. Depression is often treatable, but medication alone will not help those experiencing major life changes, such as the death of a spouse. Adequate social support and/or psychological intervention are also essential.

Alzheimer's Disease. Alzheimer's disease is an irreversible, abnormal, progressive deterioration of the brain that causes victims to steadily lose the ability to remember, reason, and comprehend. Alzheimer's disease often takes a terrible toll on the mental and eventual physical health of older people. About 5.4 million adults in the U.S. have the disease.

The 10 warning signs of Alzheimer's disease are listed in the margin. No one is sure exactly what causes this disease, but scientists have proposed various causes, including alterations in cell development or protein production in the brain, strokes, altered blood lipoprotein composition, obesity, poor blood glucose regulation (e.g., diabetes), high blood pressure, high blood cholesterol, and high free radical levels.

Early efforts at prevention are key, because the process of cognitive decline begins 10 to 20 years before warning signs appear. Preventive measures for Alzheimer's disease focus on maintaining brain activity through lifelong learning, eating a diet rich in fruits and vegetables, and taking ibuprofen. The role of nutrition in preventing or minimizing the risk of this disease is being investigated. Getting enough antioxidant nutrients, such as vitamin C, vitamin E, and selenium, helps protect the body from the damaging effects of free radicals. Adequate intakes of folate and vitamins B-6 and B-12 are especially important because elevated blood homocysteine is also a risk factor. Dietary fats, too, may play a role in keeping this disease at bay. Individuals with diets rich in omega-3 and omega-6 foods and low in saturated and *trans* fatty acids have a reduced risk of Alzheimer's disease.

The dietary intakes of those with Alzheimer's disease are poor, compared with those of a similar age without this disease. Caregivers of those who have Alzheimer's disease need to monitor the patient's weight to ensure maintenance of a healthy weight and nutritional state. Other tips are serving omega-3 rich fish in meals twice per week and making sure eating habits do not pose a health risk (e.g., holding food in one's mouth or forgetting to swallow). Regular physical activity has also been shown to improve mental status in people afflicted with this disease (see Further Reading 6).

Economic Factors. The amount of money available for purchasing food can have a great impact on the types and amounts of food one eats. Unemployment, underemployment, retirement, death of a wage earner, or anything else that limits

Ten Warning Signs of Alzheimer's Disease

1. Recent memory loss that affects job performance
2. Difficulty performing familiar tasks
3. Problems with language
4. Disorientation to time and place
5. Faulty or decreased judgment
6. Problems with abstract thinking
7. Tendency to misplace things
8. Changes in mood or behavior
9. Changes in personality
10. Loss of initiative

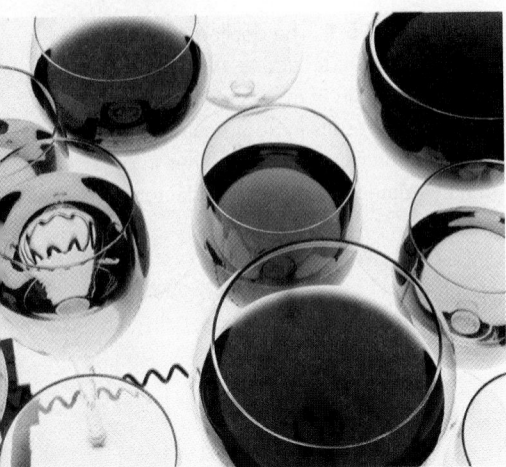

▲ Of all the alcohol sources, red wine in moderation is often singled out as the best choice because of the added bonus of the many phytochemicals present (e.g., resveratrol). These are leached out from the grape skins as the red wine is fermented. Dark beer is also a source of phytochemicals.

ethanol Chemical term for the form of alcohol found in alcoholic beverages.

income makes it difficult to get the best, most healthful foods and can diminish nutritional status and health. Insufficient income is a particular problem among those ages 65 and up and, as a result, they frequently have trouble making sure they remain well nourished. The Commodity Foods Program and Supplemental Nutrition Assistance Program are two federal U.S. programs that can help low-income individuals of all ages procure the foods they need.

CONCEPT CHECK

Physiological, psychosocial, and economic factors impact the nutritional status of older adults. The following organ systems and functions can decrease as we age: appetite; sense of taste, smell, thirst, hearing, and sight; digestion and absorption; liver, gallbladder, pancreatic, kidney, lung, and heart function; and the immune system. In addition, bone mass and muscle mass gradually decrease, the latter largely because of a deficient diet and inactivity. Appropriate dietary changes, regular physical activity, maintaining social contacts, and participating in nutrition assistance programs can often help reduce the impact of these factors.

16.5 Nutrition Implications of Alcohol Consumption

Given the wide spectrum of alcohol use and abuse, knowledge of alcohol consumption and its relationship to overall health is essential to the study of nutrition. Alcoholic beverages contain the chemical form of alcohol known as **ethanol.** Although not a nutrient *per se*, alcohol is a source of calories (about 7 kcal per gram) for approximately half of adults, constituting about 3% of total calories in the average North American diet (Table 16-4). Bear in mind that alcoholic beverages served in bars and restaurants can be 20% to 45% larger than the "standard drinks" described below.

Moderate consumption of alcohol by a person of legal age is an acceptable practice and even has some health benefits (see Further Reading 2). However, only about half

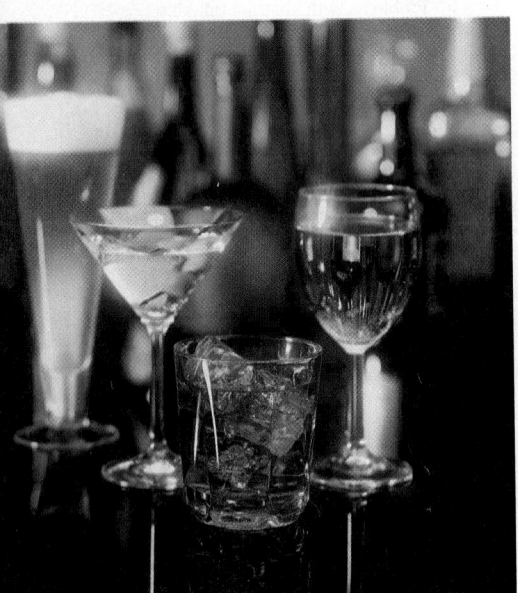

▲ One standard drink is universally defined as one 12-ounce bottle of beer or wine cooler, one 5-ounce glass of wine, 3 ounces of sherry or liqueur, or 1.5 ounces of 80-proof distilled spirits.

TABLE 16-4 Alcohol, Carbohydrate, and Calorie Content of Alcoholic Beverages*

Beverage	Amount (fluid ounces)	Alcohol (grams)	Carbohydrates (grams)	Calories (kcal)
Beer				
Regular	12.0	13	13	146
Light	12.0	11	5	99
Distilled Spirits				
Gin, rum, vodka, bourbon, whiskey (80 proof), brandy, cognac	1.5	14	—	96
Wine				
Red	5	14	2	102
White	5	14	1	100
Dessert, sweet	5	23	17	225
Rosé	5	14	2	100
Mixed Drinks				
Manhattan	3.0	26	3	191
Martini	3.0	27	—	189
Bourbon and soda	3.0	11	—	78
Whiskey sour	3.0	13	14	147

*There is little to no fat or protein contribution to calorie content.
Source: USDA.

of alcohol consumed is done so in moderation. About 17.6 million people in the United States suffer from alcohol abuse or alcohol dependence. About one in five people over the age of 12 report binge drinking in the last 30 days. Alcohol by far is the most commonly abused drug.

How Alcoholic Beverages Are Produced

The basis of alcohol production is fermentation, a process by which microorganisms break down simple sugars (e.g., glucose or maltose) to alcohol, carbon dioxide, and water in the absence of oxygen. High-carbohydrate foods especially encourage the growth of yeast, the microorganism responsible for alcohol production. Wine is formed by the fermentation of grape or other fruit juices. Beer is made from malted cereal grain. Distilled spirits (e.g., vodka, gin, whiskey) are made from any number of fruits, vegetables, and grains. Production temperatures, the composition of the food used for fermentation, and aging techniques determine the characteristics of the product.

Absorption and Metabolism of Alcohol

Alcohol requires no digestion. It is absorbed rapidly from the GI tract by diffusion, making it the most efficiently absorbed of all calorie sources. Once absorbed, alcohol is freely distributed into all the fluid compartments within the body. About 1% to 3% of alcohol is excreted via urine and about 1% to 5% evaporates via the breath, the basis for the breathalyzer test. Most alcohol (90% to 98%), however, is metabolized. The liver is the primary site for alcohol metabolism, and some may also be metabolized by the cells lining the stomach. The main pathway of alcohol metabolism involves the enzymes **alcohol dehydrogenase** and **acetaldehyde dehydrogenase.** Alcohol cannot be stored in the body, so it takes absolute priority over other energy sources for metabolism.

As a person's alcohol consumption exceeds the body's capacity to metabolize it, blood alcohol concentration rises, the brain is exposed to alcohol, and symptoms of intoxication appear (see Table 16-5). Absorption and metabolism of alcohol depend on numerous factors: gender, race, body size, physical condition, meal composition, rate of gastric emptying, the alcohol content of the beverage, use of certain drugs,

Alcohol proof represents twice the volume of alcohol in percentage terms. Thus, 80 proof vodka is 40% alcohol.

alcohol dehydrogenase An enzyme used in alcohol (ethanol) metabolism that converts alcohol into acetaldehyde.

acetaldehyde dehydrogenase An enzyme used in ethanol metabolism that eventually converts acetaldehyde into carbon dioxide and water.

alcohol abuse Excessive alcohol consumption that leads to severe alcohol-related health and other problems, such as recurrent sickness, inability to fulfill major obligations, use in hazardous situations (e.g., driving), related legal problems, or use despite social and interpersonal difficulties.

cirrhosis A loss of functioning liver cells, which are replaced by nonfunctioning connective tissue. Any substance that poisons liver cells can lead to cirrhosis. The most common cause is a chronic, excessive alcohol intake. Exposure to certain industrial chemicals also can lead to cirrhosis.

TABLE 16-5 Blood Alcohol Concentration and Symptoms

Concentration*	Sporadic Drinker	Chronic Drinker	Hours for Alcohol to Be Metabolized**
50 (party high) (0.05%)	Congenial euphoria; decreased tension; noticeable impairment in driving and coordination	No observable effect	2–3
75 (0.075%)	Gregarious	Often no effect	3–4
80 to 100 (0.08%–0.1%)	Uncoordinated; 0.08% is legally drunk (as in drunk driving) in the United States and Canada.	Minimal signs	4–6
125–150 (0.125%–0.15%)	Unrestrained behavior; episodic uncontrolled behavior	Pleasurable euphoria or beginning of uncoordination	6–10
200–250 (0.2%–0.25%)	Alertness lost; lethargic	Effort is required to maintain emotional and motor control	10–24
300–350 (0.3%–0.35%)	Stupor to coma	Drowsy and slow	10–24
>500 (>0.5%)	Some will die	Coma	>24

*Milligrams of alcohol per 100 milliliters of blood.

**For a social drinker; alcohol metabolism is somewhat faster in chronic alcohol abusers.

Modified from Wyngaarder JB, Smith LH: *Cecil Textbook of Medicine,* fourth edition, Philadelphia, 1988, WB Saunders. Used with permission.

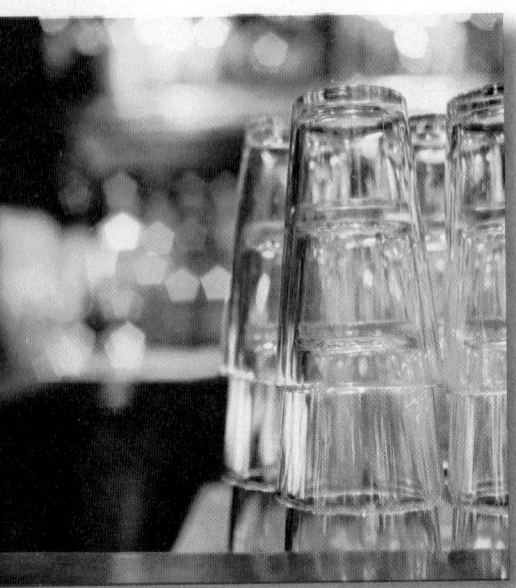

▲ There is no such thing as controlled drinking once a person has alcoholism. Total abstinence is mandatory for recovery.

chronic alcohol abuse, and even how much sleep one has had. Women absorb and metabolize alcohol differently than men. The amount of alcohol metabolized by the cells lining the stomach is greater in men than in women. Women also have less body water in which to dilute the alcohol than do men. Overall, women develop alcohol-related ailments, such as cirrhosis of the liver, more rapidly than men do with the same alcohol-consumption habits.

Benefits of Moderate Alcohol Use

When used in moderation, alcohol is linked to several health benefits. Benefits of alcohol use are associated with specific intakes of about one drink per day for men and slightly less than one for women. Socialization and relaxation are among the intangible benefits of moderate alcohol use by people of legal drinking age. In terms of physiological benefits, moderate drinkers experience lower risk of developing cardiovascular diseases and type 2 diabetes. Previous consumers of alcohol no longer experience the benefits of alcohol when consumption ceases. See Table 16-6 for additional benefits of alcohol consumption.

Risks of Alcohol Abuse

Despite the few benefits of regular, moderate use, the risks of **alcohol abuse** are more numerous and harmful. Although it is one of the most preventable health problems, excessive consumption of alcohol contributes significantly to 5 of the 10 leading causes of death in North America: heart failure, certain forms of cancer, **cirrhosis of the liver**, motor vehicle and other accidents, and suicides (review Table 16-6 for additional health risks). In the United States, about $185 billion is spent annually in terms of lost productivity, premature deaths, direct treatment expenses, and legal fees associated with alcoholism. Overall, alcohol abuse typically reduces a person's life expectancy by 15 years.

Alcoholic beverages have little nutritional value and, thus, nutrient deficiencies are a common result of alcoholism. The protein and vitamin content is extremely low, except in beer, where it is marginal. Iron content varies from drink to drink, with red wine ranking especially high in iron. Typical deficiencies seen in alcoholism arise mostly from poor nutrient intakes, but increased urinary losses and fat malabsorption (linked to poor pancreatic function) are also to blame. Vitamins most susceptible to depletion in alcoholism include vitamins A, D, E, and K; thiamin; niacin; folate; vitamin B-6 and B-12, and vitamin C. Mineral deficiencies of calcium, phosphorus, potassium, magnesium, zinc, and iron are possible. On the other hand, vitamin and mineral toxicity is also of concern. Damage to the GI tract and liver, as well as high levels of some minerals in alcoholic beverages, may lead to toxicity of vitamin A, iron, lead, or cobalt. In nutritional treatment of alcoholism, the immediate aim is eliminating alcohol intake, followed by replenishment of nutrient stores.

Alcohol dependence is the most common psychiatric disorder, affecting 13% of the North American population. Studies suggest that about 40% of a person's risk for developing alcoholism comes from genetic factors. Certainly, genetic variations coding for the enzymes of alcohol metabolism are involved, but many other genes are also under study. Therefore, people with a family history of alcoholism, particularly children of alcoholics, should be especially aware of their alcohol consumption.

Early diagnosis of **alcoholism** can prevent multiple health problems and save millions in health care costs. Asking a person about the quantity and frequency of alcohol consumption is an important means of detecting abuse and dependence (see the margin note on the CAGE questionnaire on page 642). Alcoholics may exhibit some or all of the following criteria:

- Physiological dependence on alcohol with evidence of withdrawal symptoms when intake is interrupted
- Tolerance to the effects of alcohol, prompting greater alcohol intake to achieve the desired effect

alcohol dependence The person experiences repeated alcohol-related difficulties, such as an inability to control use, spending a great deal of time associated with alcohol use, continued use of alcohol despite physical or psychological consequences, persistent desire or unsuccessful efforts to cut down or control alcohol use, and withdrawal symptoms. Tolerance is also seen.

alcoholism As defined by the American Medical Association, an illness characterized by significant impairment directly related to persistent and excessive use of alcohol.

CRITICAL THINKING

For many people, drinking and smoking go hand-in-hand. What risks and diseases could correlate with the combination of these behaviors?

TABLE 16-6 A Summary of Benefits and Risks of Alcohol Use

	Moderate Use*	Alcohol Abuse**
Coronary heart disease	Decreased risk of death in those at high risk for coronary heart disease-related death, primarily by increasing HDL-cholesterol in some people, decreasing blood clotting, and relaxing blood vessels	Heart rhythm disturbances, heart muscle damage, increased blood triglycerides, and increased blood clotting
Hypertension and stroke	Mild decrease in blood pressure; less ischemic stroke in people with normal blood pressure	Increased blood pressure (hypertension); more ischemic and hemorrhagic stroke
Peripheral vascular disease	Decreased risk due to reduced blood clotting	No benefit
Blood glucose regulation and type 2 diabetes	Decreased risk of developing type 2 diabetes; decreased risk of death from cardiovascular disease	Hypoglycemia; reduced insulin sensitivity; damage to pancreas (site of insulin production)
Bone and joint health	Some increase in bone mineral content in women, linked to estrogen output	Loss of active bone-forming cells and eventual osteoporosis (many nutrient deficiencies also contribute to this problem); increased risk of gout
Brain function	Enhanced brain function and decreased risk of dementia by increasing blood circulation in the brain	Brain tissue damage and decreased memory
Skeletal muscle health	No benefit	Skeletal muscle damage
Cancer	No benefit	Increased risk of oral, esophageal, stomach, liver, lung, colorectal, and breast cancer, to name a few (especially if the diet is deficient in the vitamin folate)
Liver function	No benefit	Fatty infiltration and eventual liver cirrhosis, especially if a person is also infected with hepatitis C; iron toxicity
GI tract disease	Decreased risk of certain bacterial infections in the stomach	Inflammation of the stomach (and pancreas); absorptive cell damage leading to malabsorption of nutrients
Immune system function	No benefit	Reduced function and increased infections
Nervous system function	No benefit	Loss of nerve sensation and nervous system control of muscles
Sleep disturbances	Some relaxation	Fragmented sleep patterns; worsens sleep apnea
Impotence and decreased libido	No benefit	Contributes to the problem in both men and women
Drug overdose	No benefit	Contributes to the problem, especially in combination with sedatives
Obesity	No benefit	Increased abdominal fat deposition, contributes to weight gain as calories from alcoholic beverages quickly add up
Nutrient intake	May supply some B vitamins and iron	Leads to numerous nutrient deficiencies: protein, vitamins, and minerals
Alcoholism	No benefit.	Increased risk of developing alcoholism, including the teenage and young adult years
Fetal health	No benefit	Variety of toxic effects on the fetus when alcohol is consumed by pregnant women (see Chapter 14)
Socialization and relaxation	Provides some benefit to socialization and leads to relaxation by increasing brain neurotransmitter activity	Contributes to violent behavior and agitation
Traffic deaths and other violent deaths	No benefit	Contributes to both traffic death and violent death

*About one drink per day for men and slightly less than one for women.

**The risks from alcohol abuse begin at an intake of more than two to three drinks per day for men or one to two drinks per day for women and all adults age 65 and older. Binge drinking (more than four drinks in a row for women or more than five drinks for men) can be especially harmful.

The CAGE questionnaire is used to identify alcohol abuse. More than one positive response suggests an alcohol problem.

C: Have you ever felt you ought to *cut* down on drinking?

A: Have people *annoyed* you by criticizing your drinking?

G: Have you ever felt bad or *guilty* about your drinking?

E: Have you ever had a drink first thing in the morning to steady your nerves or get rid of a hangover (*eye-opener*)?

Ethnicity plays an important role in both the probability of and health risks associated with alcohol dependency and abuse. Native Americans suffer the highest rates of unintentional injuries, suicide, homicide, and domestic abuse related to alcohol use. African-American alcoholics are at greater risk than other racial groups for tuberculosis, hepatitis C, HIV/AIDS, and other infectious diseases. Hispanic Americans are at particular risk for cirrhosis-related death.

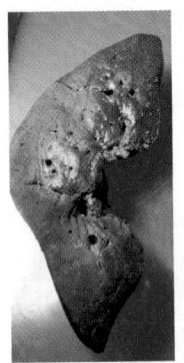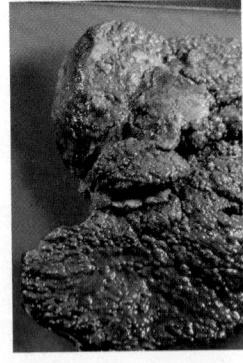

▲ Alcohol is particularly damaging to the liver. Pictured are (a) healthy liver, (b) liver with cirrhosis. There is no cure for this disease except a liver transplant.

- Evidence of alcohol-associated illnesses such as alcoholic liver disease or irreversible brain damage exhibited by memory loss, inability to concentrate, and decline in intellectual functions
- Continued drinking in defiance of strong medical and social contraindications and disruptions in normal life
- Depression, blackouts, and impairment in social and occupational functioning

Other signs of alcoholism include: alcohol odor on the breath; flushed face and reddened skin; and nervous system disorders, such as tremors. Unexplained work absences, frequent accidents, and falls or injuries of vague origin are possible signs of alcoholism. Laboratory evidence (e.g., impaired liver function, enlarged red blood cells, and elevated triglycerides) are also helpful for diagnosis of alcoholism.

Older adults are uniquely vulnerable to alcoholism, perhaps due to an abundance of free time, social events involving drinking, loneliness, or depression. Common symptoms of alcoholism—trembling hands, slurred speech, sleep problems, memory loss, and unsteady gait—can be easily overlooked as signs of old age. Slower alcohol metabolism and decreased body water allow older adults to become intoxicated from a smaller amount of alcohol than their younger counterparts. Even moderate alcohol consumption can exacerbate some chronic health conditions, such as diabetes and osteoporosis. As well, even small amounts of alcohol can react negatively with various medications used by older persons. The adverse health effects of drinking may be amplified in older adults, so people over the age of 65 should limit alcohol consumption to no more than one drink per day.

Once a diagnosis of alcohol abuse or dependence is established, a physician can arrange appropriate treatment and counseling for the person and family. Treatment of alcoholism often includes the use of certain medications, counseling, and social support. Total abstinence must be the ultimate objective. Alcoholics Anonymous (AA) or other reputable therapy programs can support alcoholics and their families as they recover from this devastating disease.

MAKING DECISIONS

Liver Cirrhosis

Alcohol is most damaging to the liver. Cirrhosis develops in up to 20% of cases of alcoholism and is the second leading reason for liver transplants, affecting about 2 million people in the United States. This chronic and usually relentlessly progressive disease is characterized by fatty infiltration of the liver. Fatty liver occurs in response to increased synthesis of fat and decreased use of it for energy by the liver. Eventually, the enlarged fat deposits choke off the blood supply, depriving the liver cells of oxygen and nutrients. Liver cells can accumulate so much fat that they burst and die and are replaced by connective (scar) tissue. At this stage, the liver is deemed cirrhotic. Early stages of alcoholic liver injury are reversible, but advanced stages are not. Once a person has cirrhosis, there is a 50% chance of death within 4 years, a far worse prognosis than many forms of cancer. While no specific level of alcohol consumption guarantees cirrhosis, some evidence suggests that damage is caused by a dose as low as 40 grams per day for men (3 beers) and 20 grams per day for women (1½ beers).

Guidance Regarding Alcohol Use

No government agencies recommend drinking alcohol. The 2010 Dietary Guidelines for Americans provide the following advice regarding use of alcoholic beverages:

- Those who choose to drink alcoholic beverages should do so sensibly and in moderation—defined as the consumption of up to one drink per day for women and up to two drinks per day for men.
- Alcoholic beverages should not be consumed by some individuals, including those who cannot restrict their alcohol intake, women who are pregnant or may

become pregnant, children and adolescents, individuals taking medications that can interact with alcohol, and those with specific medical conditions.

- Alcoholic beverages should be avoided by individuals engaging in activities that require attention, skill, or coordination, such as driving or operating machinery.
- For weight management, monitor calorie intake from alcoholic beverages.

As the understanding of the relationship between drinking alcohol and health grows, registered dietitians and other health professionals can promote healthy lifestyles—not by encouraging indiscriminate drinking, but rather by reassuring adults that moderate alcohol consumption may have beneficial health outcomes.

CONCEPT CHECK

Alcohol is not an essential nutrient but does supply calories for the body. It requires no digestion, and alcohol metabolism takes precedence over metabolism of the other energy-yielding nutrients. Alcohol is primarily metabolized in the liver by alcohol dehydrogenase and acetaldehyde dehydrogenase. A number of individual factors, such as gender, race, and body composition, determine how a person reacts to alcohol. Despite modest benefits of moderate alcohol use, alcoholism interferes with all aspects of family, professional, and social life. Excessive alcohol use increases the risk of hypertension, strokes, heart damage, birth defects, inflammation of the pancreas, brain damage, and malnutrition, to name a few. Treatment of alcoholism often includes the use of certain medications, counseling, and social support.

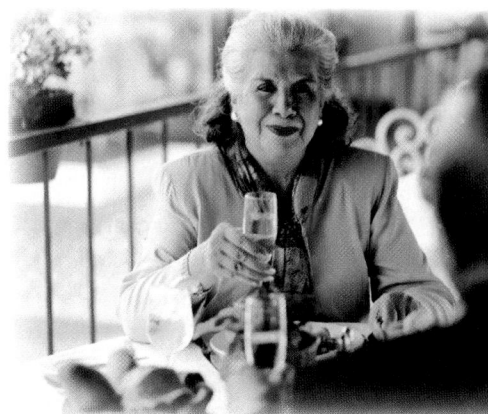

▲ The limit for alcohol intake for older adults is one drink per day.

Healthy People 2020 set an important goal regarding alcohol use: Reduce annual alcohol consumption by 10% (currently, 2.3 gallons per person ages 14 and older).

To learn more about alcoholism, visit these websites:

National Institute on Alcohol Abuse and Alcoholism; www.niaaa.nih.gov

American Society of Addiction Medicine; www.asam.org

American Self-Help Clearinghouse; www.mentalhelp.net/selfhelp.

Appendix C reviews diet planning guidelines issued by the Canadian government for Canadians. In addition, Chapter 1 discussed *Healthy People 2020*, a U.S. federal agenda aimed at disease prevention and health promotion.

16.6 Ensuring a Healthful Diet for the Adult Years

Recommended dietary practices for later years would be to increase the diet's nutrient density and to make sure fiber and fluid intakes are adequate. In addition, some protein should come from lean meats to help meet protein, vitamin B-6, vitamin B-12, iron, and zinc needs.

Singles of all ages face logistical problems with food: Purchasing, preparing, storing, and using food with minimal waste are challenging. Economy packages of meats and vegetables are normally too large to be useful for a single person. Many singles live in small dwellings, some without kitchens and freezers. Creating a diet to accommodate a limited budget and facilities and a single appetite requires special considerations. The following are some practical suggestions for diet planning for singles:

- If one owns a freezer, cook large amounts, divide into portions, and freeze.
- Buy only what one uses; small containers may be expensive, but letting food spoil is also costly.
- Ask the grocer to break open a family-sized package of wrapped meat or fresh vegetables and separate it into smaller units.
- Buy only several pieces of fruit—perhaps a ripe one, a medium-ripe one, and an unripe one—so that the fruit can be eaten over a period of several days.
- Keep a box of dry milk handy to add nutrients to recipes for baked foods and other foods for which this addition is acceptable.

Table 16-7 provides more ideas for healthful eating in later years.

Nutritional deficiencies and protein-calorie undernutrition have been identified among some aging populations, particularly those in hospitals, nursing homes, or long-term care facilities. These nutritional problems increase the risk for many diseases, including bed sores (pressure ulcers), and compromise recovery from illness and surgery. Friends, relatives, and health care professionals should monitor nutrient intake in all older people, including those who live in long-term care facilities. Family members can play a valuable role in making sure nutrient needs are met by looking for weight maintenance based on regular, healthful meal patterns. If problems arise in consuming a healthful diet, registered dietitians can offer professional and personalized advice.

TABLE 16-7 Guidelines for Healthful Eating in Later Years

Determine:

- Disease
- Eating poorly
- Tooth loss or mouth pain
- Economic hardship
- Reduced social contact and interaction
- Multiple medications
- Involuntary weight loss or gain
- Need for assistance with self-care
- Elder at an advanced age

To learn about meal programs for senior citizens in your area, call the *Administration on Aging's Elder Care Locator*, (800) 677-1116 or see www.eldercare.gov. For general information on programs for older persons, visit the following websites: *National Institute on Aging*, www.nia.nih.gov; *American Geriatrics Society*, www.americangeriatrics.org; and *Administration on Aging*, www.aoa.gov.

- Eat regularly; small, frequent meals may be best. Use nutrient-dense foods as a basis for menus.
- Use labor-saving devices and some convenience foods, but try to incorporate some fresh foods into daily menus.
- Try new foods, new seasonings, and new ways of preparing foods. Use canned goods in moderation or choose those low in sodium.
- Keep easy-to-prepare foods on hand for times when you feel tired.
- Have a treat occasionally, perhaps an expensive cut of meat or a favorite fresh fruit.
- Eat in a well-lit or sunny area; serve meals attractively; use foods with different flavors, colors, shapes, textures, and smells.
- Arrange kitchen and eating area so that food preparation and cleanup are easier.
- Eat with friends, relatives, or at a senior center when possible.
- Share cooking responsibilities with a neighbor.
- Use community resources for help in shopping and other daily care needs.
- Stay physically active.
- If possible, take a walk before eating to stimulate appetite.
- When necessary, chop, grind, or blend hard-to-chew foods. Softer, protein-rich foods (e.g., shredded meats, eggs) can be substituted for meat when poor dental function limits normal food intake. Prepare soups, stews, cooked whole-grain cereals, and casseroles.
- If your dexterity is limited, cut the food ahead of time, use utensils with deep sides or handles, and obtain more specialized utensils if needed.

NEWSWORTHY NUTRITION | Calorie restriction: Is your diet a fountain of youth?

Animal studies show that long-term calorie restriction increases longevity. Researchers for the Comprehensive Assessment of the Long-Term Effects of Reducing Intake of Energy (CALERIE) study explored the possibility that 25% calorie restriction for 6 months would alter biomarkers of longevity in humans. Forty-six overweight adults completed the study. Subjects were randomized to one of four groups: control (no caloric restriction), CR (25% calorie restriction), CREX (12.5% calorie restriction + 12.5% increased energy expenditure by structured exercise), and LCD (low-calorie diet followed by weight-maintenance diet after 15% weight loss was achieved). Subjects followed controlled diets that were deficient in calories but otherwise nutritionally adequate and underwent numerous measurements, including body composition, calorimetry (review Chapter 7), body temperature, and various blood tests. Fasting levels of insulin, energy expenditure (i.e., metabolic rate), and a marker of DNA damage decreased in all three intervention groups. Among the CR and CREX groups, core body temperature also decreased. These results indicate that prolonged calorie restriction in humans reduces metabolic rate and decreases fasting insulin and body temperature, two biomarkers of longevity. Further research is needed to distinguish effects of calorie restriction on other biomarkers and to measure life span. For this study, diet was carefully controlled and monitored frequently and all foods were provided. If calorie restriction does prove to increase longevity, could you stick with it?

Source: Heilbronn LK and others: Effect of 6-month calorie restriction on biomarkers of longevity, metabolic adaptation, and oxidative stress in overweight subjects. *Journal of the American Medical Association* 295:1539, 2006.

connect NUTRITION **Check out the Connect site** www.mcgrawhillconnect.com **to learn more about theories of aging.**

Overall, older adults benefit from good nutrition in many ways. As we discussed for younger adults, meeting nutrient needs delays the onset of some diseases; improves the management of some existing diseases; hastens recovery from many illnesses; increases mental, physical, and social well-being; and often decreases the need for and length of hospitalization. Older adults should use MyPlate as a guide to healthy meals, but emphasize nutrients of special concern (e.g., calcium, vitamin D, vitamin B-12). Daily Food Plans are available from www.ChooseMyPlate.gov for older adults, based on age, weight, height, gender, and activity level. A focus on nutrient-dense food choices, plenty of fluids, modified physical activity goals, and use of certain dietary supplements address the unique needs of older adults.

Obtaining enough food may be difficult for some older persons, especially if they are unable to drive and relatives do not live close enough to help with cooking or shopping. For an older person, a request for help may be equated to a loss of independence. Pride, or fear of being victimized by those they hire, may stand in the way of much-needed help. In these cases, friends can be a big help. Special transportation arrangements may also be available through a local transit company or taxi service.

Many eligible older people are missing meals and are poorly nourished because they don't know of available programs to help them. Irregular meal patterns and weight loss, often caused by difficulties in preparing food, are warning signs that undernutrition may be developing. An effort should be made to identify poorly nourished people and inform them of community services.

Community Nutrition Services for Older People

Health care advice and services for older people can come from clinics, private practitioners, hospitals, and health maintenance organizations. Home health care agencies, adult day-care programs, adult overnight-care programs, and **hospice care** (for the terminally ill) can provide daily care.

The Nutrition Screening Initiative, a nutrition checklist for health care workers, family members, and older persons, can be used as a tool to increase health and nutrition awareness and to plan related education of older persons (See Fig. 16-2). The Nutrition Screening Initiative uses the acronym "DETERMINE" (see margin on previous page) to help identify older people whose health needs require extra attention.

Nutrition programs for those age 60 and over in the United States include congregate meal programs, which provide lunch at a central location, and home-delivered meals (often known as Meals on Wheels if sponsored by the local private or public agencies). About 2.6 million older adults are served each year. About half of the meals use the home-delivered method.

The U.S. federal government sets specific standards for home-delivered meals and for those served in congregate feeding centers. The meals are designed to provide one-third of RDA/AI. The social aspect often improves appetite and general outlook on life.

Still, congregate meal programs generally provide one meal a day (some provide more) and usually just 5 days per week. Another problem with home-delivered meals is that the one or two meals delivered may never be eaten, and, if not eaten on delivery and left at room temperature, they may become unsafe to eat later. Thus, these programs can help older adults but probably don't meet all their nutritional needs.

In addition to congregate and home-delivered meals, federal commodity distribution is available in some areas of the United States to low-income older people. Older people whose incomes are below the poverty level can benefit from the SNAP program (food stamps) (see Chapter 12 for details on these programs). Food cooperatives and a variety of clubs and religious and social organizations provide additional aid.

▲ Immune function declines with age, so food safety become increasingly important for older adults. Chapter 13 provides advice on this topic, such as washing one's hands and work surfaces before preparing food.

hospice care A program offering care that emphasizes comfort and dignity in death.

CONCEPT CHECK

A nutrient-dense diet helps meet the unique needs of aging adults. Carefully planned use of multivitamin and mineral supplements can also help, especially for adults 70 years of age and older. Diet planning should be tailored to the individual's physiological, psychosocial, and economic status. In the United States, many nutrition services—such as congregate and home-delivered meals—are available to help the aging population obtain a healthful diet.

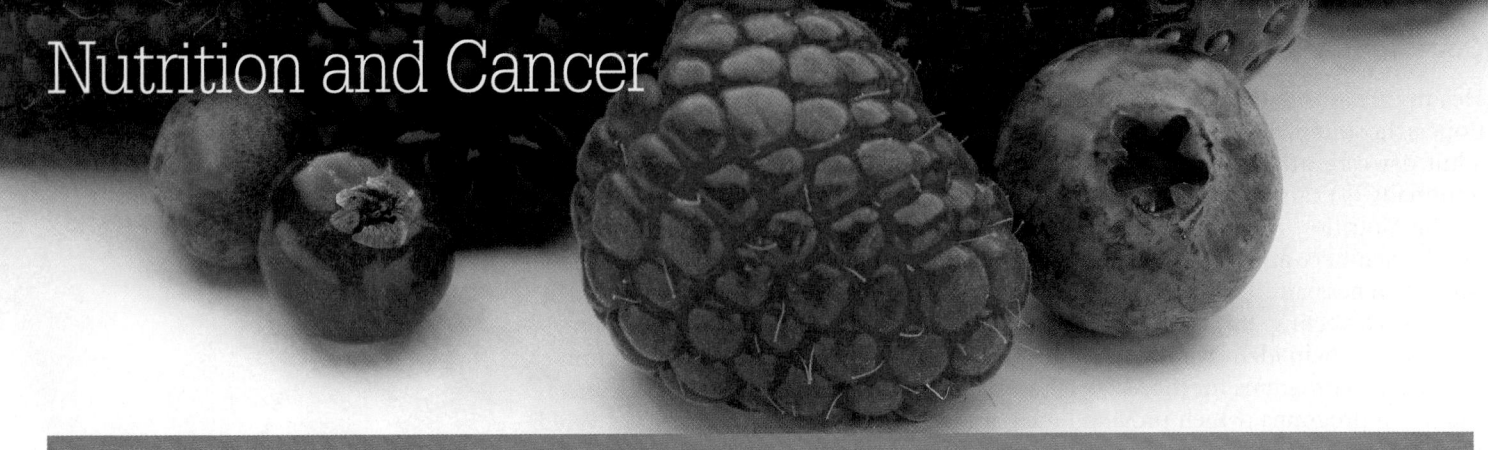

Nutrition and Cancer

Cancer is the second leading cause of death for North American adults. It is further estimated that more than 1500 people die each day of cancer in the United States. Cancer-related expenses exceed $100 billion each year. The top four cancers, causing more than 50% of cancer deaths, are lung, colorectal, breast, and prostate cancers. Of those, lung cancer in female smokers is the only form increasing on a yearly basis.

Cancer is many diseases; these differ in the types of cells affected and, in some cases, in the factors contributing to cancer development (Fig. 16-6). For example, the factors leading to skin cancer differ from those leading to breast cancer. Similarly, the treatments for the different types of cancer often vary.

Cancer essentially represents abnormal and uncontrollable division of cells that results from mutations in DNA. This initiates the cancer process. The cells then go through a variety of steps (called promotion and progression). A cancer cell is the result. Without effective treatment, cancer then typically leads to death. Most cancers take the form of tumors, although not all tumors are cancers. A **tumor** is spontaneous new tissue growth that serves no physiological purpose. It can be **benign,** like a wart, or **malignant,** like most lung cancers. The terms *malignant tumor* and *malignant neoplasm* are synonymous with cancer.

Whereas benign tumors are only dangerous if their presence interferes with normal body functions, malignant (cancerous) tumors are capable of invading surrounding structures, including blood vessels, the lymph system, and nervous tissue. Cancer can also spread, or **metastasize,** to distant sites via the blood and lymphatic circulation, thereby producing invasive tumors in almost any part of the body. Metastasis then makes the cancer much more difficult to treat. That cancer can spread explains why early detection of cancer is so important. Cancers that can be diagnosed in the early stages are those in the colon, breast, and cervix.

Genetics, environment, and lifestyle are potent forces that influence the risk for developing cancer. A genetic predisposition is especially important in development of colon cancer, some types of breast cancer (e.g., mutated BRCA1 or BRCA2 gene) and prostate cancer (35%, 27%, and 42%, respectively). About 30 cancer-susceptibility genes have been identified. However, experts estimate that only 1% to 5% of most cancers can be explained by the inheritance of a cancer gene. Overall, lifestyle and environmental exposures are also critical factors in most forms of cancer, as evidenced by the variation in cancer rates from country to country. In fact, diet likely accounts for 30% to 40% or more of all cancers.

Although we have little control over our genetic risks for cancer, we can exert a great deal of authority when making decisions about lifestyle risks, especially with regard to smoking, alcohol abuse, physical activity, and nutrient intake (food choice). It is well established that one-third of all cancers in North America are due directly to tobacco use. About half of the cancers of the mouth, pharynx, and larynx are associated with heavy use of alcohol. A combination of alcohol use and smoking increases cancer risks even higher.

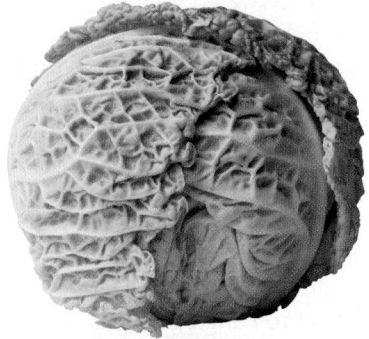

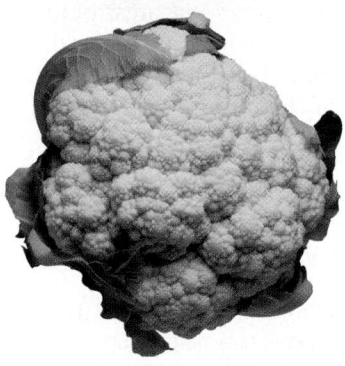

▲ Cruciferous vegetables such as cabbage and cauliflower are rich in cancer-preventing phytochemicals.

tumor Mass of cells; may be cancerous (malignant) or noncancerous (benign).

benign Noncancerous; tumors that do not spread.

malignant Malicious; in reference to a tumor, the property of spreading locally and to distant sites.

metastasize The spreading of disease from one part of the body to another, even to parts of the body that are remote from the site of the original tumor. Cancer cells can spread via blood vessels, the lymphatic system, or direct growth of the tumor.

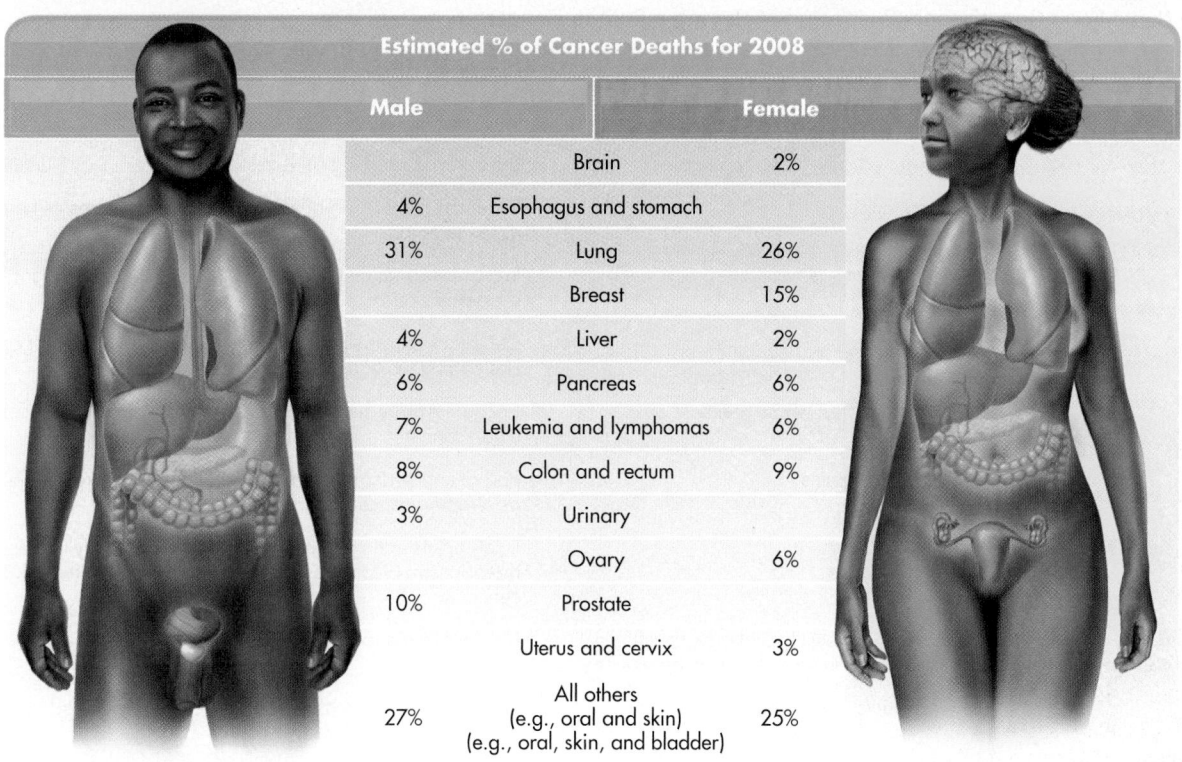

	Estimated % of Cancer Deaths for 2008	
Male		**Female**
	Brain	2%
4%	Esophagus and stomach	
31%	Lung	26%
	Breast	15%
4%	Liver	2%
6%	Pancreas	6%
7%	Leukemia and lymphomas	6%
8%	Colon and rectum	9%
3%	Urinary	
	Ovary	6%
10%	Prostate	
	Uterus and cervix	3%
27%	All others (e.g., oral and skin) (e.g., oral, skin, and bladder)	25%

FIGURE 16-6 ▶ Cancer is many diseases. Numerous types of cells and organs are its target. About one-third of all cancers arise from smoking (primarily lung cancer).

A Closer Look at Diet and Cancer

Some food constituents may contribute to cancer development, whereas others have a protective effect (Table 16-8). First the association between fat/calorie intake and cancer risk is discussed, and then some of the food constituents that may reduce the risk for cancer are presented (see Further Reading 10).

Contribution of Calorie and Fat Intakes to Cancer Risk

An excess calorie intake, leading eventually to obesity, is responsible for an estimated 14% of cancer deaths among men and as many as 20% among women. This is the main diet-cancer risk factor. This includes cancer of the breast (especially in post-menopausal women), pancreas, kidney, gallbladder, colon, **endometrium**, and prostate gland. The link probably occurs between adipose tissue and the synthesis of estrogen. High concentrations of circulating estrogen in the blood over time promote cancer. Excess insulin output resulting from an obese, insulin-resistant state is also implicated.

The National Cancer Institute (NCI) also believes there is sufficient evidence for a link between dietary fat and cancer to encourage North Americans to reduce fat intake. It recommends initially decreasing dietary fat to about 30% of total calorie intake and eventually to 20% or less of total calories if the person is at high risk and can follow such a dietary pattern.

Some scientists, however, believe that the NCI has overreacted to the fat and cancer issue. Although epidemiological evidence does link fat and certain forms of cancer, the evidence is not strong. A stronger link exists between cancer and excess calories in the diet. In animal experiments, restricting total calorie intake to about 70% of usual intake results in about a 40% reduction in tumor development, regardless of the amount of fat in the diet. Calorie restriction is the most effective technique for preventing cancer in laboratory animals.

Unfortunately, it is difficult for humans to reduce dietary calories to 70% of usual intake. So while the data obtained from laboratory animal studies are interesting, nutritionists do not see any practical way to make recommendations

on the basis of these studies. In addition, once cancer is present, calorie restriction is no longer helpful.

Cancer-Inhibiting Food Constituents

Many single nutrients may have cancer-inhibiting properties. These anticarcinogens include antioxidants and certain phytochemicals (review Table 16-8).

The antioxidant activity of vitamin C and vitamin E helps to prevent formation of **nitrosamines** in the GI tract, thus preventing formation of a potent carcinogen. Vitamin E also helps protect unsaturated fatty acids from damage by free radicals. Overall, carotenoids, vitamin E, vitamin C, and selenium function as

endometrium The membrane that lines the inside of the uterus. It increases in thickness during the menstrual cycle until ovulation occurs. The surface layers are shed during menstruation if conception does not take place.

nitrosamine A carcinogen formed from nitrates and breakdown products of amino acids; can lead to stomach cancer.

TABLE 16-8 Some Food Constituents Suspected of Having a Role in Cancer

Constituent	Dietary Sources	Action
Possibly Protective*		
Vitamin A	Liver, fortified milk, fruits, vegetables	Encourages normal cell development.
Vitamin D	Fortified milk	Increases production of a protein that suppresses cell growth, such as in the colon.
Vitamin E	Whole grains, vegetable oils, green leafy vegetables	Prevents formation of nitrosamines; general antioxidant properties.
Vitamin C	Fruits, vegetables	Can block conversion of nitrites and nitrates to potent carcinogens; likely has general antioxidant properties.
Folate	Fruits, vegetables, whole grains	Encourages normal cell development; especially reduces the risk of colon cancer.
Selenium	Meats, whole grains	Part of antioxidant system that inhibits tumor growth and kills developing cancer cells.
Carotenoids, such as lycopene	Fruits, vegetables	Likely act as antioxidants; some of these possibly influence cell metabolism. Lycopene in particular may reduce the risk of prostate cancer.
Flavonoids, indoles, phenols, and other phytochemicals	Vegetables, especially cabbage, cauliflower, broccoli, brussels sprouts, garlic, onions, tea	May reduce cancer in the stomach and other organs.
Calcium	Milk products, green vegetables	Slows cell division in the colon, binds bile acids and free fatty acids, thus reducing colon cancer risk.
Omega-3 fatty acids	Cold-water fish, such as salmon and tuna	May inhibit tumor growth.
Soy products	Tofu, soy milk, tempeh, soy nuts	Phytic acid present possibly binds carcinogens in the intestinal tract; the genistein component possibly reduces growth and metastasis of malignant cells.
Conjugated linoleic acid	Milk products, meats	May inhibit tumor development and act as an antioxidant.
Fiber-rich foods	Fruits, vegetables, whole-grain breads and cereals, beans, nuts	Colon and rectal cancer risk may be decreased by accelerating intestinal transit or binding carcinogens such that they are excreted.
Possibly Carcinogenic		
Excessive calorie intake	All macronutrients can contribute	Excess fat mass leading to obesity; linked to increased synthesis of estrogen and other sex hormones, which in excess may themselves increase the risk for cancer. Resulting excess insulin output from creation of an insulin-resistant state is also implicated.
Total fat	Meats, high-fat milk and milk products, animal fats and vegetable oils	The strongest evidence is for excessive saturated and polyunsaturated fat intake. Saturated fat is linked to an increased risk of prostate cancer.
High glycemic load carbohydrates	Cookies, cakes, sugared soft drinks, candy	Insulin surges associated with these foods may increase tumor growth, such as in the colon.
Alcohol	Beer, wine, liquor	Contributes to cancers of the throat, liver, bladder, breast, and colon (especially if the person does not consume enough folate).
Nitrites, nitrates	Cured meats, especially ham, bacon, and sausages	Under very high temperatures will bind to amino acid derivatives to form nitrosamines, potent carcinogens.
Multi-ring compounds: Aflatoxin	Formed when mold is present on peanuts or grains	May alter DNA structure and inhibit its ability to properly respond to physiologic controls; aflatoxin in particular is linked to liver cancer.
Benzo(a)pyrene and other heterocyclic amines	Charcoal-broiled foods, especially meats	Linked to stomach and colon cancer. To limit this risk, trim fat from meat before cooking, cut barbecuing time by partially cooking meat (such as in a microwave oven), and don't consume blackened parts.

*Many of the actions listed for these possibly protective agents are speculative and have been verified only by experimental animal studies. The best evidence supports obtaining these nutrients and other food constituents from foods. The U.S. Preventive Services Task Force (USPSTF) supports this statement, noting there is no clear evidence that nutrient supplements provide the same benefits.

or contribute to antioxidant protection for the body. Some of these antioxidant systems help prevent DNA mutations by electron-seeking compounds, the main way that cancer develops in the first place.

In addition, phytochemicals from fruits and vegetables, and even tea, block cancer development in some types of cells. Numerous studies suggest that fruit and vegetable intake reduces the risk of nearly all types of cancer. These foods are normally rich in carotenoids, vitamin C, and vitamin E. Adequate vitamin D intake is suspected of reducing breast, colon, prostate, and other forms of cancer. Calcium is also linked to a decreased risk for developing colon cancer. In sum, a diet that conforms to MyPlate, so that fruits, vegetables, whole grains, low-fat and fat-free dairy products, and some plant oils are eaten daily, is aimed at cancer prevention. It is likely that all of these foods have a "cocktail" effect, and that no one particular food can make as strong a claim (see Further Reading 7).

Nutrition Concerns During Cancer Treatment

Nutrition concerns during cancer treatment may vary depending on the site of the cancer, but the overall goals of medical nutrition therapy are to minimize weight loss and prevent nutrient deficiencies. Weight loss, particularly loss of muscle mass, is a major concern during cancer treatment because poor nutrition status can limit recovery from illness. Common effects of cancer and/or cancer treatments include fatigue, mouth sores, dry mouth, taste abnormalities, nausea, and diarrhea–all of which can lead to poor food intake.

During cancer treatment, the best food to eat is any food the patient can tolerate. Food choices vary based on each patient's individual symptoms, but cool, non-acidic liquids and soft, mildly-flavored foods are generally well-accepted. Small, frequent meals and foods with high nutrient density and calorie density should be emphasized to meet calorie and protein needs. Often, liquid nutritional supplements are needed. Because immunity may be suppressed during cancer treatment, safe food handling practices also are extremely important (review Chapter 13).

The Bottom Line

Given the toll of cancer treatment and lack of a definitive cure, efforts at prevention are key. A variety of dietary changes will reduce your risk for cancer. Start by making sure that your diet is moderate in calorie and fat content and that you consume many fruits and vegetables, whole-grain breads and cereals, beans, some fish, and low-fat or fat-free milk products. In addition, remain physically active; avoid obesity; consume alcohol in moderation (if at all); and limit intake of animal fat and salt-cured, smoked, and nitrate-cured foods.

Remember also that if a cancer is left untreated, it can spread quickly throughout the body. When this happens, it is much more likely to lead to death. Thus early detection is critical. Aids to early detection include the following warning signs (acronym is CAUTION):

- A Change in bowel or bladder habits
- A sore that does not heal
- Unusual bleeding or discharge
- A Thickening or lump in the breast or elsewhere
- Indigestion or difficulty in swallowing
- An Obvious change in a wart or mole
- A Nagging cough or hoarseness

Unexplained weight loss is an additional warning sign.

There are still other ways to detect cancer early. Colonoscopy examinations for middle-aged and older adults, PSA (prostate-specific antigen) tests for middle-aged and older men, and Papanicolaou tests (Pap smears) and regular breast examinations (and mammograms starting about age 40) for women are recommended by the American Cancer Society. Finally, to learn still more about cancer, review these sources of credible cancer information on the Internet:

American Cancer Society
www.cancer.org
National Cancer Institute
www.cancer.gov
Oncolink
www.oncolink.org
Harvard University Center
for Cancer Prevention
www.diseaseriskindex.harvard.edu

▶ **American Institute for Cancer Research Diet and Health Guidelines for Cancer Prevention**

1. Choose a diet rich in a variety of plant-based foods.
2. Eat plenty of vegetables and fruits.
3. Maintain a healthy weight and be physically active.
4. Drink alcohol only in moderation, if at all.
5. Select foods low in fat and salt.
6. Prepare and store food safely.

And always remember ...

Do not use tobacco in any form.

Case Study Dietary Assistance for an Older Adult

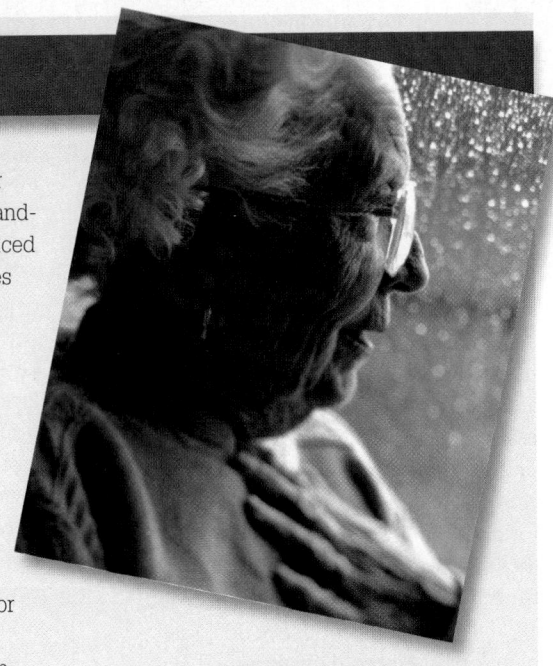

Frances is a 78-year-old woman who suffers from macular degeneration, osteoporosis, and arthritis. Since her husband died a year ago, she has moved from their family house to a small one-bedroom apartment. Her eyesight is progressively getting worse, making it hard to go to the grocery store or even to cook (for fear of burning herself). She is often lonely; her only son lives 1 hour away and works two jobs, but he visits her as often as he can. Frances has lost her appetite and, as a result, often skips meals during the week. She has resorted to eating mostly cold foods, simple to prepare but seriously limiting variety and palatability in her diet. She is slowly losing weight as a result of her dietary changes and loss of appetite.

Her typical diet usually consists of a breakfast that may include 1 slice of wheat toast with margarine, honey, and cinnamon, and 1 cup of hot tea. If she has lunch, she normally has ½ can of peaches, half of a turkey and cheese sandwich, and ½ glass of water. For dinner, she might have half of a tuna fish sandwich made with mayonnaise and 1 cup of iced tea. She usually includes one or two cookies at bedtime.

Answer the following questions, and check your responses in Appendix A.

1. What nutrients are likely to be inadequate in her current diet?
2. What potential effects will Frances' poor dietary pattern have on her health status?
3. Which physiological changes of aging will add to the effects of her poor diet (review Table 16-2)?
4. What services are available in the community that could help Frances improve her diet and possibly increase her appetite?
5. What other convenience foods could be included in her diet to make it more healthful and more varied?

Summary (Numbers refer to numbered sections in the chapter.)

16.1 Although maximum life span hasn't changed, life expectancy has increased dramatically over the past century. For many societies, this means that an increasing proportion of the population is over 65 years of age. As health care costs rise, the goal of delaying disease becomes ever important.

16.2 During adulthood, nutrients are used primarily to maintain the body rather than support physical growth. As adults get older, nutrient needs change. Adulthood is characterized by body maintenance and gradual physiological transitions, often referred to as "aging." The physiologic changes of aging are the sum of cellular changes, lifestyle practices, and environmental influences. Many of these changes can be minimized, prevented, and/or reversed by healthy lifestyles. Usual aging refers to the age-related physical and physiological changes that are commonly thought to be typical of aging. Successful aging describes the declines in physical and physiological function that occur because one grows older. Striving to have the greatest number of healthy years and the fewest of illness is referred to as compression of morbidity. The rate at which one ages is individual; it is determined by heredity, lifestyle, and environment.

16.3 A healthy diet based on MyPlate and the 2010 Dietary Guidelines for Americans can help one to preserve body function, avoid chronic disease, and age successfully. These guidelines recommend that individuals eat a variety of foods; balance the food eaten with physical activity to maintain or improve weight; choose a diet with plenty of whole grains, vegetables, and fruits; choose a diet low in saturated fat, *trans* fat, and cholesterol; limit sugars and salt; and moderate alcoholic beverage intake. Regular physical activity is also important, as is safe food preparation. American adults are fairly well nourished, although common dietary excesses are calories, fat, sodium, and for some, alcohol. Common dietary inadequacies include vitamins D and E, folate, magnesium, calcium, zinc, and fiber. People ages 65 and older, particularly those in long-term care facilities and hospitals, are at risk for malnutrition. The Nutrition Screening Initiative checklist can help identify older adults at risk of nutrient deficiencies. The DRIs for adults are divided by gender and age to reflect how nutrient needs change as adults grow older. These changes in nutrient needs take into consideration the aging-related physiological alterations in body composition, metabolism, and organ function.

16.4 The food choices and nutritional adequacy of adults' diets depend on physiological, psychosocial, and economic factors. Alterations in any of these factors can result in deteriorations in the quality of dietary intake, nutritional status, and health. Physiological factors include changes in body composition, body systems, and chronic diseases that influence dietary intake and alter nutrient needs and/or nutrient utilization. Of particular concern is sarcopenia, or loss of muscle mass that frequently accompanies aging. The use of medications and supplements can improve health and quality of life, but some also adversely affect nutritional status. Herbal products should be used with caution. Psychosocial influences on nutritional status include changes in lifestyle and social interaction and the presence of mental health issues, such as depression and Alzheimer's disease. Economic factors may also have a great impact on the types and amounts of food one eats.

16.5 Alcohol use is a complex issue because it involves psychological, social, economic, health, legal, and family issues. Alcohol is metabolized in the liver and

other tissues. The benefits of alcohol use are associated with low to moderate alcohol consumption. These benefits include the pleasurable and social aspects of alcohol use, a reduction in various forms of cardiovascular disease, increase in insulin sensitivity, and protection against some harmful stomach bacteria. Alcohol has the potential to worsen health as well. Excessive consumption of alcohol contributes significantly to five of the ten leading causes of death in North America. Alcohol increases the risk of developing certain forms of heart damage, inflammation of the pancreas, GI tract damage, vitamin and mineral deficiencies, cirrhosis of the liver, certain forms of cancer, hypertension, and hemorrhagic stroke—to name a few.

If alcohol is consumed, it should be consumed in moderation with meals. Women are advised to drink no more than one drink per day, as are adults 65 years and older; men are advised to limit intake to two drinks per day.

16.6 Diet plans for adults should be based on nutrient-dense foods and need to be individualized for existing health problems, physical abilities, presence of drug-nutrient interactions, possible depression, and economic constraints. A balanced multivitamin and mineral supplement can be used to help meet needs, especially for adults age 70 years and older. Most communities have congregate or home-delivered meal systems, food stamps, and other provisions to provide nutrition aid for those who qualify.

Check Your Knowledge (Answers to the following questions are below.)

1. Among the older population of the United States, the age of the fastest growing segment is _____ years.
   a. 65
   b. 74
   c. 79
   d. 85+

2. The diets of adults tend to be low in _____.
   a. vitamin E
   b. calcium
   c. fiber
   d. All of the above.

3. The reason the incidence of obesity increases with age is that
   a. the basal metabolic rate decreases with age.
   b. physical activity often decreases with age.
   c. energy intake exceeds energy expenditure.
   d. All of the above.

4. The immune system becomes less efficient with age, so it is especially important to consume adequate _____ and _____, nutrients that contribute to immune function.
   a. vitamin A, vitamin B-6
   b. protein, zinc

   c. zinc, iodide
   d. vitamin A, vitamin K

5. Which of the following accurately portrays a theory about the causes of aging?
   a. Increases in testosterone and estrogen affect cell processes.
   b. Blood sugar decreases, failing to supply adequate energy to brain cells.
   c. Inadequate calorie intake speeds body breakdown.
   d. Excess free radicals damage cell components.

6. To maintain optimal nutritional status and healthy weight, the diet of an older person should have a _____ nutrient density and be _____ in energy content.
   a. low, high
   b. low, low
   c. high, moderate
   d. high, high

7. Nutrition programs such as congregate meals or home-delivered meals provide which of the following?
   a. an improved nutritional status
   b. a social atmosphere

   c. an economical meal for low-income elderly
   d. All of the above.

8. During aging, the needs for vitamins and minerals
   a. continually fluctuate.
   b. greatly decrease.
   c. somewhat increase in some cases.
   d. greatly increase.

9. Alcohol is digested in the
   a. stomach.
   b. small intestine.
   c. liver.
   d. None of the above; alcohol requires no digestion.

10. Alcohol is most damaging to the
    a. brain cells because alcohol can be used as an energy source even before glucose.
    b. kidney cells because this is where alcohol is excreted.
    c. cells of the gastrointestinal tract because they are in direct contact with ingested alcohol.
    d. liver cells where alcohol is metabolized.

Answers: 1. d (LO 16.1), 2. d (LO 16.4), 3. d (LO 16.3), 4. b (LO 16.6), 5. d (LO 16.21), 6. c (LO 16.5), 7. d (LO 16.8), 8. c (LO 16.3), 9. d (LO 16.7), 10. d (LO 16.7)

Study Questions (Numbers refer to Learning Outcomes)

1. List three important points made by the Dietary Guidelines for Americans for the general population and give an example of why each one may be difficult for older adults to implement. What are some suggestions for overcoming these barriers? (LO 16.4)

2. What is the difference between life span and life expectancy? (LO 16.1)

3. List five general guidelines for cancer prevention. (LO 16.6)

4. Describe two hypotheses proposed to explain the causes of aging, and note

evidence for each in your daily life experiences. (LO 16.2)

5. List four organ systems that can decline in function in later years, along with a diet/lifestyle response to help cope with the decline. (LO 16.3)

6. Defend the recommendation for regular physical activity during older adulthood, including some resistance activity (weight training). (LO 16.5)

7. How might the nutritional needs of older people differ from those of

younger people? How are their needs similar? Be specific. (LO 16.3)

8. What three resources in a community are widely available to aid older adults in maintaining nutritional health? (LO 16.8)

9. List two benefits of moderate alcohol intake. List two risks of alcohol abuse. Should a non-drinker take up drinking for the health benefits? (LO 16.7)

10. List four warning signs of undernutrition in older people that are part of the acronym DETERMINE. Briefly justify the inclusion of each. (LO 16.6)

What Would You Choose Recommendations

Lifestyle factors, including diet, are among the most important determinants of cancer risk, so your interest in dietary changes to prevent cancer is wise. Cancer seems like a health problem that strikes mostly in older adults, but you have learned that your lifestyle choices right now will impact your health in the future. Having a genetic predisposition for a certain condition does not predetermine an adverse outcome. You can take charge of modifiable risk factors by eating well and exercising now.

Many phytochemicals are implicated in cancer prevention. For example, lycopene in tomatoes has been associated with lower risk of prostate cancer in men. Compounds in garlic and onions have been linked to reduced risk of several types of cancer. Phytochemical supplements contain isolated plant compounds with purported health benefits. As you learned in Chapter 2, dietary supplements are not tightly regulated in the United States, so the quality and composition of any dietary supplement

are questionable. In addition, there are components of whole foods that likely contribute to cancer prevention beyond the effects of an isolated phytochemical. Fruits, vegetables, and whole grains contain a variety of phytochemicals that likely work synergistically. In addition, the fiber and antioxidants (e.g., vitamins C and E) in fruits and vegetables are also beneficial for cancer prevention. In research studies, supplemental sources of certain nutrients or phytochemicals often come up short in comparison to the positive health effects of whole-food sources.

Fruit juicers are household appliances that can be used to extract juice fresh from fruits or vegetables rather than buying it in bottled or concentrated form. Freshly made juice likely does have more of some vitamins than juice that has been sitting on a shelf because, as you learned in Chapter 8, many vitamins break down over time with exposure to heat, light, or air. You can also control the amount of added sugars in the

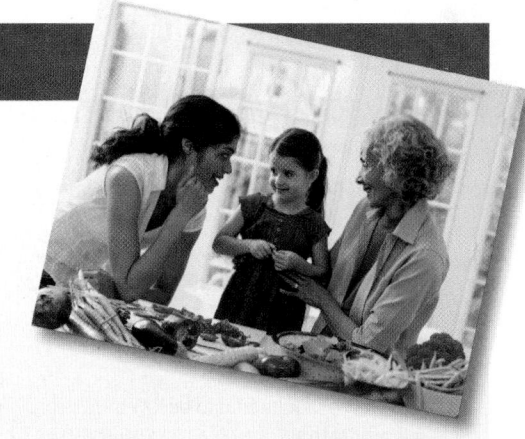

final product. Juicer manufacturers suggest using the leftover pulp as an ingredient in other foods, such as baked goods, but most of it usually ends up being discarded. Thus, much of the fiber and some healthful compounds may be lost.

When it comes to getting the most nutrients from your calories, whole fruits and vegetables offer phytochemicals, antioxidants, and fiber in a low-calorie package. Follow the suggestion of MyPlate to fill half your plate with fruits and vegetables.

Further Readings

1. ADA Reports: Position of the American Dietetic Association: Nutrition across the spectrum of aging. *Journal of the American Dietetic Association* 105:616, 2005.

Behaviors such as a healthful diet, being physically active, and not using tobacco in any form are three keys to healthful aging. The American Dietetic Association supports these

practices, as well as encourages older adults to seek medical and nutritional care to treat ongoing health problems, such as diabetes and hypertension.

2. Brannon CA: Alcohol: Functional food or addictive drug? *Today's Dietitian* 10(12):8, 2008.

   Alcohol has a long history as a functional and medicinal agent, but potential for abuse is high. This article describes the process of ethanol production, health benefits, and risks of alcohol use. A moderate intake of one to two drinks per day, particularly red wine at mealtimes, appears to be beneficial.

3. Brannon CA: Perimenopause: Nutritional management. *Today's Dietitian* 8(10):10, 2006.

   For most women, perimenopause begins in the mid-40s to early 50s. The most significant change during perimenopause is fluctuating levels of estrogen and progesterone. This article reviews several nutrition-related symptoms of this stage of the female life cycle and offers suggestions of several functional foods that contain components that may decrease these unpleasant symptoms.

4. Chodzko-Zajko WJ and others: American College of Sports Medicine Position Stand: Exercise and physical activity for older adults. *Medicine & Science in Sports & Exercise* 41:1510, 2009.

   The American College of Sports Medicine supports the advice of the 2008 Physical Activity Guidelines for Americans. Older adults should avoid inactivity and, instead, participate in physical activity for at least 150 minutes per week. A balanced routine should incorporate aerobic, strength, and flexibility exercises. Physical activity maintains physiological and cognitive functioning among aging adults.

5. De Souza Genaro P, Martini LA: Effect of protein intake on bone and muscle mass in the elderly. *Nutrition Reviews* 68:616, 2010.

   The RDA for protein for older adults is 0.8 grams per kilogram, but a growing body of research demonstrates that a slightly higher protein intake may be beneficial for preventing muscle loss (sarcopenia) and bone loss (osteopenia) during aging.

6. Eat like a Mediterranean to protect your aging brain. *Tufts University Health & Nutrition Letter* 10G:1, 2010.

   Adherence to a Mediterranean Diet is linked to lower risk of Alzheimer's disease and improved mental performance among older adults.

7. Eating to Beat Cancer. *Tufts University Health & Nutrition Letter* May Supplement:S1, 2007.

   Fruits and vegetables, especially tomatoes, cruciferous vegetables, berries, grapes, onions, and garlic, contain many phytochemicals that reduce cancer risk. Consuming fish or fish oils and adequate calcium is associated with reduced risk of colorectal cancer. The monounsaturated fats in olive oil are implicated in lowering cellular DNA damage. Green and black tea are also under study for anticancer activity.

8. Esposito K and others: Long-term effect of Mediterranean-style diet and calorie restriction on biomarkers of longevity and oxidant stress in overweight men. *Cardiology Research and Practice* 2011:1, 2010.

   After 2 years of intervention, overweight men who followed a Mediterranean-style diet with or without caloric restriction improved markers of cardiovascular health, oxidative stress, and insulin sensitivity. While long-term adherence to a calorie-restricted diet may be difficult, following a Mediterranean-style diet offers a beneficial alternative to achieving many of the same benefits as caloric restriction.

9. Grieger L: Dietary tips for baby boomers: Ageless advice for an aging generation. *Today's Dietitian* 10(3):38, 2008.

   Maintaining a healthy weight is considered to be the most important strategy for reducing chronic disease risk. Dietary practices that support and complement this advice include replacing calorie-rich, processed foods with nutrient-dense, unprocessed foods. Plant foods are emphasized because they are low in calories, yet high in vitamins, minerals, fiber, and phytochemicals. Fish is advocated as a source of omega-3 fatty acids.

10. Kushi LH and others: American Cancer Society guidelines on nutrition and physical activity for cancer prevention: Reducing the risk of cancer with healthy food choices and physical activity. *CA: A Cancer Journal for Clinicians* 56:254, 2006.

    Four general guidelines are presented as lifestyle modifications to reduce cancer risk: Maintain a healthy body weight; consume a diet low in red and processed meats and rich in fruits, vegetables, and whole grains; perform regular physical activity; and consume alcohol in moderation, if at all. ACS emphasizes the importance of a supportive social environment for incorporating such changes into a healthy lifestyle.

11. Redman LM and others: Effect of calorie restriction in non-obese humans on physiological, psychological, and behavioral outcomes. *Physiology & Behavior* 94:643, 2008.

    Although prospective, long-term studies of calorie restriction in humans are not feasible, evidence from epidemiological studies and short-term clinical trials indicate that calorie restriction decreases risk for diabetes and cardiovascular disease and improves biomarkers of aging without inducing disordered eating behaviors, constant feelings of hunger, depression, or cognitive decline. The authors point out, however, that the ability to adhere to a calorie-restricted diet will be low in an obesogenic environment. Research continues for an "anti-aging" pill that mimics the effects of calorie restriction in humans.

12. Riediger ND and others: A systemic review of the roles of n-3 fatty acids in health and disease. *Journal of the American Dietetic Association* 109: 668, 2009.

    Omega-3 fatty acids, abundant in fish, fish oils, some plant oils, and now fortified foods (e.g., eggs, spreads), have been shown to improve cardiovascular risk, cancer risk, and several mental health disorders (including depression and Alzheimer's disease). Complaints regarding consumption of fish oils include nausea and fishy burps. Megadose supplements may lead to excessive bleeding. Avoiding shark, swordfish, king mackerel, tilefish, and any fish harvested from contaminated waters can reduce the risk of consuming environmental toxins, including mercury. Typical North American diets are deficient in these healthy fats, but increased availability of fortified foods will support adequate consumption of omega-3 fatty acids.

13. Stenholm S and others: Sarcopenic obesity—definition, etiology, and consequences. *Current Opinions in Clinical Nutrition and Metabolic Care* 11:693, 2008.

    Older adults suffer from loss of muscle mass accompanied by gains in fat mass. Such body composition changes dramatically increase risks for disease and disability. The authors review potential causes for sarcopenic obesity, including changes in diet, physical activity, hormone levels, and inflammation.

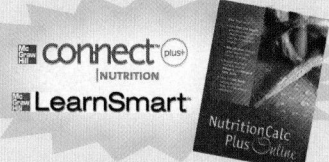

To get the most out of your study of nutrition, go to McGraw-Hill's online resources: Connect www.mcgrawhillconnect.com, where you will find NutritionCalc Plus, LearnSmart, and many other dynamic tools.

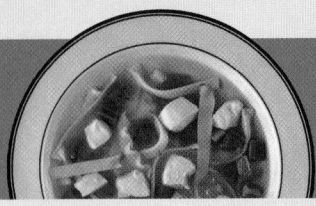

RATE YOUR PLATE

I. Am I Aging Healthfully?

Take Control of Your Aging by Dr. William B. Malarkey (Wooster Book Co., Wooster OH, 1999) includes a plan that incorporates various diet and lifestyle factors associated with successful aging. Indicate the degree to which you are following such a plan (or alternatively fill this out with a parent or another older relative in mind).

Physical: Do you eat a well-balanced diet, exercise on a regular basis, remain free of illness, abstain from smoking, refrain from drinking alcohol excessively, and experience refreshing sleep?

_____

_____

Intellectual: Are you analytical, do you read regularly, do you learn new things each day, do you engage your mental ability at work (or at school), and do you often reflect on your life?

_____

_____

_____

Emotional: Are you at peace, do you like who you are, are you optimistic, and do you laugh and relax regularly?

_____

_____

_____

Relational: Are you a good listener, do you feel supported by friends, do you attend social functions, do you talk with family members often, and do you feel close to coworkers (or fellow students)?

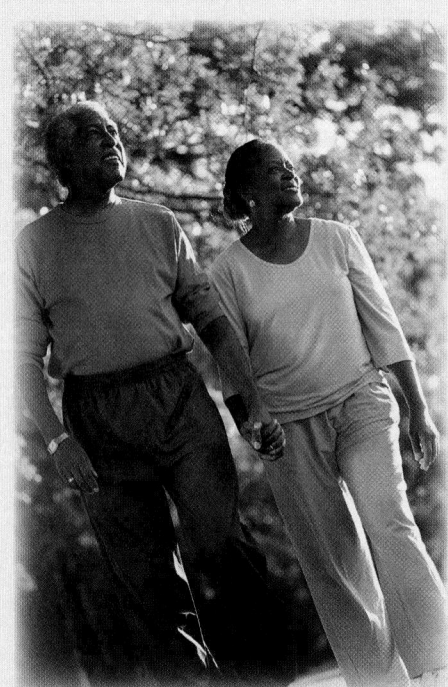

_____

_____

_____

Spiritual: Do you appreciate nature, give to or serve others, meditate or seek religious worship, and feel life has meaning?

_____

_____

_____

The more of these factors that you include in your life, the more well-rounded your plan is for maintaining overall health. Any one of the five areas in which you are not achieving success should show you characteristics to work on in the future.

II. Helping Older Adults Eat Better

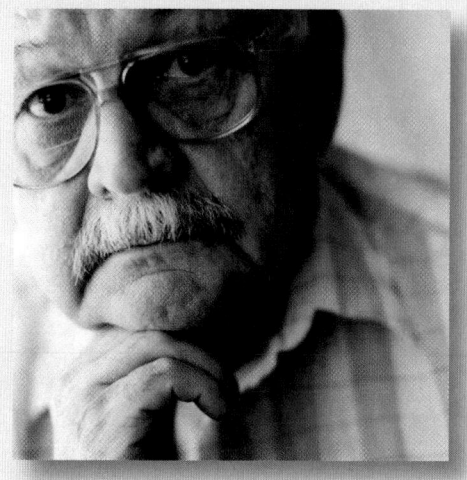

During their lifetimes, most people usually eat meals with families or loved ones. As people reach their older ages, many of them are faced with living and eating alone. In a study of the diets of 4400 older adults in the United States, one man in every five living alone and over age 55 ate poorly. One of four women between the ages of 55 and 64 years followed a low-quality diet. These poor diets can contribute to deteriorating mental and physical health. Consider the following example of the living situation of an older adult.

Neal, a 70-year-old man, lives alone in a home in a local suburban area. His wife died 1 year ago. He doesn't have many friends; his wife was his primary confidante. His neighbors across the street and next door are friendly, and Neal used to help them with yard projects in his spare time. Neal's health has been good, but he has had trouble with his teeth recently. His diet has been poor, and in the past 3 months his physical and mental vigor have deteriorated. He has been slowly lapsing into a depression and, so, keeps the shades drawn and rarely leaves his house. Neal keeps very little food in the house because his wife did most of the cooking and shopping, and he just isn't that interested in food.

If you were one of Neal's relatives and learned of Neal's situation, what six things could you do or suggest to help improve his nutritional status and mental outlook? Look back into this chapter to get some ideas.

1. _____
2. _____
3. _____
4. _____
5. _____
6. _____

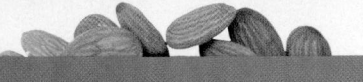

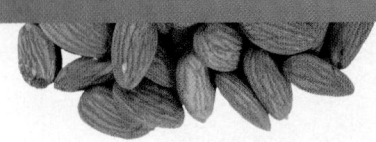

APPENDIX A Solutions: Case Studies

CASE STUDY SOLUTIONS

Chapter 1: Eating Habits in College

1. The most positive aspect of Andy's diet is that it contains good sources of protein from animal products also rich in zinc and iron. Alternating his hamburger and fries for lunch with pizza or tacos is a move in the right direction.

2.a. On the downside, Andy's diet is low in dairy products, fruits, and vegetables. This will result in a low intake of calcium, several of the vitamins and the phytochemical (plant-based) substances discussed in Chapter 1. His diet is also low in fiber because fast-food restaurants primarily use refined grain products, rather than whole-grain products and have few fruit and vegetable choices on the menu. Most of the beverages are soft drinks loaded with sugar. Many menu items, especially fries and chicken nuggets, are high in fat.

2.b. Most value menu options apply to foods rich in fat (French fries) and sugar (soft drinks) resulting in excessive amounts of these two components.

2.c. He could choose a low-fat granola bar instead of the candy bar for breakfast, or he could take the time to eat a bowl of whole-grain breakfast cereal with low-fat or fat-free milk to increase fiber and calcium (in the latter case) intake. Overall, Andy could improve his intake of fruits, vegetables, and dairy products by focusing on variety in food choice and balance among the food groups.

2.d. Andy could alternate between tacos and bean burritos to gain the benefits of plant proteins in a diet. When choosing pizza, he can replace high-fat toppings (e.g., pepperoni), and extra cheese with veggies (e.g., green peppers and onions). Many sub shops and delis offer several low-fat sandwiches, emphasizing lean meats such as turkey and vegetable toppings. For his beverages, Andy could order milk at least half of the time at his restaurant visits and substitute diet soft drinks for the regular variety. This would help moderate his sugar intake.

Chapter 2: Dietary Supplements

1. Whitney should be cautious about taking any supplement, especially one advertised as a "recent breakthrough." As you have read, dietary supplements are not closely regulated by FDA.

2. A general statement such as "increases energy" would be considered a structure/function claim and therefore does not require prior approval by FDA with regard to product labeling.

3. FDA will not have evaluated either the safety or effectiveness of such a product, and even harmful dietary supplements are difficult for FDA to recall.

4. There is a chance that the supplement, if effective, would contain little or none of the purported active ingredients.

5. Unfortunately, Whitney will find out all of this the hard way and will be out $60.

6. Whitney's hard-earned money would be better spent on a medical checkup at the Student Health Center. Consumers need to be cautious about nutrition information, especially regarding dietary supplements marketed as cure-alls and breakthroughs. Let the buyer beware!

Chapter 3: Gastroesophageal Reflux Disease

1. Overeating at mealtimes appears to bring on Caitlin's regular bouts of heart-burn.
2. Typical dietary advice includes consuming smaller, more frequent meals low in fat, not overeating at mealtimes, waiting about 2 hours after meals before lying down, and elevating the head of the bed about 6 inches (review Table 3-5). These recommendations reduce the risk of stomach contents forcing their way back up the esophagus. In addition, losing excess weight (if overweight) can alleviate GERD.
3. If dietary advice does not control symptoms, the primary medication used to control GERD inhibits acid production in the stomach (see earlier discussion on the proton pump inhibitors such as omeprazole [Prilosec] also used to treat peptic ulcers). If this and other medical therapy fails to control the problem, surgery to strengthen the lower esophageal sphincter is possible.
4. Caitlin's GERD can be treated, but most likely will be a lifelong condition. Even surgery will generally not cure the problem. Lifetime diet and lifestyle management, and most likely medications, will still be needed to manage the problem.
5. Lifelong management of GERD is important because long-standing GERD increases the risk of esophageal cancer.

Chapter 4: Problems with Milk Intake

1. Myeshia suspected that she was sensitive to milk because she developed bloating and gas when she consumed milk during one meal.
2. The disaccharide, lactose, is the most likely cause of Myeshia's symptoms.
3. When the enzyme lactase is missing or in short supply in the small intestine, undigested lactose travels to the large intestine and is fermented by bacteria there. The fermentation of lactose by bacteria produces abdominal gas, bloating, and pain. Diarrhea can also occur because the presence of lactose in the colon draws water from the blood vessels into the large intestine.
4. Lactose maldigestion is a normal pattern of physiology that often begins to develop at about ages 3 to 5 years in populations that do not rely on milk and other dairy foods as a main food source. When significant symptoms develop after lactose intake, it is then called lactose intolerance.
5. The primary form of lactose maldigestion is estimated to occur in about 75% of the world's population. Most lactose maldigesters are African-Americans (like Myeshia), Asian-Americans, and Latino/Hispanic Americans. The occurrence of lactose maldigestion also increases as people age.
6. The active bacteria cultures in yogurt digest the lactose when these bacteria are broken apart in the small intestine and release their lactase.
7. Many products, such as low-lactose milk and lactase pills, are available to enable lactose maldigesters to tolerate milk.
8. Many lactose maldigesters can consume moderate amounts of lactose with minimal or no intestinal discomfort because of the eventual lactose breakdown by bacteria in the large intestine.
9. In North America and Western Europe, milk and other dairy products are important sources of calcium and vitamin D. These are important for maintaining bone health.

10. Secondary lactose maldigestion occurs when a condition (e.g., long-standing diarrhea from a viral infection), results in a significant decline in lactase production.

Chapter 5: Planning a Heart-Healthy Diet

1. Jackie's approach to lowering blood cholesterol does not incorporate the best choices. She has excluded a great deal of fat in her diet, perhaps more than necessary, and has failed to include some key food groups that have cholesterol-lowering components.
2. Lowering fat as drastically as she has is not really necessary, especially for a physically active 21-year-old female.
3. Jackie could allow a more liberal amount of fat in her diet by including more monounsaturated fats. Canola oil and olive oil, as well as fats found in nuts and avocados, are rich sources of monounsaturated fats. These fats do not increase blood cholesterol. In addition she should include good sources of omega-3 fatty acids such as fatty fish, walnuts, flaxseeds, or soybean oil. One option is to use a canola oil-and-vinegar dressing on her salad, rather than lemon juice.
4. She has excluded a great deal of fat in her diet by merely replacing it with refined carbohydrates.
5. To make a shift to a more heart-healthy diet, Jackie would need to include at least 2 cups of fruit and 3 cups of vegetables a day, along with more whole-grain products. She should use whole-wheat bread instead of white bread for her sandwiches and eat a breakfast cereal that has at least 3 grams of fiber per serving.
6. Taking a brisk walk each morning is an excellent way to guarantee at least 30 minutes of activity on most days of the week. Exercise has been shown to increase concentration of HDL-cholesterol in the blood and decrease risk of cardiovascular disease.

Chapter 6: Planning a Vegetarian Diet

1. Studies show that the incidence of and the death rates from some chronic diseases, such as certain cardiovascular diseases, hypertension, many forms of cancer, type 2 diabetes, and obesity, are lower for vegetarians than for nonvegetarians.
2. Many components of a healthy vegetarian diet—whole grains, nuts, soy products, beans, 2 to 4 servings of fruits, and 3 to 5 servings of vegetables per day—are missing. With so few fruits and vegetables, his diet is also low in the many phytochemicals under study for numerous health benefits.
3. Protein appears to be low in the diet because Jordan has not replaced meat with a good plant source of protein. Vitamin B-12, iron, and zinc are also missing from the foods he is choosing. His diet seems to be adequate in calcium and riboflavin because he is including dairy products (milkshake and cheese).
4. Some of Jordan's food choices are high in fat (Danish pastry, milkshake, cookies) and sugar (fruit punch).
5. A healthy vegetarian diet includes whole grains, nuts, soy products, beans, 2 to 4 servings of fruits, and 3 to 5 servings of vegetables per day. It is apparent that he has not yet learned to implement the concept of complementary proteins, so the quality of protein in his diet is low. Meals that combine legumes or vegetables with grains or nuts (see Fig. 6-13) will provide the needed amounts of all amino acids.

Chapter 7: Choosing a Weight-Loss Program

1. Joe's weight has been climbing, so he has been experiencing positive energy balance.
2. When Joe is not working, his activity level is low. His time watching TV and studying does not use much energy. Joe should try to find time for physical activity after work and on weekends.

3. Balancing calorie intake with energy expenditure is the main key to weight loss and weight maintenance. Changes that Joe could make to his diet include a decrease in high-fat and -calorie items in his take-out meals. He should include more fruits, vegetables, and whole grains in his meals. A whole-grain cereal with fruit would be a healthy and convenient substitute for his pastry for breakfast. A grilled chicken sandwich or a taco salad would be a nutritious change for lunch. Grilled chicken or chili with a baked potato or salad would be healthier choices for dinner. Table 7-3 includes many ideas for food substitutions that will lower calories.

4. Joe will be wasting his money if he buys the product seen in the infomercial. Unfortunately, regulation of the supplement industry is woefully lacking. In the future, if there is a meaningful breakthrough in weight loss and weight control, health authorities such as the Surgeon General's Office or the National Institutes of Health will make North Americans aware of that fact.

5. The characteristics of a sound weight-loss diet are shown in Figure 7-15. These characteristics include a slow and steady rate of loss, flexibility relative to your habits and tastes, nutritional adequacy, behavior modification, physical activity, and maintenance of overall health.

Chapter 8: Choosing a Dietary Supplement

1. The maintenance dose of two to three tablets per day poses no risk *per se* because this dose of Nutramega does not exceed the Tolerable Upper Intake levels for vitamin A, vitamin C, niacin, or vitamin B-6.

2. a. **Vitamin A**
   33% (0.33) times the Daily Value of 1000 micrograms RAE equals 330 micrograms RAE per tablet. Sixteen tablets would yield 5280 micrograms RAE. The Upper Level is 3000 micrograms RAE for preformed vitamin A. Seventy-five percent of the vitamin A is preformed vitamin A, so this yields 3960 micrograms RAE of preformed vitamin A (5280 × 0.75 = 3960), or 1.3 times the Upper Level (3960/3000 = 1.3).

   b. **Vitamin C**
   700% (7) times the Daily Value of 60 milligrams equals 420 milligrams per tablet. 16 tablets would yield 6720 milligrams. The Upper Level is 2000 milligrams. This would then yield 3.4 times the Upper Level (6720/2000 = 3.4).

   c. **Niacin**
   200% (2) times the Daily Value of 20 milligrams equals 40 milligrams per tablet. 16 tablets would yield 640 milligrams. The Upper Level is 35 milligrams. This would then yield 18.3 times the Upper Level (640/35 = 18.3).

   d. **Vitamin B-6**
   100% (1) times the Daily Value of 2 milligrams equals 2 milligrams per tablet. 16 tablets would yield 32 milligrams. This is less than the Upper Level of 100 milligrams.

   e. The suggested use of Nutramega "at the first sign of feeling ill" poses some health risks for Amy. Taking two to three tablets every 3 hours would mean taking at least 16 tablets per day. This dosage would provide an intake of vitamin A, vitamin C, and niacin well in excess of the Upper Levels for these nutrients.

3. Nutramega is expensive compared to the cost of the typical multivitamin and mineral supplement (a 1-month supply would cost about $2 compared to about $50 for Nutramega).

4. Overall, Amy is smart to be concerned about meeting her nutrient needs, but the stress she is under does not increase nutrient needs.

5. A healthy diet as suggested by MyPlate should be Amy's primary focus. Taking a balanced multivitamin and mineral supplement is also a reasonable practice.

Chapter 9: Giving Up Milk

1. Factors contributing to her potential risk of osteoporosis include a poor dietary intake of calcium and vitamin D. Her diet also is low in protein, an important nutrient for the synthesis of connective tissue important in the skeletal system.

2. Ashley is increasing her chances of developing osteoporosis later in life because of her current high-risk lifestyle. Her new smoking habit and her low level of daily physical activity increase her risk of developing osteoporosis.

3. Ashley should rethink her rationale for avoiding milk. Fat-free milk is low in calories and provides much calcium. Dairy products such as milk do not lead to weight gain *per se*. There are even some studies suggesting that a regular intake of dairy products rich in calcium may aid in weight loss when on an otherwise calorie-restricted diet.

4. Ashley needs to find some reliable sources of calcium and vitamin D. These could include calcium-fortified juices, calcium-fortified bread and snack bars, and calcium-fortified chewable chocolate candies. Tofu (made with calcium) is another potential source, as well as calcium-fortified soy milk. Tofu and soy milk are also good sources of high-quality plant protein. Meeting the Adequate Intake of 1000 milligrams of calcium per day for her age would not be that hard if she were to make an effort to use these calcium-rich foods and/or incorporate other rich sources.

5. To decrease her risk of osteoporosis and several other chronic diseases, Ashley should stop smoking. In addition, including at least 30 minutes of physical activity on most days of the week will decrease her risk of osteoporosis and help her maintain a healthy weight.

Chapter 10: Planning a Training Diet

1. Michael is correct in following a high-carbohydrate diet.

2. In his effort to minimize his fat intake, he is probably not consuming enough calories, protein, iron, and calcium to support his training routine. He has fallen into the bagel, pasta, and pretzel routine that sports nutritionists warn is not conducive to peak performance. Low protein, iron, and overall calories may contribute to fatigue.

3. Michael's performance would improve if he also had a high-protein source at each meal. He could include milk with breakfast and possibly some low-fat yogurt or low-fat cheese at lunch. He should have a carbohydrate/protein snack before his workout, such as half a sandwich with fruit and some water. The sandwich and fruit will help provide him with fuel to support his vigorous training. In the evenings, he could substitute oil and vinegar dressing for the fat-free dressing on his salad and cheese and crackers for the pretzels to improve protein intake.

4. During his workouts, he could consume a sports drink to meet fluid needs and supply some carbohydrate, or he could consume water, along with a few graham crackers or other high-carbohydrate food.

5. Overall, it is important for Michael to fuel his body before, during, and after workouts. Before and during exercise, carbohydrates and fluid will improve athletic performance. After exercise, carbohydrates coupled with protein will enhance muscle recovery. Before and during exercise, carbohydrates and fluid will improve athletic performance. After exercise, carbohydrates coupled with protein will enhance muscle recovery.

Chapter 11: Eating Disorders—Steps to Recovery

1. Sarah has the characteristics to be diagnosed with anorexia nervosa.

2. Sarah's disordered eating habits began when she became self-conscious about her body when her peers teased her about being overweight. She began exercising each day and was successful at losing weight. Her disordered eating then

began with restricting her food intake more. She enjoyed the self-control she had over her body.

3. Sarah has the following physical symptoms of anorexia nervosa: she refuses to maintain a healthy weight-for-height, is at a weight below 85% of that expected, has a distorted view of her appearance, and has had no menstrual periods for over 3 consecutive months.

4. Her treatment would most likely consist of moderate bed rest to promote weight gain and an intake of 1000 to 1600 kcal initially, then increased by increments of about 100 to 200 kcal every few days until an acceptable rate of weight gain is achieved. The goal is to achieve a body weight that is at least 90% of an expected weight for her height, such as a BMI of at least 19.

5. Several nutrient deficiencies are likely in this case. Deficiencies of calcium and iron are probably most likely. The physician would likely prescribe a multivitamin and mineral supplement, along with an additional supplement of calcium as needed to make sure intake is in the range of 1200 to 1500 milligrams per day. Additional iron may be needed if Sarah is anemic. This overall practice will correct vitamin and mineral deficiencies that exist. The calcium in particular will contribute to bone maintenance.

6. Sarah would need to be hospitalized initially, due to her low BMI of 13.8 kg/m^2.

7. A team of health professionals, most likely consisting of a physician, registered dietitian, and psychologist, would provide therapy. Sarah's cooperation would be the most important element for therapy to be successful. She needs to realize that she has a problem and that she needs help. She must be willing to accept the assistance these professionals are willing to offer. The team, especially the psychologist, may use cognitive behavior therapy to help Sarah improve her self-image.

8. Sarah's outlook for recovery is not good unless she realizes she has a problem. Even if she is willing to accept the therapy and counseling, a relapse is likely to occur. Only 50% of anorexia nervosa patients have been found to recover fully from the disease. Sarah's disordered eating habits have been in place for about 6 years, so her problem is deep-rooted. The chances of recovery are greater if a vigorous treatment program is reinforced with close follow-up.

Chapter 12: Undernutrition During Childhood

1. Jamal should not be surprised that the children in the village were often sick and listless. The living conditions and recent natural disaster have added to the already poor conditions in this village. We know that children are especially susceptible to the effects of poverty and undernutrition.

2. Based on the reports that the children do not get enough to eat and on the outward signs of the children's health, protein, vitamin A, iron, iodide, and zinc are likely to be deficient in the diets of these children.

3. Protein, vitamin A, iron, iodide, and zinc deficiencies contribute to poor growth and stunting because of their essential functions in the body. One or more of these deficiencies is likely present in many children in the village.

4. Protein, vitamin A, iron, iodide, and zinc deficiencies may also contribute to depressed immune function, which can cause diarrhea and illness. These deficiencies are particularly risky in children.

5. The diets of these children are most likely also marginal in caloric content. A low-calorie intake during childhood will further depress the growth and overall health compromised by the protein and micronutrient deficiencies. Recall from Chapter 6 that protein-calorie malnutrition (PCM) is a form of undernutrition caused by an extremely deficient intake of calories or protein and generally is accompanied by an illness.

6. The recent storm will hopefully cause the Philippine government to send food and medicines to the village, which will be a short-term solution to some of their nutrition and health needs.

7. Poverty and undernutrition occur at much lower rates in the United States and other developed countries. Childhood nutrition concerns in developed countries are more likely to be the increasing incidence of overweight and obesity. As we discussed in Chapter 7, maintaining a healthy weight requires the proper balance of calories in and calories out. In Chapter 15 we will learn that overweight children are becoming more common because the typical number of calories they consume per day has increased at the same time that calorie expenditure in physical activity has decreased.

Chapter 13: Preventing Foodborne Illnesses at Gatherings

1. Nicole likely contracted *Clostridium perfringens*, based on the fact that she had diarrhea but did not vomit and the symptoms occurred about 8 hours after consuming the contaminated food (review Table 13-3).
2. Spores of *Clostridium perfringens* are typically present in meat. Thorough cooking will kill any of the live bacteria present, but the product may still contain spores. These can later develop into bacteria if the food is kept in a warm setting for a few hours. The beef in the empanadas was likely the bearer of the spores, and they likely germinated and produced a toxin as the beef sat in the car and on the buffet table.
3. Consuming food at large gatherings is risky for several reasons. First, foods for these events are typically cooked ahead of time and not consumed right away. Unfortunately, the foods end up remaining in the "danger zone" between 40°F and 140°F. Hot foods should be kept hot and cold foods cold. Unfortunately, proper refrigeration or heating equipment is not always available at these events. In addition, many people handle foods and serving utensils at large gatherings. It is important for anyone handling food or serving utensils to thoroughly wash their hands before and after handling food and to avoid coughing or sneezing over foods. Also, when returning to the "buffet" table, always use a clean plate to avoid cross-contamination. Finally, the focus at these events is usually on having fun and socializing and not on food safety.
4. The main precaution that was ignored was keeping the food out of the "danger zone." Overall, it is risky to leave perishable items such as meat, fish, poultry, eggs, and dairy products at room temperature for more than 1 to 2 hours.
5. Ideally, the cooked food should have remained at room temperature for no longer than 1 hour. Thus, soon after Nicole and her husband took it out of the oven, it should have been separated into a few smaller pans to speed cooling and then refrigerated because they knew it was not going to be served within 1 to 2 hours. Before leaving, they could have recombined the dish into one clean pan. Once they arrived at the party, the dish should have been refrigerated again, and then thoroughly reheated when it was time to eat.

Chapter 14: Preparing for Pregnancy

1. Lily's use of an over-the-counter vitamin and mineral supplement provides ample synthetic folic acid and can help fill some gaps between dietary intakes and requirements for various nutrients. Still, she should discuss this supplement use with her physician and would eventually benefit more from a prenatal supplement, as this will have more iron than the over-the-counter supplement. She should be sure not to exceed 100% of the Daily Value for preformed vitamin A because toxicities of this vitamin could cause birth defects. Lily is wise to avoid use of herbal supplements during pregnancy unless her physician approves of them.
2. Folate deficiency is known to be linked to neural tube defects. The synthetic folic acid in vitamin and mineral supplements is well absorbed and will certainly help to meet her needs for this nutrient. Consuming more fruits and vegetables—especially green leafy vegetables—is also a wise choice. A fortified, ready-to-eat

breakfast cereal also contributes to vitamin and mineral intake. Her physician may recommend a prenatal supplement instead of the over-the-counter supplement.

3. Many experts would say that she is consuming too much caffeine and would be wise to cut down coffee and caffeine-containing soft drinks to a total of three servings or fewer per day.

4. If Lily likes fish, she could include two servings of fish per week in her diet plan for pregnancy and breastfeeding. Fish are a good source of protein and also supply healthy fats, including omega-3 fatty acids, linked to brain and eye development in the fetus. However, Lily should avoid some types of fish that may have high mercury content, which can harm the nervous system of the developing fetus. Fish that typically have high levels of mercury include swordfish, shark, king mackerel, tile fish, largemouth bass, and canned albacore tuna.

5. The additional fruits and vegetables Lily is consuming will provide some fiber to help prevent constipation. Other ideas to increase her fiber intake include consuming a variety of whole grains and incorporating beans and legumes into her diet plan. Lily should also increase her fluid intake and be sure to maintain regular exercise, such as walking.

6. Lily expressed concern about her weight gain during pregnancy. Research clearly shows that adequate weight gain during pregnancy is critical for growth and development of the fetus. Inadequate weight gain contributes to risk for delivering a low-birth-weight or small-for-gestational-age baby. On the other hand, excessive weight gain during pregnancy can present problems as well. Excessive weight gain may promote long-term health problems and complicate the pregnancy with gestational diabetes or large-for-gestational age babies. At her pre-pregnancy weight and height, Lily's BMI (21 kg/m^2) is within the normal range, so she should aim to gain 25–35 pounds during the entire pregnancy. During the second and third trimesters, consuming an extra 350–450 kilocalories per day of nutrient-dense foods will help her to meet this goal. Regular, moderate exercise is also recommended throughout pregnancy. However, pregnancy is not a time to begin a vigorous exercise routine. Walking or riding a stationary bike are good activities to regulate weight gain. Lily should be reassured that her choice to breastfeed her baby will help her to lose those extra pounds after the baby is born.

Chapter 15: Undernutrition During Infancy

1. Ask if the formula is iron-fortified. Also, verify that Damon's caregivers are appropriately preparing his formula—adding the correct amount of powder or concentrated liquid to water. Be sure that Damon's caregivers plan to continue giving him formula until 1 year of age.

2. The scenario described puts Damon at risk for failure to thrive, likely due to his caregiver's lack of knowledge about appropriate infant feeding practices. His diet is probably lacking in total calories as well as calcium, iron, and zinc. Inadequacies may lead to stunted growth, cognitive problems, behavioral problems, and weak bones.

3. In addition to an iron-fortified infant formula, Damon should be eating fortified infant cereals, pureed fruits, vegetables, and meats, and even some table foods that are soft and cut into small pieces. After six months of age, solid foods help to meet increased nutrient demands. Processed foods, such as the hot dog described in the scenario, are usually high in sodium, fat, or sugars. These are not ideal for meeting Damon's nutritional needs. Allowing Damon to self-feed to some extent will help him to develop motor skills and build confidence.

4. Infants should not be drinking sugary beverages such as colas or fruit-flavored drinks, as these items lack the nutrient density essential to meeting Damon's needs. His caregivers should provide him no more than 4 to 6 ounces of 100% fruit juice. To prevent early childhood caries and develop self-feeding skills, Damon should be learning to drink from a cup rather than a bottle.

5. The combination of an appropriately-prepared, iron-fortified infant formula and a variety of solid foods should provide Damon all the nutrients he needs. However, if he is anemic, he may need an iron supplement.

Chapter 16: Dietary Assistance for an Older Adult

1. Frances' typical diet is low in many nutrients, including protein, calcium, iron, zinc, and vitamins B-12 and D.

2. Her poor diet will cause a more rapid decline in her lean tissue and bone mass, as well as decrease her iron status, vision, and mental function.

3. Physiological changes that will exacerbate the effects of her poor diet include increases in fat stores and decreases in her appetite; sense of taste, smell and thirst; chewing ability; bowel function; lactase production; iron status; liver, kidney, lung, cardiovascular, and immune function; vision; lean tissue; bone mass; and mental function. Review Table 16-2 for the recommended responses to these changes.

4. Frances could contact a local government office that offers congregate meal programs at a central location. She could inquire about location and availability of transportation to the site. This would give her social contact with other older persons, probably an important element missing in her life. This could help alleviate her loneliness. She could also request Meals on Wheels (if available) to provide one hot meal per day. One hot meal per day prepared for her may be what she needs to help stimulate her appetite. She could also have groceries delivered to her home if her budget could withstand the extra cost.

5. Other convenience foods that could be added to her diet include milk; assorted nuts; peanut butter; breakfast cereals; canned chicken or deli meats; yogurt; sliced cheese; cottage cheese; calcium-fortified orange juice; canned or frozen fruits and vegetables; and some fresh fruits and vegetables that do not require preparation, such as prewashed lettuce and bananas. A further possibility is a nutrition bar or a liquid nutritional supplement, such as a can of Ensure® Plus. The resulting increase in her nutrient intake would help prevent disease in the future and increase her sense of well-being.

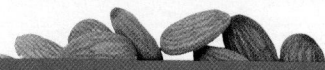

APPENDIX B   Daily Values Used on Food Labels

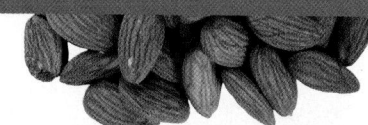

The Daily Values Used on Food Labels in the United States, with a Comparison to the Latest RDAs and Other Nutrient Standards*

Dietary Constituent	Unit of Measure	Current Daily Values for People Over 4 Years of Age	RDA or Other Current Dietary Standard	
			Males 19–30 Years Old	Females 19–30 Years Old
Total Fat[†]	g	<65	—	—
Saturated fatty acids[†]	g	<20	—	—
Protein[†]	g	50	56	46
Cholesterol[§]	mg	<300	—	—
Carbohydrate[†]	g	300	130	130
Dietary Fiber	g	25	38	25
Vitamin A	µg Retinol activity equivalents	1000	900	700
Vitamin D	International units	400	600	600
Vitamin E	International units	30	22–33	22–33
Vitamin K	µg	80	120	90
Vitamin C	mg	60	90	75
Folate	µg	400	400	400
Thiamin	mg	1.5	1.2	1.1
Riboflavin	mg	1.7	1.3	1.1
Niacin	mg	20	16	14
Vitamin B-6	mg	2	1.3	1.3
Vitamin B-12	µg	6	2.4	2.4
Biotin	µg	300	30	30
Pantothenic acid	mg	10	5	5
Calcium	mg	1000	1000	1000
Phosphorus	mg	1000	700	700
Iodide	µg	150	150	150
Iron	mg	18	8	18
Magnesium	mg	400	400	310
Copper	mg	2	0.9	0.9
Zinc	mg	15	11	8
Sodium[‡]	mg	<2400	1500	1500
Potassium[‡]	mg	3500	4700	4700
Chloride[‡]	mg	3400	2300	2300
Manganese	mg	2	2.3	1.8
Selenium	µg	70	55	55
Chromium	µg	120	35	25
Molybdenum	µg	75	45	45

Abbreviations: g = gram, mg = milligram, µg = microgram

*Daily Values are generally set at the highest nutrient recommendation in a specific age and gender category. Many Daily Values exceed current nutrient standards. This is in part because aspects of the Daily Values were originally developed in the early 1970s using estimates of nutrient needs published in 1968. The Daily Values have yet to be updated to reflect the current state of knowledge.

[†]These Daily Values are based on a 2000 kcal diet, instead of RDAs, with a caloric distribution of 30% from fat (and one-third of this total from saturated fat), 60% from carbohydrate, and 10% from protein.

[‡]The considerably higher Daily Values for sodium and chloride are there to allow for more diet flexibility, but the extra amounts are not needed to maintain health.

[§]Based on recommendations of U.S. federal agencies.

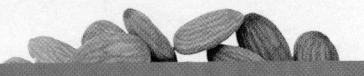

APPENDIX C   Dietary Advice for Canadians

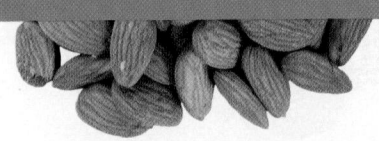

Recommended Nutrient Intake (RNI)
The Canadian version of RDA published in 1990.

▶ Excellent World Wide Web resources for Canadians are Health Canada (www.hc-sc.gc.ca), Dietitians of Canada (www.dietitians.ca), and the Institute of Nutrition, Metabolism, and Diabetes (www.cihr-irsc.gc.ca).

The information in this appendix includes advice on dietary patterns, as well as regulations that apply to food labeling. Previous **Recommended Nutrient Intakes (RNIs)** for nutrients have been replaced by the Dietary Reference Intakes (DRIs) that apply to Canadian and U.S. citizens. These are listed in the back of the text. Both Canadian and American scientists worked on the various DRI committees, coming up with a set of harmonized Dietary Reference Intakes for both countries.

SUMMARY OF THE NUTRITION RECOMMENDATIONS FOR CANADIANS

The Canadian federal department responsible for helping Canadians maintain and improve their health is Health Canada. The Office of Nutrition Policy and Promotion is within the Health Products and Food Branch of Health Canada and focuses on nutrition. Health Canada's National Dietary Guidance programs have been in existence since the 1930s and have always relied on scientific and other related evidence. Since 1977, a pattern of eating that meets nutrient needs and reduces the risk of chronic diseases has been promoted. In the 1990s, dietary guidance included *Canada's Guidelines for Healthy Eating* and *Food Guide to Healthy Eating* as well as *Nutrition for a Healthy Pregnancy* and *Nutrition for Healthy Term Infants*. The *Recommended Nutrient Intake* (RNI), a Canadian version of the RDA, was published in 1990.

In 1995, the U.S. Institutes of Medicine (IOM) brought together Canadian and American scientists to work on various committees, which came up with a set of harmonized Dietary Reference Intakes for both countries. The DRIs replaced the previous RNIs, and a new set of recommendations (EAR, AI, RDA, UL) similar to those in the United States were adopted in Canada. This led to a review and subsequent revision of *Canada's Food Guide to Healthy Eating* and *Guidelines for Healthy Eating*.

The revised *Canada's Food Guide* (Fig. C-1) was released in early 2007. The basic message to Canadians is to "Eat Well" with *Canada's Food Guide*. Learning more about *Canada's Food Guide* will help Canadians know how much food they need, what types of foods are better for them, and the importance of physical activity in their day.

In addition, if Canadians have the amount and type of food recommended and follow the tips included in *Canada's Food Guide*, this will help them:

- Meet their needs for vitamins, minerals, and other nutrients.
- Reduce their risk of obesity, type 2 diabetes, heart disease, certain types of cancer, and osteoporosis.
- Contribute to their overall health and vitality.

Canada's Food Guide places foods into four groups: vegetables and fruits; grain products; milk and alternatives; and meat and alternatives. *Canada's Food Guide* also includes information on the recommended number of Food Guide Servings per day, examples of what is one Food Guide Serving and how to make each Food Guide Serving count within each food group (Fig. C-2) and at each meal (Fig. C-3). Recommendations are also included about the types and amounts of oils and fats to consume, along with guidance to enjoy a variety of foods and to satisfy your thirst with water. Similar to the Dietary Guidelines for Americans recommendations, *Canada's Food Guide* emphasizes the combination of eating well and being active every day (Fig. C-4). The new Canadian Nutrition Facts label is also highlighted in *Canada's Food Guide* with the message to "Read the label." Finally, specific nutrition advice for different ages and stages is included (Fig. C-5). Similar to MyPlate, "My Food Guide" is a web-based interactive tool that will help you personalize the information found in *Canada's Food Guide*. Check out "My Food Guide" at http://www.hc-sc.gc.ca/fn-an/food-guide-aliment/myguide-monguide/index-eng.php.

▶ A downloadable copy of *Canada's Food Guide* is available at www.hc-sc.gc.ca

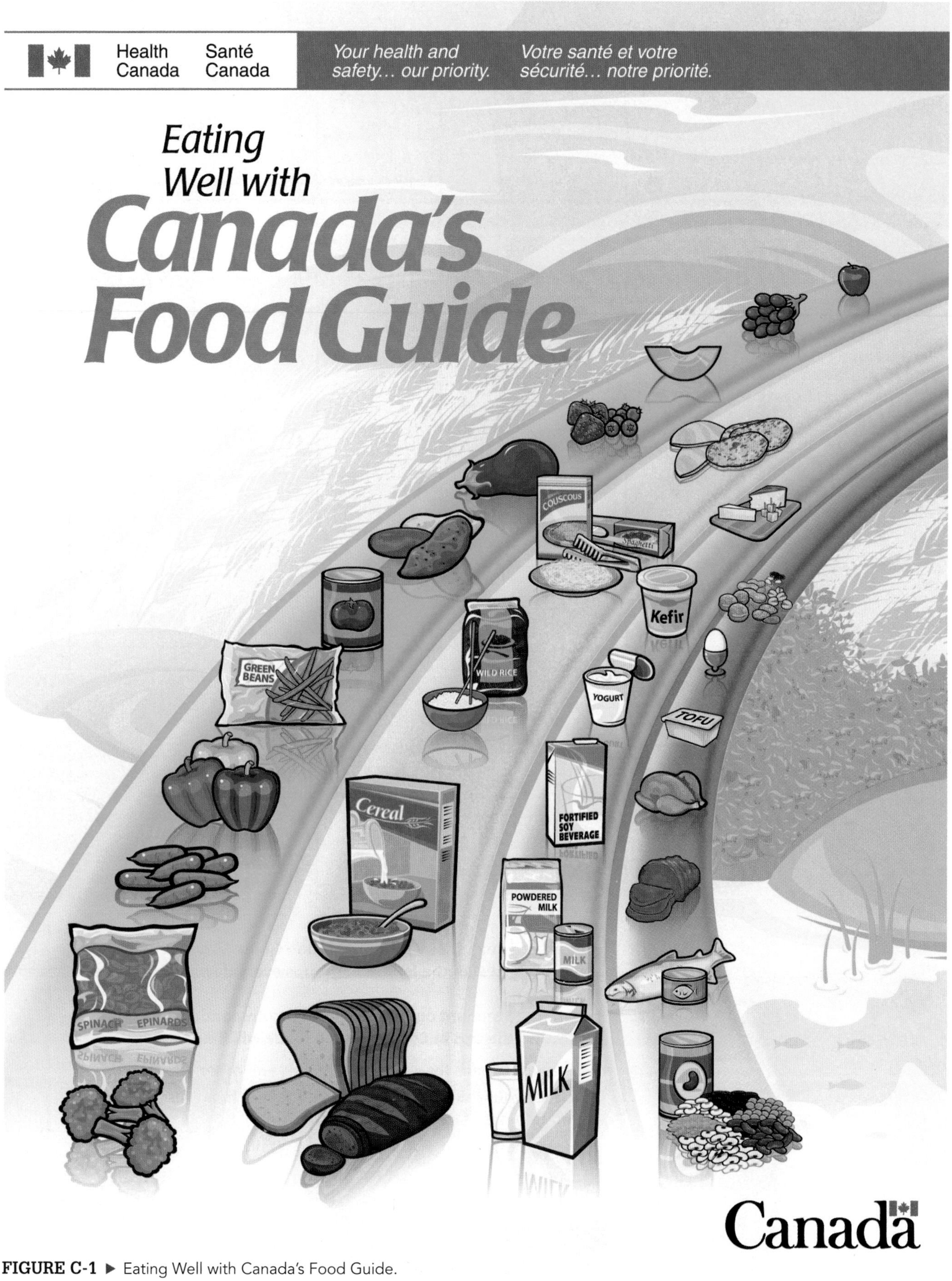

 Health Canada Santé Canada

Your health and safety... our priority. Votre santé et votre sécurité... notre priorité.

Eating Well with Canada's Food Guide

Canada

FIGURE C-1 ▶ Eating Well with Canada's Food Guide.

Recommended Number of *Food Guide Servings* per Day

	Children			Teens		Adults			
Age in Years	2-3	4-8	9-13	14-18		19-50		51+	
Sex	Girls and Boys			Females	Males	Females	Males	Females	Males
Vegetables and Fruit	4	5	6	7	8	7-8	8-10	7	7
Grain Products	3	4	6	6	7	6-7	8	6	7
Milk and Alternatives	2	2	3-4	3-4	3-4	2	2	3	3
Meat and Alternatives	1	1	1-2	2	3	2	3	2	3

The chart above shows how many Food Guide Servings you need from each of the four food groups every day.

Having the amount and type of food recommended and following the tips in *Canada's Food Guide* will help:

• Meet your needs for vitamins, minerals and other nutrients.
• Reduce your risk of obesity, type 2 diabetes, heart disease, certain types of cancer and osteoporosis.
• Contribute to your overall health and vitality.

FIGURE C-2 ▶ Information about Food Guide Servings from *Canada's Food Guide*.

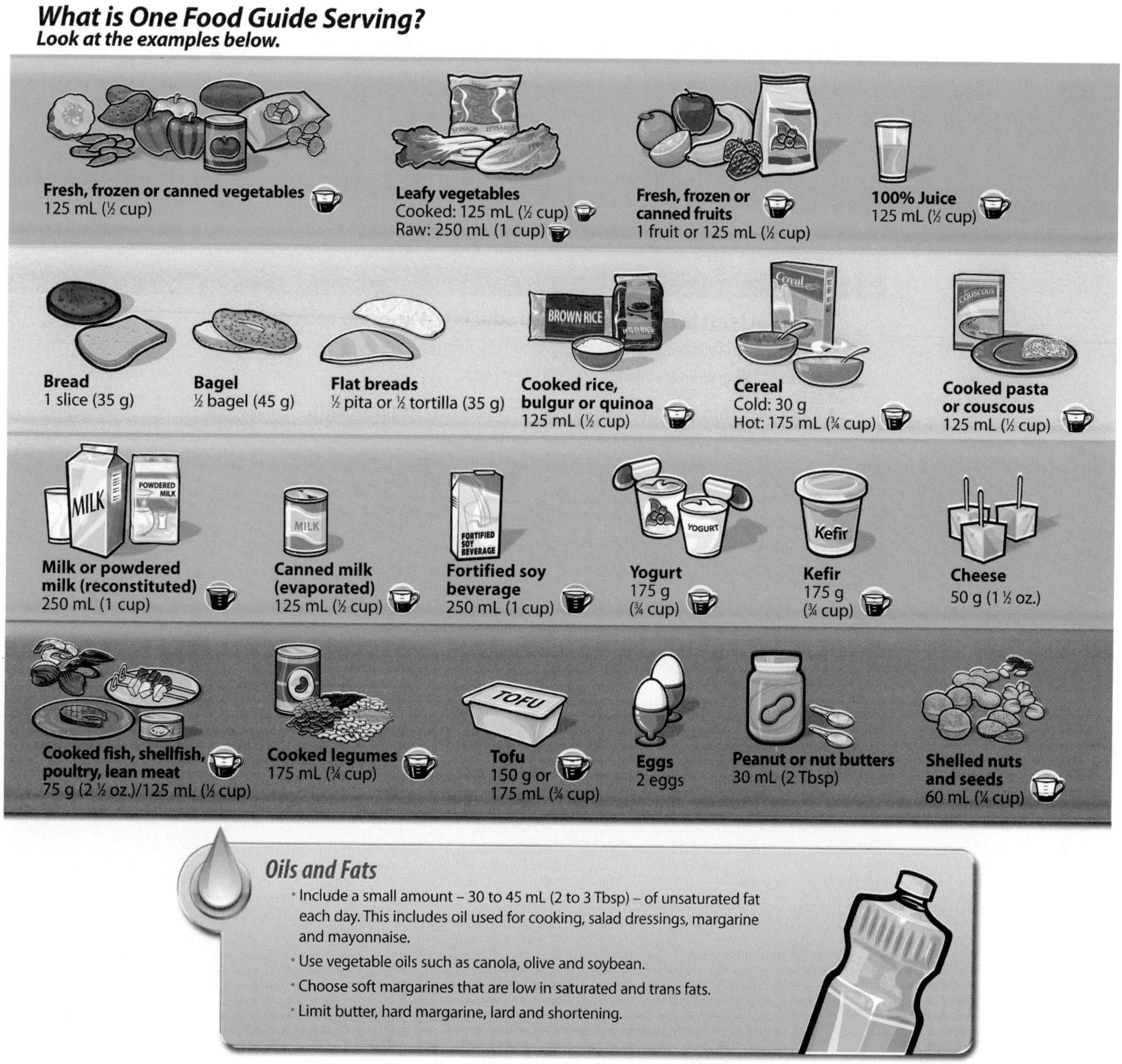
What is One Food Guide Serving?
Look at the examples below.
Fresh, frozen or canned vegetables
125 mL (½ cup)
Leafy vegetables
Cooked: 125 mL (½ cup)
Raw: 250 mL (1 cup)
Fresh, frozen or canned fruits
1 fruit or 125 mL (½ cup)
100% Juice
125 mL (½ cup)
Bread
1 slice (35 g)
Bagel
½ bagel (45 g)
Flat breads
½ pita or ½ tortilla (35 g)
BROWN RICE
Cooked rice, bulgur or quinoa
125 mL (½ cup)
Cereal
Cereal
Cold: 30 g
Hot: 175 mL (¾ cup)
Cooked pasta or couscous
125 mL (½ cup)
MILK
POWDERED MILK
Milk or powdered milk (reconstituted)
250 mL (1 cup)
MILK
Canned milk (evaporated)
125 mL (½ cup)
FORTIFIED SOY BEVERAGE
Fortified soy beverage
250 mL (1 cup)
YOGURT
Yogurt
175 g
(¾ cup)
Kefir
Kefir
175 g
(¾ cup)
Cheese
50 g (1 ½ oz.)
Cooked fish, shellfish, poultry, lean meat
75 g (2 ½ oz.)/125 mL (½ cup)
Cooked legumes
175 mL (¾ cup)
TOFU
Tofu
150 g or
175 mL (¾ cup)
Eggs
2 eggs
Peanut or nut butters
30 mL (2 Tbsp)
Shelled nuts and seeds
60 mL (¼ cup)
Oils and Fats
• Include a small amount – 30 to 45 mL (2 to 3 Tbsp) – of unsaturated fat each day. This includes oil used for cooking, salad dressings, margarine and mayonnaise.
• Use vegetable oils such as canola, olive and soybean.
• Choose soft margarines that are low in saturated and trans fats.
• Limit butter, hard margarine, lard and shortening.

FIGURE C-2 ▶ *(continued)*

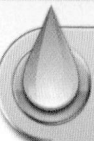

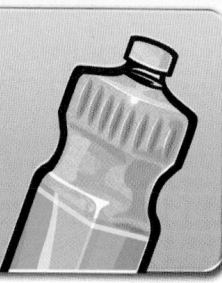

Make each Food Guide Serving count...
wherever you are – at home, at school, at work or when eating out!

▶ **Eat at least one dark green and one orange vegetable each day.**
- Go for dark green vegetables such as broccoli, romaine lettuce and spinach.
- Go for orange vegetables such as carrots, sweet potatoes and winter squash.

▶ **Choose vegetables and fruit prepared with little or no added fat, sugar or salt.**
- Enjoy vegetables steamed, baked or stir-fried instead of deep-fried.

▶ **Have vegetables and fruit more often than juice.**

▶ **Make at least half of your grain products whole grain each day.**
- Eat a variety of whole grains such as barley, brown rice, oats, quinoa and wild rice.
- Enjoy whole grain breads, oatmeal or whole wheat pasta.

▶ **Choose grain products that are lower in fat, sugar or salt.**
- Compare the Nutrition Facts table on labels to make wise choices.
- Enjoy the true taste of grain products. When adding sauces or spreads, use small amounts.

▶ **Drink skim, 1%, or 2% milk each day.**
- Have 500 mL (2 cups) of milk every day for adequate vitamin D.
- Drink fortified soy beverages if you do not drink milk.

▶ **Select lower fat milk alternatives.**
- Compare the Nutrition Facts table on yogurts or cheeses to make wise choices.

▶ **Have meat alternatives such as beans, lentils and tofu often.**

▶ **Eat at least two Food Guide Servings of fish each week.***
- Choose fish such as char, herring, mackerel, salmon, sardines and trout.

▶ **Select lean meat and alternatives prepared with little or no added fat or salt.**
- Trim the visible fat from meats. Remove the skin on poultry.
- Use cooking methods such as roasting, baking or poaching that require little or no added fat.
- If you eat luncheon meats, sausages or prepackaged meats, choose those lower in salt (sodium) and fat.

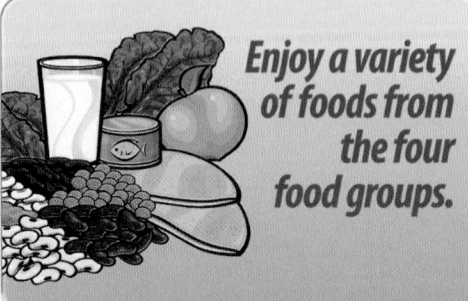

Enjoy a variety of foods from the four food groups.

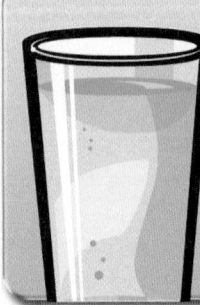

Satisfy your thirst with water!

Drink water regularly. It's a calorie-free way to quench your thirst. Drink more water in hot weather or when you are very active.

* Health Canada provides advice for limiting exposure to mercury from certain types of fish. Refer to www.healthcanada.gc.ca for the latest information.

FIGURE C-2 ▶ *(continued)*

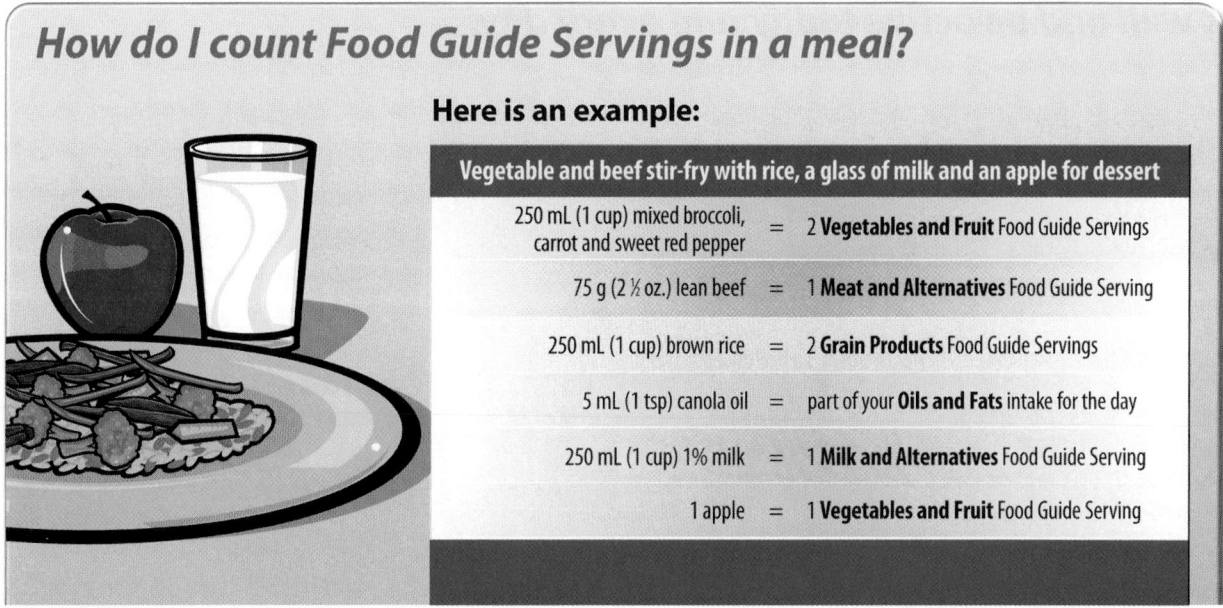

How do I count Food Guide Servings in a meal?

Here is an example:

Vegetable and beef stir-fry with rice, a glass of milk and an apple for dessert

250 mL (1 cup) mixed broccoli, carrot and sweet red pepper	=	2 **Vegetables and Fruit** Food Guide Servings
75 g (2 ½ oz.) lean beef	=	1 **Meat and Alternatives** Food Guide Serving
250 mL (1 cup) brown rice	=	2 **Grain Products** Food Guide Servings
5 mL (1 tsp) canola oil	=	part of your **Oils and Fats** intake for the day
250 mL (1 cup) 1% milk	=	1 **Milk and Alternatives** Food Guide Serving
1 apple	=	1 **Vegetables and Fruit** Food Guide Serving

FIGURE C-3 ▶ How to count Food Guide Servings in a meal.

Nutrition Labels

New labeling requirements were published on January 1, 2003. The new regulations require most food labels to carry a mandatory Nutrition Facts table listing Calories and 13 key nutrients.

How to Read the Canadian Nutrition Label

The Regulations provide for the optional declaration of the number of Calories both from fat and from saturates plus *trans*. Recommendations on the % of Calories from fat apply to the total diet rather than to an individual food. Therefore, inclusion of the % of Calories from fat in the Nutrition Facts table may be confusing and is not permitted.

The Nutrition Facts table provides information on saturated and *trans* fatty acids, shown to raise serum cholesterol levels. The declaration of the other groups of fatty acids, monounsaturates, omega-3, and omega-6 polyunsaturates, is optional unless claims are made, in which case all three must be declared.

Potassium is not included as a mandatory nutrient of the Nutrition Facts table because it is not considered to be a nutrient of general public health importance. The declaration of potassium, however, is mandatory when a claim is made for the sodium or salt content of a food that contains an added potassium salt.

Daily Value is a comparison standard comprised of
(a) vitamin or mineral amounts referred to in the definition of a recommended daily intake for that vitamin or mineral
(b) nutrient amounts referred to in the definition of reference standard for that nutrient

Serving size is stipulated for various foods.

The amount of vitamins and minerals is expressed as a percentage of the Daily Value per serving of stated size.

Nutrition Facts
Per 1 cup (264g)

Amount	% Daily Value
Calories 260	
Fat 13g	20%
Saturated Fat 3g + *Trans* Fat 2g	25%
Cholesterol 30mg	
Sodium 660mg	28%
Carbohydrate 31g	10%
Fibre 0g	0%
Sugars 5g	
Protein 5g	
Vitamin A 4% Vitamin C 2%	
Calcium 15% Iron 4%	

g = gram
mg = milligram

Eat well and be active today and every day!

The benefits of eating well and being active include:

- Better overall health.
- Lower risk of disease.
- A healthy body weight.
- Feeling and looking better.
- More energy.
- Stronger muscles and bones.

Be active

To be active every day is a step towards better health and a healthy body weight.

Canada's Physical Activity Guide recommends building 30 to 60 minutes of moderate physical activity into daily life for adults and at least 90 minutes a day for children and youth. You don't have to do it all at once. Add it up in periods of at least 10 minutes at a time for adults and five minutes at a time for children and youth.

Start slowly and build up.

Eat well

Another important step towards better health and a healthy body weight is to follow *Canada's Food Guide* by:

- Eating the recommended amount and type of food each day.
- Limiting foods and beverages high in calories, fat, sugar or salt (sodium) such as cakes and pastries, chocolate and candies, cookies and granola bars, doughnuts and muffins, ice cream and frozen desserts, French fries, potato chips, nachos and other salty snacks, alcohol, fruit flavoured drinks, soft drinks, sports and energy drinks, and sweetened hot or cold drinks.

Read the label

- Compare the Nutrition Facts table on food labels to choose products that contain less fat, saturated fat, trans fat, sugar and sodium.
- Keep in mind that the calories and nutrients listed are for the amount of food found at the top of the Nutrition Facts table.

Limit trans fat

When a Nutrition Facts table is not available, ask for nutrition information to choose foods lower in trans and saturated fats.

Nutrition Facts
Per 0 mL (0 g)

Amount	% Daily Value
Calories 0	
Fat 0 g	0 %
Saturates 0 g	0 %
+ Trans 0 g	
Cholesterol 0 mg	
Sodium 0 mg	0 %
Carbohydrate 0 g	0 %
Fibre 0 g	0 %
Sugars 0 g	
Protein 0 g	

Vitamin A	0 %	Vitamin C	0 %
Calcium	0 %	Iron	0 %

Take a step today…

✓ Have breakfast every day. It may help control your hunger later in the day.

✓ Walk wherever you can – get off the bus early, use the stairs.

✓ Benefit from eating vegetables and fruit at all meals and as snacks.

✓ Spend less time being inactive such as watching TV or playing computer games.

✓ Request nutrition information about menu items when eating out to help you make healthier choices.

✓ Enjoy eating with family and friends!

✓ Take time to eat and savour every bite!

For more information, interactive tools, or additional copies visit Canada's Food Guide on-line at: www.healthcanada.gc.ca/foodguide

or contact:

Publications
Health Canada
Ottawa, Ontario K1A 0K9
E-Mail: publications@hc-sc.gc.ca
Tel.: 1-866-225-0709
Fax: (613) 941-5366
TTY: 1-800-267-1245

Également disponible en français sous le titre :
Bien manger avec le Guide alimentaire canadien

This publication can be made available on request on diskette, large print, audio-cassette and braille.

© Her Majesty the Queen in Right of Canada, represented by the Minister of Health Canada, 2007. This publication may be reproduced without permission. No changes permitted.   HC Pub.: 4651   Cat.: H164-38/1-2007E   ISBN: 0-662-44467-1

FIGURE C-4 ▶ Recommendations to eat well and be active from *Canada's Food Guide.*

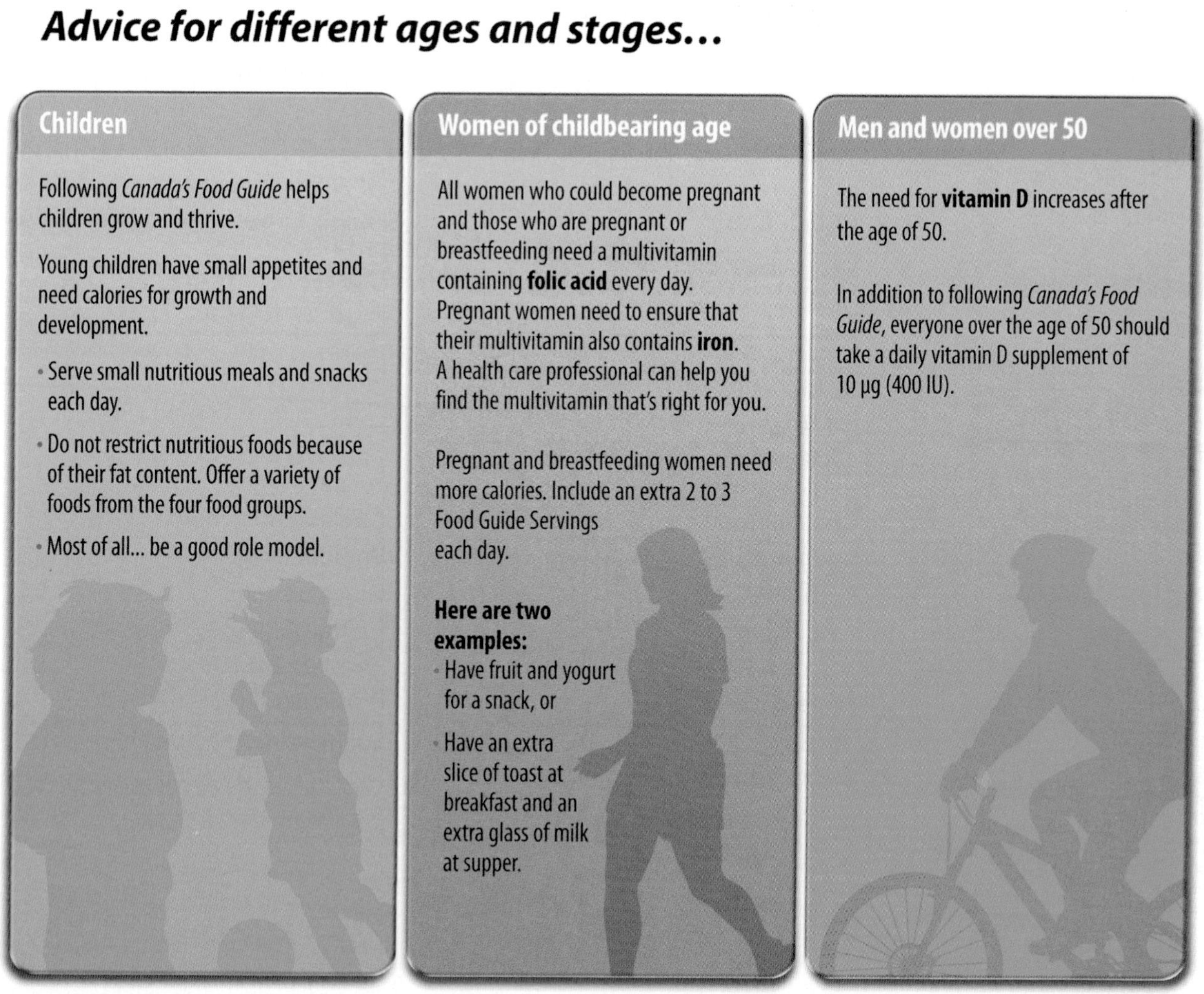

Advice for different ages and stages...

Children

Following *Canada's Food Guide* helps children grow and thrive.

Young children have small appetites and need calories for growth and development.

- Serve small nutritious meals and snacks each day.

- Do not restrict nutritious foods because of their fat content. Offer a variety of foods from the four food groups.

- Most of all... be a good role model.

Women of childbearing age

All women who could become pregnant and those who are pregnant or breastfeeding need a multivitamin containing **folic acid** every day. Pregnant women need to ensure that their multivitamin also contains **iron**. A health care professional can help you find the multivitamin that's right for you.

Pregnant and breastfeeding women need more calories. Include an extra 2 to 3 Food Guide Servings each day.

Here are two examples:
- Have fruit and yogurt for a snack, or
- Have an extra slice of toast at breakfast and an extra glass of milk at supper.

Men and women over 50

The need for **vitamin D** increases after the age of 50.

In addition to following *Canada's Food Guide*, everyone over the age of 50 should take a daily vitamin D supplement of 10 µg (400 IU).

FIGURE C-5 ▶ Advice for different ages and stages from *Canada's Food Guide.*

The new regulations make nutrition labeling mandatory on most food labels using a new format. The regulations also update requirements for nutrient content claims and permit, for the first time in Canada, diet-related health claims for foods.

Templates for Canadian "Nutrition Facts" Tables

Bilingual Label

Nutrition Facts
Valeur nutritive
Per 125 mL (87 g) / 0par 125 mL (87 g)

Amount Teneur		% Daily Value % valeur quotidienne
Calories / Calories 80		
Fat / Lipids 0.5 g		**1** %
Saturated / saturés 0 g + *Trans* / trans 0 g		**0** %
Cholesterol / Cholestérol 0 mg		
Sodium / Sodium 0 mg		**0** %
Carbohydrate / Glucides 18 g		**6** %
Fibre / Fibres 2 g		**8** %
Sugars / Sucres 2 g		
Protein / Protéines 3 g		
Vitamin A / Vitamine A		2 %
Vitamin C / Vitamine C		10 %
Calcium / Calcium		0 %
Iron / Fer		2 %

English Label

Nutrition Facts
Per 125 mL (87 g)

Amount	% Daily Value
Calories 80	
Fat 0.5 g	**1** %
Saturated 0 g + *Trans* 0 g	**0** %
Cholesterol 0 mg	
Sodium 0 mg	**0** %
Carbohydrate 18 g	**6** %
Fibre 2 g	**8** %
Sugars 2 g	
Protein 3 g	
Vitamin A 2 %	Vitamin C 10 %
Calcium 0 %	Iron 2 %

French Label

Valeur nutritive
par 125 mL (87 g)

Teneur	% valeur quotidienne
Calories 80	
Lipids 0,5 g	**1** %
saturés 0 g + trans 0 g	**0** %
Cholestérol 0 mg	
Sodium 0 mg	**0** %
Glucides 18 g	**6** %
Fibres 2 g	**8** %
Sucres 2 g	
Protéines 3 g	
Vitamine A 2 %	Vitamine C 10 %
Calcium 0 %	Fer 2 %

g = gram
mg = milligram

New Canadian Nutrition Facts Label for Children Under Two Years of Age

Nutrition Facts
Per 1 jar (126 mL)

	Amount
Calories	110
Fat	0g
Sodium	10 mg
Carbohydrate	27g
Fibre	4g
Sugars	18g
Protein	0g
% Daily Value	
Vitamin A 6% Vitamin C 45%	
Calcium 2% Iron 2%	

g = gram
mg = milligram

Recommended Daily Intakes and Reference Standards

The following are the Recommended Daily Intakes and Reference Standards used on Nutrition Labels for persons 2 years of age and older.* † ‡

Dietary Constituent	Amount	Dietary Constituent	Amount
Fat	**65 g**	Folacin	220 µg
The sum of saturated fatty acids and *trans* fatty acids	**20 g**	Vitamin B$_{12}$	2 µg
Cholesterol	**300 mg**	Pantothenic acid or pantothenate	7 mg
Carbohydrate	**300 g**	Vitamin K	**80 mg**
Fibre	**25 g**	Biotin	**30 µg**
Sodium	**2400 mg**	Calcium	1100 mg
Chloride	**3400 µg**	Phosphorus	1100 mg
Potassium	**3500 mg**	Magnesium	250 mg
Vitamin A	1000 RE	Iron	14 mg
Vitamin D	5 µg	Zinc	9 mg
Vitamin E	10 mg	Iodide	160 µg
Vitamin C	60 mg	Selenium	**50 µg**
Thiamin, thiamine or vitamin B$_1$	1.3 mg	Copper	**2 mg**
Riboflavin or vitamin B$_2$	1.6 mg	Manganese	**2 mg**
Niacin	23 NE	Chromium	**120 µg**
Vitamin B$_6$	1.8 mg	Molybdenum	**75 µg**

*RE = retinol equivalents
†NE = niacin equivalents
‡Together these constitute the Daily Values used on the Canadian Nutrition Facts Label. Reference Standards are bolded.

Approved Nutrient Content Claims for Canada

The following is a sample of approved nutrient content claims for food labels (for the complete list of regulations see the website http://gazette.gc.ca/archives/p1/2005/2005-05-07/html/reg4-eng.html).

Energy

- *Free of energy:* The food provides less than 5 Calories or 21 kilojoules per reference amount and serving of stated size.
- *Low in energy:* The food provides 40 Calories or 167 kilojoules or less per reference amount and serving of stated size.
- *Reduced in energy:* The food is processed, formulated, reformulated, or otherwise modified so that it provides at least 25% less energy per reference amount of a similar food.
- *Lower in energy:* The food provides at least 25% less energy per reference amount of a similar food.

- *Source of energy:* The food provides at least 100 Calories or 420 kilojoules per reference amount and serving of stated size.
- *More energy:* The food provides at least 25% more energy, totalling at least 100 more Calories or 420 more kilojoules per reference amount of a similar food.

Protein

- *Low in protein:* The food contains no more than 1 gram of protein per 100 grams of the food.
- *Source of protein:* The food has a protein rating of 20 or more, as determined by official method

FO-1, *Determination of Protein Rating,* October 15, 1981, (*a*) per reasonable daily intake; or (*b*) per 30 grams combined with 125 milliliters of milk, if the food is a breakfast cereal.

- *Excellent source of protein:* The food has a protein rating of 40 or more, as determined by official method FO-1, *Determination of Protein Rating,* October 15, 1981, (*a*) per reasonable daily intake; or (*b*) per 30 grams combined with 125 milliliters of milk, if the food is a breakfast cereal.
- *More protein:* The food (*a*) has a protein rating of 20 or more, as determined by official method

FO-1, *Determination of Protein Rating*, October 15, 1981, (i) per reasonable daily intake, or (ii) per 30 grams combined with 125 milliliters of milk, if the food is a breakfast cereal; and (*b*) contains at least 25% more protein, totalling at least 7 grams more, per reasonable daily intake compared to the reference food of the same food group or the similar reference food.

Fat

- *Free of fat:* The food contains less than 0.5 grams of fat per reference amount and serving of stated size.
- *Low in fat:* The food contains 3 grams or less of fat per reference amount and serving of stated size and, if the reference amount is 30 grams or 30 milliliters or less, per 50 grams.
- *Reduced in fat:* The food is processed, formulated, reformulated, or otherwise modified so that it contains at least 25% less fat than the reference amount of a similar food.
- *Lower in fat:* The food contains at least 25% less fat per reference amount of the food, than the reference amount of the reference food of the same food group.
- *100% fat-free:* The food (*a*) contains less than 0.5 grams of fat per 100 grams; (*b*) contains no added fat.
- *No added fat:* The food contains no added fats or oils set out in Division 9, or added butter or ghee, or ingredients that contain added fats or oils, or butter or ghee.
- *Free of saturated fatty acids:* The food contains less than 0.2 grams saturated fatty acids and less than 0.2 grams *trans* fatty acids per reference amount and serving of stated size.
- *Low in saturated fatty acids:* (1) The food contains 2 grams or less of saturated fatty acids and *trans* fatty acids combined per reference amount and serving of stated size. (2) The food provides 15% or less energy from the sum of saturated fatty acids and *trans* fatty acids.

- *Reduced in saturated fatty acids:* The food is processed, formulated, reformulated, or otherwise modified without increasing the content of *trans* fatty acids, so that it contains at least 25% less saturated fatty acids per reference amount of the food than the reference amount of the similar reference food.
- *Lower in saturated fatty acids:* The food contains at least 25% less saturated fatty acids and the content of *trans* fatty acids is not higher per reference amount of the food, than the reference amount of the reference food of the same food group.
- *Free of* trans *fatty acids:* The food contains less than 0.2 grams of *trans* fatty acids per reference amount and serving of stated size.
- *Reduced in* trans *fatty acids:* The food is processed, formulated, reformulated, or otherwise modified without increasing the content of saturated fatty acids, so that it contains at least 25% less *trans* fatty acids per reference amount of the food than the reference amount of the similar reference food.
- *Lower in* trans *fatty acids:* The food contains at least 25% less *trans* fatty acids and the content of saturated fatty acids is not higher per reference amount of the food compared to the reference amount of a similar food.
- *Source of omega-3 polyunsaturated fatty acids:* The food contains 0.3 grams or more of omega-3 polyunsaturated fatty acids per reference amount and serving of stated size.
- *Source of omega-6 polyunsaturated fatty acids:* The food contains 2 grams or more of omega-6 polyunsaturated fatty acids per reference amount and serving of stated size.

Cholesterol

- *Free of cholesterol:* The food contains less than 2 milligrams of cholesterol per reference amount and serving of stated size.
- *Low in cholesterol:* The food contains 20 milligrams or less of cholesterol per reference amount and serving of

stated size (if the reference amount is 30 grams or 30 milliliters or less, per 50 grams).
- *Reduced in cholesterol:* The food is processed, formulated, reformulated, or otherwise modified so that it contains at least 25% less cholesterol per reference amount of a similar food.
- *Lower in cholesterol:* The food contains at least 25% less cholesterol per reference amount of a similar food.

Sodium or Salt

- *Free of sodium or salt:* The food contains less than 5 milligrams of sodium per reference amount and serving of stated size.
- *Low in sodium or salt:* The food contains 140 milligrams or less of sodium per reference amount and serving of stated size.
- *Reduced in sodium or salt:* The food is processed, formulated, reformulated, or otherwise modified so that it contains at least 25% less sodium per reference amount of a similar food.
- *Lower in sodium or salt:* The food contains at least 25% less sodium per reference amount of the food.
- *No added sodium or salt:* The food contains no added salt, other sodium salts, or ingredients that contain sodium that functionally substitute for added salt.
- *Lightly salted:* The food contains at least 50% less added sodium than the sodium added to a similar reference food.

Sugars

- *Free of sugars:* The food contains less than 0.5 milligrams of sugars per reference amount and serving of stated size.
- *Reduced in sugars:* The food is processed, formulated, reformulated, or otherwise modified so that it contains at least 25% less sugars, totalling at least 5 grams less, per reference amount of the food.

- *Lower in sugars:* The food contains at least 25% less sugars, totalling at least 5 grams less, per reference amount of the food.
- *No added sugars:* The food contains no added sugars, no ingredients containing added sugars or ingredients that contain sugars that functionally substitute for added sugars.

Fibre

- *Source of fibre:* The food contains 2 grams or more (*a*) of fibre per reference amount and serving of stated size, if no fibre or fibre source is identified in the statement or claim; or (*b*) of each identified fibre or fibre from an identified fibre source per reference amount and serving of stated size, if a fibre or fibre source is identified in the statement or claim.
- *High source of fibre:* The food contains 4 grams or more (*a*) of fibre per reference amount and serving of stated size, if no fibre or fibre source is identified in the statement or claim; or (*b*) of each identified fibre or fibre from an identified fibre source per reference amount and serving of stated size, if a fibre or fibre source is identified in the statement or claim.
- *Very high source of fibre:* The food contains 6 grams or more (*a*) of fibre per reference amount and serving of stated size, if no fibre or fibre source is identified in the statement or claim; or (*b*) of each identified fibre or fibre from an identified fibre source per reference amount and serving of stated size, if a fibre or fibre source is identified in the statement or claim.
- *More fibre:* The food contains at least 25% more fibre, totalling at least 1 gram more, if no fibre or fibre source is identified in the statement or claim, or at least 25% more of an identified fibre or fibre from an identified fibre source, totalling at least 1 gram more, if a fibre or fibre source is identified in the statement or claim compared to reference amount of a similar food.

Light and Lean

- *Light in energy or fat:* The food meets the conditions set out for the subject "reduced in energy" or "reduced in fat."
- *Lean:* The food (*a*) is meat or poultry that has not been ground, a marine or fresh water animal or a product of any of these; and (*b*) contains 10% or less fat.
- *Extra lean:* The food (*a*) is meat or poultry that has not been ground, a marine or fresh water animal or a product of any of these; and (*b*) contains 7.5% or less fat.

Approved Health Claims for Nutrition Labels

If a manufacturer follows specific guidelines addressing both the nutrients noted in the claim as well as guidelines pertaining to other nutrients in a food, the following health claims can be made.

- A healthy diet containing foods high in potassium and low in sodium may reduce the risk of high blood pressure, a risk factor for stroke and heart disease.
- A healthy diet with adequate calcium and vitamin D, and regular physical activity, may help to achieve strong bones and may reduce the risk of osteoporosis.
- A healthy diet low in saturated and *trans* fats may reduce the risk of heart disease.
- A healthy diet rich in a variety of vegetables and fruit may help reduce the risk of some types of cancer.
- Foods very low in starch and fermentable sugars can make the following health claims:
  - Won't cause cavities;
  - Does not promote tooth decay;
  - Does not promote dental caries; or is
  - Non-cariogenic.

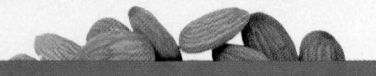

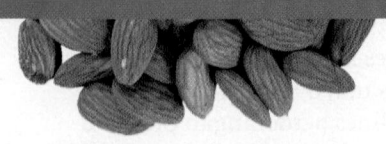

Exchange System A system for classifying foods into numerous lists based on the foods' macronutrient composition and establishing serving sizes, so that one serving of each food on a list contains the same amount of carbohydrate, protein, fat, and calorie content.

exchange The serving size of a food on a specific exchange list.

THE EXCHANGE SYSTEM

The **Exchange System** is a valuable tool for roughly estimating the calorie, protein, carbohydrate, and fat content of a food or meal. This tool organizes many details of the nutrient composition of foods into a manageable framework. By using the Exchange System, you can plan daily menus to fall roughly within specific percentages of macronutrients without having to look up or memorize the nutrient values of numerous foods, so the time you spend now becoming familiar with the Exchange System will pay off in the future.

In the Exchange System, individual foods are placed into three broad groups: carbohydrate, meat and meat substitutes, and fat. Within these groups are lists that contain foods of similar macronutrient composition: various types of milk, fruit, vegetables, starch, other carbohydrates, meat and meat substitutes, and fat. These lists are designed so that, when the proper serving size is observed, each food on a list provides about the same amount of carbohydrate, protein, fat, and calories. This equality allows the exchange of foods on each list, hence the term *Exchange System.*

The Exchange System was originally developed for planning diabetic diets. Diabetes is easier to control if the person's diet has about the same composition day after day. If a certain number of **exchanges** from each of the various lists is eaten each day, that regularity is easier to achieve. However, because the Exchange System provides a quick way to estimate the calorie, carbohydrate, protein, and fat content in any food or meal, it is a valuable menu-planning tool for people without diabetes, as well.

Becoming Familiar with the Exchange System

To use the Exchange System, you must know which foods are on each list and the serving sizes for each food.

Table D-1 gives the serving sizes for foods on each exchange list, as well as the carbohydrate, protein, fat, and calorie content per exchange. The meat and milk lists are divided into subclasses, which vary in fat content and, hence, in the amount of calories they provide. Foods on the meat and fat lists contain essentially no carbohydrate; those on the fruit and fat lists lack appreciable amounts of protein; and those on the vegetable, fruit, and other carbohydrates lists contain essentially no fat. You need to study Table D-1 and Figure D-1 to become familiar with the exchange lists, the sizes of the exchanges (that is, serving sizes) on each list, and the amounts of carbohydrate, protein, fat, and calories per exchange.

Before you can turn a group of exchanges into a daily meal plan, you must be aware of which foods are on each exchange list (Fig. D-1). The entire Exchange Lists for Diabetes (2008) is presented in Appendix D, which you should consult frequently while exploring the system to discover its various peculiarities. For example, the starch list includes not only bread, dry cereal, cooked cereal, rice, and pasta, but also baked beans, corn on the cob, and potatoes. These foods are not identical to those composing the grains group from MyPlate. The Exchange System is not concerned with the origin of a food, whether animal or vegetable. It is primarily concerned with the macronutrients carbohydrate, protein, and fat in each food on a specific list. For example, the carbohydrate composition of potatoes resembles that of bread more than that of broccoli, although potatoes are vegetables. In addition, several foods on the meat and meat substitutes list are not meats. The list of other carbohydrates includes jam, angel food cake, fat-free frozen yogurt, and foods such as frosted cake that count as both other carbohydrate exchanges and fat exchanges. Bacon appears in the fat list, rather than the high-fat meat category.

TABLE D-1 Nutrient Composition of Exchange System Lists (Based on Choose Your Foods: Exchange Lists for Diabetes, 2007)

Groups/Lists	Household Measures*	Carbohydrate (g)	Protein (g)	Fat (g)	Energy (kcal)
Carbohydrate Group					
Starch	1 slice, ¾ cup raw, or ½ cup cooked	15	3	1 or less†	80
Fruit	1 small/medium piece	15	—	—	60
Milk	1 cup				
Fat-free/very low-fat		12	8	0–3†	90
Reduced-fat		12	8	5	120
Whole		12	8	8	150
Other carbohydrates	Varies	15	Varies	Varies	Varies
Nonstarchy vegetables	1 cup raw or ½ cup cooked	5	2	—	25
Meat and Meat Substitutes Group	1 ounce				
Very lean		—	7	0–1	35
Lean		—	7	3	55
Medium-fat		—	7	5	75
High-fat		—	7	8	100
Fat Group	1 teaspoon	—	—	5	45

*An estimate; see exchange lists for actual amounts.
†Calculated as 1 gram for purposes of calorie contribution.

Reproduction of the exchange lists in whole or in part, without permission of The American Dietetic Association or the American Diabetes Association, Inc. is a violation of federal law. This material has been modified from *Choose Your Foods: Exchange Lists for Diabetes*, 2007 which is the basis of a meal planning system designed by a committee of the American Diabetes Association and The American Dietetic Association. While designed primarily for people with diabetes and others who must follow special diets, the exchange lists are based on principles of good nutrition that apply to everyone. © 2008 by the American Diabetes Association and the American Dietetic Association.

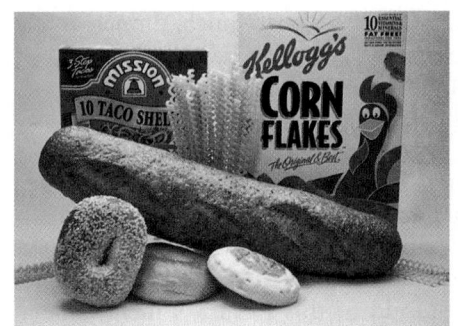

Starch exchange choices

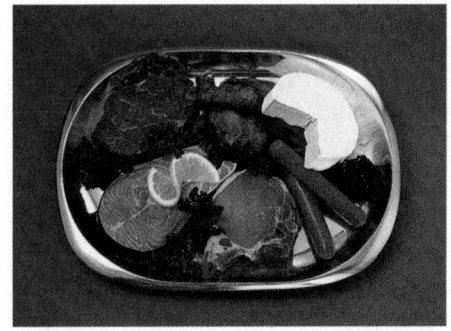

Meat and meat substitutes exchange choices

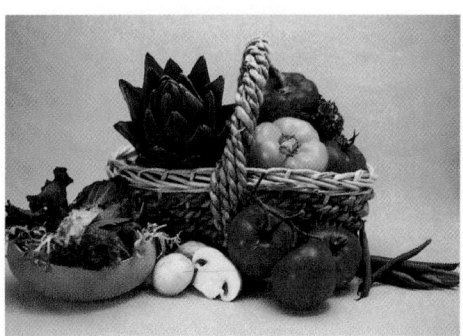

Vegetable exchange choices

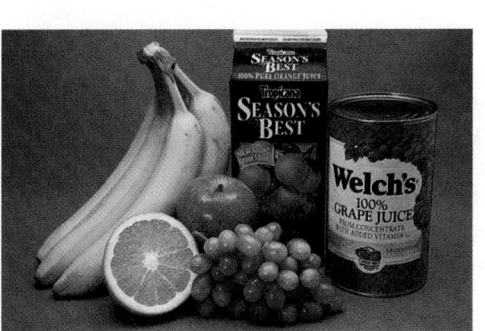

Fruit exchange choices

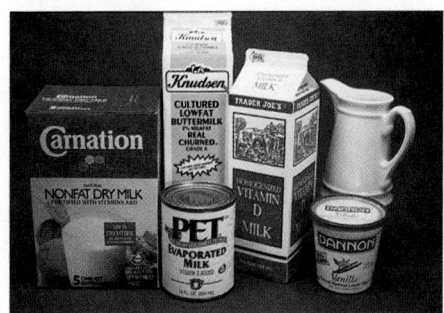

Milk exchange choices

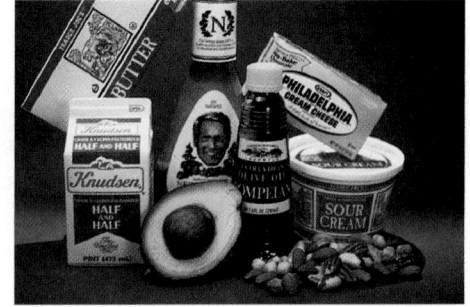

Fat exchange choices

FIGURE D-1 ▶ Foods arranged according to the Exchange Lists for Diabetes.

TABLE D-2 Possible Exchange Patterns That Yield 55% of Calories as Carbohydrate, 30% as Fat, and 15% as Protein

	kcal/Day						
Exchange List	1200*	1600*	2000	2400	2800	3200	3600
Milk (reduced-fat)	2	2	2	2	2	2	2
Vegetable	3	3	3	4	4	4	4
Fruit	3	4	5	6	8	9	9
Starch	5	8	11	13	15	18	21
Meat (lean)	4	4	4	5	6	7	8
Fat	2	4	6	8	10	11	13

This is just one set of options. More meat could be included if less milk were used, for example.

*Calorie intakes of 1200 and 1600 kcal contain 20% of calories as protein and 50% of calories as carbohydrate to allow for greater flexibility in diet planning.

Free foods (essentially calorie-free) include bouillon, diet soda, coffee, tea, dill pickles, and vinegar, as well as herbs and spices. Many vegetables, such as cabbage, celery, mushrooms, lettuce, and zucchini, also can be considered free foods; their minimal energy contribution need not count in the calculations when they are eaten in moderation (1 to 2 servings per meal or snack).

Using the Exchange System to Develop Daily Menus

Now let's use the Exchange System to plan a 1-day menu. Let's target a calorie content of 2000 kcal, with 55% derived from carbohydrates (1100 kcal), 15% from protein (300 kcal), and 30% from fat (600 kcal). This can be translated into 2 reduced-fat milk exchanges, 3 vegetable exchanges, 5 fruit exchanges, 11 starch exchanges, 4 lean meat exchanges, and 6 fat exchanges (Table D-2). This is only one of many possible combinations; the Exchange System offers great flexibility.

Table D-3 arbitrarily separates these exchanges into breakfast, lunch, dinner, and a snack. Breakfast includes 1 reduced-fat milk exchange, 2 fruit exchanges, 2 starch exchanges, and 1 fat exchange. This total corresponds to ¾ cup of a ready-to-eat breakfast cereal, 1 cup of reduced-fat milk, 1 slice of bread with 1 teaspoon margarine, and 1 cup of orange juice.

Lunch consists of 2 fat exchanges, 4 starch exchanges, 1 vegetable exchange, 1 reduced-fat milk exchange, and 2 fruit exchanges. This translates into one slice of bacon with 1 teaspoon mayonnaise on two slices of bread, with tomato—in other words, a bacon and tomato sandwich. You can also add lettuce to the sandwich. This can be considered a free vegetable choice. Add to this meal a 9-inch banana (1 exchange = 1 small banana), 1 cup of reduced-fat milk, and 6 graham crackers (2½ inches by 2½ inches). Later add a snack of ¾ ounce of pretzels for another starch exchange.

Dinner consists of 4 lean meat exchanges, 1 fruit exchange, 2 vegetable exchanges, 1 fat exchange, and 2 starch exchanges. This total corresponds to a 4-ounce broiled steak (meat only, no bone), 1 medium baked potato (1 exchange = 1 small baked potato) with 1 teaspoon of margarine, 1 cup of broccoli, and 1 kiwi fruit. Coffee (if desired) is not counted, because it contains no appreciable calories.

Finally, we have a snack containing 2 starch exchanges and 2 fat exchanges. This translates into 1 bagel with 2 tablespoons of regular cream cheese.

This 1-day menu is only one of many possible with the exchange lists. Apple juice could replace the orange juice; two apples could be exchanged for the banana. The choices are endless. An exchange diet is much easier to plan if you use individual foods, as was done here; however, the Exchange System tables list some combination foods to help you. Using combination foods, such as pizza or lasagna, however, makes it more difficult to calculate the number of exchanges in a serving. For

TABLE D-3 Sample 1-Day 2000-kcal Menu Based on the Exchange Lists for Diabetes Plan*

Breakfast

1 reduced-fat milk exchange	1 cup reduced-fat milk (some on cereal)
2 fruit exchanges	1 cup orange juice
2 starch exchanges	¾ cup ready-to-eat breakfast cereal, 1 piece whole-wheat toast
1 fat exchange	1 teaspoon soft margarine on toast

Lunch

4 starch exchanges	2 slices whole-wheat bread, 6 graham crackers (2½ inches by 2½ inches)
2 fat exchanges	1 slice bacon, 1 teaspoon mayonnaise
1 vegetable exchange	1 sliced tomato
2 fruit exchanges	1 banana (9 inches)
1 reduced-fat milk exchange	1 cup reduced-fat milk

Snack

1 starch exchange	¾ ounce pretzels

Dinner

4 lean meat exchanges	4 ounces lean steak (well trimmed)
2 starch exchanges	1 medium baked potato
1 fat exchange	1 tsp soft margarine
2 vegetable exchanges	1 cup cooked broccoli
1 fruit exchange	1 kiwi fruit
	Coffee (if desired)

Snack

2 starch exchanges	1 bagel
2 fat exchanges	2 tablespoons regular cream cheese

*The target plan was a 2000 kcal intake, with 55% of calories from carbohydrate, 15% from protein, and 30% from fat. Computer analysis indicates that this menu yielded 2040 kcal, with 53% of calories from carbohydrate, 16% from protein, and 31% from fat—in close agreement with the targeted goals.

instance, lasagna typically has meat exchanges, vegetable exchanges, and starch exchanges. With practice, you will be able to tackle such complex foods (Fig. D-2). For now, using individual foods makes learning the Exchange System much easier. Finally, you might want to prove to yourself that the food choices listed in Table D-3 really meet the Exchange plan. This demonstration will give you practice turning exchanges into food servings.

FIGURE D-2 ▶ Record the Exchange Lists for Diabetes pattern you have chosen in the left-hand column. Then distribute the exchanges throughout the day, noting the food to be used and the serving size.

Exchange List	Total Exchanges to be Consumed Daily	Exchanges Consumed at Each Meal		
		Breakfast	Lunch	Dinner
MILK				
VEGETABLE				
FRUIT				
STARCH				
MEAT AND SUBSTITUTES				
FAT				

EXCHANGE FOR DIABETES LISTS

The exchange lists are the basis of a meal planning system designed by a committee of the American Diabetes Association and the American Dietetic Association. While designed primarily for people with diabetes and others who must follow special diets, the exchange lists are based on principles of good nutrition that apply to everyone.

© 2008 by the American Diabetes Association and the American Dietetic Association.

MILK EXCHANGE LIST

Fat-Free and Low-Fat Milk

(12 g carbohydrate, 8 g protein, 0–3 g fat, 100 kcal)

Serving Size	Food
1 cup	fat-free, ½%, and 1% milk, and buttermilk
½ cup	canned, evaporated fat-free milk
1 cup	soy milk (light or regular)
⅔ cup (6 oz)	yogurt with fruit, low-fat
⅔ cup (6 oz)	yogurt, low carbohydrate (less than 6 grams), sweetened with nonnutritive sweetener and fructose

Reduced-Fat Milk

(12 g carbohydrate, 8 g protein, 5 g fat, 120 kcal)

Serving Size	Food
1 cup	2% milk, acidophilus milk, kefir
⅔ cup (6 oz)	yogurt plain, low-fat (added milk solids)
1 cup	whole milk, buttermilk, goat's milk

Whole Milk

(12 g carbohydrate, 8 g protein, 8 g fat, 160 kcal)

Serving Size	Food
½ cup	evaporated whole milk
1 cup	yogurt, plain (made from whole milk)

NON-STARCHY VEGETABLE EXCHANGE LIST

(5 g carbohydrate, 2 g protein, 0 g fat, 25 kcal)
Vegetables with small amounts of carbohydrate and calories are on the Nonstarchy Vegetables list. 1 vegetable exchange equals: ½ cup cooked vegetables or vegetable juice or 1 cup raw vegetables

artichoke
artichoke hearts
asparagus
beans (green, wax, Italian)
bean sprouts
beets
broccoli
brussels sprouts
cabbage (green, bok choy, Chinese)
carrots
cauliflower
celery

cucumber
eggplant
green onions or scallions
greens (e.g., collard, kale, mustard, turnip)
kohlrabi
leeks
mixed vegetables (without corn, peas, or pasta)
mushrooms, all kinds, fresh
okra
onions
pea pods

peppers (all varieties)
radishes
rutabaga
sauerkraut
spinach
squash (summer, zucchini)
Sugar pea snaps
Swiss chard
tomato (fresh, canned, sauce)
tomato/vegetable juice
turnips
water chestnuts

FRUIT EXCHANGE LIST

Fruit

(15 g carbohydrate, 0 g protein, 0 g fat, 60 kcal)
In general, 1 fruit choice is ½ cup of canned or fresh fruit or unsweetened fruit juice, 1 small fresh fruit (4 oz) or 2 tablespoons of dried fruit. 1 fruit exchange equals:

Serving Size	Food	Serving size	Food
1 (4 oz)	apple, unpeeled (small)	17 (3 oz)	grapes (small)
4 rings	apple, dried	1 slice (10 oz)	honeydew melon (or 1 cup cubes)
½ cup	applesauce (unsweetened)	1 (3½ oz)	kiwi
4 (5½ oz)	apricots, fresh	¾ cup	mandarin orange sections
8 halves	apricots, dried	½ (5½ oz)	mango (or ½ cup)
½ cup	apricots, canned	1 (5 oz)	nectarine (small)
1 (4 oz)	banana (small)	1 (6½ oz)	orange (small)
¾ cup	blackberries	½ (8 oz)	papaya (or 1 cup cubes)
¾ cup	blueberries	1 (4–6 oz)	peach, fresh (medium)
⅓ melon (11 oz)	cantaloupe (small)	½ cup	peaches, canned
1 cup cubes	cantaloupe	1 (4 oz)	pear, fresh
12 (3 oz)	cherries	½ cup	pear, canned
½ cup	cherries, sweet canned	¾ cup	pineapple, fresh
3	dates	½ cup	pineapple, canned
2 tbsp	Dried fruits (blueberries, cherries, cranberries, mixed fruit, raisins)	2 (5 oz)	plums (small)
		½ cup	plums, canned
2 (3½ oz)	figs, fresh (large)	3	plums dried (prunes)
1½	figs, dried	1 cup	raspberries
½ cup	fruit cocktail	1¼ cup	strawberries (raw, whole)
½ (11 oz)	grapefruit (large)	2 (8 oz)	tangerines (small)
¾ cup	grapefruit sections, canned	1 slice (13½ oz)	watermelon (or 1¼ cups cubes)

Fruit Juice

Serving Size	Food	Serving Size	Food
½ cup	apple juice/cider	½ cup	orange juice
⅓ cup	fruit juice blends, 100% juice	½ cup	pineapple juice
⅓ cup	grape juice	⅓ cup	prune juice
½ cup	grapefruit juice		

STARCH EXCHANGE LIST

(15 g carbohydrate, 0–3 g protein, 0–1 g fat, 80 kcal)
In general, 1 starch is ½ cup of cooked cereal, grain, or starchy vegetable, ⅓ cup of cooked rice or pasta, 1 oz of a bread product, such as 1 slice of bread, or ¾ oz to 1 oz of most snack foods. 1 starch exchange equals:

Bread

Serving Size	Food	Serving Size	Food
¼ (1 oz)	bagel, large (about 4 oz)	1	pancake, 4 inch across × ¼ inch thick
2 slices (1½ oz)	bread, reduced-calorie	½	pita, 6 inches across
1 slice (1 oz)	bread, white, whole-wheat, pumpernickel, grain or rye, or unfrosted raisin	1 slice (1 oz)	raisin bread, unfrosted
		1 (1 oz)	roll, plain (small)
4 (⅔ oz)	bread sticks, crisp, 4 inch × ½ inch	1	tortilla, corn, 6 inches across
½	English muffin	1	tortilla, flour, 6 inches across
½ (1 oz)	hot dog or hamburger bun	⅓	tortilla, flour, 10 inches across
¼	naan, 8 inch × 2 inch	1	waffle, 4 inches square or across, reduced-fat

Cereals and Grains

Serving Size	Food	Serving Size	Food
½ cup	bran cereal, bran	3 tbsp	cornmeal (dry)
½ cup	bulgur	⅓ cup	couscous
½ cup	cereal, cooked (oats, oatmeal)	3 tbsp	flour (dry)
¾ cup	cereal, unsweetened, ready-to-eat	¼ cup	granola, low-fat

Serving Size	Food	Serving Size	Food
½ cup	grits	⅓ cup	quinoa, cooked
½ cup	kasha	⅓ cup	rice, white or brown
⅓ cup	millet, cooked	½ cup	tabbouleh (tabouli), prepared
¼ cup	muesli	3 tbsp	wheat germ
⅓ cup	pasta, cooked	½ cup	wild rice, cooked
⅓ cup	polenta, cooked		

Starchy Vegetables

Serving Size	Food	Serving Size	Food
⅓ cup	cassava	½ cup or ½ medium (3 oz)	potato, boiled
½ cup	corn	¼ large (3 oz)	potato, baked with skin
½ (5 oz)	corn on the cob (large)	½ cup	potato, mashed with milk and fat
1 cup	mixed vegetables with corn, peas, or pasta	½ cup	spaghetti or pasta sauce, canned
½ cup	peas, green	1 cup	squash, winter (acorn, butternut, pumpkin)
½ cup	plantain, ripe	½ cup	yam, sweet potato, plain

Crackers and Snacks

Serving Size	Food	Serving Size	Food
8	animal crackers	¾ oz	pretzels
3	graham crackers, 2½-inch square	2	rice cakes, 4 inches across
¾ oz	matzoh	6	saltine-type crackers
4 slices	melba toast	15–20 (¾ oz)	snack chips, fat-free (tortilla, potato)
20	oyster crackers	2–5 (¾ oz)	whole-wheat crackers, no fat added
3 cups	popcorn (no fat added or lower-fat microwave)		

Dried Beans, Peas, and Lentils

(Counts as 1 starch exchange plus 1 very lean meat exchange)

Serving Size	Food	Serving Size	Food
⅓ cup	baked beans	½ cup	lentils
½ cup	beans and peas (garbanzo, pinto, kidney, white, split, black-eyed)	⅔ cup	lima beans
		3 tbsp	miso

Starchy Foods Prepared with Fat

(Counts as 1 starch exchange, plus 1 fat exchange)

Serving Size	Food	Serving Size	Food
1	biscuit, 2½ inches across	3 cups	popcorn, with butter
½ cup	chow mein noodles	3	sandwich crackers, cheese or peanut butter filling
1 piece (2 oz)	corn bread, 2-inch cube		
6	crackers, round butter type	9–13 (3/4 oz)	snack chips (potato, tortilla)
1 cup	croutons	⅓ cup	stuffing, bread
1 cup (2 oz)	French-fried potatoes (oven-baked) (see also the fast-foods list)	2	taco shells, 6 inches across
		1	waffle, 4-inch square or across
¼ cup	granola	4–6 (1 oz)	whole-wheat crackers, fat added
⅓ cup	hummus		

SWEETS, DESSERTS AND OTHER CARBOHYDRATES EXCHANGE LIST

One exchange equals 15 g carbohydrate, protein, fat and kcal vary.

Exchanges per Serving

Serving Size	Food	
1/12 cake (about 2 oz)	angel food cake, unfrosted	2 carbohydrates
2-inch square (about 1 oz)	brownie, unfrosted (small)	1 carbohydrate, 1 fat
2-inch square (about 1 oz)	cake, unfrosted	1 carbohydrate, 1 fat
2-inch square (about 2 oz)	cake, frosted	2 carbohydrates, 1 fat
2	cookies, fat-free (small)	1 carbohydrate
2 (about 2/3 oz)	cookies or sandwich cookies with creme filling (small)	1 carbohydrate, 1 fat
1/4 cup	cranberry sauce, jellied	1½ carbohydrates
1 (about 2 oz)	cupcake, frosted (small)	2 carbohydrates, 1 fat
1 (1½ oz)	doughnut, plain cake (medium)	1½ carbohydrates, 2 fats
3¾ inches across (2 oz)	doughnuts, glazed	2 carbohydrates, 2 fats
1 bar (1⅓ oz)	Energy, sport, or breakfast bar	2 carbohydrates, 1 fat
1 bar (2 oz)	Energy, sport, or breakfast bar	3 carbohydrates, 1 fat
½ cup (3 ½ oz)	fruit cobbler	3 carbohydrates, 1 fat
1 bar (3 oz)	fruit juice bars, frozen, 100% juice	1 carbohydrate
1 roll (¾ oz)	fruit snacks, chewy (puréed fruit concentrate)	1 carbohydrate
1½ tbsp	fruit spread, 100% fruit	1 carbohydrate
½ cup	gelatin, regular	1 carbohydrate
3	gingersnaps	1 carbohydrate
1 bar (1 oz)	granola or snack bar (regular and low-fat)	1½ carbohydrates
1 tbsp	honey	1 carbohydrate
½ cup	ice cream, low-fat	1½ carbohydrates
½ cup	ice cream	1 carbohydrate, 2 fats
½ cup	ice cream, light	1 carbohydrate, 1 fat
½ cup	ice cream, fat-free, no sugar added	1 carbohydrate
1 tbsp	jam or jelly, regular	1 carbohydrate
1 cup	milk, chocolate, whole	2 carbohydrates, 1 fat
1/4 (1 oz)	muffin, 5 oz	1 carbohydrate, ½ fat
1/6 pie	pie, fruit, 2 crusts (8 inches across)	3 carbohydrates, 2 fats
1/8 pie	pie, pumpkin or custard (8 inches across)	2 carbohydrates, 2 fats
½ cup	pudding, regular (made with reduced-fat milk)	2 carbohydrates
½ cup	pudding, sugar-free (made with fat-free milk)	1 carbohydrate
1 can (10–11 oz)	reduced-calorie meal replacement (shake)	1½ carbohydrates, 0–1 fat
1 cup	rice milk, low-fat or fat-free, plain	1 carbohydrate
1 cup	rice milk, low-fat, flavored	1½ carbohydrates
1/4 cup	salad dressing, fat-free	1 carbohydrate
½ cup	sherbet, sorbet	2 carbohydrates
1 cup (8 oz)	sports drinks	1 carbohydrate
1 tbsp	sugar	1 carbohydrate
1 (2½ oz)	sweet roll or Danish	2½ carbohydrates, 2 fats
2 tbsp	syrup, light	1 carbohydrate
1 tbsp	syrup, regular	1 carbohydrate
5	vanilla wafers	1 carbohydrate, 1 fat
⅓ cup	yogurt, frozen, fat-free	1 carbohydrate
1 cup	yogurt, low-fat with fruit	3 carbohydrates, 0–1 fat

MEAT AND MEAT SUBSTITUTES EXCHANGE LIST

Lean Meat and Substitutes List

(0 g carbohydrate, 7 g protein, 0–3 g fat, and 45 kcal)
One lean meat exchange equals:

Serving Size	Food	Serving Size	Food
1 oz	Beef: USDA Select or Choice grades of lean beef trimmed of fat: round, sirloin, and flank steak; tenderloin; roast (rib, chuck, rump); steak (T-bone, porterhouse, cubed), ground round	1 oz 6 1 oz	Fish, smoked: herring or salmon (lox) oysters (medium) Fish, fresh or frozen, plain: catfish, cod, flounder, haddock, halibut, orange roughy, salmon, tilapia, trout, tune
1 oz	Pork, lean: ham; Canadian bacon; tenderloin, center loin chop	1 oz ¼ cup	Game: buffalo, ostrich, rabbit, venison cottage cheese
1 oz	Lamb: roast, chop, leg	1 oz	cheeses with 3 g or less fat per oz
1 oz	Veal, lean chop, roast	¼ cup	egg substitute, plain
1 oz	Poultry, without skin: chicken, turkey, domestic duck or goose (well drained of fat, no skin)	2 1½ oz 1 oz	egg whites hot dogs with 3 g or less fat per oz Shellfish: clams, crab, lobster, scallops, shrimp, imitation shellfish
1 oz	processed sandwich meats with 1 g or less fat per oz, such as deli thin, shaved meats, chipped beef, turkey, ham	1 oz	sausage with 1 g or less fat per os

Medium-Fat Meat and Substitutes List

(0 g carbohydrate, 7 g protein, 4–7 g fat, and 75 kcal)
One medium-fat meat exchange equals:

Serving Size	Food	Serving Size	Food
1 oz	Beef: (ground beef; meatloaf; corned beef; short ribs; prime grades of meat trimmed (prime rib)	1 oz 1 oz	Fish: any fish product Cheese with 4–7 grams pf fat per oz: feta, mozzarella, pasteurized processed cheese spread, reduced-fat cheeses, string
1 oz	Pork: top loin, chop, Boston butt, cutlet, shoulder roast	¼ cup (2 oz)	ricotta cheese
1 oz	Lamb: rib roast, ground		**Other**
1 oz	Veal, cutlet (no breading) cubed, unbreaded	1	egg (high in cholesterol, limit to 3 per week)
1 oz	Poultry: chicken (with skin), dove, pheasant, wild duck or goose, ground turkey, fried chicken	1 oz	sausage with 4–7 grams of fat per oz

Plant-Based Proteins

(each exchange provides 7 g protein, carbohydrate, fat, and kcal vary)

Serving Size	Food	
3 strips	"bacon" strips, soy-based	1 medium-fat meat
⅓ cup	baked beans	1 starch + 1 lean meat
½ cup	beans, cooked: black, garbanzo, kidney, lima, navy, pinto, white	1 starch + 1 lean meat
2 oz	"beef" or "sausage" crumbles, soy-based	½ carbohydrate + 1 lean meat
2 nuggets (1½ oz)	"chicken" nuggets, soy-based	½ carbohydrate + 1 medium-fat meat
½ cup	edamame	½ carbohydrate + 1 lean meat
3 patties	falafel (spiced chickpea and wheat patties about 2 inches across)	1 carbohydrate + 1 high-fat meat
1 (1½ oz)	hot dog, soy-based	½ carbohydrate + 1 lean meat
⅓ cup	hummus	1 carbohydrate + 1 high-fat meat

Serving Size	Food	
½ cup	lentils, brown, green or yellow	1 carbohydrate + 1 lean meat
3 oz	meatless burger, soy-based	½ carbohydrate + 2 lean meats
1 tbsp	nut spreads: almond butter, cashew butter, peanut butter, soy nut butter	1 high-fat meat
½ cup	peas, cooked: black-eyed and split peas	1 starch + 1 lean meat
½ cup	refried beans, canned	1 starch + 1 lean meat
1 (1½ oz)	"sausage" patties, soy-based	1 medium-fat meat
¾ oz	soy nuts, unsalted	½ carbohydrate + 1 medium-fat meat
¼ cup	tempeh	1 medium-fat meat
4 oz (½ cup)	tofu	1 medium-fat meat
4 oz (½ cup)	tofu, light	1 lean meat

High-Fat Meat and Substitutes List

(0 g carbohydrate, 7 g protein, 8+ g fat, and 100 kcal)
One high-fat meat exchange equals:

Serving Size	Food	Serving Size	Food
1 oz	Pork: spareribs, ground sausage	1	hot dog (turkey or chicken) (10 per pound)
1 oz	Cheese: regular: American, bleu, brie, cheddar, hard goat, Monterey jack, queso, Swiss	2 slices	pork bacon (16 slices per pound)
1 oz	processed sandwich meats with 8 grams or more per oz, such as bologna, pastrami, hard salami	3 slices	turkey bacon (½ oz each before cooking) bacon (20 slices per pound)
1 oz	sausage with 8 grams of fat or more per oz: such as bratwurst, chorizo, Italian, knockwurst, Polish, smoked, summer	**Counts as one high-fat meat plus one fat exchange:**	
		1	hot dog (beef, pork, or combination; turkey or chicken) (10 per pound-sized package)

FAT EXCHANGE LIST

Monounsaturated Fats List

(5 g fat and 45 kcal)
One exchange equals:

Serving Size	Food	Serving Size	Food
2 tbsp (1 oz)	avocado (medium)	10 nuts	peanuts
1 tsp	oil (canola, olive, peanut)	16 nuts	pistachios
	olives:	4 halves	pecans
8	ripe, black (large)	1 tbsp	nut butters (**trans** fat-free): almond butter, cashew butter, peanut butter, smooth or crunchy
10	green, stuffed (large)		
6 nuts	almonds, cashews		
6 nuts	mixed (50% peanuts)		

Polyunsaturated Fats List

(5 g fat and 45 kcal)
One exchange equals:

Serving Size	Food	Serving Size	Food
	margarine:	1 tsp	oil (corn, cottonseed, flaxseed, grape seed, safflower, soybean, sunflower)
1 tsp	stick, tub, or squeeze (**trans** fat-free)		salad dressing:
1 tbsp	lower-fat (30% to 50% vegetable oil) (**trans** fat-free)	1 tbsp	regular
	mayonnaise:	2 tbsp	reduced-fat
1 tsp	regular	1 tbsp	seeds: flaxseed (whole), pumpkin, sesame, sunflower
1 tbsp	reduced-fat		
4 halves	nuts, walnuts, English	2 tsp	tahini or sesame paste
1 tbsp	nuts, pignolia (pine nuts)		

Saturated Fats List

(5 g fat and 45 kcal)
One exchange equals:

Serving Size	Food	Serving Size	Food
1 slice	bacon, cooked, regular or turkey	1 tsp	shortening or lard
2 tbsp (½ oz)	chitterlings, boiled		butter blends made with oil:
2 tbsp	coconut, sweetened, shredded cream	1½ tsp	regular
2 tbsp	half and half	1 tbsp	reduced-fat or light
1 tbsp	heavy		butter:
1½ tbsp	light	1 tsp	stick
2 tbsp	whipped	2 tsp	whipped
¼ cup	whipped, pressurized	1 tbsp	reduced-fat
	cream cheese:		sour cream:
1 tbsp (½ oz)	regular	2 tbsp	regular
1½ tbsp (¾ oz)	reduced-fat	3 tbsp	reduced-fat

FREE FOODS LIST

A *free food* is any food or drink that contains less than 20 kcal or less than 5 g of carbohydrate per serving. Foods with a serving size listed should be limited to three servings per day. Foods listed without a serving size can be eaten as often as you like.

Modified Fat Foods with Carbohydrate

Serving Size	Food	Serving Size	Food
1 tbsp (½ oz)	cream cheese, fat-free	1 tsp	mayonnaise, reduced-fat
1 tbsp	creamers, nondairy, liquid	1 tbsp	salad dressing, fat-free or low-fat, Italian
2 tsp	creamers, nondairy, powdered	2 tbsp	salad dressing, fat-free, Italian
1 tbsp	margarine, fat-free	1 tbsp	sour cream, fat-free, reduced-fat
1 tsp	margarine, reduced-fat	1 tbsp	whipped topping, regular
1 tbsp	mayonnaise, fat-free	2 tbsp	whipped topping, light or fat-free

Low Carbohydrate Foods

Serving Size	Food	Serving Size	Food
1 candy	candy, hard, (regular or sugar-free)		salad greens
2 tsp	jam or jelly, light or no sugar added*		sugar substitutes
		2 tbsp	syrup, sugar-free

Drinks

Serving Size	Food	Serving Size	Food
	bouillon, broth, consommé		diet soft drinks, sugar-free
	bouillon or broth, low-sodium		drink mixes, sugar-free
	carbonated or mineral water		tea, unsweetened or with sugar substitute
	club soda		tonic water, sugar-free
1 tbsp	cocoa powder, unsweetened		water
	coffee, unsweetened or with sugar substitute		water, flavored, carbohydrate free

Condiments

Serving Size	Food	Serving Size	Food
2 tsp	barbecue sauce	2 slices	pickles, sweet (bread and butter)
1 tbsp	catsup	¾ oz	pickles, sweet (gherkin)
	horseradish	¼ cup	salsa
	lemon juice	1 tbsp	soy sauce, regular or light
	mustard	1 tbsp	taco sauce
1½ tsp	miso		vinegar
1 tbsp	pickle relish	2 tbsp	yogurt, any type
1½	pickles, dill (medium)		

Seasonings

flavoring extracts
garlic
herbs, fresh or dried
nonstick cooking spray
pimento

spices
hot pepper sauce
wine, used in cooking
Worcestershire sauce

COMBINATION FOODS LIST

Serving Size	Food Desription	
	Entrées	**Exchanges per Serving**
1 cup (8 oz)	Casserole type (tuna noodle), lasagna, spaghetti with meatballs, chili with beans, macaroni and cheese	2 carbohydrates, 2 medium-fat meats
1 cup (8 oz)	stews (beef/other meats and vegetables)	1 carbohydrate, 1 medium-fat meat, 0–3 fats
½ cup (3½ oz)	tuna or chicken salad	½ carbohydrate, 2 lean meats, 1 fat
	Frozen Entrées and Meals	
1 (5 oz)	burrito (beef and bean)	
generally 14–17 oz	dinner-type meal	3 carbohydrates, 1 lean meat, 2 fats
¼ of 12-inch (6 oz)	pizza, cheese, thin crust	2 carbohydrates, 2 medium-fat meats, 1½ fats
¼ of 12-inch (6 oz)	pizza, meat topping, thin crust	2 carbohydrates, 2 medium-fat meats, 1½ fats
1 (4½ oz)	pocket sandwich	
1 (7 oz)	pot pie	2½ carbohydrates, 1 medium-fat meat, 3 fats
8–11 oz	entrée or meal with less than 340 kcal	2–3 carbohydrates, 1–2 lean meats
	Soups	
1 cup	bean	1 carbohydrate, 1 very lean meat
1 cup (8 oz)	cream (made with water)	1 carbohydrate, 1 fat
6 oz prepared	instant	1 carbohydrate
8 oz prepared	instant with beans/lentils	2½ carbohydrates, 1 very lean meat
½ cup (4 oz)	split pea (made with water)	1 carbohydrate
1 cup (8 oz)	tomato (made with water)	1 carbohydrate
1 cup (8 oz)	vegetable beef, chicken noodle, or other broth-type	1 carbohydrate

Fast-Foods

Serving Size	Food Description	
		Exchanges per Serving
1 (about 8 oz)	burritos beef and beans	3 carbohydrates, 3 medium-fat meat, 3 fat
6	chicken nuggets	1 carbohydrate, 2 medium-fat meats, 1 fat
1 each	chicken breast, breaded and fried	1 carbohydrate, 4 medium-fat meats
1	chicken sandwich, grilled	2 carbohydrates, 3 very lean meats
6 (5 oz)	chicken wings, hot	5 high-fat meats, 1½ fats
1	fish sandwich/tartar sauce	2½ carbohydrates, 2 medium-fat meats, 2 fats
1 medium serving (5 oz)	French fries	4 carbohydrates, 4 fats
1	hamburger (regular)	2 carbohydrates, 1 medium-fat, 1 fat
1	hamburger (large)	2 carbohydrates, 3 medium-fat meats, 1 fat
1	hot dog with bun	1 carbohydrate, 1 high-fat meat, 1 fat
¼ 12-inch (about 6 oz)	pizza, cheese, thin crust	2½ carbohydrates, 2 medium-fat meats, 1½ fat
⅛ 14-inch (about 4 oz)	pizza, meat, thin crust	2½ carbohydrates, 1 medium-fat meat, 1½ fat
1 (5 oz)	soft-serve cone (small)	2½ carbohydrates, 1 fat
1 sub (6 inches)	submarine sandwich	3½ carbohydrates, 2 medium-fat meats, 1 fat
1 (3–3½ oz)	taco, hard or soft shell	1 carbohydrate, 1 medium-fat meat, 1½ fat

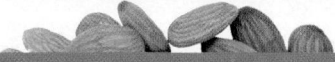
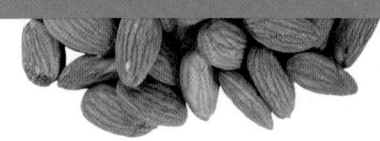

Although it may seem overwhelming at first, it is easy to track the foods you eat. One tip is to record foods and beverages consumed as soon as possible after consumption.

I. **Fill in the food record form that follows.** Appendix E contains a blank copy (see the completed example in Table E-1). Then, to estimate the nutrient values of the foods you are eating, consult food labels and use the NutritionCalc Plus software (CD or online) available with this book. If these resources do not have the serving size you need, adjust the value. If you drink ½ cup of orange juice, for example, but a table has values only for 1 cup, halve all values before you record them. Then, consider pooling all the same food to save time; if you drink a cup of 1% milk three times throughout the day, enter your milk consumption only once as 3 cups. As you record your intake for use on the nutrient analysis form that follows, consider the following tips:

- Measure and record the amounts of foods eaten in portion sizes of cups, teaspoons, tablespoons, ounces, slices, or inches (or convert metric units to these units).
- Record brand names of all food products, such as "Quick Quaker Oats."
- Measure and record all those little extras, such as gravies, salad dressings, taco sauces, pickles, jelly, sugar, catsup, and margarine.
- For beverages
  - List the type of milk, such as whole, fat-free, 1%, evaporated, chocolate, or reconstituted dry.
  - Indicate whether fruit juice is fresh, frozen, or canned.
  - Indicate type for other beverages, such as fruit drink, fruit-flavored drink, Kool-Aid, and hot chocolate made with water or milk.
- For fruits
  - Indicate whether fresh, frozen, dried, or canned.
  - If whole, record number eaten and size with approximate measurements (such as 1 apple—3 in. in diameter).
  - Indicate whether processed in water, light syrup, or heavy syrup.
- For vegetables
  - Indicate whether fresh, frozen, dried, or canned.
  - Record as portion of cup, teaspoon, or tablespoon, or as pieces (such as carrot sticks—4 in. long, ½ in. thick).
  - Record preparation method.
- For cereals
  - Record cooked cereals in portions of tablespoon or cup (a level measurement after cooking).
  - Record dry cereal in level portions of tablespoon or cup.
  - If margarine, milk, sugar, fruit, or something else is added, measure and record amount and type.
- For breads
  - Indicate whether whole wheat, rye, white, and so on.
  - Measure and record number and size of portion (biscuit—2 in. across, 1 in. thick; slice of homemade rye bread—3 in. by 4 in., ¼ in. thick).
  - Sandwiches: list all ingredients (lettuce, mayonnaise, tomato, and so on).

- For meat, fish, poultry, and cheese
  - Give size (length, width, thickness) in inches or weight in ounces after cooking for meat, fish, and poultry (such as cooked hamburger patty—3 in. across, ½ in. thick).
  - Give size (length, width, thickness) in inches or weight in ounces for cheese.
  - Record measurements only for the cooked, edible part—without bone or fat left on the plate.
  - Describe how meat, poultry, or fish was prepared.
- For eggs
  - Record as soft or hard cooked, fried, scrambled, poached, or omelet.
  - If milk, butter, or drippings are used, specify types and amount.
- For desserts
  - List commercial brand or "homemade" or "bakery" under brand.
  - Purchased candies, cookies, and cakes: specify kind and size.
  - Measure and record portion size of cakes, pies, and cookies by specifying thickness, diameter, and width or length, depending on the item.

TABLE E-1 One Day's Food Record—This Activity Can Help You Understand More About Your Food Habits

Time	Minutes Spent Eating	M or S*	H† (0–3)	Activity While Eating	Place of Eating	Food and Quantity	Others Present	Reason for Choice
7:10 a.m.	15	M	2	Standing, fixing lunch	Kitchen	Orange juice, 1 cup Crispix, 1 cup Non-fat milk, ½ cup Sugar, 2 tsp Black coffee	—	Health Habit Health Taste Habit
10:00 a.m.	4	S	1	Sitting, taking notes	Classroom	Diet cola, 12 oz	Class	Weight control
12:15 p.m.	40	M	2	Sitting, talking	Student union	Chicken sandwich with lettuce and mayonnaise (3 oz chicken, 2 slices of white bread, 2 tsp mayonnaise) Pear, 1 medium Non-fat milk, 1 cup	Friends	Taste Health Health
2:30 p.m.	10	S	1	Sitting, studying	Library	Regular cola, 12 oz	Friend	Hunger
6:30 p.m.	35	M	3	Sitting, talking	Kitchen	Pork chop, 1 Baked potato, 1 Margarine, 2 tbsp Lettuce and tomato salad, 1 cup Ranch dressing, 2 tbsp Peas, ½ cup Whole milk, 1 cup Cherry pie, 1 piece Iced tea, 12 oz	Boyfriend	Convenience Health Taste Health Taste Health Habit Taste Health
9:10 p.m.	10	S	2	Sitting, studying	Living room	Apple, 1 medium Glass mineral water, 1	—	Weight control Weight control

*M or S: Meal or snack
†H: Degree of hunger (0 = none; 3 = maximum)

Time	Minutes Spent Eating	M or S*	H† (0–3)	Activity While Eating	Place of Eating	Food and Quantity	Others Present	Reason for Choice

*M or S: Meal or snack
†H: Degree of hunger (0 = none; 3 = maximum)

II. **Now complete the nutrient analysis form as shown, using your food record.**
   A blank copy of this form for your use is on pages A-41 and A-42. NutritionCalc
   Plus will create such a table for you if you enter all food eaten.

Nutrient Analysis Form (Sample)

Name	Quantity	kcal	Protein (g)	Carbohydrates (g)	Fiber (g)	Total fat (g)	Monounsaturated fat (g)	Polyunsaturated fat (g)	Saturated fat (g)	Cholesterol (g)	Calcium (mg)	Iron (mg)
Egg bagel, 3.5-in. diameter	1 ea.	180	7.45	34.7	0.748	1.00	0.286	0.400	0.171	44.0	20.0	2.10
Jelly	1 tbsp	49.0	0.018	12.7	—	0.018	0.005	0.005	0.005	—	2.00	0.120
Orange juice, prepared fresh or frozen	1½ cup	165	2.52	40.2	1.49	0.210	0.037	0.045	0.025	—	33.0	0.411
Cheeseburger, McDonald's	2 ea.	636	30.2	57.0	0.460	32.0	12.2	2.18	13.3	80.0	338	5.68
French fries, McDonald's	1 order	220	3.00	26.1	4.19	11.5	4.37	0.570	4.61	8.57	9.10	0.605
Cola beverage, regular	1½ cup	151	—	38.5	—	—	—	—	—	—	9.00	0.120
Pork loin chop, broiled, lean	4 oz	261	36.2	—	—	11.9	5.35	1.43	4.09	112	5.67	1.04
Baked potato with skin	1 ea.	220	4.65	51.0	3.90	0.200	0.004	0.087	0.052	—	20.0	2.75
Peas, frozen, cooked	½ cup	63.0	4.12	11.4	3.61	0.220	0.019	0.103	0.039	—	19.0	1.25
Margarine, regular or soft, 80% fat	20 g	143	0.160	0.100	—	16.1	5.70	6.92	2.76	—	5.29	—
Iceberg lettuce, chopped	2 cup	14.6	1.13	2.34	1.68	0.212	0.008	0.112	0.028	—	21.2	0.560
French dressing	2 oz	300	0.318	3.63	0.431	32.0	14.2	12.4	4.94	—	7.10	0.227
Reduced-fat (i.e., 2%) milk	1 cup	121	8.12	11.7	—	4.78	1.35	0.170	2.92	22.0	297	0.120
Graham crackers	2 ea.	60.0	1.04	10.8	1.40	1.46	0.600	0.400	0.400	—	6.00	0.367
Totals		2584	99.0	300	17.9	112	44.1	24.8	33.4	266	792	15.4
RDA or related nutrient standard*		2900	58	130	38						1000	8
% of nutrient needs		89	170	230	47						79	193

Abbreviations: g = grams, mg = milligrams, µg = micrograms

*Values from inside cover. The values listed are for a male age 19 years. The number of kcal is a rough estimate. It is better to base energy needs on actual energy output.

†In RAE units. Table values generally are in RE units because the food values have not been updated to reflect the latest vitamin A standards. RAE equals RE for foods with preformed vitamin A, such as for the pork chop, but RAE are only about half the RE listed for foods with provitamin A carotenoids, such as for the peas (see Chapter 8 for details).

‡Amounts refer to actual folate content, rather than dietary folate equivalents (DFE). This difference is important to consider if the food contains added synthetic folic acid as part of enrichment or fortification. Any such folic acid is absorbed about twice as much as the folate present naturally in foods. So the total contribution of folate in the food in comparison to human needs will be greater than if all the folate was naturally in the food product. Nutrient analysis tables have yet to be updated to reflect the dietary folate equivalents of products (see Chapter 8 for more details).

Nutrient Analysis Form (Sample) Cont'd

Magnesium (mg)	Phosphorus (mg)	Potassium (mg)	Sodium (mg)	Zinc (mg)	Vitamin A (RE)	Vitamin C (mg)	Vitamin E (mg)	Thiamin (mg)	Riboflavin (mg)	Niacin (mg)	Vitamin B-6 (mg)	Folate (µg)	Vitamin B-12 (µg)
18.0	61.0	65.0	300	0.612	7.00	—	1.80	2.58	0.197	2.40	0.030	16.3	0.065
0.720	1.00	16.0	4.00	—	0.200	0.710	0.016	0.002	0.005	0.036	0.005	2.00	—
36.0	60.0	711	3.00	0.192	28.5	145	0.714	0.300	0.060	0.750	0.165	163	
45.8	410	314	1460	5.20	134	4.10	0.560	0.600	0.480	8.66	0.230	42.0	1.82
26.7	101	564	109	0.320	5.00	12.5	0.203	0.122	0.020	2.26	0.218	19.0	0.027
3.00	46.0	4.00	15.0	0.049	—	—	—	—	—	—	—	—	—
34.0	277	476	88.2	2.54	3.15	0.454	0.405	1.30	0.350	6.28	0.535	6.77	0.839
55.0	115	844	16.0	0.650	—	26.1	0.100	0.216	0.067	3.32	0.701	22.2	—
23.0	72.0	134	70.0	0.750	53.4	7.90	0.400	0.226	0.140	1.18	0.090	46.9	—
0.467	4.06	7.54	216	0.041	199	0.028	2.19	0.002	0.006	0.004	0.002	0.211	0.017
10.1	22.4	177	10.1	0.246	37.0	4.36	0.120	0.052	0.034	0.210	0.044	62.8	—
5.81	3.63	7.03	666	0.045	0.023	—	15.9	—	—	—	0.006	—	—
33.0	232	377	122	0.963	140	2.32	0.080	0.095	0.403	0.210	0.105	12.0	0.888
6.00	20.0	36.0	86.0	0.113	—	—	—	0.020	0.030	0.600	0.011	1.80	—
298	1425	3732	3165	11.7	607	204	22.5	5.52	1.79	25.9	2.14	395	3.65
400	700	4700	1500	11	900†	90	15	1.2	1.3	16	1.3	400‡	2.4
75	204	80	210	106	67	226	150	450	138	162	160	99	152

Nutrient Analysis Form

Name	Quantity	kcal	Protein (g)	Carbohydrates (g)	Fiber (g)	Total fat (g)	Monounsaturated fat (g)	Polyunsaturated fat (g)	Saturated fat (g)	Cholesterol (g)	Calcium (mg)	Iron (mg)
Totals												
RDA or related nutrient standard*												
% of nutrient needs												

*Values from inside cover. The number of kcals is a rough estimate. It is better to base energy needs on actual energy output.
†Use RAE values.
‡Use DFE values.

Nutrient Analysis Form cont'd

Magnesium (mg)	Phosphorous (mg)	Potassium (mg)	Sodium (mg)	Zinc (mg)	Vitamin A (RE)	Vitamin C (mg)	Vitamin E (mg)	Thiamin (mg)	Riboflavin (mg)	Niacin (mg)	Vitamin B-6 (mg)	Folate (µg)	Vitamin B-12 (µg)

III. **Complete the following table as you summarize your dietary intake.**

Percentage of kcal from Protein, Fat, Carbohydrate, and Alcohol

Intake

Protein (P):   ____g/day × 4 kcal per gram   =   (P)____kcal per day
Fat (F):   ____g/day × 9 kcal per gram   =   (F)____kcal per day
Carbohydrate (C):   ____g/day × 4 kcal per gram   =   (C)____kcal per day
Alcohol (A):   =   (A)____kcal per day*
                                Total kcal (T)/day   =   (T)____kcal per day

Percentage of kcal from protein:

$\frac{(P)}{(T)} \times 100 = $____%

Percentage of kcal from fat:

$\frac{(F)}{(T)} \times 100 = $____%

Percentage of kcal from carbohydrate:

$\frac{(C)}{(T)} \times 100 = $____%

Percentage of kcal from alcohol:

$\frac{(A)}{(T)} \times 100 = $____%

Note: The four percentages can total 99, 100, or 101, depending on the way in which figures were rounded off earlier.

*To calculate how many kcal in a beverage are from alcohol, first look up the beverage using the Nutrition Calc software. Then determine how many kcal are from carbohydrate (multiply carbohydrate grams times 4), fat (fat grams times 9), and protein (protein grams times 4). The remaining kcal are from alcohol.

IV. **Use the table on the following page to again record your food intake for one day, placing each food item in the correct category of MyPlate, with the correct number of servings (see Chapter 2).** A food such as a turkey and cheese sandwich contributes to three categories: grains, protein foods, and dairy. You can expect that many food choices will contribute to more than one group. Indicate the number of servings from MyPlate that each food yields.

Indicate the Number of Servings from MyPlate That Each Food Yields

Food or Beverage	Amount Eaten	Dairy	Protein	Fruits	Vegetables	Grains	SoFAS*
Group totals							
Recommended servings from www.Choose MyPlate.gov's Daily Food Plan							
Overages/Shortages in numbers of servings							

*SoFAS: solid fats and added sugars

V. **Evaluation.** Are there weaknesses suggested in your nutrient intake that correspond to missing servings in MyPlate? Consider adjusting your food choices to
comply with MyPlate standards to improve your nutrient intake.

VI. **For the same day you keep your food record, also keep a 24-hour record of
your activities.** Include sleeping, sitting, and walking, as well as the obvious
forms of exercise. Calculate your energy expenditure for these activities using
Table 7-4 in Chapter 7 or the diet analysis software available with this book. Try
to substitute a similar activity if your particular activity is not listed. Calculate
the total kcal you used for the day (total for column 3). Following is an example
of an activity record. A blank form follows for your use. Ask your professor
whether you are to turn in the form or the activity printout from NutritionCalc
Plus.

Weight (kg)*: 70 kg

Activity	Time (Minutes): Convert to Hours	Energy Cost		
		Column 1 kcal/kg/hr (from Table 7-4)	Column 2 (Column 1 × Time)	Column 3 (Column 2 × Weight in kg)
Brisk walking	(60 min) 1 hr	4.4	(× 1) = 4.4	(× 70) = 308

*lb/2.2

Weight (kg)*:

Activity	Time (Minutes): Convert to Hours	Energy Cost		
		Column 1 kcal/kg/hr (from Table 7-4)	Column 2 (Column 1 × Time)	Column 3 (Column 2 × Weight in kg)

Total kcal used (from adding all of column 3)
*lb/2.2

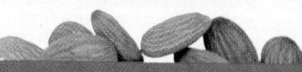
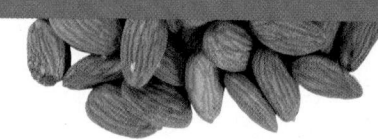

AMINO ACIDS

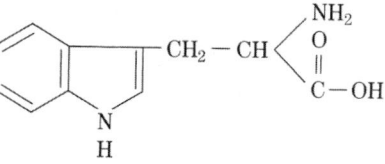

Histidine (His)
(essential)

Tryptophan (Trp)
(essential)

Glycine (Gly)

Methionine (Met)
(essential)

Leucine (Leu)
(essential)

Alanine (Ala)

Arginine (Arg)
(essential in infancy)

Lysine (Lys)
(essential)

Proline (Pro)

Glutamic Acid (Glu)

Aspartic Acid (Asp)

Serine (Ser)

Phenylalanine (Phe)
(essential)

Isoleucine (Ile)
(essential)

Tyrosine (Tyr)

Glutamine (Gln)

Asparagine (Asn)

Threonine (Thr)
(essential)

Valine (Val)
(essential)

Cysteine (Cys)

VITAMINS

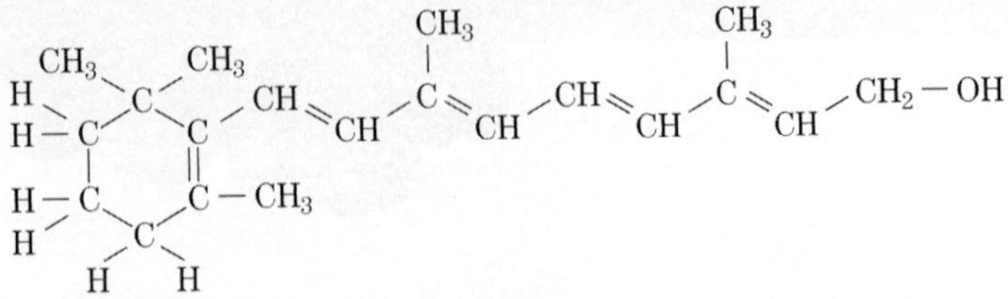

Vitamin A: retinol

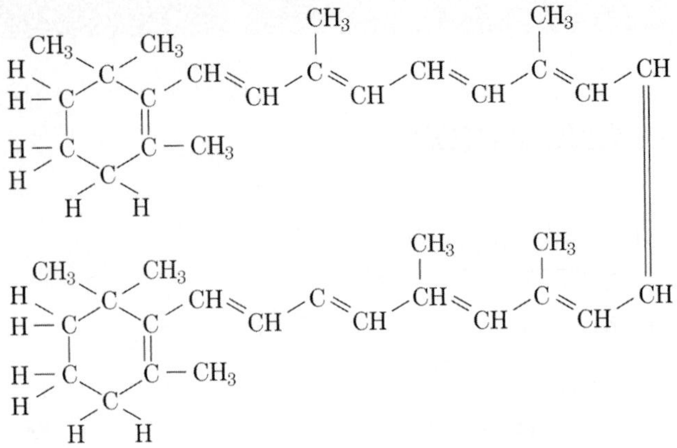

Beta-carotene

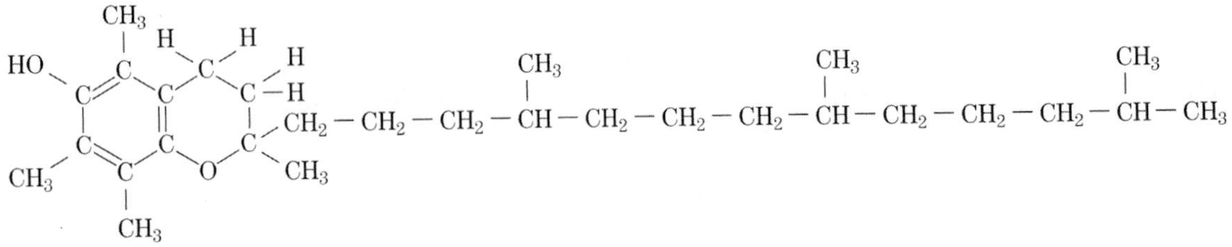

Vitamin E

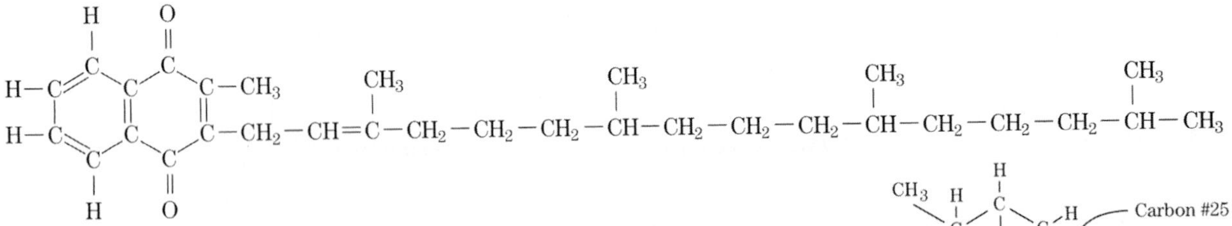

Vitamin K

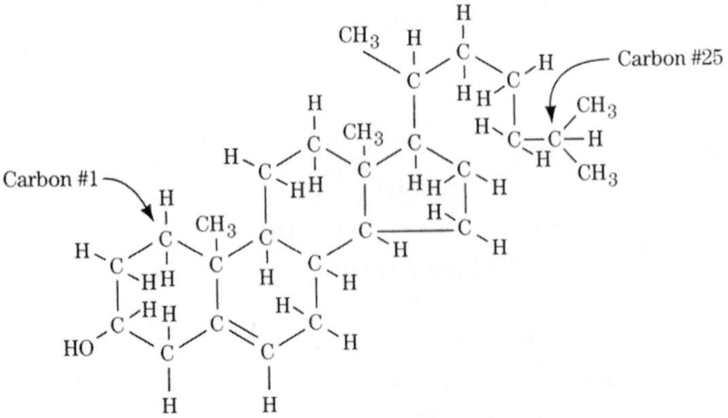

Carbon #25

Carbon #1

7-dehydrocholesterol

Carbon #25

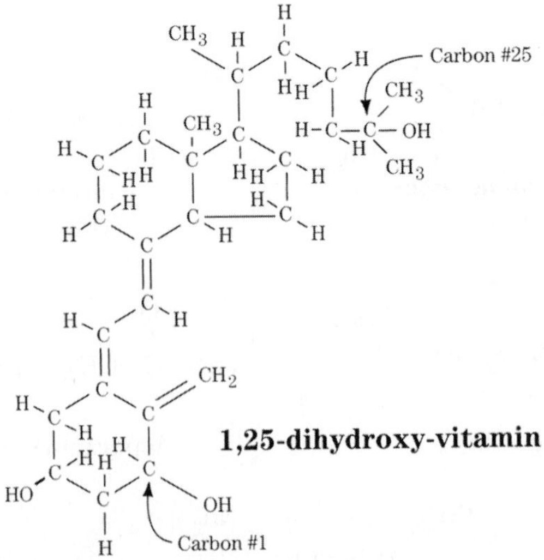

1,25-dihydroxy-vitamin D$_3$ (calcitriol)

Carbon #1

**Active vitamin D (calcitriol) and its precursor
7-dehydrocholesterol**

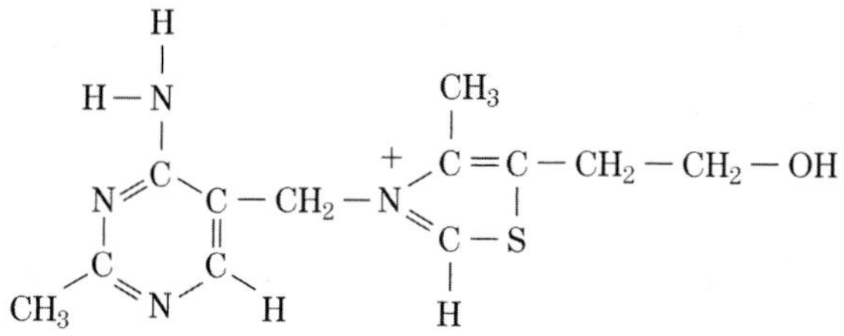

Thiamin

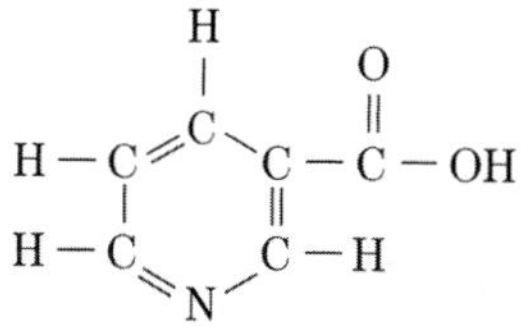

Nicotinic acid 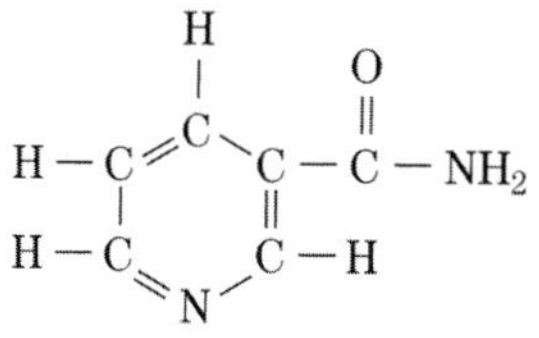   Nicotinamide

Niacin (nicotinic acid and nicotinamide)

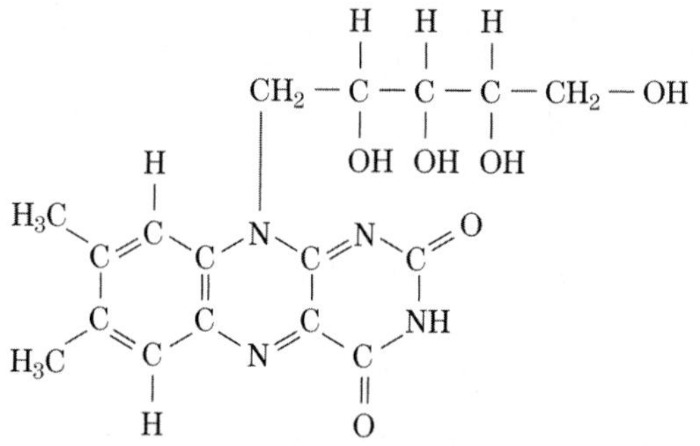

Riboflavin

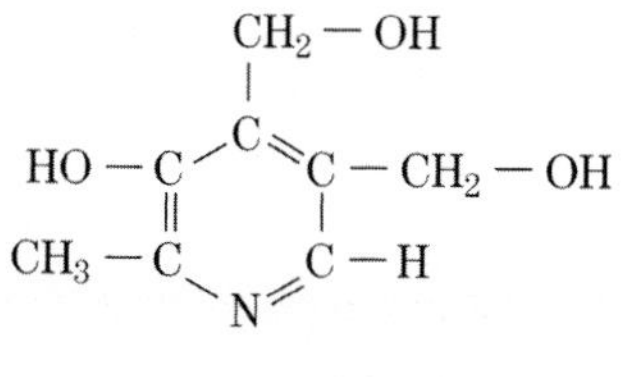

Pyridoxine 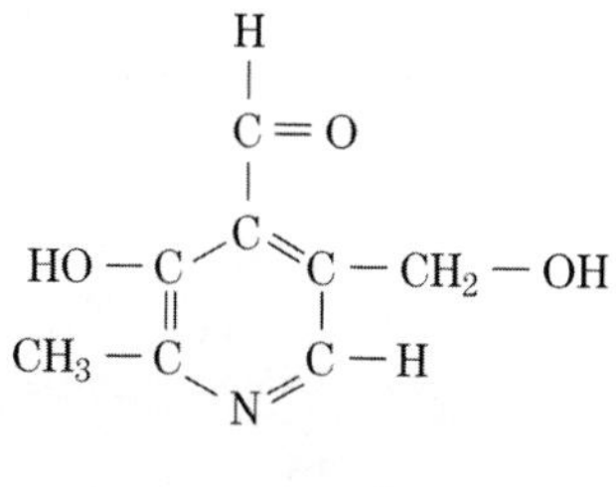   Pyridoxal 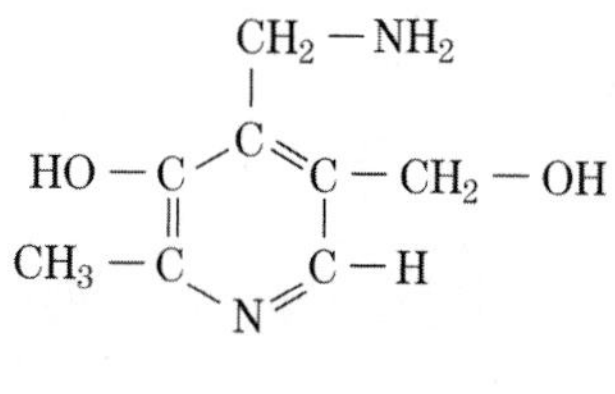   Pyridoxamine

Vitamin B-6 (a general name for three compounds—pyridoxine, pyridoxal, and pyridoxamine)

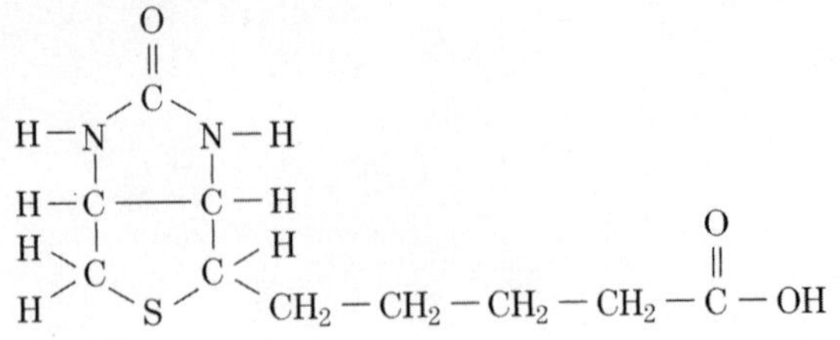

Biotin

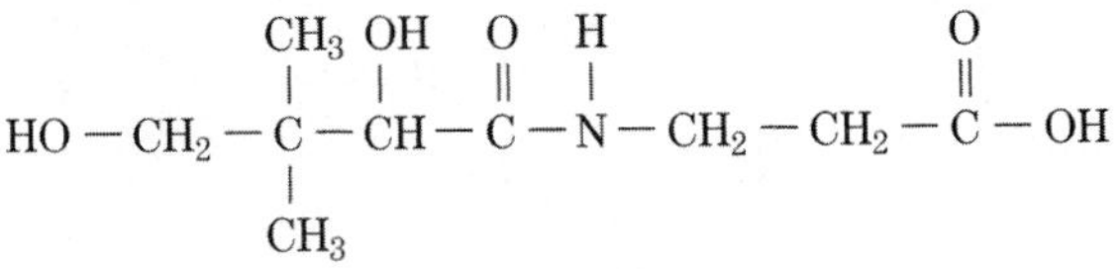

Pantothenic acid

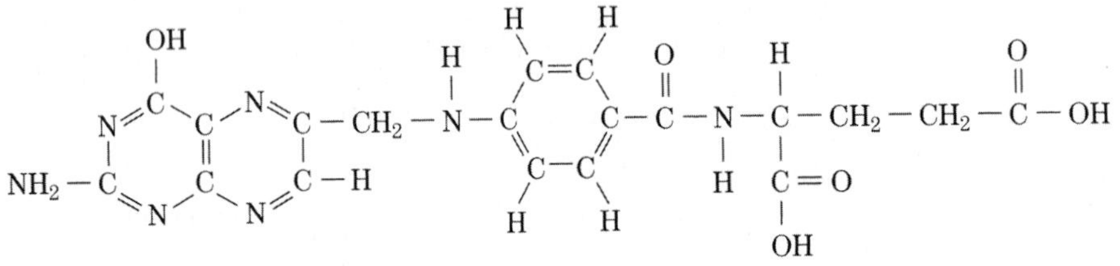

Folate (folic acid form)

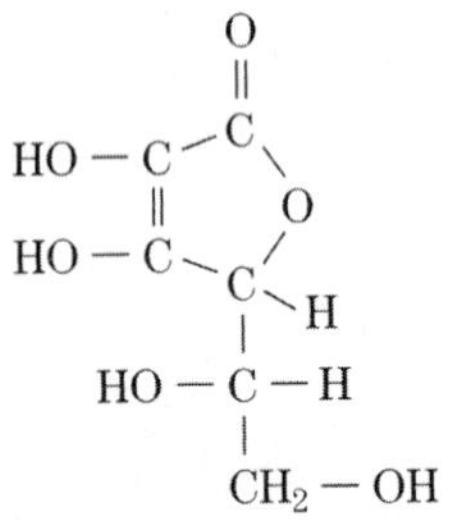

Vitamin C (ascorbic acid)

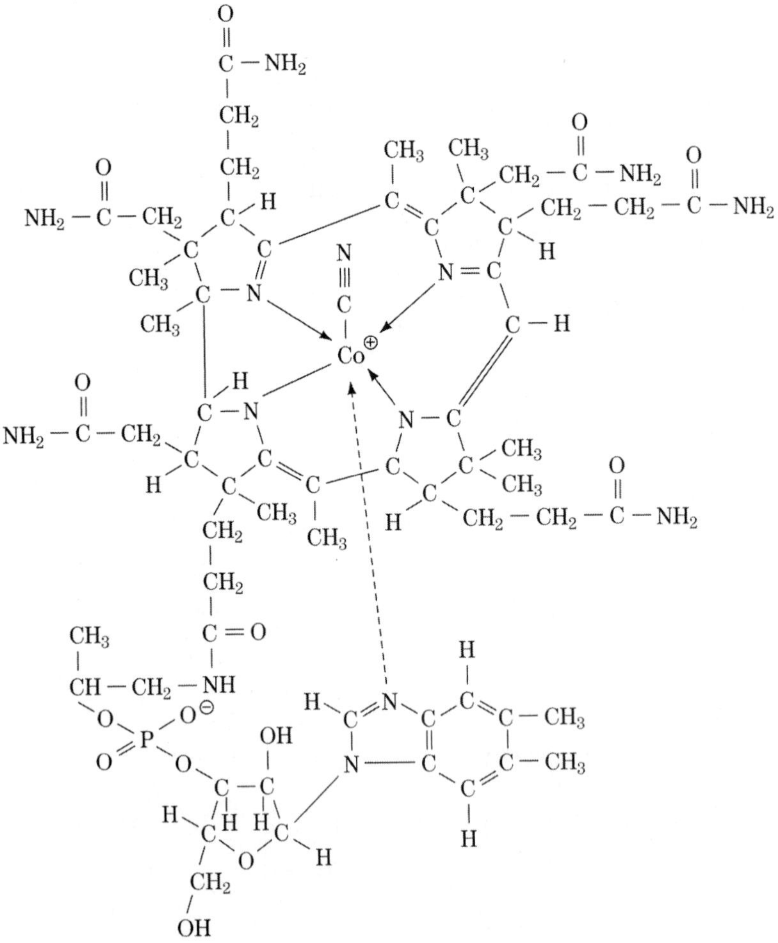

Vitamin B-12 (cyanocobalamin) The arrows in this diagram indicate that the spare electrons on the nitrogens are attracted to the cobalt atom.

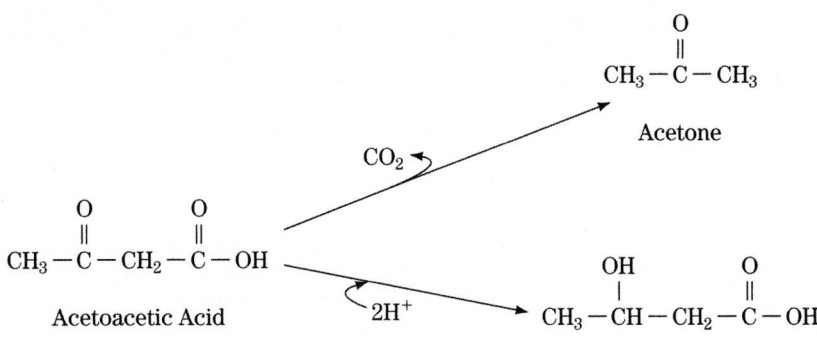

Ketone Bodies

$$CH_3-C-CH_3$$ Acetone

$$CH_3-C-CH_2-C-OH$$ Acetoacetic Acid

$$CH_3-CH-CH_2-C-OH$$ ß-Hydroxybutyric Acid

CO_2

$2H^+$

Triphosphate $\begin{cases} HO-P=O \\ HO-P=O \\ HO-P=O \end{cases}$

Point of cleavage to yield ADP and energy release

Adenine

Ribose (a sugar)

Adenosine Triphosphate (ATP)

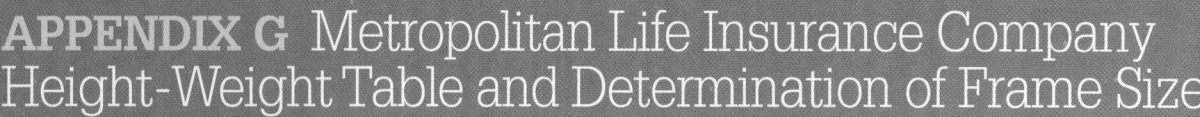

APPENDIX G Metropolitan Life Insurance Company Height-Weight Table and Determination of Frame Size

1983 Metropolitan Life Insurance Company Height-Weight Table* †

Women					Men				
Height		Frame			Height		Frame		
Ft.	In.	Small	Medium	Large	Ft.	In.	Small	Medium	Large
4	10	102–111	109–121	118–131	5	2	128–134	131–141	138–150
4	11	103–113	111–123	120–134	5	3	130–136	133–143	140–153
5	0	104–115	113–126	122–137	5	4	132–138	135–145	142–156
5	1	106–118	115–129	125–140	5	5	134–140	137–148	144–160
5	2	108–121	118–132	128–143	5	6	136–142	139–151	146–164
5	3	111–124	121–135	131–147	5	7	138–145	142–154	149–168
5	4	114–127	124–138	134–151	5	8	140–148	145–157	152–172
5	5	117–130	127–141	137–155	5	9	142–151	148–160	155–176
5	6	120–133	130–144	140–159	5	10	144–154	151–163	158–180
5	7	123–136	133–147	143–163	5	11	146–157	154–166	161–184
5	8	126–139	136–150	146–167	6	0	149–160	157–170	164–188
5	9	129–142	139–153	149–170	6	1	152–164	160–174	168–192
5	10	132–145	142–156	152–173	6	2	155–168	164–178	172–197
5	11	135–148	145–159	155–176	6	3	158–172	167–182	176–202
6	0	138–151	148–162	158–179	6	4	162–176	171–187	181–207

*Based on a weight-height mortality study conducted by the Society of Actuaries and the Association of Life Insurance Medical Directors of America, Metropolitan Life Insurance Medical Directors of America, Metropolitan Life Insurance Company, revised 1983.

†Weights in pounds (lb) at ages 25 to 59 based on lowest mortality. Height includes 1-in. heel. Weight for women includes 3 lb for indoor clothing. Weight for men includes 5 lb for indoor clothing.

Reprinted courtesy of Metropolitan Life Insurance Company, *Statistical Bulletin*.

Permission granted courtesy of Metropolitan Life Insurance Company, *Statistical Bulletin*.

USING THE METROPOLITAN LIFE INSURANCE TABLE TO ESTIMATE HEALTHY WEIGHT

The Metropolitan Life Insurance table is a common method for estimating healthy weight. The table lists, for any height, the weight that is associated with a maximum life span. The table does not tell the healthiest weight for a living person; it lists the weight associated with longevity.

There are many criticisms of this table. These stem from the inclusion of some people and the exclusion of others. For example, only policyholders of life insurance are included. In addition, smokers are included, but anyone over the age of 60 is excluded. Weight is only measured at the time of purchase of insurance, and there is no follow-up. All of these factors contribute to the fact that this table is to be used only as a rough screening tool; not meeting the exact recommendations should not be cause for alarm.

To diagnose overweight or obesity using the table, calculate the percentage of the Metropolitan Life Insurance table weight. Use the midpoint of a weight range for a specific height.

Equation: $\dfrac{(\text{Current wt.} - \text{wt. from table})}{\text{Weight from table}} \times 100$

Example: $$\frac{140 - 120}{120} \times 100 = 17\% \text{ over standard}$$

Overweight can be defined as weighing at least 10% more than the weight listed on the table. Determination of obesity is 20% more than that listed on the table. Moreover, this measure of obesity comes in degrees. Whereas mild obesity carries little health risk, severe obesity raises overall health risk twelvefold.

Degrees of Obesity	
% Over Healthy Body Weight	**Form of Obesity**
20–40%	Mild
41–99%	Moderate
100%+	Severe

DETERMINING FRAME SIZE

Method 1

Height is recorded without shoes.

Wrist circumference is measured just beyond (toward the hand) the bony (styloid) process at the wrist joint on the right arm, using a tape measure.

The following formula is used:

$$r = \frac{\text{Height (cm)}}{\text{Wrist circumference (cm)}}$$

Frame size can be determined as follows:[†]

Males	Females
$r > 10.4$ small	$r > 11$ small
$r = 9.6$–10.4 medium	$r = 10.1$–11 medium
$r < 9.6$ large	$r < 10.1$ large

[†]From Grant JP: *Handbook of Total Parenteral Nutrition.* Philadelphia: WB Saunders, 1980.

Method 2

The person's right arm is extended forward, perpendicular to the body, with the arm bent so the angle at the elbow forms 90 degrees, with the fingers pointing up and the palm turned away from the body. The greatest breadth across the elbow joint is measured with a sliding caliper along the axis of the upper arm, on the two prominent bones on either side of the elbow. This is recorded as the elbow breadth. The following tables give elbow breadth measurements for medium-framed men and women of various heights. Measurements lower than those listed indicate a small frame size; higher measurements indicate a large frame size.[‡]

Men		Women	
Height in 1" Heels	**Elbow Breadth**	**Height in 1" Heels**	**Elbow Breadth**
5'2"–5'3"	2½–2⅞"	4'10"–4'11"	2¼–2½"
5'4"–5'7"	2⅝–2⅞"	5'0"–5'3"	2¼–2½"
5'8"–5'11"	2¾–3"	5'4"–5'7"	2⅜–2⅝"
6'0"–6'3"	2¾–3¼"	5'8"–5'11"	2⅜–2⅝"
6'4" and over	2⅞–3¾"	6'0" and over	2½–2¾"

[‡]From Metropolitan Life Insurance Co., 1983.

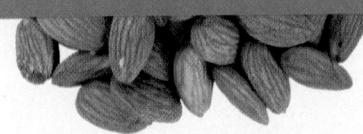

Consider the following reliable sources of food and nutrition information:

Journals That Regularly Cover Nutrition Topics

American Family Physician*
American Journal of Clinical Nutrition
American Journal of Epidemiology
American Journal of Medicine
American Journal of Nursing
American Journal of Obstetrics and Gynecology
American Journal of Physiology
American Journal of Public Health
American Scientist
Annals of Internal Medicine
Annual Review of Medicine
Annual Review of Nutrition
Archives of Disease in Childhood
Archives of Internal Medicine
British Journal of Nutrition
BMJ (British Medical Journal)
Canadian Journal of Dietetic Practice and Research
Cancer

Cancer Research
Circulation
Diabetes
Diabetes Care
Disease-a-Month
FASEB Journal
FDA Consumer*
Food and Chemical Toxicology
Food Engineering
Food Technology
Gastroenterology
Geriatrics
Gut
Journal of the American College of Nutrition*
Journal of the American Dietetic Association*
Journal of the American Geriatrics Society
JAMA (Journal of the American Medical Association)
Journal of Applied Physiology
Journal of Clinical Investigation
Journal of Food Science

JNCI (Journal of the National Cancer Institute)
Journal of Nutrition
Journal of Nutrition Education and Behavior*
Journal of Nutrition for the Elderly
Journal of Pediatrics
Lancet
Mayo Clinic Proceedings
Medicine & Science in Sports & Exercise
Nature
The New England Journal of Medicine
Nutrition
Nutrition Reviews
Nutrition in Clinical Practice*
Nutrition Today*
Pediatrics
The Physician and Sports Medicine
Postgraduate Medicine*
Proceedings of the Nutrition Society
Science
Science News*
Scientific American*

The majority of these journals are available in college and university libraries or in a specialty library on campus, such as one designated for health services or home economics. As indicated, a few journals will be filed under their abbreviations, rather than the first word in their full name. A reference librarian can help you locate any of these sources. The journals with an asterisk (*) are ones you may find especially interesting and useful because of the number of nutrition articles presented each month or the less technical nature of the presentation.

Magazines for the Consumer That Cover Nutrition Topics

Better Homes and Gardens
Good Housekeeping

Health
Men's Health

Parents
Self

Textbooks and Other Sources for Advanced Study of Nutrition Topics

Bowman BA, Russell RM: *Present knowledge in nutrition.* Vol. I and II. 9th ed. Washington DC: International Life Sciences Institute, 2006.

Brody T: *Nutritional biochemistry.* 2nd ed. San Diego: Academic Press, 1999.

Gropper SS, Smith JL: *Advanced nutrition and human metabolism.* 5th ed. Florence, KY: Wadsworth, Cengage 2009.

Mahan LK, Escott-Stump S: *Krause's food, and nutrition, therapy.* 12th ed. St. Louis: W.B. Saunders, 2008.

Murray RK and others: *Harper's illustrated biochemistry.* 28th ed. New York: McGraw-Hill, 2009.

Schils ME, Shike M, Ross AC, Caballero B, Cousins RJ: *Modern nutrition in health and disease.* 10th ed. Philadelphia: Lippincott, Williams & Wilkins, 2005.

Stipanuk MH: *Biochemical, physiological, & molecular aspects of human nutrition.* 2nd ed. Philadelphia: Elsevier Health Sciences, 2006.

Newsletters That Cover Nutrition Issues on a Regular Basis

American Institute for Cancer Research e.Newsletter
American Institute for Cancer Research
www.aicr.org

Consumer Health Digest
National Council Against Health Fraud
www.ncahf.org

The Dairy Download
National Dairy Council
www.nationaldairycouncil.org

Diabetes E-News (and others)
American Diabetes Association
www.diabetes.org

Environmental Nutrition
www.environmentalnutrition.com

Harvard Health Letter (and others)
Harvard Medical School
www.health.harvard.edu/newsletters

Health and Nutrition Letter
Tufts University
www.healthletter.tufts.edu

In-Touch
Heinz Infant Nutrition Institute
www.hini.org

Mayo Clinic House call
Mayo Clinic
www.mayoclinic.com

Nutrition Action Healthletter
Center for Science in the Public Interest
www.cspinet.org

Nutrition CloseUp
Egg Nutrition Center
www.enc-online.org

Soy Connection
United Soybean Board
www.soyconnection.com

U-Mail: Everyday Nutrition Solutions You Can Use
National Cattlemen's Beef Association
www.beefnutrition.org

Wellness Letter
University of California at Berkeley
www.wellnessletter.com

Professional Organizations

American Academy of Pediatrics
141 Northwest Point Boulevard
Elk Grove Village, IL 60007-1098
www.aap.org

American Cancer Society
1599 Clifton Road, NE
Atlanta, GA 30329
www.cancer.org

American College of Sports Medicine
PO Box 1440
Indianapolis, IN 46206-1440
www.acsm.org

American Dental Association
211 East Chicago Avenue
Chicago, IL 60611-2678
www.ada.org

American Diabetes Association
1701 North Beauregard Street
Alexandria, VA 22311
www.diabetes.org

American Dietetic Association
120 South Riverside Plaza #2000
Chicago, IL 60606-6995
www.eatright.org

American Geriatrics Society
40 Fulton Street, 18th Floor
New York, NY 10038
www.americangeriatrics.org

American Heart Association
7272 Greenville Avenue
Dallas, TX 75231
www.americanheart.org

American Medical Association
515 North State Street
Chicago, IL 60610
www.ama-assn.org

American Public Health Association
800 I Street, NW
Washington, DC 20001-3710
www.apha.org

American Society for Nutrition
9650 Rockville Pike #L-4500
Bethesda, MD 20814
www.nutrition.org

Canadian Council of Food and Nutrition
2810 Matheson Boulevard
East, 1st Floor
Mississaugo, Ontario L4W 4X7
http://www.ccfn.ca/

Canadian Diabetes Association
1400-522 University Avenue
Toronto, ON M5G 2R5
www.diabetes.ca

Canadian Nutrition Society
310-2175 Sheppard Avenue East
Toronto, Ontario M2J 1W8
www.cns-scn.ca

Dietitians of Canada
480 University Avenue #604
Toronto, ON M5G 1V2
www.dietitians.ca

Environmental Working Group
1436 U Street, NW #100
Washington, DC 20009
www.ewg.org

Food and Nutrition Board
Institute of Medicine
The National Academies
500 Fifth Street, NW
Washington, DC 20001
www.iom.edu/cMs/3788.aspx

Institute of Food Technologists
525 West Van Buren #1000
Chicago, IL 60607
www.ift.org

National Council on Aging
1901 L Street, NW, 4th floor
Washington, DC 20036
www.ncoa.org

National Osteoporosis Foundation
1150 17th Street, NW #850
Washington, DC 20036
www.nof.org

Society for Nutrition Education
9100 Purdue Road, Suite 200
Indianapolis, IN 46268
www.sne.org

Professional Organizations with a Commitment to Nutrition Issues

Bread for the World Institute
425 3rd Street SW #1200
Washington, DC 20024
www.bread.org

Food Research and Action Center
1875 Connecticut Avenue, NW #540
Washington, DC 20009 http://frac.org/

Institute for Food and Development Policy
398 60th Street
Oakland, CA 94618
www.foodfirst.org

La Leche League International
957 N. Plum Grove Road
Schaumburg, IL 60173
www.llli.org

March of Dimes
1275 Mamaroneck Avenue
White Plains, NY 10605
www.marchofdimes.com

National Council Against Health Fraud
119 Foster Street
Peabody, MA 01960
www.ncahf.org

National WIC Association
2001 S Street, NW #580
Washington, DC 20009
www.nwica.org

Overeaters Anonymous
PO Box 44020
Rio Rancho, NM 87174-4020
www.oa.org

Oxfam America
226 Causeway Street, 5th floor
Boston, MA 02114-2206
www.oxfamamerica.org

Local Resources for Advice on Nutrition Issues

Registered dietitians (RDs or in Canada also RDNs) in health care, city, county, or state agencies, as well as in private practice

Cooperative extension agents in county extension offices

Nutrition faculty affiliated with departments of food and nutrition, home economics, and dietetics

Government Agencies Concerned with Nutrition Issues or That Distribute Nutrition Information

United States

Agricultural Research Service
United States Department of Agriculture
Jamie L. Whitten Building
1400 Independence Avenue, SW
Washington, DC 20250
www.ars.usda.gov

Federal Citizen Information Center
31201 Bryan Circle
Pueblo, CO 81001
www.pueblo.gsa.gov

Food and Drug Administration
10903 New Hampshire Avenue
Silver Spring, MD 20993
www.fda.gov

Food Safety & Inspection Service
United States Department of Agriculture
331-E Jamie L. Whitten Building
1400 Independence Avenue, SW
Washington, DC 20250-3700
www.fsis.usda.gov

MyPlate
USDA Center for Nutrition Policy and
    Promotion
3101 Park Center Drive #1034
Alexandria, VA 22302-1594
www.choosemyplate.gov

National Agricultural Library
Abraham Lincoln Building
10301 Baltimore Avenue
Beltsville, MD 20705-2351
www.nal.usda.gov

National Cancer Institute
6116 Executive Boulevard #3036A
Bethesda, MD 20892-8322
www.cancer.gov

National Center for Health Statistics
1600 Clifton Road
Atlanta, GA 30333
www.cdc.gov/nchs

National Heart, Lung, and Blood
    Institute
Building 31, Room 5A52
31 Center Drive, MSC 2486
Bethesda, MD 20892
www.nhlbi.nih.gov

National Institute on Aging
Building 31, Room 5C27
31 Center Drive, MSC 2292
Bethesda, MD 20892
www.nia.nih.gov

U.S. Government Printing Office
710 North Capitol Street, NW
Washington, DC 20401
www.gpo.gov

Canada

Canadian Food Inspection Agency
1400 Merivale Road
Ottawa, Ontario K1A 0Y9
www.inspection.gc.ca

Health Canada
Brooke Claxton Building
Ottawa, Ontario K1A 0K9
www.hc-sc.gc.ca

United Nations

Food and Agriculture Organization
Liaison Office with North America
1 United Nations Plaza #DC1 - 1125
New York, NY 10017
www.fao.org

World Health Organization
Avenue Appia 20
1211 Geneva 27
Switzerland
www.who.int

Trade Organizations and Companies That Distribute Nutrition Information

Abbott Nutrition
625 Cleveland Avenue
Columbus, OH 43215-1724
www.abbottnutrition.com

American Institute of Baking
1213 Bakers Way
PO Box 3999
Manhattan, Kansas 66505-3999
www.aibonline.org

American Meat Institute
1150 Connecticut Avenue, NW,
    12th floor
Washington, DC 20036
www.meatami.com

Beech-Nut Nutrition
13023 Tesson Ferry Road
St. Louis, MO 63128
www.beechnut.com

Campbell Soup Company
1 Campbell Place
Camden, NJ 08103-1701
www.campbellsoup.com

Dannon Company
P.O. Box 90296
Allentown, PA 18109-0296
www.dannon.com

Del Monte Foods
One Maritime Plaza
San Francisco, CA 94111
www.delmonte.com

DSM Nutritional Products
45 Waterview Boulevard
Parsippany, NJ 07054-1298
www.dsm.com

General Mills/Pillsbury
PO Box 9452
Minneapolis, MN 55440
www.generalmills.com

Gerber Products Company
445 State Street
Fremont, MI 49413-0001
www.gerber.com

H.J. Heinz
90 Sheppard Avenue East #400
Toronto, ON M2N 7K5
www.heinzbaby.com

Idaho Potato Commission
661 South Rivershore Lane
Eagle, ID 83616
www.idahopotatoes.com

Kellogg Company
One Kellogg Square
Battle Creek, MI 49016
www.kelloggs.com/us/

Kraft Foods Global
1 Kraft Court
Glenview, IL 60025
www.kraftrecipes.com

Mead Johnson Nutritionals
2400 West Lloyd Expressway
Evansville, IN 47721-0001
www.meadjohnson.com

National Dairy Council
10255 West Higgins Road #900
Des Plaines, IL 60018
www.nationaldairycouncil.org

NutraSweet Company
222 Merchandise Mart Plaza
Chicago, IL 60654
www.nutrasweet.com

Sunkist Growers
14130 Riverside Drive
Sherman Oaks, CA 91423
www.sunkist.com

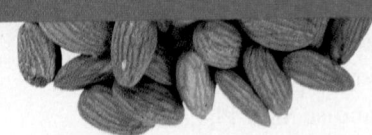

METRIC-ENGLISH CONVERSIONS

Length

English (USA)	Metric
inch (in)	= 2.54 cm, 25.4 mm
foot (ft)	= 0.30 m, 30.48 cm
yard (yd)	= 0.91 m, 91.4 cm
mile (statute) (5280 ft)	= 1.61 km, 1609 m
mile (nautical) (6077 ft, 1.15 statute mi)	= 1.85 km, 1850 m

Metric	English (USA)
millimeter (mm)	= 0.039 in (thickness of a dime)
centimeter (cm)	= 0.39 in
meter (m)	= 3.28 ft, 39.37 in
kilometer (km)	= 0.62 mi, 1091 yd, 3273 ft

Weight

English (USA)	Metric
grain	= 64.80 mg
ounce (oz)	= 28.35 g
pound (lb)	= 453.60 g, 0.45 kg
ton (short—2000 lb)	= 0.91 metric ton (907 kg)

Metric	English (USA)
milligram (mg)	= 0.002 grain (0.000035 oz)
gram (g)	= 0.04 oz ($\frac{1}{28}$ of an oz)
kilogram (kg)	= 35.27 oz, 2.20 lb
metric ton (1000 kg)	= 1.10 tons

Volume

English (USA)	Metric
cubic inch	= 16.39 cc
cubic foot	= 0.03 m³
cubic yard	= 0.765 m³
teaspoon (tsp)	= 5 ml
tablespoon (tbsp)	= 15 ml
fluid ounce	= 0.03 liter (30 ml)*
cup (c)	= 237 ml
pint (pt)	= 0.47 liter
quart (qt)	= 0.95 liter
gallon (gal)	= 3.79 liters

Metric	English (USA)
milliliter (ml)	= 0.03 oz
liter (L)	= 2.12 pt
liter	= 1.06 qt
liter	= 0.27 gal

1 liter ÷ 1000 = 1 milliliter or 1 cubic centimeter (10^{-3} liter)
1 liter ÷ 1,000,000 = 1 microliter (10^{-6} liter)
*Note: 1 ml = 1 cc

METRIC AND OTHER COMMON UNITS

Unit/Abbreviation	Other Equivalent Measure
milligram/mg	$\frac{1}{1000}$ of a gram
microgram/µg	$\frac{1}{1,000,000}$ of a gram
deciliter/dl	$\frac{1}{10}$ of a liter (about ½ cup)
milliliter/ml	$\frac{1}{1000}$ of a liter (5 ml is about 1 tsp)
International Unit/IU	Crude measure of vitamin activity generally based on growth rate seen in animals

FAHRENHEIT-CELSIUS CONVERSION SCALE

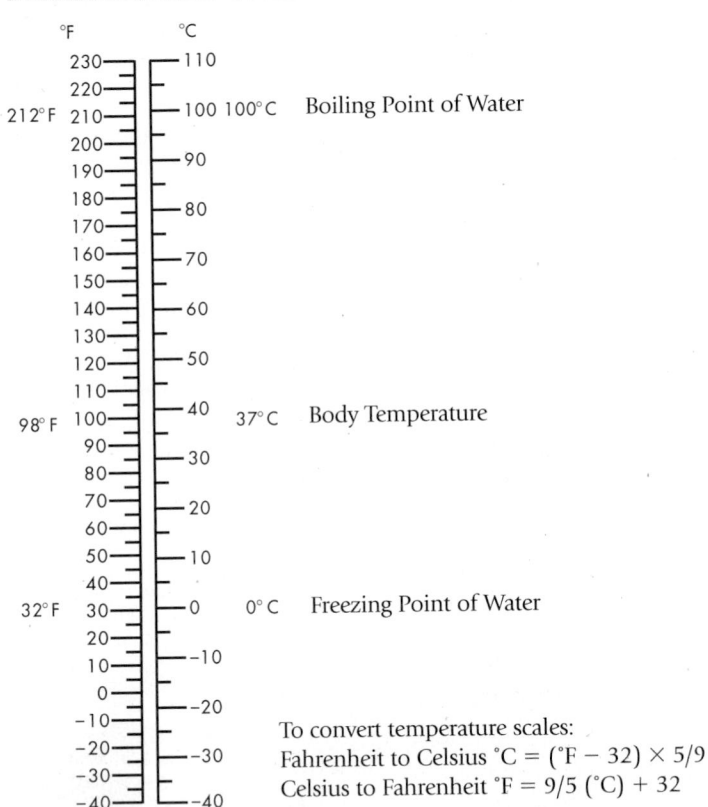

To convert temperature scales:
Fahrenheit to Celsius °C = (°F − 32) × 5/9
Celsius to Fahrenheit °F = 9/5 (°C) + 32

HOUSEHOLD UNITS

3 teaspoons	= 1 tablespoon	= 15 grams
4 tablespoons	= ¼ cup	= 60 grams
5⅓ tablespoons	= ⅓ cup	= 80 grams
8 tablespoons	= ½ cup	= 120 grams
10⅔ tablespoons	= ⅔ cup	= 160 grams
16 tablespoons	= 1 cup	= 240 grams
1 tablespoon	= ½ fluid ounce	= 15 milliliters
1 cup	= 8 fluid ounces	= 15 milliliters
1 cup	= ½ pint	= 240 grams
2 cups	= 1 pint	= 480 grams
4 cups	= 1 quart	= 960 grams = 1 liter
2 pints	= 1 quart	= 960 grams = 1 liter
4 quarts	= 1 gallon	= 3840 grams = 4 liters

absorption The process by which substances are taken up from the GI tract and enter the bloodstream or the lymph.

absorptive cells The intestinal cells that line the villi; these cells participate in nutrient absorption.

Acceptable Daily Intake (ADI) Estimate of the amount of a sweetener that an individual can safely consume daily over a lifetime. ADIs are given as mg per kg of body weight per day.

acesulfame K Alternative sweetener that yields no energy.

acetaldehyde dehydrogenase An enzyme used in ethanol metabolism that eventually converts acetaldehyde into carbon dioxide and water.

acquired immune deficiency syndrome (AIDS) A disorder in which a virus (human immunodeficiency virus [HIV]) infects specific types of immune system cells. This leaves the person with reduced immune function and, in turn, defenseless against numerous infectious agents; typically contributes to the person's death.

added sugars Sugars or syrups that are added to foods during processing or preparation.

additives Substances added to foods, such as preservatives.

adenosine diphosphate (ADP) A breakdown product of ATP. ADP is synthesized into ATP using energy from foodstuffs and a phosphate group (abbreviated P_i).

adenosine triphosphate (ATP) The main energy currency for cells. ATP energy is used to promote ion pumping, enzyme activity, and muscular contraction.

Adequate Intake (AI) Nutrient intake amount set for any nutrient for which insufficient research is available to establish an RDA. AIs are based on estimates of intakes that appear to maintain a defined nutritional state in a specific life stage.

adipose tissue A group of fat storing cells.

adjustable gastric banding A restrictive procedure in which the opening from the esophagus to the stomach is reduced by a hollow gastric band.

aerobic Requiring oxygen.

aging Time-dependent physical and physiological changes in body structure and function that occur normally and progressively throughout adulthood as humans mature and become older.

air displacement A method for estimating body composition that makes use of the volume of space taken up by a body inside a small chamber.

alcohol Ethyl alcohol or ethanol (CH_3CH_2OH) is the compound in alcoholic beverages.

alcohol abuse Excessive alcohol consumption that leads to severe alcohol-related health and other problems, such as recurrent sickness, inability to fulfill major obligations, use in hazardous situations (e.g., driving), related legal problems, or use despite social and interpersonal difficulties.

alcohol dehydrogenase An enzyme used in alcohol (ethanol) metabolism that converts alcohol into acetaldehyde.

alcohol dependence The person experiences repeated alcohol-related difficulties, such as an inability to control use, spending a great deal of time associated with alcohol use, continued use of alcohol despite physical or psychological consequences, persistent desire or unsuccessful efforts to cut down or control alcohol use, and withdrawal symptoms. Tolerance is also seen.

alcoholism As defined by the American Medical Association, an illness characterized by significant impairment directly related to persistent and excessive use of alcohol.

alcohol-related birth defects (ARBDs) One or more birth defects (e.g., malformations of the heart, bones, kidneys, eyes, or ears) related to confirmed alcohol exposure during gestation.

alcohol-related neurodevelopmental disorders (ARNDs) One or more abnormalities of the central nervous system (e.g., small head size, impaired motor skills, hearing loss, or poor hand-eye coordination) related to confirmed alcohol exposure during gestation.

aldosterone A hormone produced by the adrenal glands that acts on the kidneys to conserve sodium (and therefore water).

allergen A foreign protein, or antigen, that induces excess production of certain immune system antibodies; subsequent exposure to the same protein leads to allergic symptoms. Whereas all allergens are antigens, not all antigens are allergens.

allergy A hypersensitive immune response that occurs when immune bodies produced by us react with a protein we sense as foreign (an antigen).

alpha-linolenic acid An essential omega-3 fatty acid with 18 carbons and three double bonds.

amino acid The building block for proteins containing a central carbon atom with nitrogen and other atoms attached.

amniotic fluid Fluid contained in a sac within the uterus. This fluid surrounds and protects the fetus during development.

amphetamine A group of medications that induce stimulation of the central nervous system and have other effects in the body. Abuse is linked to physical and psychological dependence.

amylase Starch-digesting enzyme produced by the salivary glands or pancreas.

amylopectin A digestible branched-chain type of starch composed of glucose units.

amylose A digestible straight-chain type of starch composed of glucose units.

anaerobic Not requiring oxygen.

anal sphincters A group of two sphincters (inner and outer) that help control expulsion of feces from the body.

analog A chemical compound that differs slightly from another, usually natural, compound. Analogs generally contain extra or altered chemical groups and may have similar or opposite metabolic effects compared with the native compound. Also spelled *analogue*.

anaphylactic shock A severe allergic response that results in lowered blood pressure and respiratory and gastrointestinal distress. This can be fatal.

anemia Generally refers to a decreased oxygen-carrying capacity of the blood. This can be caused by many factors, such as iron deficiency or blood loss.

animal model Use of animals to study disease to understand more about human disease.

anorexia nervosa An eating disorder involving a psychological loss or denial of appetite, followed by self-starvation; related in part to a distorted body image and to various social pressures commonly associated with puberty.

anthropometric assessment Measurement of body weight and the lengths, circumferences, and thicknesses of parts of the body.

antibody Blood protein (immunoglobulin) that binds foreign proteins found in the body. This helps to prevent and control infections.

antidiuretic hormone A hormone that is secreted by the pituitary gland and that acts on the kidneys to decrease water excretion.

antigen Any substance that induces a state of sensitivity and/or resistance to microorganisms or toxic substances after a lag period; foreign substance that stimulates a specific aspect of the immune system.

antioxidant Generally a compound that stops the damaging effects of reactive substances seeking an electron (i.e., oxidizing agents). This prevents breakdown (oxidizing) of substances in foods or the body, particularly lipids.

anus Last portion of the GI tract; serves as an outlet for that organ.

appetite The primarily psychological (external) influences that encourage us to find and eat food, often in the absence of obvious hunger.

arachidonic acid An omega-6 fatty acid made from linoleic acid with 20 carbon atoms and four carbon-carbon double bonds.

artery A blood vessel that carries blood away from the heart.

aseptic processing A method by which food and container are separately and simultaneously sterilized; it allows manufacturers to produce boxes of milk that can be stored at room temperature.

aspartame Alternative sweetener made of 2 amino acids and methanol; about 200 times sweeter than sucrose.

atherosclerosis A buildup of fatty material (plaque) in the arteries, including those surrounding the heart.

atom Smallest combining unit of an element, such as iron or calcium. Atoms consist of protons, neutrons, and electrons.

bacteria Single-cell microorganisms; some produce poisonous substances, which cause illness in humans. Bacteria can be carried by water, animals, and people. They survive on skin, clothes, and hair and thrive in foods at room temperature. Some can live without oxygen and survive by means of spore formation.

bariatrics The medical specialty focusing on the treatment of obesity.

basal metabolism The minimal amount of calories the body uses to support itself in a fasting state when resting (e.g., 12 hours for both) and awake in a warm, quiet environment. It amounts to roughly 1 kcal per kilogram per hour for men and 0.9 kcal per kilogram per hour for women; these values are often referred to as *basal metabolic rate (BMR)*.

benign Noncancerous; tumors that do not spread.

beriberi The thiamin deficiency disorder characterized by muscle weakness, loss of appetite, nerve degeneration, and sometimes edema.

BHA, BHT Butylated hydroxyanisole and butylated hydroxytoluene—two common synthetic antioxidants added to foods.

bile A liver secretion stored in the gallbladder and released through the common bile duct into the first segment of the small intestine. It is essential for the digestion and absorption of fat.

binge-eating disorder An eating disorder characterized by recurrent binge eating and feelings of loss of control over eating that have lasted at least 6 months. Binge episodes can be triggered by frustration, anger, depression, anxiety, permission to eat forbidden foods, and excessive hunger.

bioavailability The degree to which an ingested nutrient is absorbed and thus is available to the body.

biochemical assessment Measurement of biochemical functions (e.g., concentrations of nutrient by-products or enzyme activities in the blood or urine) related to a nutrient's function.

bioelectrical impedance The method to estimate total body fat that uses a low-energy electrical current. The more fat storage a person has, the more impedance (resistance) to electrical flow will be exhibited.

biological pest management Control of agricultural pests by using natural predators, parasites, or pathogens. For example, ladybugs can be used to control an aphid infestation.

biotechnology A collection of processes that involves the use of biological systems for altering and, ideally, improving the characteristics of plants, animals, and other forms of life.

bisphosphonates Compounds primarily composed of carbon and phosphorus that bind to bone mineral and in turn reduce bone breakdown. Examples are alendronate (Fosamax), risedronate (Actonel), and ibandronate (Boniva).

body mass index (BMI) Weight (in kilograms) divided by height (in meters) squared; a value of 25 and above indicates overweight and a value of 30 and above indicates obesity.

bolus A moistened mass of food swallowed from the oral cavity into the pharynx.

bomb colorimeter An instrument used to determine the calorie content of a food.

bond A linkage between two atoms formed by the sharing of electrons, or attractions.

bone mass Total mineral substance (such as calcium or phosphorus) in a cross section of bone, generally expressed as grams per centimeter of length.

bone mineral density Total mineral content of bone at a specific bone site divided by the width of the bone at that site, generally expressed as grams per cubic centimeter.

branched-chain amino acids Amino acids with a branching carbon backbone; these are leucine, isoleucine, and valine. All are essential amino acids.

brown adipose tissue A specialized form of adipose tissue that produces large amounts of heat by metabolizing energy-yielding nutrients without synthesizing much useful energy for the body. The unused energy is released as heat.

buffers Compounds that cause a solution to resist changes in acid-base conditions.

bulimia nervosa An eating disorder in which large quantities of food are eaten at one time (binge eating) and then purged from the body by vomiting, or misuse of laxatives, diuretics, or enemas. Alternate means to counteract the binge behavior are fasting and excessive exercise.

capillary A microscopic blood vessel that connects the smallest arteries and veins; site of nutrient, oxygen, and waste exchange between body cells and the blood.

capillary bed Network of one-cell-thick vessels that create a junction between arterial and venous circulation. It is here that gas and nutrient exchange occurs between body cells and the blood.

carbohydrate A compound containing carbon, hydrogen, and oxygen atoms. Most are known as *sugars*, *starches*, and *fibers*.

carbohydrate loading A process in which a high carbohydrate intake is consumed for 6 days before an athletic event while tapering exercise duration in an attempt to increase muscle glycogen stores.

carbon skeleton Amino-acid structure that remains after the amino group ($-NH_2$) has been removed.

cardiovascular system The body system consisting of the heart, blood vessels, and blood. This system transports nutrients, waste products, gases, and hormones throughout the body and plays an important role in immune responses and regulation of body temperature.

carotenoids Pigment materials in fruits and vegetables that range in color from yellow to orange to red; three of the various carotenoids yield vitamin A. Many are antioxidants.

case-control study A study in which individuals who have a disease or condition, such as lung cancer, are compared with individuals who do not have the condition.

celiac disease Immunological or allergic reaction to the protein gluten in certain grains, such as wheat and rye. The effect is to destroy the intestinal enterocytes, resulting in a much reduced surface area due to flattening of the villi. Elimination of wheat, rye, and certain other grains from the diet restores the intestinal surface.

cell The structural basis of plant and animal organization. In animals it is bounded by a cell membrane. Cells contain both genetic material and systems for synthesizing energy-yielding compounds. Cells have the ability to take up compounds from and excrete compounds into their surroundings.

cell-mediated immunity A process in which certain white blood cells come in contact with the invading cells to destroy them.

cell nucleus An organelle bound by its own double membrane and containing chromosomes, the genetic information for cell protein synthesis and cell replication.

cellulose An undigestible nonfermentable straight-chain polysaccharide made of glucose molecules.

cerebrovascular accident (CVA) Death of part of the brain tissue due typically to a blood clot. Also termed a *stroke*.

chain-breaking Breaking the link between two or more behaviors that encourage overeating, such as snacking while watching television.

chemical reaction An interaction between two chemicals that changes both chemicals.

cholecystokinin (CCK) A hormone that participates in enzyme release from the pancreas, bile release from the gallbladder, and hunger regulation.

cholesterol A waxy lipid found in all body cells. It has a structure containing multiple chemical rings that is found only in foods that contain animal products.

chromosome A single, large DNA molecule and its associated proteins; contains many genes to store and transmit genetic information.

chylomicron Lipoprotein made of dietary fats surrounded by a shell of cholesterol, phospholipids, and protein. Chylomicrons are formed in the absorptive cells of the small intestine after fat absorption and travel through the lymphatic system to the bloodstream.

chyme A mixture of stomach secretions and partially digested food.

cirrhosis A loss of functioning liver cells, which are replaced by nonfunctioning connective tissue. Any substance that poisons liver cells can lead to cirrhosis. The most common cause is a chronic, excessive alcohol intake. Exposure to certain industrial chemicals also can lead to cirrhosis.

cis fatty acid A form of an unsaturated fatty acid that has the hydrogens lying on the same side of the carbon-carbon double bond.

clinical assessment Examination of general appearance of skin, eyes, and tongue; evidence of rapid hair loss; sense of touch; and ability to cough and walk.

coagulation Blood clotting; essentially a transition of blood from a liquid cell suspension into a solid, gel-like form.

coenzyme A compound that combines with an inactive enzyme to form a catalytically active form. In this manner, coenzymes aid in enzyme function.

cofactor A mineral or other substance that binds to a specific region on a protein, such as an enzyme, and is necessary for the protein's function.

cognitive behavior therapy Psychological therapy in which the person's assumptions about dieting, body weight, and related issues are confronted. New ways of thinking are explored and then practiced by the person. In this way, an individual can learn new ways to control disordered eating behaviors and related life stress.

cognitive restructuring Changing one's frame of mind regarding eating—for example, instead of using a difficult day as an excuse to overeat, substituting other pleasures for rewards, such as a relaxing walk with a friend.

colostrum The first fluid secreted by the breast during late pregnancy and the first few days after birth. This thick fluid is rich in immune factors and protein.

Community-supported agriculture (CSA) Farms that are supported by a community of growers and consumers who provide mutual support and share the risks and benefits of food production, usually including a system of weekly delivery or pick-up of vegetables and fruit, sometimes dairy products and meat.

complementary proteins Two food protein sources that make up for each other's inadequate supply of specific essential amino acids;

together they yield a sufficient amount of all nine and, so provide high-quality (complete) protein for the diet.

complex carbohydrate Carbohydrate composed of many monosaccharide molecules. Examples include glycogen, starch, and fiber.

compound A group of different types of atoms bonded together in definite proportion.

compression of morbidity Delay of the onset of disabilities caused by chronic disease.

connective tissue Protein tissue that holds different structures in the body together. Some body structures are made up of connective tissue— notably, tendons and cartilage. Connective tissue also forms part of bone and the nonmuscular structures of arteries and veins.

constipation A condition characterized by infrequent bowel movements.

contingency management Forming a plan of action to respond to a situation in which overeating is likely, such as when snacks are within arm's reach at a party.

control group Participants in an experiment who are not given the treatment being tested.

cortical bone Dense, compact bone that comprises the outer surface and shafts of bone; also called compact bone.

creatine An organic (i.e., carbon-containing) molecule in muscle cells that serves as a part of a high-energy compound (termed creatine phosphate or phosphocreatine) capable of synthesizing ATP from ADP.

cretinism The stunting of body growth and poor mental development in the offspring that results from inadequate maternal intake of iodide during pregnancy.

cystic fibrosis Inherited disease that can cause overproduction of mucus. Mucus can block the pancreatic duct, decreasing enzyme output.

cytoplasm The fluid and organelles (except the nucleus) in a cell.

Delaney Clause A clause to the 1958 Food Additives Amendment of the Pure Food and Drug Act in the United States that prevents the intentional (direct) addition to foods of a compound shown to cause cancer in laboratory animals or humans.

dementia A general loss or decrease in mental function.

denaturation Alteration of a protein's three-dimensional structure, usually because of treatment by heat, enzymes, acid or alkaline solutions, or agitation.

dental caries Erosions in the surface of a tooth caused by acids made by bacteria as they metabolize sugars.

deoxyribonucleic acid (DNA) The site of hereditary information in cells; DNA directs the synthesis of cell proteins.

diastolic blood pressure The pressure in the arterial blood vessels when the heart is between beats.

dietary assessment Estimation of typical food choices relying mostly on the recounting of one's usual intake or a record of one's previous days' intake.

dietary fiber Fiber found in food.

Dietary Guidelines for Americans General goals for nutrient intakes and diet composition set by the USDA and the U.S. Department of Health and Human Services.

Dietary Reference Intakes (DRIs) Term used to encompass nutrient recommendations made by the Food and Nutrition Board of the National Academy of Sciences. These include RDAs, EARs, AIs, EERs, and ULs.

digestion The process by which large ingested molecules are mechanically and chemically broken down to produce basic nutrients that can be absorbed across the wall of the GI tract.

digestive system The body system consisting of the gastrointestinal tract and accessory structures such as the liver, gallbladder, and pancreas. This system performs the mechanical and chemical processes of digestion, absorption of nutrients, and elimination of wastes.

diglyceride A breakdown product of a triglyceride consisting of two fatty acids bonded to a glycerol backbone.

direct calorimetry A method of determining a body's energy use by measuring heat released from the body. An insulated chamber is usually used.

disaccharide Class of sugars formed by the chemical bonding of two monosaccharides.

discretionary calories The calories allowed in a diet after the person has met overall nutrition needs. This generally small amount of calories gives individuals the flexibility to consume some foods and beverages that may contain alcohol (e.g., beer and wine), added sugars (e.g., soft drinks, candy, and desserts), or added fats that are part of moderate- or high-fat foods (e.g., many snack foods).

disordered eating Mild and short-term changes in eating patterns that occur in relation to a stressful event, an illness, or a desire to modify one's diet for a variety of health and personal appearance reasons.

diuretic A substance that increases the volume of urine.

diverticula Pouches that protrude through the exterior wall of the large intestine.

diverticulitis An inflammation of the diverticula caused by acids produced by bacterial metabolism inside the diverticula.

diverticulosis The condition of having many diverticula in the large intestine.

docosahexaenoic acid (DHA) An omega-3 fatty acid with 22 carbons and six carbon-carbon double bonds. It is present in large amounts in fatty fish and is slowly synthesized in the body from alpha-linolenic acid. DHA is especially present in the retina and brain.

double-blind study An experimental design in which neither the participants nor the researchers are aware of each participant's assignment (test or placebo) or the outcome of the study until it is completed. An independent third party holds the code and the data until the study has been completed.

dual energy X-ray absorptiometry (DEXA) A highly accurate method of measuring body composition and bone mass and density using multiple low-energy X rays.

early childhood caries Tooth decay that results from formula or juice (and even human milk) bathing the teeth as the child sleeps with a bottle in his or her mouth. The upper teeth are mostly affected as the lower teeth are protected by the tongue; formerly called *nursing bottle syndrome* and *baby bottle tooth decay*.

eating disorder Severe alterations in eating patterns linked to physiological changes. The alterations are associated with food restriction, binge eating, purging, and fluctuations in weight. They also involve a number of emotional and cognitive changes that affect the way a person perceives and experiences his or her body.

eating pattern A combination of foods and beverages that constitute an individual's complete dietary intake over time.

edema The buildup of excess fluid in extracellular spaces.

eicosapentaenoic acid (EPA) An omega-3 fatty acid with 20 carbons and five carbon-carbon double bonds. It is present in large amounts in fatty fish and is slowly synthesized in the body from alpha-linolenic acid.

electrolytes Substances that separate into ions in water and, in turn, are able to conduct an electrical current. These include sodium, chloride, and potassium.

element A substance that cannot be separated into simpler substances by chemical processes. Common elements in nutrition include carbon, oxygen, hydrogen, nitrogen, calcium, phosphorus, and iron.

elimination diet A restrictive diet that systematically tests foods that may cause an allergic response by first eliminating them for 1 to 2 weeks and then adding them back, one at a time.

embryo In humans, the developing offspring in utero from about the beginning of the third week to the end of the eighth week after conception.

empty calories Calories from solid fats and/or added sugars. Foods with empty calories supply energy but few or no other nutrients.

emulsifier A compound that can suspend fat in water by isolating individual fat droplets, using a shell of water molecules or other substances to prevent the fat from coalescing.

endocrine gland A hormone-producing gland.

endocrine system The body system consisting of the various glands and the hormones these glands secrete. This system has major regulatory functions in the body, such as reproduction and cell metabolism.

endometrium The membrane that lines the inside of the uterus. It increases in thickness during the menstrual cycle until ovulation occurs. The surface layers are shed during menstruation if conception does not take place.

endoplasmic reticulum (ER) An organelle in the cytoplasm composed of a network of canals running through the cytoplasm. Part of the endoplasmic reticulum contains ribosomes.

endorphins Natural body tranquilizers that may be involved in the feeding response and function in pain reduction.

energy balance The state in which energy intake, in the form of food and beverages, matches the energy expended, primarily through basal metabolism and physical activity.

energy density A comparison of the calorie (kcal) content of a food with the weight of the food. An energy-dense food is high in calories but weighs very little (e.g., potato chips), whereas a food low in energy density has few calories but weighs a lot, such as an orange.

enterohepatic circulation A continual recycling of compounds such as bile acids between the small intestine and the liver.

environmental assessment Includes details about living conditions, education level, and the ability of the person to purchase, transport, and cook food. The person's weekly budget for food purchases is also a key factor to consider.

enzyme A compound that speeds the rate of a chemical reaction but is not altered by the reaction. Almost all enzymes are proteins (some are made of genetic material).

epidemiology The study of how disease rates vary among different population groups.

epiglottis The flap that folds down over the trachea during swallowing.

epigenetics Inherited changes in gene expression caused by mechanisms other than changes in the DNA sequence.

epigenome The way that the genome is marked and packaged inside the cell nucleus.

epinephrine A hormone also known as *adrenaline*; it is released by the adrenal glands (located on each kidney) and various nerve endings in the body. It acts to increase glycogen breakdown in the liver, among other functions.

epithelial cells The cells that line the outside of the body and the inside of all external passages within it, such as the GI tract.

epithelial tissue The surface cells that line the outside of the body and all external passages within it.

ergogenic Work-producing. An ergogenic aid is a mechanical, nutritional, psychological, pharmacological, or physiological substance or treatment intended to directly improve exercise performance.

erythrocytes Mature red blood cells. These have no nucleus and a life span of about 120 days; they contain hemoglobin, which transports oxygen and carbon dioxide.

erythropoietin A hormone secreted mostly by the kidneys that enhances red blood cell synthesis and stimulates red blood cell release from bone marrow.

esophagus A tube in the GI tract that connects the pharynx with the stomach.

essential amino acids The amino acids that cannot be synthesized by humans in sufficient amounts or at all and therefore must be included in the diet; there are nine essential amino acids. These are also called *indispensable amino acids.*

essential fatty acids Fatty acids that must be supplied by the diet to maintain health. Currently, only linoleic acid and alpha-linolenic acid are classified as essential.

essential nutrient In nutritional terms, a substance that, when left out of a diet, leads to signs of poor health. The body either cannot produce this nutrient or cannot produce enough of it to meet its needs. Then, if added back to a diet before permanent damage occurs, the affected aspects of health are restored.

estimated Energy Requirement (EER) Estimate of the energy (kcal) intake needed to match the energy use of an average person in a specific life stage.

ethanol Chemical term for the form of alcohol found in alcoholic beverages.

extracellular fluid Fluid present outside the cells; represents about one-third of body fluid.

extracellular space The space outside cells; represents one-third of body fluid.

famine An extreme shortage of food, which leads to massive starvation in a population; often associated with crop failures, war, and political unrest.

fasting hypoglycemia Low blood glucose that follows about a day of fasting.

fat-soluble vitamins Vitamins that dissolve in fat and such substances as ether and benzene but not readily in water. These vitamins are A, D, E, and K.

fatty acid Major part of most lipids; primarily composed of a chain of carbons flanked by hydrogen.

female athlete triad A condition characterized by disordered eating, lack of menstrual periods (amenorrhea), and osteoporosis.

fermentation The conversion of carbohydrates to alcohols, acids, and carbon dioxide without the use of oxygen.

fetal alcohol effects (FAE) Hyperactivity, attention deficit disorder, poor judgment, sleep disorders, and delayed learning as a result of prenatal exposure to alcohol.

fetal alcohol spectrum disorders (FASDs) A group of irreversible physical and mental abnormalities in the infant that result from the mother's consuming alcohol during pregnancy. [NOTE: This is previous definition for *fetal alcohol syndrome (FAS)*.]

fetal alcohol syndrome (FAS) Severe form of FASD that involves abnormal facial features and problems with development of the nervous system and overall growth as a result of maternal alcohol consumption during pregnancy.

fetus The developing human life form from 8 weeks after conception until birth.

fiber Substances in plant foods not digested by the processes that take place in the human stomach or small intestine. These add bulk to feces. Fiber naturally found in foods is also called dietary fiber.

food desert An area where 33% or 500 people, whichever is less, live more than a mile from a grocery store in an urban area or more than 10 miles away in a rural area.

food insecure Condition in which the quality, variety, and/or desirability of the diet is reduced and there is difficulty at times providing enough food for everyone in the household.

food insecurity A condition of anxiety regarding running out of either food or money to buy more food.

food intolerance An adverse reaction to food that does not involve an allergic reaction.

food sensitivity A mild reaction to a substance in a food that might be expressed as slight itching or redness of the skin.

foodborne illness Sickness caused by the ingestion of food containing harmful substances.

fructose A six-carbon monosaccharide that usually exists in a ring form; found in fruits and honey; also known as *fruit sugar*.

fruitarian A person who primarily eats fruits, nuts, honey, and vegetable oils.

functional fiber Fiber added to foods that has been shown to provide health benefits.

functional foods Foods that provide health benefits beyond those supplied by the traditional nutrients they contain. For example, a tomato contains the phytochemical lycopene, so it can be called a functional food.

fungi Simple parasitic life forms, including molds, mildews, yeasts, and mushrooms. They live on dead or decaying organic matter. Fungi can grow as single cells, like yeast, or as a multicellular colony, as seen with molds.

galactose A six-carbon monosaccharide that usually exists in a ring form; closely related to glucose.

gallbladder An organ attached to the underside of the liver; site of bile storage, concentration, and eventual secretion.

gastroesophageal reflux disease (GERD) Disease that results from stomach acid backing up into the esophagus. The acid irritates the lining of the esophagus, causing pain.

gastrointestinal (GI) tract The main sites in the body used for digestion and absorption of nutrients. It consists of the mouth, esophagus, stomach, small intestine, large intestine, rectum, and anus. Also called the digestive tract.

gastroplasty Gastric bypass surgery performed on the stomach to limit its volume to approximately 30 milliliters. Also referred to as stomach stapling.

gender and development (GAD) approach Understanding the roles and responsibilities of both men and women in the process of sustainable development.

gene A specific segment on a chromosome. Genes provide the blueprint for the production of cell proteins.

gene expression Use of DNA information on a gene to produce a protein. Thought to be a major determination of cell development.

generally recognized as safe (GRAS) A list of food additives that in 1958 were considered safe for consumption. Manufacturers were allowed to continue to use these additives, without special clearance, when needed for food products. FDA bears responsibility for proving they are not safe, but can remove unsafe products from the list.

genetic engineering Manipulation of the genetic makeup of any organism with recombinant DNA technology.

genetically modified organism (GMO) Any organism created by genetic engineering.

gestation The period of intrauterine development of offspring, from conception to birth; in humans, gestation lasts for about 40 weeks after the woman's previous menstrual period.

gestational diabetes A high blood glucose concentration that develops during pregnancy and returns to normal after birth; one cause is the placental production of hormones that antagonize the regulation of blood glucose by insulin.

ghrelin A hormone made by the stomach that increases the desire to eat.

glucagon A hormone made by the pancreas that stimulates the breakdown of glycogen in the liver into glucose; this ends up increasing blood glucose. Glucagon also performs other functions.

glucose A six-carbon sugar that exists in a ring form; found as such in blood, and in table sugar bound to fructose; also known as *dextrose*, it is one of the simple sugars.

glycemic index (GI) The blood glucose response of a given food, compared to a standard (typically, glucose or white bread). Glycemic index is influenced by starch structure; fiber content; food processing; physical structure; and macronutrients in the meal, such as fat.

glycemic load (GL) The amount of carbohydrate in a serving of food multiplied by the glycemic index of that carbohydrate. The result is then divided by 100.

glycerol A three-carbon alcohol used to form triglycerides.

glycogen A carbohydrate made of multiple units of glucose with a highly branched structure. It is the storage form of glucose in humans and is synthesized (and stored) in the liver and muscles.

glycosylation The process by which glucose attaches to (glycates) other compounds, such as proteins.

goiter An enlargement of the thyroid gland; this is often caused by insufficient iodide in the diet.

Golgi complex The cell organelle near the nucleus that processes newly synthesized protein for secretion or distribution to other organelles.

green revolution This refers to increases in crop yields that accompanied the introduction of new agricultural technologies in less-developed countries, beginning in the 1960s. The key technologies were high-yielding, disease-resistant strains of rice, wheat, and corn; greater use of fertilizer and water; and improved cultivation practices.

gruels A thin mixture of grains or legumes in milk or water.

gums A viscous fiber containing chains of galactose, glucuronic acid, and other monosaccharides; characteristically found in exudates from plant stems.

H2 blocker Medication, such as cimetidine (Tagamet®), that blocks the increase of stomach acid production caused by histamine.

heart attack Rapid fall in heart function caused by reduced blood flow through the heart's blood vessels. Often part of the heart dies in the process. Technically called a myocardial infarction.

heat cramps A frequent complication of heat exhaustion. They usually occur in people who have experienced large sweat losses from exercising for several hours in a hot climate and have consumed a large volume of water. The cramps occur in skeletal muscles and consist of contractions for 1 to 3 minutes at a time.

heat exhaustion The first stage of heat-related illness that occurs because of depletion of blood volume from fluid loss by the body. This increases body temperature and can lead to headache, dizziness, muscle weakness, and visual disturbances, among other effects.

heatstroke Heatstroke can occur when internal body temperature reaches 104°F. Sweating generally ceases if left untreated, and blood circulation is greatly reduced. Nervous system damage may ensue, and death is likely. Often the skin of individuals who suffer heatstroke is hot and dry.

helminth Parasitic worm that can contaminate food, water, feces, animals, and other substances.

hematocrit The percentage of blood made up of red blood cells.

heme iron Iron provided from animal tissues in the form of hemoglobin and myoglobin. Approximately 40% of the iron in meat is heme iron; it is readily absorbed.

hemicellulose A nonfermentable fiber containing xylose, galactose, glucose, and other monosaccharides bonded together.

hemochromatosis A disorder of iron metabolism characterized by increased iron absorption and deposition in the liver and heart tissue. This eventually poisons the cells in those organs.

hemoglobin The iron-containing part of the red blood cell that carries oxygen to the cells and some carbon dioxide away from the cells. The heme iron portion is also responsible for the red color of blood.

hemolysis Destruction of red blood cells. The red blood cell membrane breaks down, allowing cell contents to leak into the fluid portion of the blood.

hemorrhage An escape of blood from blood vessels.

hemorrhagic stroke Damage to part of the brain resulting from rupture of a blood vessel and subsequent bleeding within or over the internal surface of the brain.

hemorrhoid A pronounced swelling of a large vein, particularly veins found in the anal region.

high-density lipoprotein (HDL) The lipoprotein in the blood that picks up cholesterol from dying cells and other sources and transfers it to the other lipoproteins in the bloodstream, as well as directly to the liver; low HDL increases the risk for cardiovascular disease.

high-quality (complete) proteins Dietary proteins that contain ample amounts of all nine essential amino acids.

histamine A breakdown product of the amino acid histidine that stimulates acid secretion by the stomach and has other effects on the body, such as contraction of smooth muscles, increased nasal secretions, relaxation of blood vessels, and changes in relaxation of airways.

hormone A compound secreted into the bloodstream by one type of cell that acts to control the function of another type of cell. For example, certain cells in the pancreas produce insulin, which in turn acts on muscle and other types of cells to promote uptake of nutrients from the blood.

hospice care A facility offering care that emphasizes comfort and dignity in death.

human immunodeficiency virus (HIV) The virus that leads to acquired immune deficiency syndrome (AIDS).

hunger The primarily physiological (internal) drive to find and eat food, mostly regulated by internal cues to eating.

hydrogenation The addition of hydrogen to a carbon-carbon double bond, producing a single carbon-carbon bond with two hydrogens attached to each carbon. Hydrogenation of unsaturated fatty acids in a vegetable oil increases its hardness, so this process is used to convert liquid oils into more solid fats, used in making margarine and shortening. *Trans* fatty acids are a by-product of hydrogenation of vegetable oils.

hyperglycemia High blood glucose, above 125 milligrams per 100 milliliters of blood.

hypoglycemia Low blood glucose, below 40 to 50 milligrams per 100 milliliters of blood.

hypothalamus A region at the base of the brain that contains cells that play a role in the regulation of hunger, respiration, body temperature, and other body functions.

hypotheses Tentative explanations by a scientist to explain a phenomenon.

identical twins Two offspring that develop from a single ovum and sperm and, consequently, have the same genetic makeup.

ileocecal sphincter The ring of smooth muscle between the end of the small intestine and the large intestine.

immune system The body system consisting of white blood cells, lymph glands and vessels, and various other body tissues. The immune system provides defense against foreign invaders, primarily due to the action of various types of white blood cells.

immunoglobulins Proteins found in the blood that bind to specific antigens; also called antibodies. The five major classes of immunoglobulins play different roles in antibody-mediated immunity.

incidental food additives Additives that appear in food products indirectly, from environmental contamination of food ingredients or during the manufacturing process.

indirect calorimetry A method to measure energy use by the body by measuring oxygen uptake. Formulas are then used to convert this gas exchange value into energy use.

infrastructure The basic framework of a system of organization. For a society, this includes roads, bridges, telephones, and other basic technologies.

inorganic Any substance lacking carbon atoms bonded to hydrogen atoms in the chemical structure.

insulin A hormone produced by the pancreas. Among other processes, insulin increases the synthesis of glycogen in the liver and the movement of glucose from the bloodstream into body cells.

intentional food additives Additives knowingly (directly) incorporated into food products by manufacturers.

international unit (IU) A crude measure of vitamin activity, often based on the growth rate of animals in response to the vitamin. Today IUs have largely been replaced by more precise milligram or microgram measures.

intracellular fluid Fluid contained within a cell; it represents about two-thirds of body fluid.

intrinsic factor A proteinlike compound produced by the stomach that enhances vitamin B-12 absorption.

ion An atom with an unequal number of electrons and protons. Negative ions have more electrons than protons; positive ions have more protons than electrons.

irradiation A process in which radiation energy is applied to foods, creating compounds (free radicals) within the food that destroy cell membranes, break down DNA, link proteins together, limit enzyme activity, and alter a variety of other proteins and cell functions of microorganisms that can lead to food spoilage. This process does not make the food radioactive.

isomers Different chemical structures for compounds that share the same chemical formula.

ketone bodies Partial breakdown products of fat that contain three or four carbons.

ketosis The condition of having a high concentration of ketone bodies and related breakdown products in the bloodstream and tissues.

kidney nephrons The units of kidney cells that filter wastes from the bloodstream and deposit them into the urine.

kilocalorie (kcal) Heat energy needed to raise the temperature of 1000 grams (1 L) of water 1 degree Celsius; also written as *Calories*.

kwashiorkor A disease occurring primarily in young children who have an existing disease and consume a marginal amount of calories and insufficient protein in relation to needs. The child generally suffers from infections and exhibits edema, poor growth, weakness, and an increased susceptibility to further illness.

lactase An enzyme made by absorptive cells of the small intestine; this enzyme digests lactose to glucose and galactose.

lactation The period of milk secretion following pregnancy; typically called *breast-feeding*.

lactic acid A three-carbon acid formed during anaerobic cell metabolism; a partial breakdown product of glucose; also called *lactate*.

Lactobacillus bifidus **factor** A protective factor secreted in the colostrum that encourages growth of beneficial bacteria in the newborn's intestines.

lactoovovegetarian A person who consumes plant products, dairy products, and eggs.

lactose intolerance A condition in which symptoms such as abdominal gas and bloating appear as a result of severe lactose maldigestion.

lactose maldigestion (primary and secondary) Primary lactose maldigestion occurs when production of the enzyme lactase declines for no apparent reason. Secondary lactose maldigestion occurs when a specific cause, such as long-standing diarrhea, results in a decline in lactase production. When significant symptoms develop after lactose intake, it is then called lactose intolerance.

lactose Glucose bonded to galactose; also known as *milk sugar*.

lactovegetarian A person who consumes plant products and dairy products.

lanugo Down-like hair that appears after a person has lost much body fat through semi-starvation. The hair stands erect and traps air, acting as insulation for the body to compensate for the relative lack of body fat, which usually functions as insulation.

laxative A medication or other substance that stimulates evacuation of the intestinal tract.

lean body mass Body weight minus fat storage weight equals lean body mass. This includes organs such as the brain, muscles, and liver, as well as bone and blood and other body fluids.

lecithin A group of phospholipid compounds that are major components of cell membranes.

leptin A hormone made by adipose tissue in proportion to total fat stores in the body that influences long-term regulation of fat mass. Leptin also influences reproductive functions, as well as other body processes, such as release of the hormone insulin.

let-down reflex A reflex stimulated by infant suckling that causes the release (ejection) of milk from milk ducts in the mother's breasts; also called *milk ejection reflex.*

life expectancy The average length of life for a given group of people born in a specific year (such as this year).

life span The potential oldest age a person can reach.

lignins A nonfermentable fiber made up of a multiringed alcohol (noncarbohydrate) structure.

limiting amino acid The essential amino acid in lowest concentration in a food or diet relative to body needs.

linoleic acid An essential omega-6 fatty acid with 18 carbons and two double bonds.

lipase Fat-digesting enzyme produced by the salivary glands, stomach, and pancreas.

lipid A compound containing much carbon and hydrogen, little oxygen, and sometimes other atoms. Lipids do not dissolve in water, and include fats, oils, and cholesterol.

lipoprotein A compound found in the blood-stream containing a core of lipids with a shell composed of protein, phospholipid, and cholesterol.

lipoprotein lipase An enzyme attached to the cells that form the inner lining of blood vessels; it breaks down triglycerides into free fatty acids and glycerol.

lobules Saclike structures in the breast that store milk.

locavore Someone who eats food grown or produced locally or within a certain radius such as 50, 100, or 500 miles.

long-chain fatty acid A fatty acid that contains 12 or more carbons.

low birth weight (LBW) Referring to any infant weighing less than 2.5 kilograms (5.5 pounds) at birth; most commonly results from preterm birth.

low-density lipoprotein (LDL) The lipoprotein in the blood containing primarily cholesterol; elevated LDL is strongly linked to cardiovascular disease risk.

lower esophageal sphincter A circular muscle that constricts the opening of the esophagus to the stomach. Also called the *gastroesophageal sphincter.*

lower-body obesity The type of obesity in which fat storage is primarily located in the buttocks and thigh area. Also known as gynoid or gynecoid obesity.

lower-quality (incomplete) proteins Dietary proteins that are low in or lack one or more essential amino acids.

lymph A clear fluid that flows through lymph vessels; carries most forms of fat after their absorption by the small intestine.

lymphatic system A system of vessels and lymph that accepts fluid surrounding cells and large particles, such as products of fat absorption. Lymph eventually passes into the blood-stream from the lymphatic system.

lysosome A cellular organelle that contains digestive enzymes for use inside the cell for turnover of cell parts.

lysozyme An enzyme produced by a variety of cells; it can destroy bacteria by rupturing their cell membranes.

macronutrient A nutrient needed in gram quantities in a diet.

macular degeneration A painless condition leading to disruption of the central part of the retina (in the eye) and, in turn, blurred vision.

major mineral A mineral vital to health that is required in the diet in amounts greater than 100 milligrams per day.

malignant Malicious; in reference to a tumor, the property of spreading locally and to distant sites.

malnutrition Failing health that results from long-standing dietary practices that do not coincide with nutritional needs.

maltase An enzyme made by absorptive cells of the small intestine; this enzyme digests maltose to two glucoses.

maltose Glucose bonded to glucose.

marasmus A disease resulting from consuming a grossly insufficient amount of protein and calories; one of the diseases classed as protein-calorie malnutrition. Victims have little or no fat stores, little muscle mass, and poor strength. Death from infections is common.

megadose Intake of a nutrient beyond estimates of needs to prevent a deficiency or what would be found in a balanced diet; 2 to 10 times human needs is a starting point for such a pharmacological dosage.

megaloblast A large, immature red blood cell that results from the particular cell's inability to divide normally.

megaloblastic anemia Anemia characterized by the presence of abnormally large red blood cells.

menarche The onset of menstruation. Menarche usually occurs around age 13, 2 or 3 years after the first signs of puberty start to appear.

menopause The cessation of the menstrual cycle in women, usually beginning at about 50 years of age.

metabolic syndrome A condition in which a person has poor blood glucose regulation, hypertension, increased blood triglycerides, and other health problems. This condition is usually accompanied by obesity, lack of physical activity, and a diet high in refined carbohydrates. Also called Syndrome X.

metabolism Chemical processes in the body by which energy is provided in useful forms and vital activities are sustained.

metastasize The spreading of disease from one part of the body to another, even to parts of the body that are remote from the site of the original tumor. Cancer cells can spread via blood vessels, the lymphatic system, or direct growth of the tumor.

methyl group CH_3

micronutrient A nutrient needed in milligram or microgram quantities in a diet.

microorganism Bacteria, virus, or other organism invisible to the naked eye, some of which cause diseases. Also called *microbes.*

mineral Element used in the body to promote chemical reactions and to form body structures.

mitochondria The main sites of energy production in a cell. They contain the pathway for oxidizing fat for fuel, among other metabolic pathways.

moderate-intensity aerobic physical activity Aerobic activity that increases a person's heart rate and breathing to some extent (5–6 on RPE scale). Examples include brisk walking, dancing, swimming, or bicycling on level terrain.

monoglyceride A breakdown product of a triglyceride consisting of one fatty acid attached to a glycerol backbone.

monosaccharide Simple sugar, such as glucose, that is not broken down further during digestion.

monounsaturated fatty acid A fatty acid containing one carbon-carbon double bond.

motility Generally, the ability to move spontaneously. It also refers to movement of food through the GI tract.

mottling The discoloration or marking of the surface of teeth from fluorosis.

mucilages A viscous fiber consisting of chains of galactose, mannose, and other monosaccharides; characteristically found in seaweed.

mucus A thick fluid secreted by many cells throughout the body. It contains a compound that has both carbohydrate and protein parts. It acts as a lubricant and means of protection for cells.

muscle dysmorphia psychological condition in which a person preceives him-or herself as too thin or small, despite normal or above-average muscularity. People with this condition engage in disordered eating and extreme exercise practices in the pursuit of hypermuscularity.

muscle tissue A type of tissue adapted to contract to cause movement.

muscle-strengthening activity Physical activity, including exercise, that increases skeletal muscle strength, power, endurance, and mass. Examples include strength training, resistance training, and muscle strength and endurance exercises.

myelin sheath A lipid and protein combination (lipoprotein) that covers nerve fibers.

myocardial infarction Death of part of the heart muscle. Also termed a *heart attack.*

myoglobin Iron-containing protein that binds oxygen in muscle tissue.

negative energy balance The state in which energy intake is less than energy expended, resulting in weight loss.

negative protein balance A state in which protein intake is less than related protein losses, such as often seen during acute illness.

neotame General-purpose, non-nutritive sweetener that is approximately 7000 to 13,000 times sweeter than table sugar. It has a chemical structure similar to aspartame's.

nervous system The body system consisting of the brain, spinal cord, nerves, and sensory receptors. This system detects sensations, directs movements, and controls physiological and intellectual functions.

nervous tissue Tissue composed of highly branched, elongated cells, which transport nerve impulses from one part of the body to another.

neural tube defect A defect in the formation of the neural tube occurring during early fetal development. This type of defect results in various nervous system disorders, such as spina bifida. Folate deficiency in the pregnant woman increases the risk that the fetus will develop this disorder.

neuron The structural and functional unit of the nervous system. Consists of a **cell body, dendrites,** and an **axon.**

neuropeptide Y A chemical substance made in the hypothalamus that stimulates food intake. The hormone leptin inhibits neuropeptide Y production.

neurotransmitter A compound made by a nerve cell that allows for communication between it and other cells.

night blindness A vitamin A deficiency condition in which the retina (in the eye) cannot adjust to low amounts of light.

night eating syndrome Eating a lot of food in the late evening and nocturnal awakenings with ingestion of food.

nitrosamine A carcinogen formed from nitrates and breakdown products of amino acids; can lead to stomach cancer.

non-specific immunity Defenses that stop the invasion of pathogens; requires no previous encounter with a pathogen.

nonessential amino acids Amino acids that can be synthesized by a healthy body in sufficient amounts; there are 11 nonessential amino acids. These are also called *dispensable amino acids.*

nonfermentable fiber A fiber that is not easily metabolized by intestinal bacteria.

nonheme iron Iron provided from plant sources and animal tissues other than in the forms of hemoglobin and myoglobin. Nonheme iron is less efficiently absorbed than heme iron; absorption is closely dependent on body needs.

norepinephrine A neurotransmitter from nerve endings and a hormone from the adrenal gland. It is released in times of stress and is involved in hunger regulation, blood glucose regulation, and other body processes.

NSAIDs Nonsteroidal anti-inflammatory drugs; includes aspirin, ibuprofen (Advil®), and naproxen (Aleve®).

nutrient density The ratio derived by dividing a food's nutrient content by its calorie content. When the food's contribution to our nutrient need for that nutrient exceeds its contribution to our calorie need, the food is considered to have a favorable nutrient density.

nutrients Chemical substances in food that contribute to health, many of which are essential parts of a diet. Nutrients nourish us by providing calories to fulfill energy needs, materials for building body parts, and factors to regulate necessary chemical processes in the body.

nutrigenomics Study of how food impacts health through its interaction with our genes and its subsequent effect on gene expression.

nutritional state The nutritional health of a person as determined by anthropometric measurements (height, weight, circumferences, and so on), biochemical measurements of nutrients or their by-products in blood and urine, a clinical (physical) examination, a dietary analysis, and economic evaluation; also called nutritional status.

obesogenic Tending to promote obesity by encouraging excessive calorie intake and/or discouraging physical activity.

oleic acid An omega-9 fatty acid with 18 carbons and one double bond.

omega-3 (ω-3) fatty acid An unsaturated fatty acid with the first double bond on the third carbon from the methyl end (CH_3).

omega-6 (ω-6) fatty acid An unsaturated fatty acid with the first double bond on the sixth carbon from the methyl end (CH_3).

organ A group of tissues designed to perform a specific function—for example, the heart, which contains muscle tissue, nerve tissue, and so on.

organ system A collection of organs that work together to perform an overall function.

organelles Compartments, particles, or filaments that perform specialized functions within a cell.

organic Any substance that contains carbon atoms bonded to hydrogen atoms in the chemical structure.

osmosis The passage of a solvent such as water through a semipermeable membrane from a less concentrated compartment to a more concentrated compartment.

osteomalacia Adult form of rickets. The weakening of the bones seen in this disease is caused by low calcium content. A reduction in the amount of the vitamin D hormone in the body is one cause.

osteoporosis Decreased bone mass related to the effects of aging, genetic background, and poor diet in both genders, and hormonal changes at menopause in women.

ostomy Surgically created short circuit in intestinal flow where the end point usually opens from the abdominal cavity rather than the anus—for example, a colostomy. Short circuiting the intestinal flow means more water is lost in fecal matter than would be if the intestinal tract were intact.

overnutrition A state in which nutritional intake greatly exceeds the body's needs.

ovum The egg cell from which a fetus eventually develops if the egg is fertilized by a sperm cell.

oxalic acid (oxalate) An organic acid found in spinach, rhubarb, and other leafy green vegetables that can depress the absorption of certain minerals present in the food, such as calcium.

oxidize In the most basic sense, the loss of an electron or gain of an oxygen by a chemical substance. This change typically alters the shape and/or function of the substance.

oxytocin A hormone secreted by the pituitary gland. It causes contraction of the musclelike cells surrounding the ducts of the breasts and the smooth muscle of the uterus.

parasite An organism that lives in or on another organism and derives nourishment from it.

parathyroid hormone (PTH) A hormone made by the parathyroid glands that increases synthesis of the vitamin D hormone and aids calcium release from bone and calcium conservation by the kidneys, among other functions.

pasteurizing The process of heating food products to kill pathogenic microorganisms and reduce the total number of bacteria.

pectin A viscous fiber containing chains of galacturonic acid and other monosaccharides; characteristically found between plant cell walls.

pepsin A protein-digesting enzyme produced by the stomach.

peptide bond A chemical bond formed between amino acids in a protein.

percentile Classification of a measurement of a unit into divisions of 100 units.

peristalsis A coordinated muscular contraction used to propel food down the gastrointestinal tract.

pernicious anemia The anemia that results from a lack of vitamin B-12 absorption; it is pernicious because of associated nerve degeneration that can result in eventual paralysis and death.

peroxisome A cell organelle that destroys toxic products within the cell.

pH A measure of relative acidity or alkalinity of a solution. The pH scale is 0 to 14. A pH of 7 is netural; a pH below 7 is acidic; a pH above 7 is alkaline.

phagocytes Cells that engulf substances; include neutrophils and macrophages.

phagocytosis A process in which a cell forms an indentation, and particles or fluids entering the indentation are then engulfed by the cell.

pharynx The organ of the digestive tract and respiratory tract located at the back of the oral and nasal cavities, commonly known as the throat.

phenylketonuria (PKU) Disease caused by a defect in the liver's ability to metabolize the amino acid phenylalanine into the amino acid tyrosine; untreated, toxic by-products of phenylalanine build up in the body and lead to mental retardation.

phosphocreatine (PCr) A high-energy compound that can be used to re-form ATP. It is used primarily during bursts of activity, such as lifting and jumping.

phospholipid Any of a class of fat-related substances that contain phosphorus, fatty acids, and a nitrogen-containing component. Phospholipids are an essential part of every cell.

photosynthesis Process by which plants use energy from the sun to synthesize energy-yielding compounds, such as glucose.

physical fitness The ability to perform moderate to vigorous activity without undue fatigue.

physiological anemia The normal increase in blood volume in pregnancy that dilutes the concentration of red blood cells, resulting in anemia; also called *hemodilution*.

phytic acid (phytate) A constituent of plant fibers that binds positive ions to its multiple phosphate groups.

phytochemical A chemical found in plants. Some phytochemicals may contribute to a reduced risk of cancer or cardiovascular disease in people who consume them regularly.

pica The practice of eating nonfood items, such as dirt, laundry starch, or clay.

placebo Generally a fake medicine or treatment used to disguise the treatments given to the participants in an experiment.

placenta An organ that forms in the uterus in pregnant women. Through this organ, oxygen and nutrients from the mother's blood are transferred to the fetus, and fetal wastes are removed. The placenta also releases hormones that maintain the state of pregnancy.

plaque A cholesterol-rich substance deposited in the blood vessels; it contains various white blood cells, smooth muscle cells, various proteins, cholesterol and other lipids, and eventually calcium.

plasma The fluid, extracellular portion of the circulating blood. This includes the blood serum plus all blood-clotting factors. In contrast, serum is the fluid that remains after clotting factors have been removed from plasma.

polypeptide A group of amino acids bonded together, from 50 to 2000 or more.

polysaccharide Class of complex carbohydrates containing many glucose units, from 10 to 1000 or more.

polyunsaturated fatty acid A fatty acid containing two or more carbon-carbon double bonds.

pool The amount of a nutrient stored within the body that can be mobilized when needed.

portal circulation The portion of the circulatory system that uses a large vein (portal vein) to carry nutrient-rich blood from capillaries in the intestines and portions of the stomach to the liver.

portal vein Large vein leaving the intestine and stomach and connecting to the liver.

positive energy balance The state in which energy intake is greater than energy expended, generally resulting in weight gain.

positive protein balance A state in which protein intake exceeds related protein losses, as is needed during times of growth.

prebiotic Substance that stimulates bacterial growth in the large intestines.

pregnancy-induced hypertension A serious disorder that can include high blood pressure, kidney failure, convulsions, and even death of the mother and fetus. Although its exact cause is not known, an adequate diet (especially adequate calcium intake) and prenatal care may prevent this disorder or limit its severity. Mild cases are known as *preeclampsia*; more severe cases are called *eclampsia* (formerly called *toxemia*).

preservatives Compounds that extend the shelf life of foods by inhibiting microbial growth or minimizing the destructive effect of oxygen and metals.

preterm An infant born before 37 weeks of gestation; also referred to as *premature*.

probiotic Product that contains specific types of bacteria. Use is intended to colonize the large intestine with the specific bacteria in the product. An example is yogurt.

prolactin A hormone secreted by the pituitary gland that stimulates the synthesis of milk in the breast.

prostate gland A solid, chestnut-shaped organ surrounding the first part of the urinary tract in the male. The prostate gland secretes substances into the semen.

protease Protein-digesting enzyme produced by the stomach, small intestine, and pancreas.

protein equilibrium A state in which protein intake is equal to related protein losses; the person is said to be in protein balance.

protein turnover The process by which cells break down old proteins and resynthesize new proteins. In this way the cell will have the proteins it needs to function at that time.

protein-calorie malnutrition (PCM) A condition resulting from regularly consuming insufficient amounts of calories and protein. The deficiency eventually results in body wasting, primarily of lean tissue, and an increased susceptibility to infections.

protein Food and body compounds made of amino acids; proteins contain carbon, hydrogen, oxygen, nitrogen, and sometimes other atoms, in a specific configuration. Proteins contain the form of nitrogen most easily used by the human body.

proton pump inhibitor A medication that inhibits the ability of gastric cells to secrete hydrogen ions. Low doses of this class of medications are also available without prescription (e.g., omeprazole [Prilosec]).

protozoa One-celled animals that are more complex than bacteria. Disease-causing protozoa can be spread through food and water.

provitamin/precursor A substance that can be made into a vitamin, if the body needs it.

pyloric sphincter The ring of smooth muscle between the stomach and the small intestine.

pyruvic acid A three-carbon compound formed during glucose metabolism; also called *pyruvate*.

radiation Literally, energy that is emitted from a center in all directions. Various forms of radiation energy include X-rays and ultra-violet rays from the sun.

rancid Containing products of decomposed fatty acids that have an unpleasant flavor and odor.

reactive hypoglycemia Low blood glucose that follows a meal high in simple sugars, with corresponding symptoms of irritability, headache, nervousness, sweating, and confusion; also called *postprandial hypoglycemia*.

receptor A site in a cell at which compounds (such as hormones) bind. Cells that contain receptors for a specific compound are partially controlled by that compound.

recombinant DNA technology A test tube technology that rearranges DNA sequences in an organism by cutting the DNA, adding or deleting a DNA sequence, and rejoining DNA molecules with a series of enzymes.

Recommended Dietary Allowance (RDA) Nutrient intake amount sufficient to meet the needs of 97% to 98% of the individuals in a specific life stage.

rectum Terminal portion of the large intestine.

registered dietitian (R.D.) A person who has completed a baccalaureate degree program approved by the American Dietetic Association, performed at least 1200 hours of supervised professional practice, passed a registration examination, and complies with continuing education requirements.

relapse prevention A series of strategies used to help prevent and cope with weight-control lapses, such as recognizing high-risk situations and deciding beforehand on appropriate responses.

reserve capacity The extent to which an organ can preserve essentially normal function despite decreasing cell number or cell activity.

resting metabolism The amount of calories the body uses when the person has not eaten in 4 hours and is resting (e.g., 15 to 30 minutes) and awake in a warm, quiet environment. It is roughly 6% higher than basal metabolism due to the less strict criteria for the test; often referred to as *resting metabolic rate (RMR)*.

retinoids Chemical forms of preformed vitamin A; one source is animal foods.

ribonucleic acid (RNA) The single-stranded nucleic acid involved in the transcription of genetic information and translation of that information into protein structure.

ribosomes Cytoplasmic particles that mediate the linking together of amino acids to form proteins; may exist freely in the cytoplasm or attached to endoplasmic reticulum.

rickets A disease characterized by poor mineralization of newly synthesized bones because of low calcium content. This deficiency disease arises in infants and children from insufficient amounts of the vitamin D hormone in the body.

saccharin Alternative sweetener that yields no energy to the body; 300 times sweeter than sucrose.

saliva Watery fluid, produced by the salivary glands in the mouth, that contains lubricants, enzymes, and other substances.

salivary amylase A starch-digesting enzyme produced by salivary glands.

salt Compound of sodium and chloride in a 40:60 ratio.

sarcopenia In general, loss of muscle tissue. Among older adults this loss of lean mass greatly increases their risk of illness and death.

sarcopenic obesity Loss of muscle mass accompanied by gains in fat mass.

satiety A state in which there is no longer a desire to eat; a feeling of satisfaction.

saturated fatty acid A fatty acid containing no carbon-carbon double bonds.

scavenger cells Specific form of white blood cells that can bury themselves in the artery wall and accumulate LDL. As these cells take up LDL, they contribute to the development of atherosclerosis.

scurvy The deficiency disease that results after a few weeks to months of consuming a diet that lacks vitamin C; pinpoint sites of bleeding on the skin are an early sign.

secretory vesicles Membrane-bound vesicles produced by the Golgi apparatus; contain protein and other compounds to be secreted by the cell.

self-monitoring Tracking foods eaten and conditions affecting eating; actions are usually recorded in a diary, along with location, time, and state of mind. This is a tool to help people understand more about their eating habits.

sequestrants Compounds that bind free metal ions. By so doing, they reduce the ability of ions to cause rancidity in foods containing fat.

serotonin A neurotransmitter synthesized from the amino acid tryptophan that affects mood (sense of calmness), behavior, and appetite, and induces sleep.

set point Often refers to the close regulation of body weight. It is not known what cells control this set point or how it functions in weight regulation. There is evidence, however, that mechanisms exist that help regulate weight.

sickle cell disease (sickle cell anemia) An illness that results from a malformation of the red blood cell because of an incorrect structure in part of its hemoglobin protein chains. The disease can lead to episodes of severe bone and joint pain, abdominal pain, headache, convulsions, paralysis, and even death.

simple sugar Monosaccharide or disaccharide in the diet.

small for gestational age (SGA) Referring to infants who weigh less than the expected weight for their length of gestation. This corresponds to less than 2.5 kilograms (5.5 pounds) in a full-term newborn. A preterm infant who is also SGA will most likely develop some medical complications.

solid fats Fats that are solid at room temperature, such as butter and margarine. Foods containing solid fats tend to be high in saturated fatty acids or *trans* fatty acids.

solvent A liquid substance in which other substances dissolve.

sorbitol Alcohol derivative of glucose that yields about 3 kcal/g but is slowly absorbed from the small intestine; used in some sugarless gums and dietetic foods.

specific immunity Function of lymphocytes directed at specific antigens.

spontaneous abortion Cessation of pregnancy and expulsion of the embryo or nonviable fetus prior to 20 weeks gestation. This is the result of natural causes, such as a genetic defect or developmental problem; also called *miscarriage* .

spores Dormant reproductive cells capable of turning into adult organisms without the help of another cell. Various bacteria and fungi form spores.

starch A carbohydrate made of multiple units of glucose attached together in a form the body can digest; also known as *complex carbohydrate*.

sterol A compound containing a multi-ring (steroid) structure and a hydroxyl group (–OH). Cholesterol is a typical example.

stevia Alternative sweetener derived from South American shrub; 100 to 300 times sweeter than sucrose.

stimulus control Altering the environment to minimize the stimuli for eating—for example, removing foods from sight and storing them in kitchen cabinets.

stress fracture A fracture that occurs from repeated jarring of a bone. Common sites include bones of the foot.

stroke A decrease or loss in blood flow to the brain that results from a blood clot or other change in arteries in the brain. This in turn causes the death of brain tissue. Also called a *cerebrovascular accident*.

subclinical Stage of a disease or disorder not severe enough to produce symptoms that can be detected or diagnosed.

sucralose Alternative sweetener that has chlorines in place of 3 hydroxyl (–OH) groups on sucrose; 600 times sweeter than sucrose.

sucrase An enzyme made by absorptive cells of the small intestine; this enzyme digests sucrose to glucose and fructose.

sucrose Fructose bonded to glucose; table sugar.

sugar A simple carbohydrate with the chemical composition $(CH_2O)_n$. The basic unit of all sugars is glucose, a six-carbon ring structure. The primary sugar in the diet is sucrose, which is made up of glucose and fructose.

sustainable agriculture Agricultural system that provides a secure living for farm families; maintains the natural environment and resources; supports the rural community; and offers respect and fair treatment to all involved, from farm workers to consumers to the animals raised for food.

sustainable development Economic growth that will simultaneously reduce poverty, protect the environment, and preserve natural capital.

symptom A change in health status noted by the person with the problem, such as stomach pain.

synapse The space between one neuron and another neuron (or cell).

systolic blood pressure The pressure in the arterial blood vessels associated with the pumping of blood from the heart.

teratogen A substance that may cause or increase the risk of a birth defect. Exposure to a teratogen does not always lead to a birth defect; its effects on the fetus depend on the dose, timing, and duration of exposure.

tetany A body condition marked by sharp contraction of muscles and failure to relax afterward; usually caused by abnormal calcium metabolism.

theory An explanation for a phenomenon that has numerous lines of evidence to support it.

thermic effect of food (TEF) The increase in metabolism that occurs during the digestion, absorption, and metabolism of energy-yielding nutrients. This represents 5% to 10% of calories consumed.

thermogenesis This term encompasses the ability of humans to regulate body temperature within narrow limits (thermoregulation). Two visible examples of thermogenesis are fidgeting and shivering when cold.

thyroid hormones Hormones produced by the thyroid gland that among their functions increase the rate of overall metabolism in the body.

tissues Collections of cells adapted to perform a specific function.

tocopherols The chemical name for some forms of vitamin E. The alpha form is the most potent.

Tolerable Upper Intake Level (UL) Maximum chronic daily intake level of a nutrient that is unlikely to cause adverse health effects in almost all people in a specific life stage.

total fiber Combination of dietary fiber and functional fiber in a food. Also just called *fiber*.

total parenteral nutrition The intravenous feeding of all necessary nutrients, including the most basic forms of protein, carbohydrates, lipids, vitamins, minerals, and electrolytes.

toxins Poisonous compounds produced by an organism that can cause disease.

trabecular bone The spongy, inner matrix of bone, found primarily in the spine, pelvis, and ends of bones; also called spongy or cancellous bone.

trace mineral A mineral vital to health that is required in the diet in amounts less than 100 milligrams per day.

trans fatty acids A form of an unsaturated fatty acid, usually a monounsaturated one when found in food, in which the hydrogens on both carbons forming that double bond lie on opposite sides of that bond, rather than on the same side, as in most natural fats. Stick margarine, shortenings, and deep fat-fried foods in general are rich sources.

transcription Information on DNA needed to make a protein is copied onto RNA.

transgenic Organism that contains genes originally present in another organism.

translation The information contained in RNA is used to determine the amino acids in a protein.

triglyceride The major form of lipid in the body and in food. It is composed of three fatty acids bonded to glycerol.

trimesters Three 13- to 14-week periods into which the normal pregnancy (the length of a normal pregnancy is about 40 weeks, measured from the first day of the woman's last menstrual period) is divided somewhat arbitrarily for purposes of discussion and analysis. Development of the offspring, however, is continuous throughout pregnancy, with no specific

physiological markers demarcating the transition from one trimester to the next.

trypsin A protein-digesting enzyme secreted by the pancreas to act in the small intestine.

tumor Mass of cells; may be cancerous (malignant) or noncancerous (benign).

type 1 diabetes A form of diabetes prone to ketosis and that requires insulin therapy.

type 2 diabetes A form of diabetes characterized by insulin resistance and often associated with obesity. Insulin therapy can be used but is often not required.

ulcer Erosion of the tissue lining, usually in the stomach (gastric ulcer) or the upper small intestine (duodenal ulcer). As a group these are generally referred to as peptic ulcers.

umami A brothy, meaty, savory flavor in some foods. Monosodium glutamate enhances this flavor when added to foods.

undernutrition Failing health that results from a long-standing dietary intake that is not enough to meet nutritional needs.

underwater weighing A method of estimating total body fat by weighing the individual on a standard scale and then weighing him or her again submerged in water. The difference between the two weights is used to estimate total body volume.

underweight A body mass index below 18.5. The cutoff is less precise than for obesity because this condition has been less studied.

unsaturated fatty acid A fatty acid containing one or more carbon-carbon double bonds.

upper-body obesity The type of obesity in which fat is stored primarily in the abdominal area; defined as a waist circumference more than 40 inches (102 centimeters) in men and more than 35 inches (89 centimeters) in women; closely associated with a high risk for cardiovascular disease, hypertension, and type 2 diabetes. Also known as android obesity.

urea Nitrogenous waste product of protein metabolism; major source of nitrogen in the urine.

ureter Tube that transports urine from the kidney to the urinary bladder.

urethra Tube that transports urine from the urinary bladder to the outside of the body.

urinary system The body system consisting of the kidneys, urinary bladder, and the ducts that carry urine. This system removes waste products from the circulatory system and regulates blood acid-base balance, overall chemical balance, and water balance in the body.

vegan A person who eats only plant foods.

vein A blood vessel that carries blood to the heart.

very-low-calorie diet (VLCD) Known also as *protein-sparing modified fast (PSMF)*, this diet allows a person 400 to 800 kcal per day, often in liquid form. Of this, 120 to 480 kcal is carbohydrate, and the rest is mostly high-quality protein.

very-low-density lipoprotein (VLDL) The lipoprotein created in the liver that carries cholesterol and lipids that have been taken up or newly synthesized by the liver.

vigorous-intensity aerobic physical activity Aerobic activity that greatly increases a person's heart rate and breathing (7–8 on RPE scale). Examples include jogging, singles tennis, swimming continuous laps, or bicycling uphill.

villi (singular, **villus**) The fingerlike protrusions into the small intestine that participate in digestion and absorption of food.

virus The smallest known type of infectious agent, many of which cause disease in humans. A virus is essentially a piece of genetic material surrounded by a coat of protein. They do not metabolize, grow, or move by themselves. They reproduce only with the aid of a living cellular host.

viscous fiber A fiber that is readily fermented by bacteria in the large intestine.

vitamin Compound needed in small amounts in the diet to help regulate and support chemical reactions and processes in the body.

water The universal solvent; chemically, H_2O. The body is composed of about 60% water. Water (fluid) needs are about 9 (women) or 13 (men) cups per day; needs are greater if one exercises heavily.

water-soluble vitamins Vitamins that dissolve in water. These vitamins are the B vitamins and vitamin C.

white blood cells One of the formed elements of the circulating blood system; also called *leukocytes*. White blood cells are able to squeeze through intracellular spaces and migrate. They phagocytize bacteria, fungi, and viruses, as well as detoxify proteins that may result from allergic reactions, cellular injury, and other immune system cells.

whole grains Grains containing the entire seed of the plant, including the bran, germ, and endosperm (starchy interior). Examples are whole-wheat and brown rice.

xerophthalmia Literally "dry eye." This is a cause of blindness that results from a vitamin A deficiency. A lack of mucus production by the eye, which leaves it at a greater risk of damage from surface dirt and bacteria.

xylitol Alcohol derivative of the 5-carbon monosaccharide xylose.

zygote The fertilized ovum; the cell resulting from the union of an egg cell (ovum) and sperm until it divides.

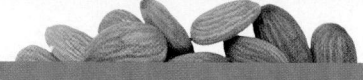
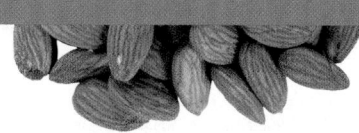

PHOTO CREDITS

Design Elements

Part One(apple): © Ingram Publishing/SuperStock/RF; Two(yellow pepper): © Getty Images/Stockbyte RF; Three(Onions): © Dynamic Graphics/PunchStock/RF; Four(Tomatoes): © Getty Images/Stockbyte/RF; Part Five(Pear): © Getty Images/Stockbyte/RF; "Nutrition and your Health"(banner of berries): © David Cook/blueshiftstudios/Alamy RFJ; "Rate your Plate"(Choose Your Plate.gov): Courtesy USDA; (soup bowl): © Burke/Triolo Productions/Getty Images RF.

Front Matter

(kebab): © The McGraw-Hill Companies, Inc., Kevin May Photography; (tomato): © Burke Triolo Productions/Getty Images RF; (radishes): © C Squared Studios/Getty Images RF; (cherries): © Burke Triolo Productions/Getty Images RF; (title page): © The McGraw-Hill Companies, Inc., Kevin May Photography.

Chapter 1

Opener: © Corbis/Punchstock RF; 1-1: © BananaStock/PunchStock RF; p. 5: © Stockbyte/PunchStock; p. 8: Reproduction with permission. © Culinary Hearts Kitchen; p. 9: © Photodisc/Getty Images RF; p. 12: © Royalty Free/Corbis; p. 13: Lifesize/Getty Images RF; p. 15 (both): Brand X RF; p. 19: Steve Cole/Getty Images RF; p. 20: U.S. Department of Health and Human Services. Office of Disease Prevention and Health Promotion. Healthy People 2020. Washington, DC; p. 22: RF/Getty Images; p. 23: © Digital Vision/PunchStock RF; p. 24: © Stockbyte/PunchStock RF; p. 25 (bottom): Punchstock RF; p. 26: © BananaStock/PunchStock RF; p. 27: © Blue Moon Stock/PunchStock RF; p. 28: © Image 100/Corbis RF; p. 30: © Stockbyte/Getty Images RF.

Chapter 2

Opener: © Plush Studios/Blend Images LLC RF; p. 36: © The McGraw-Hill Companies, Inc./Ken Karp, photographer; p. 38: Courtesy of U.S. Rice Federation; p. 39: © Comstock/PunchStock RF; p. 40: © Steve Allen/Getty Images RF; p. 41: © Photodisc/Vol. 67 RF; p. 42: © The McGraw-Hill Companies, Inc./Lars A. Niki, photographer; 2-3(Anthropometric): © The McGraw-Hill Companies, Inc./Lars A. Niki, photographer; (Biochemical): © Photodisc/Vol. 29 RF; (Clinical): © Photodisc Website RF; (Dietary): © Mike Kemp/Rubberball/Getty Images RF; (Environmental): © Comstock/PunchStock RF; p. 45: © Comstock/PunchStock RF; p. 49: © Corbis/Vol. 130 RF; 2-7 (women on scale): © David Buffington/Getty Images RF; (salt shaker): © Photodisc/Getty Images RF; (women w/ child in cart): © RF Getty Images; p. 53: © Karl Weatherly/Getty Images LLC RF; 2-9: © JGI/Blend Images LLC RF; p. 55 (top): © Peter Cade/Getty Images RF; (bottom): © Comstock/PunchStock RF; p. 56: Canada's Food Guide. Health Canada, 2007. Reproduced with the permission of the Minister of Health, 2011; 2-11: USDA; 2-12 (golf ball): © Corbis/Vol. 127 RF; (tennis ball): © Photodisc/OS25 RF; (cards): © The McGraw-Hill Companies, Inc./Jacques Cornell photographer; (baseball): © PhotoDisc/OS25 RF; p. 60: © Imagestate Media (John Foxx)/Imagestate RF; p. 61 (cereal): © Mitch Hrdlicka/Getty Images RF; (apple/sandwich): © Getty Images RF; (salmon): © C Squared Studios/Getty Images RF; p. 62: Office of Disease Prevention and Health Promotion, U.S. Department of Health and Human Services; p. 64: © Steve Cole/Getty Images RF; p. 66: © Ryan

McVay/Getty Images RF; p. 69, 70: © The McGraw-Hill Companies, Inc./Jill Braaten, photographer; p. 73 (dietitian): © liquidlibrary/PictureQuest RF; (pill): © Royalty Free/Corbis; p. 75: © Ingram Publishing RF.

Chapter 3

Opener: © Getty Images/Jonelle Weaver RF; 3-1: © Dynamic Graphics/JupiterImages RF; p. 86: © Photodisc RF; p. 99: © Ingram Publishing/SuperStock RF; p. 107: © PhotoDisc/Vol. 83 RF; p. 109: © Royalty Free/Corbis; p. 110: © Rob Meinychuk/Getty Images RF; 3-22b: © J. James/Photo Researchers, Inc.; p. 115: © C Squared Studios/Getty Images RF; p. 117 (top): © Gladden Willis, M.D./Visuals Unlimited; (bottom): © Stockdisc/Becky Denzin RF; p. 119 (top): © Getty Images/Jonelle Weaver RF; (bottom): © Royalty Free/Corbis.

Chapter 4

Opener: © Getty Images/Jonelle Weaver RF; p. 125: © Imagestate media (John Foxx)/Imagestate RF; p. 128: © C Squared Studios/Getty Images RF; p. 131: © Jupiterimages/ImageSource RF; 4-7(grains): Keith Weller/USDA; (vegetables): © Mitch Hrdlicka/Getty Images RF; (fruits): © Ingram Publishing/SuperStock RF; p. 132: © Ken Karp/McGraw-Hill Companies; p. 133: © BananaStock/PunchStock RF; p. 134(top): © BananaStock/PunchStock RF; (bottom): © Ryan McVay/Getty Images RF; p. 135: © Nancy R. Cohen/Getty Images RF; p. 136(top): © The McGraw-Hill Companies, Inc./Jill Braaten, photographer; (bottom): © Burke/Triolo Productions/Getty Images RF; p. 138: © Ingram Publishing/SuperStock RF; p. 139: Beano is a registered trademark of AkPharma Inc.; p. 140: © PhotoDisc/Getty Images RF; p. 142: © Royalty Free/Corbis; p. 143: © BananaStock/PunchStock RF; p. 145 (top): © John A. Rizzo/Getty Images RF; (bottom): © Nancy R. Cohen/Getty Images RF; p. 146: © Getty Images; p. 147: © Nancy R. Cohen/Getty Images RF; p. 148: © Brand X/Punchstock RF; p. 149: © BananaStock/PunchStock RF; Table 4-5(cart): © Photodisc/Getty Images RF; (kitchen utensils): © CMCD/Getty Images RF; (silverware): © The McGraw-Hill Companies, Inc./Jack Holtel photographer; p. 153: © Stockdisc/PunchStock RF; p. 154: © Ariel Skelley/Blend Images LLC RF; p. 155: Dynamic Graphics/JupiterImages RF; p. 157: © Getty Images/Eyewire RF; p. 159: © Real Food by Warren Diggles/Alamy RF; Table 4-7(Breakfast): © Image Source/Corbis RF; (Lunch): © BananaStock/PunchStock RF; (Dinner): © Getty Images/Jonelle Weaver RF; p. 162: © Kevin Sanchez/Cole Group/Getty Images RF.

Chapter 5

Opener: © Ingram Publishing/SuperStock RF; p. 167: © Tetra Images/Getty Images RF; p. 169: © The McGraw-Hill Companies, Inc./Elite Images; 5-5 (Avocado): © Ingram Publishing/SuperStock RF; (chicken & fries): © BananaStock/PunchStock RF; (cheese): © Pixtal/age fotostock RF; p. 172 (bottom): © Jamie Grill/Corbis RF; p. 173: © Burke/Tiolo Productions/Getty Images RF; p. 174: © Allan Rosenberg/Cole Group/Getty Images RF; p. 176(top): © D. Hurst/Alamy RF; (bottom): © The McGraw-Hill Companies Inc./Ken Cavanagh Photographer; p. 177: © Ingram Publishing/Alamy RF; p. 178: © The McGraw-Hill Companies, Inc./Eilte Images; p. 179: © Getty Images/Digital Vision RF; p. 186: Courtesy National Fisheries Institute; p. 187: © Jack Star/PhotoLink/Getty Images RF; p. 188: © SW Productions/Getty Images RF; p. 190: Royalty

Free/Corbis; p. 192: © Digital Vision/Getty Images RF; p. 193: RF/Getty Images; p. 194 (top): © John A. Rizzo/Getty Images RF; (bottom): Royalty Free/Corbis; p. 196: © image100/PunchStock RF; p. 197: © The McGraw-Hill Companies, Inc./Photo by Erick Misko, Elite Images Photography; p. 198: © The McGraw-Hill Companies, Inc./Gary He, photographer; p. 200: © The McGraw-Hill Companies, Inc./Mark Dierker, photographer; p. 201, 203: trbfoto/Brand X Pictures/Jupiterimages RF; p. 206(donut): © Jules Frazier/Getty Images RF; (bagel): © Ingram Publishing/Alamy RF.

Chapter 6

Opener: © The McGraw-Hill Companies; p. 212: © PhotoLink/Getty Images RF; p. 213: © Corbis/PictureQuest RF; p. 214: © Comstock/Jupiterimages RF; 6.3: © Dr. Stanley Flegler/Visuals Unlimited; p. 216(Panini): © Ingram Publishing/SuperStock RF; (eggs): © IT Stock/PunchStock RF; (milk): © Ingram Publishing/SuperStock RF : (beans): © IT Stock/PunchStock RF; p. 217: © Creatas/Punchstock RF; 6.6: © Corbis/Vol. 130 RF; p. 221: © Dynamic Graphics/JupiterImages RF; 6-11a: © Photodisc RF; 6-11b: © Stockbyte/Punchstock Images RF; 6-11c: © Dynamic Graphics/JupiterImages RF; Table 6.2(breakfast): © Image Source/Corbis RF; (lunch): © John A. Rizzo/Getty Images RF; (dinner): © Kevin Sanchez/Cole Group/Getty Images RF; (snack): © Comstock/Punchstock RF; p. 227: © Ingram Publishing/SuperStock RF; 6-12(left): © Kevin Fleming/Corbis; (right): © Peter Turnley/Corbis; p. 230: © The McGraw-Hill Companies/Barr Barker, photographer; p. 231: © Getty Images/Jonelle Weaver RF; p. 233(top): Walnut Marketing Board; (bottom): © Getty Images/Vol. 49 RF; p. 234: © Comstock/PunchStock RF; p. 235: © Getty Images/Jonelle Weaver RF; p. 236: © Image Source/JupiterImages RF; p. 238: © Ingram Publishing/SuperStock RF; p. 241: © Ryan McVay/Getty Images RF.

Chapter 7

Opener: © Ingram Publishing/SuperStock RF; p. 247: © Mitch Hrdlicka/Getty Images RF; p. 249: © Corbis/Vol. 130 RF; 7-5: © Samuel Ashfield/SPL/Photo Researchers, Inc.; p. 252: © Steve Mason/Getty Images RF; p. 254: © The McGraw-Hill Companies/Jill Braaton, photographer; 7-9: © Paul Efland University of Georgia; 7-10: Courtesy of Life Measurement Inc.; 7-11: © FotoSearch Stock Photography RF; 7-12: Maltron International Ltd; 7-13: Custom Medical Stock Photo; p. 258: © Corbis/RF website; p. 260(top): © Ingram Publishing/SuperStock RF; (bottom): © Jack Hollingsworth/Getty Images RF; p. 261: © Getty Images/SW Productions RF; p. 262: © PhotoDisc/Getty Images RF; 7-16(1): © Jon Feingersh/Blend Images LLC; (2): © Jose Luis Pelaez Inc/Blend Images LLC; (3): © Picture Net/Getty Images RF; p. 263: © Jose Luis Pelaez Inc/Blend Images/Jupiter Images RF; p. 265: © Zefa RF/Alamy; p. 266: © PhotoDisc/Vol. 20 RF; p. 268: © PhotoDisc/Vol. 20 RF; p. 269: © Royalty Free/Corbis Vol. 306; p. 270: © Dynamic Graphics/JupiterImages RF; p. 274: © Dynamic Graphics Group/Creatas/Alamy RF; p. 277: © Ernie Friedlander/Cole Group/Getty Images RF; p. 278: © Ryan McVay/Getty Images RF; p. 280(top): © Ingram Publishing/SuperStock RF; (bottom): © Comstock Images RF.

Chapter 8

Opener: © Royalty Free/Corbis; p. 291: © Liquid library/ Picture Quest RF; p. 292: © PhotoLink/Getty Images RF; p. 293: © PhotoDisc/OS49 RF; 8-1: A Colour Atlas and Text of Nutritional Disorders by Dr. Donald D. McLaren/ Mosby-Wolfe Europe Ltd.; 8-2: National Eye Institute, National Institute of Health; p. 295: Kevin Sanchez/ Cole Group/Getty Images RF; p. 297(broccoli): © Image Source/PunchStock RF; (cantaloupe): © Jupiterimages/ ImageSource RF; (eggs): © IT Stock/PunchStock RF; p. 297: © Kevin Sanchez/Cole Group/Getty Images RF; p. 298: © Royalty Free/Corbis; 8-6: © Jeffrey L. Rotman/ Corbis; p. 301: © Gregg Kidd and Joanne Scott; p. 303: © C Squared Studios/Getty Images RF; p. 304(cabbage): © Isabelle Rozenbaum & Frederic Cirou/PhotoAlto/ PunchStock RF; (apple): © Photodisc/Getty Images RF; (nuts): © Stockbyte/Corbis RF; p. 304: © Banana Stock/ Punchstock RF; p. 305: Visuals Unlimited; p. 306, 309: © Royalty Free/Corbis; p. 310: © Blue Moon Stock/ PunchStock RF; 8-18a: A Colour Atlas and Text of Nutritional Disorders by Dr. Donald D. McLaren/Mosby-Wolfe Europe Ltd.; 8-18b: © Dr. P. Marazzi/Science Photo Library/Photo Researchers, Inc.; 8-20a: © Dr. M.A. Ansary/Photo Researchers, Inc.; 8-20b: © Lester V. Bergman/Corbis; p. 314: © Getty Images/Jonelle Weaver RF; p. 318: © Corbis/Vol. 130 RF; p. 319(potatoes): © Ingram Publishing/SuperStock RF; (watermelon): © Siede Preis/Getty Images RF; (raw chicken): © Ingram Publishing/SuperStock RF; p. 319: © Getty Images/Jonelle Weaver RF; p. 320: © C Squared Studios/Getty Images RF.

Chapter 9

Opener: © Burke Triolo Productions/Getty Images RF; p. 350: © Royalty-Free/Corbis; 9.3(tomato): © Getty Images/Stockbyte RF; p. 352: © Royalty-Free/ Corbis; p. 355(top): © Getty Images RF; (bottom): © Corbis/Vol. 83 RF; p. 357: © Burke Triolo Productions/ Getty Images RF; p. 358: MHHE Image Library; p. 359: © Royalty Free/Corbis; p. 360: © Corbis/Vol. 43 RF; p. 362: © C Squared Studios/Getty Images RF; p. 363(tomatoes) © Brand X Pictures/PunchStock RF; (Pears) © Corbis RF; (Shrimp) © Comstock Images/ Jupiterimages RF; p. 364: © Stockdisc/PunchStock RF; p. 365: MHHE Image Library; p. 366: © Getty Images/ PhotoDisc RF; p. 367(reading milk label): McGraw-Hill Companies, Inc./Andrew Resek, photographer; p. 367(beans): © Image Source/PunchStock RF; (yogurt): © Mitch Hrdlicka/Getty Images RF; (nuts): © Image Source/PunchStock RF; p. 368: © The McGraw-Hill Companies, Inc./Jill Braaten; p. 369: © Corbis/Vol. 43 RF; p. 371(gourds): © Burke/Triolo/Getty Images RF; (peaches): © Jupiterimages/ImageSource RF; (beans): © Image Source/PunchStock RF; p. 372(top): © Corbis/ RF website; (bottom): © Michael Lamotte/Cole Group/ Getty Images RF; p. 374: © Royalty Free/Corbis; p. 376(peas): © Ingram Publishing/SuperStock RF; (apricots): © Image Source/PunchStock RF; (meats): © Brand X Pictures/PunchStock RF; p. 377: Courtesy National Cattlemen's Beef Associations; p. 378(top): © Keith Brofsky/Getty Images RF; (bottom): Photo courtesy of Harold H. Sandstead, M.D.; p. 379: © Corbis/Vol. 130 RF; p. 380(milk): © Pixtal/SuperStock RF; (asparagus): © Brand X Pictures/PunchStock RF; (chicken): © Ernie Friedlander/Cole Group/Getty Images RF; p. 381: © Ingram Publishing/SuperStock RF; p. 382: © Scott Camazine/Photo Researchers, Inc.; p. 384: Courtesy of Fishery Products International, Denver, MA; p. 386 (top): © Paul Casamassimo, DDS, MS; (bottom): © PhotoDisc/Vol. 02 RF; p. 387(top): © Corbis/RF website; (bottom): © C Squared Studios/Getty Images RF; 9-23: © Ryan McVay/Getty Images RF; p. 392(left): © PhotoDisc/Vol. 40 RF; (right): © Rob Melnychuk/Getty Images RF; p. 393: © Ryan McVay/Getty Images RF; p. 396: © Yoav Levy/Phototake; p. 398: © Royalty Free/Corbis; p. 399: © Royalty Free/Corbis; p. 401(top): © Comstock Images RF; (bottom): © JGI Blend Images LLC RF.

Chapter 10

Opener: © Getty Images; 10.1: © Rubberball/Getty Images RF; p. 411: © John Lund/Sam Diephuis/Blend Images LLC RF; 10.2: © Tetra Images/SuperStock RF; p. 413: © PhotoDisc/Sports Metaphors RF; p. 414: © Royalty Free/Corbis; p. 416: © JupiterImages RF; p. 417: © Corbis/Vol. 20 RF; p. 418: © James Mulligan; p. 419: © Corbis/RF website; p. 422(top): © IngramPublishing/SuperStock RF; (bottom): © Royalty Free/Corbis; p. 423(top): © Gordon Wardlaw; (bottom): © Royalty Free/Corbis; p. 425: © PhotoDisc/ Vol. 51 RF; p. 428(top): © Getty Images/Jonelle Weaver RF; (bottom): © John A. Rizzo/Getty Images RF; p. 429: © PhotoDisc/Vol. 51 RF; p. 434 (top): © Corbis/Vol. 20 RF; (bottom): © Comstock Images RF; p. 436: © Stockbyte/Getty Images RF; p. 438: © JupiterImages RF.

Chapter 11

Opener: © Corbis/Vol. 75 RF; p. 447: © The McGraw-Hill Companies, Inc./Lars A. Niki, photographer; p. 448: © Photodisc website RF; p. 449: © Royalty Free/Corbis; p. 450: © Mark Andersen/Getty Images RF; p. 451: © Stockbyte/PunchStock RF; p. 452: © PhotoDisc website RF; p. 455: © Tom Stewart Photography/Corbis; p. 456: © Comstock Images RF; 11-2: © Brand X Pictures/ PunchStock RF; p. 458: © Royalty Free/Corbis; p. 459: © PhotoDisc Website RF; p. 460: © Jack Star/PhotoLink/ Getty Images RF; p. 462: © BananaStock/PunchStock RF; 11-3: © Photodisc/Vol. 45 RF; p. 463: © The McGraw-Hill Companies, Inc./Lars A. Niki, photographer; p. 464: © PhotoDisc website RF; p. 465: © Digital Vision/Getty Images RF; p. 466: © Corbis/RF website; p. 467: © BananaStock/PunchStock RF; p. 469: © Don Manson/Blend Images LLC RF; p. 471: © Digital Vision/PunchStock RF.

Chapter 12

Opener: © Nicholas Pitt/Digital Vision/Getty Images RF; p. 474: © Corbis/RF website; p. 478: USDA photo by Peter Manzelli; p. 480: © Royalty Free/Corbis; p. 481: © PhotoDisc/Vol. 25 RF; p. 483: © The McGraw-Hill Companies, Inc./Barry Barker, photographer; p. 484: © Getty Images/Digital Vision RF; p. 485: © The McGraw-Hill Companies, Inc./Barry Barker, photographer; p. 486(both): © The Ohio State University Communications Photo Service; p. 487: © Corbis/RF website; p. 489: © Corbis/Vol. 25 RF; p. 491: © Erin Koran RF; p. 494: © Corbis/Vol. 609 RF; p. 495: © The Ohio State University Communications Photo Service, Jodi Miller; 12-7(child mortality): © Corbis/RF website; (human suffering, loss of parents, exploitation of women): AP Wide World Photos; p. 498: © Corbis/RF website; p. 499: © Digital Vision/PunchStock RF; p. 501: © Getty Images RF.

Chapter 13

Opener: © Lifesize/Getty Images RF; p. 507: © Royalty Free/Corbis; p. 508: © The Ohio State University Communications Photo Service; p. 511: © John A. Rizzo/ Getty Images RF; Table 13-3(Salmonella species): © Photodisc/Getty Images RF; (Campylobacter jejuni): © I. Rozenbaum/F. Cirou/Photo Alto RF; (Escherichia coli): © John A. Rizzo/Getty Images RF; (Shigella species): © Comstock Images/PictureQuest RF; (Staphylococcus aureus): © Michael Lamotte/Cole Group/Getty Images RF; (Clostridium perfringens): © Ingram Publishing/Fotosearch RF; (Listeria monocytogenes): © Digital Vision/Getty Images RF; (Clostridium botulinum): Photo provided by Jarden Home Brands, marketers of Ball® and Kerr® fresh preserving products. Jarden Home Brands is a division of Jarden Corporation (NYSE: JAH); (Vibrio): © I. Rozenbaum/F. Cirou/Photo Alto RF; (Yersinia enterocolitica): © Foodcollection/Getty Images RF; p. 514(top): © Royalty Free/Corbis; (bottom): © Image Source/Corbis RF; Table 13-5(Trichinella spiralis): © Ingram Publishing/Alamy RF; (Anisakis): © Image Source/Corbis RF; (Tapeworms):

© I. Rozenbaum/F. Cirou/Photo Alto RF; (Toxoplasma gondii): © The Ohio State University Communications Photo Service; (Cyclospora cayetanensis): © Don Farrall/ Getty Images RF; (Cryptosporidium): © John A. Rizzo/ Getty Images RF; p. 517: © Corbis/Vol. 83 RF; p. 518: © Corbis/Vol. 192 RF; p. 520: © Bob Montesciaros/Cole Group/Getty Images RF; p. 521(top): © Rob Melnychuk/ Getty Images RF; (bottom): © The Ohio State University Communications Photo Service; p. 522: © Image Source/ Corbis RF; p. 523: © Corbis/Vol. 43 RF; p. 525: © The Ohio State University Communications Photo Service; p. 526: © PhotoDisc website RF; p. 527(basket): © Corbis/Vol. 49 RF; (facet): © Comstock Images/PictureQuest RF; (USDA seal): USDA; p. 528: © C Squared Studios/Getty Images RF; p. 529: © The McGraw-Hill Companies, Inc./Christopher Kerrigan, photographer; p. 530: © Iconotec.com RF; p. 532(top): USDA; (bottom): © Greg Wolff; p. 533: © PhotoDisc/Vol. 48 RF; p. 535: © PhotoDisc/Vol. 58 RF; p. 537: © The McGraw Hill Companies, Inc.; p. 538: © Jess Alford/Getty Images RF; p. 539(top): © Digital Vision/Getty Images RF; (bottom): © David Buffington/Getty Images RF.

Chapter 14

Opener: © Getty Images RF; p. 543: © BananaStock/ PunchStock RF; p. 546: © Gordon Wardlaw, photographer Greg Wolff; p. 547: © Blend Images/Getty Images RF; p. 549: USDA; p. 550: © Tanya Constantine/Blend Images LLC RF; p. 552: © Getty Images RF; p. 555: © Photodisc Collection/Getty Images RF; p. 556: © Getty Images/ Jonelle Weaver RF; p. 558: © Corbis/Vol. 83 RF; p. 560: © Getty Images RF; p. 563: © Scott T. Baxter/Getty Images RF; p. 564: © PhotoDisc/Vol. 192 RF; p. 565: © PhotoDisc/ EP039 RF; p. 566: © 2008 Medela AG; p. 567: © Corbis/ Vol. 52 RF; p. 569: © Getty Images RF; p. 572: © Digital Vision/PunchStock RF; p. 574: © Hill Street Studios/Blend Images LLC RF; p. 577: © Andersen Ross/Getty Images RF.

Chapter 15

Opener: © Banana Stock/PunchStock RF; p. 583(top): World Health Organization; (bottom): © PhotoDisc/Vol. 113 RF; p. 584: © PhotoAlto/PictureQuest RF; p. 589(top): © PhotoDisc/Vol. 58 RF; (bottom): © Corbis/PictureQuest RF; p. 591: © PhotoDisc/Vol. 113 RF; p. 592(top): © Corbis/PictureQuest RF; (bottom): © Paul Casamassimo, DDS, MS; p. 593: © Corbis/Vol. 9 RF; p. 594: © Digital Vision/Getty Images RF; p. 595: Joanne Scott; p. 596: © Banana Stock/PunchStock RF; p. 597: USDA Photo by Ken Hammond; p. 598: © Ablestock/Alamy RF; p. 600: © Banana Stock/ PunchStock RF; p. 602: © Corbis/Vol. 552 RF; p. 603: © Ingram Publishing/SuperStock RF; p. 604: © Stockbyte/ PunchStock; p. 605: © Corbis/RF website; p. 606: © PhotoDisc/Vol. 95 RF; p. 607: © Corbis/Vol. 124 RF; p. 609: © The McGraw-Hill Companies, Inc./Ken Karp photographer; p. 611: © PhotoDisc/Vol. 61 RF; p. 613: © Dynamic Graphics/JupiterImages RF; p. 615: © The McGraw-Hill Companies, Inc./Jill Braaten, photographer.

Chapter 16

Opener: © Digital Vision/PunchStock RF; p. 621: © Royalty Free/Corbis; p. 622: © Corbis/RF website; p. 628: © Blend Images/Getty Images RF; p. 629: © Image Source/Corbis RF; p. 632: © PhotoDisc Vol. 15 RF; p. 633: © Stockbyte/Punchstock RF; p. 635: © Ingram Publishing RF; p. 638(top): © PhotoDisc/Vol. 20 RF; (bottom): © Corbis/Vol. 192 RF; p. 640: © PhotoDisc website RF; p. 642(both): © Arthur Glauberman/Photo Researchers, Inc.; p. 643: © PhotoDisc/Vol. 48 RF; p. 644: © RF/Corbis; p. 646(both): © PhotoDisc/OS49 RF; p. 650: © PhotoDisc website RF; p. 652: © Ingram Publishing RF; p. 654: © RF/Corbis; p. 655: © PhotoDisc/SS45 RF.

Appendix

Figure D-1(all): © Greg Kidd & Joanne Scott. Appendix, Glossary, Index (Almonds): © Getty Images/ Stockbyte

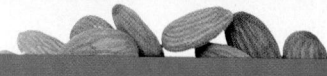
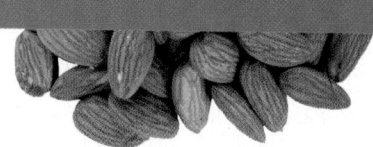

INDEX

A

Dietary Reference Intakes (DRIs): Recommended Intakes for Individuals, Vitamins
Food and Nutrition Board, Institute of Medicine, National Academies

Life Stage Group	Vitamin A (µg/d)[a]	Vitamin C (mg/d)	Vitamin D (µg/d)[b,c]	Vitamin E (mg/d)[d]	Vitamin K (µg/d)	Thiamin (mg/d)	Riboflavin (mg/d)	Niacin (mg/d)[e]	Vitamin B-6 (mg/d)	Folate (µg/d)[f]	Vitamin B-12 (µg/d)	Pantothenic Acid (mg/d)	Biotin (µg/d)	Choline (mg/d)[g]
Infants														
0–6 mo	400*	40*	10	4*	2.0*	0.2*	0.3*	2*	0.1*	65*	0.4*	1.7*	5*	125*
7–12 mo	500*	50*	10	5*	2.5*	0.3*	0.4*	4*	0.3*	80*	0.5*	1.8*	6*	150*
Children														
1–3 y	300	15	15	6	30*	0.5	0.5	6	0.5	150	0.9	2*	8*	200*
4–8 y	400	25	15	7	55*	0.6	0.6	8	0.6	200	1.2	3*	12*	250*
Males														
9–13 y	600	45	15	11	60*	0.9	0.9	12	1.0	300	1.8	4*	20*	375*
14–18 y	900	75	15	15	75*	1.2	1.3	16	1.3	400	2.4	5*	25*	550*
19–30 y	900	90	15	15	120*	1.2	1.3	16	1.3	400	2.4	5*	30*	550*
31–50 y	900	90	15	15	120*	1.2	1.3	16	1.3	400	2.4	5*	30*	550*
51–70 y	900	90	15	15	120*	1.2	1.3	16	1.7	400	2.4[h]	5*	30*	550*
>70 y	900	90	20	15	120*	1.2	1.3	16	1.7	400	2.4[h]	5*	30*	550*
Females														
9–13 y	600	45	15	11	60*	0.9	0.9	12	1.0	300	1.8	4*	20*	375*
14–18 y	700	65	15	15	75*	1.0	1.0	14	1.2	400[i]	2.4	5*	25*	400*
19–30 y	700	75	15	15	90*	1.1	1.1	14	1.3	400[i]	2.4	5*	30*	425*
31–50 y	700	75	15	15	90*	1.1	1.1	14	1.3	400[i]	2.4	5*	30*	425*
51–70 y	700	75	15	15	90*	1.1	1.1	14	1.5	400	2.4[h]	5*	30*	425*
>70 y	700	75	20	15	90*	1.1	1.1	14	1.5	400	2.4[h]	5*	30*	425*
Pregnancy														
≤18 y	750	80	15	15	75*	1.4	1.4	18	1.9	600[j]	2.6	6*	30*	450*
19–30 y	770	85	15	15	90*	1.4	1.4	18	1.9	600[j]	2.6	6*	30*	450*
31–50 y	770	85	15	15	90*	1.4	1.4	18	1.9	600[j]	2.6	6*	30*	450*
Lactation														
≤18 y	1200	115	15	19	75*	1.4	1.6	17	2.0	500	2.8	7*	35*	550*
19–30 y	1300	120	15	19	90*	1.4	1.6	17	2.0	500	2.8	7*	35*	550*
31–50 y	1300	120	15	19	90*	1.4	1.6	17	2.0	500	2.8	7*	35*	550*

mg = milligram, mg = microgram

NOTE: This table (taken from the DRI reports; see www.nap.edu) presents Recommended Dietary Allowances (RDAs) in **bold type** and Adequate Intakes (AIs) in ordinary type followed by an asterisk (*). RDAs and AIs may both be used as goals for individual intake. RDAs are set to meet the needs of almost all (97 to 98%) individuals in a group. For healthy breastfed infants, the AI is the mean intake. The AI for other life stage and gender groups is believed to cover needs of all individuals in the group, but lack of data or uncertainty in the data prevents being able to specify with confidence the percentage of individuals covered by this intake.

[a]As retinol activity equivalents (RAEs). 1 RAE = 1 µg retinol, 12 µg β-carotene, 24 µg α-carotene, or 24 µg β-cryptoxanthin. To calculate RAEs from REs of provitamin A carotenoids in foods, divide the REs by 2. For preformed vitamin A in foods or supplements and for provitamin A carotenoids in supplements, 1 RE = 1 RAE.

[b]cholecalciferol. 1 µg cholecalciferol = 40 IU vitamin D.

[c]In the absence of adequate exposure to sunlight.

[d]As α-tocopherol. α-Tocopherol includes RRR-α-tocopherol, the only form of α-tocopherol that occurs naturally in foods, and the 2R-stereoisomeric forms of α-tocopherol (RRR-, RSR-, RRS-, and RSS-α-tocopherol) that occur in fortified foods and supplements. It does not include the 2S-stereoisomeric forms of α-tocopherol (SRR-, SSR-, SRS-, and SSS-α-tocopherol), also found in fortified foods and supplements.

[e]As niacin equivalents (NE). 1 mg of niacin = 60 mg of tryptophan; 0–6 months = preformed niacin (not NE).

[f]As dietary folate equivalents (DFE). 1 DFE = 1 µg food folate = 0.6 µg of folic acid from fortified food or as a supplement consumed with food = 0.5 µg of a supplement taken on an empty stomach.

[g]Although AIs have been set for choline, there are few data to assess whether a dietary supply of choline is needed at all stages of the life cycle, and it may be that the choline requirement can be met by endogenous synthesis at some of these stages.

[h]Because 10 to 30% of older people may malabsorb food-bound B-12, it is advisable for those older than 50 years to meet their RDA mainly by consuming foods fortified with B-12 or a supplement containing B-12.

[i]In view of evidence linking folate intake with neural tube defects in the fetus, it is recommended that all women capable of becoming pregnant consume 400 µg from supplements or fortified foods in addition to intake of food folate from a varied diet.

[j]It is assumed that women will continue consuming 400 µg from supplements or fortified food until their pregnancy is confirmed and they enter prenatal care, which ordinarily occurs after the end of the periconceptional period—the critical time for formation of the neural tube.

Adapted from the Dietary Reference Intakes series, National Academies Press. Copyright 1997, 1998, 2000, 2001, 2011, by the National Academy of Sciences. The full reports are available from the National Academies Press at www.nap.edu.

Dietary Reference Intakes (DRIs): Recommended Intakes for Individuals, Elements
Food and Nutrition Board, Institute of Medicine, National Academies

Life Stage Group	Calcium (mg/d)	Chromium (µg/d)	Copper (µg/d)	Fluoride (mg/d)	Iodine (µg/d)	Iron (mg/d)	Magnesium (mg/d)	Manganese (mg/d)	Molybdenum (µg/d)	Phosphorus (mg/d)	Selenium (µg/d)	Zinc (mg/d)
Infants												
0–6 mo	200*	0.2*	200*	0.01*	110*	0.27*	30*	0.003*	2*	100*	15*	2*
7–12 mo	260*	5.5*	220*	0.5*	130*	11	75*	0.6*	3*	275*	20*	3
Children												
1–3 y	700	11*	340	0.7*	90	7	80	1.2*	17	460	20	3
4–8 y	1000	15*	440	1*	90	10	130	1.5*	22	500	30	5
Males												
9–13 y	1300	25*	700	2*	120	8	240	1.9*	34	1250	40	8
14–18 y	1300	35*	890	3*	150	11	410	2.2*	43	1250	55	11
19–30 y	1000	35*	900	4*	150	8	400	2.3*	45	700	55	11
31–50 y	1000	35*	900	4*	150	8	420	2.3*	45	700	55	11
51–70 y	1000	30*	900	4*	150	8	420	2.3*	45	700	55	11
>70 y	1200	30*	900	4*	150	8	420	2.3*	45	700	55	11
Females												
9–13 y	1300	21*	700	2*	120	8	240	1.6*	34	1250	40	8
14–18 y	1300	24*	890	3*	150	15	360	1.6*	43	1250	55	9
19–30 y	1000	25*	900	2*	150	18	310	1.8*	45	700	55	8
31–50 y	1000	25*	900	3*	150	18	320	1.8*	45	700	55	8
51–70 y	1200	20*	900	3*	150	8	320	1.8*	45	700	55	8
>70 y	1200	20*	900	3*	150	8	320	1.8*	45	700	55	8
Pregnancy												
≤18 y	1300	29*	1000	3*	220	27	400	2.0*	50	1250	60	12
19–30 y	1000	30*	1000	3*	220	27	350	2.0*	50	700	60	11
31–50 y	1000	30*	1000	3*	220	27	360	2.0*	50	700	60	11
Lactation												
≤18 y	1300	44*	1300	3*	290	10	360	2.6*	50	1250	70	13
19–30 y	1000	45*	1300	3*	290	9	310	2.6*	50	700	70	12
31–50 y	1000	45*	1300	3*	290	9	320	2.6*	50	700	70	12

NOTE: This table presents Recommended Dietary Allowances (RDAs) in **bold type** and Adequate Intakes (AIs) in ordinary type followed by an asterisk (*). RDAs and AIs may both be used as goals for individual intake. RDAs are set to meet the needs of almost all (97 to 98%) individuals in a group. For healthy breastfed infants, the AI is the mean intake. The AI for other life stage and gender groups is believed to cover needs of all individuals in the group, but lack of data or uncertainty in the data prevents being able to specify with confidence the percentage of individuals covered by this intake.

SOURCES: Dietary Reference Intakes for Calcium, Phosphorus, Magnesium, Vitamin D, and Fluoride (1997); Dietary Reference Intakes for Thiamin, Riboflavin, Niacin, Vitamin B-6, Folate, Vitamin B-12, Pantothenic Acid, Biotin, and Choline (1998); Dietary Reference Intakes for Vitamin C, Vitamin E, Selenium, and Carotenoids (2000); Dietary Reference Intakes for Vitamin A, Vitamin K, Arsenic, Boron, Chromium, Copper, Iodine, Iron, Manganese, Molybdenum, Nickel, Silicon, Vanadium, and Zinc (2001); and Dietary Reference Intakes for Calcium and Vitamin D (2011). These reports may be accessed via www.nap.edu. The full reports are available from the National Academies Press at www.nap.edu.

Adapted from the Dietary Reference Intake series, National Academies Press. Copyright 1997, 1998, 2000, 2001, and 2011 by the National Academy of Sciences.

B

Dietary Reference Intakes (DRIs): Recommended Intakes for Individuals, Macronutrients
Food and Nutrition Board, Institute of Medicine, National Academies

Life Stage Group	Carbohydrate (g/d)	Total Fiber (g/d)	Fat (g/d)	Linoleic Acid (g/d)	α-Linolenic Acid (g/d)	Protein[a] (g/d)
Infants						
0–6 mo	60*	ND	31*	4.4*	0.5*	9.1*
7–12 mo	95*	ND	30*	4.6*	0.5*	11.0
Children						
1–3 y	130	19*	ND[b]	7*	0.7*	13
4–8 y	130	25*	ND	10*	0.9*	19
Males						
9–13 y	130	31*	ND	12*	1.2*	34
14–18 y	130	38*	ND	16*	1.6*	52
19–30 y	130	38*	ND	17*	1.6*	56
31–50 y	130	38*	ND	17*	1.6*	56
51–70 y	130	30*	ND	14*	1.6*	56
>70 y	130	30*	ND	14*	1.6*	56
Females						
9–13 y	130	26*	ND	10*	1.0*	34
14–18 y	130	26*	ND	11*	1.1*	46
19–30 y	130	25*	ND	12*	1.1*	46
31–50 y	130	25*	ND	12*	1.1*	46
51–70 y	130	21*	ND	11*	1.1*	46
>70 y	130	21*	ND	11*	1.1*	46
Pregnancy						
14–18 y	175	28*	ND	13*	1.4*	71
19–30 y	175	28*	ND	13*	1.4*	71
31–50 y	175	28*	ND	13*	1.4*	71
Lactation						
14–18 y	210	29*	ND	13*	1.3*	71
19–30 y	210	29*	ND	13*	1.3*	71
31–50 y	210	29*	ND	13*	1.3*	71

NOTE: This table presents Recommended Dietary Allowances (RDAs) in **bold type** and Adequate Intakes (AIs) in ordinary type followed by an asterisk (*). RDAs and AIs may both be used as goals for individual intake. RDAs are set to meet the needs of almost all (97 to 98%) individuals in a group. For healthy breastfed infants, the AI is the mean intake. The AI for other life stage and gender groups is believed to cover needs of all individuals in the group, but lack of data or uncertainty in the data prevents being able to specify with confidence the percentage of individuals covered by this intake.
[a]Based on 0.8g protein/kg body weight for reference body weight.
[b]ND = not determinable at this time.
Sources: Dietary Reference Intakes for Energy, Carbohydrate, Fiber, Fat, Fatty Acids, Cholesterol, Protein, and Amino Acids (2002). This report may be accessed via www.nap.edu.
Adapted from the Dietary Reference Intake series, National Academies Press. Copyright 1997, 1998, 2000, 2001, by the National Academy of Sciences. The full reports are available from the National Academies Press at www.nap.edu.

Dietary Reference Intakes (DRIs): Recommended Intakes for Individuals, Electrolytes and Water
Food and Nutrition Board, Institute of Medicine, National Academies

Life Stage Group	Sodium (mg/d)	Potassium (mg/d)	Chloride (mg/d)	Water (L/d)
Infants				
0–6 mo	120*	400*	180*	0.7*
7–12 mo	370*	700*	570*	0.8*
Children				
1–3 y	1000*	3000*	1500*	1.3*
4–8 y	1200*	3800*	1900*	1.7*
Males				
9–13 y	1500*	4500*	2300*	2.4*
14–18 y	1500*	4700*	2300*	3.3*
19–30 y	1500*	4700*	2300*	3.7*
31–50 y	1500*	4700*	2300*	3.7*
51–70 y	1300*	4700*	2000*	3.7*
> 70 y	1200*	4700*	1800*	3.7*
Females				
9–13 y	1500*	4500*	2300*	2.1*
14–18 y	1500*	4700*	2300*	2.3*
19–30 y	1500*	4700*	2300*	2.7*
31–50 y	1500*	4700*	2300*	2.7*
51–70 y	1300*	4700*	2000*	2.7*
> 70 y	1200*	4700*	1800*	2.7*
Pregnancy				
14–18 y	1500*	4700*	2300*	3.0*
19–50 y	1500*	4700*	2300*	3.0*
Lactation				
14–18 y	1500*	5100*	2300*	3.8*
19–50 y	1500*	5100*	2300*	3.8*

NOTE: The table is adapted from the DRI reports. See www.nap.edu. Adequate Intakes (AIs) are followed by an asterisk (*). These may be used as a goal for individual intake. For healthy breastfed infants, the AI is the average intake. The AI for other life stage and gender groups is believed to cover the needs of all individuals in the group, but lack of data prevent being able to specify with confidence the percentage of individuals covered by this intake; therefore, no Recommended Dietary Allowance (RDA) was set.

Source: *Dietary Reference Intakes for Water, Potassium, Sodium, Chloride, and Sulfate* (2005). This report may be accessed via www.nap.edu.

Acceptable Macronutrient Distribution Ranges

Macronutrient	Range (percent of energy)		
	Children, 1–3 y	Children, 4–18 y	Adults
Fat	30–40	25–35	20–35
omega-6 polyunsaturated fats (linoleic acid)	5–10	5–10	5–10
omega-3 polyunsaturated fats[a] (α-linolenic acid)	0.6–1.2	0.6–1.2	0.6–1.2
Carbohydrate	45–65	45–65	45–65
Protein	5–20	10–30	10–35

[a]Approximately 10% of the total can come from longer-chain n-3 fatty acids.

SOURCE: *Dietary Reference Intakes for Energy, Carbohydrate, Fiber, Fat, Fatty Acids, Cholesterol, Protein, and Amino Acids* (2002). The report may be accessed via www.nap.edu.

Adapted from the Dietary Reference Intakes series, National Academies Press. Copyright 1997, 1998, 2000, 2001, 2011, by the National Academy of Sciences. The full reports are available from the National Academies Press at www.nap.edu.

Dietary Reference Intakes (DRIs): Tolerable Upper Intake Levels (UL[a]), Vitamins
Food and Nutrition Board, Institute of Medicine, National Academies

Life Stage Group	Vitamin A (µg/d)[b]	Vitamin C (mg/d)	Vitamin D (µg/d)	Vitamin E (mg/d)[c],[d]	Vitamin K	Thiamin	Riboflavin	Niacin (mg/d)[d]	Vitamin B-6 (mg/d)	Folate (µg/d)[d]	Vitamin B-12	Pantothenic Acid	Biotin	Choline (g/d)	Carotenoids[e]
Infants															
0–6 mo	600	ND	25	ND	ND	ND	ND	ND	ND	ND	ND	ND	ND	ND	ND
7–12 mo	600	ND	38	ND	ND	ND	ND	ND	ND	ND	ND	ND	ND	ND	ND
Children															
1–3 y	600	400	63	200	ND	ND	ND	10	30	300	ND	ND	ND	1.0	ND
4–8 y	900	650	75	300	ND	ND	ND	15	40	400	ND	ND	ND	1.0	ND
Males, Females															
9–13 y	1700	1200	100	600	ND	ND	ND	20	60	600	ND	ND	ND	2.0	ND
14–18 y	2800	1800	100	800	ND	ND	ND	30	80	800	ND	ND	ND	3.0	ND
19–70 y	3000	2000	100	1000	ND	ND	ND	35	100	1000	ND	ND	ND	3.5	ND
>70 y	3000	2000	100	1000	ND	ND	ND	35	100	1000	ND	ND	ND	3.5	ND
Pregnancy															
≤18 y	2800	1800	100	800	ND	ND	ND	30	80	800	ND	ND	ND	3.0	ND
19–50 y	3000	2000	100	1000	ND	ND	ND	35	100	1000	ND	ND	ND	3.5	ND
Lactation															
≤18 y	2800	1800	100	800	ND	ND	ND	30	80	800	ND	ND	ND	3.0	ND
19–50 y	3000	2000	100	1000	ND	ND	ND	35	100	1000	ND	ND	ND	3.5	ND

[a]UL = The maximum level of daily nutrient intake likely to pose no risk of adverse effects. Unless otherwise specified, the UL represents total intake from food, water, and supplements. Due to lack of suitable data, ULs could not be established for vitamin K, thiamin, riboflavin, vitamin B-12, pantothenic acid, biotin, or carotenoids. In the absence of ULs, extra caution may be warranted in consuming levels above recommended intakes.

[b]As preformed vitamin A only.

[c]As α-tocopherol; applies to any form of supplemental α-tocopherol.

[d]The ULs for vitamin E, niacin, and folate apply to synthetic forms obtained from supplements, fortified foods, or a combination of the two.

[e]β-Carotene supplements are advised only to serve as a provitamin A source for individuals at risk of vitamin A deficiency.

[f]ND = Not determinable due to lack of data of adverse effects in this age group and concern with regard to lack of ability to handle excess amounts. Source of intake should be from food only to prevent high levels of intake.

SOURCES: Dietary Reference Intakes for Calcium, Phosphorus, Magnesium, Vitamin D, and Fluoride (1997); Dietary Reference Intakes for Thiamin, Riboflavin, Niacin, Vitamin B-6, Folate, Vitamin B-12, Pantothenic Acid, Biotin, and Choline (1998); Dietary Reference Intakes for Vitamin C, Vitamin E, Selenium, and Carotenoids (2000); and Dietary Reference Intakes for Vitamin A, Vitamin K, Arsenic, Boron, Chromium, Copper, Iodine, Iron, Manganese, Molybdenum, Nickel, Silicon, Vanadium, and Zinc (2001). These reports may be accessed via www.nap.edu.

Adapted from the Dietary Reference Intakes series, National Academies Press. Copyright 1997, 1998, 2000, 2001, 2011, by the National Academy of Sciences. The full reports are available from the National Academies Press at www.nap.edu.